AF327159

MULTIDISCIPLINARY MANAGEMENT OF CLEFT LIP AND PALATE

JANUSZ BARDACH, M.D.
Professor of Plastic Surgery
Chairman, Division of Plastic and Reconstructive Surgery of the Head and Neck
Department of Otolaryngology—Head and Neck Surgery

Professor of Plastic Surgery
Division of Plastic Surgery
Department of Surgery

Director, Cleft Palate Surgical Research Laboratory
University of Iowa Hospitals and Clinics
Iowa City, Iowa

HUGHLETT L. MORRIS, Ph.D.
Professor of Speech Pathology
Director, Division of Speech and Hearing
Department of Otolaryngology—Head and Neck Surgery

Professor of Speech Pathology
Department of Speech Pathology and Audiology

Director, University of Iowa Cleft Palate Research Program
The University of Iowa
Iowa City, Iowa

1990
W.B. SAUNDERS COMPANY
Harcourt Brace Jovanovich, Inc.
Philadelphia ■ London ■ Toronto ■ Montreal ■ Sydney ■ Tokyo

W. B. SAUNDERS COMPANY
Harcourt Brace Jovanovich, Inc.

The Curtis Center
Independence Square West
Philadelphia, PA 19106

Library of Congress Cataloging-in-Publication Data

Multidisciplinary management of cleft lip and palate /
[edited by] Janusz Bardach, Hughlett L. Morris.

p. cm.

Includes index.

ISBN 0–7216–2951–2

1. Cleft lip—Surgery.   2. Cleft palate—Surgery.
   3. Cleft lip.   4. Cleft palate.   I. Bardach, Janusz.
   II. Morris, Hughlett L.
[DNLM: 1. Cleft lip—therapy.   2. Cleft palate—therapy.
WV 440 M957]

RD524.M85   1990
617.5′22—dc20
DNLM/DLC
for Library of Congress   89–10168

Editor: Richard Zorab
Designer: W. B. Saunders Staff
Production Manager: Bill Preston
Manuscript Editor: Ruth Low
Illustration Coordinator: Brett MacNaughton
Indexer: Julie Figures

Multidisciplinary Management of Cleft Lip   ISBN 0–7216–2951–2
and Palate

© 1990 by W. B. Saunders Company.

All rights reserved.   No part of this publication may be reproduced
or transmitted in any form or by any means, electronic or mechanical,
including photocopy, recording, or any information storage or retrieval
system, without written permission from the publisher.

Printed in the United States of America.

Last digit is the print number:
9   8   7   6   5   4   3   2   1

*WE WOULD LIKE TO DEDICATE THIS BOOK
TO THE IMPROVEMENT OF THE CARE
OF CHILDREN BORN WITH CLEFT LIP AND PALATE*

Howard Aduss, D.D.S., M.S.
Professor, Center for Craniofacial Anomalies, Department of Pediatrics, College of Medicine, University of Illinois at Chicago, Chicago, Illinois; Professor, Division of Plastic Surgery, Department of Surgery, Rush Medical College, Chicago, Illinois; Attending Staff, University of Illinois Hospital and Rush Presbyterian–St. Luke's Medical Center, Chicago, Illinois
Stages of Orthodontic Treatment in Complete Unilateral Cleft Lip and Palate

K. Anastasov, M.D., D.Sci.
Bulgarian Medical Academy Institute of Surgery, Clinic of Plastic and Reconstructive Surgery, Sofia, Bulgaria
Multidisciplinary Management of Cleft Lip and Palate in Bulgaria

H. Anderl, M.D.
University Professor for Plastic and Reconstructive Surgery, University of Innsbruck, Innsbruck, Austria; Head of the University Hospital for Plastic and Reconstructive Surgery, Innsbruck, Austria
Primary Unilateral Cleft Lip and Nose Reconstruction

Marc W. Anderson, D.D.S., M.S.D.
Affiliate Associate Professor, Department of Pediatric Dentistry, University of Washington, Seattle, Washington; Attending Staff, Children's Hospital and Medical Center, Seattle, Washington
Prosthetic Treatment of Velopharyngeal Incompetence

Catherine Asher, B.D.S., F.D.S.R.C.S., D. Orth. R.C.S.
Honorary Lecturer in Orthodontics, University Dental Hospital of Manchester, Manchester, England; Consultant Orthodontist, Bolton and Blackburn Health Authorities and University Dental Hospital of Manchester, Manchester, England
Multidisciplinary Management of Cleft Lip and Palate in the United Kingdom

Janusz Bardach, M.D.
Professor of Plastic Surgery, and Chairman, Division of Plastic and Reconstructive Surgery of the Head and Neck, Department of Otolaryngology—Head and Neck Surgery; Professor of Plastic Surgery, Division of Plastic Surgery, Department of Surgery, University of Iowa Hospitals and Clinics, Iowa City, Iowa; Director, Cleft Palate Surgical Research Laboratory, University of Iowa Hospitals and Clinics, Iowa City, Iowa
The Iowa-Hamburg Project: Late Results of Multidisciplinary Management at the Iowa Cleft Palate Center; Anatomy of the Unilateral and Bilateral Cleft Lip and Nose; Secondary Correction of the Unilateral and Bilateral Cleft Lip Nasal Deformity: Bardach Technique; Cleft Palate Repair: Two-Flap Palatoplasty, Research, Philosophy, Technique, and Results; Surgical-Orthodontic Correction of the Protruded Premaxilla; Directions for Future Research

R. Christopher Barden, Ph.D.
Research Professor of Medicine, W. T. Grant Faculty Scholar, University of Utah School of Medicine, Gustavus Adolphus College, Salt Lake City, Utah
Psychosocial Aspects of Cleft Lip and Palate: The Family

Ladislav Barinka, M.D., Dr. Sc.
Head Professor, Medical Faculty, J. E. Purkyně University, Brno, Czechoslovakia; Clinic of Plastic Surgery, University of Brno, Brno, Czechoslovakia
Multidisciplinary Management of Cleft Lip and Palate in Brno, Czechoslovakia

K. Behlfelt, D.D.S.
Orthodontist and Assistant Professor, Department of Orthodontics, University Hospital Eppendorf, Hamburg, Federal Republic of Germany
The Iowa-Hamburg Project: Late Results of Multidisciplinary Management at the Iowa Cleft Palate Center

Ruth A. Bentler, Ph.D.
Assistant Professor, Department of Speech Pathology and Audiology, University of Iowa, Iowa City, Iowa
Audiologic Considerations for Cleft Patients

Samuel Berkowitz, D.D.S., M.S.
Clinical Professor of Pediatrics, University of Miami School of Medicine, Miami, Florida; Co-Director, Craniofacial Anomalies Program, Miami, Florida; Malman Center for Child Development and Miami Children's Hospital, Miami, Florida
The Complete Unilateral Cleft Lip and Palate: Serial Three-Dimensional Studies of Excellent Palatal Growth

Henrik Borchgrevink, M.D.
Consultant Plastic Surgeon, University Hospital of Oslo, Oslo Cleft Lip/Palate Team, Oslo, Norway
Multidisciplinary Management of Cleft Lip and Palate in Oslo, Norway

Raymond O. Brauer, M.D.
Clinical Professor of Plastic Surgery, Baylor College of Medicine, Houston, Texas; Active Staff, St. Joseph Hospital, and Teaching Staff, St. Joseph Hospital Plastic Surgery Residency Program, Houston, Texas
Augmentation of the Posterior Pharyngeal Wall

Hillary Broder, Ph.D.
Clinical Associate Professor, Department of Dental Ecology, School of Dentistry, University of North Carolina at Chapel Hill, Chapel Hill, North Carolina; Oral-Facial and Communicative Disorders Program, University of North Carolina and North Carolina Memorial Hospital, Chapel Hill, North Carolina
Psychological and Sociocultural Aspects of Cleft Lip and Palate

M. Brousilová, M.D.
Scientific Research Worker, Laboratory of Congenital Defects, Czechoslovak Academy of Sciences, Prague, Czechoslovakia
Multidisciplinary Management of Cleft Lip and Palate in Prague, Czechoslovakia; Development of the Maxillary Arch in Cleft Patients Treated by the Schweckendiek Technique

Robert M. Bumsted, M.D.
Professor, Department of Otolaryngology–Head and Neck Surgery, University of Chicago–Pritzker School of Medicine, Chicago, Illinois; Attending Staff, University of Chicago Medical Center, Chicago, Illinois
Evaluation and Management of Nasal Airway Obstruction in the Cleft Patient

Martin D. Cassell, B.Sc. (Hons), Ph.D.
Associate Professor, Department of Anatomy, University of Iowa, Iowa City, Iowa
Anatomy and Physiology of the Velopharynx

M. Černý, M.D., C.Sc.
Associate Professor, Charles University, Institute of Plastic Surgery, Prague, Czechoslovakia
Multidisciplinary Management of Cleft Lip and Palate in Prague, Czechoslovakia

Kathy L. Chapman, Ph.D.
Assistant Professor, Case Western Reserve University, Cleveland, Ohio
Communicative Competence in Children with Cleft Lip and Palate

Linda Chase, R.N., B.S.N.
Clinical Nursing Specialist I, Pediatric Nursing Division, University of Iowa Hospitals and Clinics, Iowa City, Iowa
Comprehensive Nursing Care for Cleft Patients

Marilyn Cohen, B.A.
Speech Consultant, The Children's Hospital of Philadelphia, Philadelphia, Pennsylvania
The Furlow Double Reversing Z-Plasty for Cleft Palate Repair: The First Ten Years of Experience

Shirley Cohen, M.S.
Formerly Coordinator, Regional Craniofacial Center of Northern New Jersey, Saint Barnabas Medical Center, Livingston, New Jersey
Two-Stage Palatoplasty and Evaluation of Speech Results

Steven Cohen, M.D.
Assistant Clinical Professor, Craniofacial Fellow, UCLA Medical Center, Los Angeles, California
The Furlow Double Reversing Z-Plasty for Cleft Palate Repair: The First Ten Years of Experience

Dennis M. Crockett, M.D.
Assistant Professor, Department of Otolaryngology–Head and Neck Surgery, University of Southern California School of Medicine, Los Angeles, California; Department of Otolaryngology–Head and Neck Surgery, University of Southern California and Children's Hospital of Los Angeles, Los Angeles, California

Evaluation and Management of Nasal Airway Obstruction in the Cleft Patient

Ernest D. Cronin, M.D., F.A.C.S.
Assistant Clinical Professor in Plastic Surgery, Baylor School of Medicine, Houston, Texas; Teaching Staff, St. Joseph Hospital Plastic Surgery Residency Program and Chief of Plastic Surgery, St. Joseph Hospital, Houston, Texas
Correction of Secondary Unilateral and Bilateral Nasal Deformities: Cronin Technique

Thomas D. Cronin, M.D., F.A.C.S.
Clinical Professor of Plastic Surgery, Baylor College of Medicine, Houston, Texas; Active/Honorary Staff, St. Joseph Hospital; Consultant, St. Luke's Hospital and Texas Children's Hospital, Houston, Texas
Correction of Secondary Unilateral and Bilateral Nasal Deformities: Cronin Technique

John W. Curtin, M.D.
Professor and Chairman, Department of Plastic and Reconstructive Surgery, Rush Medical College and Presbyterian–St. Luke's Medical Center, Chicago, Illinois; Plastic Surgery Consultant, Center for Craniofacial Anomalies of the University of Illinois, Chicago, Illinois
Early Cleft Palate Repair and Speech Outcome: A Ten-Year Experience

Court B. Cutting, M.D.
Assistant Professor of Plastic Surgery, New York University Hospital, New York, New York; Attending Surgeon, New York University Hospital and Bellevue Hospital, New York, New York; Chief of Plastic Surgery, Manhattan Veterans Hospital, New York, New York
Anatomy of the Unilateral and Bilateral Cleft Lip and Nose; Scientific Evaluation of Facial Surfaces in Craniofacial Malformations Using Computer Graphics Methods

Arlene P. Dagys, D.D.S., D.Orth.
Senior Instructor, Surgical-Orthodontic Programme, Graduate Orthodontic Department, Faculty of Dentistry, University of Toronto, Toronto, Ontario; Staff Orthodontist, Craniofacial Treatment and Research Centre, Division of Orthodontics, Department of Dentistry, Hospital For Sick Children, Toronto, Ontario
Management of Jaw Deformities in the Cleft Patient

Rodger M. Dalston, Ph.D.
Associate Professor of Surgery and Dental Ecology, University of North Carolina at Chapel Hill, Chapel Hill, North Carolina
Communication Skills of Children with Cleft Lip and Palate: A Status Report

Keith A. Denkler, M.D.
Clinical Instructor in Plastic Surgery, University of California Medical School at San Francisco, San Francisco, California; Active Staff, San Francisco General Hospital and Marin General Hospital, San Francisco, California
Correction of Secondary Unilateral and Bilateral Nasal Deformities: Cronin Technique

Debra Susan Dorf, M.A.
Instructor, Department of Pediatrics, University of Illinois at Chicago, College of Medicine, Chicago, Illinois; Speech Pa-

thologist, Center for Craniofacial Anomalies, Department of Pediatrics, University of Illinois at Chicago, College of Medicine, Chicago, Illinois
Early Cleft Palate Repair and Speech Outcome: A Ten-Year Experience

Craig R. Dufresne, M.D., F.A.C.S.
Assistant Clinical Professor in the Division of Plastic Surgery and Department of Neurosurgery at the Johns Hopkins Medical Institutions, Baltimore, Maryland; Attending Staff, The Johns Hopkins Hospital and Children's Hospital, Baltimore, Maryland; Attending Staff, Fairfax Hospital, Fairfax, Virginia, and Sibley Hospital, Washington, D.C.
Oronasal and Nasolabial Fistulas

Michele J. Eliason, Ph.D.
Assistant Professor, College of Nursing, University of Iowa, Iowa City, Iowa
Neuropsychological Perspectives on Cleft Lip and Palate

Hani Elkadi, M.D.
Assistant Research Scientist, Department of Surgery, University of Iowa, Iowa City, Iowa
Anatomy and Physiology of the Velopharynx

Miroslav Fára, M.D., D.Sci.
Professor of Plastic Surgery, Charles University, Institute of Plastic Surgery, Prague, Czechoslovakia; Head of Institute of Plastic Surgery, Charles University, Prague, Czechoslovakia
Multidisciplinary Management of Cleft Lip and Palate in Prague, Czechoslovakia; Anatomy of Unilateral and Bilateral Cleft Lip; Presurgical Orthopedic Treatment in Unilateral Cleft Lip and Palate; Development of the Maxillary Arch in Cleft Patients Treated by the Schweckendiek Technique

Leslie G. Farkas, M.D., F.R.C.S. (C), C.Sc., D.Sc.
Associate Professor, Department of Surgery, University of Toronto, Toronto, Ontario; Staff (Research), Division of Plastic Surgery; Consultant, Research Institute; and Director, Craniofacial Measurement Laboratory (Division of Plastic Surgery), The Hospital for Sick Children, Toronto, Ontario
Anthropometry of the Face in Cleft Patients

Alvaro A. Figueroa, D.D.S., M.S.
Assistant Professor, Center for Craniofacial Anomalies, Department of Pediatrics, College of Medicine, University of Illinois, Chicago, Illinois; Assistant Professor, Department of Orthodontics, College of Dentistry, University of Illinois, Chicago, Illinois; Attending Staff, University of Illinois Hospital, Rush Presbyterian–St. Luke's Medical Center, and Cook County Hospital, Chicago, Illinois
Stages of Orthodontic Treatment in Complete Unilateral Cleft Lip and Palate

John W. Folkins, Ph.D.
Professor and Chair, Department of Speech Pathology and Audiology, University of Iowa, Iowa City, Iowa
Approaches to the Study of Speech Production

Raymond J. Fonseca, D.M.D.
Dean, University of Pennsylvania School of Dental Medicine, Philadelphia, Pennsylvania; Attending Staff, Hospital of The University of Pennsylvania, Philadelphia, Pennsylvania
Bone Grafting of the Cleft Maxilla

Donna R. Fox, Ph.D.
Professor of Communication Disorders, University of Houston, Houston, Texas; Allied Health Professional and Assistant Clinical Professor, Methodist Hospital, Houston, Texas
Augmentation of the Posterior Pharyngeal Wall

B. Fricke, D.D.S.
Resident at the Department of Orthodontics, University Hospital Eppendorf, Hamburg, Federal Republic of Germany
The Iowa-Hamburg Project: Late Results of Multidisciplinary Management at the Iowa Cleft Palate Center

E. Georgiev, M.D., D.Sci.
Bulgarian Medical Academy Institute of Surgery, Clinic of Plastic and Reconstructive Surgery, Sofia, Bulgaria
Multidisciplinary Management of Cleft Lip and Palate in Bulgaria

Wanda M. Gnoinski, Dr. Med. Dent.
Senior Lecturer, Department of Orthodontics, Zürich University Dental Institute, Zürich, Switzerland; Consultant, Zürich University Children's Hospital, Zürich, Switzerland
Infant Orthopedics and Later Orthodontic Monitoring for Unilateral Cleft Lip and Palate Patients in Zürich

Rosalie B. Goldberg, M.S.
Senior Associate in Department of Pediatrics and Plastic Surgery, Albert Einstein College of Medicine, Bronx, New York; Coordinator of Genetic Counseling, Center for Congenital Disorders, Montefiore Medical Center, Bronx, New York
Genetic Counseling of Cleft Lip and Palate

Siena M. Goorhuis-Brouwer, Ph.D.
Assistant Professor of Speech Pathology, University Hospital of Groningen, Groningen, The Netherlands; Head of the Department of Speech Pathology, University Hospital of Groningen, Groningen, The Netherlands
Cleft Palate Repair: The Von Langenbeck Technique

Lynn Marty Grames, M.A., C.C.C.
Pediatric Speech Pathology, Cleft Palate and Craniofacial Deformities Institute, Washington University Medical Center, St. Louis, Missouri
Intravelar Veloplasty: A Prospective Study

Steven D. Gray, M.D.
Assistant Professor and Pediatric Otolaryngologist, University of Iowa Hospitals and Clinics, Iowa City, Iowa
The Iowa-Hamburg Project: Late Results of Multidisciplinary Management at the Iowa Cleft Palate Center; Airway Obstruction and Apnea in Cleft Palate Patients

Barry H. Grayson, D.D.S.
Associate Professor of Clinical Surgery (Orthodontics), New York University School of Medicine; Associate Professor of Orthodontics, New York University Dental School, New York, New York; Institute of Reconstructive Plastic Surgery, University Hospital, New York, New York
Tensor and Three-Dimensional Cephalometric Method of Anthropometric Analysis; Planning Orthognathic Surgery

Haskell Gruber, D.D.S.
Professor of Clinical Plastic Surgery, Division of Plastic Surgery, Department of Surgery, Baylor College of Medicine,

Houston, Texas; Attending Staff, The Methodist Hospital, Texas Children's Hospital, St. Luke's Episcopal Hospital, Lyndon B. Johnson Hospital, and Ben Taub General Hospital, Houston, Texas
Presurgical Maxillary Orthopedics

Wolfgang Gubisch, M.D.

Chief Surgeon, Clinic for Plastic and Reconstructive Surgery, Marienhospital, Stuttgart, Federal Republic of Germany
Cleft Septorhinoplasty: Free Septum Replantation for Secondary Correction

K. K. H. Gundlach, M.D., D.D.S., M.S.D.

Professor of Maxillofacial Surgery, Department of Oral and Maxillofacial Surgery, Plastic Surgery of Head and Neck, Nordwestdeutsche Kieferklinik, Hamburg University, Hamburg, Federal Republic of Germany
The Iowa-Hamburg Project: Late Results of Multidisciplinary Management at the Iowa Cleft Palate Center; Two-Stage Palatoplasty

K. Güler Gürsu, M.D.

Professor and Chairman of Plastic and Reconstructive Surgery Department, Hacettepe University Medical School, Ankara, Turkey; University Hospitals of Hacettepe University Medical School, Ankara, Turkey
Multidisciplinary Management of Cleft Lip and Palate in Turkey

W. Michael Hairfield, D.D.S., M.S.

Associate Professor, Department of Dental Ecology, School of Dentistry, University of North Carolina, Chapel Hill, North Carolina; Attending, University of North Carolina Hospitals, Department of Hospital Dentistry, Chapel Hill, North Carolina
The Nasal Airway in Cleft Palate

James W. Hanson, M.D.

Professor, Department of Pediatrics, University of Iowa College of Medicine, Iowa City, Iowa; Director, Division of Medical Genetics, Department of Pediatrics, University of Iowa Hospitals and Clinics, Iowa City, Iowa
Genetic Aspects of Cleft Lip and Palate

Mary A. Hardin, Ph.D.

Assistant Professor, Case Western Reserve University, Cleveland, Ohio
Communicative Competence in Children with Cleft Lip and Palate; Speech Therapy for the Child with Cleft Lip and Palate

Gunilla Henningsson, Ph.D.

Senior Lecturer, Department of Logopedics and Phoniatrics, Karolinska Institutet, Stockholm, Sweden; Speech Pathologist, Department of Logopedics and Phoniatrics, Huddinge University Hospital, Stockholm, Sweden
Oronasal Fistulas and Speech Production

John M. Hiebert, M.D.

Professor and Chairman, Plastic Surgery, University of Kansas Medical Center, Kansas City, Kansas; Kansas University Medical Center and Kansas City VA Hospital, Kansas City, Kansas
Correction of Secondary Unilateral and Bilateral Cleft Lip Deformities

Barbel Holtman, M.D.

Assistant Professor of Anesthesiology, Washington University School of Medicine, St. Louis, Missouri; Assistant Anesthesiologist, Barnes Hospital, St. Louis, Missouri
Intravelar Veloplasty: A Prospective Study

J. Hrivnáková, M.D., D.Sci.

Deputy Head and Professor of Plastic Surgery, Charles University, Institute of Plastic Surgery, Prague, Czechoslovakia
Multidisciplinary Management of Cleft Lip and Palate in Prague, Czechoslovakia

C. Shing Huang, B.D.S., Ph.D.

Codirector, Craniofacial Center, Department of Plastic Surgery, Chang Gung Memorial Hospitals, Taipei, Taiwan
Multidisciplinary Management of Cleft Lip and Palate in Taiwan

A. G. Huddart, B.D.S., F.D.S., D.Orth., R.C.S., L.D.S.

Consultant Orthodontist, West Midlands Regional Plastic Unit, Wordsley Hospital, Wordsley, Stourbridge, West Midlands, England
Presurgical Orthopedic Treatment in Unilateral Cleft Lip and Palate

Donald V. Huebener, D.D.S., M.S., M.A. Ed.

Professor of Pediatric Dentistry, Washington University School of Dental Medicine, St. Louis, Missouri; Director, Division of Pediatric Dentistry, St. Louis Children's Hospital, St. Louis, Missouri
Alveolar Molding Appliances in the Treatment of Cleft Lip and Palate Infants

David Humphreys, M.D.

Active Staff, Memorial Mission Hospital, Asheville, North Carolina; Section Chief Plastic Surgery and Active Staff, St. Joseph Hospital, Asheville, North Carolina
Augmentation of the Posterior Pharyngeal Wall

Dennis J. Hurwitz, M.D.

Clinical Associate Professor of Surgery (Plastic), University of Pittsburgh School of Medicine, Pittsburgh, Pennsylvania
Unilateral Cleft Lip-Nose Repair

Annika Isberg, D.D.S., Ph.D.

Associate Professor, School of Dentistry, Karolinska Institutet, Stockholm, Sweden; Associate Professor, Department of Oral Radiology, School of Dentistry, Stockholm, Sweden
Oronasal Fistulas and Speech Production

Ian T. Jackson, M.D., F.R.C.S., F.A.C.S., F.R.A.C.S. (Hon.)

Director, Institute for Craniofacial and Reconstructive Surgery, Providence Hospital, Southfield, Michigan
Pharyngoplasty: Jackson Technique; Treatment of Skeletal Deformities in the Cleft Patient

D. L. Jones, Ph.D.

Assistant Research Scientist, Department of Otolaryngology—Head and Neck Surgery, College of Medicine, University of Iowa, Iowa City, Iowa; Adjunct Assistant Professor, Depart-

ment of Speech Pathology and Audiology, University of Iowa, Iowa City, Iowa
The Iowa-Hamburg Project: Late Results of Multidisciplinary Management at the Iowa Cleft Palate Center

Donald I. Kapetansky, M.D.

Late Clinical Associate Professor, Department of Surgery, Plastic Surgery Section, University of Michigan Medical School, Ann Arbor, Michigan; Late Clinical Associate Professor, Plastic and Reconstructive Surgery, Wayne State University Medical School, Detroit, Michigan; Late Director, Sinai Hospital of Detroit, Craniofacial Team, Detroit, Michigan
Bilateral Transverse Pharyngeal Flaps for Hypernasal Speech

Michael P. Karnell, Ph.D.

Assistant Professor, Otolaryngology–Head and Neck Surgery, Pritzker School of Medicine, University of Chicago, Chicago, Illinois; Director, Center for Speech and Swallowing Disorders, University of Chicago Medical Center, Chicago, Illinois
Measurement Problems in Estimating Velopharyngeal Function

E. Keller, D.D.S., M.S.D.

Associate Professor, Mayo Graduate School of Medicine, Rochester, Minnesota; Mayo Medical Center, Consultant in Oral and Maxillofacial Surgery, Rochester, Minnesota
Treatment of Skeletal Deformities in the Cleft Patient

Kevin M. Kelly, Ph.D.

Assistant Research Scientist, Department of Otolaryngology—Head and Neck Surgery, College of Medicine, University of Iowa, Iowa City, Iowa; Adjunct Assistant Professor, Department of Anthropology, University of Iowa, Iowa City, Iowa
The Iowa-Hamburg Project: Late Results of Multidisciplinary Management at the Iowa Cleft Palate Center; Cleft Lip and Palate Research: Approaches at the Cellular and Molecular Level; Expanding the Perception of Cleft Morphology: Anthropometric Studies of Body Growth, Size, and Form; Surgical-Orthodontic Correction of the Protruded Premaxilla

Susan I. Kemp-Fincham, M.A.

Doctoral Candidate, Department of Speech and Hearing Science, University of Illinois at Urbana-Champaign, Champaign, Illinois
Speech Development and the Timing of Primary Palatoplasty

Otto Kriens, M.D., D.D.S.

Professor, University of Hamburg, Bremen, Federal Republic of Germany
Documentation of Cleft Lip, Alveolus, and Palate; Anatomy of the Cleft Palate

Julia Kruk-Jeromin, M.D.

Professor and Chief of Department of Plastic Surgery, Medical Academy of Łódź, Łódź, Poland; Chief of Department of Plastic Surgery, Hospital No. 1, Medical Academy of Łódź, Łódź, Poland
Multidisciplinary Management of Cleft Lip and Palate in Łódź, Poland

Eberhard Kruse, M.D.

Assistant Professor, Department of Phoniatrics and Pedaudiology, Philipps-University Marburg/Lahn, Federal Republic of Germany
Two-Stage Palatoplasty: Schweckendiek Technique

Stan A. Kuczaj, II, Ph.D.

Professor of Psychology, Southern Methodist University, Dallas, Texas
Psychosocial Aspects of Cleft Lip and Palate: The Family

David P. Kuehn, Ph.D.

Associate Professor, Department of Speech and Hearing Science, University of Illinois at Urbana-Champaign, Champaign, Illinois
Speech Development and the Timing of Primary Palatoplasty

Don La Rossa, M.D.

Associate Professor of Surgery (Plastic), Hospital of the University of Pennsylvania, University of Pennsylvania School of Medicine, Philadelphia, Pennsylvania; Director, Cleft Lip and Palate Program, Children's Hospital of Philadelphia, and Hospital of the University of Pennsylvania, Philadelphia, Pennsylvania
The Furlow Double Reversing Z-Plasty for Cleft Palate Repair: The First Ten Years of Experience

Malcom A. Lesavoy, M.D., F.A.C.S.

Associate Professor of Surgery, Division of Plastic and Reconstructive Surgery, UCLA Medical Center, Los Angeles, California; Chief of Plastic and Reconstructive Surgery, Harbor/UCLA Medical Center, Torrance, California
Lip Adhesion in Unilateral and Bilateral Cleft Lip Repair

William K. Lindsay, M.D., B.Sc. (Med.), M.S. (Tor), F.R.C.S. (C), F.A.C.S.

Professor Emeritus, University of Toronto, Toronto, Ontario; Consultant in Surgery, The Hospital for Sick Children, Toronto, Ontario
Cleft Palate Repair: Von Langenbeck Technique

Jerilyn A. Logemann, Ph.D.

Professor and Chair, Communication Sciences and Disorders, Northwestern University, Evanston, Illinois; Professor in Otolaryngology, Head and Neck Surgery, Neurology and Communication Sciences and Disorders, Northwestern Memorial Hospital, Northwestern University, Chicago, Illinois
Early Speech Development in Cleft Palate Babies

R. Malek, M.D.

Chief of Surgery, Professor of College de Médécine des Hôpitaux de Paris, Paris, France; Hospital Jean Rostand, Sèvres-Paris Ouest, Paris, France
Multidisciplinary Management of Cleft Lip and Palate in Paris, France

W. M. Manchester, K.B.E., F.R.C.S., F.R.A.C.S., F.A.C.S.

Former Professor of Plastic and Reconstructive Surgery, University of Auckland, Auckland, New Zealand; Retired Head of the Plastic Surgical Unit, Middlemore Hospital, Auckland, New Zealand
Bilateral Cleft Lip and Palate Repair

Karin Manzari, M.D.

Resident at the Clinic for Plastic Surgery, Marienhospital, Stuttgart, Federal Republic of Germany
Twenty-five Years of Experience with Primary Bone Grafting

Jeffrey L. Marsh, M.D.

Professor of Surgery, Plastic and Reconstructive, and Professor of Surgery in Pediatrics (Plastic and Reconstructive), Washington University School of Medicine, St. Louis, Missouri; Director of Cleft Palate and Craniofacial Deformities Institute, St. Louis Children's Hospital, St. Louis, Missouri
Intravelar Veloplasty: A Prospective Study; Alveolar Molding Appliances in the Treatment of Cleft Lip and Palate Infants

H. Martinez, M.D.

Orthodontist, Hospital Jean Rostand, Sèvres, Paris, France
Multidisciplinary Management of Cleft Lip and Palate in Paris, France

Harold McComb, F.R.C.S., F.R.A.C.S, F.A.C.S.

Clinical Lecturer in Surgery, University of Western Australia, Perth, Australia; Emeritus Consultant Plastic Surgeon, Royal Perth Hospital; Emeritus Consultant Plastic Surgeon, Princess Margaret Hospital for Children, Perth, Australia
Anatomy of the Unilateral and Bilateral Cleft Lip Nose; Primary Unilateral and Bilateral Cleft Lip Nose Reconstruction

Carl O. McGrath, Ph.D.

Clinical Assistant Professor, Speech and Hearing Sciences, University of Washington, Seattle, Washington; Attending Staff, Children's Hospital and Medical Center, Seattle, Washington
Prosthetic Treatment of Velopharyngeal Incompetence

Betty Jane McWilliams, Ph.D.

Professor of Communication Disorders and Director, Cleft Palate-Craniofacial Center, University of Pittsburgh, Pittsburgh, Pennsylvania
The Long-Term Speech Results of Primary and Secondary Surgical Correction of Palatal Clefts

Robby Meijer, M.D., F.A.C.S.

Attending Plastic Surgeon, St. Barnabas Medical Center, Livingston, New Jersey; Director, Craniofacial Treatment Center, St. Barnabas Medical Center, Livingston, New Jersey
Two-Stage Palatoplasty and Evaluation of Speech Results

Ignacio Trigos Micolo, M.D.

Chief of the Plastic and Reconstructive Surgery Unit of the Hospital General Manuel Gea González; Associate Professor of Plastic Surgery, Graduate Division of the Medical School, Universidad Nacional Autónoma de Mexico, Mexico City, Mexico
Multidisciplinary Management of Cleft Lip and Palate in Mexico

Karlind T. Moller, Ph.D.

Professor and Director, Cleft Palate Maxillofacial and Craniofacial Anomalies Clinics, School of Dentistry, University of Minnesota, Minneapolis, Minnesota
Early Speech Development: The Interaction of Learning and Structure

Fernando Ortiz-Monasterio, M.D.

Professor of Plastic Surgery, Graduate Division of the Medical School, Universidad Nacional Antónoma de Mexico, Mexico City, Mexico
Multidisciplinary Management of Cleft Lip and Palate in Mexico

Jerald B. Moon, Ph.D.

Assistant Research Scientist, Adjunct Assistant Professor, Department of Speech Pathology and Audiology, University of Iowa, Iowa City, Iowa
Anatomy and Physiology of the Velopharynx; Approaches to the Study of Speech Production

Hughlett L. Morris, Ph.D.

Professor of Speech Pathology, Department of Otolaryngology–Head and Neck Surgery, Department of Speech Pathology and Audiology, University of Iowa, Iowa City, Iowa
The Iowa-Hamburg Project: Late Results of Multidisciplinary Management at the Iowa Cleft Palate Center; Clinical Assessment by the Speech Pathologist; Directions for Future Research

M-R. Mousset, Ph.D.

Speech Therapist, Hospital Jean Rostand, Sèvres-Paris Ouest, Paris, France
Multidisciplinary Management of Cleft Lip and Palate in Paris, France

Ž. Müllerová, M.D., C.Sc.

Scientific Research Worker, Head, Laboratory of Congenital Defects, Czechoslovak Academy of Sciences, Prague, Czechoslovakia
Multidisciplinary Management of Cleft Lip and Palate in Prague, Czechoslovakia; Presurgical Orthopedic Treatment in Unilateral Cleft Lip and Palate

Ian R. Munro, M.A., M.B., B. Chir., F.R.C.S. (C)

Director, Craniofacial Institute, Humana Advanced Surgical Institutes, Dallas, Texas
Orthognathic Surgery for Patients with Cleft Lip and Palate

Jeffrey C. Murray, M.D.

Associate Professor, Department of Pediatrics, University of Iowa College of Medicine, Iowa City, Iowa; Associate Professor, Department of Pediatrics, Division of Medical Genetics, University of Iowa Hospitals and Clinics, Iowa City, Iowa
Genetic Aspects of Cleft Lip and Palate

David Netscher, M.D.

Assistant Professor, Division of Plastic Surgery, Baylor College of Medicine, Houston, Texas; Attending Staff, Veterans Administration Hospital, Texas Children's Hospital, and The Methodist Hospital, Houston, Texas
Unilateral Cleft Lip Repair

M. Samuel Noordhoff, M.D., F.A.C.S.

Professor of Surgery, Chang Gung Medical College, Taipei, Taiwan; Chairman, Department of Plastic Surgery, Chang Gung Medical Hospitals, Taipei, Taiwan
Multidisciplinary Management of Cleft Lip and Palate in Taiwan; Bilateral Cleft Lip Repair

Peter Oblak, M.D., D.Sc.

Professor of Oral and Maxillofacial Surgery, University "Edvard Kardelj," Ljubljana, Yugoslavia; University Clinical Centre, Department of Oral and Maxillofacial Surgery, Ljubljana, Yugoslavia
The Importance of Nasal Airways in Cleft Patients

Mary M. O'Gara, M.A.
Assistant Professor, Team Coordinator, and Speech Language Pathologist, Northwestern University Dental School, Chicago, Illinois
Early Speech Development in Cleft Palate Babies

William H. Olin, D.D.S.
Professor, College of Medicine, Department of Otolaryngology–Head and Neck Surgery; Professor, College of Dentistry, Department of Orthodontics, University of Iowa, Iowa City, Iowa; Orthodontist, University of Iowa Hospitals and Clinics, Iowa City, Iowa
The Iowa-Hamburg Project: Late Results of Multidisciplinary Management at the Iowa Cleft Palate Center; Surgical-Orthodontic Correction of the Protruded Premaxilla; Orthodontic Treatment in Different Stages of Growth and Development

Miguel Orticochea, M.D.
Professor and Head, Plastic Surgery Division, School of Medicine, Pontificia Universidad Javeriana, Bogotá, Colombia
The Dynamic Muscle Sphincter of the Pharynx

Wiesława Perczyńska-Partyka, D.D.S.
Professor and Chief of Department of Maxillofacial Surgery, Medical Academy of Łódź, Łódź, Poland; Chief of Department of Maxillofacial Surgery, Hospital No 1, Medical Academy of Łódź, Łódź, Poland
Multidisciplinary Management of Cleft Lip and Palate in Łódź, Poland

Milivoj Perko, M.D.
Professor of Maxillofacial Surgery, University of Zürich, Zürich, Switzerland; Surgical Clinic University Children's Hospital, Zürich, Switzerland
Two-Stage Palatoplasty

Sally J. Peterson-Falzone, Ph.D.
Clinical Professor, University of California at San Francisco, San Francisco, California
A Cross-Sectional Analysis of Speech Results Following Palatal Closure

Betty Jane Philips, Ed.D.
Director, Special Clinical Services and Coordinator, Cleft Palate and Craniofacial Program, Boys Town National Institute, Omaha, Nebraska; Professor, Department of Otolaryngology and Human Communication, Medical School, Creighton University, Omaha, Nebraska
Early Speech Management

Jeffrey C. Posnick, D.M.D., M.D., F.R.C.S.C.
Assistant Professor, University of Toronto, Toronto, Ontario; Medical Director, Craniofacial Program, Department of Surgery; Consultant, Division of Plastic Surgery, The Hospital for Sick Children, Toronto, Ontario
Management of Jaw Deformities in the Cleft Patient

Tore Ramstad, B.D.S.
Prosthodontist, Oslo Cleft Lip/Palate Team, National Center of Logopedics, Oslo, Norway
Multidisciplinary Management of Cleft Lip and Palate in Oslo, Norway

Peter Randall, M.D., F.A.C.S.
Professor of Plastic Surgery, University of Pennsylvania School of Medicine, Philadelphia, Pennsylvania; Senior Surgeon, Children's Hospital of Philadelphia, Philadelphia, Pennsylvania
The Importance of Muscle; Lip Adhesion for Wide Unilateral and Bilateral Clefts of the Lip; Long-Term Results with the Triangular Flap Technique for Unilateral Cleft Lip Repair; The Furlow Double Reversing Z-Plasty for Cleft Palate Repair: The First Ten Years of Experience

Reijo Ranta, D.D.S.
Assistant Professor, Department of Pedodontics and Orthodontics, University of Helsinki, Helsinki, Finland; Senior Orthodontist, Cleft Center, Helsinki University Central Hospital, Helsinki, Finland
Orthodontic Treatment Alternatives for Unilateral Cleft Lip and Palate Patients

Heinz Reichert, M.D., D.M.D.
Professor of Surgery, Plastic Surgery, University of Ulm, Stuttgart, Federal Republic of Germany; Head and Chief Surgeon of the Clinic for Plastic and Reconstructive Surgery, Marienhospital, Stuttgart, Federal Republic of Germany
Twenty-five Years of Experience with Primary Bone Grafting; Cleft Septorhinoplasty: Free Septum Replantation for Secondary Correction

John F. Reinisch, M.D., F.A.C.S.
Associate Professor of Clinical Surgery (Plastic), and Chief of Plastic Surgery, University of Southern California School of Medicine, Los Angeles, California; Head, Division of Plastic Surgery, Children's Hospital Los Angeles; Attending Surgeon, Hospital of the Good Samaritan; Los Angeles County–University of Southern California Medical Center, Los Angeles, California
Complications of Cleft Lip Repair

Marcy T. Rogers, M. Ed.
President, International Craniofacial Foundations, Dallas, Texas
Psychosocial Aspects of Cleft Lip and Palate: The Family

M. Röhrs, M.D.
Otolaryngologist and Speech Pathologist, Department of Otolaryngology, Speech Pathology and Audiology, Hamburg University, Hamburg, Federal Republic of Germany
The Iowa-Hamburg Project: Late Results of Multidisciplinary Management at the Iowa Cleft Palate Center

Inger-Lise Saether, M.A.
Speech Pathologist, Oslo Cleft Lip/Palate Team, National Center of Logopedics, Oslo, Norway
Multidisciplinary Management of Cleft Lip and Palate in Oslo, Norway

Kenneth E. Salyer, M.D., F.A.C.S., F.A.A.P., F.I.C.S.
Director, International Craniofacial Institute, Humana Medical City, Dallas, Texas
Unilateral Cleft Lip and Cleft Lip Nasal Reconstruction; Orthognathic Surgery for Patients with Cleft Lip and Palate

Harm K. Schutte, M.D., Ph.D.
Professor of Phoniatrics, University Hospital, Groningen, The Netherlands; Chief of the Voice Research Laboratory, University Hospital, Groningen, The Netherlands
Cleft Palate Repair: The Von Langenbeck Technique

Wolfram Schweckendiek, M.D.
Professor of Otolaryngology and Maxillofacial Surgery, Klinik Dr. Schweckendiek, Hals-, Nasen- und Ohrenkrankheiten Lippen-, Kiefer-, Gaumenspalten, Marburg, Federal Republic of Germany
Two-Stage Palatoplasty: Schweckendiek Technique

Earl J. Seaver, Ph.D.
Associate Professor, Department of Communicative Disorders, Northern Illinois University, DeKalb, Illinois; Adjunct Professor, University of Illinois College of Medicine at Rockford, Rockford, Illinois, and University of Chicago, Pritzker School of Medicine, Chicago, Illinois
Measurement Problems in Estimating Velopharyngeal Function

Gunvor Semb, D.D.S.
Head of Odontological Department, National Center of Logopedics, Oslo Cleft Lip/Palate Team, Oslo, Norway
Multidisciplinary Management of Cleft Lip and Palate in Oslo, Norway; The Influence of Pharyngeal Flap on Facial Growth; Influence of Alveolar Bone Grafting on Facial Growth

William Shaw, B.D.S., M.Sc.D., Ph.D., F.D.S., D.Orth., D.D.Orth.
Professor of Orthodontics and Dentofacial Development, University Dental Hospital of Manchester, Manchester, England; Chairman, Department of Oral Health and Development, and Consultant to North West Regional Health Authority, Manchester, England
Multidisciplinary Management of Cleft Lip and Palate in the United Kingdom; The Influence of Pharyngeal Flap on Facial Growth; Influence of Alveolar Bone Grafting on Facial Growth

Robert J. Shprintzen, Ph.D.
Professor of Plastic Surgery and Otolaryngology, Albert Einstein College of Medicine, Bronx, New York; Director, Center for Craniofacial Disorders, Montefiore Medical Center, Bronx, New York
The Conceptual Framework for Pharyngeal Flap Surgery

V. Simecek, M.D.
Orthodontist, Medical Faculty, J. E. Purkyně University, Brno, Czechoslovakia; Clinic of Plastic Surgery, University of Brno, Brno, Czechoslovakia
Multidisciplinary Management of Cleft Lip and Palate in Brno, Czechoslovakia

Gerald M. Sloan, M.D., F.A.C.S.
Assistant Professor of Surgery (Plastic), University of Southern California School of Medicine, Los Angeles, California; Attending Surgeon, Children's Hospital Los Angeles, Hospital of the Good Samaritan, and Los Angeles County-University of Southern California Medical Center, Los Angeles, California
Complications of Cleft Lip Repair

Z. Šmahel, M.D., C.Sc.
Scientific Research Worker, Laboratory for Congenital Defects, Czechoslovak Academy of Sciences, Prague, Czechoslovakia

Multidisciplinary Management of Cleft Lip and Palate in Prague, Czechoslovakia; Presurgical Orthopedic Treatment in Unilateral Cleft Lip and Palate

Paul H. M. Spauwen, M.D., Ph.D.
Assistant Professor of Plastic Surgery, University Hospital, Groningen, The Netherlands; Consultant, Department of Plastic Surgery, University Hospital, Groningen, The Netherlands
Cleft Palate Repair: The Von Langenbeck Technique

Melvin Spira, M.D.
Professor and Head, Division of Plastic Surgery, Baylor College of Medicine, Houston, Texas; Chief of Plastic Surgery Service at The Methodist Hospital, Houston, Texas
Unilateral Cleft Lip Repair

Christopher A. Squier, Ph.D., Dr. Sc.
Professor, Oral Pathology, and Director, Dows Institute for Dental Research, Iowa City, Iowa; Assistant Dean for Research, College of Dentistry, University of Iowa, Iowa City, Iowa
Cleft Lip and Palate Research: Approaches at the Cellular and Molecular Level

Samuel Stal, M.D.
Associate Professor, Division of Plastic Surgery, Baylor College of Medicine, Houston, Texas; Chief of Plastic Surgery, Texas Children's Hospital; Chief of Plastic Surgery, Texas Institute for Research and Rehabilitation, Houston, Texas
Unilateral Cleft Lip Repair

Clark D. Starr, Ph.D.
Professor, Department of Communication Disorders, University of Minnesota, Minneapolis, Minnesota; Consultant, University of Minnesota Cleft Palate Maxillofacial Clinic, Minneapolis, Minnesota
Treatment by Therapeutic Exercises

Deb Starr, R.N., B.S.N.
Cleft Nurse Specialist, Otolaryngology–Head and Neck Surgery Clinic, University of Iowa Hospitals and Clinics, Iowa City, Iowa
Comprehensive Nursing Care for Cleft Patients

Ronald P. Strauss, D.M.D., Ph.D.
Professor, Department of Dental Ecology, School of Dentistry, University of North Carolina at Chapel Hill, Chapel Hill, North Carolina; Oral-Facial and Communicative Disorders Program, University of North Carolina Memorial Hospital, Chapel Hill, North Carolina
Psychological and Sociocultural Aspects of Cleft Lip and Palate

David A. Stringer, B.Sc., M.B.B.S., F.R.C.R., F.R.C.P.C.
Associate Professor, Faculty of Medicine, University of Toronto, Toronto, Ontario; Head, Sections of Gastrointestinal Radiology and Ultrasound, Department of Radiology, The Hospital for Sick Children, Toronto, Ontario
Methods of Assessing Velopharyngeal Function

Sylvan E. Stool, M.D.
Professor of Otolaryngology and Pediatrics, University of Pittsburgh School of Medicine, Pittsburgh, Pennsylvania; Children's Hospital of Pittsburgh, Pittsburgh, Pennsylvania
Ear Disease in Children with Cleft Palate: State of the Art

Richard Sturm, L.P.N.

Nurse Coordinator, Plastic Surgery, University of Kansas Medical Center, Kansas City, Kansas
Correction of Secondary Unilateral and Bilateral Cleft Lip Deformities

J. Daniel Subtelny, D.D.S., M.D.

Chairman, Department of Orthodontics, Eastman Dental Center, Rochester, New York; Professor of Clinical Dentistry, University of Rochester, Rochester, New York; Consultant, The Genesee Hospital, Rochester, New York; Professor of Clinical Dentistry, Strong Memorial Hospital, Rochester, New York
Orthodontic Principles in the Treatment of Cleft Lip and Palate

Joyce M. Tobiasen, Ph.D.

Associate Professor of Pediatrics and Surgery, and Key Investigator, Smith Research Center, University of Kansas Medical Center, Kansas City, Kansas; Attending Staff, University Hospital, University of Kansas, Kansas City, Kansas
Psychosocial Adjustment to Cleft Lip and Palate

Marie Tolarova, M.D., Ph.D., D.Sc.

Head, Clinical Genetics Laboratory, Institute of Experimental Medicine, Czechoslovak Academy of Sciences, Prague, Czechoslovakia
Genetic Findings in Cleft Lip and Palate in the Czech Population

C. Trichet, M.A.

Speech Therapist, Hospital Jean Rostand, Sèvres-Paris Ouest, Paris, France
Multidisciplinary Management of Cleft Lip and Palate in Paris, France

William C. Trier, M.D.

Professor of Surgery, School of Medicine, University of Washington, Seattle, Washington; Attending Staff, University Hospital, Children's Hospital and Medical Center, and Harborview Medical Center, Seattle, Washington
Pharyngoplasty

Judith E. Trost-Cardamone, Ph.D.

Associate Professor, Department of Communicative Disorders, California State University at Northridge, Northridge, California
Speech Development and the Timing of Primary Palatoplasty

Timothy A. Turvey, D.D.S.

Professor, Department of Oral and Maxillofacial Surgery, University of North Carolina, Chapel Hill, North Carolina; Attending Staff, The University of North Carolina Hospitals, Chapel Hill, North Carolina
Bone Grafting of the Cleft Maxilla

Cindy Tvedte, R.N., B.S.N.

Head Nurse, Otolaryngology–Head and Neck Surgery Clinic, University of Iowa Hospitals and Clinics, Iowa City, Iowa
Comprehensive Nursing Care for Cleft Patients

D. R. Van Demark, Ph.D.

Professor, Department of Otolaryngology–Head and Neck Surgery and Speech Pathology-Audiology, University of Iowa, Iowa City, Iowa; Professor, Department of Otolaryngology, Coordinator of Cleft Palate Clinic, University Hospitals, Iowa City, Iowa
Speech Therapy for the Child with Cleft Lip and Palate

Karin Vargervik, D.D.S.

Professor and Director, Center for Craniofacial Anomalies, School of Dentistry, University of California, San Francisco, California
Orthodontic Treatment of Cleft Patients: Characteristics of Growth and Development/Treatment Principles

Katherine W. L. Vig, B.D.S., M.S., F.D.S., D. Orth.

Associate Professor, Department of Orthodontics and Pediatric Dentistry, University of Michigan School of Dentistry, Ann Arbor, Michigan; University Hospital, Michigan Medical Center, Ann Arbor, Michigan
Bone Grafting of the Cleft Maxilla

M. Vohradník, M.D., C.Sc.

Assistant Professor, Charles University, Institute of Plastic Surgery, Prague, Czechoslovakia
Multidisciplinary Management of Cleft Lip and Palate in Prague, Czechoslovakia

Takeshi Wada, D.D.S., Ph.D.

Professor and Chairman, Division for Oral-Facial Disorders, Osaka University Faculty of Dentistry, Osaka, Japan; Professor and Chairman, Division for Oral-Facial Disorders, Hospital, Osaka University Faculty of Dentistry, Osaka, Japan
Multidisciplinary Management of Cleft Lip and Palate in Osaka, Japan

Bonnie Wagner, R.N., B.S.N.

Nurse Clinician II, Pediatric Nursing Division, University of Iowa Hospitals and Clinics, Iowa City, Iowa
Comprehensive Nursing Care for Cleft Patients

Donald W. Warren, D.D.S., M.S., Ph.D.

Kenan Professor and Director, Oral-Facial and Communicative Disorders Program, University of North Carolina at Chapel Hill School of Dentistry, Research Professor of Otolaryngology, School of Medicine, University of North Carolina at Chapel Hill, Chapel Hill, North Carolina; Attending, Hospital Dentistry, University of North Carolina Hospitals, Chapel Hill, North Carolina
The Nasal Airway in Cleft Palate

Libby Wilson, M.D.

Associate Clinical Professor of Surgery, University of Southern California, Los Angeles, California; Chief, Cleft Palate Service, Rancho Los Amigos Medical Center, Downey, California
Evaluation of Late Results of Cleft Palate Repair

Mary Anne Witzel, Ph.D.

Associate Professor, Faculty of Medicine; Associate Member, School of Graduate Studies; Associate in Dentistry, Faculty of

Dentistry, University of Toronto, Toronto, Ontario; Director, Department of Speech Pathology, The Hospital for Sick Children, Toronto, Ontario
Cleft Palate Repair: Von Langenbeck Technique; Management of Jaw Deformities in the Cleft Patient; Methods of Assessing Velopharyngeal Function

Jorie Wu, M.A.
Director, Speech Pathology, Craniofacial Center, Department of Plastic Surgery, Chang Gung Memorial Hospitals, Taipei, Taiwan
Multidisciplinary Management of Cleft Lip and Palate in Taiwan

There is a vast amount of literature on cleft lip and palate treatment today. The abundance of information in this field has created the impression that we know enough, or nearly enough, about the various treatment procedures developed by the individual disciplines in order to manage clefts successfully. We also have been under the impression that the various treatment procedures have been carefully investigated and that we are now able to achieve consistently satisfactory results if we apply these procedures properly. Finally, we have assumed that multidisciplinary management, interaction among various specialists, and the functioning of the cleft palate team have been well established and analyzed from different aspects.

If we take a critical look at the papers published or presented at national and international conferences and congresses, we find that relatively few sutudies have been designed to evaluate the effectiveness of various treatment procedures using the proper methods of clinical research. Perhaps such studies would not be so necessary if we were consistently getting very good or even satisfactory results. But the effectiveness of current treatment strategies is not as high as one would expect, and this should motivate us to design more comprehensive studies for evaluation of our treatment techniques.

Cleft lip and palate is one of the most common congenital anomalies. Treatment of this deformity presents a serious problem for health delivery systems all over the world, and its prevention seems unlikely in the near future. Multidisciplinary management, therefore, will be necessary for many years to come. It is imperative that we increase our efforts to improve treatment in order to achieve more accurate, comprehensive results.

These considerations, the existence of many unanswered questions, and the observation that management of patients with clefts presents more diverse facets and intricate controversies than one can imagine stimulated us to design this book as a compilation of the state-of-the-art management procedures. To accomplish our goal of producing a book that focuses on multidisciplinary treatment, long-term results, and controversial problems, we invited leading specialists in the field to participate in its preparation. Representatives from 21 countries and from the foremost centers for treatment of cleft lip and palate in the United States have contributed.

For the first time, an international review of the multidisciplinary team approach is presented and the applications of that approach are discussed. Some authors have presented new ideas for treatment, some describe the evolution of their treatment centers, and others review their treatment philosophies and the long-term results of their procedures. There are clear indications that the concept of team management, as understood and practiced at one center, may differ quite substantially from that followed at other centers. Reports from different centers demonstrate that rehabilitation of cleft patients is well organized in some countries, whereas other centers are in earlier stages of development. To get an idea of the present situation in various countries and in various centers within a country, when planning this book, we asked the contributors to present their philosophies of treatment, their clinical and research activities, and available data.

Evaluation and accurate presentation of the long-term results of multidisciplinary treatment are essential to proper assessment of our treatment strategies and techniques. For many years, we have questioned the absence of publications focusing specifically on long-term results. These results may serve as the most important information about our successes and failures. In reviewing the literature, it is almost impossible to find well-documented, long-term studies that analyze various treatment procedures. This lack of information is evident, even for those techniques that seem to be widely accepted. There are several reasons why there are few attempts to evaluate long-term results of particular treatment procedures. The primary reason seems to be that the treatment results are neither highly satisfactory nor consistently good. Many treatment procedures were never scientifically assessed, and there is no information as to how advantageous they really are. Since we strongly believe that there are many roads leading to Rome, we are not trying to select the best concept of multidisciplinary management or even the best concept for one particular procedure. We do believe that many different treatment strategies and techniques produce good results, and this is documented in the book.

The authors have compiled these strategies with quantitative documentation, which indicates that their results are satisfactory despite differing treatment philosophies and techniques. This observation supports an important possibility, which for many years escaped our attention when searching for the "best" treatment techniques: a variety of techniques may be considered the "best," since the final results may be highly acceptable even though different approaches were used. Perhaps we do not need to establish a single, uniformly accepted management strategy for treatment of cleft patients. Choosing from more than one approach may open the door to a better understanding of the various treatment strategies and their applications. This option should encourage us to explore more unorthodox ideas and approaches.

In many chapters, cooperation among specialists is emphasized, and many chapters include quantitative documentation and analysis. This part of the book is especially important because it presents the diversity of treatment strategies and techniques and emphasizes the importance of well-organized interdisciplinary collaboration. Many specialists express their opinions on the basis of their clinical observations and impressions. However, the majority of specialists in this book have presented quantitatively analyzed results to substantiate their hypotheses. In many chapters, new criteria and principles for treatment are introduced. New diagnostic techniques have been emphasized, since they facilitate planning of the overall treatment. Some chapters exemplify how a difficult and controversial problem can be approached more scientifically and expansively by involving several cooperating disciplines. Other chapters discuss the questions, problems, and controversial issues that remain and that require further and better investigation.

In this book, we present a broad spectrum of various problems related to the diagnosis and multidisciplinary treatment of patients with clefts. This spectrum includes genetics, a variety of surgical procedures, different approaches to orthodontic treatment, a multiplicity of topics related to speech pathology, problems of psychosocial aspects in cleft patients, and finally nursing care. We wish to emphasize the innovative ideas, new diagnostic and treatment techniques, and critical analyses of results that appear in each section. Over the years, it has become more and more evident that we can best learn about our weaknesses and shortcomings through comprehensive analysis of long-term results. We believe that this approach will lead us to more consistent and more successful results.

There is a paramount question to be asked: How much do we know, and how much do we have to learn to be able to provide the best treatment possible for individuals affected by clefts? Human nature and intellectual curiosity motivate us to pursue answers, explore new techniques, and define unsolved problems. To achieve this, we need an analytical approach. We believe that this book offers this to a much greater extent than ever before in the area of cleft treatment. Since we cannot yet prevent cleft deformities, we must strive to perfect their treatment.

ACKNOWLEDGMENTS. For many years, both of us cultivated the idea of this book, even though our visions differed. Use of discussions made the idea clearer, and we finally agreed on the present format. This book presents a tremendous amount of effort from an international group of outstanding cleft specialists. The editors would like to express their deep gratitude and appreciation to all of the contributors for the time and effort spent in preparation of this book.

Very special words of gratitude and deep appreciation are directed to Susan Sharkey, past research assistant at the Iowa Cleft Palate Research Center, who helped immensely in the preparation of this book by working with 109 manuscripts and organizing them for publication. We also want to express our gratitude to the members of our team, who helped with galley proofs, illustrations, and references: research assistants Kerry Johanssen and Keverley Swantz, and former research assistant, Michael Newton. Very special words of gratitude are directed to one essential person, without whom this book would not be prepared as accurately and deliberately as it is, a super secretary, Pamela Culver.

Special thanks to Mrs. Ruth Low, freelance editor, for her meticulous editorial work.

In the preparation and assembling of this book, there were many factors essential to successful accomplishment. Perhaps the most important one was coordination and mutual understanding with the publisher. This book was started in close cooperation with Diana McAninich, to whom we are indebted for her professional advice and encouragement. We are also grateful to senior medical editor Albert E. Meier, who participated in the editorial process, supplying us with his experience and expertise. A very good professional relationship established with senior medical editor Richard Zorab was very helpful in the final stages of preparation, when very serious decisions were made concerning this book. A very special gratitude is directed to Hazel A. Hacker, assistant development editor—Medical Books, for her help in coordinating chapters and organizing all of the details in every chapter. This book would not have been produced in such an elegant form without great input from the Saunders Production Department, especially by Mr. William Preston, production manager, and Mr. Brett MacNaughton, illustration coordinator.

Janusz Bardach, M.D.
Hughlett L. Morris, Ph.D.

CONTENTS

SECTION I
International Review of Management of Cleft Lip and Palate 1

SECTION II
Genetic Aspects and Classification 113

SECTION III
Primary Surgical Treatment of Cleft Lip and Nose 134

SECTION IV
Secondary Surgical Treatment of Cleft Lip and Nose 247

SECTION V
Primary Surgical Treatment of Cleft Palate 287

SECTION VI
Secondary Surgical Treatment of Cleft Palate

SECTION VII
Techniques for Evaluation of Craniofacial Morphology

SECTION X
Nasal Airway, Otologic, and Audiologic Problems Associated with Cleft Lip and Palate

SECTION XI
Speech and Language Diagnosis and Treatment

International Review of Management of Cleft Lip and Palate

CHAPTER 1

Multidisciplinary Management of Cleft Lip and Palate in Paris, France

R. Malek, H. Martinez, M-R. Mousset, and C. Trichet

Our team is based on the school of Pierre Petit, who has had vast experience in the area of clefts. During his 30 years of service he treated approximately 16,000 cleft patients. He followed Veau's technical principles.[1, 2] Like Veau, he advocated a multidisciplinary approach to cleft anomalies. With Borel-Maisonny, Veau's collaborator, Petit tried to improve the speech results of the classic method, introducing a pharyngoplasty technique to correct the residual velopharyngeal insufficiency.[3]

Petit also paid great attention to the growth of the facial skeleton and dental problems. With his pupil, Jean Psaume[4] (an orthodontist), he made several improvements in the treatment procedures. Lip surgery was delayed until 6 months of age to avoid disturbing the growth of the premaxilla. Palate repair was carried out at 18 months of age. Additionally, orthodontic treatment was systematically started during the permanent dentition phase.

Although some improvements in treatment had been made, dental results were not entirely satisfactory. In 1975, we took into account the new idea that elevating the mucoperiosteum at the time of palate repair might be detrimental to the development of the maxilla. When a technique was developed for cleft palate closure, without undermining of the mucoperiosteum, we then thought, with Psaume, that the timing and sequence of surgical procedures could be changed.[5–8] Our speech therapists, pupils of Borel-Maisonny, argued for early palate repair.

Our treatment approach is, thus, a perfect illustration of the advantages of a multidisciplinary team for the management of these cleft patients.

Method

In patients with complete clefts of the lip, alveolus, and palate, veloplasty is performed when the patient is 3 months of age. Lip repair is done at 6 months. During lip repair, the hard palate is closed as well without raising mucoperiosteal flaps. A palatal plate is applied for a short period before and after surgical repair.

The surgical treatment of cleft lip and palate is completed by the time the patient is 6 months of age (8 months for bilateral clefts, the two sides of the lip being repaired separately with an interval of 2 months between procedures). We emphasize that veloplasty should be performed prior to lip repair. *Thus, complete repair of the cleft lip, alveolus, and palate* is achieved by 6 to 8 months of age.

Physiopathologic Rationale

There are three reasons for implementation of this new therapeutic approach:

1. Skeletal and dental. The role of muscular imbalance is an important factor in maxillary growth and dental malformations.

2. Functional. Complete early repair may result in normal development of various functions.

3. Iatrogenic. The consequences of surgical techniques are now better known and understood so that harmful factors can be precluded.

Skeletal and Dental Factors

Molding of the facial skeleton during the growth and alignment of the maxillary segments depends on the muscular forces applied to their superficial and deep surfaces. On one side there are the facial muscles; on the other, the lingual muscular mass. The harmonious growth of the midface and maxillary arch depends on the balance between these forces. The cleft disrupts this equilibrium.

Lingual Musculature

Tongue physiology is disturbed. The tongue is an extremely mobile and sensitive organ, which continuously explores the roof of the oral cavity. In the presence of a cleft, the tip or the lateral surface of the tongue tends to reach between the palatal shelves (Fig. 1–1). During swallowing (and this starts very early because the fetus swallows amniotic fluid before birth), successive contractions take place in the tongue. The surface resembles a wave progressing backward to push the liquids down the esophagus. When there is a cleft palate, the tongue positions itself within the cleft, making contact with the upper part of the posterior pharyngeal wall to accomplish swallowing. Cineradiography of swallowing also has confirmed the presence of the tongue in the nasopharynx. P. Oblak has also noted it.[9–10]

The posture of the tongue (passive or dynamic), therefore, is more posterior compared with the normal position. As a consequence, there is less normal pressure against the maxillary segments. Furthermore, the tongue has a lateral position in unilateral cleft. This leads to a deviation of the vomer and a slope of the palatal shelves in addition to a lateral deviation of the mandible (Fig. 1–2).

The presence of the tongue in the nasopharynx plays a significant role in its transverse widening at the level of the pterygoid process. This is further exacerbated by the absence of the normal muscle continuity in the cleft width (Fig. 1–3). Measurements of the nasopharynx with computed tomography (CT) scans have documented this widening as reported by Peyton,[11] Wardill,[12] Psaume,[13] Subtelny,[14] and others.

Facial Musculature

The imbalance of the facial musculature plays a major role in the morphology of the cleft. The orbicularis ring is disrupted by the cleft, but the sphincteric action still occurs owing to the continuity of the facial muscles at the level of the nose and chin. The division of the orbicularis oris is responsible for the classic distortion

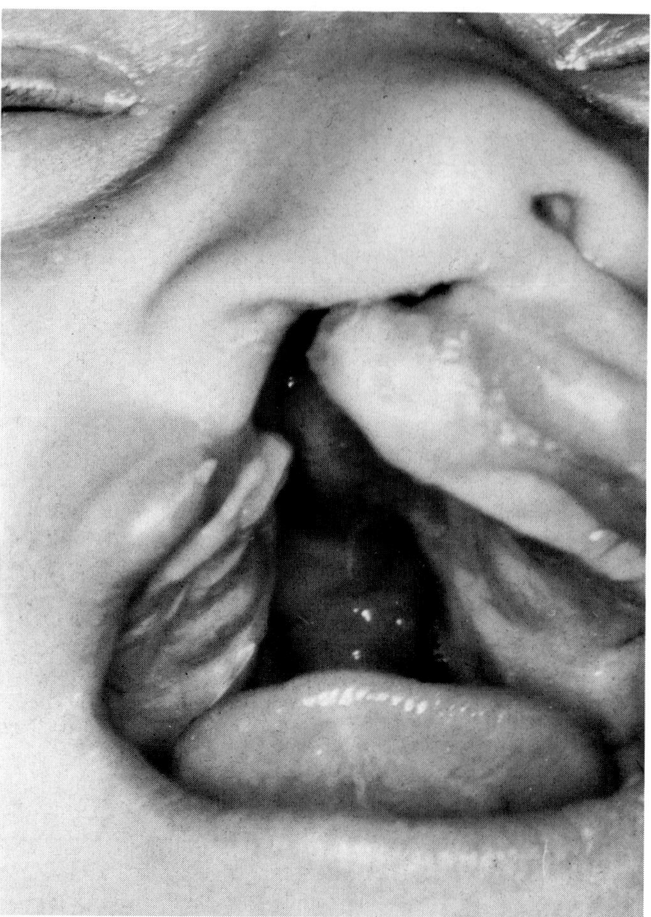

Figure 1–2 The slope of the palatal shelves and the distortion of the vomer in a unilateral cleft.

including deviation of the premaxilla and nasal spine toward the noncleft side (Fig. 1–4). The reduced pressure on the premaxilla allows it to move anteriorly, probably because it is pushed by the vomerian growth.

Imbalance of Muscle Actions

Prior to repair, there is a lack of balance between the tongue and the facial musculature, the latter being stronger. In unilateral clefts, this imbalance may be one of the factors leading to spontaneous collapse of the maxillary arch involving the smaller maxillary segment and resulting in narrowing of the arch (Fig. 1–5). This collapse can occur early and is sometimes difficult to diagnose because it is hidden by retrognathism. On the contrary, one can assume that there may be unfavorable occlusion because of the lateral deviation of the mandible, which is due to the lateral displacement of the tongue.

Based on this logic and understanding of the muscle imbalance and forces we can argue that (1) *if the lip is repaired first* (or if a lip adhesion is performed), the concentric superficial muscular forces are increased, and the risk of anterior collapse of the smaller maxillary segment is higher, or that (2) on the contrary, *if the soft palate is repaired first*, the tongue will settle into a

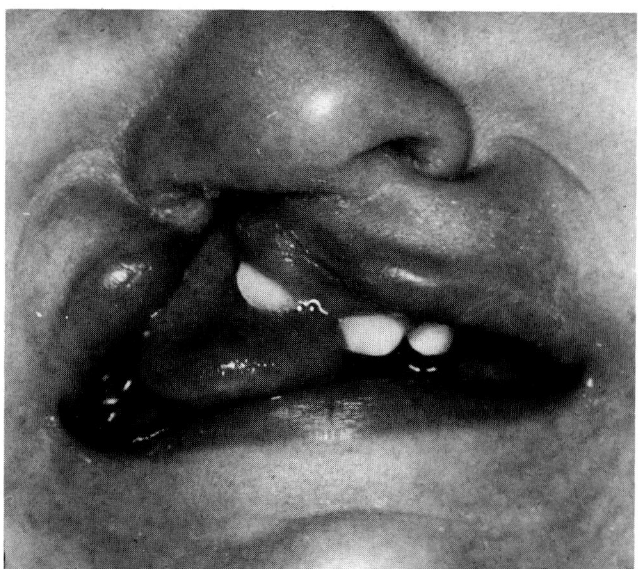

Figure 1–1 The lateral position of the tongue between the maxillary segments.

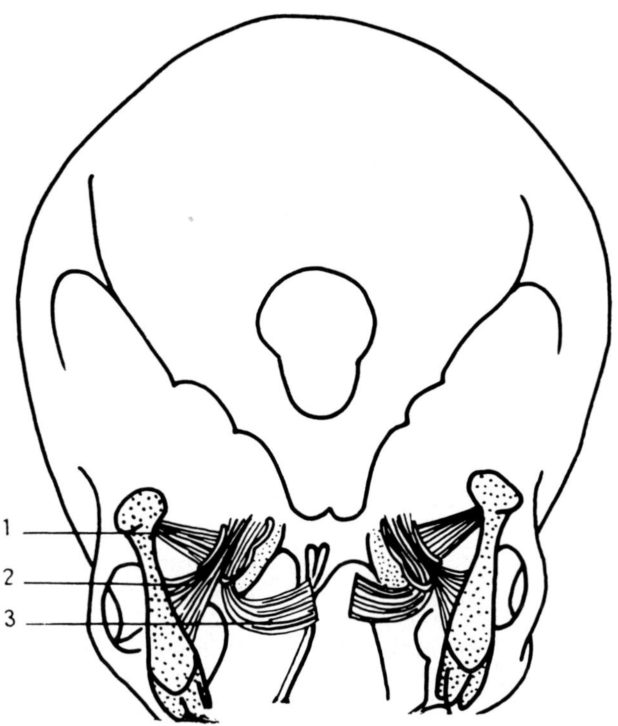

Figure 1–3 The lateral deviation of the pterygoid processes due to the palatal muscle imbalance (3), and the predominant action of the lateral (1) and medial (2) pterygoid muscles.

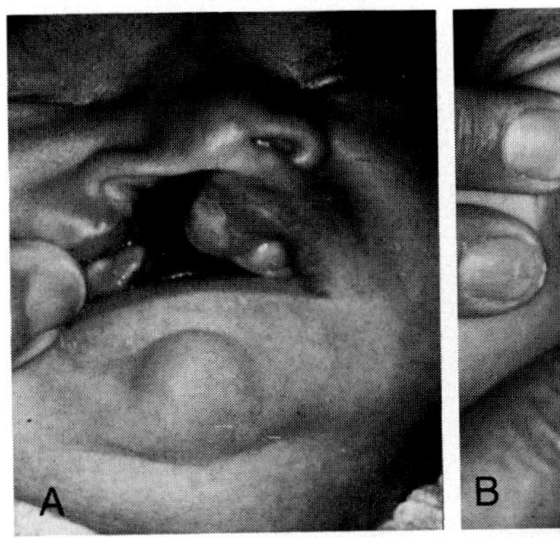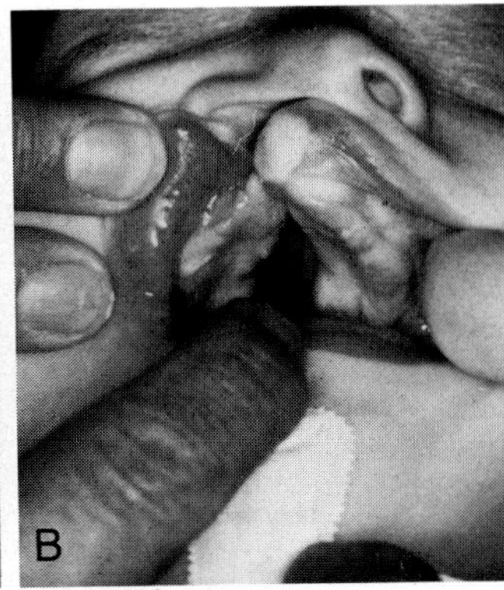

Figure 1–5 The spontaneous narrowing of the cleft (A) at birth and (B) three months later.

more anterior position, creating a counter pressure on the maxillary segments to oppose the pressure resulting from the lip repair. This hypothesis has led us to change the classic sequence of surgical treatment: *veloplasty first, lip repair second.* Our timing is as follows: (1) veloplasty is performed at 3 months of age; (2) lip repair is done at 6 months of age.

In our opinion, veloplasty logically should be performed immediately after birth; however, the cleft is often very wide at that time, and surgery may be difficult and risky. During the first 3 months, a preoperative appliance is used to prevent spontaneous narrowing of the maxillary segments and medial collapse of the lesser

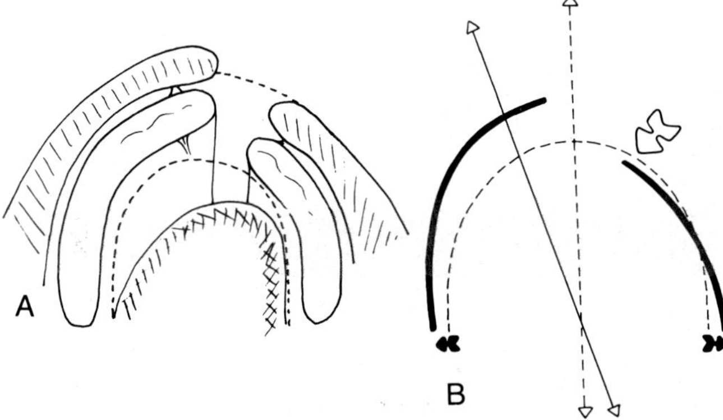

Figure 1–4 *A,* The classic position of the maxillary segments. Exterior dotted line represents superficial muscle action; interior dotted line represents deep muscle action. *B,* The imbalance between superficial and deep muscle action. Dashed line shows normal anatomic position. Clear blade arrow indicates a retropositioning of the small maxillary segment.

segment. Lip repair is performed simultaneously with closure of the hard palate at 6 months of age. Hard palate closure is easier at this time because the cleft edges are closer together owing to the effects of the veloplasty. Also, the cleft can be closed in two layers, decreasing the risk of an oronasal fistula. Another reason to delay lip repair is that early lip repair may disturb the growth of the premaxilla.[15] Furthermore, we speculate that a delay is necessary for the tongue to contract and exert more anterior pressure.

Functional Reasons

Early repair is advocated for functional reasons as well. Generally, in any growing system, the first utilizations of neural circuits and motor patterns are established by the brain in a preferential way. It is easy to imagine that when a function is learned in conjunction with an abnormal anatomy at the beginning, a pathologic impairment of this function is possible. The neuromotor patterns may be difficult to change if the correction is performed too late.

It is well known that phonetic patterns develop very early.[16] Babbling begins at about 6 months of age and is essential to further speech development. As a matter of fact, it is preceded by two successive clinical stages: (1) at 6 weeks of age an infant produces glottal stops. (2) at 3 months an infant practices anterior articulation movements. These stages must be taken into account. When veloplasty is performed at 3 months and complete closure of the hard palate at 6 months, we meet necessary requirements for the child's phonetic development. Early cleft palate repair increases the chances for normal speech. Reconstructing the muscular balance strengthens the velar and pharyngeal musculature and stimulates growth of the structures, decreasing hypoplasia. Narrowing the transverse dimension of the nasopharynx after veloplasty helps the patient achieve better velopharyngeal closure. We have shown with CT scans that enlargement of the nasopharynx can be corrected (measuring the interior interpterygoid distance at the time of the veloplasty and 3 months later).

When we compare the interpterygoid distance with the distance between the mandibular rami at the same level (we call this ratio the *pterygomandibular index*) we find that 3 months after veloplasty it approaches the normal ratio. In the normal child, this ratio of 0.33 changes little if at all (Fig. 1–6).[17]

Early repair also normalizes other essential functions that are disrupted by the cleft. These functions include (1) respiration—by restoring the oronasal partition; (2) swallowing—by changing the action of the tongue; (3) sucking—an infant cannot create negative pressure in the oral cavity when closure is impossible; (4) hearing—as the mechanism of the eustachian tube is disturbed by the cleft.

Iatrogenic Factors

The iatrogenic effects of surgical treatment support our choice of techniques and timing. The first iatrogenic factor, raising the mucoperiosteum during cleft palate repair as was classically done, has a deleterious effect (Fig. 1–7), a notion that is relatively recent (Schweckendiek's method).[18, 19] When this dissection is avoided, dentomaxillary development is improved. We are now aware of the poor speech results that are obtained with late repair of the hard palate. Therefore, in our opinion, complete, early closure of the palatal cleft is important. However, this repair is technically difficult and carries a risk of creating residual fistulas.

Another iatrogenic factor could be related to the effects of lip repair. Petit and Psaume suggested that when the lip is repaired before 6 months of age the resulting pressure on the maxillary segments may inhibit facial growth.[15] Such an assertion was probably true with the previously used techniques. We are not sure that this is presently the case because we have adopted less traumatic lip repair techniques.

In conclusion, it seems that our approach is justified in view of the anatomic and physiologic problems discussed. Yet it is true to say that surgery often has preceded reasoning. Arguments may remain theoretical; however, the study of results will demonstrate their consistency according to the principles of the experimental method.

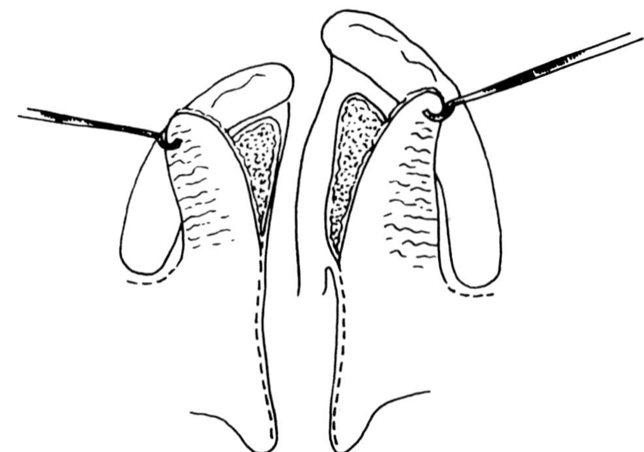

Figure 1–7 Raising of mucoperiosteum should be avoided.

Materials and Methods

We started treating complete cleft patients with this new approach in 1976. Currently, 451 children have been treated since birth. All children have been operated on by the same surgeon, giving good homogeneity to our series. The distribution of cleft types was as follows:

190 complete left unilateral clefts	42%
110 complete right unilateral clefts	24%
119 complete bilateral and symmetrical clefts	26%
32 complete bilateral and asymmetrical clefts	7%

A total of 1053 primary operations were performed; 451 veloplasties were initially performed followed by

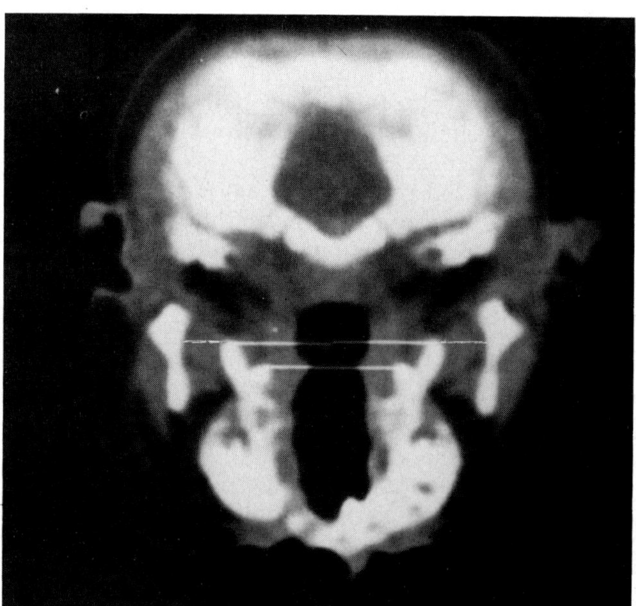

Figure 1–6 The pterygomandibular index measured by horizontal CT scan. In this example it is 0.64 instead of 0.33 (normal).

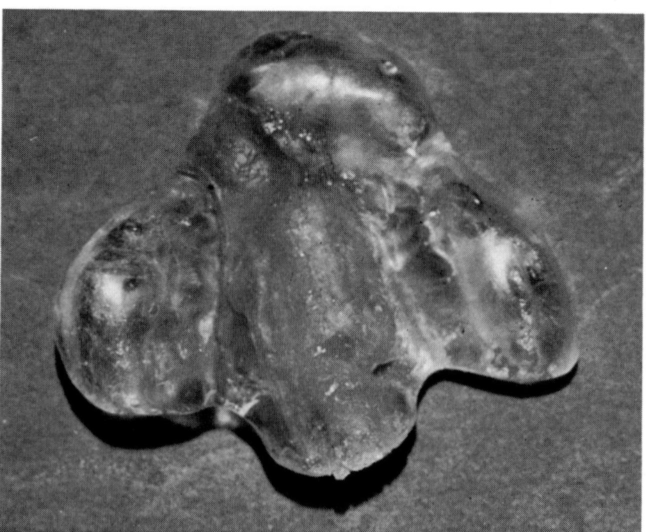

Figure 1–8 The appliance used before veloplasty with its velar extension.

602 lip repairs, including 570 closures of the hard palate during primary lip repair.

Initially, we believed that use of a palatal appliance was important prior to surgery (Fig. 1–8). We expected it to prevent the tongue interposition and to facilitate horizontalization of the palatal shelves, narrowing the cleft. We found that horizontalization of the palatal shelves did not occur (when documented with coronal CT scans); however, the width of the cleft did decrease following soft palate closure. Therefore, we thought that a certain degree of collapse of the lesser maxillary segment took place, but after the teeth erupted we did not find any significant collapse. Before we started using early repair and a palatal plate preoperatively, we sometimes observed narrow maxillary arches at 6 months of age in children who had not been operated on.

Veloplasty is performed at 3 months of age.[20] The mouth gag (Dott-Gillies type) had to be changed to fit the dimensions of the oral cavity at that age. Using a transverse incision at the level of the posterior edges of the palatal shelves, the muscles of the soft palate are detached, and the hamulus is fractured (Fig. 1–9A). The dissection is done posterior to the neurovascular bundles. The mucoperiosteum is left untouched (this is essential). A small mucosal vomer flap is raised, rotated 180 degrees, and sutured to the nasal mucosa of the velum. This allows for easier closure of the cleft, at the level of the posterior margin of the shelves where tension is the greatest (Fig. 1–9B). In bilateral clefts, this flap allows a true attachment of the inferior edge of the vomer to the palatal shelves.

Lip repair is performed at 6 months of age, using a double or single equilateral triangular flap technique (Fig. 1–10).[21] During the same operation, the hard palate is repaired (Fig. 1–11). The nasal layer is closed using mucoperiosteum from the nasal side of the palatal shelf, and a mucoperiosteal flap is raised from the vomer (Fig. 1–12A). Sometimes closure may be technically difficult, especially in narrow clefts. The nasal layer has to be lined on the oral side to decrease the risk of occurrence of a fistula. In the majority of patients the

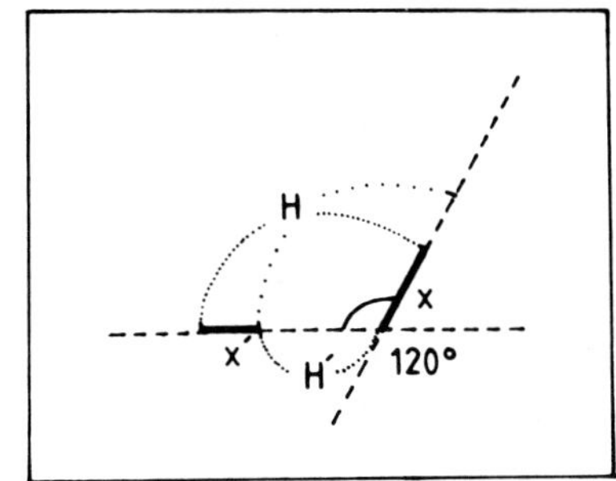

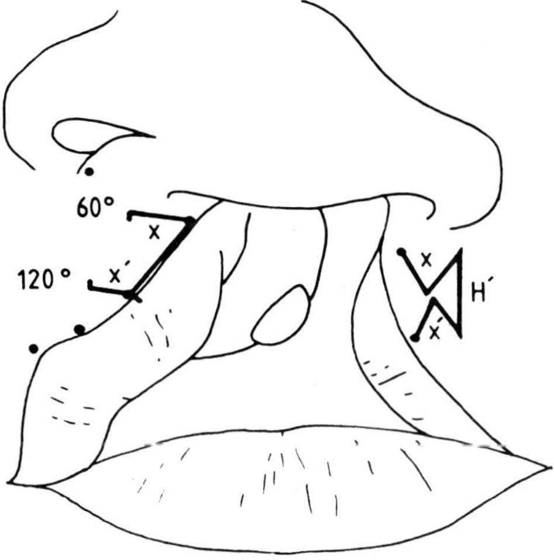

Figure 1–10 The labial incisions of the double triangular equilateral flap.[20]

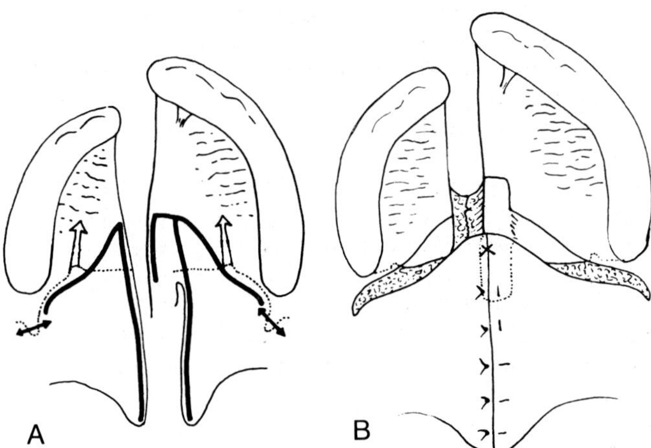

Figure 1–9 Technique of primary veloplasty. *A*, Note the vomerian mucosal flap. *B*, End of operation.

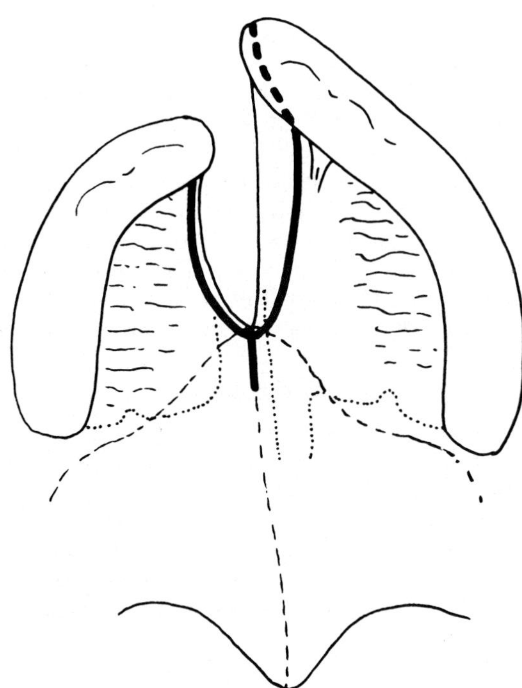

Figure 1–11 The incisions on the margins of the hard palate.

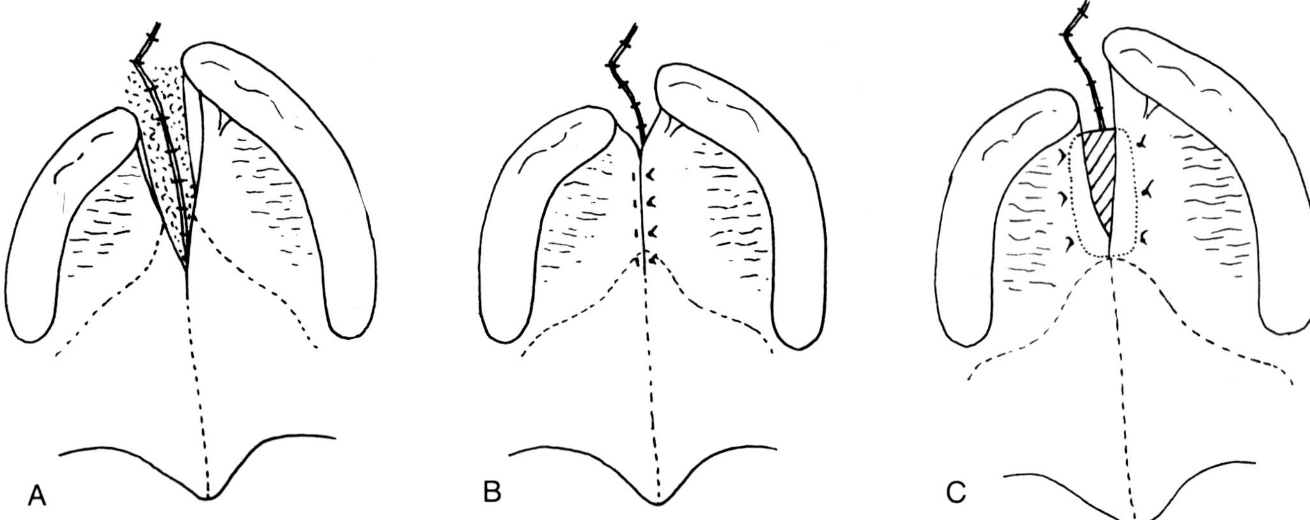

Figure 1–12 Closure of the hard palate. *A*, Closure of the nasal layer only. *B*, Two-layer closure when the cleft is narrow. *C*, Periosteal graft in the hard palate.

oral layer can be closed with minimal undermining. If this is not possible, a periosteal graft from the tibia is used as an oral layer. This material has been the most secure tissue able to survive in the oral cavity (Fig. 1–12*B*, *C*).[22] A second palatal appliance protects the sutures for 1 month and counteracts the pressure from the repaired lip that may affect the position of the maxillary segments.

Results

Following lip and palate repair, the child is seen every 6 months by the multidisciplinary team. We will not discuss the aesthetic estimation of lip and nose surgery, although these results are extremely important too. We prefer to focus on the advantages of a supple lip for good dental, facial growth, and speech development results. However, before discussing results, we must consider the difficulty in comparing results of other techniques with ours. The clinical evaluations are subjective, and there have been few statistical evaluations of the classic techniques. Furthermore, other factors, such as the surgeon's skill, cannot be compared. Nevertheless, we will try to compare some aspects of our results with those of the results generated from Veau's and Petit's vast experience and their methods.

Dental Results

The origin of our treatment change was a quest to improve the dental results. We evaluated the dental occlusion and growth of the superior maxillary complex. We can appreciate the state of the occlusion only after substantial dental development (Fig. 1–13). The position of the deciduous canine is usually measured because collapse of the small segment has been the main concern with the classic treatment. Clinical evaluation is difficult because we have to take into account the typical lingual position that leads to malocclusion in the presence of a normal bony relationship. Also, the deviation of the mandible due to the lateral position of the tongue, a consequence of "slipping planes," may result in crossbite.

In 1986 Psaume reported on the dental status of our oldest patients (6 to 10 years of age).[8] He noted that 85% of these patients had satisfactory canine occlusion. This was considered an exceptional result compared with his own observation of patients operated on by Petit. Dental results were observed to be markedly improved. We regret that there are no objective criteria nor quantitative studies of this comparison (Fig. 1–14). Pruzansky reported satisfactory occlusion in 40%.[17] Anterior collapse of the lesser maxillary segment rarely occurs, but lingual tilting of the deciduous canine is relatively common (57%). This condition requires a short period of orthodontic treatment.

Growth evaluation is more objective owing to the use of cephalometric studies (Fig. 1–15). We do this systematically as soon as the permanent incisors appear. We have now 59 cephalograms of 22 girls and 37 boys (average age 9 years). These included 46 patients with complete unilateral clefts and 13 with complete bilateral clefts. Using Tweed's[23] analysis technique, the sella, nasion, subspinale (SNA) angle reflects anteroposterior maxillary growth. The subspinale, nasion supramentale (ANB) reflects anteroposterior maxillary growth as well as helps to assess the role of disharmony of the maxilla and/or the mandible. Cephalometric measurements revealed that the SNA angle was normal in 25 patients (42%, group I), decreased in 26 patients (44%, group II), and increased in 8 patients (14%, group III).

In comparison with normal children, there was underdevelopment of the maxilla in 44% of the patients. The study of the ANB angle was undertaken to measure the maxillomandibular relationships. In group I (25 patients) we found that
1. In 13 patients the angle was normal (0–4 degrees)— class I.
2. In 11 patients the angle was increased (>4 degrees)— class II.

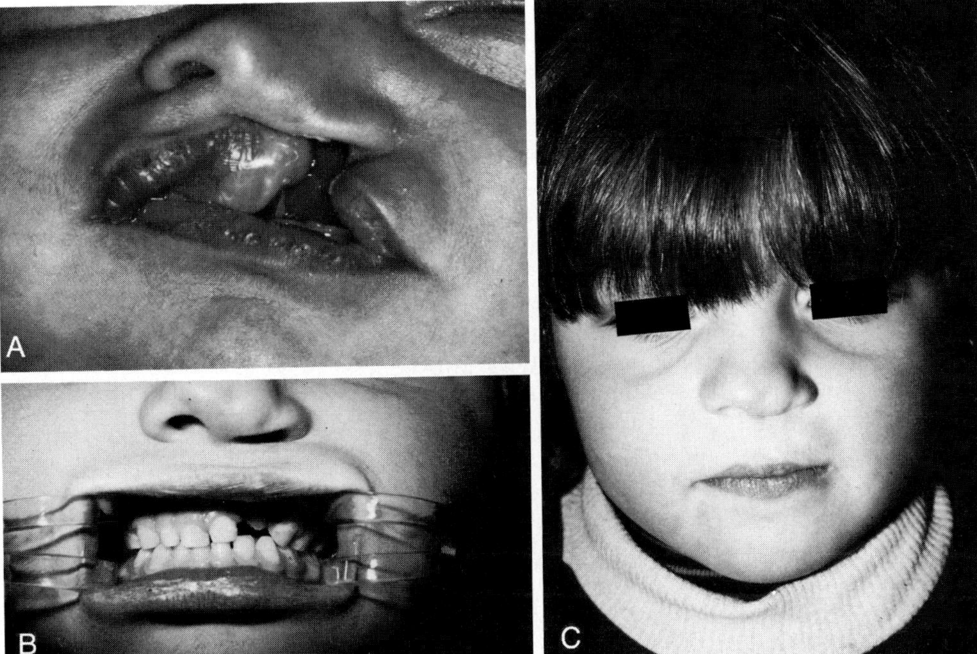

Figure 1–13 Results of a unilateral cleft repair.

3. In one patient the angle was decreased (<0 degrees)—class III.

The class III patient underwent fistula closure with undermining of the mucoperiosteum.

In group II (26 patients) we found that

1. In 14 patients the angle was normal (0–4 degrees)—class I.
2. In nine patients the angle was increased (>4 degrees)—class II.
3. In three patients the angle was decreased (<0 degrees)—class III.

Among the three class III patients, one underwent undermining of the periosteum during secondary repair, and the other two had a true prognathism.

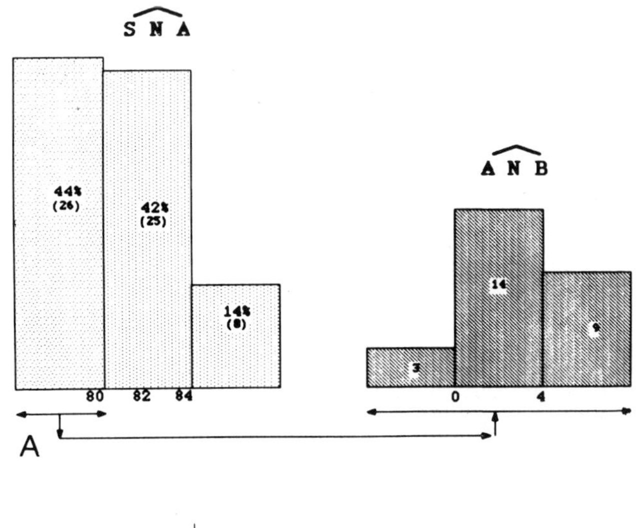

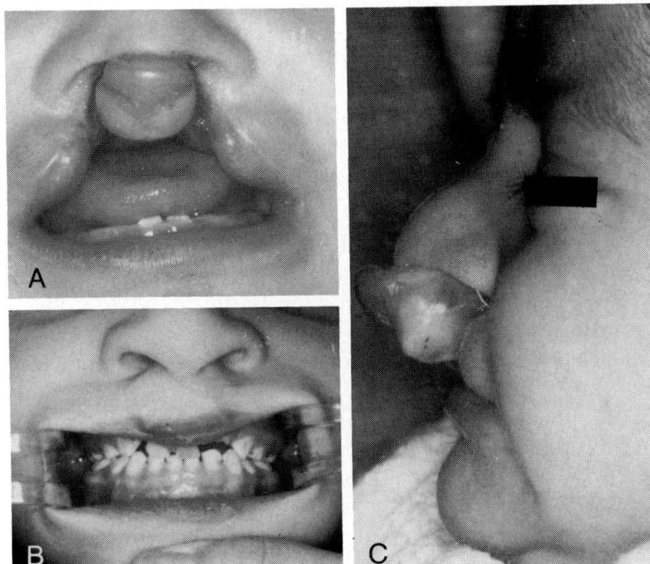

Figure 1–14 Results of a bilateral cleft repair.

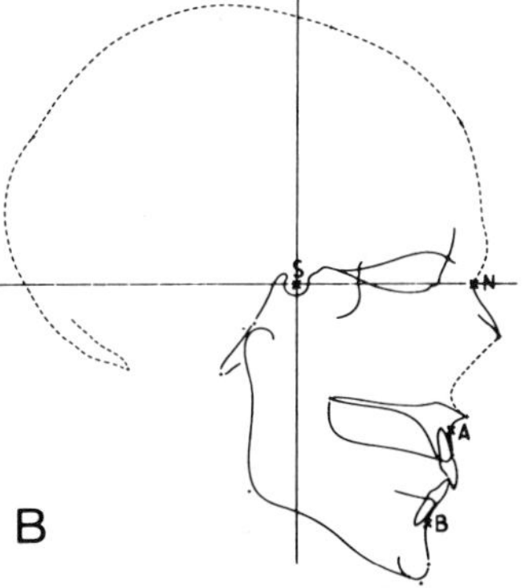

Figure 1–15 *A* and *B*, Growth evaluation by cephalometric analysis. S = Sella: center of sella turcica; N = nasion: most anterior point on the frontonasal suture; A = subspinale: deepest point on the anterior contour of the upper alveolar arch; B = supramentale: deepest point on the anterior contour of the lower alveolar arch.

In group III (eight patients) all patients had a normal or increased angle; therefore, no class III malocclusions were found. Consequently, our results indicate that our surgical technique of palate repair does not appear to be detrimental to maxillary growth.

Study of the vertical size using the Frankfort mandibular angle in Tweed's analysis allows a prognosis to be made. If this angle measures from 16 to 28 degrees, growth is directed downward in a normal way. This was the case for 40 of our patients (67%). If the angle measures from 28 to 35 degrees, growth is not as favorable but is still good. Sixteen patients (27%) were in this range. In our patients, vertical growth was satisfactory in 94%. Three patients exhibited unsatisfactory growth with no good explanation.

Phonology

Our patients are seen every 6 months starting from the time they are 1 year of age. We distinguished two features of our method that clearly demonstrated its advantages: (1) early surgery facilitated early speech development, and (2) there was improved quality of velopharyngeal function.

Just after the veloplasty at 3 months of age, normal signs of speech development appeared. Compared with children with clefts who have not had an operation, vocal emissions were longer. Vocalizations were more varied and included velar contoids /k, g, j/. Also, the pitch of the voice seemed to be higher and clearer. During the weeks following veloplasty, the tongue actively explored its new configuration in the oral cavity.

The following stage, "babbling," is very important because the syllabic structure of speech begins to take place. The plosives /p, t, k/ that require good nasopharyngeal occlusion were produced. The child without operation will try to reproduce what he perceives but cannot do so. Because he is unable to produce the oral plosives, he substitutes a laryngeal plosive or glottal stop. The whole development of the phonologic system is disturbed by that distorted starting point.[24] When the palate is entirely repaired before 10 months of age, the speech sounds and the phonologic system can be acquired in a normal way.

In our series, repaired children spoke *earlier*. About 83% uttered at least two of the three unvoiced plosives before they were 18 months of age. This fact allowed us to register meaningful words and ensured good verbal communication. Glottal stops were produced rarely. Before introduction of the new approach, 9% of our patients used glottal stops. Currently, we have less than 2%. Production of pharyngeal fricatives is no longer observed.

Because velopharyngeal function is a major concern following cleft palate repair, children are followed regularly by clinical examinations (Borel-Maisonny's scale, Table 1–1 and mirror testing). We evaluated 218 children who were followed for more than 5 years. At 1 year of age, 72.5% had a grade I or a grade I–II phonation. The grade I–II children required training in blowing to improve the efficacy of the velum and to develop pharyngeal contractions to compensate for the

Table 1–1. The Phonation Scale According to Borel-Maisonny

Grade I	Normal speech without any nasal flow
Grade I–II	Intermittent velopharyngeal closure
Grade II	Permanent nasal flow
	2b: Intelligible speech
	2m: Difficult to understand
Grade III	Important nasal flow; glottal stops, pharyngeal fricatives

shortness of the palate. More or less severe nasal escape (grade II to III phonation) was observed in 17.5% of patients. Secondary surgery (pharyngoplasty) was performed in 10% of our patients. This percentage was very similar to the number of flaps performed with the classic technique, but at the present time we expect better phonetic results and recommend secondary flap surgery for milder velopharyngeal incompetence.

Fistulas of the hard palate also may impair speech. Such fistulas have been observed more frequently in our new approach compared with the classic technique. In 451 patients we observed 120 fistulas (26.5%). This high percentage indicates that the technique must be further refined. We believe that the cause is probably the increased intraoral pressure that follows lip and palate repair.

Since we introduced two-layer closure of the hard palate, the number of fistulas has decreased markedly, from 42% to 13%. A fistula in the hard palate causes nasal air escape. It is important to distinguish nasal escape due to a fistula from that possibly due to a short palate. In the first case, closure of the fistula is sufficient. In the second case, pharyngeal flap surgery should be recommended. With a precise phonetic analysis of stop consonants articulated anterior to the fistula and of audible air passage through the fistula, indications for surgery can be established. After closure of the fistula, we obtained good phonetic results in 84.5% without performing a pharyngeal flap and without any speech therapy. This figure can be compared with the 62% that we obtained previously with Veau's technique (staphylorrhaphy at 18 months of age).[3] Thus, the phonetic benefit of early repair affects the acquisition of language as well as velopharyngeal competence.

Other advantages cannot be quantified, although they are quite perceivable by the clinician, for example, respiration and swallowing. Otitis media seems as frequent now as it was before, but we do not have statistics for quantitative comparative purposes.

Discussion

We changed our method initially to search for a technique that permitted complete closure of the palate without raising the mucoperiosteum. The advantages of avoiding this dissection have been amply demonstrated by many authors who followed Schweckendiek's recommendations. Our approach should be discussed relative to this method. Discussion will focus on three points: early veloplasty, sequence of surgical procedures, and complete hard palate closure.

Schweckendiek performed early veloplasty on patients who were 6 or 7 months of age. Many authors have expressed their opinion that early closure of the soft palate or entire palate may be advantageous.[25–28] Our experience concurs with those opinions. Presently, we do not have the data to show whether there is a significant difference between surgery at 6 months of age and surgery at 3 months. Without comparative studies we cannot answer definitively, but we have observed progress in development of speech following early velar closure. Our results demonstrate the importance of the speech improvement we have seen. Also, we have shown that enlargement of the nasopharynx between 3 and 6 months of age can be prevented. It would be desirable if other teams operating on patients at a later age would analyze the development of the transverse size of the nasopharynx with CT scans.

The change in the operative timing is characteristic of our timing and approach. We have explained the reasons for our choice of sequence of surgical procedures—physiologic reasons (interpretation of pressures) and technical reasons have been established. We would like to compare our results with those obtained by Schweckendiek's method. However, long-term use of appliances to occlude the residual hard palate cleft, as used by Schweckendiek, may interfere with dental results. On the contrary, we do not use any appliances after closure of the hard palate, and this is an advantage of our method.

We have considered closure of the entire cleft (lip and palate) at 3 months of age; however, the duration of the surgical procedure would be lengthy and would create risks for the child, and closure would be difficult if mucoperiosteal flaps were not undermined.

Finally, one of the major arguments used to justify our method is total closure of the palate at 6 months of age. The speech results attest to an indisputable advantage over the results of Schweckendiek's method.[29] Initially, one of the disadvantages of our technique was a high incidence of fistulas in the hard palate. With our new surgical technique, this risk has significantly decreased. After 13 years of experience with this approach, we are confident that this dissection does not impair development because we have not observed maxillofacial growth inhibition due to the use of a vomer flap.

Conclusion

Results of the follow-up study of our patients justify our use of early complete closure of the lip and palate when a new timing for and sequence of the surgical procedures are employed (Fig. 1–16). Marked improvements were observed in speech and dental results compared with our previously used techniques and these procedures used by other authors.

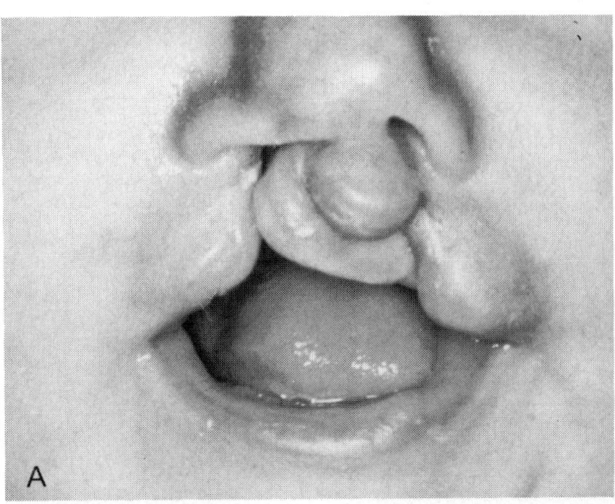
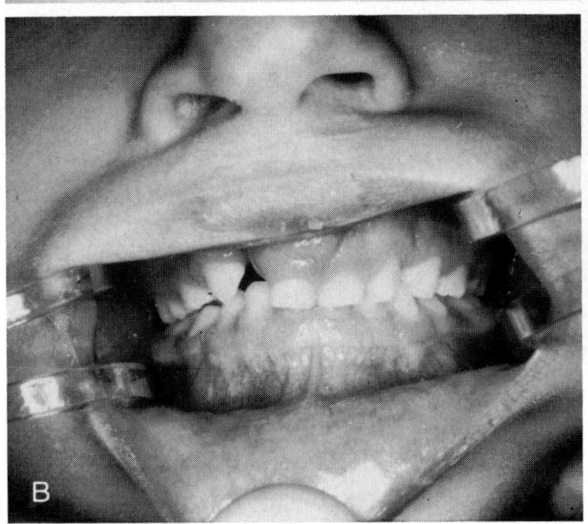
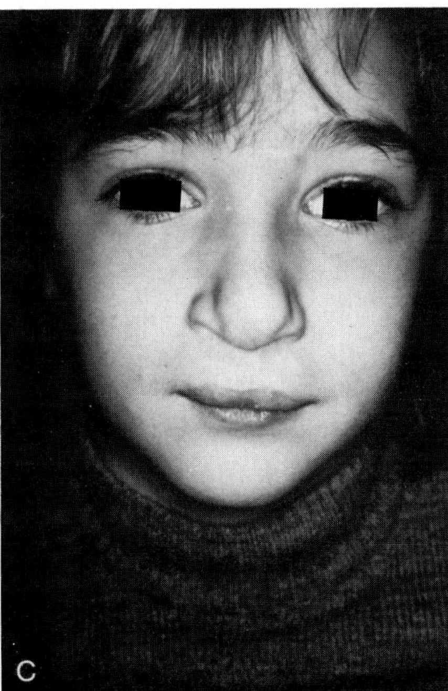

Figure 1–16 Result of asymmetric complete bilateral cleft.

ACKNOWLEDGMENTS. We wish to express our gratitude to Mrs. B. Landier, M.D., who helped us with the analysis of our series and for the illustrations and to Mrs. L. Laberge, M.D., from Montreal, who advised us on our English. And, last but not least, our thanks go to Mrs. E. Menguy, secretary, who worked hard typing the manuscript.

References

1. Veau V: Division Palatine. Paris: Masson, 1931.
2. Veau V: Bec de Lièvre. Formes cliniques—Chirurgie. Paris: Masson, 1938.
3. Oger P: Etude Critique de 2000 Divisions Palatines et Insuffisances Velaires. These, University of Paris VII, 1976.
4. Petit P, Borel-Maisonny S, Psaume J: Intérêt et résultats de pharyngoplasties à but phonétique. Rev Prat 15:2789, 1965.
5. Malek R, Psaume J: Nouvelle conception de la chronologie et de la technique chirurgicale du traitement des fentes labio-palatines. Ann Chir Plast 28:237, 1983.
6. Malek R, Psaume J, Martinez H, et al: Early treatment of cleft lip and palate. In Hotz M, et al (eds): Proceedings of the Third International Symposium on Cleft Lip and Palate. Zurich: Huber, 1986.
7. Psaume J, Malek R: Must cleft palate be repaired before cleft lip? Read before the Fourth International Congress of Cleft Palate and Related Craniofacial Anomalies, Toronto, 1971.
8. Psaume J, Malek R, Mousset MR, et al: Technique et résultats du traitement total précoce des fentes labio-palatines. Folia Phoniatr 38:176, 1986.
9. Oblak P: New concept of morphogenesis of cleft in the lip alveolus and palate. J Maxillofac Surg 3:182, 1975.
10. Oblak P: New guiding principles in the treatment of clefts. J Maxillofac Surg 3:231, 1975.
11. Peyton WT: Dimensions and growth of the palate in the normal infant and in the infant with gross maldevelopment of the upper lip and palate. Arch Surg 22:704, 1931.
12. Wardill WEM: Cleft Palate. Br J Surg 26:61, 1928.
13. Psaume J: Contribution à l'étude des déformations osseuses du bec de lièvre non opéré, thèse de médecine. University of Paris, 1950.
14. Subtelny JD: Width of the nasopharynx and related anatomic structures in normal and unoperated cleft palate children. Am J Orthod 41:12, 1955.
15. Petit P, Psaume J: Le Traitement du Bec de Lievre. Paris: Masson, 1962.
16. Morley ME: Cleft Palate and Speech. Edinburgh: E.S. Livingstone, 1958.
17. Brunelle F, Oger P, Malek R: CT evaluation of CLP. The pterygomandibular index. Read before the Fifth International Congress on Cleft Palate and Related Craniofacial Anomalies. Monaco, September, 1985.
18. Schwekendieck H: Ergebnisse bei Lippen-Kiefer-Gaumans palatoperationen mit der primaren Veloplastik. Fortsch Kiefer Gesichtschi 4:167, 1958.
19. Schwekendieck H: Primary veloplasty. Long term results without maxillary deformity. A 25 year report. Cleft Palate J 15:268, 1978.
20. Malek R: Technique de la staphylorraphie précoce. Chir Pediatr 24:286, 1983.
21. Malek R, Grossmann JAI: Cleft lip repair by a systematic Z-plasty. Clin Plast Surg 11:739, 1984.
22. Stricker M, Raphael B: Le périoste dans les fentes labio-palatines. Chir Pediatr 24:274, 1988.
23. Tweed CH: The Pranofort mandibular plane angle (FNIA) in orthodontic diagnosis, treatment, planning, and prognosis. Angle Orthod 24:121 1954.
24. Mousset MR: L'acquisition du langage par l'enfant porteur d'une fente palantine. Thèse DEA linguistique générale. University Sorbonne Nouvelle Paris III, Paris, 1979.
25. Pruzansky S: Description, classification and analysis of unoperated clefts of the lips and palate. Am J Orthod 39:590, 1953.
26. Slaughter WS, Brodie AG: Velar closure. In Grabb WC, Rosenstein SW, Broch KR (eds): Cleft Lip and Palate. Boston; Little, Brown, 1971.
27. Dorf DS, Curtin JW: Early cleft palate repair and speech outcome. Plast Reconstr Surg 70:74, 1982.
28. Kaplan EN: Cleft palate repair at 3 months? Ann Plast Surg 7:3, 1981.
29. Bardach JB, Morris HL, Olin W: Late results of primary veloplasty: The Marburg project. Plast Reconstr Surg 73:207, 1984.

CHAPTER 2

Multidisciplinary Management of Cleft Lip and Palate in the United Kingdom

Catherine Asher and William Shaw

Until the second decade of the twentieth century, correction of cleft deformity was seen in the United Kingdom as a surgical problem alone. In the 1920s, surgeons started to collaborate with speech therapists, and as a result, great improvements occurred in regard to both the appearance and the speech of the patient. However, a comprehensive service was available only to the privileged few. Great attempts were made to equalize the services offered when the National Health Service Act was passed in 1946, and from this time onward, health care became universally available. The team approach to care of the cleft palate also evolved from this period.

All areas of the country are now served by consultant plastic surgeons, speech therapists, and hospital-based orthodontists who treat cleft patients as part of their wide-ranging daily workload. However, because individual clinicians in the United Kingdom have a high degree of clinical freedom within the National Health Service, considerable diversity has resulted in the types of clinical management offered throughout the country.

Historical Aspects

During the nineteenth century, breakdown of the repaired cleft was common, speech was often poor, and the growth of the jaws was severely impeded by traumatic surgery. Understanding of the anatomy of the oral musculature was limited, and thus no attempt could be made to restore normal anatomy or function to the lip and palate. Many theories were put forward and differing surgical techniques were devised in an attempt to reduce the failure rate.[1]

With the recognition of the need for speech assessment by specialist therapists, the beginnings of a team approach were occurring as early as 1915. At this time speech therapy was judged on many occasions to be a "hopeless struggle against insuperable odds to achieve intelligible speech."[2]

Surgical Advances

Following World War I, general surgeons gained experience in the treatment of the war wounded, and flap surgery became more sophisticated and successful. These new skills were subsequently applied to the treatment of congenital facial deformities such as cleft lip and palate.[3]

In 1921 Sir Harold Gillies criticized contemporary methods of cleft closure and noted that current closure techniques caused a scarred and tight, anteriorly placed soft palate, disrupted eruption of the teeth, narrowing of the nasal passages, and poor appearance. In London, he collaborated with a dental surgeon, Kelsey Fry, who constructed obturating plates that were used following Gillies' closure of the lip and soft palate only. Such obturating plates were worn for life.[4] In Newcastle, Wardill recognized the need for a velopharyngeal seal for good speech and devised a method for elongation of the soft palate, sometimes known as the "pushback" procedure, that in modified forms is still in use today by approximately 50% of plastic surgeons in the United Kingdom.[5] He advocated early closure of the lip and soft palate and emphasized the need for a functioning speech mechanism prior to speech development. Wardill claimed that his VY advancement procedure combined "the advantages of the Veau operation with Gillies and Dorrance's at one sitting."[5, 6]

During the 1930s and 1940s, follow-up of cleft lip and palate patients was more thorough, and severe maxillary deformities and dental arch problems were recognized. Variations of surgical timing and technique were seen to be crucial, and a need for surgical specialization became apparent. This became possible with the establishment of the National Health Service in 1946. The first specialists involved in the majority of cases were either pediatric surgeons or individuals in the new specialty of plastic surgery. New appointments of consultant plastic surgeons were made steadily until the present number of around 130 was reached. A few pediatric surgeons continue to work in the cleft lip and palate field.

Like other countries after World War II, Britain benefited from improved control of infection with antibiotics. Modern anesthetic techniques meant that primary repairs could be carried out safely and reliably in the early months of life.

McNeil Technique

Until the middle of the century, the dentist's role in cleft lip and palate care was confined largely to the provision of obturators and dentures. Although the concept of presurgical alignment of the maxillary fragments was not new,[7] such techniques had largely been forgotten when surgeons such as Veau demonstrated that even wide clefts could be closed without the benefit of preoperative narrowing. In 1947, research into presurgical treatment was commenced by McNeil, a Glasgow prosthodontist.[8] McNeil's reports aroused widespread interest, particularly his claims that nonsurgical closure of the palatal cleft was possible. Variations of his technique were adopted in subsequent years in most British units. Such work was performed by hospital-based orthodontists, and, together with alignment of the erupted dentition, it continues to be part of the workload of the 175 consultants who presently hold such posts.

Treatment of Cleft Patients within the National Health Service

Administration

Every child born with a cleft of the lip and/or palate in the United Kingdom is treated within the framework of the National Health Service (NHS). A unique and complex organization, the NHS is the country's largest employer with 1.25 million employees. Comprehensive care is provided for every citizen, and 97% of care is free at the first point of contact (3% of costs are met by patient charges for medicines, dental care, and ophthalmic consultations); 87% of patient services are funded through direct taxation, so payment by individuals is graded by income. This differs from social and private insurance schemes, in which citizens' contributions vary according to their personal risk. Funding through direct taxation has a fundamental bearing on the philosophy of health care, because the health profession makes the main decision about the need for treatment, not the patient nor his ability to pay.

Underfinancing of the National Health Service is, however, a chronic problem and is largely within the hands of the government. Britain spends less on health care per capita than any other Western country (Table 2–1). This is reflected in the salaries of health personnel and the poor state of many of the hospitals. On the positive side, a comprehensive service is available to the cleft infant from the time of birth, regardless of geographic location, social class, or family finances.

England is divided geographically into 14 regions, which are further divided into a total of 212 districts. Similar divisions are made in Wales, Scotland, and Northern Ireland. Administration is undertaken within each district in individual units (hospitals), each unit being managed by an administrator, a doctor, and a director of nursing services.

Personnel

These arrangements facilitate the establishment of teams and associations between specialists within and between districts to the extent that there is commonly a duplication of services, especially in the larger urban districts. For example, in a region sufficiently large to generate a case load of 60 new cleft cases per year, there may be as many as six consultant plastic surgeons, six consultant orthodontists, and six consultant maxillofacial surgeons. Because there are no particular directives as to who does what, there is commonly a considerable fragmentation of the case load, and patterns of

Table 2–1. Percentages of Gross National Product Spent on Health

Country	Percentage
Sweden	9
West Germany	8
Canada	8.5
United States	11
France	9.5
Britain	6.2

From Organization for Economic Cooperation and Development's latest available data, The Economist, July 1988.

referral are developed along informal lines. In a survey we conducted in the spring of 1988, we found 45 orthodontists working in teams with a total of 66 plastic surgeons, seeing an average of 10.2 new cases each year (Table 2–2). On an arithmetical average, each surgeon would perform primary closure on only three or four neonates with complete unilateral or bilateral clefts. There is, however, wide variation in the individual annual case load from 2 to 80 infants with cleft deformities.

The majority of cleft patients in the United Kingdom are treated by unspecialized speech therapists in local community clinics or hospital departments as part of a heavy general workload. In the authors' district, there are 10.1 full-time equivalent speech therapists for a district with a population of 217,000. The official target for the district would be a minimum of 13 therapists. Thus, many therapists have extremely heavy commitments.

Current Cleft Lip and Palate Management in the United Kingdom

Reports of the incidence of cleft lip and palate in Britain range from 1.3 to 1.9 per thousand.[9] The disparity between estimates undoubtedly reflects underreporting, since arrangements for recording congenital deformities are somewhat loose.

In the spring of 1988, we conducted a survey for the purposes of the present chapter. Responses were received from 45 of 51 centers (a response rate of 88%). The main points of interest are summarized in Tables 2–2, 2–3, and 2–4.

Neonatal Care

Feeding methods throughout the United Kingdom vary, but most commonly involve the use of bottles with long soft nipples and enlarged holes. Advice on feeding is given to the parents by the pediatric nursing staff or the orthodontist. In many centers, a simple acrylic feeding plate may be provided by the orthodontist (Table 2–4). The baby is generally seen by the plastic surgeon or the consultant orthodontist within 24 to 48 hours of the birth, when reassurance and information are given to the parents. In most centers, impressions are taken within the first few days for study models, and photographs are taken for documentation purposes. Once the mother is confident about feeding her baby, mother and child are discharged and are seen thereafter as outpatients. At present, no national system of home visiting for cleft infants exists. An outreach program similar to the scheme used in Denmark is currently being piloted in the authors' region.

Table 2–2. 45 Cleft Teams Surveyed March 1988

Total new cleft patients seen per year	676
Total number of surgeons within teams	66
Average number of new cases per year per surgeon	10.2
Range of number of new cases per year	2–80

Table 2–3. Surgery for Cleft Lip and Palate

	Percentage
Type of lip surgery	
Millard or modified Millard rotation flap procedure	92.3
Other (including Le Mesurier flap procedure)	7.7
Timing of lip surgery (by age of patient)	
24 hours–1 week	4.9
3 months	90.2
4–6 months	4.9
Type of palatal surgery	
von Langenbeck simple closure	50
Other flap procedures	50
Timing of palatal surgery (by age of patient)	
0–6 weeks	5.1
6–12 months	12.9
9–12 months	56.4
13–18 months	25.6
Secondary bone grafting	70.5

Primary Surgery

In the majority of centers in the United Kingdom, the lip is closed surgically at the age of 3 months (Table 2–3), although a small number of surgeons close the lip during the neonatal period when the infant is 48 hours to 1 week old. The latter approach remains controversial and is often limited by the availability of the appropriate anesthetic service at short notice. However, at least one center has adopted the approach consistently over 15 years, performing lip closure in the first days of life and palate repair before the sixteenth week.[10, 11] The most favored method of lip closure at present is the rotation-advancement procedure of Millard,[12] although a number of other techniques including those based on the method advocated by Tennison[13] are in use.

In over 50% of the 45 centers surveyed the palatal cleft is closed between the ages of 9 and 12 months (Table 2–3). In a majority of the remaining centers the palate is repaired when the child is between 12 and 18 months old. The two most popular palatal closure techniques in the United Kingdom are modifications of the Wardill-Kilner operation[5] and various modifications of the simple von Langenbeck closure.[14]

Presurgical Orthopedic Treatment

Active presurgical orthopedic alignment of the alveolar segments is carried out in a majority of British centers prior to closure of the lip (Table 2–4). An acrylic plate may be constructed on a model previously sectioned and rotated to encourage forward and mesial growth of the segments (Fig. 2–1). Extra-oral strapping

Table 2–4. Presurgical Orthopedic Treatment

	Percentage
Simple obturating/feeding plates	51
Correction appliances for all complete unilateral and bilateral clefts	56.8
Correction appliances provided if requested by surgeon	31.5
No presurgical orthopedic treatment	11.7

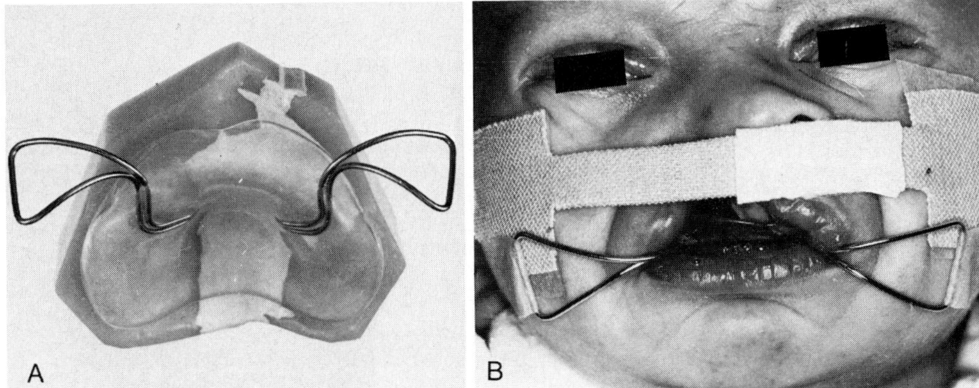

Figure 2–1 Appliances for active presurgical orthopedics as commonly used in the United Kingdom. *A,* Intraoral plate. The cleft region of the work model has been reduced to allow approximation of the anterior ends of the segments. *B,* Extraoral strapping is applied under tension by drawing the cheeks forward to receive the ends of the tape.

is often used in conjunction with these plates to reduce the width of the cleft of the lip and, in bilateral clefts, to align the premaxilla (Figs. 2–2 and 2–3). Expansion appliances are commonly used to widen the segments in complete bilateral clefts of the lip and palate.

Although the practice of presurgical orthopedic treatment in the United Kingdom has been widespread and generally favored by British surgeons for more than 30 years (and is still used in 39 of 45 centers we surveyed), its efficacy in terms of later outcome is now widely doubted. In an increasing number of centers, orthodontists are confining the employment of orthopedic plates to bilateral and wide unilateral complete clefts or discontinuing their use altogether. Primary bone grafting, which enjoyed some popularity in the 1960s, has now been completely discontinued.

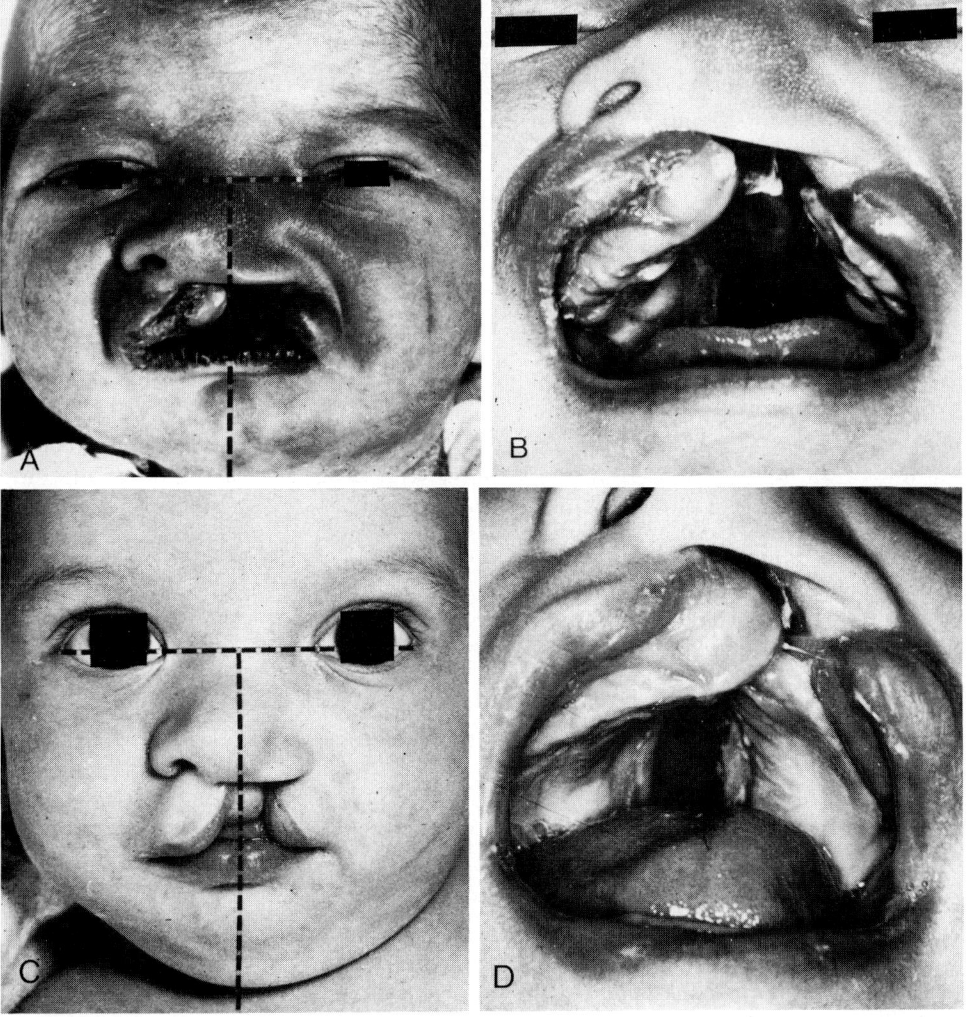

Figure 2–2 Presurgical alignment in a complete unilateral cleft (*A* and *B,* before; *C* and *D,* after presurgical orthopedic treatment). The effect of treatment is mainly confined to a medial rotation of the anterior ends of the segments. (From Shaw WC. Early orthopaedic treatment of unilateral cleft lip and palate. Br J Orthodont 5:119–132, 1978. With permission.)

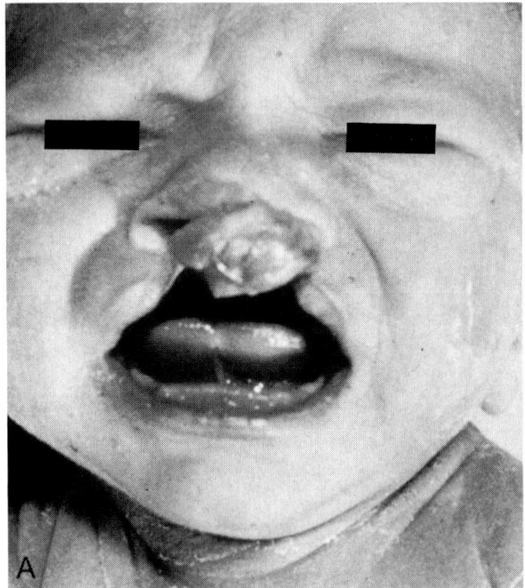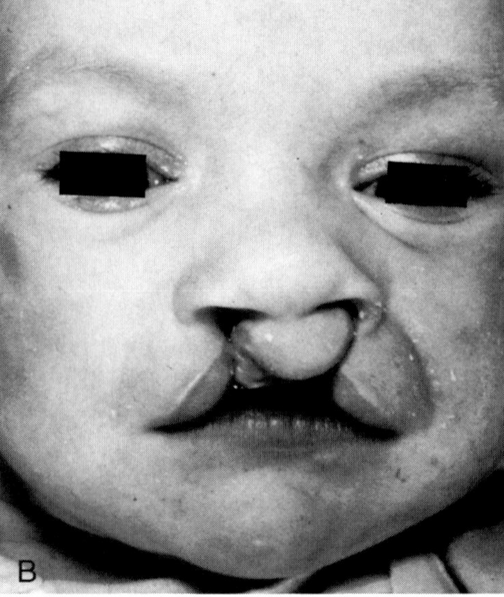

Figure 2–3 A and B, Presurgical alignment of the premaxilla in a complete bilateral cleft. The effect of treatment is to restrain the premaxilla allowing catch-up of the rest of the face. (From Robertson NRE, Shaw WC, and Volp CR. The changes produced by presurgical orthopaedic treatment of bilateral cleft lip and palate. Plast Reconstr Surg 59:86–93, 1977. With permission.)

Speech and Hearing

All cleft patients are seen by their first birthday by a chief speech therapist, who is notified directly by the clinical staff or via a computerized birth notification system. A routine hearing test is carried out on all British children at the age of 8 months. At the first speech assessment, the infant's level of language development and verbal comprehension is recorded. Following the initial assessment, the child is monitored regularly every 6 months, and at the age of 2 years a further major assessment is made. At this stage the quantity and quality of speech are noted in addition to the child's general comprehension. The nasality of speech is generally assessed by ear. The Exeter Nasal Anemometry System is routinely used in the authors' district to assess nasal escape for patients from the age of 3 years, but this is by no means in general use throughout the country.

An appropriate program is selected to correct problems of speech quality, depending on each child's needs. The patient may attend the program weekly during an extended period so that the speech therapist can deal with poor development of the speech-sound system. Alternatively, the child may be given a home-based program and assessed approximately every 2 months by the speech therapist. Naturally, the home-based program depends on excellent family support and commitment. Patients with good speech require periodic review only throughout their childhood.

If insufficient velopharyngeal function is suspected to be contributing to residual speech problems, the speech therapist, in joint consultation with the surgeon, decides whether secondary surgical intervention is advisable. Pharyngoplasty is carried out when possible before the child starts school or soon after, between the ages of 4 and 6 years.

Intensive programs are available to children with special difficulties in a small number of cleft units. The child attends a hospital department daily or lives residentially for a period of 2 to 6 weeks. It is found that children make significant progress during this period, and the experience is highly motivating for both the patient and therapist. However, the treatment is expensive and labor intensive and is not generally available throughout the country.

Speech assessments are most commonly made without the use of technologic aids, although nasal anemometry and the electropalatograph are in use in a limited number of centers.

After the age of 8 years each child's progress is monitored regularly, the speech therapist intervening if residual speech problems require correction. If further communication difficulties are encountered, management may involve referral to other members of the team, notably the plastic surgeon, the otolaryngologist, the educational psychologist, the orthodontist, or the audiologist.

Orthodontic Treatment

Of the 45 centers surveyed, none practices orthodontic treatment during the deciduous dentition phase. Preliminary alignment of the permanent maxillary incisors and arch expansion, as appropriate, are generally performed in anticipation of cancellous alveolar bone grafting around 10 years of age. This approach to arch management has been widely adopted following presentations made by the Oslo team in England during the early 1980s.[15]

As orthodontists, the authors still find themselves confronted with patients whose maxillary growth and development has been seriously disturbed by previous surgery. In the majority of children with complete clefts, we find it necessary to expand the arch transversely before bone grafting, and in a significant proportion, the degree of skeletal maxillary retrusion precludes establishment of a normal incisal relationship without surgical maxillary advancement.

When arch expansion is required, the use of the quadhelix appliance has superseded rapid expansion plates (Fig. 2–4). In our clinic, we find some use for

Figure 2–4 *A* and *B*, Prebone graft maxillary arch expansion using quad helix appliance.

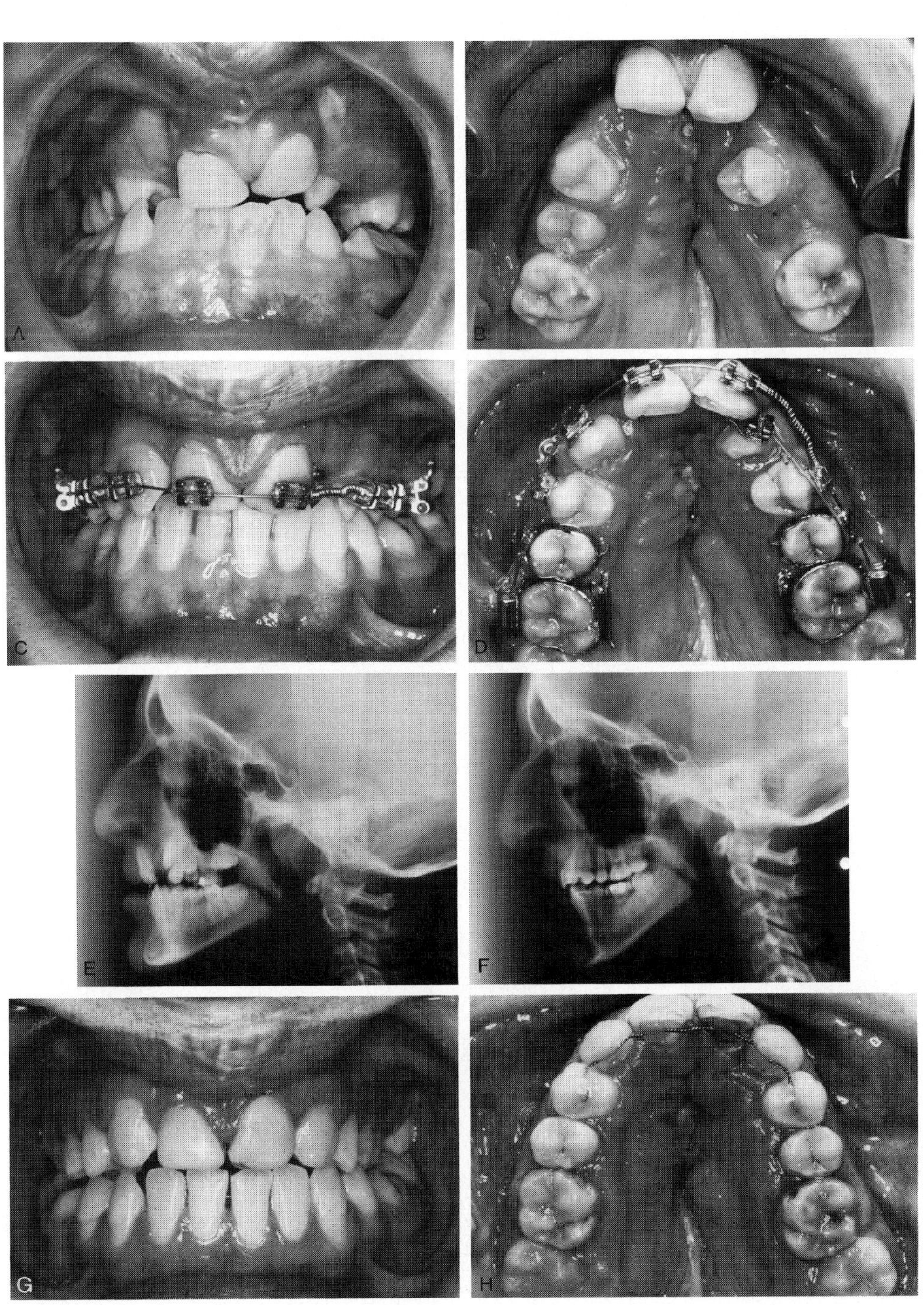

Figure 2–5 Complete bilateral cleft treated by bone grafting and orthodontic alignment. *A*, Pretreatment frontal view. *B*, Pretreatment occlusal view. *C* and *D*, Orthodontic treatment following bone grafting shows alignment of canines into grafted sites. *E*, Lateral cephalogram shows marked pretreatment incisor retroclination. *F*, After treatment. *G*, Frontal view following treatment. *H*, Occlusal view shows bonded retainer.

reverse headgear for maxillary protraction but regard this as an adjunct to advancement of the maxillary dentition rather than as a means of achieving actual skeletal change. Following bone grafting, conventional fixed appliances are used to complete alignment when the remaining permanent teeth have erupted, and in the majority of cases, orthodontic space closure is undertaken to avoid the need for artificial teeth. We regard the advent of a reliable technique of alveolar bone grafting as the most significant advance in treatment of children with clefts of the lip and palate in recent decades (Fig. 2–5).

Secondary Procedures

The timing of secondary adjustments of the lip, nose, and palatal defects is generally discussed at interdisciplinary team clinics, and a wide range of common techniques is practiced. Palatopharyngeal incompetence is mainly treated by superiorly based pharyngeal flaps, although a number of surgeons favor the operation described by Orticochea.[16]

A significant proportion of patients with complete clefts require maxillary osteotomy. This is normally performed by a consultant in maxillofacial (oral) surgery and planned in collaboration with the orthodontist. Surgical maxillary advancement is generally preceded by orthodontic treatment to level and coordinate the arches so that a satisfactory occlusion is established. The fixed appliance is also used for intermaxillary fixation. Surgery is generally deferred until at least the midteens. In the past we have found it necessary to apply protraction headgear to the maxillary dentition to resist relapse

in the postsurgical period, but with the advent of bone plates this problem has been eliminated (Fig. 2–6).

Counseling

Regrettably, few teams include a psychologist experienced in counseling cleft patients. However, genetic counseling is readily available. Also, there is an active parent association that raises funds and provides local support groups.

Cleft Lip and Palate Research in the United Kingdom

Clinical Research

As in most other countries, clinicians in the United Kingdom have rarely submitted their techniques to the rigors of the randomized, controlled trial. There have been, however, some exceptions. Jolleys and Robertson matched 14 infants who received rib grafts to the alveolus with 14 control subjects and found clear evidence of growth disturbance associated with grafting.[17] Robertson and Jolleys also compared study casts and cephalometric records taken at 11 years of age in two groups of 20 unilateral cleft lip and palate subjects, one of which had had their palate repairs delayed until 4.5 to 5 years. They found no advantage for delayed closure.[18] In a controlled trial of 45 infants, the effect of McNeil stimulation plates was tested.[19] A similar amount of palatal cleft reduction occurred in two groups of infants treated from birth to 9 months; one group was

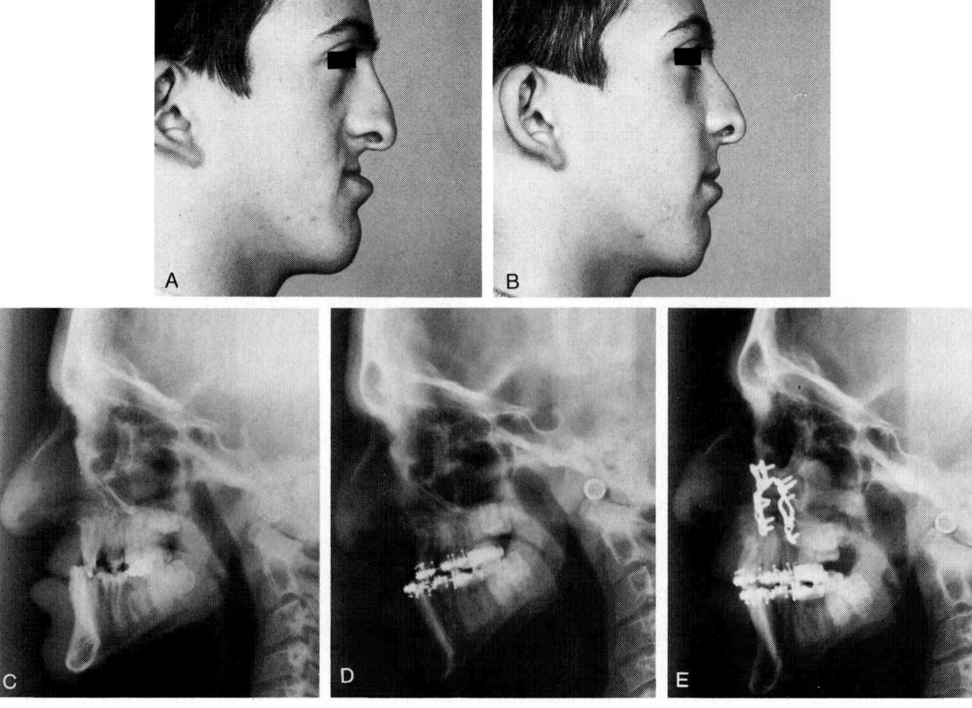

Figure 2–6 Le Fort I maxillary advancement in a patient with unilateral cleft lip and palate who was treated at a center that had practiced early bone grafting. *A* and *B*, Lateral views before and after surgery. *C*, Pretreatment cephalogram. *D*, Orthodontic alignment prior to surgery. *E*, Postsurgical cephalogram showing bone plates.

provided with McNeil stimulation plates and the other with simple obturators. In a third untreated group significantly less reduction occurred.

Huddart compared maxillary arch development in 40 unilateral cleft lip and palate subjects treated by presurgical orthopedics with 13 controls and found that crossbites were equally prevalent in both groups.[20] Numerous British studies have evaluated the nature of the changes produced by presurgical orthopedic appliances,[7, 21–23] and Pigott and associates have made a series of reports on velopharyngeal incompetence.[24]

An ambitious project led by a London team has made a series of visits to Sri Lanka and provided surgical care and speech therapy for large numbers of subjects with previously unrepaired clefts. To date, preoperative records of 400 patients with varying types of clefts and no previous surgery have been obtained, and these demonstrate a remarkable potential for maxillary growth unhindered by surgical scarring.[25]

Finally, the present authors are coordinating a six-center European comparative study of facial growth, arch development, facial appearance, and speech for a cohort of children with unilateral cleft lip and palate born during the years 1976–1979.[26]

Craniofacial Biology

Several British anatomists have contributed to the descriptive anatomy of fetal growth and development and have presented theories on growth mechanisms in cleft patients, particularly the influence of the septal cartilage.[27–29] The advent of more sophisticated techniques for the investigation of cell and structural biology and cleft inheritance has led to a number of major new initiatives in the United Kingdom, and the reader is referred to a collection of review papers describing this work.[30]

A broad range of enquiry includes the investigation by Ferguson and coworkers of developmental mechanisms during normal secondary palate development and how such mechanisms may be disrupted to cause cleft palate. Current studies have focused on the mechanism of signaling epithelial-mesenchymal interactions during terminal epithelial differentiation, the effects of various growth factors on the behavior of extracellular matrix biosynthesis, and the identification of susceptibility genes that could be used in population screens. Investigations of cellular interactions during embryonic wound healing suggest possible avenues for manipulation of postnatal wound healing and the construction of living dermal substitutes that may have an important role in clinical practice.

Various investigations of neural crest cell migration and pattern formation are being pursued by Thorogood, Tickle, and Morris-Kay, and teratogenic studies are being explored by Poswillo. Different teams led by Moore and Williamson are studying the molecular genetics of cleft palate, and cell lineage analysis in facial development is being investigated by Lumsden.

Discussion

Over the years British clinicians have made significant contributions to the body of knowledge concerning the treatment of clefts of the lip and palate. Arguably, the prime need today is to establish services that are more centralized and standardized because at present small numbers of cases are often absorbed as part of the general workload of busy surgical and orthodontic units in which a specific focus on the cleft problem is lacking. Furthermore, these arrangements and the shortage of adequate numbers of ancillary staff arising from chronic underfunding of the National Health Service contribute to a history of haphazard record keeping.

Sadly, British clinicians are as guilty as their counterparts abroad of working with imprecise treatment protocols that incorporate a host of confounding variables in the vain hope that they or someone else will be able to reach conclusions about the efficacy of their care at some future date. Yet the United Kingdom is an ideal setting for well-structured analytic prospective research. There is a high population density, the clinicians are salaried and have the same employer, and their training is uniform. Thus, it would not be difficult to generate substantial case loads of cleft subtypes treated by small groups of specialists within scientifically defined prospective trials. This is the challenge for the new generation of British clinicians.

References

1. Holdsworth WG: Cleft Lip and Palate. London: Heinemann, 1963.
2. Morley ME: Cleft Palate and Speech. London: E and S Livingstone Ltd, 1970.
3. Edwards M, Watson ACH: Advances in the Management of Cleft Palate. London: Churchill Livingstone, Longman Group, 1980.
4. Gillies HD, Kelsey-Fry W: A new principle in the surgical management of congenital cleft palate and its mechanical counterpart. Br Med J 1:335–338, 1921.
5. Wardill WEM: Technique of operation for cleft palate. Br J Surg 25:117–130, 1937.
6. Dorrance GM: Lengthening of the soft palate in cleft palate operations. Ann Surg 82:208–211, 1925.
7. Shaw WC: Early orthopaedic treatment of unilateral cleft lip and palate. Br J Orthod 5:119–132, 1978.
8. McNeil CK: Orthopaedic principles in the treatment of lip and palate clefts. In R. Hotz (ed): Early Treatment of Cleft Lip and Palate. Berne: Huber, 1964, p. 59.
9. Vanderas AP: Incidence of cleft lip, cleft palate and cleft lip and palate among races: A review. Cleft Palate J 24:216–225, 1987.
10. Desai SN: Primary cleft lip repair in newborn babies. In: Transactions of the Seventh International Congress of Plastic and Reconstructive Surgery, Rio de Janeiro, 1979.
11. Desai SN: Early cleft palate repair completed before the age of 16 weeks, observations. A personal series of 100 children. Br J Plast Surg 36:300–304, 1983.
12. Millard DRA: A radical rotation in single harelip. Am J Surg 95:318–321, 1958.
13. Tennison CW: The repair of the unilateral cleft lip by the stencil method. Plast Reconstr Surg 9:115, 1952.
14. Von Langenbeck B: Operation der angeborenen totalen Spaltung des harten Gaumens nach einer neuen Methode. Dtsch Klin 8:231–239, 1861.
15. Bergland O, Semb G, Abyholm F: Elimination of the residual alveolar cleft by secondary bone grafting and subsequent orthodontic treatment. Cleft Palate J 23:175–195, 1986.
16. Orticochea M: Construction of a dynamic muscle sphincter in cleft palate. Plast Reconstr Surg 41:323–327, 1968.
17. Jolleys A, Robertson NRE: A study of the effects of early bone-grafting in complete clefts of the lip and palate—five year study. Br J Plast Surg 25:229–237, 1972.

18. Robertson NRE, Jolleys A: A further look at the effects of delaying repair of the hard palate. In AG Huddart and MWJ Ferguson (eds): Proceedings of the First International Meeting of the Craniofacial Society of Great Britain. Manchester University Press, in press, 1989.
19. Fish J: Growth of the palatal shelves of post-alveolar cleft palate infants. Br Dent J 132:492–501, 1972.
20. Huddart AG: An evaluation of presurgical treatment. Br J Orthod 1:21–25, 1974.
21. Huddart AG: An analysis of the maxillary changes following presurgical dental orthopaedic treatment in unilateral cleft lip and palate cases. Trans Eur Orthod Soc 299–314, 1967.
22. Huddart AG: Presurgical changes in unilateral cleft palate subjects. Cleft Palate J 16:147–157, 1979.
23. Robertson NRE, Shaw WC, Volp CR: The changes produced by presurgical orthopaedic treatment of bilateral cleft lip and palate. Plast Reconstr Surg 59:86–93, 1977.
24. Pigott R: Objectives for cleft palate repairs. Ann Plast Surg 19:247–258, 1987.
25. Mars M: The Sri Lankan Project 1987. Summary available from The Hospital for Sick Children, Great Ormond Street, London.
26. Shaw WC: The European cleft lip and palate project 1987. Unpublished protocol available from the author.
27. Scott JH: The cartilage of the nasal septum. Br Dent J 95:37–43, 1953.
28. Latham RA: Development and structure of the premaxillary deformity in bilateral cleft lip and palate. Br J Plast Surg 26:1–11, 1973.
29. Atherton JD: The natural history of the bilateral cleft. Angle Orthod 44:269–278, 1974.
30. Thorogood P, Tickle C (eds): Craniofacial development. Development 103 (Suppl.), 1988.

CHAPTER 3

Multidisciplinary Management of Cleft Lip and Palate in Taiwan

M. Samuel Noordhoff, C. Shing Huang, and Jorie Wu

Establishing a cleft palate center in Taiwan, a developing country, posed problems different from those in a developed country. Major problems included a lack of funds for patient care and equipment, lack of trained personnel and specialists in all areas, no educational system for training qualified personnel, and a large patient load. Some of these problems and their solutions are presented here. Of great overall benefit was the gradual emergence of an improved economy.

Establishing a Cleft Palate Center in Taiwan

Personnel

Initially, a plastic surgeon who had had experience with a cleft team organized and directed the center. Such leadership also could have been provided by an orthodontist, pediatrician, or other specialist. Most important was the deep desire to organize, train, and persevere to establish a team to work together in the interest of the cleft child.

The first team member chosen was a social worker experienced in charity work. She evaluated patients' financial needs and helped with patient and family education. This was a primary concern because of the financial status of the families and the lack of a health insurance program. The second member selected for the team was a native who taught Chinese as a foreign language. She acted as a speech therapist because she had the ability to hear correct sounds and knew how to teach the reproduction of these sounds. Dental treatment was provided by a general dentist who used a simple removable plate to correct crossbite.

Education

In all major areas (social work, orthodontics, speech pathology, and craniofacial surgery), a general plan to improve expertise and training was initiated. Specialists from established foreign cleft centers were invited to come to our institution periodically to train our staff. Eventually, team members were sent abroad for 3 to 12 months of observation and training in recognized cleft palate centers. During the past 10 years, all our personnel have received accredited postgraduate degrees and training in their special fields, including research. Further assistance in establishing standards and protocols for research was obtained from specialists in other countries to ensure that the programs were properly executed.

Current Problems in Taiwan

Although our institution is generous in providing financial help, improved standards and the cost of medical care and research programs require outside assistance. Establishing a foundation is one of our goals. Many patients refuse orthodontic treatment, secondary bone grafting, or speech therapy because of the extra cost. Private funding is necessary to provide this care because the government does not offer financial assistance for the care of these children.

Public and patient education has improved but still needs to be emphasized so that both the public and patients can understand what can be done to rehabilitate the cleft patient. Education is provided through television, family seminars, educational brochures, and posters.

Although Taiwan is a small, densely populated island with good transportation, it is often very difficult to get patients to return for proper treatment and evaluation. This problem is due to economic factors and inadequate patient education. A recently computerized program for scheduling follow-up visits should help to correct this problem partially.

Rampant caries and poor oral hygiene are prevalent in most of our cleft patients. Fluoridation treatment is used but requires too much patient cooperation to be successful. Patients are now undergoing more orthodontic treatment, and they better accept and understand the value of this type of care.

The Chinese educational system is so demanding and competitive that children in elementary school attend special classes after regular school. Because of this, it is mandatory that school-age children have acceptable speech by the age of 4 to 6 years of age, since they have no time for speech therapy, and no speech pathology services are provided in the schools.

Objectives of the Multidisciplinary Approach

Simply stated, the purpose of the multidisciplinary approach is to rehabilitate the cleft child so that he or she can lead as normal a life as possible. Morris clearly outlined the objectives and criteria.[1] Dalston et al have well defined the minimal standards for reporting the results of surgery and treatment.[2] These include a good aesthetic result based on minimal growth disturbance and development of normal speech and hearing. To achieve this, the psychosocial aspects of the child's development become salient. It is readily apparent that many specialists must work together and record their data and results in such a way that treatment can be assessed, evaluated, and changed to improve the final results. This multidisciplinary approach and evaluation is the basis of the treatment strategy used at our center.

Delayed Hard Palate Treatment Procedure

Hotz and colleagues[3, 4, 5] introduced a program of delayed hard palate surgery, which we adopted after visiting the Zurich cleft center. The goal of delayed closure is to reduce growth deformities and achieve acceptable speech. A combined hard and soft acrylic plate is inserted over the cleft as early as possible, usually at the age of 1 month. The dental plate is passive and is used before and after lip repair. An adhesion cheiloplasty is done when the patient is 3 months of age (Fig. 3–1) and is followed by a rotation-advancement cheiloplasty at 6 months.[6] A one-stage Millard rotation-advancement cheiloplasty is performed at 3 to 6 months when enough good tissue is available for repair or if the

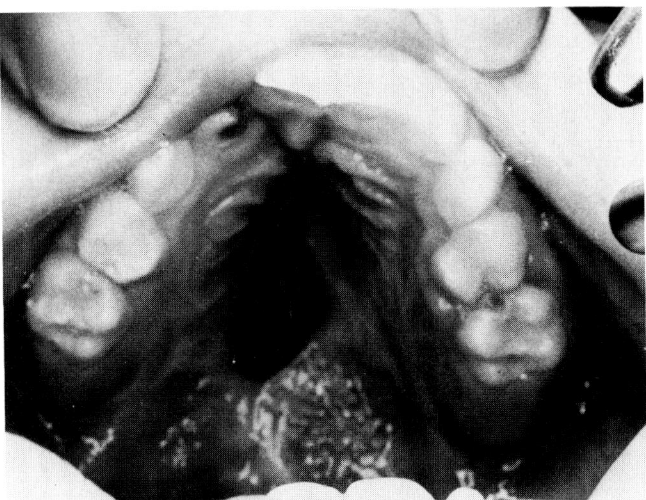

Figure 3–2 Palate after posterior palatoplasty (Perko) at 19 months of age showing remaining anterior hard palate fistula.

cleft is narrow. In patients with a complete bilateral cleft lip and palate, a banked, forked-flap cheiloplasty is used with lengthening of the columella.[7] A posterior, levator-repositioning soft palate repair without mucoperiosteal flap elevation is done at 18 months, leaving the hard palate open until the age of 5 to 7 years.[8] Usually the hard palate openings remain very large and are difficult to close with a rotational mucoperiosteal flap as described by Perko (Fig. 3–2).[9] To close the hard palate without extensive wide elevation of mucoperiosteal flaps, a vomer flap covered with a full-thickness skin graft[10] or mucosal graft is used to prevent contracture and facilitate primary healing (Figs. 3–3 and 3–4).

Results of Delayed Hard Palate Closure

Orthodontic Results

An infant dental plate was selectively constructed to guide further growth of the maxillary segments, make

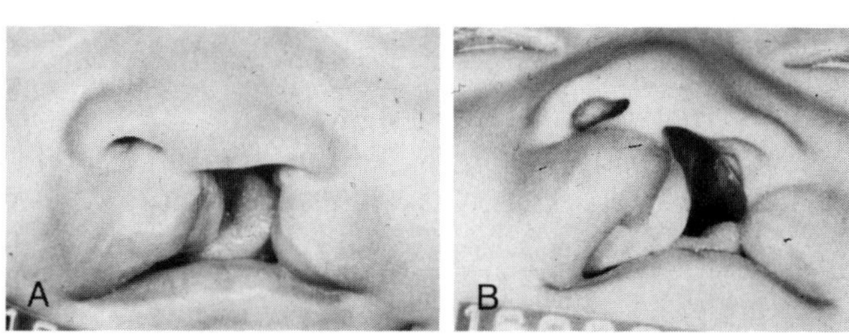

Figure 3–1 Delayed hard palate closure. *A* and *B*, Complete left cleft of primary and secondary palate, preoperative views. Adhesion cheiloplasty is planned at 3 months, rotation-advancement cheiloplasty at 14 months.

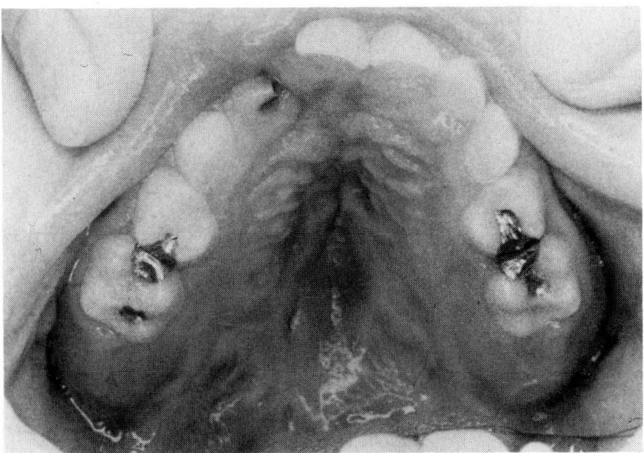

Figure 3–3 Palate after anterior closure at age 5 years with vomerine flap and full-thickness skin graft.

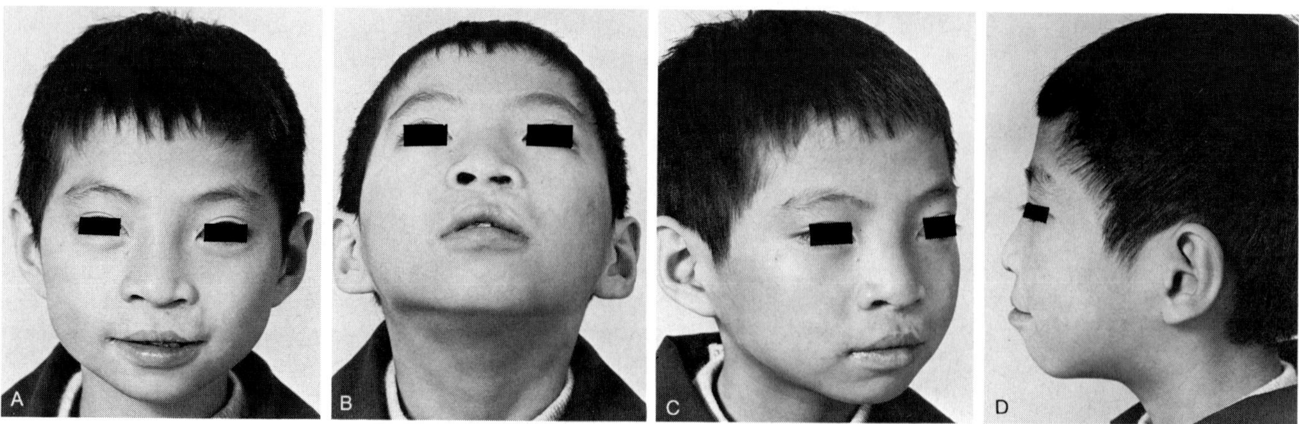

Figure 3–4 *A* to *D,* Appearance at age 10 after alveolar bone grafting at age 9.

surgery less extensive at the time of lip repair, facilitate feeding, and encourage proper tongue placement. It was difficult to assess whether tongue posture improved as reported by Hotz.[11] Our clinical impression was that the plate prevented the tongue from obturating the cleft, allowing the maxillary segments to approximate and making feeding easier. When the lip adhesion was done in conjunction with use of the infant dental plate, the maxillary segments approximated each other without collapse. Following definitive cheiloplasty at the age of 6 months, the increased tension of the lip generated enough force to disturb the surrounding orofacial structures and caused a greater degree of remodeling (or in some cases collapse) of the anterior maxillary arch. The infant dental plate usually did not fit well right after lip repair. Sometimes the plate could be used continuously after lip repair; however, prolonged use resulted in rampant caries in spite of extensive oral hygiene instruction and dietetic counseling. This observation led us to discontinue using the dental plate subsequent to lip repair.

Preliminary study of the development of the dental arch in the patient with complete unilateral cleft lip and palate has indicated that at 3 years of age the frequency of anterior and posterior crossbite was lower in patients using the infant dental plate than in patients who did not use the plate.[7] By the age of 5 years, about 50% of the patients (n = 61) using the infant dental plate had anterior crossbite, and this increased to 56% after anterior palate closure. The incidence of anterior crossbite was not less than that in patients who did not use the infant dental plate. Consequently, these findings led to a reassessment of our treatment methods and their long-term results. Currently, the infant dental plate is used in combination with gentle, extraoral, elastic traction in patients with severely malpositioned segments (for example, in patients with bilateral cleft lip and palate with a protruding premaxilla or wide unilateral clefts) to provide better alignment of segments before lip repair and to allow less extensive tissue undermining when reconstructing the lip.

After soft palate closure at 18 months of age, facial growth and development were evaluated annually. Orthodontic treatment in the primary dentition was not attempted unless the patient exhibited a functional shift of mandibular movement, that is, occlusal interference causing anterior mandibular movement. The use of speech plates to obturate the anterior hard palate cleft before surgical closure has been discontinued after 4 years of gathering and analyzing results because they had no effect on articulation and contributed to severe dental caries.[7]

The anterior cleft of the hard palate was surgically closed after the first permanent molars reached occlusion at the age of 5 to 7 years. Cephalometric analysis (Table 3–1) of the delayed, hard palate closure group at 7 years of age showed that there were no significant differences in facial growth between the early and late closure patients[12] except for a steeper mandibular plane in the early closure group and a smaller ANB (subspinale-nasion-supramentale) angle in the males of the early closure group.[13] Whether there is better facial growth in delayed closure patients will not be clear until the patients reach maturity.

The period of mixed dentition has been found to be the most advantageous time for orthodontic correction of malpositioned permanent incisors, anteroposterior discrepancy of the maxillary arch, maxillary width constriction, dental crowding, and notching in the dentoalveolar ridge. A partial fixed orthodontic appliance combined with rapid palatal expansion has commonly been used to correct dental problems at this stage. Secondary alveolar bone grafting[14] was carried out prior to emergence of the permanent canine to provide a bony base for canine eruption, arch stability, improvement of alveolar contour, and alar base support (Fig. 3–4). Extraoral orthopedic force (face masks, chin cap) occasionally has been used in patients who showed a strong angle class III tendency with questionable results.

Full orthodontic correction in the permanent dentition has usually been indicated in the majority of patients. If patients responded well to treatment in the mixed dentition stage, treatment in the permanent dentition is less complicated and is similar to ordinary orthodontic procedures. Patients with a severe maxillomandibular growth discrepancy require orthognathic surgery in conjunction with preoperative and postoperative orthodontic treatment.

Table 3–1. Cephalometric Data from Delayed and Early Hard Palate Closure Groups

	Delayed Closure[a]		Early Closure[b]	
	Male	*Female*	*Male*	*Female*
Angular Measurement (degrees)				
NSBa	132.3 ± 4.8	133.4 ± 4.6	132.3 ± 3.1	133.2 ± 4.0
SNA	78.1 ± 4.4	77.3 ± 2.9	75.4 ± 4.4	74.9 ± 4.9
SNB	75.3 ± 4.4	75.1 ± 3.0	74.9 ± 3.1	73.8 ± 4.0
ANB	2.8 ± 2.9	2.2 ± 1.6	0.5 ± 3.3[c]	41.2 ± 4.4[c]
SN-MP	36.8 ± 5.4	38.2 ± 3.2	41.5 ± 5.5[c]	41.2 ± 4.4[c]
Linear Measurement (mm)				
S-N	62.5 ± 3.0	62.2 ± 2.5	63.4 ± 2.6	62.0 ± 2.3
A'-PTM'	44.2 ± 2.8	41.9 ± 2.1	42.0 ± 3.5	40.5 ± 3.0
Ar-Me	88.4 ± 3.2	89.2 ± 4.3	90.0 ± 4.2	86.8 ± 3.5
N-Me	104.0 ± 5.9	104.5 ± 4.6	108.6 ± 5.2[c]	105.5 ± 3.2

[a]Delayed hard palate closure group.[13]
[b]Early hard palate closure group.[12]
[c]$p < 0.05$, student t-test.

Speech Results

Speech in patients in the delayed closure group was generally inferior to that of noncleft children of the same age. A 5-year-old cleft palate child with an unrepaired hard palate had poorer articulation skills than a 2-year-old noncleft child.[15] In a longitudinal study of 30 delayed closure patients aged 3 to 7 years, 21% had adequate or fair articulation skills, and only 39% had normal or slight nasality prior to palate repair. Speech improved after hard palate closure. At the age of 7, 67% had adequate to fair articulation skills and 92% had normal to slight hypernasality. Pharyngeal flaps were performed in 23.3% of the group.[16] In a cross-sectional group of 70 patients (aged 6 to 7) after hard palate closure, 80.4% had adequate velopharyngeal closure; 29% of this group had had a pharyngeal flap. Only 37% of the group had had speech therapy (usually considered inadequate in amount). A pharyngeal flap was done only after videofluoroscopic evaluation confirmed that there was velopharyngeal incompetence.

Children with large oronasal fistulas greater than 50 mm^2 had poorer articulation than those with smaller fistulas.[15] Although obturation of the fistula was attempted, most children did not tolerate the speech plate or it was discontinued because of dental caries. The presence of a hard palate fistula or dental plate resulted in a different type of sensory feedback, making anterior palatal sounds difficult to achieve. Consequently, anterior sounds were produced posteriorly, either in the mid-area of the palate or in the velar area. This posterior substitution was one of the two most common erroneous patterns occurring in the speech of children with delayed palate closure, and it was difficult or impossible to change with speech therapy.[15, 17]

In a detailed analysis of articulation proficiency in children with delayed closure, affricates were found to be the most difficult phonemes for Chinese cleft palate children to acquire. By age 5, proficiency in producing affricates was achieved by only 3%, fricatives by 39%, plosives by 62%, and nasals by 100%. Fricatives and affricates comprise almost 50% of Mandarin consonants and are usually acquired by normal children by the age of 5 years.[18]

Most of the children who needed speech therapy had poor motivation prior to closure of the hard palate. Only 36% had had speech therapy before hard palate closure, and this definitely helped articulatory placement. All children needed speech therapy after closure of the hard palate at the age of 6 to 7 years to correct their long-habitual, posterior articulation errors. Unfortunately, because of financial hardship, lack of speech pathologists in the school system, and heavy scholastic demands on the children, very few have been able to get adequate help with their speech problems.

Middle Ear Evaluation

Standard tympanograms were done during outpatient visits. If results were abnormal, medical treatment was instituted. If the tympanogram did not return to normal after 2 to 4 weeks of treatment, the patient was referred to the otorhinolaryngologist for insertion of ventilating tubes. A retrospective review of 274 patients of mixed cleft types at different stages of repair showed that serous otitis media existed in 41% to 95% of children ranging from 6 months to 6 years of age. The highest prevalence of 95% was found in the age group of 13 to 18 months (N = 44). Of the 548 ears examined, 331 had a type B tympanogram.

Early Closure of the Palate

To evaluate the problem of poor speech effectively, the treatment protocol was reversed, and complete closure of the palate was performed by 18 to 24 months. An adhesion cheiloplasty with minimal dissection and undermining was done at the age of 3 months if the cleft was wide. If not, a definitive rotation-advancement Millard cheiloplasty was done subsequent to the lip adhesion when the edges of the alveolar arches were approximated; usually this occurred by 6 to 9 months of age. The hard palate was closed at 1 year of age using a vomer flap covered with a full-thickness skin graft. Closure of the soft palate[8] was performed at the age of 18 to 24 months.

Orthodontic Results

Children in this group now are approximately 5 years of age and are in the process of being evaluated for occlusion and cephalometric studies.

Speech Results

A preliminary cross-sectional study of 52 children (aged 2 to 5 years) with complete cleft of the lip and palate who had had palate closure before 2 years of age revealed that 90% had normal to slight hypernasality. Adequate to marginal velopharyngeal function was noted in 92% of the children, and none had a pharyngeal flap. Adequate to fair articulation skills were noted in 67% of the group compared with corresponding developmental norms. These speech results were significantly better than those for the delayed hard palate closure group.

Evaluation Protocol

There is a great need for more and better data to identify factors that influence the results of treatment. The multidisciplinary approach requires a great deal of cooperation among the specialists, development of comprehensive protocols, and adherence to scientific methods of research. Our current protocol includes a multidisciplinary evaluation of patients with complete clefts of the primary palate, median dysgenesis,[19] complete bilateral and unilateral clefts of the primary and secondary palates, and postalveolar clefts. Some of the more important aspects of data collection are presented in Table 3–2, which presents a diagrammatic scheme of our protocol. Instrumentation is used only when it is required for diagnosis.

Classification of Clefts

Clefts anterior to the incisive foramen are classified as complete-incomplete, right-left clefts of the primary palate; clefts posterior to the incisive foramen are classified as complete-incomplete, right-left clefts of the secondary palate, a total of 24 possible combinations. A modified Y (Table 3–3) describes all clefts of the primary and secondary palates, allowing easy diagrammatic visualization and record-keeping in a computer program.[20] Any special patients or research programs are classified under a special code for easy recall.

Orthodontic Treatment

The major purpose of orthodontic evaluation is to assess the long-term surgical effects on facial growth and dental occlusion. Dental models and photographs (intraoral and extraoral) are taken at the age of 3 years and every 2 years thereafter. Cephalometric radiographs and dental panoramic radiographs are taken every 2 years from the age of 5 years. Dental model analysis allows for a better understanding of dental arch changes that occur after various surgical procedures. Cephalometric radiography provides further information about the growth of the cranial base, maxilla, and mandible and their relationships to each other. Other than conventional angular and linear measurements between landmarks, the projecting areas of the cranial base, maxilla, mandible, soft palate, and nasopharynx also are measured to reveal the absolute size change throughout the growth period. Functional movements of the lips, mandible, and soft palate are also monitored during various stages of development to understand the dynamic aspects of orofacial function in cleft patients.

Table 3–2. Data Collection Protocol

SPECIALTY	AGE (YR) →	1/4	1/2	1	1½	2	3	4	5	6	7	8	9	10	11	13	15
PLASTIC	EXAM					✓		✓		✓		✓		✓			
PLASTIC	PHOTO					✓		✓		✓		✓		✓			
ORTHOD	CEPH	✓	✓	✓	✓	✓	✓	✓		✓		✓		✓			
ORTHOD	EXAM							✓		✓		✓		✓			
ORTHOD	CAST				✓		✓		✓		✓		✓				
ENT	EXAM	✓	✓							✓							
ENT	TYMPANO	✓	✓														
SPEECH	EXAM	✓	✓	✓	✓	✓						✓		✓			
SPEECH	NPS	✓	✓	✓	✓	✓	✓	✓	✓	✓							
SPEECH	VFS	✓	✓			✓											
PSYCHO	EXAM				✓	✓	✓		✓	✓		✓					
SOCIAL	EXAM				✓	✓	✓		✓		✓		✓				

Table 3–3. Y *Classification*

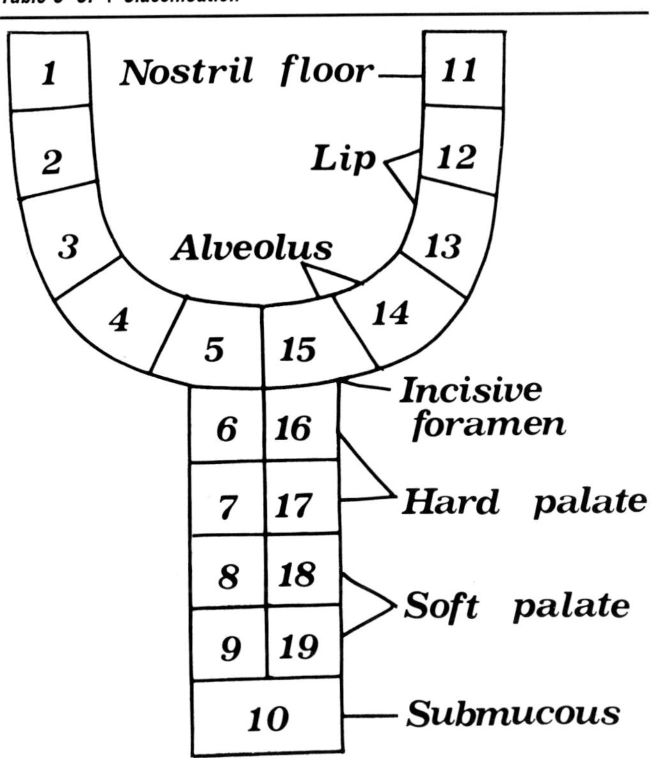

Kernahan's Y was modified into a double Y, which allows easy computer classification of all right- and left-sided clefts of both the primary and secondary palates.

Speech

Five specific areas are evaluated: (1) nasal emission; (2) resonance; (3) voice quality; (4) articulation; and (5) intelligibility (as modified by Subtelny).[21]

The presence of emission (Table 3–4) is tested by placing a mirror beneath the nostrils and by perceptual listener judgments of speech sounds other than nasals. Tasks include blowing through the mouth and producing isolated sounds, single words, and connected discourse containing bilabials /p, p^h/, affricates /tɕ ^{h}/, and/or fricatives /ɕ/.

Resonance

Resonance rating tests (Table 3–5) include bilateral single word production and sentences containing plo-

Table 3–4. Nasal Emission Rating

Absent	No air flow on nasal sounds
Reduced	Reduced or inconsistent air flow on nasal sounds
Normal	No air flow on non-nasal sounds; appropriate air flow on nasals
Mild	Inconsistent and barely perceptible air flow on nasals; perceptible to trained ear
Moderate	Air flow on most pressured sounds; perceptible to layperson
Severe	Continual air flow and consistent audible perception at all times

Table 3–5. Resonance Rating

Hyponasal	Severe	Consistent absence of nasal resonance
	Slight	Perceptible to trained ear
Normal		Normal nasal and oral resonance
Hypernasal	Mild	Inconsistent hypernasality on some sentences, generally in connected discourse; perceptible to trained ear.
	Moderate	Slight reduction in intraoral pressure, slight to moderate perceptible nasal air flow; perceptible to lay person but not offensive
	Severe	Marked reduction in intraoral pressure; prominent nasal air flow; most consonants grossly distorted; perceptible and offensive.

sives, affricates, fricatives, and connected discourse. For younger children, a hypernasality cul-de-sac test is used.[22] This involves asking the patient to repeat a word loudly and then to repeat the same word with the nares pinched. If a shift in tone quality occurs when the nares are closed, hypernasality and velopharyngeal incompetence are suspected.

Voice Quality

Voice quality is rated subjectively according to the degree of hoarseness (normal, mild, moderate, and severe). Patients with marginal velopharyngeal function have a higher incidence of hoarseness than do those with normal velopharyngeal function.[23] Hoarseness, in association with mild hypernasality, may be an early indicator of an incompetent velopharyngeal mechanism.

Articulation

A Mandarin articulation test with 21 consonants has been designed (Table 3–6). The test is similar to the Templin-Darley Articulation Test,[24] which takes developmental articulation errors into account. Articulation errors are classified as distortions, substitutions, or omissions, and a weighted score is assigned according to the type of error produced. Distortions are considered the least severe of the error types and are given a score of 1; substitutions are given a 2 and omissions a 3. This system of scoring errors is similar to that used in the Bzoch error pattern diagnostic articulation test.[22] Determination of articulation adequacy is based on clinical experience and a study of 150 normal Chinese kindergarten children aged 3 to 6 years.[18] It was found that pronunciation of vowels is acquired before age 3. Plosives /p, p^h, t, t^h, k, k^h/; nasals /m, n/; and the fricative /h/ are acquired by 90% of children by age 3. Affricates /ts, tɕ^h, ts^h/ are acquired between 3 and 4.5 years of age.

By the age of 6 years the rest of the fricatives /ɕ, ʂ/ and the affricate /tɕ/ have been acquired except for the retroflexes, which are acquired after age 6. The apical-dental affricates /ts, ts^h/ and fricates /ʂ/ and lateral /l/ are commonly substituted for the retroflexes /tʂ, tʂ^h, ʂ/ and /ʐ/. This pattern of substitution has become a well-accepted trend in the local dialogue. The general con-

Table 3–6. Mandarin Articulation Test

Mandarin Articulation Test

音 素	語 詞 1		語 詞 2		語 詞 3	
ㄅ	杯　子		爸　爸		冰　棒	
ㄆ	螃　蟹		葡　萄		皮　球	
ㄇ	貓		媽　媽		饅　頭	
ㄉ	蛋　糕		弟　弟		大　象	
ㄊ	兔　子		糖　果		踢　皮　球	
ㄋ	牛　奶		鳥		泥　巴	
ㄌ	老　師		喇　叭		樓　梯	
ㄏ	蝴　蝶		花		喝　水	
ㄍ	狗		哥　哥		國　旗	
ㄎ	筷　子		可　樂		卡　通	
ㄐ	剪　刀		姊　姊		機　器　人	
ㄑ	氣　球		青　蛙		鉛　筆	
ㄒ	西　瓜		謝　謝		學　校	
ㄗ	嘴　巴		走　路		早　安	
ㄘ	草　莓		擦　擦　手		彩　虹	
ㄙ	傘		賽　跑		掃　地	
ㄓ	鐘		桌　子		蜘　蛛	
ㄔ	船		吃　飯		吹　喇　叭	
ㄕ	書		刷　牙		睡　覺	
ㄖ	人		熱　熱　的		軟　軟　的	
ㄈ	飛　機		風　箏		肥　皂	

cept is that by the age of 5 to 6, children should have acquired the ability to pronounce all Chinese vowels and consonants.

Intelligibility

The intelligibility rating (Table 3–7) is determined by sentence repetition, paragraph reading, and spontaneous speech. Velopharyngeal competence (Table 3–8) is based on the evaluation of nasal emission and resonance tested in connected discourse. This information concerning velopharyngeal competence determines the need for speech therapy or further diagnosis. A speech evaluation graph (Table 3–9) provides a quick visualization of speech before and after various surgical procedures or treatment.

Instrumentation

Whenever velopharyngeal function is marginal or worse, videofluoroscopy and/or nasopharyngoscopic examinations are performed to evaluate the velopharyngeal function objectively. Nasopharyngoscopic examination[25] is a convenient method of assessing velopharyngeal func-

Table 3–7. Intelligibility Rating

Normal	Speech normal for age and sex
Mildly reduced	Mild difficulty in understanding, repetition not required
Moderately reduced	Moderate difficulty, repetition required infrequently
Unintelligible	Speech unintelligible even with repetition

Table 3–8. Velopharyngeal Competence Rated According to Speech Evaluation

Definitely adequate	Normal resonance and nasal emission
Probably adequate	Normal resonance and mild nasal emission
Marginal	Slight hypernasality and mild moderate nasal emission
Probably inadequate	Moderate hypernasality and moderate nasal emission
Definitely inadequate	Moderate or severe hypernasality and severe nasal emission

tion without the risk of radiation and usually can be performed when the child is 4 years old. It is felt that videofluoroscopy provides a better assessment of the velopharyngeal mechanism; however, there is a high correlation between the judgments of the pathologist and the results of videofluoroscopy and nasopharyngoscopy.[26] Table 3–10 lists the criteria for a combined rating of all three modalities of speech evaluation.

Psychosocial Aspects

The child is evaluated through developmental screening and evaluation of adjustment in school, which includes peer relations and teacher-student relations. Our evaluations of mother-child interaction and maternal satisfaction have helped us understand and treat the cleft lip and palate patient and family.[27] We also consider parental concerns and economic problems that may prevent adequate treatment.

Conclusion

Establishing a cleft center in Taiwan, a developing country, has presented some unique problems, which have been overcome with persistence, time, and the help of other established worldwide centers and specialists. The multidisciplinary approach to treatment of cleft children has been beneficial in highlighting problems that required treatment. Certain management protocols and procedures may not be directly applicable to all centers, racial groups, or countries because of local situations and factors. In our experience, speech in the delayed hard palate closure group was not acceptable and demanded improvement to meet the child's needs in school, particularly because speech therapists are not available. Also, facial growth at 7 years of age was no better in the delayed hard palate closure group than in the early closure group.

Table 3–9. Speech Evaluation Graph

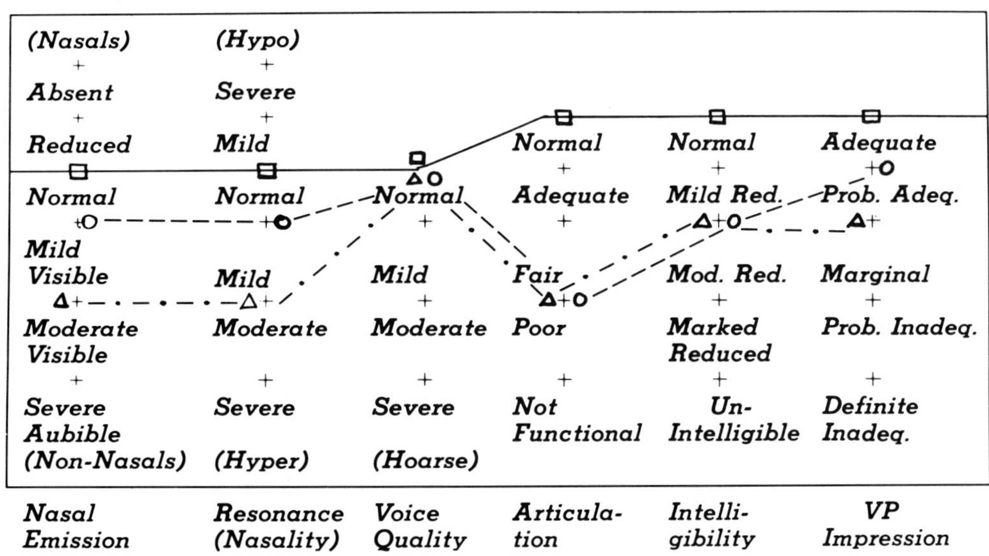

Δ: *Before hard palate closure*
O: *After hard palate closure*
□: *After speech therapy*

The graph provides a quick visualization of the speech examination and can be used to plot different types of treatment or stages of surgery and results.

Table 3–10. Combined Velopharyngeal Competence Rating: Speech, Videofluoroscopy and Nasoendoscopy

Velopharyngeal Competence	Speech	Videofluoroscopy	Nasoendoscopy
Adequate	Normal resonance and normal nasal emission	Good seal of velum and posterior pharyngeal wall (PPW), 75% or more of lateral pharyngeal wall (LPW) movement medially, closure consistently	Closure all the time
Probably adequate	Normal resonance and mild nasal emission	Good seal of velum and PPW, 50%–75% of LPW movement medially	Port closed most of the time; open port area < 25 mm^2
Marginal	Slightly hypernasal; mild to moderate nasal emission	Contact of velum and PPW, LPW movement less than 50%; or 1–3 mm gap between velum and PPW but LPW movement $>$ 50%	Closed most of the time; open port area 26–50 mm^2
Probably inadequate	Moderately hypernasal and moderate nasal emission	Velum–PPW gap > 3 mm	Port open most of the time; open port area < 50 mm^2
Definitely inadequate	Moderately or severely hypernasal and severe audible nasal emission	Short velum and gap > 3 mm	Failure of port closure; opening > 50 mm^2

This chapter has clearly pointed out the need for a multidisciplinary approach and evaluation. Further studies will undoubtedly help prevent growth disturbances, improve speech, and produce a normal-appearing, well-adjusted individual.

References

1. Morris HL, Jakobi P, Harrington D: Objectives and criteria for the management of cleft lip and palate and the delivery of management services. Cleft Palate J 15:1–5, 1978.
2. Dalston RM, Marsh JL, Vig KW, et al: Minimal standards for reporting the results of surgery on patients with cleft lip, cleft palate, or both: A proposal. Cleft Palate J 25:3–7, 1988.
3. Hotz MM: Pre- and early postoperative growth guidance in cleft lip and palate cases by maxillary orthopedics (an alternative procedure to primary bone grafting). Cleft Palate J 6:368–372, 1969.
4. Hotz MM, Gnoinski W: Comprehensive care of cleft lip and palate children at Zurich University: A preliminary report. Am J Orthod 70:481–504, 1976.
5. Hotz MM, Gnoinski WM, Nussbaumer H, et al: Early maxillary orthopedics in CLP cases: Guidelines for surgery. Cleft Palate J 15:405–411, 1978.
6. Millard DM Jr: Cleft Craft—The Evolution of Its Surgery. Vol. I. The Unilateral Deformity. Boston: Little, Brown, 1976.
7. Noordhoff MS: Delayed closure of the hard palate. In Hotz M, Gnoinski W, Perko M, et al (eds): Early Treatment of Cleft Lip and Palate. Bern: Hans Huber, 1986.
8. Perko MA: Two-stage closure of cleft palate. J Maxillfac Surg 7:76, 1979.
9. Perko M: Closure of the hard palate in unilateral cleft palate cases following previous closure of the soft palate according to Widmaier-Perko. Chir Testa Collo 1:9, 1984.
10. Stenstrom S, Thilander B: Management of cleft palate cases. Scand J Plast Reconstr Surg 8:67–72, 1974.
11. Hotz M, Gnoinski W, Perko M, et al: The Zurich approach: 1964–1984. In Hotz M, Gnoinski W, Perko M, et al (eds): Early Treatment of Cleft Lip and Palate. Bern: Huber, 1986.
12. Hayashi I, Sakude M, Takimoto K, et al: Craniofacial growth in complete unilateral cleft lip and palate: A roentgenocephalometric study. Cleft Palate J 13:215–237, 1969.
13. Wang F, Cheng WS, Huang CS, et al: Roentgenocephalometric study of complete unilateral cleft lip and palate patients treated with delayed closure of the hard palate—a preliminary report. Ann Acad Med Singapore 17:3, 1988.
14. Abyholm FE, Bergland O, Semb G: Secondary bone grafting of alveolar clefts. Scand J Plast Reconstr Surg 15:127–140, 1981.
15. Noordhoff MS, Kuo J, Wang F, et al: Development of articulation before delayed closure in children with cleft palate. A cross-sectional study. Plast Reconstr Surg 80:518–524, 1987.
16. Kuo J, Noordhoff MS, et al: Speech results in delayed closure of hard palate. Read before the Fifth International Congress on Cleft Palate and Related Craniofacial Anomalies. Monte Carlo, September, 1985.
17. Cosman B, Falk AS: Delayed hard palate repair and speech deficiencies: A cautionary report. Cleft Palate J 17:27, 1980.
18. Wang FNM, Phillips P, et al: Articulation development in Mandarin speaking preschool children, ages 3 to 6, in Taiwan. Chang Gung Med 9:68–75, 1986.
19. Noordhoff MS, Cheng WS: Median facial dysgenesis in cleft lip and palate. Ann Plast Surg 8:83–92, 1982.
20. Kernahan DA: The striped Y—a symbolic classification for cleft lip and palate. Plast Reconstr Surg 47:469–470, 1971.
21. Subtelny JD, Van Hattum RJ, Myers BB: Ratings and measures of cleft palate speech. Cleft Palate J 9:18–27, 1972.
22. Bzoch KR: Measurement and assessment of categorical aspects of cleft palate speech. In Bzoch KR (ed): Communicative Disorders Related to Cleft Lip and Palate. Boston: Little, Brown, 1971.
23. McWilliam BJ, Bluestone CD, Musgrave RH: Diagnostic implications of vocal cord nodules in children with cleft palate. Laryngoscope 79:20–27, 1969.
24. Templin M, Darley F: Screening and Diagnostic Tests of Articulation. Iowa City: Bureau of Educational Research and Service Extension Division, State University of Iowa, 1960.
25. Skolnick ML: Velopharyngeal function in cleft palate. Clin Plast Surg 2:285–297, 1975.
26. Noordhoff MS, Tsai YC, Hwang D: Comparison of videofluoroscopy, nasopharyngoscopy and speech evaluation in cleft palate patients. Southeast Asian J Surg 3:22–27, 1980.
27. Chen YR, Chen SH, Wang CY, et al: Combined cleft palate and craniofacial team. Ann Acad Med Singapore 3, 17:339–342, 1988.

CHAPTER 4

Multidisciplinary Management of Cleft Lip and Palate in Oslo, Norway

Gunvor Semb, Henrik Borchgrevink, Inger-Lise Saether, and Tore Ramstad

Norway is a long and mountainous country with only 4 million inhabitants. The geographical distance from north to south is comparable to the distance from Oslo to Rome. Most of the people live in small communities at some distance from the principal towns: Oslo (the capital), Bergen, and Trondheim (Fig. 4–1).

Historical Perspective

Before 1930 cleft lip and palate treatment in most countries was provided by surgeons, speech therapists, and prosthodontists—all independent of each other. The latter were required to fill, restore, and camouflage most of the defects following primary treatment. In Scandinavia, the prosthodontist often pioneered the establishment of interdisciplinary collaboration in cleft management. This initially included teaming with the speech therapist.

In Oslo, the Granhaug Speech Therapy Institute from as early as 1930 specialized on a small scale in treating cleft patients who had been operated on at Rikshospitalet, the University hospital. In 1939 the prosthodontist Arne Bohn began to provide dental treatment for these patients in his private practice and in 1963 he completed his thesis on dental anomalies associated with cleft lip and palate.[1]

During the early 1940s the orthodontist Egil Harvold began his pioneer work on the expansion of the maxillary segments and joined the cleft treatment group in Oslo in 1945. He collaborated with Bohn and developed a treatment plan for segment repositioning and retention.[2–4] This surprisingly late appearance of the orthodontist on the scene was typical of the times. However, the advent of cephalometry and biometric research and the deleterious effect of surgery on facial growth and development aroused orthodontic interest in facial clefts. Until this time, cleft surgery in Norway was performed by general surgeons. The first two Norwegian plastic surgeons to start practicing in 1948 after training in England were Wilhelm Loennecken, who settled in Oslo, and Halfdan Schjelderup, who began his work in Bergen. Soon after, most patients with clefts were referred to these two specialists for surgery. Consequently, management of cleft patients became central-

ized in these two towns, and this remains the case today.

Cleft teamwork for many years was managed primarily within the individual clinician's private clinics; however, in 1953, Loennecken was appointed head of a newly established plastic surgery unit at the University Hospital in Oslo, and cleft treatment underwent further organization. Still, it was not until 1968 that the dental specialists were offered a dental department at a new speech therapy center, where an audiologist and otolaryngologist also worked. After the establishment of the National Center for Logopedics in 1968, all cleft patients operated on at the Plastic Surgery Unit were routinely referred to the other team specialists, and the cleft palate team in Oslo gained its official status. At about the same time (1967), the medical registration of births, including information on congenital malformations, was introduced by law in Norway. This virtually ensured that all newborn cleft babies were referred to one of the two cleft centers.

The continuity of personnel and characteristics of the Oslo team have sustained a high level of experience. Furthermore, the basic principles established by the pioneers have undergone only minor adjustments. In 1952 Olav Bergland took over Harvold's orthodontic routines, and his devoted work on cleft pathology and treatment for over 35 years has been an enormous stimulus to the other team members. His death in 1987 was a great loss, but his assistant for 13 years, Gunvor Semb, took over his tasks and maintained the continuity.

When Arne Bohn retired in 1965, Tore Ramstad replaced him as the present team prosthodontist, and in speech therapy, Lorang Hansen, the first head of the National Center for Logopedics, was succeeded by Oddlaug Myklebust, the present head. Wilhelm Loennecken's surgical principles were continued by Henrik Borchgrevink, who joined the team in 1963 and has done cleft work at the Plastic Surgery Unit ever since, together with Gunnar Eskeland, who succeeded Loennecken as head of the department. Younger plastic

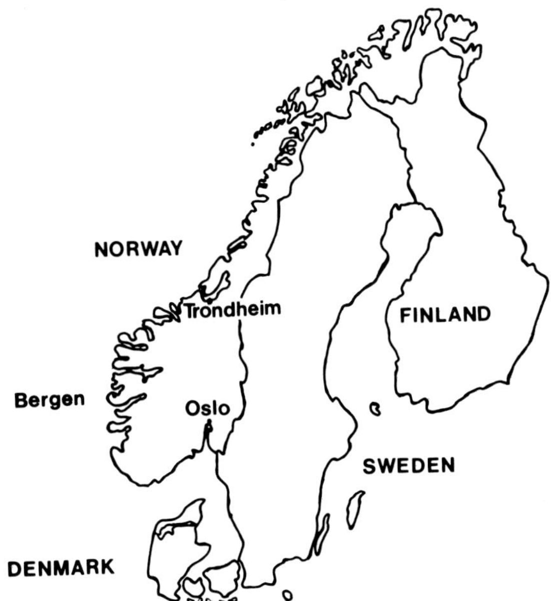

Figure 4–1 Norway and neighboring countries.

surgeons have also participated: Frank Abyholm, now professor in plastic surgery in Bergen, and Alain Ogaard.

Case Load

The incidence of cleft lip and palate in Norway is 2.08 per 1000 births.[5] About 60% of these are referred to the Oslo team, making the annual number of new cleft patients about 60 to 70. The national health system covers all expenses for hospital treatment, orthodontics, prosthodontics, speech therapy, and accommodation and transportation for the patient and parents.

Surgery

Cleft Surgery in Oslo—General Principles

Loennecken's plan for cleft surgery procedures and management was developed in 1948 in close collaboration with Harvold and Bohn. The procedures introduced comprised no new surgical interventions but rather a choice among an available variety of methods, modified to fit with a total program in accordance with a strong respect for tissue handling and conservation.

The main elements in Loennecken's operative plan in 1948 were:
1. No preoperative orthopedics
2. Closure of the cleft lip in infancy
3. Closure of the alveolar cleft region by a one-layer vomer flap during primary lip repair
4. Closure of the remaining (or isolated) cleft palate in early childhood by a von Langenbeck pattern palatoplasty
5. Secondary operations when required based on the current treatment plan and requirements of the orthodontist, prosthodontist, and speech therapist, all aiming at a final rehabilitation of the patient by 18 to 20 years of age
6. All surgery to be done meticulously; no parts—soft or hard—to be unnecessarily harmed or removed.

Surgical conservatism was applied by the team during the following decades, and thus the general approach to surgical management has been relatively consistent with only minor modifications (Fig. 4–2), partly due to Olav Bergland's general satisfaction with the dental arch form.[6] The general policy has been to keep the treatment program simple and to resist the introduction of new techniques or modalities of treatment. Thus when 1555 consecutive cleft patients treated by the Oslo team were reviewed, this was a relatively uniform group, and the results in all respects proved to be acceptable in comparison with those of well-established cleft centers of the time.[7–9]

Lip Closure—Unilateral and Incomplete Clefts

Lip closure at first was done with a Le Mesurier modification, which Loennecken used for 13 years until he changed to Millard's procedure (Fig. 4–3) in 1961. This has since been the standard for all unilateral cleft lip repairs, with an emphasis on optimal muscle rearrangement underneath a one-layer, anterior nasal floor reconstruction by mucoperiosteal flaps (vomer flaps in complete clefts). The abnormal lip muscle attachment to the bone lateral to the maxillary cleft and to the inside of the alar base is carefully dissected and transposed to the correct position anterior to the premaxilla, toward the anterior nasal spine, and to the medial lip segment. Transverse cuts in the mucosal edges, designed to release tissues during closure of the anterior nasal floor, are not made, to avoid unnecessary scarring in a region of important future bone growth and repositioning. Transverse cuts are not considered necessary when the mucoperiosteum is properly undermined on each side. Primary alar rearrangement[10, 11] is not routinely performed but is currently used when considered appropriate. No particular effort is made to elongate short unilateral cleft lip edges more than is achieved by the Millard procedure because they appear to grow over the years following the muscle union. When a tissue-saving cleft lip repair does not correct all deformities, secondary corrections are performed at later stages. This is one of the advantages of centralization: Each cleft patient "belongs" to one and the same treatment team from infancy to adulthood.

The primary operative closure of the lip and nasal floor in a combined cleft lip and palate leaves the posterior defect like an isolated cleft palate, to be repaired accordingly at a later stage.

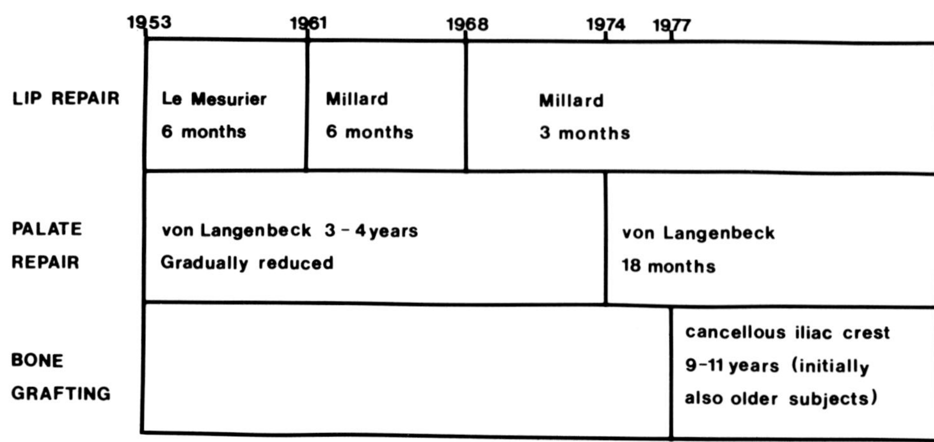

Figure 4–2 Summary of surgical management 1953–1988.

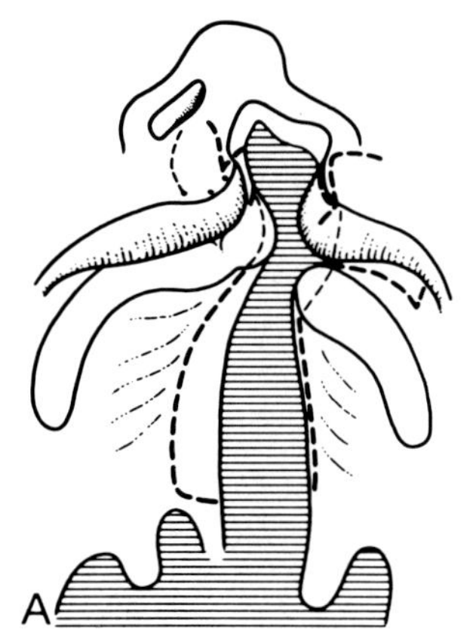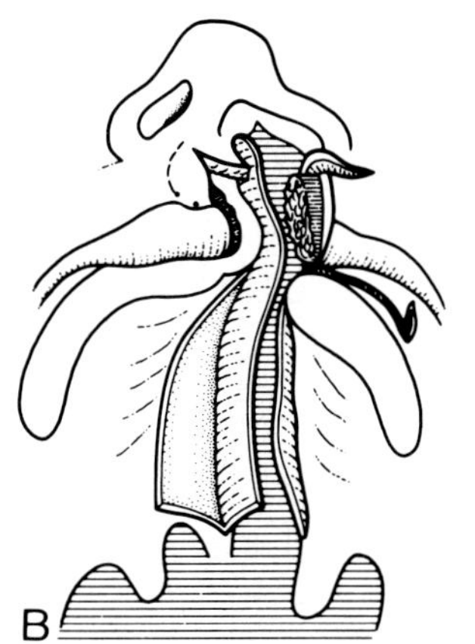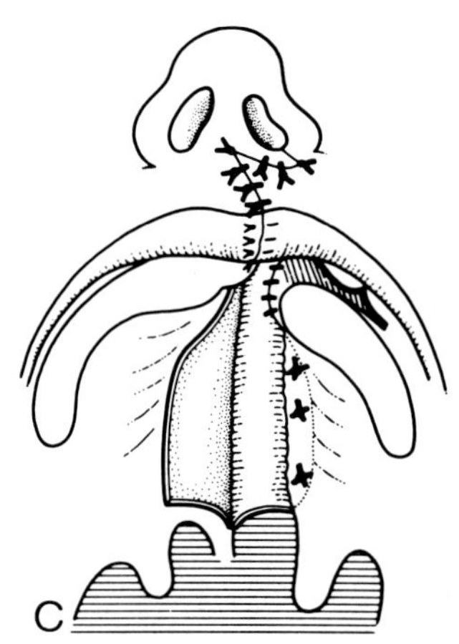

Figure 4–3 Principles of a Millard primary cleft lip repair combined with a vomer flap closure of an anterior palatal cleft. *A,* Incision lines. *B,* Lip flaps dissected out with direct continuation in vomer flap and lateral palatal cleft edge incisions. *C,* Vomer flap sutured as a one-layer nasal floor in continuation with the closure of the nostril sill in the lip repair.

Lip Closure—Bilateral Clefts

Incomplete bilateral cleft lip cases (without a bilateral cleft alveolus) are repaired in one operation, most often with a straight-line skin closure or, alternatively, using the procedure used for unilateral repair.

In complete bilateral cleft cases primary closure was initially performed on both sides at one time. Since 1962 the combined lip-vomer flap closure has been done in two operations (Fig. 4–4) to prevent ischemic insult to the growth and development of bone and teeth in the premaxilla as a result of vascular deprivation in bilateral subperiosteal soft tissue stripping. In a review of the Oslo material,[7] one group of patients who had had bilateral closure (before 1962) showed more oronasal fistulas and some cases of secondary premaxillary atrophy compared with a later group who had had a two-stage closure in which the number of fistulas was decreased by 25% and no premaxillary atrophy was seen.

Presurgical orthopedic treatment has never been used because the surgeons have found that any cleft, unilateral or bilateral, can be closed without it. The vomer flap procedure is easier, that is, less traumatic, in a wide cleft. The lip muscle reconstruction may be difficult, but even in a severe bilateral cleft it is always possible to transpose the muscles onto the anterior part of the premaxilla. Further advancement can be done at a later stage, for example, during a columella lengthening operation.

The straight-line closure in a bilateral cleft lip is easier to do (hence, less harmful) than the Millard Z-plasty because the prolabium is often very small and vulnerable. The elongation effect of a Millard procedure is not as necessary here as it is in unilateral clefts. The Millard "banking" of the flaps for future columellaplasty is not done either. The "resting" growth potential of the small prolabium is released by the lip closure, and during columellaplasty some years later, the philtrum lip skin has generally grown "too wide," providing ample skin for a biforked flap.

Palatoplasty

The posterior cleft palate, whether the residual defect following a lip-vomer flap repair in a complete cleft lip, alveolus, and palate, or an isolated cleft palate, is closed at 18 months of age using a modified von Langenbeck technique (Fig. 4–5). This procedure was introduced by Loennecken and fits well into the general principles and treatment plan of the Oslo team. The incisions along the medial margins of the cleft and the lateral incisions next to the alveolar process are based on von Langenbeck's technique. The lateral incisions are brought forward to the canine region. The same procedure is performed in incomplete and submucous palatal clefts.

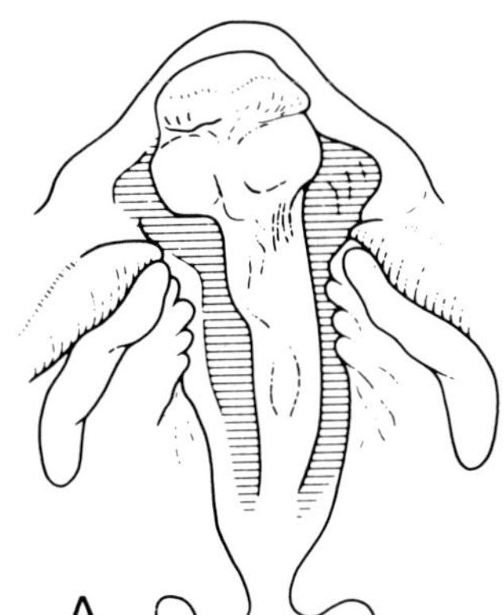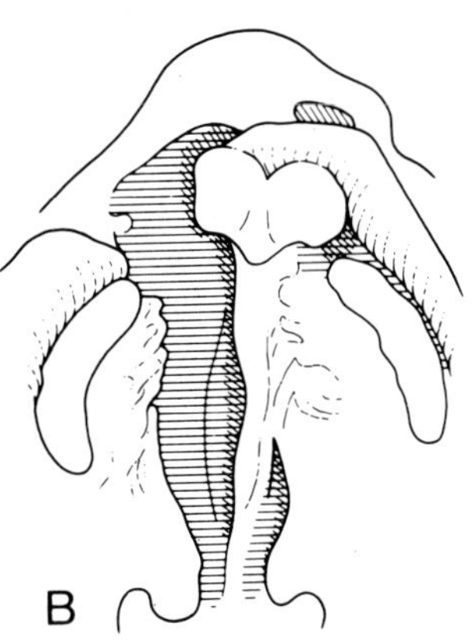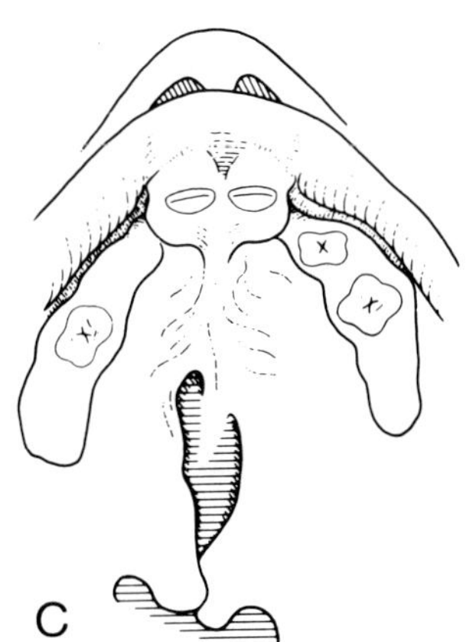

Figure 4–4 Drawings after photographs of a patient with a complete bilateral cleft of the primary and secondary palate. *A,* Preoperatively at 3 months of age. *B,* Six weeks after unilateral lip and vomer flap repair of the hard palate. *C,* Fourteen months later, before repair of the soft palate. No pre- or postoperative orthopedic treatment was given.

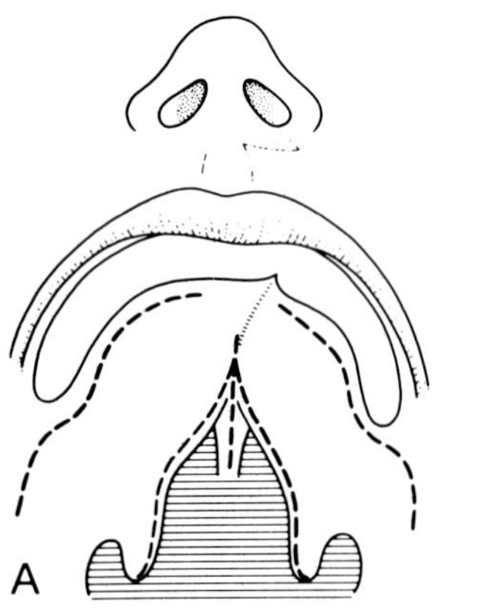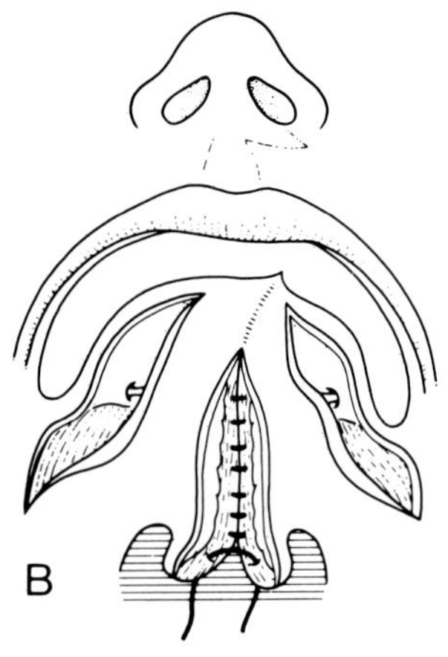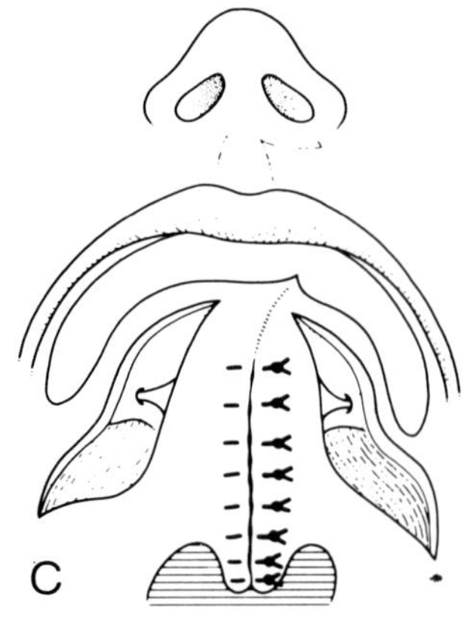

Figure 4–5 The principles of a von Langenbeck cleft palate repair. *A,* Incision lines. *B,* Bipedicled flaps mobilized; nasal mucosa sutured. *C,* Muscular and oral mucosal layers sutured; note greater palatine neurovascular bundles.

The mucoperiosteal flaps are elevated from the palatal shelves, and the muscles of the soft palate are carefully detached from the posterior edge of the bony palate. The soft tissues are detached from the lateral walls of the bony nasopharynx. The hamulus is fractured on each side; however, the tendon of the tensor muscle is kept intact. The neurovascular bundles are freed but not severed.

Following this preparation, the entire block, including the tissue of the soft palate and mucoperiosteal flap of the hard palate, can be moved medially and approximated with the other side at the midline.

Closure of the nasal mucoperiosteum starts anteriorly and continues to the tip of the uvula. Separate sutures are used to approximate the muscles of the soft palate, and mattress sutures approximate the mucoperiosteal flaps and oral mucosa of the soft palate (Fig. 4–6). The lateral releasing incisions are left open for drainage and spontaneous wound closure, which appears to be virtually complete when the patient leaves the hospital 6 days postoperatively.

No transverse incisions in the nasal mucoperiosteum are made during dissection. This ensures tissue viability and avoids transverse scar contraction and a raw surface on the nasal side with its subsequent scar contracture. For the same reasons, no transverse incisions are made anteriorly on the mucoperiosteal flaps of the palate. Since mucoperiosteal flaps remain attached anteriorly, this procedure does not allow for palatal push-back. As a matter of fact, according to our observations, the extent of real elongation of the palate following push-back procedures is considered of marginal value.[12]

Middle ear effusion occurs often in children with clefts. Many require myringotomies and tubes. Ear problems are treated by a local otolaryngologist. At the time of hospitalization all children with clefts are referred to the Department of Otolaryngology prior to surgical repair of the lip or palate.

Bone Grafting of the Alveolar Defect

This procedure was introduced in Oslo in 1977 according to principles established by Boyne and Sands[13, 14] and is thoroughly described in previous publications.[15–18] The main features are summarized in Figure 4–7.

Mucoperiosteal flaps are raised labially and lingually on both sides of the alveolar defect. Incisions are made

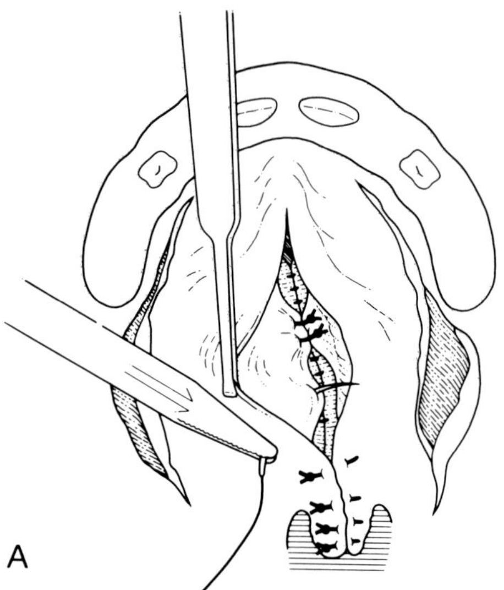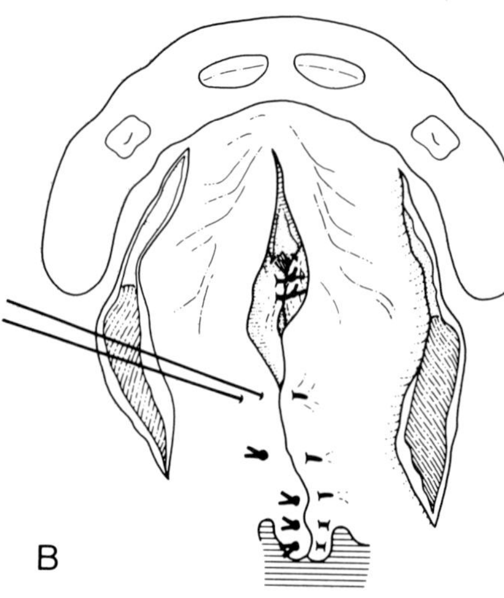

Figure 4–6 Final closing sutures. *A,* Deep generous bite of mucosa and velar muscle. *B,* Tightening of mattress sutures, just enough for approximation.

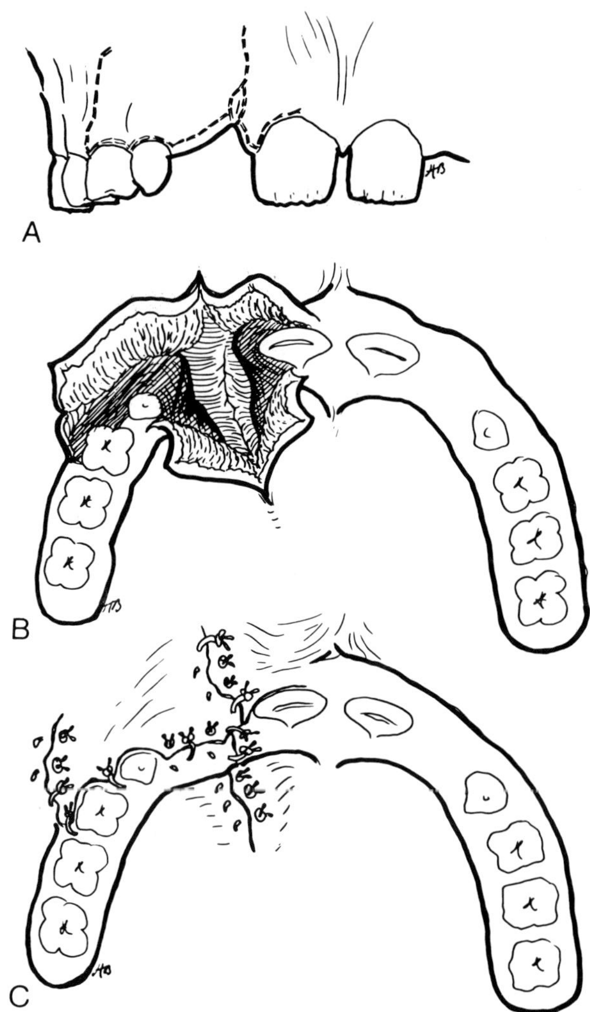

Figure 4–7 Secondary bone grafting of the alveolar defect. *A,* Incision lines for flaps of attached gingiva. *B,* Cavity dissected; no soft tissue is left on bone surfaces. The defect is now ready for packing with cancellous bone. *C,* Sutured.

on the alveolar ridge and cleft margins and in the gingival pockets buccally, along the erupted teeth from the central incisors to the first or second premolar. The alveolar cleft is fully cleared of all fibrous scar tissue (Fig. 4–7B). The mucoperiosteal flap on the buccal aspect of the lateral segment is mobilized by a vertical relaxing incision in the premolar region and is further freed by incising the periosteum along the base of the flap. Great emphasis is placed on keeping attached gingiva as the marginal tissue of all flaps, so that this specialized tissue will cover the grafted bone on the reconstructed alveolar ridge. The graft is composed of pure cancellous bone from the iliac crest.

Small bone chips are packed into the alveolar bony defect to its full height and depth and then fully enclosed as the flaps are sutured (Fig. 4–7C). In bilateral clefts both sides are grafted during the same operation. Supernumerary or malformed teeth are removed as advised by the orthodontist, who also does the postoperative follow-up after discharge from the hospital.

Timetable of Primary Operations

Timing of the primary operations has been subject to a few alterations (Fig. 4–2) since Loennecken introduced the initial protocol. Timing is often a compromise between many interests, and within the Oslo team, a point has been made of offering the same fundamental treatment to all cleft patients, without irrelevant individual variations. The geography of Norway (some patients live thousands of miles from Oslo) was one reason why Loennecken operated on the cleft lip as late as the age of 6 months. Other factors include psychosocial interests, views on general operability, availability of an anesthetic service, and so on. The age at operation for a cleft palate repair was originally 3 to 4 years, mainly to comply with the speech therapist's beliefs at that time. However, in 1969, it was agreed to change the age of the operation for a cleft lip to 3 months and for a cleft palate to 18 months. It took some years to fully effect this change, but since 1974, the age of 18 months for palatal closure has been routine (Fig. 4–2).

For the reasons discussed below, the age for alveolar bone grafting has been standardized at 8 to 11 years.

Secondary Surgery

Secondary operations are carried out in an established sequence and usually are completed when the patient is in his or her teens. Two to three times a year, a joint team conference is held to discuss complicated cases. Otherwise, most routine patient evaluation and treatment is done individually by the specialists, all working within the established protocol.

At the age of 5 to 6 years most patients who have had unilateral cleft lip repair performed in infancy are readmitted to the hospital for correction of the secondary lip deformity. When necessary, a sulcoplasty is performed to improve lip function and for orthodontic purposes. Sulcoplasty also may benefit speech production and physical appearance. Almost all cases of bilateral cleft lip and alveolus require lengthening of the columella at about 5 to 6 years of age using biforked flaps according to Millard's technique. In many patients, this operation is performed simultaneously with sulcoplasty and a lip muscle advancement. Previously, oronasal fistulas were closed at the same age. Since 1977, however, it has been found that fistulas occur infrequently, and they are closed during the bone grafting procedure performed in the patient at 8 to 11 years of age.

Indications for pharyngoplasty for correction of velopharyngeal insufficiency are established by the team speech therapists. In our center, about 15 to 20% of cleft palate patients are offered pharyngoplasty. The superiorly based pharyngeal flap is used. Timing for pharyngoplasty is decided by the patient's speech status. We prefer to perform this operation before the patient begins school.

After completion of orthodontic treatment following bone grafting, secondary lip and nose correction is done in almost all patients with clefts involving the primary palate.[19] This may involve minor procedures such as a lip scar or nostril rim revision or major reconstructive operations with deeper lip scar and muscle rearrangement and nasal skin and framework corrections (Fig. 4–8O, P). Because the primary operations have improved, there is a reduced need for major reconstructions such as extensive rhinoplasties, Abbe flaps, and complicated procedures to close large palatal defects.

We have observed an increasing demand for minor aesthetic refinements, and these are provided as long as an obvious reconstructive indication is present. We find that centralization, collaboration, and continuity within a team approach are appreciated by both parents and patients, who see their care as a stepwise program, with active treatment periods alternating with periods of growth. This attitude also enables the surgeon, in close contact with the other team members, to limit the extent of surgery at each age to a level that he feels will serve the ultimate result most favorably.

Currently, the treatment of most patients is completed when they are in their early teens (Fig. 4–8U, V) apart from the few cases requiring dental bridgework. All patients, however, are encouraged to contact the team at any later time if some corrective surgical or other procedures may be indicated.

Orthodontic Management

Objectives

The goal of orthodontic treatment is to provide an aesthetically acceptable and healthy dentition for life and to contribute positively to the general facial form and appearance. Distortions of facial growth and development with subsequent severe malocclusions in patients with repaired cleft lip and palate have, at least in the past, required many cleft lip and palate patients to wear some type of orthopedic or orthodontic appliance from birth to adulthood. Thus, for many cleft lip and palate patients, orthodontic treatment has been the most time-consuming and demanding part of the rehabilitation process. To strive for a reduction of the actual treatment periods, using appliances that are as simple as possible, seems to us to be of great advantage to our patients, provided the achievement of an optimal end-result is not jeopardized.

These principles were established by Professor Bergland, who was of the firm conviction that new forms of treatment should not be adopted unless there was clear evidence that long-term benefits would be achieved. He was also of the opinion that only orthodontists with experience in cleft lip and palate management should perform the orthodontic treatment of complete clefts. This has resulted in centralized treatment of unilateral and bilateral complete clefts at the Oslo clinic. Patients with cleft lip and isolated cleft palate are referred to local orthodontists, but advice on the treatment plan is provided if requested. However, all cleft patients are scheduled for routine follow-ups to ensure that the best possible treatment plan for a particular individual is being followed and to allow for collection of research data and documentation.

Presurgical Period

When preoperative orthopedic treatment was introduced at many cleft centers in the 1950s, it was also discussed within the Oslo team. In light of the above principles and objectives, its adoption was resisted for the following reasons:

1. The surgeons felt that they did not need it.
2. At the time presurgical orthopedic treatment was introduced, it usually meant keeping the child hospitalized and thus separate from his or her family. This was considered unacceptable (especially in a country like Norway with long distances to travel and rather poor communications, at least in the 1950s and 1960s).
3. The team, particularly the orthodontist, was worried that presurgical orthopedics might have an adverse effect on maxillary growth.
4. After instructions from the nurses at the maternity hospitals, no lasting feeding problems were encountered. When the babies came to the plastic surgery unit at 3 months of age for lip closure, they were well fed and thriving. (A booklet with information about cleft lip and palate and the treatment plans was produced in collaboration with the cleft palate team in Bergen and is available in all maternity hospitals. Mothers get the advice and support they need from the nurses, who show them how to use a special nipple for the feeding bottles before leaving the hospital.)

Presurgical orthopedic treatment has now been used extensively in Europe and the United States for over 30 years, but no report has yet appeared in the literature to demonstrate any long-term advantage for facial growth, appearance, speech, or occlusion.

Deciduous Dentition

We have never undertaken orthodontic treatment in the deciduous dentition because we find that dental irregularities are usually minor. We do not believe that treatment at this stage of dental development offers any lasting benefits.[6, 20] Correction of the deciduous teeth does not ensure normal eruption of permanent teeth.

Mixed Dentition (Preparation for Bone Grafting)

Orthodontic treatment has always been initiated in the early mixed dentition, and the following outline will emphasize the management of patients with complete clefts of the lip and palate. At all times, fixed appliance therapy alone has been used.

When Boyne and Sands presented their results of cancellous alveolar bone grafting, we recognized the potential advantages for our patients, and the first alveolar bone graft *ad modum* Boyne and Sands was performed in Oslo in January 1977 (Fig. 4–8).[14]

Careful evaluation of a large number of patients who have received cancellous bone grafts at our center revealed it to be a safe and reliable procedure.[17, 18] The height of the interdental septum in the grafted area was

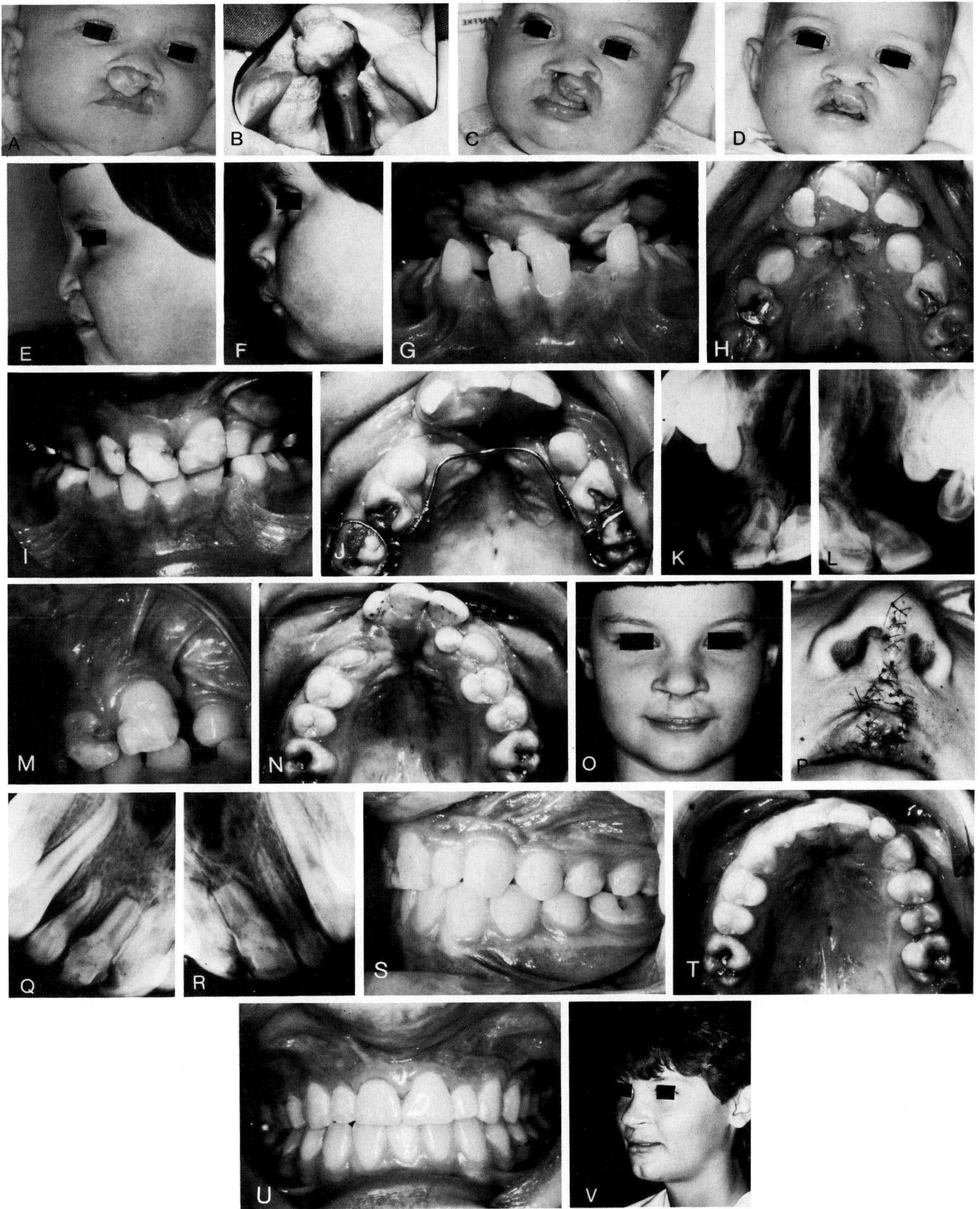

Figure 4–8 Different stages of treatment according to the Oslo principles, shown in a girl born with a complete bilateral cleft. *A* and *B*, The cleft prior to surgery. *C*, After closure of one side, age 3 months. *D*, After closure of second side, 5 weeks later. *E* and *F*, Before and after columella/sulcoplasty, age 5 years. *G* and *H*, After eruption of permanent incisors, which are usually hypoplastic. *I*, After correction of incisors.

J, Transverse maxillary expansion started. *K* and *L*, Radiographs of the two alveolar clefts prior to grafting at age 8 years. *M*, Alveolar cleft area prior to bone grafting. *N*, Spontaneous eruption of canines in the grafted region.

O and *P*, Before and after secondary lip/nose trimming, age 14 years. *Q* and *R*, Radiographs of the grafted area 8 years postoperatively. *S* and *T*, Occlusion and maxillary arch, 2 years after completion of orthodontic treatment. *U*, Porcelain laminates fitted on hypoplastic central incisors. *V*, The girl at 16 years of age.

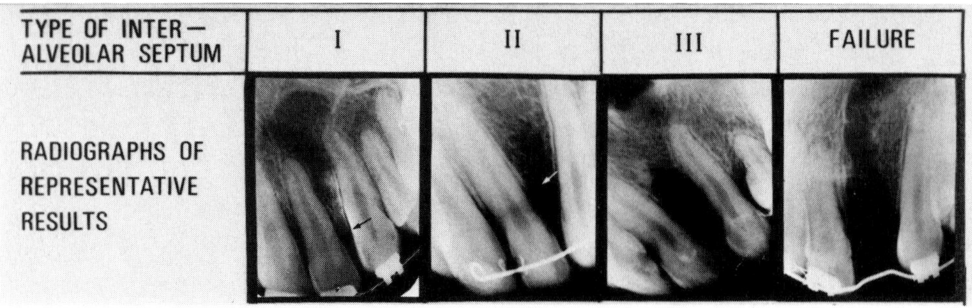

Figure 4–9 The basis for the evaluation of the height of the interdental septum formed after bone grafting. Type I: Height approximately normal; type II: Height at least three-fourths of normal height; type III: Height less than three-fourths of normal height; Failure: No bony bridge across the cleft.

assessed on intraoral radiographs (Fig. 4–9). The latest evaluation of 441 patients clearly demonstrated that the best results were achieved when grafting was performed prior to the eruption of the permanent canine teeth (Figs. 4–10, 4–11). This factor largely determines the sequence of orthodontic treatment.

The maxillary incisors, which often erupt rotated, retroinclined, and possibly in anterior crossbite (Fig. 4–8G, H), are corrected for aesthetic reasons and to facilitate oral hygiene (Fig. 4–8I). This is done with a labial archwire. Treatment generally lasts 3 to 4 months. The appliance is then removed, and a small bonded retainer is placed on the palatal surfaces of the central incisors. Approximately 25% of our complete cleft lip and palate patients have buccal crossbite attributable to segmental displacement. This is corrected simultaneously with the anterior corrections using a palatal arch auxiliary spring (Fig. 4–8J) or quad-helix arch. The correction of any remaining lateral crossbite of dentoalveolar origin is postponed until the permanent dentition.

Segmental repositioning is done just prior to the bone grafting procedure, and the lingual arch is kept on for 3 months postoperatively to retain the arch form. After this time, the bone graft is able to maintain the transverse dimension of the basal bone (any dentoalveolar

relapse is corrected later). In patients with bilateral clefts, a mobile premaxilla (which may jeopardize the immediate healing process) is stabilized with a heavy rectangular archwire to ensure immobility for 3 months postoperatively. All appliances are removed 3 months after bone grafting. In the few patients in whom the anterior maxillary teeth need retention, a sectional archwire is inserted, extending from the molar on the noncleft side to the frontal segment. This enables the teeth posterior to the cleft to migrate mesially, facilitating subsequent space closure.

Permanent Dentition

Two to three years after bone grafting, usually when the cleft-side canine has erupted spontaneously (Fig. 4–8N) or has been surgically exposed (necessary in approximately 15% of patients), orthodontic treatment is resumed. The alignment of the permanent teeth follows different principles, depending on whether orthodontic or prosthodontic space closure is planned. If at all

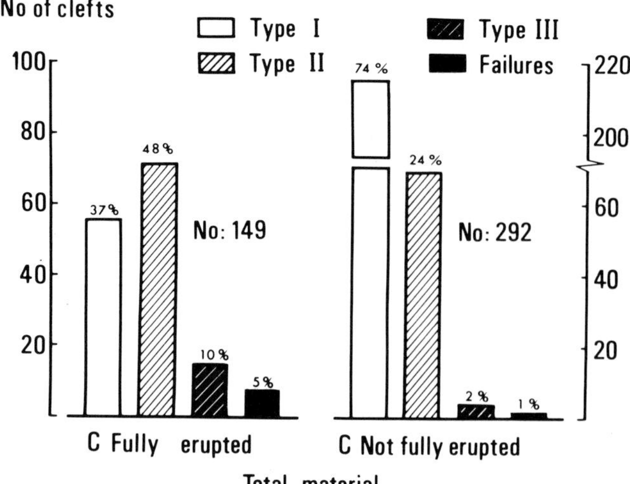

Figure 4–10 The total sample is divided into two groups according to the stage of eruption of the cleft side canine at bone grafting. The results are significantly more favorable in patients who received bone grafts prior to canine eruption compared to those receiving bone grafts after canine eruption.

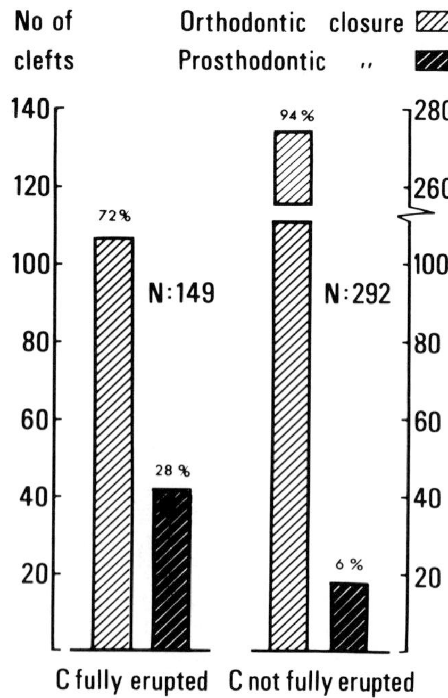

Figure 4–11 Closure of the cleft space. Orthodontic cleft space closure proved to be easier in patients who received bone grafts prior to canine eruption.

possible, we prefer orthodontic space closure because we consider bridgework in young adults to be undesirable for a number of reasons. Long-term evaluation in noncleft patients has demonstrated the superiority of orthodontic closure over restorative treatment for oral health.[21] Furthermore, bridgework calls for follow-up appointments for life (typically bridge modifications and replacements) and means, in effect, that the individual can never stop being a patient.

In all patients with a missing lateral incisor in whom orthodontic space closure seems to be possible, every effort is made to move the posterior teeth forward. For these patients, we have found protraction headgear (Delaire face mask) to be useful.[22] The forces used are intended to move teeth within the alveolar bone to help maintain a positive overjet, while the distal teeth are being pulled mesially. Thus we regard it as an adjunct to orthodontics and not as a means of achieving clinically significant skeletal change.

In most patients, the treatment period in the permanent dentition lasts 2 years and is completed by the age of 15. A bonded palatal retainer is placed so that it extends to two teeth on either side of the cleft. Until this time, the retainer is kept in place as long as the patient will accept it. Such retainers are unobtrusive and do not interfere with oral hygiene.

In patients in whom space closure is not possible owing to aplasia or a Class III occlusion, the anterior space is restored with an acrylic tooth on a fixed lingual arch or a bonded bridge until a permanent bridge can be placed at age 18.

Prosthodontic Management

When cleft repairs were undertaken by inexperienced surgeons, severe maxillary retrusion and collapse was common, and a typical cleft patient required an overlay prosthesis for the correction of horizontal and vertical growth deficiencies. When it became possible to correct the transverse discrepancy by orthodontic expansion, as described by Harvold,[3] heavy dependence was placed on prosthodontic appliances to resist the inevitable tendency to relapse. From the beginning, fixed bridgework, as opposed to removable partial dentures, has been preferred in Oslo.

Improvements in surgery subsequently led to less distorted maxillary arches, but until the mid-1970s, when alveolar bone grafting was introduced, provision of a palatal arch was still the routine means of retaining the expanded arch during the early teens. When the patient was assessed for definitive prosthodontic treatment at 17 years, it was often necessary to recorrect minor deviations of tooth position (such as a distolabial rotation of the cleft side central incisor) because its abnormal shape and pulp anatomy made abutment preparation difficult. The final design of bridgework was determined on the basis of the original malocclusion, the cleft space, the condition of the abutment teeth, periodontal status, establishment of the desired overbite and overjet, degree of premaxillary mobility in bilateral

cases, aesthetic considerations, and requirements of tooth replacement elsewhere in the arch. Experience has led to a number of refinements of traditional bridge design to suit the special requirements of cleft patients.[23]

Current treatment programs have reduced the need for bridgework to about 10% of our young adult patients,[17] but those requiring prosthetic reconstructions still present challenges. Bridgework is necessary in these patients either to correct multiple aplasia or because an underlying skeletal Class III pattern precludes full advancement of the buccal teeth into the anterior space(s) without jeopardizing a positive overjet and good lip support.

Generally speaking, bone grafting, by rebuilding the alveolar ridge and eliminating fistulas and recesses, simplifies bridge construction. Even in those patients in whom a normal interdental septum has not been obtained, better bone support for the teeth adjacent to the cleft allows better uprighting and parallelism of the abutments. Dental hygiene in the former cleft area is facilitated, and the pontic can be shaped normally without having to obturate the cleft space. In bilateral cleft cases, stabilization of the "floating" premaxilla by the graft greatly reduces the risk of bridge failure and allows the bridge to be less extensive.

The marked reduction in numbers of new bridgework patients now permits full attention to be given to follow-up of a large number of adult patients requiring complex prosthetic revisions and replacements and allows time for the cosmetic restoration of hypoplastic incisors in teenagers with composite or porcelain laminates.

Speech Therapy

Before 1968, speech pathology services were not well organized. The goal of treatment was intelligible speech, and obturation was used only for severe cases of hypernasality. In the initial years following the opening of The National Center for Logopedics, patients came for assessment at 3 to 4 years of age. Speech therapy was provided at the center, but because the speech service in previous years had been so inadequate, therapy was mainly reserved for children aged 6 to 7. Throughout the 1970s the speech service caught up with the need and was directed more toward earlier contact with parents and children.

Routines

Since the end of the 1970s the routines of the speech pathology service include the following:

1. Initial meeting with the parents as they accompany their child for the primary cleft palate repair.
2. Initial assessment of the child at 2 years. The child is evaluated by a speech pathologist, an otolaryngologist, and an audiologist.
3. Further reviews are arranged annually or according to individual needs.
4. At the age of 6 years, a year before the child starts school, formal language and articulation tests are performed.

Table 4–1. Frequency of Hypernasality

Level of Hypernasality Age 6 Years	1	2	3	4
CLP	67	19	13	4
CP	42	21	12	8
Number of children	109	40	25	11
	(58.9%)	(21.6%)	(13.5%)	(6%)

1 = Normal speech, 2 = slight variation from normal but without influence on intelligibility, 3 = moderate variation from normal, intelligibility is influenced, 4 = severe variation from normal, intelligibility is severely influenced.

From Myklebust O: Ekspressiv sprakferdigheter hos 6-aringer med leppe/kjeve/ganespalte. Unpublished thesis, 1981.

During the first years of the child's life, language development is stressed. If a child is language–delayed, therapy is recommended locally as soon as possible and is offered in the home or in preschool facilities. In these cases, the speech pathologist from the team will act as a consultant for the local therapist.

During recent years, we have found that approximately 35% of patients need direct speech therapy. For these children, therapy is started at the age of 4 to 4½ years. This is done at The National Center for Logopedics in Oslo. The child and an accompanying person (normally the mother) come to stay at the center for a period of 2 weeks. During this time, speech therapy is provided daily, two to three times a day. The number of sessions are offered according to individual needs. Approximately 22% of the children come for one to three sessions between the ages of 4 and 6 years. Ten to twelve percent need from four to eight sessions. Speech therapy is offered according to individual needs beyond 6 years of age.

During treatment at the center, the speech therapists have the opportunity to establish good rapport with the parents and provide a better understanding of the child's speech and language development. The mother and child also have the advantage of meeting others with the same problem. We consider this to be important because in the small communities of Norway, cleft lip and palate has a scarce representation.

When the child needs to be followed up locally by a speech therapist in the preschool or school, the speech therapists from The National Center for Logopedics are responsible for providing the necessary information and guidance, and good cooperation with local professionals is normally established.

Pharyngeal Flap

The pharyngeal flap operation was introduced in Oslo around 1960, and during the 1970s it became the most

Table 4–2. Articulation Ability

Articulation Ability Age 6 Years	1	2	3	4
CL	9	9	—	—
CLP	34	54	11	8
CP	43	26	8	1
Number of children	86	89	19	9
	(42.4%)	(43.8%)	(9.4%)	(4.4%)

1–4, See footnote to Table 4–1 for explanation.

From Myklebust O: Ekspressiv sprakferdigheter hos 6-aringer med leppe/kjeve/ganespalte. Unpublished thesis, 1981.

Table 4–3. Frequency of Hypernasality

Level of Hypernasality Age 6 Years	1	2	3	4
CLP	46	16	6	—
CP	27	12	4	—
Number of children	73	28	10	—
	(65.8%)	(25.2%)	(9%)	

1–4. See footnote to Table 4–1 for explanation.

From Saether IL: A study on hypernasality and articulation ability in cleft children. Preliminary unpublished data, 1988.

frequently used technique for the correction of velopharyngeal incompetence. Initially, the operation was performed at 8 to 9 years of age or even later, but it is now generally performed at around 5 years of age, once the patient is conscious of the placement of the tongue for correct articulation. The operation generally produces an improvement of velopharyngeal competence, giving the child an impetus in the process of articulation acquisition. Pharyngoplasty is now recommended in about 15 to 20% of cleft patients as our definition of acceptable speech becomes more critical.

Speech Results

In 1981 speech and language were assessed in patients who were 6 years old (Tables 4–1 and 4–2).[24] Hypernasality and articulation were judged on a four-point scale. It was found that approximately 59% of the patients had normal nasality, whereas 21% had a slight variation from normal (Table 4–1). About 42% had normal articulation, and 44% had a slight variation from normal (Table 4–2).

A preliminary review of 6-year-old patients born between 1978 and 1982 indicated that an improvement in outcome has occurred, the corresponding values for nasality being 66% and 25% (Table 4–3), and for articulation, 62% and 23% (Table 4–4).[25] A pharyngeal flap had been performed in 17% of this group.

Parental Counseling

A special counseling service for parents at the time of birth of a cleft infant is provided by speech therapists at maternity units in the Oslo region. Given the geographic dispersion of the population, the provision of such a service on a national scale is an important challenge for the years ahead.

Table 4–4. Articulation Ability

Articulation Ability Age 6 Years	1	2	3	4
CLP	37	16	9	2
CP	26	7	3	1
Number of children	63	23	12	3
	(62.4%)	(22.8%)	(11.9%)	(2.9%)

1–4. See footnote to Table 4–1 for explanation.

From Saether IL. A study on hypernasality and articulation ability in cleft children. Preliminary unpublished data, 1988.

References

1. Bohn A: Dental anomalies in harelip and cleft palate. Acta Odontol Scand 21:Suppl 37, 1963.
2. Harvold EP: Observations on the development of the upper jaw by harelip and cleft palate. Odontologisk Tidsskrift 55:289, 1947.
3. Harvold EP: Prinsippene for den kjeveortopediske behandling av overkjeven ved ensidig total ganespalte. Nor Tannlaegeforen Tid 59:395, 1949.
4. Bohn A: Nye protetiske oppgaver i behandlingen av pasienter med hareskar og ganespalte. Nor Tannlaegeforen Tid 59:403, 1949.
5. Abyholm FE: Cleft lip and palate in Norway. I. Registration, incidence and early mortality of infants with cleft lip and palate. Scand J Plast Reconstr Surg 12:29, 1978.
6. Bergland O: Changes in cleft palate malocclusion after the introduction of improved surgery. Eur Orthod Soc Trans 43:383, 1967.
7. Abyholm FE, Borchgrevink HC, Eskeland G: Palatal fistulae following cleft palate surgery. Scand J Plast Reconstr Surg 13:295, 1979.
8. Eskeland G, Borchgrevink HC, Abyholm FE: Columella lengthening in bilateral cleft lip patients. Experience with the forked flap procedure. Scand J Plast Reconstr Surg 13:429, 1979.
9. Abyholm FE, Borchgrevink HC, Eskeland G: Cleft lip and palate in Norway. III Surgical treatment of CLP patients in Oslo 1954–75. Scand J Plast Reconstr Surg 15:15, 1981.
10. Anderl H: Simultaneous repair of lip and nose in the unilateral cleft (a long term report). In Jackson IT, Sommerlad BC (eds.): Rec Adv Plast Surg no 3. London: Churchill Livingstone, 1985.
11. McComb H: Primary correction of unilateral cleft lip nasal deformity: A 10-year review. Plast Reconstr Surg 75:791, 1985.
12. Borchgrevink HHC: Cleft palate repair. In Muir IFK (ed): Current Operative Surgery, Plastic and Reconstructive Surgery. London: Bailliere Tindall, 1986.
13. Boyne PJ, Sands NR: Secondary bone grafting of residual alveolar and palatal clefts. J Oral Surg 30:87, 1972.
14. Boyne PJ, Sands NR: Combined orthodontic-surgical management of residual alveolar cleft defects. Am J Orthod 70:20, 1976.
15. Abyholm FE, Bergland O, Semb G: Secondary bone grafting of alveolar clefts. Scand J Plast Reconstr Surg 15:127, 1981.
16. Eskeland G, Bergland O, Borchgrevink H, et al: Management of the cleft alveolar arch. In Jackson IT, Sommerlad BC (eds.): Rec Adv Plast Surg no 3. London: Churchill Livingstone, 1985.
17. Bergland O, Semb G, Abyholm FE: Elimination of the residual alveolar cleft by secondary bone grafting and subsequent orthodontic treatment. Cleft Palate J 23:175, 1986.
18. Bergland O, Semb G, Abyholm FE, et al: Secondary bone grafting and orthodontic treatment in patients with bilateral complete clefts of the lip and palate. Ann Plast Surg 17:460, 1986.
19. Borchgrevink HHC: The rotation-advancement operation of Millard as applied to secondary cleft lip deformities. Cleft Palate J 7:161, 1970.
20. Bergland O, Sidhu SS: Occlusal changes from the deciduous to the early mixed dentition in unilateral complete clefts. Cleft Palate J 11:317, 1974.
21. Nordquist GG, McNeill RW: Orthodontic vs restorative treatment of the congenitally absent lateral incisor. Long term periodontal and occlusal evaluation. J Periodontol 46:139, 1975.
22. Delaire J: La croissance maxillaire. Déductions thérapeutiques. Trans Eur Soc Orthod 47:81, 1971.
23. Ramstad T: Post-orthodontic retention and post-prosthodontic occlusion in adult complete unilateral and bilateral cleft subjects. Cleft Palate J 10:34, 1973.
24. Myklebust O: Ekspressiv sprakferdigheter hos 6-aringer med leppe/kjeve/ganespalte. Unpublished thesis, 1981.
25. Saether IL: A study on hypernasality and articulation ability in cleft children. Preliminary unpublished data, 1988.

CHAPTER 5

Multidisciplinary Management of Cleft Lip and Palate in Osaka, Japan

Takeshi Wada

The incidence of cleft lip and/or palate in Japan, 0.19%, is one of the highest reported in the world and thus is a major problem in our country.[1] Oral and maxillofacial manifestations of cleft lip and palate touch the very heart of the interest and activities of dentistry, since the entire anatomy and oral function are involved in the defect. Feeding, speaking, occlusion, mastication, maxillofacial growth, and psychological problems all are affected as a result of clefting. Treatment should begin at the appropriate time during the development of the patient and in many cases should include long-term follow-up.

The concept of multidisciplinary management for the treatment of patients with cleft lip and palate comprises the need to provide maximal care and shared responsibility for problems in widely differing fields and to exchange investigative materials for better service. It is obvious that many of these areas are of considerable interest to the dental profession, and the Osaka University Cleft Palate Team, located within the School of Dentistry, has played a continuing role in an effort to find a solution.

The Origin of the Cleft Palate Team in Osaka

Surgery for cleft lip and palate was begun first in 1939 by Professor Iwao Nagai of the Department of Oral and Maxillofacial Surgery, Osaka University Medical School. He devoted himself primarily to surgery of the cleft lip and palate in more than 20,000 patients during his service of 30 years. Also, he conducted studies to improve cleft surgery and speech results.

In 1968, Professor Tadashi Miyazaki, associate of Nagai, who had studied speech science at the Institute of Logopedics (directed by Dr. Martin Palmer) in Wichita, Kansas from 1960 to 1962, was appointed head of the Department of Oral and Maxillofacial Surgery at the Osaka University School of Dentistry. The traditional treatment at that time was lip repair at 6 months of age using Millard's procedure and palate repair at 2 to 2½ years of age with a palatal push-back procedure. Using this treatment, it became evident that 34% of patients had velopharyngeal incompetence following surgery that required secondary palate procedures such as pharyngeal flap surgery.[2] Dental arch collapse also was common. Miyazaki promoted projects related to cleft palate speech pathology and therapy and applied the principle of a team approach for the multidisciplinary management of cleft lip and palate.

In an effort to establish a multidisciplinary management program, the cleft palate clinic, with branch status in the department, was founded at the School of Dentistry in 1972. In this clinic oral surgeons and speech therapists cooperated in evaluating surgical results and speech treatment. Other problems of feeding, secondary deformities, and velopharyngeal incompetence following primary surgery were also of interest to the members team. Among many outstanding studies by was the development of a nasopharyngeal that is now commonly used for evaluation of velopharyngeal competence and for visual speech training.[3–5]

Professor Tokuzo Matsuya succeeded Miyazaki in 1986 as professor in the department. Currently, he is conducting surgery and research projects on cleft lip and palate.

In 1986, the cleft palate clinic was elevated to the status of Division for Oral-Facial Disorders in the School of Dentistry, and I was appointed as head. The Division was created to facilitate management of the multidisciplinary approach for a total care program in cooperation with other related departments. This is the current status of the cleft palate team in Osaka.

Role of the Cleft Palate Team Members

The cleft palate team offers the services of oral and maxillofacial surgeons, orthodontists, prosthodontists, speech therapists, pediatricians, pedodontists, dentist/ speech scientists, otolaryngologists, anesthesiologists, nurses, and researchers in a coordinated, individualized treatment program designed to achieve the best possible results.

Oral and Maxillofacial Surgeon

All surgical management of the cleft lip and palate patient is performed by these surgeons. They evaluate the effects of lip and palate surgery and do extensive planning in surgical procedures, including secondary corrections of the lip–nose and palate deformities, bone grafting, and surgical-orthodontic treatment. Since most of the morphologic and functional corrections needed depend on the results of primary surgery, and since these surgeons are major team members, they play important roles not only as clinicians but also as geneticists, physiologists of oral function, and researchers.

Orthodontist

The orthodontists are responsible primarily for correction of malocclusion. They analyze maxillary retrusion and mandibular prognathism relative to craniofacial growth. They play an important role in integrating surgical and orthodontic treatment.

Pedodontist

The pedodontists are responsible for the prevention of dental caries. When patients are admitted for lip or palate surgery, the pedodontist counsels the parents about oral hygiene and arranges regular check-up examinations.

Prosthodontist

The prosthodontists usually are concerned with the permanent replacement of missing teeth or severe tissue defects following surgical and orthodontic treatment.

Speech Therapist

The speech therapist evaluates speech and language development. Examinations include analysis and evaluation of speech intelligibility, audiometry, intelligibility quotient, and sound spectrograph analysis, among other factors.

Dentist/Speech Scientist

Some of the dentists in our division are especially concerned with speech therapy and speech physiology. They not only participate in specific areas of speech therapy, such as devising speech appliances and visual speech training with the nasopharyngeal fiberscope, but also perform oral examinations and speech science investigations using electromyography, aerodynamic systems, sound spectrography, and the nasopharyngeal fiberscope.

Pediatrician

The pediatricians advise on nutrition and physical condition. Also, they make recommendations for the appropriate timing for surgery.

Otolaryngologist

The otolaryngologists may recommend hearing testing or place the patient under observation when hearing impairment or middle-ear effusion is suspected.

Multidisciplinary Treatment Program

The conventional course of treatment is carried out in four phases.

Phase I. Presurgical management including parent orientation, feeding practice, and presurgical orthopedic treatment.

Phase II. Surgical management of the cleft lip at 4 to 5 months of age and repair of the palate at 14 to 24 months of age.

Phase III. Management of speech and language development. Speech therapy after cleft palate repair to 6 years of age. Management of dental care and secondary procedures for velopharyngeal incompetence with speech appliances.

Phase IV. Management of secondary correction for upper lip and nose deformity and velopharyngeal incompetence, e.g., pharyngeal flap. Management of orthodontic, prosthodontic, and surgical-orthodontic treatments.

Currently, approximately 15 newborn patients with cleft lip and/or palate are referred each month to the Department of Oral and Maxillofacial Surgery or the Division for Oral-Facial Disorders by obstetricians, pediatricians, parent groups, and social workers.

During the patient's first visit, the examining resident completes the chart file, which contains a description of the birth and maternal history, a diagram of anomalies showing the type and extent of the defect, full-face and profile photographs, and evaluations by the obstetrician and/or pediatrician. The patient is then referred to the next step of the treatment program according to the routing sheet. Some of our specific approaches to the several problems in each phase of the treatment program are described below.

Phase I: Presurgical Management

Parent Orientation

When a baby is born with a cleft of the lip and/or palate, the parents may have feelings of confusion, fear, and guilt. By the time of the first visit, most parents already have had discussions with their physician or with a parent group and understand the problem more fully. However, more information, and in greater detail, is needed about the treatment requirements. For that purpose, we present a brochure to the parents that includes information about genetics, classification, general treatment programs, routing sheet, and treatment records. We also tell them the estimates for medical and dental care costs and answer any questions that they may have.

Genetic counseling is perhaps the most serious discussion for the parents because of its implications not only for the newborn with the cleft but also for the risk that other children born might have a cleft as well.

Treatment costs (surgery, dental care, speech therapy, and orthodontic treatment) are also a special concern of the parents. Obviously, the cost of treatment varies with the patient's requirements. In 1988, cleft lip and palate surgery costs were $7000 (United States dollars)—$3500 for each operation. Speech therapy costs are $50 per visit. Team visits are $20. Orthodontic treatment usually requires a period of at least 2 to 3 years, and estimated costs range from $6000 to $8000.

Fortunately, families are assisted in meeting these costs as a result of participation in either the national health insurance program or one of the private insurance programs in Japan. Standard treatment procedures and costs for cleft lip and palate (and other diseases and disorders) are determined by the federal health insurance committee. Coverage by either the federal or a private program is 100% for the employee/worker and 70% for family members. There is an additional welfare program (IKUSEI IRYO) for handicapped children that is supported by local public funds. Many of the treatment costs described above for cleft lip and palate can be covered by this program. We provide all available information about these programs to the families and assist them in making necessary applications.

Feeding Practice

Feeding is the first behavior of the newborn, sucking and swallowing activities being the result of coordination of the lips, tongue, cheek, and palate. Early acquisition of these efficient and rhythmic feeding movements is important not only for physical growth but also for the development of oral skills that are important in the later development of oral function and speech.[6] Within the Division for Oral-Facial Disorders there is also a special feeding clinic for infants with feeding problems.

Our routine examination includes gathering information about feeding time and intake, tongue position and activity, and other sucking parameters such as the sucking counts, rhythms, suction pressure (production of intraoral negative pressure), and expression pressure exerted to the nipple by the tongue and mandible. The goals of our feeding clinic are to provide a comprehensive feeding assessment, to determine the choice of nipple and/or use of the dental feeding plate, and to indicate methods for stimulating oral skills during feeding.

A new type of nipple for cleft palate feeding has been developed.[7,8] The nipple is designed to be flat and hard on the top, hemispherical and soft on the bottom, and have a crosscut opening. The shape and softness of the nipple allow better adaptation to the palatal anatomy and better oral sensation to encourage proper feeding practice.

The feeding clinic is used for training not only dental students but also students in dental hygienics and nursing. These students have the opportunity to see maxillofacial anomalies, learn how to approach a child, perform an extraoral and intraoral examination, and gain experience in recognizing when a feeding referral is necessary.

Presurgical Orthopedics

For many years, surgeons and orthodontists have been concerned about segmental displacement, arch collapse in the dental arch form, and underdevelopment of the maxilla. Several clinicians advocate the achievement of arch alignment soon after birth.[9,10] Their work has demonstrated that molding of the alveolar segments is easily accomplished by conventional methods. However, questions remain about the long-term results of moving the alveolar segments.

We do not employ presurgical orthopedic treatment routinely. Rather, our philosophy is to allow development of the alveolar segments without restriction. It seems probable that the modern technique of lip repair achieves sufficient cosmetic results in most instances. The repaired lip appears to mold the greater segment into alignment with the minor segment in the majority of patients with complete unilateral cleft lip and palate. In complete bilateral cleft patients with excessive premaxillary protrusion, we use an elastic band appliance on the labial side of the premaxilla until it rotates back into close approximation with the lateral alveolar segments.

Phase II: Surgical Management

Cleft Lip

Primary cleft lip repair in unilateral cleft patients is usually scheduled at approximately 4 to 5 months of age. Two-stage lip repair is preferred in most bilateral clefts to control the premaxillary protrusion by repairing one side at 4 months of age and the other at 7 months of age. According to the policy of our hospital, the infant can be accompanied by the parents so that they can better understand instructions about the needed pre- and postsurgical care as provided by the medical staff. Parents also are able to share experiences with other families with the same problem. Thus, parents are relieved and encouraged to be an integral part of the bedside care.

The patient is hospitalized 4 days prior to surgery for appropriate preoperative preparation including a complete blood count analysis, urine and serum analyses, a chest x-ray, electrocardiogram, and so on. Visits from the pediatrician and anesthesiologist complete the preoperative work-up 1 day before surgery. At each weekly conference, all of the presurgical reports for the scheduled surgery and the brief follow-up reports on current cases are presented and followed by general discussion.

There has been continuing improvement in the surgical repair of cleft lip during the past decade. Millard's rotation-advancement method or Tennison's triangular flap technique, with our modifications, is most often used for cleft lip repair. After completion of the lip repair, the suture line is sealed by adhesive skin closure tape. We use elbow restraints to prevent the child from disturbing the sutured wound. The sutures usually are removed on the third to fifth postoperative day, and the infant may be discharged 10 days after surgery when the wound is healing well. Since the parents accompany the infant, they understand well the instructions for home care regarding feeding and care of the suture line. Follow-up visits to the surgeon are continued for several weeks for evaluation of wound healing and the appearance and shape of the lip–nose area subsequent to repair.

Cleft Palate

Palate closure usually is scheduled at 18 to 24 months of age, prior to the development of speech. The operation we have used for a number of years is a modification of a V/W-Y mucoperiosteal palatal push-back operation with nasal mucosal lining flaps.[11] Our basic procedure includes:

1. Dissection and preservation of the neurovascular bundles.
2. Detachment of the aponeurotic connection and muscle from the posterior border of the hard palate.
3. Dissection of the ligament around the hamulus and detachment of the tensor veli palatini muscle for releasing tension.
4. Closure of the palate in layers, starting with the nasal mucosa, then the levator veli palatini muscles (to create a muscle sling), and finally, the palatal flaps.

An advantage of this procedure is that the actual gain in palatal length is relatively large, and there is a success rate for velopharyngeal competence of 76% at 4 years of age. However, a review of our investigations of maxillary growth indicated problems of maxillary growth and dental arch collapse.[12–14]

Some effects of palatal surgery on maxillary growth are suggested in an experimental animal study, which indicated that growth inhibition of the maxilla could result from surgical intervention of the periosteal tissue, leading to severe wound contracture and scar formation in the denuded area on the hard palate after V-Y palatoplasty simulations.[15] Growth inhibition also was observed following surgical trauma to the area of the vomer in beagles.[16]

Use of supraperiosteal mucosal flaps in palatal surgery was introduced first by Perko in a two-stage procedure.[17] The express purpose of his technique was to leave the periosteal layer intact on the hard palate. Preliminary results of Perko's study showed minimal maxillary growth restriction and sufficient velar function for satisfactory speech. The general interest in a two-stage palatal closure and Perko's encouraging results prompted us, in 1980, to treat some patients with complete clefts with primary veloplasty and delayed hard palate closure. Our procedure was based on Perko's technique and was performed at 18 months of age. The procedure was designed to achieve:

1. Dissection of palatal mucosal flaps from the posterior third of the hard palate to minimize surgical intervention, leaving periosteal tissue intact and the neurovascular bundles in place.
2. Sufficient retropositioning of the soft palate with a Z-plasty on the nasal mucosa.
3. Construction of a levator veli palatini muscle sling.
4. Delayed hard palate closure with the palatal hinge-flap technique at 5 to 6 years of age with no surgical trauma to the area of the vomer.

Results of a follow-up study to determine whether any difference in effects between the patients with different types of cleft palate repair have been reported.[18,19] After lip repair, patients were randomly selected for either the two-stage closure or the single-stage mucoperiosteal push-back procedure as described previously. Table 5–1 presents the distribution of the subjects.

Patients in the unilateral two-stage group (Unil-T) had a complete unilateral cleft lip and palate; in these patients lip repair was performed at 5 months of age using Tennison's procedure, primary veloplasty at 20 months, and hard palate closure at 5 years 10 months. Patients in the unilateral single-stage group (Unil-S) also had complete unilateral cleft lip and palate and had lip repair at 5 months of age (Tennison's procedure) and single-stage palatal push-back at 20 months of age. Patients in the bilateral two-stage (Bil-T) group had complete bilateral cleft lip and palate with primary lip repair (Manchester technique) at 5 months of age, primary veloplasty at 20 months, and hard palate closure at 5 years 10 months. Patients in the bilateral single-stage group (Bil-S) also had complete bilateral cleft lip and palate and had lip repair at 5 months of age using Manchester's technique and a single-stage palatal push-back operation at 20 months of age. A group of noncleft subjects served as controls.

The subjects were studied at 5 months of age, just prior to lip repair (stage A); at 20 months prior to

Table 5–1. Distribution of Subjects

| | Cleft Groups | | | | Noncleft |
Stage	Unil-T	Unil-S	Bil-T	Bil-S	Control
A: at lip repair					
Number patients	16	14	7	7	11
Body weight (kg)	7.1 ± 0.6	7.5 ± 0.5	7.2 ± 0.9	6.6 ± 0.5	7.2 ± 0.5
Age in months	4.9 ± 0.5	4.8 ± 0.4	5.1 ± 0.8	4.5 ± 0.2	5.5 ± 0.3
B: at palate surgery					
Number patients	16	14	7	7	11
Body weight (kg)	11.3 ± 0.9	11.1 ± 0.8	11.8 ± 1.9	11.3 ± 0.5	11.9 ± 0.7
Age in months	20.5 ± 0.6	20.4 ± 0.7	20.5 ± 1.6	20.1 ± 0.5	21.3 ± 1.8
C: at 4 years					
Number patients	16	14	7	7	11
Body weight (kg)	16.4 ± 1.5	16.2 ± 1.3	16.4 ± 2.8	16.5 ± 1.2	17.6 ± 1.8
Age in months	51.1 ± 3.2	50.5 ± 2.4	51.1 ± 4.2	49.5 ± 2.6	48.8 ± 3.3
D: at 6 years					
Number patients	16	14	7	7	11
Body weight (kg)	19.1 ± 3.6	18.2 ± 1.4	19.0 ± 3.6	18.9 ± 2.9	19.3 ± 2.1
Age in months	73.3 ± 3.8	72.1 ± 3.2	74.0 ± 4.8	73.5 ± 4.6	73.3 ± 3.8

Means and standard deviation given for body weight and age. There were no significant differences in the mean body weight and in the mean age between the groups of the same stage at 5% level of confidence (using student's t-test).

primary palate repair (stage B); at 4 years of age (stage C); and at 6 years of age (stage D), which was 2 months after hard palate closure for the two-stage groups. Three-dimensional maxillofacial impressions were obtained from each patient, and growth was followed using Wada's method.[14] Figures 5–1 and 5–2 demonstrate mean patterns of growth changes in depth and height at the incisor and canine points. Since the incisor point of bilateral cleft groups is located on the premaxilla, the growth in depth and height at this point indicates forward protrusion and upward rotation at stage A. However, there were no growth differences in these dimensions between the unilateral cleft groups and the control group at stage A. These findings confirm the view that patients with complete clefts of the lip and palate may have maxillary growth potential comparable to that in noncleft subjects.

After lip repair, growth increases in these dimensions in both unilateral and bilateral cleft groups showed smaller increments compared with the control group by stage B. This suggests that growth inhibition in the downward and forward directions appeared to result from the molding action immediately placed on the lip after lip repair.

The maxillary growth difference between Unil-T and Unil-S groups became distinctive after primary cleft palate surgery. The growth inhibition in depth and height, which occurred after lip repair, was compensated in the Unil-T group by catch-up in the subsequent stages, resulting in no difference from the control group at stage D. However, this did not occur in the Unil-S group. It was also interesting to note that there were no growth differences between the Bil-T and Bil-S groups in any dimension studied, and that the growth

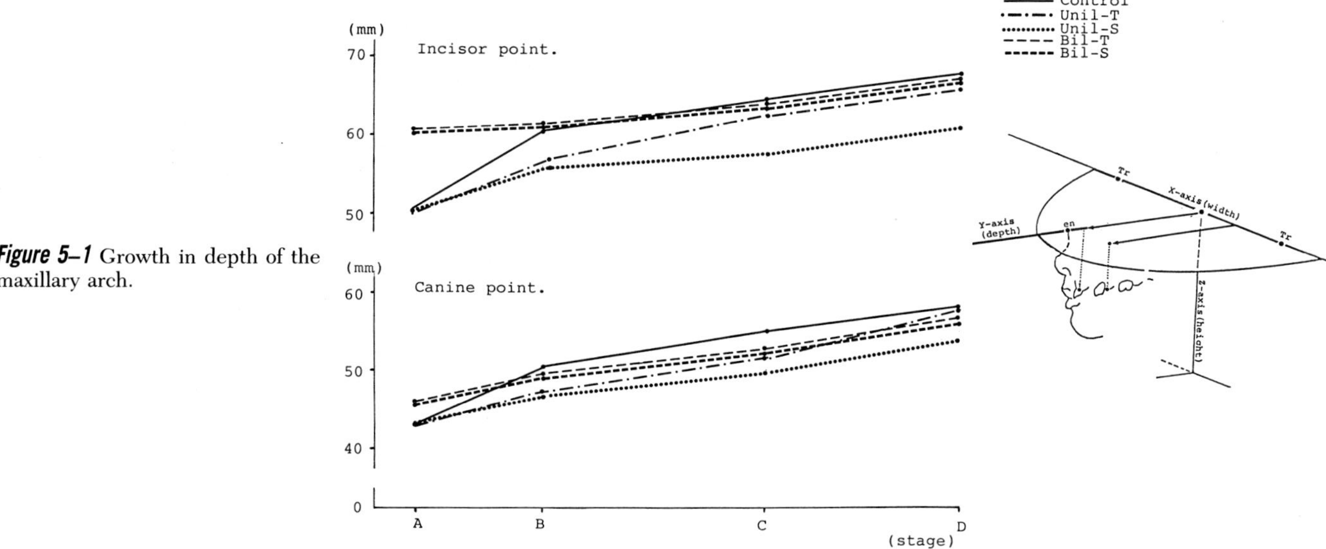

Figure 5–1 Growth in depth of the maxillary arch.

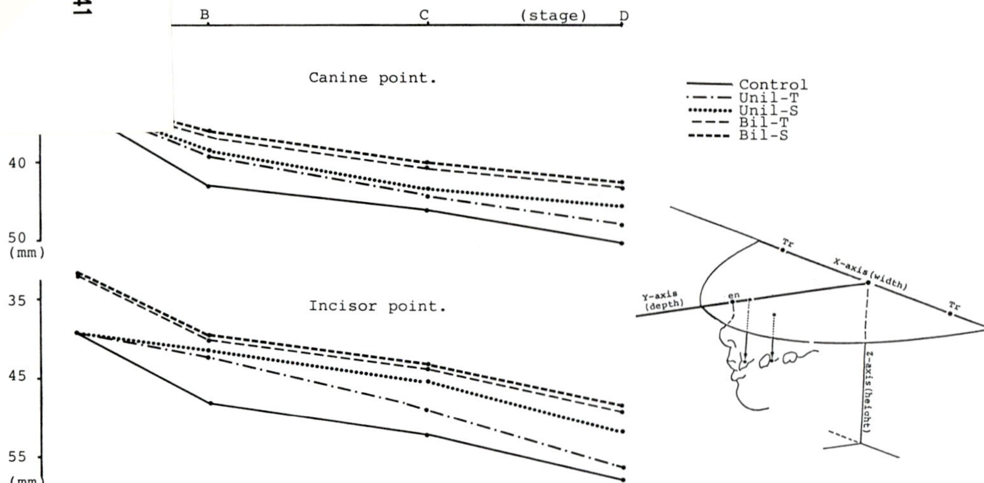

Figure 5–2 Growth in height of the maxillary arch.

in height at incisor and canine points of both bilateral groups was evident compared with the control group at stage D. A study of dental occlusion in the cleft groups at stage D revealed that 36% of patients in the Unil-S and 75% of patients in the Unil-T groups showed near-normal edge-to-edge incisor relationships. Lateral cross-bite was shown in 72% of patients in the Unil-S and Bil-S groups and 76% of patients in the Unil-T and Bil-T groups.

All of the patients had speech therapy in our speech clinic every three months, beginning from 2 years of age. An obturator was used in the patients who underwent two-stage repair of the palate following primary veloplasty until hard palate closure (Fig. 5–3). The obturator was remade every 6 months to accommodate the maxillary growth changes. Velopharyngeal function at 7 years of age was determined from clinical observations, use of a nasopharyngeal fiberscope, and lateral cephalograms. Results showed that 85% of patients in the Unil-S and Bil-S groups and 81% of the patients in the Unil-T and Bil-T groups achieved velopharyngeal competence during phonation.

Although the study has not had sufficient time at this point to evaluate the additional effect of hard palate closure on maxillary growth, it has suggested that two-stage palate repair with the present technique was more beneficial than the single-stage procedure in unilateral cleft patients. However, perhaps it is not so good for patients with complete bilateral clefts. This is an ongoing project and we expect to make a final evaluation when the patients are approximately 15 years of age.

Phase III: Management of Speech Following Cleft Palate Repair

After cleft palate repair, all patients are referred to the speech clinic in our Division where speech therapists and speech scientists are engaged in both therapy and research. The speech therapy program is designed to teach blowing skills, maintain intraoral air pressure control, foster muscle training, stimulate speech development, and prevent undesirable compensatory articulations. Many of our patients might acquire normal articulation and phonologic patterns spontaneously by preschool to early school age without speech therapy; however, to ensure the best results, all patients are placed under this service subsequent to palate repair (about 18 months of age) until 4 years of age. During this period, the patient is seen in the clinic every 2 to 3 months.

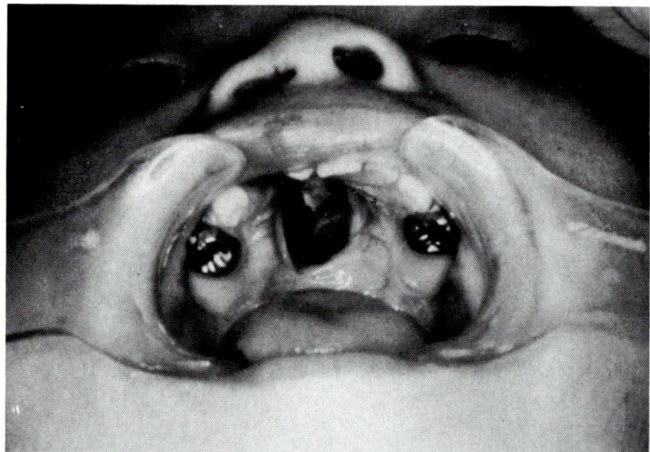

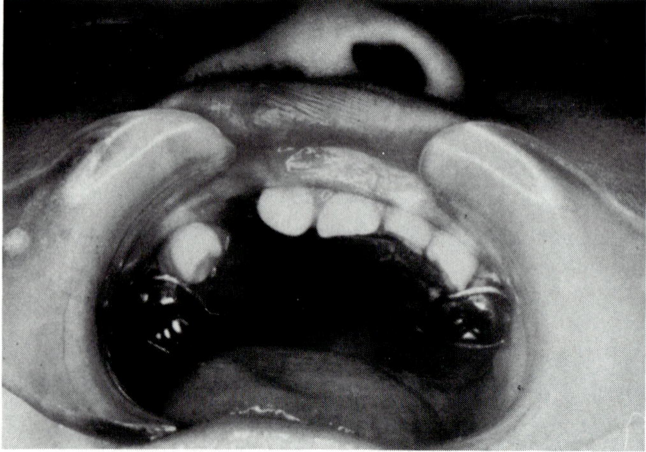

Figure 5–3 Cleft of the hard palate after primary veloplasty (top); placement of an obturator until the time of hard palate closure (bottom).

Procedures include practice in blowing and easy phonations or articulations according to the patient's level of speech development (Fig. 5–4). The majority of patients 3 and 4 years of age can cooperate with early articulation training, in which emphasis is placed on development of the ability to produce plosives and fricatives. Parents always are present during the therapy and their understanding is a great help for achieving better behavior of the children and providing appropriate speech stimulation at home.

Speech development, articulation skills, and velopharyngeal function are evaluated when the patient is 4 years of age. Evaluation includes an articulation test, radiographic evaluation of the nasopharyngeal configuration, assessment of nasal air emission, an oral examination, sound spectrography, and intelligence testing. Our findings indicate that 76% of those who have had a one-stage push-back procedure for palate repair achieve acceptable speech results; however, the remaining 24% demonstrate velopharyngeal incompetence and require a continuation of speech therapy, secondary palate procedures, or both. The initial step in a secondary palate procedure in our clinic is a prosthetic speech appliance to stimulate palatal movements and promote velopharyngeal closure for correct sound production.

We use two categories to judge velopharyngeal incompetence: relative and absolute. Relative incompetence is defined as poor function or mobility in spite of adequate tissue in the velopharynx. Absolute incompetence is defined as an organic tissue deficiency such as a short palate. The judgment is based on the oral examination, lateral head films, and observation through the nasopharyngeal fiberscope. A palatal lift prosthesis usually is used in the former and a speech aid prosthesis is employed in the latter. The prosthesis is adjusted (reduction of a pharyngeal bulb or extension of the velar lift) according to the development of compensatory movements of the velopharyngeal musculature. Speech therapy should be provided with such an appliance and the correct articulation should be maintained with marked reduction of nasal air emission. In selected patients with marginal velopharyngeal closure, it has

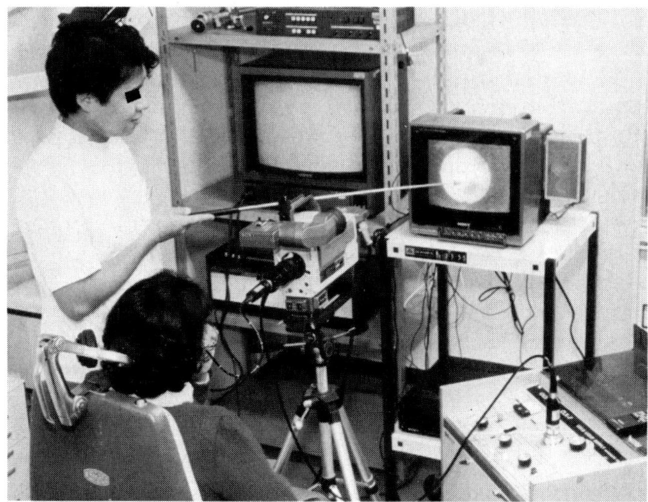

Figure 5–5 "Visual speech training" with nasopharyngeal fiberscope system in our speech clinic.

been our experience that good velopharyngeal function can be achieved with the palatal lift prosthesis, and that eventually this good function can be retained after removal of the prosthesis.

We also have had considerable success using combined speech therapy with a speech appliance and simultaneous nasopharyngeal fiberscopic observation for individuals who demonstrate absolute velopharyngeal incompetence. When these patients are 5 to 6 years of age, they can cooperate for insertion of the nasopharyngeal fiberscope through the nostril into the upper pharynx. The actual velopharyngeal movements during speech are recognizable on the video monitor by means of the nasopharyngeal fiberscope and video camera. Thus, it is possible to see the adaptability of the speech appliance in the velopharynx and analyze the modes of velopharyngeal closure during speech. Not only the patient but also the instructors and parents are able to view the movements and the immediate response at the velopharynx according to instruction (Fig. 5–5). We have named the system a "visual speech training system," and regard it as an effective tool for stimulating the patient's feedback mechanism in speech. It is used not only for our main speech treatment method but also as a recorded progress record, for which it is quite effective. The nasopharyngeal fiberscope examination gives us considerable information for diagnosis and designing of the pharyngeal flap procedure.

Phase IV: Secondary Surgical Correction and Orthodontic-Prosthodontic Procedures

In the majority of our patients, the secondary surgical correction of the lip, nose, and palate is usually postponed until the patient is 6 years of age because speech therapy is our main treatment during that time and following primary surgery. In addition, the period from 1 to 6 years of age is a time of rapid craniofacial growth.[20]

Children with malocclusion are referred before school age to the Department of Orthodontics, mainly for

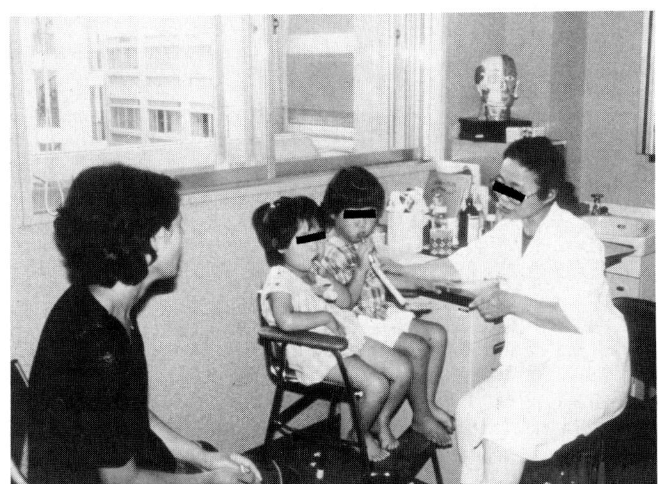

Figure 5–4 Practice of blowing during early speech therapy.

registration. Currently, in the majority of patients, orthodontic treatment starts around 10 years of age and is completed within 2 or 3 years. The patient who may require surgical-orthodontic treatment, final prosthodontic treatment, or pharyngeal flap surgery is presented to the team during conference for further treatment planning.

The pharyngeal flap operation usually is postponed until the patient is 10 years of age to lessen the growth effects in the velopharynx in regard to the pharyngeal flap and size of the lateral ports. Until that time, special emphasis is placed on correction of misarticulations with a speech appliance, so that only the nasality remains to be corrected surgically. The pharyngeal flap procedure is based on our technique. It is designed to construct a feasible and functional pharyngeal flap without leaving a raw surface on any portion of the flap. We also unite the muscles at the base of the pharyngeal wall.[21] The procedure includes:

1. Placement of a through-and-through incision along the midline on the soft palate.
2. Separation of the soft palate into two layers of nasal mucosa and palatal flaps.
3. Placement of a transverse incision on each side of the nasal mucosa to elongate the soft palate, allowing it to reach the posterior pharyngeal wall.
4. Dissection of a superiorly based pharyngeal flap, consisting of the entire width of the posterior pharynx extending downward into the hypopharynx, with a length equal to the distance from the pharyngeal wall at the level of the atlas to the posterior margin of the hard palate.
5. Approximation of the nasal mucosa and the lateral margins of the pharyngeal flap.
6. Construction of a small muscle union with the superior constrictor pharyngeal muscle and the posterior third of the levator muscle at the base of the pharyngeal flap, leaving lateral pharyngeal ports 5 mm in diameter on each side, and construction of a levator muscle sling with the remaining anterior two thirds of the levator veli palatini muscle at the middle portion of the soft palate.
7. Approximation of the palatal flaps and complete closure of the wound on the palate and pharyngeal wall.

The basic premise of the procedure is construction of double muscle unions. One is the union of the major part of the levator muscle for the velopharyngeal closure of the soft palate and the other is the posterior muscle union, which is the small muscle union around the ports. We have used this procedure in more than 120 patients. Many show denasality for 1 or 2 weeks after surgery, but this is reduced to normal within 1 month. The procedure serves to fix the base of the pharyngeal flap at the desired level following postsurgical healing. Approximately 4 weeks after the pharyngeal flap operation, we again treat the patient with visual speech training using the nasopharyngeal fiberscope. A considerable amount of success is achieved within 6 months after surgery.

Conclusions

The cleft palate team in Osaka is proud of its contribution in the field of cleft lip and palate, although we do not claim to have originated any specific method of treatment. Our contribution, rather, has been to demonstrate the problems with which the cleft lip and palate patient has to struggle and to identify the needs for medical, dental, and speech care in a lifelong program. Based on our clinical and research activities, we expect the treatment program to continue to improve and become more available to a greater number of patients and their families.

References

1. Miyazaki T, Kohama G, Ohashi Y: The incidence of cleft lip and/or palate in Japan: Records of 1981 and 1982. J Jpn Cleft Palate Assoc 10:191, 1985 (in Japanese).
2. Tsuji T, Mimura T, Matsuya T, et al: Speech rehabilitation of cleft palate patients. J Jpn Oral Maxillofac Surg 18:560, 1972 (in Japanese).
3. Matsuya T, Miyazaki T, Yamaoka M: Fiberscopic examination of velopharyngeal closure in normal individuals. Cleft Palate J 11:286, 1974.
4. Matsuya T, Yamaoka M, Miyazaki T: A fiberscopic study of velopharyngeal closure in patients with operated cleft palates. Plast Reconstr Surg 63:497, 1979.
5. Miyazaki T, Matsuya T, Yamaoka M: Fiberscopic methods for assessment of velopharyngeal closure during various activities. Cleft Palate J 12:107, 1975.
6. Wada T, Ishi T, Sugai T, et al: Mandibular traction for relieving respiratory distress in the Pierre Robin anomaly. J Maxillofac Surg 11:187, 1983.
7. Wada T, Tachimura T, Yakushiji N, et al: A new type of nipple for cleft palate feeding. J Jpn Cleft Palate Assoc 11:213, 1986 (in Japanese).
8. Wada T, Tachimura T, Yakushiji N, et al: Clinical evaluation on the effect of a new type of nipple for cleft palate feeding. J Jpn Cleft Palate Assoc 11:221, 1986 (in Japanese).
9. Hotz M, Gnoinski W: Effects of early maxillary orthopedics in coordination with delayed surgery for cleft lip and palate. J Maxillofac Surg 7:201, 1979.
10. Gnoinski W: Early maxillary orthopedics as a supplement to conventional primary surgery in complete cleft lip and palate cases. J Maxillofac Surg 3:165, 1982.
11. Miyazaki T: Cleft palate treatment. In Sakakibara S (ed): Clinical Surgery Today. Vol 30, Tokyo: Medical View, 1980.
12. Wada T, Miyazaki T: Growth and changes in maxillary arch form in complete unilateral cleft lip and palate children. Cleft Palate J 12:115, 1975.
13. Wada T, Miyazaki T: Treatment principles for the changing arch form in children with complete unilateral cleft lip and palates. Cleft Palate J 13:273, 1976.
14. Wada T, Mizokawa N, Miyazaki T, et al: Maxillary dental arch growth in different types of cleft. Cleft Palate J 21:180, 1984.
15. Kremenak CR, Huffman WC, Olin WH: Maxillary growth inhibition by mucoperiosteal denudation of palatal shelf bone in non-cleft beagles. Cleft Palate J 7:817, 1970.
16. Wada T, Miyazaki T: Midfacial growth effects of surgical trauma to the area of the vomer in beagles. J Osaka Univ Dent Sch 20:241, 1980.
17. Perko NM: Two-stage closure of cleft palate. J Maxillofac Surg 7:76, 1979.
18. Wada T, Yakushiji N, Tachimura T, et al: Late results of two-stage palatal closure in complete unilateral cleft lip and palate. J Osaka Dent Sch 27:253, 1987.
19. Wada T, Yakushiji N, Tachimura T, et al: Effect of two-stage palatal closure on the maxillary growth in complete bilateral cleft lip and palate. J Jpn Cleft Palate Assoc 12:210, 1987 (in Japanese).
20. Krogman WM, Jain RB, Oka SW: Craniofacial growth in different cleft types from one month to ten years. Cleft Palate J 19:206, 1983.
21. Imai J, Matsuya T, Mimura T, et al: A new velopharyngeal fixation method. J Jpn Cleft Palate Assoc 2:40, 1977.

CHAPTER 6

Multidisciplinary Management of Cleft Lip and Palate in Prague, Czechoslovakia

M. Fára, Ž. Müllerová, Z. Šmahel, M. Brousilová, J. Hrivnáková, M. Černý, and M. Vohradník

The incidence of clefting in Czechoslovakia is almost 2 in 1000 live births. This high incidence stimulated us to devise some means that could prevent the birth of children with these malformations. Also, within the scope of the free health services in Czechoslovakia, an adequate and effective therapy could help to rehabilitate children with clefts.

The Institute of Plastic Surgery at Charles University in Prague, in addition to a variety of other services, also provides complex multidisciplinary treatment of patients with facial clefts for the whole territory of Bohemia, which has a population of approximately 6 million. Every year approximately 140 primary cleft lip repairs and 140 cleft palate repairs are performed here.

The Czechoslovak National Health Care policy promotes this complex treatment in several ways.

1. A uniform registry of these patients is maintained.
2. Traveling expenses are reimbursed, and work leave is granted to relatives accompanying the patient.
3. Surgical and other procedures and tests are free of charge.
4. All specialized departments that participate in treatment of cleft patients are situated in our institute.

Clinical Genetics and Teratology

Clinical genetics and teratology services are provided by a professor in genetics, a clinical teratologist, and a laboratory assistant. The laboratory cooperates with the departments of gynecology, immunology, and epidemiology at the university.

Family members are examined during their first visit to the institute, usually 3 to 4 weeks after the birth of a cleft infant. They receive information about the heredity of clefting, empiric risks, and a preconceptional and prenatal protection program. Etiologic factors are investigated, and a genetic register is kept, which at the present time includes more than 4500 families from Bohemia recorded since 1964. Our detection rate is approximately 80 to 90% of children born with cleft deformities, not including stillborn or deceased infants or those operated on elsewhere.[1]

Genetic Studies

During the first visit to the institute, the parents of the cleft infant complete a genealogic questionnaire that seeks information about the course of pregnancy with special reference to the period of teratogenesis. Examination of the child focuses on detection of any associated malformations or syndromes. A blood sample from the mother is tested for the presence of antibodies against infection with the TORCH group of microorganisms or any other agents (Epstein-Barr virus, Lyme disease). The blood sample is also used for biochemical studies and research (determination of HLA antigens and ABO blood groups). If antibody studies are positive, a pediatrician is informed, and the child is subjected to further pertinent tests to prevent postoperative complications. Suspicious chemicals to which the mother was exposed during pregnancy are tested for teratogenic activity on chick embryos in our laboratory.[2,3]

Preconceptional Program

If a high-risk family wishes to have more children, we endeavor to determine the optimal conditions for conception and the subsequent development of the fetus.[3–5] We use the information provided in the medical history and by etiologic investigations for this purpose. Studies aimed at detection of chronic infections are repeated and are supplemented if necessary by tests for the diagnosis of various types of anemia and thyreopathies, and so on. Despite sophisticated laboratory tests, many questions concerning the genetics of clefts still cannot be answered at the present time.

An effort is made to eliminate as much as possible any potential teratogenic effects disclosed in the medical history. It is determined whether the mother has uterine hypoplasia or any atypic changes, gynecologic inflammatory disorders, or deviations of estrogen or gestagen levels. Two months prior to conception and during the first trimester of pregnancy, the mother's diet should be rich in proteins, minerals, vitamins, and folic acid. Fetoscopy is indicated if the recurrence risk exceeds 10% (without hormonal premedication). Sometimes we attempt to influence the sex of the child prior to conception. Artificial insemination from a donor is rarely advised. These preventive measures are associated with some risks because of the reduced prenatal selection (spontaneous abortion) and possible increase of fertility in high-risk families. However, they could be effective in women with a low genetic predisposition. In high-risk cases, we consider termination of the pregnancy if it is desired by the pregnant female.

Investigation of Etiologic Factors

Analysis of suspected factors is based on the notion that an "inflow" of the etiologic factor into a group of embryos (malformed due to its embryotoxic action) is compensated for by its "outflow" due to the increased lethality of malformed embryos. After birth, we failed to demonstrate increased levels of this factor in children with malformations compared with the levels in control patients (Fig. 6–1).[1,4–7] Therefore, we have attempted to devise some measures that would be helpful in predicting these situations. In a population of embryos between the threshold of teratogenesis and the threshold of lethality, changes (modifications) could develop in the severity of the malformation that could be used for testing.

1. The ascertained differences in the amount of suspected factors in individual subtypes of clefts suggested possible activity of the factor, but they were not sufficient to determine the line along which this activity proceeds (etiologic, modifying, lethal, protective).

2. Comparison in males and females in different subtypes of clefts (determination of the sex ratio) was carried out. Thus, there was a highly significant negative correlation between the sex ratio of cleft lip and palate (CLP) and cleft palate (CP) according to year of birth and, in subseries, also according to geographic region (Fig. 6–2). A certain intensity of embryotoxic activity in male embryos led to CLP (with an increase of sex ratio in CLP), whereas in female embryos it produced only CP (decrease of sex ratio) (Fig. 6–3).[5–8]

3. In another subseries of individual subtypes of clefts a correlation was found between the numbers of probands and the frequency of malformations in their first-degree relatives and the investigated factor.[1,4–7] A positive correlation usually was found in the following subseries: incomplete cleft lip (CL), complete CL, unilateral cleft lip and palate (UCLP), bilateral cleft lip and palate (BCLP), hard CP, and soft CP, or in the six subseries according to the type of cleft (CL, CLP, CP) and sex. A positive correlation could be due to genetic predisposition, whereas a negative correlation could be present in the case of an opposite action.

4. In individual subseries, the interactions of two or more factors were determined. In a family with a positive medical history of malformations, the birth of the first child was associated with a semilethal

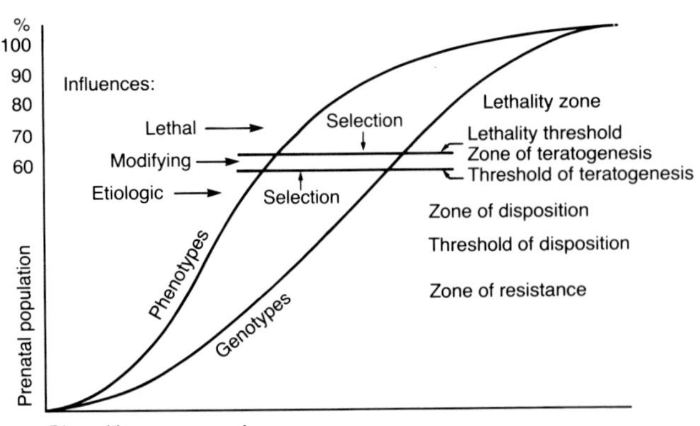

Figure 6–1 Cumulative curve illustrates the population of human embryos, of which 30 to 40 percent are eliminated by lethal factors. The zone of teratogenesis (and modifications) forms a narrow boundary between the threshold of teratogenesis and lethality. An embryotoxic factor reduces the teratogenetic zone (with an increase in lethality), yet the distance between the two thresholds is maintained.

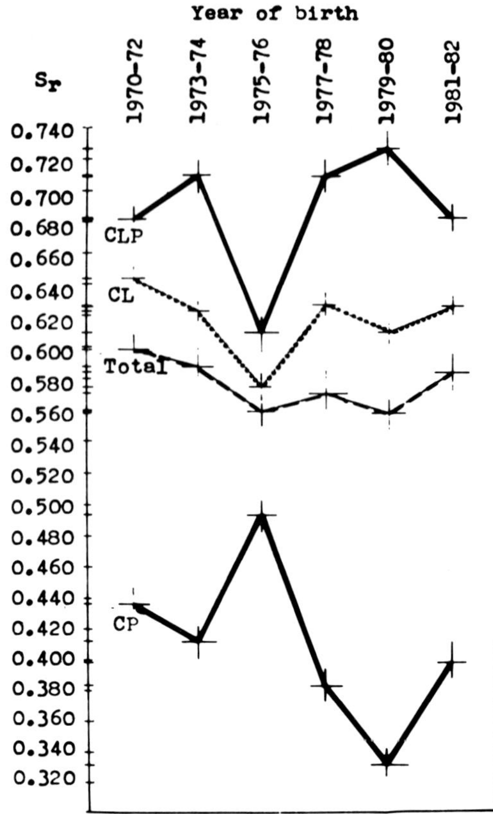

Figure 6–2 Sex ratio (Sr) in cleft lip and palate (CLP), cleft lip (CL), and cleft palate (CP) in the series as a whole and in subseries according to year of birth. Note the marked negative correlation between the sex ratio in CLP and CP.

effect.[4] The observation that blood group A (ABO system) reduced this effect suggested its protective action, unlike the effect of blood group B.

In our material, an embryotoxic action probably appears in genetically predisposed male embryos and is influenced by regional differences, effects of blood groups B and AB, action of HLA B17 antigen in primiparous women, and multiple pregnancies as well as by older age of the mother and cytomegalovirus infections. The Epstein-Barr virus infection of the mother most probably increases the lethality of embryos with more severe clefts (CLP). It is assumed that a protective action is exerted in female embryos by the blood group A, and the HLA A9, A11, and B35 antigens and in younger multiparous women without a familial history of malformations. However, we are well aware that in semilethal malformations, we find ourselves on unstable ground due to interrelated variables and factor complexes. Therefore, interpretation is not always quite uniform.[6,7]

Psychology

Services in the Department of Psychology are provided by a psychologist and a nurse. After the mother has given birth to a malformed child, she usually is psychologically unstable and anxious. The mother and

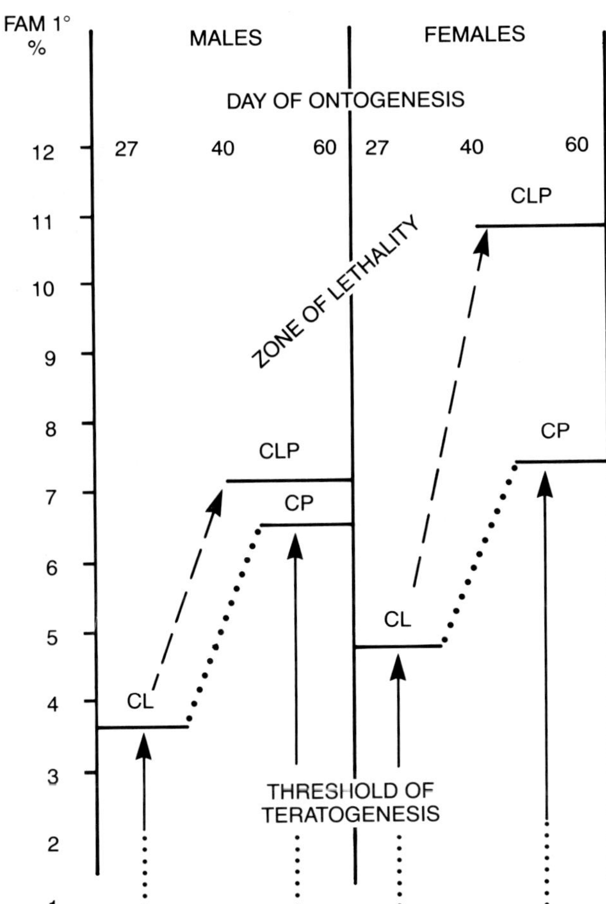

Figure 6–3 The thresholds of teratogenesis in cleft lip (CL), cleft lip and palate (CLP), and cleft palate (CP) in males and females plotted in percentages according to the positive familial history of malformations in first-degree relatives (FAM 1°). CLP in males requires the same quantitative predisposition as CP in females; CL can be modified to CLP.

other family members ask questions about the causes of development of the cleft; however, these cannot be ascertained. This uncertainty inevitably leads to the question of culpability, and if this notion is accepted, family relationships may be impaired. Rationalization and the desire for an optimum outcome for both child and family then follow, as does desire for future parenthood.

During the first visit 3 to 4 weeks after delivery, the parents are interviewed by a psychologist and counseled about the course of treatment and potential problems of raising a child with a cleft.[9] In our opinion, if in early infancy the child is deprived of oral-tactile stimulation, the relationship between the mother and child may be impaired, leading to deficient social adaptability of the child. Therefore, the mother is advised to promote an affectionate relationship between herself and her child, augmented by tactile stimulation.

Cleft children tend to have lower scores on socialization tests, to remain in the background within a group of normal children, and to be less assertive. Parents are more tolerant of cleft children. These tendencies can be corrected within the family by affectionate behavior,

higher demands on the cleft child's performance, and rewards for the child's activities and successes. Including cleft children in groups of normal children (e.g., in kindergarten) earlier than 3 years of age is not recommended. Children with cleft palate are included in groups of normal children only after successful rehabilitation of speech, at approximately 5 to 6 years of age.

During the school years, cleft children have a higher absence rate and are affected by persistent speech, hearing, and orthodontic abnormalities. These may cause discriminating behavior of normal children toward patients with clefts. The birth of a cleft infant may even instigate a divorce, which severely affects the cleft child. For this reason, our psychology department cooperates with the marital advisory office.[9]

A child with a malformation influences family life. Cooperation of the family is a prerequisite for effective therapeutic care. Therefore, as many family members as possible should be informed about the requirements and risks of the prospective method of management.[3] This protocol is designated the familial protective program.[9–12]

Pediatrics

Every infant with a facial cleft born in Bohemia is referred to our institute by the hospital where it was born or by the local pediatrician. Subsequently, the infant is scheduled for the first pediatric examination at 3 to 4 weeks of age. During this visit, a definite diagnosis is established (extent of the cleft, associated malformations, etc.) and the child is entered in our registry.

Independent of the child's registration at the Laboratory of Genetics and Teratology, the pertinent data from the family medical history are recorded, and the parents are educated about the prospective therapeutic measures and the individual stages of multidisciplinary treatment. The parents are given written instructions about how to manage the cleft infant that highlight the harmful effects of finger sucking, allowing the child to lie in a prone position, and so on. Also stressed is the importance of a healthy lifestyle, including fresh air and proper diet. Parents are shown how to massage the lip segments prior to lip repair. Repeated blood counts are necessary because the hemoglobin value should not be allowed to fall below 70%.

Infants with cleft palate are seen in the phoniatric department at approximately 12 to 15 months of age. The phoniatrician evaluates and refers the child to a local speech therapist for logopedic speech therapy prior to palate repair. The pediatrician examines every child before each surgery to ensure that the child is in good health.

Lip Repair

More than 60 years of experience with almost 9000 cleft patients have provided us the opportunity to evaluate the merits of various surgical techniques and develop our own approach. At the Institute of Plastic Surgery in Prague, primary lip repair is carried out in infants with unilateral or bilateral clefts between 5 and 7 months of age. In infants with severe unilateral clefts, the Tennison-Randall technique is used,[13] whereas incomplete clefts are repaired according to Millard's technique.[14]

The primary procedure is based on three principles:

1. The muscle stumps are turned down and joined end to end.
2. The bony cleft is bridged with a periosteal flap.
3. The cartilaginous septum is repositioned toward the midline.

In bilateral cleft lip, both sides are operated on simultaneously. A broad triangular flap of prolabium is preserved and incorporated into the lateral portion of the vermilion. The muscle stumps are joined by a catgut suture behind the skin of the prolabium. In wide bilateral clefts, the muscle stumps are rotated downward into the margin of the prolabium. Creation of a deep vestibular sulcus at the time of primary lip repair facilitates orthodontic treatment and normal lip function.

Our histologic studies indicate that muscle fibers from the lateral muscle stumps grow into the prolabium, producing satisfactory function of the lip. Pressure of the reconstructed lip on the premaxilla substantially reduces premaxillary retropositioning (less than 4% compared with earlier numbers of 8.3%).[15]

Primary Repair of the Alveolar Cleft

In our opinion, a facial cleft represents an actual deficiency of the involved tissues. This deficiency affects the skeletal framework of the maxilla most severely. To prevent postoperative collapse of the maxillary segments, bone grafting of the maxillary and alveolar clefts is performed. Reconstruction of the orbicularis oris muscle, use of various orthodontic appliances, and bone grafting of the alveolus are important factors in preventing postoperative collapse of the maxillary segments.

Primary osteoplasty with a bone graft from the rib or tibia, or a periosteal flap from the maxilla, may be used as part of the primary lip repair procedure. Both procedures have been used in our institute for many years and have been compared with each other with respect to results of long-term growth and development of the maxilla. Follow-up examinations, radiographs, and dental casts were used for the assessment.

Initially, we were apprehensive about the idea of primary bone grafting because we feared that bone grafts in infants would result in improper fixation of the maxillary segments, complicating orthodontic treatment. However, encouraged by results from other centers, we began primary bone grafting in unilateral cleft patients using rib grafts (Fig. 6–4). Full-thickness rib grafts were implanted at the lower margin of the piriform aperture and covered with a mucoperiosteal flap from the vomer with mucous membrane and a mucosal flap from the lip. This technique was used only for unilateral cleft patients because in bilateral cleft patients we

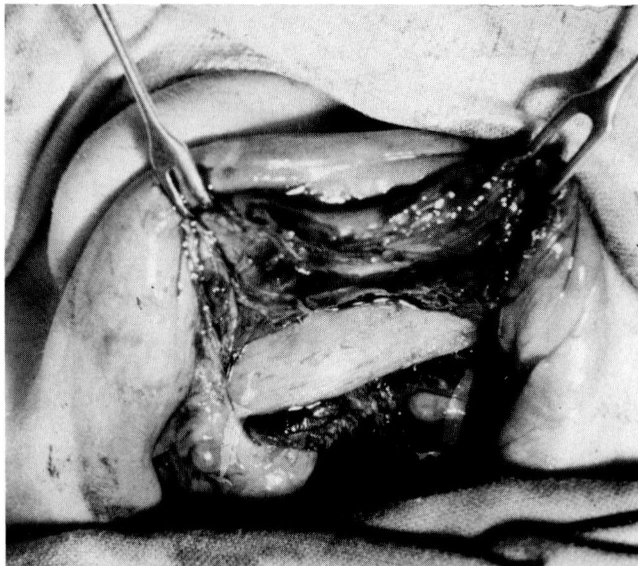

Figure 6–4 Rib graft placed at the lower margin of the piriform aperture.

wanted to avoid locking the protruding premaxilla in front of the maxillary segments.

A follow-up study of our primary bone graft results was done in 245 patients with complete unilateral cleft lip, alveolus, and palate.[16] Orthodontic examination revealed a favorable alignment of the alveolar arch. The edges of the alveolar processes were closely approximated. However, the width of the process was somewhat reduced in the canine region. The width of the alveolus in the region of the molars remained within normal limits. At the time of eruption of the primary dentition, lateral crossbite was observed on the side of the larger maxillary segment in many cases. Occlusion on the cleft side usually was within normal limits. In some patients, anterior or lateral crossbite was present. Sagittal occlusion was not impaired.

Primary lip repair resulted in shortening and narrowing of the dental and alveolar arches. In patients who prior to surgery had lateral displacement of the larger maxillary segment, improvement in alignment and occlusion was observed postoperatively. In conclusion, our study indicated that primary bone grafting with a rib graft in patients with unilateral cleft lip, alveolus, and palate reduced the deformity in the region of the dental and alveolar arches during the time of early mixed dentition (Fig. 6–5).[16]

Use of Periosteal Flaps

Because we avoid extensive exposure of the anterior side of the maxilla in infants during the creation of a large periosteal flap (Skoog method), we use a narrower periosteal flap. Justification for this precaution was demonstrated by histologic studies aimed at detection of the assumed new bone formation from the periosteum at the site of the defect. Histologic examination of three specimens obtained from this site at intervals of 3 to 4

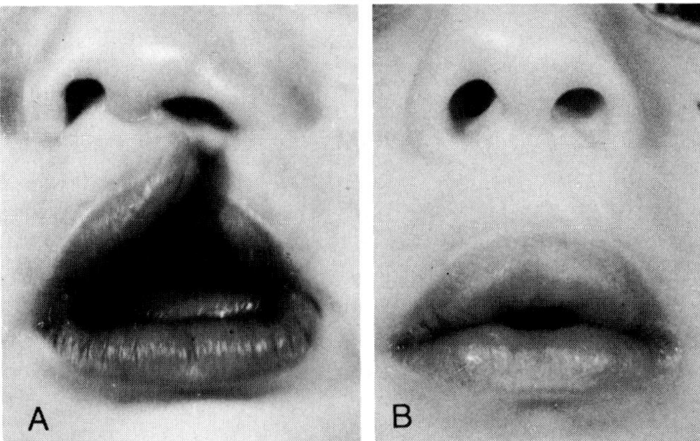

Figure 6–5 *A*, Left cleft lip and palate. *B*, Following primary lip repair using the Tennison-Randall technique and primary bone grafting.

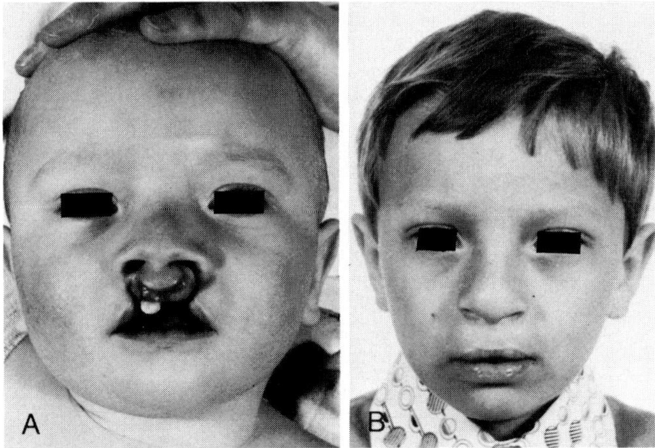

Figure 6–7 *A*, Bilateral cleft lip, alveolus, and palate with a Simonart's band on the right side. *B*, Following one-stage straight line closure with a periosteal flap on each side.

years after the surgical procedure revealed only scar tissue.

The periosteal flap used in our institute is 5 to 7 mm wide and about 20 mm in length so that it can be extended over the maxillary and alveolar clefts. After its dissection, the flap is turned toward the defect with its pedicle situated on the edge of the piriform aperture. The free edge of this flap is sutured to the periosteum of the premaxilla. We believe that our modification prevents possible damage to the infraorbital nerve and induces new bone formation across the bony cleft defect.

Follow-up observations indicate that the periosteal flap proved to be sufficient for growth of a bony bridge between the maxillary segments within a few months. Conceivably, the newly formed bone might not be sufficient to fill the entire alveolar and maxillary bone defect; however, it definitely exerts a beneficial effect on the dynamics of maxillary growth and development. In patients with unilateral clefts, proper alignment of the maxillary arch occurred earlier than in those with bilateral clefts.

Unlike the firm, postoperative connection of the maxillary segment due to the rib graft, a periosteal flap and its subsequent new bone formation provides flexibility of the segments that may be influenced by the function of the orbicularis oris muscle and tongue (Figs. 6–6 and 6–7).

Our series of 183 patients treated with a periosteal flap was divided so that 33 had unilateral cleft lip and alveolus, 107 had unilateral cleft lip and palate, and 43 had bilateral cleft lip and palate. Documentation consisted of clinical observations, photographs, radiographic films, and dental casts obtained during treatment and follow-up.

Among these 183 patients, no complications were observed following lip repair (Figs. 6–8 and 6–9). Within the first two weeks after the operation, enhanced rounding of the anterior part of the maxillary arch was evident in patients with both unilateral and bilateral clefts (Figs. 6–10 and 6–11). Elevation of the base of the ala due to the tension of the periosteal flap stretched underneath helped position the alar base at the same level as the normal side.

When using periosteal flaps, there is no need to create a special pocket to cover the flap as for bone grafts. Our observations indicated that new bone for-

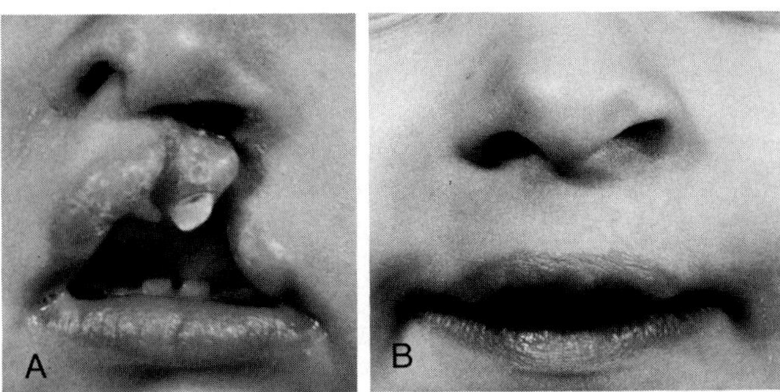

Figure 6–6 *A*, Complete left cleft lip, alveolus, and palate. *B*, Following primary lip repair using the triangular flap technique (Tennison-Randall) with a simultaneous periosteal flap.

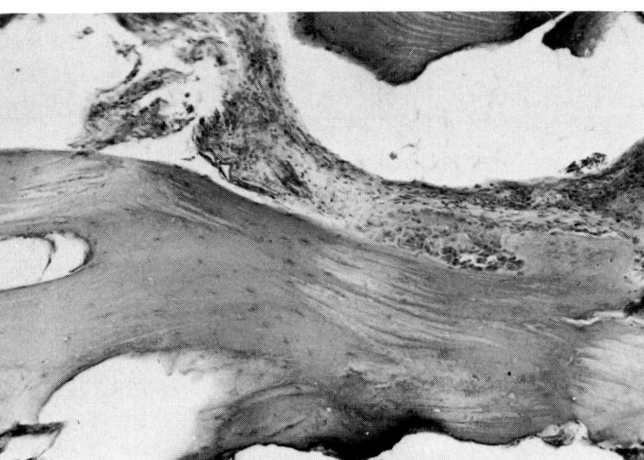

Figure 6–8 New bone formation at the site of the periosteal flap 4 years after operation. Bony tissue with osteoblasts is visible in the central part of the figure.

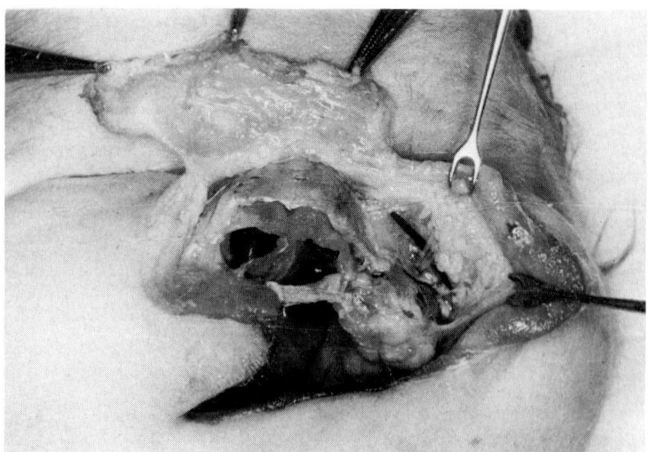

Figure 6–9 Periosteal flap reconstruction in a stillborn infant.

mation following transposition of the periosteal flap amounted to 3 to 4 mm in thickness, whereas in rib grafts, much more solid bone developed within the alveolar and maxillary clefts.

During evaluation of the growth and development of the maxillary complex, attention is paid to the status not only of the skeletal structures but also of the soft tissues. We believe that primary lip repair should be performed free of tension because even moderate tension is transferred as pressure on the maxilla and may lead to collapse of the maxillary segments, resulting in malocclusion.[17]

Results of the use of a periosteal flap were evaluated in 183 children 7 to 9 years subsequent to lip repair. Results in this group were compared with those in a control group that had lip repair without periosteoplasty. Compared with the group of controls, patients with periosteoplasty exhibited a more marked rounding of the alveolus, no protrusion of the premaxilla, and no oral inclination of the lateral cleft segment.

Use of the periosteal flap did not result in impairment of the growth potential of the maxilla. New bone formation within the region of the implanted periosteal flap was ascertained with radiographic studies in 75% of the patients. In patients with unilateral clefts, intense growth of the anterior region of the lateral segment was observed. This allowed gradual contact to be established between both segments. On the edge of the alveolar segment on the noncleft side, no new bone formation was detected. Transverse growth of the maxilla was not affected. During primary dentition and at the beginning of the period of mixed dentition, orthodontic anomalies were markedly reduced compared with control patients.

In patients with bilateral clefts, the periosteal flap contributed to improvement of the relationships between the three segments of the maxilla. Periosteoplasty had a particularly favorable effect on the premaxilla with gradual elimination of its protrusion. There was also spontaneous correction of premaxillary asymmetry in the mediosagittal plane of the face.

Primary Repositioning of the Cartilaginous Nasal Septum

Another important prerequisite for normal development of the middle face is normal growth of the nasal septum. In patients with unilateral clefts the septum usually is deviated, whereas in bilateral clefts a marked shortening of the columella interferes with development of the septum.

In bilateral clefts the development of the nasal septum has been enhanced by early lengthening of the columella with a forked flap procedure.[18] Little is known about the importance of primary repositioning of the cartilaginous nasal septum in unilateral clefts because the cartilaginous septum is deviated in its distal insertion, together with a large segment of the maxilla, toward the unaffected side. In the tip of the nose the cartilaginous septum may be deviated into a horizontal position. Mobilization from the maxilla requires blunt separation about halfway up the cartilaginous septum without the use of scalpel incisions. At the nasal tip, the upper edge of the septum is detached completely from the lower lateral cartilage, straightening the deformed upper segment of the septum (Figs. 6–12 and 6–13).[19] Early straightening of the nasal septum prevents secondary nasal deformities and airway obstruction related to the deviated septum. It also ensures better conditions for midfacial growth and development.

Palatoplasty

Cleft palate repair is performed at the age of 4 years. Timing of this repair is based on our conviction that a

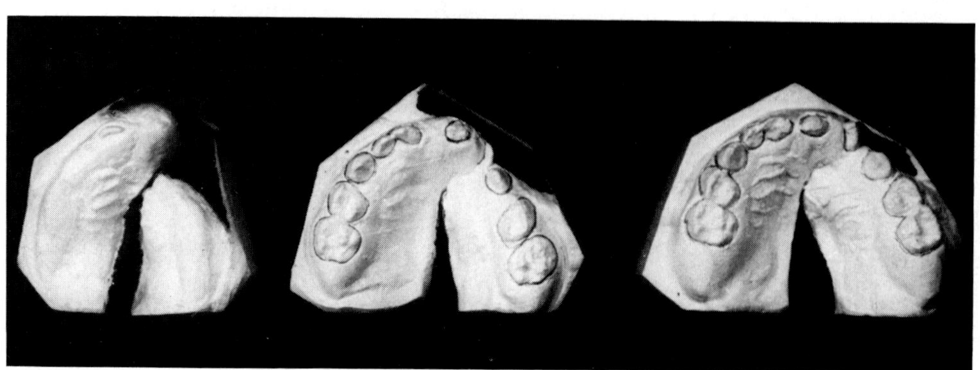

Figure 6–10 Complete left cleft lip, alveolus, and palate. Dental casts taken at age 8 months, 2.5 years, and 5 years. No orthodontic therapy was performed. A periosteal flap was created during primary repair.

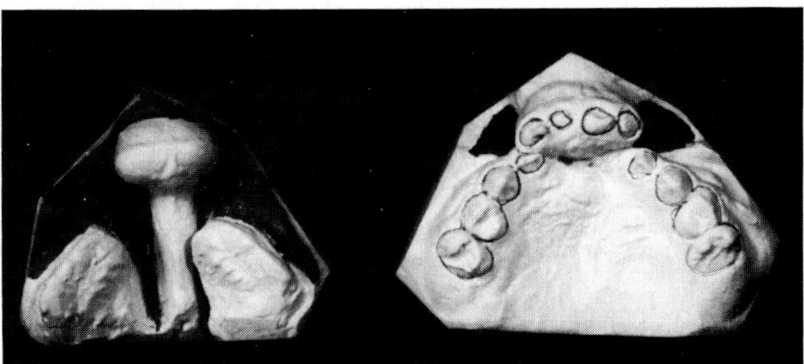

Figure 6–11 Complete bilateral cleft. Dental casts taken at age 8 months and 6.5 years. No orthodontic treatment was used. Bilateral periosteal flaps were created during primary repair.

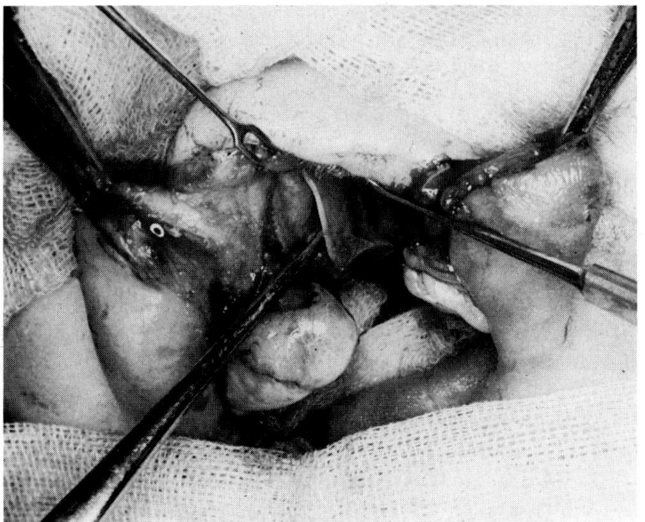

Figure 6–13 Deviated cartilaginous septum after mobilization.

large proportion of growth in the maxillary width has taken place by this age. Furthermore, abnormal speech patterns have not developed to the extent that they are uncorrectable.

On the oral side of the cleft, three mucoperiosteal flaps (occasionally two) are created. The neurovascular bundles remain intact and are shifted backward toward the midline. Good functional results are ensured owing to (1) detachment of the soft palate muscles from their improper insertions on the posterior borders of the palatal plates, suturing them in their normal positions, and (2) simultaneous pharyngeal flap surgery with use of the superiorly based tubulated pharyngeal flap (Fig. 6–14).

The palatal part of the palatopharyngeus, the palato-glossus, and the anterior bundles of the levator are detached from the posterior edge of the palatal shelf, from the posterior nasal spine, and from the cleft margin of the hard palate. Near the last-named, the sling-shaped tendinomuscular link between the tensor and levator is severed. This facilitates push-back of the muscles of the soft palate. Only the greater part of the tensor, fixed to the developed part of the aponeurosis, remains in place. As a result of this maneuver, the retropositioned ends of the muscles turn slightly toward the midline, facilitating their end-to-end suture.

In less severe clefts of the soft palate only, closure without tension is obtained without mobilizing the mucoperiosteal flaps. To lengthen the soft palate, Z-plasty or a transverse incision through the nasal mucoperiosteal margin of the palatal shelves is used. This opens a diamond-shaped defect, which serves as a bed for insertion of a superiorly based pharyngeal flap.

Pharyngeal Flap Surgery

Primary pharyngeal flap surgery is used at our institute as a routine procedure in the majority of palate repairs. It is omitted only when simple retropositioning creates excellent velopharyngeal closure.

Long-term follow-up of our patients indicates that the quality of speech, given the phonetic characteristics of the Czech language, in which perfect velopharyngeal closure is a major feature, is much better in patients who had primary pharyngeal flaps than in those who underwent the procedure later. Results also show that

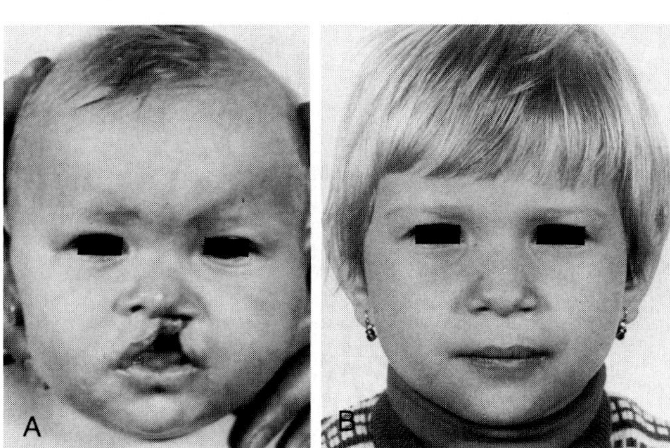

Figure 6–12 *A,* Complete left cleft. Note marked deviation of the nasal septum. *B,* After operation using the Tennison-Randall technique with simultaneous repositioning of the nasal septum.

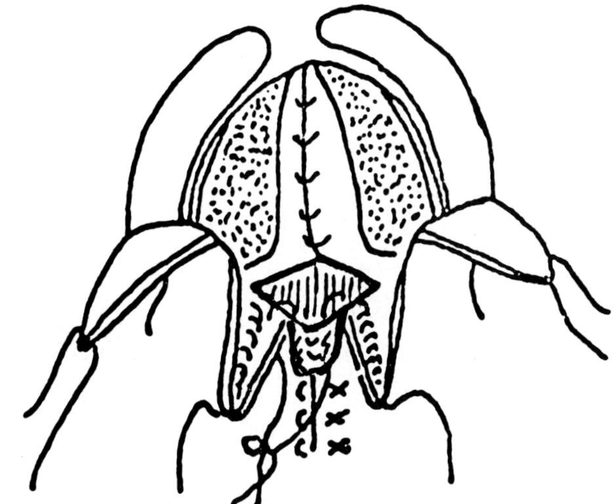

Figure 6–14 Superiorly based pharyngeal flap is sutured in front of the retropositioned velar muscles in complete cleft palate.

the superiorly based tubulated pharyngeal flap produces better velopharyngeal closure than a pharyngeal flap with a raw surface exposed. The superiorly based tubed pharyngeal flap is anchored in front of the retropositioned velar muscles.

Primary pharyngeal flap surgery has the following advantages:

1. The pharyngeal hiatus is diminished by the flap, and its transverse diameter is narrowed by suturing of the secondary defect.
2. Postoperatively, the muscular fibers retain a certain ability to contract and create traction on the soft palate.[20]
3. Functional activity is preserved for a longer period of time than an open flap, which is exposed to severe scarring and contraction.[21]
4. It facilitates the operation by adding tissue to the palate and by filling the defect caused by unfolding of the transverse incisions on the nasal side of the retropositioned velum.

Secondary Corrective Procedures

The following secondary procedures are most frequently used for correction of remaining deformities. In bilateral cleft patients, lengthening of the columella with a forked-flap procedure is performed at approximately 5 years of age. When creating the forked flap, a large triangular skin flap is dissected at the threshold of the nostril, shifted upward, and inserted into the defect created behind the columella (Fig. 6–15).

In unilateral cleft patients, secondary procedures have been reduced substantially owing to the primary repositioning of the nasal septum. We rarely perform osteotomies of the nasal bones and septum or corrective procedures on the alar base; however, there is still a need for final repair of the tip of the nose. When

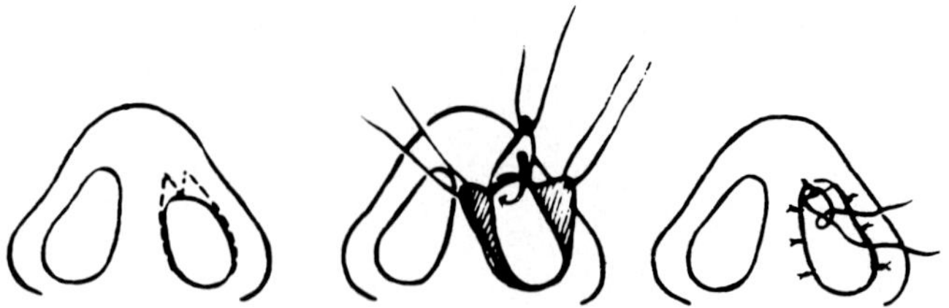

Figure 6–16 Excision of excessive skin from the fornix of the nostril using our modification.

necessary, the deformed lower lateral cartilage is lifted or supplemented by transposition of the alar cartilage from the normal side on a pedicle across the nasal tip to the affected side. Excision of excessive skin is performed in a way that preserves the shape of the ala, especially its free margin. Excessive lining also may be removed and the lower lateral cartilage transposed (Figs. 6–16 and 6–17).[22]

Over the past two years, we have modified the rotation of the alar cartilage from the normal side across the tip of the nose for augmentation of the deformed lower lateral cartilage on the cleft side. The transposed cartilage is sutured to the edge of the nostril (not the alar cartilage), which elevates and maintains the cartilage in a higher position.

After orthodontic treatment is finished in patients with unilateral and bilateral clefts, a residual defect in the maxilla or alveolus is filled with a bone graft from the iliac crest. We usually use a whole piece of bone, shaped so that it can be anchored under the periosteum and fixed in this position. The bone graft is covered from the nasal side by mucoperiosteum from the vomer and on the oral side by a mucosal flap from the oral vestibule. With regard to the requirements of the prosthetician, the bone graft is placed at the level of the ridge of the alveolar process. Cancellous bone is used to fill the alveolar cleft because we believe it allows migration of the marginal tooth.[23]

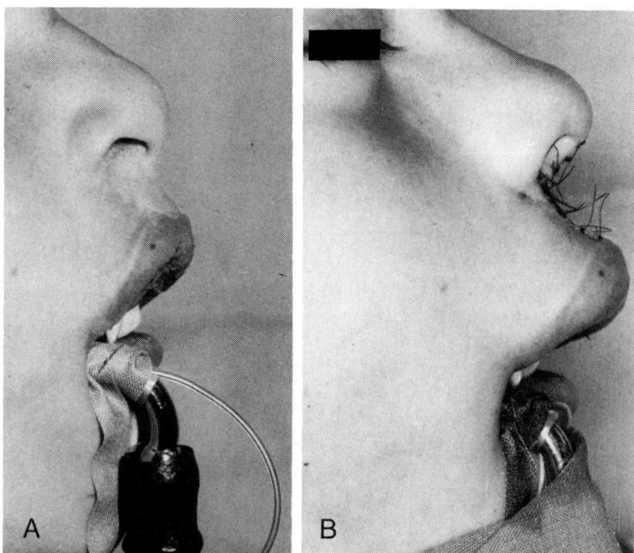

Figure 6–15 *A,* Lengthening of the columella in bilateral cleft. *B,* Lenghtening of the columella using the forked-flap technique.

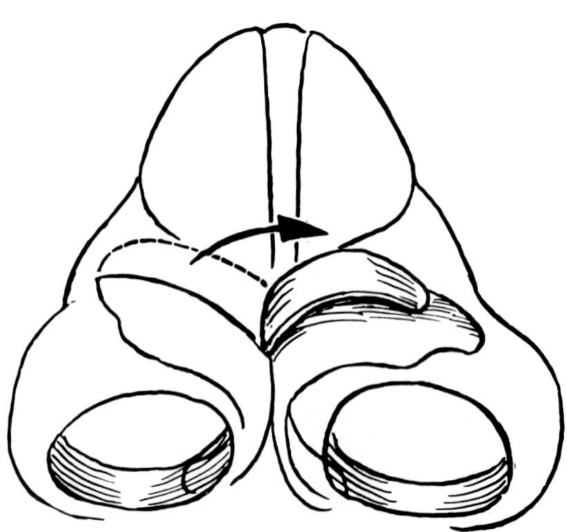

Figure 6–17 Rotation of the alar cartilage and fixation to the margin of the affected nostril.

Rationale of Our Surgical Treatment

The effects of various treatment techniques on facial growth and development have been evaluated in morphologic and growth studies using roentgencephalometry, direct cephalometry, and measurements taken from dental casts. Particular attention is devoted to the prepubertal period, when it is possible already to observe maxillofacial changes. Our long-term studies have revealed that postoperative facial development proceeds in a uniform way. The insignificant correlation coefficients between the extent of deviation at the age of 10 years and subsequent changes up to the age of 15 years showed that a less favorable situation at 10 years of age does not mean a more marked impairment of development during puberty.

In spite of the intense orthodontic treatment, the period of puberty is associated with further deterioration of maxillary development. Between the ages of 10 and 15 years anteroposterior occlusal relationships deteriorated in 75% of the patients with primary bone grafts, and facial convexity deteriorated in 90% of patients. Improvement occurred in virtually no cases.

The effects of surgical techniques on subsequent facial growth can be assessed as early as 10 years of age. We concluded that when deficient development of the maxillary complex is observed prior to puberty, it cannot be expected to improve after puberty. Therefore, in patients with evidence of more deficient maxillary growth, it is neither necessary nor desirable to delay decisions about changes of surgical treatment until facial growth is completed.

Comparison of the effects of surgical techniques used at our institute on maxillofacial growth in complete unilateral cleft lip and palate is described and documented in the chapter on presurgical orthopedic treatment (see Chapter 72).

During the early 1960s, the Schweckendiek palatoplasty technique was used. The series of patients was followed longitudinally through adolescence (see Chapter 80). Using our modification of this technique, we did not observe enhanced maxillofacial development (Table 6–1; Fig. 6–18).

More recently, primary osteoplasty has been used simultaneously with primary cleft lip repair. This technique was carefully evaluated after longitudinal follow-up of 35 males and 25 females aged 10 years with unilateral cleft lip, alveolus, and palate. Results of this study are presented in Chapter 72. Furthermore, results suggested that periosteoplasty had beneficial effects on facial growth and development; however, definite conclusions will be possible only when these patients have reached approximately 15 years of age. Currently, use of cancellous bone for bone grafts to the alveolar cleft has been introduced, but no data are available yet to evaluate this approach.

The effect of primary repositioning of the nasal septum on nasal configuration in patients with complete unilateral cleft lip and palate was assessed prior to surgical correction (at about 10 years of age). After primary repositioning of the nasal septum, deviation of the nose in these patients was reduced by more than 50% compared with individuals who did not undergo this procedure. This change also resulted in markedly less asymmetry of the length of the nasal ala between the cleft and noncleft sides as well as less flattening of the nasal tip.

Table 6–1. Mean Values of Radiographic Cephalometric Characteristics in Complete Unilateral Cleft Lip and Palate Patients Treated with Two-Stage Palate Closure Compared with Individuals with One-Stage Closure (10 years)

Cephalometric Variable	Two-Stage Closure	One-Stage Closure
N-S-Ba	132.6	131.9
N-S-Pgn	70.5	70.6
ML-NSL	38.5	38.0
S-N-Ss	76.0	75.1
S-N-Sm	74.2	73.7
S-N-Pg	75.1	74.9
ANB (Ss-N-Sm)	1.8	1.4
N-Ss-Pg	178.1	179.3
Is-Ii	0.3[a]	−08.[a]
I_1-PL	99.3	96.9
Ls-Li	0.9	0.6
N-Sp%N-Gn	42.5	42.9
S-Go%N-Gn	60.4	60.5
N	24	27

ML-NSL = angle between the slope of mandibular body and NSL; I_1-PL = angle between the axis of central incisors and PL; N-Sp%N-Gn = N-Sp in terms of percent of N-Gn, etc.; Ls-Li = upper lip prominence; Is-Ii = overjet (see Fig. 6–18)

[a]p <0.1 difference

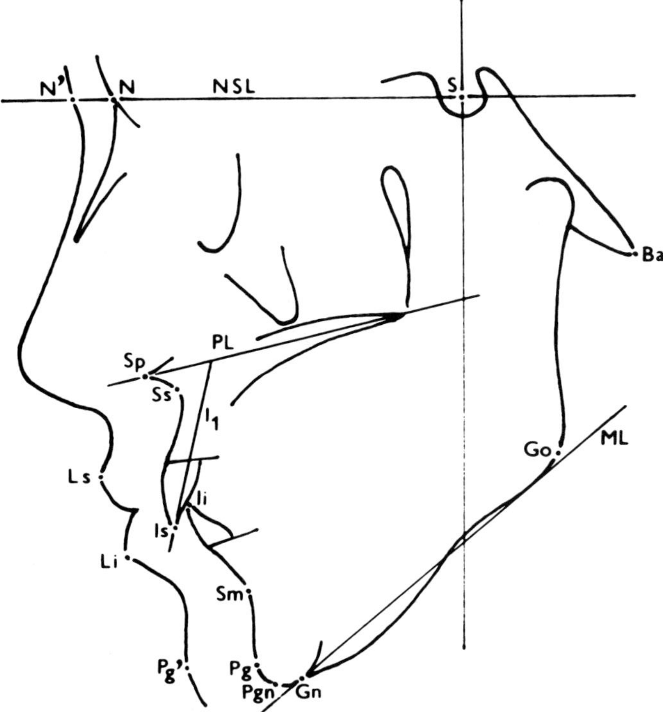

Figure 6–18 Cephalometric points referred to in Table 6–1. Overjet (Is-Ii) was measured parallel to occlusal plane. Lip prominence was measured as projective distance between Ls and Li perpendicular to the line connecting N' and Pg'.

The effect of the timing of palatoplasty on maxillofacial growth was assessed in adult male cleft patients. None of the patients had primary bone grafting or periosteoplasty. The patients were divided according to age at time of surgery. Results failed to disclose any differences in facial growth and development between patients with cleft of the palate only who were operated on at mean ages of 2.8 and 6.5 years.[24] Also, there were no significant differences in patients with cleft lip and palate operated on at the ages of 4 and 6 years.

A separate assessment of patients with the most severe cleft types, i.e., complete cleft lip and palate, revealed more favorable results in those who were operated on at a later date. Individuals operated on at a mean age of 6.5 years had a slighter retrusion of the maxilla, edge-to-edge occlusion, and an almost normal ANB angle compared with patients who had had surgery at the age of 4 years and who had a negative ANB angle (-2.3 degrees), reversed overjet, and more marked retrusion of the maxilla (by 1.4 degrees). Results support delayed surgery in patients with the most severe clefts and demonstrate the utility of a differentiated approach for timing of palatoplasty according to the type and severity of the cleft defect.

A roentgencephalometric comparison of two groups of adult males with unilateral cleft lip and palate with and without pharyngeal flap surgery (both with a push-back palatoplasty) revealed that the pharyngeal flap exerted no negative effect on the anteroposterior position or depth of the maxilla. The length of the dentoalveolar arch measured on dental casts was unchanged as well. Similar conclusions were drawn in patients with isolated cleft palate. However, pharyngeal flaps promoted mouth breathing and posterior growth rotation of the face, especially in wide flaps. Therefore, we prefer narrow, tubulated flaps.

Assessment of adult patients with complete bilateral cleft lip and palate treated during childhood with the use of premaxillary recession without stabilization of the premaxilla by bone grafting revealed marked retrusion of the middle face compared with individuals who had had no premaxillary retropositioning.[25] Consequently, these procedures are used only in the most difficult clefts and are supplemented by stabilization of the premaxilla with bone grafts fixed to the lateral maxillary segments.

Orthodontic Management and Treatment Philosophy

Dental care at the institute is part of the multidisciplinary cleft treatment. A group of orthodontists and a clinical anthropologist provide services for cleft patients. In addition to dental care, this team performs research in the area of maxillofacial growth following various surgical and orthodontic treatment techniques. Results are documented by data obtained through evaluation of dental casts, intraoral and facial photographs, lateral and frontal cephalometric radiographs, and extra- and intraoral radiographs.

Long-term orthodontic therapy is divided into four stages according to the development of dentition.

Stage I

Predentition treatment includes the time before and after primary lip repair. In our opinion, presurgical orthopedic treatment is indicated only rarely, after consultation with a surgeon. Various appliances are used; however, pressure bands are contraindicated in children with bilateral clefts because they cause retrusion of the middle face. Presurgical orthopedic treatment is described in detail in Chapter 72.

Stage II

Treatment of the primary dentition in children with unilateral and bilateral clefts is initiated after the child is 3 years of age. Therapeutic procedures include treatment of severe maxillary constrictions, marked asymmetries of the dental and alveolar arches that produce severe functional mandibular shift, severe disorders of occlusion, and, at the request of the phoniatrician, addition of supplementary teeth within the region of the cleft. We use removable appliances with a screw, functional appliances, and appliances with teeth exclusively. Follow-up of the development of dentition is carried out. Occasionally, extraction of supernumerary and malpositioned teeth is necessary.

During this period, most of our patients with unilateral cleft lip and palate have rounded upper dental and alveolar arches with or without a contact between the alveolar arches. The length of the alveolar arches is reduced, and occasionally a medial shift of the cleft segment occurs. In bilateral clefts, there may be some degree of protrusion and oral inclination of the premaxilla. More commonly, the width of the arches is reduced, and a medial shift of the cleft segments is encountered. Anterior and posterior crossbite are not common; rather an edge-to-edge occlusion or crossbite of the canines is observed.

Studies of the facial skeletal framework in unilateral cleft lip and palate revealed that prior to palatoplasty at 5 years of age, most of the basic craniofacial changes observed at an adult age are present—for example, reduced upper face height, dentoalveolar retroinclination of the maxilla, displacement of the maxillary segments posteriorly, widening of the maxillary complex, and shortening of the mandible associated with changes of mandibular shape.[26] Shortening of the anteroposterior dimension of the maxilla was observed after palatoplasty. These changes affect other facial parameters including facial proportions, reduction of the anterior growth of the midface, occlusion, and so on. At this age, prominence of the upper lip remains satisfactory. In cases of cleft of the palate only, slight shortening of the maxilla and mandible was recorded preoperatively.[27] We did not observe posterior displacement and dentoalveolar retroinclination of the maxilla with a reduction of the upper facial height in children and adults.

The craniofacial and dentoalveolar changes described above confirm that during this stage, indications for orthodontic therapy should be precisely defined. In cases of cleft lip only or cleft palate only, treatment at this stage is not indicated. In complete clefts, therapy is initiated as described above.

Stage III

In the majority of our cleft patients, orthodontic therapy is initiated during the period of mixed dentition. The most common problems consist of malposition of the permanent incisors as well as of their lingual eruption and rotation. Anterior crossbite is observed frequently, and maxillary constriction is rather common as well. The anteroposterior skeletal imbalance results in abnormalities of molar relationships (class III). There are also many other dental problems such as supernumerary teeth, congenitally missing teeth, malformed teeth, and malpositioned teeth.

The most important objective during this phase is restoration of the overjet. The protrusion and derotation of lingually erupted permanent incisors should begin immediately when they are sufficiently erupted to allow the use of an appliance. The restoration of overjet is of decisive importance because it exerts an action on the ultimate position of the mandible and on development of favorable anteroposterior relations. This was confirmed by analysis of 64 adult males with isolated cleft palate and restored positive overjet. The patients were divided into three groups according to the degree of maxillary retrusion. In a positive overjet, the increasing retrusion of the maxilla displaced the mandible backward, and the anteroposterior relations remained almost unchanged (Fig. 6–19). Similar results, although in a smaller number of cases, were obtained after division of the patients into five groups. Analysis confirmed the high correlation coefficient between the degree of the protrusion of the maxilla and mandible. A similar relationship was ascertained in a control group of adult males.

These findings indicate that restoration of the overjet is an effective mechanism that acts favorably on the configuration of the facial profile in cleft patients. Therefore, patients with unilateral cleft lip and palate without orthodontic treatment differed as adults from individuals with the same type of cleft and adequate therapy in the position of their mandible, but there was no difference in the retrusion of the maxilla. In patients in whom the overjet was not restored, the mandible was displaced anteriorly. Radiographic cephalometric analysis of patients 12 to 15 years old with unilateral cleft lip and palate and a prognathic mandible revealed that this deviation was due to the anterior displacement of the mandible rather than to the marked retrusion of the maxilla. Data analysis showed that the anterior mandibular displacement occurred because the positive overjet was not restored at an early age. Thus, it is mandatory to restore positive overjet as soon as possible after eruption of the permanent incisors.

Treatment procedures include use of removable and fixed intra- and extraoral appliances. Usually, plates with a screw are used. Functional appliances are used occasionally to treat patients with Pierre Robin syn-

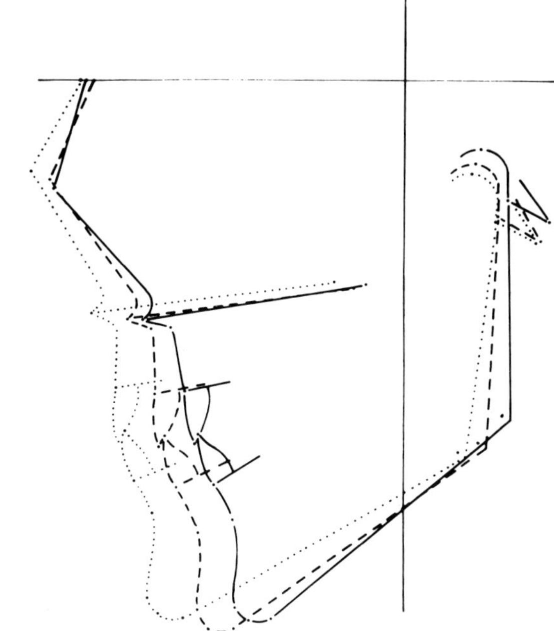

Figure 6–19 Faciograms in adult males with isolated cleft palate divided into three categories according to the degree of maxillary retrusion. Mean values of S-N-Ss and ANB angles are presented in Table 6–1. In the second table (shown here at bottom right), patients are divided into five groups.

drome and temporarily in cases of severe mandibular displacement. In children with class III growth tendencies, intraoral elastic forms, headgear, extraoral forces, and face masks are used. Orthodontic extractions may be helpful if there is insufficient space in the arches. For dentoalveolar compensation of a reversed overjet, extraction of teeth in the lower jaw is performed.

During the period of mixed dentition orthodontic therapy is mandatory, and the primary goal is to restore and maintain overjet and limit class III growth tendencies.

Stage IV

During the period of permanent dentition, orthodontic treatment is usually completed, and the period of retention begins. If the patient requires continued orthodontic therapy, fixed appliances and similar treatments used in normal children are employed. Our studies demonstrate that fixed appliances are more effective than removable ones during this stage.

The relationship of the development of the overjet to the changes in anteroposterior jaw relations between the ages of 10 and 15 years while using removable and fixed appliances is illustrated by Fig. 6–20. Use of fixed appliances improved occlusion even in the presence of marked impairment of anteroposterior relationships of the maxilla and mandible.

Assessment of the same relationship in the prepubertal period (8 to 11 years of age) and the pubertal period (11 to 14 years of age) after use of removable appliances in patients without bone grafting disclosed that children in the pubertal period had the same relationships as those seen in individuals with bone grafts (Fig. 6–21). During the prepubertal period, owing to dentoalveolar compensation, the degree of overjet was maintained in spite of a deterioration in anteroposterior jaw relations. However, the compensatory mechanism gradually wore out, resulting in an impairment of overjet during the period of puberty.

The retention period may be associated with some problems. Specifically, overjet may change into an edge-to-edge occlusion or into reversed overjet. An overbite may change into an anterior open bite. In these cases and if there is severe primary growth deficiency, skeletal surgery is considered. However, the ultimate goal of orthodontic treatment is aimed at reducing the need for surgical intervention.

Studies of the incidence of mandibular prognathism demonstrated that this developed most frequently in patients with unilateral cleft lip and palate (36%) followed by those with bilateral cleft lip and palate (30%) and isolated cleft of the palate only (10%). However, after introduction of orthodontic therapy with fixed appliances, it was possible to reduce by 50% the need for skeletal surgery. These procedures were indicated in approximately 15% of individuals with complete cleft lip, alveolus, and palate compared with 2 to 3% of patients with cleft of the palate only.

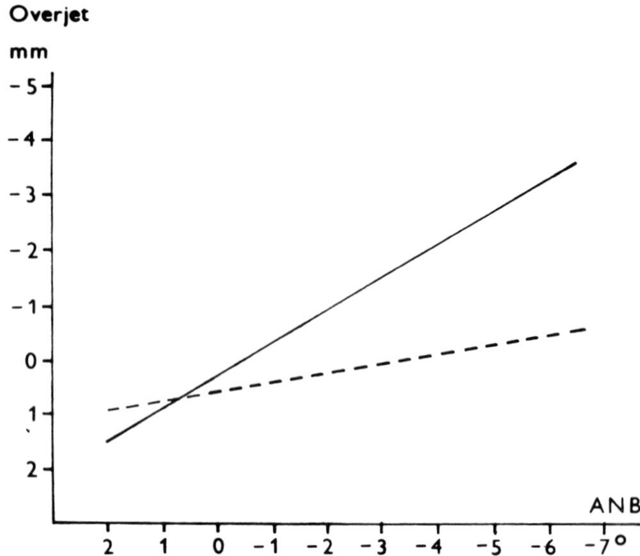

Figure 6–21 Relationship between changes of anteroposterior jaw relations (ANB) and changes in overjet during prepubertal (dashed line) and pubertal (solid line) periods in patients with complete unilateral cleft treated with removable appliances only.

Orthodontic treatment is completed in cooperation with a prosthodontist, who may supplement the dentoalveolar arch with a permanent fixed bridge after the patient is 18 years of age. Dental care is based mostly on the use of effective intra- and extraoral fixed orthodontic appliances, which, in association with adequate treatment strategy, reduce facial malformations and restore and maintain overjet and posterior displacement of the mandible.

Speech and Voice Problems

The most important changes in children with velopharyngeal insufficiency (VPI) are those affecting speech development and resonance characteristics. The care of our patients at the institute is organized by the phoniatric departments in hospitals. All stages of diagnostics, therapy, and rehabilitation are provided by a staff that consists of a phoniatrician, psychologist, speech pathologist, and nurse. Such a team exists in each district.

Rehabilitation begins at approximately 18 months of age and is focused on stimulating proprioceptive feedback of the articulatory organs. All types of toys requiring air flow from the mouth are used. Parents work with their children daily on these tasks. Special speech training to encourage correct articulation begins later depending on the psychological development of the child. Palatoplasty is usually performed when the child is 4 years of age. At this time, very intense speech therapy is provided with weekly consultations at a phoniatric department. All activities of the district phoniatric departments are coordinated with the Phoniatric Laboratory in the Institute of Plastic Surgery in Prague.

The goal of speech and voice therapy is to facilitate almost normal speech production before the child enters

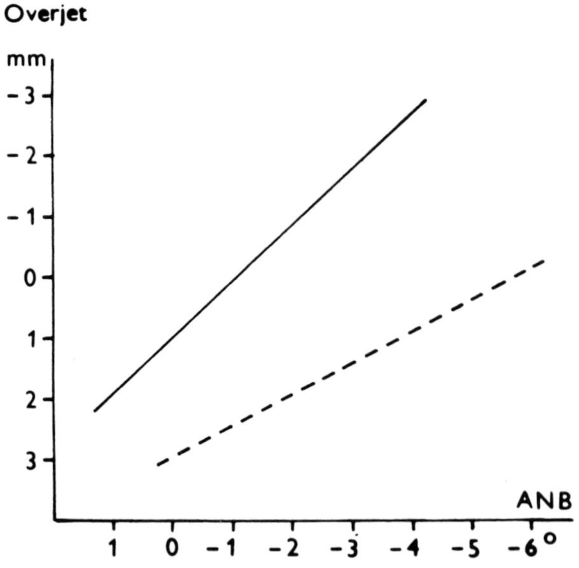

Figure 6–20 Relationship between changes of anteroposterior jaw relationships (ANB) and changes of overjet during the ages 10 to 15 years in patients with complete unilateral cleft who were treated with removable (solid line) and fixed (dashed line) appliances.

school at 6 years of age. The delayed timing of palatoplasty and intensive speech rehabilitation allow this goal to be attained. In the Czech language, the function of the velopharyngeal mechanism must be very precise. Pronunciation is characterized by a binary unit of nasality–non-nasality—a distinctive feature in the phonologic system. Any trace of nasality (with the exception of nasals) is perceived by the listener as a pathologic sign.

Velopharyngeal insufficiency is evaluated by two methods: listener judgments and acoustic analysis (computerized long-term average spectra, or LTAS). Acoustic analyses are used for speech samples longer than 20 seconds so that the global individual timbre can be assessed. The LTAS parameters that indicate the subjective perception of palatophony and its changes are:[28]

1. Percentage of fundamental tone energy.
2. Difference of the first and second harmonic zones.
3. Dip of antiresonance in the border of the fundamental tone zone and of the formant zone.
4. Loss of energy from the fundamental zone to this antiresonance dip.

The LTAS method has shown its wide versatility in acoustic analysis of VPI patients and is used in our daily practice, especially in borderline cases (persons with submucous clefts, short velum, and so on). Close cooperation among the plastic surgeon, phoniatrician, orthodontist, and others of the cleft team is most important to the successful treatment of VPI patients.

References

1. Černý M, Fára M, Hrivnáková J, et al: Cleft lip and palate: Variability in the Czech population, sex ratio, and familial incidence. Acta Chir Plast 29:1, 1987.
2. Jelínek R, Dostál M, Peterka M: Cleft Lip and Palate in an Experiment (in Czech). Prague: Charles University Press, 1983.
3. Fára M, Peterka M, Černý M, et al: Are we capable of preventing inborn defects? (in Czech). Čas Lék čes 123:1406, 1984.
4. Černý M, Fára M, Hrivnáková J, et al: Cleft lip and palate: Influence of parity and multiple pregnancy (in Czech). Čs Gynekol 52:417, 1987.
5. Černý M, Fára M, Hrivnáková J, et al: Cleft lip and palate: Relationship with cytomegalovirus infection (in Czech). Čas Lék čes 126:469, 1987.
6. Černý M, Fára M, Hrivnáková J, et al: HLA antigens in mothers of children with a cleft lip and palate (in Czech). Čas Lék čes 126:1001, 1987.
7. Černý M, Fára M, Hrivnáková J, et al: ABO blood groups in cleft lip and palate (in Czech). Čas Lék čes 127:236, 1988.
8. Černý M, Fára M, Hrivnáková J, et al: Reciprocal equilibrium in clefts (in Czech). Rozhl Chir 64:127, 1985.
9. Černý M, Fára M, Hrivnáková J: Familial protective regimen in cleft lip and palate (in Czech). Prakt Lék 68:320, 1988.
10. Černý M: Family and Heredity (in Czech). Prague: Avicenum, 1971.
11. Fára M: Theory and empiricism in surgical treatment of orofacial clefts. Teratology 8:210, 1973.
12. Hájek Z, Melková J, Vančurová V, et al: Postnatal development of children after gravidity following preconceptional genetic care (in Czech). Čs Gynek 49:171, 1984.
13. Randall P: A triangular flap operation for the primary repair of unilateral cleft of the lip. Plast Reconstr Surg 23:331, 1959.
14. Millard DR, Jr: Cleft Craft: The Evolution of its Surgery. I. The Unilateral Deformity. Boston: Little, Brown, 1976.
15. Fára M, Hrivnáková J: The problem of protruding premaxilla in bilateral total clefts. Acta Chir Plast 7:281, 1965.
16. Hrivnáková J, Fára M, Müllerová Ž: Maxillary development in facial clefts after primary bone implantation and after bridging the gap with a periosteal flap: A comparison. Acta Chir Plast 25:57, 1983.
17. Fára M: Principles of physiological approach to complex management of facial clefts (in Czech). Rozhl Chir 52:439, 1973.
18. Peskova H, Fára M: Lengthening of the columella in bilateral clefts. Acta Chir Plast (Praha) 2:18, 1960.
19. Hrivnáková J, Fára M: Nasal septum reposition in unilateral clefts as an integral part of primary suture of the lip. Acta Chir Plast 29:15, 1987.
20. Fára M, Véle F: The histology and electromyography of primary pharyngeal flaps. Cleft Palate J 9:64, 1972.
21. Fára M, Sedláčková E, Klásková O, et al: Primary pharyngofixation in cleft palate repair: A survey of 46 years experience with an evaluation of 2,073 cases. Plast Reconstr Surg 45:449, 1970.
22. Hrivnáková J, Fára M: Correction of the overhanging (or thickened) alar rim in unilateral clefts by a marginal excision with a triangular flap. Acta Chir Plast 17:177, 1975.
23. Eskeland G, Bergland O, Borchgrevink H, et al: Management of the cleft alveolar arch. In IT Jackson, BC Sommerlad (eds): Recent Advances in Plastic Surgery. New York: Churchill Livingstone, 1985.
24. Šmahel Z: Effects of certain therapeutic factors on facial development in isolated cleft palate. Acta Chir Plast 31:35, 1989.
25. Šmahel Z: Craniofacial morphology in adults with bilateral complete cleft lip and palate. Cleft Palate J 21:159, 1984.
26. Šmahel Z, Müllerová Ž: Craniofacial morphology in unilateral cleft lip and palate prior to palatoplasty. Cleft Palate J 23:225, 1986.
27. Šmahel Z, Brousilová M, Müllerová Ž: Craniofacial morphology in isolated cleft palate prior to palatoplasty. Cleft Palate J 24:200, 1987.
28. Vohradník M: Phoniatric documentation in cleft palate children. Proceedings of Union of European Phoniatricians Congress (XIV), Dresden, 1987.

CHAPTER 7

Multidisciplinary Management of Cleft Lip and Palate in Mexico

Fernando Ortiz Monasterio and Ignacio Trigos Micolo

The first multidisciplinary clinic for the care of cleft lip and palate patients was started in our country at the Hospital General de Mexico in Mexico City in 1958. We were faced with a large number of patients of all ages with untreated clefts who arrived at our institution not only from the capital and its surrounding area but also from very distant geographic locations. One orthodontist, one speech pathologist, and the staff of the plastic surgery service formed a group that met once a week to study and discuss the cleft patients. As time went on, specialists from other disciplines were incorporated. The interest of some of the early members decreased, but many younger, well-trained professionals joined the team, which continues to treat cleft patients today.

During the early stages, the interest of the group was maintained by the fascinating experience of learning from each other. The opportunity to discover the possibilities of a coordinated interdisciplinary team stimulated our imaginations and provided the motivation to continue our work. Further interest was developed later when the late results of patients were evaluated and showed a clear improvement in the quality of care.[1–3]

As a logical consequence of the clinic and the continuing interest of the team, numerous clinical research projects were developed to provide some answers and to ask new questions. More than thirty years later, we continue to learn every day from our colleagues in other disciplines. We are pleased to see that the standards of care and the final results are improving, and we still are excited by new research projects.

Clinical Material

From 1958 to 1988 we treated 11,200 patients with clefts of the lip and/or palate at our clinic. During the early stages, infants represented 2% of the series, children from 2 to 12 years 50%, teenagers from 13 to 19 years 30% and adults from 20 to 60 years the remaining 18%. Time has altered these proportions. At this time the first group represents 52% of our patients, the second group 33%, the third 12%, and the last 3%. Sixty percent of our patients come from Mexico City and 40% from rural areas.[4-6]

At this time, patients of all ages with untreated clefts represent 82% of our series. The rest have received some form of treatment, usually surgical treatment requiring secondary correction for aesthetic and functional problems.

Unilateral clefts of the primary palate (lip and alveolus) are found in 7%, and unilateral complete clefts of the primary and secondary palates occur in 73%. Bilateral cleft of the primary palate comprises 1%. Bilateral complete clefts are found in 16% and clefts of the secondary palate alone in 3%.[5, 7]

The prevalence of clefts that had not been surgically treated after infancy was further investigated in 1960; this study indicated that 85% of these patients came from distant locations, most of them from rural areas with limited or difficult access to medical facilities and with a cultural background in which deformities were socially acceptable.[5, 8]

As an outgrowth of this study, we organized our first mobile unit. We planned initially to use a true mobile surgical facility with a small operating room, dental unit, x-ray equipment, cephalometric equipment, photographic facilities, and sterilization equipment. We soon found that our "dream boat" was difficult to operate and had complicated logistics, and we decided to use the hospitals available in the area instead. Our team provided extra surgical, anesthetic, and dental material as well as the professional help needed. With some variations of the original model, we have worked for periods of 3 days, six to eight times a year, in the rural areas during the last 20 years. A total of 5800 patients have been treated in this manner in addition to the series treated in our clinic in Mexico City.

Because of the characteristics of our patient population, follow-up in our series is irregular. In the series treated at our institution during the late 1950s and early 1960s, evaluation after 5 years was obtained only in 15% of the series. At the present time, periodic revision is possible. We have a 5 year follow-up of 85% and a 10 year follow-up of 65% of the patients. Evaluation of the group operated on in the rural areas is considerably lower in spite of the fact that our team worked at least 5 years in each geographic area.[8, 9]

The Multidisciplinary Team

Our cleft palate clinic is part of the plastic surgery department. It involves the following disciplines: plastic surgery, orthodontics, speech pathology, psychology, otorhinolaryngology, genetics, pediatrics, and social work. Only patients with clefts of the lip and palate are seen; other persons with craniofacial anomalies go to the Craniofacial Clinic. The initial work-up is done by the plastic surgery residents; the patients are then seen by the different specialists and referred to the cleft clinic, which meets twice a month. The average number of patients seen at each clinic is 42. All the problem patients are presented for discussion before surgery when a comprehensive therapeutic plan is decided by the whole team. Postoperatively, all patients, regardless of the severity of their deformity, are evaluated periodically at the Clinic.[1, 10]

Treatment Plan

Surgical Treatment

Surgical closure of the primary palate is done at 2 to 3 months of age. This includes lip repair, closure of the nasal floor with a vomer flap, and extensive subcutaneous nasal dissection and alignment of the alar cartilages, and myringotomy.[2, 11-16] A rotation-advancement technique is used in most cases of unilateral cleft palate. Triangular flap closure is selected for the severe perialveolar clefts with unequal lengths of the lip segments.

The refinements of surgical techniques have improved the results of lip repair. It is now reasonable to expect symmetry of the upper lip with minimal scarring and good muscle alignment in practically all patients operated on at an early age. The correction of the nasal deformity, however, has been postponed in many centers to a later age on the assumption that surgery would interfere with growth of the nose. The nasal asymmetry remains as a permanent stigma during the early years of life and affects the self-image of the patients during that critical stage.

The idea that nasal correction in infancy would interfere with growth was transmitted through several generations of surgeons; however, it was never supported by any scientific evidence. Observations based on long-term follow-up of a small number of patients after early nasal surgery were accepted as valid. Furthermore, many of the procedures used for the correction of the nose were inadequate and often unnecessarily aggressive. It has been shown that surgery performed on the nose during infancy does not affect growth if the anatomic structures are carefully preserved and scars are avoided or kept to a minimum.

Nasal correction has been carried out in all of our cleft patients at the time of primary lip repair for more than 18 years. To achieve consistently good results, some anatomic observations must be considered. Except in the extremely rare cases, the dimensions of the alar cartilage on the cleft side are similar to those of the normal side. The cartilage is located in a lower position in relation to the upper lateral cartilage and to the skin coverage of the ala and the rim of the nostrils. The lateral crus is displaced laterally to the other side of the maxillary cleft. Its relation to the medial crus of the normal side is also altered by the lateral displacement, so that the dome of the nostril is asymmetric not only in relation to the midline but also in the anterior projection. These alterations cannot be corrected unless the alar cartilage is freed from the surrounding structures and repositioned in a proper anatomic location.

For early correction of the nasal deformity we follow the principles described by McComb.[11] The procedure begins in the conventional manner with incisions on both sides of the cleft. At this point the dissection of the alar cartilage is carried out with fine scissors introduced through the incision on the lateral lip segment. The cartilage is freed from the skin, and undermining is extended superiorly over the upper lateral cartilage to the free edge of the nasal bones. Caudally, the dissection extends around the alar rim and into the nasal mucosa to the inferior edge of the alar cartilage. The lateral crus is separated from the soft tissues of the ala and freed from its abnormal insertion beyond the bony cleft.

The scissors are then introduced through the incision in the prolabium, and the medial crus is separated from its contralateral. The dissection extends to the rim and the alar dome at the cleft side and to the dome in the normal side. At this stage, the alar cartilage is free from all its surrounding structures except the mucosal lining, which is carefully preserved. It can be mobilized without any tension to a position identical to that of the normal ala (Fig. 7–1).

The lip is closed in the conventional manner, and the alar cartilage on the cleft side is stabilized in the proper position. To achieve symmetry of the lower lateral cartilages and domes, we insert two or three pull-out sutures using a straight needle introduced through the skin at the root of the nose. The suture takes a cephalic edge of the cartilage and comes out through the skin at the root of the nose (see Fig. 7–4H). Exerting gentle tension on the sutures, the ala is repositioned, and the loose ends are taped to the skin. These sutures may not be necessary. The results depend on the complete separation of the cartilage from the skin, but we find them helpful for hemostasis.

We have followed our results with this nasal correction in a large number of patients for 5 to ten years and for as long as 12 years in an initial group of 20 patients. No alterations of growth have been observed in this series (Figs. 7–2 and 7–3).

For bilateral clefts, we use a modified Manchester procedure, including vomer flap closure of the floor of the nose and realignment of the alar cartilages.

We use a straight line technique designed to obtain a narrow philtrum and to construct an adequate buccal sulcus.[17] The prolabium incisions extend from the base of the columella to the peak of the Cupid's bow on each

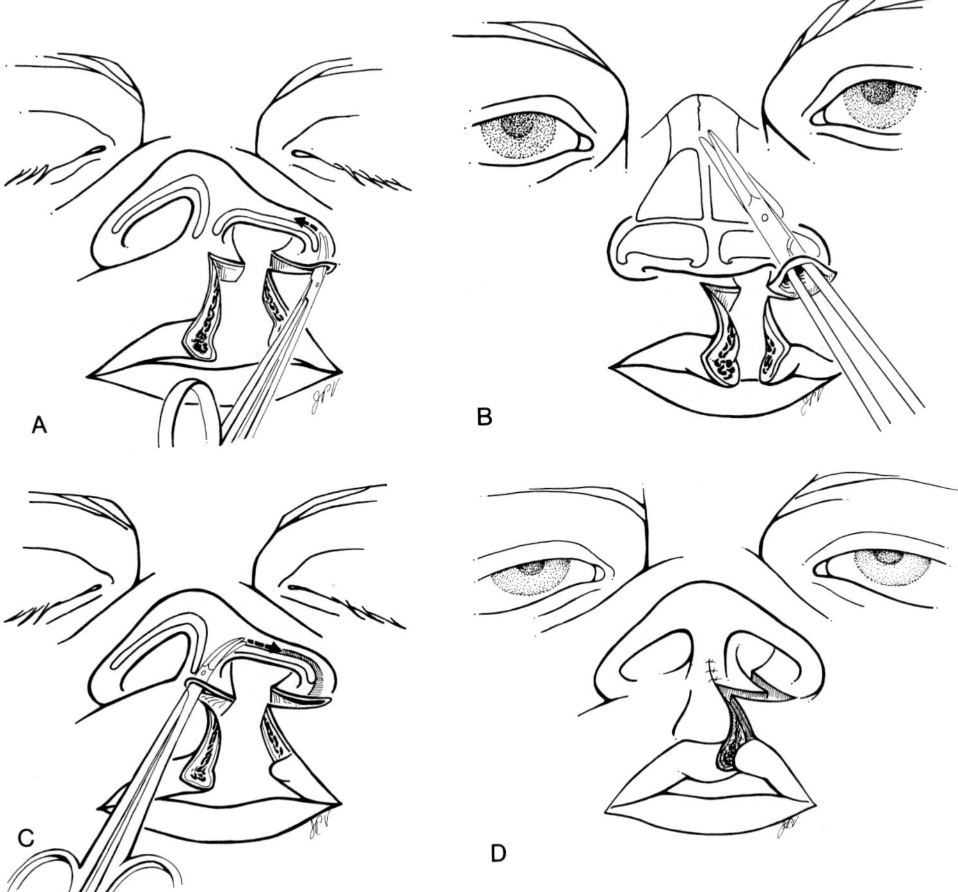

Figure 7–1 *A*, The lateral crus is dissected from the edge of the piriform aperture and from the skin around the rim. *B*, The skin dissection extends to the nasal bone. *C*, The medial crus is separated from the contralateral alar cartilage and from the skin of the alar dome, extending the dissection around the rim to the caudal edge of the alar cartilage. *D*, Lip closure is completed in the usual manner. Elongation of the columella on the cleft side added to the cartilage dissection produces a symmetric nose.

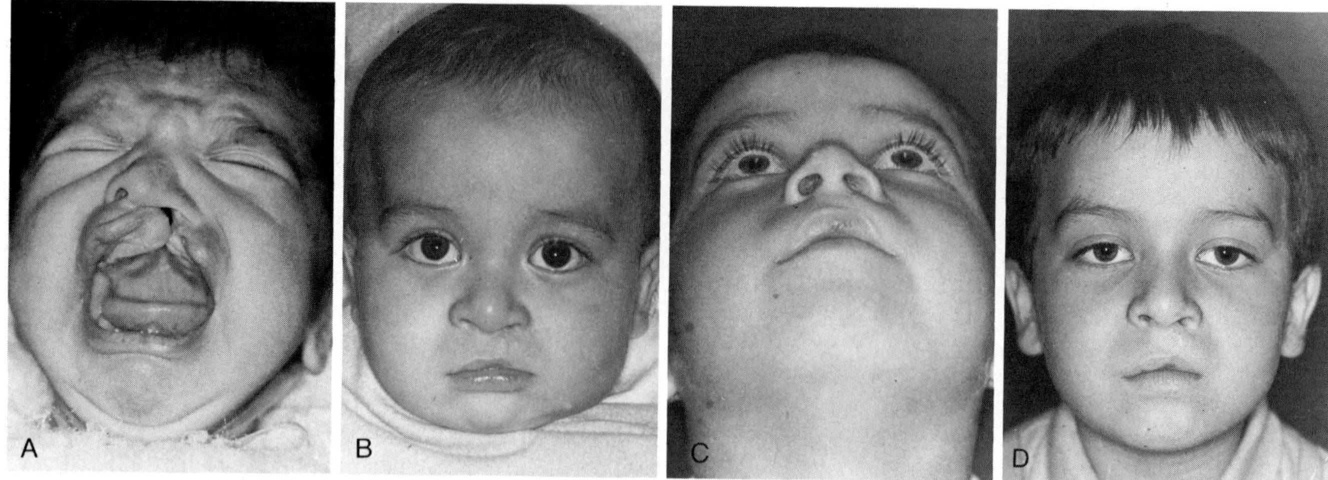

Figure 7–2 *A*, Preoperative view of a 2-month-old baby with a wide unilateral cleft and considerable nose distortion. *B*, One year postoperatively, acceptable symmetry of the nose is present. *C* and *D*, Seven years after lip closure there is no alteration of nasal growth. Symmetry is maintained.

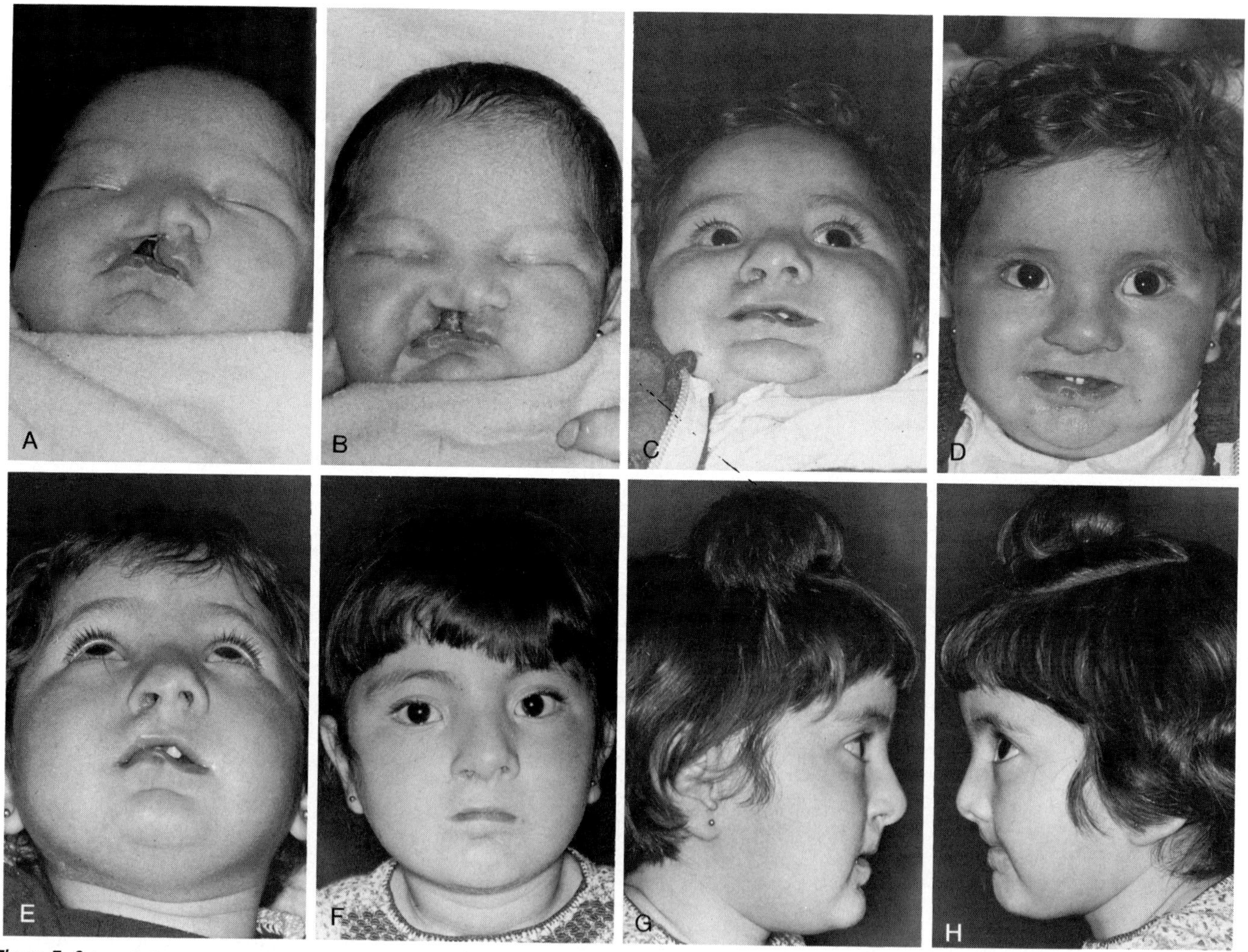

Figure 7–3 *A* and *B*, Preoperative view of a wide unilateral cleft with severe nasal deformity. *C* and *D*, Postoperative view at 18 months of age. *E* and *F*, Same patient at 6 years of age. *G* and *H*, The two profiles at age 6 demonstrate permanent symmetry and normal growth.

side. The maximum width of the philtrum is 6 mm. This is separated completely from the premaxilla and rotated cephalad temporarily. The two lateral mucosal and skin flaps are advanced medially and sutured at the midline over the premaxilla.

The incisions on the lateral segments are then carried out, rotating the mucosal skin flaps medially so that the ephithelialized side is in contact with the mucosa covering the prolabium. They are then sutured to each other at the midline, creating the labial mucosa of the buccal sulcus. The prolabial flap is returned to its normal position and sutured to the lateral segments.

As in unilateral clefts, the alar cartilages are freed entirely from the skin, from each other, and from the upper lateral cartilages so that they remain attached only to the mucosa inside the nose. The medial crura are sutured to each other to achieve anterior projection, and the same percutaneous sutures described for the unilateral nose correction are then applied to elevate the alae to their proper position. The lateral crura are also dissected from their attachments lateral to the cleft on each side and are rotated medially with the base of the alae closing the base of the nostrils (Fig. 7–4).

This nasal correction has improved our early results by creating a narrower nasal base and increased anterior projection of the lip. This, however, is not enough to correct the shortness of the columella inherent to this particular malformation. Secondary columellar elonga-

tion, usually performed at the time of the palatal closure, is necessary in most patients (Figs. 7–5 and 7–6).

Closure of the nasal floor is done in patients with both unilateral and bilateral clefts at the time of the primary operation. A superiorly based vomer mucoperichondrial flap is dissected on the cleft side (two flaps are used in bilateral clefts) and rotated laterally. Another short flap is elevated from the lateral wall of the nose and sutured to the vomer flap (Figs. 7–7 and 7–8). This maneuver has decreased the incidence of oronasal fistulas from 35 to 7%. The complete palatal clefts are converted at this time into incomplete posterior clefts, making the palatal closure a simpler procedure.

Preoperative orthopedic treatment is used in 2% of those with unilateral clefts and 40% of those with bilateral defects.

Palatal repair is performed at 1 year of age. A modified Wardill push-back procedure is used with meticulous dissection and suturing of the palatal muscles at the midline.[20] A simultaneous Sanvenero-Roselli pharyngoplasty is done routinely by some of the surgeons in our team.[21] Others prefer the Furlow Z-plasty in selected cases.[22–24] As stated before, some form of elongation of the columella is done in patients with bilateral clefts at the time of palatal closure.

Middle ear examination is carried out at the time of lip repair in all of our patients. Because of the high incidence of middle ear effusions, myringotomy is done routinely in all patients.

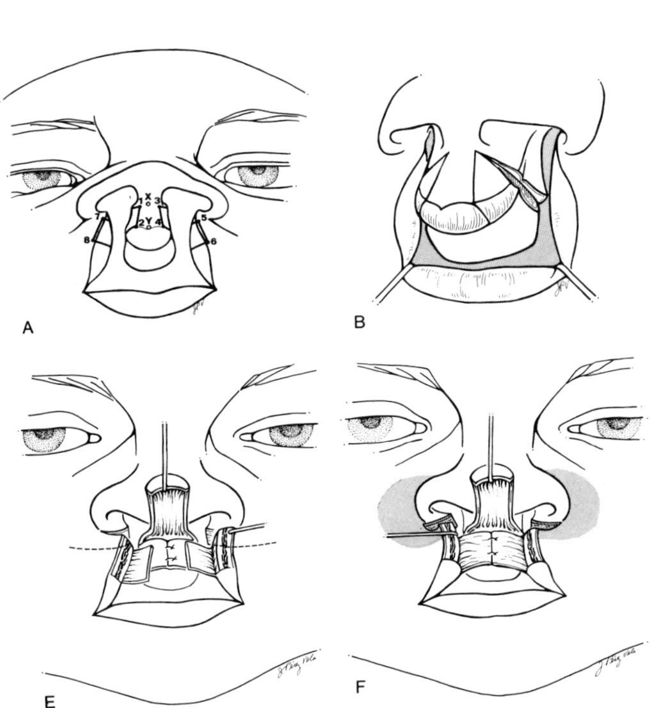
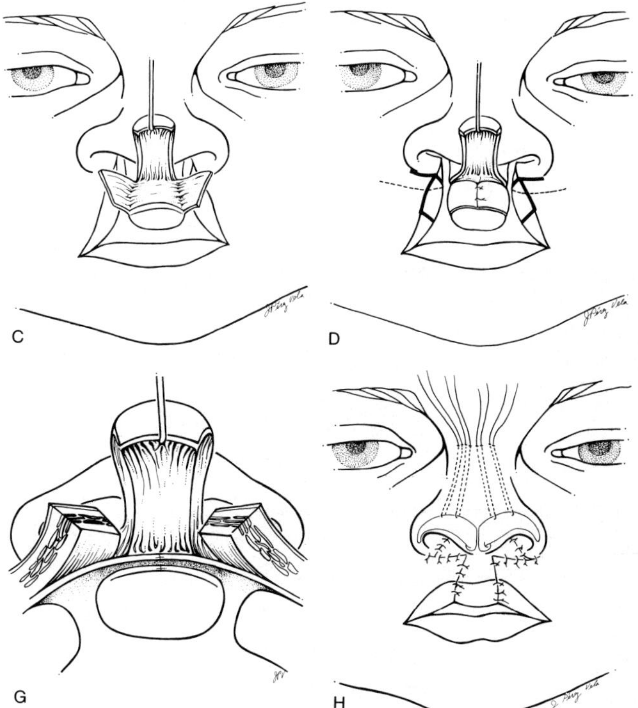

Figure 7–4 *A,* Tracing of the incisions for bilateral lip repair. Maximum width of the philtrum is 6 mm. *B,* The transverse incision at the base of the columella is extended to the premaxilla and then medially to the vomer to dissect the vomer flap (see Fig. 7–5A, B). *C,* The philtrum is dissected superiorly. *D,* The prolabial flaps 1–2 and 3–4 are sutured at the midline over the premaxilla. *E,* The labial flaps 5–6 and 7–8 are dissected from the lip segments and rotated so that the epithelial side completes the buccal sulcus. *F* and *G,* The labial mucosal flaps are sutured at the midline. The raw surface is ready to receive the philtrum. *H,* Lip closure completed. The alar cartilages have been freed from their skin attachments and maintained in position with pull-out sutures of nonabsorbable material.

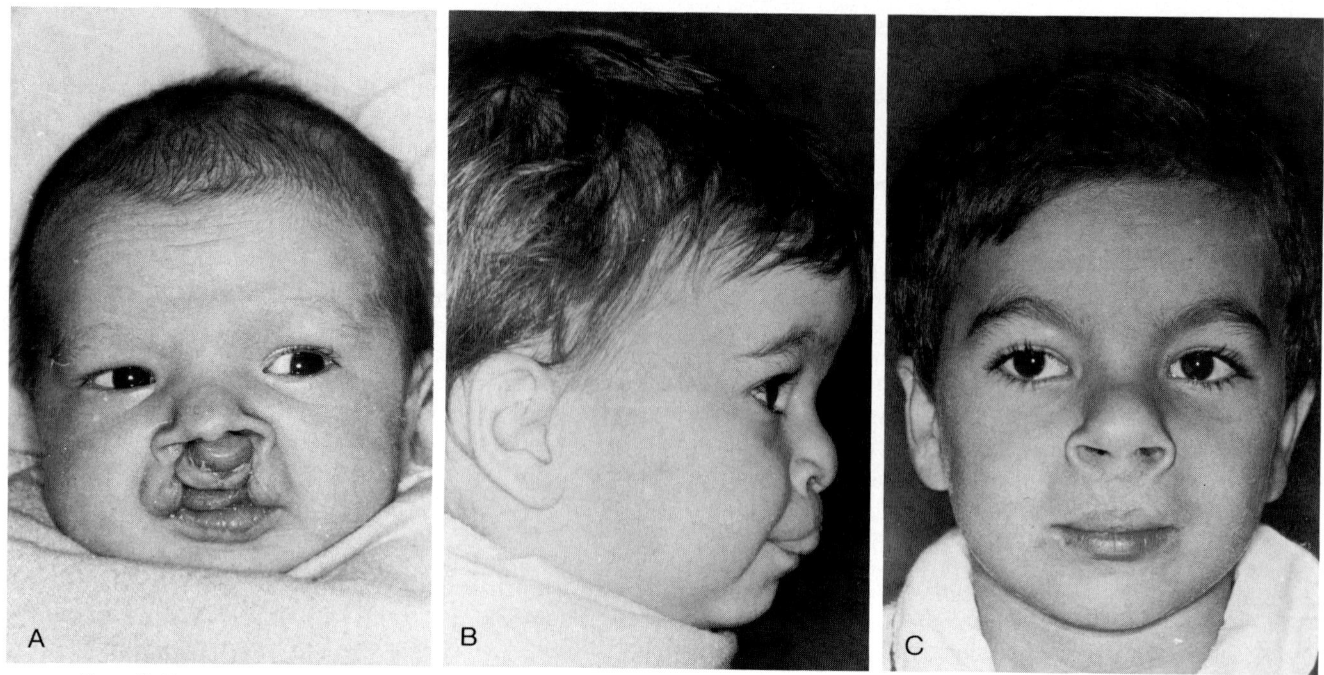

Figure 7–5 *A*, Preoperative view of bilateral cleft. *B*, Postoperative view at age 2 years. *C*, Postoperative view at age 10 years.

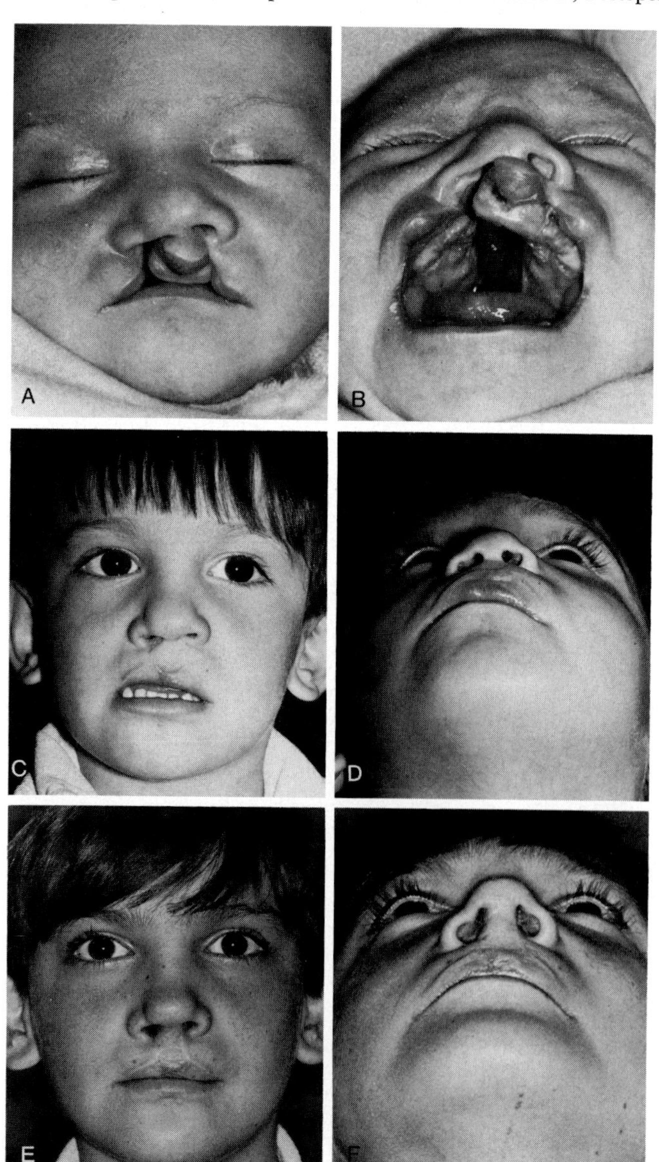

Figure 7–6 *A* and *B*, Preoperative views of bilateral cleft. *C* and *D*, Three years after the initial repair before columellar elongation. *E* and *F*, Result at age 14 years.

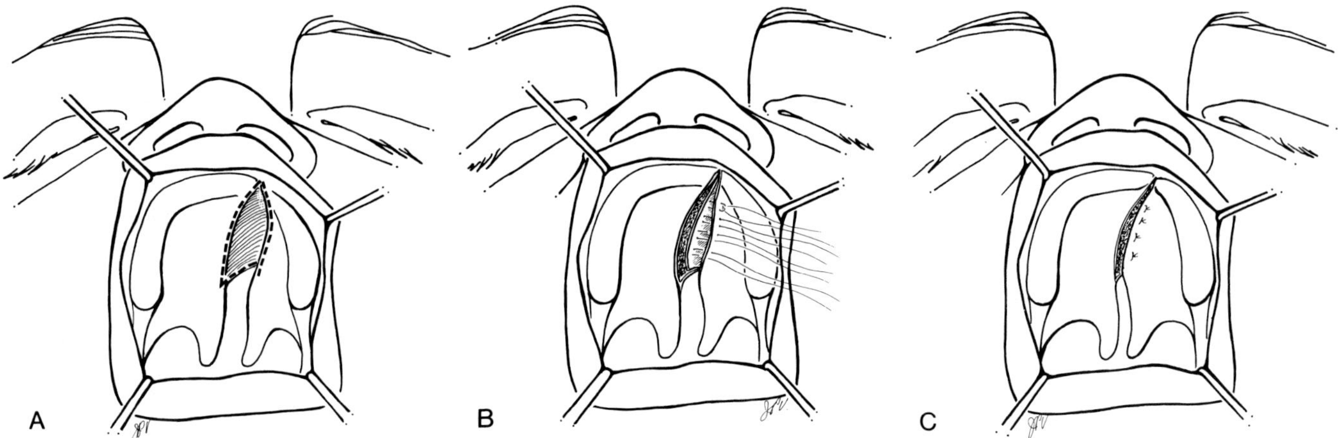

Figure 7–7 *A*, Closure of the nasal floor. Tracing of an incision for the vomer flap in a unilateral cleft. *B*, The mucoperichondrial flap is rotated laterally and sutured to the nasal mucosa. *C*, Sutures completed. This is done simultaneously with lip closure to prevent oronasal fistulas.

Speech Pathology Treatment and Indications for Pharyngoplasty

Speech and velopharyngeal closure are evaluated by the speech pathologist every 6 months after surgery. Articulatory problems are treated by the speech therapist in our unit or are referred to a speech clinic near the patient's home. Velopharyngeal insufficiency is routinely evaluated by rhinopharyngoscopy and multiview fluoroscopy to assess sphincter activity and to determine the pattern of closure. Seventeen percent of our patients require a secondary operation to correct velopharyngeal incompetency. Superiorly based pharyngeal flaps are used in most of our patients in this group. Our recent observations on sleep apnea associated with pharyngeal flap have changed the indications for this procedure. Based on the degree of velopharyngeal incompetency and the type of sphincter closure present, we use a modified Orticochea-Jackson pharyngoplasty or a cartilage graft in the posterior pharygneal wall when indicated.[24–29] Tailor-made pharyngeal flaps are used in a smaller group[21, 30–32] (Figs. 7–9 and 7–10).

Orthodontic Treatment

Orthodontic care is provided as needed after lip repair when a plate is used to prevent collapse of the maxillary segments and also later after palatal surgery to control the position of these segments. Bone grafting of the alveolar cleft is done only in selected patients at the beginning of the permanent dentition to provide a base for the eruption of the teeth. In most patients, it is done around the age of 12, after expansion, to obtain a solid stable arch when the permanent dentition is complete.

Because of the large number of patients and our limited orthodontic facilities, cleft patients are divided into three groups. Group I comprises patients with a high IQ who live in Mexico City or close by who have highly motivated parents who are willing and able to give the time to keep all their appointments. This group receives complete orthodontic care. Group II is formed of patients who are not able to keep their appointments either because of family problems or because they live too far away. Only basic orthopedic treatment, such as expansion or retention plates, are provided, and general directives are given for them to be treated elsewhere. Group III includes untreated adults and patients who, because of their cultural background or very distant location, cannot keep periodic appointments for treatment. No orthodontic care is provided for this group.[7, 8, 30, 33]

Secondary Surgical Procedures

For secondary nasal correction, we follow the same principles outlined for primary correction. The abnor-

Figure 7–8 *A*, Tracing of the incisions for closure of the nasal floor at the initial operation in a bilateral cleft. *B*, The two vomer flaps sutured to the nasal mucosa.

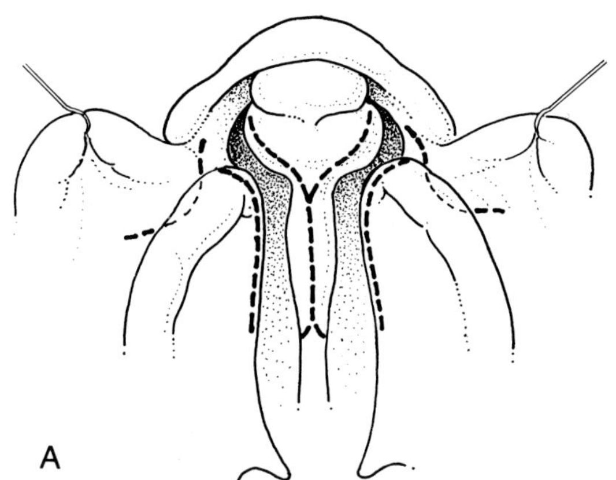

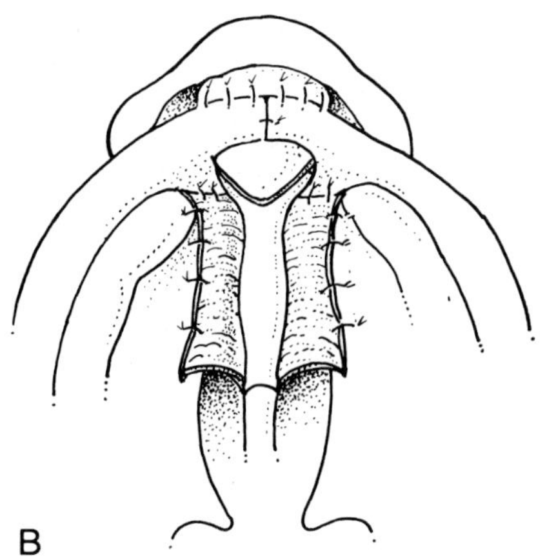

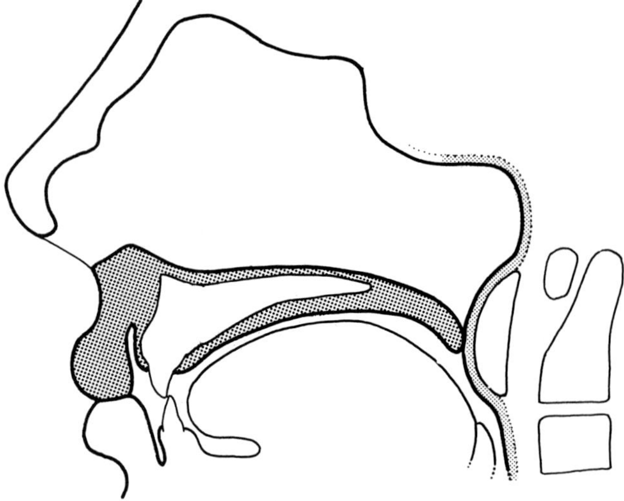

Figure 7–9 Diagrammatic representation of autogenous cartilage graft inserted into the posterior pharyngeal wall for the correction of moderate velopharyngeal incompetency.

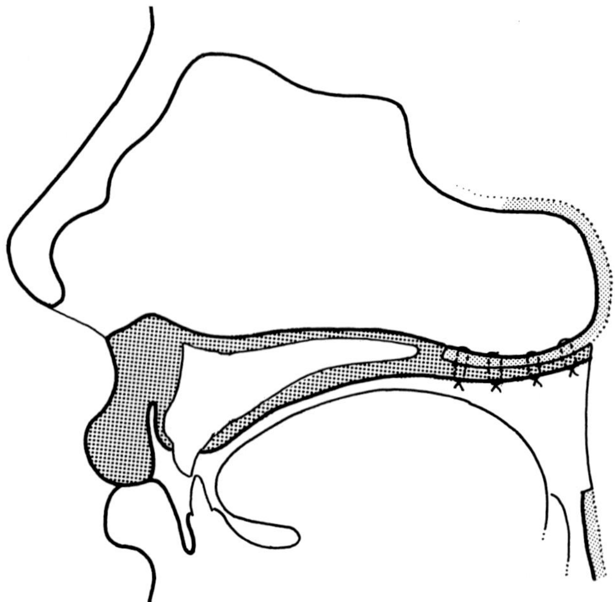

Figure 7–10 Diagrammatic representation of the superiorly based pharyngeal flap used to correct velopharyngeal incompetency. A flap of nasal mucosa of the soft palate is used to cover the raw surface of the pharyngeal flap.

mally located alar cartilages on the cleft side must be repositioned to produce symmetry. Intranasal mucosal incisions are necessary in this case. The first incision starts at the nasal rim in the upper third of the columella and follows the caudal edge of the alar cartilage near the piriform fossa. The skin is extensively dissected from the cartilage and from the upper lateral cartilage to the nasal bones. Medially, the lower lateral cartilages are separated from each other up to the dome of the ala on the normal side. A back cut is then made at the lateral

end of the incision, forming a medially based mucosal and cartilage flap, which is rotated. Then the alar cartilages are sutured together at the midline. The incision is closed in a **V-Y** fashion. The alar base is elevated and advanced medially to achieve symmetry.

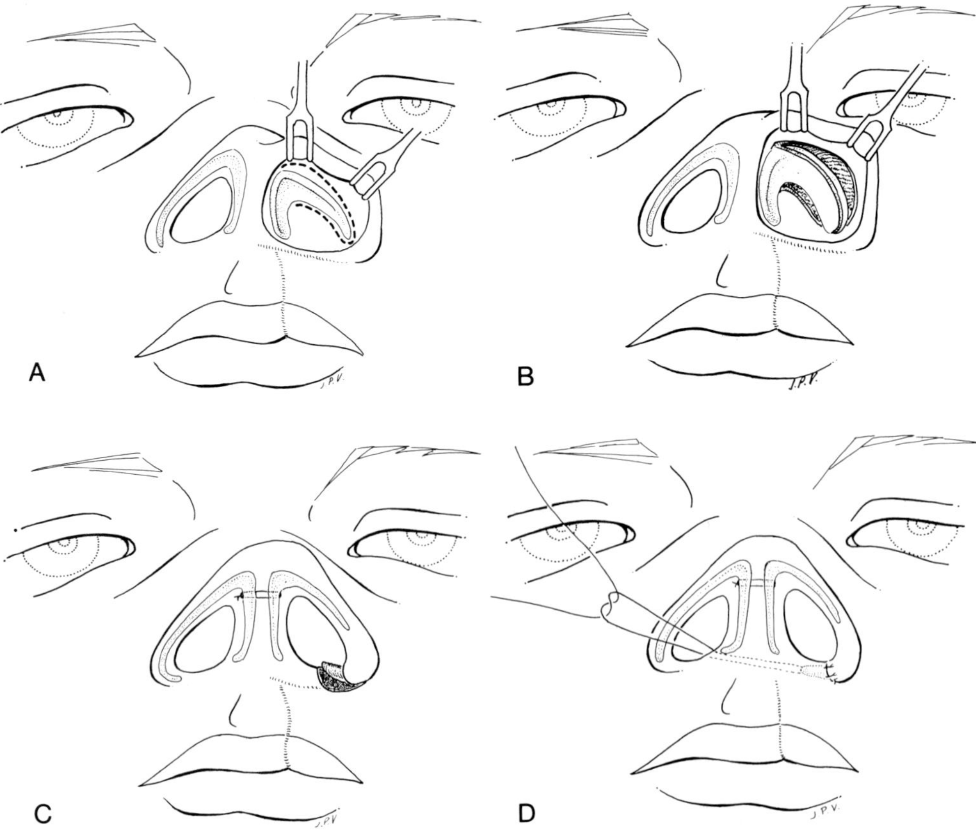

Figure 7–11 A, Incision used for the secondary correction of nasal asymmetry. B, A medially based flap of mucosa including the whole alar cartilage is elevated and displaced medially. C, The alar dome is sutured to the contralateral side in the proper position. The alar base is elevated, and the tip of the flap is deepithelialized. D, The denuded tip of the alar flap is buried at the base of the columella.

The excess tissue at the base of the nostrils can be excised or deepithelialized and introduced at the base of the columella to provide the volume usually lacking in this area (Fig. 7–11).

We use this type of correction for both unilateral and bilateral clefts during childhood but do not hesitate to do medial and lateral osteotomies when the bony skeleton is deviated in children 5 or 6 years of age. Ear cartilage grafts also are used to increase nasal tip projection in some patients in this age group. In adults, this procedure is always combined with osteotomies and septoplasty (Figs. 7–12 and 7–13).

Secondary midfacial hypoplasia presents a variety of deformities that must be treated according to the particular problem presented by each patient. In patients with normal dental occlusion, the main problem is the lack of volume in the piriform fossa corresponding to the site of the bony cleft. In this group, we use an autogenous rib cartilage graft introduced through a small incision in the upper buccal sulcus. The graft is carved in a semicircular shape to follow the contour of the piriform aperture and to fill the depression of the bone.

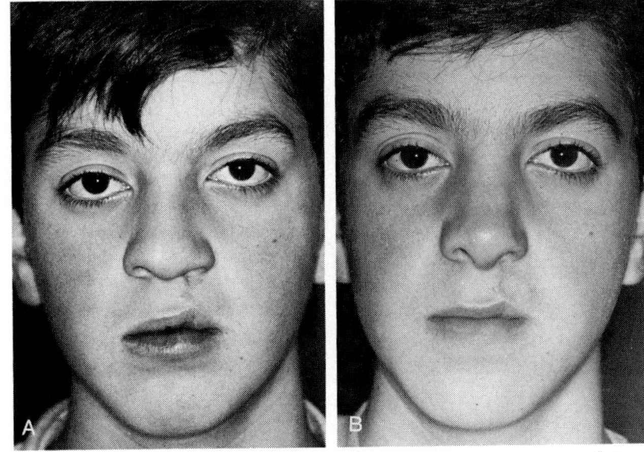

Figure 7–12 *A,* Preoperative view of a cleft nasal deformity that alters the whole facial symmetry. *B,* Postoperative view after repositioning of the alar cartilages using the technique shown in Figure 7–11.

The dissection is limited to provide a snug pocket for the graft and to prevent its displacement. Bone grafts obtained from the cranium or from other areas also can

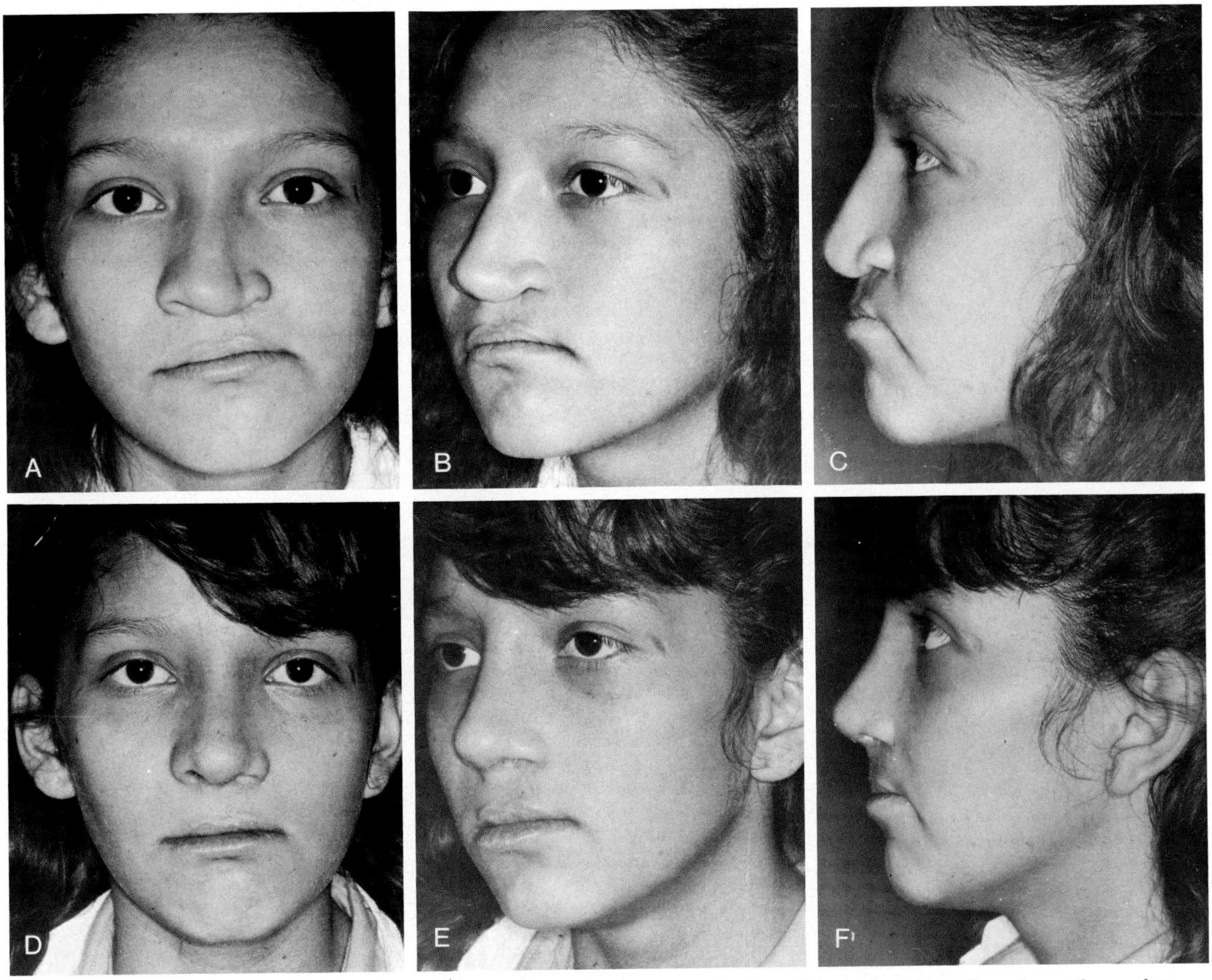

Figure 7–13 *A–C,* Preoperative views of a 16-year-old girl with severe cleft nose deformity. *D–F,* Postoperative views after rhinoseptoplasty combined with cartilage graft to the piriform fossa. The nasal tip was corrected using the technique shown in Figure 7–11.

be used, but partial or total resorption may occur, whereas cartilage will maintain its volume permanently (Fig. 7–13).

Secondary operations such as rhinoplasty, midface advancement, segmental osteotomy, and soft tissue revision are done at the final stage in patients originally treated in our clinic and in others who were referred after primary surgery performed elsewhere.[12]

Maxillomandibular discrepancy occurs as a result of maxillary hypoplasia, collapse of the maxillary segments, or a combination of both factors. Other elements contribute to exaggerate the facial deformity associated with this problem. The lack of space in the upper half of the oral cavity forces the tongue inferiorly, exerting constant pressure on the mandible and producing prognathism. In fact, the incidence of true prognathism confirmed by cephalometric studies in this group of patients is much higher than in the normal population. The maxillary hypoplasia is not limited to the alveolar ridge. The whole structure of the maxilla is often small in relation to other facial structures.

Functional and aesthetic objectives must be considered to correct this deformity. Maxillary advancement improves the convexity of the face and provides an adequate dental occlusion but in many patients fails to restore the normal contour of the paranasal area. We also have found that the osteocartilaginous framework of the lower half of the nose is inadequate in many of these patients, requiring other procedures to achieve facial harmony.

For the advancement of the midface, we perform maxillary osteotomy following the general pattern of the LeFort I fracture. The level of the horizontal osteotomy is determined by the type of deformity. This procedure is performed after the secondary dentition is complete and requires previous orthodontic treatment to obtain a stable dental occlusion postoperatively. For this it is often necessary to mobilize the maxillary segments in a lateral direction at the same time as the advancement procedure.

Permanent postoperative stability in this multifragment extensive mobilization can be obtained only by solid fixation with miniplates. We use metallic fixation in all of our patients and fill the gap with bone grafts. When a significant maxillary advancement is required and when there is preoperative marginal velopharyngeal insufficiency, we routinely do a pharyngeal flap during the same procedure.

The midface advancement restores the facial convexity and the normal occlusion but must often be complemented with bone or cartilage grafts in the paranasal area. Optimal results, however, can only be achieved when the nose is corrected during the final stage of the treatment. We prefer to do the rhinoplasty whenever possible at the same surgical procedure. The use of miniplates has eliminated the need for intermaxillary fixation in most cases, so once the osteotomy is finished we change from nasal to oral intubation and proceed to correction of the nose. This is simplified by cutting the endotracheal tube at the level of the nostril and extracting it through the mouth. The refinements of aesthetic rhinoplasty are important in this group of patients. Cartilage grafts to the dorsum, the tip, or the columella are very frequently used in these patients (Figs. 7–14 and 7–15).

The same principles are used for secondary nasal correction in patients with bilateral clefts. The alar cartilages are freed from the skin and rotated medially to increase the anterior projection. This procedure is usually complemented by cartilage grafts to the tip and columella to reinforce the structural support and to achieve definition. We consider septal cartilage the optimal material for these procedures. Rib cartilage is used when a large amount of material is required for support and for restoration of the nasal and paranasal contour.

Total replacement of the skin coverage of the upper lip with a scalp flap is often used in adult males with very severe scars. Because of poor color match of free skin grafts in patients with a relatively dark complexion, this procedure is rarely used in our patients (Fig. 7–16).

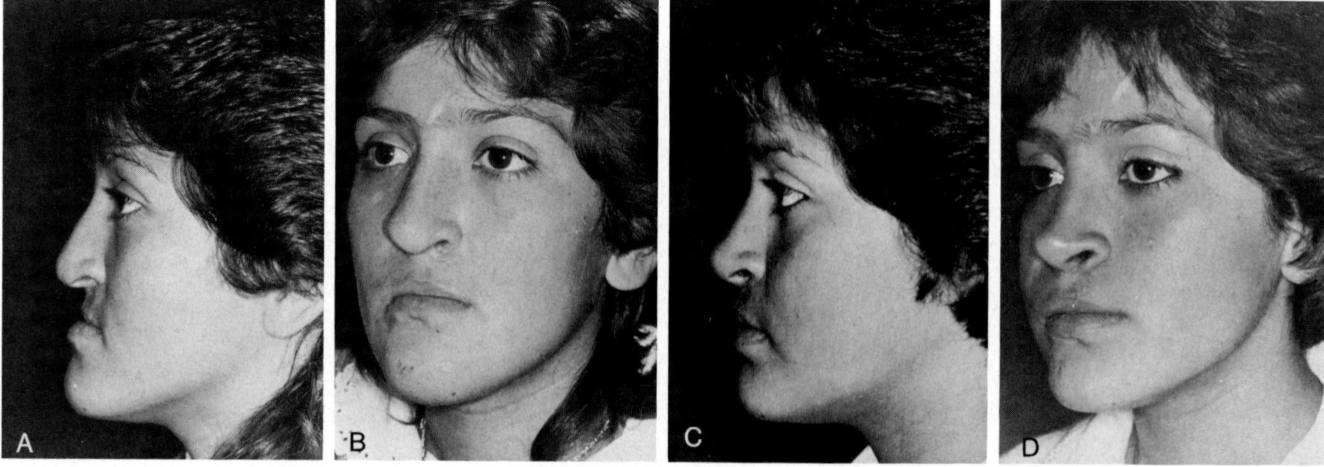

Figure 7–14 *A* and *B*, Preoperative views of an 18-year-old girl with severe nasal deformity and maxillary hypoplasia. *C* and *D*, Postoperative views after simultaneous midface advancement (Le Fort I) and rhinoplasty.

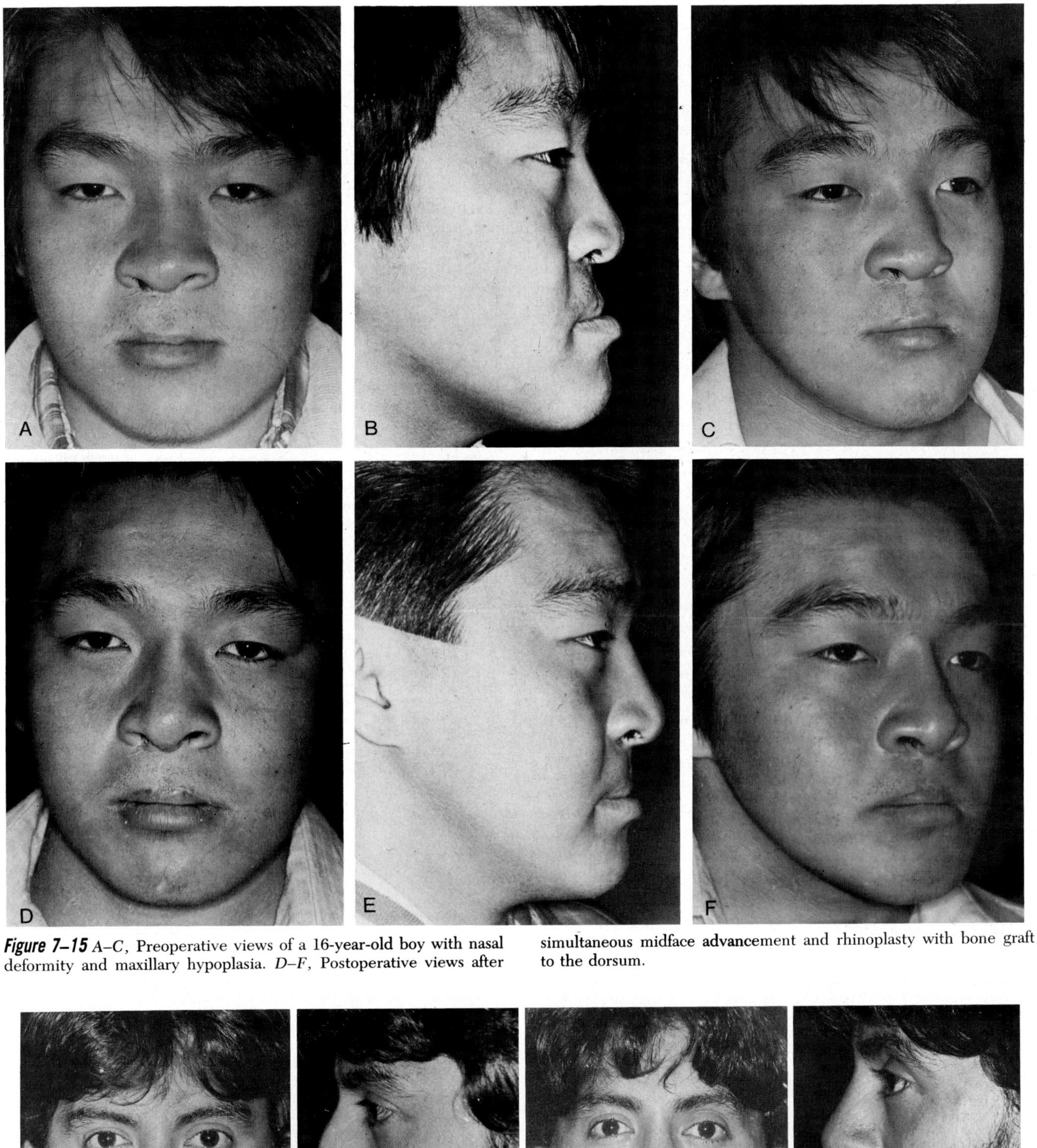

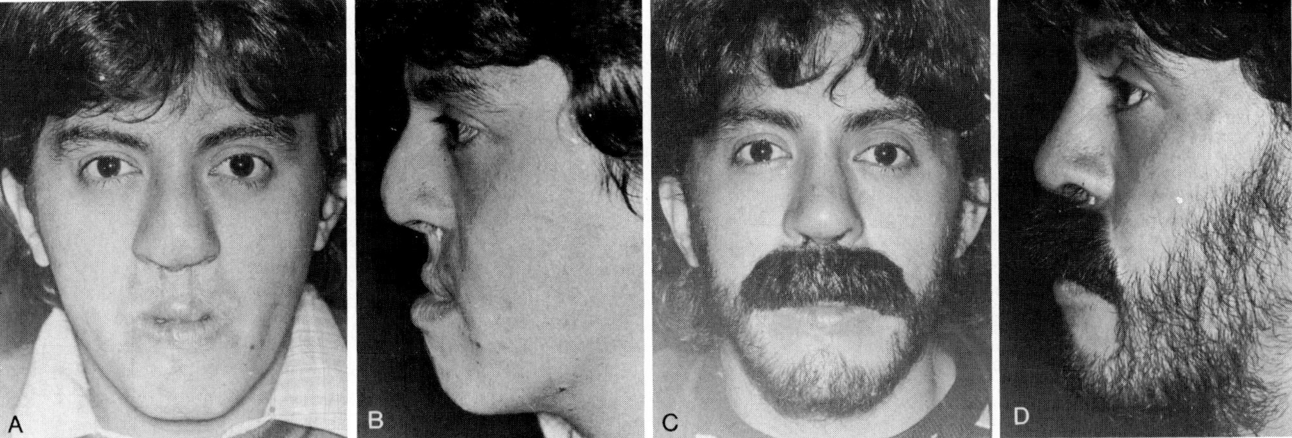

Figure 7–15 *A–C*, Preoperative views of a 16-year-old boy with nasal deformity and maxillary hypoplasia. *D–F*, Postoperative views after simultaneous midface **advancement** and rhinoplasty with bone graft to the dorsum.

Figure 7–16 *A* and *B*, Preoperative views of a 20-year-old man with severe nasal deformity and scarring of the upper lip. *C* and *D*, Postoperative views after rhinoplasty with a cartilage graft to the nose and island scalp flap to replace the skin of the whole upper lip.

Research

Our research projects have focused mainly on clinical research. Three areas have been investigated. Growth has been evaluated in unoperated patients by means of a cross-sectional study in adults and as a longitudinal project in other age groups. These projects include evaluation of maxillary and nasal growth in relation to age at correction and soft tissue development and to the several surgical techniques used throughout the years.[14, 25, 34–43]

Sociologic studies have been done in both our urban and rural groups in regard to the concept of the deformity, cultural influences, and belief in magic as an influence on thinking. These studies have been applied, along with psychological studies, to classify patients in several groups receiving different types of treatment in an effort to optimize the utilization of limited resources.

Other projects have been directed toward the evaluation of results using different technical procedures in relation to both functional and aesthetic outcome.

During the last 3 years, we have worked on making intrauterine repairs of clefts. The initial part of the project was carried out in rats and our findings coincide with the reports of Hallock and others regarding the absence of scarring both macroscopically and microscopically.[44] Growth in rats as measured by x-ray cephalometry, dental casts, and dry skull measurements has shown no alterations when compared to controls in spite of major resections of the lip in the fetuses.

Studies have also been carried out in a series of monkeys. Our results were similar to those in rats when intrauterine surgery was performed early. This part of our study, which was also designed to refine surgical techniques, has been completed, and operations on human fetuses are being considered as our next possible step.

References

1. Fuente del Campo A, Ortiz Monasterio F, Yudovich M: Organizacion de la Clinica de Cirugia Craneofacial. Special supplement Rev Cir Plast Iberolatinoamericano, 1979.
2. Navarro R, Ortiz Monasterio F, Trigos I: Un metodo didatico para la practica del cierre de las fisuras del paladar primario. Rev Cir Plast Iberolatinoamericano 5:17, 1979.
3. Ortiz Monasterio F, Serrano AR, Barrera G, et al: A study of untreated adult cleft palate patients. Plast Reconstr Surg 38:1, 1966.
4. Ortiz Monasterio F, Serrano AR, Valderrama M, et al: Cephalometric measurements of adult patients with non-operated cleft palate. Plast Reconstr Surg 24:1, 1959.
5. Ortiz Monasterio F, Olmedo A, Trigos I, et al: Final results from the delayed repairs of patients with clefts of the lip and palate. Scand J Plast Surg 8:1, 1974.
6. Ortiz Monasterio F: Mobile unit for detection and care of craniofacial anomalies. Plast Reconstr Surg 55:2, 1975.
7. Ortiz Monasterio F, Serrano AR, Barrera G, et al: A study of untreated adult cleft palate patients. Plast Reconstr Surg 38:1, 1966.
8. Ortiz Monasterio F, Serrano AR: Cultural aspects of cleft lip and palate treatment. In Grabb WK, Rosenstein SW, Bzoch KR (eds): Cleft Lip and Palate. Boston: Little, Brown, 1971.
9. Trigos I, Ruenes R, Ortiz Monasterio F: La radiografia en la fisura palatina. Rev Mex Radiologia 21:3, 1967.
10. Ortiz Monasterio F, Vasquez A: La integracion y el adiestramiento de un equipo multidisciplinario para cirugia craneofacial. La Prensa Med Mex 39:3, 1974.
11. McComb H: Primary correction of unilateral cleft lip nasal deformity: A 10 year review. Plast Reconstr Surg 75:791, 1985.
12. Ortiz Monasterio F, Olmedo A: Corrective rhinoplasty before puberty. Plast Reconstr Surg 68:3, 1981.
13. Ortiz Monasterio F: Correccion secundaria del esqueleto facial y la nariz. Manejo y tratamiento integral de la fisura labio palatina. Mexico City: Department of Medical Editions, Hospital Infantil de Mexico, 1987.
14. Ortiz Monasterio F: Crecimiento facial en pacientes operados con labio y paladar hendido. Manejo y tratamiento integral de la fisura labio palatina. Mexico City Department of Medical Editions, Hospital Infantil de Mexico, 1987.
15. Ortiz Monasterio F, Olmedo A: Cleft lip nose. In Rees and Baker (eds): Controversies and Complications of Rhinoplasty. St. Louis: Mosby, 1987.
16. Randall DR, Jr: Refinements in rotation-advancement cleft lip technique. Plast Reconstr Surg 23:331, 1959.
17. Garcia-Velasco M, Nahas A: Surgical repair of the bilateral cleft of the primary palate. Ann Plast Surg 20:1, 1988.
18. Manchester WM: The repair of double cleft lip as part of an integrated program. Plast Reconstr Surg 45:207, 1970.
19. Viale-Gonzalez M, Barreto F, Ortiz Monasterio F: Surgical management of the bilateral cleft lip. Plast Reconstr Surg 51:6, 1973.
20. Wardill WEM: The technique of operation for cleft palate. Br J Plast Surg 25:117, 1937.
21. Trigos I, Ysunza A, et al: San Venero Roselli pharyngoplasty. Electromyographic study of the palatopharyngeus. Cleft Palate J, 25:385, 1988.
22. Furlow LT, Jr: Cleft palate repair: Preliminary report on lengthening and muscle transposition by Z-plasty. Presented at the Annual Meeting of the Southeastern Society of Plastic and Reconstructive Surgery, Boca Raton, Florida, May 16, 1978.
23. Garcia-Velasco M, Galvez F, Ysunza A, et al: Paladar hendido submucoso. Rev Med Hosp Infantil Mex 42:657, 1985.
24. Garcia-Velasco M, Ysunza A, Hernandez X, et al: Diagnosis and treatment of submucous cleft palate: A review of 108 cases. Cleft Palate J 25:2, 1988.
25. Garcia-Velasco M, Ysunza A, Ruiz Primo E, et al: Sindrome de apnea obstructiva secundaria a anomalias craneofaciales y cirugia de insuficiencia velofaringea. Rev Cir Plast Iberolatinoamericano 14:3, 1988.
26. Hynes W: Pharyngoplasty by muscle transplantation. Br J Plast Surg 3:128, 1950.
27. Jackson IT, Silverton JS: Sphincter pharyngoplasty as a secondary procedure in cleft palates. Plast Reconstr Surg 59:518, 1977.
28. Orticochea M: Results of the dynamic sphincter operation in cleft palates. Br J Plast Surg 23:108, 1970.
29. Orticochea M: A review of 236 cleft palate patients treated with dynamic muscle sphincter. Plast Reconstr Surg 71:180, 1983.
30. Serrano AR, Ortiz Monasterio F, Barrera G, et al: El colgajo retrofaringeo en la rehabilitacion del lenguaje en el paladar hendido. Gac Med Mex 95:4, 1965.
31. Trigos I, Ysunza A, et al: Surgical treatment of border line velopharyngeal insufficiency using homologous cartilage implantation with videonasopharyngoscopic monitoring. Cleft Palate J 25:167, 1988.
32. Trigos I, Ysunza A, et al: A comparison of palatoplasty with and without primary pharyngoplasty. Cleft Palate J 25:163, 1988.
33. Trigos I, Ortiz Monasterio F: Otologic evaluation of cleft palate patients. (Special reference to an untreated adult group). Rev Cir Plast Iberolatinoamericano 17:2, 1973.
34. Amaya Reza S: Estudios del crecimiento del tercio medio de la cara y determinacion de normales en el mexicano (adulto). Mexico, DF: Universidad Nacional Autonoma de Mexico, Facultad de Medicina, 1963.
35. Fuente-del-Campo A, et al: Estudios comparativo de dos tecnicas para cierre de labio. Rev Med Hosp Gral 35:1, 1972.
36. Martinez Perez JJ: Determinacion de crecimiento del maxilar superior en el mexicano mediante antropometria radiologica. Mexico City, DF: Universidad Nacional Autonoma de Mexico, Facultad de Medicina, 1962.
37. Shubich I, Trigos I, Ysunza A: Diagnosis y tratamiento de apnea del sueno obstructiva. Bol Med Hosp Infantil Mex 43:384, 1988.
38. Velazquez A, Ortiz Monasterio F: Primary simultaneous correction of the lips and nose in the unilateral cleft lip. Plast Reconstr Surg 54:5, 1974.
39. Viale-Gonzalez M, Ortiz Monasterio F: Observations of growth of the columella and prolabius in the bilateral cleft lip. Plast Reconstr Surg 46:2, 1970.
40. Ysunza A: Chasquidos por conduccion osea versus enmascaramiento por via osea para valoraciones audiologicas con potenciales evocados auditivos en pacientes pediatricos. Bol Med Hosp Infantil Mex, 42:99, 1985.
41. Ysunza A, Trigos I: Nasofaringoscopia y videofluoroscopia en el diagnostico de la insuficiencia velofaringea. Rev Cir Plast Iberolatinoamericano 12:7, 1986.
42. Ysunza A, Cone-Wesson BK: Bone-conduction masking for BAEO pediatric audiological evaluation. Validation of the test. Int J Ped Oto Rhin Laryngol 12:291, 1987.
43. Ysunza A, Baldizon N, Trigos I: Sustituciones articulatorias gruesas en el diagnostico y tratamiento de las insuficiencias velofaringeas. Bol Med Hosp Infantil Mex 44:81, 1987.
44. Hallock GG: In utero cleft lip repair in A/J mice. Plast Reconstr Surg 75:785, 1985.

CHAPTER 8

Multidisciplinary Management of Cleft Lip and Palate in Turkey

K. Güler Gürsu

The first printed *Turkish Surgical Manuscript* by Sherafeddin Sabuncuoglu[1] in the fifteenth century has several miniature illustrations of different plastic surgery procedures that range from mandibular fractures to a possible case of hypospadias. Figure 8–1 shows a miniature entitled Repair of a Lip Fissure.

In spite of this early surgical awareness little plastic surgery was performed in Turkey until the 1920s, when the pioneers of plastic surgery in this country began to perform several procedures. Professor Halit Ziya Konuralp was one of the founding members representing Turkey at the first meeting of the International Federation of Plastic and Reconstructive Surgery in 1955 in Stockholm. At that time, cleft lip and palate patients were recognized and treated by doctors who were referred to as jaw surgeons or dentists. Jaw surgery was a specialty available at Gülhane Military Academy. Also, there was one small plastic surgery unit at the General Surgery Department of Istanbul University Medical School. There were no training centers for plastic surgery in universities or in other institutions. The Turkish Plastic Surgery Society, which was founded in 1961 by the pioneers, did not act as an instrument for the establishment of this specialty and initially was rather slow in structuring the foundation for education and training. In 1965 the society reorganized its by-laws to meet the standards of the International Federation of Plastic and Reconstructive Surgery, bringing very strict regulations to the standards for plastic surgery training. Until 1965, the situation in Turkey resembled the situation elsewhere in the 1940s.

In this setting, Hacettepe was founded first as the Children's Center in 1958; it became a medical school in 1963 and finally was established as a university with several faculties (colleges) in 1967. Presently, the university has a total of ten faculties and 25,767 students. The medical school has two divisions: One presents the curriculum in English, the other in Turkish. The total number of medical students is 2495. The medical school has two hospitals with a total of 1229 beds; of these, 350 beds are strictly for children.

The Hacettepe Plastic and Reconstructive Surgery Department officially opened in March, 1965, as a small unit within the Department of General Surgery. In 1967 it was separated from the general surgery department and became an independent department with 22 beds.

At present, there are 50 beds, half of which are reserved for children and infants.

When plastic and reconstructive surgery became a new department reactions varied. In some medical circles, plastic surgery was perceived as a luxury; plastic surgery meant aesthetic surgery only. In the military academy the name of the department was still Jaw Surgery, and as a result, most of the patients treated there needed head and neck surgery. Nevertheless, this department trained general surgeons as specialists in surgery of clefts of the lip and palate. They were, in one sense, the pioneers of cleft lip and palate treatment in Turkey.

Owing to a lack of proper anesthesiology, current philosophy of treatment, and knowledge of congenital anomalies, cleft lip and palate patients were treated at a very late age. At Hacettepe these patients were treated by an otolaryngologist before my arrival.

Since my training with Barsky in the principles of cleft lip and palate repair was quite different from that in the existing program in Turkey at that time, a sort of crusade had to be started regarding the timing of lip and palate repair and the methods used. Starting a department in a new medical school had its advantages and disadvantages. The main advantage was the number of available patients. Having a very large pediatric department within the school certainly was an advantage, and initially it was quite easy to encourage pediatricians to make early referrals.

A series of conferences was organized for all departments with special emphasis on congenital anomalies. Consequently, a large number of patients began to be seen in the Department of Plastic and Reconstructive Surgery. The understanding and cooperation of my colleagues, who were all trained in the United States in their own fields, was another advantage. Among other advantages was the immediate availability of instruments and books on plastic surgery, which was not the case

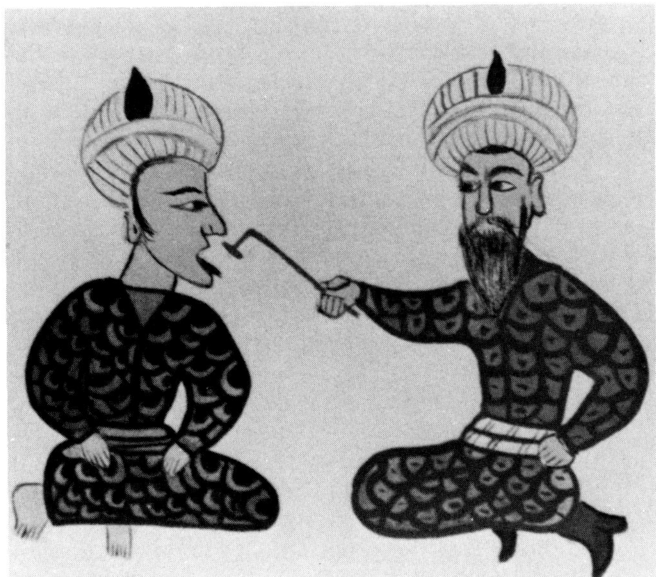

Figure 8–1 Miniature illustration reproduced from a fifteenth century surgical manual.[1]

Table 8–1. Analysis of 174 Patients Seen Between March 1965 and September 1966

	CL	CL (%)	CP	CP (%)	CL+CP	CL+CP (%)	MC	MC (%)	Total	Total (%)
Total	40	23	36	20.7	94	54.1	4	2.2	174	100
Unilateral	35	20.1			61	35.1				
Incomplete	23	13.2	11	6.3	20	11.5				
Left	15	65.2			16	60				
Male										
Female										
Right	6	34.6			4	20				
Male										
Female										
Complete	12	6.9	13	7.5	41	23.6				
Left	7	56.3			31	75.6				
Male										
Female										
Right	5	41.7			10	24.4				
Male										
Female										
Bilateral	5	2.9			33	19				
Complete	2	1.2			26	16.1				
Incomplete	3	1.7			5	2.9				
Male										
Female										
Submucosa			12	6.9						

CL = cleft lip; CP = cleft palate; MC = median cleft.

for other institutions. The base of medical knowledge within the medical school staff made my work much easier. Most of my colleagues at the University Hospital began to refer patients soon after birth. However, it was not the same story with the outside medical world. They had to be convinced not only about the need or place of plastic surgery but also about its training, requirements, and wide range of practice.[2,3]

However, there were disadvantages in starting a new department as well. The entire department consisted of only one person. During the first 3 years, I had to function with the help of only one technician. There were a few rotating residents from other departments until our own training program started in 1968. Also, because we lacked some of the proper instruments we had to operate with those that were available, making surgery very difficult.

Soon after the Department of Plastic Surgery in the Hacettepe Medical School was established in 1965, I was invited to the Congress on Plastic Surgery held in Bratislava, Czechoslovakia. There I had the chance to operate again with Dr. Ralph Millard; I had worked with him previously as part of my training in Kingston, Jamaica, before completing my residency program in the United States.

During the same congress I met for the first time Professors Paul Fogh-Anderson of Denmark, Eric Peet of England, Bardach of Poland, and Demejien of Czechoslovakia. This was my first opportunity to discuss the kinds of cases I had begun to see at our Department of Plastic Surgery in Hacettepe. These individuals all gave me the kind of courage and self-confidence one needs from his or her seniors.

When I won a scholarship in 1967 from the Dr. Noel Foundation, I had the opportunity to work with Professors Peet, Fogh-Anderson, and Dufferental and to observe plastic surgery techniques in Europe and England. During this period, I met Professor Tord Skoog

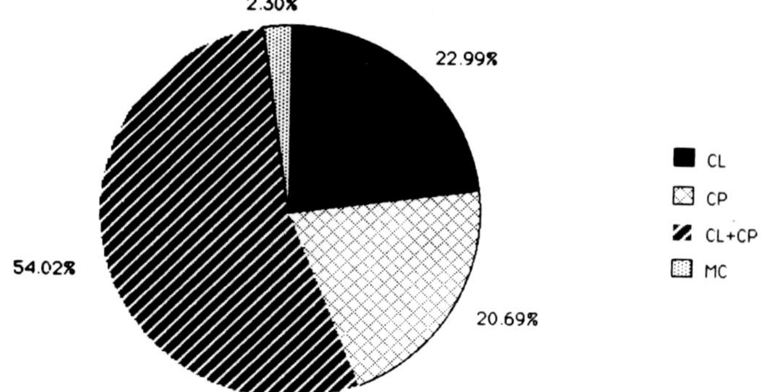

Figure 8–2 Distribution of 174 patients seen between March 1965 and September 1966 according to cleft type. CL-cleft lip; CP-cleft palate; CL+CP-cleft lip & palate; MC-median cleft.

at the University of Uppsala. This tour of 3 months gave me a greater understanding of the wide variety of techniques used in plastic surgery. All of my postgraduate training in plastic surgery took place in the United States, and I had very little knowledge of what techniques were used in Europe. This scholarship allowed me to learn a great deal about these techniques.

The first analytical report of cleft lip and palate patients from Hacettepe was given as a scientific exhibition at the Fourth International Congress of Plastic and Reconstructive Surgery in Rome in October, 1967. This was a report of 174 patients who were seen during an 18-month period (Table 8–1 and Fig. 8–2). Of the 174 patients, a total of 40 had cleft lip only; 35 of these were unilateral clefts. Of these 35 unilateral cleft lips, 23 were incomplete. We had 94 cleft lip and cleft palate patients. These comprised 54.1% of the 174 cases. There were also four median cleft cases in this first report.[4-6] The incidences reported in this first study were comparable with those reported in other international studies presented at the Congress.

Table 8–2. Analysis of 724 Patients Seen Between March 1965 and March 1970

	CL	CL (%)	CP	CP (%)	CL+CP	CL+CP (%)	MC	MC (%)	Total	Total (%)
Total	159	21.9	206	28.5	351	46.5	6	1.1	724	100
Unilateral	82	11.3			146	20.2				
Incomplete	57	7.9	107	14.8	27	3.7				
Left	33	4.6			14	1.9				
Male	21	2.9	56	7.7	11	1.5				
Female	12	1.7	51	7.1	3	0.4				
Right	26	3.3			13	1.6				
Male	12	1.65			7	1.0				
Female	12	1.65			6	0.6				
Complete	25	3.4	17	7.5	119	16.5				
Left	15	2			69	12.3				
Male	9	1.2	10	1.3	63	6.7				
Female	6	0.6	7	1	26	3.6				
Right	10	1.4			30	4.2				
Male	3	0.4			16	2.5				
Female	7	1.0			12	1.7				
Bilateral	17	23			61	8.4				
Complete	5	0.7			52	7.2				
Male	2	0.3			41	5.7				
Female	3	0.4			11	1.5				
Incomplete	9	1.2			7	0.9				
Male	5	0.8	12	6.9	6	0.8				
Female	3	0.4			1	0.1				
Mix	3	0.4			2	0.3				
Male	3	0.4			2	0.3				
Female										
Submucosa			12	1.7						
Unclassified	60	8.3	70	9.7	144	19.9				
Male	35	4.8								
Female	25	3.5								

CL = cleft; CP = cleft palate; MC = median cleft.

One year later, the First National Congress of the Turkish Plastic Surgery Society was held in Ankara, Turkey in June, 1968. I again presented a statistical report on cleft lip and cleft palate patients. This time the total number of patients was 223.[5] The third report followed in April, 1970, and covered a 5-year period beginning March, 1965.[7] The total number of patients reached 724 (Table 8–2, Fig. 8–3).

Between April, 1970, and January, 1987, an additional 1482 patients were seen, which meant that over a period of 22 years we had seen a total of 2206 patients.[8] An analysis of this final number is given in Figure 8–4.

Of these 2206 patients, 301 had cleft lip only, 1013 had cleft palate only, 876 had cleft lip and cleft palate, and 16 had median clefts.

A special data collection form for cleft patients was developed and we began to record information about the patients in regard to the intermarriage of parents, the presence of cleft lip and palate or any other congenital anomaly in the family, number of siblings, geographic location, and socioeconomic situation of the family, among other items. These important points were studied and later reported[9–11] as the first specialty thesis from this department (Tables 8–4 through 8–7).[12]

In one study, 550 patients with cleft lip were found to have multiple additional malformations (2.73%) (Fig. 8–5). However, another study of 1482 patients with cleft lip and palate revealed 157 patients (11%) with additional malformations. Of these patients, 80 were females. The largest group with additional malformations (107) was patients with cleft palate only (Table 8–8).

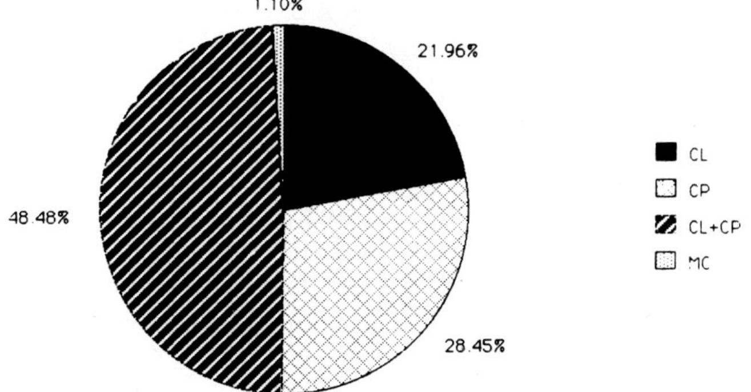

Figure 8–3 Distribution of 724 patients seen between March 1965 and March 1970 according to cleft type.

In the same study of 1482 patients, a blood relationship between the parents was found in 244. This analysis is shown in Table 8–9. An interesting finding in this study was that the most frequent anomaly was isolated cleft palate (139 patients), and the most affected group was females (78 patients). Further research on multiple congenital anomalies was carried out in the Department of Pediatrics. A postmortem study of 1000 infants showed that 104 had congenital heart disease[13]; 72 (68.2%) of these 104 had various other cardiac malformations. Interestingly, the second most common anomaly was cleft lip and cleft palate (six infants) among those with cardiac malformations (Table 8–9 and Fig. 8–6).

Table 8–3. Analysis of 2206 Patients Seen Between March 1965 and January 1987

	CL	CL (%)	CP	CP (%)	CL+CP	CL+CP (%)	MC	MC (%)	Total	Total (%)
Total	301	13.6	10013	45.9	676	39.7	16	0.07	2206	100
Unilateral	204	9.2			461	20.9				
Incomplete	126	5.8	706	32.1	70	3.7				
Left	56	3.9			44	2				
Male	45	2.1	303	13.7	33	1.5				
Female	40	1.8	405	15.4	11	0.05				
Right	42	1.9			26	1.2				
Male	21	0.95			16	0.07				
Female	21	0.95			10	0.05				
Complete	76	3.4	193	9	391	17.7				
Left	44	2			268	12.1				
Male	15	0.65	36	3.9	199	9				
Female	29	1.35	112	5.1	69	3.1				
Right	32	1.4			123	5.6				
Male	15	0.65			60	3.6				
Female	17	0.75			43	2				
Bilateral	37	1.7			260	11.8				
Complete	12	0.6			185	8.4				
Male	6	0.4			132	6				
Female	4	0.2			53	2.4				
Incomplete	16	0.8			24	1.1				
Male	12	0.6			22	1				
Female	6	0.2			2	0.01				
Mix	7	0.3			51	2.3				
Male	5	0.2			36	1.5				
Female	1	0.1			15	0.07				
Submucosa		2.7	37	1.7						
Unclassified	60		70	3.2	155	7				
Male	35	1.6			94	4.3				
Female	25	1.1			61	2.7				

CL = cleft lip; CP = cleft palate; MC = median cleft.

Surgical Management of Cleft Lip and Palate

It is difficult to discuss multidisciplinary management strategies including surgical, orthodontic, and speech treatment of cleft lip and palate patients in a country where plastic surgery was not a board certified or an officially acknowledged specialty until 1968. Consequently, orthodontists, speech pathologists, and speech therapists were unavailable. Thus, all patients were evaluated pre- and postoperatively by a surgeon only, and the following findings are based on clinical observations. However, for the past few years we have had the help and support of the Department of Orthodontics at Hacettepe Dental School. The results of this collaboration, however limited, also will be presented.

Initially, the most important strategy was establishment of the timing and preferred method of repair. Timing was a new issue, and most physicians favored surgical repair at a later age (puberty), mostly due to the status of anesthesia services. But, Hacettepe Med-

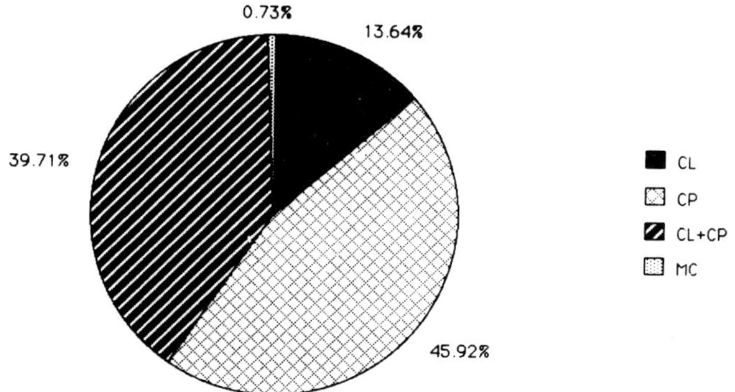

Figure 8–4 Distribution of 2206 patients seen between March 1965 and January 1987 according to cleft type.

ical School was very fortunate to have a staff of extremely well-trained anesthesiologists, and as a result of this collaboration, it was possible to introduce an "early repair" principle.

We began to treat patients when they first came to the clinic, but very soon we started to see patients soon

Table 8–4. Analysis of the Family History of 327 Cleft Lip Patients Seen Between January 1965 and June 1971

	Patients with CL		Control Group (Normal Population) x^2		
No Relation	240	73.4%	6972	78.8%	1.166
Close Relative	66	20.2%	495	5.6%	109.710
Distant Relative	21	6.4%	1386	15.6%	17.440
Total	327	100.0%	8853	100.0%	128.417

CL = cleft lip.

Table 8–5. Analysis of the Family History of 434 Cleft Lip Patients Seen Between January 1965 and June 1971

	Number of Patients	%
Positive family history	29	6.68
Affected sibling	14	3.22
Positive family history + affected sibling	3	0.70
No family history or affected sibling	388	89.40
Total	434	100.00

Table 8–6. Analysis of Mother's Age in 304 Cleft Lip Patients Seen Between January 1965 and June 1971

Mother's Age	Mean Age of the Mother	Number of Patients
15–19	17	34
20–24	22	102
25–29	27	72
30–34	32	51
35–39	37	35
40–44	42	10
Total	26.68	304

Table 8–7. Analysis of Birth Sequence of 444 Cleft Lip Patients Seen Between January 1965 and June 1971

Patients with CL	Control Group (Normal Population)				
Sequence of Birth	*Number*	*%*	*Number*	*%*	x^2
1st	111	25.0	3108	35.7	13.642
2nd	90	20.3	1908	21.91	0.530
3rd	87	19.6	1306	15.1	5.580
4th	65	14.7	843	9.7	10.532
5th	45	10.1	586	6.7	6.420
6th or more	46	10.2	955	11.0	0.191
Total	444	100	8706	100.0	36.895

CL = cleft lip.

Table 8–8. Distribution of Cleft Type and Sex in 157 Cleft Patients with Additional Malformations

	CL	CP	CL+CP	Total
Male	3	43	31	77
Female	4	64	12	80
Total	7	107	43	157

CL = cleft lip; CP = cleft palate.

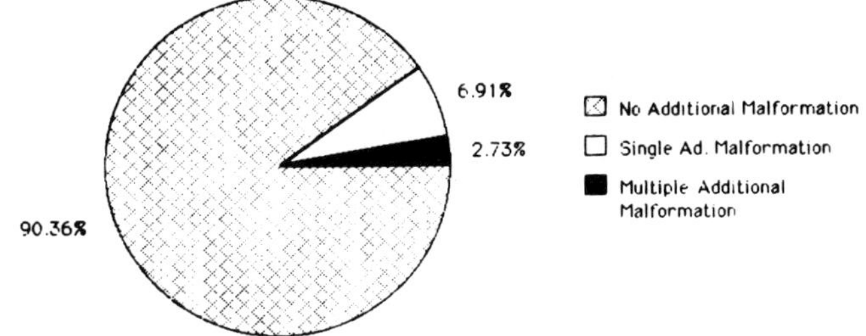

Figure 8–5 Distribution of 550 patients with malformations in addition to cleft lip between 1957 and 1971.

Table 8–9. First- and Second-Degree Blood Relation of Parents in 244 Cleft Patients

	CL	CP	CL+CP	MC	Total
Male	6	61	63	0	130
Female	13	78	21	2	114
Total	19	139	84	2	244

CL = cleft lip; CP = cleft palate; MC = median cleft.

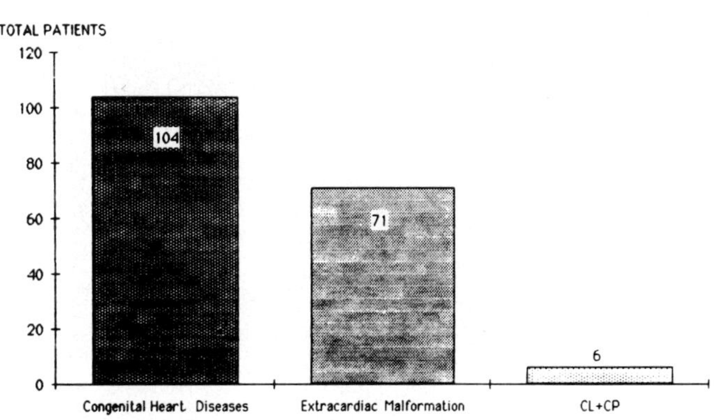

Figure 8–6 Total patients with additional malformations.

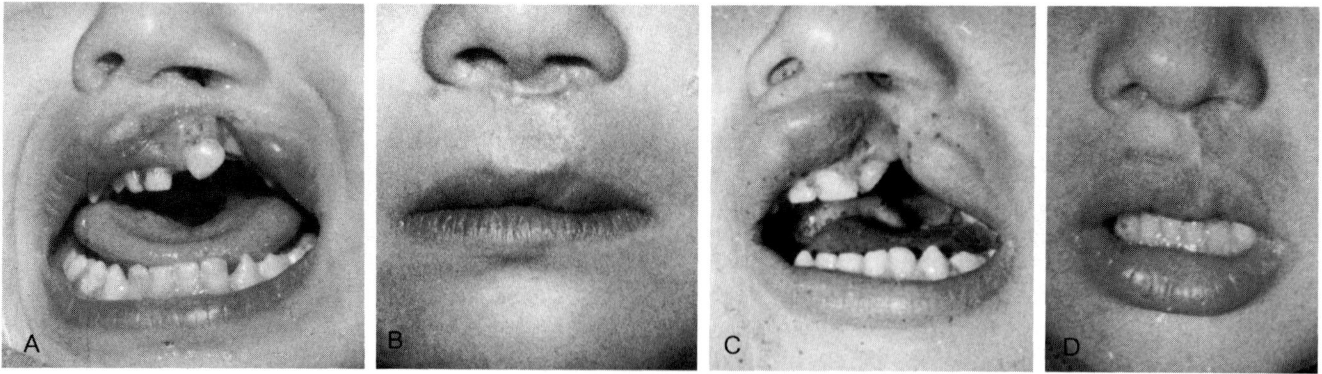

Figure 8–7 *A* and *B*, Pre- and postoperative views of a patient with an incomplete unilateral cleft lip. *C* and *D*, A second patient with the same deformity.

after birth. In a short period of time, it became standard practice to operate on cleft lip patients at the age of 3 months and on cleft palate patients at the age of 18 months. We have not had one mortality that was due to anesthetic complications during the past 24 years. Our success has influenced other medical schools and institutions, and currently, early repair has become a nationally accepted principle. About 75 to 80% of all patients still come to Hacettepe Medical School. Currently, there are more than 12 medical schools with independent plastic surgery departments, and at least an equal number of state hospitals and several social security hospitals also have plastic surgery departments that treat cleft lip and cleft palate patients. We believe that the incidence of clefting still approximates 1 in 1000.

Surgical technique was also another important issue. Although I trained with Barksy at Mount Sinai Medical School in New York City, I also had the opportunity to observe and work with Millard. Like other trainees during the 1960s, I was impressed by his rotation-advancement cheiloplasty, which I found much simpler to perform and teach with good overall results. Consequently, all patients in our department were operated on using the Millard technique.[14,15] The modifications by Millard were adopted, and some of our own modifications have been incorporated as well. Some of the results achieved in unilateral cleft lip patients are presented in Figures 8–7 and 8–8.

In 1974, an article entitled "A New Modified Method for Bilateral Cleft Lip Repair" was published by our department.[16] In this paper we described a combined method that was based on the Millard rotation-advancement technique with some additional techniques borrowed from both the Barsky and Veau methods. As seen in Figure 8–9, the principal modification was the addition of D flaps. This method later was modified. Results achieved in some of our patients with bilateral clefts are presented in Figures 8–9 through 8–11.

Regarding cleft palate patients, initially we operated on a very large number of patients for secondary closures or fistula repairs. However, as time went on, most patients were primary cases who had been treated in our clinic.

All patients were operated on using the V-Y pushback and lengthening technique.[17] No early closure of the soft palate with delayed hard palate closure was carried out. In a very small group of patients, the palate was closed before the lip owing to their age (between 8 and 18 years); even then, however, no primary pharyngoplasty was performed. All patients were given endotracheal anesthesia. The mean age at operation was 24 months. Whenever possible, our general policy has been to operate at the age of 18 months. There have been no major postoperative complications, and less than 3 to 4% received blood transfusions during surgery. The mean length of hospital stay was 1 week.

In Turkey, one of the most difficult problems is

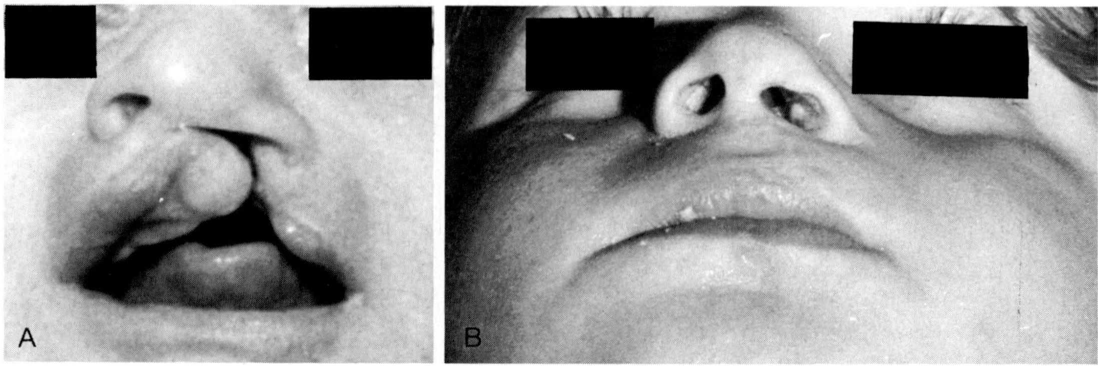

Figure 8–8 *A* and *B*, Pre- and postoperative views of a patient with a complete unilateral cleft lip.

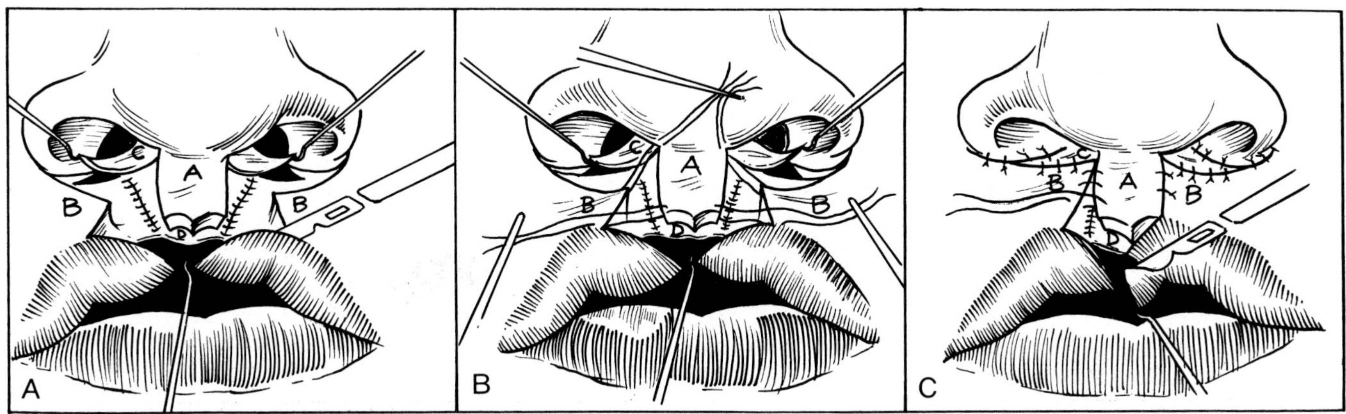

Figure 8–9 Surgical technique for bilateral cleft lip. *A*, Mucosa of flap B is sutured to the lateral edge of flap D. *B*, Rotation of flap C. *C*, Following all muscle and skin suturing, excess tissue from the vermilion border is excised. The tissues are sutured in three layers.

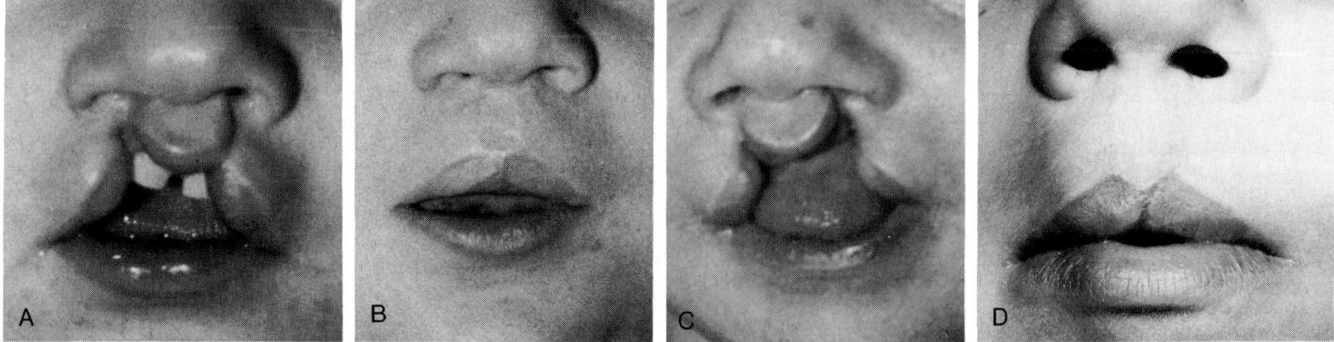

Figure 8–10 *A* and *B*, Pre- and postoperative views of a patient with an incomplete bilateral cleft lip. *C* and *D*, A second patient with bilateral cleft lip.

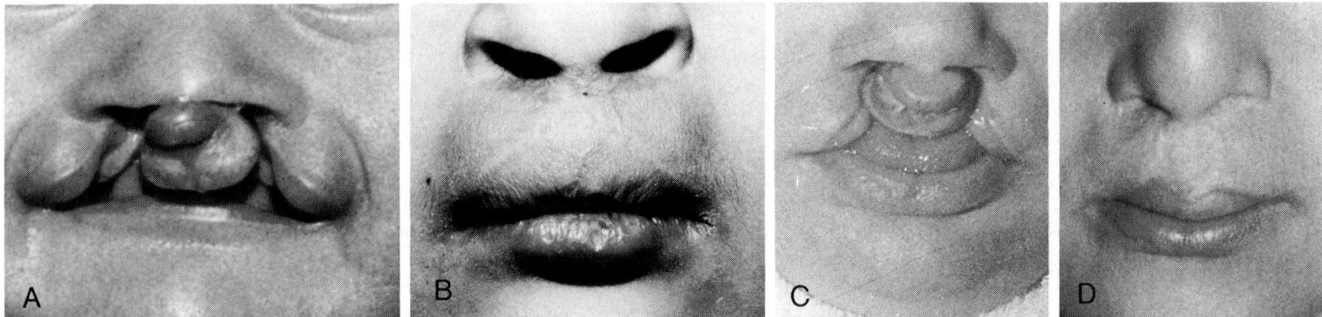

Figure 8–11 *A* and *B*, Pre- and postoperative views of a patient with complete bilateral cleft lip. *C* and *D*, Another bilateral cleft patient.

patient follow-up. When the lip is repaired, the patient comes back for palate repair. Following palate repair, the patient typically is lost after a few postoperative visits. Consequently, we are not able to follow these patients with regard to speech results or the occurrence of fistulas. I can only state that we do not see very many fistulas. The ones we see are closed with secondary procedures. There have been only five patients with fistulas that could not be closed surgically. They are wearing obturators, and all were operated on elsewhere. The surgeons try to advise patients on speech therapy and to give genetic counseling because there are no other team members.

Several studies were carried out in this department on the subject of cleft lip and palate as specialty theses, which are equivalent to board certification examinations in the United States.[18–22] Each thesis is a printed, booklike document. Highlights of some of these studies will be presented because each examines a particular problem. One study was entitled Evaluation of Partial Nose-Lip Measurements in Normal and Post-Repair Cleft Lip Individuals in Regard to Millard's Method.[23] Several age groups among 1000 normal and 36 postoperative cleft lip individuals were examined. Nine measurements (three for the nose and six for lip) were recorded and then compared (Fig. 8–12). The measurements taken included:

1. Width of the columella.
2. Height of the columella.
3. Width of the alar bases.
4. Ala to tip of Cupid's bow.
5. Columellar base to tip of Cupid's bow.
6. Columellar base to center of Cupid's bow.
7. Width of Cupid's bow.
8. Tip of Cupid's bow to commissure.
9. Intercommissural distance.

This study showed no significant differences between normal and surgically treated groups.

Another study that compared the Millard and Dibbell methods in cleft lip-nose repair showed no significant difference between the two techniques in correction of this deformity.[24] In 1984 the Cronin and Millard techniques were compared in the correction of bilateral cleft lip-nose deformity.[25] This study showed that both techniques were satisfactory for columella lengthening and narrowing of the alar bases as well as for adjustment of the nostrils and nose-lip angle. All three studies concerned secondary cleft lip-nose deformities. In 1985 another specialty thesis was published on primary cleft lip-nose repair. This study compared the Millard and Skoog techniques. Again, no significant differences were reported.[26]

One of the most recent studies focused on new bone formation following cleft palate repair.[27] Radiologic and scintigraphic investigation of cleft palate patients who were operated on with a V-Y push-back and lengthening technique demonstrated osteoblastic activity as early as 4 to 6 weeks postoperatively.

A tissue expanderlike device was designed by one of the members of this department in cooperation with the orthodontics department for correction of the cleft lip-nose deformity.[28] We believe that it eliminates many problems associated with surgery. Its application is simple and is not discomforting for the child or the parents. The length of the columella can be adjusted by increasing or decreasing the application period. An example of this device in use is shown in Figure 8–13.

Maxillary Orthopedic and Orthodontic Management

As stated earlier, we recently have had the help and collaboration of the dental school. The following section is contributed by Ayhan Enacar, Ph.D.

In the treatment of cleft lip and palate patients, we support the principle of early maxillary orthopedic treatment in terms of efficacy. We prefer to initiate this therapy as early as possible.

The following are our goals for early maxillary orthopedic treatment:

1. Prevention of displacement of maxillary segments.
2. Repositioning of the abnormally positioned maxillary segments into proper alignment.
3. Establishment of a proper skeletal base for surgical correction of soft tissues.
4. Establishment of ideal conditions for the growth of the maxillary segments.

When the maxillary segments are not displaced, we maintain the position of the segments by using a passive

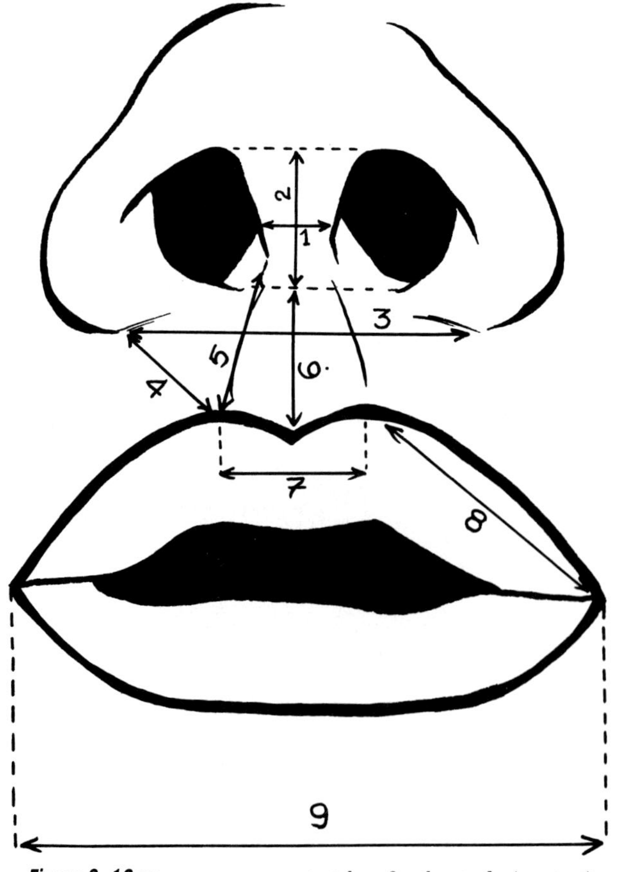

Figure 8–12 Nine measurements taken for the study (see text).

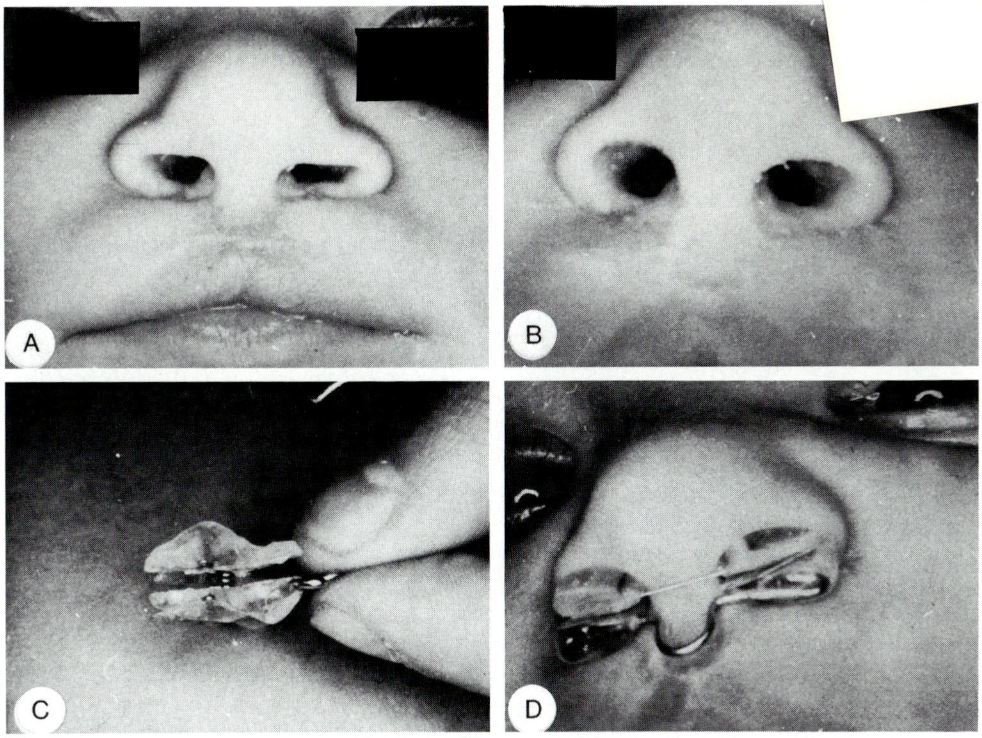

Figure 8–13 Patient with bilateral cleft lip who underwent correction using a tissue expanderlike device designed by Erk-Enacar. *A*, View of nasal deformity following bilateral cleft lip repair. *B*, Nasal deformity corrected by using tissue expanderlike device. *C*, Lateral view of tissue expander prosthesis. *D*, Application of prosthesis.

acrylic appliance. On the contrary, when the segments are displaced, we employ corrective methods according to type of malposition found.

We utilize Hotz's "selective grinding plate" in patients with complete unilateral cleft lip and palate when rotation of the maxillary segments results in overexpansion of the maxilla and an abnormal cleft width. Application of these plates enables us to direct these segments into their proper positions (Fig. 8–14). In unilateral cleft lip–palate cases we no longer use extraoral elastic bands.

In patients with complete bilateral cleft lip and palate, we apply expansion plates to improve collapsed lateral maxillary segments, a common finding. When premaxillary protrusion is not severe, we use light-pull, extra-

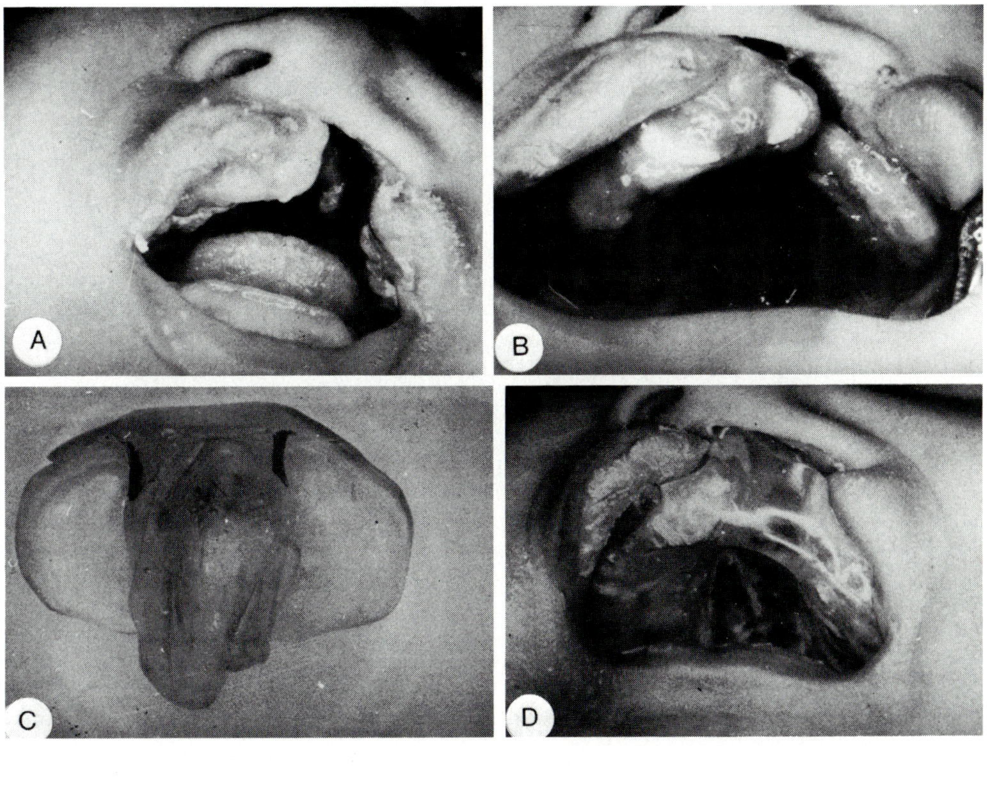

Figure 8–14 *A* and *B*, Complete unilateral cleft lip patient treated with the Hotz selective grinding plate. *C* and *D*, Shaded area indicates where the appliance has been ground progressively.

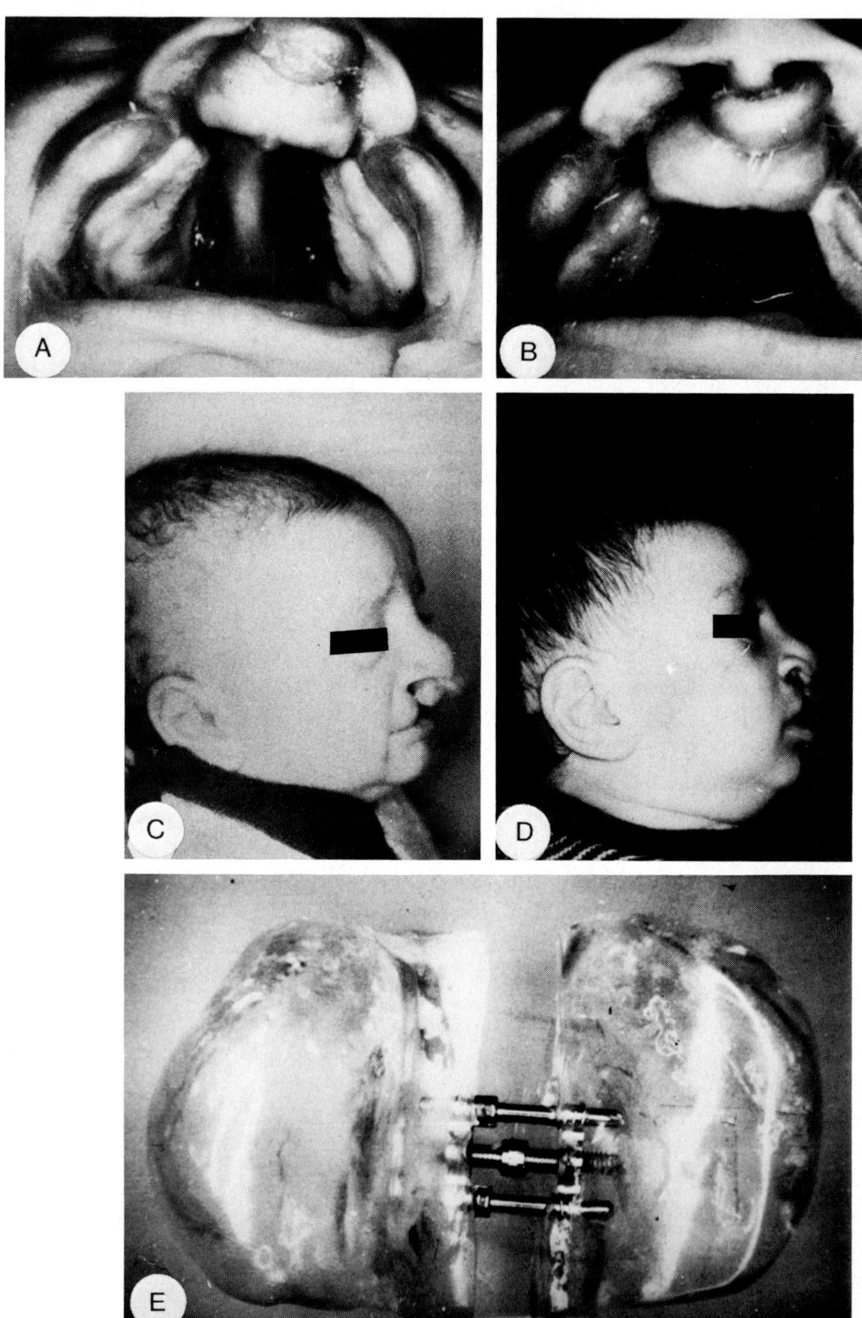

Figure 8–15 *A* and *B*, Bilateral cleft lip and palate patients treated by a combined application of an expansion plate and extraoral elastic bands. *C* and *D*, Pre- and post-treatment profile changes. *E*, Expansion plate used in the patient.

oral elastic traction to reposition the segments (Fig. 8–15).

The quad-helix expansion appliance is used postoperatively to treat maxillary expansion. We also utilize the Hickam or Delaire-type maxillary protraction headgear to stimulate development of the maxilla. Figure 8–16 shows a patient wearing this device who was operated on elsewhere.

Currently, we defer postsurgical orthodontic treatment until 12 years of age because of the difficulties in retention and the long duration of the treatment period. A major problem in the treatment of cleft lip and palate deformities in Turkey is the low ratio of orthodontists to the patient population. In addition to this, the geographic and socioeconomic conditions of the country do not allow us to follow-up such patients.

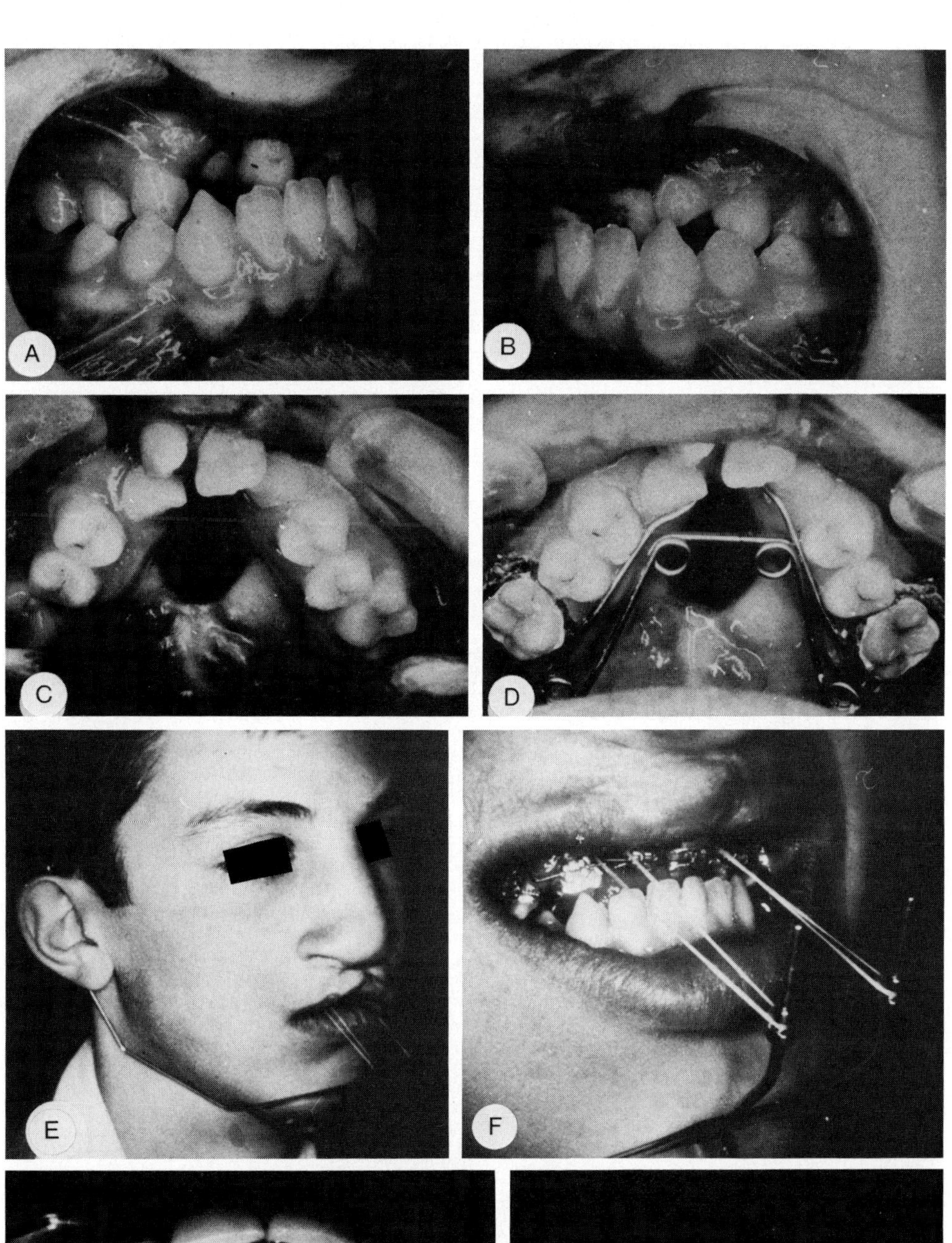

Figure 8–16 *A–C*, Occlusion in a 14-year-old patient with bilateral cleft lip and palate displaying maxillary collapse, an oronasal fistula, and maxillary retrusion. *D*, Quad-helix appliance. *E* and *F*, Hickman maxillary protraction head gear. *G* and *H*, Treatment completed with prosthesis.

References

1. Sabuncuoglu, S: Cerrahiyet al-Haniye Paris: Les Editions Roger Dacosta, 1960 (Paris, Bibliotheque National, Suppl Turc, 693:27, Le Premier Manuscript Chirurgical Turc, p. 23.)
2. Gursu KG, Hoffman S: Problems in reconstruction of a short columella. Plast Reconstr Surg 33:182, 1964.
3. Gursu KG: Dudak damak yariklarinin siniflandirilmasi. Ankara Univ Tip Fak Dis Hekimligi Bulteni-Plastik Cerrahi Ozel Sayisi. Cilt:1, Sayi: 4, 1966.
4. Gursu KG: Median cleft deformity. Trans Fourth Int Cong Plast Reconstr Surg, Rome, October, 1967.
5. Gursu KG: Dudak damak yariklarinin siniflandirilmasi ve Tedavisi. Istanbul Univ Dis Hekimligi Fakultesi Dergisi. Cilt:3 Sayi:1, 1968.
6. Gursu KG: Median cleft deformity. Hacettepe Bull Med/Surg 1:3, 1968.
7. Gursu KG: A statistical report on cleft lip and cleft palate deformities in Turkey. Hacettepe Bull Med/Surg 7:2, 1974.
8. Gursu-Hazarli KG: Analysis of the cleft lip and palate cases in Hacettepe University Medical School (report of 22 years). Presentation at the State of the Art Conference on Multidisciplinary Management of the Unilateral Cleft Lip and Palate, Iowa City, Iowa, October, 1987.
9. Erol OO; Gursu KG: Dudak yarigi (primer damak yarigi) ile Beraber gorulen ek malformasyonlar. Hacettepe Tip Cerrahi Bulteni. Cilt: 7, Sayi:2, 1974.
10. Erol OO, Gursu KG: Bolumumuzde gorulen dudak yariklarinda etiyolojik bazi faktorlerin klinik arastirmasi. Hacettepe Tip Cerrahi Bulteni. Cilt:7, Sayi:2, 1974.
11. Erol OO, Gursu KG: Millard metodu ile dudak yarigi Tamirinden alinan Sonuclar. Hacettepe Tip Cerrahi Bulteni. Cilt:7, Sayi:3, 1974.
12. Erol OO: Dudak yarigi sorunu. Hacettepe Univ Tip Fak Plastik ve Rek Cer. Uzmanlik Tezi, 1971.
13. Kural N, Tinaztepe K, Saraclar M, et al: Konjenital kalp hastaliklariyla birlikte gorulen ekstrakardiak malformasyonlar. Cocuk Sagiligi ve Hastaliklari Dergisi. Cilt:19, Sayi:4, 1976.
14. Millard DR: Refinements in rotation-advancement cleft lip technique. Plast Reconstr Surg 33:26, 1964.
15. Millard DR: Cleft Craft: The Evolution of Its Surgery. Boston: Little, Brown, 1980.
16. Gursu KG, Erol OO: Bilateral dudak yariklarinin onariminda modifie yeni bir yontem. Hacettepe Tip Cerrahi Bulteni. Cilt:7, Sayi:4, 1974.
17. Peet E: The Oxford technique of cleft palate repair. Plast Reconstr Surg 28:282, 1961.
18. Erk Y: Fare embriolarinda cortison, dexamethazon, endantoinle damak yarigi meydana getirilmesi. Hacettepe Univ Tip Fak Plast ve Rek Cer. Uzmanlik Tezi, 1973.
19. Gursu KG: Hamartoma of the soft palate. Hacettepe Bull Med/Surg 7:1, 1974.
20. Erol OO, Gursu KG: Velo-farengeal yetmezlige bagli konusma bozukluklarinin farengeal flap ile Tedavisi. Hacettepe Tip Cerrahi Bulteni. Cilt:7, Sayi:3, 1974.
21. Erk Y: Embriyolojik donemde prostaglandinlerin damak fuzyonuna etkileri. Hacettepe Univ Tip Fak Plast ve Rek Cer. Docentlik Tezi, 1977.
22. Erk Y: The effects of prostaglandins on the development of cleft palate in mice embryos. First prize, Plastic Surgery Education Foundation scholarship contest (Investigator Class), Am Coll Surg Surgical Forum Vol. XXXIII pp. 576–579, 1982.
23. Celebi C: Normal ve dudak yarigi onarimi yapilmis kisilerde parsiyel burundudak olcumlerinin Millard yontemi acisindan degerlendirilmesi. Hacettepe Univ Tip Fak Plast ve Rek Cer. Uzmanlik Tezi, 1979.
24. Barutcu A: Yarik dudak burnu onariminda Millard ve Dibbell yontemlerinin karsilatirilmasi. Hacettepe Univ Tip Fak Plast ve Rek Cer. Uzmanlik Tezi, 1983.
25. Uysal A: Iki tarafli dudak yarigi burun deformitesi onariminda Cronin ve Millard yontemlerinin degerlendirilmesi. Hacettepe Univ Tip Fak Plast ve Rek Cer. Uzmanlik Tezi, 1984.
26. Kivanc O: Yarik dudak burun deformitesi primer onariminda Millard ve Skoog yontemlerinin karsilastirilmasi. Hacettepe Univ Tip Fak Plas ve Rekonstruktif Cer. Uzmanlik Tezi, 1985.
27. Ozgur F: Tam damak yariklarinin onarimindan sonra yeni kemik olusumunun radyolojik ve sintigrafik olarak incelenmesi. Hacettepe Univ Tip Fak Plast ve Rek Cer. Uzmanlik Tezi, 1987.
28. Erik Y, Spira M, Enacar A, Gürsu KG: Tissue expander for short columella: A new nonsurgical approach to cleft lip nose deformity. Presentation at the State of the Art Conference on Multidisciplinary Management of the Unilateral Cleft Lip and Palate, Iowa City, Iowa, October, 1987.

CHAPTER 9

Multidisciplinary Management of Cleft Lip and Palate in Łódź, Poland

Wiesława Perczyńska-Partyka and Julia Kruk-Jeromin

The rehabilitation of children born with cleft lip and palate involves the participation of many specialists because of the multiplicity of anatomic and structural changes and the variety of functional problems associated with these changes. Specialists participating in cleft treatment may work independently or as part of a team. Our experience indicates that a consolidated team located within one health center is the best option for effective organization of multidisciplinary treatment and productive implementation of the management principles designed by the members of the cleft team. The presence of all cleft team members within one center facilitates comprehensive planning for each patient, taking into consideration the recommendations of each specialist. With this arrangement the specialists are able to perform periodic examinations, charting the patient's growth, development, and treatment progress. Furthermore, consultation and discussion among specialists can take place on a daily basis so that no important changes concerning the patient and his treatment are overlooked.

The well-organized cleft palate team interacts closely throughout the entire treatment and rehabilitative period. Having all specialists based at one center is beneficial for the patients and their families as well because time, energy, and travel costs are saved. Furthermore, greater interaction between families and treatment specialists is promoted, which seems to alleviate problems caused by psychological distress.

In 1962, the first center for congenital maxillofacial deformities in Poland was initiated by Bardach, who at that time was chairman of the Department of Maxillofacial Surgery at the Medical Academy of Łódź. Later, this department was divided into the Department of Plastic Surgery (chaired by Bardach) and the Department of Maxillofacial Surgery (chaired by Perczyńska-Partyka). Currently, the Department of Plastic Surgery is headed by Kruk-Jeromin. The Center for Congenital Maxillofacial Deformities remains within the Department of Plastic Surgery.

Since 1972, the activity of the center has been expanded to include treatment of patients with congenital deformities other than clefts.[1–6] During the past 25 years, over 3300 children with cleft lip and/or palate deformities have been treated at the center. Each year approximately 150 new cleft patients are added to the center's registry.

Analysis of the patients treated in our center shows that clefts occur more frequently in males than in females and that the incidence of clefts is higher on the left side than on the right. Unilateral cleft defects are more common than bilateral deformities. In 18% of our patients, clefting coincided with at least one other congential defect. The patient's family histories confirmed a hereditary factor in 24% of cases. On further investigation of these cases, no other causes that could be associated with the development of clefting were found. According to our observations, the fact that a pregancy was the first or a subsequent one had no influence on the incidence of clefting.

Cleft lip only or cleft lip and alveolus was observed in 20% of our patients, of whom 4% had bilateral defects. Cleft lip, alveolus, and palate occurred in 57% of the patients, including 6% who had bilateral defects. Children with a cleft palate constituted only 23% of our patients.

The organization of multidisciplinary treatment of children with clefts is based on a precisely executed information system between the neonatal wards and the Center for Congenital Defects. Each newborn with a deformity in Łódź and its surrounding regions is reported to the center within 24 hours after birth. Thus, all newborns in the area are automatically referred to the center for management. The center designates a nurse specialist or a physician, in special cases, to inform the parents and medical personnel about the special care needed—especially feeding techniques—and the plan for multidisciplinary treatment.

The infant's initial visit to the center is scheduled for the second or third week of life. During the first visit, precise etiopathogenetic data and information concerning the development of the child are obtained from the parents. Next, the child is examined by specialists including a pediatrician, surgeon, and orthodontist. An individualized course of treatment is planned, taking into consideration the type and severity of the cleft as well as the physical and psychological development of the patient.

Stages of Multidisciplinary Treatment

The general schedule of treatment can be divided into five stages, which begin at birth and continue until the patient is approximately 16 years of age. Patients are under the care of a pediatrician throughout this period. As treatment progresses, the roles of some specialists are more dominant than others. The five stages of multidisciplinary treatment are:

1. Presurgical orthopedic treatment, from 3 weeks of age.
2. Surgical treatment. Cleft lip repair is done at 6 months of age.
3. Orthodontic treatment.
4. Surgical treatment. Cleft palate repair is done at 18 to 24 months of age.
5. Phoniatric, orthodontic, and surgical treatment. Correction of secondary lip and/or nasal deformities, correction of skeletal deformities, and pharyngeal flaps.

Stage I

During the time preceding cleft lip repair, the pediatrician takes care of the infant by tracking his or her growth and development and preparing the infant for surgery.[7, 8] When presurgical orthopedic treatment is indicated (particularly in cases of patients with complete unilateral cleft lip, alveolus, and palate), the orthodontist starts treatment when the infant is 2 to 3 weeks old. At this time, the goal of orthodontic treatment is to reposition the maxillary segments and create an alveolar arch that is as normal as possible. Treatment also focuses on stimulating growth of the maxillary segments, especially at the margins of the cleft. During this period of orthodontic treatment prior to surgery, periodic examinations are performed jointly by the orthodontist and the surgeon. The patient's overall progress is evaluated, and the optimal time for surgery is planned.

Since 1965, an individual vestibulopalatal appliance, designed by Perczyńska-Partyka, has been used at our center.[1, 6, 9] The appliance consists of a vestibular plate joined to a palatal plate with steel wire. This appliance redirects the position of the maxillary segments and stimulates their growth. In addition to these advantages, this orthodontic appliance plays the role of an obturator, separating the oral and nasal cavities and greatly improving the conditions for feeding and breathing. The palatal plate also prevents the tongue from entering the palatal cleft. Since pressure from the tongue may prevent approximation of the maxillary segments, separation of the tongue from the cleft using the palatal appliance improves the alignment of the segments. Furthermore, the appliance prevents development of inflammatory diseases of the upper respiratory tract and middle ear and precludes hyperplastic changes in the nasal and nasopharyngeal cavities. Presurgical orthopedic treatment, in conjunction with use of the vestibulopalatal appliance, improves the position of the maxillary segments, narrows the distance between the alveolar segments, improves the position of the skeletal platform for the alar base, and improves the overall conditions for lip and nose repair (Figs. 9–1, and 9–2).

Children who are referred too late for presurgical orthopedic treatment undergo cleft lip repair without the benefits of orthodontic preparation. Nevertheless, a well-executed, precise surgical procedure often results in aesthetic and functional results that are no different from those seen in infants who undergo presurgical orthopedic treatment. This observation has suggested that well-designed comparative studies are needed to re-evaluate critically the role and advantages of presurgical orthopedic treatment.

Stage II

Cleft lip repair, in our opinion, is an essential element in the overall treatment of this congenital defect. Seem-

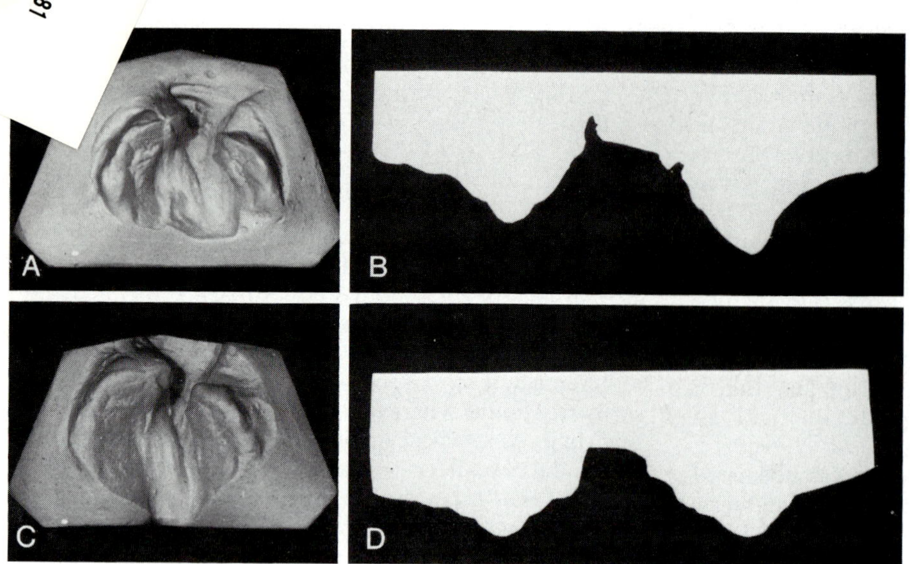

Figure 9–1 Presurgical orthopedic treatment. *A* and *B*, At 3 weeks of age. *C* and *D*, At 3 months of age.

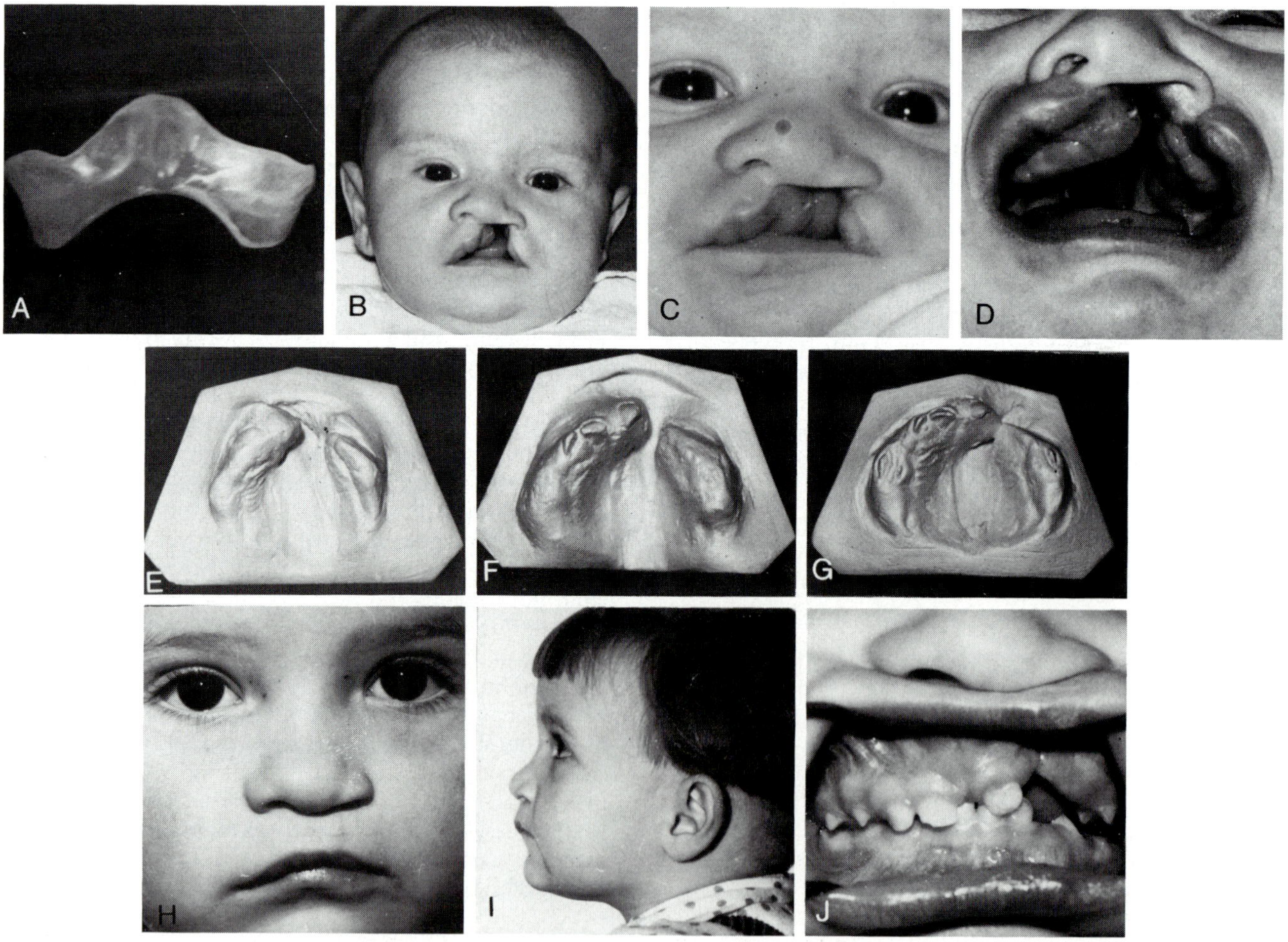

Figure 9–2 *A*, Individualized vestibular-palatal appliance designed by Perczynska-Partyka. *B–D*, Complete unilateral cleft lip, alveolus, and palate at age 3 months. *E–G*, Changes in position of the maxillary segment following presurgical orthopedic treatment at 6 months of age. *H–J*, At age 3 years following lip and palate repair.

ingly not a complicated procedure, cleft lip repair requires vast surgical experience, extensive knowledge of the anatomy and developmental disorders of the midportion of the face, and a thorough understanding of the influence of the reconstructed lip on the underlying maxillofacial skeleton. Much controversy surrounds the decision of when to perform cleft lip repair. Determining the optimal time to operate is important to the final result. At our center, the recommendations of all specialists involved in treatment of the cleft patient are considered; however, we have found that 6 months of age is generally the most appropriate time for cleft lip repair in light of the needs of the patient before and after surgery.

During the infant's first 6 months of life, proper pediatric care ensures that the child will undergo surgery in optimal condition. By the time the infant is 6 months old and ready for cleft lip repair, the maxillary segments are properly aligned as a result of orthodontic treatment, and typically there is new bone formation at the cleft margins of the alveolar processes. These conditions allow the surgeon to produce a better aesthetic and functional result. Reconstruction of the lip without excessive tension promotes normal healing, harmonious growth of the midportion of the face, and development of normal occlusal relations.

The technique of choice for reconstruction of the cleft lip also remains a subject for discussion. The large number of methods available and the continuous development of new techniques reflects the difficulties encountered by surgeons performing this operation. Review of the literature indicates that many surgeons prefer a technique based on precise calculation of measurements and design. Creation and transposition of tissue flaps to obtain symmetry and an acceptable shape of the lip are also important components of the technique. Knowing how to design, create, and transpose various flaps of tissue contributes to lip repair that produces very good results.

During the past 25 years, we have used various surgical techniques for cleft lip repair. The choice of repair depends on the form of the cleft, its severity and width, and the position of the maxillary segments (Figs. 9–3 to 9–8).[10] Our basic goal is to reconstruct the lip with all of its anatomic features, including the Cupid's bow, sulcus, and a continuous orbicularis oris muscle. At the time of primary lip repair we also attempt to reconstruct the floor of the nose and correctly position the columella and alar base. We do not use bone grafting of the alveolar cleft during primary repair.

In both partial and complete narrow clefts, we most frequently use the single triangular flap repair described by Tennison and Randall.[11, 12] The double triangular flap technique designed by Bardach and Perczyńska-Partyka[1, 6, 13, 14] is used for complete wide clefts. During the 1960s, we used the LeMesurier technique;[15] however, we abandoned this procedure because of unfavorable late results. In recent years, we have frequently used the rotation-advancement technique designed by Millard[16] for all but very wide clefts.

Many serious problems are associated with bilateral

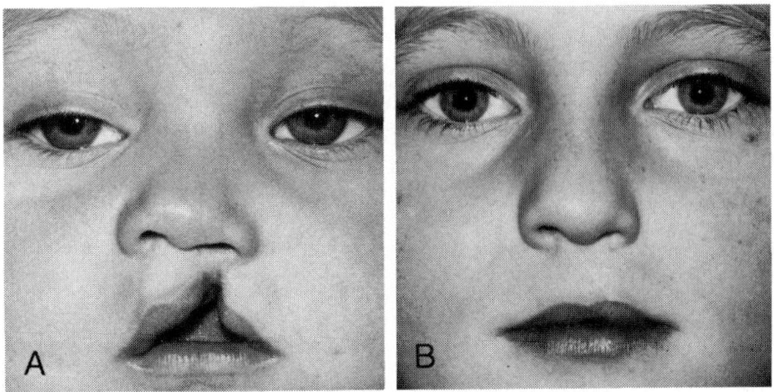

Figure 9–3 *A*, Partial unilateral cleft lip. *B*, Subsequent to repair using the Tennison technique.

clefts of the lip. We routinely use the entire prolabium for reconstruction of the midportion of the lip. The lip is repaired in two stages with 6 to 8 weeks between operations. We are conservative in our management of the protruding premaxilla—that is, we use orthodontic treatment only with no surgical intervention. In patients with partial bilateral clefts, lip repair typically is performed in one stage (Fig. 9–9). Reconstruction of the full thickness of the vermilion in the midsection of the lip involves rotating flaps of the vermilion from the lateral lip portions. Lengthening of the columella and narrowing of the nasal tip is performed when the child is of preschool age.

In the 1960s, a large series of cleft patients with complete unilateral and bilateral clefts of the lip, alveolus, and palate had primary lip repair performed simultaneously with primary soft palate repair according to the technique described by Schweckendiek.[17] When

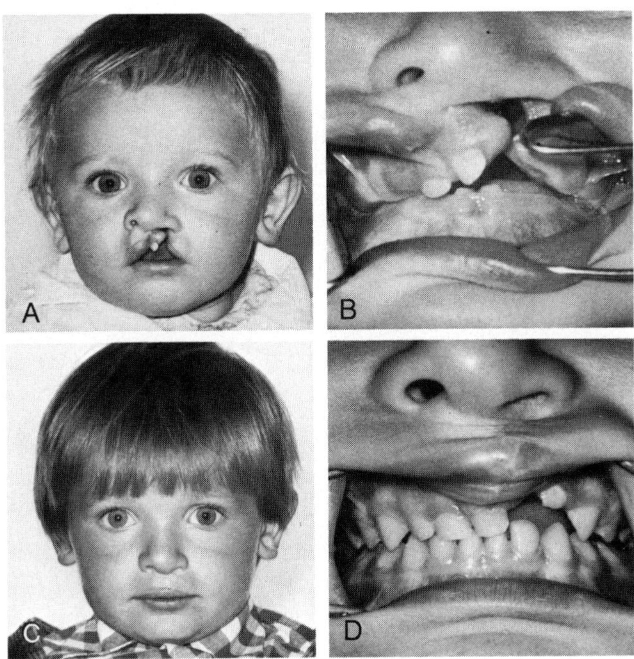

Figure 9–4 *A* and *B*, Complete unilateral cleft lip and alveolus. *C* and *D*, After repair using the Millard technique.

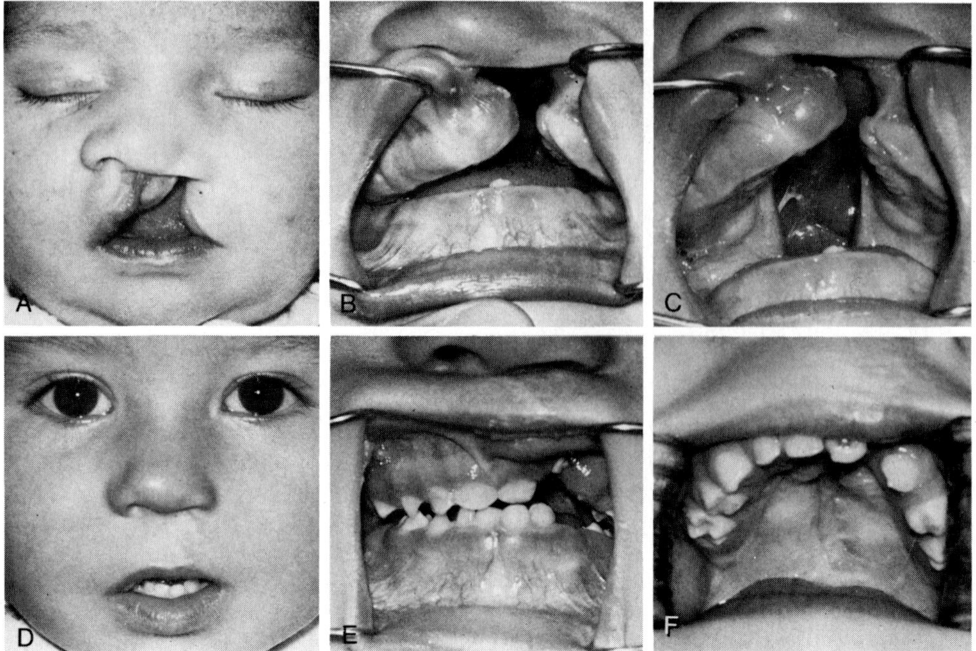

Figure 9–5 A–C, Complete unilateral cleft lip, alveolus, and palate. D–F, After repair using the Bardach technique.

patients were selected to undergo this procedure, determination of the palatal index (ratio of the width of the palate to the length of the palate) was most important. This technique has since been abandoned owing to the poor speech results and discomfort caused by the opening left in the hard palate for several years.

Stage III

This stage of multidisciplinary treatment is defined by the time that elapses between lip repair and palate repair. During this stage, the patient is followed by the surgeon, orthodontist, and pediatrician. The surgeon observes changes in alignment of the maxillary segments and in the width of the cleft to help determine the optimal time for surgery. The pediatrician follows the general growth and development of the patient and prepares him for the next major operation—palatoplasty. The orthodontist plays a less active role in treatment during this stage. We believe that subsequent to lip repair the reconstructed orbicularis oris muscle func-

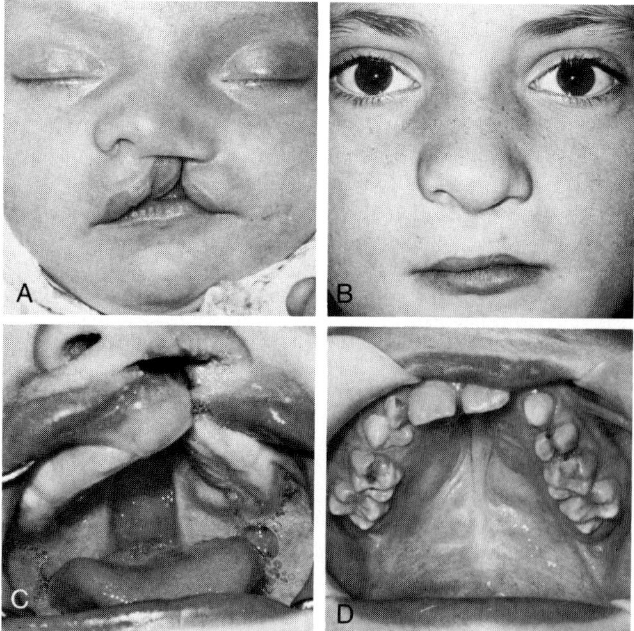

Figure 9–6 Complete unilateral cleft lip, alveolus, and palate. A and B, Lip repair using the Perczynska-Partyka techique. C and D, Two-flap palatoplasty using Bardach's approach.

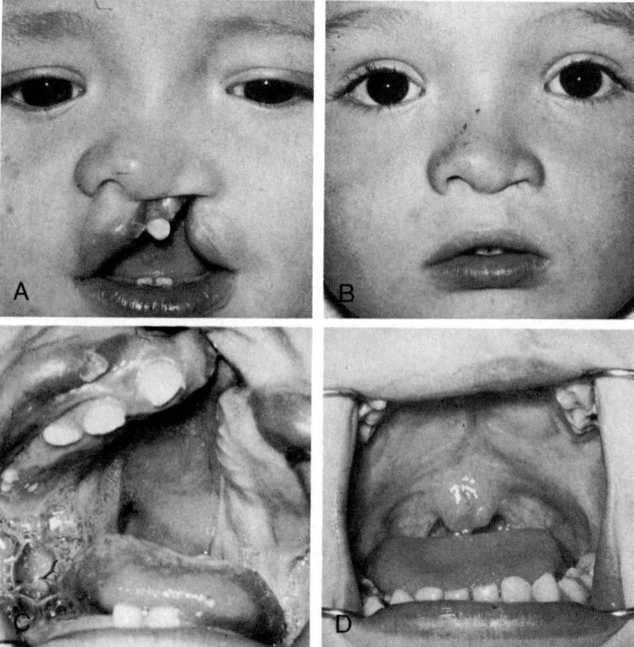

Figure 9–7 Complete unilateral cleft lip, alveolus, and palate. A and B, Lip repair using Millard's technique. C and D, Palate repair using the two-flap palatoplasty.

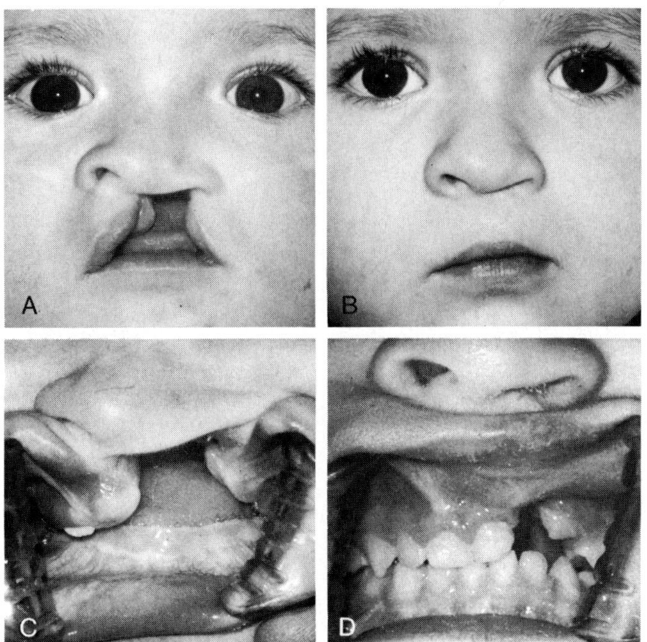

Figure 9–8 Complete unilateral cleft lip, alveolus, and palate. *A* and *B*, Cleft lip repair using Tennison's technique. *C*, Extremely wide alveolar cleft. *D*, Occlusion following lip and palate repair.

tions like an orthodontic appliance worn 24 hours a day. A properly repaired lip has a beneficial effect on facial growth and occlusion. Conversely, a lip repaired with excessive tension or with poor alignment of the orbicularis oris muscle may be detrimental to facial growth and occlusion.

Stage IV

There are many differing opinions concerning the optimal time for cleft palate repair. Our experience has shown that cleft palate repair performed between 18 and 24 months of age enables the surgeon to create an adequate velopharyngeal mechanism for normal speech production. Only in children with Pierre Robin syndrome is palate repair delayed until approximately 3 years of age.

In surgical management of cleft palate, we attempt to reconstruct a long, mobile soft palate with its posterior

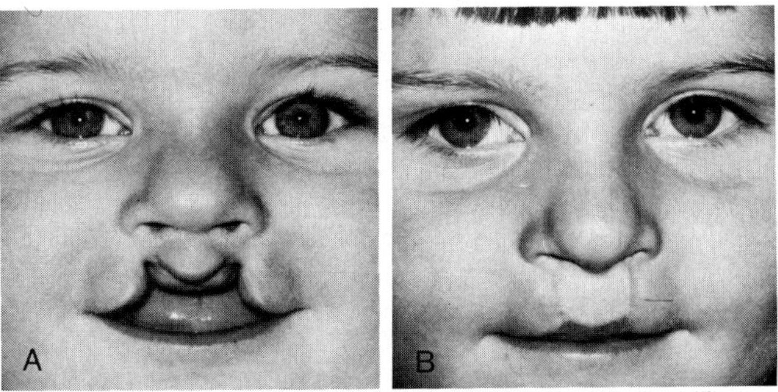

Figure 9–9 *A*, Partial bilateral cleft lip and alveolus. *B*, Subsequent to lip repair using Millard's technique.

edge close to the posterior pharyngeal wall. This narrows the velopharyngeal port during phonation, resulting in more normal speech production. The major highlight of our surgical procedure is two-layer closure of the hard palate and three-layer closure of the soft palate. The surgical procedure is performed according to Veau's design, modified by Bardach.[1, 3, 6, 18] Special attention is given to mobilizing the mucoperiosteal flaps, freeing of the neurovascular bundles, and wide undermining of the mucoperiosteum on the nasal side of the palatal shelves. There is no intervention in the bony structures of the palatal shelves. Furthermore, no grafts of any kind are used for closure of the palatal cleft (Figs. 9–5 to 9–7, 9–10 to 9–12).

In cases of marked underdevelopment of the soft palate we create a superiorly based pharyngeal flap during the palatoplasty operation (Fig. 9–13). Marked underdevelopment is defined as (1) a distance between the posterior edge of the soft palate and the posterior pharyngeal wall that is greater than 2 cm; (2) a minimal Passavant's pad; and (3) weak lateral movement of the pharyngeal walls. To avoid airway obstruction following this surgery, the pharyngeal flap is created no wider than 1.5 cm.[1, 18, 19] The success of palatoplasty and pharyngoplasty is evaluated by an otolaryngologist, phoniatrician, and surgeon. To test further the efficacy of this procedure we perform an analysis of articulation and measure air flow during phonation using a manometer.

Stage V

Stage V is the longest stage of multidisciplinary treatment. The main role in this stage is played by the orthodontist and phoniatrician; however, the surgeon may correct secondary defects during this period. The orthodontist continues to manage occlusion, usually with a screw-type acrylic appliance. The phoniatrician offers speech therapy if needed; however, for the majority of patients, speech is judged to be within normal limits.[1, 18] If indicated, a pyschologist or even a psychiatrist may be consulted to treat the patient.

Despite the constant progress of surgical techniques and better cooperation among specialists, optimal aesthetic and functional results are not always obtained. We have observed that secondary deformities may appear or increase in severity around the time of puberty. Secondary maxillofacial deformities are more difficult to treat than primary ones. This is true of both soft tissue and skeletal defects. Secondary defects may affect the lip, nose, palate, occlusion, maxilla, and mandible. The type and extent of the secondary deformity are related to the primary defect and its treatment. Insufficient planning, poor surgical technique, postoperative complications, and inadequate orthodontic and/or speech treatment have a definite influence on the outcome of primary procedures.

Procedures used to correct secondary deformities on the lip may include scar revision, partial or total reoperation, augmentation of the vermilion, and correction of asymmetries. On the palate, secondary procedures

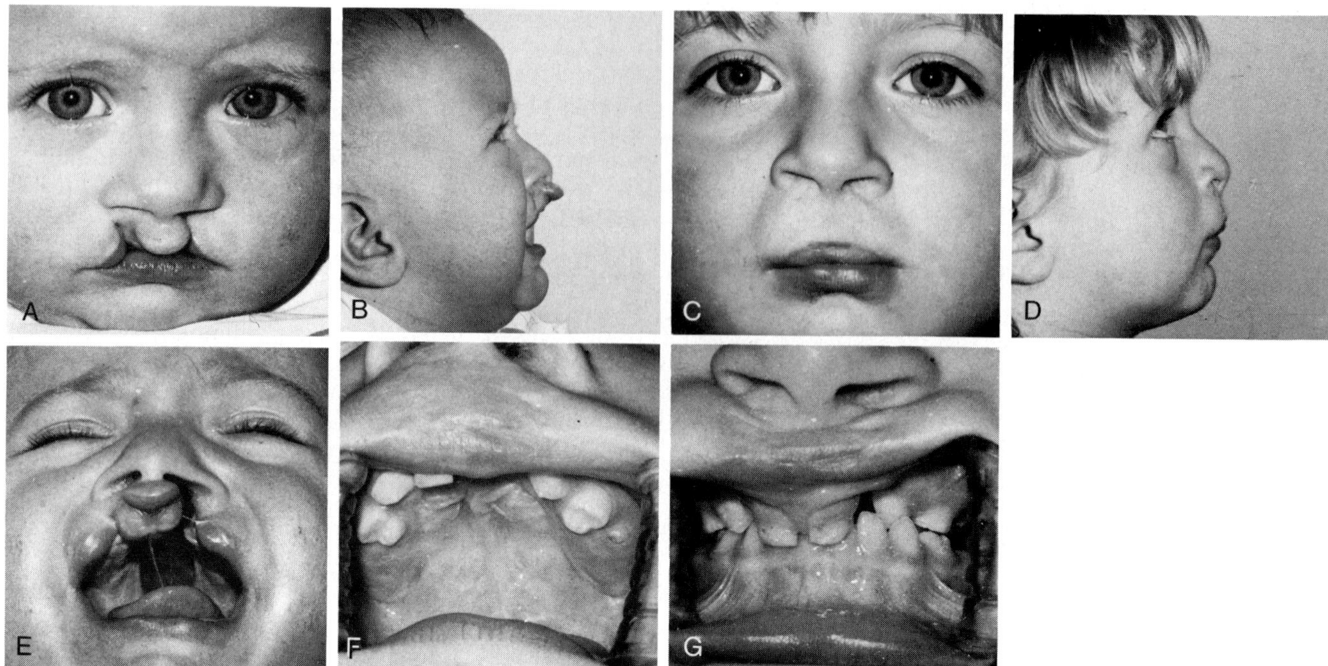

Figure 9–10 *A* and *B*, Asymmetric bilateral cleft lip, alveolus, and palate. *C* and *D*, Following lip repair using the Tennison technique. *E* and *F*, Palatal cleft before and following two-flap palatoplasty. *G*, Occlusion subsequent to lip and palate repair.

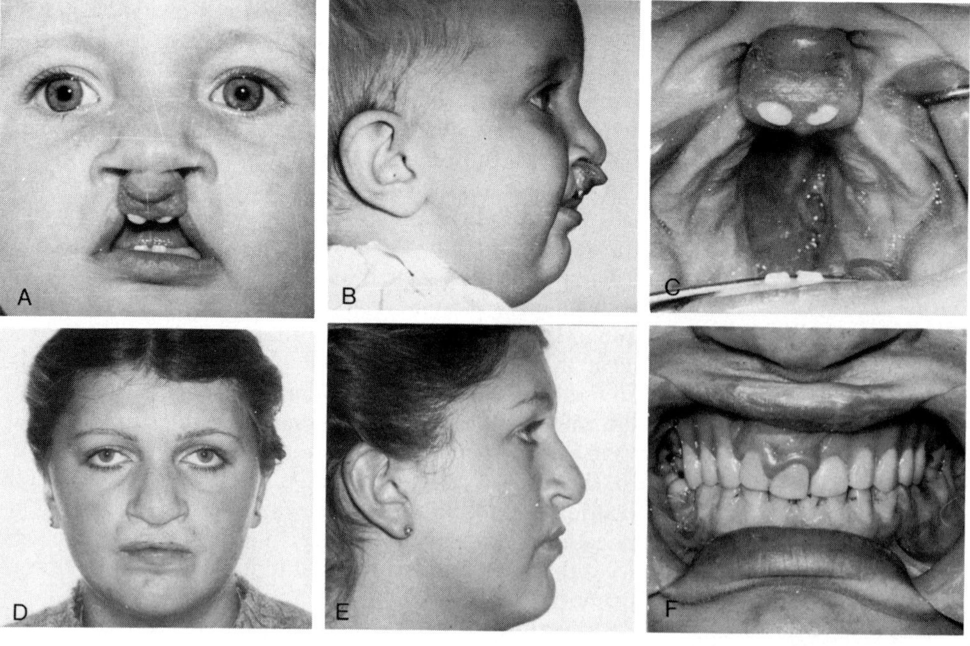

Figure 9–11 *A–C*, Complete bilateral cleft lip, alveolus, and palate. *D–F*, Following lip repair using the Perczynska-Partyka technique, two-flap palatoplasty, and orthodontic-prosthetic treatment.

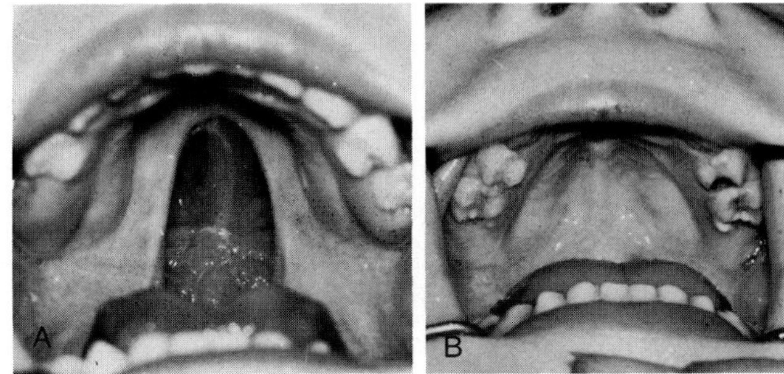

Figure 9–12 *A*, Cleft of the soft palate and partial cleft of the hard palate. *B*, Following two-flap palatoplasty.

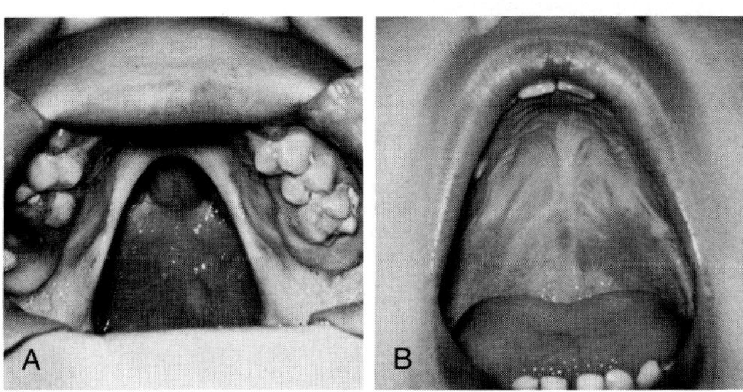

Figure 9–13 *A*, Complete cleft of the palate only. *B*, Following palatoplasty and a superiorly based pharyngeal flap.

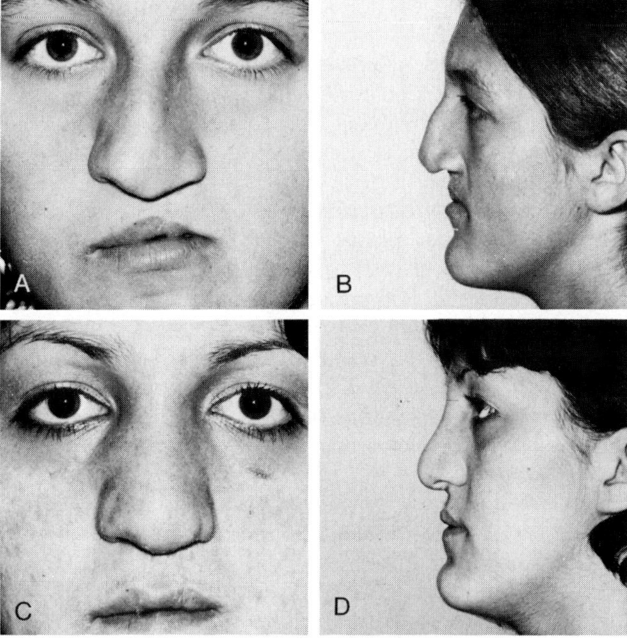

Figure 9–14 *A* and *B*, Secondary deformity of the lip and nose following repair of the unilateral cleft lip and palate. *C* and *D*, Subsequent to correction of the lip and nose deformity.

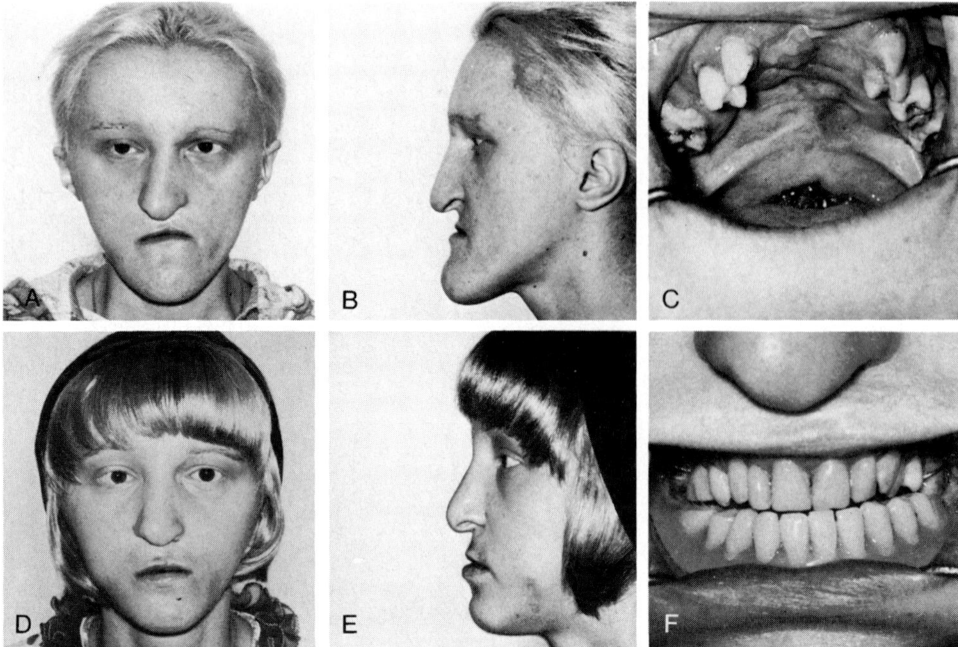

Figure 9–15 *A–C*, Secondary facial deformity associated with complete unilateral cleft lip, alveolus, and palate. *D–F*, Following correction of the nose, lip, and mandible and prosthetic treatment.

may include repair of oronasal fistulas and pharyngoplasty. Nasal deformities may require correction of the nasal tip, ala, septoplasty, and/or total rhinoplasty including osteotomies. Osteotomies on the maxilla or mandible depend on changes in the skeletal structures (Figs. 9–11, 9–14, 9–15).

Results of Multidisciplinary Treatment

Results of treatment of children with clefts continue to improve due to the long-term experience gained by our cleft team, earlier multidisciplinary interventions, and more active cooperation of the parents. The best results are obtained in management of unilateral cleft lip, alveolus, and palate. In these patients, very good or good aesthetic and functional results are achieved in 75% of cases. However, nasal deformities, especially flattening of the ala, may persist. Correction of the nasal deformity associated with unilateral cleft lip, alveolus, and palate is very difficult.

Results of palatoplasty in patients with cleft palate only and unilateral cleft lip and palate are rated as very good or good in 95% of cases. Of this 95%, 50% of patients have speech production judged to be within normal limits. In the remaining patients (45%), marked improvement of speech production is seen following speech therapy. Only 5% of patients require secondary palatoplasty to correct oronasal fistulas or velopharyngeal incompetence.

Various degrees of malocclusion are found in all patients with alveolar clefts. Treatment results depend on the method of lip surgery and orthodontic intervention. Almost normal occlusion is obtained in only 50% of patients with unilateral clefts who undergo routine orthodontic treatment.

The worst aesthetic and functional results are seen in patients with bilateral clefts of the lip and palate. In this group, very good or good results of multidisciplinary treatment are obtained in only 20% of cases.

References

1. Bardach J: Rozszczepy Wargi Górnej i Podniebienia. Warszawa: Państwowy Zakład Wydawnictw Lekarskich, 1967.
2. Bardach J, Januszewska W, Partyka W, et al: Działalność ośrodka leczenia wad rozwojowych twarzy od 1.01.1962 do 1.07.1964 r. Czas Stomat 18:927, 1965.
3. Perczyńska-Partyka W: Nowoczesne poglady na leczenie rozszczepów wargi górnej, wyrostka zebodołowego i podniebienia. Czas Stomat 26:547, 1973.
4. Goldstein J, Kruk J, Januszewska W: Complex treatment of cleft lip and cleft palate. Acta Chir Plast 22:134, 1980.
5. Kruk-Jeromin J: Zespołowe leczenie dzieci z rozszczepami wargi i podniebienia. Chir Szczek Twarz Stomat 1:69, 1985.
6. Perczyńska-Partyka W: Rozszczepy wargi, wyrostka zebodołowego i podniebienia. In Kryst L (ed): Chirurgia Szczekowo-twarzowa. Warszawa: Państwowy Zakład Wydawnictw Lekarskich, 1987.
7. Januszewska W: Przygotowanie dziecka z rozszczepem wargi i podniebienia do zabiegu operacyjnego. Czas Stomat 17:931, 1965.
8. Januszewska W: Rola lekarza pediatry w leczeniu dzieci z rozszczepem wargi górnej i podniebienia. Czas Stomat 12:641, 1968.
9. Perczyńska-Partyka W: Przedoperacyjne leczenie rozszczepów wargi, wyrostka zebodołowego i podniebienia płytka przedsionkowo-podniebienna własnej modyfikacji. Czas Stomat 20:1055, 1967.
10. Kruk-Jeromin J: Experiences in surgical treatment of unilateral cleft lip. Read before the State-of-the-Art Conference on Multidisciplinary Management of the Unilateral Cleft Lip and Palate, Iowa City, Iowa, October 14–17, 1987.
11. Tennison CW: The repair of unilateral cleft lip by the stencil method. Plast Reconstr Surg 9:115, 1952.
12. Randall P: A triangular flap operation for the primary repair of unilateral cleft of the lip. Plast Reconstr Surg 23:331, 1959.
13. Bardach J, Salyer K: Surgical Techniques in Cleft Lip and Palate. Chicago: Year Book, 1987.
14. Perczyńska-Partyka W: Wlasny sposób operacji jednostronnego rozszczepu wargi górnej. Czas Stomat 18:969, 1965.
15. LeMesurier AB: A method of cutting and suturing the lip in the treatment of complete unilateral clefts. Plast Reconstr Surg 4:1, 1949.
16. Millard DR, Jr: Cleft Craft: The Evolution of Its Surgery. I. The Unilateral Deformity. Boston: Little, Brown, 1976.
17. Schweckendiek H: Zur zweiphasigen Gaumenspalten-operation bei primarem Velumverschub. Fortschr Kiefer Gesichtschir 1, 1944.
18. Buehl A, Kruk J: Leczenie chirurgiczne rozszczepów podniebienia z zastosowaniem płata gardłowego. Czas Stomat 30:177, 1977.
19. Tronczyńska J, Perczyńska-Partyka W: Wskazania do płastyki platem podniebienno-gardłowym w leczeniu rozszczepów podniebienia. Czas Stomat 18:947, 1965.

CHAPTER 10

Multidisciplinary Management of Cleft Lip and Palate in Brno, Czechoslovakia

Ladislav Barinka and V. Simecek

Early Lip Repair: Barinka Technique

A modification of Veau's lip repair was applied in principle at the Department of Plastic Surgery in Brno from 1949 to 1974 in 3800 patients with cleft lip. Twenty-five years of monitoring these patients revealed satisfactory functional results. However, the aesthetic results did not meet our expectations. A section of the upper lip as complex and dominant as the philtrum and its typical prominence, the Cupid's bow, could not be reconstructed satisfactorily using Veau's method.[1] The height of the lip on the cleft side was shorter owing to scar contracture that pulled the vermilion upward. This "curtain" of red vermilion unfavorably influenced the general aesthetic impression of the lip.

In our department, the main focus was to continue the Czechoslovak tradition in the treatment of clefts, which we believe to be rich and of long standing. Barinka established the principle of restoring lip function, not concentrating exclusively on the aesthetic effect, which might change during the patient's continued development. He emphasized delicate manipulation of the tissues and their proper functional integration.

Barinka's main principles are as follows:

1. To maintain the continuity of the orbicularis oris muscle and align it in a horizontal position.
2. To reconstruct, during primary lip repair, a deep sulcus to achieve good fixation of orthodontic appliances when indicated.
3. To partially correct the nasal deformity during the primary lip repair procedure. This includes closure of the nasal floor and creation of symmetrical nostrils. A vomerine flap has been found to be most useful in this respect (Figs. 10–1 and 10–2).

A mucosal flap from the vomer is used to close the nasal floor and the anterior portion of the hard palate. Incisions along the vestibular fold, along which the flap is turned, ensure proper shaping of the alar base and shift the musculature medially, allowing suturing of all layers without tension. Another advantage of this method, in comparison to Veau's, is the perfect conformation and resulting shape of the lip, eliminating the undesirable prospect of secondary corrections, which previously were very frequent.

Early Repair and Secondary Management

The surgical technique used for reconstruction of cleft lip and palate is not discussed as frequently as the timing of the surgery, which always has been of prime interest to the various specialists involved in treatment of cleft patients. There is pressure from parents as well to have the defect corrected as soon as possible. It has become apparent that treatment of orofacial clefts cannot be left to one branch of medicine but must involve a multidisciplinary approach. Satisfactory results depend not only on the extent of knowledge in each of these specialties but also on perfect coordination and collaboration among the specialists.

Specialists in facial growth have studied and evaluated the effects of surgical procedures, restoration of function, and effects of orthodontic treatment on the development and growth of the maxillofacial complex. Longitudinal studies have shown that restitution of normal function is important to further growth. Conclusions drawn by specialists in the evaluation of growth processes and disturbances have been used by plastic surgeons in Brno to establish new criteria for lip and palate repair.

The primary lip repair operation, previously carried out at 6 to 12 months of age, is now performed at 3 months of age. The change in the timing of procedures was implemented in October, 1985. Present evaluation of the results of these early lip repair operations indicates that results are much improved over those seen in patients who were operated on at later ages. The lip is aesthetically pleasing and functionally adequate. The alveolar process of the maxilla is properly aligned and rounded, and the maxillomandibular occlusal relationship is correct. Facial aesthetics are improved by better nasal symmetry, including correct positioning of the alar base on the cleft side. We did not observe maxillofacial growth inhibition or collapse of the maxillary segments. Thus, we concluded that "heavy-handed" surgery has been a major contributing factor in the incidence of anteroposterior maxillary growth inhibition and secondary maxillofacial deformities.

Another important topic of discussion is timing of cleft palate repair. Dentists prefer that palate repair be undertaken after the completion of skeletal growth, which contradicts the demands of the phoniatrician, who would like the palate to function appropriately early, that is, by 1 year of age. Schweckendiek proposed a compromise in which the soft palate was sutured at an early stage and repair of the hard palate was postponed until the age of 12 years or later.[2, 3] Some specialists have indicated that this method does not benefit the growth and development of the maxilla and speech as Schweckendiek suggests.[4–7]

Palate repair used to be performed at 3 years of age. However, since the end of 1985, we have operated on the palate at the age of 12 to 18 months. We believe that healing is better at this age than in 3-year-olds, and we have observed no growth inhibition in the 18-month

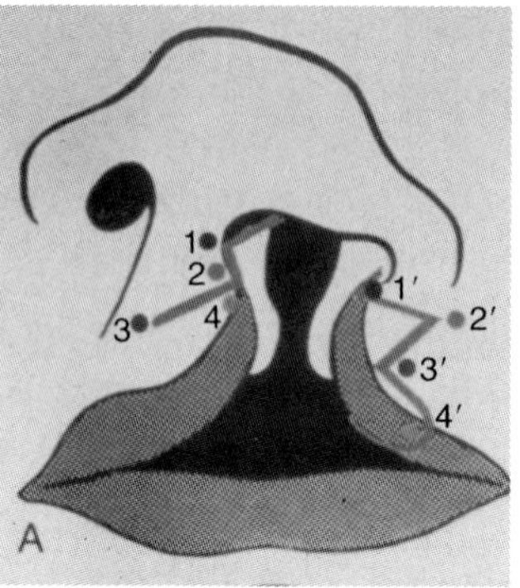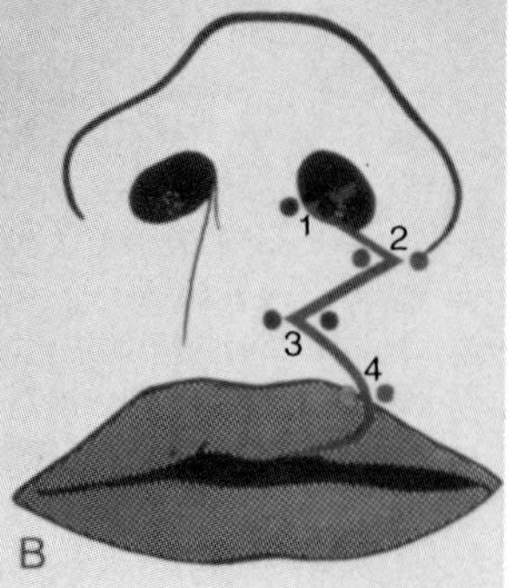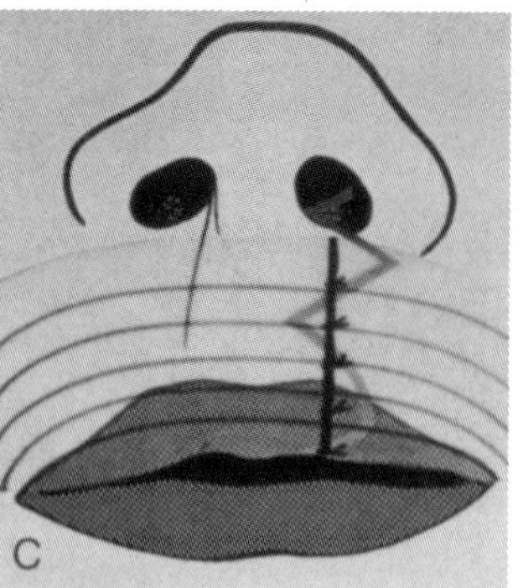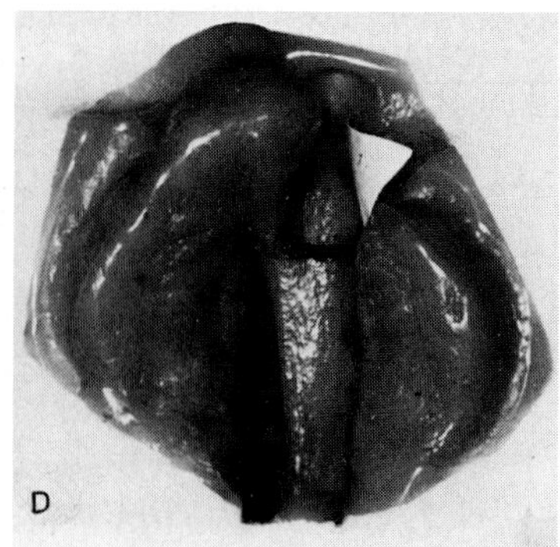

Figure 10–1 *A* and *B*, Design of the triangular flap technique for lip repair used (Barinka's technique). *C*, Suturing of the lip musculature. *D*, Vomerine flap: design, extent, and transposition.

period following the operation. Speech development was found to be close to normal. Speech pathologists found no indication for pharyngoplasty, even in patients with the more severe forms of clefts. In some patients (when indicated), we operated on both the lip and the palate simultaneously at the age of 6 to 12 months.

Currently, the number of early lip repair patients in our clinic has reached 55. The oldest child studied was 3 years 3 months of age. Based on a follow-up period of 24 months, maxillofacial growth has been observed to be normal in this patient. Early palate repair has been performed 53 times, the longest period of follow-up being 32 months. There have been 17 simultaneous lip and palate repairs. The longest follow-up period in these patients has been 28 months (Figs. 10–3 and 10–4).

Early Cleft Lip and Palate Repair: Speech Results

The development of speech in children with cleft lip and/or palate may be characterized by rhinophonia, articulation defects, and facial grimaces. Early operation on the cleft palate has the following advantages:

1. Avoidance of speech defects, that is, rhinophonia. In patients operated on at 3 years of age or later, rhinophonia did not improve after surgery. Correction of speech takes several years of cooperative work with the patient by the speech pathologist and speech therapist.

2. Avoidance of palatal dysfunction. Cleft palate repair performed in patients 3 years old or older cannot ensure proper function and results in an improperly functioning velopharyngeal mechansim. Massage of the soft palate is not always effective, and pharyngoplasty may be indicated.

3. Aural pathology, mostly middle ear infection, is avoided. We recommend and consider early palatal surgery, by 24 months of age at the latest, an effective means of prevention of aural pathology in children with cleft palate. Infections of the middle ear occur mainly after the age of 3 years. Hearing impairment due to middle ear infection may cause speech delays. Our data indicated that the following percentages of patients had some degree of hearing loss secondary to middle ear infection: slight deafness, 31%; medium deafness, 25%; serious deafness, 10%

4. Mimic defects and facial grimaces do not develop.

Secondary Correction of the Cleft Lip

Secondary correction of the cleft lip builds on the foundation established by restoration of lip function and by maximum preservation of the growth and development of the affected region. These are always impaired, and it is essential to tackle the effects of impairment on the patient's defect. The intensity of these effects depends on the extent of the cleft. In less severe clefts, orthodontic measures to correct dentition may be suffi-

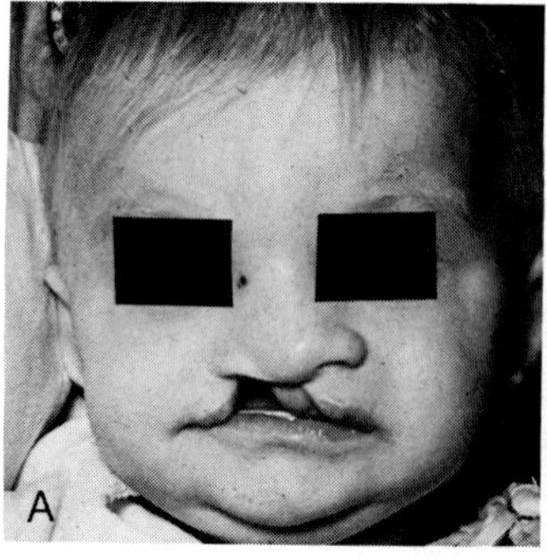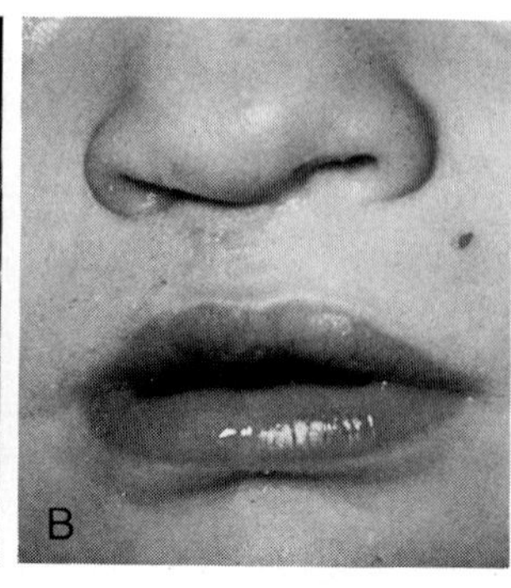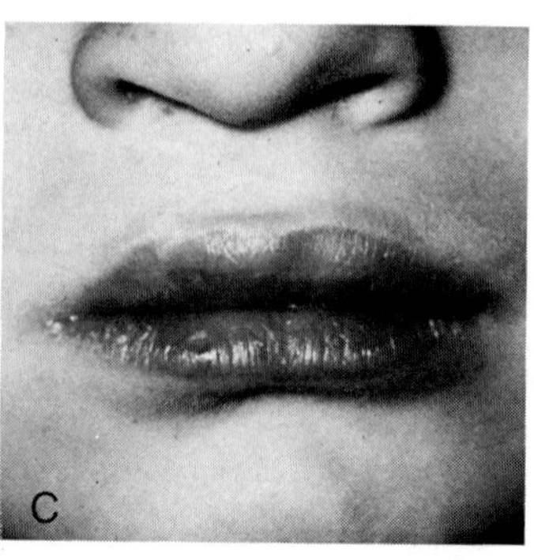

Figure 10–2 *A*, Complete right unilateral cleft lip, alveolus, and palate. *B* and *C*, Six months and 14 years after cleft lip repair using Barinka's technique.

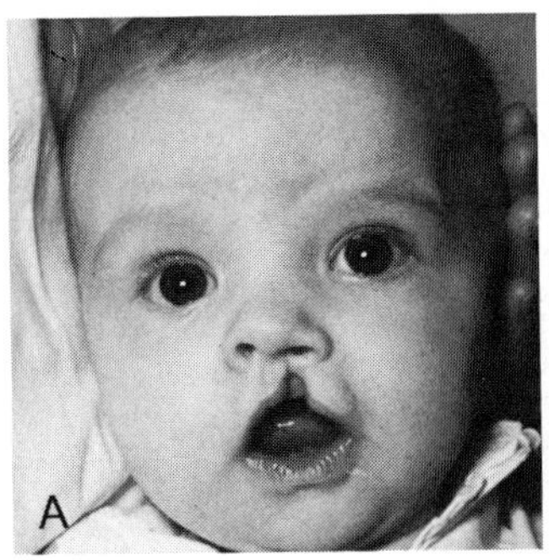 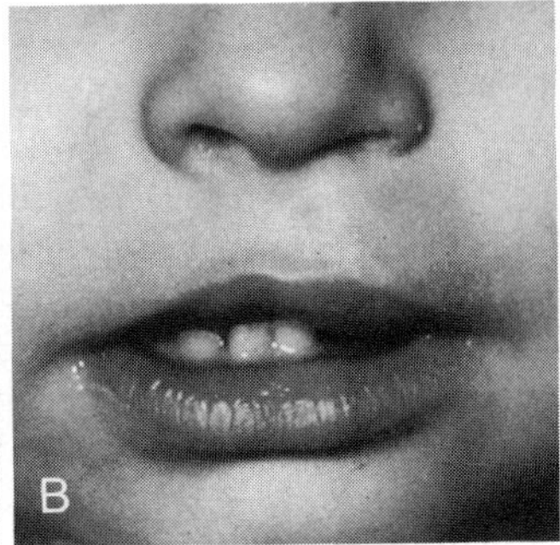 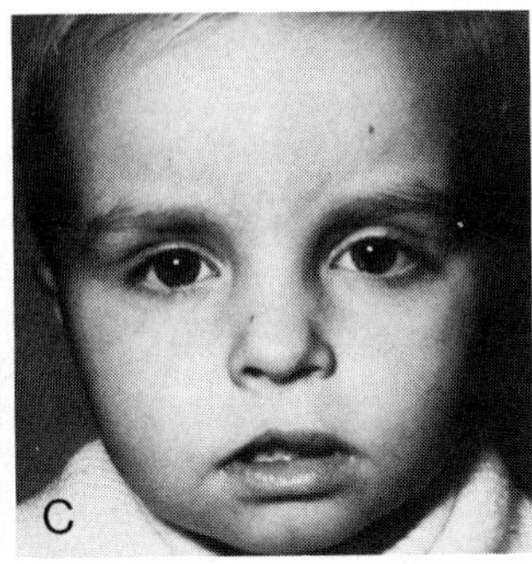

Figure 10–3 A, Incomplete cleft lip on the left side. Three months of age. *B* and *C,* Result 3 years later following use of Barinka's technique.

cient; however, in severe clefts, complicated orthognathic procedures may be indicated for correction of soft and bony tissues.

Soft Tissue

During primary lip repair, we intentionally leave a slightly excessive length of the lip on the affected side to compensate in advance for less intensive growth on that side. Later correction may be needed. The sulcus may need to be deepened or nasolabial fistulas may need to be closed. Correction of the nose during primary lip repair usually precludes the need for later secondary repair.

Alveolar Process

Tissue defects are invariably met with in the hard tissues of the maxillary process. These not only are detrimental to maxillomandibular relationships and further development of the dentition as a whole but also impair the development of teeth, which are supported by the alveolar process. One of the most serious possible consequences is deformation of the canines, which, because of the defect in the alveolar bone, cannot properly erupt, remaining in infraocclusal and mesial inclination. Thus, the teeth that are of most value in stomatologic prosthetics lose much of their quality as pillars.

Maxilla and Maxillary Dental Arch

The maxilla is the structure most affected by the cleft. Its growth and development are affected in different degrees of severity, which cannot always be attributed to surgical intervention. The maxillomandibular mal-

alignment in the frontal and lateral regions of the dental arch, owing to the underdeveloped maxilla, is further complicated by retroinclination of the anterior segment of the alveolus and its dentition. Left untreated, this condition may, through the mandibular orthopedic forces, aggravate factors that are detrimental to growth and development. A specific problem is the development and growth of the premaxilla in cases of complete bilateral clefts. Anterior growth and irregular development of the premaxilla are uninhibited in the prenatal period; however, this changes after cleft lip repair. The muscular pressure of the repaired lip leads to retroinclination of the tooth germs in the premaxilla. This excessive pressure also may lead to curvature of the vomer, which results in serious distortion in the occlusal plane and major supraocclusion of the alveolar process and the teeth of the premaxilla.

Dentition

The dentoalveolar shelf, which provides a foundation for the deciduous and permanent dentition, cannot escape the effects of cleft deformities. The extent of the defects covers a broad spectrum, from irregular shape and size of teeth to numerous anomalies. Planning the course of treatment in such cases forms the most intimate point of contact in multidisciplinary treatment.

Therapeutic Aims

Careful decisions about the optimal goals of treatment maximize the functional and aesthetic results in patients with clefts. The good of the patient is the first priority, and this principle must guide the efforts of all specialists participating in treatment of cleft patients.

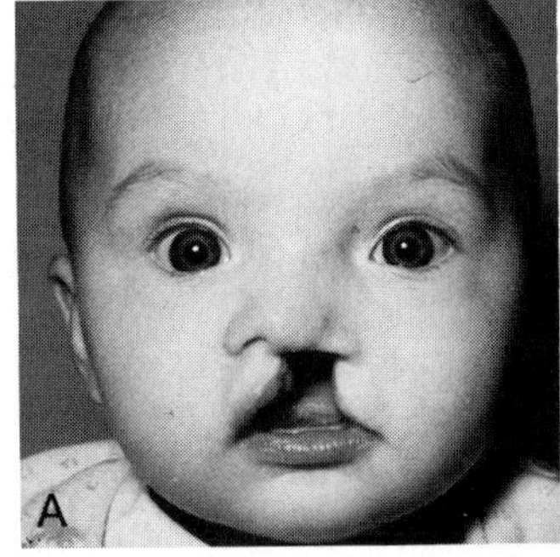 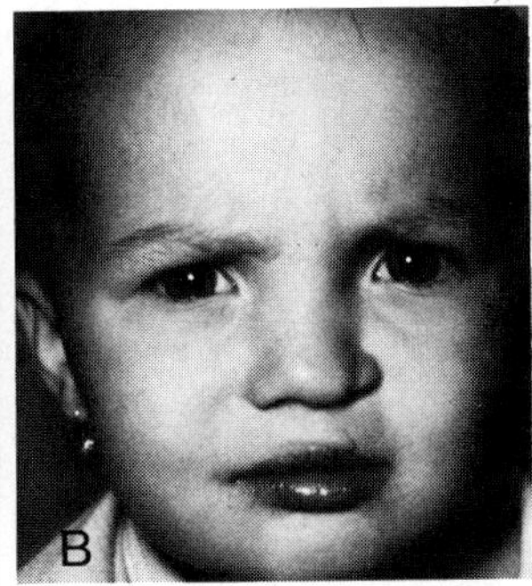 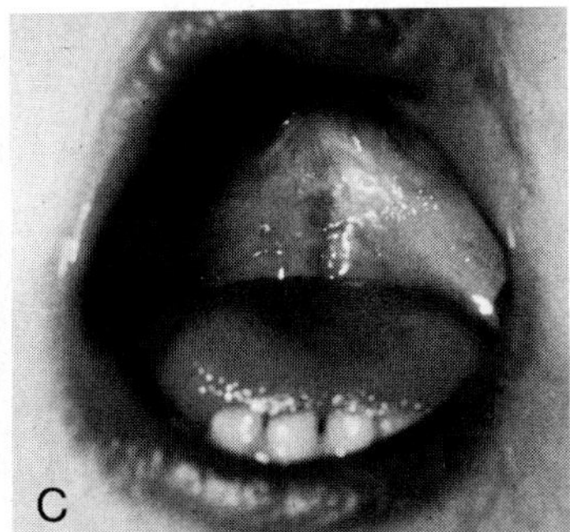

Figure 10–4 A, Wide unilateral cleft lip, alveolus, and palate on the left side. Four months of age. *B* and *C,* lip and palate 3 years after the operation.

Soft Tissue

In reconstruction of the soft tissues immediately adjacent to the alveolar process, the nasolabial fistula must be closed. Oronasal fistulas in the anterior portion of the palate must always be repaired. The fistula must be closed without creating a bulk of tissue or shallowing the sulcus. Great attention is directed to reconstructing a deep sulcus so that orthodontic and prosthodontic appliances can be used if needed. The fistula is closed using a mucoperiosteal flap transposed from the alveolar process with the incision carried up to the first molar on the cleft side. We have found this method satisfactory, because it does not affect tooth eruption or disturb the periodontal system.

Alveolar Process

The alveolar process forms the basis for the anchorage of the dentition. The alveolar defect associated with a cleft usually impairs tooth development. One of the most serious problems is deformation of the canines, which may not erupt in their proper position. Thus, the teeth that are most valuable are functionally useless.

Reconstruction of the alveolar process sets the conditions for further improvement of the maxillofacial system affected by the cleft. Its reconstruction is important to facilitate proper growth and development of the maxillofacial region. There are two possible approaches for bone grafting in this area. The first uses a solid graft of cancellous bone. The second approach involves small chips of cancellous bone.

Depending on the specific conditions of the patient, either approach may be indicated. A solid graft is indicated when development of the maxillary dental arch is completed and further growth is not anticipated. In such patients, the bone graft fixes the condition that has been achieved. Cancellous bone chips are used when further development and growth are expected. Following closure of any fistulas, bone chips form the basis of the alveolar bone, allowing development of the dentition to take place in this grafted area. By filling the alveolar ridge with cancellous bone, we create conditions for a mesial shift in the lateral teeth to avoid prosthetic rehabilitation of the dentition. The chief advantage of our approach is that it allows for eruption of the upper canine in the dental arch. Righting of the root restores the canine on the cleft side to the quality of a first-class pillar. Any inclusion of teeth between the permanent upper first incisor and the canine is advantageous, even if not permanent, since it defers the need for a definitive denture.

Dentition

The upper second incisors are almost always affected in some way. A frequent finding is anodontia of the second incisors together with supernumerary canines, that is, precanines. However, the first maxillary incisors also are likely to change in shape. These changes affect not only the root section but also the crowns. In planning therapy one must not concentrate on a particular aspect.

The value of a tooth is determined not only by its own morphology but also by its position in relation to the other teeth. The relation to the remaining dentition of the anterior part of the maxilla (whether the second incisors or supernumerary anterior teeth in patients with unilateral clefts, or the anterior teeth in those with bilateral clefts), morphology, and the shape and quality of the alveolus are the main criteria used in considering the prognosis.

Decisions must be made not on the basis of the short-term effect but according to the long-term prognosis, particularly for the functional fitness of the dentition. This calls for careful and responsible assessment of the quality of the anterior teeth. On one hand, one must not hesitate to perform extractions or to align the alveolar process when the premaxilla is in extreme protrusion and supraocclusion. On the other hand, full attention should be paid to the preservation even of supernumerary teeth with a well-developed root, good position in the dental arch, and a good quality alveolar process. Current techniques for alveolar bone grafting should be considered among the treatment options.

Timing of Secondary Reconstruction

Period of Deciduous Dentition

Following primary reconstruction of the lip and palate and throughout the period of the deciduous dentition, no orthodontic treatment is indicated. We prefer not to disturb the development of the jaws. During this time, the speech pathologists and speech therapists work on promotion of good speech habits.

Period of Early Mixed Dentition

Surgical intervention during this period depends on favorable conditions for the further development of the germs of the second incisors and supernumerary canines. Subsequent to eruption of the first incisors, the quality of the second incisors and any precanines that might take over their function is considered. Where necessary conditions exist—that is, good quality root formation and suitable positioning—cancellous bone chips are implanted to ensure the eruption of precanines in place of second incisors. If the quality of the germs of these teeth is inadequate, a decision is deferred.

Period of Late Mixed Dentition

During this period, a strategy must be formulated for the frontal part of the dentition. Eruption of the upper premolars and the start of eruption of the upper canines is assumed. At the last examination, the possibility of preserving teeth that have been formed between the first incisors and the canines was considered and rejected. The aim of treatment is either to wait for the eruption of the permanent canines so that they may take the place of the second incisors, or to reduce the gap between the canines and the first incisors with a dental appliance.

Period of Permanent Dentition

Treatment in this period is reserved for patients who were first examined at a time when the optimal period for treatment had passed. Although there is a minimum number of such patients, they must be taken into account. Their treatment generally is orthodontic-surgical in nature. For closure of the defect in the alveolar process, a solid cancellous bone graft is used and the dentition is reconstructed using a flat-anchored fixed bridge or a removable prosthesis.

Management of the Premaxilla in Bilateral Clefts

Therapeutic Goals

Functionally and aesthetically, one of the most disturbing structures in patients with bilateral cleft lip and palate is the prominence of the premaxilla with retroinclination and supraocclusion of the first maxillary incisors. Other striking characteristics are the short columella, flat nasal tip, broad nostrils, and deficiency of the upper lip in its midportion.

The aim of current orthodontic surgical treatment is preservation of the maximum number of teeth in the maxillary arch. The *biologic quality* of the maxillary incisors in patients with bilateral clefts is, in most cases, however, unfavorable. They may be atypical in shape, with dysplasia of the enamel, which is susceptible to caries. The malformed roots are short and are set in sockets composed only of a thin bony lamella. Prominence of the premaxilla is partly due to protrusion of the alveolar process, which covers the labially dislocated roots of the first maxillary incisors. By remodeling it, correct anatomical conditions can be restored in the anterior section of the maxillary arch without surgical correction of the basic structure of the maxilla (Fig. 10–5).

Extraction of the upper first incisors, remodeling of the alveolar process of the premaxilla, and closure of the oronasal fistulas allow:

1. Creation of an aesthetically more satisfactory denture.
2. Release of the tension in the upper lip, improvement of its configuration, and creation of closure for the oral cavity.
3. Sagittal growth of the mandible without retroinclination or secondary crowding of the anterior mandibular dentition, which is possible because of the removal of the impediment to growth.
4. Removal of traumatization of the periodontum of the anterior teeth.
5. Improvement of oral hygiene and comfort of the patient by closure of the oronasal fistulas.

Prominence of the premaxilla, which is striking in early infancy, has attracted the attention of plastic surgeons. Retropositioning of the premaxilla has been advocated by some surgeons and orthodontists, whereas excision has been considered detrimental to maxillofacial growth.[8–12] Long-term study of maxillofacial growth of cleft patients revealed a pattern of growth in which there was an uneven intensity with a compensating spurt following operation and a dependence of growth on function. It is our opinion that retropositioning is not necessary because correction of the shape of the alveolar process creates favorable conditions for a dental prosthesis.[13, 14]

On the basis of the dental evaluation of the premaxilla and possible surgical-orthodontic-prosthodontic solutions for the mobile and protruding premaxilla, we designed and introduced a new operative procedure. When considering the best time to perform the procedure, we did not want to disturb the growth and development of the maxilla. Also, we felt it was important to consider not the age of the patient but the stage of growth of the maxilla and its dentition. Some have recommended surgical intervention after 13 years of age.[11, 15] Others believe that the operation should be done during the period of eruption of the maxillary second incisors.[14, 16] We consider the age of 9 to 10 years to be ideal, when for the most part maxillary growth is completed, the maxillary first incisors are fully erupted, and the upper canines have not yet begun to erupt.[13, 17, 18] The condition of the upper second incisors and the presence, shape, and position of supernumerary maxillary canines also are important criteria for deciding the optimal time for the operation.

Operating Procedure and Results

Following is a summary of the steps of our new procedure for management of the protruding premaxilla.

1. The maxillary incisors are extracted along with any supernumerary anterior teeth not suitable for use as pillars.
2. By shortening the alveolar process of the premaxilla, we level the alveolar ridge. By removing some alveolar bone, we can model the labial surface of the

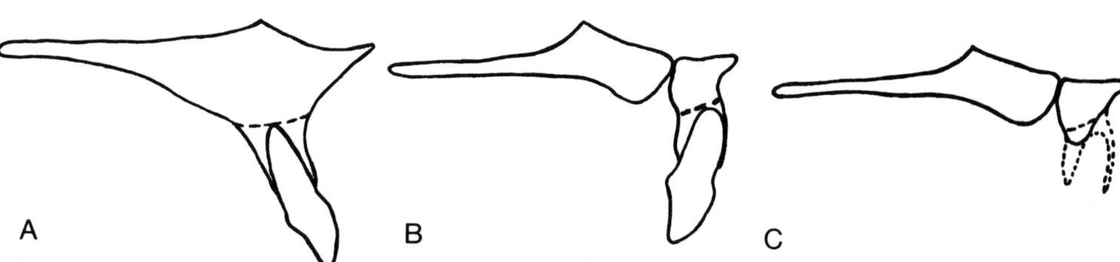

Figure 10–5 *A*, Diagram of normal maxilla. *B*, Cleft maxilla. *C*, Principle of premaxillary correction.

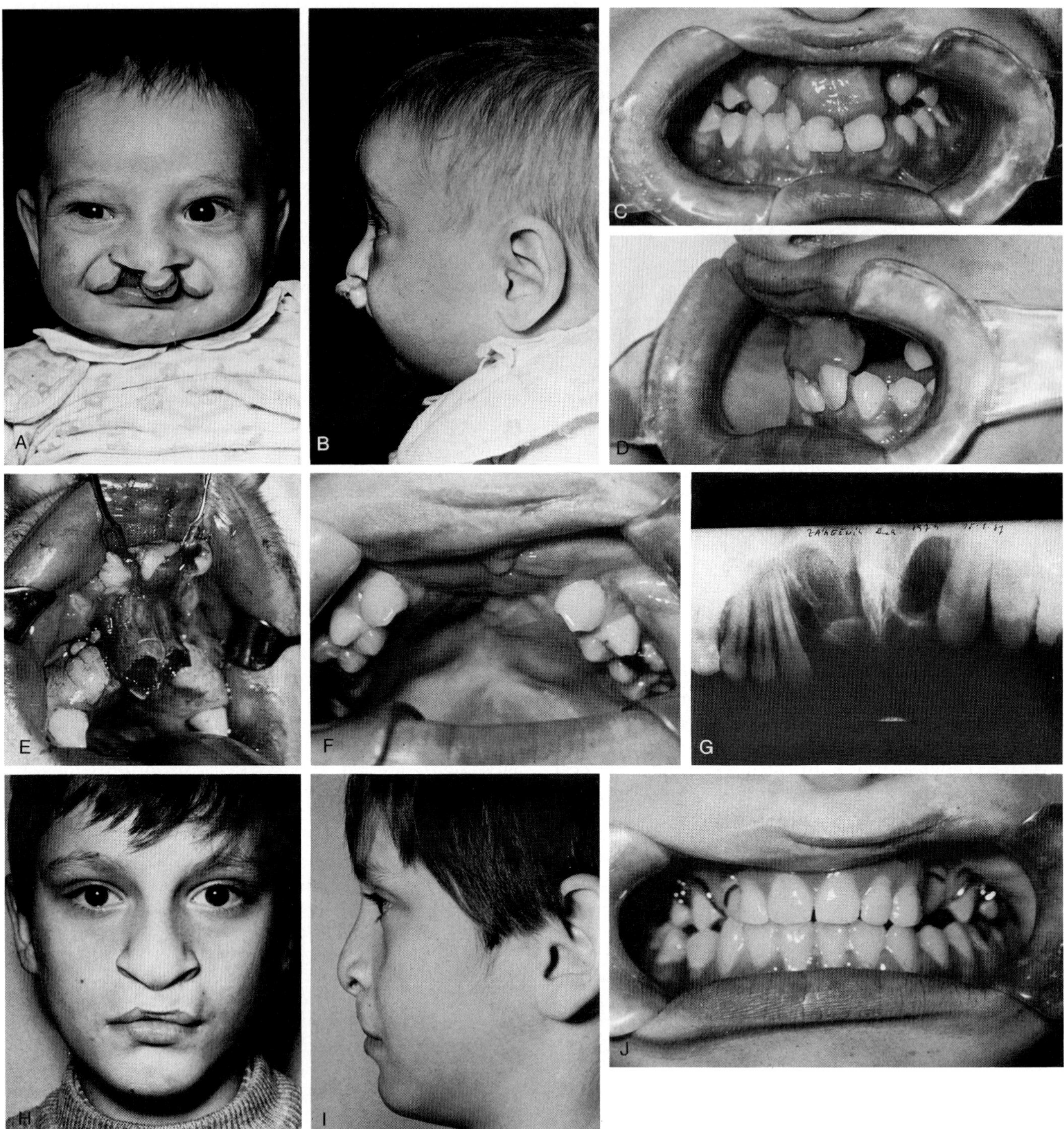

Figure 10–6 *A* and *B*, Complete bilateral cleft prior to operation in 6-month-old infant. *C* and *D*, Condition of dentition at 12 years of age before correction of the premaxilla. *E*, Maxillary incisors are extracted and shortened. Alveolar process of the premaxilla is leveled near the alveolar ridge. *F*, Condition following operation. *G*, X-ray subsequent to operation. *H–J*, Result 6 months following operation with temporary removable denture.

alveolus of the premaxilla to the desired extent. The bone structure of the premaxilla is left in its original state.

3. Mucoperiosteal flaps are used to close the oronasal fistulas. The mucoperiosteum from the palatal surface is used for the nasal lining.

4. Cancellous bone is used to graft the alveolar clefts on each side of the premaxilla.[14, 16, 18]

Our results have indicated that following this operation, all vestibular fistulas were closed in all patients. Oronasal fistulas were closed in 76% of the patients studied. In patients with early mixed dentition, formation of new bone was observed 6 months after surgery. A solid bony bridge had formed across the cleft defect. The mesially inclined germs of the maxillary incisors shifted mesially and straightened up. It was possible to make temporary removable dentures for all patients. At the age of 18 years, the temporary appliances were replaced by permanent bridges. Both temporary and permanent prostheses fulfilled their functional and aesthetic roles well (Fig. 10–6).

Remodeling of the alveolar process of the premaxilla restored the regular anatomic relations in the region of the maxillary alveolar ridge. The excess soft tissue allowed closure of oronasal fistulas with good quality mucoperiosteal flaps. This improved oral hygiene, prevented food from passing into the nasal cavity, and increased patient comfort. The upper lip, which was no longer under tension, had normal tone.

References

1. Veau V: Bec-de-Lievre. Paris: Masson, 1938.
2. Schweckendiek H: Zur zweiphasigen Gaumenspalten-operation bei primaremVelumverschub. Fortschr Kiefer Gesichtschir 1, 1944.
3. Schweckendiek H: Zur Frage der Frish- und Spatoperation der angeborenenLippen-Kiefer-Gaumenspalten. Z Laryngol 30:51, 1951.
4. Fara M, Brousilova M: Experiences with early closure of velum and later closure of hard palate. Plast Reconstr Surg 43:129, 1969.
5. Cosman B, Falk AS: Delayed hard palate repair and speech deficiencies: A cautionary report. Cleft Palate J 17:27, 1980.
6. Jackson I, McLennan G, Scheker L: Primary veloplasty or primary palatoplasty: Some preliminary findings. Plast Reconstr Surg 72:153, 1983.
7. Witzel M, Salyer KE, Ross B: Delayed hard palate closure: The philosophy revisited. Cleft Palate J 21:4, 1984.
8. Fara M, Hrivnakova J: Zkusenosti s chirurgickym zasunovanim mezicelisti u celkovych oboustrannych rozstepu. Rozhledy r Chirurgii 49:276, 1970.
9. Friede H, Pruzansky S: Long-term effects of premaxillary setback on facial skeletal profile in complete bilateral cleft lip and palate. Cleft Palate J 22:97, 1985.
10. Narula JK, Ross RB: Facial growth in children with complete bilateral cleft lip and palate. Cleft Palate J 7:239, 1970.
11. Pruzansky S: Pre-surgical orthopedics and bone grafting for infants with cleft lip and palate: A dissent. Cleft Palate J 1:164, 1964.
12. Zilberman Z, Poulton DR: Identical twins with bilateral and unilateral clefts: A 20-year study. Am J Orthod 86:14, 1984.
13. Johanson B, Ohlsson A, Friede H, Ahlgren J: Secondary bone grafting and prosthetic rehabilitation. A follow-up study of cleft lip and palate patients treated with orthodontics. Scand J Plast Reconstr Surg 8:121, 1974.
14. Wolfe SA, Berkowitz S: The use of cranial bone grafts in the closure of alveolar and anterior palatal clefts. Plast Reconstr Surg 72:659, 1983.
15. Ross RB: The clinical implications of facial growth in cleft lip and palate. Cleft Palate J 7:37, 1970.
16. Boyne PJ, Sands NR: Combined orthodontic-surgical management of residual palato-alveolar cleft defects. Am J Orthod 70:20, 1976.
17. Jarabak JR, Fizzel JA: Technique and Treatment with Light Wire Edgewise Appliances. St. Louis: Mosby, 1972.
18. Turvey TA, Vig K, Moriarty J, et al: Delayed bone grafting in the cleft maxilla and palate: A retrospective multidisciplinary analysis. Am J Orthod 86:244, 1984.

CHAPTER 11

Multidisciplinary Management of Cleft Lip and Palate in Bulgaria

K. Anastasov and E. Georgiev

In the Department of Plastic and Reconstructive Surgery in Sofia (Bulgaria) a total of 1119 children with cleft lip and palate have been treated. Of this total, 731 had cleft lip and palate and 388 had cleft palate only. An assessment was made of the different aspects of the multidisciplinary approach, treatment policy, and associated problems specific to this country. In this chapter, the authors review multidisciplinary treatment of cleft lip and palate in Bulgaria keeping in mind its future organization and development.

Today, there is no doubt that the treatment of cleft lip and palate should be performed by a team consisting of a plastic or pediatric surgeon, orthodontist, and speech pathologist. In some instances, these professionals may be assisted by a psychologist, pediatrician, or social worker. Treatment is begun as early as possible after birth and is considered completed when all aesthetic and functional defects have been corrected. In some cases, the therapeutic steps are complex, and not infrequently, treatment may last 10 to 20 years.

Each specialist participates in treatment; however, during the various phases, one specialist may play a more dominant role. Surgeons definitely play the primary role during lip and palate repair and other surgical corrective procedures. The orthodontist and speech pathologist also may dominate the rehabilitation process. Indeed, many times all specialists may be simultaneously involved.

In our opinion, there are three main issues underlying the management of cleft lip and palate:
1. Prophylactic measures to prevent the birth of children with such malformations.
2. Determination of the optimal age for surgery.
3. Development of a universal protocol for multidisciplinary management of cleft lip and palate.

The great progress of plastic surgery in the last decades, the advances of modern anesthesiology, and the practical implementation of the surgical techniques proposed by Veau,[1] Millard,[2] Tennisson,[3] Wynn,[4] Obukhova,[5] Limberg,[6] and many others, have set forth and emphasized the issues listed above. The qualified and well-trained plastic surgeon uses a surgical technique based on his own experience rather than one based on presentations at meetings or published in the literature.

Clinical Research

The history of cleft lip and palate surgery in Bulgaria dates back to 1895, when a child was operated on with the Giraldes-Tilleaux[7] technique. Thereafter, general surgeons, maxillofacial surgeons, pediatric surgeons, otorhinolaryngologists, and others, based on the experience of various clinics in Europe, introduced the procedures of von Langenbeck,[8] Limberg,[6] Veau,[1] Millard,[2] Kavrakirov,[9] and others. It is very difficult to assess the late results because purposeful follow-up studies on the variables in question have not been carried out in Bulgaria. At the present time, some of these patients have needed corrective operations of the nose, palate, lips, maxilla, and mandible. Since 1944, the health care services in Bulgaria have been free of charge. This has facilitated development of a multidisciplinary approach to the treatment of malformations among newborns, including cleft lip and palate. In the early postwar years, cleft lip and palate repair, as performed by highly qualified plastic surgeons or maxillofacial surgeons, definitely improved the aesthetic and functional results and effectively prevented development of serious secondary postoperative deformities.

The national program for multidisciplinary treatment of cleft lip and palate after World War II up to 1971 was based on the following main principles:

1. Primary lip repair is performed at approximately the sixth month of age.
2. The palate is repaired between 5 and 10 years of age.
3. Orthodontic treatment is conducted in regional dental (stomatologic) clinics.
4. Speech rehabilitation has not been provided because we lack specialized centers for speech pathology that specialize in treatment of cleft palate. Some children have been trained in special schools for general speech disturbances or by their parents after instruction by the surgeon.

The earliest studies on the incidence of cleft lip and palate were performed from 1951 to 1962 (see Table 11–1). Jekov,[10] in 1966, and later Koev,[11] Iovtchev,[12] and others proposed a national program for outpatient care and complete management of cleft lip and palate under the guidance of a maxillofacial surgeon and an orthodontist. The small number of patients per district (there were 30 districts in a population of 9 million, or about 4 patients with clefts per 300,000 patients per year) was the reason the problem was not considered a serious one. For this reason, some of the patients were omitted from systematic follow-up studies. It has been very difficult to obtain objective data on the outcome of multidisciplinary management of cleft lip and palate.

Since 1960, Georgiev[13] has initiated studies of etiologic factors such as vaccination, influenza, use of drugs, exposure to the effect of insecticides, toxicosis, abortion, mental trauma, ionizing radiation factors, and so on. Results have informed and alerted medical workers and future mothers about the potential factors that create favorable conditions for the development of malformations.

In a joint research project with genetic centers in Bulgaria, we investigated the presence of cytogenetically induced chromosomal abnormalities in patients with an isolated cleft, but no correlation was demonstrated. For this reason cytogenetic investigations are performed only in patients with multiple abnormalities. In each child the genealogic tree is studied. Based on our data (Georgiev),[13] 20.6% of patients with cleft lip and palate and 16% with cleft lip only had a positive family history. The incidence of familial inheritance was consistent with the polygenic hereditary theory. In a study covering southwest Bulgaria, a positive familial history was found in 22.9% of the carriers of cleft lip and palate. In a study carried out in Campeche by one of the authors (Anastasov),[14] hereditary factors were documented in 40% of the Mayas in Campeche, Mexico. The likely explanation of this finding was the fact that more than 50% of the families had more than five children.

In Bulgaria, no relationship has been established between blood specificity (ABO and Rh) and cleft lip and palate. Regarding the age of parents, mothers over 35 run a higher risk of giving birth to children with cleft lip and palate deformity. Georgiev[13] confirmed the role of this factor for the father. Investigations also have been conducted on the developmental aspects of cleft lip and palate children, namely postnatal weight, nutrition, morbidity, and so on.

The clinical studies outlined above clarify certain aspects of the problem discussed on a nationwide scale, which in turn serve as a basis for development of a national program for the prevention and treatment of cleft lip and palate deformities. For nearly 10 years, the Department of Plastic and Aesthetic Surgery in Sofia has been the only specialized center for cleft lip and palate treatment in Bulgaria.

Multidisciplinary Treatment Strategy

Primary cleft lip repair is performed when the patient is approximately 2 to 3 months of age and has adapted to living without the mother, and before the occurrence of rickets. The following conditions must be met before surgery is performed:

1. Body weight is at least 4.5 kg.
2. Hemoglobin value is at least 10 gm/100 ml.
3. The child is in good health.

Consultation with a pediatrician and anesthesiologist takes place prior to the operation. In some cases, preparation of the infant for surgery is done in the Clinic of Plastic Surgery or in the Clinic of Pediatrics. The

Table 11–1. Incidence of Cleft Lip and Palate in Bulgaria

Jekov 1951–1962	1:1417
Kuiyumdjiev 1959–1969 (Pazardjik)	1: 916
Jordanova 1964–1972 (Pleven)	1:1282
Guergieff 1963–1975 (Sofia)	1: 850

methods for repair used at the present time include those developed by Mirault,[15] Tennisson,[3] Millard,[2] Kavrakirov,[9] and Wynn.[4] The technique selected depends on the form and character of the lip deformity.

During the past year, we have considered the possibility of operating within 48 hours after birth in the maternity home using local anesthesia. Evidently, this approach has many benefits from the psychosocial point of view, but no definitive conclusions have yet been drawn.

All children undergoing operation for cleft lip are examined at least once per year. Corrective operations for the asymmetric vermilion, notch of the vermilion, excessive vermilion, nasolabial fistulas, broad scars, and so on are performed 1 year after the primary operation. To date, a total of 731 children with cleft lip and palate have been operated on. Analysis of the results, using Bardach's protocol from the Iowa Cleft Palate Conference for secondary deformities evaluation, is currently in progress.

Regarding the operation on the palate, an individual approach has been adopted. Whenever the cleft is less than 10 mm wide, we operate at 1 year of age, using the modified method of Schweckendiek.[16, 17] To date, a total of 200 children aged 1 to 2 years have been treated using this technique. If the cleft involves only the soft palate, this operation is definitive. Whenever the cleft involves the hard palate, the second operation for closure of the anterior portion is done at 5 to 6 years of age, that is, when the maxilla is three-fourths the size of that in adults. Measurements are done on dental models periodically by the orthodontist. When the cleft is wider than 10 mm, we operate on the palate after 5 to 6 years of age, using the procedure of Limberg[6] or von Langenbeck,[8] depending on the size of the defect.

The last reports indicate that the method of von Langenbeck[8] produces good results in terms of speech. We have failed to estimate speech results by the Schweckendiek technique[16, 17] because closure of the hard palate cleft is delayed. Limberg's[6] procedure (radical retrotranspositioning with mesopharyngeal constriction by interlaminary osteotomy) invariably yields good anatomic reconstruction, although speech production is not satisfactory. Analysis of the underlying causes for the poor speech results is forthcoming. Subsequent to palate repair, follow-up examination is done within 1 month and once or twice again within the year. The goal of examination is to detect eventual orthodontic, speech, and/or auditory defects.

We intend to study the proposed evaluation techniques of Bardach et al[18] and Dalston et al[19] to establish minimum standards for surgical results in patients with cleft lip, cleft palate, or both. However, we feel that such standards are rather complicated and have more of a research application than a clinical one.

To evaluate primary lip repair and subsequent deformities, the following criteria are used: asymmetric vermilion, notch at the vermilion, deficient vermilion, excessive vermilion, and broad scars.

Secondary deformities of the nose may include asymmetric nose, asymmetric tip, asymmetric nostrils, nostril too large or too small, deviated columella, short columella, depressed ala, absence of the nasal floor, caudal septal dislocation, and deviated septum.

Secondary deformities of the palate may include oronasal fistulas, short palate, and narrowing of the maxillae.

Speech evaluation by the Iowa Pressure Articulation Test[20] seems to be most useful when performed in a specialized laboratory and by a highly competent specialist. In the near future, we intend to carry out a comparative assessment of 50 children—25 with radical palatorrhaphy and 25 with fissurorrhaphy only.

On the whole, the fact that Bardach et al[18] reported that only 16% of patients from 14 to 22 years of age had treatment completed by three specialists indicates the real situation even in advanced countries. If we analyze the probable factors, it is reasonable to assume that the lack of a national program involving various specialists within a single institution and the dispersion of patients in different regions distant from the center interfere with outpatient observation and multidisciplinary management of cleft lip and palate patients.

Conclusions

1. In our opinion, the staff of maternity homes should be thoroughly familiar with the care of infants born with congenital clefts of the lip and palate, and should instruct and comfort the parents, assuring them that correction of the anomaly will be accomplished gradually.

2. During the next few years, we plan to continue to improve the organization of the operative management of cleft lip, with surgery being performed within the first 24 to 48 postnatal hours, provided that there are no contraindications.

3. Operation on the cleft lip is performed routinely at the age of 2 to 3 months. The choice of technique depends on the type and degree of severity of the cleft.

4. Whenever the width of the cleft palate does not exceed 10 mm, the operation is done between the first and second years of life, using the modified technique of Schweckendiek.[16, 17]

5. Operation on larger clefts is done after the fourth year of life by radical palatoplasty according to Limberg[6] or in combination with the technique of Schweckendiek.[16, 17] We intend to introduce Bardach's method[21] and compare it with the other procedures.

6. The principles of orthodontic treatment should include the following: the specialist in plastic surgery should analyze and prognosticate the changes needed in occlusion and articulation, and treatment should be carried out in specialized orthodontic clinics throughout the country.

7. Follow-up examinations in our clinic by various specialists are done at about 6-month intervals to coordinate the treatment approach based on examination results.

8. Logopedic treatment is recommended at 4 years of age and even prior to cleft palate repair in certain cases. It should be directed by qualified logopedists in the respective regional facilities.

9. In conjunction with the center of genetics, fami-

lies with a positive history for cleft deformities and children presenting associated anomalies are subjected to follow-up to be sure that these factors will be considered in future family planning.

10. Analysis of our data and pertinent literature gives us sufficient justification to propose development of a working group of experts that will handle the problems posed by clefts of the lip and palate and will be affiliated with the World Health Organization. This group will work out a comprehensive, multidisciplinary program to serve the needs of cleft lip and palate patients in the best way possible.

References

1. Veau V: Bec-de-Lievre. Paris: Masson, 1938.
2. Millard DR, Jr: Cleft Craft: The Evolution of Its Surgery. I. The Unilateral Deformity. Boston: Little, Brown, 1976.
3. Tennisson CW: The repair of unilateral cleft lip by the stencil method. Plast Reconstr Surg 9:115, 1952.
4. Wynn SK: Correction of secondary cleft lip and nasal deformities. In Georgiade NG, Hagerty RF (eds): Symposium on Management of Cleft Lip and Palate and Associated Deformities. St. Louis: Mosby, 1974.
5. Obukhova LM: Correction plasty of the cleft lip and nostril. Nauchni Tr Samarkandskova Med Inst 15:363, 1957.
6. Limberg AA: The Planning of Local Plastic Operations on the Body Surface: Theory and Practice. A Handbook for Surgeons. Leningrad: Government Printing for Medical Literature (Medgiz), 1963.
7. Giraldes MJ: Bec-de-Lievre complique operation. Bull Soc Chir Paris 6:407, 1866.
8. von Langenbeck B: Die uranoplastik mittelst Ablosung des mucos-periostalen Gaumenuberzuges. Langenbecks Arch Klin Chir 2:205, 1861.
9. Kavrakirov V: Congenital Clefts of the Lip. Sofia: Med Fisk, 1961.
10. Jekov CHR: To the question of the frequency of congenital clefts in the maxillo-facial region. Stomatol 48:98, 1966.
11. Koev J: Dento-maxillary Deformities. Sofia: Med Fisk, 1961.
12. Iovtchev V: For the complex treatment of the cleft lip and palate. Stomatol 47:81, 1965.
13. Georgiev E: Congenital clefts of the upper lip. M.D. dissertation. Bulgarian Medical Academy, Sofia, 1978.
14. Anastasov K: Cleft lip and palate among the Mayas in Campeche-Mexico. Personal investigation, 1980–1981.
15. Mirault G: Lettre sur le bec-de-lievre. Malgaigne. J Chir (Paris) 2:257, 1844.
16. Schweckendiek H: Zur zweiphasigen Gaumenspalten-operation bei primarem Velumverschub. Fortschr Kiefer Gesichtschir 1, 1944.
17. Schweckendiek H: Zur Frage der Frish- und Spatoperation der angeborehen Lippen-Kiefer-Gaumenspalten. Z Laryngol 30:51, 1951.
18. Bardach J, Morris HL, Olin W, et al: Late results of multidisciplinary management of unilateral cleft lip and palate. Ann Plast Surg 12:235, 1984.
19. Dalston RM, et al: Minimal standards for reporting the results of surgery on patients with cleft lip, cleft palate or both: A proposal. Cleft Palate J 25:3, 1988.
20. Morris HL, Spriestersbach DC, Daily FL: An articulation test for assessing competency of velopharyngeal closure. J Speech Hear Res 4:48, 1961.
21. Bardach J: Unilateral cleft palate repair. In Gates GA (ed): Current Therapy in Otolaryngology—Head and Neck Surgery, 1984–1985. St. Louis: Mosby, 1984.

CHAPTER 12

The Iowa-Hamburg Project: Late Results of Multidisciplinary Management at the Iowa Cleft Palate Center

IOWA TEAM: J. Bardach, H. L. Morris, W. H. Olin, S. D. Gray, D. L. Jones, and K. M. Kelly
HAMBURG TEAM: K. K. H. Gundlach, M. Röhrs, K. Behlfelt, and B. Fricke

During May of 1987 members of The University of Iowa Cleft Palate Team were invited to visit the cleft palate center at the University of Hamburg to evaluate late results of multidisciplinary treatment as performed by the Hamburg team. Findings from that study were reported at the Fourth International Symposium on Craniofacial Anomalies and Clefts of Lip, Alveolus, and Palate, held August 31 through September 4, 1987, in Hamburg, Germany, and will be published in the transactions of that symposium.[1]

In October, 1987, the Hamburg team, led by Gundlach, was invited to visit The University of Iowa Cleft Palate Center to evaluate patients treated there. The Hamburg group included a surgeon, orthodontist, and otolaryngologist. The speech pathologist could not join the team, so no speech results are presented in the Hamburg section. The cooperation between the Hamburg and Iowa cleft palate centers exemplifies our long-term efforts to establish a series of comparative studies encompassing various cleft centers in the United States and abroad. Studies of the late results of multidisciplinary management for cleft lip and palate may help us to learn more about the diversity of treatment strategies and techniques and the current state of the art. In the past, we have conducted similar comparative studies abroad; however, this study represents the first time that both participating teams have analyzed and reported their results together.

Typically, it has been assumed that multidisciplinary management and collaboration among specialists has been well established and evaluated from different perspectives. Furthermore, many specialists have been under the impression that we have sufficient information to support the validity and efficacy of the treatment techniques used. Currently, it is very difficult to assess the techniques used in multidisciplinary management of the cleft patient owing to their diversity and the lack of scientific data. There may be more than one treatment strategy that is highly effective; however, we need to report the evidence that justifies use of a particular technique. In our opinion, this information can only be generated through controlled evaluations of the late results from various cleft centers.

Review of the literature revealed that among an abundance of published studies on clefts, only a few have been designed to evaluate the relative effectiveness of various treatment procedures through the use of proper methods of clinical research. Perhaps such studies would not be so clearly necessary if we were consistently getting very good, or even satisfactory, results. But current treatment strategies and techniques are not as effective as one would expect, and this should stimulate us in our efforts to evaluate long-term results to determine our weaknesses and successes.

PART I
EVALUATION BY THE IOWA TEAM

In 1984 we published the findings of our first study on late results of multidisciplinary management of unilateral cleft lip and palate.[2] This pilot study was conducted by a plastic surgeon, a speech pathologist, and an orthodontist. The findings were surprising and even somewhat shocking. We found that of 45 patients in the age group of 14 to 22 years with unilateral cleft lip, alveolus, and palate, only 16% were judged by all three specialists to have completed treatment with satisfactory results. We chose 14 years as the lower limit for this group because we expected that treatment would be completed by this age for the great majority of patients. It also was surprising that in any one of these specialties, satisfactory results were achieved in less than 50% of the patients.

These findings stimulated us to initiate a series of studies to analyze our late results in various age groups and in various cleft forms. These results also stimulated us to widen the scope of investigation by adding an otolaryngologist and a speech physiologist to the team.

Materials and Methods

Fifty-eight patients, all treated by The University of Iowa Cleft Palate Team, were included in this study. These patients were randomly selected from the larger population treated by the Iowa Cleft Palate Team. All patients participating in this study had unilateral cleft lip, alveolus, and palate. Two age groups of patients were studied: those aged 5 to 10 years, and those aged 11 to 19 years (Table 12–1) to allow comparison of results at two stages of treatment. Presumably, a larger number of older children would be more nearly finished with treatment than the younger patients. Also, we wondered how the younger children looked and sounded.

The distribution of clefts on the left and right sides in the 58 patients was similar to the distribution within each age group (Table 12–2). Thirty-nine had a cleft on

Table 12–2. Distribution of Study Group by Age, Sex, and Cleft Side

	Ages 5–10		Ages 11–19		
	Male	*Female*	*Male*	*Female*	**Totals**
Cleft side					
Right	5	5	4	5	19
Left	13	7	15	4	29
Totals	18	12	19	9	58

the left side, and 19 had one on the right side (ratio 2:1). In the 5- to 10-year-old age group there were 20 clefts on the left side and 10 on the right; in the 11- to 19-year-old age group there were, respectively, 19 and 9.

We are well aware that despite selection of patients representing the same cleft form, there may be substantial differences and considerable individual variations in terms of congenital dysmorphogenesis, cleft width, position of the maxillary segments, and severity of the nasal deformity. Thus, even though all patients had unilateral cleft lip, alveolus, and palate, the group cannot be considered homogeneous. Nevertheless, we decided to consider the patients in this group as a whole because the multiplicity of important variables made it impossible to devise truly homogeneous groups.

We used the same procedures in this study, with some exceptions, as were used in the 1984 study.[2] All data were gathered within the period of 1 week. Each patient in the study was evaluated by a plastic surgeon, orthodontist, speech pathologist, speech physiologist, and an otolaryngologist. Still photographs, cephalometric and Panorex films, and dental study models were obtained for each patient. Oral and nasal aerodynamic measurements, rhinomanometry, and audiograms also were performed. Information from hospital records, photographs, clinical materials, study models, tapes, and other research files was used to describe both the original defect and the treatment provided.

Evaluation by the Plastic Surgeon

Primary cleft lip repair was performed at an average age of 3.2 months. In the younger age group, 28 patients had triangular flap repair (Bardach's modification), and two patients had the Millard type of repair. All 30 patients were operated on by one surgeon (Bardach). In the older age group, 17 patients had triangular flap repair, and 11 had the Millard type of repair. Seventeen patients were operated on by Bardach, and 11 were operated on by three other surgeons. Measured blood loss for lip surgery in the younger group was 12.5 ml, whereas for the older group it was 19.8 ml.

Out of 58 patients with unilateral cleft lip repair, 38 (65.5%) required correction of the secondary lip deformity. Of these 38, 29 patients (76%) had one correction, 8 (21%) had two corrections, and 3 (8%) had three corrective procedures. Usually, we delay correction of the secondary lip deformity until the patient is 2 to 3 years of age or later. In our experience, the repaired lip improves with age because of its function. Immedi-

Table 12–1. Study Group Age Statistics (in years)

	Median Age	Average Age (± SD)
Total sample	9	10.64 (±3.78)
Ages 5–10	7	7.43 (±1.36)
Ages 11–19	14	14.07 (±2.14)

ately after surgery, massage of the scar with vitamin E cream is recommended to soften the scar. Conversely, some asymmetries become more evident with age because of the different growth tendencies on both sides of the cleft.

In the younger group (5 to 10 years), 18 patients had lip revision—17 had it done once, and 1 twice. In the older group (11 to 19 years), 20 patients had lip revision—14 once, 4 twice, and 2 three times. For correction of the secondary lip deformity, usually the same technique is used as in the primary repair. If there is only a notch in the vermilion, unequal Z-plasty is usually performed.

Closure of the nasolabial fistula was performed in 33 of the 58 patients (57%). In 27 patients it was performed once, in 6 patients twice. At the time of primary cleft lip repair, we always attempt to close the nasolabial fistula; however, the postoperative result is not always successful. In many patients, even after the fistula has been closed, maxillary expansion at approximately 3½ to 4 years of age may cause the fistula to reopen. Of 33 patients, closure of the nasolabial fistula was performed in 29 between 5 and 13 years of age. Closure of a nasolabial fistula is always performed in two layers and may be combined with alveolar and maxillary bone grafting.

Two-flap palatoplasty, as described in 1967 and 1984 by Bardach[3, 4] and in 1987 by Bardach and Salyer,[5] is designed to obtain complete closure of the palatal cleft and create an adequate velopharyngeal mechanism. In this technique no push-back is performed. The details of this operation are further described in Chapter 46.

Cleft palate repair was performed at an average age of 19 months. In the younger age group two-flap palatoplasty was performed by the same surgeon (Bardach) in all 30 patients. In the older group, two-flap palatoplasty was performed by the same surgeon (Bardach) in 17 patients, while three different surgeons performed the four-flap Oxford technique in 11 patients. Estimated blood loss for palate repair in both groups was 95.0 ml. There were no postoperative complications and no oronasal fistulas in the younger group. In the older group, in one patient there was partial necrosis of the mucoperiosteal flap following the four-flap technique. In another there was a fistula in the anterior portion of the hard palate following two-flap palatoplasty.

Oronasal fistulas in the anterior palate appeared following maxillary expansion in eight patients in the older group. Six were operated on once, and two twice. In one patient, closure was performed at 3 years of age. In the remaining patients, the average age at closure was 10.2 years. Closure in these 11 patients was performed with alveolar bone grafting. Closure of oronasal fistulas is performed in two layers using mucoperiosteal flaps to cover the oral layer.

Pharyngeal flaps were created in 11 of the 58 patients studied (19%). Three underwent the pharyngeal flap procedure at 4 years of age, three at 5 years, two at 6 years, one at 7 years, one at 10 years, and one at 11 years. In 10 patients Hogan's technique was used, and in one patient the fish-mouth technique was performed.

None of the patients required secondary procedures and none developed sleep apnea or other complications.

Alveolar bone grafting was performed in 11 of the 58 (19%) patients at an average age of 10.2 years. A cancellous bone graft was obtained from the iliac crest using a split incision through the crest without elevating muscles from the bone. This approach greatly reduces postoperative morbidity. In some patients bone grafting was performed simultaneously with closure of nasolabial and/or oronasal fistulas. Only one patient had indications for skeletal surgery—Le Fort I maxillary osteotomy.

Correction of a cleft nasal deformity was performed in 13 of the 58 (22%) patients. Bardach's technique for correction of the unilateral cleft lip nasal deformity was used in all. One patient underwent this operation twice. In 7 of the 13 patients septoplasty was performed simultaneously with cleft rhinoplasty; in 6, septoplasty was performed prior to rhinoplasty. Four patients also had turbinectomies, and four required some additional procedures for correction of the cleft nasal deformity (narrowing of the ala).

The distribution of secondary deformities found at the time of examination is presented in Table 12–3. In both groups most secondary deformities were related to the nose. In the younger group the most common nasal deformities were flat ala (60%), asymmetric tip (57%), asymmetric nostrils (53%), and caudal-septal dislocation (53%). The most common secondary lip deformities in the younger group were asymmetric vermilion (17%) and notch in the vermilion (13%). Four patients in the younger group had nasolabial fistulas, and two had oronasal fistulas in the anterior portion of the hard palate.

In the older group, the most common nasal deformities were asymmetric nostrils (50%), caudal-septal dislocation (35.7%), asymmetric tip (28.5), and flattened ala (28.5%). A notch in the vermilion was found in six

Table 12–3. Distribution of Patients with Secondary Cleft Deformities

	Age Group (yr)	
Cleft Deformity	*5–10*	*11–19*
Notch of the vermilion	4	6
Elevated vermilion	5	1
Asymmetric vermilion	0	1
Short upper lip	0	1
Pouting lower lip	0	1
Broad scar	4	1
Deviated columella	6	2
Hanging columella	0	2
Orientation of nostrils	17	0
Nostril too small	0	1
Flat ala	18	8
S-Shaped ala	11	3
Alar base depression	5	3
Hooding tip	12	6
Asymmetric tip	17	8
Caudal-septal dislocation	16	10
Asymmetric nasal pyramid	2	4
Nasolabial fistula	4	2
Oronasal fistula in hard palate	3	6
Sluggish palate	0	1
Nasal airway obstruction or deviated septum	0	2
Nostrils asymmetric	16	14
Nostrils too large	3	0

patients; two nasolabial fistulas and four oronasal fistulas in the anterior portion of the hard palate were found at the time of examination.

Sixteen patients (27.6%) did not have any secondary nasal deformities: nine were in the older group, and seven were in the younger group. Another 12 patients had only one secondary deformity. Six were in the older group and six in the younger. Only 2 of these 12 patients required correction of secondary deformities. Although ten did not require any more surgery, seven had a slight asymmetry of the nostrils, and three had a slightly flattened ala.

Overall, in 26 (44.8%) of the 58 patients evaluated, there was general agreement by the patient, the family, and the examining surgeon that surgical treatment was completed. Sixteen of the twenty-six patients in the older group and 10 of the 30 younger patients were judged to have completed surgical treatment.

The 26 patients judged to have treatment completed had either no secondary deformities or a single, rather insignificant deformity that required no further surgical correction. The remaining 32 patients had two or more secondary deformities. Twenty-six of these had more than five secondary deformities; 17 were in the older group and 9 were in the younger group.

Evaluation by the Speech Pathologist

Treatment Program

Speech pathology services for our patients are provided by both specialists at the Iowa Cleft Palate Center and local practitioners. The speech pathologists on the cleft team provide early counseling to the family about language and speech development and instruct parents on methods for stimulating language. Speech production and speech physiology are evaluated and diagnosed as well at yearly intervals for as long as is necessary. Diagnostic findings and recommendations are reported to the local speech pathologists, who provide most of the therapy because the majority of our patients live too far from Iowa City to be treated by our staff with sufficient frequency to be effective. The local personnel then report back to the team about therapy methods and progress. The nature of therapy depends on the nature of the disorder, but in most cases it is focused on articulatory and phonologic aspects of speech and language. In some locales, speech pathology treatment is available to preschool children with special needs; in others it is not available until the child enters school.

Of the 58 patients in this study, 47 had speech therapy; 34 of the 47 had one or two years of therapy, another 11 patients had three years or more, and no reliable information was available for the remaining two. Eleven had no therapy.

Method of Evaluation

The speech pathologist (HLM) examined all patients in a quiet setting during the week-long examination period. All protocols were scored and clinical judgments made at the time of examination. The protocol was similar to that used in our previous clinical investigations and included the following evaluations:[2, 6–9]

1. The 43-item Iowa Pressure Articulation Test (IPAT)[10] was used to record error by type (nasal, distortion, oral, glottal, or pharyngeal fricative).
2. Stimulability test of /p/ and /s/ to determine whether the patient could produce these sounds correctly with audiovisual stimulation.
3. A clinical judgment of overall articulation defectiveness made on a seven-point rating scale (1 = least defective, 7 = most defective).
4. A clinical judgment of severity of nasality made on the basis of connected speech during the clinical examination on a seven-point rating scale (1 = least defective, 7 = most defective).
5. Judgment of nares constriction or facial contortion during the clinical examination.
6. A clinical judgment of denasality made on the basis of connected speech during the clinical examination using a five-point classification system (1 = mild, 2 = moderate, 3 = severe, 4 = mixed hyper- and hyponasal, 5 = none).
7. A physical examination of the oral cavity with specific reference to occlusion, orthodontic appliances, and oronasal and nasolabial fistulas.

From these tests and evaluations, three clinical judgments were made: adequacy of velopharyngeal function for speech (function within normal limits, marginally normal function, and dysfunction); dental hazards to speech production (yes or no); and functional or learning factors (yes or no).

Information about the reliability of the speech pathology tests and ratings is presented in Table 12–4. Examinations for six subjects selected at random were audiotaped and used as a basis for evaluating intrajudge and interjudge reliability. With one exception, agreement for both IPAT scoring and clinical judgments was relatively high. The exception was IPAT scoring according to error type, for which case the two judges were in agreement only 34% of the time.

Information about the reliability and validity of the clinical ratings of velopharyngeal function is available in Table 12–5. Of particular interest is the data from the post hoc ratings, a strategy used in an earlier study in which we determined the extent of agreement between the clinical ratings and the post hoc ratings, made independently after data collection, on the basis of predetermined criteria sets.[2] As in the earlier study, the criteria sets used in this study were as follows:

1. Velopharyngeal function within normal limits: Pressure consonants on the IPAT were oral or /p/ or /s/ stimulable; no nares constriction; nasality rating 1 or 2.
2. Marginally normal function: Oral or nasal pressure consonants on the IPAT were either oral or nasal; /p/ and /s/ may or may not be stimulable; nasality ratings of 3 or 4.
3. Dysfunction: Nasal pressure consonants on the IPAT were consistently nasal; /p/ and /s/ were not stimulable; nasality rating was 5 to 7.

Table 12–4. Summary of Information About Scoring Reliability of Speech Pathology Measures in Six Patients Selected at Random

IPAT Score—43 Items	Intrajudge (HLM Live/HLM Taped)	Interjudge (HLM Live/DRV Taped)
1. Differences between obtained scores:		
Mean	4.1	4.0
Range	2–8	0–10
2. Percentage agreement on right/wrong basis:		
Mean	84.2	77.2
Range	69.7–93.0	62.7–88.7
3. Percentage agreement about error type on responses identified as wrong by both judges or in both conditions:		
Mean	86.2	34.0
Range	71–100	0–83
Clinical Judgments (no. of patients)		
1. Severity of articulation defectiveness (seven-point scale)		
Agreement	3	4
Differ by:		
One value	3	2
Two values	0	0
More than two values	0	0
2. Severity of nasality (seven-point scale)		
Agreement	3	3
Differ by:		
One value	3	2
Two values	0	1
More than two values	0	0
3. Severity of denasality (five-point scale)		
Agreement	6	4
Differ by:		
One value	0	2
Two values	0	0
More than two values	0	0

As indicated in Table 12–5, there was high agreement between the two data sets. Subjects for whom there was disagreement (9 of 58) were categorized by one or the other procedure as marginally normal.

Two additional types of data were obtained to provide information about speech physiology. Lateral still radiographs were available for 46 of the 47 no-flap subjects during rest, occlusion, and sustained production of /s/. These films were rated for relationships among the velopharyngeal structures in the midsagittal plane in the method described by Van Demark et al.[11]

Also, nasal air flow rate and nasal-oral differential pressure measurements were obtained for 49 of the 58 subjects (by author DLJ). These data were used to estimate the area of the velopharyngeal port in a manner similar to that described by Warren and Dubois.[12] Velopharyngeal area estimations were determined at the peak differential pressure of the nasal-plosive blend in the words *hamper* and *pamper*. Using the criteria established by Warren,[13] the status of velopharyngeal function for each subject was classified as follows: adequate "within normal limits" function (0–9.9 mm²); marginally normal function (10.0–19.9 mm²), and dysfunction (area greater than 19.9 mm²).

Results of Speech Evaluation

Tables 12–5 and 12–6 show data from the speech pathology examination findings and the various estimates of velopharyngeal function. In both tables, data are reported separately for the 47 patients who had not had pharyngeal flap surgery at the time of examination, and for the 11 patients who had. In addition, data in Table 12–5 are reported separately for the two age groups: 5 to 10 years of age and 11 to 19 years.

Data in Table 12–5 indicate that differences between the two age groups for the no-flap subjects are small. The patients who had had previous pharyngeal flap surgery also were evenly distributed between the two age groups; five in the younger group and six in the older. Thus, age at examination does not appear to be a discriminating factor.

The data also indicate that speech production skills in all three groups were generally good, with high test scores and low connected speech ratings of overall defectiveness. Only 3 of the 58 patients showed speech sound substitutions on the IPAT that might be considered grossly compensatory. Only 1 of the 58 subjects showed nares constriction.

Data in item 8 in Table 12–5 present information from the speech pathology findings about the effectiveness of providing velopharyngeal function for speech of both primary palatoplasty alone and primary palatoplasty performed together with any subsequent pharyngeal flap surgery. In the first case, patients with pharyngeal flap surgery were combined with the four no-flap patients who showed velopharyngeal dysfunction at the time of examination. The resulting distribution was as follows: 37 (63.8%) of the 58 patients had function judged to be within normal limits; six (10.3%) had marginally normal function; and 15 (25.9%) had previous pharyngeal flaps or were judged to be suitable candidates for flaps.

In the second case, the focus is on velopharyngeal function at the time of examination for both the no-flap and flap groups. The resulting distribution was 47 (81.0%) of the 58 patients had function judged to be within normal limits; seven (12.1%) had marginally normal function; and four (6.9%) showed velopharyngeal dysfunction or had previous pharyngeal flaps.

The data shown in Table 12–6 indicate that, by aerodynamic assessment, 46 of the 47 (97.9%) no-flap patients had velopharyngeal function within normal limits, whereas one (2.1%) had marginally normal function. By the same assessment, all 11 of the patients with pharyngeal flaps had normal function.

Assessment based on the lateral still radiographs showed more variability. Of the 46 patients for whom films were available, 30 (65.2%) showed midsagittal velar-pharyngeal contact; 10 (21.7%) showed touch contact; and 6 (13.0%) showed no contact. No films were taken of the pharyngeal flap patients.

Two additional observations regarding nasopharyngeal obstruction were made about the 11 pharyngeal flap patients (Table 12–7): a clinical rating of denasality (mild, moderate, severe, mixed, none) and information

Table 12–5. Data on Speech Production for 47 Two-Flap Patients Without Pharyngeal Flap by Age Group and for 11 Two-Flap Patients with Pharyngeal Flap

1. IPAT Score (43 Items)

| | No. Patients (% Group) | | |
| | No Pharyngeal Flap | | Pharyngeal Flap |
Distribution of Scores	5–10 Yr	11–19 Yr	7–16 Yr
36–43	3 (12.0)	3 (13.6)	2 (18.1)
26–35	15 (60.0)	14 (63.6)	7 (65.6)
16–25	4 (16.0)	4 (18.1)	2 (18.1)
6–15	2 (8.0)	0	0
0–5	1 (4.0)	1 (4.5)	0
Range	3–43	0–43	24–41
Mean score	26.2	29.0	30.0
SD	8.9	9.3	5.0

2. Nasal/Oral Errors on the IPAT

| | No Pharyngeal Flap | | | | Pharyngeal Flap | |
| | 5–10 Yr | | 11–19 Yr | | 7–16 Yr | |
No. of Errors (43 Possible)	Nasal	Oral	Nasal	Oral	Nasal	Oral
0–10	17	15	15	19	9	8
11–30	5	10	6	3	2	3
31–43	3	0	1	0	0	0
Range	0–34	0–20	0–43	0–17	0–14	0–13
Mean number	8.8	11.1	8.6	4.7	5.6	5.8
SD	7.9	6.2	10.4	4.4	4.6	4.7

3. Glottal/Pharyngeal Substitutions on IPAT

| | No Pharyngeal Flap | | Pharyngeal Flap |
No. Substitutions (43 possible)	5–10 Yr	11–19 Yr	7–16 Yr
None	23	22	10
1–5	2	0	0
6–15	0	0	1
15+	0	0	0

4. Clinical Ratings of Connected Speech:
Articulation Defectiveness and Severity of Hypernasality
(On a scale of 1 to 7, 1 = least defective, 7 = most defective)

| | No Pharyngeal Flap | | | | Pharyngeal Flap | |
| | 5–10 Yr | | 11–19 Yr | | 7–16 Yr | |
Rating	Artic	Nasal	Artic	Nasal	Artic	Nasal
1	4	17	2	14	3	7
2	10	3	11	5	4	3
3	7	4	9	3	3	1
4	3	0	0	0	1	0
5	1	1	0	0	0	0
6	0	0	0	0	0	0
7	0	0	0	0	0	0

5. Stimulability of /p/ or /s/

| | No Pharyngeal Flap | | Pharyngeal Flap |
	5–10 Yr	11–19 Yr	7–16 Yr
Both stimulable	20	19	10
Only /p/	3	1	1
Only /s/	0	0	0
Neither	2	2	0

6. Palatal Fistulas: None in any of the 58 subjects

7. Nares Constriction on the IPAT: Only one subject in the no-flap, 11 to 19-year-old group who also showed other symptoms of velopharyngeal dysfunction

8. Clinical Judgments of Velopharyngeal Function for Speech Production

| | No. Subjects (% Group) | | |
| | No Pharyngeal Flap | | Pharyngeal Flap |
	5–10 Yr	11–19 Yr	7–16 Yr
Velopharyngeal function within normal limits	20 (80.0)	17 (77.3)	10 (90.9)
Marginally normal	3 (12.0)	3 (13.6)	1 (9.1)
Velopharyngeal dysfunction	2 (8.0)	2 (9.1)	0

IPAT = Iowa Pressure Articulation Test
Note: Of the patients without pharyngeal flap, 25 were 5–10 years old, and 22 were 11–19 years old. The patients with pharyngeal flap were not divided by age because their number was so small.

Table 12–6. Comparisons of Clinical Ratings of Velopharyngeal Function for Speech with Aerodynamic Estimates of Velopharyngeal Area, Midsagittal Velar-Pharyngeal Relationships During Production of /s/ from Still Lateral Radiographs, and Post Hoc Ratings for the No-Flap and Flap Groups

	Aerodynamic			Lateral Radiographs			Post Hoc		
	WNL	MN	DYS	WNL	MN	DYS	WNL	MN	DYS
47 Subjects Without Pharyngeal Flap Surgey									
WNL	37	0	0	29[a]	6	1	36	1	0
MN	6	0	0	1	3	2	1	1	4
DYS	3	1	0	0	1	3	0	2	2
11 Subjects with Pharyngeal Flap Surgery									
WNL	10	0	0				10	0	0
MN	1	0	0				1	0	0
DYS	0	0	0				0	0	0

Categories are velopharyngeal function within normal limits (WNL), marginally normal (MN), and dysfunction (DYS). Entries are number of subjects in each two-way comparison.

[a]No film for 1 subject.

about observed mouth breathing during the speech pathology examination. Only one of the 11 showed more than mild denasality. He also showed chronic mouth breathing by observation and history and was reported by his mother to make more sleep noises than she thought normal. However, she did not consider the disturbances so significant that she wanted to take the risk of the child returning to hypernasal speech as a result of surgical revision of the velopharyngeal mechanism. For comparison, only 1 of the 47 patients without a pharyngeal flap was judged to demonstrate mildly denasal speech.

Shown also in Table 12–7 is the finding that approximately one-third of the patients were observed to breathe through the mouth during the examination regardless of whether they had had pharyngeal flap surgery or whether they were younger or older than 10 years of age.

As indicated earlier, judgments were made during the speech pathology examination about whether there were dental hazards to normal speech production and whether speech therapy seemed indicated. As expected, because these patients had unilateral cleft lip and palate and thus the dento-occlusal disorders associated with alveolar clefts, a large majority (40 of 58) were judged to have dental occlusion and/or orthodontic appliances that were hazardous to speech production, most likely, sibilants.

Table 12–7. Clinical Ratings of Denasality and Observed Mouth Breathing for 47 No-Flap and 11 Pharyngeal Flap Subjects

	No Flap (47 Subjects)		Flap (11 Subjects)	
Denasality				
None	46		7	
Mild	1		3	
Moderate	0		1	
Severe	0		0	
Mixed	0		0	
Observed mouth breathing	5–10 yr (25 subjects)	11–19 yr (22 subjects)	5–10 yr (5 subjects)	11–19 yr (6 subjects)

From the speech pathology viewpoint, nearly all (93%) of the 58 patients had satisfactory status regarding velopharyngeal function. The majority of them, from both age groups, continued to show oral distortions, particularly of sibilants. Some of these distortions were probably related to malocclusion factors, particularly for those not yet finished with orthodontic treatment. Still others appeared to be "functional" in nature, that is, not the result of physiologic limitations. Twelve patients were still in speech therapy. Another 12 could probably benefit but were not interested because the disorder was mild.

Evaluation by the Orthodontist

Fifty-six patients (21 female, 35 male) were evaluated by the orthodontist. Two patients who did not complete the orthodontic protocol were excluded from the analysis. Thus, the number of patients analyzed in this section is 56, not 58. The examination consisted of panoramic x-rays, cephalometric x-rays, plaster study models, photographs, and a complete intraoral examination. All patients had been treated at the Iowa Cleft Palate Center or by a local orthodontist in conjunction with our program.

Stages of Treatment

We feel that it is very important to establish a normal dental arch at an early age. Early treatment will influence development of the dental arches and aid in eliminating many of the problems confronting the orthodontist at a later date. Most patients undergo three phases of orthodontic treatment:

Phase I: This phase starts when the patient is 3 to 4 years of age to correct lingually positioned teeth.

Phase II: Mixed dentition treatment is given to correct rotations and molar relations (crowding, for example).

Phase III: Final treatment follows eruption of permanent teeth.

Results

Deformed, Congenitally Missing, and Supernumerary Teeth. In the present study, the entire group of subjects was found to have some degree of irregularity of one or more anterior maxillary teeth. The teeth involved usually were the central and/or lateral incisors on the cleft side. The central incisor on the unaffected side and both canines were not affected. In most cases, the severity of the problem corresponded to the severity of the original cleft defect. These findings were consistent with those from our previous studies.[2, 14, 15]

Supernumerary teeth frequently were found in the cleft area. The exact number of supernumerary teeth was difficult to determine because some had been extracted and in some patients it was difficult to distinguish primary from permanent teeth.

Twenty, or 36%, of the 56 patients were found to have one or more missing premolars. The most frequently missing tooth was the maxillary second premolar. Three patients had missing mandibular premolars, four had maxillary and mandibular premolars missing, and 13 had maxillary premolars missing. Six of the patients in the older age group (11 to 17 years) had missing third molars.

It is important to identify missing, malformed, and supernumerary teeth at an early age to facilitate and provide the best possible treatment as early as possible. By the time the patient is 4½ to 5 years of age, we usually are able to determine the presence or absence of premolars and the presence of deformed or supernumerary teeth.

Crossbite. Another area that we investigated was crossbite. Our definition of crossbite was any maxillary tooth or teeth that were in lingual or end-to-end occlusion with the mandibular teeth. Results revealed that of the 27 patients in the 11- to 17-year age group, 12 had a posterior crossbite of one or more teeth (canine, primary molars, premolars, and first and second permanent molars). Three had a crossbite of the canine only. All patients with crossbite were still undergoing treatment.

In the 29 patients 5 to 10 years of age, eight had a posterior crossbite involving one or more teeth. Five patients had a crossbite of the canine only. All patients in this age group were still in active orthodontic treatment as well.

Of the 56 patients, 12 had an anterior crossbite, and 2 had anterior open bite. Of the 12 with anterior crossbite, 6 had true crossbite with a bony discrepancy, whereas 6 had a one- or two-tooth crossbite as a result of faulty tooth position that will be corrected easily with further orthodontic treatment. Results are summarized in Table 12–8.

Cephalometric Results. Figure 12–1 shows the major points used in our cephalometric evaluation. Tables 12–9 and 12–10 present the data for the two main age groups and for males versus females.

The cephalometric data indicated that the middle third of the face was slightly underdeveloped; however, the mandible also was found to be smaller, resulting in a favorable relationship between the mandible and the maxilla. These results produced very little adverse effect on facial proportions and appearance.

Critical observation of the cephalometric data, plus

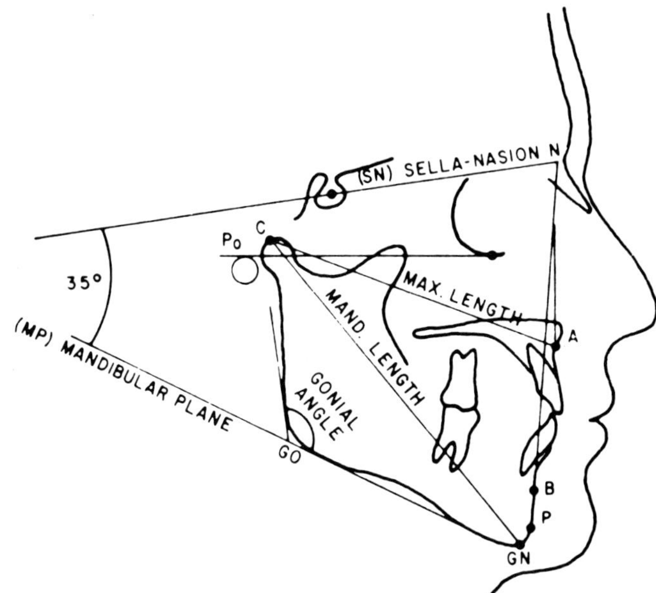

Figure 12–1 Points used for cephalometric evaluation.

frontal and lateral photographs, revealed only three patients with an aesthetically unsatisfactory facial appearance from a growth standpoint. These patients will in all probability require major orthognathic surgery at a later date. All had negative ANB angles; one was −06 degrees and the other two were −02 degrees. The value of the negative ANB angle in three other patients was −01 degree.

An overall view of the 56 patients revealed reasonably good facial growth and satisfactory facial aesthetics. The one problem that appeared frequently was posterior crossbite.

Evaluation by the Otolaryngologist

The focus of the otolaryngologic evaluation centered on two aspects: (1) otologic disorders, and (2) nasal disorders. In addition, audiologic findings are reported.

Audiologic Findings

All patients were tested by pure tone audiogram in a sound-treated environment. By air conduction, all but two patients had normal hearing, defined as better than a 20 dB threshold for the speech frequencies. One of the two patients had conductive bilateral thresholds at 30 dB. The other showed a sensorineural loss bilaterally, ranging from 30 to 50 dB for the speech frequencies. In both patients, speech reception thresholds were between 20 and 35 dB.

Otologic Disorders

The most common otologic procedure performed was placement of pressure equalization tubes (PET). Indications for PET placement included:

1. Persistent middle ear effusion of longer than 10 to 12 weeks' duration.

Table 12–8. Changes in Occlusion (percentages with numbers in parentheses)

	5–10 Yr (N = 29)	11–17 Yr (N = 27)	Combined (N = 56)
Anterior crossbite	37.9 (11)	11.1 (3)	25 (14)
Posterior crossbite	27.6 (8)	44.4 (12)	35.7 (20)
Canine crossbite	51.7 (15)	22.2 (6)	37.5 (21)
Normal occlusion	20.7 (6)	40.7 (11)	30.4 (17)

Patients listed with anterior crossbite include two patients (one in each age group) with anterior open crossbite. Patients listed with canine crossbite include three patients (one in the 5–10 year age group and two in the 11–17 year age group) with bilateral canine crossbite.

Table 12–9. Comparison of Cephalometric Data of Male Patients with Normative Data from the Iowa Growth Study

	Males 5–10 Years (N = 17) Mean ± SD	Norms Mean ± SD	Males 11–17 Years (N = 18) Mean ± SD	Norms Mean ± SD
SNA	77.97 ± 2.84	80 ± 4.0	77.25 ± 3.73	81 ± 3.8
SNB	73.38 ± 3.88	76 ± 3.4	75.17 ± 2.29	78 ± 3.3
ANB	4.56 ± 3.07	4 ± 1.6	2.14 ± 2.55	3 ± 1.7
NAPog	8.62 ± 7.38	9 ± 3.8	1.33 ± 5.44	7 ± 4.3
SNPog	73.65 ± 4.20	76 ± 3.5	77.00 ± 2.61	78 ± 3.7
FHNPog	80.47 ± 4.43	83 ± 2.8	79.97 ± 4.59	83 ± 3.7
MPSN	37.00 ± 4.43	35 ± 4.6	35.14 ± 5.69	32 ± 5.2
MPFH	30.29 ± 5.18	27 ± 4.3	32.03 ± 7.79	28 ± 4.9
NSGn	69.70 ± 3.78	68 ± 2.8	69.30 ± 3.12	68 ± 3.2
FHSGn	62.91 ± 4.56	61 ± 2.6	66.14 ± 3.40	63 ± 3.3

2. Recurrent acute otitis media not controlled by medical therapy.
3. Pathologic changes in the middle ear structures thought to be due to negative middle ear pressure such as severe atelectasis of the tympanic membrane, retraction pockets, and ossicular injury.

The older group of patients received a total of 98 PETs (each PET represents one pair of tubes in this study) for an average of 3.5 PETs per patient. For this group only, because four PETs were placed after the subjects had reached 11 years of age, 94 of the 98 PETS were placed between 0 and 10 years of age. This finding is consistent with previous reports indicating that age is an important factor in assessing eustachian tube function. Six patients (21%) never required PETs. If those patients are excluded, the average number of PETs received by each patient was 4.45 per patient.

The younger group of patients received a total of 80 PETs for an average of 2.67 per patient. Only one patient (3%) in this group had not received PETs. Some individuals in this group continue to experience eustachian tube dysfunction, so it is likely that the average number of PETs per patient for this group will increase. It is unlikely that the average will reach that of the older group because the rate of PETs placement in the younger group of patients is decreasing rapidly as a function of their increasing age.

A comparison of the two groups allows assessment of a change in treatment philosophy during the last 20 years. It appears that more cleft children are receiving PETs than those of earlier decades. This may be due to better diagnosis and detection of the disease and a better awareness of the otologic care needed in cleft children. Although 97% of the younger patients received PETs as compared with 79% of the older group, the average number of PETs per patient is smaller for the group of younger patients. Since the technique of palate repair was similar in both groups, this difference is unlikely to be due to the method of palatal closure. It has been suggested that this difference represents the effect of earlier intervention with PETs, and consequently earlier prevention. Without a doubt, a major contributing factor that has led to fewer PETs per patient in the latter group has been use of PETs that are designed to stay in the tympanic membrane for a longer time.

The results of this study confirm the findings of Graham[16] and Severeid[17] that the most important variable in evaluating eustachian tube–related disease in cleft patients is age. In this study, only 4% of the 98 PETs placed in the older patients were placed after the age of 11 years. Only 3 of 28 older patients still have significant eustachian tube–related disease requiring surgical intervention.

Review of the findings seems to indicate that PETs are now used more often than in the past at the Iowa Cleft Palate Center. Only 1 of 30 patients in the older group did not receive PETs compared with the group of younger patients, in which 6 of 28 did not receive PETs. This increase may reflect a heightened awareness of the prevalence of otitis media with effusion in the younger patients. In 1969, Paradise reported that 96% of 100 infant tympanic membranes in cleft patients were abnormal.[18] Stool and Randall reported that 47 of 50 cleft children had mucoid middle ear effusion at the time of lip or palate repair.[19]

Certainly, one must ask if we are overtreating these patients. Although the indications for tubes have been

Table 12–10. Comparison of Cephalometric Data of Female Patients with Normative Data from the Iowa Growth Study

	Females 5–10 Years (N = 12) Mean ± SD	Norms Mean ± SD	Females 11–16 Years (N = 9) Mean ± SD	Norms Mean ± SD
SNA	78.88 ± 4.38	80 ± 4.0	77.67 ± 6.50	80 ± 3.8
SNB	75.54 ± 3.58	76 ± 3.4	76.11 ± 5.68	77 ± 3.3
ANB	3.33 ± 3.58	4 ± 1.6	1.56 ± 1.63	3 ± 2.1
NAPog	4.29 ± 10.64	9 ± 3.8	−1.22 ± 3.52	6 ± 5.6
SNPog	76.83 ± 4.31	76 ± 3.5	78.28 ± 5.37	77 ± 3.3
FHNPog	83.42 ± 5.01	83 ± 2.8	83.39 ± 7.21	84 ± 2.5
MPSN	34.25 ± 5.64	35 ± 4.6	34.44 ± 7.95	34 ± 4.2
MPFH	27.71 ± .87	27 ± 4.3	29.33 ± 9.46	28 ± 4.9
NSGn	66.88 ± .53	68 ± 2.8	68.11 ± 5.68	68 ± 3.0
FHSGn	60.42 ± .24	61 ± 2.6	62.94 ± 7.40	62 ± 2.9

refined since their revival by Armstrong,[20] the indications as defined above have not changed significantly enough since 1968 to affect the change between the two groups. It is likely that the difference between groups represents a lower tolerance for middle ear disease in these patients in the last decade. Because many of the PETs placed in the younger group were done by local otolaryngologists, it may be that this low tolerance for middle ear disease reflects a change in the attitude of practicing otolaryngologists toward cleft patients.

The most common otologic conditions seen in these patients were persistent middle ear effusion and recurrent acute otitis media. The third most common condition was tympanic membrane perforation. Of the 58 patients (116 total ears), 11 had tympanic membrane perforations (unilateral) present at the time of investigation. Six of the eleven perforations were present in the 11- to 19-year-old group. The 11 patients with perforations accounted for 55 PET placements, for an average of 5.0 PETs per patient. No tympanoplasties had been performed at the time of the study in any of the patients. Only one patient did not have a previous history of PET placement, and it appeared that most of the perforations were a result of permanent perforation following PET extrusion.

Only one other otologic operation, a canal up mastoidectomy, was noted. No other significant otologic disease was encountered. No cholesteatomas were found in this patient group. Harker found two cholesteatomas in 150 patients with repaired cleft palates.[21]

Nasal Disorders

Unilateral cleft lip and palate patients may experience nasal obstruction for a variety of reasons. Anatomic nasal obstruction may occur from a small nostril, rotated lower lateral cartilage, valving, nasal-septal deviation, or hypertrophy of the turbinates. Crockett and Bumsted (see Chapter 81) extensively describe the intranasal deformities present in cleft patients, so this problem will not be described here. Nasal obstruction may also result from turbinate mucosal congestion. Crockett and Bumsted address the issue of whether the patient felt he was experiencing nasal obstruction, whether the otolaryngologist thought nasal obstruction was present, and whether there was abnormal air flow resistance as determined by rhinomanometry.

In the older group of patients, 21 of 28 patients (75%) felt that they had normal nasal breathing without obstruction. This group had undergone four partial inferior turbinectomies and seven septoplasties (two combined with partial inferior turbinectomies and three with rhinoplasty) to relieve nasal obstruction. On clinical examination, the nasal passage was rated as obstructive in 16 of 28 patients (57.1%). When the examination was rated as showing obstruction, the obstruction was evaluated as anatomic (septal deviation or large turbinate resistance to decongestion with 0.2 ml xylometazoline hydrochloride, 0.05%), mucosal (decongestion with relieved nasal obstruction), or both. Eight nasal obstructions were attributed to anatomic factors, eight to both

anatomic and mucosal factors, and none to mucosal only.

Of considerable interest is the agreement rate between the physician and the patient. Agreement was considered present when both the physician and the patient felt that nasal obstruction was or was not present. Agreement occurred in 18 of 28 (64%) in the older group.

In the younger group of patients, 28 of 30 (93.3%) felt that they had normal nasal breathing. This group had experienced three partial inferior turbinectomies and one septorhinoplasty. The nasal examination was rated as showing obstruction by the physician in 19 of 30 patients (63.3%). Anatomic factors contributed to the nasal obstruction in ten of these patients, whereas both anatomic and mucosal factors contributed in nine other patients. Agreement between physician and patient was present in only 13 of 30 patients or 43%.

Agreement between physician and patients improves as a function of the patient's age. Bumsted has suggested that many cleft patients are unaware of the nasal obstruction from which they suffer until they either have the obstruction corrected or learn that they should be able to breathe more freely through both sides of the nose. When nasal surgery is taken into account in the older patients, the number of patients who suffer from nasal obstruction as determined by the physician is similar for both groups. It would appear that as the young cleft patients grow older, they become more symptomatic. Also, it is suggested that if nasal surgery is considered to relieve nasal obstruction, one should not perform this surgery until the patient is an adolescent because agreement between physician and patient is higher then.

Discussion

The findings of the present study must be analyzed from various viewpoints. Are the results of treatment obtained by the Iowa Cleft Palate Team satisfactory in terms of aesthetic appearance, maxillofacial growth, occlusion, speech, hearing, and nasal physiology? Was the sample adequately selected to represent the outcome of treatment techniques in patients with unilateral cleft lip and palate? How well did the criteria evaluate the variables that cannot readily be measured? Some of the above questions can be answered with a high degree of reliability, while others cannot because the measurement techniques are inherently subjective.

These questions are also difficult to answer because we could find no comparable studies in the literature (except our own from 1984). Others have published late results; however, compared results would not be reliable because of the number of different variables that were not constant between studies (for example, different surgeons and techniques, various standards of evaluation, and so on). Therefore, we can only present our findings to provide the data that can be used for comparative studies later if a study with a similar design is followed.

Table 12–11 summarizes the number of patients

Table 12–11. Distribution of Patients Judged to Have Treatment Completed

Types of Treatment	5–10 Yr		11–19 Yr	
	No.	*%*	*No.*	*%*
Surgery	10	33.3	16	57.1
Orthodontics	0	0.0	8	28.6
Speech	9	30.0	15	51.7

judged to have treatment completed. Evaluation of surgical results revealed that 44.8% of patients did not require further surgical treatment. Of these 26 patients, 16 were in the older group and 10 were in the younger group. Patients judged to have treatment completed had either no deformity or a single slight secondary deformity that did not require further surgical intervention. Treatment was judged completed not only by the surgeon but also by the patient and his or her family.

In the remaining 32 patients, further surgical correction was recommended. Six patients had two secondary deformities. The deformities were minimal, and the patient expressed satisfaction with the present status; however, in the opinion of the surgeon, further improvement could be achieved.

Completed surgical treatment provides no indication of the acceptability of the aesthetic results. Aesthetics were judged subjectively by the examining physicians and nursing staff involved in the project. Function and aesthetics of the lip and nose were judged apart from overall aesthetics. A rating scale of 1 to 4 was used, with 1 signifying optimal results and 4 representing poor results. In analyzing the results, it seemed that lip repair and correction of the nasal deformity as currently performed produced better results than those reported in our 1984 study, even though the group of patients in the 1984 study were 14 years of age and older.[2] Use of the two-flap palatoplasty as performed by one surgeon yielded considerably better results than results found in patients who had other types of repairs performed by other surgeons.

The major weakness of surgical treatment was considered to be primary correction of the nasal deformity. Definitely, we are not radical enough to correct the nasal deformity during primary repair. Therefore, the majority of secondary deformities found in our patients were related to the nose. We concluded that late alveolar and maxillary bone grafting was indicated only in patients with hypoplasia of the maxilla beneath the base of the ala. Patients with proper occlusion and no sign of bony deficiency did not require bone grafting. Most of the patients with complete unilateral clefts had a septal deviation; however, we are reluctant to operate on the septum early because it may interfere with growth. Typically, septoplasty is performed in our patients after they are at least 14 years old.

In general, these 58 patients are doing well in their speech production. Of these 58, 54 (93%) showed oral-nasal balance of speech that is within normal limits, or nearly so. Of the 54, 43 had had only primary palatoplasty and a moderate amount of speech therapy; 11 also had had pharyngeal flap surgery. The remaining four showed clear indications of velopharyngeal dys-

function at this examination and should be considered for secondary surgery.

A fair number continue to show minimal oral distortion of sibilants. Since even the older subjects (who presumably are finished with orthodontic treatment) show these distortions, it may be that this kind of mild speech distortion is characteristic of the group. A review of the available findings about the problem seemed to indicate that is the case.[22] One suspects that such minimal oral distortion of sibilants is the combined effect of dental factors and learning-articulator placement factors and is relatively difficult to correct even with extensive therapy. On the other hand, it probably constitutes a very minor hazard to oral communication.

As we have reported previously, very few patients in our population show glottal stops and pharyngeal fricatives, two speech articulation patterns that are generally considered compensatory to velopharyngeal dysfunction.[2,6] We have attributed this to two factors. First, the majority of our patients can achieve velopharyngeal function within normal limits relatively early in life (between 12 and 18 months). Second, our program of speech and language stimulation by the parents and preschool therapy, when available, is generally effective in preventing the development of such abnormal speech production patterns.

The issue has been raised whether there are other, more subtle articulator placement "errors" that also may be compensatory in nature.[23] This seems reasonable, considering the variety of oral structure malformations (or deviations from normal) with which the young child must contend in his effort to learn proper speech articulation patterns. However, there is not yet any consensus about the identification of or the significance of such "errors." At any rate, we have not attempted such fine phonetic transcription, and so we considering comments about the issue.

The findings from this study indicate a higher success rate for velopharyngeal function than we have reported for our patients previously. Using similar but not identical criteria, we reported 52% normal or near normal velopharyngeal function in a series of patients with a von Langenbeck procedure and 70% for a series with V-Y push-back.[7] In a later study, we reported results, also with comparable measures, of 46% for a group of patients who had had a variety of procedures, but the majority (76%) had had the von Langenbeck procedure.[2] Thus, these combined data sets are consistent in showing better results for the two-flap and V-Y techniques than for the von Langenbeck. All data referred to here are for patients with unilateral cleft lip and palatal clefts only.

The 75% "success rate" from primary palatoplasty is consistent with estimates from a literature review stating that 60% to 70% of results can reasonably be expected to be successful from contemporary methods for cleft palate repair.[24]

The small data set in regard to the 11 patients with pharyngeal flaps cannot be interpreted as definitive, but the findings indicate the relative success of the procedure with regard to oral-nasal balance of speech and, generally, show few indications of the hazards of overclosure of the nasopharynx. More extensive investigation of this patient group is planned.

The extent of agreement among the various estimates of velopharyngeal function is pretty much that expected on the basis of the present understanding about the measures and similar comparisons from other studies, notably the study by McWilliams et al.[25] The limitations of midsagittal, still radiographs in predicting patterns of oral-nasal balance during functional speech are obvious and pertain mostly to sampling problems. Sampling problems are to be expected as well in making such predictions based on the limited aerodynamic data that result from the two speech tasks of saying the words *hamper* and *pamper*. As with the data reported by McWilliams et al,[25] most of the disagreements among measures are found in patients who, by one definition or another, show velopharyngeal function that is marginally normal. The case can be made that the size of the velopharyngeal opening alone is not a good indicator of how speech will be perceived in regard to oral-nasal balance, but that spatiotemporal factors in the entire speech production system must also be considered.[26,27] If this is true, those factors could easily be the determinants for patients with these marginal mechanisms.[22]

Orthodontic evaluation revealed that of 56 patients, 8 (14.3%) had treatment completed. By completed treatment, we understand that the patient requires no further orthodontic treatment, facial growth is within normal limits, and optimal results for occlusion and dentition have been achieved. It is our opinion that orthodontic treatment cannot be considered complete as long as facial growth continues to develop. However, if normal occlusion and facial growth are found at an early age, it indicates that normal occlusal relationships and facial growth can be expected in the future. Thus, the treatment plan is geared toward obtaining optimal occlusal relationships during the period of mixed dentition, anticipating that this relationship will be maintained during the phase of permanent dentition.

As we anticipated, less malocclusion was found in the older group than in the younger patients. In the older group, 11 of 27 patients had normal occlusion, whereas in the younger, only 6 of 30 had normal occlusion. Anterior crossbite was observed in three patients in the older age group; one patient also had an open bite. In the younger group, anterior crossbite was found in nine patients, one of whom also had an open bite. Posterior crossbite was observed in 11 patients in the older group. Three of these eleven showed bilateral posterior crossbite. Eight patients in the younger group had posterior crossbite, one of which was bilateral. The most typical crossbite observed was a canine crossbite. This was found in eight patients in the older group (two were bilateral) and in 16 patients in the younger group (one bilateral).

Cephalometric findings revealed slight underdevelopment of the midface and the mandible that resulted in a favorable maxillary-mandibular relationship in the majority of patients. Of the 56 patients examined, only three (5.3%) will require orthognathic surgery. All three were in the older group of patients. All other patients exhibited facial growth that was judged to be within normal limits and acceptable facial proportions and appearance.

Audiologic findings revealed that all but two patients had normal hearing. This indicated that persistent middle ear effusion and recurrent otitis media, the most common otologic conditions in cleft children, do not affect hearing significantly. Placement of PETs is done early and is repeated as indicated. The need for tube placement decreases rapidly as a function of increasing age.

Patients with unilateral clefts have a high degree of nasal obstruction. This is due mainly to nasal-septal deviations and hypertrophy of the inferior turbinates. Currently, we delay correction of the septal deformity until the patient is 12 to 14 years of age, anticipating that radical intervention on the septum may affect growth adversely.

Conclusion

Evaluation of late results has led us to several conclusions. Overall, treatment of these patients seemed to be satisfactory. However, better treatment results should be expected, especially in the older group, in which treatment programs were completed by all specialists—surgery, speech, and orthodontics—in less than 50%. Critical analysis also led us to conclude that we may need to revise our approach to multidisciplinary management.

In regard to surgical treatment, more attention should be directed toward primary correction of the nasal deformity at the time of primary lip repair. It seems reasonable to perform septoplasty at an earlier age as well to reduce nasal obstruction. Also, indications for secondary bone grafting should be modified to allow for eruption of the permanent teeth in the cleft area and to create a better skeletal platform for the base of the ala to improve the configuration of the nose. Presently, we are satisfied with our results of lip and palate repair and secondary correction of the nasal deformity.

Concerning speech treatment, we are highly satisfied with the degree of velopharyngeal competence achieved in the patients. However, we feel that more effort should be directed at reduction of the minor oral distortions that persist following both primary and secondary surgical repairs for speech purposes.

The results of orthodontic treatment were favorable in the patients studied. The average age for completion of orthodontic treatment in noncleft patients is 14 to 15 years of age. Given that the age of eruption is delayed in cleft children, our results were comparable to those seen in normal children.

PART II
EVALUATION BY THE HAMBURG TEAM

The initial purpose of this cooperative investigation was to examine patients born with cleft palate only as well as patients with complete unilateral cleft of the lip, alveolus, and palate. At the Hamburg center, we invited patients representing these two categories to participate in the evaluation. Patients were either 8 or 16 years of age. Of the 79 patients invited, over half did not respond. Therefore, the cleft palate only group was excluded from the study because the number of patients was too small for meaningful investigation.[1] Subsequently, when we traveled to the Iowa center for a comparative study, only patients with complete unilateral cleft lip, alveolus, and palate who were 5 to 19 years of age were invited to participate.

As mentioned previously, the speech pathologist from the Hamburg team did not make the trip to the Iowa center for the investigation. Therefore, no speech results are reported in the Hamburg analysis of the patients.

Materials and Methods

To facilitate future comparison of the patients, we selected only those belonging to specific age groups: 7 to 9 and 15 to 17 years of age. Our data for surgical, orthodontic, and otolaryngologic evaluations are based on a total of 29 patients from the Iowa Cleft Palate Center with complete unilateral cleft lip, alveolus, and palate. Fourteen patients (nine males, five females) represented the older age group (referred to as UCLAP 16 years) and 15 children (seven males, eight females) comprised the younger age group (referred to as UCLAP 8 years). The mean age for the two groups was 15.7 and 8.6 years, respectively (Table 12–12). For rhinomanometry evaluation, 53 patients (33 males, 20 females) were included. Mean age for this group was 11.4 years.

Examination and evaluation of the patients were performed independently. The results reported represent another perspective and a different interpretation of the findings from those reported by the Iowa team.

Evaluation by the Plastic Surgeon

The number of lip and nose revisions was found to be relatively high (Table 12–13). Minor revisions of the lip were performed mostly in the younger groups of patients. Columella lengthening, septoplasty, trimming of the turbinates, and rhinoplasty procedures were performed mainly in the older group of patients.

In almost all patients, the orbicularis oris muscle was repaired perfectly. Two-thirds of the patients had a symmetric repaired lip, and in approximately 50% of the patients, minor irregularities of the vermilion border and/or the Cupid's bow were observed.

Evaluation of aesthetics involved comparison of color

Table 12–12. Number and Age of Investigated Groups of Iowa Children with Complete Unilateral Clefts of Lip, Alveolus, and Palate as Discussed by the Hamburg Team

Group	N	$\bar{x}$	SD
UCLAP 8 yr	15	8.6	0.80
UCLAP 16 yr	14	15.7	0.79

N = number of cases; $\bar{x}$ = arithmetic mean of age; SD = standard deviation

Table 12–13. Analysis of the Nose and Lip in 29 Patients with Complete Unilateral Clefts of Lip, Alveolus, and Palate

	~ 8 Years	~ 16 Years
Total no. of patients	15	14
No. patients with nose revisions	1	7
No. nose revisions	1	13
No. patients with intranasal surgery	1	7
No. patients with lip revisions	8	10
No. lip revisions	11	18
No. high nasal floors at cleft side	1	3
No. anterior obstructions by valve or ala nasi	4	4
No. posterior obstructions by dislocated or deviated septum	10	7
No. intranasal synechial scars	0	1
No. asymmetric lip heights	5	6
No. asymmetric Cupid's bows	5	7
No. incontinuous vermilion borders	9	8
No. incomplete muscular rings	0	1

photographs of the patients. However, evaluation of the appearance of the nose and lip seemed to favor patients from one center only, thus we discarded these parameters. Specialists apparently have become so accustomed to the facial appearance of their patients that they tend to become biased in their judgments of others.

Evaluation by the Orthodontist

Posterior crossbite on the cleft side was found in approximately 33% of the patients in both age groups (Table 12–14). On the noncleft side, no posterior crossbite was observed in the younger group. In the older group, eight patients (57%) had a crossbite. Bilateral posterior crossbite was found in only four of the patients in the older group.

The frequency of canine crossbite on the cleft side was higher in the younger group as compared with the older group, that is, 64.3% and 28.6%, respectively. With the exception of one younger patient, no patients had canine crossbite on the noncleft side. Four patients in the younger group and one in the older displayed bilateral crossbite of the central incisors.

Anterior open bite, as assessed for the central incisors, was found bilaterally in one child and on the noncleft side in another in the younger group (Table 12–15). In the older group, three children had an anterior open bite bilaterally, one had an open bite on the cleft side, and one had an open bite on the noncleft side.

Evaluation by the Otolaryngologist

Only results from 14 patients in the younger group are reported here because not all patients were evaluated or would not cooperate with the evaluation. The audiologic findings are presented in Table 12–16. The history of ear, nose, and throat infections did not differ between the two age groups.

Middle ear function improved with age. Only 7% of the older age group patients had PETs in situ at examination compared with 79% in the younger age group. In 82% of the older patients, hearing acuity was

Table 12–14. Frequency of Crossbite in the Posterior Segments, for Canines, and Central Incisors on Cleft Side, Healthy Side, and Bilaterally in 8- and 16-Year-Old Children with Unilateral Clefts of Lip, Alveolus, and Palate

| | UCLAP 8 Years | | UCLAP 16 Years | |
Site of Crossbite	N	Crossbite	N	Crossbite
Posterior; cleft side	15	5 (33.3)	14	5 (35.7)
Posterior; healthy side	15	0 (0.0)	14	8 (57.1)
Posterior; bilaterally	15	0 (0.0)	14	4 (28.6)
Canine; cleft side	14	9 (64.3)	14	4 (28.6)
Canine; healthy side	14	1 (7.1)	14	0 (0.0)
Canine; bilaterally	14	0 (0.0)	14	0 (0.0)
Central incisor; cleft side	14	4 (28.6)	13	1 (7.7)
Central incisor; healthy side	14	4 (28.6)	14	1 (7.1)
Central incisor; bilaterally	14	4 (28.6)	13	1 (7.7)

N = number of cases investigated; crossbite expressed in absolute numbers and in percent (parentheses).

Table 12–16. Otologic Disorders in 28 Patients with Unilateral Clefts of Lip, Alveolus, and Palate

	~ 8 Years	~ 16 Years
Number of patients	14	14
Number of ears	28	28
History of recurrent rhinitis, otitis or allergic rhinitis	6	8
Drum appearance		
Normal or light scarring	15	21
Perforation	2	5
Acute otitis	1	0
Cholesteatoma	0	0
PET in situ	11	1
Mastoidectomy/myringoplasty	0	1
Audiologic findings		
No audiogram	1	0
Hearing level at speech frequencies 0.5–4 kHz		
0–20 dB	24	23
> 20 dB conductive loss	3	3
> 20 dB sensorineural loss	0	2

normal. The good hearing in the younger group was partly due to the PETs. Repeated tube insertion (in two patients up to 14 times) resulted in scarring of the tympanic membrane in only a few patients, generally not impairing their hearing level. In the older patients, persistent perforation following tube extrusion worked like tubal aeration, normalizing hearing.

Rhinomanometric Evaluation

Rhinomanometry was performed using the anterior method (Rhinomanometer A 440, Allergopharma Joachim Ganzer KG, Reinbek bei Hamburg). One tube was attached to one nostril with an airtight seal. This allowed recording of the pressure at the posterior nasal aperture. The other tube measured the pressure in the mask. Air flow was measured at the same time at a pressure differential of 1.47 mbar, providing results for the turbulent air flow. Pressure difference was measured on the left and right sides before and after application of a vasoconstricting agent (0.2 ml xylometazoline hydrochloride 0.05%). The latter values reflect the gross morphology of the nasal cavity (Figs. 12–2 and 12–3).

The arithmetic mean of the turbulent airflow in 51 patients evaluated prior to the application of the nasal spray was 53.5 ml/sec/1.47 mbar with a standard deviation of 66.9. Subsequent to the application of the nasal spray, the mean was 82.3 ml/sec/1.47 mbar with a standard deviation of 96.4.

Discussion

In our evaluation of the Iowa patients with complete unilateral cleft lip, alveolus, and palate, four major

points of interest were noted: number of therapeutic interventions, status of the nasal airway, symmetry and harmony of the upper lip, and occlusion.

We observed a high incidence of insertion of PETs in the patients in the younger age group. Also, there seemed to be a large number of lip revisions in the younger patients and of nose revisions in the older group of patients.

We found it interesting that the triangular flap lip repair technique as performed by Bardach did not result in producing a lip that was too long. However, minor deficiencies in lip height were encountered in some of the patients. Normally, this would be expected in techniques that involved linear scar closure [28–30] rather than a Z-plasty type scar. Reconstruction of the orbicularis oris muscle was achieved in all but one patient.

The functional results of nasal surgery were not as satisfactory. As indicated by rhinomanometry, the obvious anatomic improvement may not imply functional improvement. In some patients, the airway on the cleft side was occluded despite the use of a vasoconstricting nasal spray. Therefore, the obstruction consisted of hard tissue (scars or bone). This nasal airway impairment may be due to the technique of closing the anterior nasal

Table 12–15. Frequency of Anterior Open Bite as Assessed for the Central Incisors on the Cleft Side, Healthy Side, and Bilaterally in the 8- and 16-Year-Old Children with Unilateral Clefts of Lip, Alveolus, and Palate

| | UCLAP 8 years | | UCLAP 16 years | |
Site of Open Bite	N	Open Bite	N	Open Bite
Central incisor; cleft side	14	1 (7.1)	13	4 (30.8)
Central incisor; healthy side	14	2 (14.3)	14	4 (28.6)
Central incisor; bilaterally	14	1 (7.1)	13	3 (23.1)

N = number of cases investigated; open bite in absolute numbers and in percent (parentheses).

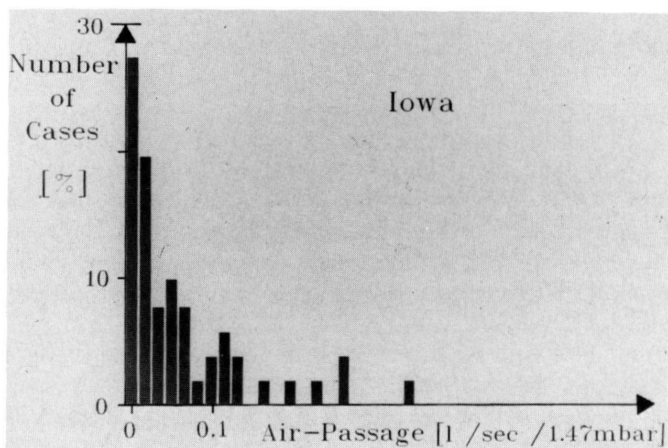

Figure 12–2 Distribution of turbulent air flow measurements on the cleft side prior to application of the vasoconstricting nasal spray.

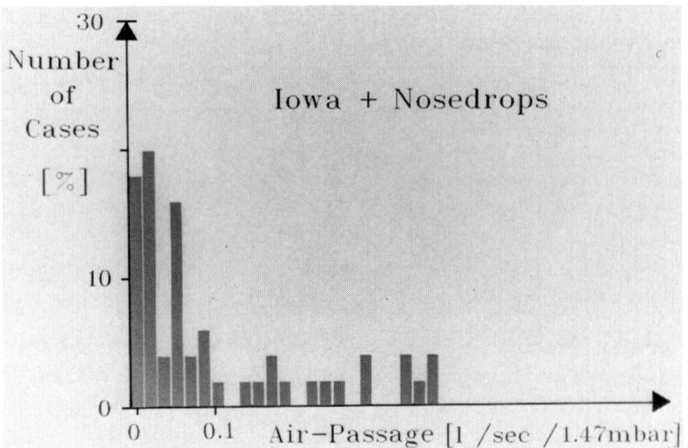

Figure 12–3 Distribution of turbulent air flow measurements on the cleft side after application of the vasoconstricting nasal spray.

floor. Also, contact between the inferior turbinate on the cleft side and the septum may prevent medial movement of the cleft segment.[31] Straightening of the septum and trimming of the turbinate may result in alveolar collapse, consequently narrowing the nasal airway further.

None of the patients in the younger group had posterior crossbite on the noncleft side; however, this was found in 57% of the patients in the older age group. On the cleft side, approximately one-third of the patients in both age groups had posterior crossbite. Canine crossbite was noted with one exception only on the cleft side in both groups. Thus, it seems that posterior crossbite and canine crossbite on the cleft side represented the major dentoalveolar treatment problems in regard to orthodontics.

The reason for the high incidence of crossbite may be the early closure of the hard palate, since this is known to result in a high frequency of anterior and posterior crossbites.[31] Furthermore, controlling orthodontic therapy in a rural population could be more difficult than in an urban area.

According to the data reported in the literature, middle ear function improved with age in the children we evaluated.[33] Because we follow a more conservative treatment philosophy influenced by the Scandinavian point of view,[34, 35] we found the high rate of PET insertion to be of interest. We were surprised by the low rate of complications associated with repeated tube placement. Early and repeated tube insertion may be favored in a rural and geographically widespread region where follow-up is not easily done.

This multidisciplinary investigation conducted by specialists from two cooperating cleft centers presents results that differ from each other, demonstrating the objectivity and utility of a combined approach for treatment evaluation. The results document that treatment of cleft patients at the Iowa Center produced satisfactory results; however, there is also some room for improvement in all areas. Results also indicate that the present state of all specialties involved in multidisciplinary management must be perfected to achieve optimal results in patients.

ACKNOWLEDGMENTS. Portions of this paper were critically read by Shirley Cohen, St. Barnabas Medical Center, and Rodger Dalston, University of North Carolina. We thank them for their assistance.

References

1. Gundlach KKH: Two-stage palatoplasty. In preparation, 1989.
2. Bardach J, Morris HL, Olin W, et al: E: Late results of multidisciplinary management of unilateral cleft lip and palate. Ann Plast Surg 12:235, 1984.
3. Bardach J: Rozszczepy Warg; Gornej; Podniebienia. Warszawa: Panstwowy Zaklad Wydawn, Le Karskich, 1967. (346 pp in Polish.)
4. Bardach J: Unilateral cleft palate repair. In Gates GA (ed): Current Therapy in Otolaryngology—Head and Neck Surgery, 1984–1985. St. Louis: Mosby, 1984.
5. Bardach J, Salyer KS: Surgical Techniques in Cleft Lip and Palate. Chicago: Year Book, 1987.
6. Van Demark DR: Assessment of velopharyngeal competency for children with cleft palate. Cleft Palate J 11:310, 1974.
7. Krause CJ, Tharp R, Rosemary F, et al: A comparative study of results of the Von Langenbeck and V-Y pushback palatoplasties. Cleft Palate J 13:11, 1976
8. Morris HL: Cleft palate. In Wallace HM, Oglesby AC, Biehl FR, et al (eds): Handicapped Children and Youth. New York: Human Sciences Press, 1987.
9. Bardach J, Morris HL, Olin WH: Late results of primary veloplasty: The Marburg project. Plast Reconstr Surg 73:207, 1984
10. Morris HL, Spriestersbach DC, Darly FL: An articulation test for assessing competency of velopharyngeal closure. J Speech Hear Res 4:48, 1961.
11. Van Demark DR, Kuehn DP, Tharp RF: Prediction of velopharyngeal competency. Cleft Palate J 12:5, 1975.
12. Warren DW, DuBois AB: A pressure-flow technique for measuring velopharyngeal orifice area during continuous speech. Cleft Palate J 1:52, 1964.
13. Warren DW: PERCI: A method for rating palatal efficiency. Cleft Palate J 16:279, 1979.
14. Olin WH: Cleft Lip and Palate. Springfield, IL: CC Thomas, 1960.
15. Olin WH: Dental anomalies in cleft lip and palate patients. Angle Orthod 34:119, 1964.
16. Graham MD: A longitudinal study of ear diseases and hearing loss in patients with cleft lips and palates. Ann Otol Rhinol Laryngol 73:34, 1964.
17. Severeid LR: Development of cholesteatoma in children with cleft palate: A longitudinal study. In McCabe BF, Sade J, Abramson M (eds): Cholesteatoma. First International Conference. Birmingham, AL: Aesculapius Publishing, 1977.
18. Paradise JL, Bluestone CD, Felder H: The universality of otitis media in 50 infants with cleft palate. Pediatrics 44:35, 1969.
19. Stool SE, Randall P: Unexpected ear disease in infants with cleft palate. Cleft Palate J 4:99, 1967.
20. Armstrong BW: A new treatment for chronic secretory otitis media. Arch Otolaryngol 59:653, 1954.
21. Harker LA, Severeid LR: Cholesteatoma in the cleft palate patient. In Sade J (ed): Cholesteatoma and Mastoid Surgery: Proceedings of the Second International Conference on Cholesteatoma and Mastoid Surgery. Amsterdam: Kugler, 1982.
22. McWilliams BJ, Morris HL, Shelton R: Cleft Palate Speech. Philadelphia: BC Decker, 1984.
23. Trost JE: Articulatory additions to the classical description of the speech of persons with cleft palate. Cleft Palate J 18:193, 1981.
24. Morris HL: Velopharyngeal competence and primary cleft palate surgery, 1960–1971: A critical review. Cleft Palate J 10:62, 1973.
25. McWilliams BJ, Glaser ER, Philips BJ, et al: A comparative study of four methods of evaluating velopharyngeal adequacy. Plast Reconstr Surg 68:1, 1981.
26. Curtis JF: Acoustics of speech production and nasalization. In Spriesterbach DC, Sherman D (eds): Cleft Palate and Communication. New York: Academic Press, 1968.
27. Folkins JW: Issues in speech motor control and their relation to the speech of individuals with cleft palate. Cleft Palate J 22:106, 1985.
28. Millard DR, Jr: Cleft Craft: The Evolution of Its Surgery. I. The Unilateral Deformity. Boston: Little, Brown, 1976.
29. Veau V: Division Palatine. Paris: Masson, 1931.
30. Pfeifer G: The wave-line procedure for primary cleft lip. Abstracts of the Second International Congress on Cleft Palate. Copenhagen, 1973, p. 190.
31. Aduss H, and Pruzansky S: The nasal cavity in complete unilateral cleft lip and palate. Arch Otolaryngol 85:53–61, 1967.
32. Rood SR, Stool SE: Current concepts of the etiology, diagnosis, and management of cleft palate related otopathologic disease. Otolaryngol Clin North Am 14:865–884, 1981.
33. Møller P: Hearing, middle ear pressure and otopathology in a cleft palate population. Acta Otolaryngol 92:521–528, 1981.
34. Rintala A, and Ranta R: Primary treatment of cleft lip and palate at the Finnish Red Cross Cleft Center from 1966 to 1980. In Hotz M, Gnoinski W, Perko M, Nussbaumer H, Hof E, Haubensak R (eds): Early treatment of cleft lip and palate. Toronto-Lewiston-Bern-Stuttgart, H. Huber, 1986, pp 140–143.
35. Tos M: Epidemiology and spontaneous improvement of secretory otitis. Acta Otorhinolaryngol Belg 37:31–43, 1983.

Genetic Aspects and Classification

CHAPTER 13

Genetic Findings in Cleft Lip and Palate in the Czech Population

Marie Tolarova

In 1965, Professor F. Burian established a clinical genetic unit in the Laboratory of Plastic Surgery within the Czechoslovak Academy of Sciences in Prague. Under his leadership, this research laboratory concentrated on several special fields that required specific and detailed research.[1] Professor Burian directed my first steps in the unexplored area of clinical genetics of orofacial clefts. Shortly before his death, he outlined very clear directions for further research in this area.

As a geneticist, I was very lucky to be able to work closely with plastic surgeons for many years. Our genetic unit was located in the same building as the Department of Plastic Surgery. During the past 23 years, we have seen a large number of patients with morphologic malformations who have been treated by plastic surgeons.

Currently, there are more than 10,000 families with probands with a morphologic malformation or syndrome who have been genetically examined and registered in our Clinical Genetics Laboratory. Families with a history of orofacial clefts represent the majority of these patients.

Material and Methods

Since 1965 we have collected 8952 pedigrees of probands affected by orofacial clefts. The sample consists of 8502 nonsyndromic cases, from which 2231 are probands with cleft lip (CL); only 3491 are probands with cleft lip and palate (CLP); and 2780 are probands with isolated cleft palate (CP) (Table 13–1). The dates of birth of our probands extend over one century—our oldest proband was born in 1886 and our youngest in 1986. The sample of 8952 orofacial cleft pedigrees, on which our present results are based, is one of the largest samples in the world (probably it is the largest one).

Since 1965 we have examined all these probands in our Clinical Genetics Laboratory. I have now observed the second generation, children of our patients from the 1960s, and even the third generation—grandchildren of our oldest patients. Currently, we are conducting a detailed study of these patients.

We also have been able to evaluate the majority of the first-degree relatives of our probands. We have looked carefully for minor manifestations or microforms. We have examined all of our probands, looking for associated malformations, symptoms of syndromes, and so on. In my opinion, this fact is crucial to the quality and completeness of the data as well as to the validity of our results.

Several genetic and epidemiologic analyses of cleft data have been published in the literature.[2–19] Unfortunately, a weak point of some of these studies is the incompleteness of the basic data. Our sample was evaluated with respect to incidence, sex ratio, severity and laterality, birth order, age of parents, seasonal incidence, associated malformations, twin analysis, proband's birth weight and length, proportion of familiar and solitary cases, hereditary empiric risk figures, genetic counseling, syndromes and multiple malformations associated with clefts, atypical clefts, model of inheritance, and effectiveness of primary prevention.

All results of this detailed analysis are presented in our monograph.[20] The facts that are of importance for multidisciplinary management of this serious congenital anomaly are presented here.

Results

Not all of our results will be discussed here. Some have been presented previously,[21, 22] and analysis of others is still in progress and will be published in the near future.

In my opinion, the two most important results that could influence further research in this field are:
1. A hypothesis of a *four-threshold model of liability* of orofacial clefts.
2. A hypothesis and results of *primary prevention* of the cleft lip and palate.

For both hypotheses, the crucial results were obtained from an analysis of incidence, sex ratio, severity of the affliction, and a genealogic study.

One of the most important basic characteristics of any kind of genetic and epidemiologic analysis is a precise estimate (as precise as possible) of the population incidence. The incidence of orofacial clefts has been calcu-

Table 13–1. Sample of 8952 Probands with Orofacial Clefts Born Between 1886 and 1986 in Bohemia by Type of Cleft and Period of Birth

		Male	Female	Total	Cleft in Multiple Malformations	Cleft in Syndromes	Total
CL	1886–1963	748	523	1271	+	+	1271
	1964–1986	589	371	960	17	5	982
	total	1337	894	2231	17	5	2253
CLP	1886–1963	1258	586	1844	+	+	1844
	1964–1986	1095	552	1647	126	22	1795
	total	2353	1138	3491	126	22	3639
CP	1886–1963	632	843	1475	+	+	1475
	1964–1986	547	758	1305	90	190	1585
	total	1179	1601	2780	90	190	3060
Total		4869	3633	8502	233	217	8952

CL = cleft lip, CLP = cleft lip and palate, CP = cleft palate, + = not registered.

lated from the most valuable part of our sample, which is represented by 4362 probands born between 1964 and 1986 in Bohemia (see Table 13–1). We have registered and seen all children born with an orofacial cleft between 1964 and 1983 and the majority of the remaining ones. Before calculation of the incidence, all syndromes and multiple malformations were excluded (Table 13–2). Our estimation of the incidences of the cleft types is

1:2243 (0.4458‰) for cleft lip
1:1307 (0.7607‰) for cleft lip and palate
1:1650 (0.6038‰) for cleft palate
1:826 (1.2104‰) for cleft lip plus cleft lip and cleft palate

To precisely estimate the incidence of clefting, it is necessary to collect data from the same region for several years because the incidence varies owing to the differences in exogenous factors. In our 23-year study, significant differences in some values of incidence have been found compared to the average value for the whole period (Fig. 13–1).

Interesting results were obtained when the relationship between stillbirth and the incidence of each type of cleft was evaluated. The results suggested that during a certain period, reciprocal relations between the incidence of cleft lip and the frequency of stillbirth might exist. That is, a decreasing cleft lip incidence corresponded with an increase in stillbirth frequency. It was assumed that exogenous factors in a certain combination or dose caused one type of birth defect (for example, cleft lip), whereas in a different combination or in a lower or higher dose, the same factors caused another type of anomaly that led to the death of the fetus before birth (Fig. 13–2).

Table 13–2. Incidence of Nonsyndromic Orofacial Clefts in Czech Population During 1964 to 1986

Type of Cleft	Total Number	Incidence ‰	Proportion
CL	960	0.4458 ± 0.0572	1 : 2243
CLP	1647	0.7607 ± 0.0878	1 : 1307
CL + CLP	2607	1.2104 ± 0.1094	1 : 826
CP	1305	0.6038 ± 0.0787	1 : 1650

CL = cleft lip, CLP = cleft lip and palate, CP = cleft palate.
Note: Total number of live births = 2,153,221 individuals.

A higher incidence of cleft lip and a lower incidence of cleft lip and palate occurring in some periods (for example, from 1966 to 1970) could also be explained by differences in a set of exogenous factors involved (Fig. 13–1). The same explanations had been suggested previously.[23, 24] When a hypothesis of independent fluctuations near a mean value was tested, no relation between incidence of the individual cleft types was found.

However, if exogenous factors are considered as a cause of differences between yearly incidences, it has to be pointed out that even the different sets of exogenous factors in a small geographic region like Bohemia that includes smaller regions (districts) may cause variation in the incidence values. In the case of the yearly incidence in the whole region, either an extreme local value of the incidence could influence the value for the whole region, or the exogenous factor could affect the whole region (for example, a viral epidemic). In this way, extremely high incidences of all types of clefts, especially cleft lip in 1975, can be explained. We found that cleft lip is the most variable type of cleft with respect to its incidence. This finding is in agreement with findings in other populations.[23, 25–27] Therefore, in our opinion, cleft lip seems to be the cleft type that is most sensitive to exogenous factors.

The incidences of cleft lip, cleft lip and palate, and cleft palate were compared, and some interesting features were revealed. Districts with significantly high incidences of cleft palate (two standard deviations above the mean) did not have significantly different values for the incidence of cleft lip or cleft lip and palate. However, districts with a significantly lower incidence of cleft palate had a significantly higher incidence of cleft lip or cleft lip and palate. This finding can be explained by an observation by Leck, who noted an increasing cleft lip incidence and a decreasing incidence of spontaneous abortions following an influenza epidemic.[25] It also could be that a more or less permanent exogenous factor (probably a geofactor) exists in this region. This factor could act as a teratogen causing cleft lip and cleft palate. It would either increase resistance of cleft lip embryos to spontaneous abortions or decrease resistance to spontaneous abortions in cleft palate embryos.

These findings formed a base for further detailed analysis of these regions in respect to the incidence of

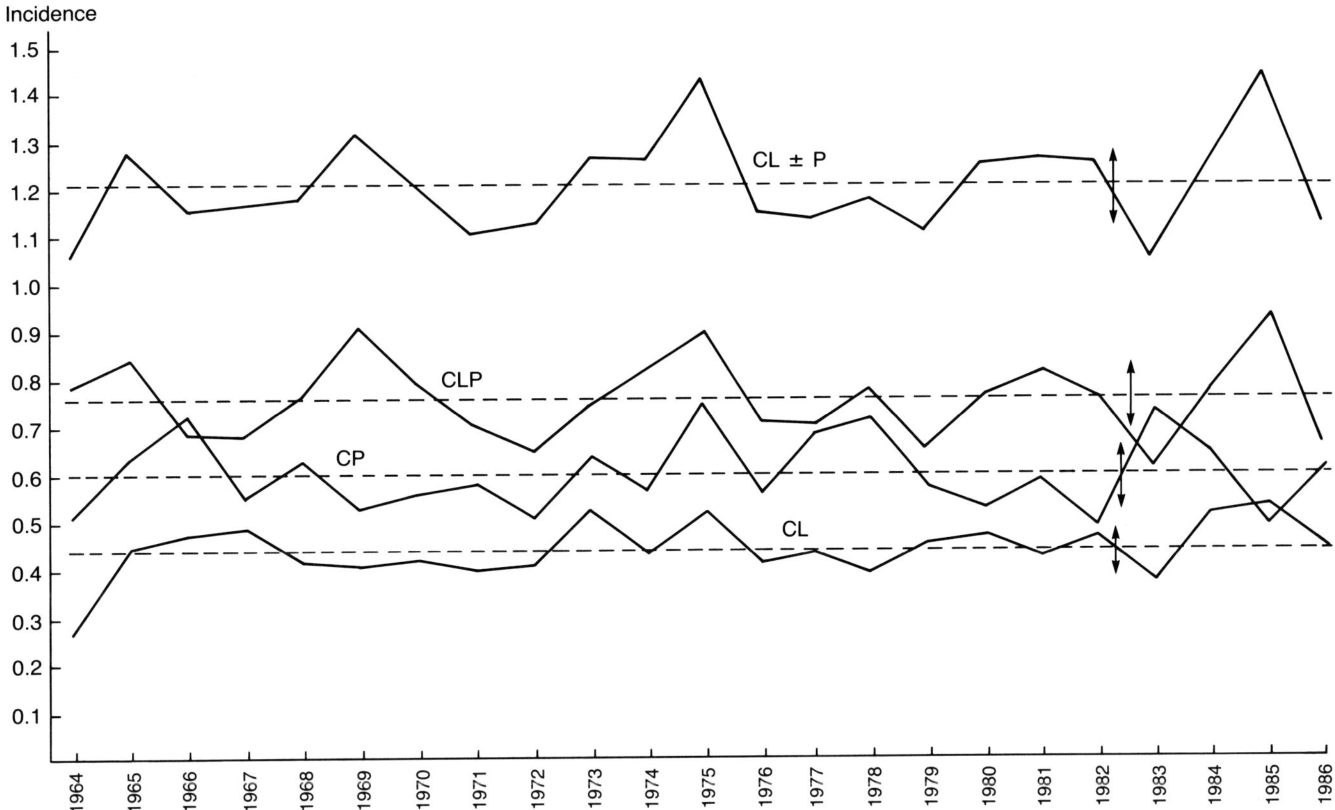

Figure 13–1 Incidence of clefting, 1964 to 1986. CL ± P = cleft lip plus cleft lip and palate; CLP = cleft lip and palate; CP = cleft palate; CL = cleft lip.

clefts and the incidence of other birth defects, as well as the incidence of spontaneous abortions. The *phenotype of the individual with orofacial cleft* was analyzed with regard to such characteristics as sex ratio, laterality, severity of the cleft lip and cleft lip and palate, associated malformations, birth weight and length, occurrence of microforms, and the season of birth of the cleft proband.

The sex ratio belongs to the main characteristics of a

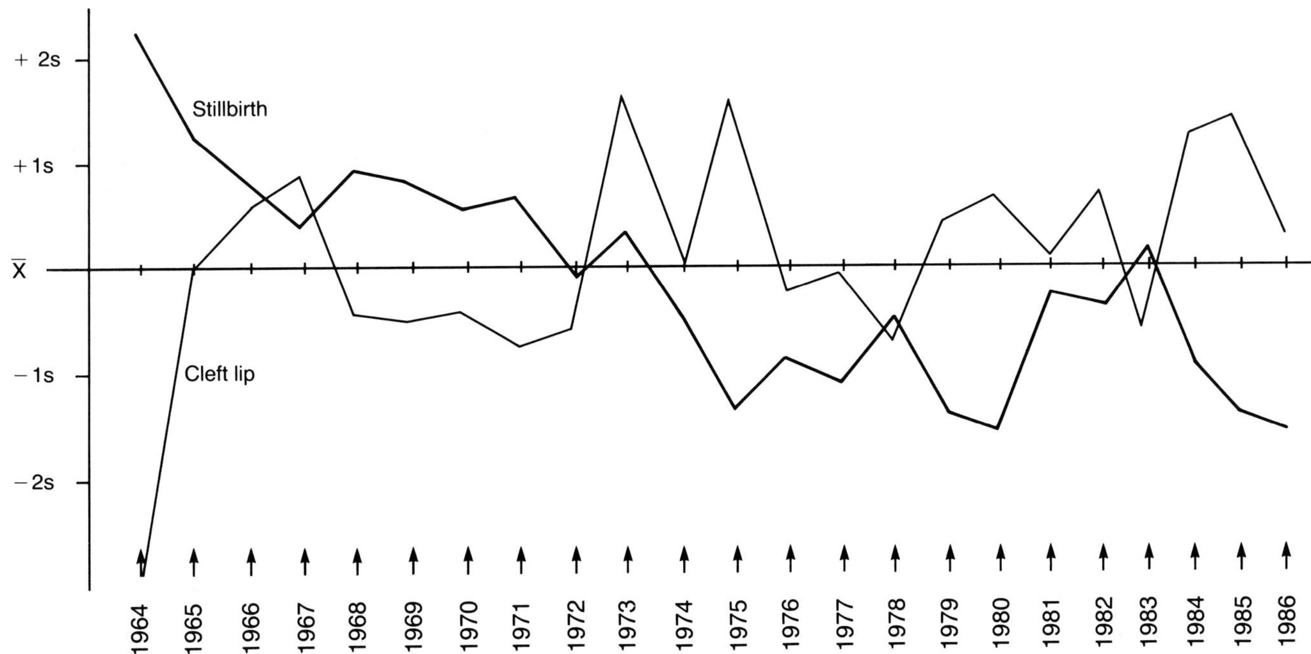

Figure 13–2 Incidence of cleft lip related to stillbirth.

cleft population. It is well known that significant differences in incidence in males and females are found in both cleft lip with or without cleft palate and cleft palate. Although a predominance of males over females is found in cleft lip and cleft lip and palate, the opposite situation, a significantly higher incidence of females compared to males, is found in cleft palate. In our study, the following incidences were found: 0.5337 in males and 0.3534 in females with cleft lip; 0.9923 in males and 0.5259 in females with cleft lip and palate; and 0.4957 in males and 0.7221 in females with cleft palate.

The sex ratio values of 1.59 in cleft lip, 1.98 in cleft lip and palate, and 0.72 in cleft palate were found for nonsyndromic cases in a subsample of patients born between 1964 and 1986. For the whole sample (1886 to 1986), the sex ratio values did not differ from those found in the sample of the complete register: for cleft lip, 1.50 (2231 individuals); for cleft lip and palate, 2.07 (3491 individuals); and for cleft palate, 0.74 (2780 individuals). Comparisons of annual sex ratio values during the entire 23-year period confirmed that sex ratio was a very sensitive parameter that could be influenced by a variety of factors (Fig. 13–3).

Results of our analysis indicated that only a sample that is great enough (coming from a large geographic region and over a long time period) could indicate a precise general value in the sex ratio. On the other hand, it should be pointed out that these average values conceal all year varieties of sex ratio values, which probably correspond to a changed spectrum of exogenous factors.

Table 13–3. The Value of Sex Ratio in Orofacial Clefts

	CL	CLP	CP
1886–1986	1.50	2.07	0.74
1964–1986	1.59	1.98	0.72
Isolated cases	1.68	2.07	0.74
Cleft + one associated anomaly	0.93	1.53	0.67
C isolated and C + one assoc. anomaly	1.61	2.01	0.73
C + two or more assoc. anomalies	0.88	1.53	1.00
C in syndromes	1.00	0.54	0.81
C + 1 or more assoc. anomalies	0.91	1.53	0.76
C right	1.71	2.26	—
C left	1.71	1.91	—
C bilat	1.00	2.14	—

CL = cleft lip, CLP = cleft lip and palate, CP = cleft palate, C = cleft.

The greatest differences again were found in cleft lip, which ranged from 0.73 in 1965 to 2.91 in 1978. Also, in cleft palate, the values of sex ratio varied, but the differences were not so extreme. In 1965, 1973, and 1975, the values of sex ratio corresponded to the average values. The most stable values were found in cleft lip and palate. Significant differences existed between isolated cases and cases that were associated with two or more other malformations, especially in the cleft lip and cleft palate types, counted in a subsample of the complete register from 1964 to 1986 (Table 13–3).

The prevalence of unilateral (left-sided) types is a usual finding in children with cleft lip as well as in those with cleft lip and palate. The left side is affected twice as often as the right side. The same thing has been

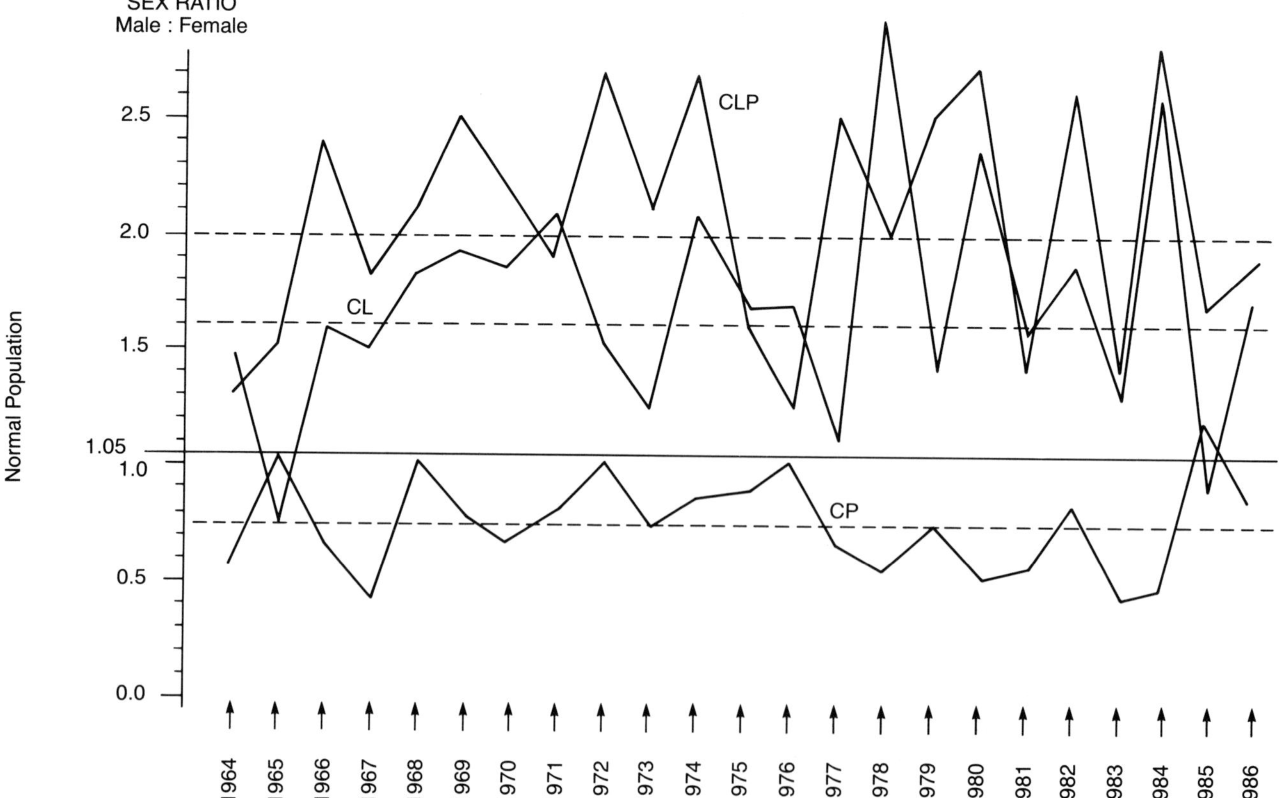

Figure 13–3 Sex ratio values in a cleft population, 1964 to 1986. CP = cleft palate; CLP = cleft lip and palate; CL = cleft lip.

observed in experimental animals. It was suggested that major blood vessels supplying the right side of the head of the fetus exited from the aortic arch closer to the head and more in line with blood flow than those going to the left side.[28]

Our analysis of laterality has been done from several points of view. A prevalence ratio of left unilateral cases of 1.3:1 (left to right) in cleft lip and cleft lip and palate was a very stable finding, corresponding neither to severity of the cleft nor to the sex of the proband.

Sex ratio divided by laterality in individual subgroups yielded the highest value in right-sided cleft lip (2.26) and lower values in bilateral cleft lip and palate (2.14), left-sided cleft lip and palate (1.19), and left- or right-sided cleft lip (1.71). In a rather small group of bilateral cleft lip patients (although it was the largest group of such patients reported in the literature), the same proportion of males and females was found.

The ratio of unilateral to bilateral cases was almost the same in both the whole sample of 8952 cases (persons born between 1886 and 1986) and the subsample of the complete register from Bohemia (4362 children born between 1964 and 1986). A unilateral-to-bilateral ratio of 11.1 was found in cleft lip, and the unilateral-to-bilateral ratio of 2.5 was found in cleft lip and palate. In the literature, this ratio of unilateral to bilateral cases varies and is probably also influenced by race; for example, in blacks, the bilateral form is described more frequently than in the Caucasian population.[11]

It is important to know for further analysis that expression of unilaterality or bilaterality of the cleft is a significant indicator of the degree of severity. This factor is much more significant and specific for degree of severity than occurrence of a cleft of the secondary palate—that is, the ratio of cleft lip to cleft lip and palate.

The ratio of cleft lip to cleft lip and palate is probably influenced by a variety of different factors, even when we consider that the less severe forms of cleft lip may be under-represented in some studies. The racial factors play a significant role too (the highest proportion of cleft lip was found in Japanese studies). There could exist etiologically different types of cleft lip, as suggested by an experimental study of Trasler and Fraser,[29] or, alternatively, the differences could be related to different morphologic shapes of the face as determined by racial factors.[30] Morphologic features of the skull and face in man may include characteristics that are "predisposing" or may serve as "markers" for orofacial clefts in their offspring. This also has been suggested in patients with cleft palate.[31] In our sample, the ratios of cleft lip to cleft lip and palate were 0.64 and 0.59 in the subsample of the complete register.

To evaluate the role of genetic factors in the etiology of orofacial clefts, genealogic analysis, and estimation of heritability, 87 cleft twin pairs were evaluated, and a model of liability of cleft lip with or without cleft palate was designed. The incidence of clefts among 21,147 first-, second-, and third-degree relatives was evaluated in two subsamples. The first subsample was formed by 798 probands born between 1970 and 1974. An assumption of closed sibship (very low chance of further pregnancy of the mother) served as the criterion for inclusion in this subsample. In this group, the proportion of affected individuals in sibship, parents, and second- and third-degree relatives was evaluated. The second sample was formed by our 837 older probands. The proportion of affected individuals among children, grandchildren, and siblings was evaluated.

The results of this part of the analysis provided empiric risk figures suitable for many kinds of counseling situations with regard to type of cleft, sex of proband, degree of relationship to proband with cleft, and so on (Table 13–4). In cleft lip with and without cleft palate, a higher proportion of affected individuals among first-degree relatives was found in the subgroup of patients with bilateral clefts (10.14 ± 2.62%) compared with unilateral clefts (3.68 ± 0.72%). Important results were obtained when combinations of sex and affection of parents and children were analyzed; more children of affected mothers (5.35 ± 1.30%) had clefts than children of affected fathers (4.47 ± 0.91%). The highest risk was found for sons of affected mothers (6.83 ± 2.06%) and the lowest for daughters of affected fathers (2.68 ± 1.01%).

A reversed situation was found in cleft palate. The highest risk (8.57 ± 3.50%) was obtained for daughters of fathers affected with cleft palate and the lowest risk (0.79 ± 0.79%) for sons of mothers affected with cleft palate.

The fact that risk figures were higher in subgroups, which were more rare in the population, suggested a higher proportion of genetic factors. This supposition was confirmed by an estimation of heritability. For first-degree relatives of cleft lip with or without cleft palate patients, the value of heritability was 0.7302 ± 0.0242 standard error (SE). It was a little higher for children (0.8267 ± 0.0442 SE) compared to siblings (0.7302 ± 0.0306 SE).

A higher value of heritability also was found for bilateral cases than for unilateral ones, and for females compared with males. In cleft palate, the value of

Table 13–4. Risk of Recurrence in Orofacial Clefts

Type of Cleft of Proband		In Sibs			In Children			Other Relatives	
		Brother	*Sister*	*Not Distinguished*	*Son*	*Daughter*	*Not Distinguished*	*2nd Degree*	*3rd Degree*
Unilateral CL ± P	Male	2.99 ± 0.80	1.02 ± 0.51	2.09 ± 0.49	4.91 ± 1.48	2.27 ± 1.02	3.60 ± 0.90	0.44 ± 0.13	0.61 ± 0.13
	Female	6.09 ± 1.63	3.66 ± 1.22	4.83 ± 1.01	4.55 ± 1.86	3.05 ± 1.53	3.80 ± 1.20	0.87 ± 0.28	0.44 ± 0.17
Bilateral CL ± P	Male	4.63 ± 2.07	4.44 ± 2.22	4.54 ± 1.51	11.54 ± 4.71	4.88 ± 3.45	8.60 ± 3.04	1.20 ± 0.45	0.10
	Female	2.04	8.00 ± 4.00	5.05 ± 2.26	17.24 ± 7.71	7.69 ± 5.44	12.73 ± 4.81	0.32	0.24
Isolated CP	Male	1.69 ± 0.98	1.68 ± 0.97	1.69 ± 0.69	2.94 ± 2.08	8.57 ± 3.50	5.80 ± 2.05	0.33 ± 0.19	0.36 ± 0.16
	Female	2.70 ± 1.20	2.25 ± 1.13	2.48 ± 0.83	0.79 ± 0.79	2.86 ± 1.65	1.73 ± 0.87	1.03 ± 0.31	0.33 ± 0.15

heritability for first-degree relatives was 0.7482 ± 0.0376 SE. It was again higher for children (0.7990 ± 0.0726 SE) than for siblings (0.6872 ± 0.0606 SE). We used the classic method of Falconer.[32]

The results presented above revealed significant differences among the four basic subgroups. These findings led us to suggest a multifactorial model of liability with four different thresholds related to the sex of the proband and the severity of the anomaly.[21, 22]

According to Carter,[3, 4] although opposed by Melnick and his associates, who reanalyzed the classic Danish data,[14, 15] the most economical hypothesis of the etiology of most cleft lip with or without cleft palate cases was the multifactorial threshold model. Liability was dependent on the sum of the genetic and nongenetic exogenous factors and was represented by a curve of normal distribution and the threshold, beyond which individuals were affected with cleft lip with or without cleft palate.

Different values of population incidence in males and females subdivide the population above the threshold into two subgroups. A similar situation is found when a division is made according to severity of clefts; bilateral clefts are rarer than unilateral ones. Therefore, the risk of transmitting the cleft to offspring is higher in females and bilateral cleft patients than in males and unilateral cleft patients.

A combination of both characteristics results in the four-threshold model of liability (Fig. 13–4) with different thresholds for individual subgroups:

1. Male with unilateral cleft lip ± cleft palate.
2. Female with unilateral cleft lip ± cleft palate.
3. Male with bilateral cleft lip ± cleft palate.
4. Female with bilateral cleft lip ± cleft palate.

The main characteristics distinguishing these four subgroups are presented in Table 13–5. From the first (unilateral male) to the fourth (bilateral female) groups, the incidence in the general population decreases and the risk of recurrence and the value of heredity increase. Also, the results of our method of primary prevention of orofacial clefts seem to support our hypothesis of the four-threshold model of liability.

Table 13–5. Main Characteristics of Our Subgroups of CL ± P

	Unilateral		Bilateral	
	Male	*Female*	*Male*	*Female*
Incidence in general population	0.0601	0.0320	0.0188	0.0099
Risk in sibs or children (in %)	2.85	4.32	6.57	8.89
Heritability (first degree)	0.6385	0.7682	0.8749	0.8779
Effectivity of primary prevention[a]	−2.76	−2.09	−1.18	−0.04

[a]The difference between number of expected and observed cases in treated group.

The problem of prevention of congenital malformations is one of the most important in contemporary genetics. Although the scan technique enables us to recognize individual structures in the craniofacial region of the fetus in utero (and this method is still developing rapidly), the only method of prenatal diagnosis by which orofacial clefts can be safely diagnosed is visualization fetoscopy. We recommend that high-risk families with clefts (families in which the risk is above 10%) and those with autosomal dominant and autosomal recessive syndromes of morphologic malformations undergo this procedure. This preventive method should be called a secondary method of prevention and depends on prenatal diagnosis.

More efficient, because it could affect a larger group of individuals at risk, is a "primary" mode of prevention that acts on the embryo before the cleft develops. The possibility of purposefully influencing the genetic background in patients at risk is far in the future. The only recently discovered possibility of preventing clefts is to preclude the summation of genetic and environmental factors, or at least to exclude some of them (Fig. 13–5).

It has been known for some time that there is a connection between the composition of the mother's diet in pregnancy and the health status of her offspring. An association between nutritional deficiency in pregnant animals and birth defects in their offspring was

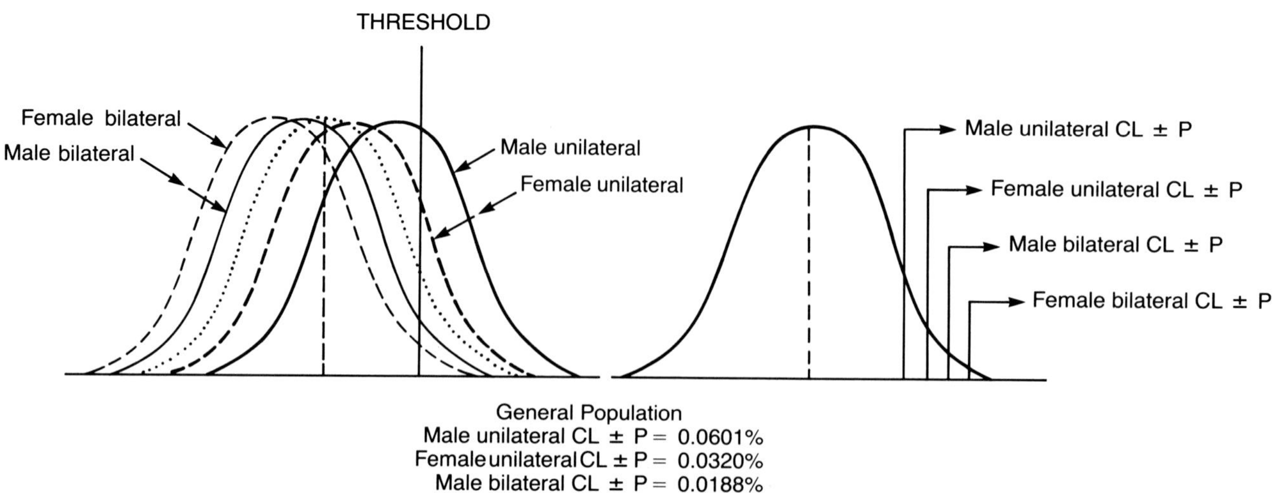

Figure 13–4 Four-threshold model of liability (see text for further discussion).

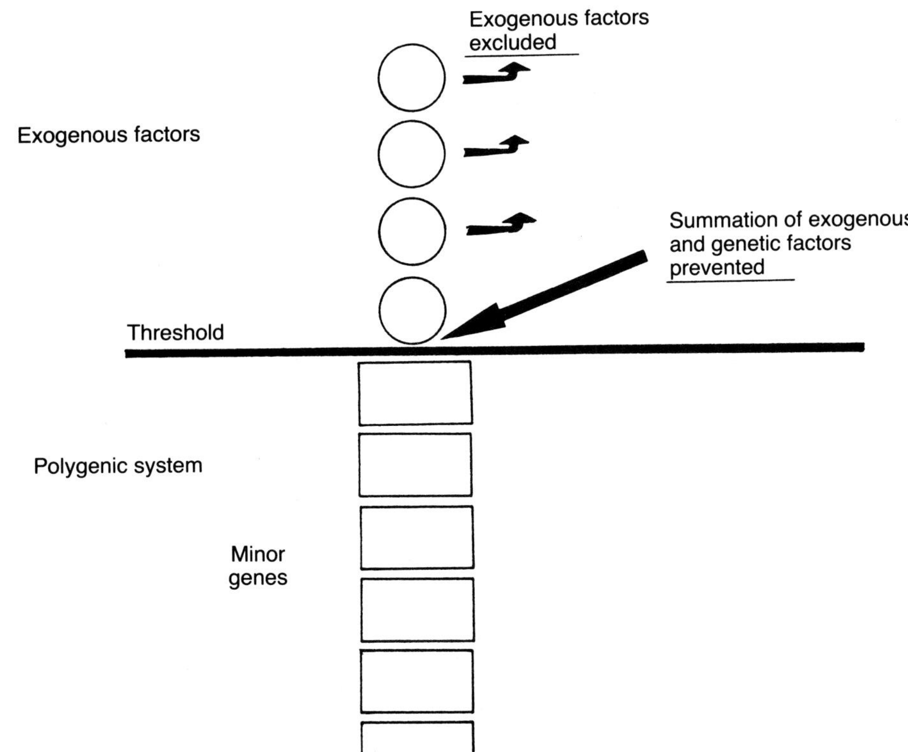

Figure 13–5 Hypothesis of primary prevention of orofacial clefts using periconceptional supplementation by vitamins and folic acid.

probably first recorded in 1940 by Warkany and Nelson[32] and by Warkany and Schraffenberger in 1943.[27] Since that time, several attempts at dietary prevention of birth defects in man have been carried out. Vitamins and folic acid were used for prevention of orofacial clefts by Peer and associates,[34] and later by Douglas, Conway, Briggs, Gabka, von Kreybig,[35–39] and recently these components were used for prevention of neural tube defects (NTD) by Laurence and colleagues and Smithells and associates.[40, 41]

Our method of primary prevention corresponds to our hypothesis of different thresholds based on different proportions of genetic and exogenous factors in the four individual subgroups of clefts. It also is based on another hypothesis: that environmental triggers, which probably play a very important role in the etiology of clefts, may be suppressed or inhibited by diet.

We have used periconceptional supplementation with the multivitamin preparation SPOFAVIT (three times daily) vitamin A (2000 IU), vitamin B_1 (1 mg), vitamin B_2 (1 mg), vitamin B_6, vitamin C (51 mg), vitamin D_3 (1000 IU), nicotinamide (PP) (10 mg), calcium phosphate (1 mg), and folic acid (10 mg daily). Our present results, based on the evaluation of 280 pregnancies in which primary prevention was applied, have reconfirmed our positive results published previously in 1980.[42] In agreement with the four-threshold model, the best results have been obtained in the most frequently encountered subgroup, that of male probands with unilateral clefts, in which there is the highest proportion of exogenous

Table 13–6. Results of Primary Prevention of CL $\pm$ P by Polyvitamin and Folic Acid Periconceptional Supplementation in 275 Families

		Unilateral		Bilateral			Cleft in
		Male	*Female*	*Male*	*Female*	*Total*	Pedigree
Supplemented group	Total number	96	68	34	16	214	61
	Number with cleft	—	1	1	1	3	1
	% with cleft	—	1.47	2.94	6.25	1.40 ± 0.81	1.64
Control group	Total number	973	593	218	117	1901	
	Number with cleft	28	27	14	8	77	
	% with cleft	2.88 ± 0.54	4.55 ± 0.88	6.42 ± 1.72	6.84 ± 2.42	4.05 ± 0.46	
Evaluation of effectivity	Number of expected cases	2.76	3.09	2.18	1.04	8.67	
	Number of observed cases	—	1	1	1	3	
	Difference	− 2.76[a]	− 2.09[b]	− 1.18[c]	− 0.04	5.67[d]	

+ = Not evaluated statistically
Fisher's exact one-tailed test X^2
[a] p = 0.1006   p = 0.05975
[b] p = 0.2897   p = 0.1678
[c] p = 0.4361   p = 0.2529
[d] p = 0.0659   p = 0.0514

factors (Table 13–6). Still, more data are necessary to confirm our hypothesis conclusively. However, if we consider the results of cleft prevention by this method, the prevention of neural tube defects seems to be one of the most promising ways by which the frequency of cleft lip and palate can be decreased in risk families.

Conclusion

Our research deals with one of the most common groups of anomalies—orofacial clefts. Their epidemiologic and genetic characteristics were evaluated, and possible ways of prevention were critically discussed. Our sample consisted of 8952 probands with cleft lip (CL), cleft lip and palate (CLP), and isolated cleft palate (CP) who were born between 1886 and 1986. Data were collected during the time period from 1965 to 1986 in the Clinical Genetics Laboratory of the Institute of Experimental Medicine of the Czechoslovak Academy of Sciences.

A valuable part of this sample consists of 4362 individuals with clefts born from 1964 to 1986 in Bohemia. These probands represent a complete register of all children with clefts born in Bohemia during the period 1964 to 1986. The incidence of orofacial clefts calculated from this sample was 1 in 2243 for cleft lip, 1 in 1307 for cleft lip and palate, 1 in 1650 for cleft palate, and 1 in 826 for cleft lip with or without cleft palate. A comparison of stillbirth and incidence of clefting showed a reciprocal relationship between the incidence of cleft lip and the incidence of stillborn children.

The features of the proband's phenotype as sex ratio, laterality, and clinical severity were evaluated. The genealogic analysis of 21,147 first-, second-, and third-degree relatives resulted in an estimation of the proportion of individuals affected with a cleft in different groups of probands, divided according to the type of cleft, laterality, clinical severity, and age of the parents. The obtained values represented empiric risk figures in corresponding categories of relatives.

A dependence of the value of the risk of recurrence on the combination of sex of the parents and their children may be considered a new finding. The highest figure was found for sons of mothers with cleft lip with or without cleft palate, and the lowest was found for daughters of fathers with this defect. In cleft palate cases, a completely opposite situation was found—the highest risk occurred in daughters of male probands and the lowest in sons of female probands.

The results of our study suggested a multifactorial four-threshold model of liability to cleft lip with or without cleft palate according to the severity of the cleft and the sex of the proband. Four groups of probands that are significantly different in several characteristics (such as incidence of the anomaly, risk of recurrence, heritability, and efficacy of the primary prevention method) are situated behind the threshold in the following order, progressing from those with least risk of recurrence to those with the highest risk:

1. Male with unilateral cleft lip ± cleft palate.
2. Female with unilateral cleft lip ± cleft palate.
3. Male with bilateral cleft lip ± cleft palate.
4. Female with bilateral cleft lip ± cleft palate.

The results of our method of primary prevention of orofacial clefts by vitamin and folic acid supplementation in 275 pregnancies are presented. The best results were obtained in the subgroup of male probands with unilateral clefts. With this method of primary prevention, the risk of recurrence decreased by 50% of the expected value in the experimental group. This result corresponds well with our multifactorial four-threshold model of liability.

References

1. Peskova H: Professor Frantisek Burian and Czechoslovak Plastic Surgery. Plast Reconstr Surg 79:823, 1987.
2. Bixler D, Fogh-Anderson P, Conneally PM: Incidence of cleft lip and palate in the offsprings of cleft parents. Clin Genet 2:155, 1971.
3. Carter CO, Evans K, Coffey R, et al: A three generation family study of cleft lip with or without cleft palate. J Med Genet 19:246, 1982.
4. Carter CO, Evans K, Coffey R, et al: A family study of isolated cleft palate. J Med Genet 19:329, 1982.
5. Fogh-Andersen P: Inheritance of harelip and cleft palate. Copenhagen: Busck, 1942.
6. Fujino H, Tanaka K, Sanui Y: Genetic study of cleft lips and cleft palates based upon 2829 Japanese cases. Kyushu J Med Sci 14:317, 1963.
7. Fujino H, Tashiro Y, Sanui Y, et al: Empirical genetic risk among offsprings of cleft lip and palate patients. Jap J Hum Genet 12:62, 1967.
8. Henriksson TG: Cleft lip and palate in Sweden. A genetic and clinical investigation. Institute for Medical Genetics, University of Uppsala, 1971.
9. Chung CS, Ching GHS, Morton NE: A genetic study of cleft lip and palate in Hawaii. II. Complex segregation analysis and genetic risks. Am J Hum Genet 26:177, 1974.
10. Ingalls TH, Taube IE, Klingberg MA: Cleft lip and palate: Epidemiologic considerations. Plast Reconstr Surg 34:1, 1964.
11. Iregbulem LM: The incidence of cleft lip and palate in Nigeria. Cleft Palate J 19:201, 1982.
12. Koguchi H: Population data on cleft lip and cleft palate in Japanese. (Progress in Clinical and Biological Research, Vol 46) 1980.
13. Lowry RB, Renwick DHD: Incidence of cleft lip and palate in British Columbia Indians. J Med Genet 6:67, 1969.
14. Melnick M, Shields ED, Bixler D: Studies of cleft lip and palate in the population of Denmark. (Progress in Clinical and Biological Research, Vol 46) 1980.
15. Melnick M, Bixler D, Fogh-Andersen P, et al: Cleft lip ± cleft palate: An overview of the literature and an analysis of Danish cases born between 1941—1968. Am J Med Genet 6:83, 1980.
16. Niswander JD, Adams MS: Oral clefts in the American Indians. Public Health Rep 82:807, 1967.
17. Saxen I, Lathi A: Cleft lip and palate in Finland: Incidence, secular, seasonal, geographical variations. Teratology 9:217, 1974.
18. Shields ED, Bixler D, Fogh-Andersen P: Cleft palate: A genetic and epidemiologic investigation. Clin Genet 20:13, 1981.
19. Woolf CM, Woolf RM, Broadbent TR: Cleft lip and palate in parent and child. Plast Reconstr Surg 44:436, 1969.
20. Tolarova M, Cervenka J: Cleft Lip and Palate in Man. New York: Oxford University Press, in press, 1989.
21. Tolarova M: Spontaneous abortions and facial clefts. Clin Genet 26:77, 1984.
22. Tolarova M: Orofacial clefts in Czechoslovakia. Incidence, genetics and prevention of cleft lip and palate over a 19-year period. Scand J Plast Reconstr Surg 21:19, 1987.
23. Knox EG, Braithwaite F: Cleft lips and palates in Northumberland and Durham. Arch Dis Child 38:66, 1963.
24. Pleydell MJ: Anencephaly and other congenital abnormalities. An epidemiological study in Northamptonshire. Br Med J 1:309, 1960.
25. Leck I: Further tests of the hypothesis that influenza in pregnancy caused malformations. HSMHA Health Reports 86:265, 1971.
26. Leck I: The etiology of human malformations. Insights from epidemiology. Teratology 5:303, 1972.
27. Warkany J, Schraffenberger E: Congenital malformations induced in rats by maternal nutritional deficiency. V: Effects of a purified diet lacking riboflavin. Proc Soc Exp Biol Med 54:92, 1943.
28. Johnston MC, Sulik K: Discussion to Section V. In Pratt RL, Christiansen GA (eds): Current Research Trends in Prenatal Craniofacial Development. North Holland: Elsevier, 1980.
29. Trasler DG, Fraser FC: Time-position relationship with particular reference to cleft lip and palate. In Wilson JG, Fraser FC (eds): Handbook of Teratology, Vol 2. New York: Plenum Press, 1977, P. 271.

30. Fraser FC: Evolution of a palatable multifactorial threshold model. Am J Hum Genet 32:796, 1980.
31. Prochazkova J, Tolarova M: Craniofacial morphological features in parents of children with isolated cleft palate. Acta Chir Plast 28:194, 1986.
32. Falconer DS: The inheritance of liability to certain diseases, estimated from the incidence among relatives. Ann Hum Genet (London) 29:51, 1965.
33. Warkany J, Nelson RS: Appearance of skeletal abnormalities in the offspring of rats reared on a deficient diet. Science 92:383, 1940.
34. Peer I, Gordon HW, Bernard WG: Effects of vitamins on human teratology. Plast Reconstr Surg 34:358, 1964.
35. Briggs RM: Vitamin supplementation as a possible factor in the incidence of cleft lip/palate deformities in human. Clin Plast Surg 3:647, 1976.
36. Conway H: Effect of supplemental vitamin therapy on the limitation of incidence of cleft lip and cleft palate in humans. Plast Reconstr Surg 22:450, 1958.
37. Douglas B: The role of environmental factors in the etiology of "so called" congenital malformations. Part I. Plast Reconstr Surg 22:94, 1958; Part II 22:214, 1958.
38. Gabka J: Zur Ätiologie der Lippen-Kiefer-Gaumen-Spalten. Dtsch Zahn-, Mund- Kieferheilke 20:381, 1954.
39. von Kreybig T, Stoeckenius M: Fehlbildungen beim Menschen: Lippen-Kiefer-Gaumenspalten. Entstehung, Ursachen und Praventionmassnahmen. Med Mo Pharm 1/8:243, 1978.
40. Laurence KM, James N, Miller M, et al: Double-blind randomized controlled trial of folate treatment before conception to prevent recurrence of neural tube defects. Br Med J 282:1509, 1981.
41. Smithells RW, Sheppard S, Schorah CJ, et al: Apparent prevention of neural tube defects by a periconceptional vitamin supplementation. Arch Dis Child 56:911, 1981.
42. Tolarova M: Periconceptional supplementation with vitamins and folic acid to prevent recurrence of cleft lip. Lancet 2:217, 1982.

CHAPTER 14

Genetic Aspects of Cleft Lip and Palate

James W. Hanson and Jeffrey C. Murray

Cleft lip and/or cleft palate are among the most common congenital malformations. Although the frequency varies by racial or ethnic group, cleft lip with or without cleft palate occurs in approximately 1 in 1000 term newborns, and cleft palate alone occurs in about 1 in 2000. These disorders carry with them the necessity for significant surgical, medical, and psychological intervention as discussed elsewhere in this volume. Beginning with the pioneering work of Fogh-Anderson,[1] these disorders have been recognized as etiologically heterogeneous. In this chapter we will review the genetic and environmental influences on the occurrence of cleft lip and palate, discuss recurrence risks, summarize syndromes and associated anomalies, and provide an outline for the genetic evaluation of affected individuals.

Cleft Classification

Fogh-Anderson's family studies of the ethnically homogeneous population in Denmark demonstrated that cleft lip, with or without cleft palate (CL ± CP), occurs in families distinct from isolated cleft palate (CP) alone. Additional studies identified a wide range of anomalies associated with cleft lip with or without cleft palate that have been subsequently subcategorized into a variety of patterns (syndromes). Syndromic forms are those in which a medically or surgically relevant abnormality is identified for an organ system outside the anatomic cleft region and may include mental retardation. At the present time cleft lip with or without cleft palate can be broadly divided into four general categories:

1. Nonsyndromic cleft lip with or without cleft palate (NS CL ± CP).
2. Nonsyndromic cleft palate alone (NS CP).
3. Syndromic cleft lip with or without cleft palate (S CL ± CP).
4. Syndromic cleft palate (S CP).

The occurrence of cleft lip and/or cleft palate was reported in over 150 recognizable conditions by Cohen.[2] In 1987, the London Dysmorphology Database listed 215 nonchromosomal syndromes that can include one or more of cleft lip, cleft palate, or bifid uvula. Facial clefts have been reported in association with abnormalities of every human chromosome (including X/Y rearrangements). Nonetheless, in the aggregate, the majority of individuals with cleft lip with or without cleft palate appear to have nonsyndromic forms. Estimates of syndromic forms vary from as high as 60% of the cleft population[3] studied in a high-risk cleft lip and palate clinic (which may have ascertainment bias due to referral of more complicated cases) to studies that suggest that nonsyndromic forms make up 85% of cases in more randomly ascertained populations.[4] Either way, a substantial portion of CL ± CP will result from recognizable syndromes whose identification has important prognostic and genetic implications. We will discuss each of the groups in more detail.

Nonsyndromic Cleft Lip and Palate

Cleft lip, with or without cleft palate, is classified as nonsyndromic when affected individuals have no other associated anomalies, no family history identifying single gene causes of cleft lip or palate, no environmental or teratogenic exposures known to predispose to clefting, and normal cognitive and physical development. Work by Fraser[5] and Carter et al[6] in the 1950s and 1960s has been subsequently expanded by Melnick et al,[7] Chung et al,[8] Marazita et al,[9] and others to provide statistical evidence of the complex etiology of this form of cleft. Striking sex differences have been noted, with males affected about twice as frequently as females. Segregation analysis initially suggested that cleft lip with or without cleft palate fits the multifactorial threshold model in which a variety of genetic predisposing factors combine with environmental influences to raise the liability for clefting across a certain threshold, beyond which an individual would develop the clinical features of clefting. Recently, Chung et al[8] and Marazita et al[9] have reanalyzed previous data using more powerful computer algorithms. In the Caucasian population the data best fit a model that would implicate a single major gene with autosomal recessive inheritance as the cause of 30% to 40% of all cases of nonsyndromic clefting. Data on the Japanese population, however, suggest that a single major locus does not explain the cases of clefting in this population. Because a substantial portion of NS CL ± CP may still not be inherited in an autosomal recessive fashion and because at present we are unable to distinguish recessive forms from sporadic forms, empiric recurrence risk estimates are still necessary to provide families with counseling information. Table 14–1 lists the empiric recurrence risk estimates for Caucasians with nonsyndromic cleft lip and palate. These data are drawn from a summary of data presented by Williams.[10] His data were drawn from studies of Caucasians in the United States, Canada, England, Denmark, and Australia. In this pooled group there was a population incidence of CL ± CP of 0.1%, which broke down into 0.14% for males and 0.06% for females. As the specific genes involved in CL ± CP are identified, it will be possible to identify risks more explicitly for particular families and individuals. Such studies are now underway.

Nonsyndromic Cleft Palate

Nonsyndromic cleft palate alone occurs in approximately 50% of all cases of cleft palate. The proportion is lower (25%) for velopharyngeal insufficiency.[4] As will be discussed below, a number of syndromic disorders that include cleft palate as part of their manifestations may present with very subtle clinical features. Because of this, it is important to have an individual skilled in identification of such associated findings examine all children with cleft palate so that accurate recurrence risks and prognosis data can be provided to the family.

Segregation analysis on cleft palate families has been more difficult to perform, but data, nonetheless, suggest that the multifactorial threshold model may still be relevant for this group. However, the application of more powerful analytic algorithms may in the future change our understanding of the genetics of this disorder. Recurrence risk estimates for individuals with nonsyndromic cleft palate in the Caucasian population are presented in Table 14–2.[10] Again, these are pooled data on several Caucasian populations in which cleft

Table 14–1. *Empiric Risk for Nonsyndromic Cleft Lip With or Without Cleft Palate in Caucasians*

Affected Individual/ At Risk Individual	% At Risk Individuals Affected with CL ± CP	No. At Risk Studied
Parent/child	2.9	1290
Sibling/sibling	4.0	5751
Uncle or aunt/nephew or niece	0.7	8794
First cousin/first cousin	0.2	3942
Grandparent/grandchild	0.3	365

Table 14–2. *Empiric Recurrence Risks for Nonsyndromic Cleft Palate in Caucasians*

Affected Individual/ At Risk Individual	% At Risk Individuals With CP	No. At Risk Studied
Parent/child	3.8	585
Sibling/sibling	2.6	2067
Uncle or aunt/nephew or niece	0.4	4638
First cousin/first cousin	0.2	8191
Grandparent/grandchild	0.1	705

palate alone had an overall incidence of 0.045%, which was divided into 0.037% for males and 0.054% for females. This reversal in the male-female ratio for CP compared to CL ± CP is unexplained. In addition, because many early studies of CL ± CP and CP undoubtedly overlooked or preceded awareness of many syndromic forms, the true incidence of nonsyndromic forms is probably lower than stated.

Syndromic Cleft Lip With or Without Cleft Palate

As noted above, syndromic forms of cleft lip with or without cleft palate may represent anywhere from 15% to 60% of all patients seen in an active referral clinic. The mechanism for identifying particular syndromic varieties is described below. Over 200 disorders are known to include cleft lip or cleft palate as part of their manifestations. These disorders can be divided into Mendelian causes (autosomal recessive, autosomal dominant, and X-linked) as well as chromosomal, sporadic, and environmental. Mendelian or single gene causes of S CL ± CP have well-established recurrence risks depending on the particular mode of inheritance. Thus, autosomal recessive disorders occur in 25% of siblings of affected individuals with the sexes affected equally, but they have a low risk of recurrence in the offspring of affected individuals unless the spouse of the affected has the same disorder or is a close relative. Autosomal dominant disorders affect 50% of the siblings and 50% of the offspring of affected individuals. An exception to this rule occurs when the first affected individual appears to be a new mutation. In this case, his or her future siblings will have a low risk, but his or her offspring will still have a 50% risk. Since it may be difficult to distinguish truly unaffected parents from parents with nonpenetrant or nonexpressing genes or gonadal mosaicism, a low empiric risk estimate (3% to 5%) for siblings in such cases may be justified. X-linked disorders affect 50% of the male offspring of carrier females, and 50% of the female offspring are carriers. Lyonization (the unequal inactivation of the normal X chromosome) may result in some affected females. A similar difficulty in distinguishing new mutations from unaffected carriers found in autosomal dominant disorders is also common in X-linked disorders. A trained clinical geneticist may help to identify the particular probabilities. Table 14–3 lists a sampling of several of the more common disorders associated with cleft lip with or without cleft palate and their inheritance patterns.

Table 14–3. Common Single Gene (Mendelian) Forms of CL ± CP

Disorder	Type of Cleft	Mode of Inheritance
Apert's	CP	AD
Ectrodactyly-ectodermal dysplasia—clefting	CL ± CP	AR
Cryptophthalmos	CL ± CP	AR
Diastrophic dysplasia	CP	AR
Meckel-Gruber's	CL ± CP	AR
Oro-facial-digital I	CL ± CP	X-linked
Oro-facial-digital II	CL ± CP	AR
Opitz's	CP	AD
Shprintzen's	CP	AD
Stickler's	CP	AD
Treacher-Collins's	CP	AD
Van der Woude's	CL ± CP	AD
Waardenburg's	CL ± CP	AD

AD = autosomal dominant; AR = autosomal recessive.

We might particularly stress that disorders such as the Van der Woude syndrome (VDWS), which includes lip pits as the only additional manifestation of the clefting syndrome, may be overlooked or not present in all affected individuals. This disorder is of particular importance because as many as 3% of all cases of CL ± CP may have VDWS.[11] It is imperative that affected individuals be closely examined, a family history obtained, and examination of appropriate other family members be performed to rule out this genetic form. Given the recurrence risk of 50% for Van der Woude syndrome, it may considerably change the statistical data provided to families as well as their own outlook on future pregnancies.

Teratogenic influences that may predispose to cleft lip and palate include a wide variety of drug and chemical agents, physical agents, and maternal health conditions. These are summarized in Table 14–4. The diagnosis of these conditions can be difficult because the frequency and severity of physical and functional

Table 14–4. Teratogenic Agents Associated with Facial Clefts

Agent	Cleft Lip ± Cleft Palate	Cleft Palate	Other Systemic Abnormalities
Drug and Chemical Agents			
Ethanol	?	+	+
Vitamin A congeners	?	+	+
Folate antagonists	−	+	+
Alkylating agents	−	+	+
Phenytoin	+	+	+
Trimethadione	−	+	+
Valproic acid	+	−	+
Barbiturates	?	?	+
Benzodiazepines	?	?	−
Meprobamate	−	?	?
Physical agents			
Fetal constraint	−	?	+
Amniotic bands	+	+	+
Maternal health conditions			
Diabetes mellitus	+	+	+
Myotonic dystrophy	−	+	+
Vitamin deficiency	?	−	+

+ = Associated with this agent, − = not known to be associated, ? = possibly associated but data insufficient to warrant definitive conclusion.

abnormalities found among prenatally exposed individuals vary owing to differences in dosage, developmental timing of exposure, differences in maternal or fetal genetic or developmental susceptibility, and interactions with other environmental exposure. A more complete description of the phenotypic consequences of such prenatal exposures can be found elsewhere.[12] These conditions are of particular importance because they are preventable. Furthermore, the recurrence risk is negligible unless the exposure occurs again during a subsequent pregnancy.

Syndromic Cleft Palate

Syndromic forms of cleft palate have been identified in more than 70 different disorders. In a few cases these disorders may overlap with cleft lip and palate syndromes as well as with the Van der Woude syndrome noted above. However, cleft palate occurs more commonly in syndromes distinct from those identified with cleft lip just as there is an apparent genetic separation between the nonsyndromic forms of cleft lip with and without cleft palate, and cleft palate alone. Table 14–3 lists a number of the single gene disorders more commonly associated with cleft palate, and Table 14–4 lists teratogenic causes. Again, we emphasize that disorders such as Stickler's syndrome and Shprintzen's syndrome may have relatively mild additional manifestations that can be overlooked or not appreciated. Because of this, a thorough evaluation of affected individuals, and their parents and additional family members when indicated, is imperative so that accurate recurrence risks can be provided. Given the high frequency of Stickler's syndrome, one author[4] recommends that all infants with isolated CP have an ophthalmologic examination in early childhood to look for the ocular manifestations of this disorder (myopia, glaucoma, retinal detachment). In addition, an X-linked form of cleft palate that occurs with ankyloglossia has also been identified and, although rare, may be established only through appropriate pedigree analysis.[13–15] This form is of particular interest because gene mapping work has identified the position of its gene on the X chromosome, opening the door to the eventual identification of a specific molecular abnormality causing CL ± CP.[16] Finally, the Pierre-Robin complex, which includes micrognathia and glossoptosis in addition to a U-shaped cleft palate, is frequently associated with syndromes. However, in 34 affected individuals with no identified syndromic cause, there were no siblings affected out of a total of 65 studied.[17]

Genetic Evaluation

Genetic evaluation of an infant or child with cleft lip with or without cleft palate should be undertaken during the first visit of the child for overall medical and surgical treatment. This evaluation will begin with an accurate prenatal history including evidence of exposure to known teratogens (alcohol, phenytoin, vitamin A, and so on). A family history should be obtained to look for relatives with clefting disorders and also individuals who might have lip pits, mental retardation, congenital heart disease, limb abnormalities, ocular abnormalities, arthritis, bone dysplasias or short stature, or other birth defects known to arise in occurrence with clefting syndromes.

A complete physical examination of the affected child is then undertaken, placing particular emphasis on the presence of associated craniofacial anomalies. During the general physical examination the physician should pay close attention to the cardiac evaluation and abnormalities of the limbs including polydactyly, syndactyly, or evidence of dwarfing conditions. Cleft palate is found with a number of conditions that cause short stature that may be overlooked in the newborn period. Finally, an examination of siblings and both parents should be carried out to look for minor features such as lip pits or submucous clefts that may provide hints that Mendelian disorders are segregating in the family. Relevant genetic laboratory tests, particularly chromosomal analysis, should be obtained when indicated. Chromosomal analysis is essential for cases in which major organ system involvement outside of the cleft or evidence of developmental delay is found that is not explained by a known nonchromosomal syndrome. Trisomy 13, trisomy 18p-, and trisomy 4p- are relatively common chromosome disorders in which clefting may occur with great frequency. Such chromosome disorders need to be characterized prior to undertaking surgical correction of the cleft(s) because associated anomalies may present increased hazards or special treatment needs. For some chromosome disorders (triploidy, trisomy 13, trisomy 18) and other syndromes (e.g., Meckel-Gruber syndrome), parents need to understand the long-term prognosis before assenting to surgical intervention.

The genetic evaluation is not complete until appropriate medical records have been obtained on family members with disorders of potential interest, particularly those with clefting conditions, and evaluations have been completed by other appropriate consulting specialties such as ophthalmology or cardiology. When all the information has been gathered and thoroughly reviewed, a diagnosis of syndromic or nonsyndromic cleft lip with or without cleft palate can be made. If a particular syndromic form is identified, the parents should then be counseled about its etiology, recurrence risk, and long-term prognosis.

Artificial insemination may be an option for some families with autosomal recessive forms of clefting or for those with autosomal dominant types in which the father is affected. Some syndromic forms of cleft lip and palate may be amenable to prenatal diagnosis. Such diagnosis would include the use of amniocentesis for those cases with identified chromosomal anomalies in which parents may be carriers of balanced translocations or inversions. Some syndromic forms may have associated anomalies such as dwarfing conditions, renal abnormalities, central nervous system abnormalities, or limb abnormalities that may be suitable for prenatal diagnosis using ultrasound. If such is the case, the parents should be informed prior to undertaking future pregnancies so that they may make appropriate informed decisions about

pregnancy and prenatal diagnosis. Counseling is carried out in a nondirective fashion, giving the parents information about the cause and prognosis of the clefting disorder in their child and the implications for future children.

Because the range of clinical manifestations is quite broad for many clefting disorders, parents need to fully understand that having a severely affected child does not necessarily predict severe disease in future children, nor does having a mildly affected child mean that future children will not be more involved. Legitimate decisions by the parents about future pregnancies should be supported by the involved clinicians regardless of their personal beliefs about what a family should do.

Conclusion

We have reviewed the various causes and recurrence risks for cleft lip with or without cleft palate. Clefting is an etiologically heterogeneous disorder that requires the close cooperation of geneticists with the other members of the health care team to provide the most accurate diagnosis and follow-up for the family. Particular emphasis is placed on the subtlety of a number of anomalies associated with cleft lip and cleft palate and the necessity for distinguishing syndromic from nonsyndromic forms for both prognostic and recurrence risk reasons.

References

1. Fogh-Andersen P: Inheritance of Hare-lip and Cleft Palate. Copenhagen: Munksgaard, 1942.
2. Cohen M: Syndromes with cleft lip and cleft palate. Cleft Palate J 15(4):306–328, 1978.
3. Shprintzen RJ, Siegel-Sadewitz VL, Amato J, et al: Anomalies associated with cleft lip, cleft palate, or both. Am J Med Genet 20:585–595, 1985.
4. Jones MC: Etiology of facial clefts: Prospective evaluation of 428 patients. Cleft Palate J 25:16–20, 1988.
5. Fraser FC: The genetics of cleft lip and cleft palate. Am J Hum Genet 22:336–352, 1970.
6. Carter CO, Evans K, Coffey R, et al: A three generation family study of cleft lip with or without cleft palate. J Med Genet 19:246–261, 1982.
7. Melnick M, Shields ED, Bixler D: Studies of Cleft Lip and Palate in the Population of Denmark. Etiology of Cleft Lip and Cleft Palate. New York: Alan R Liss, 1980.
8. Chung CS, Bixler D, Watanabe T, et al: Segregation analysis of cleft lip with or without cleft palate: A comparison of Danish and Japanese data. Am J Hum Genet 39:603–611, 1986.
9. Marazita ML, Goldstein AM, Smalley SL, et al: Cleft lip with or without cleft palate: Reanalysis of a three-generation family study from England. Genet Epidemiol 3:335–342, 1986.
10. Williams W: Segregation Analysis of Cleft Lip and Palate. Thesis. Honolulu, University of Hawaii, 1981.
11. Burdick AB, Bixler D, Puckett CL: Genetic analysis in families with Van der Woude syndrome. J Craniofac Genet Dev Biol 5:181–208, 1985.
12. Gorlin R, Cohen M: Syndromes of the Head and Neck, 3rd ed. New York, McGraw-Hill, 1989.
13. Rollnick BR, Kaye CI: Mendelian inheritance of isolated nonsyndromic cleft palate. Am J Med Genet 24:465–473, 1986.
14. Bixler D: X-linked cleft palate. (Letter). Am J Med Genet 28:503–505, 1987.
15. Rollnick BR, Pruzansky S: Genetic services at a center for craniofacial anomalies. Cleft Palate J 18(4):304–313, 1981.
16. Moore GE, Ivens A, Chambers J, et al: Linkage of an X-chromosome cleft palate gene. Nature 326:91–92, 1987.
17. Sheffield JA, Reiss K, Strohm CJ, et al: A genetic follow-up study of 64 patients with Pierre-Robin complex. Am J Med Genet 28:25–36, 1987.

CHAPTER 15

Genetic Counseling of Cleft Lip and Palate

Rosalie B. Goldberg

The large majority of families visiting a craniofacial or cleft palate center for the first time already have heard the words, "There is something wrong with your child." What happens to families under this type of stress is complex and personal and has been reviewed extensively in this text and in the literature.[1]

Referral to a center that specializes in the treatment of cleft lip, cleft palate, or craniofacial and dentofacial anomalies is made by a variety of different professionals, often for a variety of reasons. Some patients and families come solely for treatment, while others come for diagnosis or a second opinion. Probably the largest group comes for both multidisciplinary evaluation and subsequent treatment.

This chapter will deal with a conceptual framework that places the genetic counselor in the role of contact person for the team. This professional is the first person to have contact with the family, and is also the first professional who will introduce the family to the team concept by detailing the roles of the team's other members. At the same time, she or he serves as an ombudsman. In this context, *ombudsman* is synonymous with *mediator*. The counselor becomes the ombudsman and moves to uncomplicate a system that often does not budge to fit differing parental personality types and coping styles. She or he listens to complaints, "prophylactically" solves problems, interprets medical and dental materials and information, and serves as liaison with all other professionals while at the same time representing parental concerns.

Historically, the management of the family with an abnormal newborn is a specific and highly challenging form of genetic counseling. We usually alert inexperienced parents (first-time parents who have a child with problems) at their very first introductory session that, in order to negotiate the complicated health care system to provide the care required for their child's problem, they will probably need an advocate. The counselor who is assigned this task must have a combination of skills, as both a health professional and a psychosocial assessor, to assume this role efficiently and effectively.

For the purpose of definition in this context, a genetic counselor is a trained, master's-level graduate of an established program in human genetics and genetic counseling. There are now at least 12 programs available for genetic counselor training in the United States.[2] The person who carries the title of genetic counselor is trained to acquire a combination of skills that enable him or her to understand both the implications of genetic disease and the resulting psychosocial havoc it can play on a family system. An important factor in the training of genetic counselors is the certification examination first given by the American Board of Medical Genetics in 1981. Subsequent board examinations are given every 2 years. More than 650 people have already graduated from programs that train genetic counselors, making them eligible to sit for the board examination. Readers who wish more information may consult the excellent review article by Scott et al.[2]

Diagnosis

A diagnosis is essential to the process of genetic counseling. In an attempt to clarify the complicated process of making a diagnosis, many investigators have tabulated the frequency of minor and major anomalies that accompany clefts. The data have been inconsistent, ranging from a 3% to 64% incidence of associated anomalies in cleft patients.[3] Shprintzen et al, in a critical review of the data, analyzed various characteristics of the so-called cleft palate child.[4] They concluded that use of the term *cleft palate child* incorrectly implies homogeneity in this population of patients born with clefts. It is generally accepted that clefting is extremely variable in its expression and etiology and extremely varied in its occurrence in syndromes. One must exclude cleft syndromes from isolated cleft lip with or without cleft palate, or isolated cleft palate, prior to any attempt to give recurrence risk counseling or, for that matter, even to suggest prognosis following treatment. There are numerous conditions in which cleft lip and cleft palate occur, some genetic, some teratogenic, and some syndromic; therefore, it is incorrect and no longer acceptable to refer to a child seen at a craniofacial or cleft palate center as a cleft palate child.

Methods

So how does the team approach this complex task? I would like to take the reader through a detailed step-by-step method that has served our Montefiore team well. The method was developed first in 1975 and has been revised as new personnel join the team.

To begin with, the client or family is greeted by office staff and introduced to the genetic counselor. The counselor begins the evaluation by taking a family history. Family data can best be visualized in the form of a pedigree, a simple shorthand method of recording the family history. The reader who needs more detail is asked to consult a genetics textbook. The pedigree should record three generations of family members when information on them is available. The term *proband* is used to refer to the family member who brings the family into treatment. *Propositus* can be used instead of proband when referring to males, whereas *proposita* is an alternative term for proband when referring to females. *Sibs* (siblings) are brothers and sisters. The parent generation is designated by P, and the first generation of offspring of two parents is F_1.

While the pedigree is being constructed, the counselor asks questions about pregnancy and general physical health. This information is recorded and will be expanded by the pediatrician, who sees the patient next. The pediatrician focuses on the medical aspects of this history, expanding the history when necessary. Certain basic information is needed such as duration of pregnancy, specifics of delivery (vertex or breech presentation), illnesses during pregnancy, high fevers, medications, and consumption of alcohol, nicotine, or illegal drugs. Also needed are specifics such as weight gain, fetal movement experienced, duration of labor, type of delivery and condition of newborn (Apgar scores, and so on).

During the process of intake of data the counselor has the attention of the family and can use this time to educate the family, emphasizing the important aspects of the biology of the condition, perhaps using books and pamphlets as visual aids. Giving the chronology of normal development while at the same time explaining abnormal development is also helpful in promoting parental understanding. Experience suggests that parents who are well informed about these issues are less frightened than they otherwise would be. The goal is to treat the whole family, not just the proband. Undoubtedly, the first prerequisite is that the teacher, in this case the counselor, must be well informed. Furthermore, team members must maintain consistency in the information of this kind that they give to clients and must avoid overstepping professional boundaries. Thus, if the genetic counselor is the coordinator, she or he must be readily available as the need arises. The counselor can be especially helpful to the family when there is inconsistency in information given or when the parent or patient has questions that have not yet been satisfactorily discussed.

The astute counselor uses the interview period also to gather information about family interactions and to acquire clues about the way in which the family copes with problems. Much information can be obtained from watching the members interact and react to each other and, at the same time, manage their child. Sometimes other members of the support system are present during the interview, such as friends, clergy, or grandparents. Understanding the role of all these participants, as they help the family cope, is important.

One senses that the family arrives for the first visit with a preconceived notion about the way health care

should optimally be delivered. If the team does not meet their expectations, seems not to be trying, or does not read the family's reaction correctly, the family may become unreceptive to recommendations and generally fail to follow directions. For example, if the team suggests psychological counseling or "coping" counseling, certain parents may be unreceptive, but still others may welcome the opportunity.

Some families clearly need additional information. Yet sometimes the stressed families seems to be over-intellectualizing rather than emotionally reacting to the problem. These parents need help to work through their situation emotionally as well as intellectually. Another example is the family that craves an extraordinary amount of reassurance, even when the condition has a poor prognosis. In such a case, the counselor must emphasize this reality and the likelihood of morbidity and finally mortality (such as in the case of the cleft child with holoprosencephaly).

The need for a trained professional is essential. All families need hope, but not all families welcome the invasion of an "outsider" into their family domain, regardless of how needy they feel. Some feel that the parental role is usurped in the health care setting.

Conclusion

To summarize, counseling of this kind must take into account a multitude of considerations, not just giving recurrence risk figures. A family in crisis needs to be understood, respected for their individual style, and nurtured through a complex, difficult time. Genetic counselors, by virtue of their training and experience with the emotional issues associated with birth anomalies and their access to many individuals with the same disorder, are often uniquely qualified to reduce feelings of isolation and teach ways of coping to stressed families. As a consequence, they have an important role to play in the management system for cleft lip and palate and for craniofacial anomalies in general.

References

1. Miezio PM: Parenting Children with Disabilities. New York: Marcel Dekker, 1983.
2. Scott JA, Walker AP, Eunpu DI, et al: Genetic counselor training: A review and considerations for the future. Am J Hum Genet 42:191–199, 1988.
3. Cohen MM, Gorlin RJ, Levin S: Syndromes of the Head and Neck. Vol. 3. New York: Raven, in press, 1989.
4. Shprintzen RJ, Siegel-Sadewitz VL, Amato J, et al: Anomalies associated with cleft lip, cleft palate or both. Am J Med Genet 20:585, 1985.

CHAPTER 16

Documentation of Cleft Lip, Alveolus, and Palate

Otto Kriens

Documentation differs from registration in that it is based on an arrangement according to some systematic division into classes or groups. A sound classification system is a mandatory prerequisite of documentation. This has become evident during the history of cleft lip and palate documentation. Clefts were grouped according to morphologic and/or anatomic criteria until the embryologic classification was discovered. On the other hand, a documentation system should extend beyond mere recording. If documentation means support or proof by reference to systematically arranged subjects or items, the system itself should serve as a vehicle for further research into related fields.

Morphologic Classifications

In the 1920s, several centers for cleft lip, alveolus, and palate treated a large number of patients with different cleft forms, which called for an appropriate system of registration. Various suggestions were made. In 1922, Davies and Ritchie[1] divided their clefts into three morphologic groups: (1) cleft lip, (2) cleft palate, and (3) a combination of the two. The subdivisions used were unilateral, median, and bilateral cleft lip and palate. The palate was recorded as hard and soft palate, each being subdivided into thirds, indicating the length of the cleft. Microforms were not included.

In 1932 Veau[2] proposed four groups: (1) soft palate, (2) soft and hard palate, (3) unilateral cleft lip and palate, and (4) bilateral cleft lip and palate. Cleft lip (and alveolus), partial clefts, and microforms were not included.

In 1942, Fogh-Andersen[3] documented the alveolar process with the lip in what seemed to be just another morphologic "classification," comprising (1) cleft lip, (2) cleft lip and palate, and (3) cleft palate. In 1964, Fogh-Andersen[4] noted that "unlike Stark,[5] it was not an embryological, but simply a practical reason" to include cases with alveolar clefts in the cleft lip group.

Embryologic Classification

In 1958, Kernahan and Stark made the revolutionary discovery that the incisive foramen is the embryologic border between clefts of the phylogenetic primary and secondary palate.[5] Their embryologic classification in-

cluded the alveolus. There are three groups: (1) cleft lip and alveolus, (2) cleft hard and soft palate, and (3) combination of 1 and 2. This convincing concept immediately gained general acceptance. Classification was no longer a problem. Documentation, however, remained tedious, complicated, and not infrequently incomplete and inaccurate.

General Considerations

The documentation of cleft diagnoses in writing is time consuming. To record a "left partial cleft lip associated with a complete soft palate cleft partially extending into the left hard palate" necessitates the writing of 18 words. To type this diagnosis takes 113 taps on letter keys and the space bar. Therefore, coding has challenged several authors. Efforts for a concise documentation system have been made in two directions: (1) using abbreviations (letters or numerals) to define the cleft region(s) or the degree of clefting, and (2) designing visual symbols.

Prerequisites

An optimal documentation of a cleft lip, alveolus, and palate diagnosis should include the cleft region, the side of the cleft, and the degree of clefting. However, a documentation is not a description, although it would be appropriate to include as much morphologic information as feasible. It goes without saying that overburdening a documentation system with descriptive annotations makes it less practical or even useless. It is known from clinical experience that it does not matter very much skeletally whether a lip is cleft one-fourth, two-thirds, or any other fraction of its height. However, complete and partial clefts have different general morphologic impacts. Microforms should be recorded for genetic studies. A modern documentation system should allow the diagnoses to be typed on a keyboard for digitization into computers. Finally, codes should be plausible and not numerous.

Recent Documentation Systems

The proposals of Harkins et al in 1960[6] and 1962[7] were along the lines of the work done prior to the embryologic classification of Kernahan and Stark.[5] Nevertheless, the Subcommittee of the International Confederation for Plastic and Reconstructive Surgery accepted their classification.

Based on the embryologic classification, Vilar-Sancho proposed a code for a detailed documentation system in 1962.[8] He suggested using the first letter of Greek words to define the anatomic cleft regions—that is, K (keilos) = lip, G (gnathos) = jaw, alveolus, U (uranos) = palate, S (staphyle) = velum, uvula. This choice was not practical because Greek is not as frequently used in medical terminology as Latin or the English words of Latin origin. The side of the cleft was indicated by

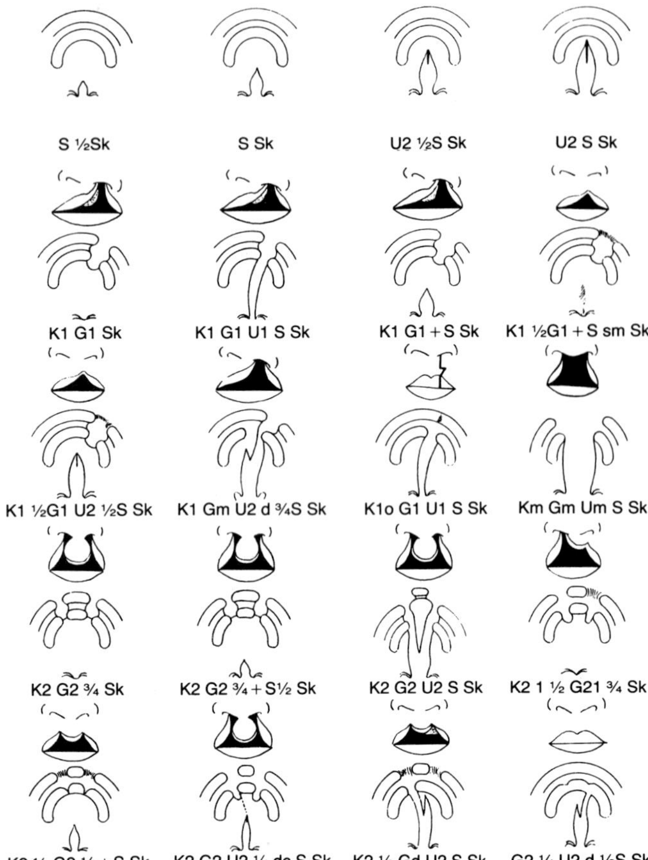

Figure 16–1 Vilar-Sancho's original illustrations of his contribution during the Second Hamburg International Symposium. (From Schuchardt K (ed.), Treatment of Patients with Clefts of Lip, Alveolus, and Palate. Stuttgart, Thieme Verlag, 1966. With permission.)

letters and numerals: d = right, 1 = left, 2 = bilateral, and m = median. At the end of the cleft formula the code Sk (skisis = cleft) separately identified the formula as pertaining to a cleft. Vilar-Sancho's documentation of a complete bilateral cleft lip, alveolus, and palate, for example, read: Ks Gs Us S Sk. According to the formula this documentation was complicated by the repetition of the side (d, 1, m, 2) in each cleft area. Like others, Vilar-Sancho followed Davies and Ritchie[1] in adding fractions behind the cleft area to indicate the linear extent of any partial clefting. K2 1/2 G2 1/4 U2 d1/2 S Sk described a bilateral partial lip cleft involving half of the lip height, a bilateral partial cleft alveolus of one-quarter in extent (three-dimensional?), a complete hard palate cleft on the left side with a partial cleft of one-half of the sagittal length of the hard palate on the right side, and a velar cleft. Besides the erroneous inclusion of median clefts and "congenital scars," the complexity of the registration has barred Vilar-Sancho's documentation system from general acceptance (Fig. 16–1).

In 1963, Koch published a similarly complex documentation, also based on the embryologic classification.[9] In 1987, Koch and Prein presented a recent version of this documentation system for the palate area during the Advanced Workshop at Bremen.[10] The bifid posterior nasal spine, which is an ontogenetic secondary cleft anomaly of the velar cleft, unfortunately was included in the documentation of the hard palate cleft.

In 1966 McCabe suggested a documentation system that was overburdened with measurement data.[11] For example, besides measuring the sagittal extent of a velar cleft in fractions in thirds, the greatest width of the cleft was identified within the limits of 2, 6, 10, 14, 18, 22, 26, and 30 mm. Moreover, there were too many subdivisions—for example, code 49 for the velar cleft (one-third to three-thirds of the sagittal dimension), code 53 for the hard palate, code 57 for the hard and soft palate cleft (sagittal extent in one-sixth fractions), and code 58 for an isolated hard and soft palate cleft. The width of velar clefts was recorded as code 52 (2, 6, 10, 14, 18, 22, 26, and 30 mm) and that of the hard palate in code 56. Users of this documentation system had to resort to a manual to record their findings.

McCabe's documentation exemplifies the overburdening of a system with too many descriptive notes of secondary importance. Some of these data may even be irrelevant, since most of these measurements would require a three-dimensional rather than a linear assessment. Many of the documentation systems proposed aim at perfection, but by including too many details they do not provide "universal intelligibility" as postulated by Pruzansky in 1953.[12]

Visual Symbols

In 1963 Pfeifer devised a system of visual symbols to index cleft lip, alveolus, and palate diagnoses (Fig. 16–2).[13] A vertical block of three rectangular pairs (right and left lip, alveolus, and hard palate) on top of a triangle (soft palate) schematically outlined the cleft areas. He showed complete clefts by blackening the areas and partial ones by cross-hatching the areas. Submucous clefts or microforms could not be recorded. The greatest disadvantage of such an appealing symbol is that it cannot be written or typed. A visual symbol may be compared with Hollerith's card and its punch holes. Once valuable, it was discarded when electronic data-retrieving systems were introduced. Lacking a written code (numerals or letters), a visual symbol may be appropriate for a small number of records but not

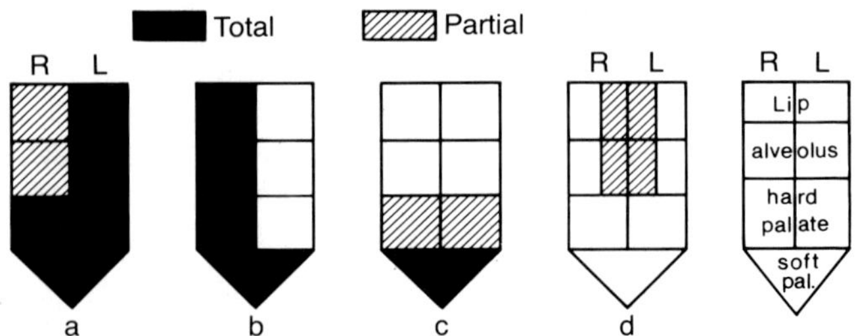

Figure 16–2 Pfeifer's original illustrations of his contribution during the Second Hamburg International Symposium. (From Schuchardt K (ed.), Treatment of Patients with Clefts of Lip, Alveolus, and Palate. Stuttgart, G. Thieme Verlay, 1966. With permission.) The median cleft lip and premaxilla (Fig. 16–2D) does not fit into Pfeifer's morphogenetic scheme and was added on the recommendations of the American Cleft Palate Association at that time.

for modern computer-aided data processing and communication.

In 1971 Kernahan published the "striped Y" system (Fig. 16–3).[14] Areas 3 and 4 as well as 7 and 8 did not correspond with specific embryologic or anatomic regions. Complete and partial clefting was indicated by shading.

In 1972, one year after Kernahan's proposal of the striped Y, Elsahy added two triangles, two circles, and two arrows to improve the striped Y.[15] He did not erase the anatomically meaningless rectangulars 3 and 4. Elsahy tried to correct the vertical (i.e., median) limb by adding two arrows to indicate a right and/or left hard palate cleft. This did not improve the logical sequence of the coded data. The addition of the two arrows impaired computer input.

LAHSHAL

The Anatomic Paraphrase of Cleft Lip, Alveolus, and Palate

In 1953 Pruzansky stated that "most classifications are insufficiently descriptive without providing universal intelligibility."[12] A code should be derived from the anatomic structures involved, otherwise it has to be memorized and will soon be forgotten. Ideally, a code should represent the anatomic region, the side, and the type of cleft (complete, partial, microform). Because recent model analyses have shown that clinical cleft width is related more to malposition of the cleft segments than to a defect, linear measurements may be irrelevant.[16, 17] Angular measurements are more appropriate and reflect positional changes during growth and treatment.

A cleft lip, alveolus, and palate is a malformation in the sagittal direction, from lip to uvula. Because clefts of the lip (L), alveolus (A), and hard palate (H) occur bilaterally and the soft palate cleft (S) is in the midline, the velar region is used as a hinge for the two sagittal prongs containing the paramedian cleft areas LAH (Fig. 16–4). Once these two bilateral cleft areas are turned laterally into the level of the velar cleft, the code of a bilateral cleft lip, alveolus, and palate reads LAHSHAL. This cleft formula is read like a radiograph: the right side of the patient is on the left side and vice versa. The soft palate area, S, is the middle of the cleft formula. Every code has to be allocated on the left or right side. If only the lip (and alveolus) is clefted, the middle portion of the LAHSHAL formula is defined by a dash (–). Thus the side of the cleft is always automatically recorded in the LAHSHAL system. L– defines a complete right cleft lip, and –L a corresponding cleft on the other side (see Table 16–1).

Three degrees of clefting (complete, partial, microform) can be documented with the LAHSHAL codes as well. Upper case letters define complete clefts and lower case letters partial ones. Microforms are written as asterisks in the particular LAHSHAL location concerned (Table 16–2).

Table 16–1. LAHSHAL Documentation System for Complete Clefts

Tabl. 1 Computer Code		Written Diagnoses of Complete Clefts		Chart Form
L	=	Complete right lip cleft	=	L –
LA	=	Complete right lip-alveolus cleft	=	LA
LAHS . . .	=	Complete right unilateral CLAP cleft	=	LAHS
. . HSH . .	=	Complete cleft of hard and soft palate	=	HSH
. . . S . . .	=	Complete velar cleft	=	S
. . . SHAL	=	Complete left unilateral CLAP cleft	=	SHAL
. . . . . AL	=	Complete left lip-alveolus cleft	=	AL
. L	=	Complete left lip cleft	=	– L
L L	=	Complete bilateral lip cleft	=	L–L
LA . . . AL	=	Complete bilateral lip-alveolus cleft	=	LA–AL
LAHSHAL	=	Complete bilateral CLAP cleft	=	LAHSHAL

In the palatal region, sss denotes a submucous velar cleft and s*s a submucous velar cleft with a bifid uvula. A submucous cleft of the hard and soft palate is hsh, and h*h defines the same submucous cleft with a bifid uvula. Combinations of embryologically different clefts are easily and concisely recorded with the LAHSHAL system as well (Table 16–3).

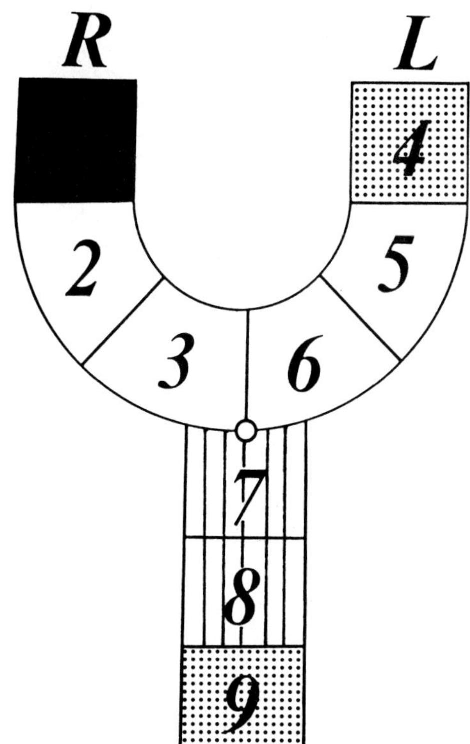

Figure 16–3 Kernahan's original illustration. A complete right and partial left cleft lip associated with a submucous cleft of the hard and soft palate with a bifid uvula have been marked. The LAHSHAL formula for this cleft is "Ls*sl." (From Kernahan DS. The striped Y—a symbolic classification for cleft lip and palate. Plast Reconstr Surg 47:469, 1971. With permission.)

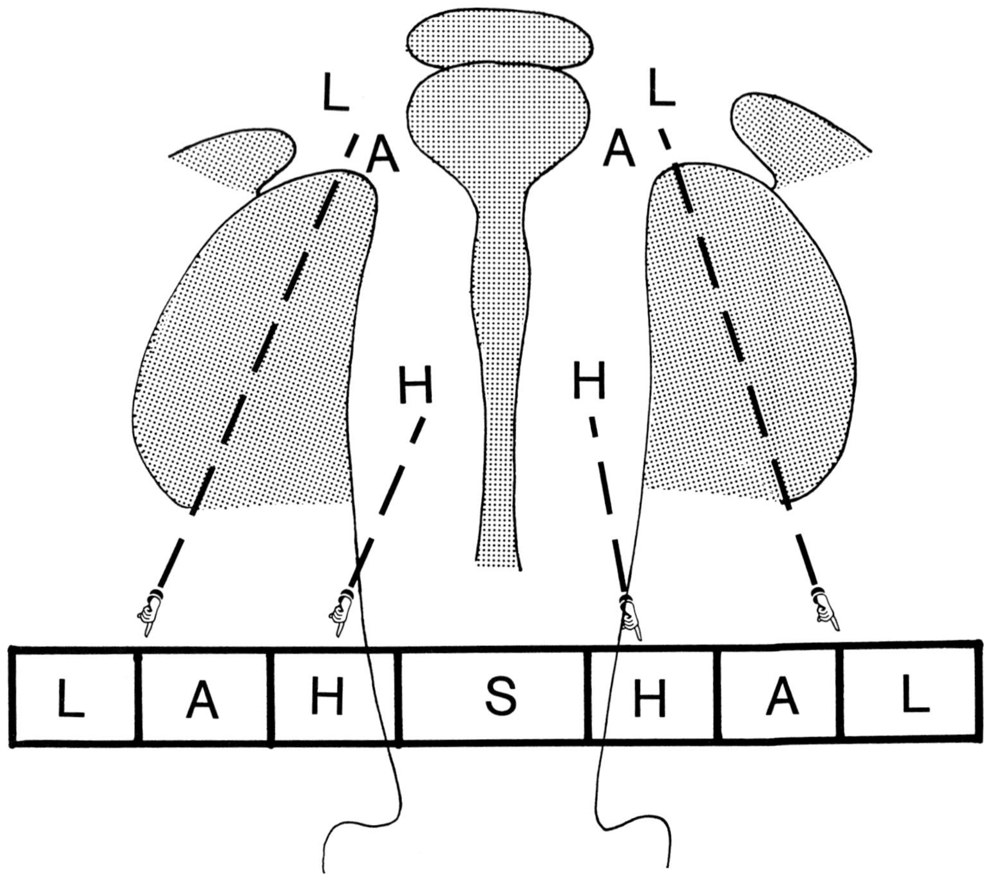

Figure 16–4 LAHSHAL, a paraphrase of the anatomic areas affected by cleft lip (L), alveolus (A), and hard (H) and soft palate (S). The paramedian cleft regions LAH are projected on a line with the median S, resulting in the LAHSHAL formula.

Table 16–2. LAHSHAL Documentation System for Partial Clefts and Microforms

Tabl. 2 Computer Code		Written Diagnoses of Partial Clefts and Microforms	Chart Code
*	=	Microform of cleft lip on right side . . . . =	* −
l	=	Partial cleft lip of the right side =	l−
l*	=	Partial right cleft lip with microform of right alveolus cleft =	l*
la	=	Partial right lip-alveolus cleft =	la
. . . . s . .	=	Partial velar cleft =	s
. . . . * . .	=	Bifid uvula =	*
. . sss . .	=	Submucous velar cleft =	sss
. . h . h . .	=	Submucous clefts of hard palate only . . . . =	hh
. . hsh . .	=	Submucous clefts of hard and soft palate . . . . =	hsh
. . h*h . .	=	Hsh with bifid uvula =	h*h
. . . . .al	=	Partial left lip-alveolus cleft =	al
. . . . . *l	=	Microform of alveolus cleft with partial lip cleft on the left side =	*l
. l	=	Partial left lip cleft =	−l
. . . . . .*	=	Microform of cleft lip on left side . . . . =	−*
l l	=	Partial bilateral cleft lip =	l—l
la . . . al	=	Partial bilateral lip-alveolus cleft =	la–al
l* . . . *l	=	Bilateral microform of lip clefts =	l*–*l

In the majority of patients, combined clefts contain partial cleft forms, as shown in Table 16–4. Even very complex cleft forms can swiftly be documented in a short and exact LAHSHAL formula. The LAHSHAL system has been effectively used for more than 10 years and was presented by us in 1987.[18]

LAHSHAL Beyond Mere Documentation

Besides providing an easy and short form of documentation, the LAHSHAL system also provides many possibilities for investigating larger groups of cleft palate patients. Two examples are described. The LAHSHAL formula allows verification of the number and types of

Table 16–3. LAHSHAL Documentation System for Combined Complete Clefts

Tabl. 3 Computer Code		Written Diagnoses of Combined Complete Clefts	Chart Form
L . . S . . .	=	Complete cleft of velum and right lip . . . . =	LS
LA . S . . L	=	Complete right lip and alveolus cleft associated with a complete left cleft lip and complete velar cleft . . . . =	LASL
LA.SAHL	=	Complete right lip and alveolus cleft associated with a complete unilateral cleft lip, alveolus and palate . . . . =	LHSHL
L.HSH.L	=	Complete bilateral cleft lip associated with a complete cleft of the hard and soft palate . . . . . =	LHSHL

Table 16–4. LAHSHAL Documentation System for Combinations of Complete and Partial Clefts

Tabl. 4 Computer Code		Written Diagnoses of Combinations of Complete and Partial Clefts	Chart Form
lahSh . .	=	Partial right lip and alveolus cleft associated with a complete velar cleft extending into the hard palate . . . . =	lahSh
LahSHAL	=	Complete right lip and partial alveolus cleft associated with a complete left unilateral CLAP extending into the hard palate on the right side . . . . =	LahSHAL
lA . S . Al	=	Partial bilateral cleft lip and complete bilateral alveolus cleft associated with a complete soft palate cleft . . . . =	lASAl

the various cleft forms among the 1285 cleft patients presently documented.[18] There are 116 different cleft forms, 94 in males and 63 in females (Fig. 16–5). The expected total number of different cleft forms can be calculated polynomially. Statistical analyses reveal that there should be 124 different cleft forms, 96 in males and 79 in females (Fig. 16–6).[19]

The simplicity and ease of use of the LAHSHAL system will certainly generate investigations into ethnic differences and the sex distribution of subgroups of certain clefts to elucidate their genetic background and the statistical analyses of problems related to cleft lip, alveolus, and palate.

Conclusion

LAHSHAL, a paraphrase of the anatomic areas of cleft lip, alveolus, and palate, provides an easy, concise, and exact system of documentation for clinical and research work on large numbers of cleft diagnoses. The LAHSHAL documentation system has effectively stood

Number of cleft forms in 1285 patients

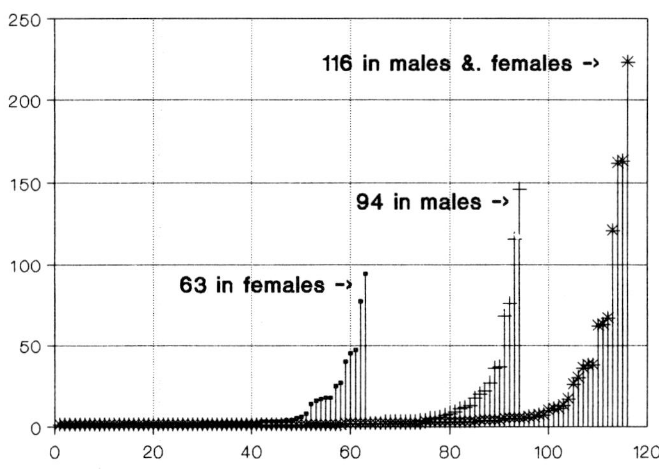

Figure 16–5 Distribution of cleft forms in males and females.

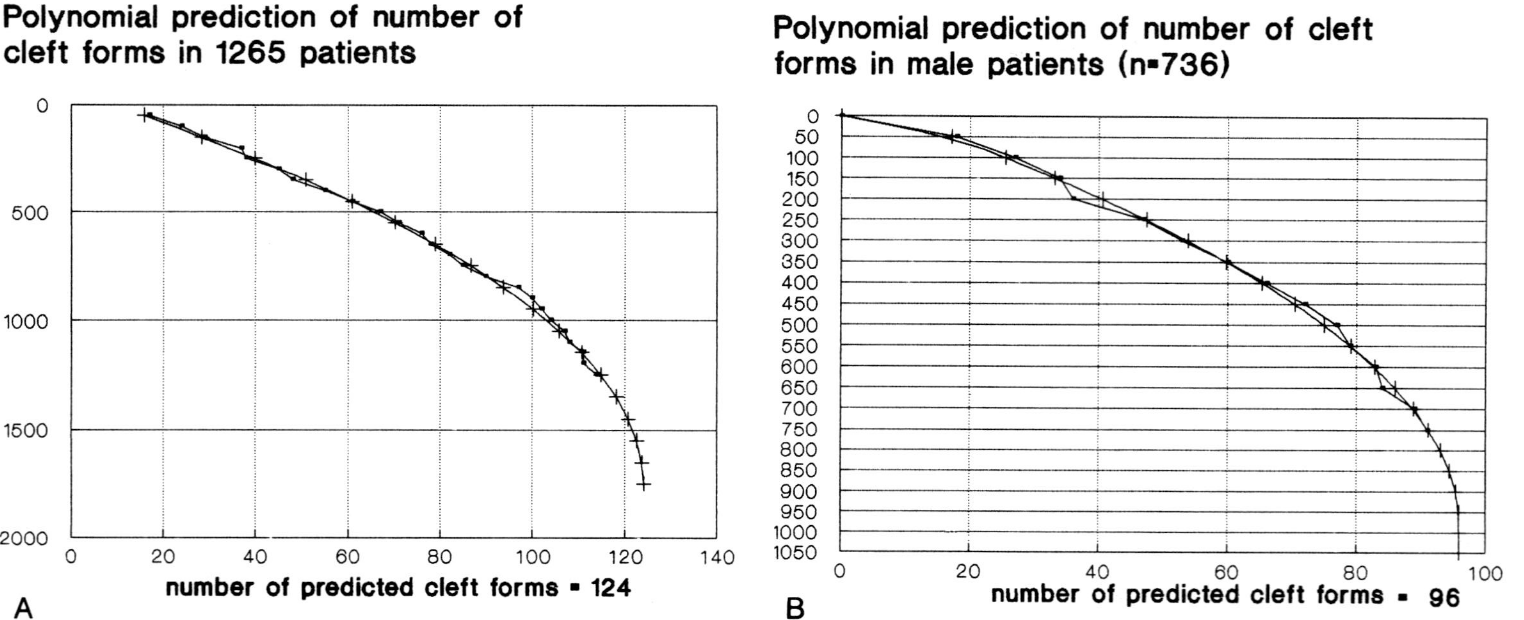

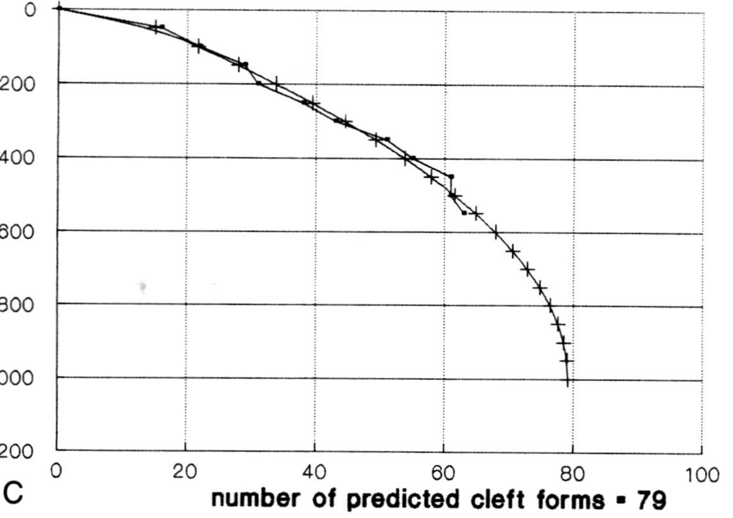

Figure 16–6 A–C, Polynomial prediction of the number of cleft forms.

the test of time for more than 10 years in more than 1280 patients. The LAHSHAL system has opened the door to a wide variety of research activities (statistical, epidemiologic, ethnic, genetic).

References

1. Davies JB, Ritchie HP: Classification of congenital clefts of the lip and palate. JAMA 79:1323, 1922.
2. Veau V: Division palatine. Paris: Masson, 1931.
3. Fogh-Andersen P: Inheritance of harelip and cleft palate. Copenhagen: Arnold Busk, 1942.
4. Fogh-Andersen P: Documentation. Discussion by Invitation. In Schuchardt K (ed): Treatment of Cleft Lip, Alveolus and Palate. Stuttgart: G. Thieme, 1966. p. 223.
5. Kernahan DA, Stark RB: A new classification for cleft lip and palate. Plast Reconstr Surg 22:435, 1958.
6. Harkins CS, Berlin A, Harding R, et al: Report on the nomenclature committee. Cleft Palate Bull 10:11, 1960.
7. Harkins CS, Berlin A, Harding R, et al: A classification of cleft lip and cleft palate. Plast Reconstr Surg 29:31, 1962.
8. Vilar-Sancho B: A proposed new international classification of congenital cleft lip and cleft palate. Plast Reconstr Surg 30:263, 1962.
9. Koch J: Zur Diagnostik der Lippen-Kiefer- und Gaumen-spalten. Dtsch Stomat 9:66, 1963.
10. Koch J, Prein J: Documentation of cleft lip and palate with regard to location and extent of the palate cleft. In Kriens O (ed): Proceedings of the Advanced Workshop: "What is a Cleft?". Stuttgart: G. Thieme, 1989.
11. McCabe PA: A coding procedure for classification of cleft lip and cleft palate. Cleft Palate J 3:383, 1966.
12. Pruzansky S: Description, classification, and analysis of unoperated clefts of lip and palate. Am J Orthod 39:590, 1953.
13. Pfeifer G: Documentation. Discussion by Invitation. In Schuchardt K (ed): Treatment of Patients with Cleft Lip, Alveolus and Palate. Stuttgart: G. Thieme, 1966, p. 226.
14. Kernahan DS: The striped Y—a symbolic classification for cleft lip and palate. Plast Reconstr Surg 47:469, 1971.
15. Elsahy NI: The modified striped Y—a systematic classification for cleft lip and palate. Cleft Palate J 10:245, 1973.
16. Kriens O: Three-dimensional measurement of maxillary models of infants with UCLAP using the reflex microscope. In Kriens O: Proceedings of the Advanced Workshop: "What is a Cleft?". Stuttgart: G. Thieme, 1989.
17. Shaw W: Communication during the discussion of the session Model Analysis. In Kriens O (ed): Proceedings of the Advanced Workshop: "What is a Cleft?". Stuttgart: G. Thieme, 1989.
18. Kriens O: LAHSHAL: An easy clinical system of cleft lip, alveolus and palate documentation. In Kriens O (ed): Proceedings of the Advanced Workshop: "What is a Cleft?". Stuttgart: G. Thieme, 1989.
19. Kriens O, Jindelt Van W: Assessment and polynomial prediction of the number of different cleft lip, alveolus and palate forms. Cleft Palate J (submitted for publication).

Primary Surgical Treatment of Cleft Lip/Nose

CHAPTER 17

Anatomy of Unilateral and Bilateral Cleft Lip

Miroslav Fára

In the reconstruction of any kind of orofacial defect, a prerequisite for success is a thorough knowledge of the anatomy of the oral and facial regions and of the variations existing in the afflicted lip and palate. During reconstruction of a cleft lip, both the faulty formation of its individual components and its incomplete or defective development must be corrected. Furthermore, the anatomic and functional relationships between the lip and the immediately adjacent facial structures, such as the expressive musculature and the nose and the more remote muscle entities of the palate and pharynx, must be respected.

The structure of the upper and lower lips is almost identical, the only striking difference being the somewhat more complicated architecture of the upper lip with its clearly differentiated medial part, the philtrum. The philtrum originates with the premaxilla from the fused nasomedial processes and is bordered laterally by distinctly protruding cristae philtri, which arise from the maxillary processes (Fig. 17–1).

The skin of the lip passes into the vermilion zone by way of a sharp and slightly elevated ridge. This line may be doubled, an important consideration for the surgeon. The vermilion zone represents a transitional area to the mucous membrane and is covered by a thin and nonkeratinized epithelium. Its red color is due to an excess of capillaries and to an increased translucency of the epithelial layers. In the central part of the lip, the depression of the philtrum, with its raised adjacent structures, the cristae philtri and medial tubercle, form a curve at the vermilion border—the Cupid's bow.

There are many sweat and mucous glands in the lip. The latter are numerous within the mucous membrane. The vermilion zone does not, as a rule, contain any glands. Hair follicles are completely absent.

The main component of the lip is the orbicularis oris muscle, which is attached firmly to the skin and mucous membrane. Because of this, there is no distinct folding of the skin, which follows the smallest movements of the muscle. The edges of a cleft lip are hypoplastic. The labial sulcus is shallow in the area adjacent to the cleft. Consideration must be given to the shape and size of the lip defect when planning reconstructive procedures. Differences in the course and state of the orbicularis oris muscle and in the blood supply to the individual segments of the cleft lip represent the major deviations from normal.

The orbicularis oris muscle provides the oral region with its function and at the same time contributes considerably to the appearance of the lip. This mutual relationship between function and shape and their reciprocal influence are important and should be constantly considered during lip reconstruction. In many cases the poor result of lip repair may be attributed to inappropriate reconstruction of the orbicularis oris muscle. Suturing the muscle stumps end to side spoils the morphologic and functional results of any method (Fig. 17–2).

The Muscles of the Lip

The musculature of the lip is represented by the musculus orbicularis oris. It originates, together with the other facial muscles, from the second branchial arch. The density of the mesenchymal cells gives origin to this muscle; even in the fourth week of gestation, the "muscle blastema" may be found. During the fifth week the main trunk of the facial nerve, supplying the area of the second branchial arch, becomes fan-shaped and

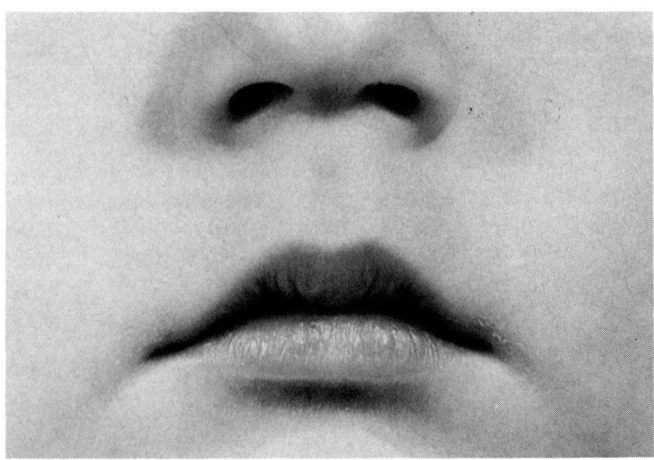

Figure 17–1 Normal lip with its philtrum, cristae, medial tubercle, and Cupid's bow.

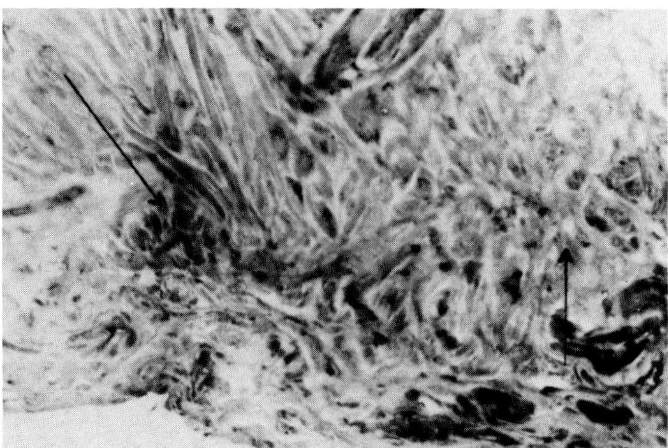

Figure 17–2 Faulty approximation of the stumps of the musculus orbicularis oris (MOO). Histologic findings from the corrective procedure of the lip.

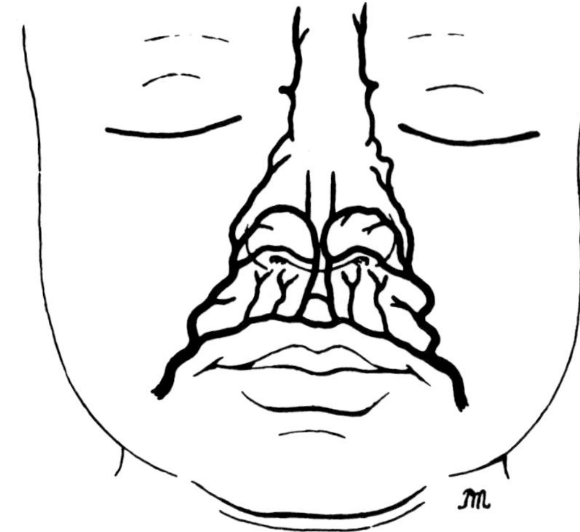

Figure 17–4 Arteries of the upper lip.

penetrates the mesenchymal formation. The tissue of this muscle blastema, innervated by the branches of the facial nerve, develops and spreads up and down, giving rise to the orbicularis oris muscle. In the course of normal embryonic development during the second month, this primitive muscle reaches the medial line of the lip, where it joins the opposite muscle (Fig. 17–3).

The orbicularis oris passes around the oral fissure. Since it is not covered by fascia, it is in contact anteriorly with the skin and posteriorly with the mucous membrane. It consists anatomically and functionally of two parts, the external and internal layers. The external part of the orbicularis oris muscle originates in the periosteum of the maxilla and mandible in the region of the frontal teeth. It is influenced by the mimical muscles passing into it and participating in its function by their dilating and/or stabilizing effect. This external part of the orbicularis oris enables the mouth to open and make expressions with the upper and lower lips. The internal part, passing between both corners of the mouth, represents the true mouth constrictor without any other function.

The circular bundles of the orbicularis oris are occasionally interspersed with a few fibers of musculi labii propii (compressor labii, musculus cutaneomucosus, and musculus rectus labii), which pass obliquely between the skin and the mucous membrane. These muscle fibers can be found more easily in the lateral parts of the lip than in the philtrum. They are supposed to draw the lip to the jaw when the child is sucking and disappear after the nursing period.

The nutritional arteries are situated on the underside of the muscle beneath the mucous membrane. The veins form a subcutaneous and submucous network.

The main artery of the upper lip is the arteria labialis superior, a branch of the a. maxillaris externa. It runs in the marginal part of the lip parallel to the bundles of the orbicularis oris and produces branches upward toward the nasal base (Figs. 17–4 and 17–5).

Arteriae labiales superiores of both sides meet at the medial line and join. After branching off the labial superior artery, just below the corner of the mouth, the a. maxillaris externa proceeds upward toward the nasolabial crease and splits into two branches at the nasal ala. One of these branches a. nasalis lateralis, supplies the area of the nasal ala and tip. The other, a. angularis, joins with a. dorsalis nasi, which is the terminal branch of a. ophthalmica. Arteria labialis superior, in the philtral part of the lip, produces a small branch for the

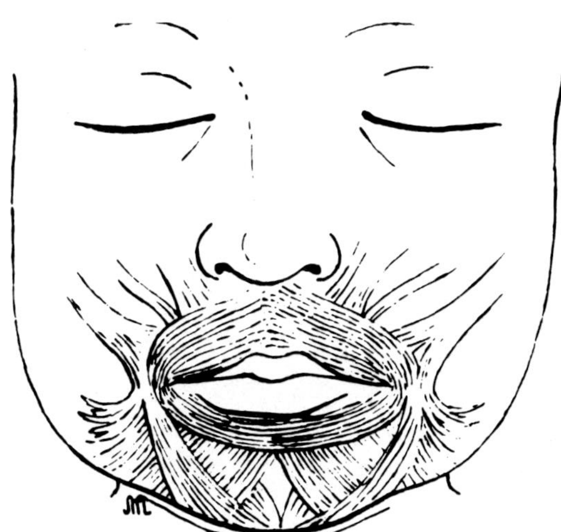

Figure 17–3 Muscles of the oral region. (From Fára M: The musculature of cleft lip and palate. In Converse JM (ed): Reconstructive Plastic Surgery, Vol. IV. Philadelphia, WB Saunders, 1977, p 1966. With permission.)

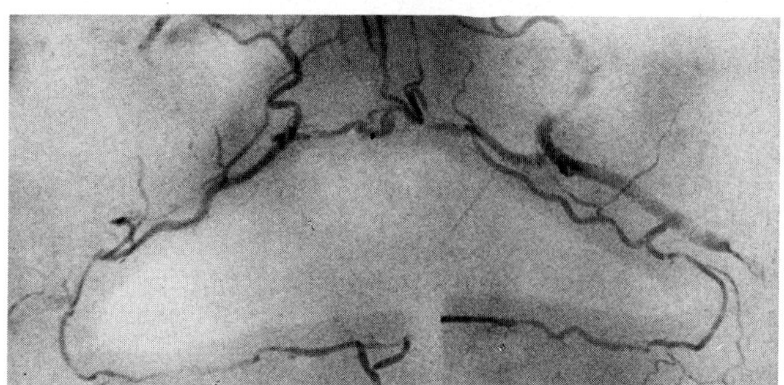

Figure 17–5 Arteriogram of the normal oral region.

lower margin of the frontal part of the nasal septum, and this joins with the terminal branches of the arteriae nasales posteriores septi.

Unilateral Clefts

In patients with complete unilateral cleft lip the fibers of the orbicularis oris muscle, proceeding horizontally from the corner of the mouth toward the midline, turn upward along the margins of the cleft. They terminate at the lateral side beneath the base of the nasal ala and at the philtral side beneath the base of the columella, where most attach to the periosteum of the maxilla. A few disappear in the subcutis (Figs. 17–6 to 17–8).

The muscle behaves in the same way in patients with an incomplete unilateral cleft lip, in whom only narrow bridges are formed. These bridges of tissue are known as Simonart's bands. In incomplete clefts, in which the cleft does not exceed two-thirds of the lip height, the muscle fibers reach over the top of the cleft and pass from the lateral to the philtral part of the lip. The muscle within the cleft is, however, interspersed by the trabeculi of the collagenous connective tissue (Figs. 17–9 to 17–12).

An excess and swelling of the lip muscle may be seen and palpated on the lateral side in patients with incomplete clefts. This is caused by a certain contraction or bulging of the muscle, which was prevented from developing to its proper length. The muscle on the philtral side, on the other hand, is underdeveloped and does not extend as far forward to the edge of the cleft as it does on the lateral side. At autopsy, as well as during surgery, we almost always see a striking thinning of the muscle layer in the entire half of the philtrum adjacent to the cleft.

In an incomplete cleft, manifested by a small coloboma in the lower part of the lip, a groove on the skin passes upward to the threshold of the nostril. This

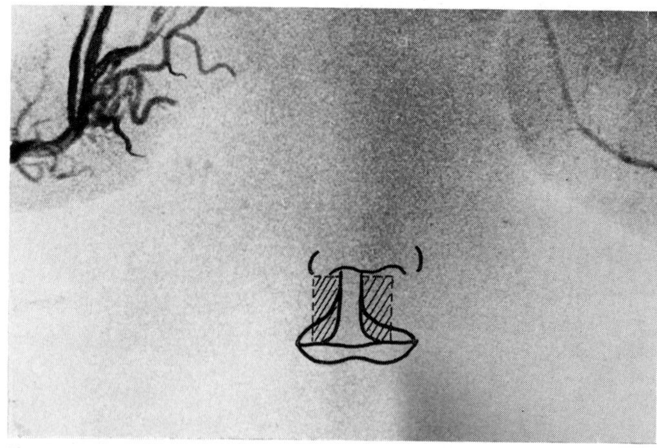

Figure 17–7 Typical arteriogram in a complete right cleft. Main branch of the superior labial artery passes along the edge of the cleft on both sides but is much more developed in the lateral segment. Inset shows orientation of the radiograph. (From Fára M: The musculature of cleft lip and palate. In Converse JM (ed): Reconstructive Plastic Surgery, Vol. IV. Philadelphia, WB Saunders, 1977, p 1967. With permission.)

external finding is manifested on the orbicularis oris muscle, which is compressed in a frontodorsal direction.

Similar findings have been seen in the arterial network. The superior labial artery on the lateral side of the cleft mostly follows the course of orbicularis oris bundles and deviates in a parallel fashion with the edge of the cleft upward to the nasal ala, where it anastomoses with the lateral nasal or angular artery. In incomplete clefts this artery is in the form of a thin terminal branch, which passes into the bridge of the nose. On the philtral side, the artery behaves in the same way, but its diameter is visibly smaller and its branches fewer than on the lateral side, corresponding to the same difference in the situation of the musculature of both cleft lip segments. The superior labial artery passes through its terminal branches into the columella, where it anastomoses mainly with the posterior septal artery.

In 3 of 42 dissected stillborn children with cleft lip,

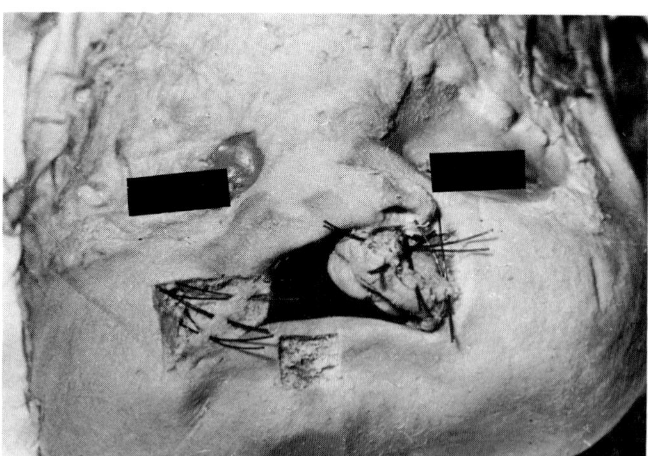

Figure 17–6 Dissection of a complete right cleft lip. Main muscle bundles are more clearly shown by the length of black nylon. Muscles pass along the edge of the cleft. (From Fára M: The musculature of cleft lip and palate. In Converse JM (ed): Reconstructive Plastic Surgery, Vol. IV. Philadelphia, WB Saunders, 1977, p 1967. With permission.)

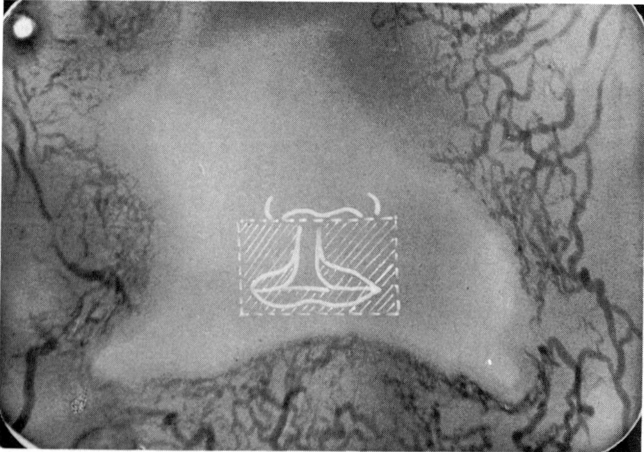

Figure 17–8 Arteriogram of complete unilateral cleft lip, demonstrating an unusually dense anastomotic network between the superior labial artery and the angular artery in both lip segments. (From Fára M: The musculature of cleft lip and palate. In Converse JM (ed): Reconstructive Plastic Surgery, Vol. IV. Philadelphia, WB Saunders, 1977, p 1967. With permission.)

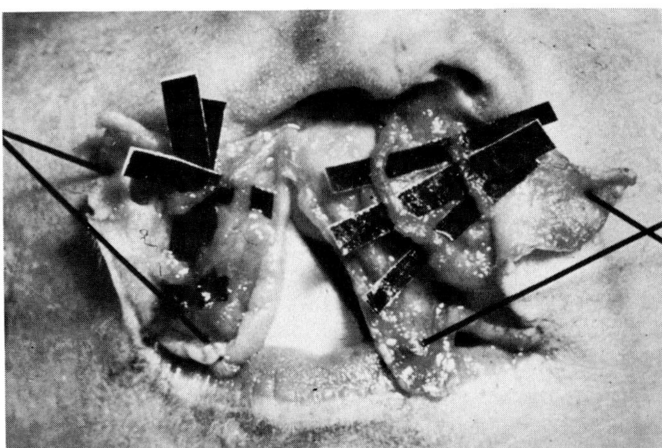

Figure 17–9 Dissection of MOO in an incomplete right cleft with a Simonart's band. Dissected main muscle bundles are placed on strips of black paper for better visibility. On the lateral side the transition of muscle fibers into the bridge can be seen. On the philtral side, however, the stronger muscle bundles only reach the medial line of the lip. (From Fára M: The musculature of cleft lip and palate. In Converse JM (ed): Reconstructive Plastic Surgery, Vol. IV. Philadelphia, WB Saunders, 1977, p 1968. With permission.)

the muscle fibers showed a tendency to run horizontally, entering the edge of the cleft and disappearing in the connective tissue there. The blood supply in these cases was also atypical, as can be seen in the arteriogram of the complete left-sided cleft.

The underdevelopment of the muscles and the poorer blood supply in the half of the philtrum facing the cleft suggests that the ability of the muscular stump of the orbicularis oris to grow across the midline of the lip, which ontogenetically represents its anatomic border, is to some extent limited. It is as though the orbicularis oris muscle of one-half of the lip is incapable of supplying musculature to the contralateral side.

Bilateral Clefts

In a complete bilateral cleft, the muscle stumps and arterial network of the lateral segments of the lip course in the same way as in a unilateral cleft (Figs. 17–13 to 17–16). The medial lip segment or the prolabium, on the other hand, is composed only of collagenous con-

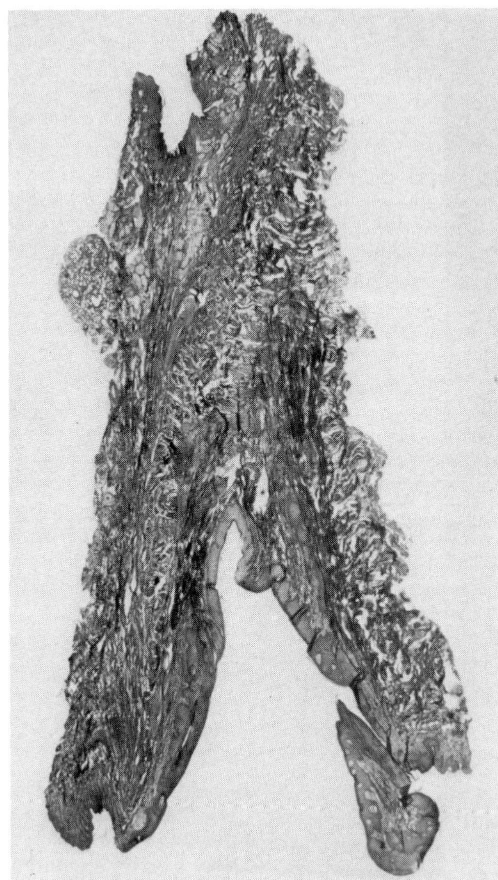

Figure 17–11 Specimen from an incomplete right cleft, frontal section. Muscle fibers follow the margins of the cleft. (From Fára M: The musculature of cleft lip and palate. In Converse JM (ed): Reconstructive Plastic Surgery, Vol. IV. Philadelphia, WB Saunders, 1977, p 1969. With permission.)

nective tissue, penetrated by a rich vascular network starting in the septal and columellar arteries, the aa. nasales posteriores septi, the terminal branches of a. ethmoidalis anterior, and the aa. nasales laterales (Figs. 17–17 and 17–18).

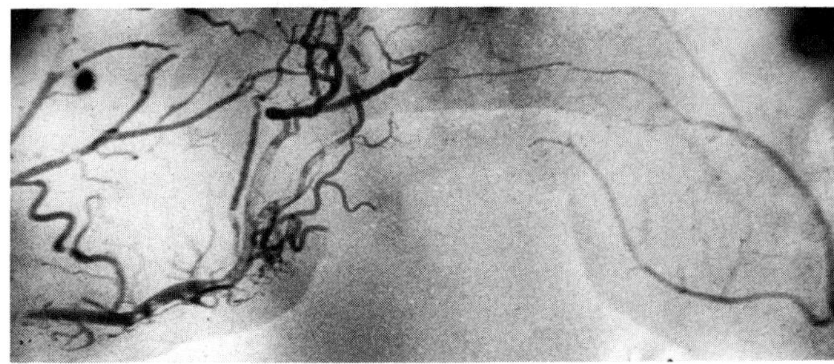

Figure 17–10 Arteriogram of an incomplete right cleft with a Simonart's band (injected with barium-formalin). Note the striking difference in the caliber of the vessels in the lateral and medial segments. A strong arterial branch penetrates into the bridge from the lateral side.

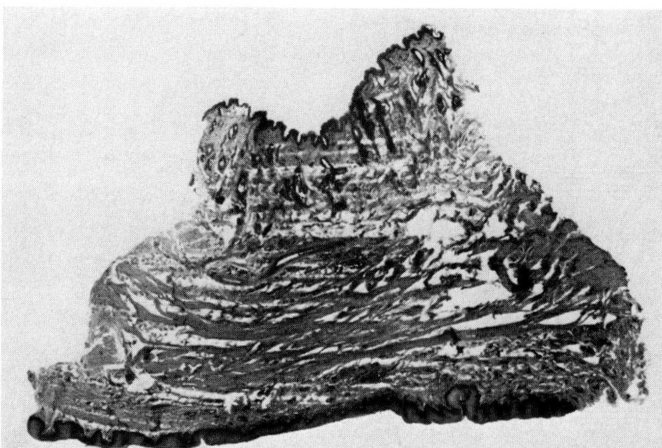

Figure 17–12 Specimen from an incomplete cleft, horizontal section. Note deviation in the course of the muscle fibers and the distinct frontodorsal compression. (From Fára M: The musculature of cleft lip and palate. In Converse JM (ed): Reconstructive Plastic Surgery, Vol. IV. Philadelphia, WB Saunders, 1977, p 1969. With permission.)

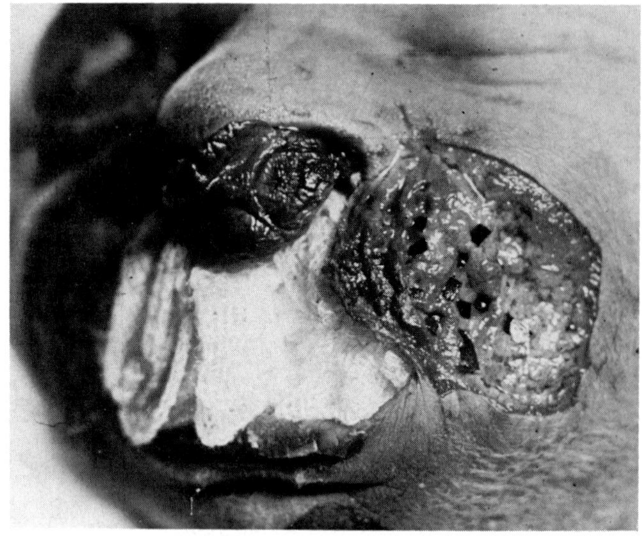

Figure 17–13 Dissection of muscle bundles of the right lateral segment (underlaid with black paper strips) in a complete bilateral cleft. (From Fára M: The musculature of cleft lip and palate. In Converse JM (ed): Reconstructive Plastic Surgery, Vol. IV. Philadelphia, WB Saunders, 1977, p 1970. With permission.)

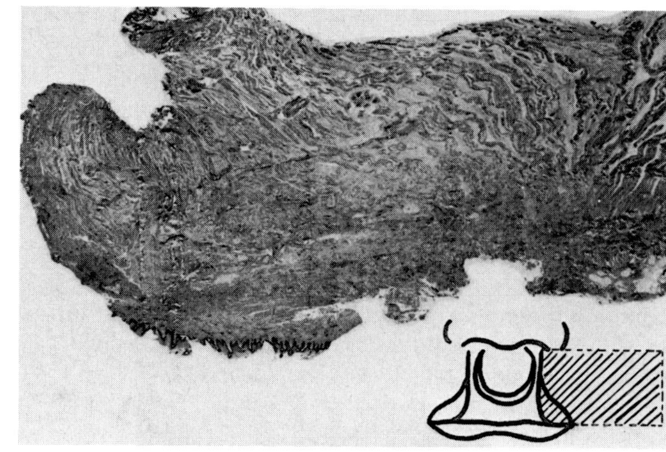

Figure 17–14 Frontal section of the lateral segment in a complete bilateral cleft (Van Gieson). Muscle fiber bundles pass upward along the edge of the cleft. At the corner of the mouth, they merge with the muscles of facial expression. (From Fára M: The musculature of cleft lip and palate. In Converse JM (ed): Reconstructive Plastic Surgery, Vol. IV. Philadelphia, WB Saunders, 1977, p 1970. With permission.)

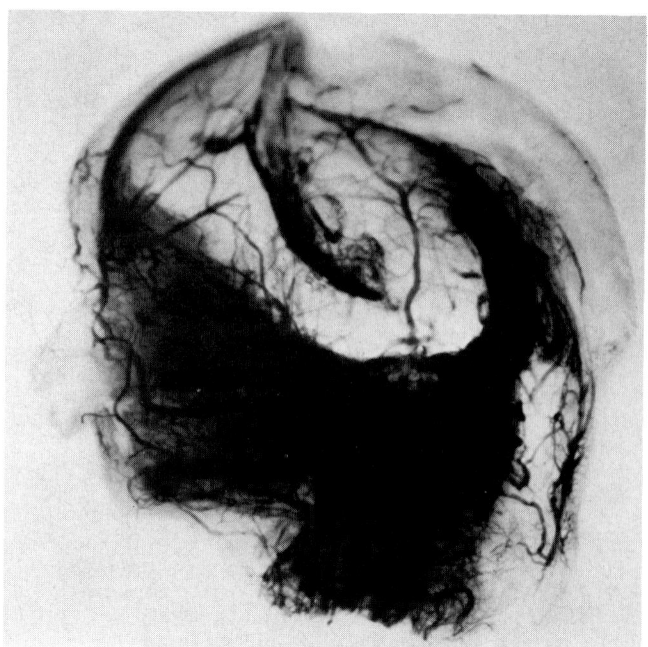

Figure 17–15 Lateral arteriogram of a complete bilateral cleft, after barium-formalin injection. (From Fára M: The musculature of cleft lip and palate. In Converse JM (ed): Reconstructive Plastic Surgery, Vol. IV. Philadelphia, WB Saunders, 1977, p 1971. With permission.)

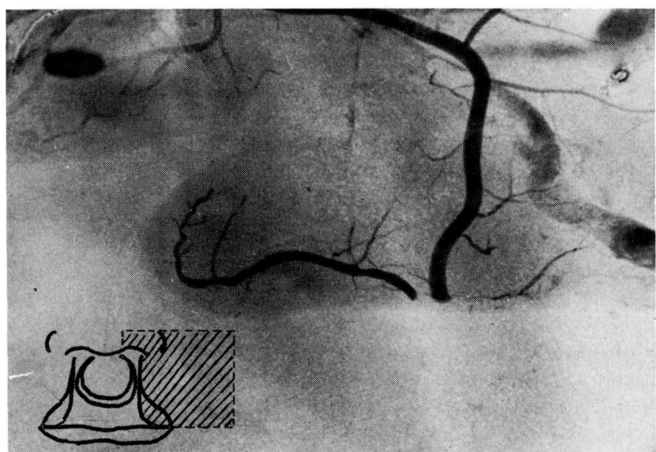

Figure 17–16 Arteriogram of lateral segment of a stillborn with complete bilateral cleft. Lip severed just above the beginning of the superior labial artery. A branch from the nasal ala can be seen at the upper left. (From Fára M: The musculature of cleft lip and palate. In Converse JM (ed): Reconstructive Plastic Surgery, Vol. IV. Philadelphia, WB Saunders, 1977, p 1971. With permission.)

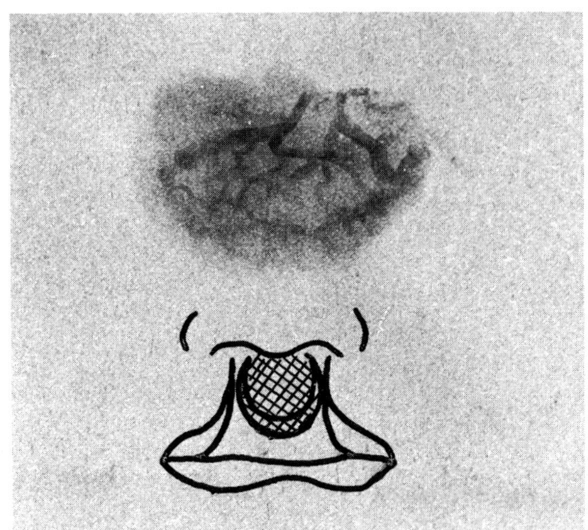

Figure 17–18 Arteriogram of an isolated prolabium of a stillborn with a complete bilateral cleft. Note the well-developed vessels originating from the nasal septum. (From Fára M: The musculature of cleft lip and palate. In Converse JM (ed): Reconstructive Plastic Surgery, Vol. IV. Philadelphia, WB Saunders, 1977, p 1971. With permission.)

In an incomplete bilateral cleft, the muscle bundles of the lateral segments cross the coloboma of the cleft quite smoothly into the medial lip segment, completely filling it (Figs. 17–19 to 17–21).

There is a striking difference between the state of the soft tissue bridges in unilateral and bilateral incomplete clefts. In the unilateral incomplete cleft, the muscles do not, as a rule, cross the cleft unless the bridge is at least one-third the height of the lip. On the other hand, in a bilateral cleft, the bridges are unusually well filled with muscle fibers, which penetrate from the lateral segments to the medial part of the lip, where they open like a fan. In contrast to unilateral clefts, this happens even when the bridges are very thin. Such bridges, in incomplete bilateral clefts, tend to be cylindrical in shape, whereas in unilateral clefts they are generally quite flat (Figs. 17–22 and 17–23).

An explanation for this different behavior of the musculature in incomplete bilateral clefts compared with incomplete unilateral clefts may be that in the former, the central part of the lip, partially isolated by the cleft and originally without any muscle fibers, can absorb the necessary tissue for each of its halves from the ontogenetically corresponding lateral, richly muscled, lip segment.

In the case of a bilateral cleft in which a bridge is formed on only one side, the muscle bundles brought in from the lateral segment adequately fill only the adjacent half of the prolabium. Not a single muscle fiber penetrates as far as the other border of the prolabium facing the complete cleft. This situation is similar to the condition of the philtrum in a complete unilateral cleft (Fig. 17–24).

Proliferation of the Musculus Orbicularis Oris into the Prolabium After Bilateral Cleft Lip Repair

For many years, the question of the tissue structure of the prolabium in complete bilateral clefts has been discussed. To help clarify this problem and at the same time attempt to ascertain possible changes in the prolabium after its fusion with lateral segments, we carried out a three-phase histologic examination of 30 children.

Phase I

During the repair of the first side of the lip, which was performed at the age of 5 to 7 months by folding down the muscle stump into the margin of the prolabium, we found in the excised parts of the prolabial

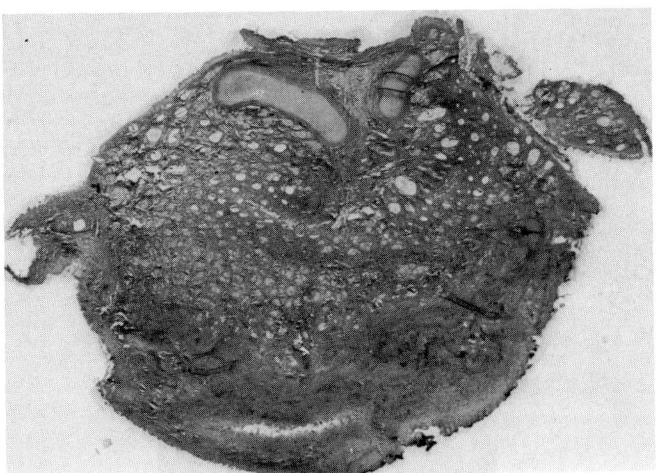

Figure 17–17 Frontal section from a prolabium. Cartilages of the nasal septum are seen in the upper part. Note the absence of muscle fibers (Van Gieson). (From Fára M: The musculature of cleft lip and palate. In Converse JM (ed): Reconstructive Plastic Surgery, Vol. IV. Philadelphia, WB Saunders, 1977, p 1970. With permission.)

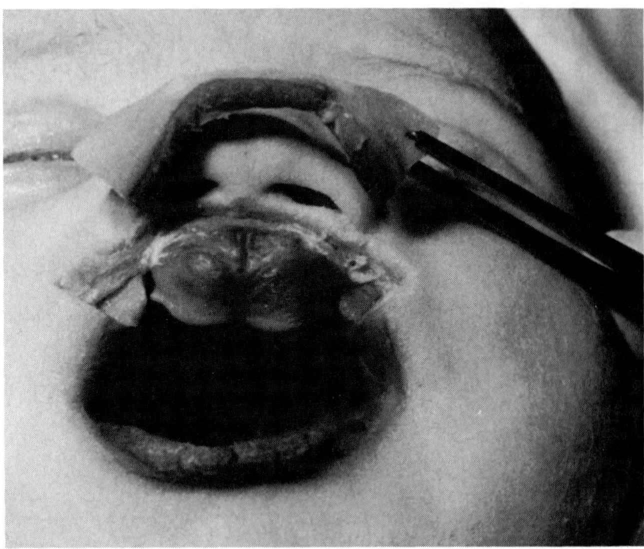

Figure 17–19 In a stillborn with incomplete bilateral cleft, the main part of the upper lip was excised and examined histologically. Muscle fibers passed through the wide bridges into the central segment. Note the excised specimen held by a surgical clamp. (From Fára M: The musculature of cleft lip and palate. In Converse JM (ed): Reconstructive Plastic Surgery, Vol. IV. Philadelphia, WB Saunders, 1977, p 1975. With permission.)

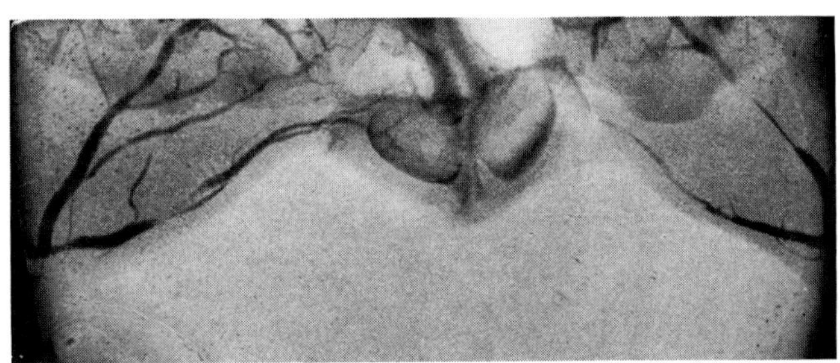

Figure 17–20 Arteriogram of the upper lip and premaxilla in an incomplete bilateral cleft, taken from a semiaxial angle. Branches of the superior labial artery pass through the soft tissue bridges into the central part of the lip. Intraoral view.

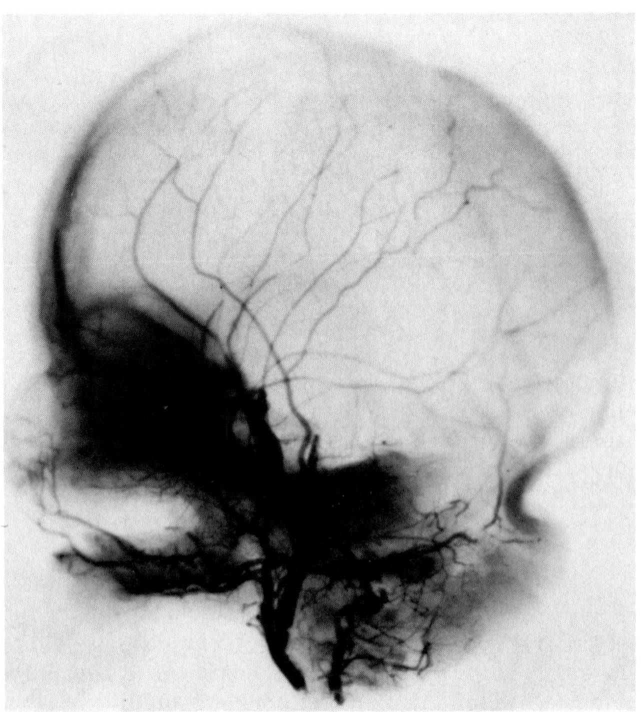

Figure 17–21 Lateral arteriogram of an incomplete bilateral cleft after barium-formalin injection. Note that the branches of the labial vessels pass into the prolabial segment. (From Fára M: The musculature of cleft lip and palate. In Converse JM (ed): Reconstructive Plastic Surgery, Vol. IV. Philadelphia, WB Saunders, 1977, p 1976. With permission.)

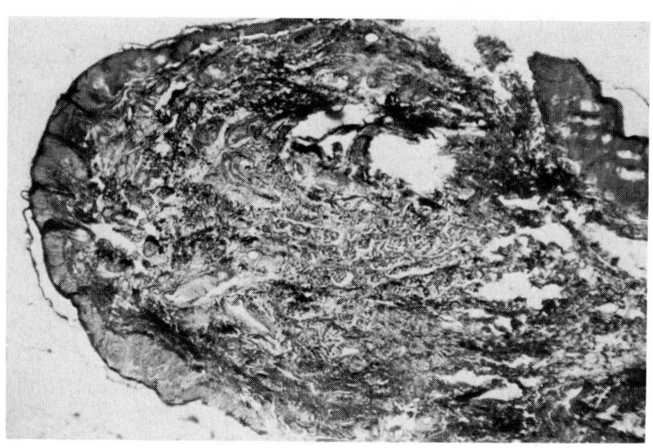

Figure 17–22 Cross section of a thin, soft tissue bridge from an operated incomplete bilateral cleft. Numerous muscle fiber bundles penetrate the collagenous tissue from the lateral segment to the central part (van Gieson). (From Fára M: The musculature of cleft lip and palate. In Converse JM (ed): Reconstructive Plastic Surgery, Vol. IV. Philadelphia, WB Saunders, 1977, p 1976. With permission.)

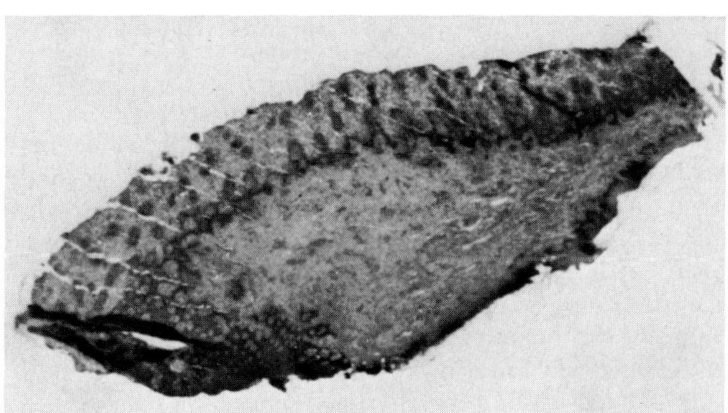

Figure 17–23 Cross section of a bridge from an operated incomplete unilateral cleft. Only collagenous tissue is seen. Muscle fibers are absent (Van Gieson). (From Fára M: The musculature of cleft lip and palate. In Converse JM (ed): Reconstructive Plastic Surgery, Vol. IV. Philadelphia, WB Saunders, 1977, p 1977. With permission.

Figure 17–24 Dissection of M00 in complete bilateral cleft with a bridge on the left side. The muscle bundles of the left lateral segment cross the bridge to the prolabium, where they fill only its left half adequately.

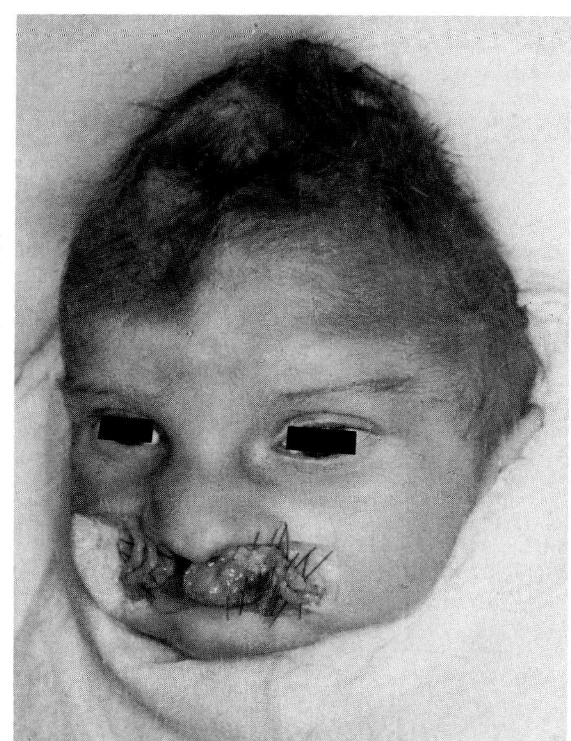

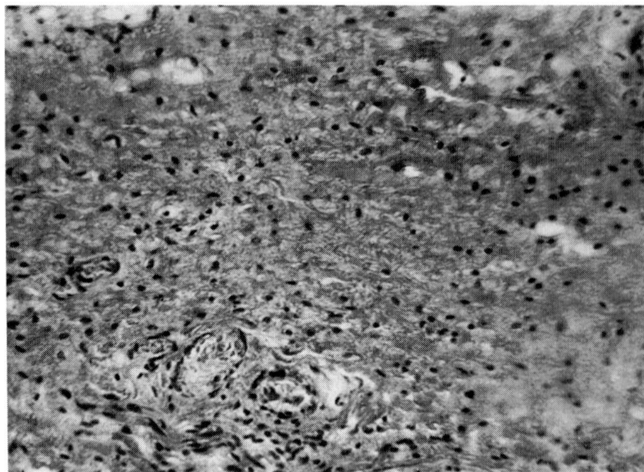

Figure 17–25 Biopsy from a prolabium. Collagenous connective tissue without any muscle fibers, either mature or in any stage of development.

tissue only collagenous fibrillar connective tissue (Fig. 17–25).

Phase II

During the repair of the second side, performed after an interval of 6 weeks to 6 months and based on a study of samples taken across the previous suture, we found a proliferation of muscle fibers running from the lateral into the medial lip segment. This proliferation appeared to be markedly dense.

The greatest number of differentiated muscular fibers proliferating from the lateral muscle stump into the prolabium was found nearest the repaired cleft. In the central portions of the prolabium, the number of said fibers decreased, and finally only isolated fibers were observed. The quantity of muscular fibers and the distance of their ingrowth into the prolabium differed with each case. To get an overall orientation, we measured the distance by which the muscular fibers passed the boundary of the two lip segments, the gauge being a millimeter scale that was placed on the slide after previously fixing the starting line. We found that the fibers had grown an average distance of 2 to 5 mm, which represented one-fourth to one-third of the width

of the prolabium at each side, or one-eighth to one-sixth of the total prolabial width (Fig. 17–26).

Phase III

More information was obtained from excisions performed on the lip during corrective surgery, usually when deepening the labial sulcus 1 to 10 years following the primary repair. In 20 patients from the original series of 30, part of these muscle fibers was found to have been gradually replaced by connective tissue. The fibers of the collagenous connective tissue were mostly parallel to the longitudinal axis of the lip and at some points suggested a tendonlike arrangement that was striking, particularly in the central part of the prolabium.

Many muscle fibers, however, were preserved and, together with the collagen fibers, grouped into horizontal rows forming a favorable elastic link between both contractile ends of the orbicularis oris muscle (Figs. 17–27 and 17–28). In this way, the restoration of the mouth constrictor was satisfactorily achieved in the wide bilateral cleft, even when approximation and suture of muscle stumps from each side could not be performed without excessive tension.

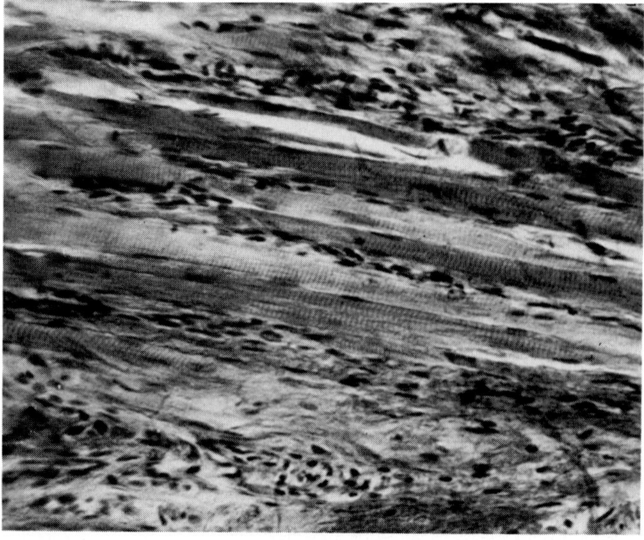

Figure 17–26 Biopsy from a prolabium 3 months after surgery. Striated muscle fibers penetrate the collagenous connective tissue (Masson's trichromatic method).

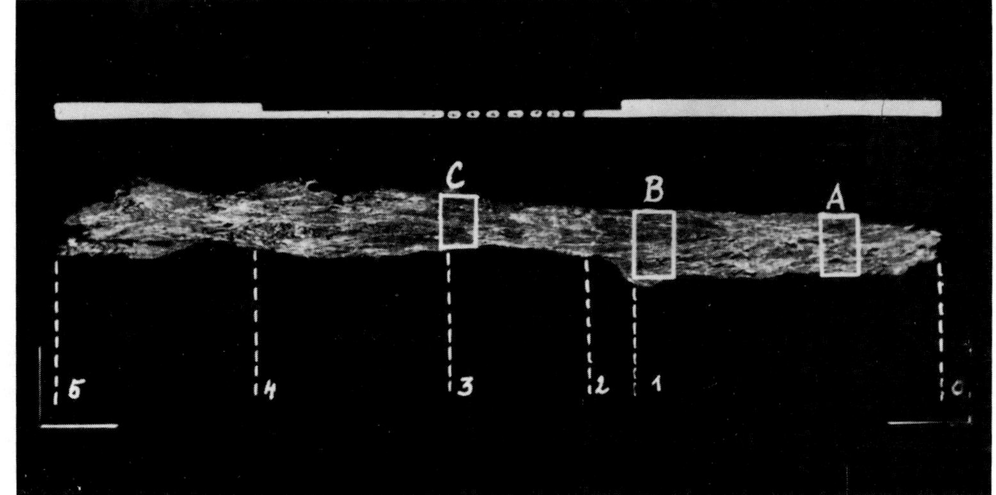

Figure 17-27. Excision across the whole lip 10 years after primary repair. The quantity of muscle fibers and the distance of the ingrowth into the prolabium was measured and evaluated in this way.

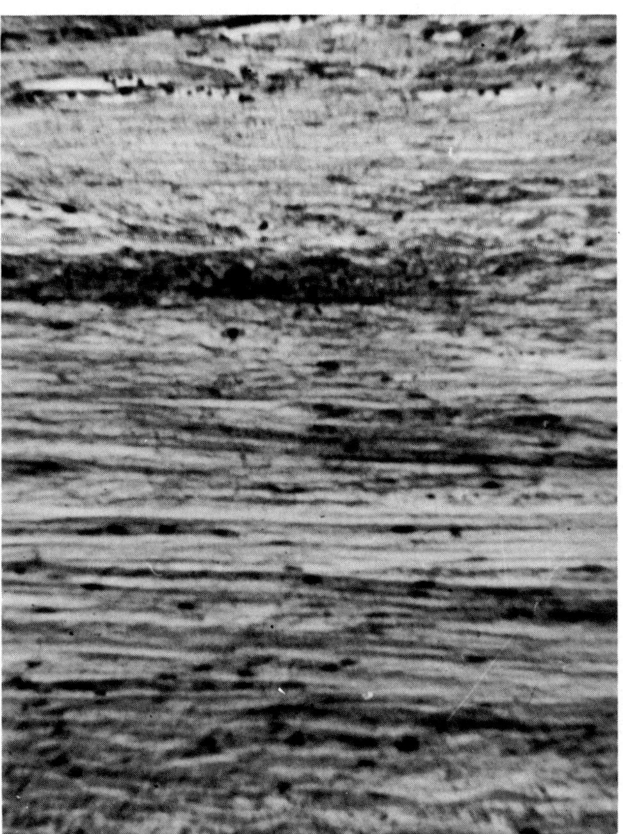

Figure 17-28 Histology of the middle portion of the lip 10 years after surgery (portion 2 to 3 in Fig. 17-27). Note parallel arrangement of collagen fibers (Masson's trichromatic method). (From Fára M: The musculature of cleft lip and palate. In Converse JM (ed): Reconstructive Plastic Surgery, Vol. IV. Philadelphia, WB Saunders, 1977, p 1974. With permission.)

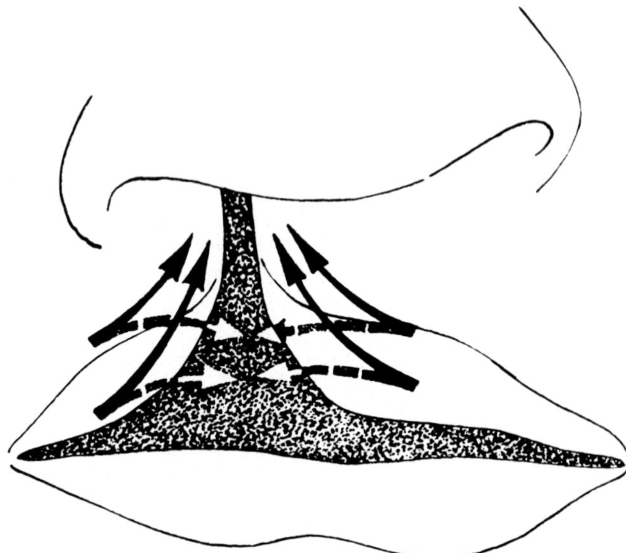

Figure 17–29 The detachment of the muscle stumps from their substitute cleft insertions and their distal folding in unilateral cleft.

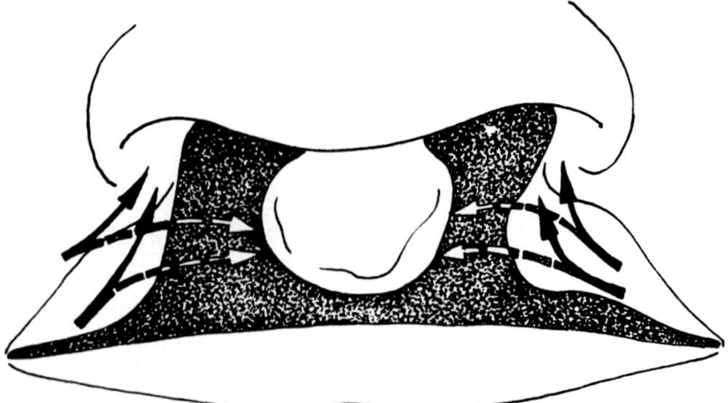

Figure 17–30 Detachment of the muscle stumps from their substitute cleft insertions and their distal folding in bilateral cleft.

Conclusions

Our research in the anatomy of cleft lip has been focused mainly on the changes in the course and state of the orbicularis oris muscle. The facial nerve fibers and lip arteries follow the course of the muscle bundles and, apart from some clinically unimportant atypical anastomoses, no basic deviations from normal are known or are likely to be expected.

Differences between the normal and cleft arrangement of the orbicularis oris are due to the fact that the muscle stumps, which extend during their embryonic growth in a lateromedial direction, fail to meet in the central line of the lip and thus seek other attachments at firm points in the immediate vicinity. These atypical insertions, however, prevent the muscle from becoming fully functional, and therefore, its development is incomplete.

The prolabium in complete bilateral clefts does not contain any musculature, but the ability of the lateral muscle stumps to grow a certain distance into its connective tissue following lip closure has been demonstrated.

On the basis of this knowledge, the detachment of the muscle stumps from their substitute cleft insertions and their distal folding become a prime condition for any successful operation on the lip because they make it possible for the muscle bundles to be brought together end to end, or, in the case of complete bilateral cleft, to grow smoothly into the prolabium. Only this step secures the proper function and further development of the lip (Figs. 17–29 and 17–30).

Reference

1. Fára M: The musculature of cleft lip and palate. In Converse JM (ed): Reconstructive Plastic Surgery. Vol. IV. Philadelphia: Saunders, 1977.

CHAPTER 18

Anatomy of the Unilateral and Bilateral Cleft Lip Nose

Harold McComb

Pathogenesis

All clefts of the lip are associated with some degree of nasal deformity. In the embryo the nose develops in conjunction with the primary palate, which contributes the premaxilla, the columella, and the anterior nasal septum. Each of these structures may show faulty development. Although the exact process of formation of the region is not completely understood, it is generally agreed that there is a deficiency of mesoderm and ectoderm in cleft formation.[1–5]

At least two factors are involved in the development of the cleft lip nose. First, there is agenesis of tissues in the region of the cleft because of the deficiencies of mesoderm and ectoderm. Second, mechanical stresses resulting from progressive separation of the sides of the cleft are applied to the developing nose. It is clear, however, that these mechanical forces are not alone responsible for the deformity. Significant displacement of the alar cartilage and drooping of the nostril rim can occur in mild clefts in which there is very little widening of the nasal floor.

The fundamental deficiency of mesoderm is seen in the lack of development of bone at the piriform margin in the floor of the cleft nostril, in the deficiency of the septal cartilage, and in the nasal spine in some cases.[6,7] The ala nasi is sometimes thinner on the side of the cleft, and the soft tissues deep in the alar base may be poorly developed. The ectodermal deficiency is represented by the dental abnormalities that underlie the cleft lip nose.[8–13]

Soon after the cleft is established in the embryo, the gap begins to widen. The premaxilla moves forward as it is pulled by the growing nasal septum, to which it is attached by the septopremaxillary ligament.[14,15] At the same time, there is a lack of forward development of the maxilla, and the region of the alar base remains retroposed.[16,17] Therefore, there is increased widening of the distance between the base of the columella and the alar base. This separation reaches an extreme degree in bilateral clefts in which the premaxilla is thrust forward.

When the medial and lateral crura of the alar cartilage are pulled apart, there is initial lowering of the alar arch in a dorsal direction. With further widening of the cleft, the fascia nasalis, which connects the upper border of the alar cartilage to the lower border of the upper lateral cartilage, is tightened. The infundibulum between the two cartilages disappears, and the alar arch is forced to tilt downward in a caudal direction. The lower edge of the alar cartilage is also displaced dorsally, and it raises a fold in the vestibular lining.[18,19]

At one time, it was hypothesized that shortening of the columella in bilateral clefts was due to lack of any restraint on movement of the premaxilla, which was no longer joined to the maxillae. Because the premaxilla was free to move forward with the septum, it was thought that there would be no differential growth of the septum beyond the premaxilla, and therefore no development of a columella.[20] However, recent dissections suggest that shortening of the columella is due to wide displacement of the alar cartilages, which are pulled away from each side of the nasal septum, commencing at the tip. The columella is therefore progressively shortened back toward its base, at the junction of the prolabium.

Anatomy of the Unilateral Cleft

The extent and nature of the nasal deformity that occurs in unilateral and bilateral cleft lips has been clarified by nasal dissections in stillborn infants. These have emphasized the basic role of the alar cartilage in the deformity.

In the unilateral cleft there is considerable deformity of the bony and cartilaginous skeleton underlying the cleft lip nose (Fig. 18–1). The cleft side of the premaxilla is displaced forward and medially toward the noncleft side and is also often tilted upward into the cleft. Laterally, on the side of the cleft, the piriform margin and the arch of the alveolus are usually in their normal position in relation to the midline. When the cleft is complete, however, the piriform margin and the anterior wall of the maxilla are retroposed. Therefore, there is considerable widening of the distance between the anterior nasal spine and the piriform margin in the region of the alar base in both the coronal and sagittal planes.

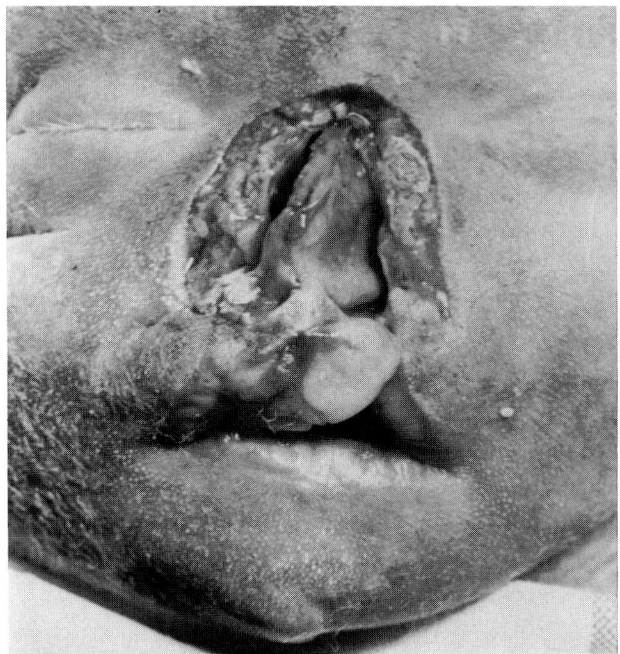

Figure 18–1 Considerable deformity of the skeletal base underlies the cleft lip nose.

The anterior part of the septum is displaced increasingly toward the noncleft side of the nose from above downward. The caudal edge of the anterior septum may in fact be dislocated laterally, beyond the anterior nasal spine, into the noncleft nostril. The septum is also convex on the side of the cleft, mainly in the horizontal plane but also to a lesser extent vertically. The nostril is increasingly stretched between its medial attachment to the anterior nasal spine at the base of the columella and its lateral attachment to the piriform margin in the region of the alar base. Fibers of the cleft orbicularis oris muscle stream over the alar cartilage and contribute to the nostril widening.[21]

The alar cartilage is the center point of the cleft lip nasal deformity. Normally, the cartilages ride quite high in the nasal tip, and the alar domes lie at the level of the junction of the middle and lower thirds of the nasal bridge (Fig. 18–2). On the cleft side, the alar cartilage is spread out and also is rotated caudally downward like a bucket handle, while the alar dome is displaced downward, backward, and laterally. The upper border of the lateral crus no longer overlaps the lower border of the upper lateral cartilage, and the infundibulum is opened out. The lower border of the lateral crus is displaced downward and tilted backward into the nostril. In the columella, the medial crus is displaced slightly caudally (Fig. 18–3).

Since there is no lessening of the distance between the lower edge of the lateral crus of the alar cartilage and the nostril rim, caudal rotation of the cartilage produces drooping of the nostril rim on the side of the cleft. The tilted edge of the lower lateral crus creates an oblique ridge within the vestibule of the nose. This oblique ridge becomes more marked as the cleft widens and the alar cartilage becomes increasingly tilted (Fig.

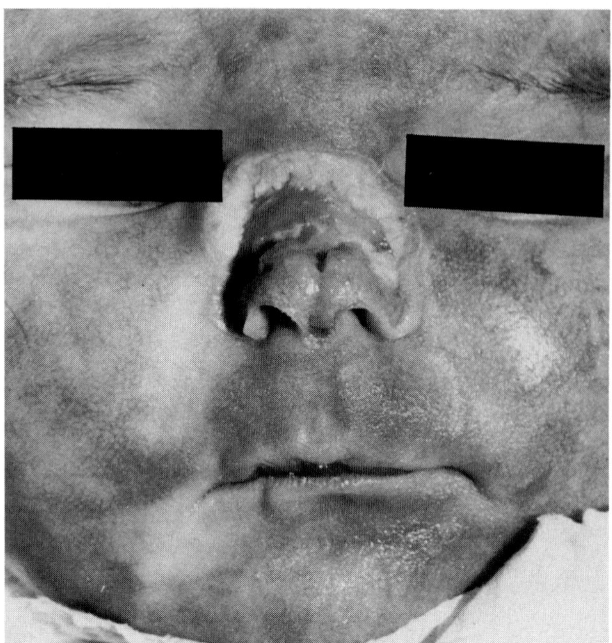

Figure 18–2 In the normal nose the alar domes lie at the junction of the middle and lower thirds of the nasal bridge.

18–4). When the alar dome and the adjacent part of the medial crus are pulled away from the nasal tip, there is some shortening of the columella on the cleft side. Although the alar cartilage is spread across the cleft, its length remains unchanged.[23]

The external appearance of the cleft lip nose reflects the deformity of its bony and cartilaginous skeleton. Measured from the level of the nasion to the nostril margin, the nose is longer on the side of the cleft (Fig. 18–5). The nostril rim is lower than on the noncleft side, and sometimes the normal upward sweep of the margin is changed to a drooping, downward convexity. The covering skin on the cleft side of the nose is lengthened from above downward. This increase in length occurs mainly over the area of separation of the upper and lower lateral cartilages.

The arch of the nostril is flattened, and the ala joins the columella at an oblique angle. The columella is tilted and is displaced away from the midline, toward the noncleft side, and lies obliquely along the edge of the displaced septum. It is shortened on the side of the cleft and lies a little more caudally on the cleft side. In wide clefts, the columella and the nostril rim are almost completely straight. The alar base joins the cheek at an oblique angle (Fig. 18–6).

The tip of the cleft lip nose is irregular and broad. There is loss of tip prominence on the cleft side because of the alar dome being moved backward, laterally, and downward. In wide clefts, there is an oblique furrow on the surface of the nose, which runs upward and laterally. It lies below and lateral to the depressed alar dome and corresponds to the ridge within the vestibule that is produced by tilting and retrodisplacement of the caudal edge of the lateral crus of the alar cartilage. This groove may extend down to the nostril rim, where it creates a dip in the margin. At this point, the nostril rim becomes concave rather than convex.

In wide clefts, the nasal wall often appears to be broadened and everted at the alar base (Fig. 18–7). This is due to the attachment of the nostril lining medially to the piriform margin, combined with lateral displacement and eversion of the alar base by the attachment of the orbicularis muscle fibers. The alar base on the side of the cleft is usually, but not always, lower than on the opposite side. In complete clefts, the width of the nose is greater than normal, but each alar base is displaced equally from the midline (Fig. 18–8).[23] In incomplete clefts, the nasal floor is widened to a variable degree. Lack of development of the underlying piriform margin causes grooving of the nasal floor, and the total circumference of the nostril is increased.

Caudal rotation of the alar cartilage is of threefold significance in relation to repair of cleft lip nasal deformity. First, the alar arch must be lifted to shorten the nose on the side of the cleft and to level the nostril rims. Second, lifting the alar cartilage with the attached nasal lining corrects the oblique fold within the vestibule. Third, when the alar cartilage is raised from its position of caudal rotation, the compound curve that produces the typical flare of the cleft lip nostril is avoided.

Anatomy of the Bilateral Cleft

In the skeletal base of the bilateral cleft lip nose, there is unbridled projection of the premaxilla and of

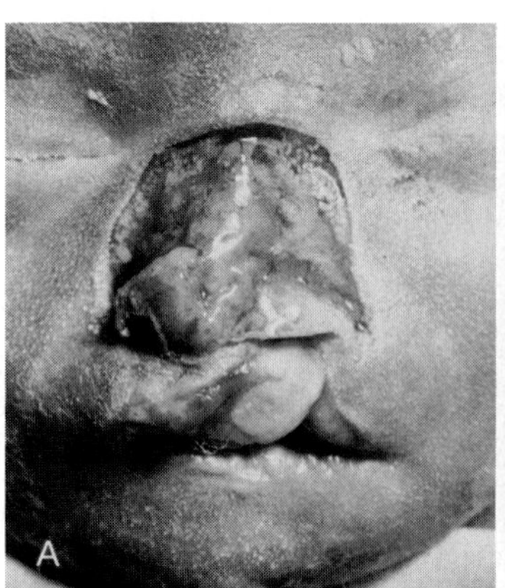
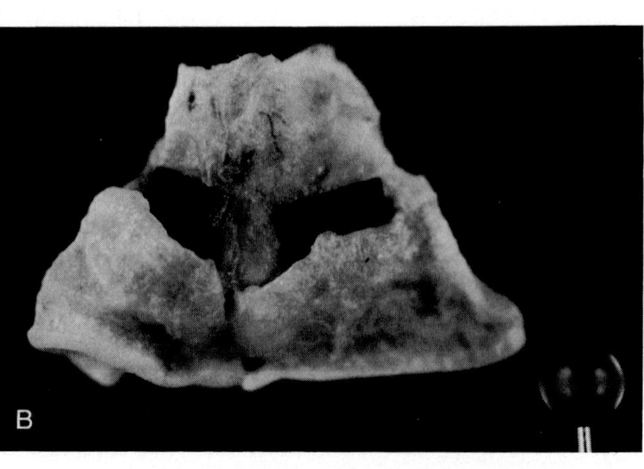

Figure 18–3 *A*, The alar cartilage on the side of the cleft is rotated caudally downward. *B*, The alar cartilage, including the columella crus, is swung downward like a bucket handle.

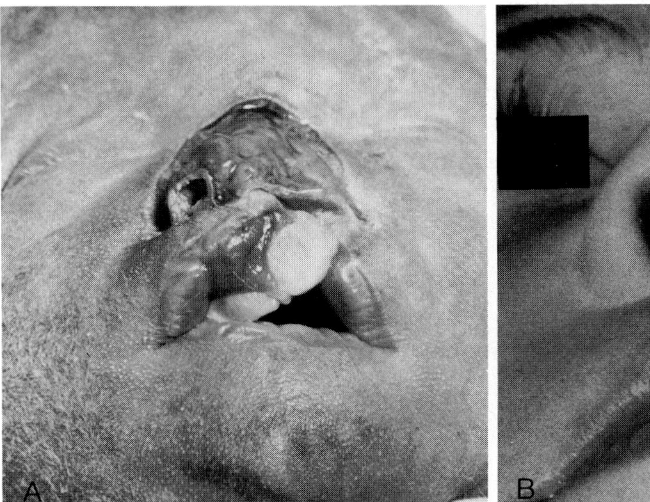

Figure 18–4 *A*, The tilted lower edge of the alar cartilage pushes up an oblique ridge within the vestibule. *B*, This oblique ridge persists if the alar cartilage is not lifted.

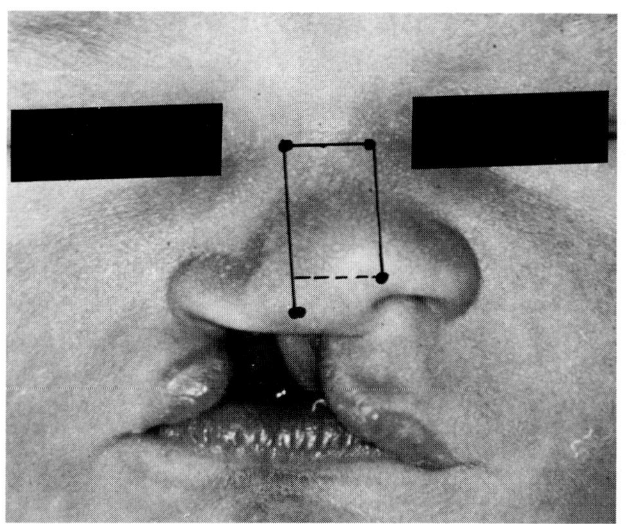

Figure 18–5 The cleft lip nose is longer on the cleft side.

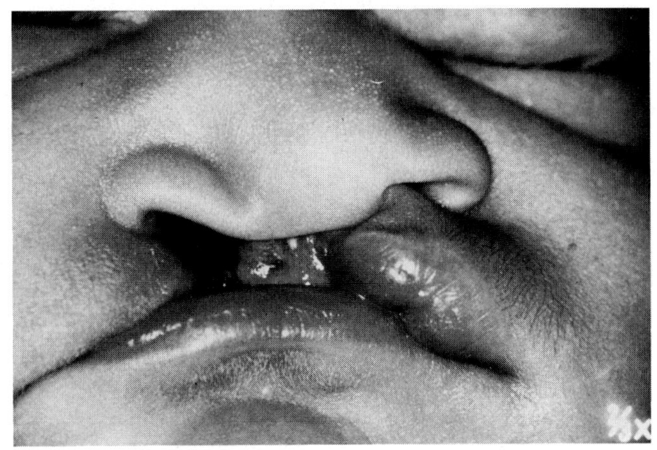

Figure 18–6 Tilting of the alar cartilage produces an oblique furrow on the surface of the nose. This corresponds to the ridge within the vestibule that is produced by the lower border of the alar cartilage. The nostril rim becomes concave and droops downward.

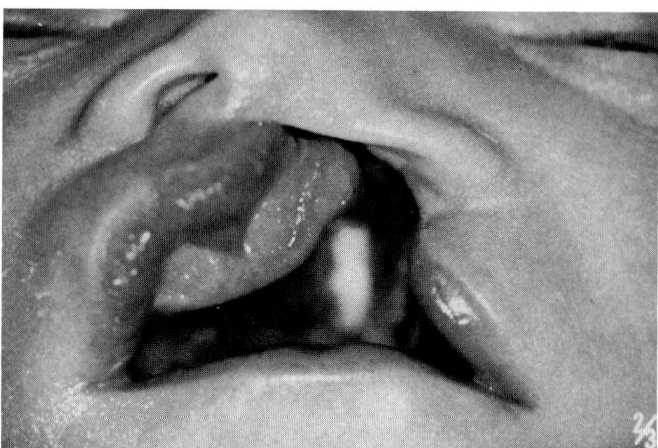

Figure 18–7 The alar base sometimes appears to be everted.

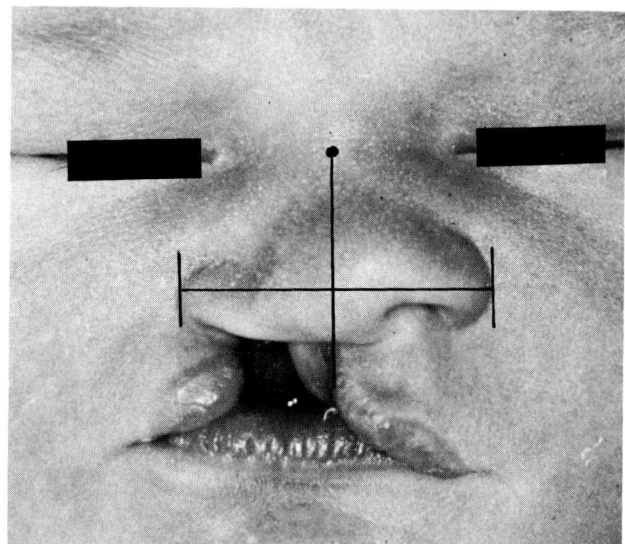

Figure 18–8 The cleft lip nose is wider than normal, but each alar base is displaced equally from the midline.

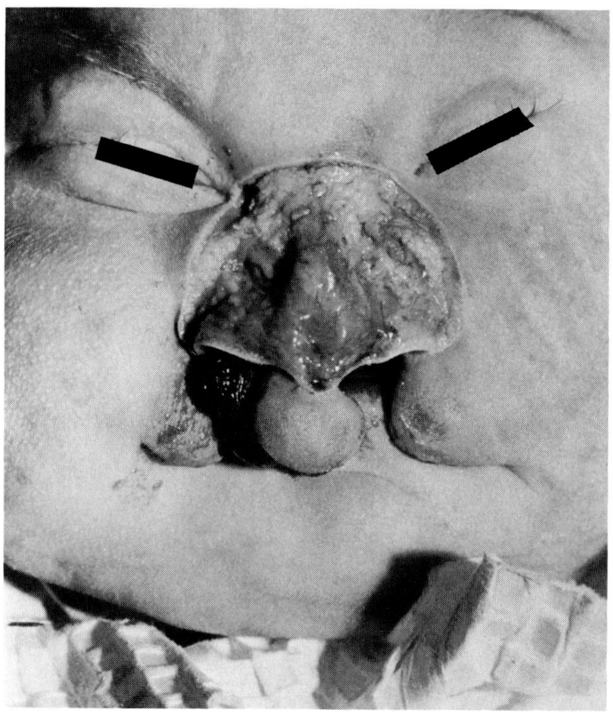

Figure 18–9 In the bilateral cleft lip nose, both alar cartilages are pulled away from the septum and are rotated caudally downward.

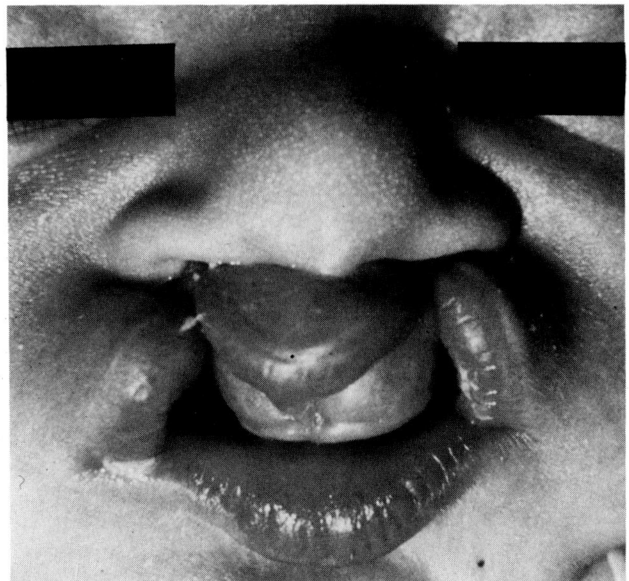

Figure 18–10 The separated alar domes and columellar crura are incorporated into the broad nasal tip. The base of the shortened columella is attached to the prolabium.

the lower part of the nasal septum. In complete clefts, both maxillae are shortened in an anteroposterior direction, and the margins of the piriform opening are retroposed to various degrees. The septum is usually in the midline, but considerable twisting and deviation of the premaxilla can occur if a Simonart's band is present on one side or if one cleft is incomplete. The nostrils are stretched between their attachments to the anterior nasal spine medially and the piriform margins laterally. Both alar cartilages are rotated caudally downward, duplicating the deformity that is found in a unilateral cleft (Fig. 18–9).

The height of the cartilaginous septum is usually normal, but the alar domes are widely separated and the medial crura are stripped away from their positions along the lower margin of the cartilaginous septum. As the alar domes and the columellar crura are pulled apart, they are incorporated into the broadened tissues of the nasal tip. The medial crura may be separated as far back as the base of the prolabium. The broad nasal tip then appears to be attached directly to the prolabial tissue.

In external appearance, the nasal tip is flat and broad, without any prominence created by the alar domes (Fig. 18–10). The nostril rims droop and may be curved convexly downward. Oblique ridges are raised within the vestibules by the lower borders of the alar cartilages,

which are in caudal rotation. Externally, these ridges may appear as oblique grooves running upward and outward over the alae.

The columella appears to be shortened or nonexistent, and the prolabium often appears to be joined directly to the tip of the nose. The medial crura, which have been pulled apart, are then incorporated into the broad nasal tip, which is pulled down toward the prolabium. At its junction with the prolabium, the base of the short columella may be the only normal (but displaced) point in the bilateral cleft lip nose.

References

1. His W: Beobachtungen zur Geschichte und Gamenbildung beim menschlichen Embryo. Kgl Akad Wiss 27, 1901.
2. Stark RB: The pathogenesis of harelip and cleft palate. Plast Reconstr Surg 13:20, 1954.
3. Patten BM: Embryology of the palate and the maxillofacial region. In Grabb WC, Rosenstein SW, Bzoch KR (eds): Cleft Lip and Palate. Boston: Little, Brown, 1971.
4. Avery JK: The nasal capsule in cleft palate. Anat Anz (Suppl) 109:722, 1962.
5. Stark RB, Kaplan JM: Development of the cleft lip nose. Plast Reconstr Surg 51:413, 1973.
6. Takahashi R, Yamazaki Y: Studies on the external nose in cases of cleft lip and their application to plastic surgery. Transactions of the Third International Congress of Plastic Surgery. Amsterdam: Excerpta Medica, 1963.
7. Noordhoff MS, Cheng W-S: Median facial dysgenesis in cleft lip and palate. Ann Plast Surg 8:83, 1982.
8. Brown RF: The cleft lip nasal deformity in the absence of cleft lip. Transactions of the Fifth International Congress of Plastic Surgery. Stoneham, MA: Butterworths, 1971.
9. Stenstrom SJ, Thilander BL: Cleft lip nasal deformity in the absence of cleft lip. Plast Reconstr Surg 35:160, 1965.
10. Cosman B, Crikelair GF: The minimal cleft lip. Plast Reconstr Surg 37:355, 1966.
11. Khoo Boo-Chai, Tange I: The isolated cleft lip nose. Plast Reconstr Surg 41:28, 1968.
12. Tulenko J: Cleft lip nasal deformity in the absence of cleft lip. Plast Reconstr Surg 41:35, 1968.
13. Brown RF: A reappraisal of the cleft lip nose with the report of a case. Br J Plast Surg 17:168, 1964.
14. Latham RA: The pathogenesis of the skeletal deformity associated with unilateral cleft lip and palate. Cleft Palate J 6:404, 1969.
15. Siegel MI, Mooney MP, Kines KR, et al: Traction, prenatal development and the labiosepto-premaxillary region. Plast Reconstr Surg 76:25, 1985.
16. Atherton JD: A descriptive anatomy of the face in human foetuses with unilateral cleft lip and palate. Cleft Palate J 4:104, 1967.
17. Dado DV, Kernahan DA: Radiographic analysis of the midface of a stillborn infant with a unilateral cleft lip and palate. Plast Reconstr Surg 78:238, 1986.
18. Stenstrom SJ, Oberg T: The nasal deformity in unilateral cleft lip. Plast Reconstr Surg 28:295, 1961.
19. Huffman WC, Lierle DM: Studies on the pathologic anatomy of the unilateral hare-lip nose. Plast Reconstr Surg 4:225, 1949.
20. Latham RA, Workman C: Anatomy of the philtrum and columella: The soft tissue deformity in bilateral cleft lip and palate. In Georgiade NG, Hagerty RF (eds): Symposium on Management of Cleft Lip and Palate and Associated Deformities. St. Louis: Mosby, 1974.
21. Kernahan DA, Dado DV, Bauer BS: The anatomy of the orbicularis oris muscle in unilateral cleft lip based on a three-dimensional histological reconstruction. Plast Reconstr Surg 73:875, 1984.
22. Cosman B, Crikelair GF: The shape of the unilateral cleft lip defect. Plast Reconstr Surg 35:484, 1965.
23. Hajinis K, Pigalova P: Shape of the nose in cheilo-gnatho-palatoschisis unilateralis before operational repair. Acta Chir Plast 15:11, 1973.

CHAPTER 19

Anatomy of the Unilateral and Bilateral Cleft Lip and Nose

Janusz Bardach and Court Cutting

Elements of the nasal deformity associated with unilateral and bilateral cleft lip and palate share certain basic characteristics, although the extent and degree of severity of the deformity vary considerably between individuals. It is necessary to discuss the nasal deformity associated with unilateral and bilateral cleft separately because the anatomy is entirely different in each cleft type. Prior to a detailed description of the anatomy of the cleft lip nose, a theoretical background for the pathogenesis of cleft deformities is presented to elucidate the factors involved.

Pathogenesis of the Cleft Lip Nasal Deformity

Some of the theories of the pathogenesis of the cleft lip nasal deformity involve tissue deficiency (especially skeletal hypoplasia), malposition of the maxillary segments, asymmetry of the skeletal base and its effect on the nasal structures, the effect of muscle imbalance, and the influence of surgical procedures on secondary nasal deformities. It is helpful for the surgeon to consider these etiologic factors, particularly at the time of primary lip and nose repair when severe secondary deformities may be prevented. Careful consideration and assessment of the nasal deformity is important in selecting the appropriate surgical approach for both primary lip repair and secondary nasal reconstruction.

The embryogenesis of the cleft lip deformity was originally thought to be due to a failure of fusion of the primary facial processes. This theory was attributed to Dursy[1] and His,[2] who described the lip as having been formed from the fusion of the lateral maxillary processes with the frontonasal process. The cutaneous lip lateral to the philtral columns and the vermilion were derived from the lateral maxillary processes, whereas the central philtrum medial to the columns was due to the contribution of the frontonasal process. These processes were believed to fuse when the segments touched owing to epithelial cell death followed by healing of the processes.

This idea was challenged by Veau,[3] based on his study of embryos with cleft lip. Veau felt that the theories of Pohlman[4] and Fleischmann[5] better explained his observations. In Fleischmann's theory, the facial processes were projections of developing mesoderm under a common epithelial layer. As these processes grew closer

together, a filmy epithelial bilayer lifted up as a meniscus between the processes. Further development of these mounds caused the mesoderm to penetrate the thin epithelial bilayer, resulting in the joining of what had originally been separate centers of mesodermal development. A structure like a Simonart's band is much easier to explain using this theory.

The general acceptance of the theory of failure of mesodermal penetration of the epithelial bilayer compared with the theory of the fusion of the facial processes has important implications for the way in which the surgeon approaches the tissue at the time of operation. If the failure of fusion of processes theory was assumed to be correct, the surgeon might erroneously proceed on the premise that all the tissue was present and that it merely required skillful rearrangement. The Fleischmann-Veau notion, on the other hand, implied a failure of full mesodermal development, which assumes tissue deficiency.

The surgeon must realize that there is tissue deficiency in the region of the cleft. This is true for the soft tissue and the facial skeleton. One of the most important defects needing correction in the secondary cleft lip nose deformity is the lack of skeletal support beneath the alar base. Anderl[6] addresses the bony deficiency under the alar base at the time of primary lip repair. Latham[7] advocates lateral maxillary advancement on the cleft side using presurgical orthopedic treatment prior to lip repair. In this way, support for the alar base is provided at the time of lip repair. Cutting believes that the salutary effects of presurgical orthopedic treatment have a positive effect on the quality of the primary nasal correction, allowing it to be performed with minimal undermining. Avery[8] reported that the nasal cartilages are deficient on the cleft side. In the clinical experience of the authors, who use an external rhinoplasty technique for the correction of severe secondary cleft nasal deformities, it is hard to discern whether or not there is any lower lateral cartilage missing; rather, it seems that it may be displaced. On the other hand, the skeletal deficiency under the alar base is often quite severe. In some patients the alar base is deficient on the cleft side. In addition to mesodermal deficiency, the alar base deficiency appears to be related to the technique of the primary surgery. This will be discussed later in the chapter.

An understanding of the mechanisms that produce the malpositioning of the maxillary segments is helpful in developing further ideas that explain the cleft nose deformity. Scott[9] originally proposed that the nasal septum was the primary force responsible for the downward and forward growth of the midface. In view of the more recent theories of Enlow[10] and Moss,[11] this idea appears somewhat simplistic. Enlow and Moss view facial growth as developing in response to the muscle forces on the facial skeleton. Although this is true, it is impossible to deny that some of the facial growth is due to the decoding of inherent genetic information.

Latham[12,13] described the "septopremaxillary ligament" as the structure that keeps the premaxilla attached to the anterior caudal edge of the septum (Fig. 19–1). When the premaxilla joins with the lateral max-

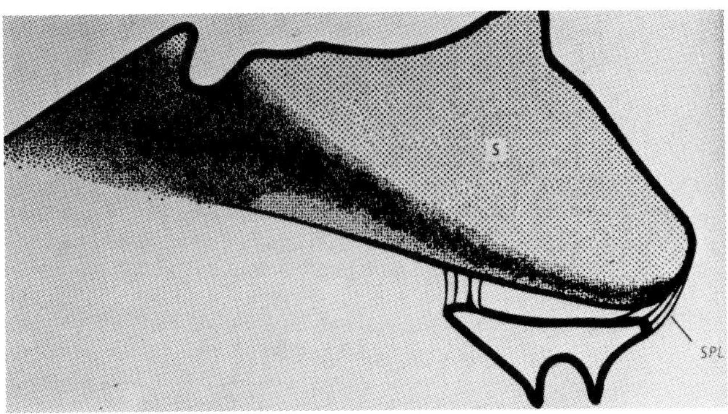

Figure 19–1 Latham's septopremaxillary ligament showing the premaxilla attached to the caudal cartilaginous septum by the ligament.

illary segments, both mesodermal development centers are favorably affected. The lateral segments are drawn anteriorly by their attachment to the premaxilla. In a similar manner, the lateral segments draw the premaxilla backward along the caudal edge of the septum. The septopremaxillary ligament stretches as the cartilaginous septum moves forward and the premaxilla is drawn back. The anterior nasal spine is the result of the premaxilla being drawn back in this manner.

King et al[14] presented a three-dimensional reconstruction from serial sections of a fetus with bilateral cleft lip and palate and compared it with normal development. Figure 19–2 demonstrates the result of the lack of fusion

of the premaxilla with the lateral maxillary segments. The unrestrained forward movement of the premaxilla results in excessive secondary bone deposition at the premaxillary-vomerine suture, causing a protruding premaxilla on a long bony stem. The mechanisms that produce the anterior nasal spine are not present. This allows the cartilages of the developing medial crura to be posteriorly positioned above the bone of the premaxilla, contributing to the development of a short columella and very little alar cartilage projection. In the unilateral cleft, it is useful to imagine the same forces acting on one side only. The premaxilla is overprojected on the cleft side, and the lateral maxillary segment is posteriorly positioned. The foot of the medial crus is posteriorly positioned on the cleft side relative to the noncleft side.

Stenstrom and Oberg[15] reported that most of the deformities of the lower lateral cartilages could be attributed to the underlying malposition of the maxillary segments. They demonstrated this by mimicking these orthopedic effects in adult cadaver noses (Fig. 19–3). By drawing the lateral foot of the lateral cartilage posteriorly and laterally, they were able to demonstrate most of the morphologic changes seen in the secondary deformities of the cleft lip nose. The foot of the medial crus was drawn posteriorly relative to the opposite side. The junction between the medial and lateral crura was pulled laterally, inferiorly, and posteriorly, resulting in the usual flattening of the dome on the cleft side. The

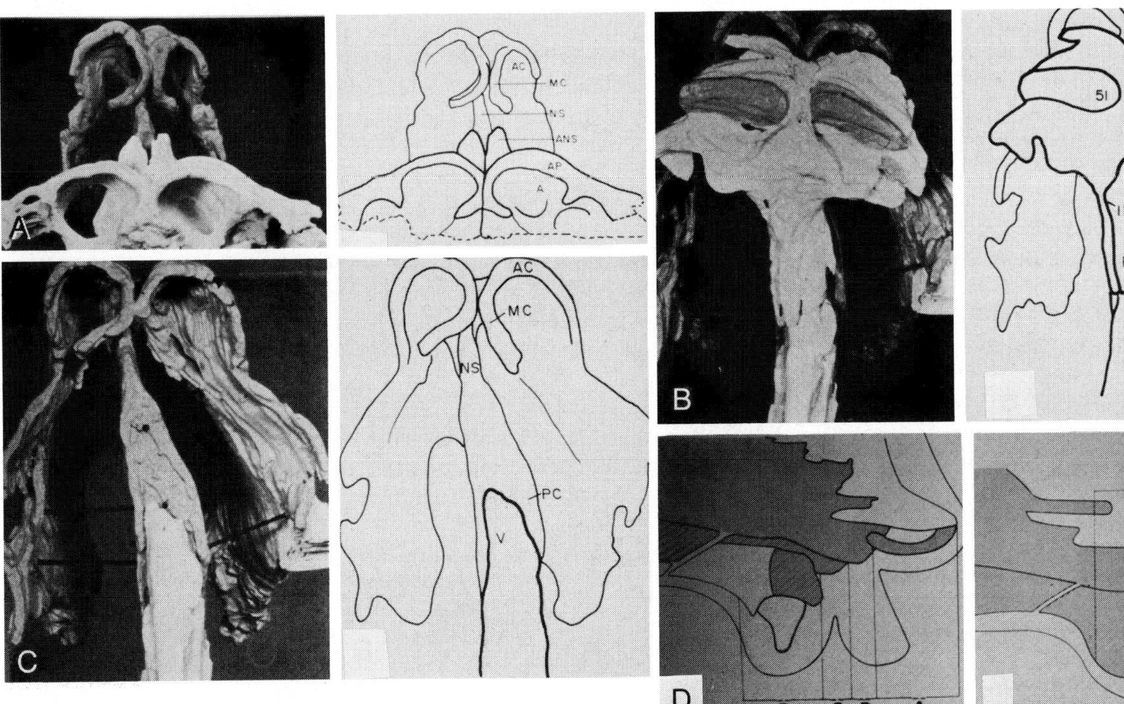

Figure 19–2 Three-dimensional models made from serial sections of a facially normal fetus and one with bilateral cleft lip and palate. *A,* Normal relationship between facial skeleton and nasal cartilages. The premaxilla has been drawn back along the caudal septum, allowing the nasal tip cartilages to assume their normal configuration. *B,* Fetus with bilateral cleft showing no "reining back" of the premaxilla by its connections with the lateral segments. Secondary bone deposition at

the premaxillary-vomerine suture has occurred. *C,* Removal of the premaxilla from the specimen shows the effect of this anterior bony protrusion on the nasal cartilages. *D,* Diagram of the view. Note that the protrusion of the premaxilla has resulted in the loss of an anterior nasal spine prominence. The foot of the medial crus is also posteriorly positioned with respect to the bone.

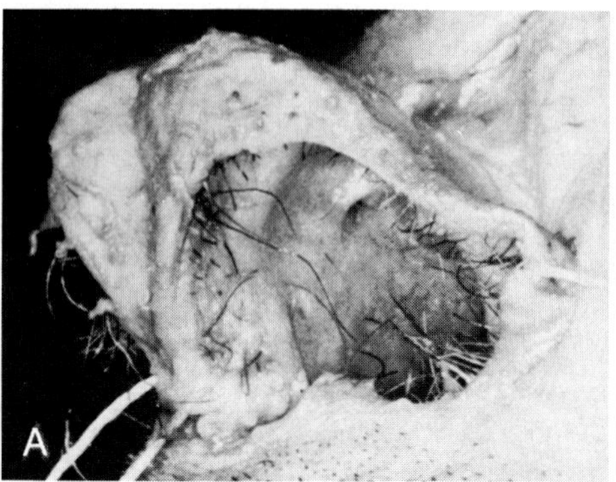

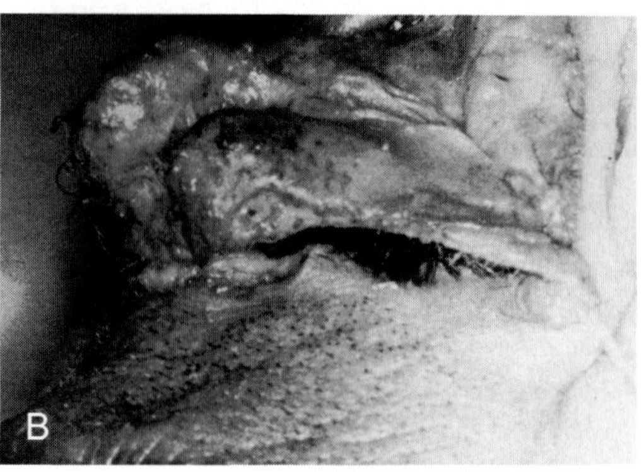

Figure 19–3 *A*, Stenstrom and Oberg's dissection of a normal cadaver nose, which has been dissected to show the nasal cartilages. *B*, The effect of simulating the orthopedic (or muscular) midpositions of the base of the lower lateral cartilage that would be present with a unilateral cleft lip, alveolus, and palate. Note that the usual secondary deformities of the cartilage in secondary cleft-lip noses are seen. The dome is pulled laterally and posteriorly on the "cleft" side, and the cartilage has been pulled into the soft triangle.

cartilage dropped vertically, down into the nasal apex, obliterating the soft triangle. The most anterior part of the medial crus was recruited into the lateral dome where the lateral crus was usually positioned. These findings will be described in further detail later in this chapter in the section on morphology of the secondary cleft lip nose deformity.

Hogan and Converse[16] described a similar mechanism for the production of the septal deviation typically seen in the unilateral cleft lip nose (Fig. 19–4). According to their concept, the cartilaginous septum is like the supporting strut in a tent. If the base of that support is pushed anteriorly and toward the noncleft side while the lateral part of the cleft side of the tent is drawn laterally and posteriorly, the typical septal deviation in the unilateral cleft lip nose can be explained.

The authors feel that the muscle imbalance on either side of the unilateral cleft lip has great influence on the production of the secondary nasal deformity through a similar mechanism. Fara[17] described the abnormal muscle insertions in the unilateral cleft lip. The medial muscle is displaced vertically and upward, inserting at the base of the columella. Contraction of the muscle pulls the base of the septum and columella toward the noncleft side. The lateral muscle is displaced vertically and upward, inserting near the foot of the alar base. Contraction of the muscle draws the ala laterally and posteriorly. The biophysical influences on the shape of the septum and lower lateral cartilages are the same as those described by Hogan and Converse, and Stenstrom and Oberg, respectively. This mechanism explains why infants with clefts of the lip only, without palatal clefts, often present severe deformities typical of the cleft lip nose.

Nasal Deformity Associated with Unilateral Clefts

Morphologic Factors

The nasal deformity in unilateral clefts is an integral part of the complex cleft syndrome that includes the lip, alveolus, palate, maxilla, and nose. Unilateral clefting, both complete and incomplete, results in a nasal deformity that may be caused by three major factors: (1) imbalance of the facial musculature, (2) hypoplasia of the skeletal base, and (3) asymmetry of the skeletal base.

Muscle imbalance affects nasal symmetry in both incomplete and complete cleft forms. Even a slight muscle imbalance distorts the position of the alar base and the shape of the nostril. Partial disruption of the orbicularis oris muscle creates a situation in which the facial muscles attached to the orbicularis oris on the cleft side pull the base of the ala more laterally than on the normal side. The greater the separation of the orbicularis oris, the more severe the cleft nasal deformity. The existing muscle imbalance results in displacement of the alar base and changes the orientation of the nostril from oblique to horizontal. This affects the position of the lower lateral cartilage. Correction of the muscle imbalance, which takes place during primary lip repair, does not necessarily alleviate the existing nasal deformity totally because displacement of the lower lateral cartilage persists, resulting in a typical unilateral cleft lip nasal deformity. Unless lip repair is combined with simultaneous repositioning of the alar base and lower lateral cartilage, the nasal deformity will not

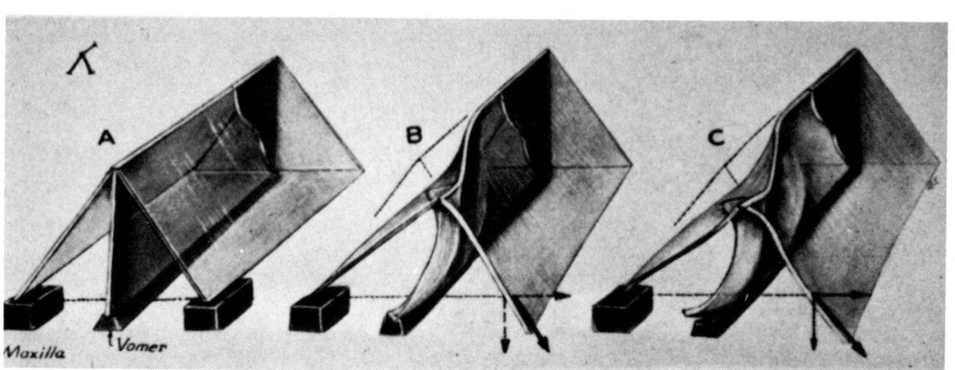

Figure 19–4 Tilted tripod concept of Hogan and Converse. As the alar base and the foot of the lateral crus of the lower lateral cartilage are displaced posteriorly and laterally, the septum is forced to deviate.

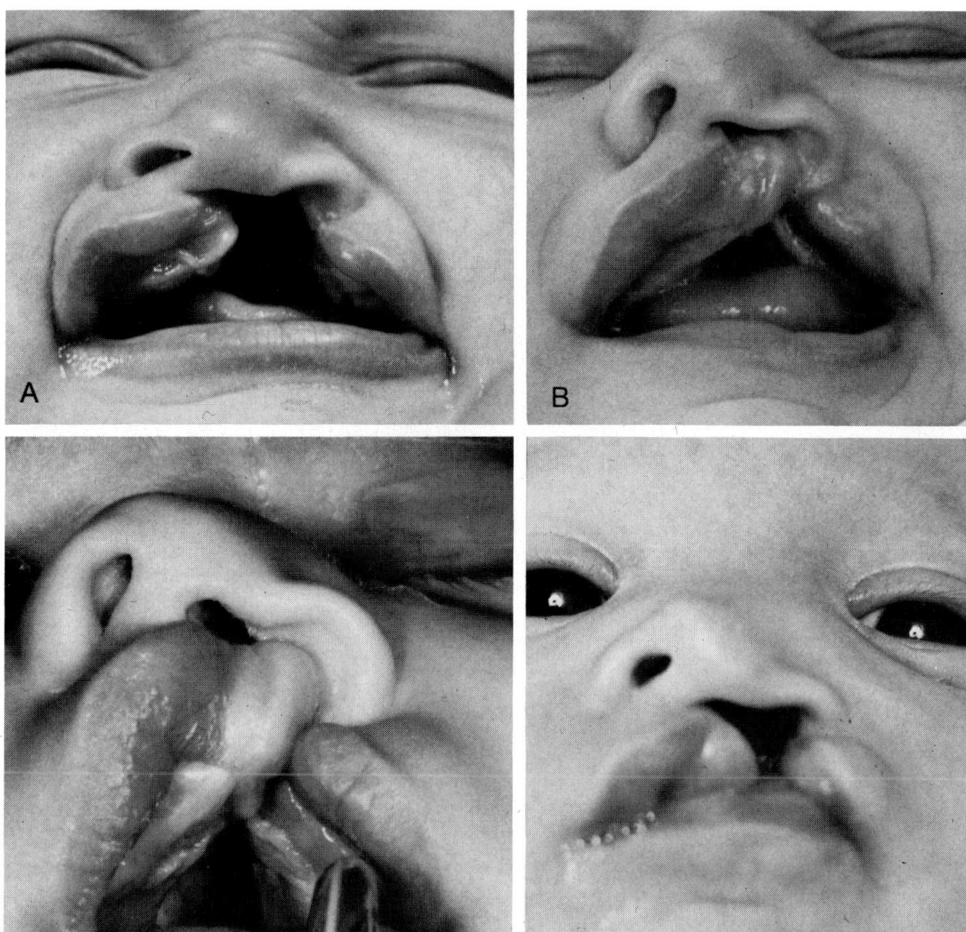

Figure 19–5 A–D, Unilateral cleft lip, alveolus, and palate with severe nasal distortion and collapse of the lesser maxillary segment.

improve with growth. The majority of patients require secondary correction to rearrange the lower lateral cartilage (Fig. 19–5).

Hypoplasia of the skeletal base may be observed not only in complete clefts but also in partial clefts in which the alveolus and palate do not seem to be affected. Hypoplasia of the lesser maxillary segment occurs most commonly along its edges and at the edge of the piriform aperture. The existing hypoplasia may accentuate the nasal deformity owing to the imbalance and asymmetry of the alar base. The most severe deformity occurs in complete unilateral clefts owing to the asymmetry of the maxillary segments. Asymmetry of these segments and the width of the cleft greatly contribute to the extent and severity of the nasal deformity.

The maxillary segments may be malpositioned in the frontal, horizontal, and vertical planes, leading to a nasal deformity affecting all structures on the cleft side, including the nasal septum. Collapse of the lesser maxillary segment leads to malpositioning of the alar base posteriorly and inferiorly, creating a severe imbalance of the entire lower portion of the nose and affecting the position of the lower lateral cartilage and the symmetry of the nasal tip. Lateral extension of the base of the ala results in flattening and elongation of the nostril with the typical downward deflection of the lateral crus of the lower lateral cartilage.

The lower lateral cartilage may be deformed in several ways. The orientation of the medial to lateral crura is changed because the ala is extended with its base pulled laterally and inferiorly. The medial crus is shorter than that on the noncleft side, whereas the lateral crus is longer than its noncleft counterpart. The domes also differ; the dome on the cleft side is obtuse and lower than the dome on the noncleft side. This cartilage also is deformed in the sense that it is rotated downward in the area of the nasal tip and drawn into an S-shaped fold because the ala is pulled laterally and the cartilage buckles. This distortion of the lower lateral cartilage, when severe, is difficult to correct during the primary operation (Fig. 19–6). Milder deformities may be corrected successfully during the primary cleft lip repair using the techniques described by Salyer, McComb, or Anderl (see Chapters 23 to 25).

The columella and nasal septum also may be affected by the morphologic changes associated with the unilateral cleft. Since the medial crus of the lower lateral cartilage is shorter on the cleft side, the columella is also shorter. The columella is pulled to the noncleft side by the muscles entering its base and joined by the orbicularis oris muscle. The septal deformity almost always is present; however, the severity of it varies greatly. The caudal edge usually is deviated to the noncleft side, and the entire septum may be deformed

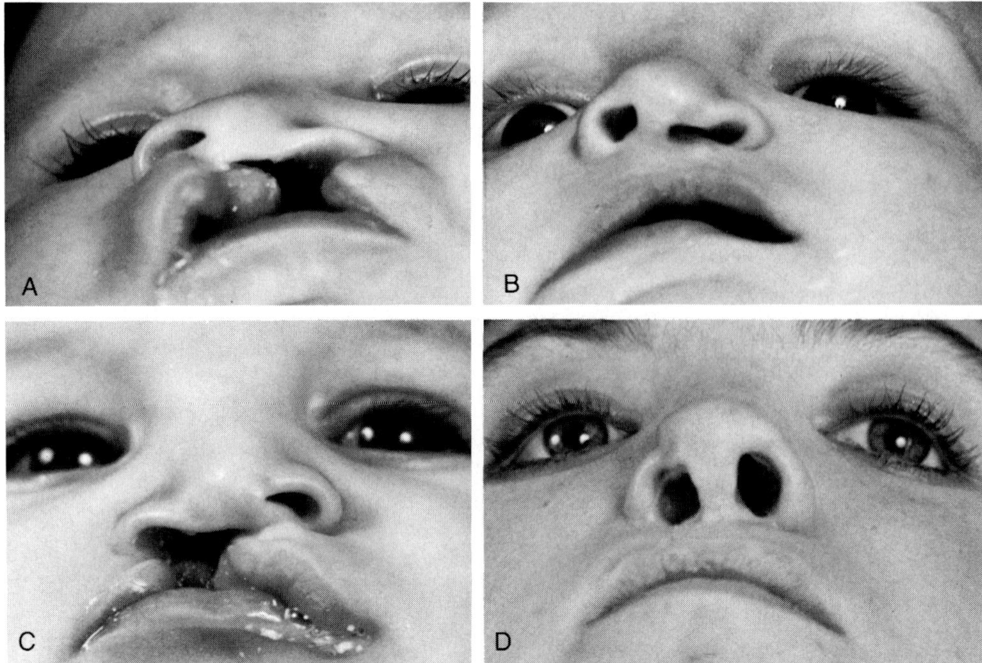

Figure 19–6 Unilateral cleft lip, alveolus, and palate with severe distortion of lower lateral cartilage. Nasal deformity remains after primary cleft lip repair. *A* and *B*, Large nostril following triangular flap repair. *C* and *D*, Small nostril following rotation-advancement repair.

in two planes—sagittal and frontal. The base of the septum is dislocated from the groove on the crest of the maxilla. The septal deviation may be so severe that it partially or completely obstructs the nasal passage on the cleft side. A more detailed description of the evaluation and management of the nasal airways is presented in Chapters 81 and 82.

There is no question that each of these factors—muscle imbalance, hypoplasia, and asymmetry of the skeletal base—results in a nasal deformity of various degrees of severity. However, a combination of these factors, which occurs in almost all patients with complete unilateral clefts, produces the most severe forms of nasal deformities.

Analysis of Nasal Deformity

For these reasons, it is important to determine which factor plays the major role so that the specialist can design ways to correct the deformity surgically, orthodontically, or, more commonly, through a combined surgical-orthodontic approach. When analyzing the nasal deformity, it must be realized that correction of one of the factors rarely suffices to alleviate the existing nasal deformity. It should be understood that the factors leading to the nasal deformity have already produced changes in the lower lateral cartilage, nostril, columella, septum, alar base, and so on. These changes should be treated while correcting the causal factors. By restoring the muscle balance through primary lip repair and surgical-orthodontic treatment, a more symmetric skeletal base can be established. Bone grafting can augment the skeletal base, but it will not improve the position of the lower lateral cartilage or the deviated septum. Surgeons who claim that a bone-cartilage graft will eliminate the nasal deformity at an early age are not

entirely correct. A graft can produce a more symmetric skeletal base, but it will not eliminate the deformity of the lower lateral cartilage, nasal tip, or septum.

The first and most complete description of the nasal deformity associated with the unilateral cleft was done by Huffman and Lierle.[18] Their findings were based on the observations of many patients over the years, allowing them to describe a "typical" nasal deformity. We felt that their description should be revised and expanded on the basis of new findings and a better understanding of the morphologic changes.[19]

The following is a list of characteristics of a typical unilateral nasal deformity; however, they are not necessarily listed in order of frequency or importance. All of them may be present prior to lip repair and subsequent to the primary operation. The degree and severity of the deformities vary greatly, and not all are present in each patient. The deformities include the following:

1. The columella is shorter on the cleft side.
2. The columella has an oblique position with its base deviated to the noncleft side.
3. The lateral crus of the lower lateral cartilage and the adherent skin are drawn into an S-shaped fold.
4. The lateral crus of the lower lateral cartilage is longer on the cleft side.
5. The lower lateral cartilage is displaced in the frontal and horizontal (backward and downward) planes.
6. The nasal tip is displaced in the frontal and horizontal planes following displacement of the lower lateral cartilage.
7. The nasal tip is asymmetric.
8. The vestibular dome is excessively obtuse.
9. The ala is flattened, resulting in a horizontal orientation of the nostril.
10. The nostril is smaller or larger than that of the opposite side.

11. The entire nostril is retropositioned.
12. The base of the ala is displaced laterally and/or posteriorly, and/or inferiorly.
13. The nasal floor is absent.
14. The nasal floor is lower on the cleft side.
15. Nasolabial fistula may be present.
16. The caudal edge of the nasal septum and the anterior nasal spine are deflected into the noncleft vestibule.
17. The nasal septum is deviated, resulting in varying degrees of nasal obstruction on the cleft side.
18. The lower turbinate on the cleft side is hypertrophic.
19. The nasal pyramid is asymmetric.
20. The maxilla is hypoplastic on the cleft side.
21. The maxillary segment is displaced on the cleft side.
22. The premaxilla and maxillary segment are displaced on the noncleft side.

Correction of the unilateral cleft lip nasal deformity presents a very difficult problem. For many years the focus was on lip and palate repair rather than on correction of the nasal deformity. Only recently have attempts been made to correct this deformity at the time of primary lip repair. Correction of the secondary nasal deformity at a later age depends on the type and severity of the deformity and may require complex surgical intervention.

Some of the deformities seen in the secondary unilateral cleft lip nose arise as a result of the technique of operation at the time of primary lip repair (Fig. 19–7).

Recently, Cutting et al[20] studied skin envelope deformities that resulted following rotation-advancement and triangular flap cleft lip repairs. In both groups, no primary nasal correction was performed. There were statistically significant differences in the skin envelope in the horizontal dimension in the two groups. In the rotation-advancement group the position of the alar base was considerably more normal, whereas in the triangular flap repair group the alar base was positioned more laterally. On the other hand, the rotation-advancement group had a greater horizontal alar base deficiency than the triangular flap repair group. This deficiency tended to result in a small nostril in the rotation-advancement group.

The cause of this difference in the horizontal aspect of the skin envelope between the two types of lip repair can be readily explained. In the rotation-advancement method, lip length is gained by the medial advancement of the upper lateral lip element. This procedure results in bringing the alar base into a more normal medial position. Unfortunately, if the columella is short and the dome is flat on the cleft side, this procedure also tends to produce a small nostril. With the triangular flap lip repair, lip length is gained by medial transposition of the inferior aspect of the lateral lip element. This results in minimal medial movement of the alar base at the time of cleft lip repair. As a result, the alar base is positioned too far laterally. In a patient with a short columella and a flattened dome, however, this procedure has a protective effect in minimizing alar

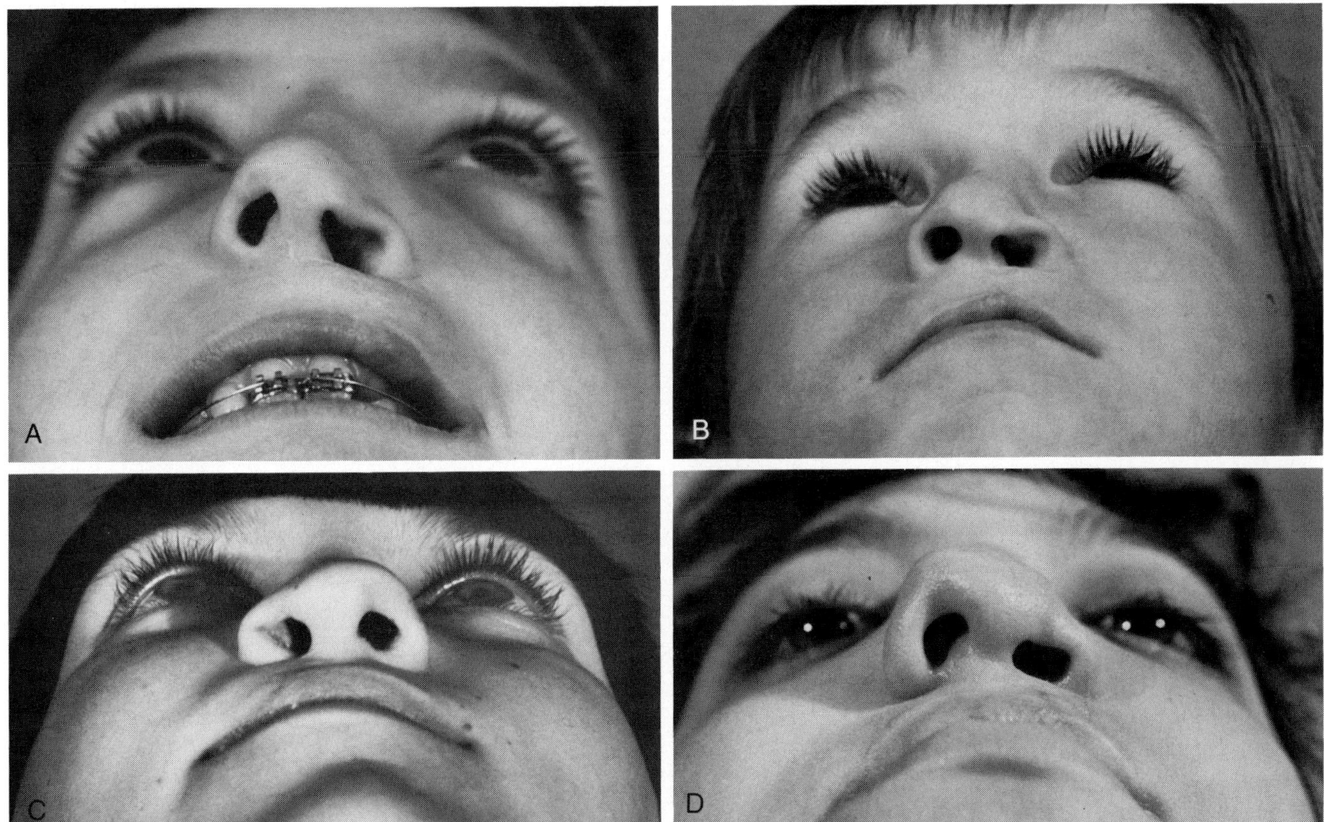

Figure 19–7 *A–D*, Various types of secondary nasal deformity.

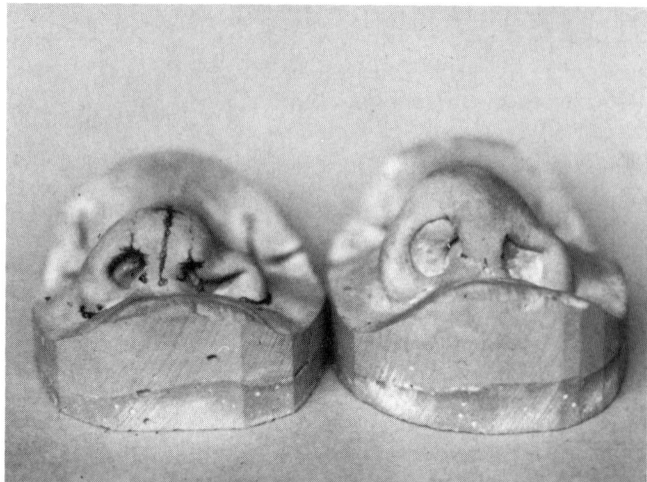

Figure 19–8 Typical secondary nasal deformities following a triangular flap lip repair on the left and a rotation-advancement repair on the right. In both cases, no primary nasal correction was performed. Note that the triangular repair left the alar base more laterally positioned but did not produce a horizontal alar base deficiency in the skin envelope. The rotation-advancement nose looks better, but there is a horizontal alar base deficiency on the cleft side that is hard to correct.

base deficiency. The nose, following triangular flap lip repair, looks worse than after rotation-advancement repair, but the nasal deformity is easier to correct. Bardach feels that this is a strong argument for the continued use of the triangular flap lip repair in a wide cleft with a severe nasal deformity. Cutting feels that primary elongation of the short columella and elevation of the depressed dome at the time of rotation-advancement lip repair is preferable in patients with wide clefts. Figure 19–8 shows a model of a typical rotation-advancement secondary nasal deformity next to a model of the nasal deformity resulting from a triangular flap lip repair.

There is currently much renewed interest in primary cleft lip nasal correction. Recently, Anderl,[6] McComb,[21] and Salyer[22] have presented long-term results of patients who have undergone nasal corrections at the time of primary lip repair. The surgical techniques employed appear to have originated with Blair in 1948[23] and were illustrated in Holdsworth's text on cleft lip and palate in 1957 (Fig. 19–9).[24] It should be noted that the technique used by each of these authors involved only

unilamellar dissection of the perichondrium of the lower lateral cartilage.

Wellisz et al[25] recently demonstrated that dissection of one side of the perichondrium from the cartilage in the ear of a newborn rabbit does not result in any decrease in growth of the surface area of the cartilage compared with the opposite ear. The shape of the ear was slightly affected; the ear appeared to bend slightly toward the side of the perichondrial dissection. Examination of the long-term results, reported by McComb,[21] suggests that a similar mechanism may be operating in the noses of his patients. In any case, there does not seem to be any decrease in the overall size of the nose following primary nasal correction, but the shape is not entirely normal either. It is possible that the scar produced on one side of the cartilage causes the growing cartilage to warp slightly on that side.

Nasal Deformity Associated with the Bilateral Cleft

The nasal deformity associated with the bilateral cleft also has some typical characteristics that vary only in degree of severity. In bilateral clefts, the initial nasal deformity may differ from the deformity appearing subsequent to primary cleft lip repair.

The nasal deformity in symmetric bilateral clefts is different from that in asymmetric bilateral clefts. The deformity may also vary depending on the position of the premaxilla. In patients with symmetric bilateral clefts with the premaxilla positioned within the alveolar arch, the shape and position of the nose may appear normal. These clefts are usually incomplete clefts of the lip only. Entirely different structural changes occur when there is a complete symmetric cleft lip and palate but the premaxilla and prolabium are isolated from the other structures. In these patients, in spite of the apparently normal shape and symmetry of the nose, the prolabium is closely attached to the nasal tip with a very short columella. This initial condition inadvertently leads to a typical secondary nasal deformity. Following lip repair, the short columella pulls the nasal tip downward, flattening it and changing the orientation of the nostrils from oblique to horizontal. Furthermore, this

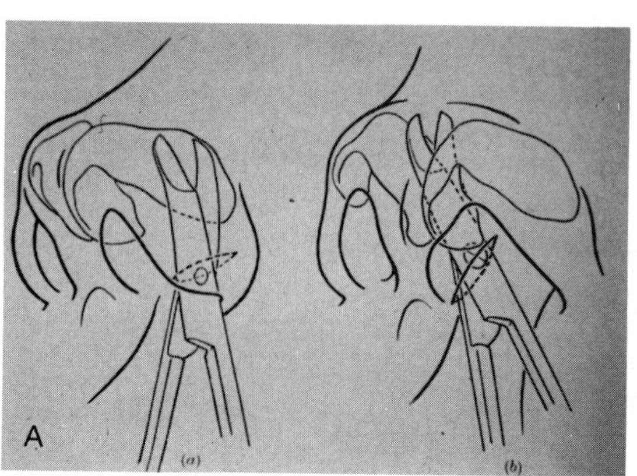

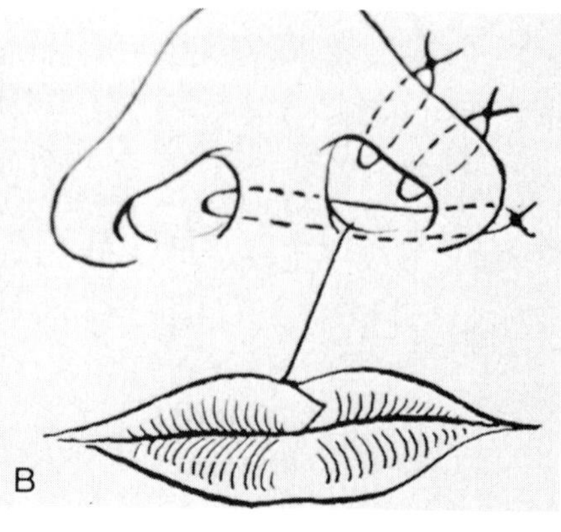

Figure 19–9 Holdsworth's illustration of Vilray Blair's method of primary nasal correction. The dissection technique is shown in A. Sutures are used to maintain position as shown in B. Note the similarity of current versions of primary nasal correction to Blair's. (From Holdsworth WG: Cleft Lip and Palate. London: William Heinemann Medical Books, Ltd., 1957.)

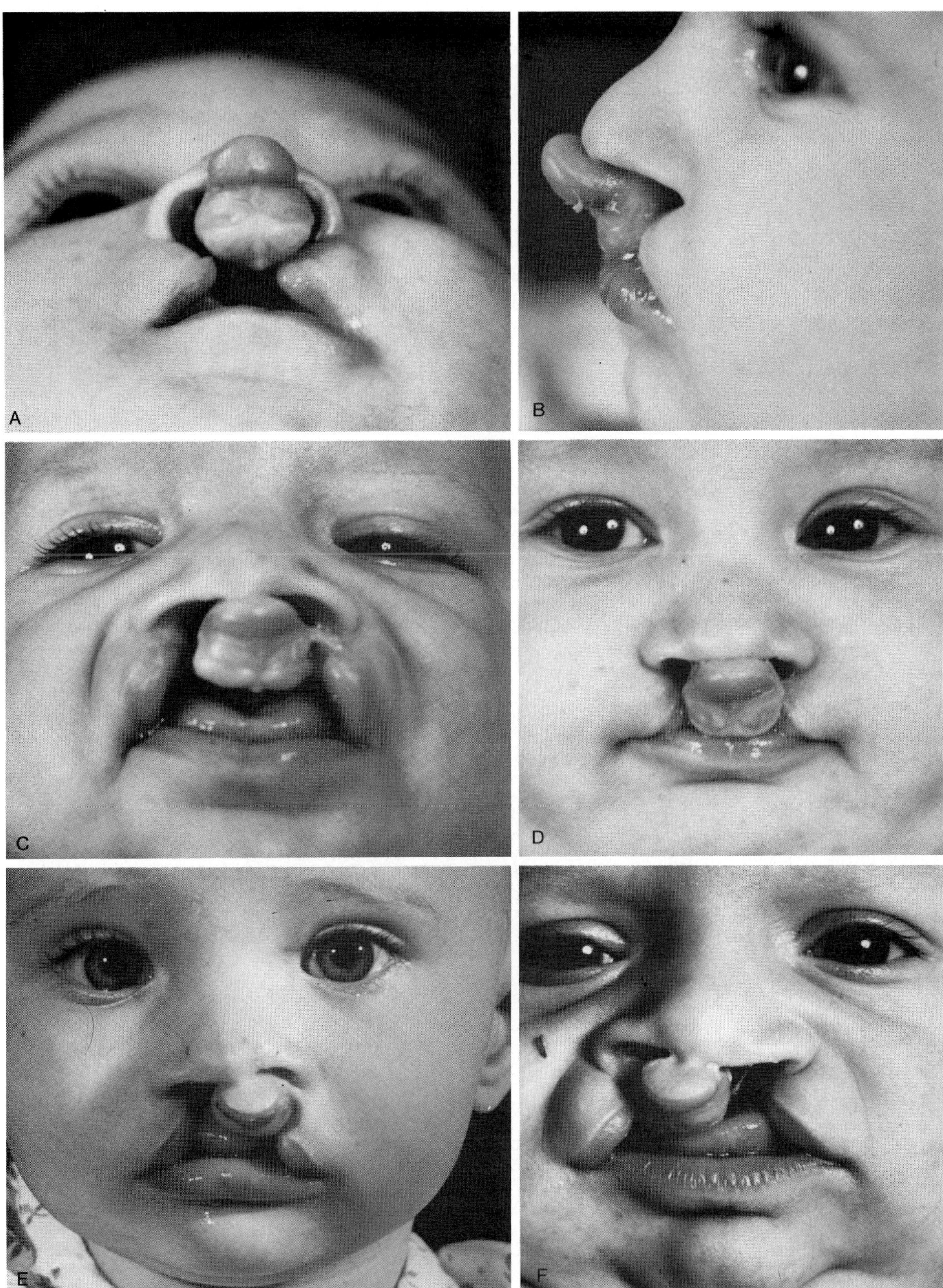

Figure 19–10 *A–F*, Nasal deformity in the bilateral symmetric and asymmetric cleft lip, alveolus, and palate.

defect leads to widening of the alar bases, creating an excessively wide and flat nose in its entire lower portion.

The lower lateral cartilages become shortened at the medial crura and elongated and displaced in the lateral crura. The domes are obtuse and flat and are quite distant from each other. Since most of the described changes result from the short columella, an attempt is made to lengthen it during primary lip repair to preclude the aforementioned secondary deformities.

McComb rearranges the lower lateral cartilages during primary lip repair to maintain an undistorted nasal tip and columella with an adequate length. The skin of the prolabium is used to lengthen the columella. However, use of the prolabium during primary lip repair to reconstruct the length of the columella may create complications for definitive lip repair. The prolabium should be used for reconstruction of the philtrum. However, if the prolabium is used for this purpose, it results in a short columella with the typical sequence of deformities described above. Nevertheless, early correction may be indicated because the prolabium usually contains more than enough tissue to create a philtrum of normal size.

The typical secondary nasal deformity occurs in asymmetric and symmetric clefts as well as in complete and incomplete clefts. The nasal deformity is corrected most successfully when it is symmetric. According to our experience with wide symmetric or asymmetric bilateral clefts or in patients with a small prolabium or a protruded premaxilla, two-stage lip repair may lead to a less severe secondary nasal deformity than a one-stage, simultaneous procedure (Fig. 19–10).

In symmetric bilateral clefts, usually the nasal septum is not affected. The deformity affects the columella, nasal tip, ala, and lower lateral cartilages. The most characteristic features of the bilateral cleft lip nasal deformity, both before and after lip repair, are the short columella, flat and broad nasal tip, a laterally displaced alar base, and horizontally oriented nostrils (Fig. 19–11).

The most severe nasal deformity occurs when the premaxilla is protruded or when the bilateral cleft is wide and asymmetric. A very small prolabium situated initially at the nasal tip makes the prognosis for good aesthetic results dubious. The most characteristic features associated with the bilateral cleft lip may include any or all of the following.

1. The columella is very short. Sometimes it seems not to exist, and the prolabium appears to be attached to the nasal tip.
2. The nasal tip is flat and broad.
3. The nasal alae are flat and sometimes drawn in an S-shaped fashion.
4. The bases of the alae are displaced laterally and sometimes inferiorly and posteriorly.
5. Both nostrils are oriented in a horizontal position.
6. The lower lateral cartilages are severely deformed: (a) The medial crura are short and widely separated at the nasal tip; (b) the lateral crura are flat and elongated; (c) the dome is angled obtusely.
7. The nasal floor is absent.
8. The columella, caudal end of the septum, and anterior nasal spine are displaced inferiorly relative to the level of the alar bases.
9. The nasal tip and nostrils are asymmetric.

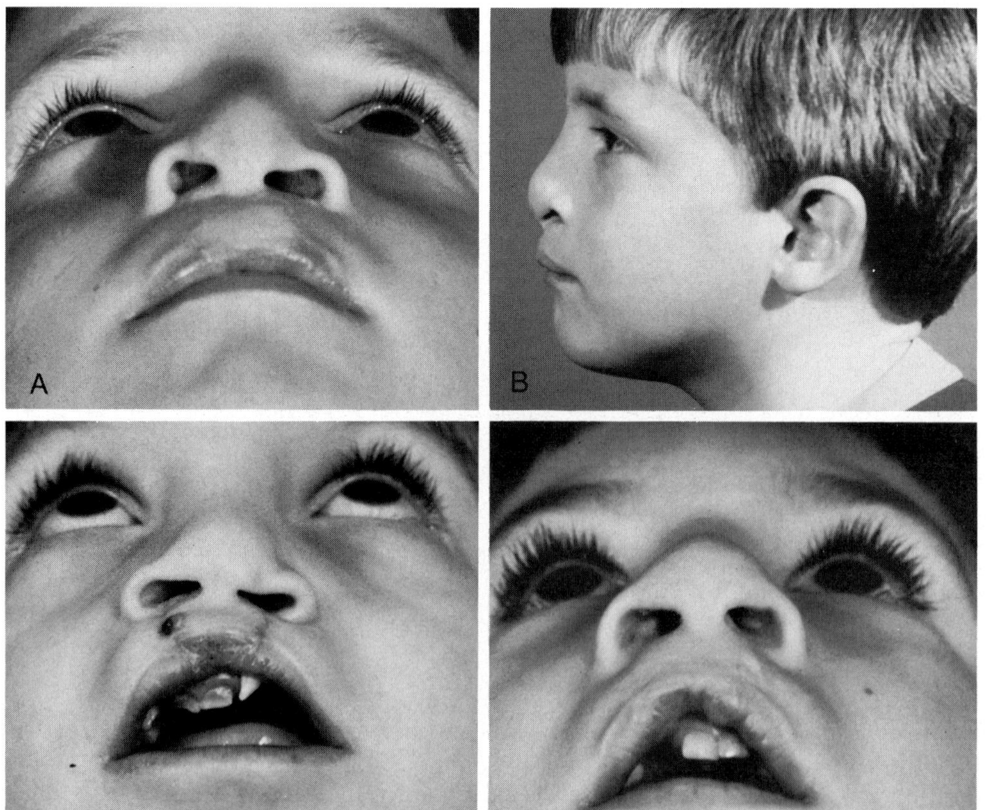

Figure 19–11 *A–D*, Secondary deformity in bilateral clefts. Note the broad and flattened nasal tip, the horizontal orientation of the nostrils, and the wide alar bases.

Correction of the bilateral cleft lip nasal deformity presents a difficult problem that only recently has been treated more successfully during the initial stages of repair as well as during secondary phases. Detailed descriptions for methods of repairing primary and secondary nasal deformities are presented in Chapters 23 to 26, 33, and 34.

References

1. Dursy E: Zur Entwicklungsgeschichte des Ropfes des Menschen und der hoheren Wirbelthiere. Tubingen: Lauppschern, 1869.
2. His E: Beobachtungen zur Geschichte und Gamenbildung beim menschlichen Embryo. Kgl Acad Wiss 27:1901.
3. Veau V: Bec-de-lievre. Hypothese sur la malformation initiale. Ann Anat Pathol 12:329, 1935.
4. Pohlman G: A Dissertation on the Embryology of the Face (dissertation). Leipzig, 1910.
5. Fleischmann A: Die Kopfregion der Amnioten. Morphology 41:615, 1910.
6. Anderl H: Simultaneous repair of lip and nose in the unilateral cleft (a longterm report). In Jackson IT, Sommerlad BC (eds): Recent Advances in Plastic Surgery, Vol. 3. Edinburgh: Churchill Livingstone, 1985.
7. Latham R: Orthopedic advancement of the cleft maxillary segment: A preliminary report. Cleft Palate J 17:227, 1980.
8. Avery J: The nasal capsule in cleft palate. Anat Anz 109:722, 1961.
9. Scott J: The cartilage of the nasal septum. Br Dent J 95:37, 1953.
10. Enlow DH: Handbook of Facial Growth, 2nd ed. Philadelphia: Saunders, 1982.
11. Moss ML: Twenty years of functional cranial analysis. Am J Orthod 61:479, 1972.
12. Latham RA: The pathogenesis of the skeletal deformity associated with unilateral cleft lip and palate. Cleft Palate J 6:404, 1969.
13. Latham RA: The septopremaxillary ligament and maxillary development. J Anat 104:584, 1969.
14. King BF, Workman CH, Latham RA: An anatomical study of the columella and the protruding premaxillae in a bilateral cleft lip and palate infant. Cleft Palate J 16:223, 1979.
15. Stenstrom S, Oberg T: The nasal deformity in unilateral cleft lip. Plast Reconstr Surg 28:295, 1961.
16. Hogan VM, Converse JM: Secondary deformities of unilateral cleft lip and nose. In Grabb WC, Rosenstein S, Bzoch K (eds): Cleft Lip and Palate. Boston: Little, Brown, 1971.
17. Fara M: The musculature of cleft lip and palate. In Converse JG, McCarthy JG (eds): Reconstructive Plastic Surgery. Philadelphia: Saunders, 1977.
18. Huffman WC, Lierle DM: Studies on the pathologic anatomy of the unilateral hare-lip nose. Plast Reconstr Surg 4:225, 1949.
19. Bardach J, Salyer K: Surgical Techniques in Cleft Lip and Palate. Chicago: Year Book, 1987.
20. Cutting C, Bardach J, Pang R: A comparative study of the skin envelope of the unilateral cleft-lip nose subsequent to rotation-advancement and triangular flap lip repairs. Plast Reconstr Surg Sept 1989.
21. McComb H: Primary correction of unilateral cleft lip-nose deformity: A 10 year review. Plast Reconstr Surg 75:791, 1985.
22. Salyer K: Primary correction of the unilateral cleft nose: A 15 year experience. Plast Reconstr Surg 77:558, 1986.
23. Blair V, Robinson R: Primary closure of harelip. Surg Gynecol Obstet 86:502, 1948.
24. Holdsworth WG: Cleft Lip and Palate. New York: Grune & Stratton, 1957.
25. Wellisz TZ, Cutting CB, McCarthy JG: The effects of unilamellar perichondrial dissection on the growth of rabbit ear cartilage. Plast Reconstr Surg 79:935, 1987.

CHAPTER 20

The Importance of Muscle

Peter Randall

Dr. James Barrett Brown of St. Louis used to say that "surgery of cleft lip is a four-dimensional problem for a two-dimensional mind."[1] This comment suggests that in our speaking and writing we are usually confined to the two dimensions of the photograph, the drawing, or the diagram, whereas we should be thinking not only of the third dimension of depth but also of the fourth dimension of movement.

Our lips are so expressive of mood—from anger to pleasure to determination to astonishment and so on—that this movement of expression is as critical as the movement needed to achieve a watertight seal or a bilabial plosive. Because the disoriented muscle in the cleft nearly parallels the cleft margins, as seen in severe unilateral or bilateral clefts, the upper end of the lateral muscle bundle, located near the alar base, is really directed superiorly and laterally, pointing toward the pupil of the eye. In the normal position, these fibers probably would be directed horizontally, near the free border of the lip, and would extend past the midline to insert in the dermis on the opposite side of the philtrum.[2–4]

With contraction of this displaced muscle, the vector of movement pulls the inferior portion of the lateral part of the cleft in a superior lateral direction, as in the normal person, with movement toward the center of the oral orifice. It is no wonder that without repositioning the muscle, contraction produces an "orbicularis bulge" laterally. Our cleft patients have great difficulty trying to whistle.

Orbicularis Oris Muscle

The "before" and "after" photographs in Figure 20–1 represent an unusual situation. This young fellow, as clearly shown, had not had a very good bilateral cleft lip repair. A Mirault-Brown-McDowell flap was used on each side, which totally destroyed the Cupid's bow. The scars in the lip are rather irregular and prominent. However, the only things that bothered him and his parents and that were noted mostly when he tried to whistle, were the lateral bulges of the orbicularis muscle. In fact, he and his parents would not let us operate on anything except these two muscle bulges.

In this patient, the only step that was done was a repositioning of the orbicularis oris muscle. This was accomplished through an incision in the buccal sulcus, dissecting laterally between the muscle and mucosa and between the muscle and skin. The muscle then was released from the alar base. The sweep upward of the displaced muscle fibers was clearly evident. When the muscle was dissected free and brought all the way down into the horizontal position, it was sutured with an overlap. These muscle fibers are not very thick, and in

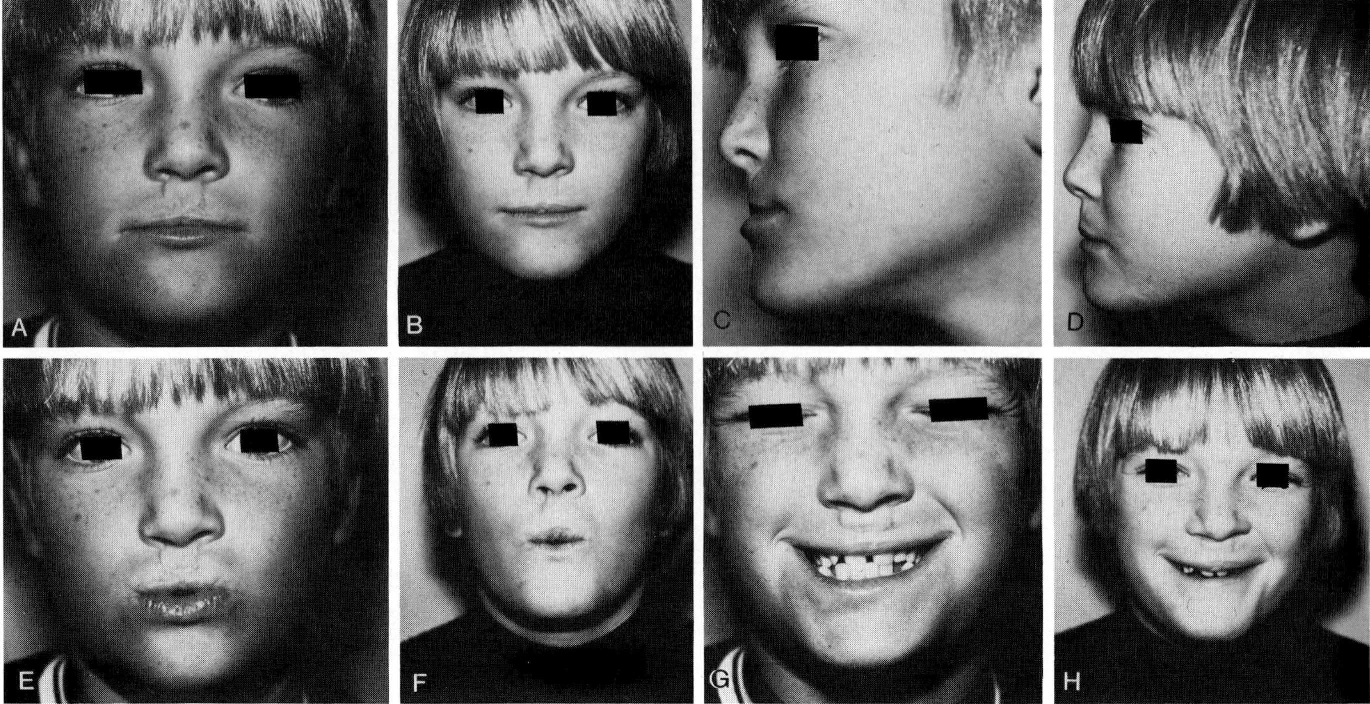

Figure 20–1 A patient with an inadequate bilateral cleft lip repair. Preoperative *(A–D)* and postoperative *(E–H)* photographs were taken following a secondary operation in which the only step taken was to reorient the orbicularis oris muscle by way of the buccal sulcus.

performing this procedure, the surgeon must be very careful not to twist the muscle because the lip needs to be inverted to gain access through the buccal sulcus incision, and twisting is not difficult to do.

Postoperatively, this patient can now whistle, whereas before, he was unable to do so. Furthermore, the entire appearance of the lip, in both the full face and the lateral photographs in repose, shows an improvement. His face now has an element of normalcy and a "softness" that was not seen preoperatively. One of the most difficult aspects of studying patients in whom this procedure has been carried out is documentation of just how much improvement has been achieved. Usually other procedures are included in a secondary operation to improve the appearance of the face and these steps may overshadow the improvement in muscle repositioning.

Nasolabialis Muscle

The normal lip, of course, includes the very fine slips of vertical fibers of the nasolabialis muscle (Fig. 20–2). This muscle is close to the midline and inserts at the base of the nasal spine. It elevates the central part of the lip to provide a little more exposure of the incisor teeth during smiling. In the complete bilateral cleft, since the nasolabialis fibers should be located in the prolabium, they are probably missing completely. This elevating action has not been restored in the patient seen in Figure 20–1. The somewhat distorted appearance of his smile really has not been improved at all by the repositioning of the orbicularis oris muscle. Fur-

thermore, I do not see how this function can reasonably be restored.

In most patients with unilateral clefts, the nasolabialis muscle is partially present, but in some patients the lack of central elevation or the asymmetric central elevation on smiling can be demonstrated postoperatively. Dado and Kernahan have stated that in their dissections of unilateral clefts, the orbicularis oris fibers have not been found in an orderly parallel pattern, as described by Fara, but are in a disorderly, "jumbled" pattern that would almost defy reorientation at the time of surgery.[5] These authors, however, for the most part, carried out their intricate studies in that portion of tissue in incomplete clefts that is usually discarded. In only one patient (a cadaver dissection) were they looking at the fibers located further laterally. Indeed, Fara, in his many dissections of stillborns, also described one such case in whom the muscle bundles laterally were in a jumbled pattern rather than an orderly array.

I have seen many of these muscles during surgery and am more inclined to agree with Fara's description than with Dado and Kernahan's. The direction of the muscle fibers is more easily seen on the mucosal side than on the dermal side, and the amount of displacement or distortion of orientation does vary from one patient to another. In general, muscle fibers are more markedly displaced in patients with the more severe clefts; indeed, the muscle pretty much parallels the lip margin, both medially and laterally. Along the cleft margin it does indeed appear to be a bit jumbled, as described by Kernahan, but further laterally the orderly disorientation is easily seen. As the muscle approaches the alar base, it becomes very attenuated and seems to be almost fibrotic.

Muscle Repair

It is still a puzzle to me as to what is the best way to handle these muscles in primary cleft lip repair. I think they should be freed up by undermining between skin and muscle and between mucosa and muscle. Then they can be cut loose from any superior attachment and brought down to the horizontal position, both on the lateral side and on the medial side. In patients with bilateral clefts, of course, there is no muscle in the prolabium that can be used except in very incomplete clefts, and there it is rather rudimentary. We used to overlap the medial and lateral muscle flaps, suturing the medial side on top of the lateral side from the vermilion to the nasal spine and suturing muscle to muscle. Kernahan divides the lateral muscle flap ("jumble" and all) into a larger superior segment, which is sutured to the nasal spine, and a smaller inferior segment, which is sutured more horizontally to the muscle on the medial side.[6]

More recently, we have been dividing both the medial and lateral muscle flaps into three or four muscle "slips" and interdigitating these slips.[7] The superior lateral slip is sutured to the nasal spine, and the superior medial slip is sutured to dermis just below the alar base. The more central slips are again crossed and sutured to dermis, and the inferior slips are sutured one on top of the other, just below the skin vermilion border. In patients with bilateral clefts this interdigitation can occasionally be done if the muscle is long enough, but more often the muscle is sutured end to end, with a superior suture securing the muscle to the nasal spine.

We have found it very frustrating to try to assess the results of this muscle reconstruction objectively. The patients seem to look better and can whistle better, although some still have a slight orbicularis bulge lat-erally. The depression frequently seen just below the nostril sill seems to be filled out much better, and some patients even have a good philtral ridge at this point. Nevertheless, it is difficult to document these impressions in an objective way.

Stark has described the etiology of prepalatal clefts as the result of mesodermal deficiency.[8] So it is not surprising that in clefts of both the lip and the palate, profound disturbances in the muscular elements are seen. Indeed, mesodermal distortion seems to be a key part of many congenital anomalies. These include cardiac anomalies, hernias, congenital limb problems, diaphragmatic problems, and pharyngeal and esophageal anomalies. Clefts of the lip and palate have their obvious epithelial distortions, but it is not difficult to imagine that the problem is probably due primarily to the underlying mesodermal structures. For example, the cleft lip nose seems to be due largely to cartilaginous displacement and distortion. Similarly, microtia and the facies of the patient with Treacher-Collins syndrome and hemifacial microsomia are basically defects in mesoderm, with the epithelial elements "following suit."

Thus it seems that in the functional repair of cleft lip and cleft palate, reconstruction of the muscular elements is the key. Many of the problems encountered in repair of both lip and palatal clefts have to do with the orientation of the muscle. It has been argued that the surgical steps needed to dissect these muscles free from the surrounding tissue and suture them into a new position must add scar tissue to the area, where a restricting scar is counterproductive. In addition, the undermining and dissection can also lead to an increased likelihood of bleeding with hematoma, sepsis, and breakdown. Hematoma has occurred three times in my lip repairs with muscle dissection, and in two of these patients there was drainage but no breakdown.

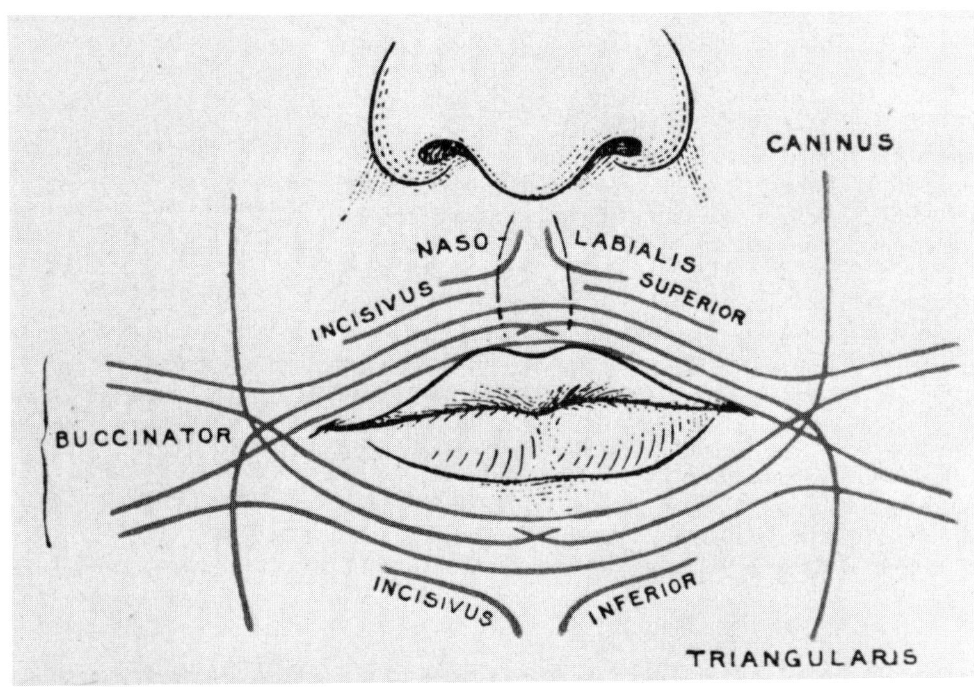

Figure 20–2 Diagrammatic representation of the muscle fibers in the lip. Note the position of the nasolabialis muscle, which elevates the central part of the lip and which is obviously missing or not working in the patient in Figure 20–1. From Lewis WH (ed): Gray's Anatomy of the Human Body. Philadelphia, Lea & Febiger, 1943. With permission.)

Muscular Movement

In the palate, the movement of the normal palate as seen on video film is well known to those interested in clefts. It is a quick, accurate, light movement that seems to be virtually effortless. I have likened it to the movement of a blink, except that continuous use of the orbicularis oculi leads to fatigue, and the levator palati seems to be able to function almost indefinitely. Shprintzen[9] has shown that velopharyngeal incompetence can occur with what would appear to be the isolated absence of the musculus uvulae.

Sommerlad has taken the dissection of the levator palati muscle one step further than we have, so that, in an intravelar veloplasty, the muscle is freed up in a virtually bloodless plane and is carried down almost all the way to the eustachean tube.[10] In doing this procedure, he reports that the muscle seems to move much more freely than it did when a more limited dissection was carried out. He further implies that if the muscle is not dissected this much, it is not completely freed and remains somewhat tethered. Perhaps nasoendoscopic observation of these muscles in action will tell us which method will give the best results.

Most of us have seen videotapes of repaired cleft palates that achieve complete velopharyngeal closure but do so in a very slow, sluggish, and ponderous way. This is not normal movement and is a far cry from the light, bouncy excursion seen in the normal palate. Weatherly-White once studied the speed with which the soft palate moves, using cineradiographs while the patient or subject was enunciating the words *simple* and *sample*.[11] Both of these words require palatal closure for the /s/ and following vowel, opening for the nasal consonant /m/, and immediate closure for the plosive /p/. By using a ruler with opaque markers, he could literally calculate the speed of palatal movement in millimeters per second. In spite of supposedly being able to achieve closure, the slowly moving palates did not always achieve closure in time and also apparently required so much effort to achieve closure that they became fatigued more easily than palates with more rapid movement. The speed of soft palate movement was seen to be directly related to its function.

There is another parameter that we should be looking into—that is, how much effort is it taking this patient to achieve complete velopharyngeal closure? If it is taking a great deal of effort and concentration, then speech will deteriorate when the person is talking rapidly or is fatigued. For example, in theory, if a child is able to achieve closure but we could show that he is exerting, let us say, ten times the normal amount of effort and concentration to do so, we should not be satisfied with this result. To achieve velopharyngeal competence in such a case through speech therapy is, indeed, a triumph for the speech pathologist, but I wonder if it is the best thing for the patient. Particularly, I wonder if there is some way that the palate can be made to achieve competence more efficiently and with less concentration and effort.

Pigott has stressed the importance of the contraction of the musculus uvuli in producing a fullness on the nasal side of the soft palate, at the point of closure with the adenoid pad.[12] In the normal palate, this muscle is easily seen, as noted by Shprintzen.[9] In the child with a cleft, it is difficult to see how it can be adquately reconstructed.

At the present time, as reported by Brown et al, we are getting better results with muscle construction in the intravelar veloplasty than we did before we used techniques utilizing reorientation of the levator palati muscle.[13] In addition, the Furlow technique, which repositions this muscle in its overlapped position with less muscular dissection, again is producing better speech results than those seen in patients who have had the intravelar veloplasty. Patients undergoing the Furlow repair were evaluated 6.9 to 9.3 years after surgery and were found to be only 40% as likely to need a secondary posterior pharyngeal flap procedure as those who had had intravelar veloplasty (p < 0.01).

It would seem that muscle reconstruction and reorientation is an extremely important factor in developing a lip that not only looks normal but also is symmetric and is capable of more normal movements for eating, speaking, and facial expression. A number of parameters in the muscular function of the soft palate need to be studied to determine not only which operations are producing the best incidence of velopharyngeal competence but also which are producing palates that can move as quickly and easily as a normal palate and with as little fatigue.

References

1. Brown JB: Personal communication, 1951.
2. Fara M: Anatomy and arteriography of cleft lips in stillborn children. Plast Reconstr Surg 42:29, 1968.
3. Randall P, Whitaker LA, LaRossa D: The importance of muscle reconstruction in primary and secondary cleft lip repair. Plast Reconstr Surg 54:316, 1974.
4. Latham RA, Deaton TG: The structural basis of the philtrum and the contour of the vermilion border: A study of the musculature of the upper lip. J Anat 121:151, 1976.
5. Dado PV, Kernahan DA: Anatomy of the orbicularis oris muscle in incomplete unilateral cleft lip, based on histological examination. Ann Plast Surg 15:90, 1985.
6. Kernahan DA: Cleft lip repair. In Barclay TL, Kernahan DA (eds): Rob and Smith's Operative Surgery: Plastic Surgery, 4th ed. London: Butterworth, 1986.
7. Randall P: Triangular flap cleft lip repair. In Barclay TL, Kernahan DA (eds): Rob and Smith's Operative Surgery: Plastic Surgery, 4th ed. London: Butterworth, 1986.
8. Stark RB: The pathogenesis of harelip and cleft palate. Plast Reconstr Surg 13:20, 1954.
9. Lewin ML, Croft CB, Shprintzen RJ: Velopharyngeal insufficiency due to hypoplasia of the musculus uvulae and occult submucous cleft palate. Plast Reconstr Surg 65:585–591, 1980.
10. Sommerlad B: Personal communication, 1988.
11. Weatherly-White RCA: Presentation to the American Cleft Palate Association.
12. Pigott RW: Musculus uvulae. Presentation to the American Cleft Palate Association, New York, 1987.
13. Brown AA, Cohen M, Randall P: Levator muscle reconstruction: Does it make a difference? Plast Reconstr Surg 72:1–6,1983.

CHAPTER 21

Lip Adhesion for Wide Unilateral and Bilateral Clefts of the Lip

Peter Randall

The lip adhesion operation, in its most simple analysis, converts a difficult wide cleft into a much less difficult incomplete cleft.[1] Lip adhesion is most useful in patients with a bilateral cleft with a protruding premaxilla and is probably the most gentle and natural way of shaping and positioning the premaxillary segment, even in patients with unilateral clefts. It can be done at any age, but we usually combine it with closure of the cleft of the soft palate at 3 to 6 months of age. It is not a difficult operation and can be performed under either local anesthesia with sedation or general endotracheal anesthesia.

History

When Johanson first started to do primary bone grafting, he performed a preliminary operation on the lip and alveolus to achieve initial closure.[2-4] He then went back at a second operation, inserted autogenous bone in the alveolar cleft, and did a definitive lip repair. We thought this sequence of events was a good plan, but in carrying it out we were surprised to see that there was frequently little or no space in the alveolar cleft where one could insert any bone. However, the alveolus had been nicely repositioned, and with the conversion of the cleft to an incomplete cleft, the lip repair was obviously much easier than it would have been otherwise. The underlying bone was much more even, the surface landmarks were more readily apparent, and closure was completed with far less tension. In addition, in bilateral cleft patients with a very small prolabium, the lip adhesion was, literally, a skin expander, and the prolabium after this procedure was significantly stretched—again making the definitive repair much easier. Accordingly, we started using Johanson's preliminary operation, not to provide a bed for a primary bone graft but to make a difficult lip operation a much easier one.

Millard had described a similar procedure in unilateral clefts using just the upper third of the lip.[5] Shortly after publication of our version of the procedure, Collito and Walker described the C-W lip adhesion.[6] In the C-W adhesion, instead of turning flaps based on the edge of the cleft from side to side, they turned down flaps consisting mostly of vermilion and based each one

inferiorly. The C-W adhesion relieves some of the tension inferiorly but exerts more tension superiorly, whereas the lip adhesion described here relieves more tension superiorly and exerts a greater amount of tension inferiorly. Otherwise, these two techniques are similar and achieve essentially the same result.

Collito insists on allowing absolutely no relaxing incisions or undermining of the lip in order to minimize scarring. We feel that limited undermining, if needed to relieve tension, is not a severe detriment. In view of Skoog's use of both wide undermining and reflection of maxillary periosteum to achieve "boneless bone grafting" in primary cleft lip repair, the amount of limited undermining that we do does not seem unreasonable.

At one time we used the lip adhesion procedure for all complete (or total) clefts, unilateral and bilateral. This now seems to be totally unnecessary, and our decision at present as to whether or not to use a lip adhesion is determined at the time of surgery, depending on whether or not it would be difficult to get the edges together in a primary closure without undue tension. Often a cleft that seems excessively wide at birth, leading one to believe that a lip adhesion would be advisable, will not be nearly so difficult when done at the age of 3 to 4 months.

Most surgeons who do not use the lip adhesion method use elastic compression on a head cap or elastic adhesive tape to achieve the same end. This strapping is often combined with presurgical orthodontic (or orthopedic) treatment to keep the lateral maxillary segment expanded. Elastic traction or compression accomplishes essentially the same goals as the lip adhesion operation while avoiding a surgical procedure. However, strapping does not have the skin stretching or "expanding" advantages that the lip adhesion has. As noted, this procedure is particularly useful in patients with bilateral clefts. Also, the intact lip seems to be a more gentle molder of the premaxilla than external compression. The flaired or protruding premaxilla is never seen unless the constricting force of the intact lip is interrupted by a cleft. So the "natural" step to reconstitute this compression would seem to be the reestablishment of the intact lip.

As noted above, we usually combine the lip adhesion procedure with closure of the soft palate, and 3 to 4 months later, when the lip tissue has softened, a definitive lip repair is done with closure of the hard palate cleft. Presently, we prefer a Furlow repair of the soft palate and a vomer closure in one or two layers in the hard palate.

A dramatic narrowing of a wide hard palate cleft can be expected to occur very quickly following a lip adhesion and closure of the soft palate. In patients with wide bilateral clefts, we do not hesitate to do a lip adhesion on just one side at a time, preferring to do the more difficult side first, if this is possible, but doing the easier side first if necessary. The tilting of the prolabium toward the repaired side has not been a problem, since it straightens out almost completely after closure of the other side.

The lip adhesion operation is also a good choice of preliminary repair to be made in a child who may have a number of other physical problems, such as cardiac anomalies, laryngomalacia, or failure to thrive.

Operation

The operation can be done at virtually any age, under either local anesthesia with sedation or endotracheal general anesthesia. After the face has been prepared and draped, the key landmarks for the desired lip repair are noted. The incisions for the lip adhesion flaps are placed in tissue that would ordinarily be discarded. The lip is injected with tiny amounts of 1% lidocaine mixed with epinephrine 1:100,000, and we then wait 7 minutes

(by the clock). Then the incisions are made and taken down to the underlying muscle. Lateral undermining with an incision in the gingival buccal sulcus may be needed but is not done routinely.

Closure is begun, using 5–0 chromic as everting mattress sutures, along the posterior mucosal margins. Several sutures of either 4–0 chromic or 4–0 polyglycolic acid are placed in the muscle layer.

A tension-relieving suture (Lane type) is placed as noted in Figure 21–1. A 3–0 or 4–0 monofilament, nonabsorbable suture is used for this. It is placed on a straight cutting (Keith) needle, started on the mucosal side of the lip, and brought out laterally in the midportion of the nasolabial fold. The needle is reintroduced

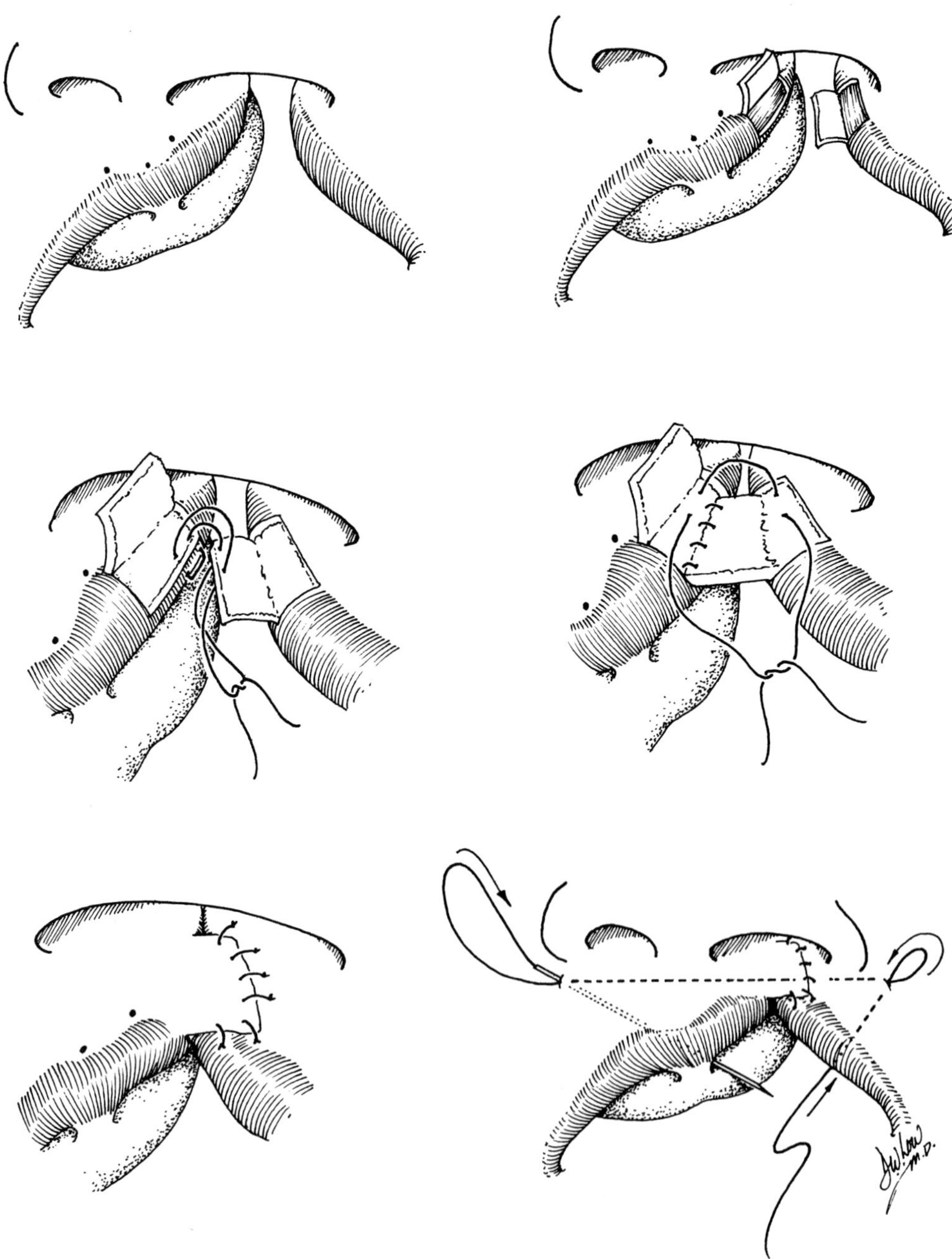

Figure 21–1 The usual lip markings are made and rectangular flaps are designed in tissue that would ordinarily be discarded. Closure is started with an absorbable suture on the posterior skin mucosal approximation. Two or three sutures of 4–0 chromic or polyglycolic acid suture are placed on the muscle layer. The exposed skin enclosure can be completed with either 5–0 chromic or a nonabsorbable stitch. A Lane-type tension suture of 3-0 or 4–0 monofilament, nonabsorbable material is inserted from the mucosal side using a straight needle, coming all the way through the lip and out through the skin near the nasolabial fold. The needle is then reintroduced into the same hole, taken through the lip adhesion, across to the opposite side, and out through the skin near the nasolabial fold. The needle is inserted back through this hole, threaded again through the entire lip, and brought through the mucosa near the original entrance. This suture is tied down sufficiently to relieve tension on the closure and is kept in place for 10 to 14 days.

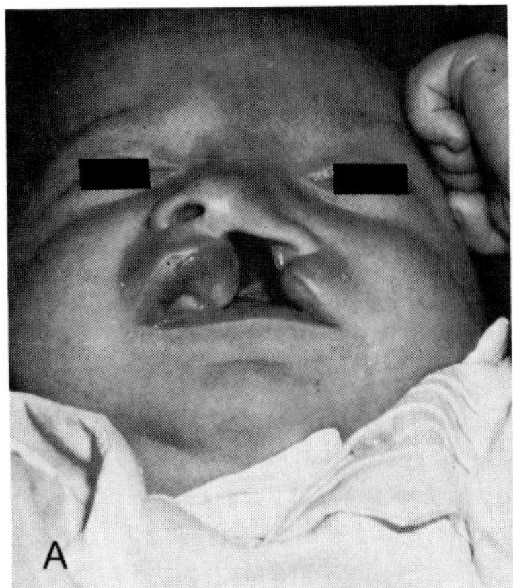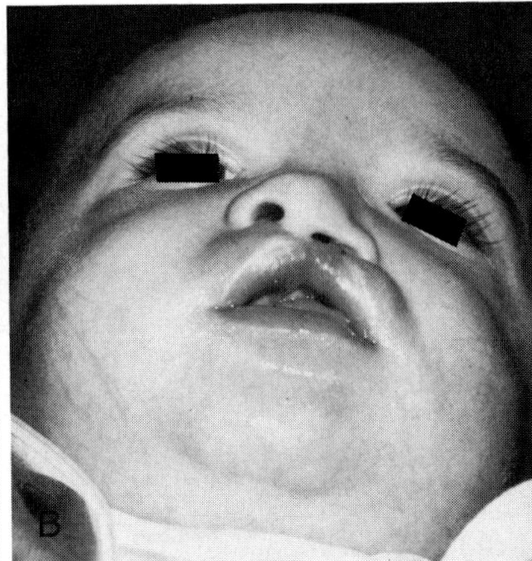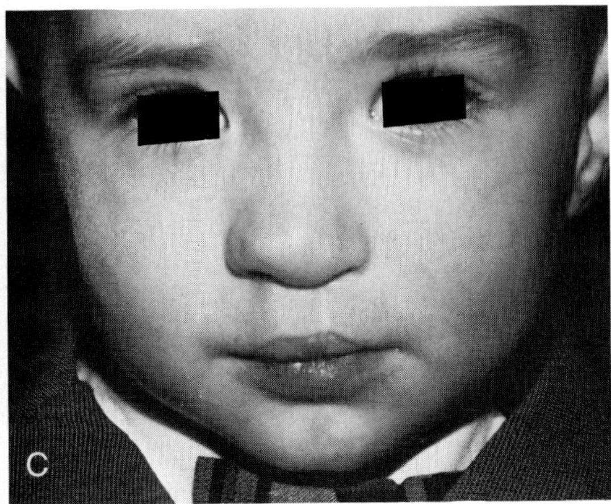

Figure 21–2 A wide unilateral cleft with considerable separation of the alveolar segments *(A)*. The lip adhesion has essentially converted a wide complete cleft into an incomplete cleft *(B)*. Definitive closure can be completed over a much more even bony foundation, with more easily identifying landmarks, and with far less tension *(C)*.

into the same hole and guided transversely through the incision of the lip adhesion, across the lip on the other side, and out again through the nasolabial fold. The needle is then reintroduced through this hole and brought back through the buccal mucosa, close to the point where the needle was first introduced. This suture is tied down, just tight enough to relieve a significant amount of tension from the surgical repair. It is tied with multiple knots, and a long end is left so that it will be easy to remove in 10 to 14 days.

Postoperatively, feeding is started on the same day as the surgery, as soon as the child is sufficiently awake to drink. The suture line is cleaned three to four times a day with soap and water. The definitive cleft lip repair can be done 3 to 4 months later if the tissues have softened completely.

Complications

Dehiscence of the lip adhesion with loss of its advantages is often mentioned as a frequent complication. In our own series, at one time this problem occurred in 18% of our patients. Since we began using the Lane retention suture mentioned above, the occurrence of dehiscence has reached almost zero.[7]

Scarring in the region of the lip repair also has been noted as a complication. It is true that some of the tissue adjacent to the area of the lip repair remains fibrotic, but this problem has usually been minor. The improvement in positioning of the alar base and the lack of tension in the definitive lip repair are far greater benefits to the eventual result, in our opinion, than trying to get a good repair with an excessive amount of tension.

Conclusions

The lip adhesion operation has been used for many years. It has been helpful in converting the difficult, wide, complete cleft into a much easier incomplete cleft in patients with both unilateral and bilateral clefts. It is an effective and probably the most gentle means of repositioning a protruding premaxilla. In patients with bilateral clefts, it also acts as an "expander" of the prolabial skin. The lip adhesion is usually combined with closure of the soft palate at the same time, and this combined procedure has been associated with a marked and dramatic narrowing of the hard palate cleft. Definitive lip repair can then be done with much greater ease, better landmarks, and less tension (Fig. 21–2). In the same way, because the hard palate defect is much narrower, closure is simpler and more effective.

In the original series of patients there was an 18% incidence of dehiscence, which has almost disappeared since we started using a Lane-type tension suture. The operation would seem to be a very worthwhile addition to the surgeon's armamentarium.

References

1. Randall P: A lip adhesion operation in cleft lip surgery. Plast Reconstr Surg 35:371–376, 1965.
2. Johanson B, Ohlsson A: Bone grafting and dental orthopaedics in primary and secondary cases of cleft lip and palate. Acta Chir Scand 122:112, 1964.
3. Johanson B, Ohlsson A: Die Osteoplastik bei Spatbehandlung der Lippen-, Kiefer-, und Gaumenspalten. Arch Klin Chir 295:876, 1960.
4. Nordin KE, Johanson B: Freie Knochen-Transplantation bei Defekten in Alveolarkammen nach kieferorthopadischer Einstellung der Maxilla bei Lippen-, Kiefer- und Gaumenspalten Fortschr Kiefer Gesichtschir 1:168, 1955.
5. Millard DR: A preliminary adhesion. In Millard DR (ed): Cleft Craft: The Unilateral Deformity, Vol. 1. Boston: Little, Brown, 1976.
6. Walker J, Collito M, et al: Physiologic considerations in cleft lip closure: The C-W technique. Plast Reconstr Surg 37:552–557, 1966.
7. Randall P, Graham WP: Lip adhesion in the repair of bilateral cleft lip. In Grabb WC, Rosenstein SW, Bzoch KR (eds): Cleft Lip and Palate. Boston: Little, Brown, 1971. Chapter 18.

CHAPTER 22

Lip Adhesion in Unilateral and Bilateral Cleft Lip Repair

Malcolm A. Lesavoy

Webster's New Collegiate Dictionary defines the word *adhesion* as a "steady or firm attachment . . . a union of bodily parts by growth . . . tissues abnormally united by fibrous tissue resulting from an inflammatory process. . . ." Aside from the surgical procedure of forming a scar between the adjacent lip elements in patients with unilateral or bilateral cleft lip, occasionally much "inflammation" has been produced by discussions and writings of plastic surgeons on the relative merits of the lip adhesion. Basically, the lip adhesion is a preliminary operative procedure that prepares a unilateral or a bilateral cleft lip deformity for the definitive repair. Advantages and disadvantages exist, and this author is biased by his training and experience toward the use of lip adhesion.

In 1954, Johanson was credited with discussing the use of lip adhesion as a preliminary procedure to be used prior to anterior palatal primary bone grafting.[1] Subsequently, Johanson and Ohlsson felt that the lip adhesion procedure allowed for a more definitive lip closure.[2] In 1964, Millard[3] reported that a "partial union of the lip will help to mould the distorted maxilla . . . " and that ". . . a simple straight first stage approximation of the superior one third of the lip cleft is a possibility. This could be carried out high enough to avoid destruction of any natural landmarks. The rotation advancement method then is available for final lip closure." This technique was popularized in 1965 by Peter Randall,[4] when he described a lip adhesion for complete clefts because "there is likely to be more concern over tension, the position of the lip segments after the bony segments have been molded in the ventral position of the alar base." Randall[5] used two triangular flaps comprising most of the vertical dimension of the cleft, whereas Millard's lip adhesion was limited to the superior portions of the cleft.

The specific techniques used to enable the attachments of the lateral lip elements to actually pull the lateral alveolar segment to a more anterior and medial position were described by Walker and Collito in 1966.[6] They felt that incision in the buccal sulcus and separation of the lip elements from the alveolus would not allow normal arch formation. Millard subsequently described, in *Cleft Craft,* the "high, half-undermined adhesion" that makes the most sense.[7] The no-cleft or medial lip element (in the unilateral cleft lip deformity) was undermined moderately so that tension on the lip adhesion

was relieved. This medial lip element was then "adhered" to the *nonundermined* lateral lip element. In this way, the intact attachments of the lateral lip to the alveolus were encouraged to provide a dynamic tension and to pull the lateral alveolus and maxilla to a more anterior and medial position, while at the same time the undermined and freed medial attachments acted as a rubber band that pushed the protruding and more prominent medial alveolus and premaxilla inferiorly and posteriorly to meet the upcoming lateral segment. This procedure provided an orthopedic force on these very malleable bony elements early in life and prepared the stage for the definitive lip repair.

Similarly, a lip adhesion provides for a type of "tissue expansion." Prior to any surgical manipulation, the lateral and medial lip elements in a complete unilateral or bilateral cleft lip are untethered. The orbicularis oris muscle is continuous. With the expression of smiling or crying the lip elements tend to contract and separate. After a lip adhesion, the lip elements as well as the muscle are tethered (although not aesthetically or anatomically perfect). Now, during smiling or crying, the medial and lateral lip elements do not separate but actually pull on themselves and are in a constant state of stretch or mild tension. In addition, both the rapid degree of growth in the 2 or 3 months intervening between a lip adhesion and the definitive lip repair and the underlying pressure of the alveolar elements pressing on the overlying soft tissue add another dimension of natural tissue expansion. Therefore, when definitive lip repair is attempted, there is more volume and substance of tissue.

Another advantage of the lip adhesion procedure is the repositioning of the nasal alar base.[8] Since the cleft lip nasal deformity is possibly one of the most difficult reconstructive procedures in plastic surgery, any procedure that will help to repair this deformity is gladly accepted. The preliminary lip adhesion procedure tends to act on the alar base in the same way as it does on the soft tissue elements of the lip. Subjectively, it seems that the alar deformity is less grotesque in its subluxation and malrotation after lip adhesion, and definitive future procedures on the nose seem to be made easier by this soft tissue manipulation.

In patients with complete bilateral cleft lip, preliminary lip adhesion, as in unilateral cleft lip patients, helps to reposition the bony arch, brings the premaxilla into a more ideal position, and allows for a type of "tissue expansion" of the soft tissue elements of the prolabium and lateral lip elements. The difference between unilateral versus bilateral lip adhesions is that in the latter no undermining is done in the medial prolabial lip element. Only a minimal amount of undermining is performed on the lateral lip element to effect closure of the soft tissues with little tension. This lack of undermining allows the soft tissue elements to exert their orthopedic forces on both the premaxilla and the lateral lip elements. When the premaxilla is severely asymmetric in bilateral cleft lip patients, a unilateral lip adhesion can be done to pull the premaxilla back into the midline.

Surgical Procedure

The surgical procedure is quite straightforward and easily reproduced. It can be done under general endotracheal anesthesia or with local anesthesia and sedation. The most important aspect of the lip adhesion procedure is first to mark the lines for the definitive lip repair completely. Regardless of the preference of the plastic surgeon for the type of definitive lip repair, the lip elements of skin and mucosa cannot be violated during the lip adhesion procedure. This author's preference of technique for all clefts is the Millard rotation-advancement repair. Therefore, at the time of the lip adhesion procedure, the rotation-advancement flaps are marked on the patient, and these lines are never violated during the lip adhesion. The lip adhesion is constructed from tissue *outside* of the definitive cleft repair markings. One must also keep in mind that the main objective of the lip adhesion is to apply adherence between the divided orbicularis oris muscle and adjacent soft tissue. The object of the procedure is to attach these elements so that there is a firm adhesion. Tiny mucosal flaps will not be effective.

A bilateral cleft lip deformity and lip adhesion procedure are shown as an example. However, one can easily extrapolate one side of the bilateral cleft lip adhesion to the unilateral cleft lip adhesion. The only difference between them is the undermining of the medial lip element (Fig. 22–1).

After marking the lines of the definitive lip repair, designing rectangular flaps on the adjacent margins seems to facilitate the procedure (Fig. 22–2).

From the lateral lip element, a superiorly based rectangular flap is elevated from the alar base to the medial portion of the vermilion (distal to the height of the Cupid's bow on the cleft-side lateral element). This flap measures approximately 4 to 5 mm in the vertical dimension by approximately 2 mm horizontally. The flap is elevated, and the muscular layer is identified and minimally undermined.

On the medial side of the cleft (prolabium and premaxilla in the bilateral cleft) a similar rectangular flap based inferiorly on the premaxilla is elevated. Once this

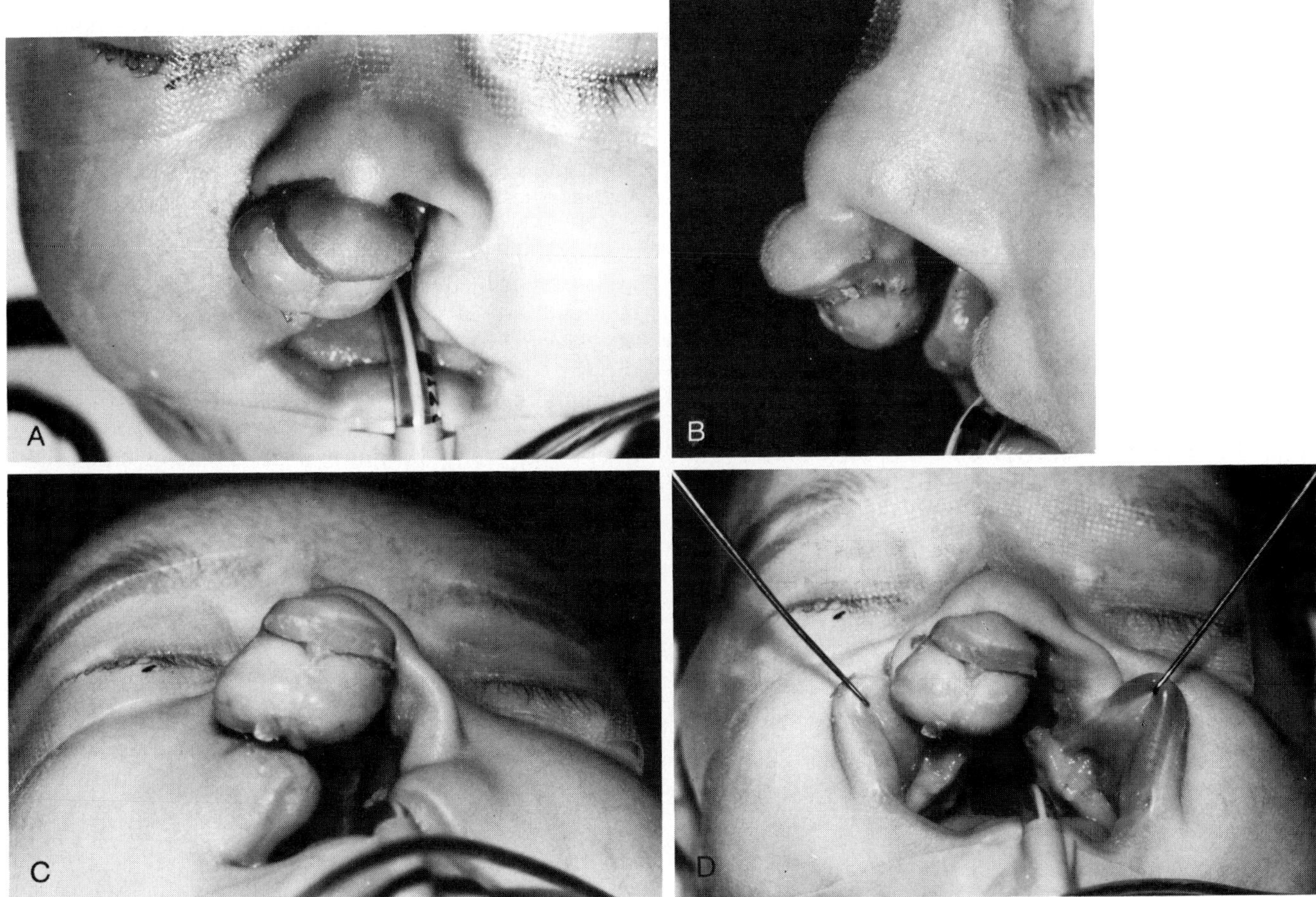

Figure 22–1 *A–D,* Severe bilateral asymmetric, complete cleft of the lip, alveolus, and palate, with protruding premaxilla.

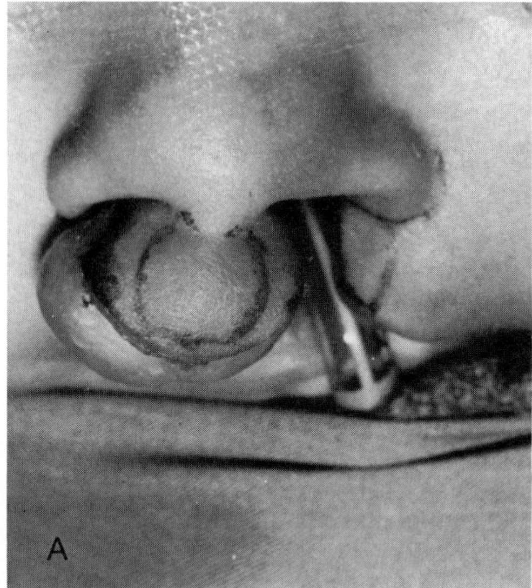
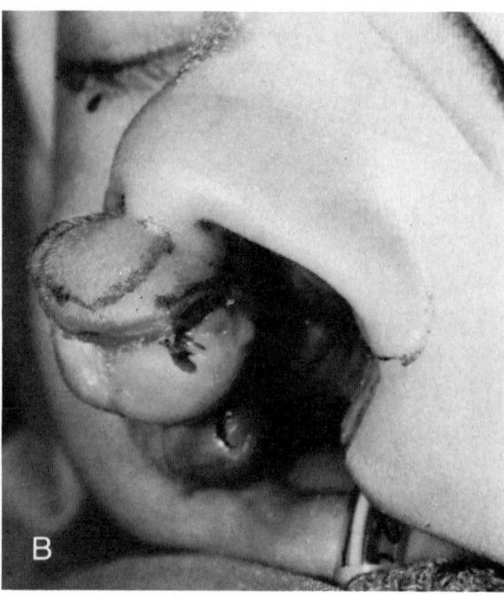

Figure 22–2 *A* and *B*, Preoperative markings for the Millard rotation-advancement technique.

is accomplished, hemostasis is achieved, and the flap is approximated to the lateral lip element advancing mucosa with 4–0 or 5–0 chromic catgut sutures. The next layer, that of the orbicularis oris muscle, is the most important and provides the most action and traction on the soft tissue and bony elements. This layer is approximated with interrupted 3–0 or 4–0 chromic sutures. In the bilateral cleft lip, the lateral muscular element is easy to identify, and this is approximated to the lesser muscular elements in the prolabium at the level of the subcutaneous tissues. One must feel certain that a good "bite" is obtained, or there will be subsequent dehiscence. If the prolabium is sufficiently small, this muscular element can be approximated to the periosteum under the prolabium (Fig. 22–3).

Following the muscular layer closure, the lateral, superiorly based rectangular flap is approximated to the wound edge of the soft tissue above the medial muscular sutures. This can be tissue that will be discarded or pared at the definitive lip repair, or it can be the lateral edges of what may be the parings of the future C-flap in the Millard rotation-advancement technique. This also corresponds to the lateral portion of the future banked forked flap that will be transposed during the definitive bilateral cleft lip repair. The sutures used also are absorbable, so suture removal is not necessary.

Once the lip adhesion is completed, a Logan bow is placed to alleviate tension on the repair (Figs. 22–4 and 22–5). Obviously, there is controversy about the use of a Logan bow; however, during a 13-year period the author has observed dehiscence in less than 2% of lip adhesion patients in whom it was used. The Logan bow is kept in place for approximately 2 weeks. Elbow restraints are applied also for the same period of time.

Discussion

The lip adhesion procedure should be done as early as possible in the neonatal period. With conjoint consultations of a pediatrician and pediatric anesthesiologist, we feel that 2 to 3 months of age is ideal. Following lip adhesion, the lip elements and maxillary segments seem to be ready for definitive lip repair after a period of 1 to 3 months.

Great time and effort must be taken to explain to the parents this entire plan and its efficacy. To the uninitiated family, the lip adhesion may represent a "poor definitive lip repair" if adequate explanation is not given prior to the operation. However, with good rapport, the family is usually quite happy because "something is finally being done," the deformity is not as grotesque as it was when the child was born, and a plan is now in progress.

It is the author's opinion that not all unilateral or bilateral clefts of the lip benefit from a lip adhesion procedure. Obviously, in the child with an incomplete unilateral or bilateral cleft lip, in which the lip and bony elements are in good alignment, a lip adhesion is not necessary (Fig. 22–6). Nature has already provided for the lip adhesion. However, in occasional children the incomplete unilateral or bilateral cleft lip deformity may still have a tremendous amount of separation of soft tissue and bone. In these patients, a lip adhesion is advisable. In patients with complete unilateral or bilateral cleft lip, it is the author's judgment that approximately 80% of these children will benefit from a lip adhesion procedure (Figs. 22–7 and 22–8).

The negative aspects of lip adhesion procedures are the obvious ones: an extra operation with the added risks of anesthesia and the manipulation of tissues. Do the means justify the ends? Is a definitive lip repair instead of a lip adhesion advisable when, 2 or 3 years later, one may "revise" the definitive lip repair? Obviously, this is a very subjective judgment. In 1984, Furnas discussed straight-line closure as a preliminary procedure to the Millard unilateral cleft lip repair.[9,10] This work added light to the entire concept of lip adhesion. Surgical principle dictates that when soft tissues are optimal in size and integrity and when

Text continued on page 173

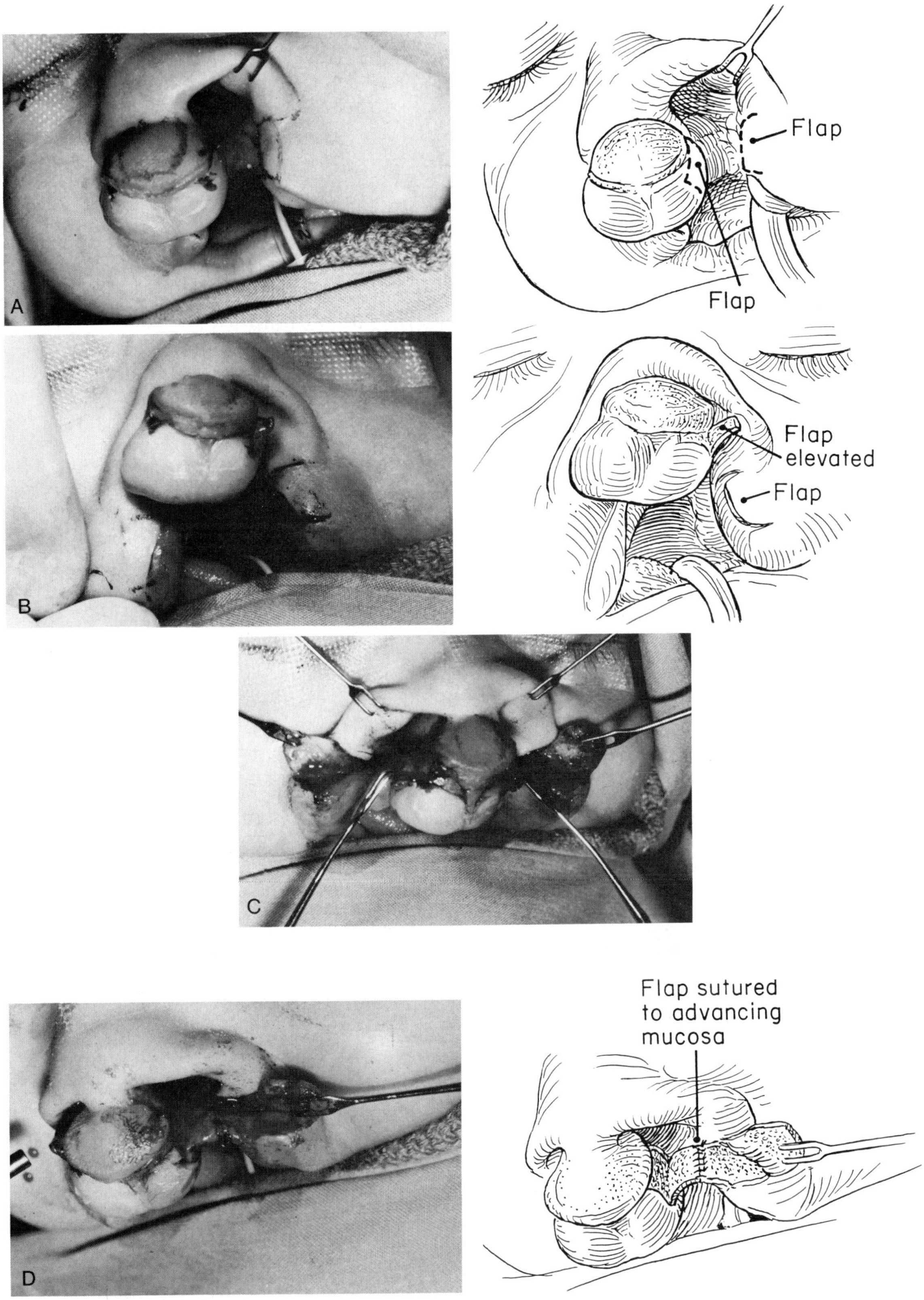

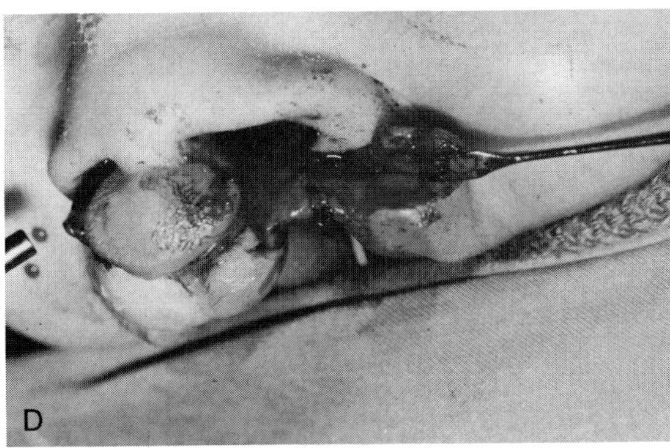

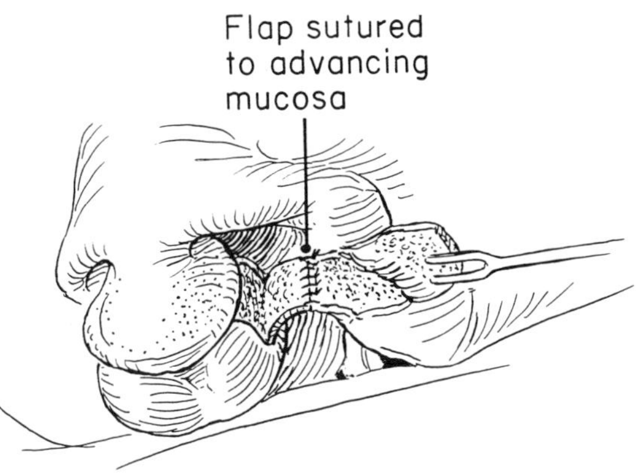

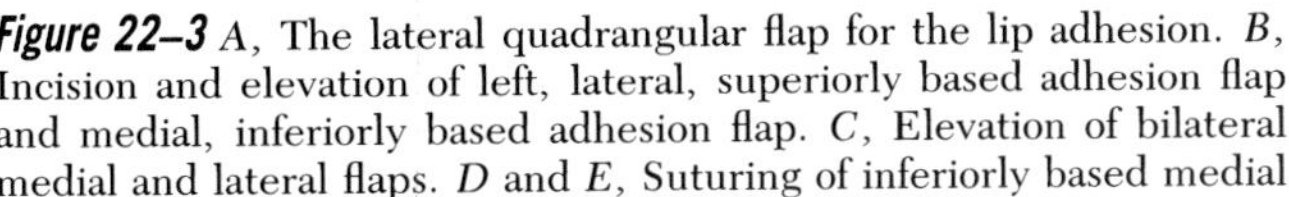

Figure 22–3 *A*, The lateral quadrangular flap for the lip adhesion. *B*, Incision and elevation of left, lateral, superiorly based adhesion flap and medial, inferiorly based adhesion flap. *C*, Elevation of bilateral medial and lateral flaps. *D* and *E*, Suturing of inferiorly based medial rectangular flap to advancing lateral mucosa. *F* and *G*, Lateral muscularis element has been attached to medial element. *H* and *I*, Lateral cutaneous flap closed bilaterally.

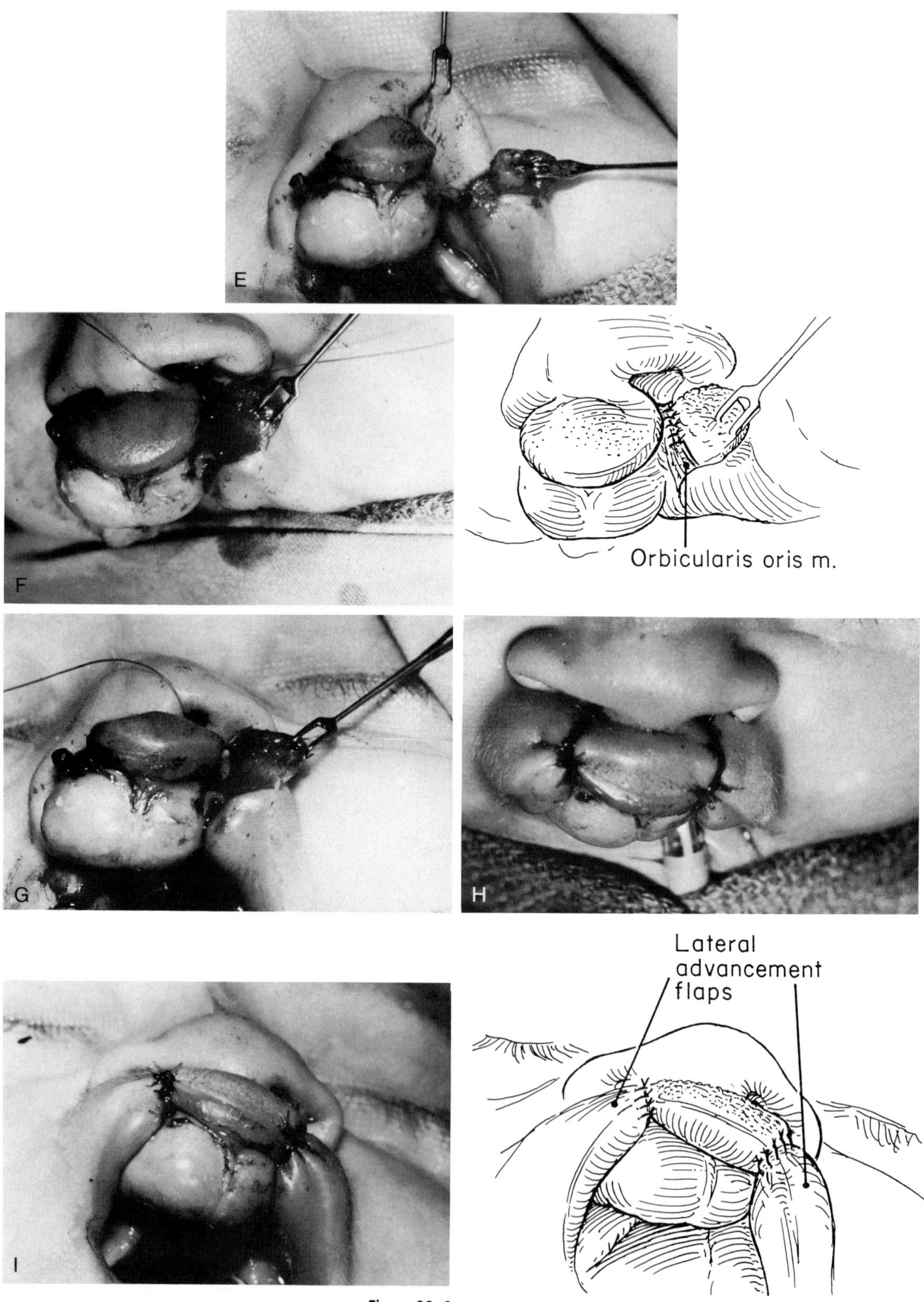

Figure 22–3 Continued

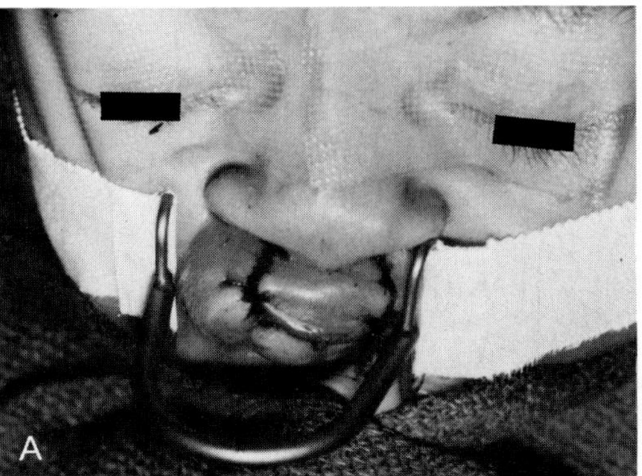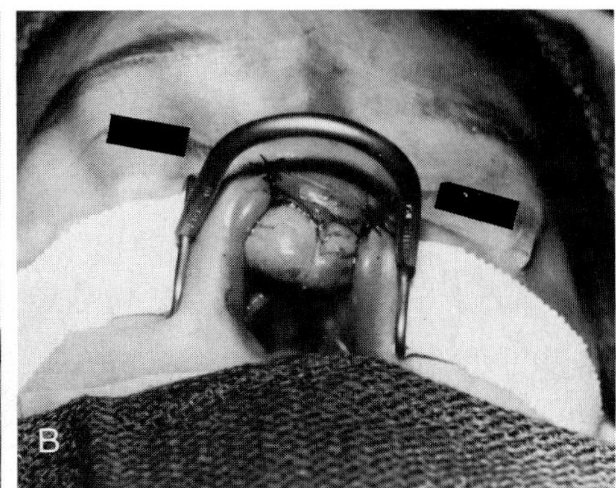

Figure 22–4 *A* and *B*, Application of Logan bow.

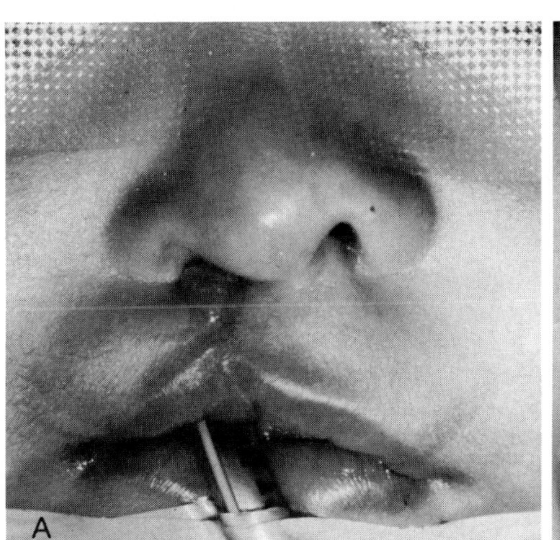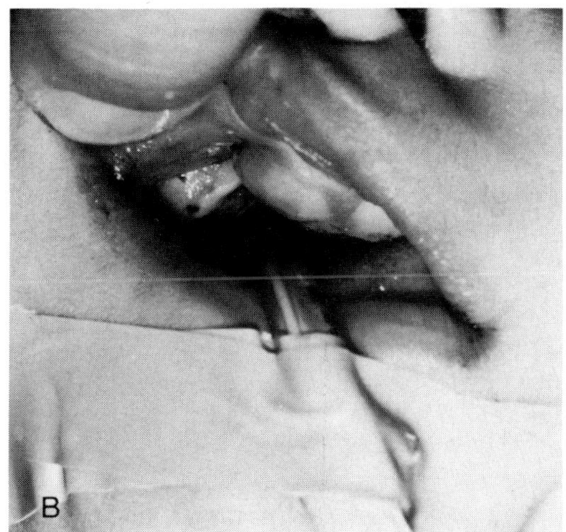

Figure 22–5 *A* and *B*, Postoperative unilateral lip adhesion with alveolar alignment.

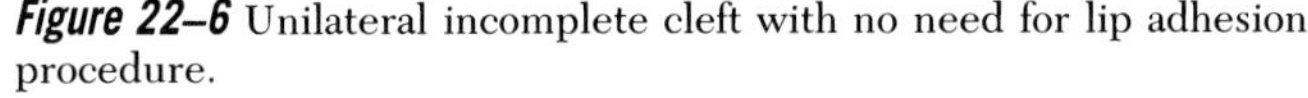

Figure 22–6 Unilateral incomplete cleft with no need for lip adhesion procedure.

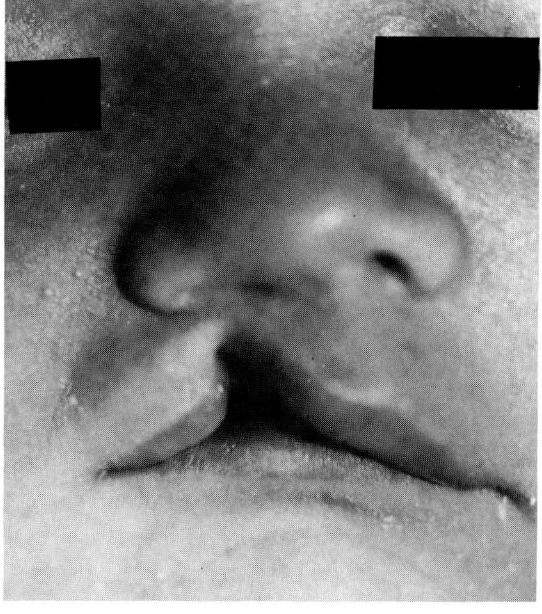

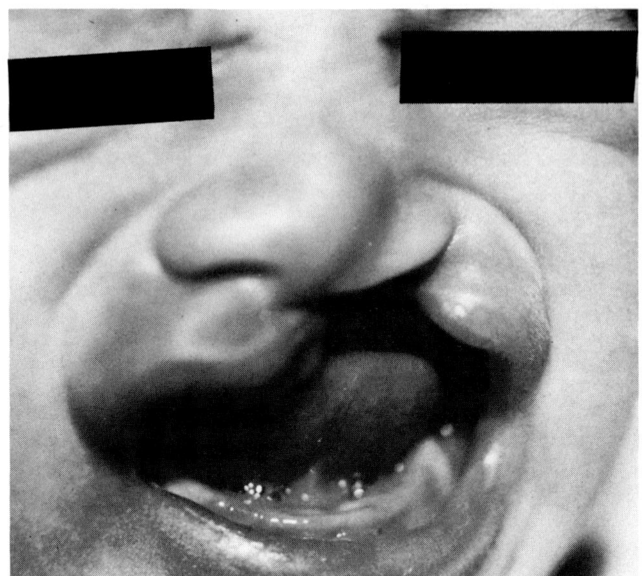

Figure 22–7 Severe unilateral cleft with nasal deformity requiring lip adhesion.

Figure 22–8 *A*, Lip adhesion with severe right alar deformity. *B*, Lip adhesion with improvement of right alar sill ready for definitive repair.

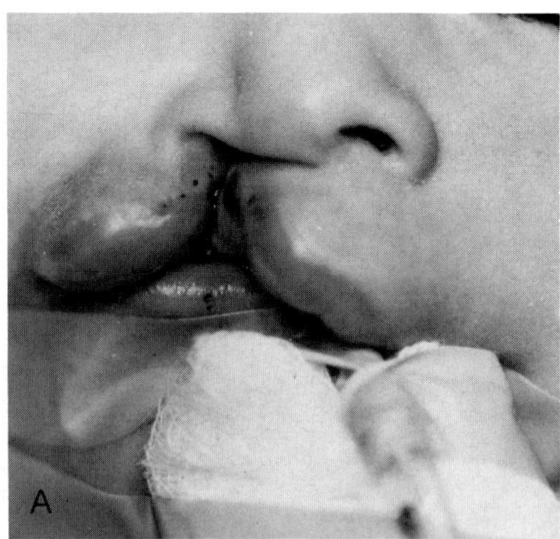

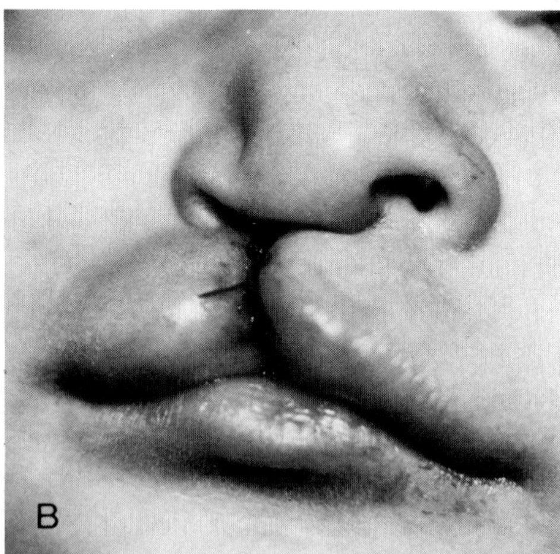

underlying bony platforms are aligned, definitive results are the outcome. There is no question that excellent results can be obtained without a lip adhesion; however, again, this conclusion is extremely subjective. It is the author's feeling that improved results are obtained with the aid of the lip adhesion procedure. The maxillary arch is improved, the final lip repair seems better, and the nasal deformity is prepared for an easier definitive reconstruction.

References

1. Johanson B, Ohlsson A: Die Osteoplastik bei Spatbehandlung der Lippen-Kiefer-Gaumenspalten. Arch Klin Chir 295:876, 1960.
2. Johanson B, Ohlsson A: Bone grafting and dental orthopaedics in primary and secondary cases of cleft lip and palate. Acta Chir Scand 122:112, 1961.
3. Millard DR, Jr: Refinements in rotation-advancement cleft lip technique. Plast Reconstr Surg 33:26, 1964.
4. Randall P: A lip adhesion operation in cleft lip surgery. Plast Reconstr Surg 35:371, 1965.
5. Randall P: The unilateral cleft lip. In Georgiade NG, Hagerty RF (eds): Symposium on Management of Cleft Lip and Palate and Associated Deformities. St. Louis: C. V. Mosby, 1974.
6. Walker JC, Jr, Collito MB, Mancusi-Ungaro A, et al: Physiologic considerations in cleft lip closure: The C-W technique. Plast Reconstr Surg 37:552, 1966.
7. Millard DR, Jr: Cleft Craft—The Evolution of Its Surgery. I: The Unilateral Deformity. Boston: Little, Brown, 1976.
8. Millard DR, Jr: Earlier correction of the unilateral cleft lip nose. Plast Reconstr Surg 70:64, 1982.
9. Furnas DW: Straight-line closure: A preliminary to Millard closure in unilateral cleft lips (with a history of the straight-line closure, including the Mirault misunderstanding). Clin Plast Surg 11:701, 1984.
10. Blair VP, Brown JB: Mirault operation for single harelip. Surg Gynecol Obstet 51:81, 1930.

CHAPTER 23

Unilateral Cleft Lip and Cleft Lip Nasal Reconstruction

Kenneth E. Salyer

Since the time of Ambroise Paré, many surgeons have directed their attention toward the surgical correction of the cleft deformity. Recently, cleft nasal repair has been emphasized (see Chaps. 24 and 34). This report is based on 21 years of experience in unilateral cleft reconstruction. The purpose of this chapter is to describe a surgical technique that I have used successfully for many years. Over the years, this technique has been refined with equal attention directed to reconstruction of the lip and nose. When I started my surgical career, attention was concentrated on lip repair only. However, greater interest in the nose and a challenge to correct the nasal deformity stimulated me to improve my technique to correct both the lip and the nose during the primary operation.

A most complete review of surgical technique for cleft lip repair can be found in Millard's *Cleft Craft*.[1] Therefore, the lip will not be reviewed here.

The single most important factor in determining good results is a proper diagnosis of the cleft, which is based on the surgeon's analysis, experience, and expertise in transforming not only theoretically but technically a given cleft deformity into an attractive normal appearance. The performance of cleft surgery is based on science but is dependent on a three-dimensional art form of visualization and a feel for the tissues as well as a mode of execution based on extensive experience in attempting to achieve excellence in repair. Many surgeons have developed the ability to achieve satisfactory results in children with the unilateral cleft deformity. It is my opinion, based on the technique presented here

and on techniques demonstrated by other surgeons, that unilateral clefts can for the most part be surgically corrected leaving minimal scarring and deformity. The problem of bilateral cleft deformity has not been resolved with the same degree of success (Figs. 23–1 and 23–2).

Assessment

It is difficult to be objective when assessing one's own surgical results. Beauty is indeed in the eye of the beholder, and frequently the surgeon becomes biased in regard to his own self-critical evaluation. I believe that the majority of the results today are good. Rarely, if ever, is it possible to achieve perfection or arrive at a totally satisfactory result. The stigma of the cleft deformity always remains, whether it is as scarring, minimal displacement of the alar base or nose, or a slight asymmetry of the alar cartilage.

Based on my experience, the majority of unilateral cleft patients require secondary surgery.[2] It is possible with the techniques described here to achieve a marked improvement in the nasal deformity and a satisfactory lip appearance with muscle continuity in most primary repair cases. The minor stigmata that remain, whether a slightly elevated peak of the Cupid's bow, an asymmetric nostril, a foreshortened columella, or a markedly deformed skeletal base, require further surgery. Today, it is not possible in children with unilateral complete cleft to achieve perfection in one operation. However, it is possible to eliminate marked deformity and to strive for standards that are comparable to those used in aesthetic surgery in general.

Surgical Orthopedic Treatment

For the last ten years, we have utilized presurgical orthopedic treatment similar to that described by McNeil[3] in 1947 and to the early orthopedic treatment used by Hotz and colleagues[4] in Zurich. I use an acrylic plate that can be expanded and held with a dental adhesive (e.g., Poligrip). This technique has been developed in collaboration with my orthodontist.[5]

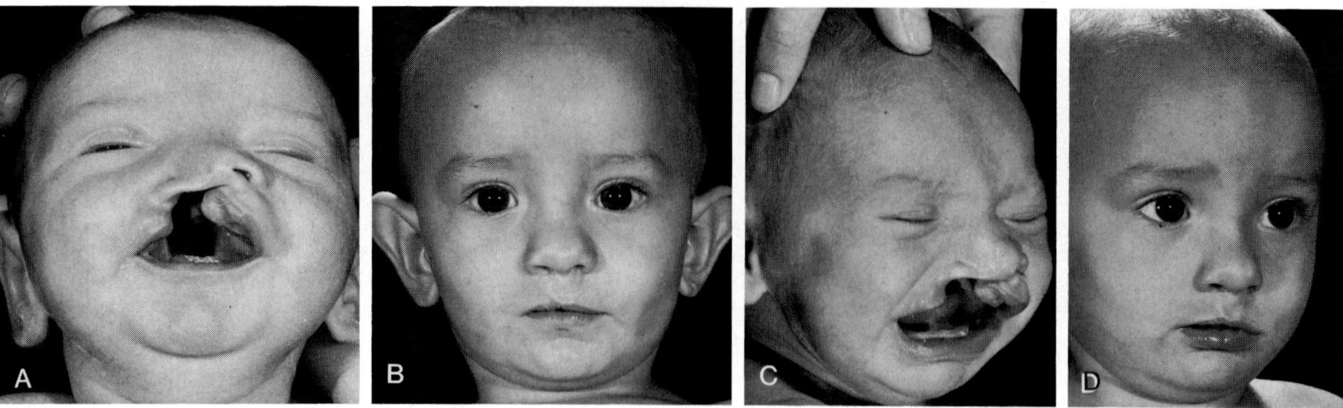

Figure 23–1 *A,* Preoperative view of a 19-day-old infant with unilateral complete right-sided cleft lip and cleft nasal deformity. *B,* One year following surgical reconstruction using technique described in this chapter. *C,* Oblique preoperative view. *D,* Oblique postoperative view.

In patients who have maxillary collapse, expansion of the lesser maxillary segment is achieved. Expansion allows control of the segments once the lip closure has been performed. Such control provides better alignment of the arch form, especially in patients with wide clefts and clefts with severe collapse of the maxillary segments. The appliance is worn until palatoplasty is performed. Although it does not facilitate closure at the time of the

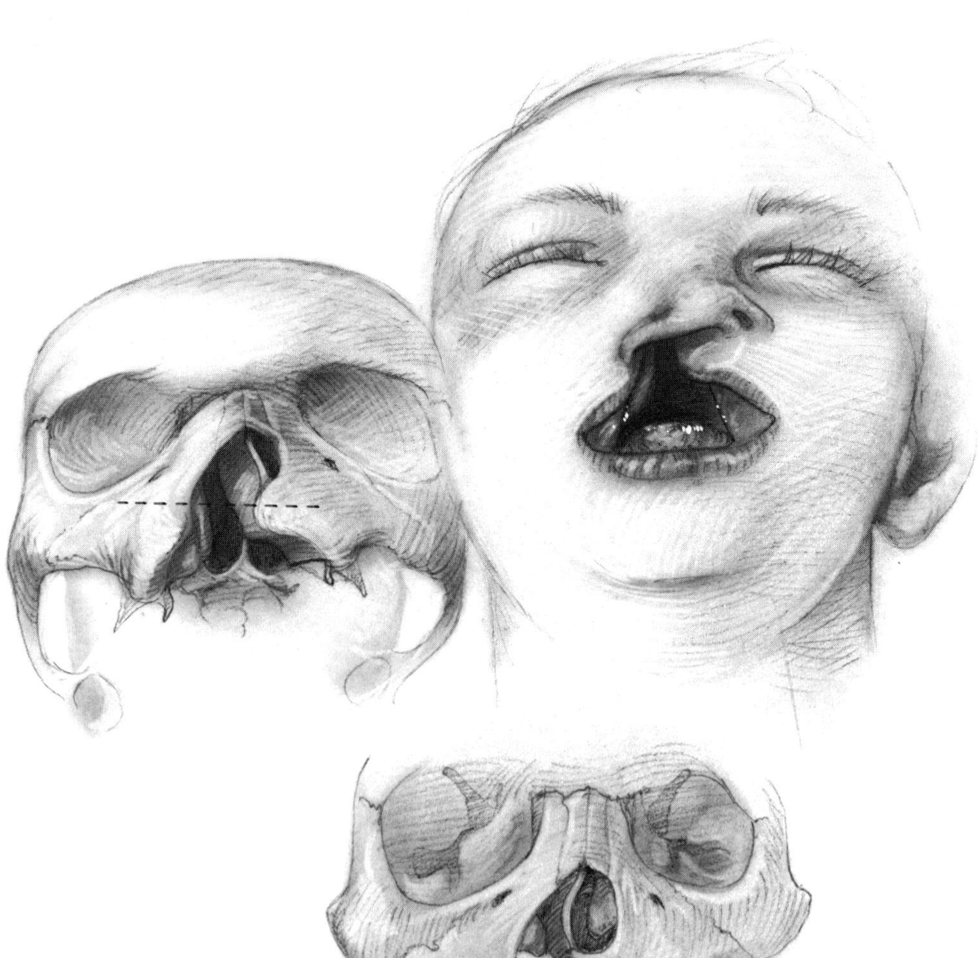

Figure 23–2 Underlying skeletal deformity as depicted by the medical illustrator.

primary lip and nose repair, it does improve alignment of the maxillary segments following lip closure. In many patients, when alignment of the maxillary segments is adequate prior to lip repair, no presurgical orthopedic treatment is necessary. Orthopedic treatment is primarily concerned with the alignment of the maxillary segments once lip closure has been performed. It is my opinion, based on evaluation of a large series of patients in whom this technique was not used, that this is a beneficial adjunctive method in the overall results of treatment of unilateral cleft lip and cleft nasal deformity.

Planning of Surgery

Many factors are important in planning cleft lip surgery. A detailed evaluation of the existing deformity including the severity and type of deformity of the lip, nose, and skeletal base is important. The unilateral cleft may be partial or complete, and there may be varying degrees of involvement of the orbicularis oris muscle.

In most partial unilateral cleft lips, the degree of clefting affects only part of the lip; however, the orbicularis oris muscle is usually divided completely. When the orbicularis oris is divided, a groove in the upper portion of the skin of the lip is evident, particularly during lip movement. During contraction on the cleft side, separation of the muscle may cause it to bulge.

In patients with complete cleft lip, the asymmetric division of the orbicularis oris causes a functional muscle imbalance that affects facial growth and development. This imbalance impairs function because different forces act on each side of the cleft. The complex skeletal and remaining soft tissue deformities may contribute to the nasal deformity. The alar base is displaced laterally, inferiorly, and posteriorly. The asymmetry caused by the functional imbalance also may be apparent in the position of the maxillary segments. Muscle forces acting on the noncleft side influence the growth and development of the larger maxillary segment and cause an upward and outward rotation of the premaxillary segment. The sooner muscle equilibrium is established following lip repair, the better the chance of achieving normal alignment of the maxillary segments and thus normal facial growth and development. In my opinion, coordinated use of surgical orthopedic treatment plus accurate, careful alignment of the musculature and soft tissue reconstruction allows for more normal facial growth and development and contributes to the elimination of deformity.

Surgical Technique

State-of-the-art surgical techniques allow surgeons to achieve good functional and aesthetic results in reconstruction of the cleft lip in most cleft patients. These results, coupled with the ability to reconstruct the nose and the underlying facial skeleton adequately, have eliminated the grotesque or severely deformed cleft patient. These are, however, tens of thousands of patients in the United States who have had or are receiving

inadequate care. Many reasons exist for this deficiency. One reason is the inadequate training and experience of surgeons who perform this type of surgery only occasionally. Another is the lack of multidisciplinary management. The development of a long-term philosophy of cleft care utilizing a multidisciplinary team approach can improve the results and care of these patients.

A modified Millard rotation-advancement technique is our procedure of choice for most lip repairs.[6] This procedure has undergone many changes since its inception. The procedure was designed and executed in various ways depending on the surgeon's preference, ingenuity, and experience. The rotation-advancement technique has many attributes that make it popular for repair of the unilateral complete and incomplete cleft lip and for coupling this with the popular cleft lip nasal operations used. The technique, when well performed, is a malleable, flexible, and fluid operation that is easily adjusted as the surgeon proceeds. Exact measurements are less important in this technique than the other techniques commonly used for cleft repair. The advantages include:

1. A camouflaged suture line.
2. Flexible and adaptable technique, allowing improvisation and artistry by the surgeon.
3. Minimal tissue is discarded.
4. Good access to the nose during primary reconstruction, and a good supply of tissue is available for deficient areas of the nose.
5. The possible creation of a normal-looking Cupid's bow is possible.
6. The alar base and nasal floor are easily reconstructed.

The disadvantages include:

1. Difficulty of execution for the inexperienced surgeon because it is a "sight method."
2. Excessive tension and undermining may produce increased scarring of the lip.
3. Extensive undermining of the cheek is necessary to perform this procedure adequately in many patients.
4. Occasional difficulty in overcoming the mismatch of the vermilion, which is much thinner on the noncleft side and thicker on the cleft side.
5. In cases of severe tissue deficiency, the gap on the noncleft side created by the downward rotation of the flap may be too extensive for the lateral advancement flap, which must be moved under great tension.
6. Frequent contracture of the vertical scar resulting in notching of the vermilion or shortening of the entire lip in the vertical dimension (Fig. 23–3).

Marking for the Rotation-Advancement Procedure

The peak of the Cupid's bow on the noncleft side is located and marked with methylene blue (Fig. 23–3A). Next, the midpoint or lowest point of the Cupid's bow is located along the vermilion (Fig. 23–3B). The distance between these two points is measured, and the point at an equal distance from the midportion to the peak of the Cupid's bow on the cleft side (point 3) is marked. Usually this is where the white roll disappears along the vermilion-cutaneous junction. Sometimes this point

Text continued on page 180

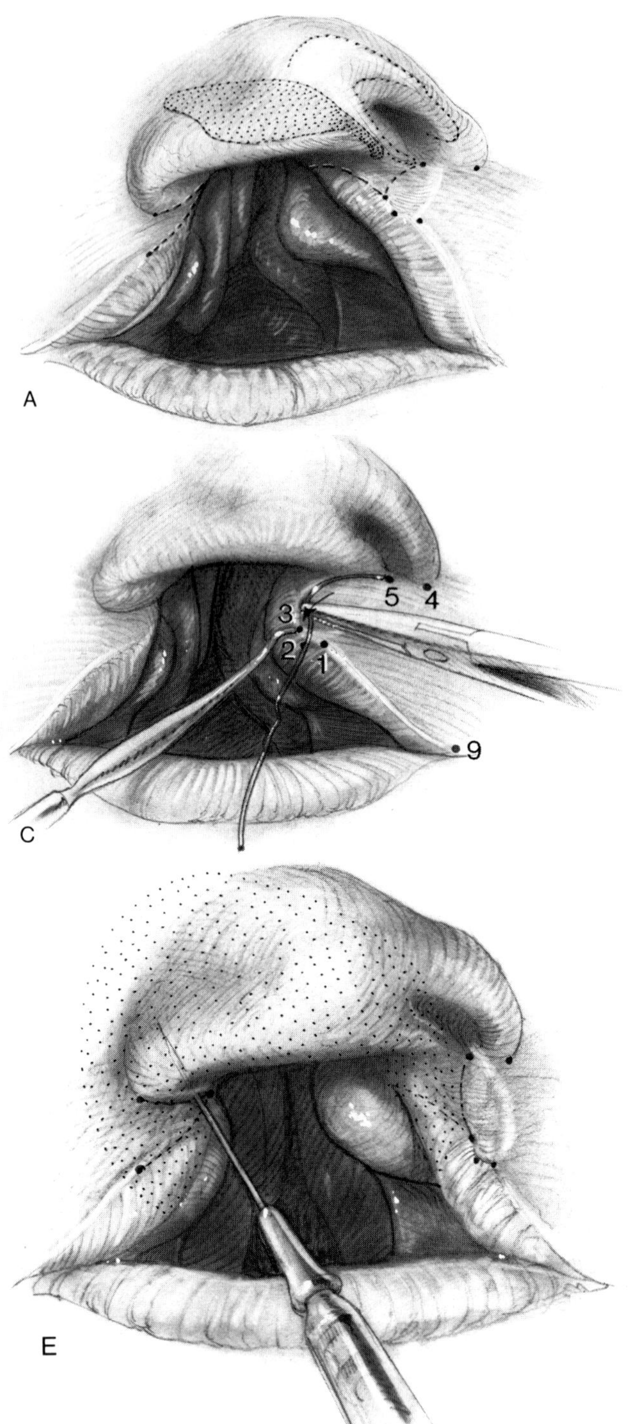

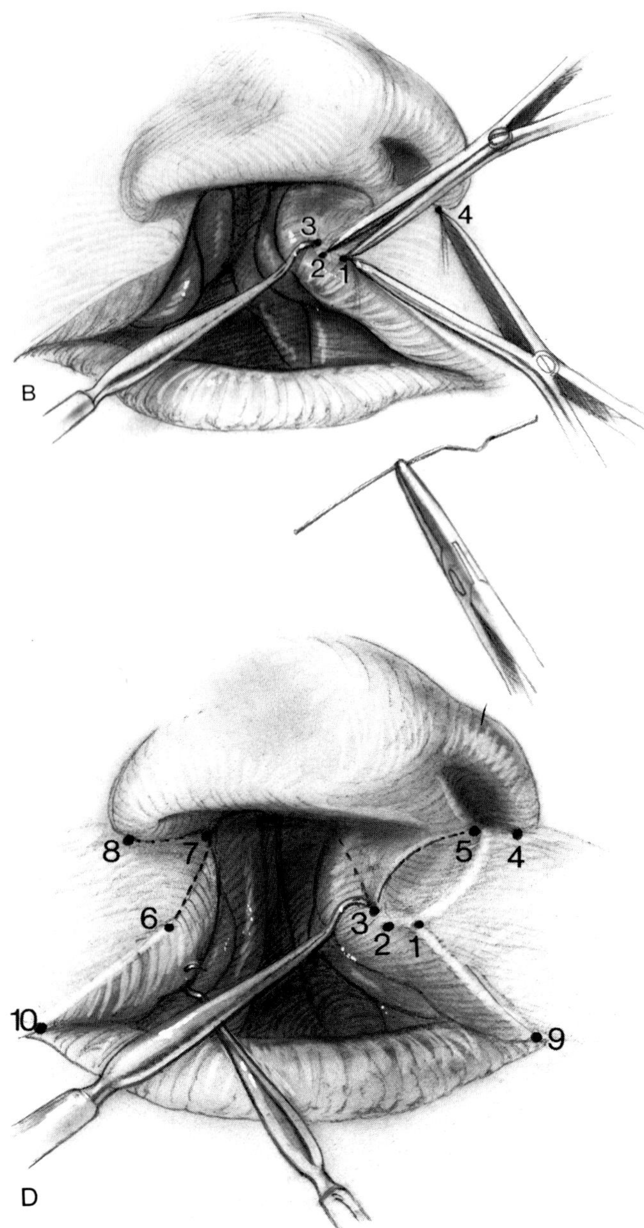

Figure 23–3 *A,* Unilateral complete cleft lip and cleft nasal deformity
showing the proposed rotation-advancement operation. The key points
of the Cupid's bow and alar base for the rotation-advancement are
marked on the lip. There is marked variation in each cleft deformity;
each patient is approached differently according to the deformity that
is present. The displaced and abnormal lower lateral cartilages on the
normal and abnormal sides are noted in this drawing.

B, The peak of the Cupid's bow on the noncleft side is located and
marked with methylene blue (1); the midportion or lowest point of
the Cupid's bow is located along the vermilion (2). The distance
between these two points is measured, and an equal distance from
the midportion of the peak of the Cupid's bow on the cleft side (3) is
marked. This point is usually where the white roll disappears along
the vermilion-cutaneous junction. The height of the lip on the noncleft
side is determined by making a mark at the base of the ala (4) and
measuring the distance from the peak of the Cupid's bow on the
noncleft side to point 4. After the height of the lip on the noncleft

side is determined, a wire is measured the length of the height of the
Cupid's bow and is bent in the curvature to be marked out on the
lip.

C, After the height of the lip on the noncleft side is determined,
the curvilinear line is drawn from the base of the columella to the
peak of the Cupid's bow using the curved wire. The distance from
the base of the columella to the peak of the Cupid's bow was previously
determined by measurement. A wire the same length as the height
of the normal side may be used. The distance from 4 to 1 is curved
to match the line from 5 to 3. The line for the new height of the lip
on the cleft side is designed to use as much of the curvilinear length
as possible, depending on the shape of the cleft.

D, The remaining points of orientation are completed. Markings on
the cleft side start at the peak of the Cupid's bow (6), the point where
the white roll of tissue disappears. The next point is marked at the
alar base (7). The distance between these two points must match the
height of the lip on the noncleft side. The base of the ala on the cleft
side (8) corresponds to the base of the ala on the noncleft side (4). An
additional measurement that helps to create a symmetric lip is the
distance from the peak of the Cupid's bow to the commissure on the
noncleft side (9). This distance should roughly equal the distance from
the peak of the Cupid's bow on the cleft side (6) to the commissure
(10).

E, A 30-gauge needle on a 1-ml tuberculin syringe is used to inject
a total of 1 ml of 1:100,000 epinephrine with 1 per cent Xylocaine.
The stippled area represents the region infiltrated with local anesthetic.

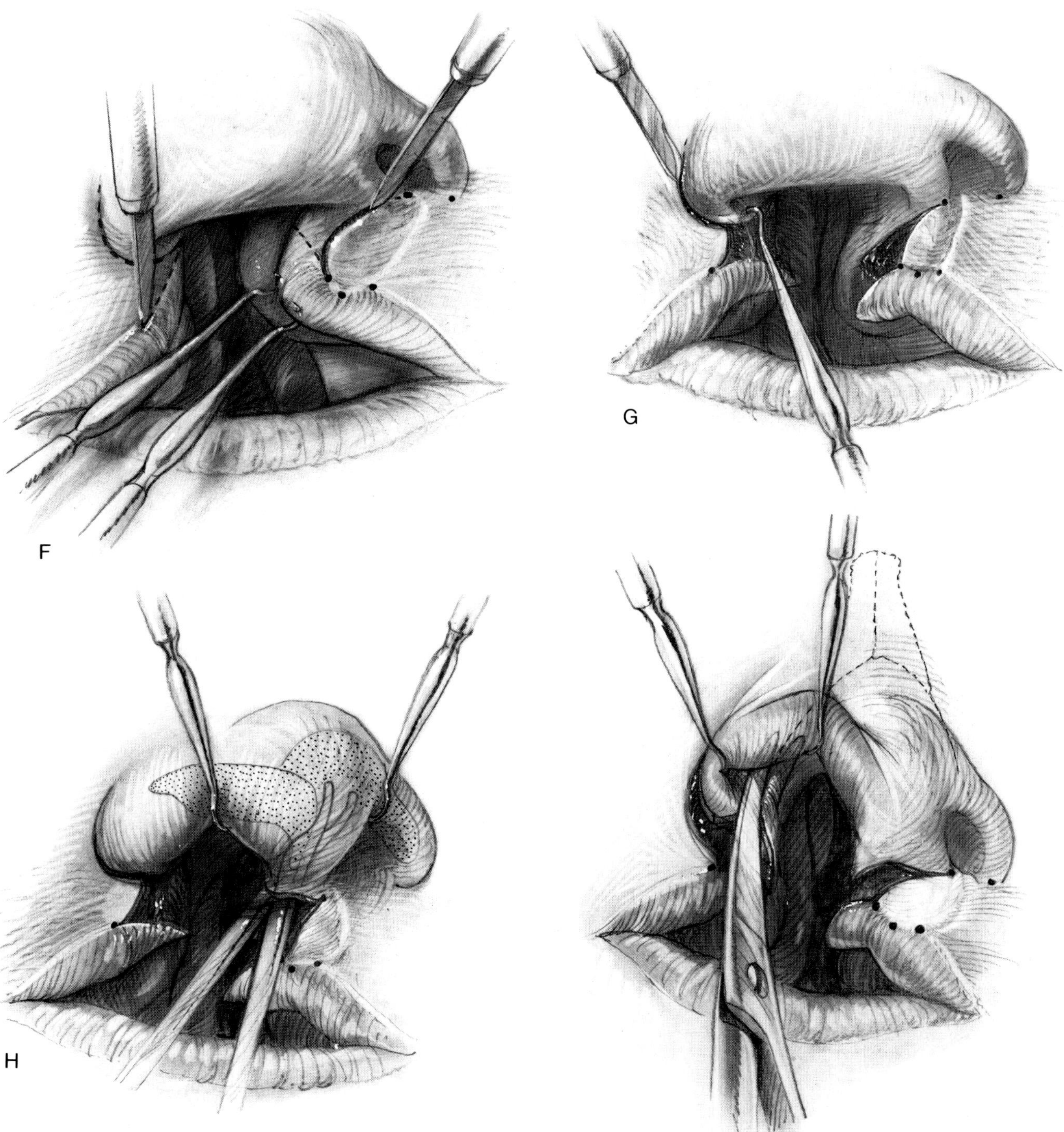

Figure 23–3 *Continued F,* The medial and lateral lip element is cut to maintain flaps of vermilion. The vermilion flaps are used to build up vermilion in the area of the tubercle of the lip. The medial lip element is cut, altering the design and size of the C-flap as needed for the columella. The lateral lip element is marked out and then cut.

G, The lateral lip element around the alar base is cut and pulled down with a hook to gain good control during dissection.

H, The C-flap is pulled cephalad, and small tonotomy scissors are used between the medial crura of the lower lateral cartilages to free the skin of the cleft and noncleft sides along the nasal dome.

I, After dissection of the alar base laterally, a cut is made high along the maxilla to separate the soft tissues from the maxilla along the attachment of the maxillary process and nasal bone. This cut is made well above the lower lateral and upper lateral cartilages.

Illustration continued on following page

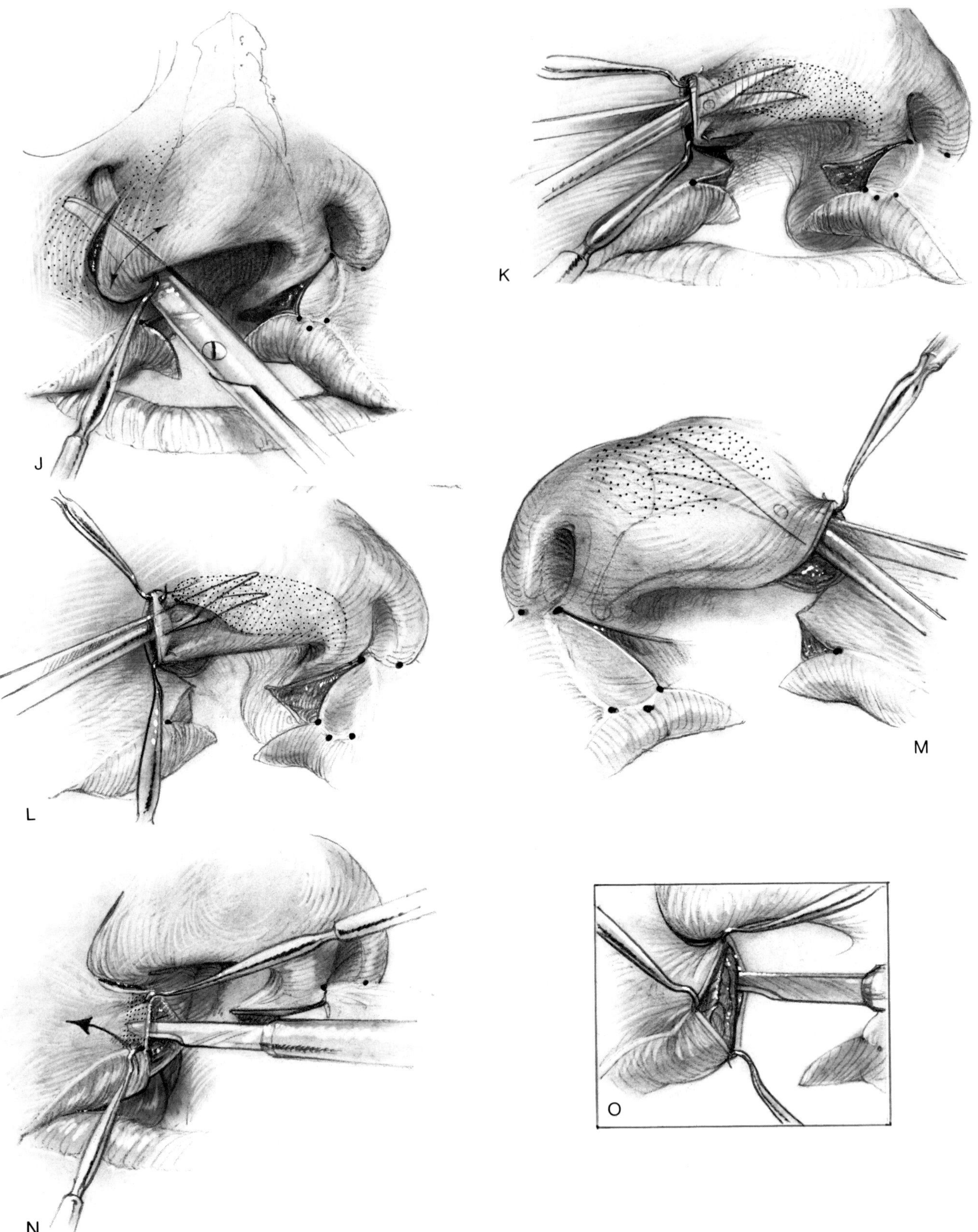

Figure 23–3 *Continued J*, The soft tissue over the maxilla is freed using the incision over the alar base and dissecting scissors in a blunt fashion at the preperiosteal level.

K, Using tonotomy scissors, the skin is separated from the lateral crus of the lower lateral cartilage connecting the incision with the previously freed skin over the dome through the medial approach.

L, Gaining access through the same alar base incision, the ala lateral crus of the lower lateral cartilage is separated from the underlying lining of the alar dome region, maintaining the lining of the alar dome.

M, Dissection is completed, freeing the skin of the entire nose over the lower lateral and upper lateral cartilages. *N*, The lateral lip element is separated from the skin. *O*, The mucosal attachment to the muscle is likewise freed for closure.

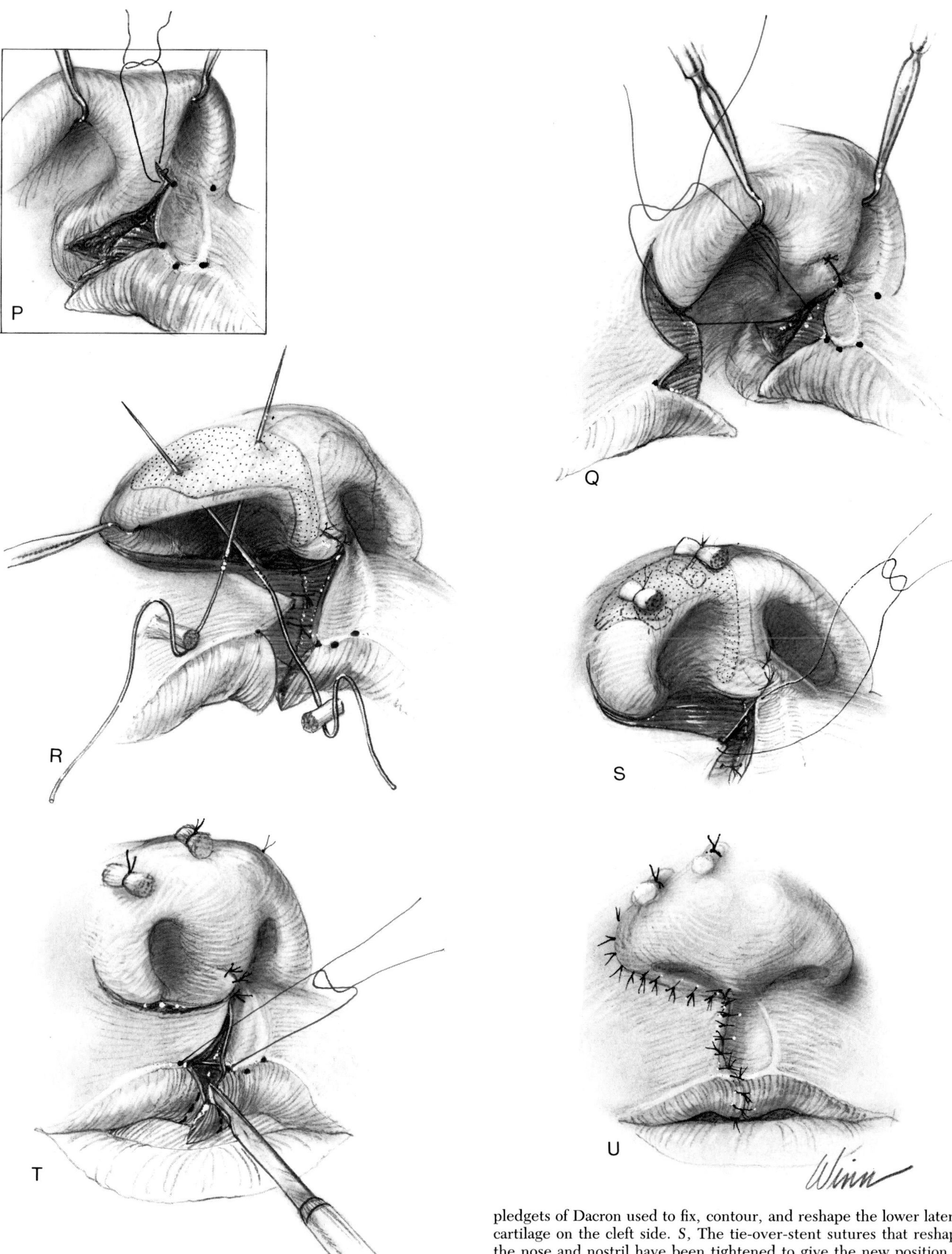

Figure 23–3 *Continued P*, Advancement flap C is sutured with 6–0 nylon, lengthening the columella on the cleft side. *Q*, The key muscle stitch that sets up the alar base and nose as well as the symmetry of the lip is now placed using 3–0 chromic catgut suture in the muscle.

R, Needles with 3–0 nylon are placed through the ala cartilage with pledgets of Dacron used to fix, contour, and reshape the lower lateral cartilage on the cleft side. *S*, The tie-over-stent sutures that reshape the nose and nostril have been tightened to give the new position of the ala cartilage. *T*, Now that the skin suturing is completed, a dey stitch is placed at the peak of the Cupid's bow on the cleft side, and the final adjustment of the vermilion is made in order to create a tubercle. This may be done with straight line or Z-plasty closure. *U*, The final skin sutures of 6–0 nylon are left in for approximately 5 to 6 days. The stents remain in the nose for the same time and sometimes remain in for 8 to 9 days.

179

must be altered or moved 1 or 2 mm to adjust the length of the rotation-advancement flap on the medial segment on the cleft side to fit the advancement flap from the lateral segment.

The height of the lip on the noncleft side is determined by marking the base of the ala (point 4) and measuring the distance to the peak of the Cupid's bow on the noncleft side (point 1). The base of the ala is used because the midportion of the nasal sill may be shifted or altered due to the distortion of the alar base and columella in the unilateral cleft lip. It must be emphasized that the markings are only a rough guide and usually are not definitive in terms of the final lip contour.

After the height of the lip on the noncleft side has been determined, a curved line is drawn from the base of the columella to the peak of the Cupid's bow, which was previously determined by measurement (point 5). This line deviates from the vermilion-cutaneous junction, creating a C-flap in the tissue between this line and the vermilion. Many factors determine the size of the C-flap. The flap is used primarily to establish the normal height of the lip and to create a cosmetically appealing contour. In some cases it is used for columellar lengthening. However, in partial clefts the nasal sill and a portion of the floor of the nose may be used for this purpose.

The more recent addition of the M-flap by Millard is, in my opinion, superfluous and is not used today. I prefer to use the vermilion to create symmetry on both sides and to prevent notching. If the vermilion is full enough it can be brought straight down from the peak of the Cupid's bow at that point. The surgeon must determine whether the fullness of the lip is adequate. If not, an advancement of the full side into the deficient side must be performed using a Z-plasty technique or a V-Y advancement. The vermilion-cutaneous junction is a key point in the proper alignment of the vermilion. Another guide for this purpose is the line that divides the vermilion into extraoral and intraoral segments. There is a distinct change in color at this point that facilitates precise alignment of the vermilion. This is a definite aid in design and alignment in cleft lip reconstruction.

Marking on the cleft side starts at the peak of the Cupid's bow (Fig. 23–3D, point 6), and a point is marked at the alar base (point 7). The distance between these two points must match the height of the lip on the noncleft side. The incision on the cleft side around the ala is designed to provide the proper amount of tissue for the advancement flap so that it can be transposed into the gap created on the noncleft side. Often tissue deficiency precludes optimal results for lip and nose repair, necessitating adjustments at the time of surgery. In patients with complete unilateral clefts, creation of the floor of the nose and alignment of the alar base improve symmetry.

The incision around the base of the ala must completely surround the ala to expose the maxilla and detach the alar base from its abnormal position. Another measurement that is helpful for creating a symmetric lip is the distance from the peak of the Cupid's bow to the commissure on the noncleft side (Fig. 23–3D, point 9). An equal distance between the commissure (point 10) and the peak of the Cupid's bow on the cleft side is determined. Usually there is a slight discrepancy between the two sides. In my experience, a 1- or 2-mm difference is insignificant and is hardly noticeable.

The use of vermilion for an L-flap has been described by Millard.[1] It was used to fill the lateral mucosal defect of the nose after releasing the entire lateral ala from the maxilla. This procedure is no longer used because it adds tissue to the deficient area but does not improve long-term results and may even, in my opinion, hinder the results.

Frequently, the length of the rotational lip element on the cleft side is inadequate. Millard recommends use of a back cut; however, surgeons must be careful when designing the lip element that is to be rotated inferiorly. Since this element is designed in a curvilinear fashion, it may not fit the advancement flap, which is designed in a straight line. Therefore, adjustment, which involves discarding some tissue, is necessary. The amount of discarded tissue varies according to the initial width and length of the lip and degree of rotation.

Despite use of a back cut, the medial lip element may still be too short relative to the lateral lip portion. Symmetric height can be established with the help of the following technique. The medial lip element is designed in a straight line. A 2- or 3-mm transverse cut is used to lengthen this element using a Z-plasty technique. This combination of rotation-advancement flap and Z-plasty is most helpful for achieving optimal symmetry of the lip without introducing a zigzag scar, which would break up the philtrum. The Z-plasty and the length of its arms are tailored individually, based on the discrepancy in height between the medial and lateral lip elements.

Less experienced surgeons frequently underrotate the medial flap. On rotation of the medial lip segment, it is determined whether or not the degree of rotation is adequate. If the height of the Cupid's bow on the noncleft side is too short, the lip will not have the desired length after the operation. Scar contracture causes some shortening of the lip postoperatively along the line of repair.

The main goal of unilateral cleft repair is to create a symmetric and pliable lip with minimal scarring. Three basic factors contribute to achievement of this goal. First, no permanent sutures are used for lip repair. Chromic sutures are used for the muscle layer because they do not cause excessive scarring. Monofilament nylon (6–0 or 7–0) is used for closure of the skin. These sutures are removed 5 days postoperatively.

The second factor is use of paper tape on the incision sites following suture removal. This technique was observed by Noordhoff in Taiwan. He has had vast experience treating Oriental patients, who are predisposed to hypertrophic scarring. Taping the scar on the lip for 3 or 4 months postoperatively successfully prevents hypertrophic scarring and seems to improve all cleft scars.

The third factor, massage of the scar following lip repair, eliminates firmness of the lip secondary to scar formation. Massage keeps the scar soft and the lip pliable.

Surgical Technique for the Rotation-Advancement Lip Repair

After the skin has been marked for the operation, the lip is infiltrated with epinephrine solution in a concentration of 1:100,000 (Fig. 23–3*E*). Even though infiltration distorts the lip tissue, epinephrine is used to decrease bleeding during the operation. The total amount of solution is approximately 2 ml for the lip and nose.

The incision is initiated on the noncleft side, and the segment is rotated inferiorly to establish the proper position of the Cupid's bow. A back cut, combined with Z-plasty, is used to rotate the medial portion of the lip. Since the rotation-advancement technique depends on visual judgment rather than on precise measurements, first attempts at achieving balance and contour may be unsatisfactory. In such cases the sutures are removed, and additional adjustments are made until a good result is obtained.

Repair of the Orbicularis Oris Muscle

In my opinion, the orbicularis oris muscle should be repaired separately. The muscle is dissected as a separate layer from the skin; however, I do not believe that a number of distinct variable muscle flaps, as described by Millard,[1] are necessary or advantageous. The muscle is released from its abnormal attachment and sutured as a separate layer (Fig. 23–3*N–R*). Dissection of both segments of the orbicularis oris muscle must be limited because wide dissection may be detrimental, resulting in increased scarring (Fig. 23–4).

Primary Unilateral Cleft Nasal Reconstruction

The goals of primary cleft lip-nose repair are to create a balanced, symmetric lip and a normal looking nose. These goals are difficult to achieve; however, we can reach these goals by modifying and improving our surgical treatments.[7]

The nasal deformity associated with complete unilateral cleft lip, alveolus, and palate involves various anatomic structures: the nasal ala, alar base, alar cartilage, columella, medial and lateral crura, nasal dome, and nasal septum. The position of the maxillary segments greatly contributes to the severity of the nasal deformity and its asymmetry. In the cleft nasal deformity, the lower lateral cartilage on the cleft side is displaced laterally and inferiorly. As a result, the alar dome is flat and turned downward. The ala on the cleft side is also flat and seems to be longer than the ala on the noncleft side. The floor of the nose is absent.

In primary cleft nasal repair, we attempt to achieve the following:

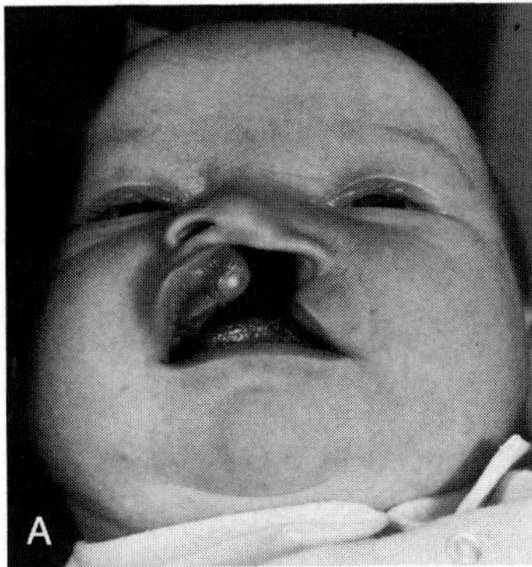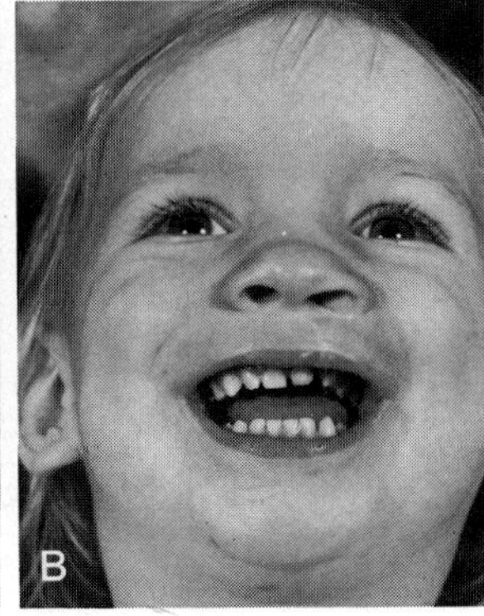

Figure 23–4 *A*, Preoperative view of 13-day-old infant with severe unilateral cleft lip, alveolus, and nasal deformity. *B*, Two years after surgery.

1. Closure of the nasal floor.
2. Symmetry of the nasal floor, ala, and dome on both sides.
3. Symmetric nasal tip projection.
4. Reshaping of the lower lateral cartilage.
5. Repositioning of the lower lateral cartilage.
6. Repositioning of the alar base.
7. Reshaping of the nasal ala.

Important steps for early reconstruction of the cleft lip nasal deformity include the following:
1. Dissection of the lower lateral cartilage from the skin and mucosa.
2. Shifting and repositioning of the lower lateral cartilage and redraping of the skin and lining.
3. Creation of a symmetric ala and nasal tip.
4. Creation of a symmetric alar base (Fig. 23–5).

Following rotation of the medial lip element, a C-flap is used to lengthen the columella on the cleft side. In many cases, the incision must be extended into the nasal mucosa, but not so far that the nasal crus of the lower lateral cartilage is exposed. Through this incision, dissection between the two medial crura is performed using small curved tonotomy dissection scissors. Dissection is carried over the alar dome, and the skin is undermined over both lower lateral cartilages in the area of the alar dome. The lower lateral cartilage is not exposed, and only the skin overlying it in the dome area is undermined. The attachment of the cartilage to the nasal mucosa in the dome area is maintained, allowing shifting of the entire lower lateral cartilage together with the attached nasal mucosa. Adjustments are made to position the lower lateral cartilage so that it is symmetric with respect to the normal side to establish normal contour and projection of the nasal tip and ala.

Laterally, access to the lower lateral cartilage is achieved through an incision in the crease around the alar base, anticipating the medial shift of the alar base. The suture line around the ala is hidden in the natural crease. The next incision is carried through the nasal mucosa, separating the entire ala from its attachment to the maxilla. Transection is carried to the nasal process of the maxilla.

Total dissection of the alar base from the underlying bony structure facilitates the approach to the lateral

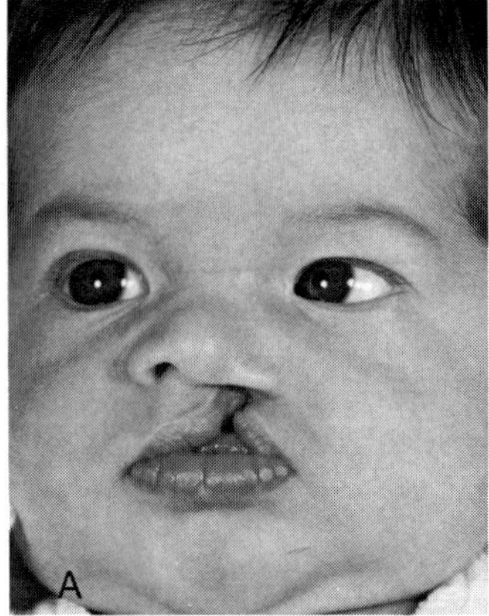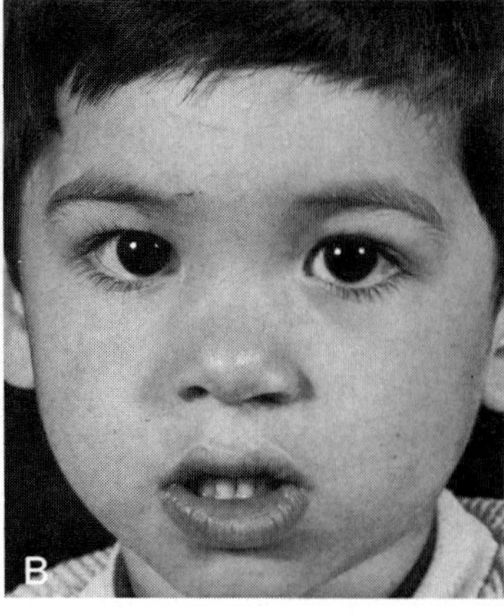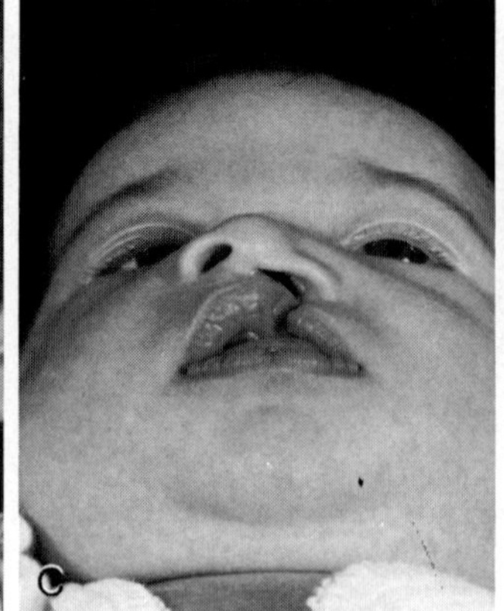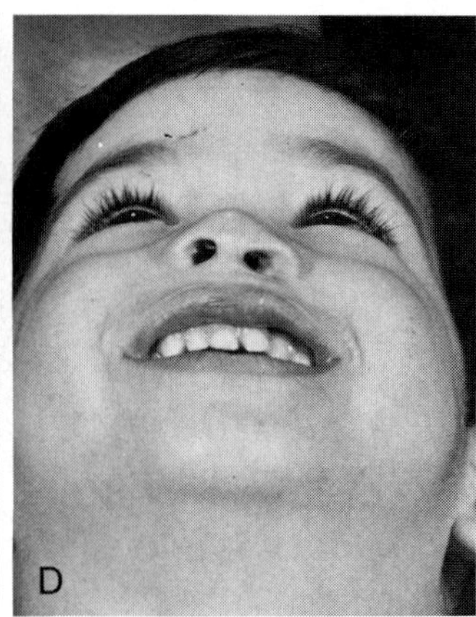

Figure 23–5 *A*, Preoperative frontal view at 1 month of age showing mild unilateral cleft lip and cleft palate with nasal deformity. *B*, Frontal view 3 years following primary surgery. *C*, Preoperative submental view. *D*, Postoperative submental view.

crus of the lower lateral cartilage. Dissection of the lip from the maxillary segments is performed in the plane above the periosteum, separating the orbicularis oris muscle attachment so that it can be repositioned and sutured together with the muscle of the medial lip element. Undermining of the lip at this level does not impair facial growth and development but does facilitate reorientation of the orbicularis oris muscle and allows better cosmetic and functional results.

I also have noted that wide dissection of the nasal ala from the bony structures does not have an adverse effect on facial growth. As indicated earlier, this incision is helpful for approaching the lateral crus and dissecting it from the skin, then proceeding toward the dorsum and the alar dome and joining the dissection of the lower lateral cartilage previously described. In this manner, the lower lateral cartilage is freed entirely from the overlying skin. Because the attachment of the lower lateral cartilage to the nasal mucosa is preserved only at the dome level, the lateral crus and the medial crus are totally separated from the skin and nasal mucosa and are easily shifted to the new position. The entire dissection of the lower lateral crus is performed without exposure.

Once the lower lateral cartilage has been dissected and mobilized from the skin and nasal mucosa, it is repositioned anteriorly and superiorly to match the position of the lower lateral cartilage on the noncleft side. Special attention is focused on creating a nasal tip and ala that are symmetric with respect to the opposite side. On the cleft side, total dissection of the lower lateral cartilage from the nasal mucosa allows the entire cartilage to be shifted. This maneuver results in a delicately curved dome and eliminates the flat, elongated shape of the lateral crus. When the alar base remains displaced following shifting of the entire lower lateral cartilage, additional lining, as described by Millard, is felt not only to be unnecessary but also possibly detrimental.

The repositioned lower lateral cartilage is stabilized with stent sutures of Dacron through the skin, cartilage, and nasal lining. This produces a contoured shape of the ala that is similar to that on the noncleft side. When the maneuvers described do not produce the desired

effect, vertical suspension sutures can be used to augment the technique for early nasal reconstruction. Suspension sutures, such as those described by McComb[8] or Anderl (see Chap. 24), are useful additions in primary reconstructive procedures. I have used variations of this procedure since 1971, and use a similar technique today that incorporates Dacron stents using straight Keith needles, as shown in Figure 23–3R–U. With adequate dissection, these sutures act to stabilize the structures in a new position, allowing healing without more radical dissection or direct exposure of the cartilage. Anderl's more radical approach incorporates a more extensive dissection as well as dissection of the septum. I defer septoplasty until the patient is older.

Another important aspect of early nasal repair is creation of the nasal floor and/or sill. This procedure is performed according to Bardach's technique, in which a mucoperichondrial flap from the septum and a mucoperiosteal flap from the lateral nasal wall are sutured together to form the nasal floor.[5]

Once the floor of the nose has been created, the alar base is positioned so that it is symmetric with respect to the noncleft side. At this stage, it is important not to overcorrect when trying to establish a curved shape of the ala. Overcorrection typically results in a nostril that is smaller than the one on the opposite side. It is much easier to decrease nostril size than to increase it. Correction of the nostril that is too small is a most difficult, if not impossible, task (Fig. 23–6).

Secondary Correction of Unilateral Cleft Nasal Deformity

The previously described procedures do not always correct the nasal deformity adequately. Typically, the lower lateral cartilage is displaced laterally and inferiorly, the alar dome is flat, and the nostril retains a horizontal orientation to a varying degree. During surgery, the surgeon may realize that satisfactory primary correction cannot be obtained for a particular patient. The decision must then be made whether or not to attempt further surgery or delay correction of the remaining nasal deformity until the patient is older. For

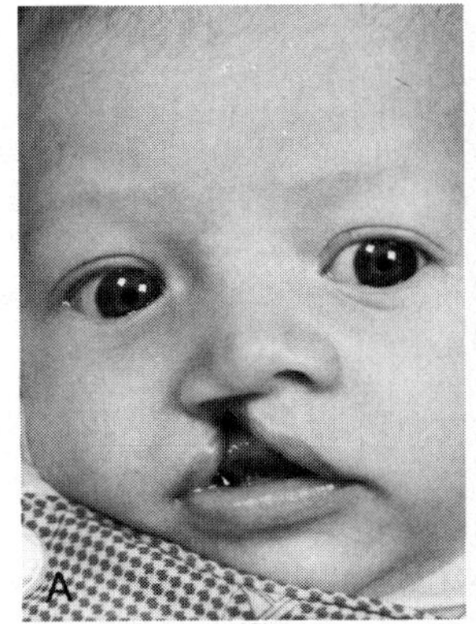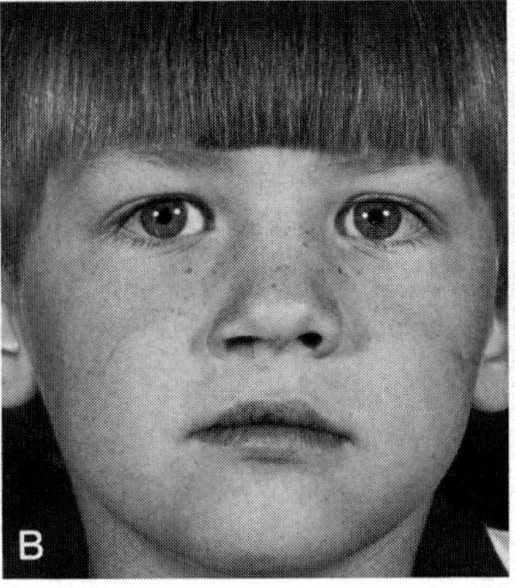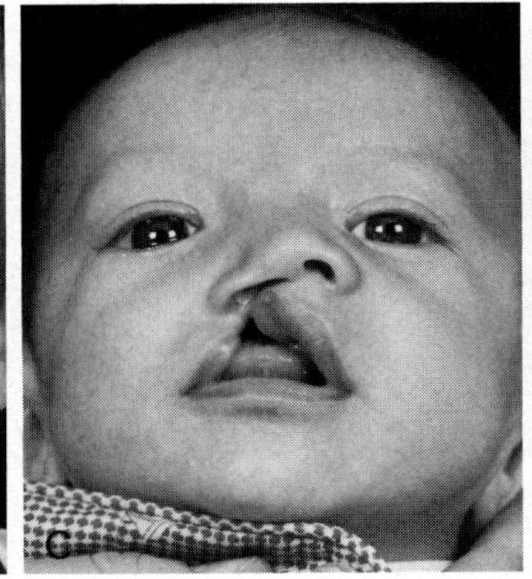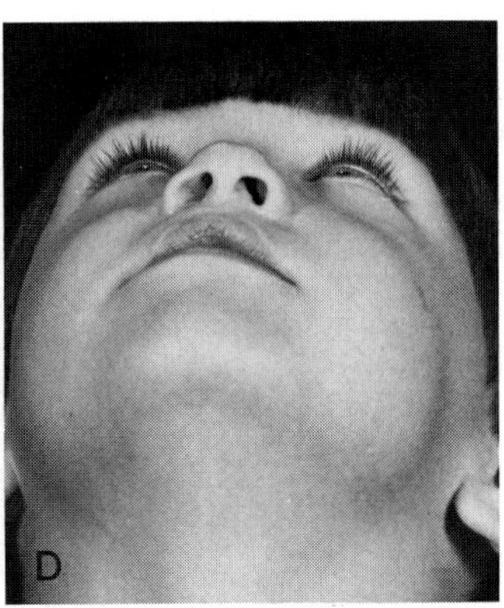

Figure 23–6 *A,* Preoperative frontal view of 3-month-old infant with incomplete unilateral cleft with minimal nasal deformity. *B,* Frontal view 5 years after surgery. *C,* Submental view showing incomplete cleft lip with nasal deformity. *D,* Five years following surgery.

most unilateral cleft nasal deformities, septorhinoplasty at a later age is indicated. Cartilage augmentation also may be necessary as a secondary procedure. In my opinion, radical surgery at the time of primary repair is not recommended (Fig. 23–7).

Secondary correction is usually performed when the child is 4 to 15 years of age. It should be emphasized that correction of the nasal deformity during primary lip repair and further secondary operations do not inhibit nasal growth; however, I have observed some patients in whom overly aggressive surgery resulted in excessive scarring and severe secondary deformities. Delicate technique is important in obtaining good results.

Optimal results for correction of a severe nasal deformity may be achieved through direct exposure of the lower lateral cartilage. The cartilage is shifted, recontoured, and sutured to the cartilage on the noncleft side. The philosophy of the surgeon influences whether this procedure is attempted at the time of primary lip repair or is done as a secondary procedure. Recontouring and reshaping of the lower lateral cartilage may be more difficult in older patients when the cartilage is firmer and less flexible. Furthermore, leaving the child with a significant secondary deformity until the age of 8

to 12 years is undesirable because the patient may experience psychological problems related to self-image. The technique described here achieves improvement at the time of primary lip repair, although it is kept in mind that some nasal asymmetry may persist. Results that appear satisfactory for the nasal deformity at the time of primary lip repair do not always continue to be satisfactory as the patient matures, and further surgery may be suggested. Fortunately, for most patients the long-term results remain satisfactory and require only minimal surgery or septal surgery when the patient is older (Fig. 23–8).

In reviewing the late results of 21 years of experience of cleft lip and cleft nose repair, I concluded that the surgical techniques described here allow marked improvement of the shape of the nose at the time of the primary repair. We must remember that because the alar cartilage is displaced in three dimensions, cartilage reshaping and repositioning is easier to perform in infants. Most patients with a unilateral cleft require repeated surgery to achieve aesthetic results that can eliminate cleft stigma. This means correction of the skeletal deformity as well as good primary and secondary soft tissue reconstruction (see Chap 63).

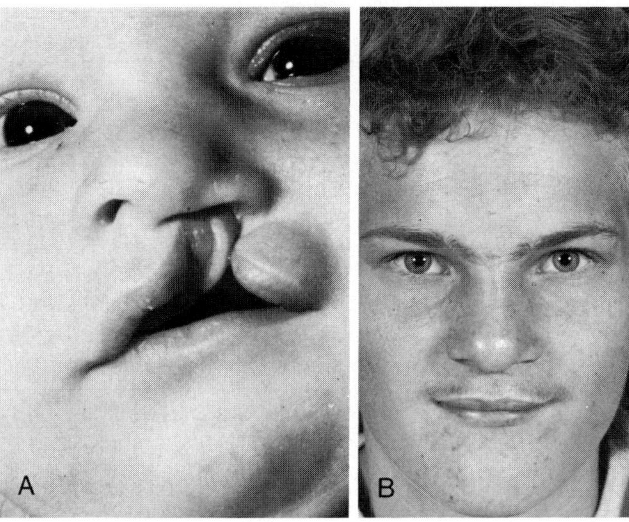

Figure 23–7 *A,* Preoperative view of first patient in whom this technique was utilized for unilateral cleft lip and palate. *B,* Twelve years after primary cleft lip and nose repair.

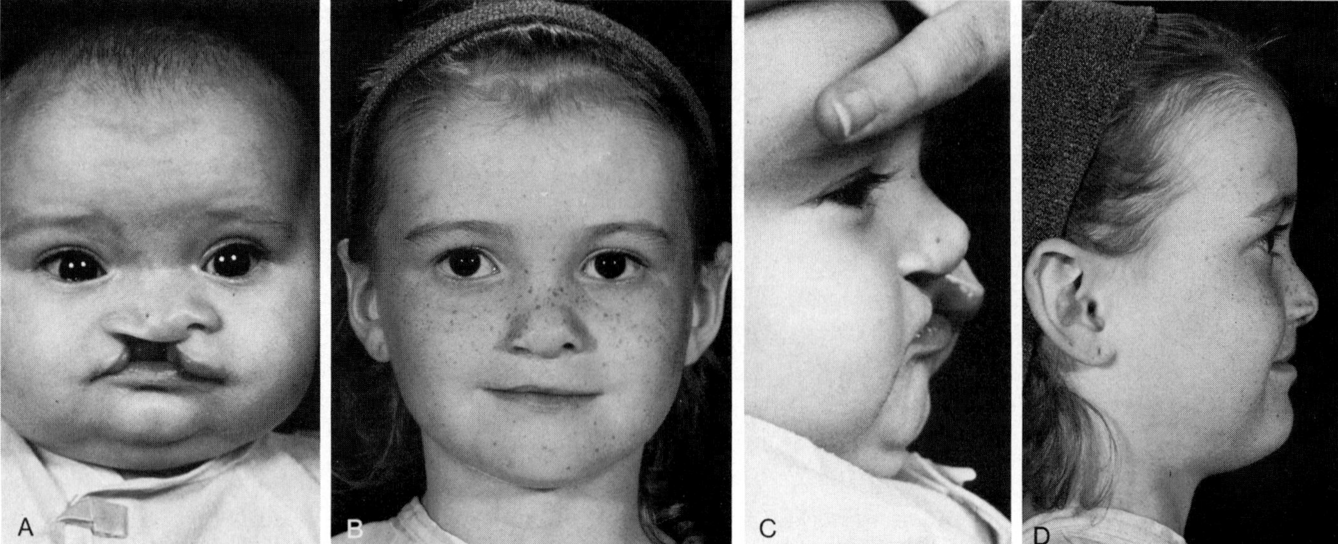

Figure 23–8 *A*, Preoperative frontal view of 1-month-old infant with wide unilateral cleft lip, palate, and severe nasal deformity. *B*, Seven years following surgery. *C*, Preoperative lateral view showing severe cleft lip and nasal deformity. *D*, Lateral view 7 years after surgical correction.

References

1. Millard DR, Jr: Cleft Craft: The Evolution of Its Surgery. I. The Unilateral Deformity. Boston: Little, Brown, 1976.
2. Salyer KE: Techniques in Aesthetic Craniofacial Surgery (Introduction). New York: Gower Medical Publishers, 1988.
3. McNeil CK: Oral and Facial Deformity. London: Pitman, 1954.
4. Hotz M, Gnoinski W, Perko M, et al: The Zurich approach, 1964–1984. In Hotz M, et al (eds): Early Treatment of Cleft Lip and Palate. Toronto: Hans Huber, 1986.
5. Bardach J, Salyer KE: Surgical Techniques in Cleft Lip and Palate. Chicago: Year Book, 1987.
6. Millard DR, Jr: A primary camouflage of the unilateral harelip. Transactions of the First International Congress of Plastic Surgery, Stockholm, Sweden, 1957.
7. Salyer KE: Primary correction of the unilateral cleft nose: A 15-year experience. Plast Reconstr Surg 77:558, 1986.
8. McComb H: Primary correction of unilateral cleft lip nasal deformity: A 10-year review. Plast Reconstr Surg 75:791, 1985.

CHAPTER 24

Primary Unilateral Cleft Lip and Nose Reconstruction

H. Anderl

In all procedures for repair of the unilateral cleft, great care is taken to achieve optimal results in the function and aesthetic appearance of the lip, taking even very minor details of the anatomy into consideration. Less attention has been directed toward correcting the deformity of the nose, even after the underlying skeletal structures were corrected. The reason for this conservative attitude was based on fear of inhibiting growth. As a result, there are considerable differences of opinion about the timing of corrective surgery for the cleft nose.

Some authors (e.g., Gelbke)[1] were very active in promoting primary repair of the nose, performing incisions and excisions and denuding the cartilage with consequently unsatisfactory results and severe distur-

bances of growth. Other surgeons, such as Blair,[2] McIndoe,[3] McDowell,[4] and Burian,[5] advocated primary construction of the shape of the nose but restricted it to the deformed ala only.

More recently, Berkeley,[6, 7] Velasquez and Ortiz-Monasterio,[8] and Randall[9] have used an external incision to better expose and reshape the alar cartilage. Although they confirm that this approach does not produce visible scars, such a stigma never can be removed. Skoog[10] and Millard[11, 12] made an incision inside the nose to allow better repositioning of the alar cartilage. From this exposure they also detached the alar base from the piriform aperture. This incision may lead to scar contracture and narrowing of the nostril. Skoog has applied external splints to avoid this complication. Salyer also uses an internal incision, but, in addition, he dissects the cartilage completely, denuding the protective and nourishing lining of the mucoperichondrium to achieve an optimal position of the cartilage.[13] McComb[14, 15] and Pigott[16] use very wide undermining of the nasal skin and have presented good results in a long-term follow-up period of 12 to 16 years.

However, none of these authors has considered every aspect of the deformity, such as the deviation of the frontal part of the septum and hypoplasia of the maxilla and piriform aperture. We have found that correction of these structures is essential for complete success in one stage.[17–20] Jackson[21] stressed this very important feature of the bony deficit some years ago.

Our approach includes all aspects of the deformity. On the other hand, we have avoided the disadvantages that may occur after internal and external incisions and complete denuding of the cartilage. Based on our long-term experience, we are firmly convinced that such procedures are not necessary to achieve good results.

Our intentions in performing primary simultaneous repair of the lip and nose are based on the following:

1. Long-term observation indicates that careful handling of the growing tissue is not detrimental.
2. In a great number of patients lip repair alone leads to the typical nasal deformity, with functional and aesthetic disorders that cause discontent in patients, parents, and the surgeon (Fig. 24–1).
3. Even the patience shown during the long waiting period until corrective operations can be performed on the adolescent patient, usually with considerable difficulty, is not always rewarded with good results.

Method and Goal of Repair

The goal of our operative procedure, which utilizes extensive but careful mobilization of tissue, is to place the different dislocated parts of the lip and nose in anatomically normal and symmetrical positions, to eliminate unphysiologic tension and pressure, and to stimulate bone growth in hypoplastic areas of the maxilla, thus ensuring fairly normal development of all structures. Furthermore, this mobilization allows easy closure of the lip without any tension and provides optimal correction of the nose.

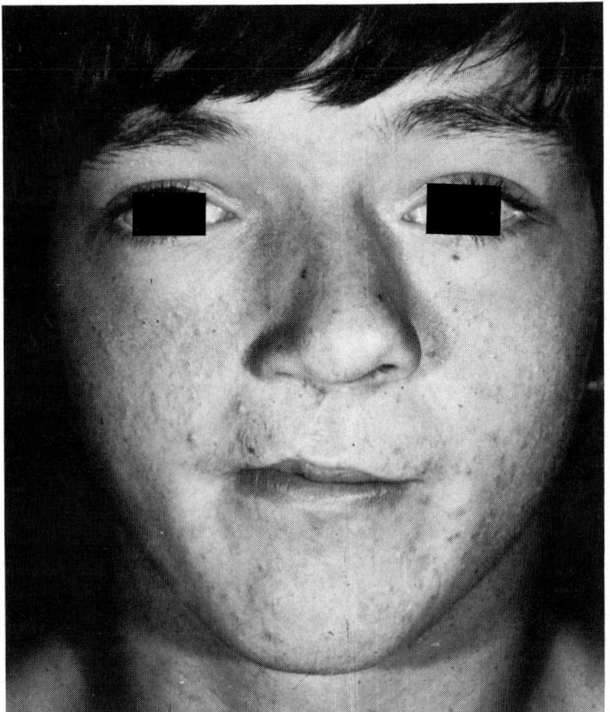

Figure 24–1 Typical nasal deformity that was not corrected during lip repair.

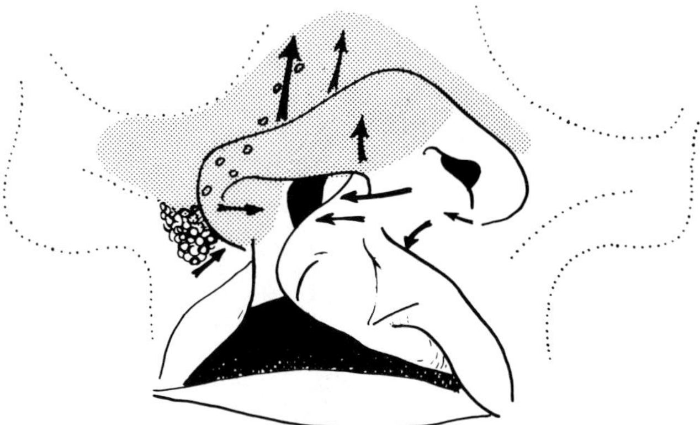

Figure 24–2 Movements of tissue on either side of the cleft (arrows). Undermining is indicated by the gray area; stimulation of growth by small circles.

To correct the lip and nose simultaneously, we perform the following procedures (Fig. 24–2):

1. The cheek with the lateral part of the lip and alar base is advanced toward the midline.
2. The medial portions of the lip and nose are moved toward the cleft side, and the lip is rotated downward. The orbicularis oris muscle is reconstructed. It supports the base of the nose as well as the columella and creates the contours for the philtrum, the Cupid's bow, and the dimple. It also repositions the rotated premaxilla by exerting continuous active pressure.
3. The frontal curved septum is shifted to a normal sagittal position. The tendency toward recurrent deviation must be reduced to a minimum.
4. The tip of the nose and the ala, with the abundance of skin on the cleft side, are raised, the columella is lengthened, and the flattened ala is curved.
5. Bone growth is stimulated under the alar base and along the margin of the piriform aperture on the cleft side.

The operation is performed at the age of 5 to 6 months. We feel that comparatively late timing is important to facilitate extensive and careful dissection and to ensure accurate reconstruction of tissue that is already better developed. The late timing of surgery sometimes leads to problems with the parents, who would prefer earlier treatment for obvious reasons, and good arguments are required to convince them. Parents seem to appreciate the results more if they have lived for a while with the child's deformity.

Operation

Undermining and Lip Repair

Simultaneous repair of the lip and nose requires that all dissections that have to be performed for repair of both are of mutual value, facilitate closure of skin and muscle without tension, and create an optimal shape of the nose. The lip is an essential part of the function and aesthetic harmony of the face and guarantees the stability of the lower nose. Our method of choice for lip closure is the rotation-advancement technique of Millard[11] with some modifications (Fig. 24–3).

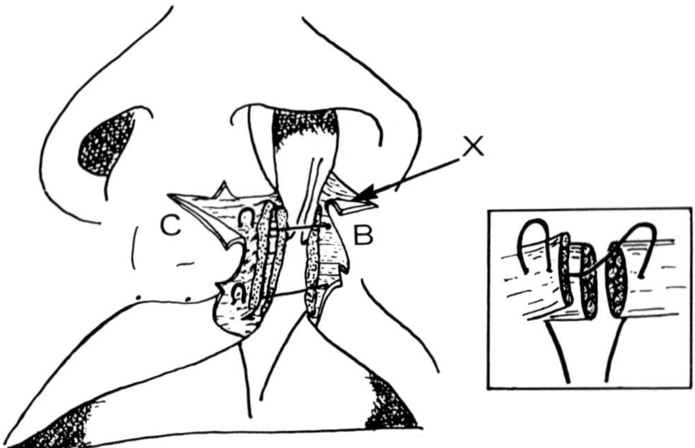

Figure 24–3 Repair of the lip using a modified Millard procedure. The muscle is joined using a suture technique. Flap B with incision X is created at the end of the operation to integrate flap C.

The curved incision on the noncleft side does not penetrate the muscle but is restricted to the skin to preserve the underlying muscle fibers. Furthermore, it crosses the midline if necessary to achieve the correct length of the lip. The incision line on the lateral segment of the cleft does not run directly along the vermilion margin but is slightly curved in the white area of the lip to provide a better adaptation to the curved skin margin on the medial lip portion. This incision also starts with a little triangle just above the point for the future Cupid's bow, which will be integrated into a tiny incision gap in the downward rotated lip in the corresponding area of that Cupid's bow. The philtrum is shaped by a special suture technique consisting of back stitches on the outer surface of the orbicularis oris muscle that produce a ridge (Fig. 24–3). The C-flap is integrated at the end of the whole operation (which will be described later). We never use the cut under and around the nasal base because the natural ridge dispersing to the lip may be spoiled. The little triangle excision in the columella that Millard has advocated to lengthen the short columella on the cleft side is also used.

Wide undermining of the cheek is of great value in allowing movement toward the midline (Fig. 24–4).

Access is achieved through the vestibulum of the cleft side, and the incision line is extended behind the maxillary tuberosity, ending with a back cut in the mucosa of about 1 cm, which allows further advancement of the cheek toward the front (Fig. 24–5). The medial part of that incision runs along the margin of the hard palate (within the alveolus cleft) just 1 cm behind the alveolar arch. Then a 1-cm perpendicular cut crosses the lower turbinate. Dissection in this area proceeds subperiostally, and a little piece of bone of the lower turbinate is removed. This maneuver makes additional mucosa available for construction of the nasal floor together with the vomerine flap of the medial side of the cleft.

In the frontal aspect of the maxilla the dissection preserves the periosteum and extends from the piriform aperture toward and behind the tuberosity of the maxilla and from the vestibular incision toward the infraorbital margin. On the noncleft side the lip incision runs around the premaxilla toward the base of the septum and provides the vomerine flap for closure of the nasal floor, as already described.

Correction of the Dislocated Septum

When straightening the septum, two points have to be considered: (1) The curved frontal part must be released from the bone, and (2) the mucosa must be detached from the cartilage in this area. Figure 24–6 demonstrates the behavior of the distorted septum. If the mucosa of the frontal dislocated part is not elevated from the cartilage on either side, the tension in this system always retracts the septum into its original position. After dissecting the mucosa on both sides of the curved septum and disconnecting it from the bone,

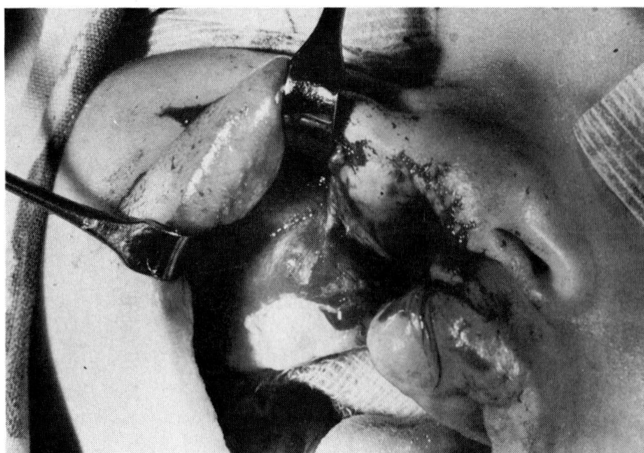

Figure 24–4 Area of undermining of the cheek. The periosteum remains intact.

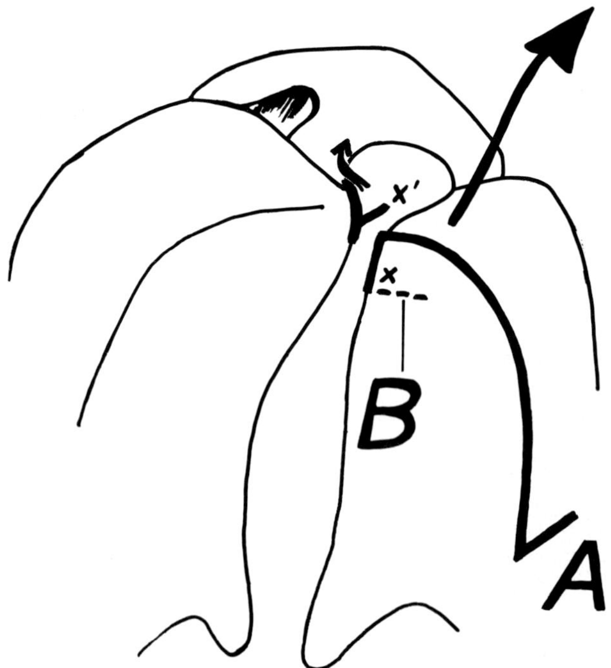

Figure 24–5 Vestibular incision and back cut A. Point B = incision in the lower turbinate (dotted line). Point X′ = incision in the frontal vomerine flap to lengthen columella. Point X is integrated into point X′.

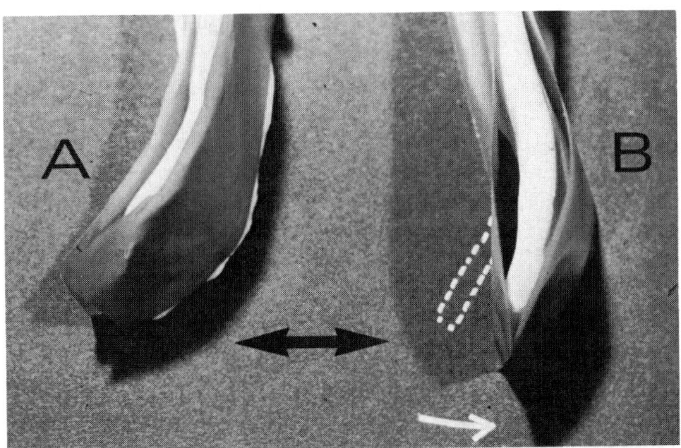

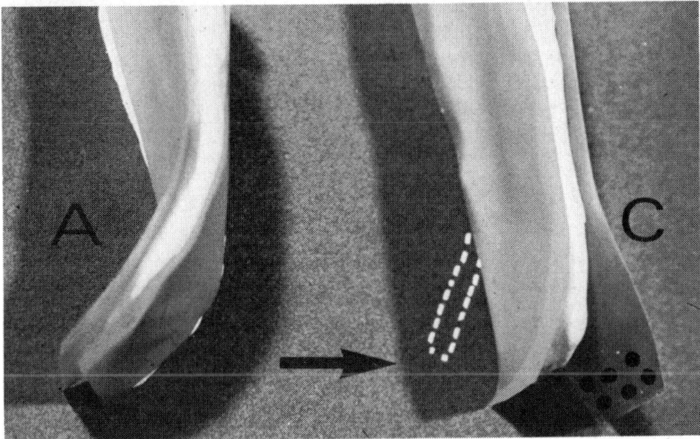

Figure 24–6 Illustration of mucoperichondrial dissection in the deviated septum. A ↔ B (upper). If the mucosa remains attached, the septal cartilage cannot stay in the straight position. A → C (lower). After the mucosa is freed from the septum in the curved area, it can be moved easily (dotted line), and there is a gain of an excess amount of mucosa (dark dots).

the septum and all other structures can be shifted to the midline (Fig. 24–7). In addition, excessive mucosa is gained on the cleft side, which is of value for lengthening the columella and raising the nasal tip. The mucosa can be attached again to the overcorrected septum by transseptal mattress stitches with chromic catgut.

Mobilizing the Dropped Ala and Forming the Nasal Tip

In this part of the operation we place the dropped ala in a symmetric position relative to the normal side and lift the nasal tip on the cleft side. This mobilization is accomplished through extensive undermining of the nasal skin and separation of the cartilages from each other within the columella and the dome (Fig. 24–8).

From the subnasal incision the medial crura of the alar cartilages are separated, and the dissection is continued between the mucosal layers of the frontal septum, which have already been freed. There is a free space between these mucosal layers, which extends from the anterior margin of the septum to the skin of the columella.

From this space, the skin of the dome and the entire nose is undermined from the underlying cartilages and bone. Mobilization of the alar skin on the cleft side,

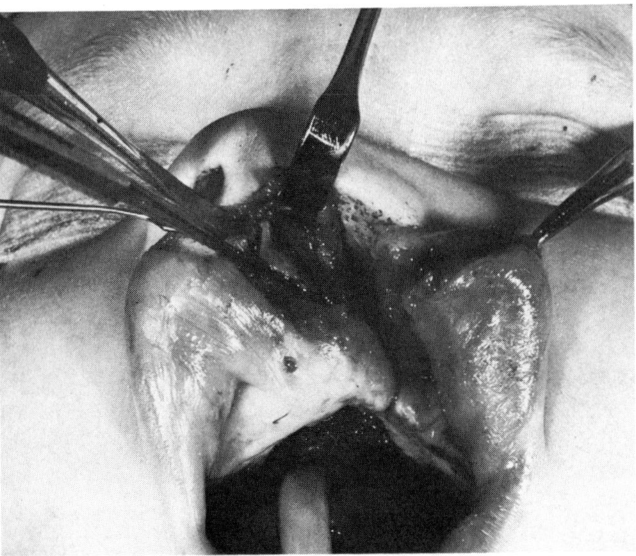

Figure 24–7 Mucoperichondrial dissection in the frontal part of the nasal septum and detachment from bone by blunt dissection.

especially in the area of the intercartilaginous space, can be supplemented by dissection from the alar base through the vestibular incision (Fig. 24–9). No mucosal incision is necessary, and the nourishing lining of the alar cartilage should not be touched. After this maneuver the elongated part of the skin on the cleft side and the ala can be shifted upward.

The nostrils are now equally wide, and there must be no narrowing inside the nose. Occasionally, the ala of the cleft shows some submucosal thickening, originating from fibrous tissue that can be excised in a later operation. In a few patients, excessive tension in the alar cartilage prevents a completely normal shaping of the nostril. In these patients later correction must be applied. Such corrections will also be necessary if some hypoplasia of the alar cartilage is present.

Stimulation of Bone Growth

It is very important to influence bone growth in the skeletal structure of the hypoplastic part of the piriform

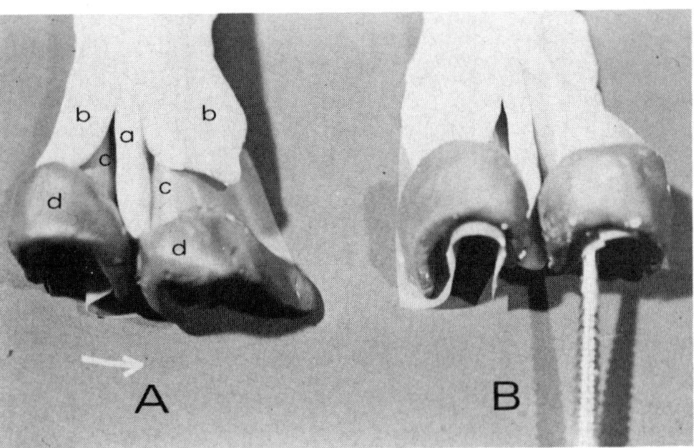

Figure 24–8 Correction of the deformed ala. *A*, The typical alar deformity on the left side; arrow indicates repositioned septum (a, septum; b, lateral cartilage; c, mucosa; d, alar cartilage). *B*, After mobilization and repositioning of the ala.

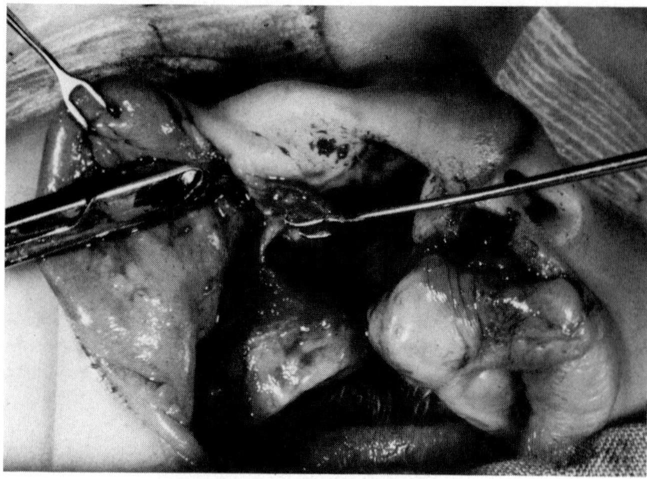

Figure 24–9 Undermining of the base of the ala between skin and cartilage from the lateral approach in the intercartilaginous space. The mucosa stays intact on the cartilage. No incision is made within the nasal cavity.

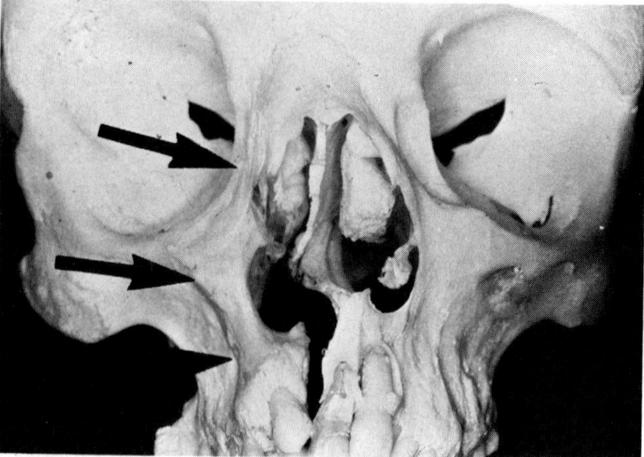

Figure 24–10 Right unilateral cleft visualized on the skull of an adult. Arrows indicate hypoplasia along the piriform aperture and under the alar base.

aperture and the platform of the alar base of the maxilla. In Figures 24–10 and 24–11 this hypoplasia is very well visualized in the skulls of an adult and a child. The morphologic consequences of this deficiency have been illustrated by Hogan and Converse.[22] In a schematic representation they compared the cleft lip nose to a tilted tripod (Fig. 24–12). The greater the deficiency of bone in these areas, the more twisted and deviated the septum.

Therefore, the alar base and lateral nose have to be completely freed from the maxilla and piriform aperture by blunt dissection. This dissection can be done after making the incision in the mucosa of the lower turbinate as previously mentioned (Fig. 24–13). In this area dissection is extended subperiosteally. The instrument is pushed along the bony margin of the aperture toward the midline, lifting the soft tissue and forming a tentlike excavation of periosteum with the bone of the maxilla

as a base (Fig. 24–14). The created space filled with clotted blood can be additionally augmented with Surgicel (Fig. 24–15). In this area between normal bone and periosteum, onlay bone is produced to restore the deficiency under the alar base and lateral nose. The osteogenic activity of periosteum, especially when vascularized, is well known.[23–25]

After these preparations, closure of the lip can be started. The mucosa in the vestibule and the nasal floor is sutured with chromic catgut. If some tension remains on the vomerine flap, preventing the columella of the cleft side from being shifted cranially, a little incision in this flap allows release of this tension (Fig. 24–5). The abundance of mucosa gained by the lower turbinate incision can be used to fill this gap. To achieve good nasal support the anatomic closure of the orbicularis oris muscle, as already described, is of great importance (Fig. 24–3).

Next, the corresponding points of the future Cupid's bow (marked with a needle and ink) are sutured with

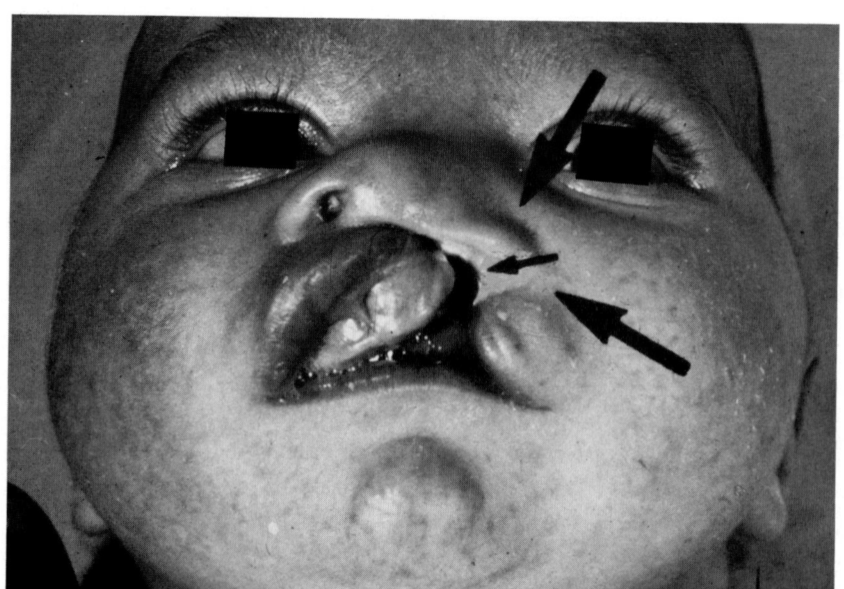

Figure 24–11 Bony hypoplasia. Smaller arrow indicates fibrotic tissue beneath mucosa.

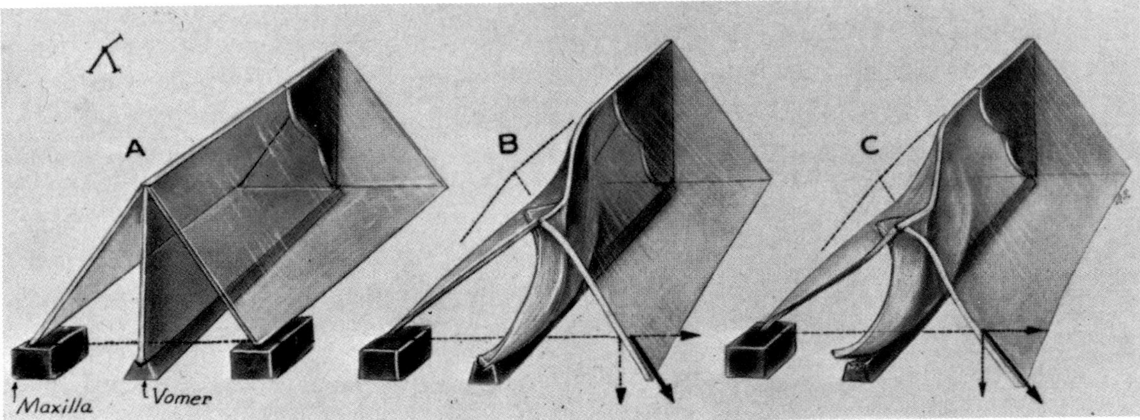

Figure 24–12 The tilted tripod. *A,* Schematic representation of the nose illustrating the basic tripod nature of the nasal structure. The tripod consists of the dorsal portion of the septum and nasal bones, and the two alar arms. *B,* The tilting effect resulting from maxillary hypoplasia with secondary deformity of the septum and cleft ala. *C,* More dramatic illustration of the convex deformity of the septum and the vertical bending of the septum posterior to the junction of the membranous and cartilaginous portions of the septum. Restriction of the caudal border of the septum in its anterior thrust causes it to bend toward the normal nostril. If there is a more severe deformity of the vomer, the septum is displaced into the normal nostril. (From Hogan, V.M., and Converse, J.M.: Secondary deformities of unilateral cleft lip and nose. *In* Grabb, W.C., Rosenstein, S.E., and Bzoch, K.R. (Eds.): Cleft Lip and Palate. Boston, Little, Brown & Company, 1971.)

6–0 nylon. The skin is closed step by step with 7–0 nylon about halfway up the lower part of the lip. At this stage of lip closure the Millard C-flap is integrated in the nasal floor at the entrance of the nostril. Flap B is constructed for this purpose (see Fig. 24–3). The incision is performed from inside the nasal floor medial to the alar base at a slightly oblique angle toward the corner of the alar ridge. This cut must be very accurate because the circumference of the nostril will otherwise become either too big or too small.

Flap C must be adjusted into the triangular gap that appears if flap B has been sutured under the columella. If flap C is too big, that part of the skin has to be deepithelialized and the abundance of tissue buried under the surface to augment a common deficit of tissue in this area.

At the end of the operation the lip and nose stay in position by themselves. Two or three percutaneous mattress sutures are placed to avoid free spaces that could lead to hematoma (Figs. 24–16 and 24–17).

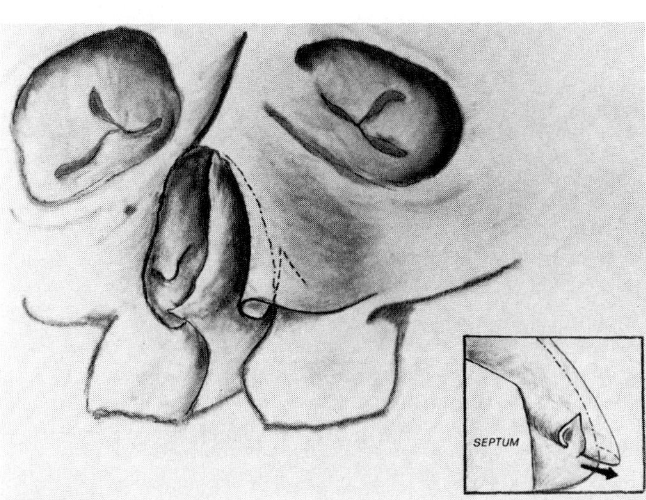

Figure 24–13 Tentlike space of periosteum along the bony aperture and under the alar base. Incision crossing the lower turbinate is demonstrated (especially in the small insert). Frontal advancement of this tentlike excavation is indicated by the arrow.

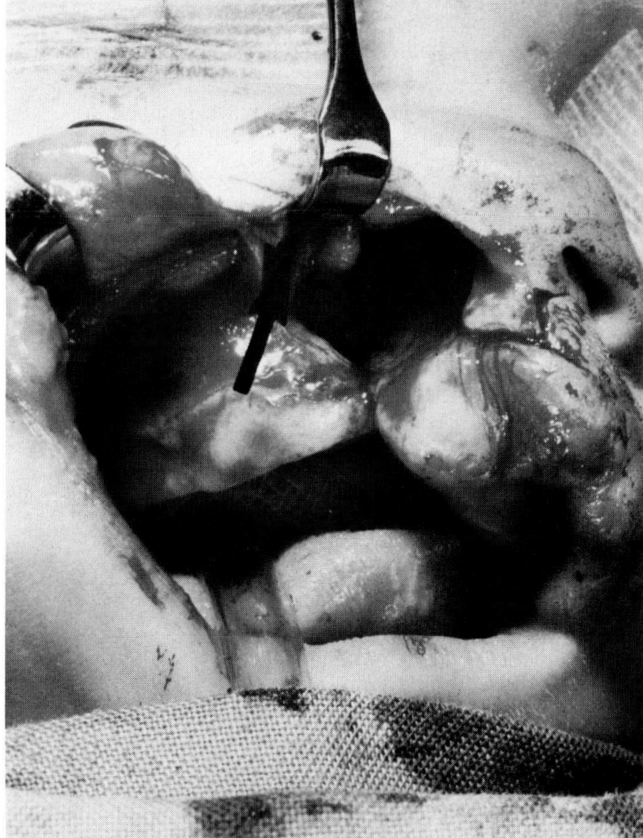

Figure 24–14 The tentlike cavity from below.

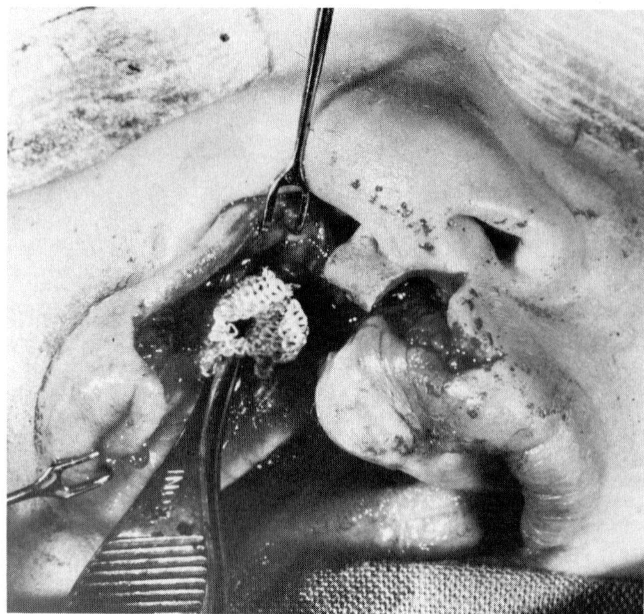

Figure 24–15 Insertion of Surgicel into the periosteal cavity.

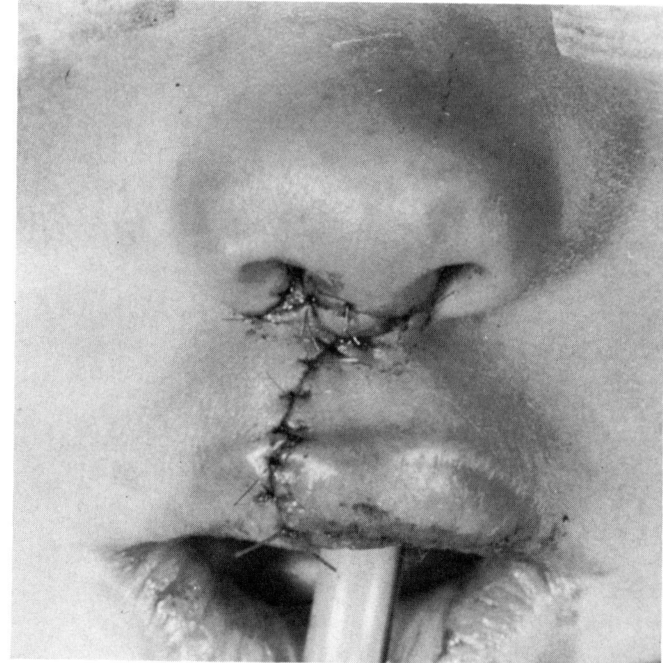

Figure 24–16 After suturing the nasal floor, muscle, and skin, all structures stay in their normal position owing to extensive mobilization.

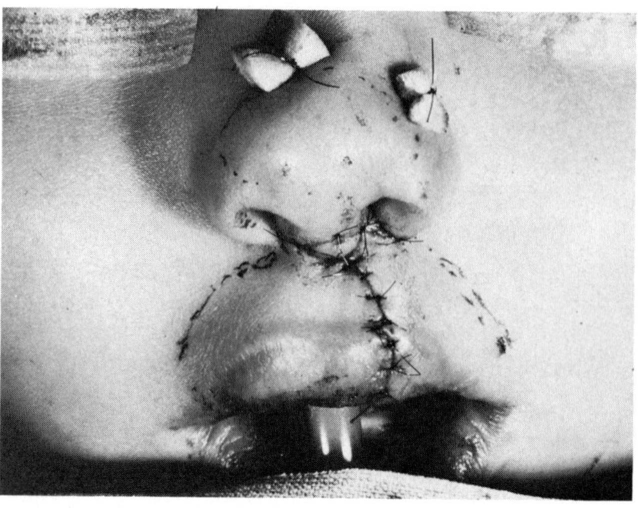

Figure 24–17 Mattress sutures are placed in the lower nose to avoid hematoma. Slight overcorrection is performed in the alar base and along the piriform aperture. Dotted line indicates orbicularis oris muscle.

Results

Summarizing our experience, three questions must be addressed:

1. What are the results and advantages that can be achieved with simultaneous lip and nose repair?
2. What negative consequences must be considered with this kind of surgery?
3. Is there any sign of growth retardation of the nose in long-term follow-up of 18 years?

Evaluation of the results of simultaneous primary lip and nose repair is based on results achieved in 266 children with unilateral clefts who were operated on since 1970. A preliminary statement of results can be presented because the first group of patients have already reached the age of 18 years.

For longitudinal evaluation the children were seen for follow-up examination every 6 months. Pre- and postoperative photographs were taken at 6-month intervals as well. In a few cases, x-ray evaluation was added (half-axial exposure of the face to demonstrate the front of the maxilla and the piriform aperture). In two patients histologic samples were taken to evaluate appositional bone growth in the maxillary area. In a few patients CT scans were used for evaluation. In the follow-up investigation the following criteria were of importance: Investigation of the lip included judgment of the height of the lip, the philtrum, the dimple, the Cupid's bow, and the vermilion scar formation and positions of the premaxilla and teeth. Investigations of the nose included the following factors:

1. Comparisons of the right and left sides of the nose and comparison with the nose of a normal child of the same age.
2. Deviation of the nose and septum.
3. Symmetry of the tip of the nose or asymmetry on the cleft side (too high or too low).
4. Shape and position of the alar cartilages.
5. Any signs of hypoplasia of the nose.
6. Shape of the nostrils (especially on the cleft side).
7. Position and length of the columella and the shape of the nasal base.
8. Evidence of hypoplasia of the underlying bone.

The advantages of our approach have led to good results in approximately 80% of patients, especially when compared to patients who were operated on before application of this concept. Wide undermining facili-

tated lip and nose repair because there was less tension on the suture line. The scars in the lip were therefore much less striking. Projection of the philtrum and appearance of a dimple were improved by our special suture technique of the muscle. Our modification of the Millard procedure could be applied to all kinds of unilateral clefts regardless of the degree of severity. A frequent objection to the Millard procedure, the short lip, was very rare in our patients.

Correction of the nasal deformity resulted in adequate and symmetric projection of the nasal tip and a curved shape of the alar rim. Because no incision was made inside the nasal vestibulum, there were no contractures of the nostrils or nasal entrance. The induced augmentation of onlay bone under the alar base provided good symmetry and prevented recurrence both of dropping of the ala and deviation of the caudal edge of the septum. Overall, we can say that no child will have a completely normal appearance, and the stigma of a cleft always will remain, even in the best cases. In some of the patients with good late results, we had to perform few corrections to improve the results. We never had to do difficult secondary operations, especially in the area of the nose as we used to do. With more experience, which we lacked in the earlier cases, more successful results were achieved (Fig. 24–18 to 24–25).

The *negative consequences* of our technique must be considered as well. They may result from technical errors or from the severity of the initial deformity. Secondary lip deformities may include a lip that is too short, a Cupid's bow that is not completely symmetric compared to the healthy side, a tissue deficiency below the columella, or a broad, hypertrophic, or asymmetric vermilion. These secondary deformities are easily corrected. Our suture technique of the muscle creates a very good philtrum and makes the dimple more visible.

We have abandoned Z-plasty in the vermilion because it always resulted in excessive thickness. Good adjustment of the V is achieved if the area just below the vermilion border of the lateral lip is integrated with the opposite side by a small semicircular vermilion flap.

In the nose we also have accepted minor imperfections, especially in patients with severe clefts or clefts in which this method was applied initially. However, increasing experience and greater attention to minor details have been rewarded with better results in about 80% of the patients. In the remaining patients, about

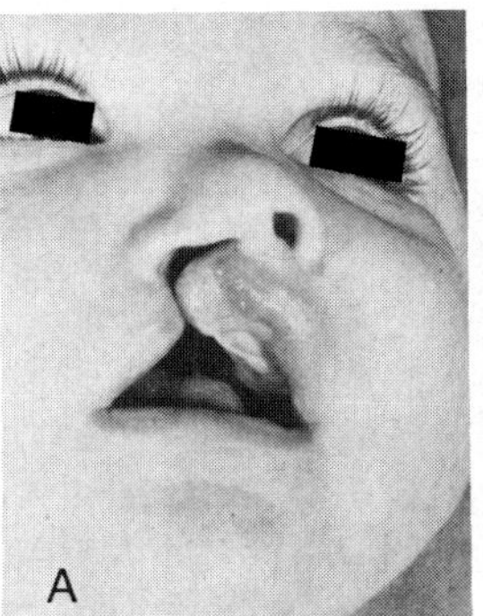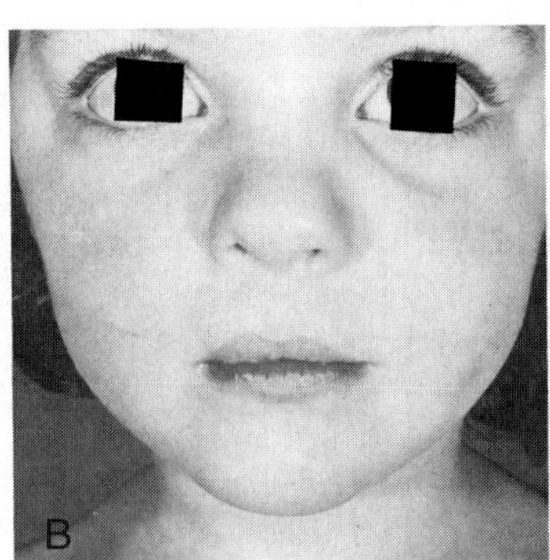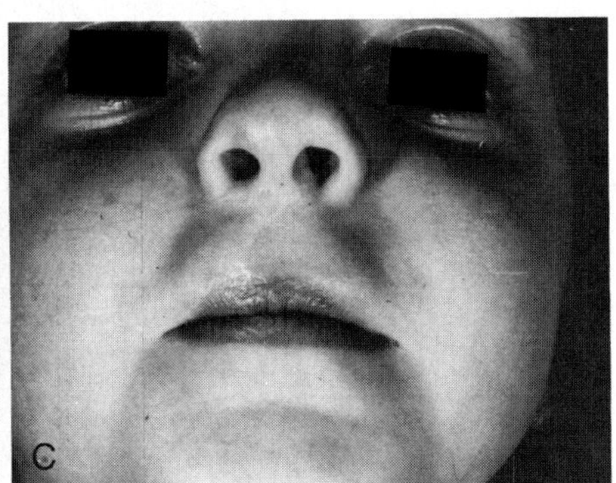

Figure 24–18 *A,* Before operation. *B,* At 6 years of age. *C,* At 7 years. Note the philtrum and the dimple.

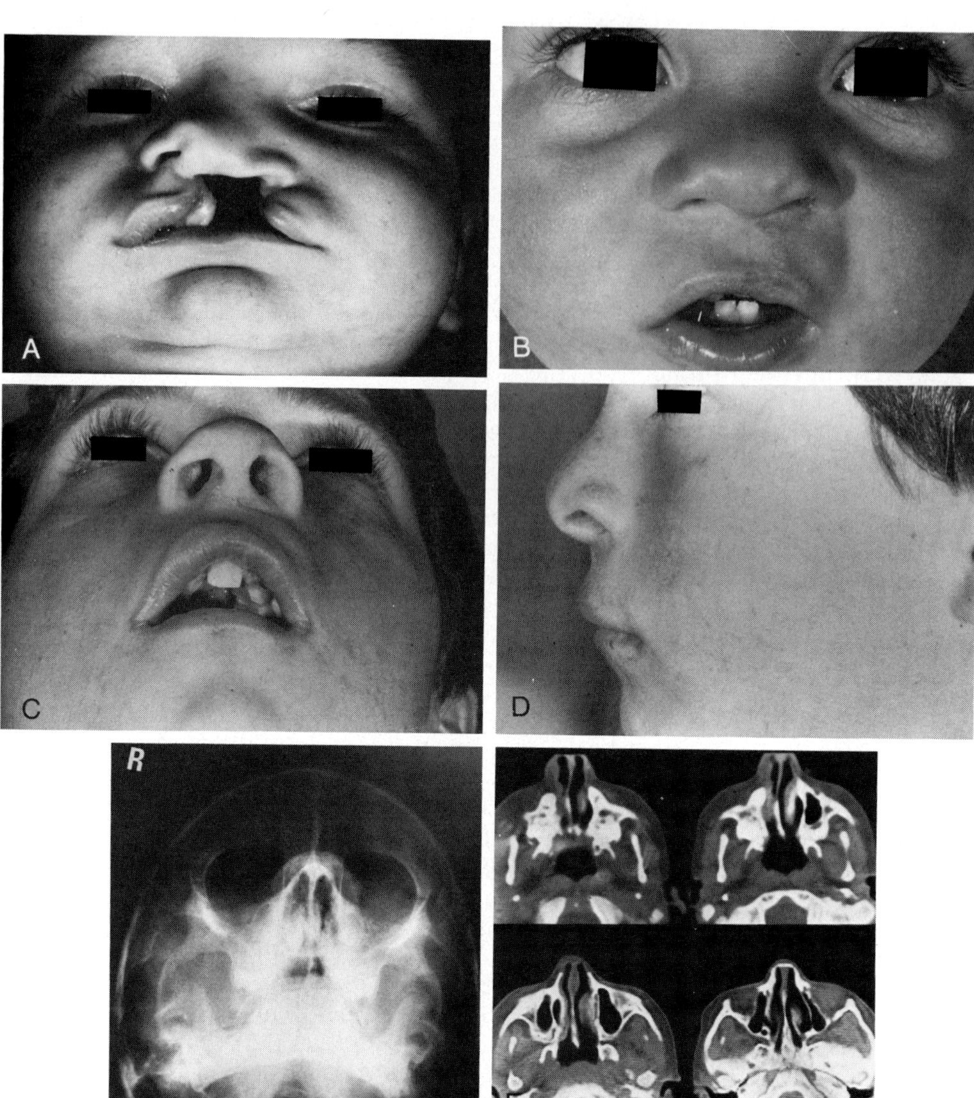

Figure 24–19 *A*, Before surgery. *B*, At 2½ years of age. *C*, At 10 years. *D*, Profile view. *E* and *F*, X-ray and CT scan showing fairly normal contours of bony structures.

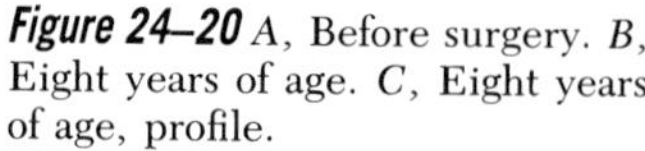

Figure 24–20 *A*, Before surgery. *B*, Eight years of age. *C*, Eight years of age, profile.

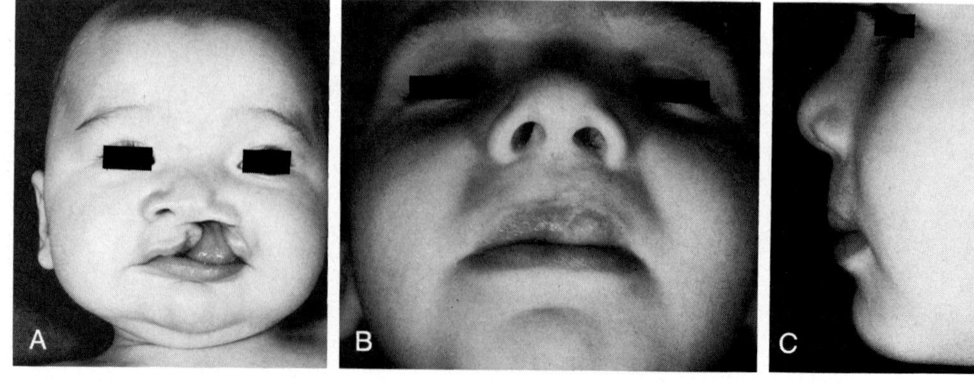

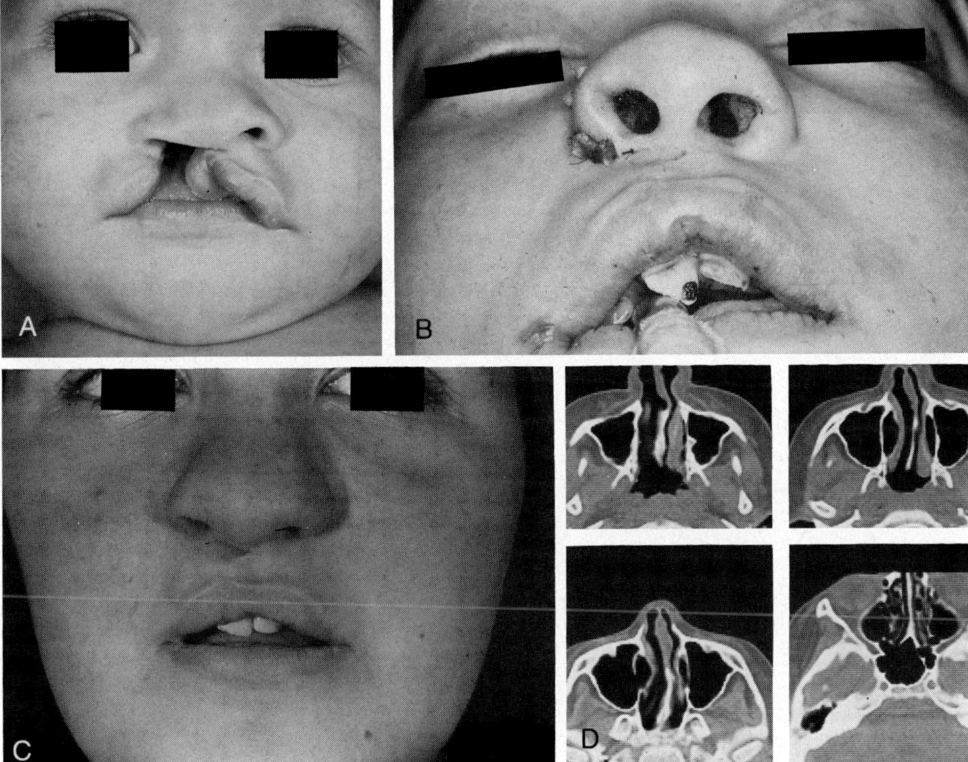

Figure 24–21 *A*, Before surgery. *B*, At 12 years of age after removal of submucosal connective tissue from the right ala. *C*, At 17 years. *D*, CT scan showing slightly curved septum and symmetric development of alar base.

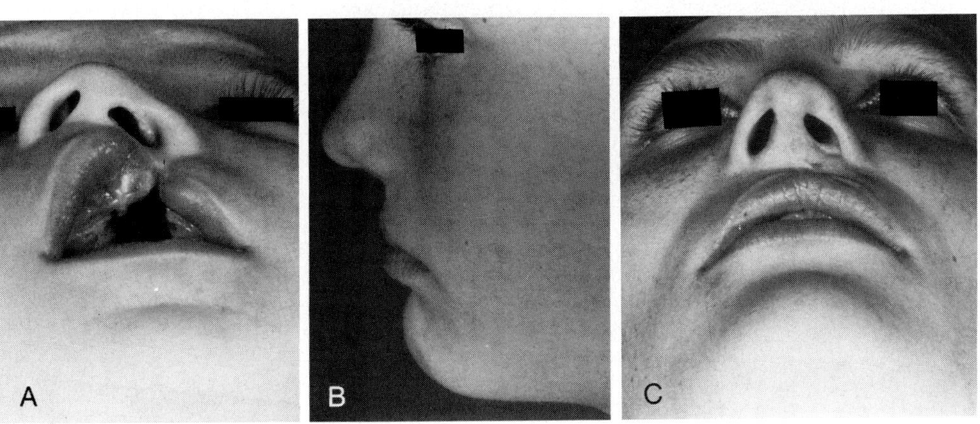

Figure 24–22 *A*, Before surgery. *B*, Profile view. *C*, 18 years of age. Note the thin configuration of the left alar rim.

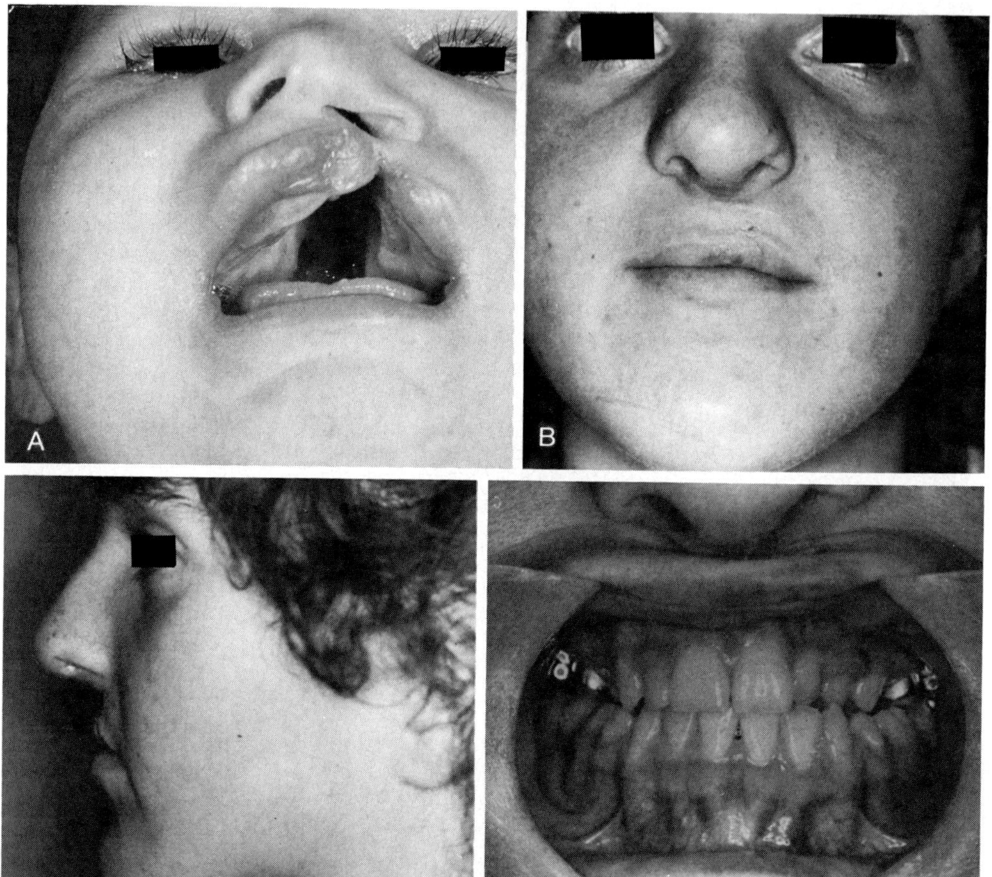

Figure 24–23 A, Before surgery. B, At the age of 18. C, Profile view. D, Dental occlusion. Good symmetry of the nostrils is evident.

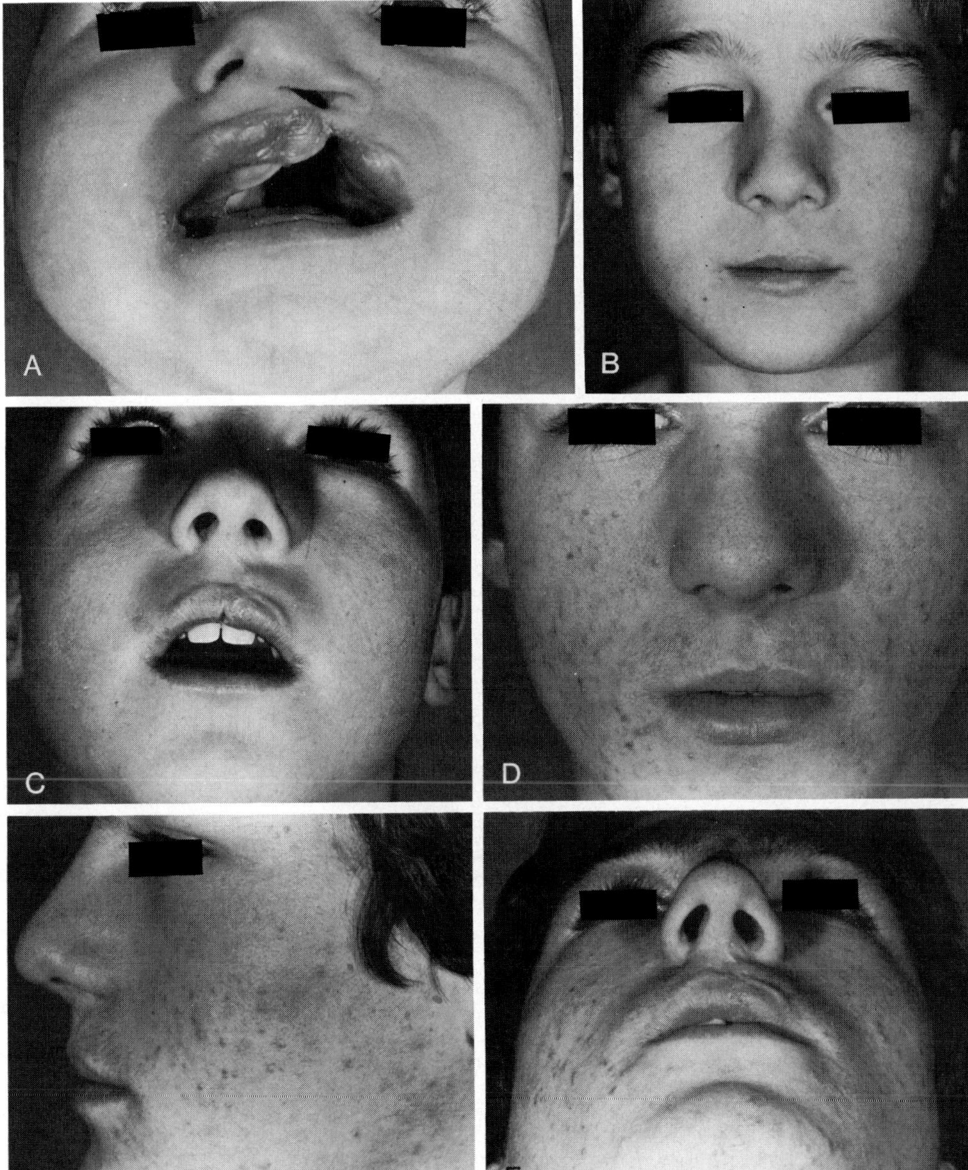

Figure 24–24 *A*, Before surgery. *B* and *C*, At 14 years of age. *D–F*, At 18 years of age.

50% have a slight asymmetry in the shape and circumference of the nostrils. This may be caused by severe deformity of the alar cartilage or, more frequently, when the asymmetry is in the circumference, by poor adjustment of the triangular C-flap to the alar base, resulting in nostrils that are either too wide or too narrow (Fig. 24–25). The impression of an abnormally narrow nostril or nose entrance can also be caused by submucosal abundance of connective tissue, which must be removed in a second operation.

In some severe deformities, the septum and even the bony nose show a tendency toward recurrent deviation even though the tip of the nose remains normal. This recurrent deformity does not become obvious until later in life, although it usually starts to develop gradually soon after primary surgery. The degree of this deviation cannot be compared with that in noses in which primary correction has not been attempted. About 3% of our patients show severe recurrent deviation of the nose and septum for reasons that we cannot explain.

In regard to the very important question of whether we could find *any growth impairment* in the nasal structure due to this kind of surgery, we are able to say that none of these patients exhibited such a retardation. The described shortcomings in the nose have been caused by technical errors, not by predictible alterations during growth. The structures of the cleft nose in all these cases correspond to the amount of tissue on the normal side as documented by x-ray and CT scan (Fig. 24–19).

In the great majority of our patients, there was symmetry of the alar bases, demonstrating corrected bone structure under the soft tissue as well as bone formation on x-rays and on CT scan. The histologic findings in the thickened new bone could not be differentiated from those in bone of the maxilla. The mobili-

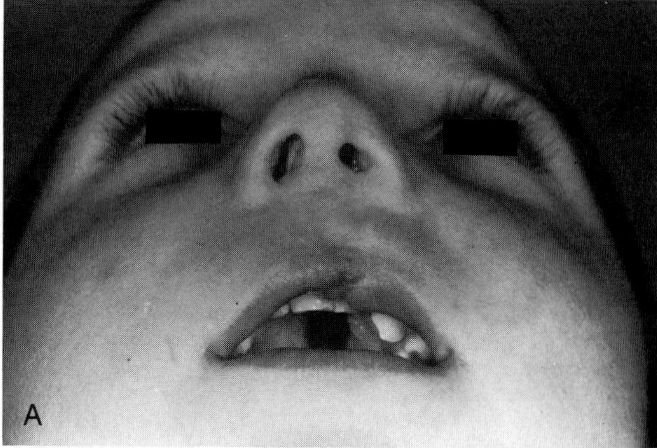

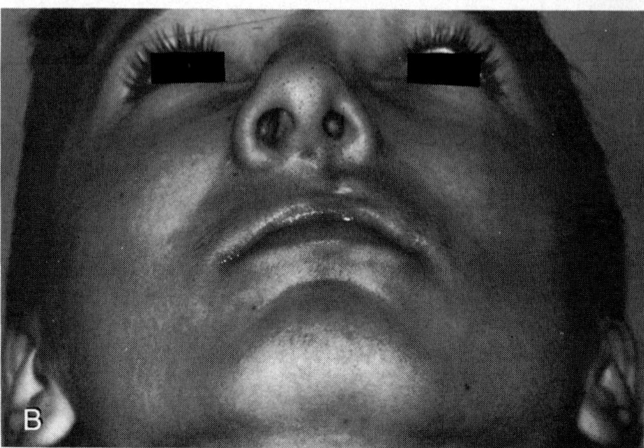

Figure 24–25 A, Small nostril at 2 years of age. *B,* At 14 years of age. Nose developed good nasal tip, but nostril remained small.

zation of the tight mucoperiosteum in the frontal curved part of the septum did not retard development of the nose, especially in regard to height.

In summary, I want to emphasize that simultaneous primary repair of cleft lip and nose by wide undermining and repositioning of all dislocated structures, together with induction of bone growth in hypoplastic areas, led to very satisfactory results in the majority of patients. The wide undermining of all dislocated structures allowed optimal repair of the lip and nose in the majority of cases.

Our findings are based on follow-up studies performed on nearly 266 children operated on since 1970. No growth impairment was observed, justifying further application of this method.

References

1. Gelbke H: The nostril problem in unilateral harelips and its surgical management. Plast Reconstr Surg 18:65–76, 1956.
2. Blair VP: Nasal deformities associated with congenital clefts of lip. JAMA 84:125, 1925.
3. McIndoe A: Correction of alar deformity in cleft lip. Lancet 1:607–609, 1938.
4. McDowell F: Late results after long-term growth in cleft lip repairs. Plast Reconstr Surg 38:444, 1966.
5. Burian F: The Plastic Surgery Atlas. Vol 2. London: Butterworths, 1967, p 165.
6. Berkeley WT: The cleft lip nose. Plast Reconstr Surg 23:567–575, 1959.
7. Berkeley WT: Correction of the unilateral cleft lip nasal deformity. In Grabb WC, Rosensteins SW, Bzoch KR (eds): Cleft Lip and Palate. Boston: Little, Brown, 1971, pp 227–242.
8. Velasquez JM, Ortiz-Monasterio F: Primary simultaneous correction of the lip and nose in the unilateral cleft lip. Plast Reconstr Surg 54:558–561, 1974.
9. Randall P: Personal communication, 1978.
10. Skoog T: Repair of unilateral cleft lip deformity: Maxilla, nose, lip. Scand J Plast Reconstr Surg 3:109–133, 1969.
11. Millard RD: Cleft Craft: The Evolution of Its Surgery. Vol 1. The Unilateral Deformity. Boston: Little, Brown, 1976.
12. Millard RD: Earlier correction of the unilateral cleft lip nose. Plast Reconstr Surg 70:64, 1982.
13. Salyer K: Primary correction of the unilateral cleft lip nose. A 15-year experience. Plast Reconstr Surg 77:556–566, 1986.
14. McComb H: Treatment of the unilateral cleft lip nose. Plast Reconstr Surg 55:596–601, 1975.
15. McComb H: Primary correction of unilateral cleft lip nasal deformity. A 10 year review. Plast Reconstr Surg 75:791, 1985.
16. Pigott R: Personal communication, 1978.
17. Anderl H: Zur Mobilisierung beim Lippenverschluß der einseitigen Lippen- und Kieferspalte. Acta Chir Austriaca 5:172–174, 1970.
18. Anderl H: Extensive primary nose repair in unilateral cleft lip. Abstracts of the Third International Congress on Cleft Palate and Related Craniofacial Anomalies, Toronto, No. 150, 1977.
19. Anderl H: Primare Formung der Lippe und Nase bei Spaltbildungen. Kongreßband der 22. Tagung der Osterreichische. Gesellschaft für Chirurgie, Linz, 1981, pp 129–130.
20. Anderl H: Simultaneous repair of lip and nose in the unilateral cleft (a long term report). In Jackson IT, Sommerlad BC (eds): Recent Advances in Plastic Surgery. Edinburgh: Churchill Livingstone, 1985.
21. Jackson I: Personal communication, 1981.
22. Hogan VM, Converse JM: Secondary deformities of unilateral cleft lip and nose. In Crabb WC, Rosenstein SE, Bzoch KR (eds): Cleft Lip and Palate. Boston: Little, Brown, 1971.
23. Cohen J, Lacroix P: Bone and cartilage formation by periosteum. J Bone Joint Surg 37A:717, 1955.
24. Skoog T: The use of periosteum and "Surgicel" for bone restoration in congenital clefts of maxila. Scand J Plast Reconstr Surg 1:113, 1967.
25. Finley J, Acland R, Wood M: Revascularized periosteal grafts—a new method to produce functional new bone without bone grafting. Plast Reconstr Surg 61:1–6, 1978.

CHAPTER 25

Primary Unilateral and Bilateral Cleft Lip Nose Reconstruction

Harold McComb

Unilateral Cleft Lip Nose

When improved methods of primary lip repair were developed, attempts were made also to correct the associated nasal deformity, but the long-term results were generally disappointing. A wide range of procedures has been described, including freeing and mobilizing the slumped alar cartilage using releasing incisions within the nostril, use of external nasal incisions, and a combination of both.[1-12] Millard corrected the nostril rim by excising a crescent of tissue from the nostril margin.[13] Longacre believed that primary correction could be achieved by simply building up the base of the nostril by implanting a rib graft.[14]

The unsatisfactory results that followed primary correction of the nasal deformity were probably due to three factors. First, caudal rotation of the alar cartilage was not recognized as a fundamental feature of the deformity. This element was responsible for the drooping nostril rim, the oblique ridge within the vestibule, and flaring of the nostril margin. Initial attempts at nasal repair were directed mainly toward the buckling and distortion of the nostril wall that occurred when the floor of the nose was closed. Attempts were also made to reestablish the nasal tip by moving the slumped alar dome medially and forward but not necessarily upward.

The second factor in failure of nasal repair was scarring, particularly of the nasal lining, that was created at the time of nasal repair. Although it has been suggested that early surgery on the infant nose alters the growth of the nasal cartilage, no specific documentation of this interference has been published.[15] On the contrary, many surgeons have observed that there is no alteration in growth of the cartilage following early surgery, although tissues can be displaced and deformed by contraction of scar tissue.[7, 12, 16-23] Circumferential scars in the lining of an infant's nose have a marked tendency to contract and cause stenosis. The intercartilaginous and paramarginal incisions that were widely used in early attempts at primary repair of the cleft lip nose probably produced significant stenosis and deformity.

The third factor contributing to unsatisfactory results in primary repair of the cleft lip nose was the relatively significant change in size and shape of the nose that occurred during growth spurts, particularly at adolescence. Unless perfect lifting and repositioning of the alar cartilage is achieved at the initial operation, subsequent growth magnifies any small discrepancy. The cleft lip nasal stigma then reappears to a greater or lesser degree.

Therefore, there are three criteria for successful primary correction of cleft lip nasal deformity:

1. Lifting and replacement of the alar cartilage into a symmetric position.
2. Avoidance of scarring within the nostril lining.
3. Accuracy in the initial repair.

Downward rotation of the alar cartilage on the cleft side was first described in 1961 by Stenstrom and Oberg, who published a method of lifting the alar cartilage in secondary correction of the cleft lip nose.[24, 25] Reynolds and Horton subsequently also described an alar lift procedure in secondary cleft lip rhinoplasty.[26]

Skoog, in 1969, first reported incorporation of an alar lift in primary repair of the cleft lip nose.[27] He used an intercartilaginous incision and moved the alar cartilage medially and upward, where it was sutured in a position overlapping the anterior surface of the lower part of the upper lateral cartilage. Skoog reported a tendency for the deformity to relapse, presumably because of contraction of the scar in the nasal lining. He tried to combat this with a nostril stent. A number of recently published papers show that careful, early primary surgery of the unilateral cleft lip nose can correct the deformity in the longer term while causing no interference with growth.[11, 12, 16-21, 27-32]

Documentation of these procedures, however, is still incomplete. Results from only two groups of consecutive but otherwise unselected patients have been published.[20, 21] These results were presented 10 years following primary repair of the nasal deformity in patients with unilateral and bilateral clefts. We are awaiting final evaluation of the average samples of patients who are fully grown.

In 1985, McComb published a 10-year follow-up of primary nasal repair in patients with unilateral clefts.[20] He used presurgical orthopedic treatment to realign the skeletal base and a hemirhinoplasty at the time of lip repair to shorten the nose on the cleft side. No incisions were made in the nasal lining. During the same year, Anderl published results of his experience with primary correction of the cleft lip nose during a period of 14 years.[17] After wide undermining, he returned all the dislocated structures, including the anterior cartilaginous septum, to their normal positions. The alar cartilage was lifted, and no incisions were made in the nasal lining. Bone growth was stimulated beneath the alar base.

Piggott radically mobilized the alar cartilage with an "alar leap-frog" technique to reposition the cartilage at the time of lip repair.[18] This technique involved the use of both external and internal nasal incisions. Some problems were reported with scar stenosis of the nostril. In 1986, Salyer published results of his 14 years of experience with primary correction of the unilateral cleft lip nose.[19] He used presurgical orthopedic treatment and repositioned the lateral crus of the alar cartilage after wide undermining. He made no incisions in the nasal lining.

None of these authors found that early primary surgery had adverse effects on growth of the nose. More harm is probably done by failing to correct the initial deformity. If the nostril floor is repaired while the alar cartilage remains in a slumped, retroposed position, the circumference of the nostril lining is shortened in a transverse direction. This tethers and fixes the alar cartilage in a deformed manner, making secondary correction difficult.

Surgical Procedure

The first step in primary correction of the cleft lip nose is preparation of a symmetric bony platform by means of presurgical orthopedic treatment. This process aligns the maxillary segments and reduces the displacement of the nasal septum. Surgical correction essentially consists in a hemirhinoplasty to reposition the displaced alar cartilage. This procedure is performed at the start of the repair to place the nasal structures in their correct position before the lip is closed. This sequence is important. The alar cartilage, together with the attached nasal lining, is lifted to re-create the vault of the vestibule and obliterate the vestibular ridge. This procedure establishes the full circumference of the nasal lining of the nostril at the start of the repair.

The following method of primary nasal correction can be combined with any type of lip repair. When the lip incisions are being marked, a flap is designed that can be turned to build up the nostril sill. In a rotation-advancement repair, this is achieved with a C-flap. In other forms of lip repair, an alar-based flap is used.

No incisions are made in the nasal lining. The nasal skin on the side of the cleft is elevated completely beginning from the nostril rim below and continuing over the nasal tip and up to the nasion above. Complete elevation is essential to allow contraction and shortening of the lengthened skin on the cleft side of the nose. This lengthening occurs particularly at the junction of the nasal cartilages, where the upper border of the alar cartilage has slipped down off the lower border of the upper lateral cartilage.

Sharp-pointed scissors are introduced through the upper buccal sulcus, deep to the base of the nostril (Fig. 25–1). The alar base is separated from its attachment near the margin of the piriform aperture, and scissor dissection continues over the subcutaneous surface of the alar cartilage, over the dome of the opposite alar cartilage, and over the remainder of the nasal skeleton on the side of the cleft. No incisions are made in the nasal lining. Scissors are also introduced through the upper buccal sulcus in the region of the anterior nasal spine; dissection continues over the subcutaneous surface of the columellar crura and joins the area of dissection over the nasal tip. The nasal lining is dissected from the lower part of the cartilaginous septum and from the lateral wall of the nose in the region of the piriform aperture.

When the dissection is complete, the alar cartilage and the nasal lining can be lifted easily. The alar cartilage can be rotated upward and forward, raising the nostril rim and forming the vault of the vestibule while obliterating the vestibular fold. The infundibulum is reestablished, and the upper edge of the alar cartilage is

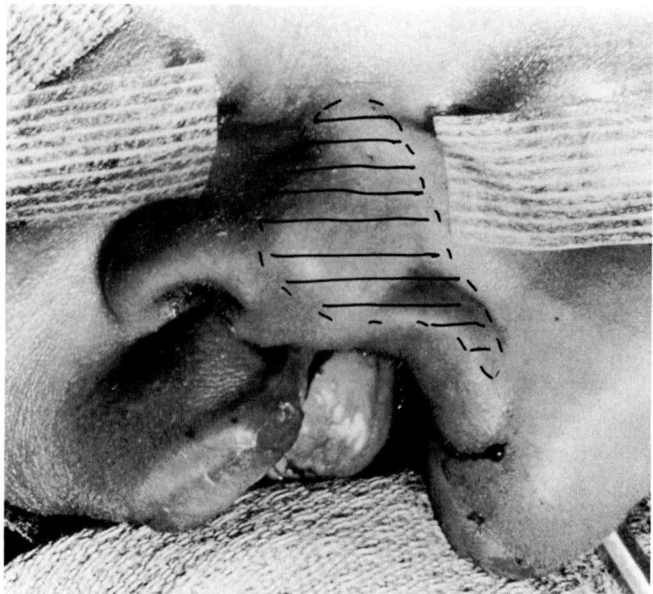

Figure 25–1 The skin of the nose on the side of the cleft is widely undermined from the nostril rim to the nasion by scissors introduced through the incisions in the upper buccal sulcus. The shading indicates the area of undermining.

positioned above and superficial to the lower part of the upper lateral cartilage.

At the completion of the lip dissection, the first sutures that are placed in the repair are long, elevating mattress sutures of 5–0 silk that will lift the alar cartilage and establish the correct position of the nasal lining before the nasal floor is closed. It is essential that the position of the alar cartilage be adjusted at the start of the repair (Fig. 25–2).

The site of the alar dome is selected by the points of forceps, which lift the alar cartilage from within the vestibule. The first lifting mattress suture is inserted at this position. It is introduced on straight needles that pass through the lining and the alar dome, then enter the dissected subcutaneous space and pass upward and slightly medially through it to emerge in the region of the nasion. A second elevating suture is also passed through the lateral crus of the alar cartilage, emerging on the upper part of the nasal bridge. These sutures are looped around small bolsters that round out the nasal vestibule. Gentle traction on the sutures lifts the alar cartilage to its correct position, and the nose immediately loses the typical cleft lip appearance. The nostril rim is on the same level as that on the opposite side, and the vestibular vault is established. The nasal floor is repaired with the alar cartilage in its correct position. The nostril sill is built up with local flaps. Sound muscle union is established beneath the nasal floor.

It is unusual for the elevating mattress sutures to lie in their correct position at the completion of the repair. Some notching or irregularity of the nostril margin may have become evident, and the nasal tip and nostril rim will probably not be positioned perfectly. It is almost always necessary to remove and replace the elevating sutures at the end of the operation to realign their position and direction. Finally, these long sutures are

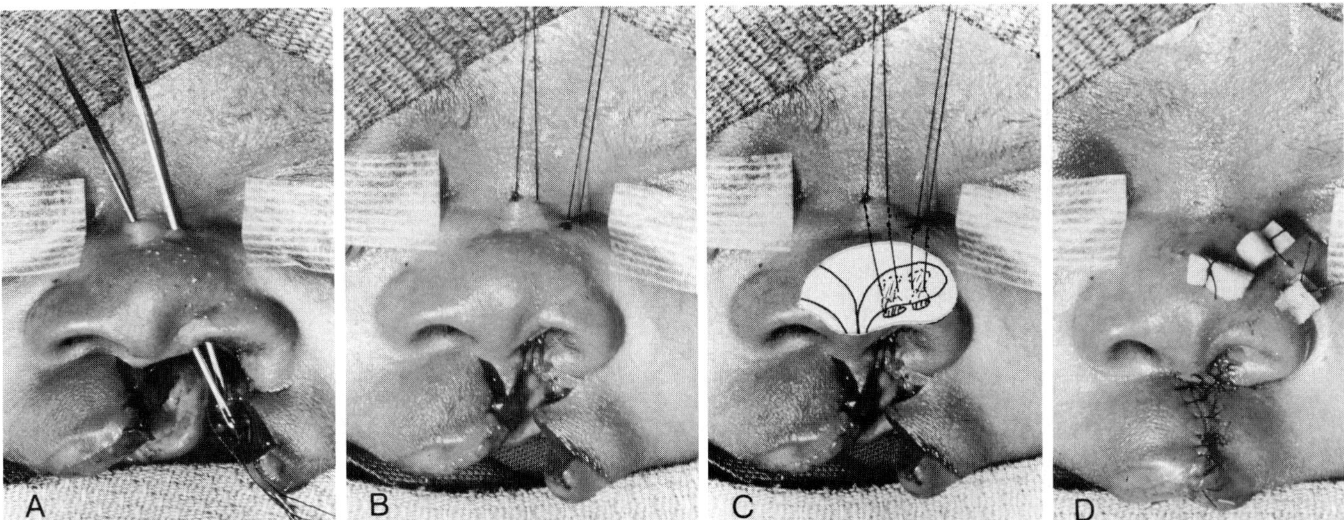

Figure 25–2 *A*, Elevating sutures are introduced through the alar dome. They pass subcutaneously upward and emerge at the nasion. *B*, Gentle traction raises the alar cartilage and lifts the nostril rim. *C*, Cutaway diagram shows the position of the lifting sutures, which pass around bolsters that round out the vestibule. *D*, The first lifting sutures are usually replaced at the completion of the operation and are tied over small bolsters.

tied over bolsters in the region of the nasion, and one or two lateral mattress sutures are inserted through the wall of the nose to obliterate the potential dead space (Fig. 25–3). One of these sutures is placed in the lateral sulcus at the base of the nostril. Although it is important that the nostril rims be at the same level on both sides, slight overcorrection is acceptable. Any mild, residual discrepancy will be accentuated by later growth of the nose.

The cartilaginous nasal septum is not dissected and realigned at the time of lip repair. Significant displacement of the anterior septum is considerably reduced by presurgical orthopedic treatment. The nasal sutures are removed with the final lip sutures on the fifth postoperative day. The covering skin has then shortened and healed, and the alar cartilage is fixed in its correct position. There has been no interference with growth following this procedure, and the position of the nasal tip and alar cartilages has been maintained (Fig. 25–4).

The cardinal points in primary correction of the unilateral cleft lip nose are presurgical alignment of the skeletal base; wide undermining of the skin on the cleft side of the nose; initial lifting and correction of the displaced alar cartilage as the first step in the surgical repair; and removal, replacement, and realignment of the long, elevating sutures at the end of the operation.

Bilateral Cleft Lip Nose

Repair of the bilateral cleft lip nose remains a difficult, unsolved problem. Although the prolabium is embryologically part of the lip, it is usually used in a convenient compromise to reconstruct the short columella. How-

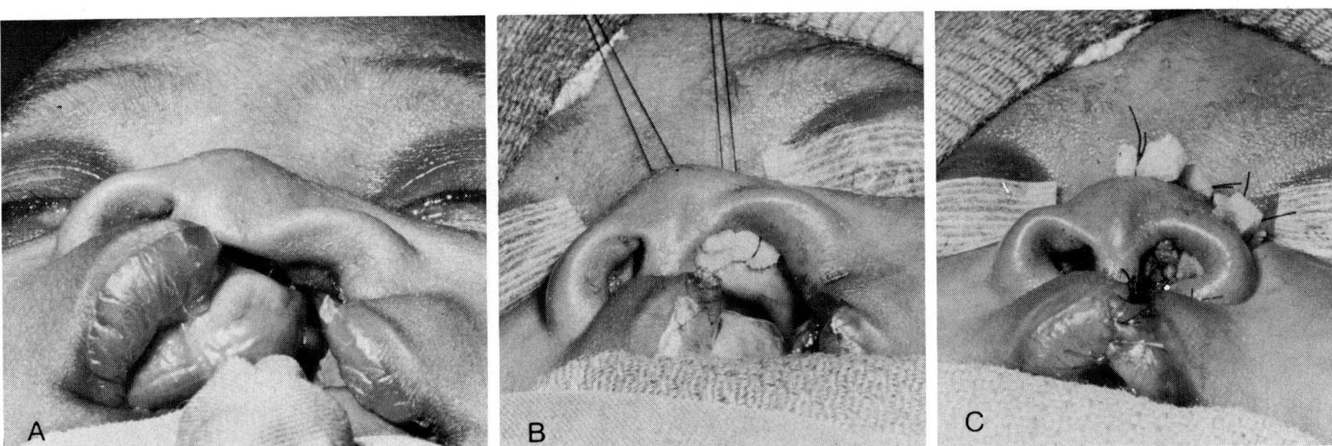

Figure 25–3 *A*, The alar cartilage is slumped and the nostril rim is concave. *B*, The long lifting sutures are the first sutures that are placed in the repair. They lift the nostril and round out the vestibule. *C*, The lifting sutures are looped around bolsters inside the nose and are tied over bolsters on the outside.

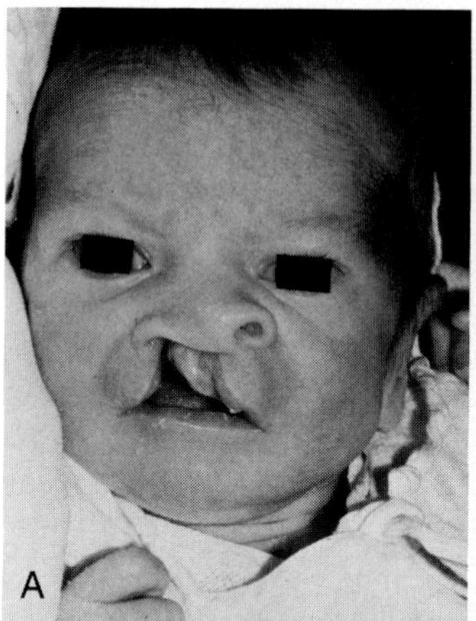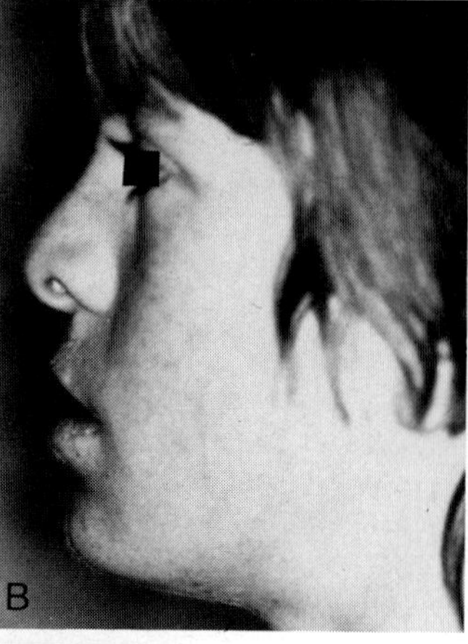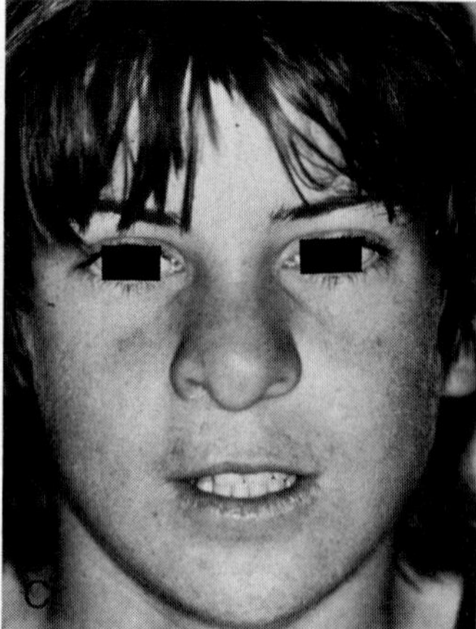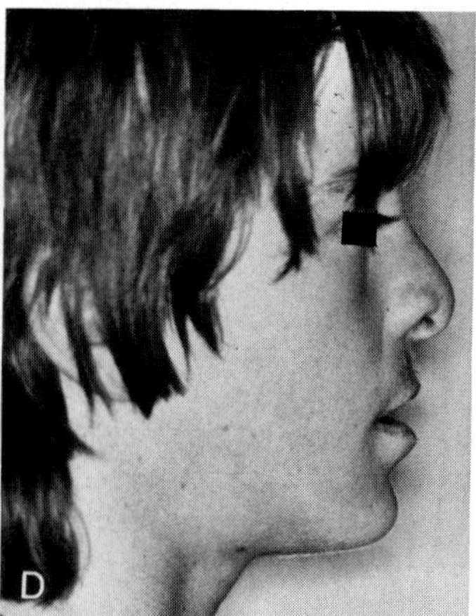

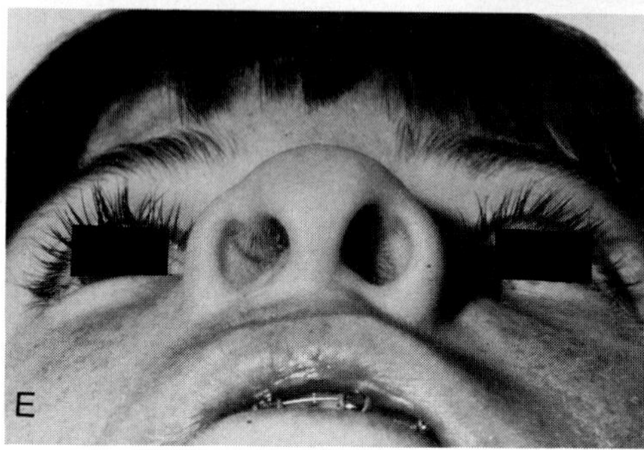

Figure 25–4 A–E, The first child who was treated by this alar lift procedure is now 15 years old. The initial correction has been maintained, and there has been no interference with growth.

ever, nasal dissections in patients with bilateral clefts have demonstrated wide separation of the alar cartilages in the nasal tip. The alar domes and the medial crura are pulled apart with consequent shortening of the columella back toward its base, where it joins the prolabium. The columellar tissues lie in the broad nasal tip. Probably the columella should be lengthened by rearrangement of the nasal tip tissues, reuniting the splayed columellar crura and joining the separated alar domes.

Morel-Fatio and Lalardrie described secondary lengthening of the columella using tissues from the nasal tip, but this procedure carries a penalty of external scarring in older patients.[33] Better scars could be expected, however, if the columella were lengthened from the nasal tip in infancy. If the columella could be reconstructed without incisions across its base and with the bony attachment of the lip-columella angle undisturbed, the blood supply of the prolabium would remain intact. This would permit simultaneous reconstruction of the columella from the nasal tip, adjustment of the alar cartilages, and repair of the bilateral cleft lip in a single stage.

Broadbent and Woolf have described primary repair of the bilateral cleft lip nose by medial advancement of the alar cartilages using intercartilaginous incisions combined with excision of the excess skin of the nasal tip.[16] They presented one patient who had been evaluated at 12 months of age.

The technical difficulty of closing wide, distorted, bilateral clefts of the lip has discouraged simultaneous correction of the associated nasal deformity. The usual plan of treatment has been to repair the lip and then release the nasal tip by reconstruction of the columella at about 3 years of age. Two-staged methods of primary repair of the bilateral cleft lip nose have been described in which closure of each lip cleft is accompanied by partial lengthening of the columella.[34, 35]

Millard described a primary forked flap for reconstructing the columella at the time of lip repair.[36, 37] However, the central prolabial element was left attached to the premaxilla, which provided its blood supply. It was therefore not possible to join the lateral mucomuscular lip flaps behind the prolabium when the lip was closed. Subsequently, a method of "banking" forked flaps was described,[38, 39] and primary columella reconstruction at the time of lip adhesion was also reported.[40–42]

In these procedures, attention was directed toward lengthening the columella at the time of, or soon after, repair of the cleft lip. However, none of the authors described the second basic fault in the bilateral cleft lip nose—namely, caudal rotation of the alar cartilages. If this is not corrected at the time of lip repair, irregularity of the nostril margins persists, together with the oblique folds within the vestibules. Noordhoff elevates the alar cartilages when the lip is repaired and subsequently lengthens the columella when the child is between 1 and 6 years of age.[43]

Stenstrom reported secondary repair of the bilateral cleft lip nasal deformity by lifting the alar cartilages after preliminary lengthening of the columella.[25] A short columella usually tethers the cartilages in caudal rotation, and it is necessary to release them by lengthening the columella before the lip and nose are repaired simultaneously.

In 1975, McComb described a method of primary

repair of the bilateral cleft lip nose in which the alar cartilages are lifted at the time of lip repair, after initial release of the nasal tip by preliminary columella lengthening using a forked flap.[30] The bilateral cleft is no exception to the rule that tissues should be placed in their normal positions before a defect is repaired. The bony platform is realigned, the nasal tip is separated from the lip by reconstructing the columella, and the alar cartilages are lifted before the clefts are closed and repaired.

Although this procedure has greatly improved the results of primary repair of the bilateral cleft deformity, it is nevertheless based on the convenient compromise of using tissue from the prolabium to lengthen the columella. The alar domes remain separated in the nasal tip, often producing a noticeably broad tip in many patients. Also, the attachment of the lip-columellar angle in the region of the anterior nasal spine is transgressed. This sometimes results in caudal drift of the base of the reconstructed columella.

Surgical Procedure

The first step in primary correction of the bilateral cleft lip nose is alignment of the bony platform by presurgical orthopedic treatment. The prominence of the premaxilla is reduced, and any twisting is corrected. Reduction of the premaxilla permits simultaneous repair of the lip clefts and incorporation of the prolabium, which has already been narrowed by migration of a forked flap into the columella.

There are two basic defects in the bilateral cleft lip nose. First, both alar cartilages are rotated caudally downward. Second, the medial crura of the alar cartilages are pulled apart, causing shortening of the columella toward its base. If the lip is repaired with the alar cartilages in downward rotation, the nostril rims droop, and oblique ridges persist within the nostrils. Twisting of the alar cartilages creates a compound curve that is responsible for the typical nostril flare. The nasal tip is flat and broad.

When the columella is subsequently lengthened as a secondary procedure, the alar cartilages remain in cau-

dal rotation because they are tethered by the attachment of the shortened nostril lining. The irregular nostril margins and the oblique vestibular ridges remain as a persisting deformity. In many patients, the broad nasal tip and nostril flare also persist after secondary lengthening of the columella.

Surgical treatment requires two stages. In the first stage, the columella is lengthened to release the nasal tip and permit subsequent elevation of the alar cartilages. Six weeks later, simultaneous repair of the lip and nose is performed.

Examination of 220 Caucasian children showed that the columella in an infant's nose is 5 to 5.5 mm in length, the distance being measured from the base of the columella to the level of the intercrural angles of the nostrils. There was no difference between males and females. Growth of the columella does not start until the child is about 18 months old.

In healthy infants, primary reconstruction of the columella is performed at 6 weeks of age using a forked flap of skin with a posterior margin of mucosa taken from the edges of the prolabium. The mucosal incision is extended up the membranous septum to allow advancement of the flap into the columella. The forks of the flaps are quadrangular in shape with pointed tips. Furthermore, they must be reasonably bulky to avoid creation of a retracted columella (Fig. 25–5). The flaps are lifted completely out of the prolabium, and their apices are carefully fixed together with a deep suture that also passes through the tissues in the region of the anterior nasal spine. This is done to avoid any later tendency for the columellar base to drift down into the prolabium.

The elastic strapping across the prolabium, which is used in presurgical orthopedic treatment, is discontinued during the phase of columellar reconstruction and healing. During this time, the premaxilla is held in its reduced position by an extension that is added to the sucking plate. As soon as the prolabium is healed, pressure from the elastic strapping is resumed. To some extent, this expands the tissues of the prolabium that have been narrowed by formation of the forked flap.

Six weeks after lengthening of the columella, simul-

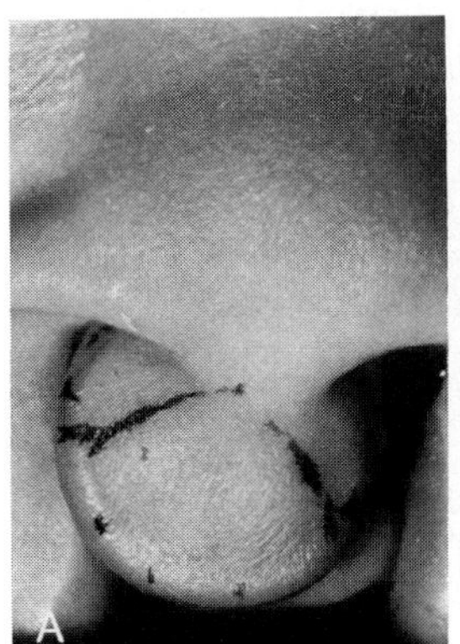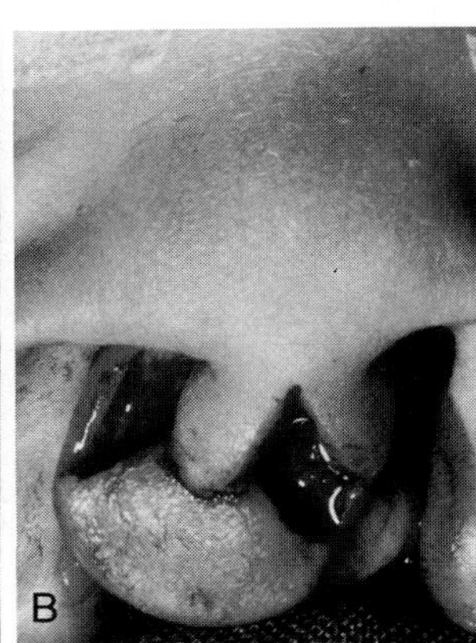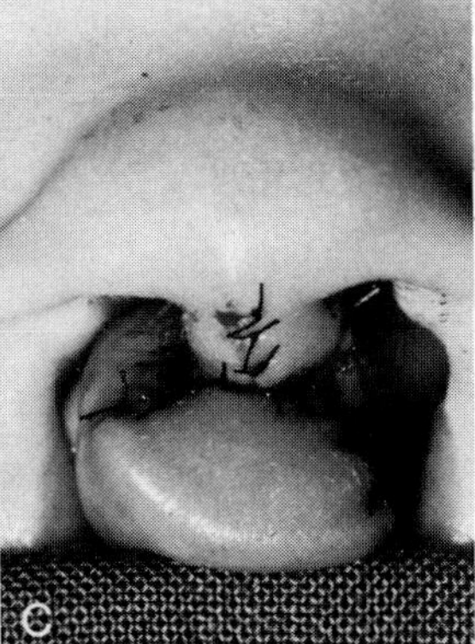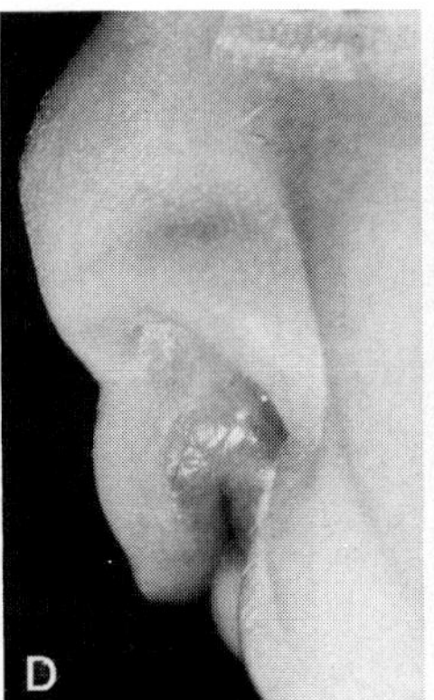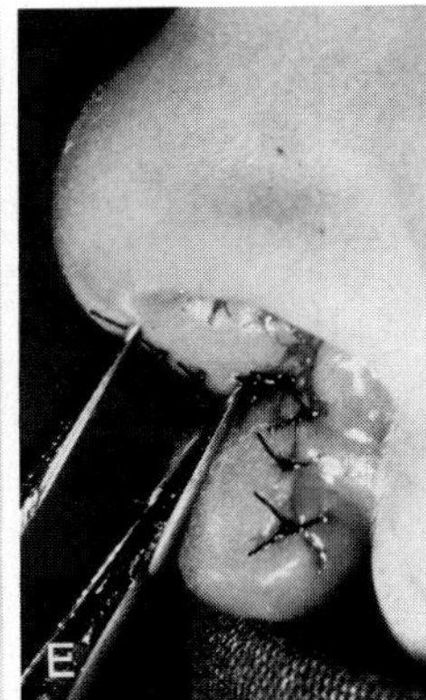

Figure 25–5 *A,* A forked flap of skin with a posterior margin of mucosa is taken from the sides of the prolabium. *B,* The flap is dissected free. *C,* The apices of the flaps are fixed in the region of the anterior nasal spine. *D,* The columella is lengthened to 5 mm measured from its base to the level of the intercrural angles of the nostrils.

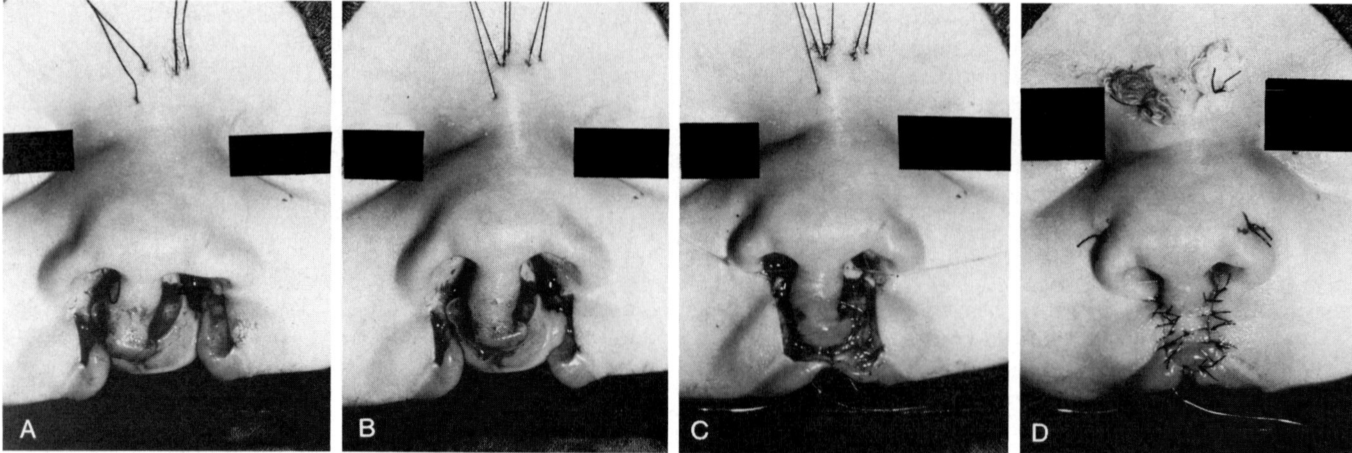

Figure 25–6 *A,* At the completion of the dissection, the first sutures placed in the repair are the long, elevating mattress sutures. *B,* Gentle traction of the sutures elevates both alar cartilages. *C,* The nostril floors are repaired with the alar cartilages in their reduced, elevated position. *D,* Lateral mattress sutures are added at the completion of the repair to obliterate the dead space.

taneous repair of the lip and nasal deformity is performed. The child is usually 3 months old at this time. The lip is repaired using a modified Manchester technique.[44] A central segment that is approximately the width of the philtrum is marked on the prolabium. Alar base flaps are also marked for construction of the nostril sills (Fig. 25–6).

The prolabial tissue is carefully dissected from the premaxilla, proceeding just far enough superiorly to allow the mucomuscular flaps, which contain the orbicularis oris muscles in the lateral lip elements, to be joined behind the prolabial philtrum in the midline. Although scars from the recently constructed columella are present across the base of the prolabium, there has

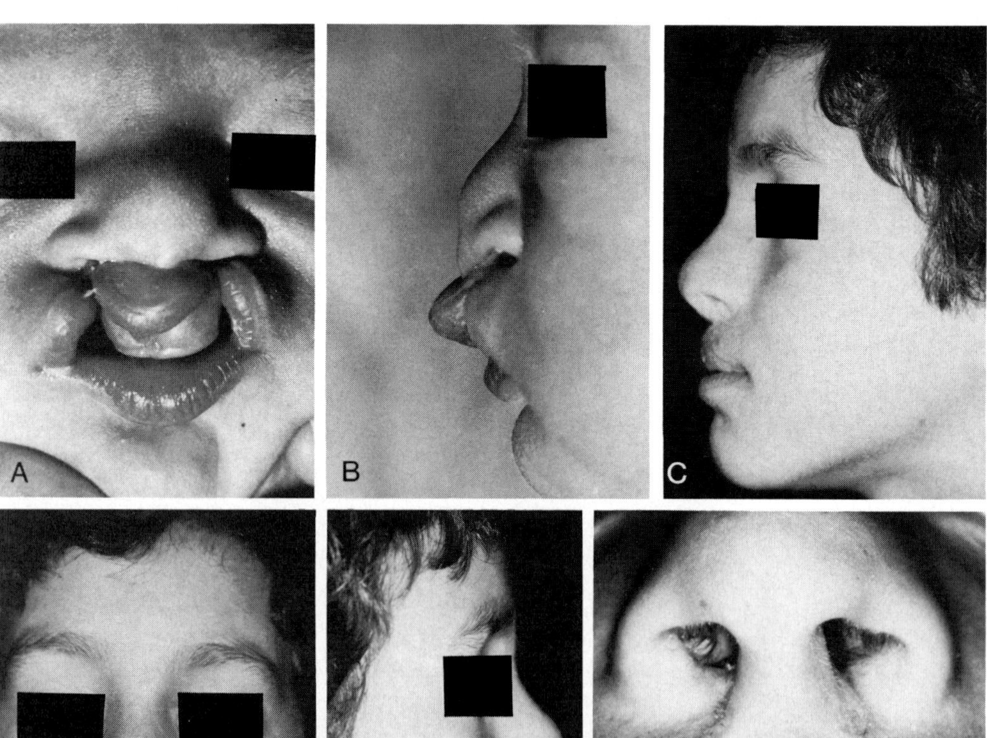

Figure 25–7 *A, B,* Infant with bilateral cleft of the lip, alveolus, and palate. *C, D,* and *E,* The same patient at 11 years of age following primary repair of bilateral cleft lip nose.

been no loss of tissue in the central segment. At the completion of the repair, tension across the lip may cause the philtral segment to become pale or dusky blue, depending on the vascular input, but this change clears quite quickly.

The nasal repair essentially involves correcting the caudal displacement of the alar cartilage, as in primary correction of the unilateral cleft lip nose. The nostril rims are lifted, and the vaults of the vestibules are established without shortage of lining, before the nostril floors are repaired. The nasal skin is completely elevated from both sides of the nose and over the nasal tip, extending from the nostril rims below to the nasion above. No dissection is performed in the region of the reconstructed columella, and no incisions are made in the nostril linings.

Both alar cartilages are lifted by one or more long, elevating mattress sutures on each side. As in the unilateral cleft, these are the first sutures placed in the repair, and they establish the position of the alar cartilages and nasal lining before the nasal floors are closed. At the completion of the operation, it is unusual to find the elevating sutures lying in an optimal position. There may be some kinking or irregularity of the nostril margins. The long sutures almost always are removed, repositioned, and realigned at the end of the operation.

Finally, the ends of the sutures are tied over small bolsters to maintain the levels of the nostril rims. One or more lateral mattress sutures also are inserted to obliterate the dead space on each side of the nose; one is always placed in the lateral groove at the base of each nostril. The mattress sutures are removed with the final lip sutures on the fifth postoperative day.

This is not the final answer to the problem of the bilateral cleft lip nose. In many patients, the alar domes remain widely spaced and produce a broad nasal tip. There is also a significant tendency for the base of the reconstructed columella to drift caudally downward (Fig. 25–7). It is likely that future procedures used for primary correction of the bilateral cleft lip nose will include reconstruction of the columella from the spread-out elements in the nasal tip.

References

1. Blair VP, Brown JB: Mirault operation for single harelip. Surg Gynecol Obstet 51:81, 1930.
2. Brown JB, McDowell F: Simplified design for repair of single cleft lips. Surg Gynecol Obstet 80:12, 1945.
3. Brown JB, McDowell F: Small triangular flap operation for the primary repair of single cleft lips. Plast Reconstr Surg 5:392, 1950.
4. McIndoe AH: Correction of alar deformity in cleft lip. Lancet 1:607, 1948.
5. Steffensen WH: A method of repair of the unilateral cleft lip. Plast Reconstr Surg 4:144, 1949.
6. Davis AD: Management of the wide unilateral cleft lip with nostril deformity. Plast Reconstr Surg 8:249, 1951.
7. Lamont E: Plastic surgery in reconstructing the primary cleft lip and nasal deformity. Am J Surg 86:200, 1953.
8. Bauer TD, Trusler HM, Glanz S: Repair of unilateral cleft lip: Advantages of Le Mesurier technique use of mucous membrane flaps in maxillary clefts. Plast Reconstr Surg 11:56, 1953.
9. Brauer RO: A consideration of the Le Mesurier technique of single harelip repair with a new concept as to its use in incomplete and secondary harelip repairs. Plast Reconstr Surg 11:275, 1953.
10. Gelbke H: The nostril problem in unilateral harelips and its surgical management. Plast Reconstr Surg 18:65, 1956.
11. Berkeley WT: The cleft lip nose. Plast Reconstr Surg 23:567, 1959.
12. Berkeley WT: Correction of the unilateral cleft lip nasal deformity. In Grabb WC, Rosenstein SW, Bzoch KR (eds): Cleft Lip and Palate. Boston: Little, Brown, 1971.
13. Millard DR: The unilateral cleft lip nose. Plast Reconstr Surg 34:169, 1964.
14. Longacre JJ, Halak DB, Munick LH, et al: A new approach to the correction of the nasal deformity following cleft lip repair. Plast Reconstr Surg 38:555, 1966.
15. McIndoe A, Rees TD: Synchronous repair of secondary deformities in cleft lip and nose. Plast Reconstr Surg 24:150, 1959.
16. Broadbent TR, Woolf RM: Cleft lip nasal deformity. Ann Plast Surg 12:216, 1984.
17. Anderl H: Simultaneous repair of lip and nose in the unilateral cleft (a long-term report). In Jackson IT, Sommerlad BC (eds): Recent Advances in Plastic Surgery. Edinburgh: Churchill Livingstone, 1985.
18. Pigott RW: Alar leapfrog. Clin Plast Surg 12:643, 1985.
19. Salyer KE: Primary correction of the unilateral cleft lip nose: A 15-year experience. Plast Reconstr Surg 77:558, 1986.
20. McComb H: Primary correction of unilateral cleft lip nasal deformity: A ten-year review. Plast Reconstr Surg 75:791, 1985.
21. McComb H: Primary repair of the bilateral cleft lip nose. Br J Plast Surg 28:262, 1975.
22. Ortiz-Monasterio F, Olmedo A: Corrective rhinoplasty before puberty: A long-term follow-up. Plast Reconstr Surg 68:381, 1981.
23. Stenstrom SJ: Follow-up clinic: The alar cartilages and nasal deformity in unilateral cleft lip. Plast Reconstr Surg 55:359, 1975.
24. Stenstrom SJ, Oberg T: The nasal deformity in unilateral cleft lip. Plast Reconstr Surg 28:295, 1961.
25. Stenstrom SJ: The alar cartilage and the nasal deformity in unilateral cleft lip. Plast Reconstr Surg 38:223, 1966.
26. Reynolds JR, Horton CE: An alar lift procedure in cleft lip rhinoplasty. Plast Reconstr Surg 35:377, 1965.
27. Skoog T: Repair of unilateral cleft lip deformity: Maxilla, nose and lip. Scand J Plast Reconstr Surg 3:109, 1969.
28. Wynn SK: Primary nostril reconstruction in complete cleft lips. Plast Reconstr Surg 49:56, 1972.
29. McComb H: Treatment of the unilateral cleft lip nose. Plast Reconstr Surg 55:596, 1975.
30. McComb H: Primary repair of the bilateral cleft lip nose: A ten-year review. Plast Reconstr Surg 77:701, 1986.
31. Sawhney CP: Nasal deformity in unilateral cleft lip. Cleft Palate J 13:291, 1976.
32. Kernahan DA, Bauer BS, Harris GD: Experience with the Tajima procedure in primary and secondary repair in unilateral cleft lip nasal deformity. Plast Reconstr Surg 66:46, 1980.
33. Morel-Fatio D, Lalardrie JP: External nasal approach in the correction of major morphological sequelae of the cleft lip nose. Plast Reconstr Surg 38:116, 1966.
34. Skoog T: The management of the bilateral cleft of the primary palate (lip and alveolus). Plast Reconstr Surg 35:34, 1965.
35. Trauner R, Trauner M. Results of cleft lip operations. Plast Reconstr Surg 40:209, 1967.
36. Millard DR: Bilateral cleft lip and primary forked flap: A preliminary report. Plast Reconstr Surg 39:59, 1967.
37. Millard DR: Cleft Craft: The Evolution of Its Surgery: II. Bilateral and Rare Deformities. Boston: Little, Brown, 1977.
38. Duffy MM: Restoration of orbicularis oris muscle continuity in the repair of bilateral cleft lip. Br J Plast Surg 24:48, 1971.
39. Millard DR: Closure of bilateral cleft lip and elongation of columella by two operations in infancy. Plast Reconstr Surg 47:324, 1971.
40. Randall P, Lynch DJ: Primary reconstruction of the columella in bilateral prepalatal clefts. Presented to the American Association of Plastic and Reconstructive Surgeons, Seattle, May 1974.
41. Randall P, Brown A: Primary reconstruction of the columella in bilateral clefts of the lip. Second International Congress on Cleft Palate, Copenhagen, 1973 (abstr).
42. Tolhurst DE: Primary columella lengthening and lip adhesion. Br J Plast Surg 38:89, 1985.
43. Noordhoff MS: Bilateral cleft lip reconstruction. Plast Reconstr Surg 78:45, 1986.
44. Manchester, WM: The repair of double cleft lip as part of an integrated program. Plast Reconstr Surg 45:207, 1970.

CHAPTER 26

Unilateral Cleft Lip–Nose Repair

Dennis J. Hurwitz

Congenital unilateral cleft lip disrupts a most conspicuous, complex, and emotionally laden facial feature. The treatment of this highly variable deformity requires an understanding of facial embryology, normal and pathologic anatomy, growth and development, and neuromuscular and visceral function. Selecting from and adapting to a variety of surgical options, the plastic surgeon must develop an artistic eye, possess fine technical skills, exhibit bursts of creativity, and endure moments of uncertainty and self-recrimination. The culmination of this 2-hour operating room exercise is an artistic rendering of mobile structure that must satisfy the most stringent critic, for residual lip and nasal deformities will spontaneously improve little, if any, during the remaining growth period of the patient. The litany of revisionary procedures attests to our shortcomings. Unfortunately, the intrusion into the fine-line scar customarily produced in infancy hazards a far more conspicuous surgical remnant.

In the increasingly competitive medical arena, the commanding presence of plastic surgeons in cleft surgery reflects their exceptionally thoughtful and talented reconstruction. Following an in-depth, multicenter study of the variables that might have an impact on vertical and anteroposterior facial growth deficiency, Ross concluded that a skilled and experienced plastic surgeon produced the best results.[1] Early alveolar closure reduced vertical facial height. Otherwise, type of lip repair, timing of surgery, delayed palate closure, and so on caused no significant variation in facial growth. Expert input from cooperating disciplines such as dentistry, otolaryngology, and speech pathology improves rehabilitation but does not fundamentally alter the anatomic result. As Ross notes, "Surgeons would do well to develop 'soft hands' when operating in this area, because that is probably the key to success." For the young and/or inexperienced plastic surgeon, a deliberate plan to achieve excellence in cleft surgery is appropriate.

Since 1977, the author's deliberate plan has taken the following outline:

1. A comprehensive description of the deformity and surgical result.
2. A sketch of the deformity.
3. Scholarly and technical mastery of a uniformly applicable technique—the Millard rotation-advancement flap.
4. Active teaching of plastic surgery residents in cleft surgery, focusing on those features of the lip and nose that are most difficult to construct in a given case.
5. Preoperative and immediate postoperative photographs.
6. An operative note that describes each aspect of the deformity and how it was treated.
7. A periodic and longitudinal review of the results.
8. Incorporation of technical modifications.
9. Review and frank discussions with colleagues regarding results.
10. Regular attendance and participation at meetings on craniofacial and cleft disorders.

Patient Evaluation

Surgical artistry in the performance of cleft lip repair begins with a comprehensive description of the deformity based on a thorough understanding of normalcy. There is a wide normal range in infant nasal tip form and projection, lip length, philtral column contour, lip convexity, Cupid's bow definition, vermilion fullness, and lip animation. The surgeon should familiarize himself with the midfacial features unique to infants. The biologic parents should be examined because when the child's face favors one of them, the lip may also. Aside from the traditional reasons for waiting 3 to 5 months to repair the lip (larger size, reduced patient morbidity, parent acceptance of the deformity, and so on), the indistinctive newborn face may be transformed into a recognizable family member by that time.

The description of the cleft recognizes the normal features and focuses on tissue deficiency and malposition. A complete description combines the findings on clinical and intraoperative examination because information on both lip dynamics and precise linear measurements should be documented. Figure 26–1 shows a patient with a complete unilateral cleft lip and palate who was photographed from the front. This is a healthy and responsive infant with good muscular tone and appropriate fat distribution. The midface is broad with a wide maxillary dental arch. The lip elements and alveolar process are widely separated by 5 mm and 4 mm, respectively. The alveolar ridge of the cleft segment is prominent, tilted, and rotated superiorly. The lesser segment is not collapsed. The Cupid's bow on the noncleft side rises so that its high point is 4 mm above the high point on the cleft side. The philtral dimple is well defined, and the noncleft philtral column is minimally convex, extending to the nostril sill just lateral to the columella. From the lip tubercle to the edge of the cleft, the vermilion tapers to a narrow wedge. The buccal labial sulcus between the philtrum and the alveolus is obliterated. The lateral cleft segment is deficient, with skin and muscle extending just medial to the alar base. There is a lateral lip bulge extending from the cleft margin to the alar base. The vermilion is well developed, and the white roll is distinct.

In general, the severity of the cleft lip nasal deformity is proportional to that of the cleft lip. Although the extent of tissue deficiency in the cleft lip is debated, there is a consensus that the nasal deformity is largely

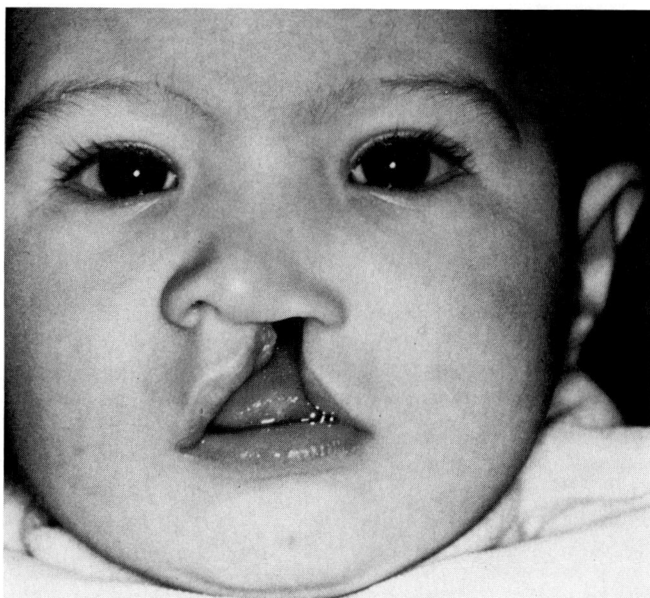

Figure 26–1 Three-month-old female with wide complete cleft lip and palate. This patient serves as a model for the operative drawing sequence that follows. The steep vertical tilt to the Cupid's bow is accentuated by the upward rotation of the underlying cleft alveolus and the slightly open-mouth posture that lowers the labial commissures.

due to malposition and distortion of normally developed structures.[2–6] The cleft side of the nose, from nasion to rim, is longer than the noncleft side. In patients with complete unilateral cleft lip (Figs. 26–1 and 26–2), the ipsilateral nasal dome is depressed and rotated toward the cleft owing to the inferior displacement of the alar cartilage. The cephalic portion of the lateral crus is displaced inferior to the upper lateral cartilage. As described by McComb, the alar cartilage lies "spread eagled" and resembles a "fallen bucket handle."[7] Its

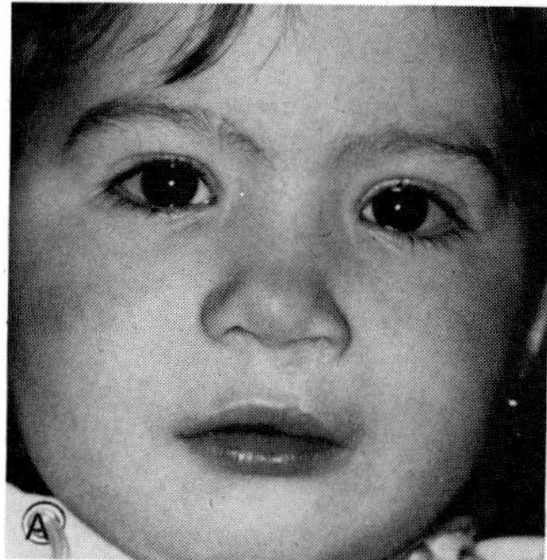
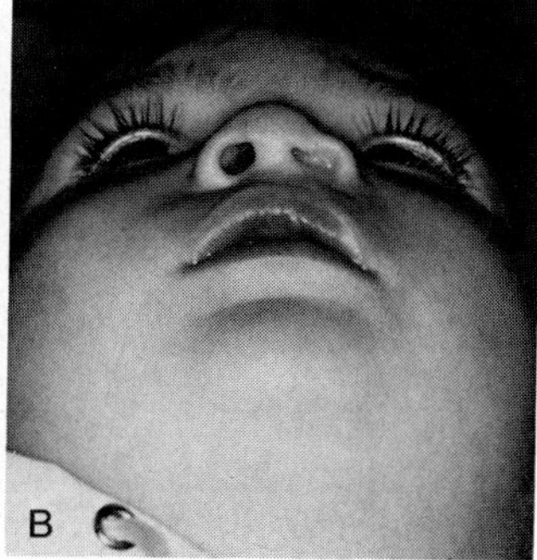

Figure 26–2 *A* and *B*, The 5-month postoperative result is shown. The flash reflex highlights the symmetric height of the nasal domes. The cleft side hemicolumella has been adequately lengthened. The ala is slightly webbed. The alar base is positioned at the same height as that on the opposite side. The nostril floor is the same level but is slightly wider than the noncleft side. The nostril floor scars have not yet resolved. The reconstructed philtral column mirrors the opposite column. Lip fullness is normal. The orbicularis muscle repair is intact. The Cupid's bow is well formed with horizontal orientation. There is appropriate width to the vermilion, and the alar base position will change little.

inferior margin forms the characteristic web of the nasal vestibule. Instead of a gentle arch forming an acute angle with the cheek, the alar base sits obliquely on the nasolabial fold. The hemicolumella on the cleft side is shortened, and the cartilaginous footplate of the medial crus lies more forward and deeper in the lip than on the other side. Along with the columella, the septal cartilage is deviated toward the noncleft nostril. The noncleft lateral crus forms an overly acute angle with its medial crus.

Goals of Cleft Lip–Nose Repair

The goal of cleft lip–nose repair is a multilayered, anatomic closure of the cleft with restoration of lip function by the realignment of the displaced lip and nasal anatomy and conservation of as much tissue as possible. In a patient with a unilateral deformity, the cleft lip–nose repair is successful when symmetry is established without leaving conspicuous scars. Complete cleft lip presents two major challenges. The first is to lengthen and align the cleft margins with minimal sacrifice of tissue in the transverse direction. The second and more controversial challenge is the nose. The displaced nasal dome, ala, and alar base need to be atraumatically aligned without causing skin webbing, folds, or vestibular stenoses.

There are other significant considerations as well. One must create an adequate buccal sulcus with release of a tethering frenulum. Symmetric vermilion fullness is most difficult to obtain below the reconstructed high point of the Cupid's bow and may require interposition of a segment of "throw away" lateral vermilion.[8] The white roll alignment at the reconstructed Cupid's bow is easily offset. The orbicularis oris muscle on both lip segments must be released and advanced to create an anatomically secure and dynamic system.[9–14]

The Millard repair can be adapted to virtually any unilateral cleft lip deformity.[15, 16] A prerequisite for adoption of the rotation-advancement technique is careful study of volume I of Millard's *Cleft Craft*.[15] In a most engaging manner, Millard describes the development of his repair. Although tissue deficiency and distortion can be severe, Millard's admonition to move "normal to normal and keep it there" remains the keystone concept.

Millard's technique recognizes the disturbance in the lip anatomy and corrects it primarily by interdigitating a large medial lip rotation flap with a lateral lip and cheek advancement flap. A long convex incision of the medial element, with the assistance of a back cut, aligns the Cupid's bow horizontally and places the only crossing scar of the lip under the shadow of the nose. Into the space opened by downward rotation of the flap, a spear-shaped lateral element is advanced. The distal 80% of the length of the scar simulates the cleft side philtral column. A skin extension of the shortened columella onto the lip includes the inferior displaced medial crus footplate and is called the C-flap. This tissue is advanced and approximated to the opposite hemicolumella. If the C-flap is long enough, it may contribute to the reconstruction of the nostril floor. The flared base of the nose is detached from a recessed piriform aperture. Following release of the nasal skin over subluxated alar cartilage, the alar base is drawn in, and the slumped nasal dome is resurrected.

With the anticipated movement of the lip tissue in mind, attention is directed to the position of the alveolus. If the palate is intact, the surgeon obviously proceeds with definitive lip repair after 3 months of age. However, if there is a complete cleft and the segments are not abutting in a sweeping, near-continuous arch, consideration is given to preliminary lip adhesion[15] or straight-line closure.[17] An uneven bony platform makes construction of a symmetric and horizontal Cupid's bow guesswork. Preliminary lip adhesion or infant orthopedic management of the arches is indicated if:

1. The cleft is more than 3 mm in width between the alveolar processes.
2. There is an anteroposterior discrepancy between a forward and rotated medial segment.
3. There is a diminutive and collapsed lateral segment.

The lip adhesion or straight-line closure succeeds because there is no attempt with it to correct the shortened lip. Lip closure and lengthening are achieved at the expense of the transverse dimension, so without lip lengthening, the closure requires less undermining. Moreover, there is rigorous experimental and tenuous clinical evidence to suggest that extensive undermining over the maxilla during lip repair causes a chronic increase in lip pressure and is detrimental to facial growth.[18] Excessive skin tension results in widened scars that are inconsequential to the first stage lip adhesion.

A preliminary lip adhesion procedure facilitates primary nasal tip correction.[16] The alar cartilage cannot be advanced to its proper position if its alar base is tied down to a deficient maxillary segment. Millard has described a lip adhesion procedure that incorporates limited alar cartilage release.

For all its touted usefulness, lip adhesion has practical and theoretical problems. It is an additional procedure, usually performed under general anesthesia in a relatively vulnerable period of the child's life. Owing to limited undermining and the considerable tension exerted by the closure, dehiscences do occur. Finally, the definitive lip repair must be performed through fresh lip scar, which must be excised completely, sacrificing some precious lip tissue.

A wide alveolar cleft is a poor indication for lip adhesion because low-tension closure can be obtained when adequate undermining of soft tissue is performed. An extensive incision along the buccal labial sulcus is required, and the facial musculature must be elevated off the maxilla and zygoma.[10] The effect of such undermining on facial growth is uncertain and controversial. Bardach cautions that such a procedure is deleterious to facial growth and has extensive animal data to support his clinical observations.[18] Conversely, Delaire argues that the facial musculature must be widely released from its abnormal attachments to the cleft margins, nose, and maxilla and then secured anatomically to the opposite muscles and nasal spine.[10] During the past 15 years, this French maxillofacial surgeon has consistently

argued that the superior nasolabial ring of musculature, which includes the transverse nasal muscle, the levator labii superioris, and the levator labii superioris alaeque nasi muscles, is intertwined with the superficial portion of the orbicularis oris muscle, and both must be reconstructed.

The ideal preparation for surgery on the wide, complete unilateral cleft lip involves sophisticated orthopedic manipulation of the alveolar margins. In lieu of that support, I reserve lip adhesion for patients with a wide and uneven arch formation.

In accordance with a University of Pittsburgh Cleft Palate Center delayed hard palate closure protocol, a dental impression is made 1 week prior to lip repair, and from this a model is fabricated. An acrylic prosthesis is made to fit the hard palate and extends to the lingual side of the alveolar arch. The lip repair will mold the arch around the prosthesis without collapsing the lesser segment.

Surgical Technique

The procedure is performed under general anesthesia with a noncuffed endotracheal tube taped to the midline of the lower lip. The table is turned so that the anesthesiologist is at the left side of the patient, allowing the surgeon and his assistant an unobstructed approach to the patient's face.

For those who are accustomed to their use, wide-field, surgical telescopes of 3- to 4-magnification power aid in identifying anatomic landmarks, dissecting muscle, and reconstructing the high point of Cupid's bow. The drawing of anatomic points and incisions is sighted through various viewing angles and with the lip and nose tugged toward their proper positions. Linear measurements, whether by caliper or ruler, are confirmatory. Because of tissue elasticity, careful artistic sighting is more reliable than the tape measure.

The sequence, strategies, and technique of correction of complete cleft lip and its nasal deformity will be described. The model patient, a 3-month-old female, is shown before the operation in Figure 26–1 and 15 months later in Figure 26–2. There are two interoperative photographs, Figures 26–3 and 26–4. Her specific operative sequence has been diagrammed in Figures 26–5 through 26–13.

The high point of the Cupid's bow on the noncleft side is easily sighted and coincides with the greatest height of the vermilion. This point is tattooed on the mucocutaneous junction with methylene blue using a 26-gauge needle. The lowest point of the Cupid's bow that overlies the midline lip tubercle is found 2 to 4 mm medially. The reconstructed high point of the Cupid's bow along the cleft margin is sighted, and that position is confirmed by the use of a Castroviejo caliper that matches the interval between the first two points.

The convexity of the rotation incision anticipates the new position of the reconstructed philtral column and determines the width of the C-flap. Too broad a sweep positions the upper portion of the scar too far laterally, requiring regrettable resection of lip skin later in the

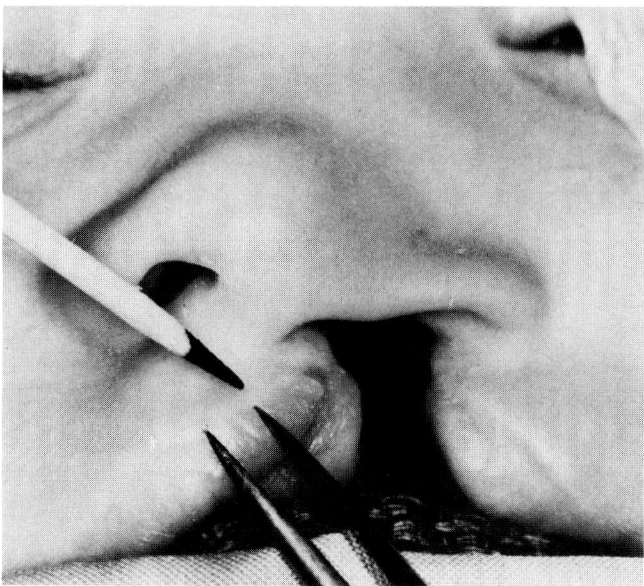

Figure 26–3 This operative photograph demonstrates the confirmation of the cleft margin high point of the Cupid's bow with the use of calipers. These points will be tattooed with a 26-gauge needle dipped in methylene blue. This single interoperative photograph was taken midway through the operation. The medial lip tissues and columella have been dissected. The lip and nasal complex have been elevated from the maxilla.

procedure. Too restricted an arch causes the scar to appear too low on the lip. A back cut, which does not cross the opposite philtral column, is necessary to lower the Cupid's bow more than 2 mm. When there is a steep tilt to the Cupid's bow and the noncleft philtral column begins lateral to the columellar base, the rotation incision should be extended into the columella.[19] Compare the different rotation incisions in Figures 26–

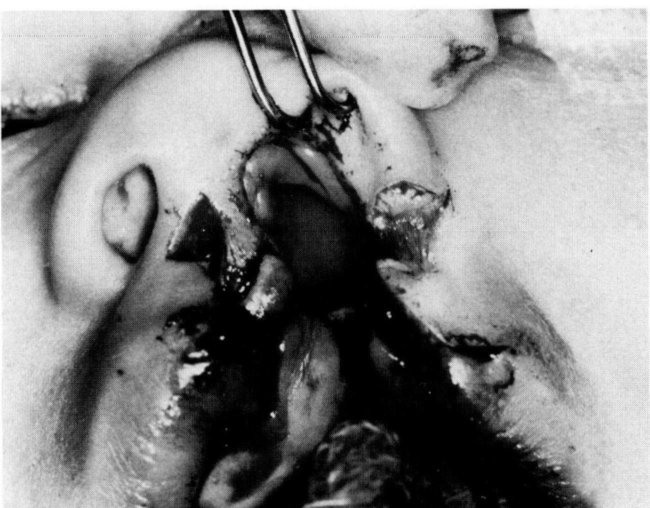

Figure 26–4 The alar base incision has just been made, allowing for visualization of aberrant musculature extending from the lip into the base of the nose. The C-flap and underlying medial crus have been dissected free from the lip, the opposite hemicolumella, and the septum. Elevation of the nostril rim with the use of a double skin hook automatically relocates the composite C-flap into its appropriate hemicolumella position.

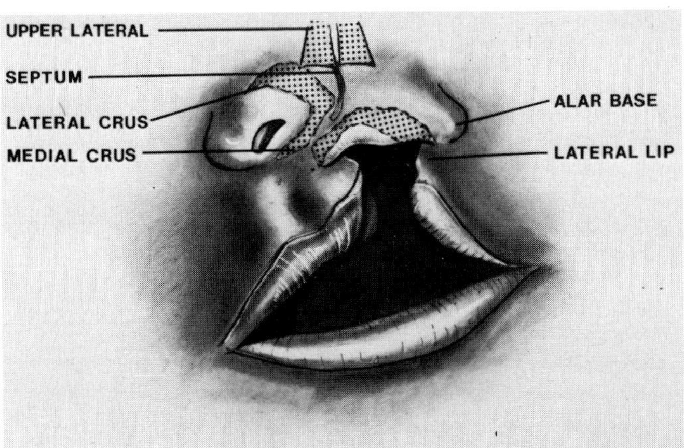

Figure 26–5 This is the first of a series of diagrams depicting the operation on the patient shown in Figure 26–1. By visual examination and palpation, the critical features can be identified. The cleft side nostril rim is consistently further from the nasion than that on the noncleft side. This is due to a downward slumping of the alar cartilage. The caudal margin of the alar cartilage forms a web across the nasal vestibule. There is a gap between the upper lateral and lateral crus of the alar cartilage. The septum is deviated toward the noncleft side. The upward tilt of the Cupid's bow is accentuated by the rotational deformity of the underlying alveolar cleft segment.

6 and 26–7. The modified rotation incision will position the transverse portion of the lip closure close to the columella and the proximal portion of the reconstructed philtral column lateral to the columella. The length of the rotation incision and its back cut is greater than the height of the intact philtral column. A confounding situation is the malrotated premaxilla, which accentuates the tilt of Cupid's bow. The surgeon/artist must imagine the effect of the restored alveolar alignment.

The rotation incision forms the medial boundary of the C-flap. The lateral incision of the C-flap hugs the mucocutaneous junction of the cleft margin from the reconstructed high point of Cupid's bow to the membranous septum and then upward along the caudal margin of the septal cartilage. The incision ends near the nasal dome. The C-flap, the medial alar crus, and membranous septum will advance as a unit to raise the heminasal dome. The distal portion of the C-flap may help fill the rotation gap and/or contribute to the nostril sill. The success of this procedure hinges on the artistic and efficient use of this tissue.

The final flap to be drawn on the medial portion of the cleft is the cleft-margined, alveolar-based, vermilion-mucosal flap. This so-called M-flap helps close septal or nasal floor defects.

The height of the vermilion below the reconstructed high point of the Cupid's bow is noted. There is often 50% less vermilion under this point on the cleft side than on the noncleft side. In such cases the junction of the vermilion with the mucosa should be incised. Into this fish-mouthed opening a V-shaped flap will be inserted from the vermilion flap on the lateral cleft edge (Figs. 26–6 and 26–7).[8] If uncorrected, the lip tubercle will have exposed mucosa that will form a flat, dry, frequently chafed area.

After completing the markings for the medial cleft segment, the surgeon indicates the high point of the

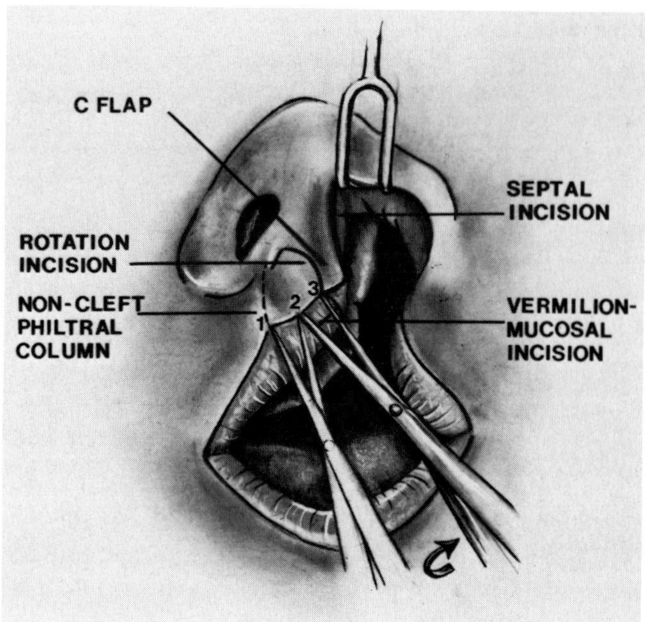

Figure 26–6 The markings on the medial cleft segment are demonstrated. With the deformed nostril held in proper position with a double skin hook retractor, the noncleft philtral column is sighted. It leads from the base of the columella to the rather obvious high point of the Cupid's bow. A dashed line is made between these two points. The artistic goal is to construct an identically curved cleft philtral column on the cleft side. The noncleft high point is designated 1 and the low point, centered over the lip tubercle, is 2. The third (3) is the high point of the Cupid's bow. The interval between 1 and 2 should equal the interval between 2 and 3, which is confirmed by calipers. The rotation incision anticipates the new philtral column and lowers 3 horizontal to 1. The 3- to 5-mm back cut angles sharply from the rotation incision. This back cut will not be made unless it is needed. The C-flap continues along the margin of the cleft edge between the skin and vermilion and extends into the membranous septum just in front of the caudal border of the septum. The vermilion incision extends from point 3 and continues along the margin of the cleft. After a short distance, it takes a right angle turn back toward the alveolus, thereby becoming a small rectangular flap. A vermilion-mucosal incision of the lip tubercle is drawn angled to the vertical limb of the M-flap if it is deemed appropriate to augment the vermilion with a lateral segment V-shaped flap.

Cupid's bow on the lateral segment. This is where the cleft edge vermilion begins to taper. From this dot a line is drawn along the cutaneous border of the cleft edge to the nostril sill. This cleft edge line is as long as the rotation incision and back cut combined. This line may have to be extended into the nasal vestibule, as indicated by the calipers in Figure 26–7. Up to 2 mm of alar base skin can be included in the flap to obtain adequate vertical lip height. Any further contribution from the nose foreshortens the ala. Positioning the high point of the Cupid's bow closer to the labial commisure also adds length to an insufficient cleft edge; however, if this point is lateralized more than 3 mm the philtrum will be reconstructed off center. The cleft edge incision then separates into the oblique arms of a Y to embrace the alar base. The lower limb separates the ala from the lip skin and should lie within the sulcus. The upper limb continues into the nasal vestibule, ending at the caudal margin of the lateral alar crus. These oblique

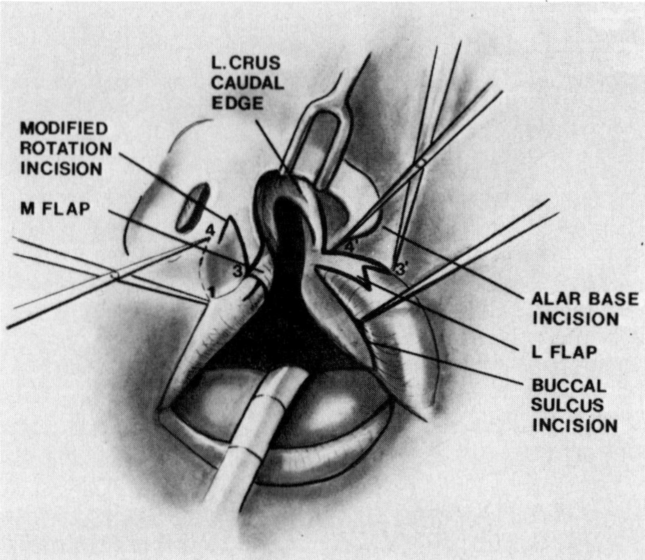

Figure 26–7 The rotation incision has been modified between points 3 and 4 because of the extraordinary high tilt of the Cupid's bow and the lateral position of the noncleft philtral column. The rotation extends into the proximal third of the columella, and the back cut forms a sharper angle. After sighting the reconstructed high point of the Cupid's bow on the lateral cleft segment, an identical distance of the noncleft philtral column is marked off with calipers along the cleft margin from 3′ to 4′. Additional length should be added to the 3′–4′ incision because the rotation incision is longer than the noncleft philtral column. The two excisional limits extending from the nasal vestibular end are made along the junction between the ala and the lip skin inferiorly and up to the caudal border of the lateral crus superiorly. The lateral cleft margin flap has been drawn with a fish tail, and this is called the L-flap. The final incision is drawn in the buccal sulcus, which in wide clefts may extend to the maxillary tuberosity.

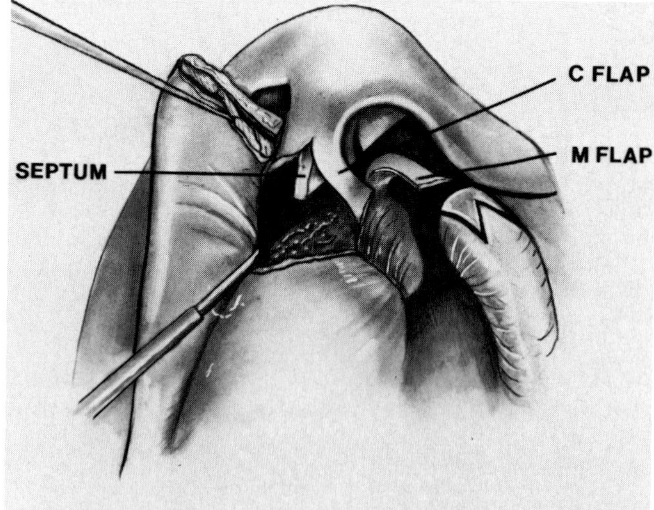

Figure 26–8 The incisions releasing the rotation C- and M-flaps have been made. The medial buccal sulcus is being incised, which releases the lip from the gingiva. The lip has been dissected to the caudal portion of the nasal septum and alar base. The C-flap, with its underlying ala and posteriorly extended membranous septum, has been freed from its septal attachments. The thin and short M-flap dangles within the nasal vestibule. The lip-mucosa muscle and skin have been separated. Do not undermine the philtral dimple from the orbicularis oris muscle.

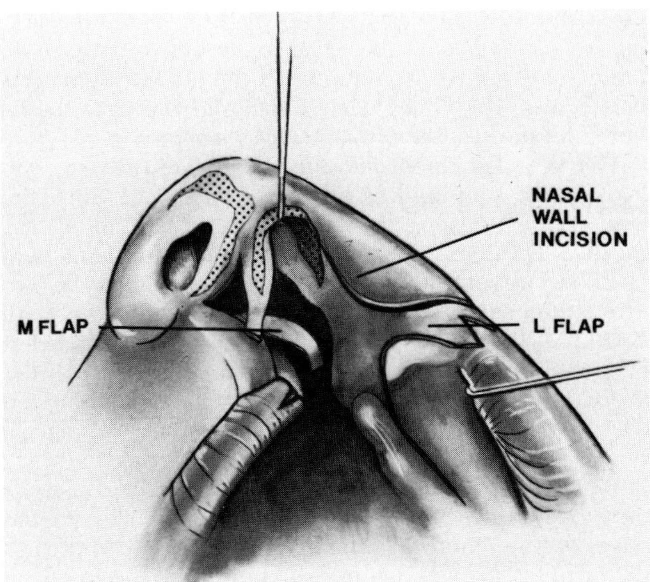

Figure 26–9 The incisions extending from the L-flap are shown. One limb goes to the piriform aperture, and the other limb extends along the buccal sulcus. The L-flap will be turned into the gap of the lateral nasal wall caused by release of the alar base. On release of the medial lip and nasal tissue, the skin hook is able to elevate the droopy alar cartilage into a better position.

limbs of the Y incision allow independent release of the alar base.

The lateral cleft-margined, vermilion-mucosal flap is drawn. This L-flap is pedicled just above the cleft alveolus. When the medial segment of the vermilion is deficient, the lateral cleft margin vermilion will have a

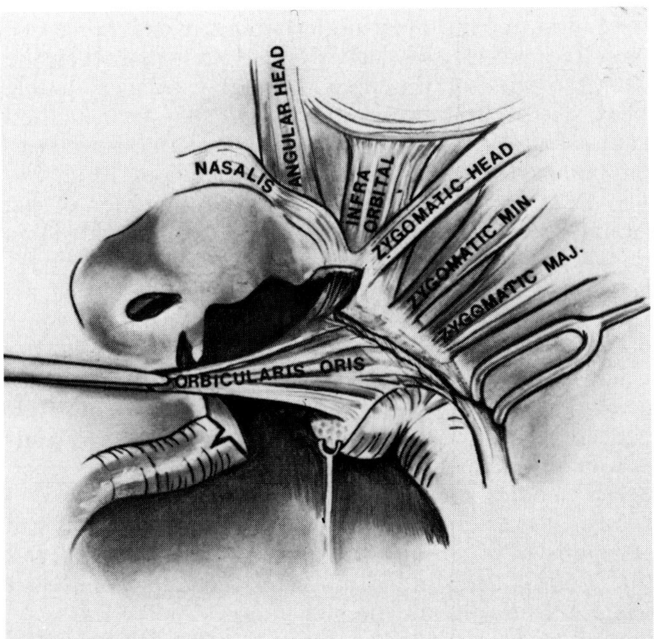

Figure 26–10 The undermining of the lip and cheek from the maxilla is completed when pull on the orbicularis oris muscle causes palpable traction on the nasolabial complex of muscles. The skin of the lip is undermined approximately 1 cm from the cleft margin. The supraperiosteal dissection extends from the nasal bones across the maxilla to the zygoma.

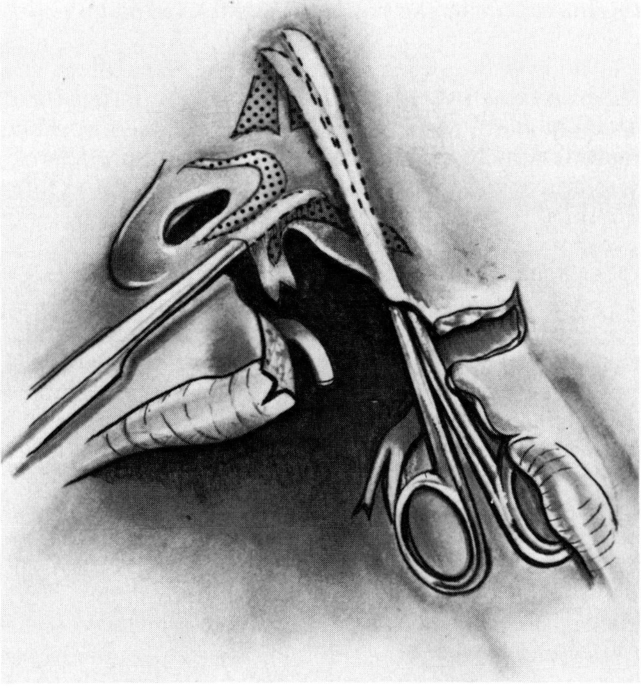

Figure 26–11 With the lip dissection completed, the surgeon dissects the soft tissues off the osseous cartilaginous framework of the nose. The alar base incision is a convenient entrance for the scissor dissection. The midcolumella incision allows for separation of the medial crura and assists in undermining of the remaining nasal skin. The mucosal surfaces of the nasal cartilages are undisturbed. The assisting fingertip helps with palpable awareness of the dissection planes, and sharp, pointed scissors seem less traumatizing than blunt-tipped ones.

V-shaped extension that will be inserted into a fish-mouth opening on the medial segment at the lip tubercle.[8] This or any other zigzag interposition along the vermilion should not be routine because it creates unnatural lip contouring. Nevertheless, interruption of straight-line lip closure may inhibit scar contracture and, if deemed appropriate, should be limited to the mucosa.

Xylocaine (several milliliters) with 1:200,000 epinephrine is infiltrated about the lip and nose. After the lip blanches (approximately 5 minutes), the operation is begun on the medial segment. The initial dissection is facilitated by placement of a medium-sized skin hook through the vermilion mucosal margin of the lip. The vermilion is pulled over the outstretched middle finger to provide a stable platform for the initial incisions. The rotation incision parallels the cleft margin, mirroring the opposite philtral column. It traverses the columella–lip junction and ends as an angled back cut that is extended as necessary. The back cut does not cross the noncleft philtral column because the entire lip will be lengthened.

The incision between the C- and M-flaps is made to the alveolus and then continued up the membranous septum along the caudal edge of the septum nearly to the nasal dome. As the C-flap is retracted with fine double hooks, the perpendicular vermilion-mucosa incision is made. The right-angle turn for the rectangularly shaped M-flap is continued to the mucosa. From there, the buccal sulcus incision transects the frenulum and is continued just beyond it (Fig. 26–8). The soft tissue is elevated off the premaxilla above the periosteum, and the dissection extends to the noncleft alar base. About 4 mm of cleft edge orbicularis muscle is freed from the philtral skin. The philtral dimple should not be violated. The mucosa and submucosal glands are dissected from the deep surface of the muscle, and the muscle release is completed when a gentle pull on the leading edge of the orbicularis muscle causes traction on the cheek muscles.

Taking care to include its underlying medial crus alar footplate, the C-flap is elevated off the premaxilla. Sharp, pointed scissors are placed in the columella, and the medial crura are separated. From this approach the nasal dome skin is undermined from the alar cartilage. Laceration or amputation of the alar cartilage during this or any other portion of the nasal tip dissection will deform the tip. A tactile sensibility, developed from performing numerous closed rhinoplasties, is critical. The rim skin blanches while the inferior portion of the cartilage is freed. With the nasal dome now free to be retracted into its proper position, the rotated medial lip flap can be finally released. The cleft edge is rotated down in order to orient the Cupid's bow horizontally. The restricting orbicularis or depressor nasal septum muscle is cut. Persistent blanching of the columella while the nose and lip are held in the proper position indicates a need to increase the back cut.

After completing the dissection of the medial seg-

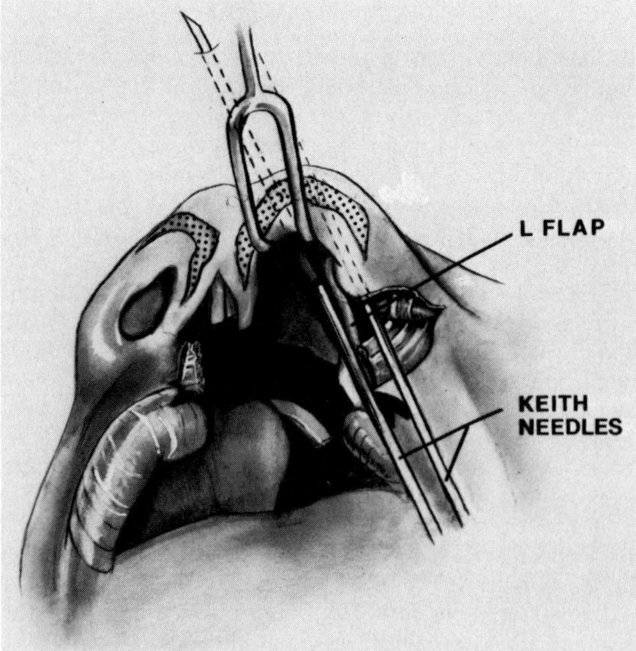

Figure 26–12 The suspension of the cleft-sided lateral crus is established by 4–0 double-armed Keith needles. This stitch is threaded through a short half segment of a No. 8 French red rubber catheter, which will be a mucosal bumper. The needles enter the nasal mucosa along the cephalic border of the alar cartilage. After piercing that structure, the needles shimmy along the undermined nasal skin to exit at the nasion. The stitch is then clamped to the head drape, causing slight overpull of the alar cartilage. The nasal tip is held in this position until the lip is closed.

ment, the surgeon can revise his lateral segment markings to accommodate the advancement of this flap to fill the gap caused by the rotation. If the lateral segment is insufficient, the C-flap can partially fill the gap. Inadequate fill of the rotation gap causes a short lip.

The lateral segment incision is facilitated by two skin hooks. One skin hook is held by an assistant along the alar rim. The second skin hook is inserted at the mucosal-vermilion junction by the operator and held over his or her middle finger. This stabilizes the lip. The lateral segment incision is begun high in the nasal vestibule. It continues along the cutaneous mucosal cleft edge margin and changes direction at the high point of the Cupid's bow (Fig. 26–9). The V-shaped vermilion dart into the L-flap is then made. The mucosal margin is incised to the buccal sulcus and continued laterally toward the maxillary tuberosity. The thin L-flap is dissected from the cleft edge and is pedicled on the edge of the gingiva. The lip-nasal-cheek complex is undermined above the periosteum from the piriform aperture and frontal process of the maxilla, under the infraorbital nerve as far as the zygoma. With the visual cues obtained by a simulated approximation of the lip-nasal complex, the incision between the alar base and lip is made precisely. The alar base is then cut free from the lateral lip element (Fig. 26–4). Aberrant nasolabial musculature is encountered that must be freed from its skin attachments. The continuity of the nasolabial and nasal musculature with the orbicularis muscle is maintained. Skin and mucosa are dissected from the orbicularis muscle for about 1 cm. The muscular dissection is completed when traction on the leading edge of the orbicularis tethers and dimples the cheek skin (Fig. 26–10).

The nasal base incision is a convenient entry for completion of the nasal undermining. Confirming that the intranasal incision has extended no further than the lateral border of the upper lateral cartilage, double sharp scissors are inserted through the alar base incision to dissect the soft tissues from the upper lateral cartilage, the nasal bones, and the opposite nasal dome (Fig. 26–11). It is important to free the caudal border of the lateral crus from the nostril rim and the nasal dome skin. The mucosal attachments of the ala and upper lateral cartilages remain undisturbed.

In anticipation of the lateral nasal wall gap created by the advancement of the alar base to the columella, the L-flap is turned about 150 degrees and sewn into this nasal vestibular opening (Fig. 26–12).

Suspension of the alar cartilages is achieved by means of a full-thickness nasal suture of 4–0 nylon. A second Keith needle is added to the end of a single-armed suture. Nasal bumpers are made by cutting small half segments of No. 8 French red rubber catheters and then placing each end of the stitch through them. First one Keith needle and then the second enter the nasal mucosa at the cephalic margin of the alar cartilage. The needles then perforate the cartilage and slither beneath the undermined nasal skin over the upper lateral cartilages and nasal bones to exit through the skin at the nasion (Fig. 26–12). A tug on these threads establishes the overlapping relationship of the alar cartilage to the upper lateral cartilage. One or two horizontal mattress sutures are placed along the nasal dome and lateral crus to optimize the skin-cartilage relationships as well as to close the dissected dead space. Several of these nasal sutures may have to be replaced after the lip is repaired, which is awkward.

Lip closure is begun by advancing the buccal sulcus flaps onto the alveolar mucosa. The M-flap can be helpful in closing the cleft space. Several sutures approximate the two lip mucosal flaps, starting at the depth of the labial sulcus and ending short of the vermilion. A Z-plasty can be placed at the junction of the vermilion and mucosa at the end of the procedure. This will interrupt the long straight-line closure. Both end-to-end[15, 20] and interdigitating[21, 22] muscle closures have been advocated. An overlapping muscle repair is recommended to avoid dehiscence that may be encountered in revision surgery of bilateral cleft lip repair.[23, 24] This technique can also be applied to primary unilateral lip repair, providing the advantages of more secure closure and improved lip contour compared with end-to-end approximation.

First, the musculature in the vermilion and mucosa is sewn end-to-end with 5–0 synthetic absorbable sutures. If inadequate muscle is present at this level, some undermining is appropriate. Some surgeons would consider this the deep portion of the orbicularis oris muscle.[13] Continuing from the cutaneous margin of the lip, the lateral segment musculature is overlapped with the medial segment using horizontal mattress sutures (Fig. 26–13). A 4–0 synthetic absorbable suture is used to enter the superficial surface of the lateral lip muscle. From its exit through the deep surface, it then enters the superficial surface of the medial muscle. After passing through the deep surface, the suture reenters

the deep surface of the medial muscle and passes through its superficial surface to enter the deep surface of the lateral muscle. As it is pulled taut, the lateral muscle is elevated over the medial. This overlap accentuates the rise of the reconstructed philtral column. The edge of the lateral orbicularis muscle crosses toward the opposite philtral column, simulating a normal midline fiber decussation when the unsatisfied orbicularis fibers heal to the dermis. As this muscle closure approaches the anterior nasal spine, the tissues are approximated under increasing tension, which accentuates lip pouting and medial cleft rotation. A high muscle closure fills the nostril floor and establishes a labionasal circuit of musculature that extends to the caudal margin of the septum.

Skin closure begins with 6–0 proline stitching of the C-flap to the normal hemicolumella. Whatever excess amount (in millimeters) of the flap is not needed at this time is left to dangle. The leading edge of the advancement flap is sewn into the defect created by the medial segment back cut. Then, a point just above the vermilion white roll border is closed with a subcuticular stitch of 5–0 chromic. If the Cupid's bow lies in a horizontal orientation, the skin between these stitches is closed in two layers. If an upward tilt persists, the rotation is increased by further releasing the orbicularis muscle from the nose and possibly extending the back cut. If the Cupid's bow is still inadequate, a small triangular flap of the lateral cleft margin skin can be interdigitated into a releasing incision above the white roll of the reconstructed high point of the Cupid's bow.

Closure of the nasal floor is postponed until adequate lip height has been constructed. The tip of the C-flap can be artfully moved to reconstruct the alar footplate bulge. The leading edge of the alar base flap is deepi-

Figure 26–13 This illustration is a completed diagram of the lip closure. The first layer is the lip mucosal repair. The second layer is the lateral to medial overlap of the orbicularis oris muscles. The inset shows this repair using horizontal mattress sutures of PDS. The final layer is the suturing of the deep dermis with 5–0 chromic and the skin with 6–0 and 7–0 Prolene. The reconstructed nostril is more vertical than the opposite one. The Cupid's bow is not quite horizontal because there is an outwardly rotated medial cleft segment that will change position and tension of the lip repair. The V-flap augmentation of the lip tubercle vermilion is shown. A long suspension suture and shorter rim transnasal suspension sutures are secured with adhesive skin strips to the nasal skin. A half-segment of red rubber catheter bolster lies within the nasal vestibule. An additional contouring suture is sometimes necessary. Compare with pre- and postoperative photographs (Figs. 26–1 and 26–2).

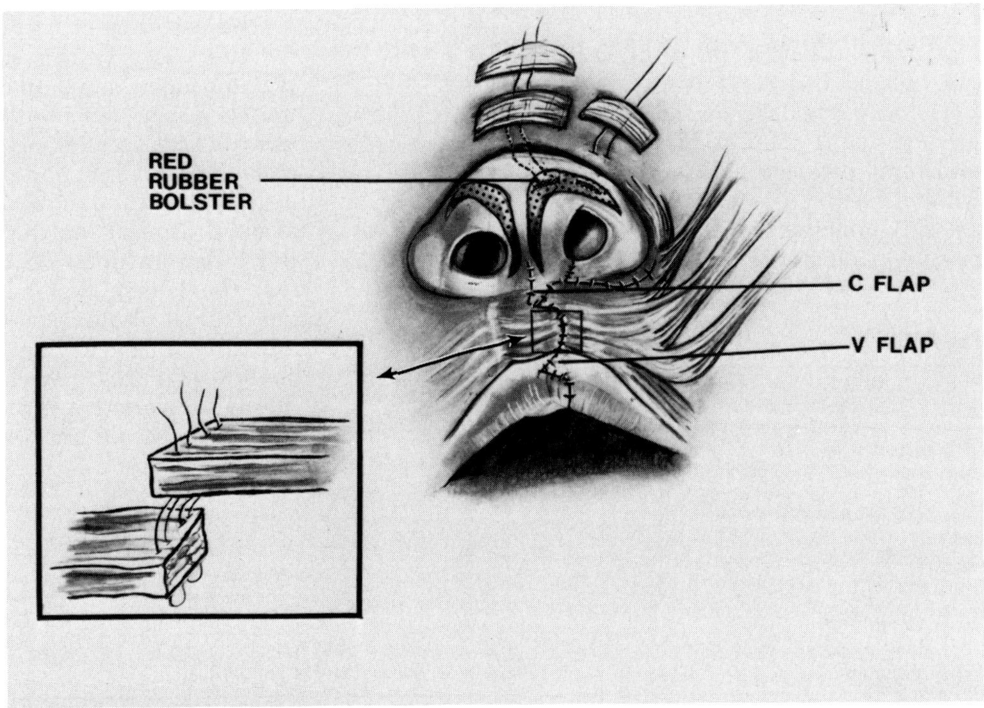

Table 26–1.

R.S. 2/84	Lip/Nose 3/85	Evaluation 3/88
Tip	9	
Ala	7	
Floor	8	31
Columella	7	
Animation	10	
Length	9	
Scar	8	
Cupid's bow	9	53
Pout/contour	8	
Vermilion	9	

thelialized and anchored to the septum with a long-lasting, absorbable suture. The reconstructed nostril sill should match the opposite side. If nostril rim webbing or irregularities have not been corrected by the cartilage repositioning, the nasal mattress sutures should be adjusted. The height of the nostril opening should be overcorrected (Fig. 26–13). Because there is no excess skin, one should be reluctant to excise webbing or bulges because nostril stenosis is a likely sequela.

The vermilion is closed directly with horizontal mattress sutures of 6–0 chromic. The V-shaped lateral vermilion flap is interdigitated with the transverse incision of the lip tubercle to correct the tubercle deficiency. Otherwise, a mucosal Z-plasty is performed.

At the completion of the procedure, the nasal skin is cleansed and benzoin is applied so that skin adhesive strips can be placed over the alar retention sutures. The common tie-over gauze bolster is avoided to prevent any chance of leaving stitch marks due to the delayed removal of these sutures. Xeroform gauze is packed into the nasal vestibule and removed in 2 days. The skin sutures should be removed 4 to 5 days following surgery. Nasal sutures are removed 10 to 14 days postoperatively.

Evaluation of Late Results

The combined repair of the lip and nose by the method just described can be applied to patients with unilateral complete or incomplete cleft lip with or without cleft of the palate. A comparison group of 33 patients underwent lip repair alone. Pre- and postoperative photographs were available for each patient.

Table 26–2.

W.H. 3/80	Lip/Repair 10/80	Evaluation 9/83
Tip	5	
Ala	5	
Floor	6	22
Columella	6	
Animation	9	
Length	9	
Scar	7	
Cupid's bow	8	48
Pout/contour	7	
Vermilion	8	

Table 26–3.

Type of Cleft	Lip Repair	Lip/Nose Repair
Incomplete cleft	15	7
Complete cleft	18	10

From these photographs and physical examination, a qualitative rating of individual features was made. Modified from the methodology of Williams, four of the items used to rate the repair related to nasal form, which included the tip, ala, floor, and columella.[25] Six factors related to the lip, including animation, length, quality of the scar, alignment of the Cupid's bow, lip pout and contour, and vermilion. The quality of these items was rated on a scale of from 1 to 10. A grade of less than 7 indicated the need for revision (Tables 26–1 and 26–2).

The two groups of patients were subdivided into those with incomplete and those with complete cleft lip. Table 26–3 lists the number of patients in each group; Table 26–4 shows the comparisons between patients with incomplete and complete cleft lip with or without nasal tip repair. Results were significantly better for patients with lip and nose repair than for those with lip repair alone (Figs. 26–14 to 26–17). The major improvement was in the appearance of the nose. The incomplete cleft lip group increased their repair rating 8 points, and the complete cleft lip group increased 10 points.

Participation in a cleft palate team with other specialists is crucial for providing the best patient care. Critical preoperative assessment and postoperative review, with the assistance of high-quality photographs, are the surgeon's best teachers.

Discussion

Optimal primary correction of cleft lip and its nasal deformity inextricably combines two procedures. The maintenance of nasal tip correction requires an anatomic muscle repair; and a lip repair that ignores the displaced alar cartilage accentuates the congenital nasal deformity, making later correction difficult and unpredictable.

The Millard rotation-advancement operation can be adapted to most unilateral clefts, bearing in mind that the C-flap includes the displaced medial footplate and that the lateral cleft edge vermilion dovetails into a deficient lip tubercle. Both the oral and nasolabial muscular slings are reconstructed after releasing all abnormal muscle attachments. The lateral-to-medial muscular overlap is a secure closure that elevates the reconstructed philtral ridge and accentuates the philtral dimple.

Table 26–4.

Type of Cleft	Lip Repair	Lip/Nose Repair
Incomplete cleft	30 + 51 = 81	38 + 55 = 93
Complete cleft	25 + 48 = 73	35 + 51 = 86

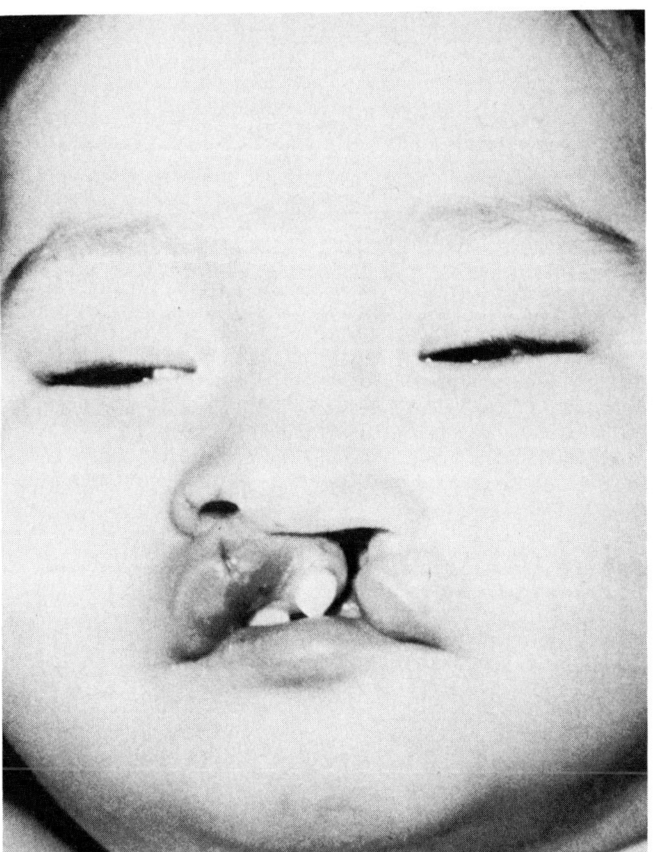

Figure 26–14 This 1-year-old has a complete unilateral cleft lip and palate. The medial segment is rotated outward.

The approach to primary repair of the wide complete cleft lip with malaligned palatal segments is unsettled. It is difficult to level a Cupid's bow on an uneven and changing platform. Preliminary manipulation of the displaced cleft segments simplifies the reconstruction and minimizes surgical interference with maxillofacial growth.

The rotation-advancement repair adapts poorly to lateral lip segment insufficiency. Lip adhesions may slightly expand the lateral lip skin. Otherwise, one can lengthen the lip by borrowing from the alar base, by interdigitating small cleft edge Z-plasties, by lateralizing the lip philtrum, or by any combination of these intrusive measures.

Moreover, a disjoined alveolar arch compromises nasal tip reconstruction because the cleft side alar base and lateral nose retract down to a depressed bony platform. Undaunted, Anderl augments the deficient piriform rim with Surgicel.[26] Nasal septoplasty[26] and nasal floor reconstruction[14] require extensive dissection when the maxilla and septum are widely displaced. Preliminary arch manipulation with orthopedic devices and/or lip repair is preferred.

The resurgent interest in primary cleft lip nasal repair has resulted in a variety of techniques.[2, 7, 14, 16, 26, 27] In cleft patients, sufficient nasal cartilage is present to allow the surgeon to improve the form of the nose. The goal is to create nasal tip symmetry without interfering with growth or complicating later surgery. The alar malposition is not limited to the lateral crus, as noted by Broadbent,[2] but also includes inferior displacement of the medial crus into the lip.[26, 27] Inadequate release of the medial crus, particularly its depressed footplate lying within the lip, has led to a shortened columella and an artificial nasolabial angle. Adequate correction can be obtained by creating a subcutaneous separation of the two medial crura. There is no need to extend the rotation incision through the columella to the nasal tip, as advocated by Pigott.[27] The undermined skin adjusts to the new position of the cartilage.

The congenital nasal vestibular band is formed by the caudal margin of the lateral crus, not the cephalic edge as diagrammed by Salyer.[14] When the cleft side of the nose rests on a hypoplastic maxilla, the elevation of the tip requires interposition of soft tissue, which can be satisfied by the L-flap. This flap should not be extended between the upper and lower lateral cartilages. Although direct exposure and suture of the lateral crus to nearby cartilage may be more exacting,[2, 16, 24, 27] wide undermining of the nasal skin from the displaced lateral crus[7] combined with release of the two medial crura[26, 27]

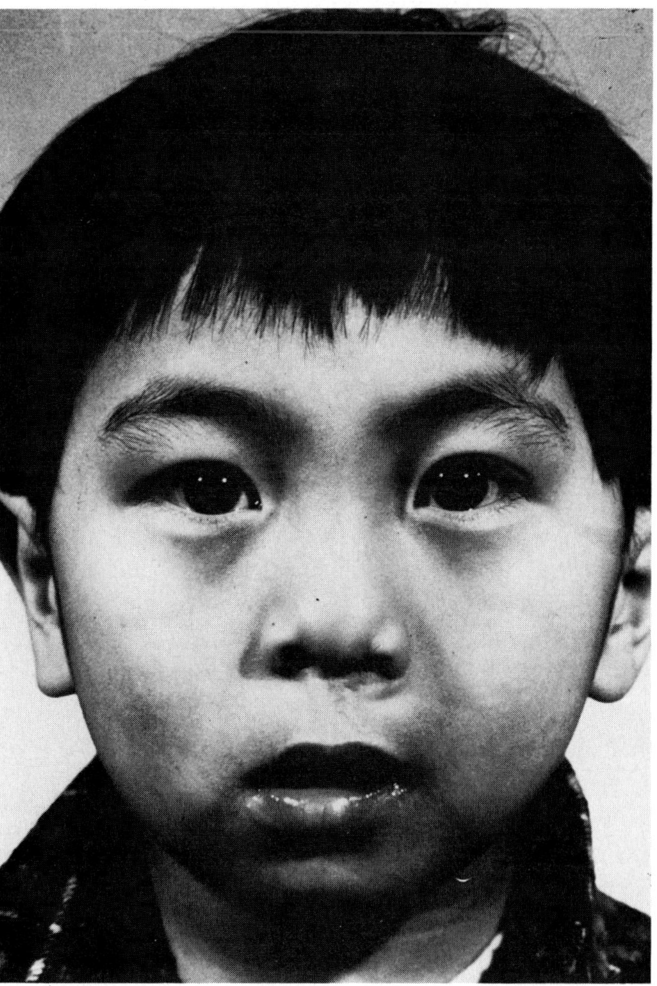

Figure 26–15 The result 3 years following the lip and nasal repair of the infant shown in Fig. 26–14. The scar is faint, and there is slight webbing of the alar columella angle.

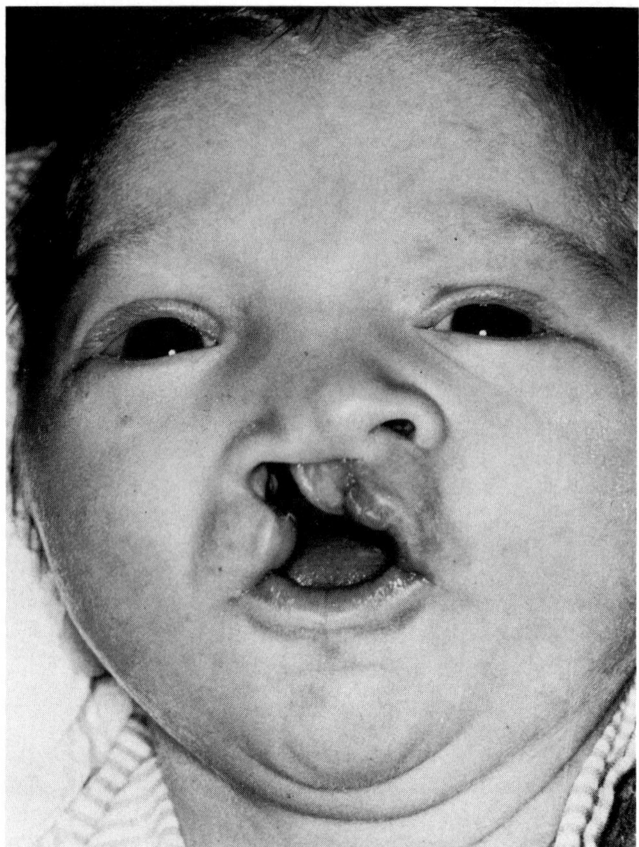

Figure 26–16 This 3-month-old infant has a complete unilateral cleft lip and palate. The lesser maxillary segment is collapsed.

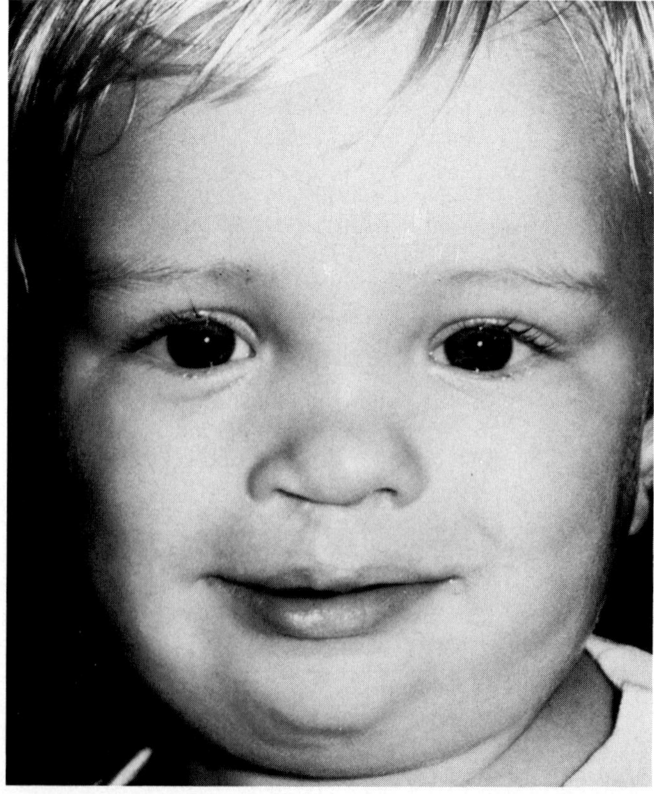

Figure 26–17 The 3-year result of lip repair without nasal tip correction in infant shown in Fig. 26–16. Notice the flattening and distortion of the right alar cartilage.

is sufficient for repositioning the cephalic edge of the lateral crus over the upper lateral cartilage. Dissection of the mucosa from the alar cartilage is unnecessary and possibly deleterious.

Transnasal retention sutures slightly overcorrect the alar position, causing a well-defined, soft, triangle dimple. The sutures are secured to the nasal skin adhesive strips because tie-over dressings left in longer than 1 week may leave suture marks.

In comparing a series of patients with lip and nasal repair with those who have had lip repair only, this author notes that not only was there significant improvement in the nasal tip symmetry in the former, but also to a lesser extent the lip repair was improved. Improved lip repair resulted from a more extensive muscle dissection, followed by secure overlapping of the orbicularis edges from the vermilion margin to the caudal septum. This repair improved lip pout, length, contour, ·and animation.

The rotation incision may be extended into the columella to keep the transverse lip scar high. The C-flap should be made as large as possible because this tissue may have to be used to help fill the rotation gap. The back cut should be extended as far as necessary without crossing the opposite philtral column to allow for tension-free rotation. All adherent muscle is dissected from the columella and noncleft nostril sill. Also, the lip is slightly lengthened by a complete muscle dissection and by overlapping this repair.[28]

The major deficiencies in my cleft lip nasal repair are webbing at the alar rim–columellar junction, the alar base to cheek angle and the roll of the alar base into the nostril sill. Direct alar rim recontouring should be considered. Strategically placed retention sutures may be helpful. Additional attention has to be given to the vestibular and sill reconstruction. Because this region is somewhat hidden, it has a low priority for the allocation of scar tissue. This is the location most likely to experience delayed healing and hypertrophic scarring.

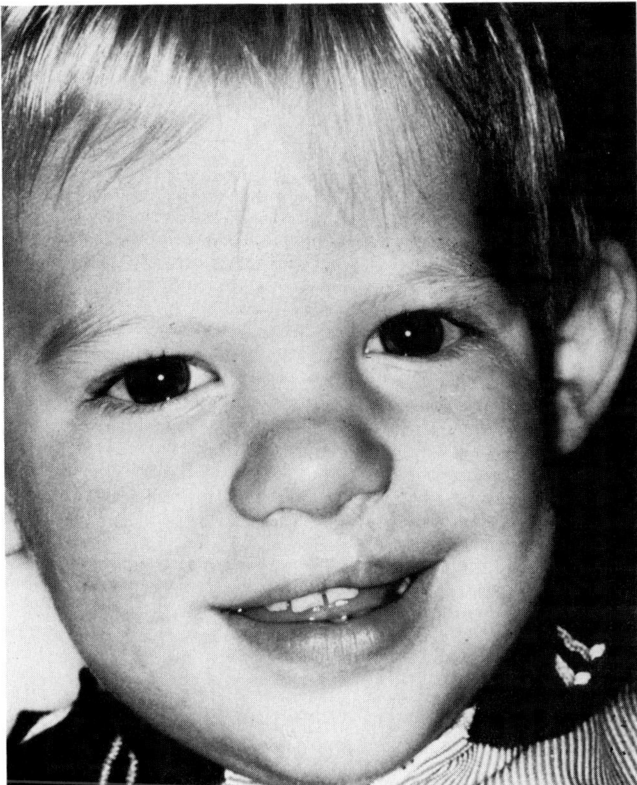

Figure 26–19 Postoperative result 3 years following surgery. Good nasal tip and alar base symmetry is present. The lip scar remains somewhat thickened.

The small nostril is a preventable complication (Figs. 26–18 to 26–20). Lateral nasal webbing can be minimized and nostril stenosis avoided by nasal vestibular to cheek and nasal vestibular to buccal sulcus retention sutures as well as by nasal packing. Also important are the fill of the lateral nasal wall advancement with the L-flap, limited intranasal incisions, closure of all nasal wounds, and undercorrection of the nostril floor. In other words, the alar base should be left a little further laterally than symmetry would suggest because scar contracture may pull it toward the columella.

Incomplete clefts are less difficult to repair than complete clefts because there is more tissue and a less distorted anatomy. The extent of dissection is less. At times, primary rhinoplasty is unnecessary. Accurate evaluation of the deformity will dictate the extent of dissection and repair.

Radical correction of the cleft lip nasal deformity often entails thorough mobilization of displaced skin, muscle, and cartilages of the mid-face. When performed by the method described, the surgical trauma is well tolerated. There is minimal increase in blood loss and postoperative swelling compared with the traditional lip repair. None of the patients required a transfusion.

The early restoration of a normal anatomic relationship has become an accepted principle in craniofacial surgery. This principle should be applied to cleft surgery as well. This method of lip and nasal repair violates no recognized growth centers. On the contrary, follow-up of 1 to 5 years of the author's 17 patients has shown

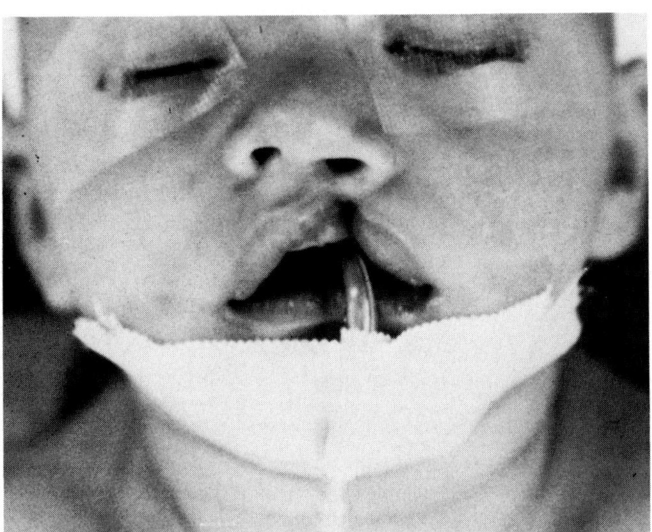

Figure 26–18 Intraoperative photograph of a child with incomplete cleft lip and cleft lip nasal deformity.

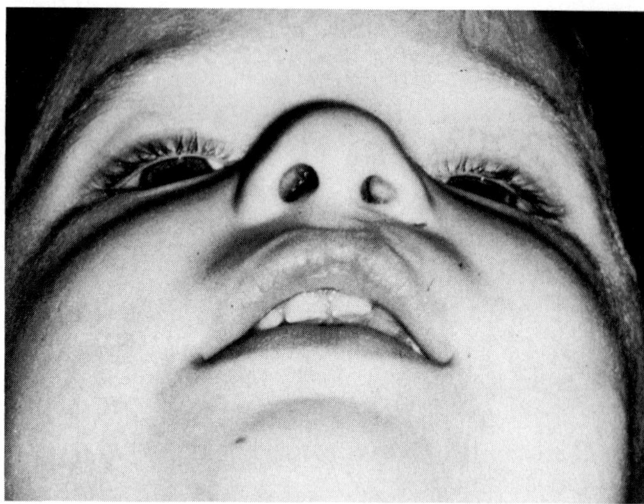

Figure 26–20 This view shows the slightly smaller nares on the operated side than on the noncleft side, which is representative of our experience in three patients. The measures described in the text are likely to prevent this problem.

maintenance of early postoperative relationships. Reported results of similar techniques with over 10 years of follow-up show no adverse sequelae.[14, 15]

Conclusions

Multidisciplinary cleft management creates an opportunity for the surgeon to work closely with the other specialists involved in treatment of this congenital deformity. Only through close collaboration of the various disciplines can improved results be achieved. The surgeon bears most of the responsibility because he or she makes and carries out the decisions concerning surgical repair. This responsibility is unique to the surgeon; however, the other specialists may influence the timing for surgery and the choice of repair.

At the present time, advances in surgical technique enable the surgeon to achieve good results in cleft lip repair. However, we feel strongly that more improvement can be achieved at the time of the primary operation. Correction of the nasal deformity at the time of primary lip repair is the newest and most valuable addition to the wide array of operations described for treatment of cleft lip.

References

1. Ross RB: Treatment variables affecting facial growth in complete unilateral cleft lip and palate. Part 7: An overview of treatment and growth. Cleft Palate J 24:71, 1987.
2. Broadbent TR, Woolf RM: Cleft lip nasal deformity. Ann Plast Surg 12:216, 1984.
3. Huffman WC, Lierle DM: Studies on the pathologic anatomy of the harelip nose. Plast Reconstr Surg 4:225, 1949.
4. McComb H: Treatment of the unilateral cleft lip nose. Plast Reconstr Surg 55:596, 1975.
5. Mooney MP, Siegel MI, Kimes KR, et al: Development of the orbicularis oris muscle in normal and cleft lip and palate human fetuses using three-dimensional computer reconstruction. Plast Reconstr Surg 81:336, 1988.
6. Sadove R, Ladaga L, Magee WP: Cartilaginous histology of the cleft lip nose: Proving the extrinsic etiology. Plast Reconstr Surg 81:655, 1988.
7. McComb H: Primary correction of unilateral cleft lip nasal deformity: A ten-year review. Plast Reconstr Surg 75:791, 1985.
8. Noordhoff MS: Reconstruction of vermilion in unilateral and bilateral cleft lip. Plast Reconstr Surg 73:52, 1984.
9. Delaire J: The potential role of facial muscles in monitoring maxillary growth and morphogenesis. In Carlson R, McNamara J (eds): Muscle adaptation in the craniofacial region. University of Michigan Growth and Developmental Series. Ann Arbor: University of Michigan Press, 1976.
10. Delaire J: Theoretical principles and techniques of functional closure of the lip and nasal aperture. J Maxillofac Surg 6:105, 1978.
11. Delaire J, Precious D: Influence of the nasal septum on maxillofacial growth in patients with congenital labiomaxillary cleft. Cleft Palate J 23:270, 1986.
12. Kernahan DA, Bauer SB: Functional cleft lip repair: A sequential layered closure with orbicularis muscle alignment. Plast Reconstr Surg 72:459, 1983.
13. Nicolau PJ: The orbicularis oris muscle: A functional approach to its repair in the cleft lip. Br J Plast Surg 36:141, 1983.
14. Salyer KE: Primary correction of the unilateral cleft lip nose: A fifteen-year experience. Plast Reconstr Surg 77:558, 1986.
15. Millard DR: Cleft Craft. Vol. I. Boston: Little, Brown, 1976.
16. Millard DR: The unilateral cleft lip. In Serafin D, Georgiade NG (eds): Pediatric Plastic Surgery. Vol. I. St. Louis: C. V. Mosby, 1984.
17. Furnas DW: Straight-line closure: A preliminary to Millard closure in unilateral cleft lips. Clin Plast Surg 11:701, 1984.
18. Bardach J: Facial growth following cleft lip and palate repair. Experimental studies in rabbits and beagles. In Jackson IT, Sommerlad BC (eds): Recent Advances in Plastic Surgery. Edinburgh: Churchill Livingstone, 1985.
19. Mohler LR: Unilateral cleft lip repair. Plast Reconstr Surg 80:511, 1987.
20. Musgrave RH, Garrett WS: Surgery for cleft lip and nostril. In Goldwyn RM (ed): The Unfavorable Result in Plastic Surgery: Avoidance and Treatment. Boston: Little, Brown, 1984.
21. Kernahan DA, Dado DV, Bauer SB: The anatomy of the orbicularis oris muscle in unilateral cleft lip based on a three-dimensional histologic reconstruction. Plast Reconstr Surg 73:875, 1984.
22. LaRossa DD, Randall P: The Unilateral Cleft Lip. In Georgiade NG, et al (eds): Essentials of Plastic, Maxillofacial, and Reconstructive Surgery. Baltimore: Williams & Wilkins, 1987. Chapter 25.
23. Berkeley WT: The cleft lip nose. Plast Reconstr Surg 23:567, 1959.
24. Blair VP, Brown JB: Mirault operation for single harelip. Surg Gynecol Obstet 51:81, 1930.
25. Williams HB: A method of assessing cleft lip repairs: Comparison of LeMesurier and Millard techniques. Plast Reconstr Surg 41:103, 1968.
26. Anderl H: Simultaneous repair of lip and nose in the unilateral cleft (a long-term report). In Jackson IT, Sommerlad BC (eds): Recent Advances in Plastic Surgery. Edinburgh: Churchill Livingstone, 1985.
27. Pigott RW: Alar leapfrog—A technique for repositioning the total alar cartilage at primary cleft lip repair. Clin Plast Surg 12:643, 1985.
28. Dado DV: Analysis of the lengthening effect of the muscle repair in functional cleft lip repair. Plast Reconstr Surg 82:594, 1988.

CHAPTER 27

Unilateral Cleft Lip Repair

Samuel Stal,
David Netscher, and
Melvin Spira

Cleft lip and palate continues to be a significant public health problem. The reported incidence of 1 in 800 live births by Linwood Grace is undoubtedly higher now.[1] Fogh-Anderson in Denmark has shown a progressive increase in frequency and has suggested several reasons for this trend, foremost of which is improved operative results, which have encouraged propagation among cleft patients.[2] We certainly have come a long way since the time when Brown in frustration was forced to remark, "Only God can make a Cupid's bow." However, each surgeon must analyze his own results very critically and honestly in the pursuit of perfection. Since the descriptions of the repairs by Tennison[3] and Millard,[4] no major further developments have occurred, but there have been many significant contributions, each of which in its own small way has enhanced the final outcome.

Preoperative Analysis

Treatment of the patient with cleft lip starts with the preoperative evaluation, when the child is seen at the first consultation. Randall advocates performing lip repair in the first 10 days of life, or as soon as the general health of the child permits.[5] We agree that the second to sixth weeks of life should be avoided because of the usual decline in hemoglobin levels during this time. We, however, prefer to wait until the patient is 10 to 12 weeks old before performing lip repair. As Millard advocated, we still adhere to the "rule of tens"—10 weeks, 10 grams hemoglobin, and 10 pounds weight.[6] Some have suggested a psychological advantage to waiting, saying that it enables the parents to become more fully aware of the defect, so that they can better appreciate the results of surgery. A more important reason for the delay in performing lip repair is that the landmarks for repair are more visible than they are in the newborn.

We also feel more comfortable delaying surgery because we incorporate the expertise of an in-office orthodontist. We feel that maxillary orthopedic treatment plays a major role in the treatment of the cleft patient.[7] Maxillary collapse can be treated using a simple spring-loaded device. Preventive therapy is preferred. In the patient with a complete unilateral cleft, if the arch is normal at birth, prevention of the almost inevitable collapse is achieved by means of a maxillary retainer. If there is protrusion or collapse of the maxillary segment at birth, restoration must be undertaken. However, in the patient with a very wide cleft, some early collapse of the maxillary segments may be advantageous to subsequent lip repair (Fig. 27–1).

Finally, in the preoperative assessment, one should attempt to make a broad classification of the type of cleft. The purists will, no doubt, continue to insist that the surgeon should become familiar with only one type of lip repair and perfect that technique. Musgrave has suggested that a Millard repair is more suitable for an incomplete cleft, while the Tennison repair is best suited to the wide cleft.[8] It is interesting that even though several authors allude to the fact that no two clefts are alike and that although both the Millard and Tennison repairs allow a certain amount of freehand adjustment, no real classification exists for the types of unilateral clefts. The unilateral cleft lip may be incomplete or complete. In turn, complete clefts may be wide or narrow. The width of the cleft has generally been based on the width of the alveolar cleft. We have arbitrarily defined a wide cleft as one in which the arch segments are separated by a gap of 10 mm or greater (Fig. 27–2). Undoubtedly, there are unilateral cleft lips in which the arch gap is wide but the soft tissue cleft is relatively narrow. Thus, complete clefts in general differ greatly in appearance, but individual differences are related more to degree than to type.

Choice of Lip Repair

As Marcks et al. have noted, the Cupid's bow is normally present on the medial side of the cleft.[9] It is simply displaced upward and may be so distorted by tension that it is not recognizable. Both the Tennison and Millard repairs are modified Z-plasties. Clifford and Pool have clearly shown that the cleft is deficient in its vertical element but that the horizontal elements are all present.[10] The quadrilateral flap of LeMesurier discards some vermilion and drags the lateral lip element across to the midline. The lip repaired with this procedure ends up too long in its vertical height and somewhat tight with a flat horizontal contour. The Tennison repair does not discard full-thickness vermilion, so natural lip pout is restored.

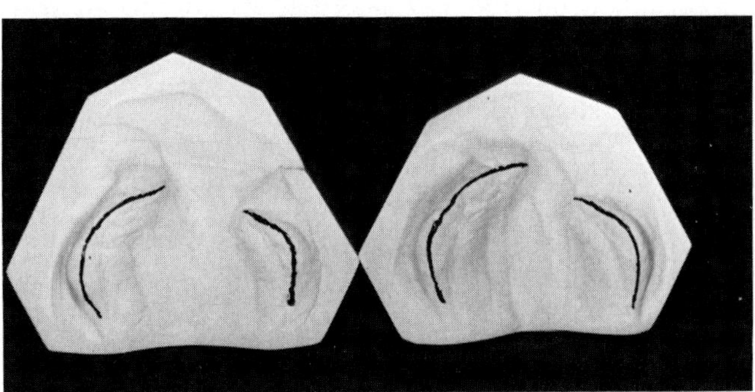

Figure 27–1 Collapse of a wide alveolar cleft in the period before lip repair.

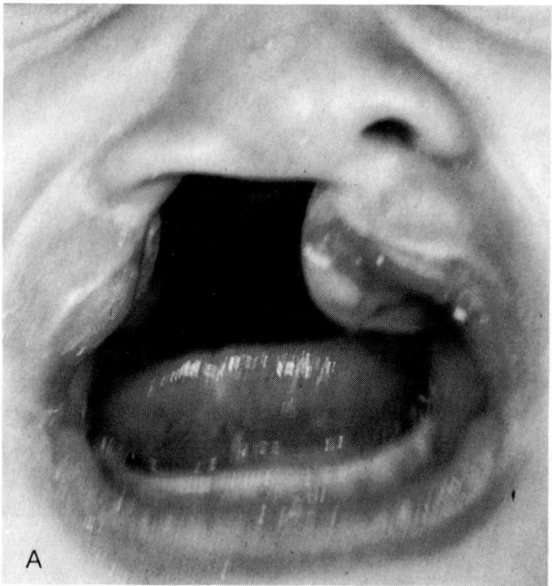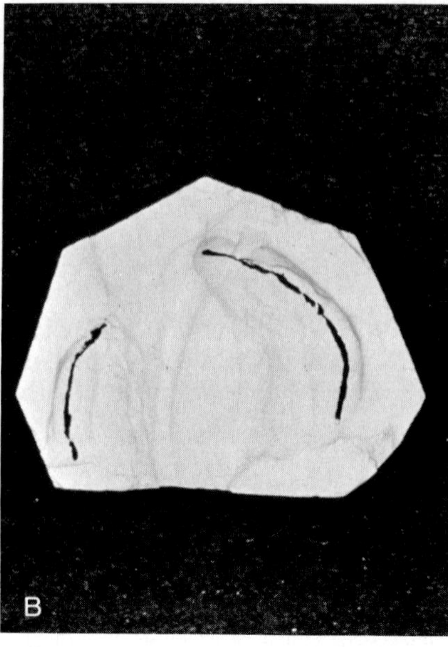

Figure 27–2 Wide cleft lip. *A,* Soft tissue deformity of approximately 16 mm. *B,* Alveolar cleft of approximately 12 mm.

In the Millard repair, because the Z-plasty is at the top of the cleft, the greatest tension is at the base of the nares—that is, the point of maximum tension is along the horizontal limb of the Z where the greatest amount of inward mobilization must occur. In the very wide lip, this inward mobilization may not be possible or may be done at the expense of creating a notch in the floor of the nose. An advantage of the flap procedures that are done at the lower half of the cleft is that they put the line of maximum tension below the alveolar ridge at the point where the lip normally begins to pout.

Millard has offered several refinements to help close wide clefts.[11, 12] These include:

1. Extension of the lateral flap into the vestibule. This provides "extra skin" to bridge the defect across the wide nasal floor and to place in the rotation defect.
2. Back cutting the rotation flap allows the peak of the Cupid's bow on the cleft side to be repositioned to achieve symmetry with the opposite side.
3. Extension of the advancement flap around the ala allows the alar and lip-cheek flaps to move independently and to achieve better nasal symmetry. It also allows wide soft tissue undermining of both the ala and cheek up to the infraorbital nerve.
4. In a patient with a particularly tight closure, lateral vermilion on the cleft side may be attenuated with "bunching" medially. This should be corrected at the primary operation with a vermilion transposition flap from medial to lateral.

Finally, Millard admits that in certain cases when the cleft is exceptionally wide, lip adhesion in the upper third of the cleft (so as not to destroy any of the recognizable landmarks) may be necessary as a preliminary procedure. We feel that lip adhesion has several disadvantages and that the Tennison repair can be used for wide clefts without preliminary adhesion. Disadvantages of lip adhesion are (1) resulting scar tissue may interfere with definitive repair, and (2) two procedures are necessary.

We do, however, feel that in the incomplete cleft lip (and perhaps for the complete narrow cleft), the Millard repair is probably unsurpassed by any other type of repair. This repair more readily addresses nasal symmetry and also helps to re-create the philtral column on the cleft side. Some of the refinements suggested by Millard apply specifically to early correction of the associated nasal deformity.

1. The rotation incision not only allows the Cupid's bow-dimple complex to drop but also allows the C-flap to rise and contribute to unilateral columellar lengthening.
2. The curve around the alar base enables the alar position on the cleft side to be reset to achieve symmetry.
3. The C-flap also can be freed along the membranous septum and the vermilion M-flap inserted here. This enables greater columellar lengthening.
4. A vestibular incision in the intercartilaginous plane allows the alar complex to be advanced forward and medially. The vermilion L-flap can be used to fill in this gap.

For wide unilateral clefts, we advocate the Tennison repair. This repair also has the advantage of being readily taught to others using the system of measurements introduced by Randall[5] and refined by Brauer.[6, 13] The marking of our incisions is modified from the method of Goulian et al.[14] We believe that attention should be directed to the following details:

1. In a wide cleft, maxillary release is required through a sublabial incision, enabling the lateral lip element to be unfurled and the anatomic landmarks to be delineated prior to marking. Maxillary release is often performed before marking the lip (Fig. 27–3).
2. As Cronin advocated, the oblique incision of the triangular flap is terminated 1 mm above the vermilion.[15] This simplifies adjustment of the vermilion. The offset above the vermilion interrupts the oblique scar of the lower margin of the triangular

flap so that it does not appear that the vermilion ridge extends into the skin of the lip.

3. Since there is a tendency for the lip on the cleft side to become too long in the vertical direction, the repaired side is made 1 mm shorter than the noncleft side.[16] That is, the minor vertical distance is obtained by subtracting the major distance from the vertical height on the noncleft side minus 1 mm.

4. A skin hook is placed in the ala on the cleft side and lifted so that it is level with the normal side. This helps to identify points 5 and 6. Placement of points 5 and 6 is a judgment decision. These points are placed at the bases of the columella and ala, respectively; they should be in the lip itself and not in the nose.[6] Thus, the surgeon should err on the side away from the columella to preserve its already decreased length.

5. Point 4 is placed on the vermilion of the lateral lip segment where the "white roll" begins to disappear and where the vermilion is of normal thickness.[6]

6. Angle 9–3–6 approximates 90 degrees. However, this angle varies depending on the height discrepancy that must be made up. If point 1 must be lowered more than 4 mm—that is, if the minor vertical distance is greater than 4 mm—then this angle becomes more obtuse.[6, 13]

7. The length of line 9–3 depends on the lengths of the sides of the isosceles triangle of the triangular flap. Length of line 9–3 should initially extend to the midpoint of the philtrum. It should not extend beyond **xy** or this will "open up" the noncleft side, lengthening the opposite lip.

8. In the patient with a wider cleft, the triangular flap will be significantly larger (and less tissue will be sacrificed) and will be positioned more parallel and closer to the cleft edges (Fig. 27–4).[13]

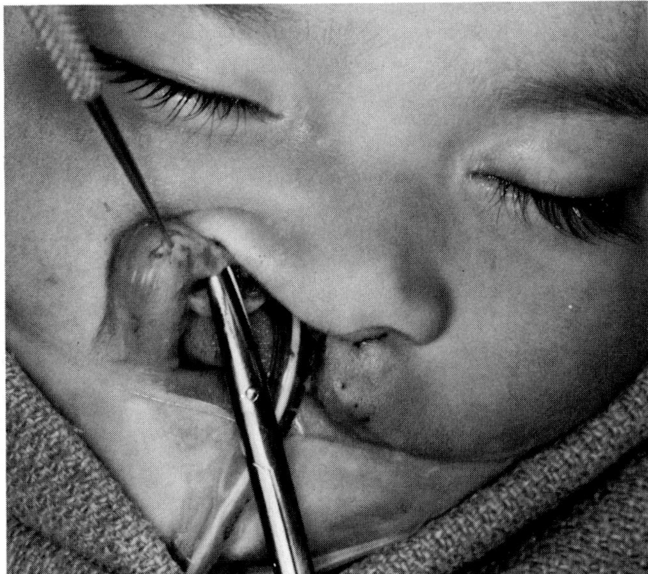

Figure 27–3 Releasing the lip from the cleft before definitive lip marking.

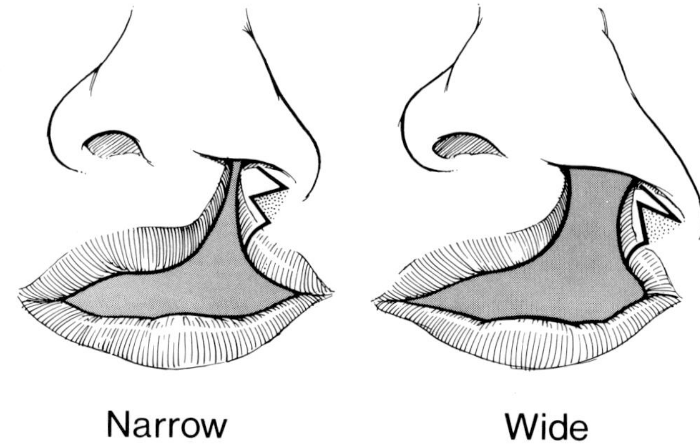

Figure 27–4 Size and position of the triangular flap relative to the size of the cleft. The wider the cleft, the larger the flap and the more oblique its orientation.

9. Appropriate beveling is necessary to minimize redundant tissue, and the superiorly based lateral vermilion flap should not be discarded but utilized to reinforce reconstruction of the nasal flow. Careful beveling also preserves adequate dermis for a precise, less tension-free subcutaneous closure (Fig. 27–5).

10. To allow the lip and nose to move independently, a perialar incision is used, and the tethering fibrous bands between the lateral alar cartilage and maxilla must be freed (Fig. 27–6). The nostril on the cleft side should be purposely created larger. It is easier to correct a nostril that is too large than one that is too small (Fig. 27–7).

11. Lateral undermining of the cheek to the infraorbital nerve allows greater advancement of the lateral lip element (Fig. 27–8).

Problems with the Tennison repair include the following:

1. The philtral column is not restored.

2. Because revisions are difficult the initial repair must be meticulous and must recognize the subtle varieties of cleft lip.

3. A lip that is too short results when the surgeon places point 6 too far medially into the cleft.

4. The Tennison repair does not address the nasal deformity as well as the Millard repair.

5. It may produce a lip that is too long. However, attention to several details will avoid this problem.

6. Although some object to the "unanatomic" placement of the scar, this has not been a problem for us even in our dark-skinned patients (Fig. 27–9).

It was initially felt that growth of the realigned muscle fibers produced the increase in lip length seen with the Tennison repair. This is no longer felt to be the reason for a long lip.[16] However, a lip that is too long is a distinct possibility if the following factors are not observed:

1. In patients with an incomplete cleft, the surgeon should be aware that the lateral lip element is too long and that it is necessary to excise a full-thickness triangle along the alar base.

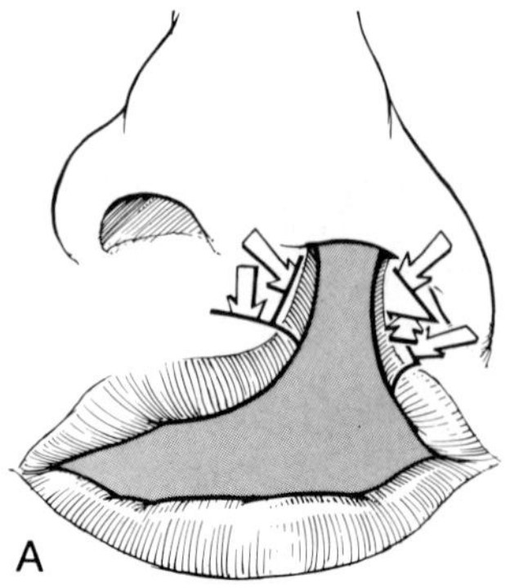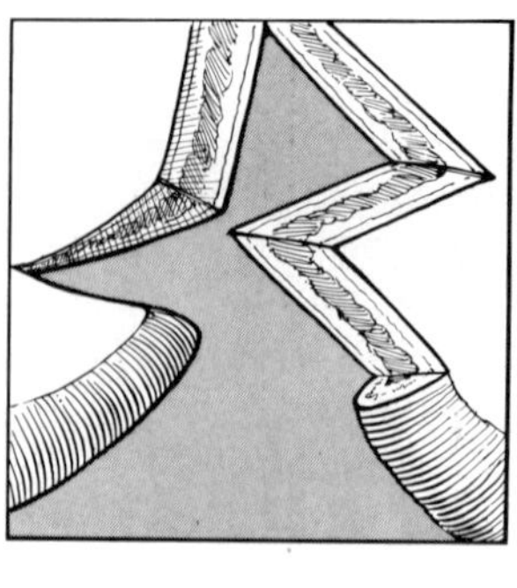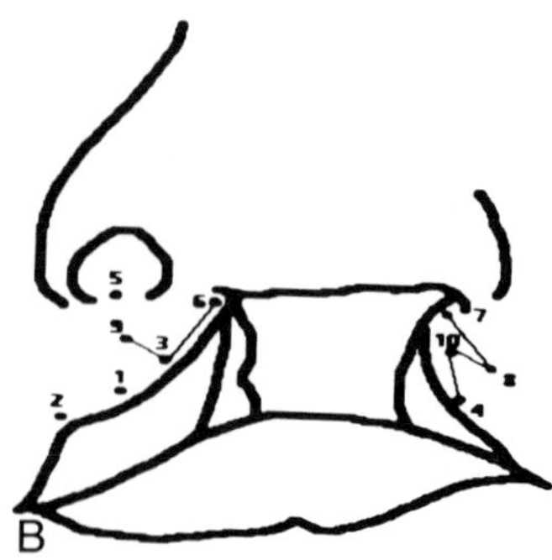

Figure 27–5 *A,* Areas where appropriate beveling is necessary in a triangular flap repair. *B,* Operative markings for triangular flap lip repair. A 27-gauge needle dipped in methylene blue is used to mark the lip after appropriate anesthesia has been given. The numbering system is modified from the traditional Tennison-Randall system to reflect the sequence in which the surgery is done.[14]

0 = Oral commissures.
1 = Midline of the philtrum at the vermilion.
2 = Normal height of Cupid's bow.
3 = Cupid's bow on the medial cleft side where the white roll fades. This is determined using a caliper so that the distance from 1 to 2 equals the distance from 1 to 3.
4 = The peak of the Cupid's bow on the lateral side, which is confirmed by measurement from the oral commissure to points 2 and 4. This should be relatively equal and is used only as a rough estimate. Anatomically, point 4 corresponds to the point where both the white roll and the vermilion thin out.
5 = Middle of the nostril still on the normal side.

6 = Medial aspect of the nostril still on the normal side.
7 = Medial aspect of the lateral nostril still on the cleft side.
8 = The length of the lip on the normal side is measured and the distance of 5 to 2 is then recorded. The vertical distance of the lip between points 6 and 3 is then measured. The difference in the length of 5 to 2 minus 6 to 3 is the amount that the lip needs to be lengthened. This distance is set on the first of the calipers used to draw an arched line from point 4. A second caliper is based on the length of line 6 to 3 and is swung from point 7. The point where the arcs intersect becomes point 8.
9 = The middle of the philtrum at a right angle to point 3 (6 to 3). The length of the line 3 to 9 equals the amount that the lip needs to be lengthened to accommodate the triangle.
10 = Using the length of line 3 to 9 as the length of the triangle's limb, an arc is swung from 4 and 8. The intersecting point determines point 10. In a very wide cleft, points 4, 8, and 10 can be subjectively modified depending on the width of the cleft.

2. The second cause for a long lip is furling of the lateral element by its attachments to the maxilla. The lip must be released from the maxilla before any markings are made for the repair.
3. The lateral lip should be purposely created 1 mm shorter than the medial side.[15]

The original description of the Tennison repair does not address correction of the nasal deformity. However, certain modifications do enable preliminary work on the nose:

1. The perialar incision allows the ala to be positioned medially (Fig. 27–10).
2. Brauer recommends saving the triangular flap at the alar base so that it can be rotated into a small incision made at the junction of the columella and membranous septum.[6] This procedure allows some columellar lengthening. Randall[5] also has alluded to this possibility by adding a small triangular flap to the alar side within the nose.

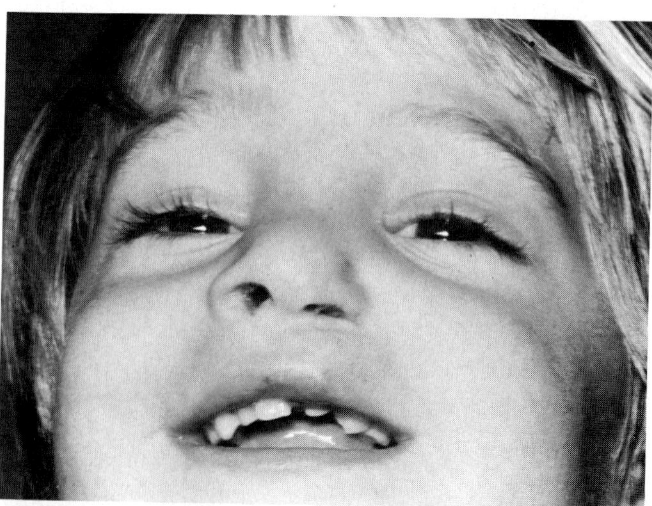

Figure 27–6 Perialar incision used to allow the lip and nose to move independently.

Figure 27–7 Nostril that was made too small with subsequent aesthetic and functional deformity.

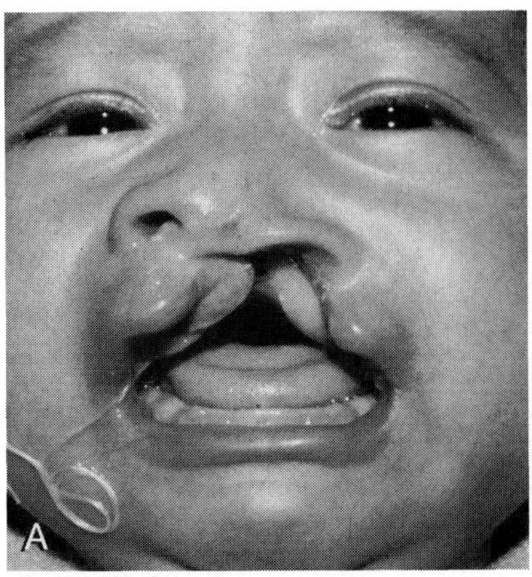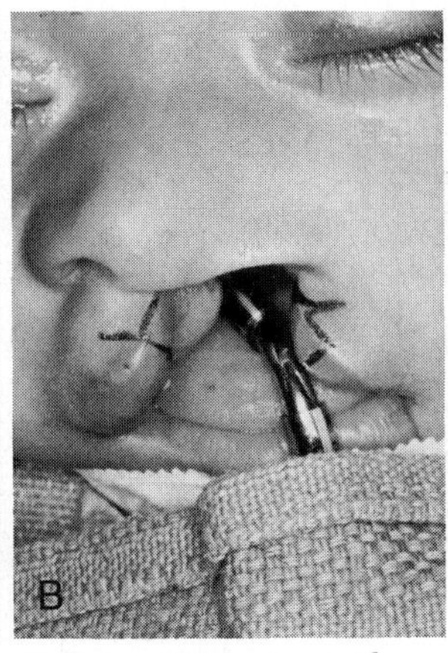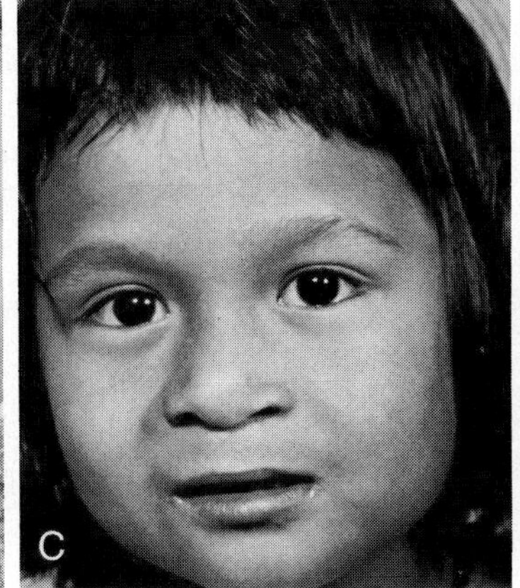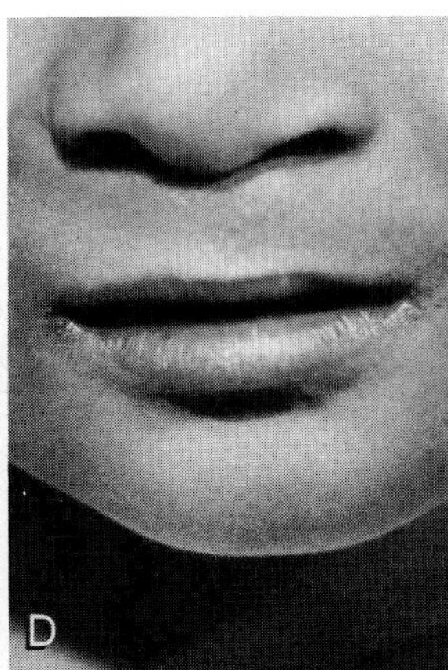

Figure 27–8 Very wide unilateral cleft lip. *A*, Preoperative view with prosthesis in place at 3 months. *B*, Preoperative markings showing the large triangular flap. *C*, Five years postoperatively. *D*, Close-up of lip. Nasal tip repair is usually done at age 5 years.

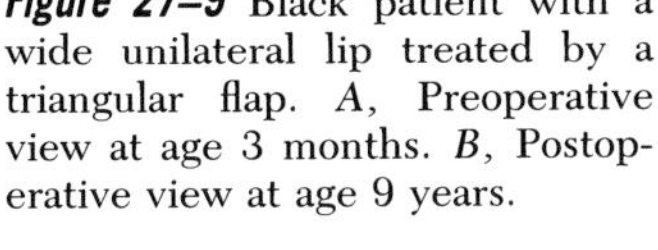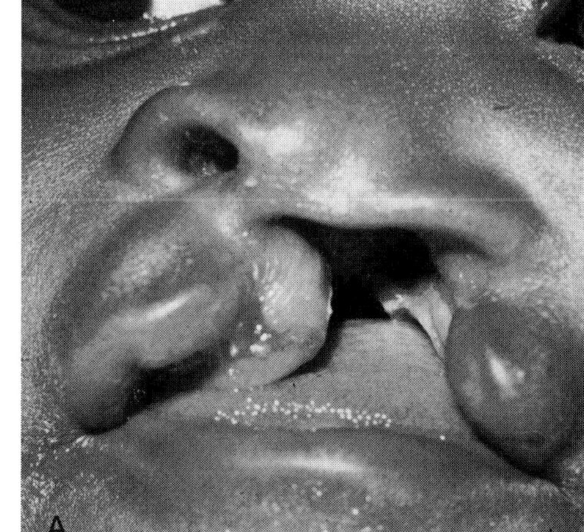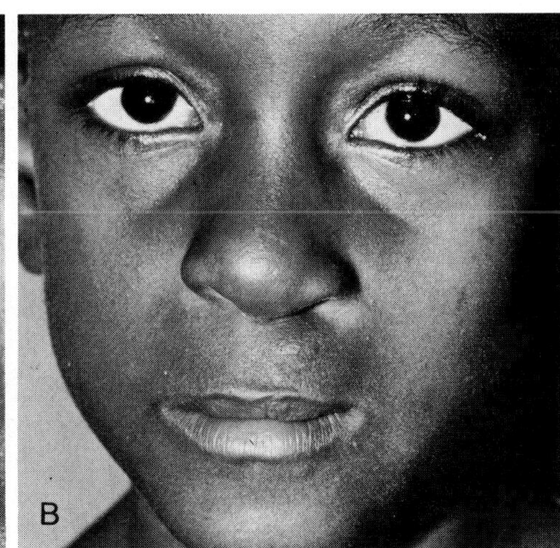

Figure 27–9 Black patient with a wide unilateral lip treated by a triangular flap. *A*, Preoperative view at age 3 months. *B*, Postoperative view at age 9 years.

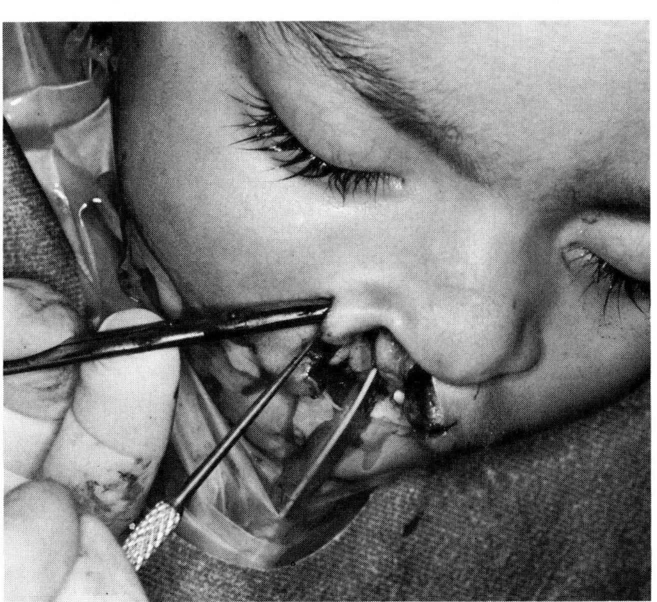

Figure 27–10 Access from the perialar incision is used to free the alar cartilage and aberrant attachments to the cleft.

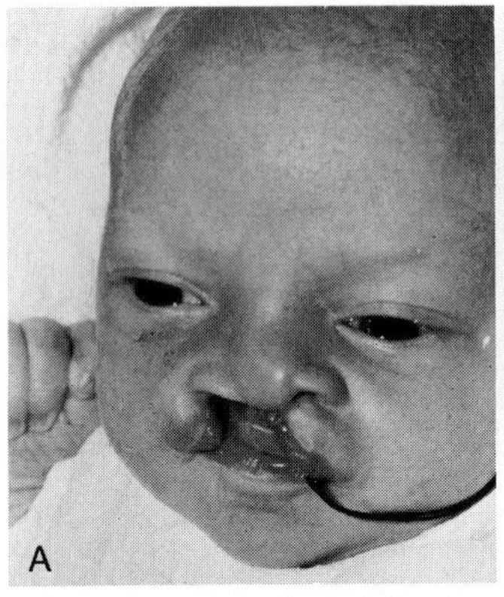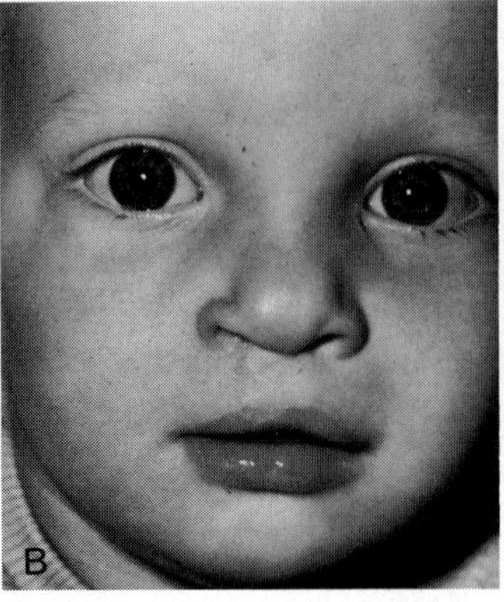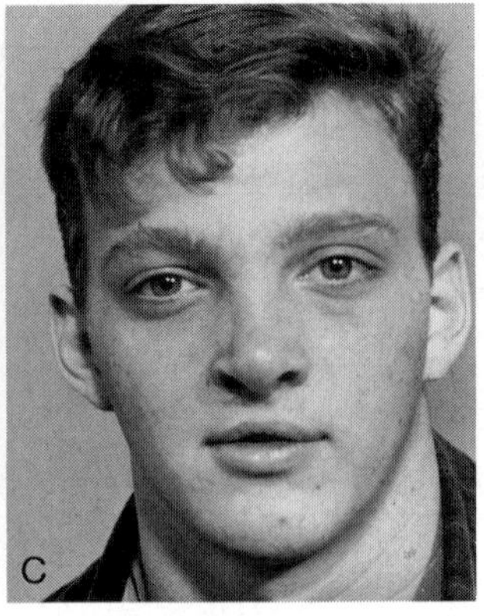

Figure 27–11 Wide unilateral cleft. *A*, Preoperative view at 3 months of age. *B*, Postoperative view at age 1 year. *C*, Postoperative view at age 18.

In 1968, Millard advocated radical correction of the nasal deformity during primary lip repair.[12] There has been a resurgence of interest in radical primary correction of the nasal deformity as shown by recent publications by Salyer[17] and McComb.[18] We have not yet had experience with such radical undermining, but our preliminary data favor a primary Kilner crescent-shaped excision and one or two alar suspension sutures.

Conclusion

We believe that both the Millard and Tennison repairs should be incorporated into the armamentarium of the cleft lip surgeon and used appropriately in selected cases. The primary repair is the most significant and sets the stage for the patient (Fig. 27–11). We generally avoid lip adhesions. Now that we are able to re-create the Cupid's bow and the normal lip pout successfully, we still need to address the associated nasal deformity. Further long-term follow-up of patients who have had radical primary nasal correction is required to determine if any growth disturbances result from the surgery. A useful addition would be the universal adoption of a standardized evaluation system that assesses both the residual nasal deformity and the lip deformity.[19] Standard soft tissue x-rays and cephalometric evaluation also may be incorporated into such a system.

References

1. Grace L: Frequency of occurrence of cleft palates and harelips. J Dent Res 22:495, 1963.
2. Fogh-Anderson P: Incidence of cleft lip and palate: Constant or increasing? Acta Chir Scand 122:106, 1961.
3. Tennison CW: The repair of the unilateral cleft lip by the stencil method. Plast Reconstr Surg 9:115, 1952.
4. Millard DR: Complete unilateral clefts. Plast Reconstr Surg 25:595, 1960.
5. Randall P: A triangular flap operation for the primary repair of unilateral clefts of the lip. Plast Reconstr Surg 23:331, 1959.
6. Brauer RO, Cronin TD: The Tennison lip repair revisited. Plast Reconstr Surg 71:633, 1983.
7. Brauer RO, Cronin TD, Reaves EL: Early maxillary orthopedics, orthodontics, and alveolar bone grafting in complete clefts of the palate. Plast Reconstr Surg 29:625, 1962.
8. Musgrave RH: Observations on the repair of the unilateral cleft lip. Bull Am Cleft Palate Assoc 13:4, 1963.
9. Marcks KM, Trevaskis AE, Da Costa A: Further observation in cleft lip repair. Plast Reconstr Surg 12:392, 1953.
10. Clifford RH, Pool R: The analysis of the anatomy and geometry of the unilateral cleft lip. Plast Reconstr Surg 24:311, 1959.
11. Millard DR: Refinements in rotation advancement cleft lip technique. Plast Reconstr Surg 33:26, 1964.
12. Millard DR: Extensions of the rotation-advancement principle for wide unilateral cleft lips. Plast Reconstr Surg 42:535, 1968.
13. Brauer RO: Repair of unilateral cleft lip: Triangular flap repairs. Clin Plast Surg 12:595, 1985.
14. Goulian D, et al: Further refinements on the triangular flap closure of the cleft lip. Plast Reconstr Surg 80:29, 1987.
15. Cronin TD: A modification of the Tennison-type lip repair. Cleft Palate J 3:376, 1966.
16. Saunders DE, Malek A, Karandy E: Growth of the cleft lip following a triangular flap repair. Plast Reconstr Surg 77:227, 1986.
17. Salyer KE: Primary correction of the unilateral cleft lip nose: A 15-year experience. Plast Reconstr surg 77:558, 1986.
18. McComb H: Primary correction of unilateral cleft lip nasal deformity: A ten-year review. Plast Reconstr Surg 75:791, 1985.
19. Williams HB: A method of assessing cleft lip repairs: Comparison of LeMesurier and Millard techniques. Plast Reconstr Surg 41:103, 1968.

CHAPTER 28

Long-Term Results with the Triangular Flap Technique for Unilateral Cleft Lip Repair

Peter Randall

History

Prior to using the triangular flap operation for unilateral cleft lip repair this author had been trained to use the Brown-McDowell-Mirault technique.[1] This pattern produced symmetry in a predictable way but destroyed the natural Cupid's bow and produced a central high spot at the skin vermilion junction that was very abnormal.

The LeMesurier modification of the Hagedorn procedure gave fine results in some cases but asymmetric results in many others.[2, 3] Soon thereafter, Tennison described his "paper clip stencil operation" using a large triangular flap.[4] The same year that Tennison described his operation, Cardoso pointed out that the medial half of the Cupid's bow on the cleft side is usually present and should be preserved.[5] It is not entirely clear from Tennison's publication whether he was aware of Cardoso's work or not, but he quickly included this valuable addition to his presentations.

I first saw this technique used by Dr. Kirwin Marcks of Allentown, Pennsylvania.[6] Marcks had been trained by Kilner at Oxford, England, and had a large practice of children with clefts. His results with this new technique were superb. He preserved the Cupid's bow, created good symmetry without the central high point of the Mirault flap, and had good fullness in the vermilion. This technique preceded Millard's 1957 publication of his rotation-advancement technique in his Korean patients.[7]

Measurements

In trying to put logic and reason into Tennison's operation, it did not make very good sense to use an incision with three equal length segments in all patients no matter whether the Cupid's bow was displaced a little or a great deal. The solution to the system of measurement, which was presented in 1958 and published in 1959, came from looking at postoperative patients.[8] In virtually all of these patients, the superior edge of the triangular flap was placed horizontally and usually was bisected by a line from the base of the columella to the peak of the Cupid's bow. Furthermore, it was obvious that this vertical distance should be the same on the cleft as on the noncleft side and that the measurement across the triangular flap should be equal to the vertical height on the normal side minus the distance from the columella base to the midpoint of the philtrum incision on the medial side of the cleft. That is, the vertical width of the triangular flap should equal the distance that the Cupid's bow should be moved down to match its height on the noncleft side (Fig. 28–1).

Choice of Operation

At one time, this operation seemed to have taken the place of the Mirault flap and the LeMesurier technique in worldwide use. Yet it appears that the Millard rotation-advancement flap is now more popular in European and American clinics. I have difficulty (more difficulty than Millard) in getting the rotation-advancement flap to work well in clefts in which the Cupid's bow has to be moved a long distance, that is, 3 to 5 mm in an infant. By the same token, poor cleft lip repairs using the triangular flap technique are in my hands usually too long on the repaired side. Lip repairs with poor results using the rotation advancement-technique, however, are usually too short on the repaired side. For these reasons, I prefer to use the rotation-advancement technique for clefts with little upward displacement of the Cupid's bow and the triangular flap procedure for clefts with greater displacement of the Cupid's bow. Greater displacement is usually present in wider clefts and lesser displacement in incomplete clefts, though this may not be absolutely true.

Lip Adhesion

If the cleft is very wide and difficult to close, I prefer to do a lip adhesion operation first (often in conjunction with a soft palate closure) and then, 3 to 4 months later when the tissues have softened, go ahead with the definitive cleft lip repair and closure of the hard palate.[9] At the time of cleft lip repair, the choice between these two operations is based on the same factors mentioned earlier.

Further Development

Saunders et al have shown that if discrepancies in vertical height are seen at the end of the lip repair or in the early postoperative period, they probably will continue to exist.[10] Cronin added a very short vertical limb between the triangular flap and the skin vermilion border that helps to break up the appearance of the lateral vermilion and extends up into the diagonal incision.[11] Borde et al have used the same triangular principle but calculate the dimensions by using a clever measurement of angles.[12]

Originally, my technique for cleft lip repair included a small flap placed across the nostril floor into the base

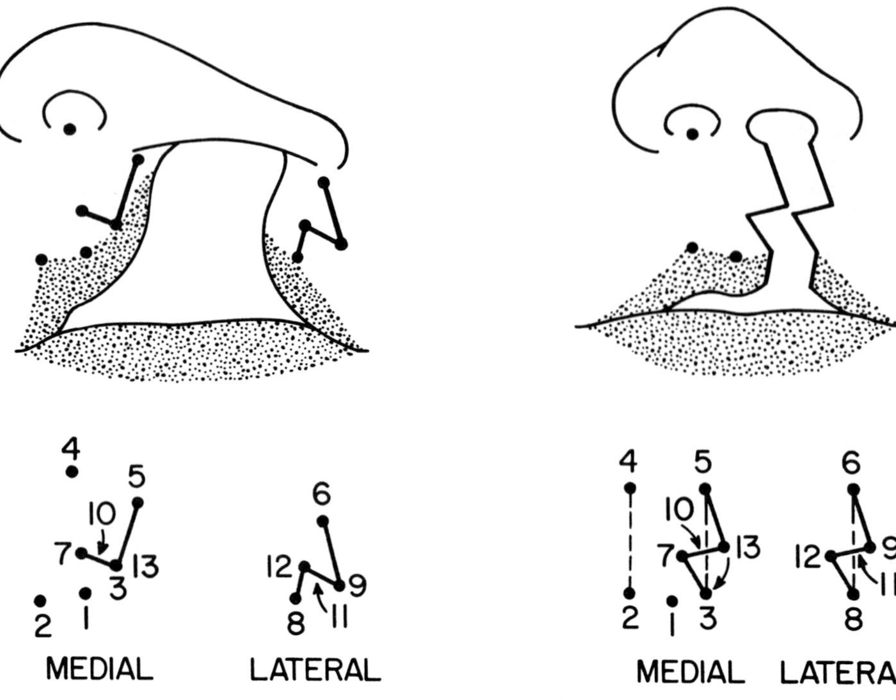

Figure 28–1 Original diagram of the measurements for the triangular flap repair. The vertical distance across the triangular flap equals the height on the normal side minus the distance from the columella base to the midpoint of the incision into the philtrum. This flap is not made larger than 4 mm in a 3-month-old child. (From Randall P. A triangular flap operation for the primary repair of unilateral clefts of the lips. Plast Reconstr Surg, 23:331–347, 1959. With permission.)

of the columella[8] (Fig. 28–2). I first saw this used by Lewis in Galveston, Texas. This flap has a tendency to build up the nostril sill, prevent a notch in the nostril floor, and provide a little fullness in the columellar "shoulder." At that time, Skoog was using two triangular flaps, one placed just above the skin vermilion junction as in the triangular flap technique and the other placed in the upper part of the lip just below the columella.[13] I visited Skoog in Upsala in 1959 and we discussed these two flaps. He was sure that I would like the "outside" flap, and I felt that the "inside" flap had advantages. Before I left Upsala, Skoog said, "Peter, why don't you try the outside flap and I will try the inside flap, and we will see which we like best." I must confess that I never kept my part of this bargain, but at the present time in most places, the inside flap is referred to as the "Skoog flap."

The original design and measurements in my hands have remained pretty much as first described except for one modification. In an effort to prevent the lip from being too long on the cleft side, I do not make the flap any larger than 4 mm in the 3- to 4-month-old infant. In older children and adults with unrepaired clefts, a larger flap can be used (Fig. 28–3).

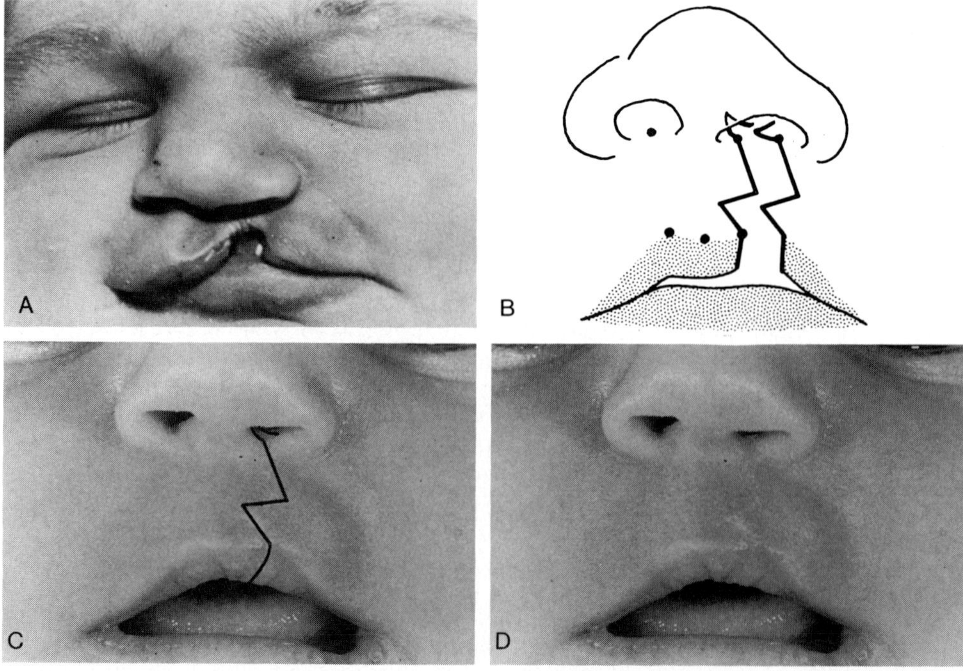

Figure 28–2 A small flap is placed on the base of the columella to fill out the columella "shoulder" and produce a nostril sill. (From Randall P. A triangular flap operation for the primary repair of unilateral clefts of the lip. Plast Reconstr Surg 23:331–347, 1959. With permission.)

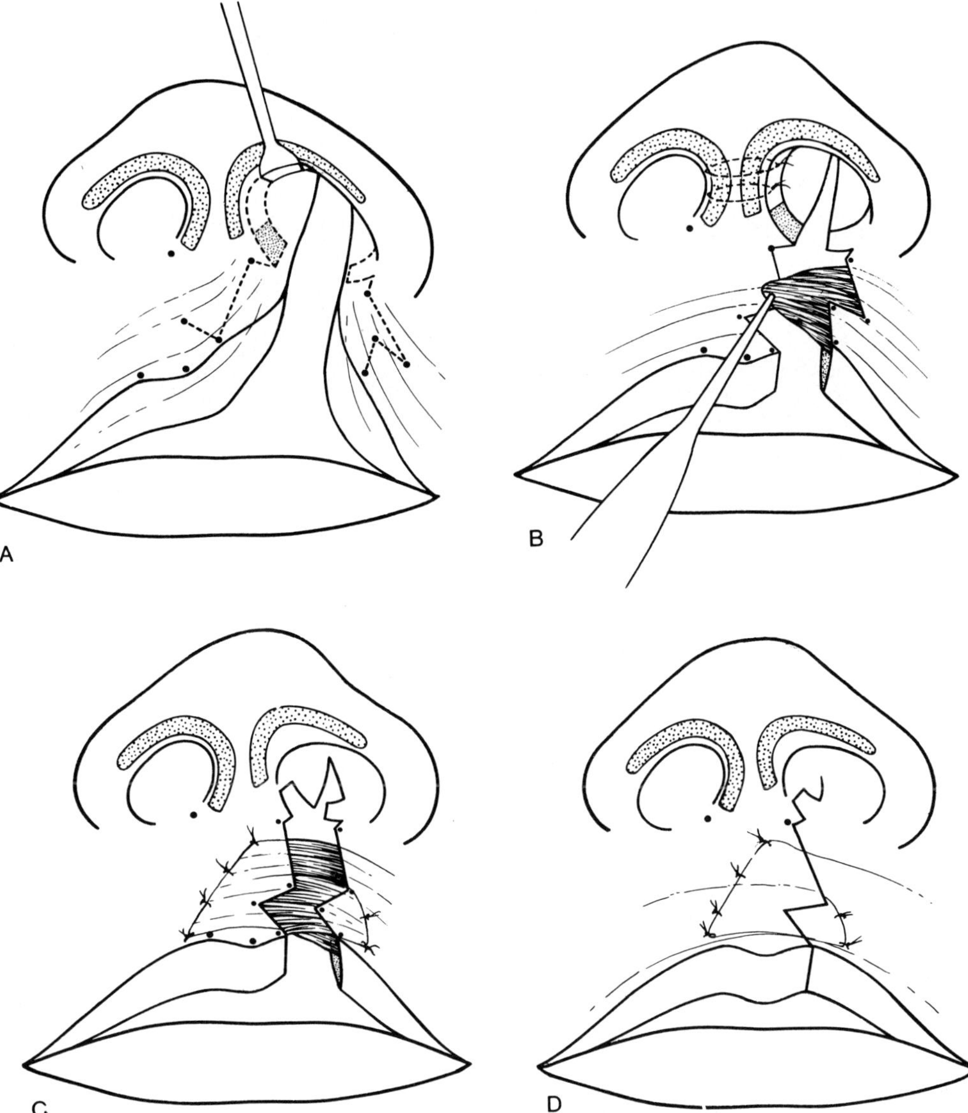

Figure 28–3 The misplaced orbicularis oris fibers paralleling the cleft margin *(A)*. The misplaced orbicularis muscle was dissected free of the overlying skin and underlying mucosa *(B)*. The lateral and medial muscle flaps were overlapped *(C)*. The muscles were sutured to each other and to the nasal spine, taking much tension off the skin closure *(D)*. (From Randall P. Triangular flap repair of the unilateral cleft lip. *In* Brent B (ed): The Artistry of Plastic Surgery. St. Louis: CV Mosby, 1987. With permission.)

Results

The question now is whether this technique has withstood the test of time. In the beginning nothing was done to reorient the orbicularis oris muscle. Incisions were simply carried all the way through the skin muscle and mucosa. I even had a mucosal triangular flap directly below the skin triangular flap until it was obvious that this produced excessive fullness in the free border of the vermilion. The incisions were closed in three layers, and many of these patients had a persistent lateral bulge, or "orbicularis muscle bulge." Some have had secondary reorientations of the orbicularis muscle using an incision in the buccal sulcus. I have more recently reoriented the displaced orbicularis and am now trying to interdigitate the medial and lateral slips of muscle in an attempt to reconstruct the sphincter action of the muscle and its insertion into the dermis.[14, 15, 16]

Changes in vertical height to make the Cupid's bow more symmetric can be achieved either at the time of surgery or at a secondary procedure. Should the repaired side be too long vertically at the time of surgery, the triangular flap can simply be shifted laterally a little bit, thereby closing the incision in the philtrum as a Y instead of a V and doing the same laterally. Reduction in vertical length also can be achieved by removing a small amount of tissue from either the superior or the inferior edge of the horizontal incision (along the superior edge of the triangular flap). When doing this excision as a secondary operation, it is necessary to remove about twice as much in width as the distance needed to bring up the Cupid's bow so it will be even with the noncleft side.

A "bow-shaped" excision also can be carried out in the upper part of the lip starting beneath the columella and continuing to the nostril floor, then coursing laterally just a short distance around part of the alar base. However, the width of this excision should be about three times the amount the Cupid's bow is to be shifted. In making this excision, I think it is helpful to suture the deeper tissues on the medial side of the cleft to the

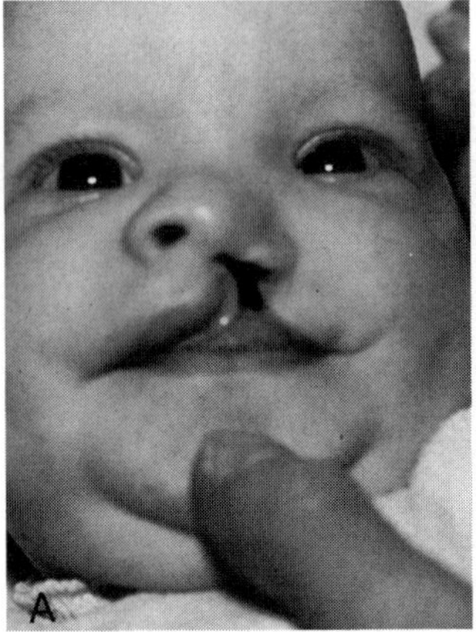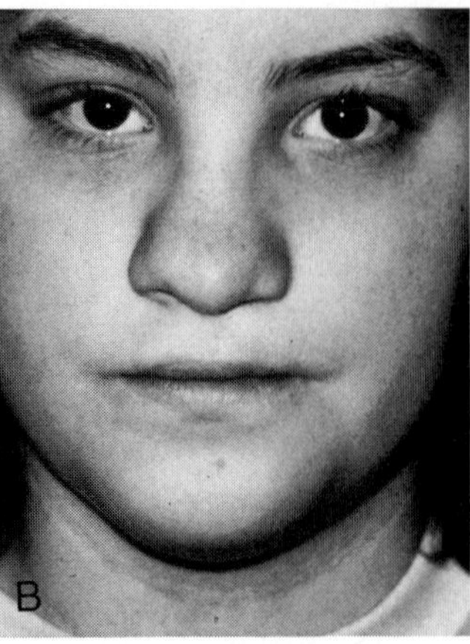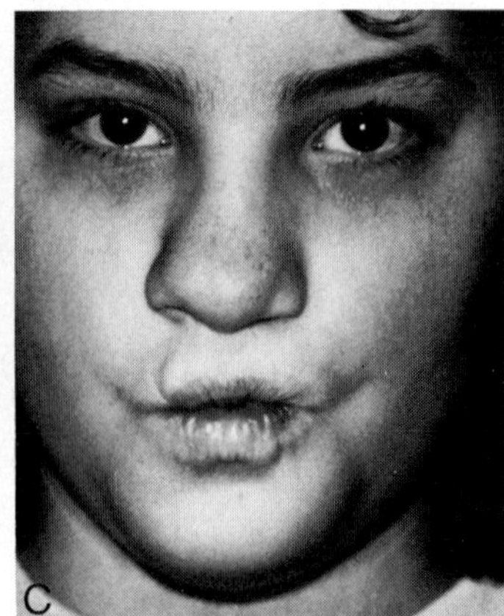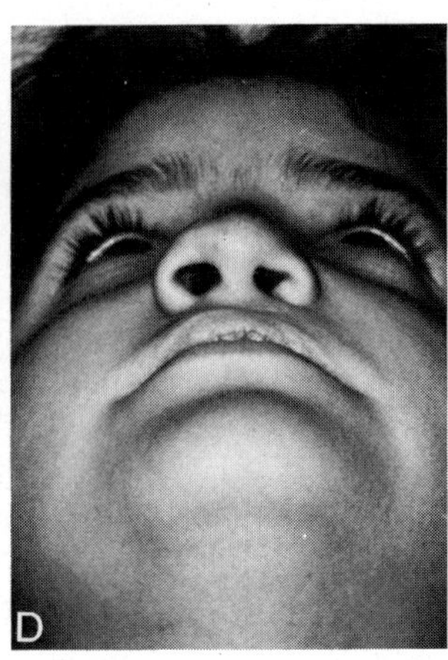

Figure 28–4 Pre- and postoperative photographs of a patient with a complete left unilateral cleft repaired with a triangular flap technique and muscle reconstruction. At the time of the initial repair the medial crus was advanced toward the nasal tip into a slightly overcorrected position. The nose has had no further external work. A small midline vermilion tubercle has been constructed with a V-Y advancement at a secondary operation, and the left lateral vermilion was reduced during a recent operation.

periosteum of the nasal spine and to the nostril floor laterally to take the tension off the skin closure.

Should the height have to be increased, either at the time of the initial surgery or as a secondary procedure, the triangular flap can be advanced medially, thus increasing its effective width. Further excision may have to be done in the vermilion lateral to the initial incision to facilitate closure (Fig. 28–4).

Discussion

Dr. James Barrett Brown used to say that in facial reconstruction it is better to fit the pieces together as though they were pieces of wood rather than pieces of rubber. This statement indicates a basic philosophy quite different from the principles of "pull," "stretch," and "undermine," yet it indicates that if the pieces fit together easily and exactly without the need to pull and stretch, the end results both immediately and for years to come will avoid tension and an abnormal appearance. This concept applies to the triangular flap repair very well because these pieces should fit together accurately.

Many patients lack a midline vermilion tubercle. The technique I use most frequently to construct a tubercle is simply a V–Y advancement of a mucosal flap with the base of the V at the free border of the lip and the width about equal to the distance between the midportion of each central incisor (Fig. 28–4). With realignment of the orbicularis muscle, better contour and motion of the lips are achieved when using the V–Y advancement flap with either the rotation-advancement operation or the triangular flap. However, a high percentage of these patients with muscle reconstruction have fullness in the vermilion lateral to the lip repair on the cleft side. This is corrected by excising a wide elliptical band of mucosa just inside the free border of the lip. In doing this, I usually take out some of the underlying muscle as well.

A few male patients have grown mustaches but lack hair follicles, not only in the scar but also often in the skin adjacent to the scar, particularly on the medial side. Individual, 1- to 2-mm micro hair plugs taken from the scalp and placed in round holes, usually made with a 1- or 2-mm skin biopsy punch, have helped to overcome this problem.

Conclusions

On the whole, this operation has been a reliable technique for repairing the more severe clefts. This technique is more a matter of how far the Cupid's bow is displaced upward than the width of the cleft, although more severe displacement is usually associated with more severe clefts. I have preferred the triangular flap operation to the Millard rotation-advancement operation in patients who need to have the Cupid's bow brought down 3 mm or more.

If the cleft is very wide (particularly if it is bilateral) a lip adhesion procedure has helped by converting the difficult, wide, complete cleft into a much easier incomplete cleft with better alignment of the alveolar segments. The lip adhesion procedure achieves virtually the same positioning of the premaxillary alveolar segment as elastic strapping of the wide cleft. I usually combine lip adhesion with closure of the soft palate when the infant is 3 to 4 months old, and then in 3 or 4 months' time (when the tissues have softened) I do a definitive lip repair with a vomer flap closure of the hard palate.

References

1. Brown JB, McDowell F: A small triangular flap operation for the primary repair of single cleft lips. Plast Reconstr Surg 5:392–402, 1950.
2. LeMesurier AB: The quadrilateral Mirault flap for harelip. Plast Reconstr Surg 16:422–433, 1955.
3. Hagedorn WH: Über eine Modifikation der Hasemschartenoperation. Centralb R Chir 11:756, 1884.
4. Tennison CW: The repair of the unilateral cleft lip by the stencil method. Plast Reconstr Surg 9:115–120, 1952.
5. Cardoso, AD: New technique for harelip. Plast Reconstr Surg 10:92–95, 1952.
6. Marcks KM, Trevaskis AE, daCosta A: Further observations in cleft lip repair. Plast Reconstr Surg 12:392–402, 1953.

7. Millard DR: A primary camouflage of the unilateral harelip. In Transactions of the First International Congress of Plastic Surgery. Baltimore: Williams & Wilkins, 1957, pp 160–166.

8. Randall P: A triangular flap operation for the primary repair of unilateral clefts of the lip. Plast Reconstr Surg 23:331–347, 1959.

9. Randall P: A lip adhesion operation in cleft lip surgery. Plast Reconstr Surg 35:371–376, 1965.

10. Saunders DE, Malek A, Karrandy E: Growth of the cleft lip following a triangular flap repair. Plast Reconstr Surg 77:227–237, 1986.

11. Cronin TD: A modification of the Tennison-type lip repair. Cleft Palate J 3:376–382, 1966.

12. Borde J, Bedonelle J, Malek R: Traitement du bec-de-lievre par un procede plastique utilisant un lambeau triangulaire equilatéral. Ann Chiv Inf 2:111–115, 1961.

13. Skoog T: A design for the repair at the unilateral cleft lip. Am J Surg 95:223–225, 1958.

14. Fará M: Anatomy and arteriography in cleft lips in stillborn children. Plast Reconstr Surg 42:29–36, 1968.

15. Randall P, Whitaker LA, LaRossa D: The importance of muscle reconstruction in primary and secondary cleft lip repair. Plast Reconstr Surg 54:316–323, 1974.

16. LaRossa DD, Randall P: The unilateral cleft lip. In Georgiade NA, Georgiade GS, Riefkoh R, et al (eds): Essentials of Plastic, Maxillofacial and Reconstructive Surgery. Baltimore: Williams & Wilkins, 1987, pp. 241–250.

CHAPTER 29

Bilateral Cleft Lip and Palate Repair

W. M. Manchester

The Philosophy Behind the Repair

I believe the philosophy behind this technique can best be stated by quoting verbatim the introduction to the first paper I published on this subject in the *British Journal of Surgery* in November, 1965.[1]

No greater problem exists in the whole field of surgery than the successful treatment of a patient suffering from complete, bilateral, cleft lip and palate. The responsibility resting on the shoulders of anyone attempting this repair is an onerous one, as failure to achieve its objectives represents a lifelong human tragedy which later surgery can only partially correct.

The objectives are easily stated, but not so easily achieved. They are—to produce a normal appearance, normal speech and normal dental occlusion. Of the three, the last is probably the least important. The first and second are both very important, but perhaps normal speech requires just a little more emphasis than normal appearance if a choice has to be made. The three are to some extent interdependent and also, to some extent, mutually exclusive. In producing a comprehensive, integrated programme the best we can hope for is some kind of compromise in which certain sacrifices have to be made to accomplish something that is regarded as more desirable.

This present work, though more concerned with the repair of the lip, cannot altogether ignore the question of palatal repair, dental orthopaedics and orthodontics. The author believes therefore that at the same time as both sides of the lip are repaired, at the age of five months, the anterior palate must also be repaired on both sides. There are two reasons for this. Firstly, the avoidance of fistulae in the anterior part of the palate—it is believed that this can be achieved satisfactorily only at this first operation on the lip—and secondly, the result of the first operation should be to convert a bilateral cleft of the lip into a simple cleft of little more than the soft palate. In order to do this it is necessary to use the whole of the vomerine mucosa on both sides to make good the repair of the anterior palate in sufficient length to allow the second stage, which is performed at the age of nine months, to produce the longest possible palate with the shortest possible suture line. In this way shrinkage is cut down to a minimum. It is for this reason that, if bone grafting of the alveolar defect is to be carried out, it is preferred as a secondary rather than a primary procedure. This is simply because if the vomerine mucosa is used to cover the bone graft at a primary operation, it is not then available to make its proper contribution to the achievement of normal speech. *It is further believed that the first operation on the lip should, as far as possible, be the only one.* This seldom seems to be possible with primary bone grafting of the alveolar ridge.

This discussion has been necessary to explain the belief that the lip repair cannot be considered apart from these other factors and to emphasize the fact that the lip repair is only a part of the total plan.

After developing this technique for a further quarter of a century I still believe this basic philosophy to be sound, although of course many refinements have been introduced as a result of careful study of the results in the follow-up clinic.

The Evolution of the Present Technique

Forty-nine years ago, when I first started training in the surgery of cleft lip and palate, the results in patients with bilateral clefts were simply appalling. In many patients, dental occlusion was nonexistent, speech was unintelligible, and physical appearance was grotesque. In some patients, the blood supply to the premaxilla had been cut off, resulting in its complete loss. In almost every patient, the lateral lip elements were sewn to each other in the midline below the prolabium, which itself had usually been pushed upward in an attempt to lengthen the columella. The finished lip was therefore too tight from side to side, lacking its central element, and this converted it into an orthopedic device acting in exactly the opposite direction to what was required. The result was that premaxillary development did not occur properly, and a class III relationship almost always developed.

With this kind of skeletal defect, no matter how skillful the lip surgery nor how beautiful the scars, the end result is always bad, and the stigma of bilateral cleft lip is recognizable across the street. This is because the upper lip lies behind its proper plane and often behind that of the lower lip itself.

Examination of a normal baby's lip at the age of 5 months reveals the philtral dimple in the midline, flanked on either side by its two columns. The vermilion border, separated from the skin by the mucocutaneous

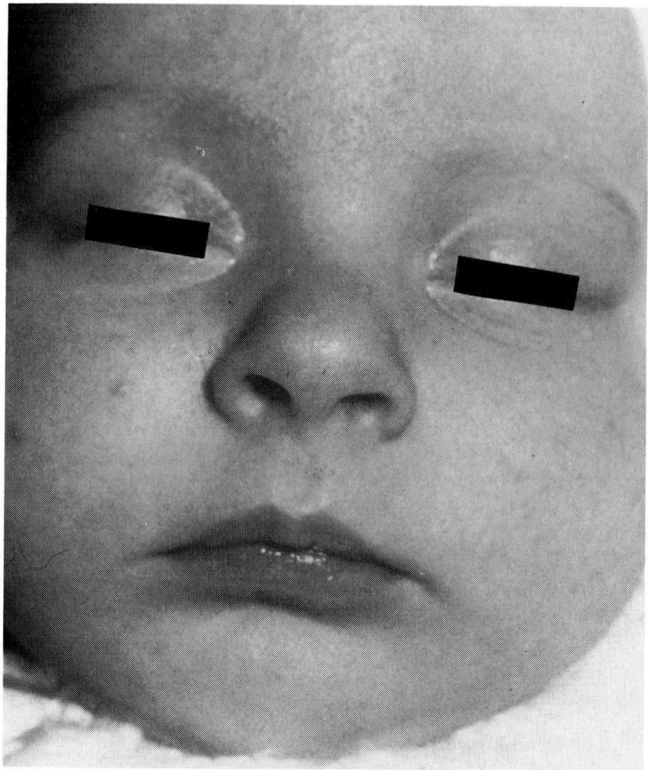

Figure 29–1 Normal baby's lip. The vermilion is fullest at the center where it forms the median tubercle. It tapers toward the commissures.

ridge, is narrowest at the two sides and tapers to the commissure, whereas in the middle it is at its fullest, forming the pouting median tubercle of the lip (Fig. 29–1).

In patients with bilateral cleft lip and palate, on the other hand, the prolabium, which ought to have formed the philtrum, is quite different in shape. Its vermilion border is very small and the vermilion of the lateral elements is very full, and they themselves are thick and muscular. The prolabium, or central part, has no muscle in it at all (Fig. 29–2A).

It is quite clear that if these three elements were simply joined together the result would be the opposite of normal—a narrow vermilion in the middle and a wider vermilion on either side producing what is commonly known as a "whistle" deformity (Fig. 29–2B).

The Need for Presurgical Orthopedic Treatment

Normal development of the premaxilla depends on normal soft tissue stresses during fetal life. When there is a bilateral cleft of the lip and palate these soft tissue stresses are in a state of gross imbalance. At birth the outward signs of this are seen in a very prominent premaxilla (Fig. 29–3A).

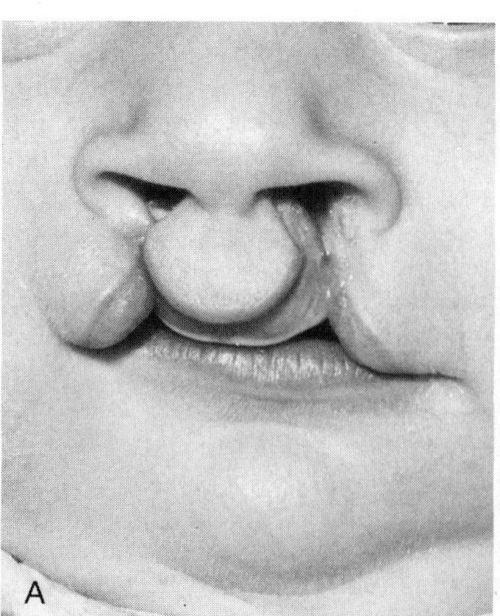

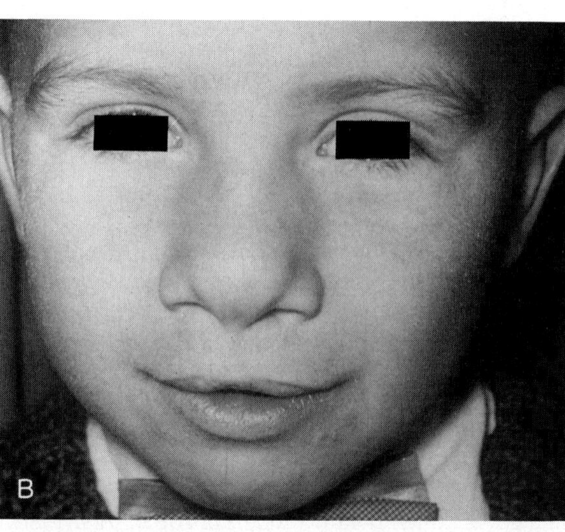

Figure 29–2 A, Complete bilateral cleft. In the center of the prolabium only the narrowest strip of vermilion is visible from the front in contrast to the lateral lip elements, which show much wider areas of vermilion. Simply uniting these three elements would produce a whistle deformity. B, Whistle deformity resulting from earlier methods of repair. (From Manchester WM: The repair of bilateral cleft lip and palate. Br J Surg 52(11):878–882, 1965.)

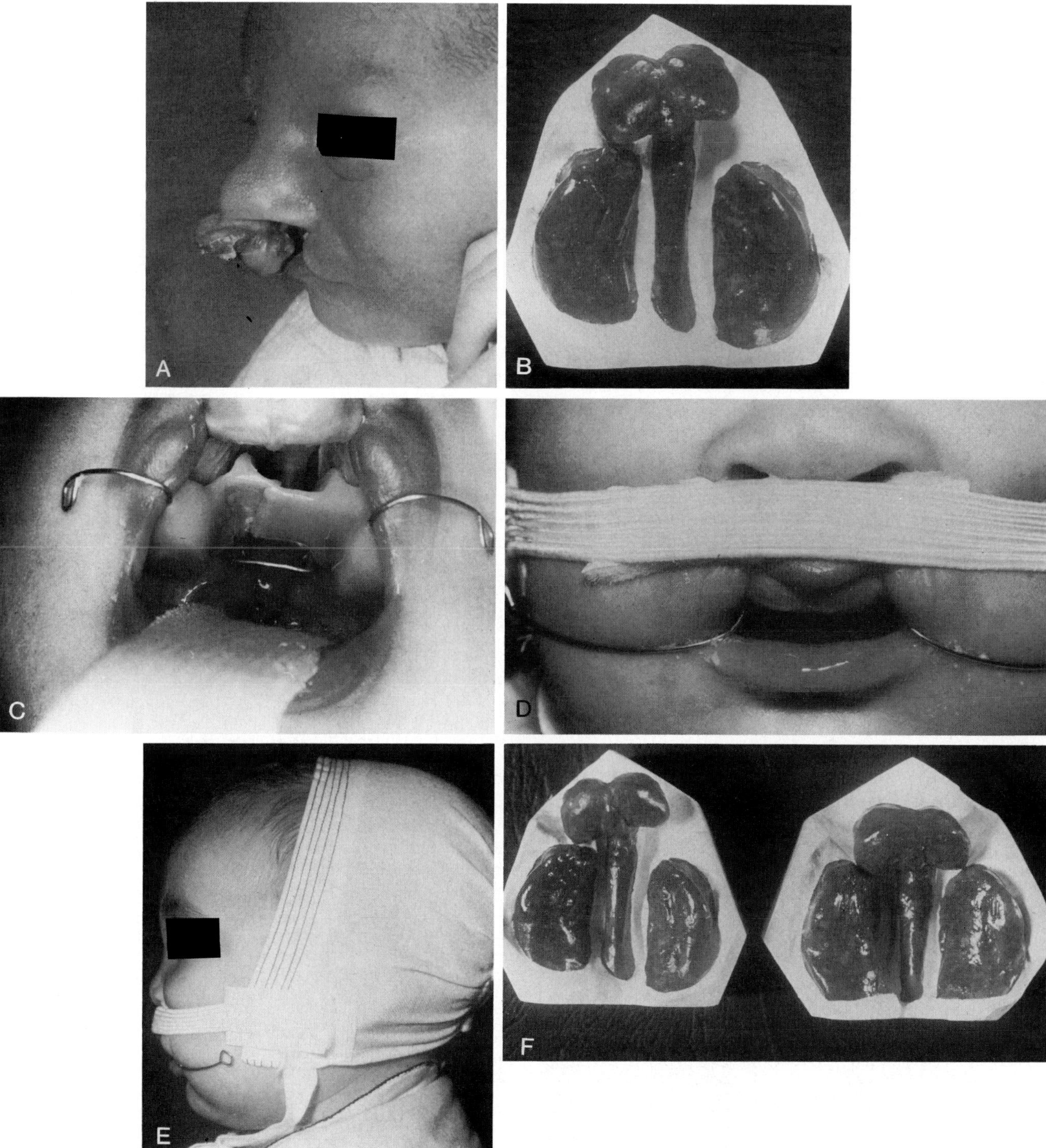

Figure 29–3 *A*, Prominent premaxilla resulting from gross imbalance of soft tissue structures during fetal life. *B*, Model of the same patient. The premaxilla is much too anterior. *C*, Appliance being introduced to the cleft, with the spring at the back under slight tension. *D*, Elastic traction on the central structures to simulate normal lip pressures. *E*, Velcro patches and a cap are used for easy management of the elastic. *F*, Model on the left shows the state of affairs at birth. The model on the right shows that the parts have grown well and that the premaxilla is in a more normal position and forms a keystone to the dental arch. (*A* to *F* from Manchester WM: The repair of double cleft lip as part of an integrated programme. Plast Reconstr Surg 45:207, 1970. By permission of Williams & Wilkins.)

Examination of a model of the upper jaw in such cases shows what has happened. The tongue has been able to get up into the cleft, thrust on the back of the premaxilla, and encourage its forward growth. The imbalance is further aggravated by the lack of continuity of the muscle of the upper lip, which would otherwise have restrained it (Fig. 29–3B).

The scar tissue resulting from repair of the lip and palate in this condition would cause collapse of the lateral maxillary segments behind the premaxilla, and later treatment could never correct it.

All this can be prevented only by a program of presurgical orthopedic treatment that starts at birth and continues for the next 5 months. Its objective is to change the anatomy to make it more suitable for surgery and for the ultimate goal of normal dental occlusion. Its aim is not the forcible thrusting of displaced segments into a more normal position, but influencing the growth of the premaxilla and maxilla in such a way that a more normal configuration of their segments results, making them more suitable for surgery.

It is my belief that if the maxillary segments can be encouraged to grow laterally and the forward growth of the premaxilla diminished, we will have a situation that subsequent scar tissue shrinkage will not affect too adversely. The premaxilla will then form a keystone to the arch.

J. H. Peat, the senior orthodontist on the team, devised an appliance consisting of an upper dental plate in two halves with a spring joining them. It has two segments that overlap each other so that when the apparatus spreads under its own slight spring tension there is still an effective roof to the mouth that prevents the tongue thrusting on the back of the premaxilla and encouraging its forward growth (Fig. 29–3C–D).

At the same time, elastic traction is exercised on the prolabium to simulate normal lip pressures.

Provided that the components of the upper jaw grow at the normal rate, comparison of models taken at birth and 5 months later—just before surgery—will show an alveolar arch that forms a continuous horseshoe with the premaxilla acting as a stable keystone between the maxillary segments (Fig. 29–3F).

Twenty-five years ago the author and his colleagues became so dissatisfied with the methods then in use for bilateral cleft lip repair that they decided to see how this unpromising material could be used:

1. To fashion a normal looking lip with a Cupid's bow and a full median tubercle.
2. To produce a lip that was not too tight and therefore did not contribute to poor premaxillary development.
3. To contribute at a second operation to the development of normal speech.

The Main Problem

One of the basic problems was that the central prolabial vermilion was not large enough to make a full central tubercle. This difficulty was overcome by incising transversely the mucosal side of the prolabium near the upper labial sulcus, everting the vermilion and lining mucosa, thus enlarging the area of the central vermilion as seen from the front (Fig. 29–4A–C).

This maneuver naturally leaves a raw surface on the back of the prolabium that is made good by making flaps of the vermilion bordering the cleft on the lateral lip elements. *This is bonus tissue because it is there only because there is a cleft.* These flaps are rotated toward each other so as to meet in the midline in front of the premaxilla with their raw surface facing forward, thus filling the gap on the back of the prolabium without undue tension on the premaxilla. The upper edges of these flaps fit along the mucoperiosteal cut edge on the premaxilla, thus reestablishing the upper labial sulcus (Fig. 29–5).

Program of Treatment

The child is seen by the cleft lip and palate team very soon after birth. If there is a prominent premaxilla or other abnormality the orthodontist begins his presurgical orthopedic program, which has been described briefly earlier and in detail elsewhere.[2–4]

Provided that the child grows at a proper rate, by the

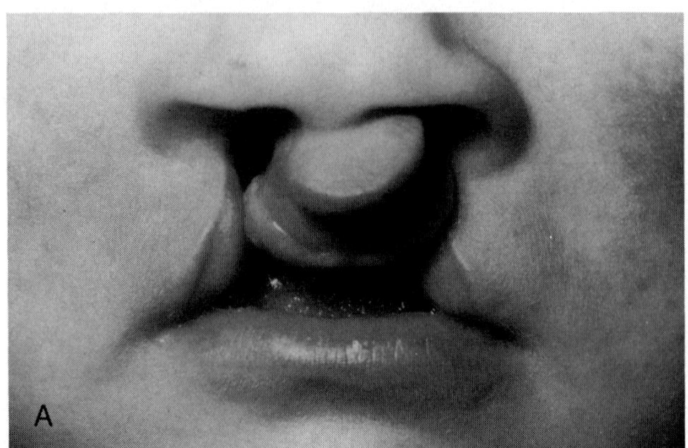

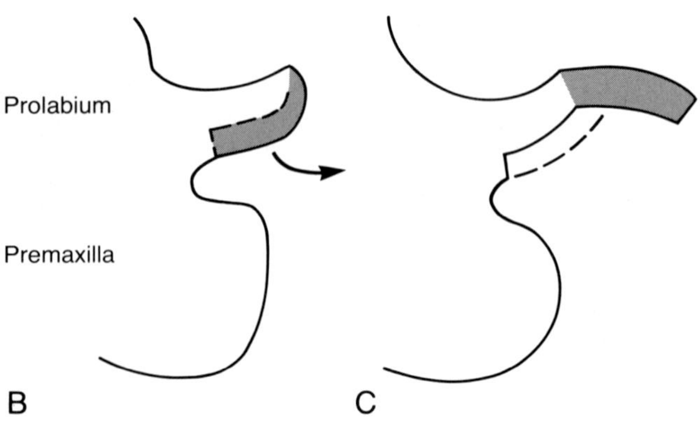

Figure 29–4 *A*, The amount of central prolabial vermilion is not enough to make a full central tubercle. *B*, Diagrammatic view of the incisions needed to evert the prolabial mucosa and vermilion. *C*, Mucosa and vermilion everted but at the expense of a raw surface on the oral side.

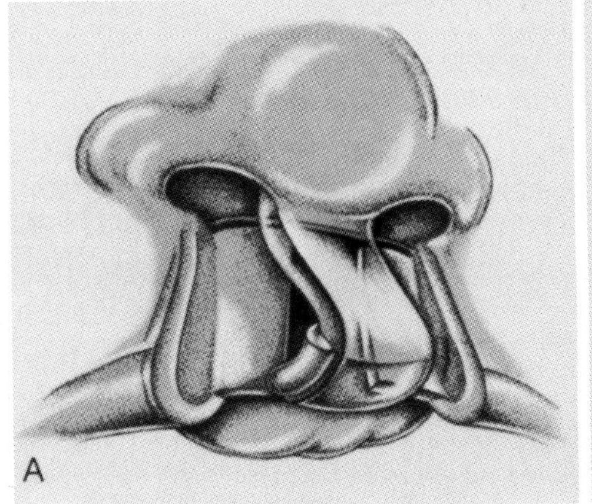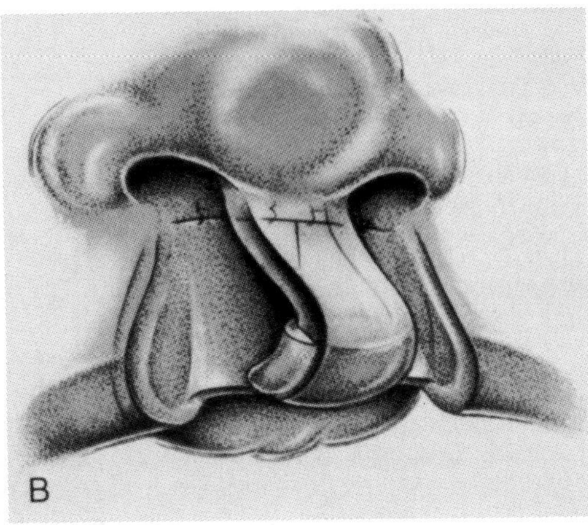

Figure 29–5 Flaps from the lateral lip elements have been rotated through 180 degrees to cover the raw surface on the back of the prolabium and to reconstitute the upper labial sulcus. *B,* These flaps have been united along their upper edge in the region of the upper labial sulcus and to each other in the midline.

age of 5 months a much better configuration of the segments will have been established, and the child is then admitted for surgery.

The aim of the first operation is to repair the lip and the floor of the nose on both sides and the hard palate as far back as the junction with the soft palate.

The Markings

The markings are very simple. At the vermilion border the midline of the lip is marked on the mucocutaneous ridge of the prolabium. On either side of this, but very close to it, the points that will become the peaks of the Cupid's bow are marked. Similar points are marked on the prolabium at the columellar base. These are also kept very close to the midline to reduce the widening of the prolabium that tends to occur after surgery. On the lateral lip elements matching points at the alar base are marked, as is the point that will become the peak of the Cupid's bow at the vermilion border on the mucocutaneous ridge. This latter point is easily established because it is the point where the mucocutaneous ridge peters out and the vermilion begins to taper up alongside the cleft. The pairs of points on either side of the cleft are joined by marks representing the incisions to be made. These marks are made on the skin just beyond the vermilion bordering the cleft in each case.

On each lateral lip element points also are marked on the mucosal side of the lip directly behind those at the alar base and the peak of the Cupid's bow. A line is then drawn from each cutaneous point horizontally around the vermilion to the corresponding point on the back. These lines represent the upper and lower borders, and the space between them is the vertical height of the vermilion flap, which will thus be exactly the same as the distance between the two points on the skin side (Fig. 29–6A and B).

Injection of Adrenalin

Adrenalin, 1:100,000, is then injected into the prolabium, both lateral lip elements, and the upper buccal sulci. Inside the mouth it is injected under the mucoperiosteum of the vomer, the premaxilla, and the palatal mucoperiosteum covering the palatal processes.

Preparation of Mucosal Flaps

The operation is begun on one of the lateral lip elements by making an incision along the line previously marked on the skin and another parallel with it, just inside the vermilion border near the mucocutaneous ridge. These two incisions allow the mucocutaneous ridge to be excised. Incisions are then made above and below along the lines previously marked, joining the points at the alar base and at the peak of the Cupid's bow, around the vermilion to the corresponding points on the mucosal side. These incisions give the outline of the vermilion flap, and only the slightest dissection is necessary to free it and develop it (Fig. 29–6C).

Freeing of the Lateral Lip Elements

The alar base and lip are fixed to the relatively retroposed lateral maxillary segment and must be freed from it if they are to come forward and rest medially without tension in front of the premaxilla, adjacent to the columella. An incision is therefore made along the upper buccal sulcus and the lip and alar base and freed from the facial surface of the maxilla and from the frontal process of the maxilla on both its facial and nasal sides (Fig. 29–6D and E). Even with successful presurgical orthopedic treatment and extensive freeing, the alar base is often still not quite free enough. This freeing is completed by making a reentrant cut into the free edge of the nasal lining for a short distance along the intercartilaginous line. As the alar base is brought forward onto the premaxilla, this cut opens up to leave a triangular gap in the nostril floor and lateral wall. We will see later how this gap is filled to avoid a raw surface. *All this is repeated on the opposite side. Incisions are not made at this stage in the prolabial part because it is very vascular and bleeds a great deal.*

Attention is now directed to the repair of the hard palate.

Preparation of Vomerine-Premaxillary Flaps

Gags are inserted, and an incision is made from behind forward along the greater part of the length of the vomer. At the point where it reaches the back of the premaxilla the incision changes direction sharply

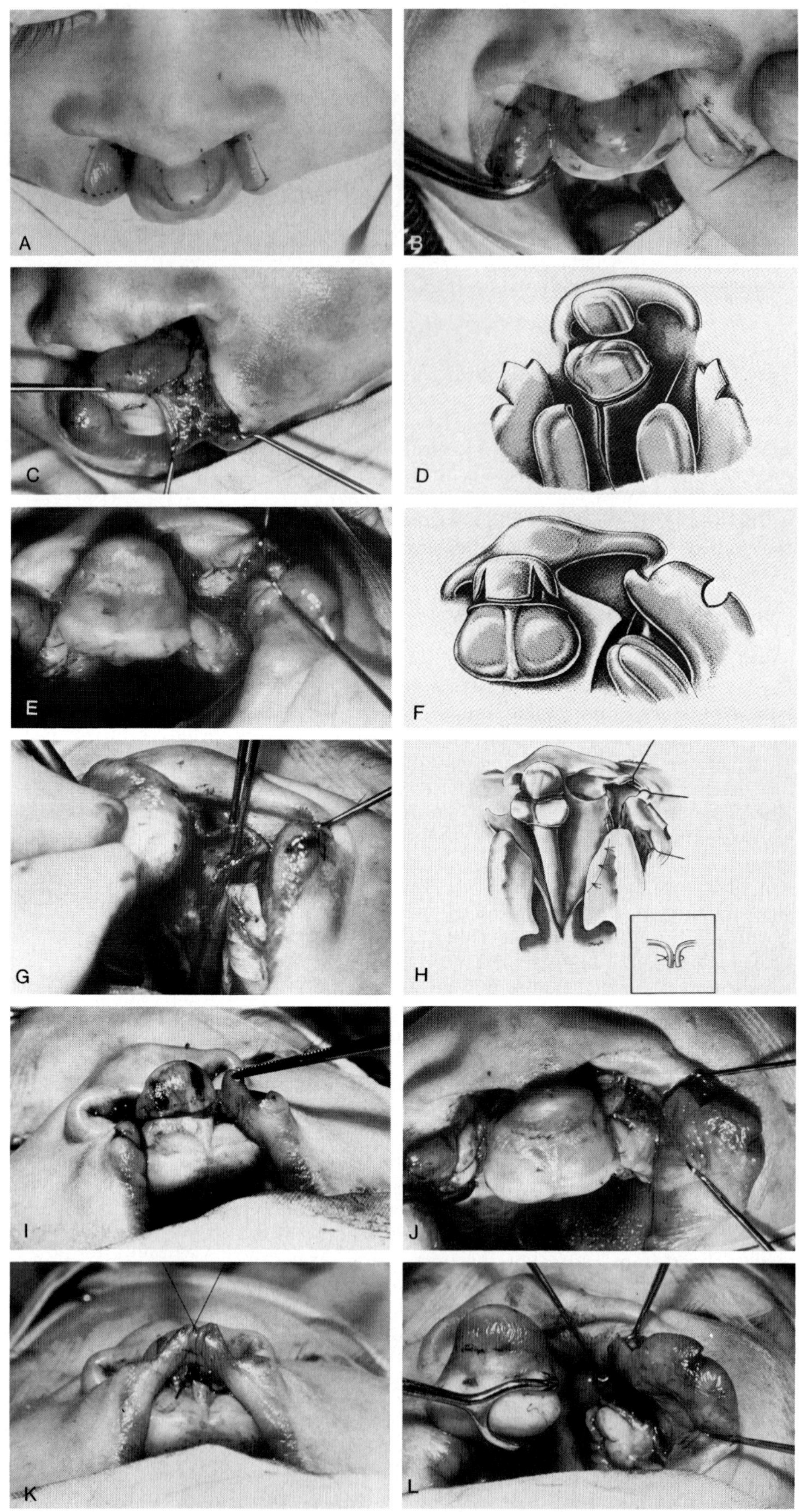

Figure 29–6 *A*, Lip markings. Note the horizontal lines on the patient's lateral lip elements outlining the vermilion and mucosal flaps. *B*, Adrenalin has been injected. On the patient's left, incisions have been made on both sides of the mucocutaneous ridge, which will be excised. *C*, The horizontal incisions previously marked have been made, and the vermilion and mucosal flap has been developed and rotated through 180 degrees. It is sitting almost in its final position, and, with its fellow of the opposite side, will recreate the lining of the central part of the upper lip.

D, An incision has been made in the upper buccal sulcus. The alar base and the vestibular lining have been cleared from the facial and nasal surfaces. The most medial single hook is in the cut free edge of the mucosa of the inferior meatus as it moves forward toward the alar base. *E*, A re-entrant cut has been made into the free edge seen in Figure 29–6*D* and continued along the intercartilaginous line of the nostril wall, pulling forward on the alar base and opening up a triangular defect here. *F*, The position of the incision to prepare the vomerine and premaxillary mucoperiosteal flaps. Note the point in the midline on each side where the two parts of the incision join. *G*, The mucoperiosteal and premaxillary flap has been freed, and the point shown in *F* has moved out toward the lateral nostril wall. The cut free edge of mucosa at the inferior meatus is visible near the point of the flap. *H*, Same maneuver as shown in *G*. The point of the vomerine premaxillary flap is opposite the free margin of the mucosa and skin of the inferior meatus and vestibule; further back its free edge is approaching the hard palatal margin. *I*, The hard palatal mucoperiosteum has been elevated laterally and the vomerine flap tucked under it and united there by mattress stitches. Further forward the edge of the flap is united to the inferior meatal mucosa by mattress stitches. Further forward still it is clear how the point of the vomerine premaxillary flap will easily fit into the raw surface on the nostril wall to make good the raw surface there. Between these two areas a single layer closure is needed using mattress stitches, as shown in the inset.

J, The point of the vomerine premaxillary flap seen from the front, with a catgut stitch in the apex of the flap and at the apex of the re-entrant cut. The right-angled point between this catgut stitch and the hook in the alar base is rounded off. When the repair of these two edges is complete, the alar base will be joined to the columellar base. *K*, The upper margin of the mucosal flap derived from the lateral lip elements has been sewn to the cut edge on the front of the premaxilla as far as the frenum of the lip. Two parallel marks on the mucosa of the prolabium, when incised, will outline the central flap that will become the median tubercle of the lip. *L*, The right-hand flap has been similarly sewn and the medial edges of the flap united to each other in the midline. The upper labial sulcus is now complete at its original level. No incisions have yet been made in the prolabium to reduce blood loss.

232

and skirts around the premaxilla at about the level of the upper labial sulcus. The incision on the other side is similar and meets its fellow at the frenum of the lip in front of the premaxilla. Thus the premaxilla is completely encircled. The mucoperiosteal flaps on each side are elevated, and at the point where the incisions change direction there will be a point on each flap (Fig. 29–6F–H). We will see the fate of this point later.

Repair of the Hard Palate

A split is then made in the mucoperiosteum of the free edge of each palatal process. The mucoperiosteum of the hard palate is then elevated laterally for a short distance along its whole length. The mucoperiosteal flap derived from the vomer is then tucked under it so as to produce a two-layer closure, which is completed with mattress stitches. As this part of the repair is traced forward, the hard palatal mucoperiosteum runs out, and the repair is completed in the region of the floor of the nose and premaxilla by uniting, in single-layer fashion but with a broad surface of apposition, the premaxillary part of the central flap and the nasal mucoperiosteum of the inferior meatus and, finally, a little further forward, the skin of the vestibule of the nose. Mattress stitches are used for this purpose (Fig. 29–6I).

Repair of the Floor of the Nose and Nostril

It is, however, a little more complicated than this because of the triangular gap in the nasal floor and nasal wall resulting from the opening up of the reentrant intercartilaginous incision used to free up the alar base. As the single layer closure of the premaxillary part of the mucoperiosteal flap to the inferior meatal mucosa flap proceeds forward, the point of this flap, described above, fits neatly into the triangular gap so that raw surface here is avoided. The repair proceeds until the alar base is joined to the columellar base (Fig. 29–6H–J).

If this is done properly, absolutely no fistula results and there is almost always a small area of bony union between the lateral maxillary segment and the premaxilla. This results in a premaxilla that is solid and immobile.

The hard palate is now complete, and the stage is set to finish the lip repair.

Re-creation of the Upper Labial Sulcus

The upper borders of the vermilion and mucosal flaps from the lateral lip elements prepared at the beginning of the operation are sewn to the cut edge on the front of the premaxilla on each side, in each case as far as the frenum of the lip in the midline where they meet. Their free margins are joined to each other in front of the premaxilla. This reconstitutes the upper labial sulcus at its original level. *There is no need to deepen it, as some authors suggest* (Fig. 29–6K and L).

This procedure also completes the lining of the central prolabial part of the upper lip. No incisions have yet been made in the prolabium except in the region of the upper labial sulcus. These prolabial incisions have been delayed until just before their final suturing to reduce blood loss (Fig. 29–7A).

Preparation of the Central Prolabial Skin

Incisions are now made in the prolabium, and these join the upper and lower points previously planned on each side. Only a very narrow strip of prolabial skin should remain when these skin incisions are completed down to the vermilion border (Fig. 29–7B).

Formation of the Central Vermilion and Mucosal Flap

On the mucosal side corresponding parallel incisions are made downward from the transverse incision at the upper labial sulcus toward the free margin of the prolabium. These incisions outline the flap that will become the full median tubercle. It is freed up to a sufficient degree to allow it to be everted.

The result of these prolabial skin and mucosal incisions is to produce two lateral tags of tissue attached at the free margin of the lip but free at their upper ends (Fig. 29–7B). These lateral tags are deepithelialized but not discarded (Fig. 29–7C and D). The deepithelialized flaps are then turned inward and overlapped to add bulk to the median tubercle (Fig. 29–7E).

It is now time to make the final assembly of the components of the lip.

Repair of the Muscle Layer

The muscle bundles are joined to each side of the dermis of the central prolabial skin using catgut stitches. Thus, the muscle bundles have not been united to each other across the front of the premaxilla (Fig. 29–7F).

Should the Muscle Be Joined in Front of the Premaxilla?

The question now arises as to whether the muscle bundles in the lateral lip elements should be joined to each other in front of the premaxilla. It would of course be desirable to free up and unite the muscle bundles in the lateral lip elements to each other in the midline, but *I believe there is a significant defect in the musculature of the lip corresponding to the muscle that is absent in the prolabium.*

I also believe that if the two lateral muscular elements are joined to each other across the front of the premaxilla, the soft tissues will be too tight from side to side and will inhibit premaxillary growth and development. Such a joining is likely to result in a class III incisor relationship with disastrous results in appearance and dental occlusion. Not joining these muscular elements has disadvantages, of course. The muscle sometimes has a bunched-up look, and the prolabium has a tendency to widen somewhat. If long-term experience of joining them (not yet available) results in class III occlusion, nothing will have been gained and much will have been

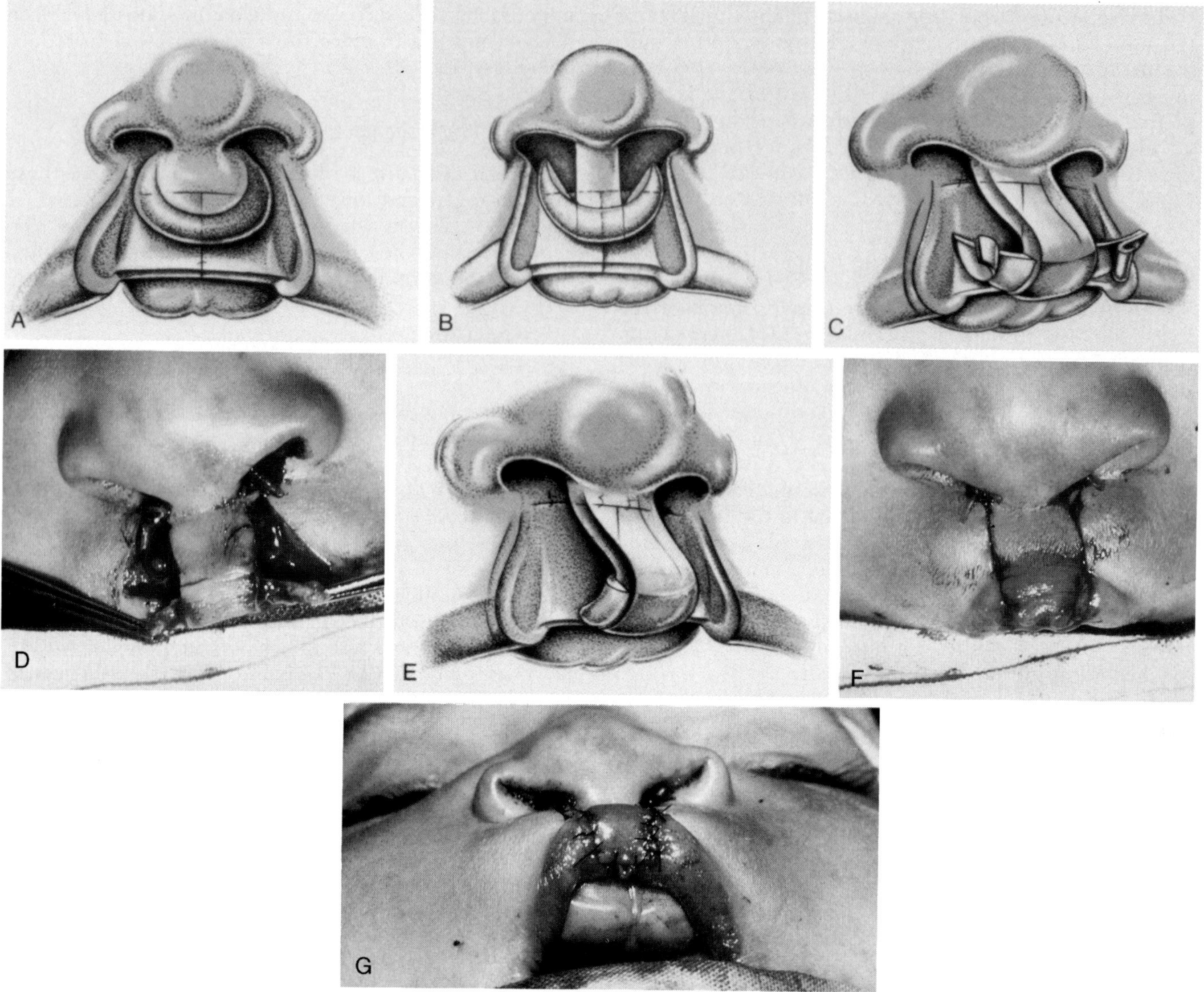

Figure 29–7 *A*, The situation at this stage, as seen from the front. *B*, The skin and mucosal incisions have been made in the prolabium, the lateral tags have been pulled laterally, and the central vermilion that will become the median tubercle has been outlined. *C*, The central vermilion flap has been everted, and the lateral tags are being de-epithelialized. *D*, Same view as shown in *C*, with the lateral tags de-epithelialized. *E*, The de-epithelialized flaps have been turned inward and overlapped to add bulk to the median tubercle. *F*, The whole lip has been assembled with subcuticular catgut stitches. The skin stitches merely provide apposition, without tension. *G*, The two vermilion mucosal flaps are united in the midline just in front of the frenum on the premaxilla, and the central everted prelabial flap is united.

lost. We know already that not joining them is compatible with normal premaxillary development, at least until the pubertal growth spurt. For these reasons, I have until now refrained from joining these muscles to each other and have been content simply to sew the musculature on each side to the dermis of the prolabial skin.

Completion of the Repair

This brings the three parts of the repair together as far down as the mucocutaneous ridges. The final apposition of the skin and vermilion is completed using 6–0 silk sutures. These sutures carry no tension because tension is taken by the subcuticular stitches. The repair is now complete (Fig. 29–7*G*).

Removal of Stitches

The skin stitches are removed on the fifth postoperative day, and the stitches in the hard palate are removed on the tenth day.

Result

The result is a lip with a natural central tubercle, a convincing Cupid's bow, and a fistula-free repair in the nostril floor and hard palate as far back as its junction with the soft palate, leaving only a cleft of the soft palate to be repaired at the final operation at the age of 9 months.

If I were still doing this work,[5–8] I would be dissecting the muscle bundles of the lateral lip elements and uniting them to each other in the midline at the level of the floor of the nose but not at the free margin. A long period of follow-up would be needed to observe the results of this procedure, and a decision as to whether more complete union would be compatible with normal premaxillary development would then be made. The answer to this question is not yet known for certain, and I believe great caution should be used.

Follow-up Treatment—Soft Palate Repair

The patient is seen at the multidisciplinary follow-up clinic at a meeting in which the surgeons, orthodontists, and speech pathologist are all present in the same room, so that proper consultation can occur at least once a year. If an earlier appointment is needed, it is decided then. The orthodontist then makes whatever independent appointments are needed.

I have asked Dr. Peat, the senior orthodontist on the team, to give the following more detailed account of the postoperative orthodontic management.

Orthodontic Management Following Surgery

After the surgical reconstruction of the bilateral cleft lip and palate, the child is examined annually by the combined clinic of specialists. At this clinic the orthodontist monitors the child's dental development and facial growth.

During the deciduous dentition period, that is, up to 5 to 6 years of age, no active orthodontic treatment is initiated apart from the extraction of any teeth that may be producing a traumatogenic occlusion such as malposed or supernumerary teeth. It is considered a very important concept that, because these children will be undergoing extensive treatment during many years by many specialists, there must be rest periods, free of treatment, when they can live normal lives. Such a period is the first 5 years of life only. Only basic records in the form of dental study models, cephalometric radiographs, and photographs are obtained at 4 to 5 years of age to permit future comparisons of facial and dental development.

With the advent of the mixed dentition period, signaled by the eruption of the upper and lower permanent incisor teeth, full records, consisting of dental study models and full mouth and cephalometric radiographs and photographs, are obtained. At this time, if an incisor crossbite has developed, orthodontic correction is instituted if such a correction will be self-retaining. This depends on the skeletal base difference and the degree of overbite.

Long-term mechanical retention of the overbite at this age is not justified. At approximately 8 to 9 years of age, while the permanent canine is still in its dental crypt, lateral expansion of the dental buccal segments is carried out when necessary, followed by alveolar bone grafting into the cleft area. This is followed by another rest period until the eruption of all the permanent teeth occurs.

When all the permanent teeth have erupted, that is, at 12 to 13 years of age, full orthodontic treatment is commenced to align the teeth and correct the occlusion. With the Manchester technique, a good incisor relationship can usually be obtained, and therefore treatment is directed mainly at correcting any medial collapse of the buccal segments and closing spaces where teeth are missing. If the space in the alveolar cleft area is too great to be closed orthodontically or if a bone graft is inappropriate, a prosthetic solution is justified—either a chrome-cobalt partial denture or a dental bridge of the conventional or Maryland type.

A final assessment of the dental occlusion and facial form is made near the end of the growth period. If there is an obvious midface deficiency that occurs in all three planes of space, then surgical correction is recommended; depending on the severity of the malrelation, such surgery may range from a single Le Fort I advancement to a three-piece maxillary expansion and advancement combined with a mandibular reduction. The use of bone grafts and miniplates assists the stability of the result, but it is still advisable to plan for overcorrection of the deficiency.

At the cessation of growth, the patient is discharged following collection of final study models, radiographs, and photographs. Records have thus been obtained longitudinally from birth until maturity.

The Manchester technique usually results in normal premaxillary development with a class I incisor relationship until the pubertal growth spurt begins. As this proceeds, not uncommonly, premaxillary development lags somewhat, and orthodontic treatment is necessary to restore a class I relationship. It is also necessary in many cases to supply some kind of retention device.[8]

Results

A series of photographs illustrates the long-range results in 11 patients (Figs. 29–8 through 29–14).

Conclusions

After 46 years of cleft lip and palate surgery I have come to the following conclusions:

1. In most patients with bilateral clefts there should be presurgical orthopedic treatment.
2. Both sides of the lip and the hard palate should be repaired simultaneously to avoid fistulas in the alveolar region. This treatment usually gives a solid premaxilla with a small area of bony union on each side.
3. There should be a central part of the lip derived from the prolabium whose vermilion and mucosa should form the central tubercle.
4. As I pointed out in 1965, I believe that the first operation on the lip should be the only one. Revisional surgery always achieves something, but some of the charm of the result is always lost.

Text continued on page 240

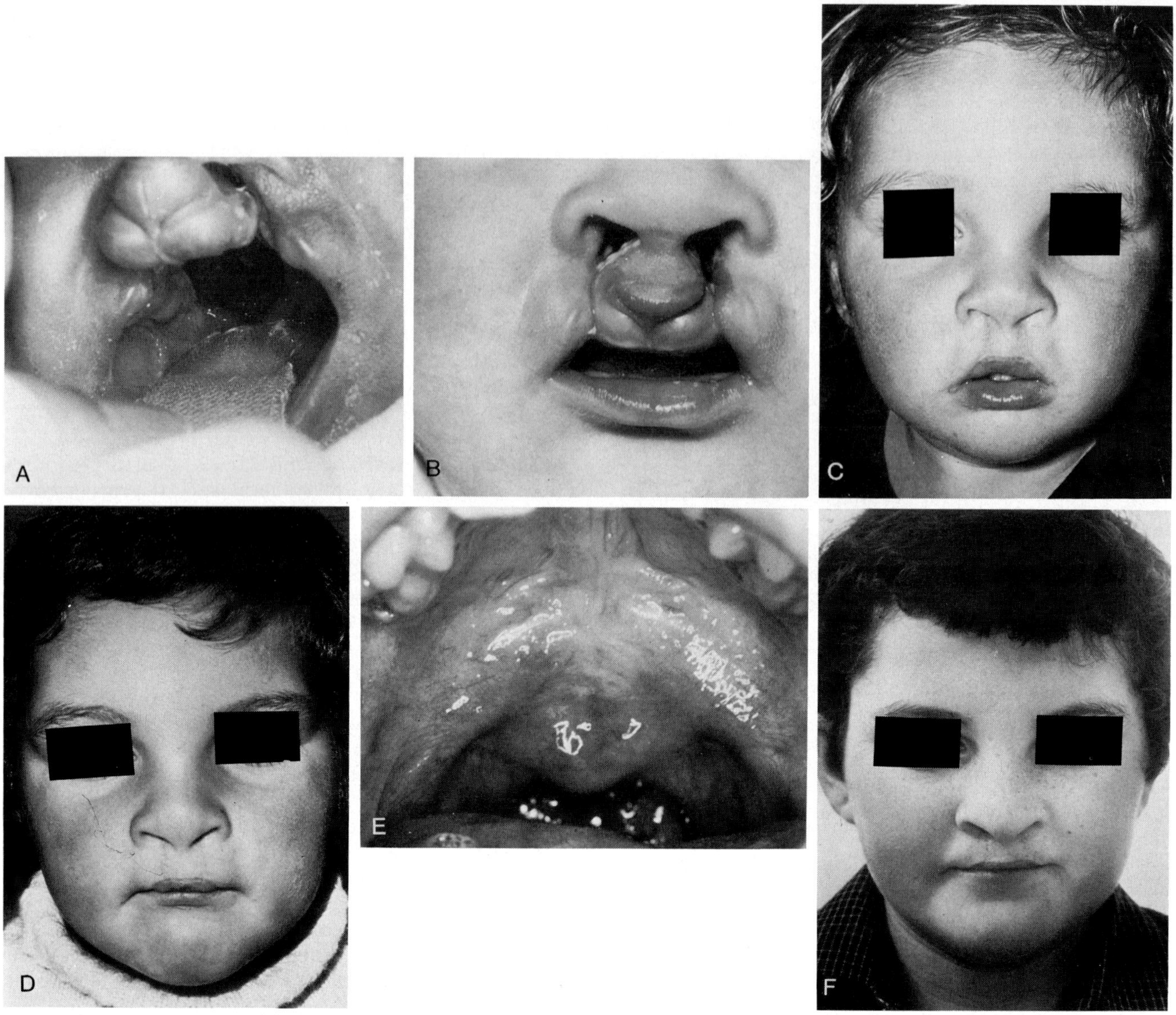

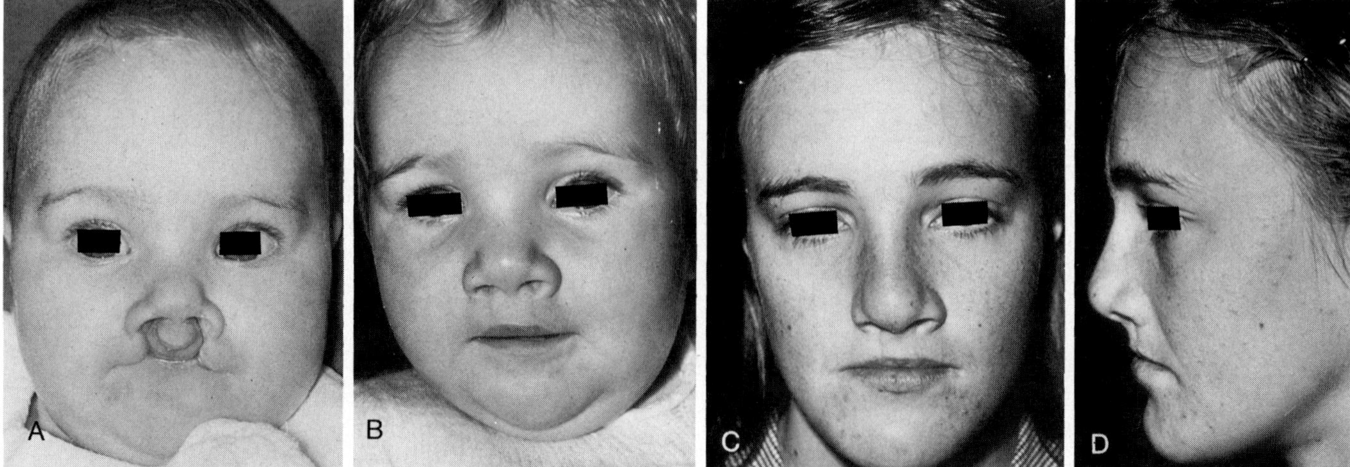

Figure 29–8 *A*, Complete bilateral cleft. A very prominent premaxilla with a very wide cleft. *B*, After 5 months of growth with presurgical orthopedics, the premaxilla is much less prominent with left lateral lip element in front of the premaxilla. *C*, At 18 months. *D*, At 4 years. No revisional surgery has been done. *E*, The soft palate at 11 years: long, mobile, and close to the posterior pharyngeal wall. *F*, At 11 years of age.

Figure 29–9 *A*, Complete bilateral cleft, but premaxilla is less prominent than in the previous patient. *B*, At 6 months. *C*, At 16 years. No revisional surgery has been done. *D*, Satisfactory development of the nasal tip even though no surgery has ever been performed on it.

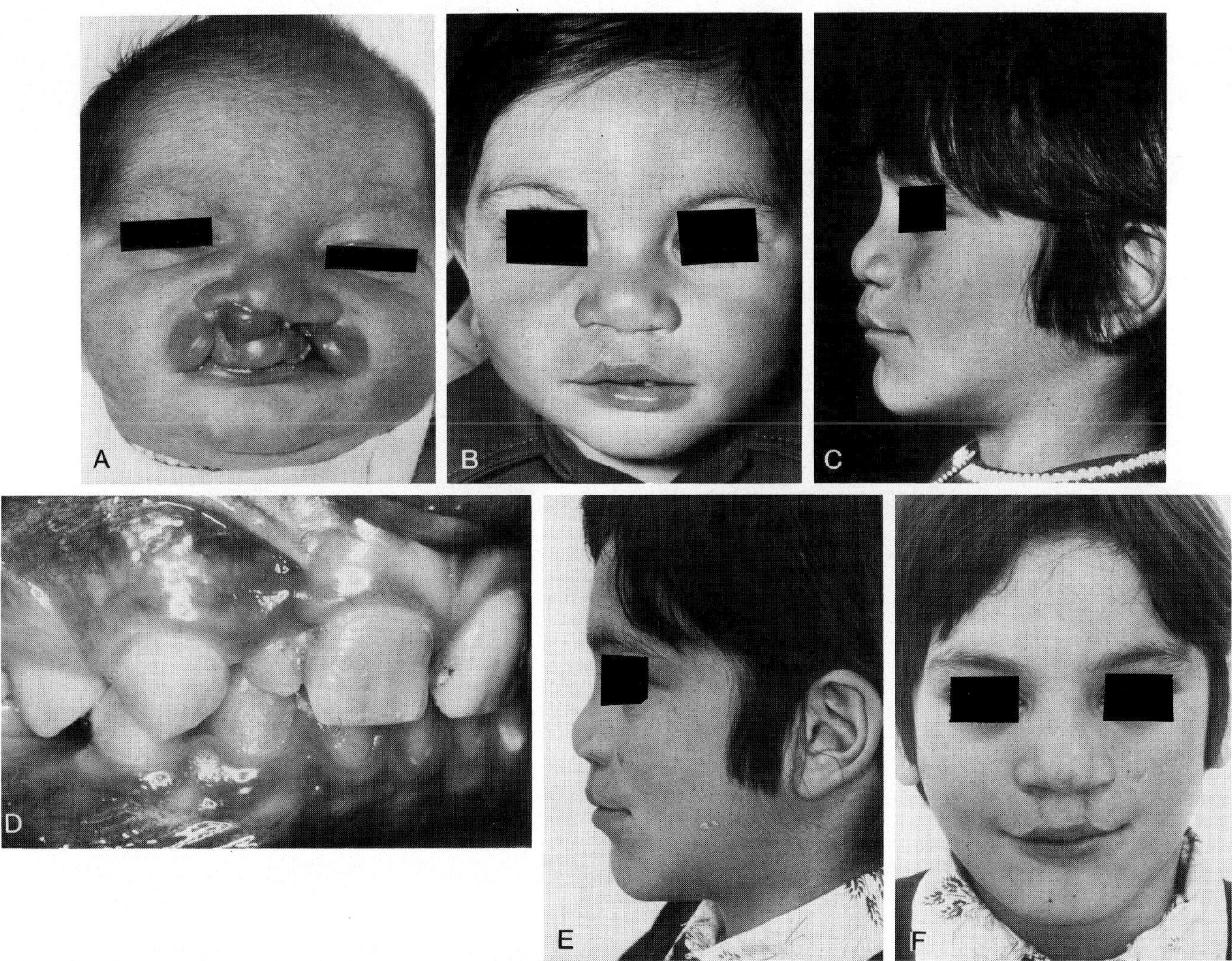

Figure 29–10 *A*, Complete bilateral cleft. Small prolabium. *B*, At 1 year. The peak of the Cupid's bow on the patient's right is not quite accurately aligned. *C*, At 9 years. In profile. Good premaxillary development. *D*, Dental occlusion at 11 years. No orthodontic treatment has been carried out. The incisor relationship is class I, as is the canine. *E*, At 12 years. *F*, At 12 years. The only revisional surgery has been an adjustment of the right peak of the Cupid's bow.

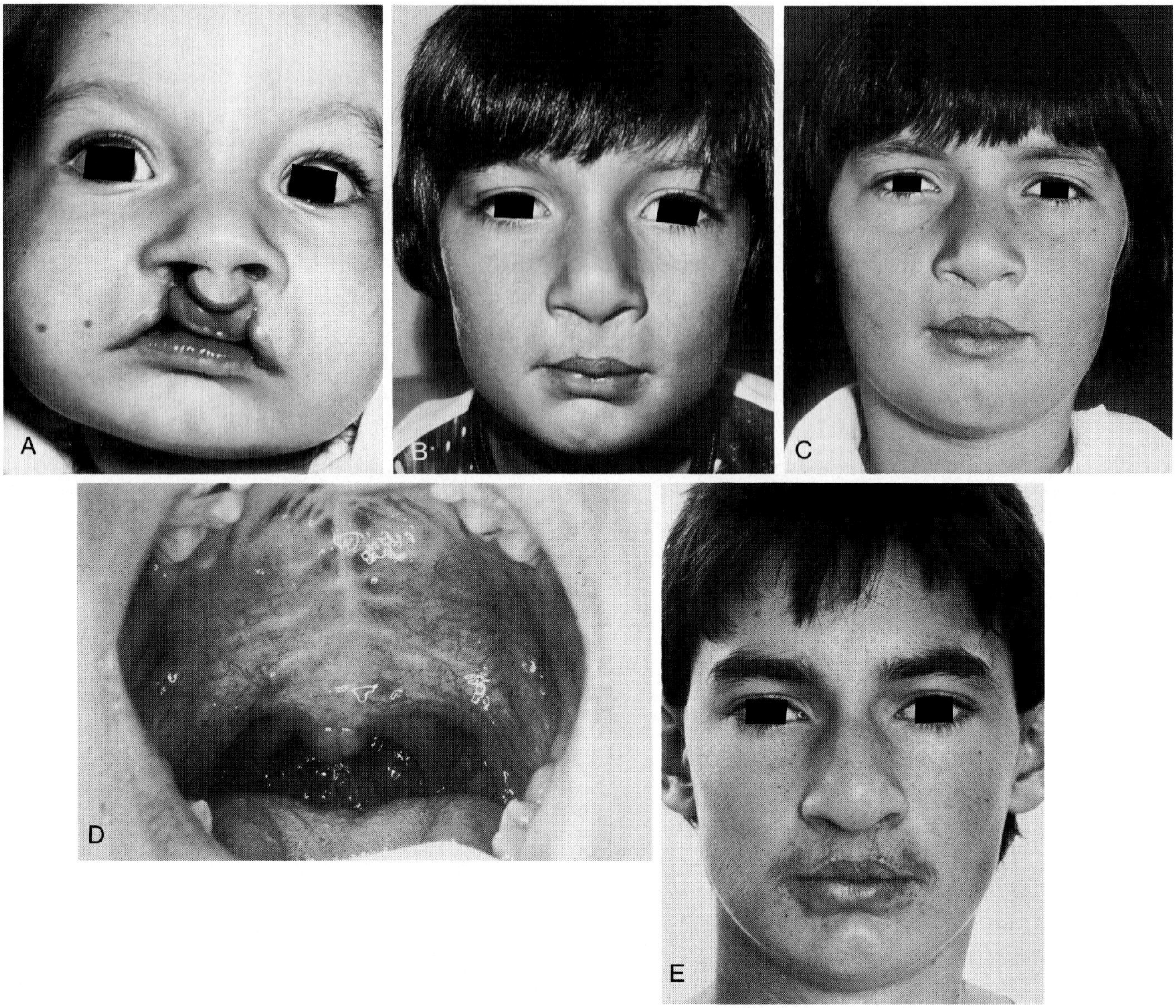

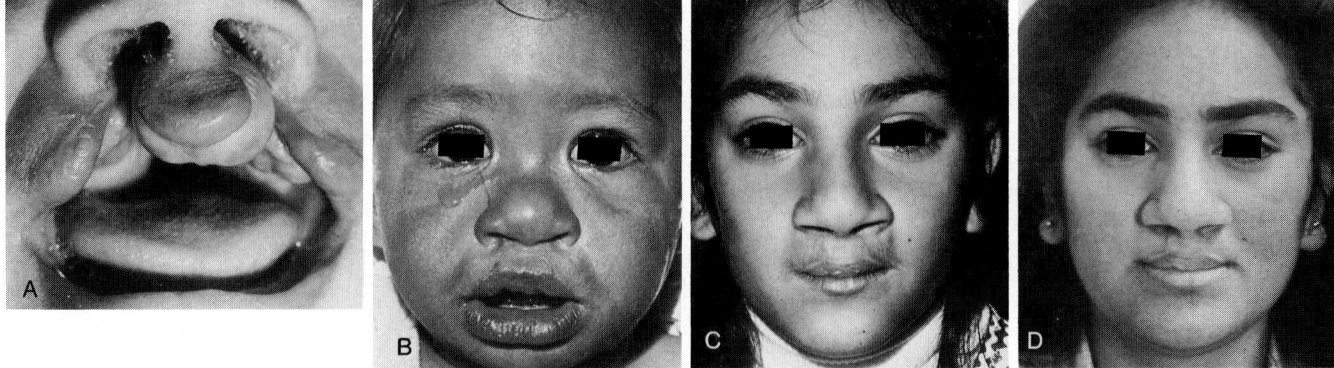

Figure 29–11 *A*, At 5 months. a bilateral complete cleft but with a small Simonart's band on the left. *B*, At 8 years. *C*, At 10 years. The original operation is the only one that has ever been done on the lip. *D*, The soft palate at 10 years. Long and mobile and almost touching the posterior pharyngeal wall. *E*, At 17 years. Dental occlusion has a class I relationship. No revisional surgery has ever been done on the lip.

Figure 29–12 *A*, Presurgical orthopedic treatment just completed at the age of 5 months. *B*, At 9 months. *C*, At 8 years. *D*, At 17 years. Orthodontic treatment complete, Class I relationship. Only one operation has ever been done on the lip. Rhinoplasty still has to be done.

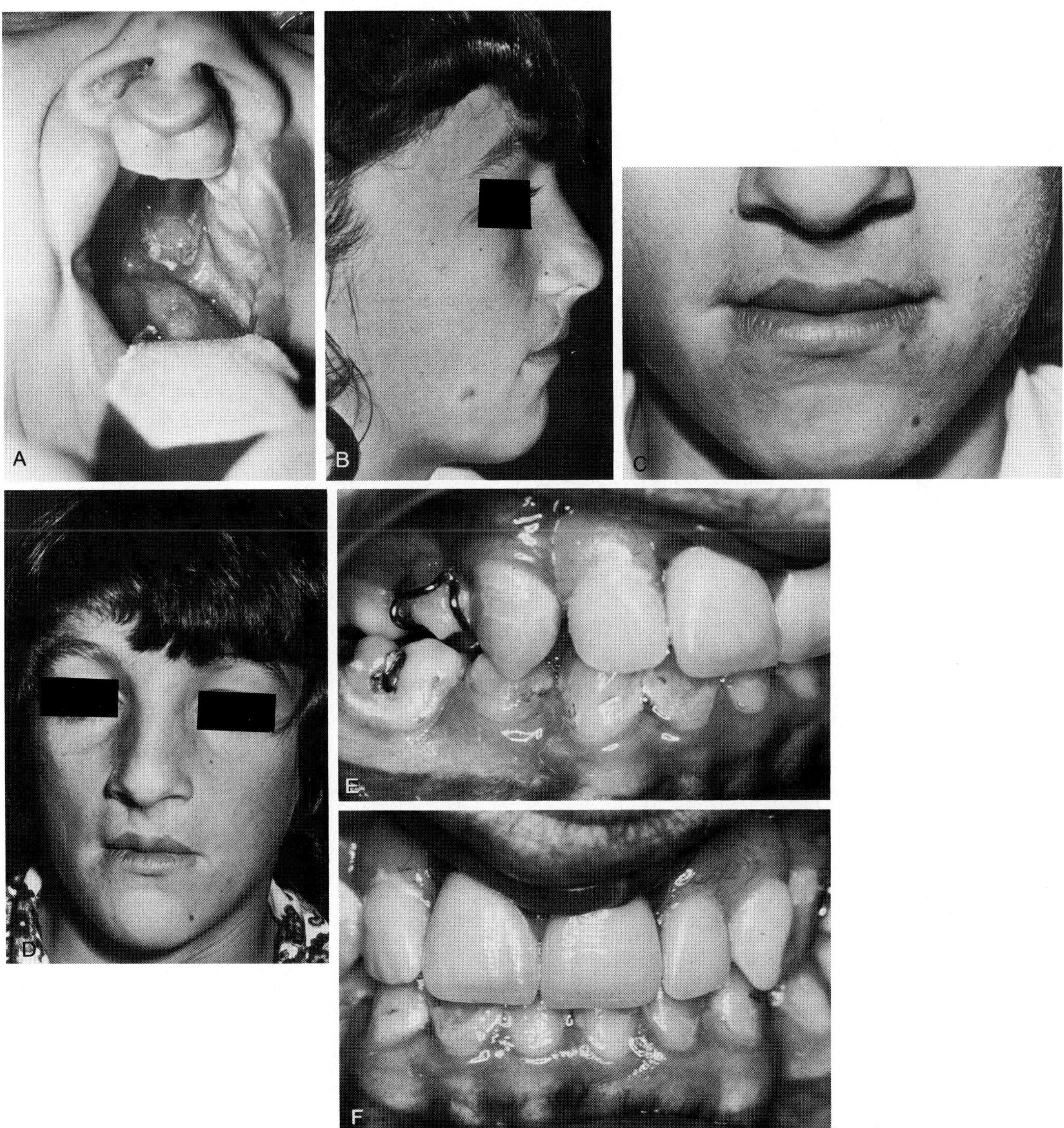

Figure 29–13 *A*, Complete bilateral cleft at 5 months. *B*, At 14 years. Proper relationship between upper and lower lips. *C*, Detail of lip at age 14. *D*, At 14 years. No revisional surgery. *E*, Dental occlusion at age 19. The incisor teeth were lost through neglect by the patient but have been restored by chrome-cobalt partial skeleton denture. *F*, Class I relationship at age 19. (*A* and *C* from Manchester WM: How I do it colloquium. Surgical management of bilateral cleft lip. Ann Plast Surg 1:509, 1978. Reproduced with permission of Little, Brown, Inc.)

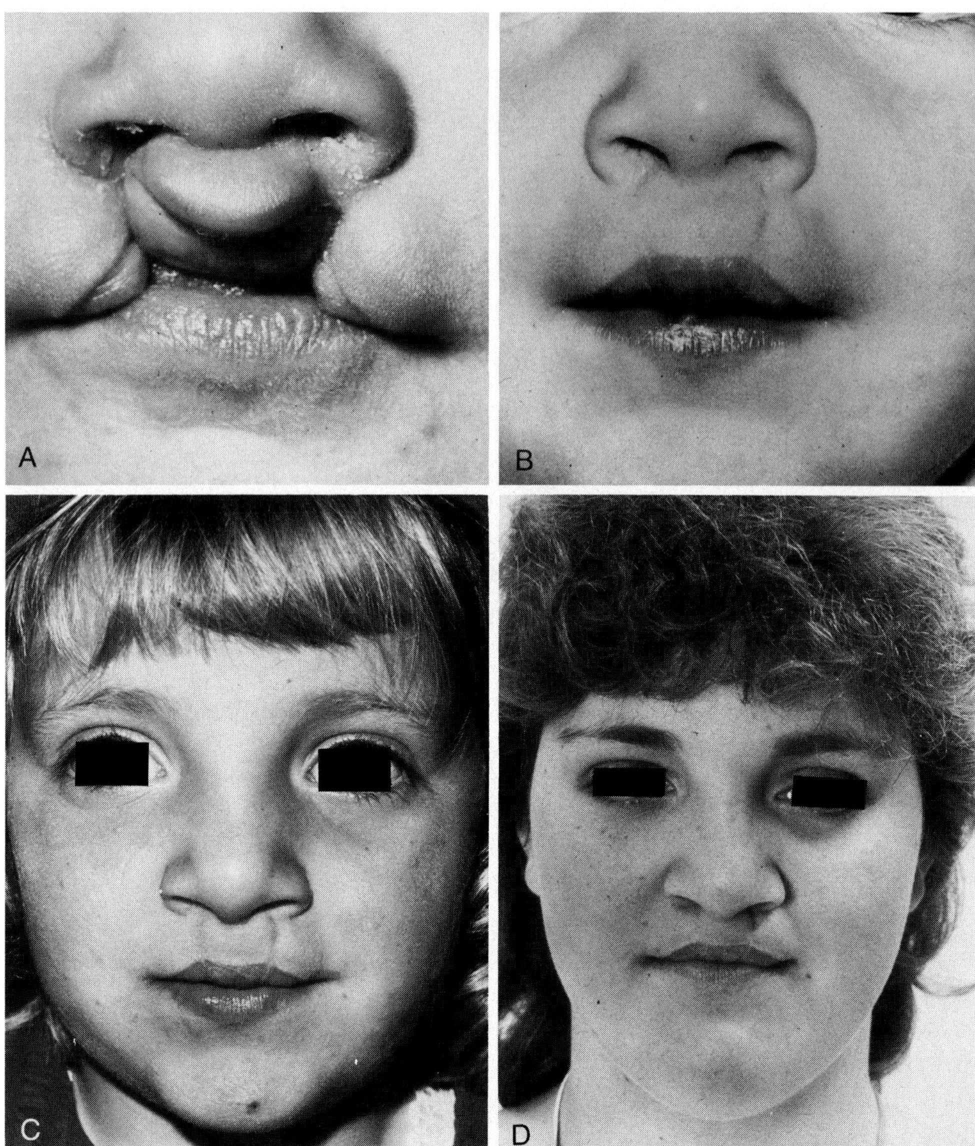

Figure 29–14 *A*, Bilateral complete cleft but with a Simonart's band on the left. At 5 months. *B*, At 1 year. *C*, At 4 years. *D*, Full face at 14 years. Full, lax lip, pleasing median tubercle and Cupid's bow, and slight depression of the scar on the left, which is easily corrected by a minor revisional operation.

5. I am still not sure whether the muscles in the lateral lip elements should be joined to each other in front of the premaxilla at the primary operation. The absence of the central segment of the muscle means that the lip might be far too tight. Further study is necessary to determine whether such a procedure produces anterior crossbite before puberty; I think there is a good chance that it will in many cases.

References

1. Manchester WM: The repair of bilateral cleft lip and palate. Br J Surg 52:878, 1965.
2. Peat JH: Early orthodontic treatment for complete clefts. Am J Orthod 65:238–246, 1974.
3. Peat JH: The dental management of children with clefts of the lip and palate. NZ Dent J 70:109–117, 1974.
4. Peat JH: Effects of presurgical oral orthopaedics on bilateral complete clefts of the lip and palate. Cleft Palate J 19:100–103, 1982.
5. Manchester WM: Integrated cleft lip and palate repair. In Transactions of the Fourth International Congress of Plastic and Reconstructive Surgery, Rome, October, 1967. Amsterdam: Excerpta Medica, 1967, pp 362–367.
6. Manchester WM: The repair of double cleft lip as part of an integrated programme. Plast Reconstr Surg 45:207, 1970.
7. Manchester WM: A method of primary double cleft lip repair. In Transactions of the Fifth International Congress of Plastic and Reconstructive Surgery, Melbourne, Australia, February, 1971. Melbourne: Butterworths, 1971, pp. 193–205.
8. Manchester WM: How I do it/colloquium. Surgical management of bilateral cleft lip. Ann Plast Surg 1:509, 1978.

CHAPTER 30

Bilateral Cleft Lip Repair

M. Samuel Noordhoff

Satisfactory reconstruction of the bilateral cleft lip seems an elusive goal. Some factors over which we have minimal control such as racial differences, genetic variations, and social and economic factors influence the end-result. Stark and Ehrmann[1] noted a "horrendous deficiency" of nasal germ plasm in the bilateral cleft lip embryo. This factor might explain the wide anatomic variations seen in the premaxilla, prolabium, and nasal cartilages. The reconstructive surgeon must be aware of these deficiencies and choose procedures that give the best results with the least growth disturbance. The procedure to be described has been reported previously,[2] and the presented modifications are the result of experience gained from over 160 bilateral cleft lip operations.

Preoperative Care

An orthopedic plate is used when indicated to prevent maxillary collapse. Gentle traction on the premaxilla using orthodontic rubber bands attached to a nonallergic Micropore tape allows the premaxilla to be repositioned posteriorly. Presurgical orthopedic treatment is beneficial[3] but is not always used because of poor patient cooperation. Lip repair is done at 3 months of age if the baby is gaining weight and in good health.

Surgical Technique

Prolabial markings are described in Figure 30–1. The vertical limb 3–2 goes from point 3 at the base of the columella to point 2 on the prolabium. This results in a 5- to 6-mm width of the columella, which is average in the Chinese race at the age of 3 months. It is technically difficult to make the distance between points 1 and 2 smaller than 2 to 3 mm. The ideal width of the Cupid's bow should be determined by racial characteristics but should rarely exceed 6 mm.

Lateral Lip Markings

The white and red lines have been previously described[2, 4] and refer to the cutaneovermilion and mucosalvermilion junction lines, respectively. On the lateral lip these two lines always converge medially at the cleft edge. Starting at this point and moving laterally, point 2' is placed where the vermilion is widest. This corresponds to the base of the philtral column, which

usually is 3 to 4 mm lateral to the point of junction of the converging white and red lines.

Vertical lip length is measured from the alar base to point 2'. This measurement indicates whether the lip needs to be shortened on one side or the other. Lengthening the prolabium with interdigitating flaps is not indicated. The prolabium, even when short, always stretches. Line 2'–3' shows the prolabial length on the lateral lip; however, it is not an incision line.

The vermilion medial to point 2' is used for reconstruction of the central prolabial vermilion. Point 2' on the white line can be moved 1 or 2 mm medially or laterally as needed. Moving point 2' medially increases the horizontal width of the lip (leaving less vermilion for reconstruction of the central portion of the vermilion under the prolabium) and shortens the vertical height of the lip. There must be enough vermilion medial to point 2' to give parallel white and red lines (see Fig. 30–8) and prevent a peaking effect (see Fig. 30–9). Moving point 2' laterally shortens the horizontal width of the lip, leaves more vermilion for reconstruction of the central portion of the vermilion under the prolabium, and increases vertical lip length from the alar base to the white skin roll.

Lateral Lip Incision

A buccal mucosal flap (L) and inferior turbinate flap (T) are elevated with an intercartilaginous incision to allow release of the alar base and lateral lip. Dissection is minimal along the edge of the maxilla; periosteum is left intact (Fig. 30–2). The orbicularis marginalis (OM)

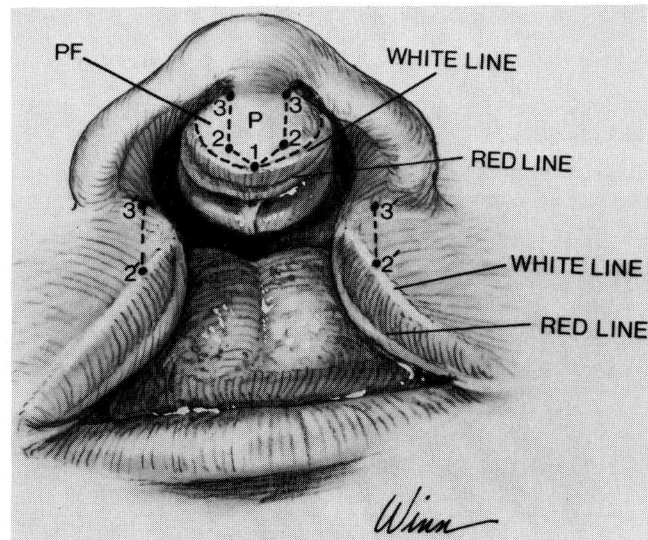

Figure 30–1 The white line is the cutaneovermilion junction, and the red line is the mucosal vermilion junction. Point 1 is centrally placed on the prolabial white line. Point 2 is placed 2 mm higher on a line dropped from point 3 at the base of the columella. This divides the prolabium into a central prolabial flap (P) and two lateral forked flaps (PF). The prolabial length 2–3 is transferred to the lateral lip with the base of the future philtral column point 2' placed where the vermilion first becomes widest and point 3' placed near the ala. Line 2'–3' is not an incision line. (From Noordhoff MS: Plast Reconstr Surg 78:45–54, with permission.)

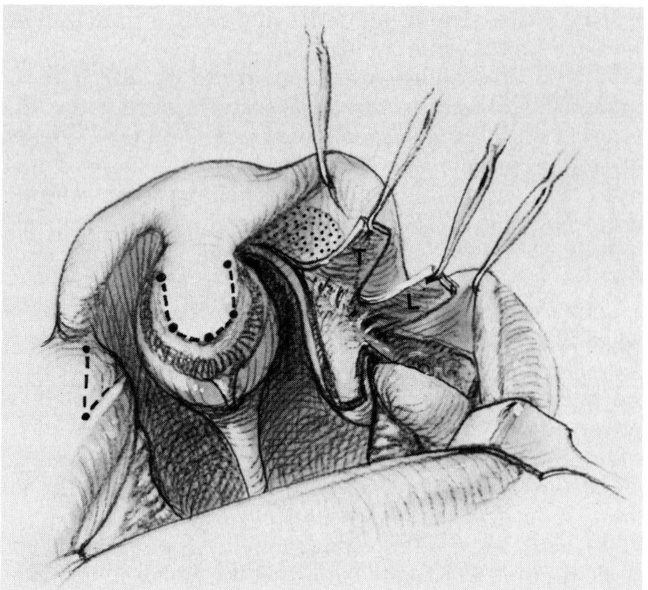

Figure 30–2 A buccal alveolar mucosal flap (L) is raised on the vestibular skin. An additional inferior turbinate mucosal flap (T) is elevated by extending the incision line from the piriform fossa on the inferior border of the inferior turbinate across to its superior border, continuing as an intercartilaginous incision to the dome of the alar cartilage.

flap (Fig. 30–3) for reconstruction of the central portion of the lip is incised along the edge of the white line (Fig. 30–2). The remaining free edge is opened (Fig. 30–3). Subdermal dissection of the orbicularis peripher-

alis (OP) from the skin allows it to be mobilized medially, leaving mucosa attached posteriorly.

Prolabial Incisions

Prolabial incisions (see Fig. 30–1) are made, and the prolabium is elevated (Fig. 30–3). The lateral forked-flap incision line is extended behind the columella at the junction of the skin and mucosa to release the prolabium (see insert in Fig. 30–3). The premaxilla is covered with the remaining prolabial mucosa (PM) for creation of the buccal alveolar sulcus.

Vestibular Reconstruction

The alar cartilage is elevated by a traction suture in its dome (Fig. 30–4), where it is held with one inter-cartilaginous suture and a McComb[5] suspension suture, the latter being placed at the end of the procedure (see insert in Fig. 30–4). The inferior turbinate mucosal flap (T) and the buccal mucosal flap (L) are sutured as described (Fig. 30–4), resulting in complete mucosal closure of all incisions, additional mucosa in the vestibule and piriform area, and reconstruction of a good nostril floor (Fig. 30–5).

Nasal Floor Reconstruction

The folded-over L-flap (Figs. 30–4 and 30–5) is swung over and sutured to the apex of the incision behind the columella and to the exposed open free edge of the

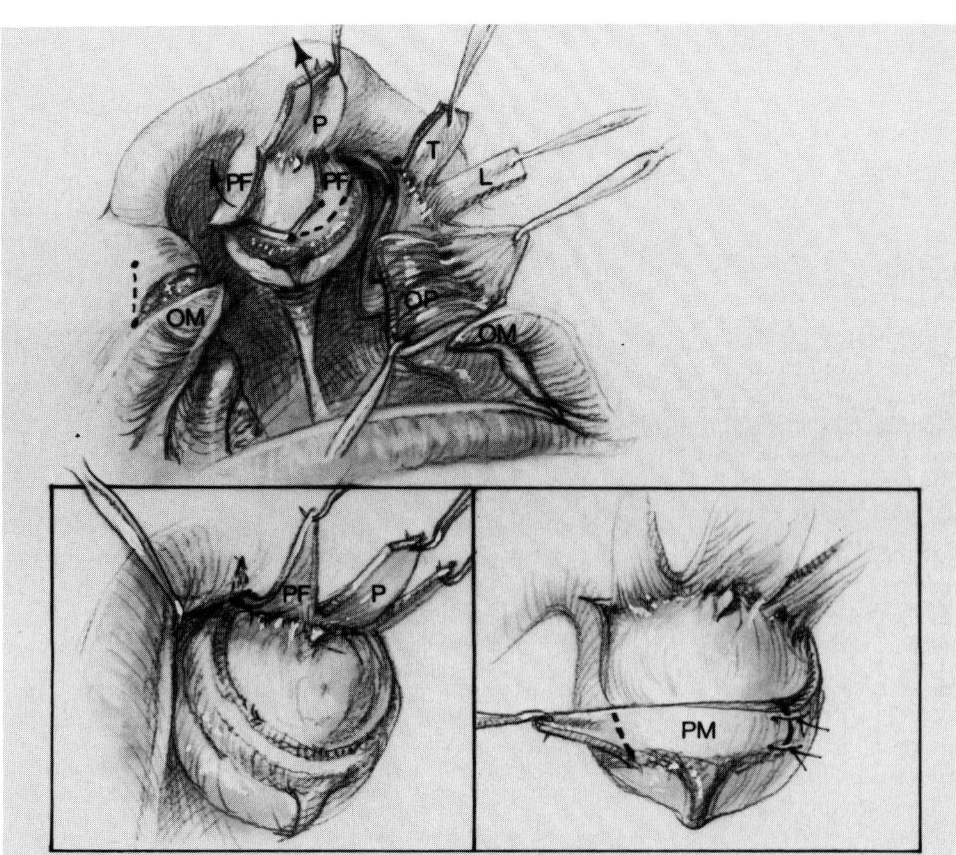

Figure 30–3 The orbicularis marginalis flap (OM) is cut on the dotted line (see Fig. 30–2) to include a 1-mm white skin roll, vermilion, and orbicularis and mucosal flaps. After incising the OM flap the incision extends on the edge of the skin to the edge of the L-flap, allowing for mobilization and dissection of the orbicularis peripheralis (OP). The central prolabial flaps P and PF have been incised, freeing the prolabium. The premaxilla is lined with remaining prolabial mucosa (PM) (see insert).

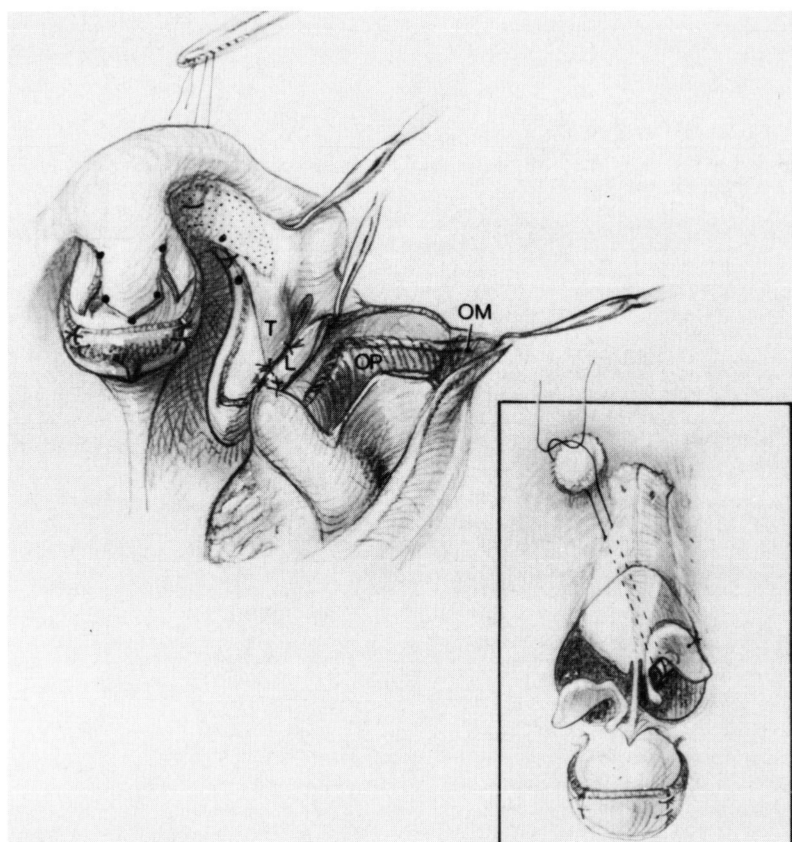

Figure 30–4 A traction suture is placed in the dome of the alar cartilage, and the alar cartilage is elevated superiorly. The inferior turbinate flap T is rotated into the piriform area, usually reaching the edge of the alveolus, where it is sutured. The L-flap is folded on itself attached to the alveolus and the edge of the T-flap. Its advancing edge is sutured laterally at the base of the columella (see Fig. 30–5). The alar cartilage is fixed with one intercartilaginous suture at its base. At the completion of the procedure the alar cartilage is supported with a traction suture emerging from the skin and tied over a bolster (see insert).

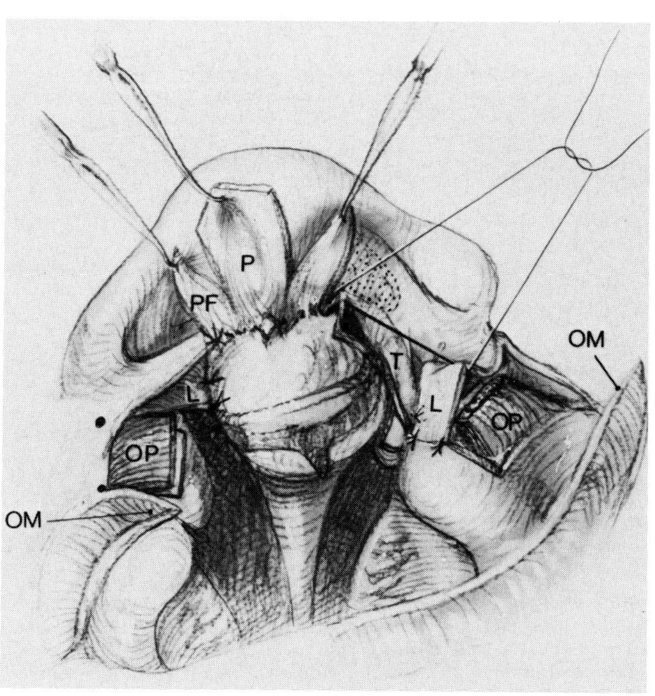

Figure 30–5 On the left side the L-flap is folded on itself and sutured laterally to the base of the columella and to the free edge of the premaxilla, which is devoid of covering mucosa on its upper half bridging the alveolar gap and providing a good nostril floor as seen on the completed right side. The OP muscle flap with attached mucosa has been dissected from the skin and maxilla as far as necessary to allow approximation without tension. (OM = orbicularis marginalis; P and PF = prolabial flaps.)

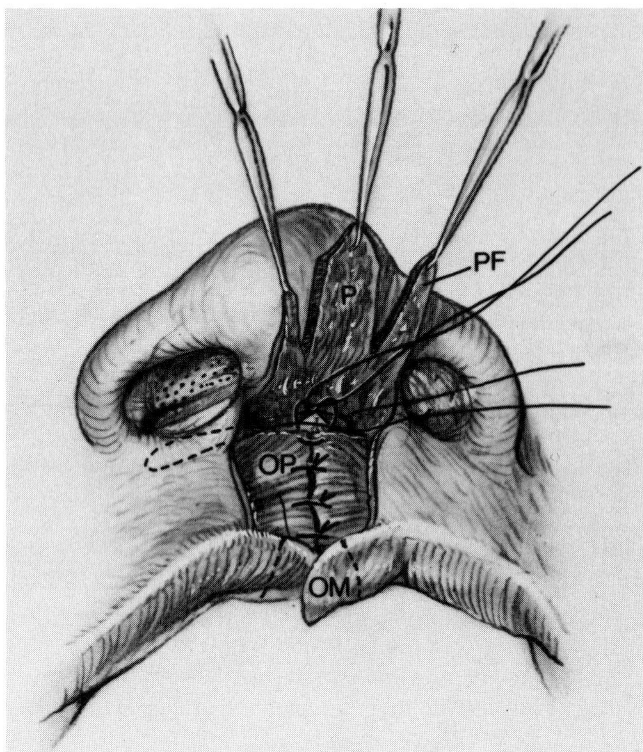

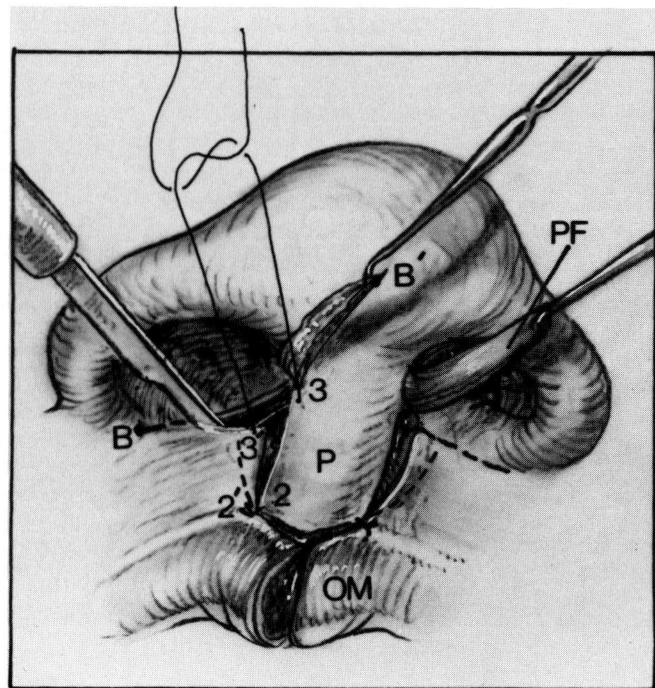

Figure 30–6 The orbicularis peripheralis (OP) is sutured in front of the premaxilla and anchored to the nasal spine. An additional traction suture from the alar base to the nasal spine helps to hold the alar base in as narrow a position as possible. (From Noordhoff MS: Plast Reconstr Surg 78:45–54, with permission.)

Figure 30–7 Points 2′–2 are approximated with subcuticular sutures, and the orbicularis marginalis flaps OM are trimmed to fit under the prolabial flap (P). The vertical length of the lateral skin margin is measured so that 2′–3′ corresponds to the prolabial vertical length 2–3. The horizontal incision is then made from points 3–3′ lateral to point B, and the tip of the prolabial forked flap B′ is inserted to point B.

premaxilla not covered with prolabial mucosa (see insert Fig. 30–3). The suturing of this flap (Fig. 30–5) provides complete posterior mucosal closure and a good nostril floor.

Muscle Reconstruction

The orbicularis peripheralis muscle is sutured together in the midline along with the attached underlying mucosa (Fig. 30–6). This muscle is also sutured to the nasal spine.

Prolabium

The prolabial flap (P) is sutured at points 2–2′. Orbicularis marginalis flaps are trimmed to fit beneath the prolabium (Fig. 30–7). Usually a forked flap from the lateral lip is not elevated because the skin is too tight. The remaining incision lines are closed (Fig. 30–7).

Cupid's Bow

Closing the OM flaps with a slight eversion fills the central tubercle and produces parallel red and white lines with a full vermilion centrally (Fig. 30–7). The placement of point 2′ on the white skin roll (see Fig. 30–1) is important in creating a full central vermilion

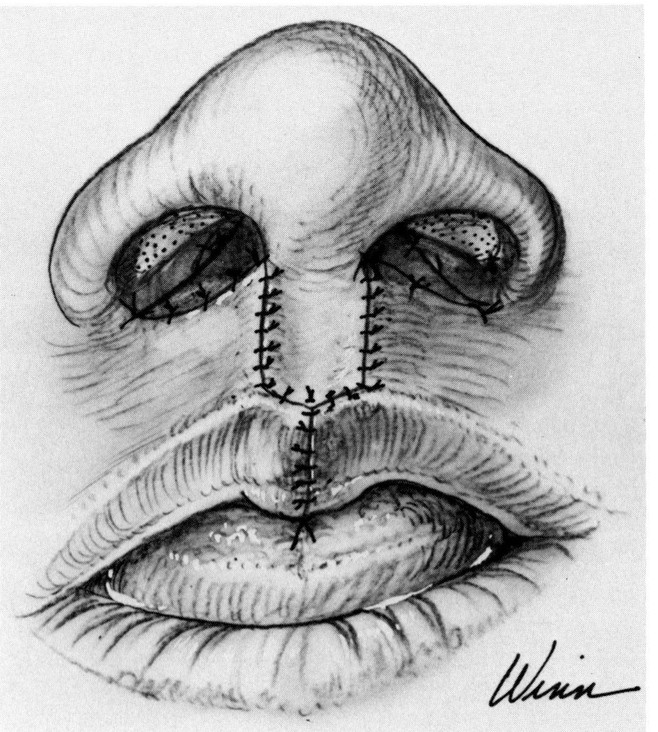

Figure 30–8 At the completion of the procedure there should be parallel white and red lines with the vermilion width widest at the base of the philtral column. This gives uninterrupted free-flowing white and red lines with a full vermilion.

(Fig. 30–8). If point 2′ is placed too far medially, there is inadequate vermilion in the OM flap (see Fig. 30–3, Fig. 30–7), resulting in a peaking effect (Fig. 30–9) that does not look good.

Lip Asymmetry

All bilateral clefts of the lip and palate have some degree of asymmetry. It is important to measure these differences preoperatively, particularly the distance from the alar base to the new philtral column on the lateral lip (point 2′, see Fig. 30–1). At the time of muscle closure, any significant excessive vertical length of muscle can be corrected by excising the excess. The final vertical lip length is corrected at the time of skin closure by excising excess skin (Fig. 30–7).

Postoperative Care

Fine, 7–0 absorbable sutures are used in the skin; they loosen after about 7 to 10 days and can be removed in the outpatient clinic. The wound is supported with a strip of Micropore tape. The parents are instructed to start gentle finger massage at 2 to 3 weeks as recommended by Schultz.[6] This is continued until the wound matures.

Elongation of Columella

Columellar lengthening is done at the age of 2 to 6 years as recommended by Cronin and Upton.[7] Nasal

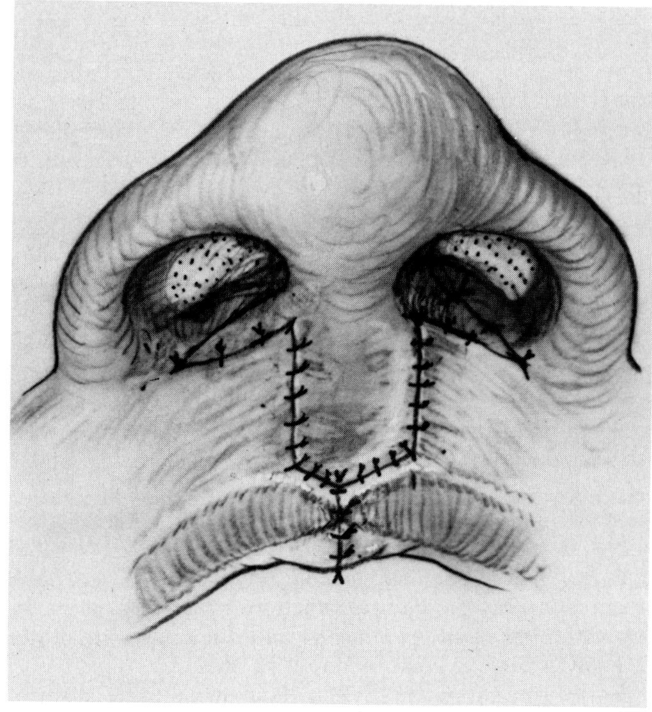

Figure 30–9 An undesirable peaking effect of the red line will occur centrally if point 2′ (see Fig. 30–1) is placed too far medially.

floor flaps should be thin and the orbicularis muscle left attached to the nasal spine to prevent drifting of the columella and lip down onto the premaxilla. Use of a cartilage strut taken from the ear and advanced flaps

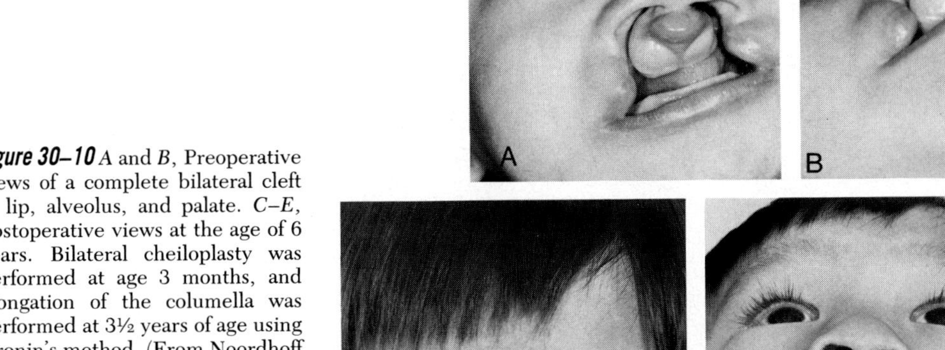

Figure 30–10 *A* and *B*, Preoperative views of a complete bilateral cleft of lip, alveolus, and palate. *C–E*, Postoperative views at the age of 6 years. Bilateral cheiloplasty was performed at age 3 months, and elongation of the columella was performed at 3½ years of age using Cronin's method. (From Noordhoff MS: Plast Reconstr Surg 78:45–54, with permission.)

secured to the septum helps prevent columellar drift. Lower lateral cartilage repositioning also is done at this time (see Fig. 30–4). If inadequate tissue is available on the nostril floor, a composite ear graft is used to elongate the columella.[2, 8] A patient treated by this technique of bilateral cheiloplasty and elongation of the columella is shown in Figure 30–10.

Discussion

The bilateral cheiloplasty has been modified from that previously described by the author[2] and is similar to the one used by Millard.[9–10] It is important to stress the need to reconstruct the lip in such a way that it is never reentered.[11] This requires that the buccal alveolar sulcus be reconstructed as shown in Figure 30–3.[12] The importance of good muscle continuity is emphasized to give a full upper lip.[13] Preliminary active recession of the premaxilla has been advocated[14]; however, this is not necessary because gentle traction provides adequate repositioning of the premaxilla and does not contribute to growth disturbances as noted by Peat.[3]

Repositioning of the premaxilla allows muscle closure without excess tension and can always be achieved without extensive soft tissue undermining as sometimes advocated.[15] Minimal soft tissue undermining appears to be important because growth disturbances in the rabbit have been reported with extensive soft tissue undermining.[16]

Use of the buccal mucosal flap and inferior turbinate mucosal flap provides additional tissue in the vestibule and piriform area. Use of these flaps also allows easy closure of the nostril floor without tension and provides additional tissue that facilitates subsequent elongation of the columella as a separate procedure.

References

1. Stark RB, Ehrmann NA: The development of the center of the face with particular reference to surgical correction of bilateral cleft lip. Plast Reconstr Surg 21:177–192, 1958.
2. Noordhoff MS: Bilateral cleft lip reconstruction. Plast Reconstr Surg 78:45–54, 1986.
3. Peat JH: Effects of presurgical oral orthopedics on bilateral complete clefts of the lip and palate. Cleft Palate J 19:100–103, 1982.
4. Noordhoff MS: Reconstruction of vermilion in unilateral and bilateral cleft lips. Plast Reconstr Surg 73:52–61, 1984.
5. McComb H: Primary repair of the bilateral cleft lip nose: A 10 year review. Plast Reconstr Surg 77:701–713, 1986.
6. Schultz LW: Bilateral cleft lips. Plast Reconstr Surg 1:338–343, 1946.
7. Cronin TD, Upton J: Lengthening of the short columella associated with bilateral cleft lip. Ann Plast Surg 1:75–95, 1978.
8. Meade RJ: Composite ear grafts for reconstruction of columella. Plast Reconstr Surg 23:134–147, 1959.
9. Millard DR, Jr: Closure of bilateral cleft lip and elongation of columella by two operations in infancy. Plast Reconstr Surg 47:324–331, 1971.
10. Millard DR, Jr: Cleft Craft. Vol. 2. Boston: Little, Brown, 1977, pp 32, 359.
11. Broadbent TR, Woolf RM: Bilateral cleft lip and palate: One stage primary repair. In Georgiade NG, Hagerty RT (eds): Symposium on Management of Cleft Lip and Palate and Associated Deformities. Vol. 8. St. Louis: C. V. Mosby, 1974, pp. 134–138.
12. Horton CE, Adamson JE, Mladick RA, et al: The upper lip sulcus in cleft lips. Plast Reconstr Surg 45:31–37, 1970.
13. Randall P, Whitaker LA, LaRossa D: The importance of muscle reconstruction in primary and secondary cleft lip repair. Plast Reconstr Surg 53:316–323, 1974.
14. Georgiade NG, Latham RA: Maxillary arch alignment in the bilateral cleft lip and palate infant, using the pinned coaxial screw appliance. Plast Reconstr Surg 56:52–60, 1975.
15. Mulliken JB: Principles and techniques of bilateral complete cleft lip repair. Plast Reconstr Surg 75:477–486, 1985.
16. Bardach J, Mooney M, Giedrojc-Juraha ZL: A comparative study of facial growth following cleft lip repair with or without soft-tissue undermining: An experimental study in rabbits. Plast Reconstr Surg 69:745, 1982.

CHAPTER 31

Complications of Cleft Lip Repair

John F. Reinisch and Gerald M. Sloan

The goal of cleft lip surgery is the creation of a normal appearance and normal function. The less experienced cleft surgeon occasionally may obtain excellent results, particularly in patients with less severe initial deformities. More severe initial deformities require experienced surgical skills and a deep understanding of cleft morphology. However, even experienced surgeons may face complications following lip repair. Fortunately, many of these complications can be prevented. The experienced surgeon learns to avoid the technical errors that can lead to complications, poor results, and multiple revisions. With proper attention to detail, the actual complication rate of unilateral and bilateral cleft lip repair should be low.

The emphasis of this chapter is on *avoiding* complications. In systematically reviewing the many potential complications of cleft lip surgery, our recurring theme is that proper surgical planning and execution can prevent most of them. Although attention to detail and planning are important in all types of surgery, they are critical in cleft lip repair, which is particularly unforgiving of even minor errors. Although major complications are rare, even minor complications can result in deformities on the most noticeable part of the face. These become a permanent record of the surgeon's success or failure.

In this chapter, we have divided complications into early and late entities. Early complications are those that are most likely to occur in the first two weeks following surgery, such as bleeding, infection, flap necrosis, airway obstruction, and wound disruption. Late complications may not appear initially but become obvious with time. These include asymmetry, nostril stenosis, vermilion defects, orbicularis oris discontinuity, alveolar collapse, and persistent premaxillary protrusion.

Early Complications

Bleeding

Bleeding is a very uncommon complication following cleft lip repair. We have never seen significant postoperative bleeding or hematoma formation with cleft lip surgery. In the absence of a history of any bleeding abnormalities, we do not routinely test clotting parameters before surgery. Similarly, we do not type and cross-match blood for possible transfusion. We do obtain a complete blood count and prefer that the patient have a preoperative hemoglobin value of 10.0 gm per 100 ml or greater. If the hemoglobin value is significantly lower than this, we wait 2 to 3 weeks for it to rise to an acceptable level. Intraoperative blood loss usually is 30 ml or less. We inject the lip with 0.5% lidocaine containing 1:200,000 epinephrine 5 to 10 minutes before making the incisions to help minimize blood loss. Any bleeding points seen during surgery are immediately coagulated using electrocautery. All incisions are closed securely in layers. Layered closure prevents potential dead space and hematoma formation.

Infection

Infection following cleft lip repair is uncommon. In our most recent 132 operations for primary cleft lip repair, we have had three wound infections (2.3%). All three resolved rapidly with oral antibiotics. None resulted in wound separation or unsatisfactory scarring.

At the time of surgery, we administer prophylactic antibiotics just before making our incisions. In a patient not allergic to cephalosporins, we routinely administer a single intravenous dose of cephazolin. A similar dose may be given every 6 to 8 hours for 24 to 48 hours, but we consider the intraoperative dose the most important one. Since most of our patients go home on the day of their operation after the surgery, the intraoperative antibiotic dose is often the only one that they receive. We do not send patients home with oral antibiotics unless we are treating a specific infection (usually otitis media). Patients are routinely seen 4 to 6 days following surgery, and the parents are instructed to call us if significant swelling or erythema is noted. Significant erythema in the first 24 to 72 hours following surgery may represent streptococcal cellulitis. Rapidly progressing erythema would be treated in the hospital with penicillin, with further antibiotics added if improvement is not rapid.

Erythema, induration, warmth, swelling, and fever,

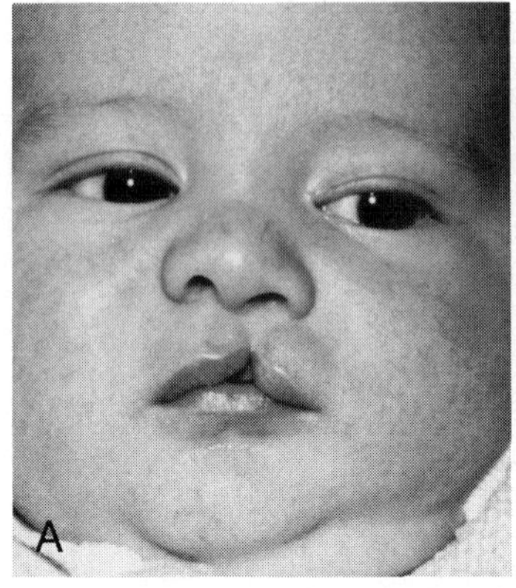
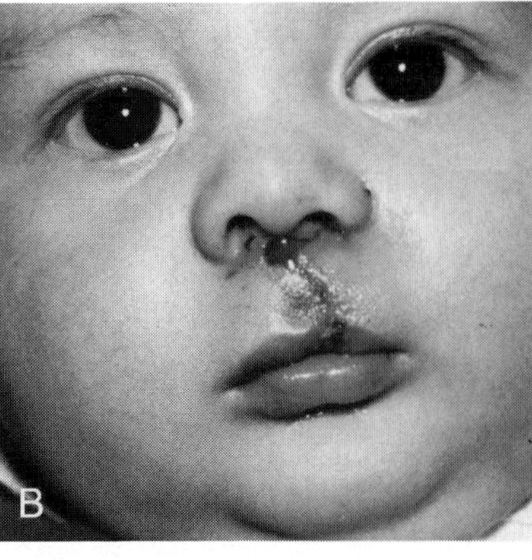

Figure 31–1 *A*, A 2-month-old boy with an incomplete unilateral cleft lip on the left side prior to repair. *B*, The same patient 6 days following lip repair. There is moderate erythema, and a purulent discharge is seen at the upper aspect of the incision. The infection quickly resolved with oral antibiotics.

particularly if they are increasing more than 2 days following surgery, suggest a wound infection. With an infection, purulent drainage is often seen adjacent to the nostril (Fig. 31–1). A sample should be sent for culture and antibiotic sensitivities. While these results are pending, we begin antibiotic therapy with dicloxacillin. The most likely responsible organism is *Staphylococcus aureus*, although almost any organism found in the mouth or on the skin may be the cause. Fortunately, these infections tend to resolve rapidly, usually without causing any tissue necrosis or wound dehiscence. However, the increased inflammation can result in some degree of scar hypertrophy.

Flap Necrosis

For patients with unilateral cleft lip, we use a rotation-advancement repair. We have never seen necrosis of any of the flaps used in this type of repair. For patients with bilateral cleft lip, we use a one-stage lip repair. Simultaneous repair of both sides produces better symmetry. Our experience has been that the philtrum will spread following surgery. To avoid a philtrum that is too wide later, we design the flap to be only 2 to 3 mm in width superiorly and 4 mm inferiorly. We have had necrosis of one such flap (Fig. 31–2). In that case, the philtrum had been excessively thinned in an attempt to produce a philtral dimple. We still advocate a very narrow philtrum but avoid excessive thinning of the philtral skin. We also avoid a dermal suture to create a philtral dimple, feeling that this is a potential source of flap compromise. When faced with flap necrosis we recommend topical antibiotics (bacitracin ointment or

silver sulfadiazine cream) until the flap has completely demarcated. If there has been significant skin loss, a full-thickness postauricular skin graft may be very helpful in replacing the missing tissue. In older patients, an Abbe flap may also be used.

Wound Disruption

Reported rates of wound dehiscence following cleft repair range from 1% to 7.4%.[1-4] In our experience, wound disruption has been limited to repair of bilateral cleft lip almost exclusively. We have seen only one wound disruption following unilateral cleft lip repair. This low rate occurs in spite of the fact that we repair even the widest complete unilateral cleft lip in a single stage without prior lip adhesion. On the other hand, among our primary bilateral cleft lip repairs, we encountered six postoperative separations (Fig. 31–3). Five of these occurred in children older than 9 months of age. The disruptions could be directly related to trauma in all of these cases—for example, one child fell while attempting to walk and another was struck by a sibling.

Based on our experience, we advise particular caution when performing bilateral lip repair in patients older than 9 months. Families should be informed of the risk of lip trauma and wound disruption in these patients. We do not feel that a longer hospital stay would prevent this problem because our disruptions occurred 1 week or more following surgery. We find it difficult to justify routinely keeping these patients in the hospital for that long following surgery.

Following disruption, if the patient is seen soon after

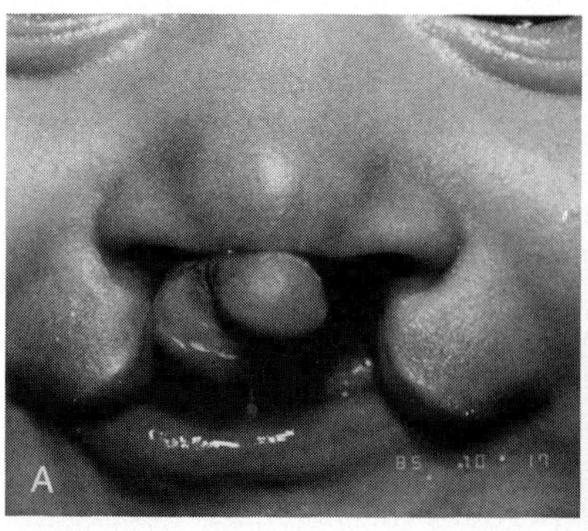
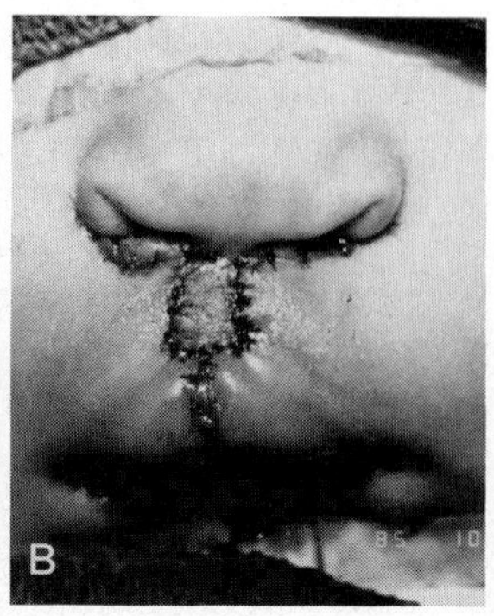
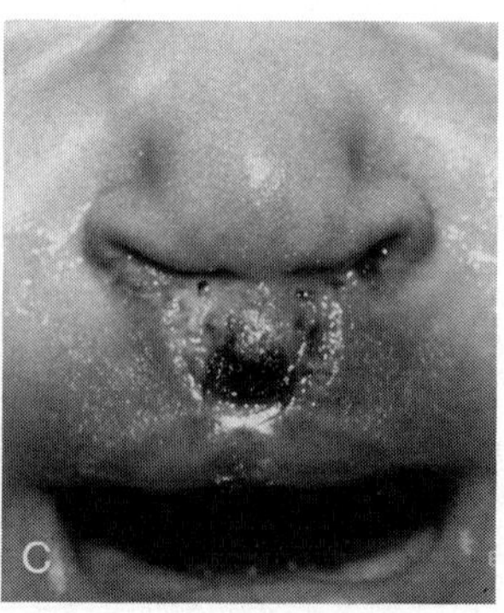

Figure 31–2 *A*, A 3-month-old girl with an unrepaired complete bilateral cleft lip and palate. *B*, Immediately following completion of repair, with the patient still on the operating table, the distal portion of the philtral flap already shows some ischemic changes. *C*, Six days later there is necrosis of the distal 40% of the philtral flap.

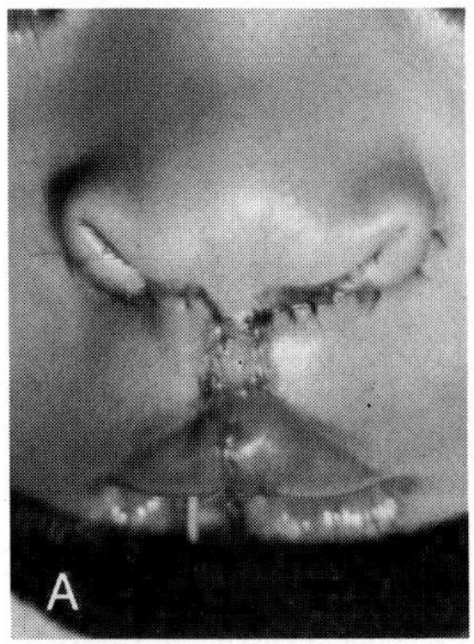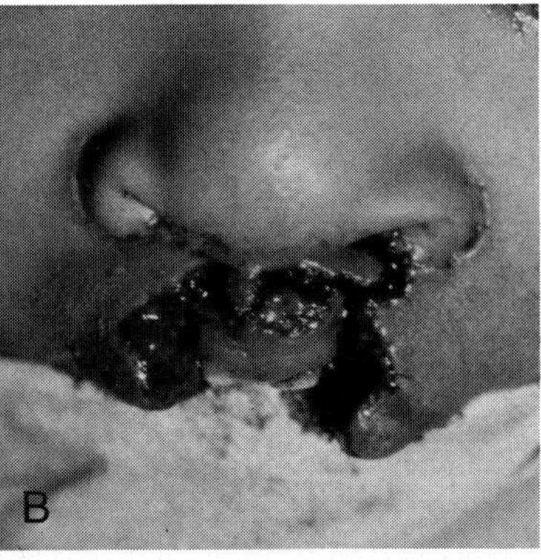

Figure 31–3 *A,* A 4-year-old boy, who had never undergone previous surgery, is shown immediately following completion of bilateral cleft lip repair. *B,* Seven days later the patient is again on the operating table for repair of traumatic wound disruption.

a traumatically caused disruption, surgical reclosure is indicated. If seen later, or if the cause of the disruption is in doubt, we recommend conservative management with topical antibiotics followed by delayed surgical reclosure using the original incisions and flaps as far as possible.

Nasal Airway Obstruction

It is not unusual for cleft lip repair to cause nasal airway obstruction. Not only does the surgical re-arrangement narrow one or both nostrils, but also there is postoperative edema in that area. In almost all cases, the infant quickly adapts to a change from nasal breathing to mouth breathing without incident.

Occasionally, however, significant respiratory distress may be noted, particularly in repair of bilateral clefts. This problem immediately responds to gentle insertion of a short nasal cannula of a relatively stiff material, such as a cut segment from an endotracheal tube. Because of their small diameter, these cannulas must be cleaned frequently to maintain their patency. Sullivan has reported two infants who had respiratory distress due to nasal obstruction following cleft lip repair.[5] Both were successfully treated with insertion of nasal cannulas.

Late Complications

The late complications of cleft lip repair are the residual or iatrogenic deformities resulting from avoidable errors of planning or execution. The surgeon must learn to avoid these late complications and achieve near normal appearance. With cleft repair, the surgeon's shortcomings are worn by the patient. They are seen as displeasing alterations in lip configuration, nasal shape, and jaw relationships.

Deformities of the Lip

Late complications of cleft repair are seen in the lip as either asymmetries or disproportions. Ideally, the reconstructed cleft lip will closely resemble the normal appearance of the lip. The human eye is extremely sensitive to and critical of asymmetry. A normal appearing lip blends with the other features of the face and escapes unusual scrutiny. However, a poorly executed lip reconstruction draws the eye to the lip and disrupts the normal harmony of facial features.

Of the upper lip structures, the vermilion is the most noticeable. Along its superior edge, it stands in sharp contrast to the cutaneous portion of the upper lip. Inferiorly, the whiteness of the teeth silhouettes the lip's lower border. To achieve a normal appearing lip, one must create a symmetric vermilion-cutaneous junction as the upper border of a balanced vermilion width. In addition, separation of the orbicularis oris muscle should not distract from the appearance of the lip, and the scar should be thin and its position well camouflaged.

Failure to achieve balance of the vermilion-cutaneous junction is the most common late complication of lip reconstruction and is most often seen as a vertical height discrepancy. It is critical in repair of the unilateral cleft lip to place the peak of the Cupid's bow on the cleft side, level with the peak on the noncleft side. A 1-mm discrepancy is a significant deformity. In our experience, a short lip on the repaired side is far more common than excessive length. Scar contracture in the first few months following lip repair is not uncommon and may be marked. Softening and relaxation of the scar will return the lip to its immediate postrepair position. However, if the lip repair is short on the operating table, it will always remain short. It is wishful thinking to expect improvement with time or massage.

In the bilateral cleft lip, vertical height symmetry is extremely difficult to achieve if the lip repair is done in two stages. Matching the height of the second side to the height of the previously repaired and possibly contracted opposite side may be difficult. Central vermilion thinness (whistle deformity) is also commonly seen after the two-stage approach. The single-stage bilateral repair, in which the vermilion of the lateral segments replaces the prolabial vermilion, results in better symmetry and a fuller vermilion tubercle.

Although horizontal asymmetry may be a less obvious lip deformity than vertical height asymmetry, it also is an important deformity. It is our feeling that the repaired cleft lip, both unilateral and bilateral, frequently exhibits a philtrum that is too wide. In the rotation-advancement repair of a unilateral cleft lip, a wide philtrum directly affects a surgeon's ability to rotate the lip inferiorly. The wider one marks the philtrum, the higher up the cleft margin one places the new peak of the Cupid's bow. Therefore, a wide philtrum results in a greater vertical discrepancy between the normal peak of the Cupid's bow on the unaffected side and the new height of the Cupid's bow on the cleft side.

Adequate downward rotation is far easier to achieve if a narrow philtrum is designed. In the rotation-advancement repair, the philtral width is determined by the distance between the depth of the Cupid's bow and its peak on the normal side. This measurement then pivots on the depth of the Cupid's bow to determine the peak of the Cupid's bow along the cleft margin. Unfortunately, the depth of the Cupid's bow is not an easily identifiable point. It frequently is closer to the peak of the Cupid's bow on the normal side than initially estimated. If the mark for the depth of the Cupid's bow is moved 1 mm toward the normal side, the width of the "hemiphiltrum" on that side is narrowed. Using this same width to mark the peak of the Cupid's bow along the cleft margin, the peak on the cleft side is now marked 2 mm more medial than it would have been.

Using this modification, we have found it far easier to obtain vertical symmetry and have rarely needed to use a backcut, which results in a noticeable lowering of the oblique lip scar. We do not feel that altering the depth of the Cupid's bow is an artificial technique to make the rotation easier. If one studies repaired clefts by bisecting the philtra, the area between the bisecting line and the philtrum on the repaired side is frequently significantly larger than the corresponding area on the opposite side. Scar revisions to improve the vertical height of the lip are often accomplished not so much by rerotating the lip as by removing the old scar and a portion of the adjacent normal lip. This essentially places the peak of the Cupid's bow on the cleft side closer to the opposite side, narrowing the philtrum.

In the bilateral cleft, good vertical symmetry is often spoiled by the unnaturally wide appearance of the philtrum. Although this excess width can eventually be used to lengthen the columella, the secondary nasal procedure requires reentering the lip and producing new scars. If the philtrum can be narrowed at the time of the initial bilateral reconstruction, the lip need not be reentered. Extra tissue can be banked in the nostril floor at the time of the initial repair and later used for columellar reconstruction. In addition, the narrower one makes the philtrum at the time of the initial bilateral repair, the more vermilion is available for central tubercle construction.

A narrow philtrum and an adequate vermilion tubercle go a long way in preventing the stigmata normally associated with a bilateral cleft repair. We have found that methylene blue tattooing of the superior and inferior margins of the white roll prior to injection of an infiltrating solution allows the most accurate alignment of this structure. The superior and inferior margins of the white roll are best seen with the bright operative lights turned away. The alignment of two points, as opposed to the usual single mark, also has been helpful in the occasional instances in which one tattoo mark is difficult to see or has been inadvertently excised.

Vermilion Irregularities

Vermilion irregularity is a common residual deformity in the cleft-lip patient. This deformity can occur superiorly at the vermilion-cutaneous junction or along the inferior border of the vermilion as a notch or excess of tissue. The most common irregularity of the vermilion in the unilateral repair is a notch at the site of the repair. If recognized at the time of the initial repair, this can be treated with a vermilion Z-plasty. One of the causes of the notched vermilion is incising the lip

beyond the fullest portion of the vermilion. Coaptation of the vermilion then leaves a narrow portion at the point of repair, the immediate adjacent areas being thicker. This results in the notched appearance (Figs. 31–4 and 31–5). By taking care to incise the vermilion at its fullest portion, one can prevent notching and obviate the need for Z-plasty.

In the bilateral cleft lip, the vermilion of the prolabium is deficient, in both volume and character. The use of prolabial vermilion generally results in a central deficiency or whistle deformity. Later attempts at plumping the central portion rarely produce a natural vermilion tubercle. The character of the epithelium lining the prolabial vermilion is also different from that of the vermilion of the lateral segments. Peeling is commonly observed when it is incorporated into the tubercle. For the above reasons, one can obtain a better central vermilion by utilizing the lateral cleft vermilion, which is brought beneath the cutaneous portion of the prolabium and sutured in the midline.

To obtain sufficient vermilion volume in the central portion of the lip, one needs to overcorrect this area at the time of the initial repair. The overcorrection rapidly reduces in volume. With experience one finds that it is difficult to place too much vermilion in the central portion of the upper lip. The inexperienced surgeon need not be timid in this regard. Excess vermilion can be more easily removed than added. We have never

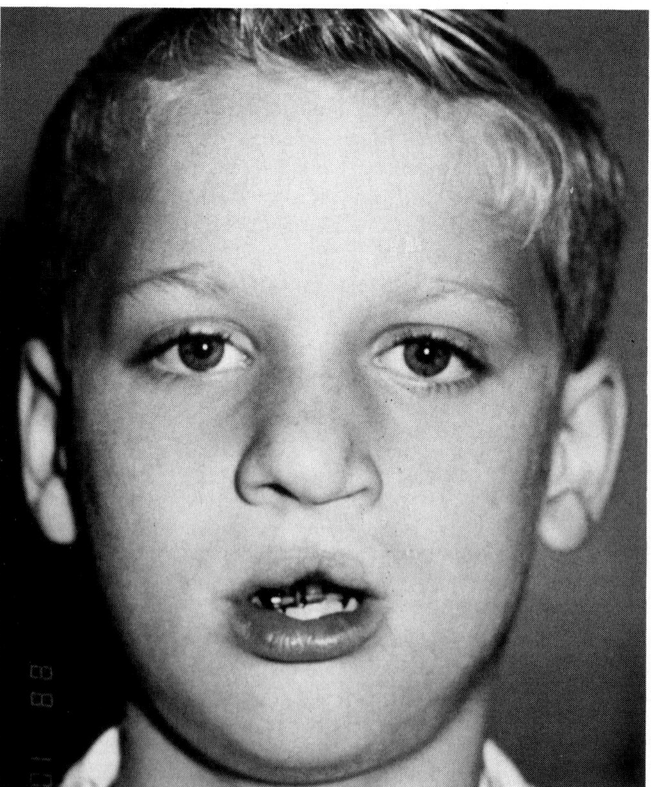

Figure 31–4 The typical notched vermilion that is seen following unilateral cleft lip repair in which the vermilion incisions have been made too far toward the cleft. If the fuller vermilion, on either side of the notch, had been approximated, the notching could have been prevented.

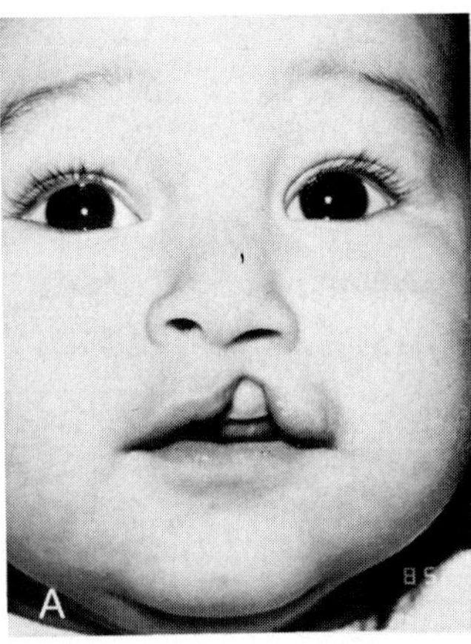 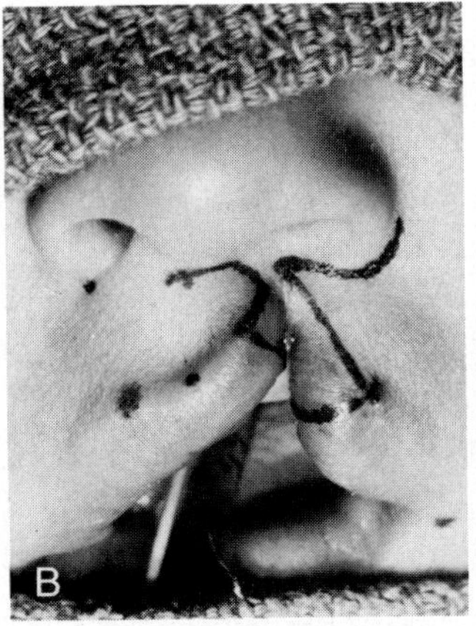 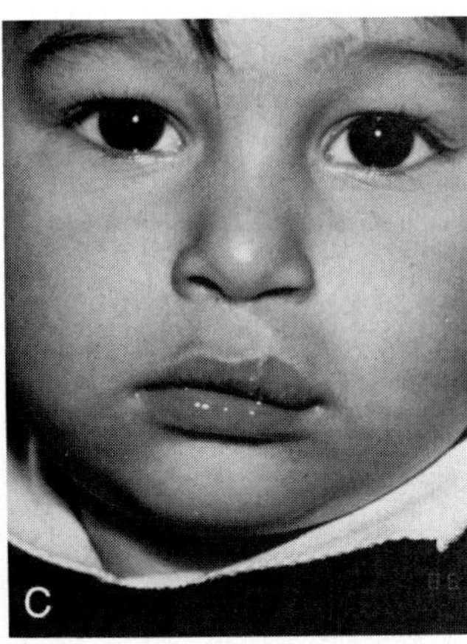

Figure 31–5 A, A 5-month-old boy with an unrepaired unilateral cleft lip on the left side. *B,* The surgical skin markings demonstrate placement of the vermilion incisions too far toward the cleft. Particularly on the lateral segment, notice that the fullest portion of the vermilion is approximately 4 mm lateral to the planned incision. *C,* The same patient 1 year later has excess vermilion fullness laterally because of the placement of the original incisions.

found it necessary to reduce the too prominent central tubercle.

Muscle Deformity

The disrupted orbicularis oris muscle requires proper reconstruction in cleft repair. Muscle discontinuity, either because of failure to join the muscle segments at the time of repair or because of subsequent muscle dehiscence, leads to an unnatural appearing lip. Muscle discontinuity is less commonly seen in unilateral repairs. When present, a groove or trough appears beneath the cutaneous scar. Muscle discontinuity in the bilateral lip is seen more frequently. The resulting deformity is more noticeable with lip animation. The muscle segments appear as bulges laterally (Fig. 31–6). This complication is prevented by adequate muscle dissection and suture. We utilize permanent suture material, feeling that even late dissolving sutures lose their strength too rapidly.

External Scars

Complications involving scars due to cleft lip repair are related to the position and thickness of the scar. Scar formation in the lip is generally quite good and is certainly more forgiving than in some other areas of the body. The vermilion is consistent in its minimal scar

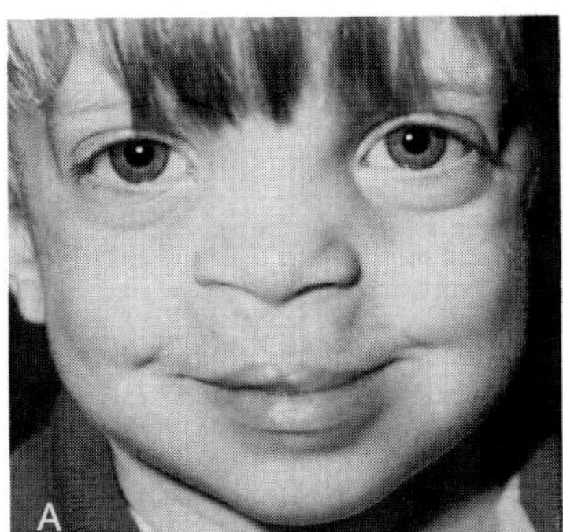 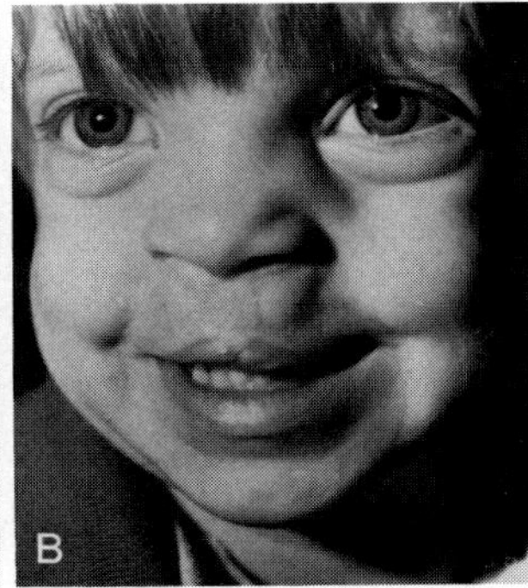

Figure 31–6 A, Following bilateral cleft lip repair, a bulge is seen to the left of the midline. This suggests orbicularis oris discontinuity. *B,* With animation, the bulge is more prominent, confirming muscle discontinuity.

formation. Marked hypertrophic scarring following lip repair is very rare but does occasionally occur.

A more minor degree of scar hypertrophy may be seen and persist as a red, firm, shortened scar that tents the vermilion and contributes to lip asymmetry. To minimize the incidence of scar hypertrophy, we try to keep skin manipulation to a minimum. There is a great temptation to place deep dermal sutures to help coapt and align the skin edges and to minimize tension. These buried sutures cause greater dermal trauma and can be a persistent focus of inflammation if they work themselves to the surface. In an attempt to minimize untoward scar formation, we like to avoid the buried dermal suture. By resecting 3 to 4 mm of orbicularis oris muscle from each lip segment prior to suturing, we can achieve good skin approximation with muscle closure alone. Suturing of the shortened muscle does not allow a gap between the cutaneous portion of the lip segments. This technique minimizes the need for buried dermal sutures and reduces the number of skin sutures required.

It is our opinion that the initial repair heals with a more consistently acceptable scar than subsequent revisions. For this reason, we attempt to achieve final symmetry with the initial surgery and to avoid reopening the lip with subsequent procedures such as a columella lengthening.

Placement of the advancement flap to fill the rotation defect is the cornerstone of the rotation-advancement repair. We have found that a better scar results if the C-flap is used to fill the rotation defect. By utilizing the C-flap in the rotation defect, the advancement flap can be oriented in a more vertical direction to better match the opposite philtral column (Fig. 31–7). The appearance of a lip repair utilizing this technique is significantly better than the oblique scar crossing the philtra, seen when the advancement flap is used to fill the entire rotation defect.

Another late complication of the rotation-advancement technique of unilateral repair is the late appearance of hair on the lip. The hair generally appears at the tip of the advancement flap. It is a direct result of taking skin from the nasal vestibule to obtain a sufficient length of advancement flap. This complication occurs a number of years following the initial repair, with the subsequent development of vestibular hair growth. By

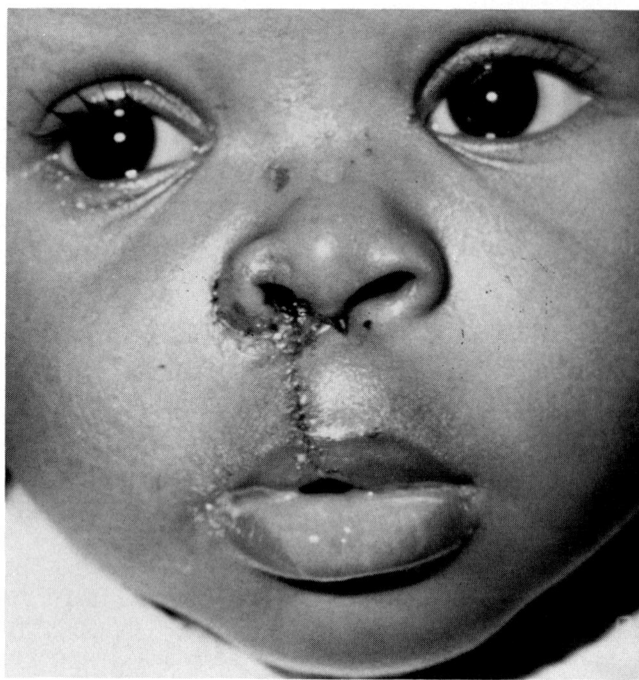

Figure 31–7 Using the C-flap to fill in the rotation defect allows placement of the tip of the advancement flap in the nostril sill; however, it may cause decrease in nostril size and asymmetry of the nostrils.

utilizing the C-flap to fill the rotation defect, one does not need to achieve extra length for the advancement flap. This helps to confine the flap to lip tissue and will prevent the complication of later hair growth.

Nasal Deformity

The nasal deformity associated with clefting is discussed elsewhere in this book. Athough nasal deformity is certainly the result of the initial clefting process, it can be compounded by the cleft lip repair itself.

Repair of the cleft lip will uniformly improve the nasal appearance. The degree to which surgeons address the problem of nasal reconstruction at the time of the initial repair varies. Excellent nasal appearance can be obtained either by repairing the nose at the time of the initial lip repair[6] or by postponing this repair until later.

Nostril Stenosis

The most difficult late nasal complication associated with cleft lip repair is that of nostril stenosis. Because stenosis is so difficult to correct, great care should be taken by the surgeon to avoid this complication. A minor degree of nostril narrowing is not unusual following cleft lip repair. It is far easier to narrow a nostril than it is to enlarge it. For this reason, one should err

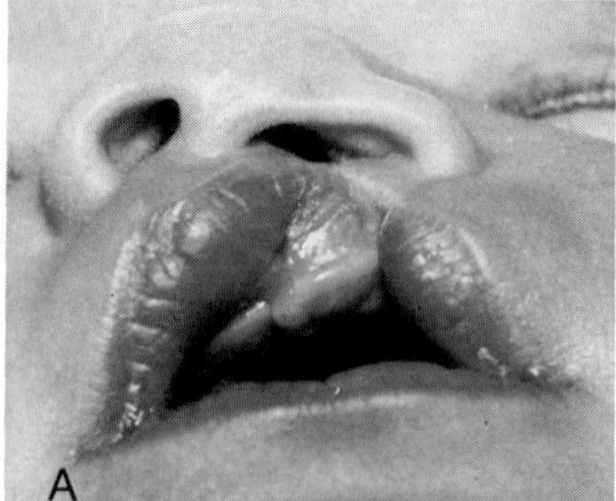
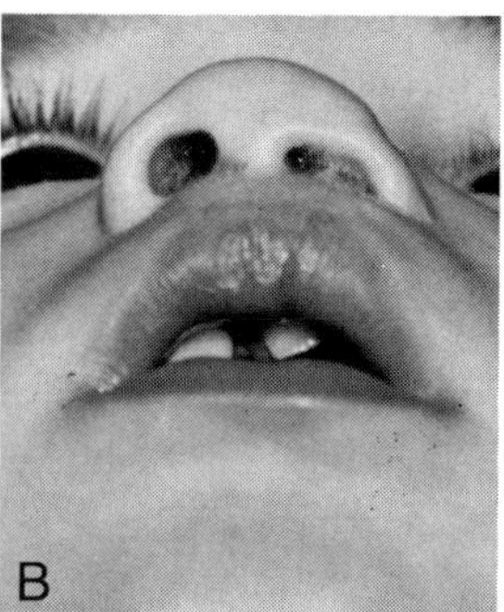

Figure 31–8 *A*, An incomplete unilateral cleft lip on the left side prior to repair. An intercartilaginous incision was used for nasal reconstruction at the time of primary lip repair. *B*, The same patient, 1 year following surgery, has a web that is nearly occluding the left nostril.

on the side of making too large a nostril on the repaired side.

Fortunately, tight stenosis is relatively uncommon. Although certain technical considerations make this occurrence less likely, it cannot be completely avoided if one chooses to perform definitive nasal reconstruction at the time of primary lip repair. In our experience, a circumferential nasal lining incision has been associated with a higher incidence of nostril stenosis. These intercartilaginous or rim incisions have also been associated with a more severe degree of stenosis (Fig. 31–8). With rotation-advancement repair, placement of the L-flap in the nasal vestibule helps to provide adequate nasal lining and reduce the likelihood of stenosis. We recently have favored the nasal reconstruction technique described by McComb.[6] Since using this technique, we have seen much less nostril stenosis, although it still occurs occasionally.

Conclusion

Acute complications of cleft lip repair fortunately are rare. As in most surgery, they can be avoided by good technique. The late complications cause persistent deformity and result in the need for multiple revisions. With experience, the cleft surgeon can reduce complications to a minimum and improve the final results for his patients.

References

1. Bromley GS, Rothaus KO, Goulian D: Cleft lip: Morbidity and mortality in early repair. Ann Plast Surg 10:214, 1983.
2. Schettler D: Intra- and post-operative complications in surgical repair of clefts in infancy. J Maxillofac Surg 1:40, 1973.
3. Weatherley-White RCA, Kuehn DP, Mirrett P, et al: Early repair and breast-feeding for infants with cleft lip. Plast Reconstr Surg 79:879, 1987.
4. Wilhelmsen HR, Musgrave RH: Complications of cleft lip surgery. Cleft Palate J 3:223, 1966.
5. Sullivan WG: Respiratory distress following cleft lip repair: The role of obligatory nasal breathing in the infant. Ann Plast Surg 20:590, 1988.
6. McComb H: Primary correction of unilateral cleft lip nasal deformity: A 10-year review. Plast Reconstr Surg 75:791, 1985.

CHAPTER 32

Correction of Secondary Unilateral and Bilateral Cleft Lip Deformities

John M. Hiebert and
Richard Sturm

Need for Secondary Repair

Recent improvements in the understanding and technical execution of the primary cleft lip repair have significantly reduced secondary sequelae and the consequent need for heroic secondary surgical execution. However, although improvement exists, perfection is elusive. Numerous factors may condition the need for secondary surgical intervention in patients with both unilateral and bilateral cleft lip. Such factors begin with the severity of the initial deformity but also include the planning, precision of execution of the primary repair, and success of the postoperative management. This management includes the numerous nonsurgical elements such as effective dental orthopedics, treatment, prosthodontics, and timely integration of the surgical and dental components. Despite the most favorable surgical treatment, the severity of the problem and postoperative complications can result in unacceptable results that command secondary intervention. The most important operation in lip surgery is the primary repair, and every effort should be made to accomplish excellent results with the first operation. However, "perfection is the enemy of good," and there is no substitute for sound clinical judgment in operative decisions. In patients with complicated cleft lips, particularly complicated bilateral cleft lips, staged surgical procedures are required.

When secondary lip deformities exist, associated nasal, maxillary, and dental deformities often distort the facial appearance. This chapter will deal with secondary deformities of the lip because methods for correction of nasal, maxillofacial, orthognathic, and dental deformities are discussed in other chapters. It should be emphasized, however, that often contiguous deformities are interactive. An alteration of one component may significantly alter another.

Despite the diversity of opinions regarding the importance and timing of repair of given deformities, general principles of lip function and aesthetics should guide the surgeon in his choices of surgical procedures and timing. This chapter presents an approach to secondary lip repair and offers a rationale and philosophy supporting this approach.

Goals of Secondary Repair

Goals for secondary lip reconstruction must combine a recognition of the deformity with a reasonable expectation for its improvement. Steffensen[1] has outlined reasonable requirements for lip repair, which include:
1. Accurate skin, muscle, and mucous membrane union.
2. Proper rotation of the deflected lateral orbicularis oris muscle into a horizontal position with its medial components (if present).
3. A symmetric nostril floor and nostril tip.
4. An even vermilion border with reproduction of the Cupid's bow (if possible).
5. Slight eversion or pouting of the central upper lip.
6. A minimal scar that by its contraction will not interfere with the accomplishment of the other stated requirements.

Significant deviations from these requirements suggest a need for secondary repair. These six requirements provide reasonable goals for secondary repair. Although restoration of a "normal" anatomy (including dimension, proportion, and symmetry) is an expected goal of secondary reconstruction, it must be tempered if the patient or his or her family has an unrealistic expectation for perfection.

Indications for Surgery

Anatomic Factors

Malalignment or displacement of lip elements often persists following even the most exact lip repairs. This deviation may become more obvious with facial growth or may improve with time. Surgical indications depend *first* on the anatomic abnormalities as identified by the surgeon. *Second* (in the older patient) is the patient's "realistic" perception of the anatomic distortions. *Third* is the recognition of the anatomic factors and desire for improvement by the family (generally the parents).

Detailed anatomic factors involving the lip have been reviewed elsewhere in this book (see Chap. 17). However, simple elements of the normal surface anatomy are important to provide clarity in defining the degree of deformity (Fig. 32–1). A rule of thumb for lip proportion (height) in the upper lip is one-half the length of the lower lip. A symmetric proportionate philtrum with a central dimple, equal philtral lines, and a full tubercle with a slight pout are key elements in the normal upper lip. A symmetric, even white roll frames the lip vermilion. Symmetric vermilion shape and lip length should provide a slight show (1 to 2 mm) of upper teeth when the lip is in repose, and symmetric lateral elements of the commissure contribute some of the essential features of an aesthetically formed lip. Identification of specific and measurable variations in these general features justifies secondary repair. This is a reconstructive, not cosmetic, justification because the variation is not normal. The factors accounting for the variability from the normal anatomy provide the foun-

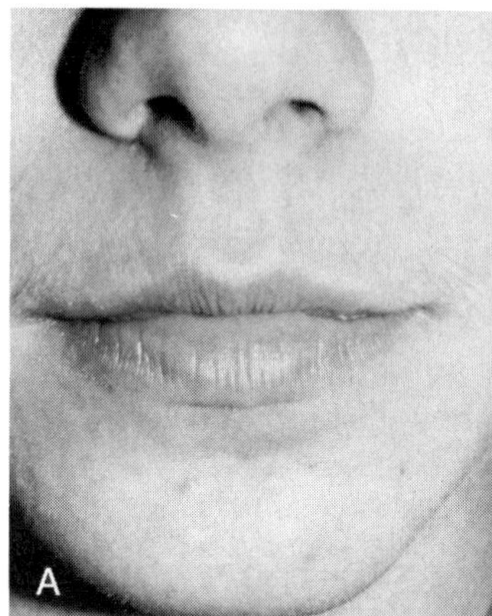
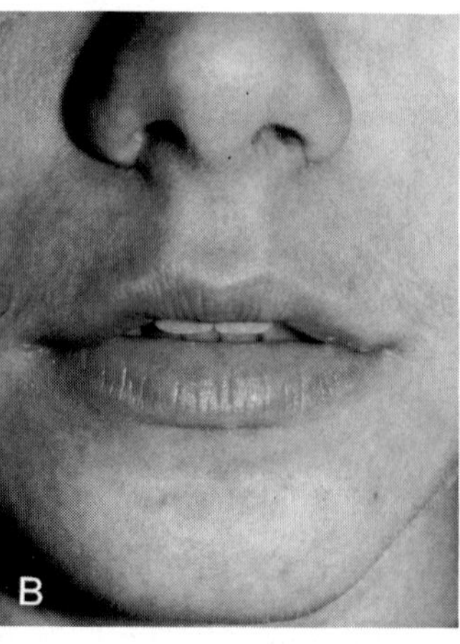
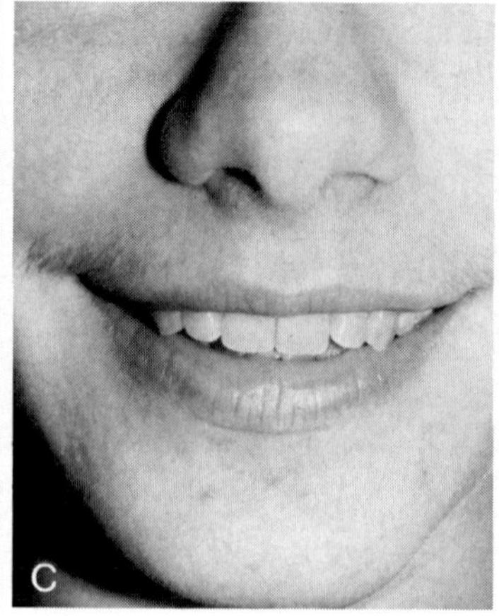
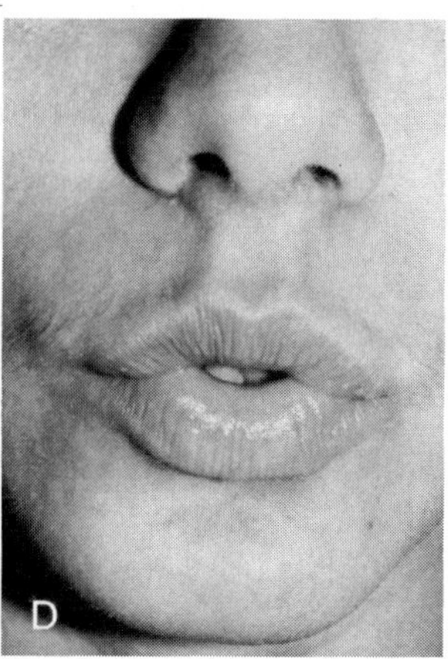

Figure 32–1 Essential features of a normal lip in a young adult female showing the important aspects of structure, symmetry, and proportion. *A*, With the lips closed, the length of the base of the nose to the tip of the tubercle is one-half that of the length of the upper central margin to the base of the chin of the lower lip. The philtral lines accentuate the philtral dimple present in the lower third of this philtrum. The white roll frames the upper lip, accentuating the symmetry and fullness of the tubercle and vermilion. *B*, Lip in repose during relaxation. Two mm of dental "show" is visible beneath the upper lip. *C*, Increased lip elevation in the smile position. *D*, Accentuation of the central tubercle during pucker. The philtrum is accentuated and the central dimple brought into greater relief.

dation for surgical planning but may require more complex integrated care (dental and orthognathic factors of lip support and facial proportion). Indications for surgery, however, must be tempered by a reasonable understanding of scarring and the process of wound healing. A contracture occurs in nearly all repairs, resulting in a temporary notch that, with time and patience, will generally improve. Table 32–1 displays important linear measurements that provide norms for comparison.[2] Perhaps more important than linear measures, however, are aspects of proportion and symmetry. Significant deviations from these norms in terms of millimeters provide the most important anatomic indications for surgical reconstruction.

Amaratunga[3] has applied the criteria of Steffensen[1] and Musgrave[4] in developing a quantitative index for determining the symmetry of the features of the lip. This interesting method, the Cleft Lip Component Symmetry Index (CLCSI), may have utility not only in comparing the results of surgical methods but also in identifying specific components of the lip that require secondary revision (Fig. 32–2) and providing an objective assessment of improvement following revision.

Table 32–1. Linear Measurement Norms Comparing Vertical and Horizontal Dimensions of the 5-Year-Old and Adult Lip

| | Normal Lip Dimensions in Caucasians (cm) | | | |
| | 5 Years | | Adult | |
Mean Lip Measurements	**M**	**F**	**M**	**F**
Vertical length (columella base to tubercle)	2.1	2.1	2.4	2.0
Vertical length (nasal base to peak of Cupid's bow)	1.6	1.4	2.2	1.5
Width (Cupid's bow to commissure)	2.3	2.3	3.2	2.9
Width (philtrum)	1.0	1.0	1.5	1.3
Width (mouth)	5.6	5.3	6.3	5.7

Patient Desires

Satisfying patient desires in the infant means providing adequate physiologic sucking with lip closure. Young children, however, at about the age of 3 are able to recognize aesthetic variances from the norm. Indeed, early measures of intelligence incorporate this discriminate ability in young children.[5] Although the young child may recognize his abnormality, the child seldom indicates concern about this perceived abnormality prior to school age. The imposed socialization of school, however, takes on new significance in that it is an important aspect of social rejection.[6] This evidence provides a compelling motivation to complete reconstruction of some deformities by the time the child reaches school age.

During the periods of childhood and adolescence, more definitive secondary procedures can be carried out. Clearly, by this time the child or young adult is able to enter more actively into the decision making concerning his or her treatment. The patient's desire for improvement, however, is frequently moderated by fear of hospitalization and the pain and discomfort of the surgical experience as well as by reluctance to adhere to limitations on postsurgical activities.[7] Reconstruction at this time must be undertaken cautiously. Honest preoperative counseling is essential. False hope for perfection and inadequate preparation for the operative and postoperative experience can lead to bitter disappointment, often compromising the anatomic improvement that surgery has accomplished. Concomitant counseling with a knowledgeable counselor of the multidisciplinary team may enhance the operative result.[8]

Family and Social Considerations

In the early years, up to age 5, the parents' wishes, expectations, and fears are paramount and must be dealt with in an honest yet compassionate way. Failure to do so will doom an excellent surgical result to a mediocre

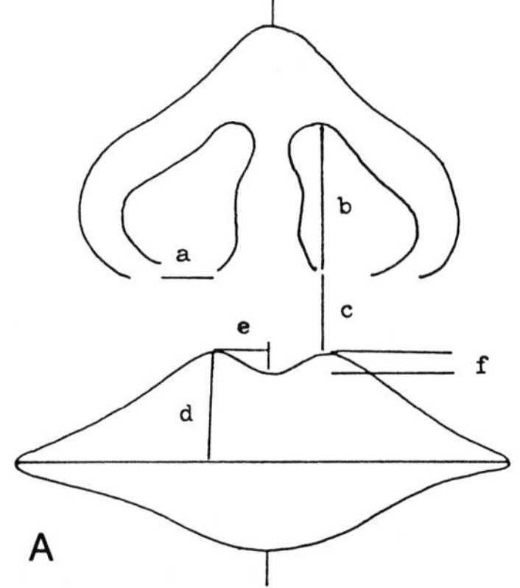

Figure 32–2 Quantitative method comparing symmetry of important lip features as described by Amaratunga. This method can be used to compare one operative method of repair with another. (From Amaratunga ND. J Oral Maxillofacial Surg 46:834, 1988. With permission.)

Cleft Lip Component Symmetry Index for Nostril Floor Width =

$$\frac{\text{Nostril Floor Width on the Cleft Side}}{\text{Nostril Floor Width on the Normal Side}} \times 100 = \frac{a_2}{a_1} \times 100$$

A value of 100 would indicate perfect symmetry

reception at best. At the same time, a noncompliant family, unable to carry out the necessary nonsurgical instructions for dental, orthopedic, or orthodontic care, should serve as a red flag to the surgeon wishing to improve a secondary deformity. Assertive yet patient counseling is helpful in overcoming these pitfalls. Honest financial planning and assistance with financial support should be discussed with the parents before an elective secondary procedure is performed.

Surgical Timing

The Deformity

Surgical timing for repair of secondary deformities is less clear-cut than that for primary repairs. The nature of the deformity itself, scar formation, and the effect of surgical trauma on facial growth are important factors in the optimal timing of secondary repair.[9] Surgery on the more straightforward component deformities (for example, lip scars, muscle bulging, white line irregularity, and so on) generally can be carried out as early as 12 months following the initial lip repair. Structural deformities such as the long, tight, or short lip are conditioned by interactive structural growth factors. Definitive repair of structural deformities generally fares better when the dental, orthognathic, and maxillary components have been managed. In both unilateral and bilateral clefts, untreated skeletal and dental asymmetry significantly impairs a favorable lip result, particularly in bilateral clefts in which the premaxilla is unstable or malpositioned. A malpositioned or unstable premaxilla will change with time and affect the results of lip revision.

Integration of Surgery with Other Components of Care

Integrated care in the management of secondary cleft lip provides the best rehabilitative results. Thus, the timing for a secondary surgical procedure may be delayed so that more pressing problems can be addressed. For instance, a pharyngeal flap may be required as a result of velopharyngeal incompetence and may command priority to allow more effective utilization of speech therapy. Dental or orthopedic bony manipulation may rightfully delay lip surgery until a reasonable

orthodontic goal has been accomplished. Although this delay may be counter to the patient's or the family's priorities, the decision for surgical correction should be made to achieve the most favorable long-term result. Individual or family counseling is helpful in providing emotional support during presurgical preparation. The desire to accomplish "everything at once" in correction of the secondary deformity is generally unrealistic, and the potential risks are high.

Classification

A classification system (Table 32–2) is presented that combines numerous methods of approaching secondary cleft lip repair. Often the repair of a lip deformity is complicated by foundational problems involving bone, teeth, and so on. In these cases, attention to the deformity requires an understanding of the integration of numerous factors that influence decisions on surgical timing.

Surgical Approaches to Structural Deformities

Structural deformities generally consist of several components that, if not thoughtfully analyzed prior to surgical intervention, will result in disappointing out-

Table 32–2. Classification of Secondary Cleft Lip Repair

I. Structural deformities
A. Long lip
B. Short lip
C. Tight lip
II. Component deformities
A. Mucous membrane
B. Vermilion
C. Skin deformity
D. Muscle deformity
E. Bone deformity
F. Dental deformity

Note: This proposed classification system focuses on major structural deformities (composite) and specific components of the lip. More than one deformity may exist in a given lip, and more than one technique may be employed to improve the deformity.

comes. The causes of these deformities are multiple, and no single solution fits all patients.

Long Lip

This deformity may be apparent or absolute (Fig. 32–3). It is seen more commonly in patients with bilateral clefts, but also may occur (generally with less severity) in unilateral anomalies. The long lip is conditioned by the severity of the cleft and may be associated with concomitant maxillary retrusion and poor dental support of the lip. Often, however, it occurs as a result of the original lip repair. Although the methods of repair vary, Musgrave[4] has cautioned that the triangular and especially the quadrangular flap repairs have a greater tendency to produce a long lip than the straight-line or rotation-advancement methods. The deformity becomes more obvious as untreated facial growth and dental deficiencies develop and scar relaxation occurs. This may be an unfair indictment because the former techniques are sometimes chosen for treatment of the more severe unilateral clefts. It does, however, challenge advocates of these repairs to give careful consideration to facial growth and lip length in designing the original flap repairs.[10] It is unusual to achieve "over-rotation" using the rotation-advancement method, although it has been reported.[11]

Evaluation of the *unilateral* long lip should include a careful physical examination including precise bilateral measurements of the philtral lines, tubercle, and central lower lip to chin dimension. Examination of the vestibule, dental occlusion, and cephalometric measurements should be routine. If the long lip is minimal and a primary quadrangular repair has been used, orthodontic or orthognathic treatment alone should be considered because revision by lip shortening is difficult. If a Millard or straight-line repair was originally employed, a take-down procedure can be carried out to shorten the lip and improve symmetry. Millard has advocated ignoring the previous scars and converting the imbalanced lip to a rotation-advancement design if the defor-

mity is moderate to severe (when there is a total imbalance of length or asymmetry of 2 mm or more between the medial and lateral dimensions).[12]

In the *bilateral* anomaly, a long lip may result when laterally based skin and vermilion flaps are placed below the prolabium in the primary repair. This often becomes more apparent with time and is particularly aggravated by an unstable premaxilla. It also occurs when the prolabium has been cut free from the columella during columellar advancement, thus directing the premaxillary vector downward.[13] The net effect of these factors sacrifices upper lip width for height and also may be associated with a tight lip.

Although numerous methods have been described to shorten the lip, these results can be disappointing if the premaxilla, maxilla, or vestibule is not adequately treated. Early lip-shortening procedures by Teale,[14] Erich,[15] Vaughan,[16] and others produced a shorter lip, but objectionable scars or an isolated ring about the prolabium may have overshadowed the improvements made by shortening the lip.

Four general approaches characterize recent surgical procedures used to shorten the long lip:
1. Subalar resection (upper lip shortening).
2. Supravermilion resection (lower lip shortening).
3. Combined upper and lower resections.
4. Combined lip shortening with other corrections.

Holdsworth described a bilateral subalar resection procedure (Fig. 32–4).[17] This is useful when the philtral tubercle unit is not excessive. Millard,[13] Austin,[18] and others have proposed a more extensive full-thickness, transverse, subalar, subcolumellar skin resection if other nasal-labial features are satisfactory.

Supravermilion shortening by resection of skin flaps beneath the prolabium has been advocated by Gillies and Kilner.[19] Specific designs to create a Cupid's bow vary depending on the details of the deformity. However, skin resection alone seldom accomplishes satisfactory results. Vermilion advancement and appropriate muscle resections are important modifications (Fig. 32–4). If the columella is short and the lip is tight, this procedure may give disappointing long-term results.[13]

Harding[20] and others have described excisional procedures that combine both upper and lower full-thickness skin excisions by re-creating the prolabial scar along the philtral lines into a "bull's head" configuration. This procedure may be used in patients in whom the tubercle is particularly long (Fig. 32–4).

Combining shortening procedures with other techniques allows several associated components of the long lip to be repaired. Peterson et al.[21] incorporated an abbreviated Abbe flap utilizing only the lower lip vermilion, orbicularis marginalis, and mucosa into an upper and lower lip shortening procedure. This design shortens the long lip yet provides a supple tubercle. Use of the abbreviated Abbe flap also can be effective in correcting a tight sulcus or whistle deformity associated with a long lip.[22] Millard[23] described a two-staged procedure that involved switching the lateral based rectangular flaps below the prolabium into a vertical position parallel to the prolabium, thus elevating the vermilion and shortening the lip. These flaps are then used

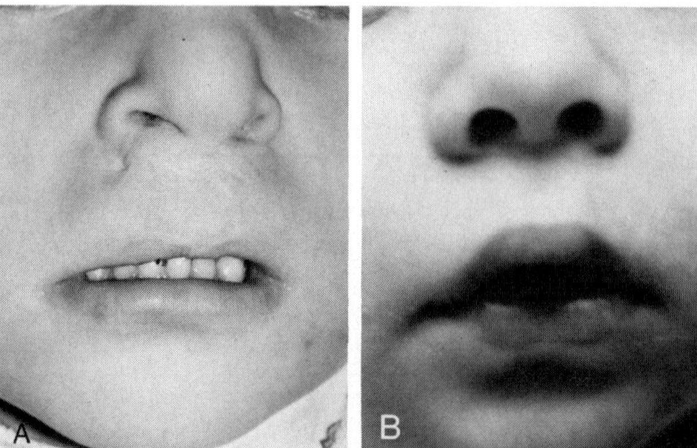

Figure 32–3 Excessively long lip in this 3-year-old with a bilateral cleft. Note that the 1:2 proportion of upper to lower lip has been lost because the upper lip is nearly as long as the lower lip. Also, in the relaxed state, no upper dental show can be seen below the upper lip margin. This contrasts with the normal 3-year-old lip (B).

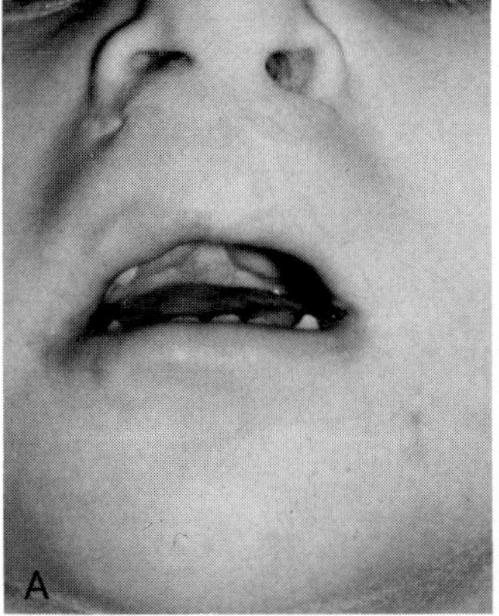
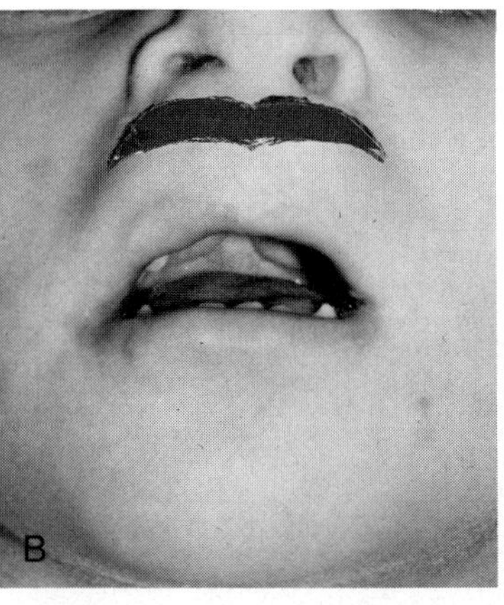
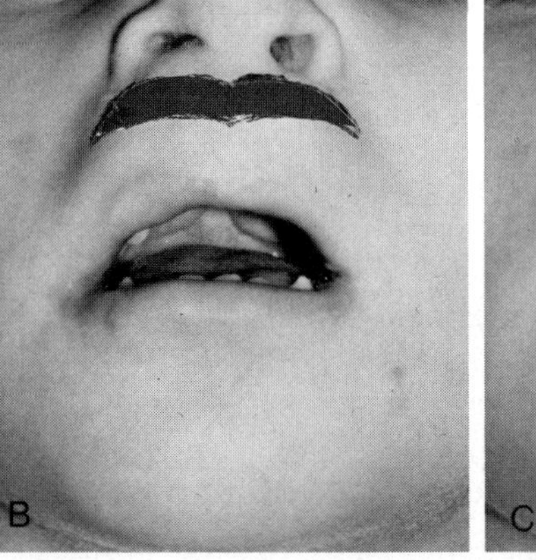
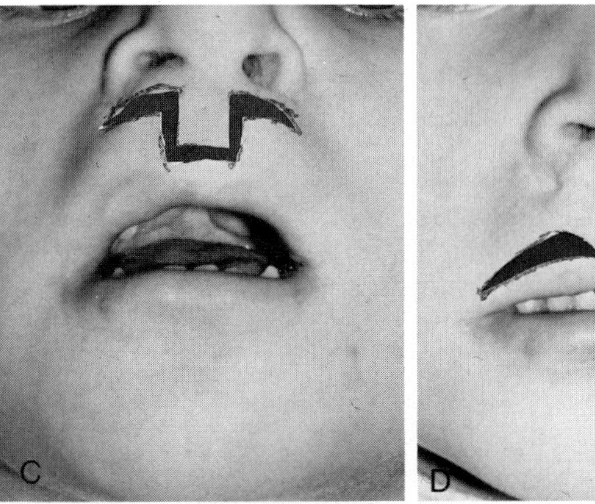

Figure 32–4 Methods of shortening of the long upper lip are shown in this 3-year-old child with a bilateral cleft. *A,* An excessively long repaired bilateral cleft lip. *B,* Upper subalar resection methods as proposed by Holdsworth[17] and Millard.[13] *C,* Vermilion shortening method as proposed by Gillies.[20] *D,* The "bull's head" method of resection as described by Harding.[25]

secondarily to elongate the columella, using the switch flaps as forked flaps. When considerable lip scarring has occurred in the long lip, an abbreviated Abbe flap can be incorporated into the Ragnell bull's head shortening procedure. The columella can be lengthened by elevating the abbreviated prolabium.

Regardless of the methods employed to correct the long lip, slight overcorrection may be necessary to overcome a postoperative tendency to sag and may produce sustained improvement.

Short Lip

The short lip is seen more commonly when unilateral straight-line and rotation-advancement methods have been used for the primary procedures. Like the long lip deformity, it is difficult to correct because several components may be involved such as a protruded premaxilla, excessive dental or maxillary height, inadequate sulcus, small prolabium, excessive scarring, or an inadequate tubercle. Thus, several treatment options must be considered. Repair of the short lip, however, involves not only an aesthetic insult but also adds a significant dental risk because of tooth exposure from impaired lip closure.[20]

In a short unilateral cleft lip, an asymmetry generally exists. This can often be corrected by a take-down procedure of the primary Millard repair and by precise realignment. In unilateral straight-line repairs that have resulted in shortness, scar excision and a variety of Z-plasty techniques are useful.[24] If additional length is required after a triangular flap primary repair, further Z-plasties may be used.[25] The short lip is unusual following the quadrangular repair. An inadequate tubercle or sulcus frustrates any lengthening procedure; thus, an independent or combined vestibuloplasty may be essential.

Corrective structural lip lengthening procedures can be classified as follows, and their general principles apply in all upper lip reconstructions.
1. Rotation-advancement flaps.
2. Z-plasty.
3. V-Y or forked flaps.
4. Muscle advancement.
5. Abbe flaps.

Advancement flaps can be placed low, which produces an unnatural horizontal line at the caudal margin of the prolabium and presents the reverse of the frequent problems seen with the long lip. High advancement flaps follow the Millard principle and can be used effectively to correct slightly short lips. Laterally placed cheek flaps as proposed by Webster may be useful in treatment of severely shortened lips.[26]

In patients with bilateral clefts with secondary short lips, a protruded premaxilla may produce a relatively tight lip, and premature lengthening of the lip may result in an eventual long lip. Thus, secondary lip lengthening may be delayed until dental and bony treatment have been accomplished (Fig. 32–5). Scar excision and Z-plasty can achieve 2 to 3 mm of length or more if multiple Z-plasties are used.[27] These are effective for length but produce abnormally placed scars that may require further treatment (dermabrasion or dimple reconstruction procedures). V-Y advancement of the philtrum can lengthen the lip but may produce an unnatural dimple at the base of the columella. If the V-Y is created by use of a forked flap columellar advancement, the dimple problem can be minimized (Fig. 32–6). If the vertical shortness is minimal and lateral muscle diastasis is present, correction of the muscle deformity by properly joining the orbicularis oris muscle will add some vertical lip height. If the philtrum and tubercle are inadequate, significantly scarred, or absent, or if the lip is tight in the horizontal dimension, a carefully designed, centrally placed Abbe flap is the procedure of choice.

A slightly short lip may be due to an inadequate central vermilion or tubercle. Methods of repair for this problem will be discussed later in the chapter.

It should be emphasized that total deficiencies of lip tissue nearly always exist in the repaired cleft lip. Procedures designed to lengthen the vertical dimension are accomplished at the sacrifice of horizontal length. Thus, a tight lip may result, and a cross-lip flap or

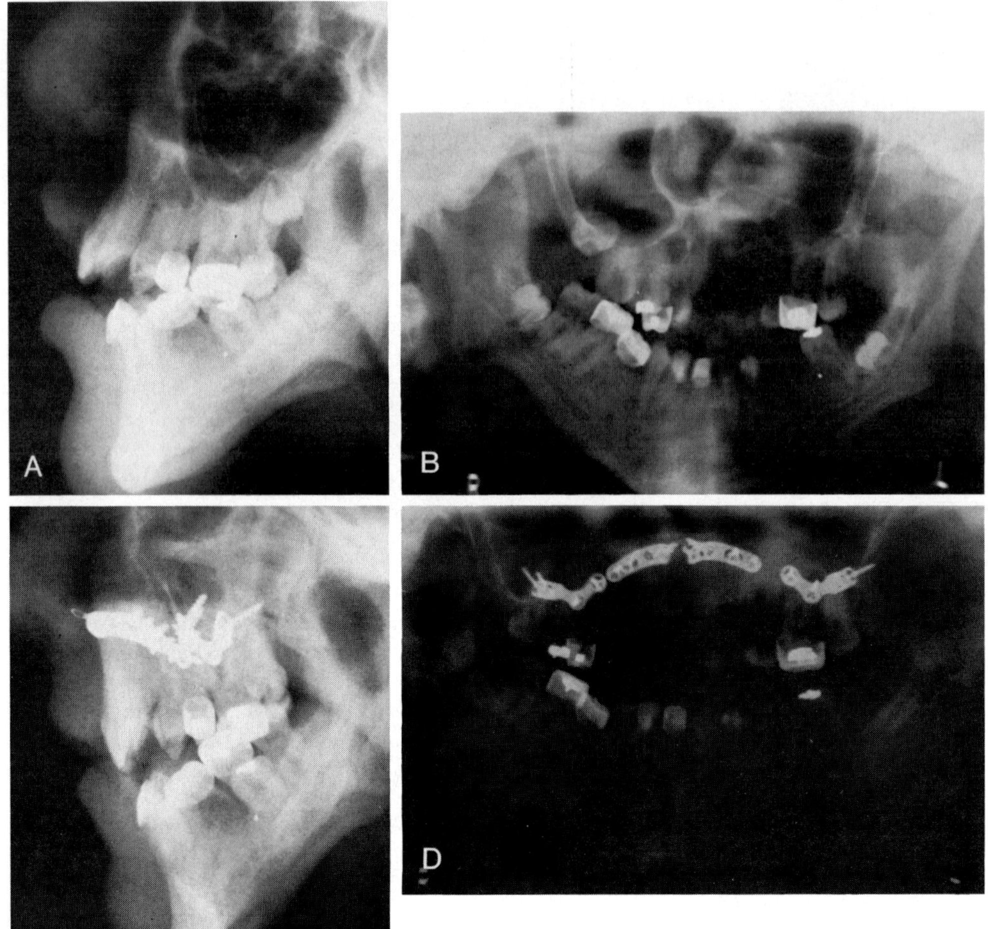

Figure 32–5 This x-ray series demonstrates bony and soft tissue abnormalities in a 15-year-old white girl with a wide unilateral cleft lip. *A* and *B*, Preoperative open bite and class II malocclusion. The soft tissue shadow shows a short upper lip that is approximately one-third the soft tissue shadow of the lower lip. *C* and *D*, Improved relationship of the lips following orthognathic surgery. Three millimeters of real length in the lip was gained after maxillary surgery alone.

Figure 32–6 V-Y advancement of the central tubercle in limited tubercle deficiencies. *A*, Deficient central tubercle in a 6-year-old with a repaired bilateral cleft lip. *B*, V-Y advancement technique. *C*, Postoperative result showing some increased lip pout projection of the tubercle.

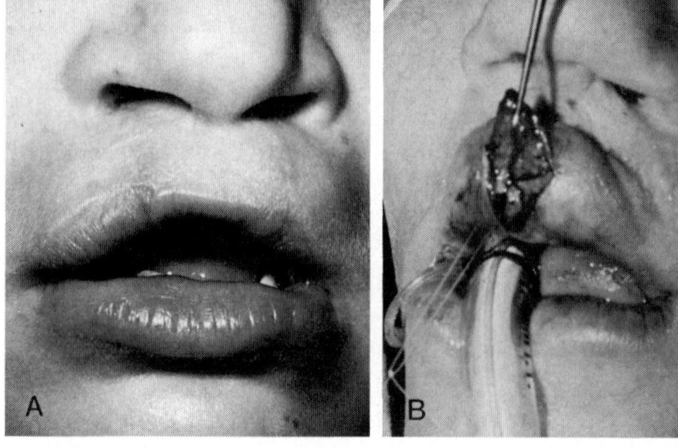
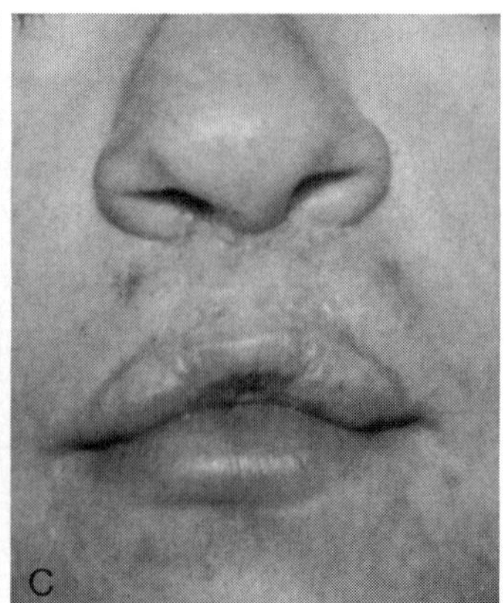

composite graft may be needed as proposed by Gillies and Millard.[28]

Tight Lip

The tight upper lip is short in the horizontal dimension and most frequently is seen in patients with a bilateral cleft. It may be associated with a long lip as well but invariably places strain on the developing premaxilla and midface. This may further compound the deformity by restricting anteroposterior facial growth.[20]

The basic problem is inadequate soft tissue. Correction requires the addition of new tissue (Fig. 32–7). The use of a cross-lip flap or composite graft provides the best tissue. Available prolabium can be used when needed to augment a deficient columella using the forked flap method or other prolabial advancement methods in a single or staged procedure. As opposed to the long lip alone, however, it is advisable to release the tight lip before performing bony advancement or a bone graft. Bone graft resorption has been observed in the presence of a tight lip.[20]

The cross-lip flap provides comparable tissue to the deficient upper lip without significantly compromising the horizontal length of the lower lip. Robert Abbe first described in 1889 the staged, central, lower to upper lip flap for augmentation procedures in cleft lip deformities.[29] Others, however, used and described this principle of tissue transfer before Abbe. Sabattini[30] in 1838 and years later Stein[31] described use of the cross-lip principle for correction of the lip deformity following resection of the lip for cancer. Estlander[32] described his modification in 1872, which was designed to repair lateral defects in the upper lip. Many modifications of this procedure have been described. It is the "workhorse" for repair of upper lip deficiencies. The composite cross-lip graft described by Flanagin[32] and others eliminates the necessity and delay of a pedicle but is less predictable than the pedicle flap.

Several physiologic features of transferred tissue have been reported. Smith[33] observed that sensory reinner-vation developed in a certain sequence, with pain first appearing in the periphery of the flap followed by light touch and temperature over a period of 2 years. Muscle function returned in 1 year together with autonomic functions (e.g., sweating).

Anatomic placement of the flap in the midline or eccentrically remains controversial. In the unilateral tight lip, satisfactory release of lip tightness has been achieved by placing the flap in the cleft defect centrally, ignoring the original scar.[34] Others place the flap in the original scarred defect.[35] The choice depends partly on the original method of repair and partly on the nature of the deformity. Eccentrically placed flaps, however, will never produce normal anatomic landmarks. In the bilateral cleft, the question of central placement is seldom an issue. Rather, the anatomic questions deal with the width and height of the flap design.

The Abbe flap can be utilized to:

1. Correct upper lip deficiencies (central or eccentric placement) (Fig. 32–7);
2. Correct vermilion or tubercle deficiencies (shaved Abbe flap) (see Fig. 32–10);
3. Correct components of the lip deformity in combination with other techniques (long tight lip).

Operative Technique of the Abbe Flap

Cannon and Murray[36] as well as McGregor[34] have described the technical features of the construction and inset of the Abbe flap. The design begins with the height and width requirements of the upper lip. Cannon and Murray have suggested that the flap width measurement should be 1 to 2 mm greater than the difference between the horizontal length of the upper and lower lips measured commissure to commissure at the level of the white line. This can produce a wide philtrum. The adult philtrum normally measures 0.8 to 1.2 cm at the vermilion and 0.6 to 0.9 at the root of the columella. In the bilateral cleft lip, in which the natural philtrum is used for the columella, flap length is very important. It should measure no longer than that needed to produce a sufficient tubercle while allowing 1 to 2 mm of dental "show." In the unilateral cleft lip, it should be no longer than the shortest distance between the apex of the Cupid's bow and the nostril floor on the normal side.

General anesthesia is advised, at least in children, using an oral or nasal endotracheal tube. The flap is designed on the lower lip, and a shelf of muscle can be incorporated beyond the limits of the skin incision to reduce scar depression at the line of inset. Identification and careful preservation of the labial coronary artery is accomplished by observing its position on the cut edge. A three-layer closure is recommended, and careful attention is directed to placing the white line alignment.

Postoperatively, a Barton's dressing can be helpful during the extubation period to prevent flap disruption. Feeding is facilitated by a straw or bulb syringe, and suture line care is essential. The flap can be safely divided 10 days after the operation and precise inset of the mucosa surface carried out.

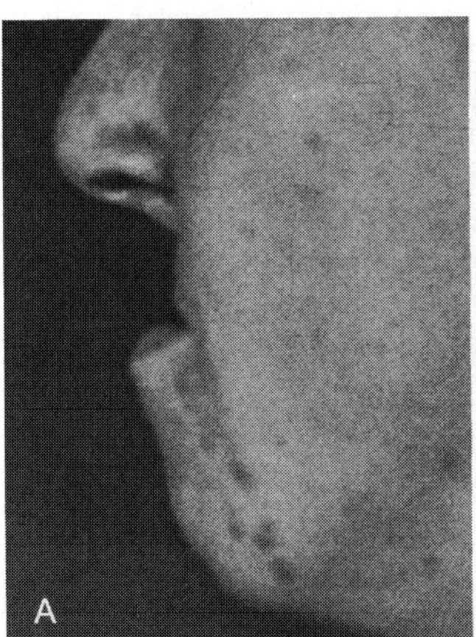
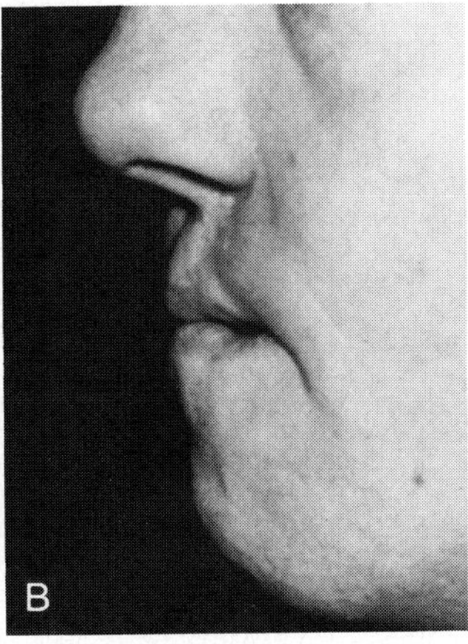

Figure 32–7 A 14-year-old white boy with a tight lip resulting from a bilateral cleft. *A,* Preoperative lip tightness in horizontal length. *B,* Postoperative improvement following an Abbe flap.

If a dental prosthetic device is used, it should be in place during the operative procedure. Healing is generally complete in 1 to 2 years.

Surgical Approaches for Component Deformities

Component deformity describes specific anatomic features of the lip that may occur in isolation or in combination with other components. Since each component is interdependent, it is helpful to identify carefully the deformities in each of the components during preoperative surgical planning.

Mucous Membrane

Tight Sulcus. An upper lip sulcus is essential for the creation of normal lip mobility and lip pout. It also allows access into the mouth for orthodontic and prosthodontic treatment. This sulcus may be lost when sulcal flap construction is ignored in the primary repair, but generally it results from necrosis, infection, or disruption of the mucous membranes postoperatively. In the unilateral cleft, an abnormal restricting band or tight frenulum can be divided and elongated by Z-plasty. When the sulcus is obliterated by prolabial attachment to the premaxilla, complete release of the lip and creation of a sulcus by a variety of mucosal flaps or free skin grafts are indicated.

Esser utilized a skin graft to create the lip sulcus.[37] Cosman and Crikelair were successful in using a mucosal graft to create the sulcus.[38] The extent of the dissection can be extended to free the nose and columella elongated from prolabial tissue with the sulcus release as described by von Reilen.[39] Although graft take is excellent, maintenance of the sulcus depends on adequate obturation because early contraction will limit the release and produce an unacceptable cul-de-sac.

In an effort to reduce this problem, mucosal flaps have been used to create a sulcus. Falcone used a mucosal flap lifted off the premaxilla and elevated on the labial surface.[40] The exposed bone on the premaxilla reepithelializes. A variety of geometric flaps have been proposed by Horton and his associates in sulcus reconstruction.[41]

Release of the tight sulcus is an essential first step in secondary lip revision. Failure to release the sulcus will limit the success of the revision and may further restrict maxillary and dental growth.

Nasolabial Fistula. It is desirable to avoid a nasolabial fistula in the primary repair. When it occurs, the timing of its closure will depend on the significance of patient symptoms. In many cases, symptoms are quite limited, and therefore there is no urgent need for closure. The nasolabial fistula can be closed at the time of alveolar bone grafting, if indicated, or it can be closed independently. If adequate sulcus tissue is present, the fistula's lining is turned inward, thus creating a nasal lining. Advancement or rotation flaps of the oral sulcus can then be used to complete the closure.

Vermilion Deformities

Vermilion Asymmetry. In the unilateral cleft, an asymmetric irregularity that has developed at the skin vermilion border can be revised by excision; precise reunion is generally sufficient. This procedure is particularly useful when skin has violated the vermilion or when a pink vermilion stains the skin incision line and the philtrum. Small irregular notching at the vermilion cutaneous junction can be corrected by a balanced or unbalanced Z-plasty (Fig. 32–8). An unbalanced Z-plasty can further augment a deficient tubercle, or more than one Z-plasty can be added at the free-lip border or on the mucous membrane surface.

Lateral vermilion asymmetry, which is not associated with significant muscle irregularity, can be improved with a unilateral, full-thickness skin excision and vermilion advancement as proposed by Gillies and Kilnar.[19] If the asymmetry is caused by excessive or redundant vermilion, a unilateral Z- or W-plasty excision at the mucovermilion junction produces improved balance (Fig. 32–9). When minor notching deficiencies exist at the free lip border, a vermilion V-Y advancement is an effective technique.

Whistle Deformity. In the bilateral cleft lip, a true whistle deformity is common. Duffey[42] attributed this deformity to the failure of intrinsic tissue development and suggested that advancement of the orbicularis oris to the midline is a solution. Thus, whistle deformity is a multicomponent problem and requires attention to the vermilion, muscle, and mucous membrane as demonstrated by Randall et al.,[43] Robinson et al.,[44] Pucket et al.,[45] and others.

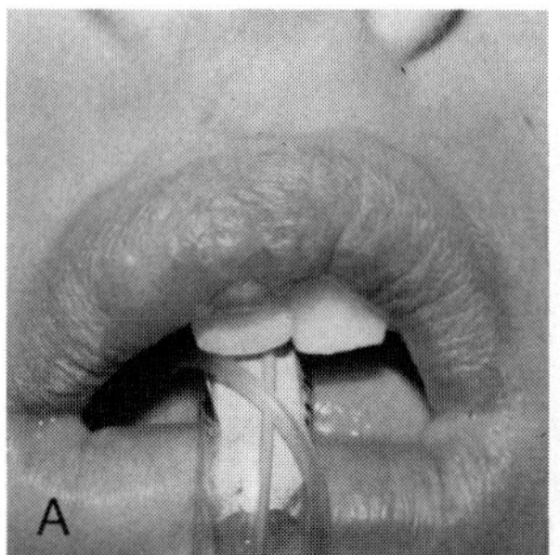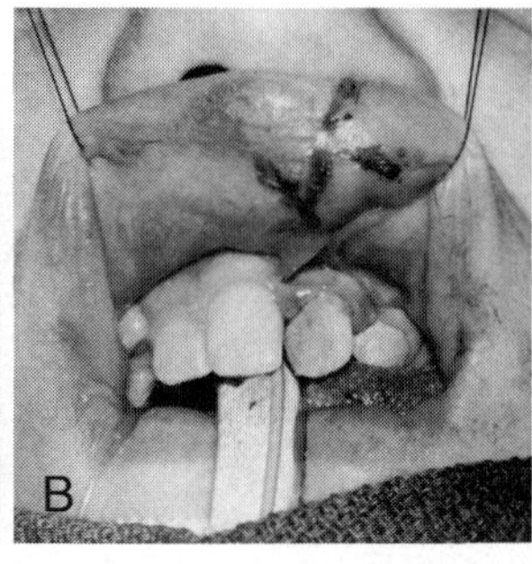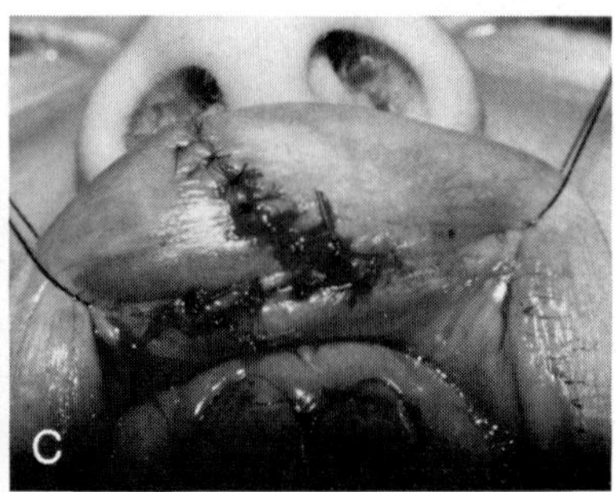

Figure 32–8 A–C, Use of an eccentric Z-plasty to improve a vermilion irregularity with notching in a 12-year-old white boy.

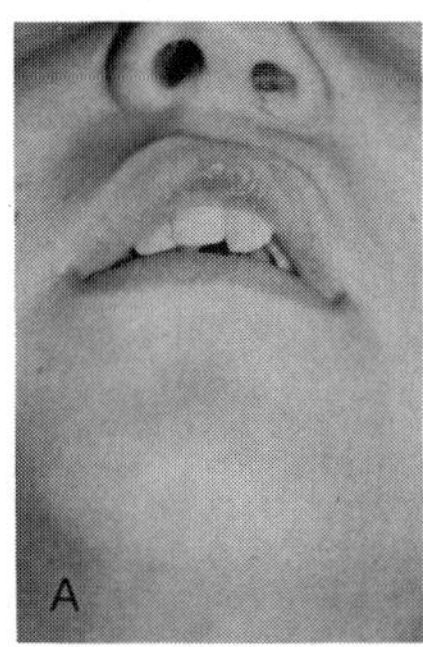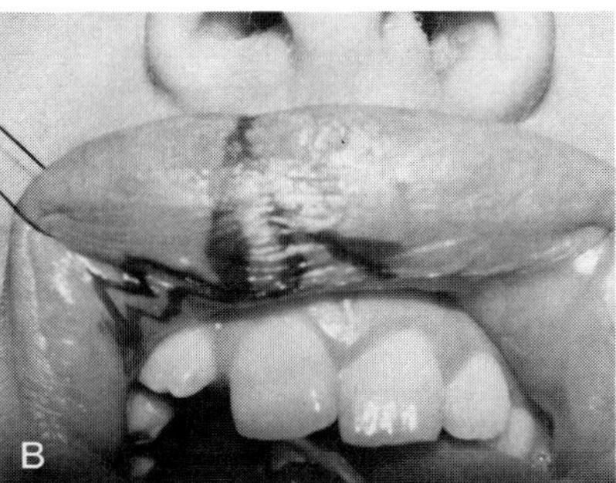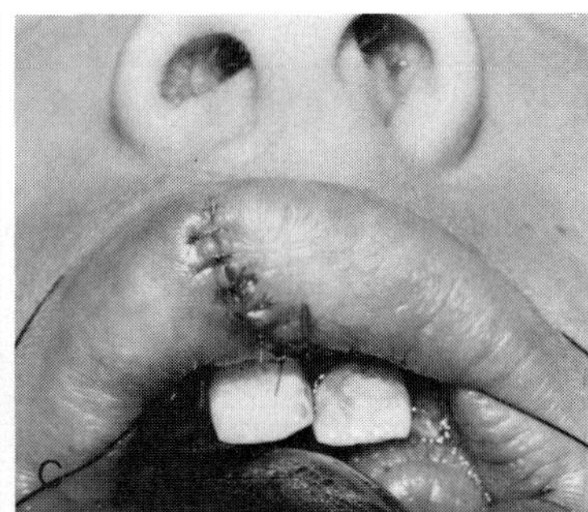

Figure 32–9 *A–C,* Methods of Z-plasty and W-plasty for correction of vermilion asymmetry in this 12-year-old boy with a unilateral cleft lip.

Inadequate Tubercle. Deformities of the tubercle occur as a result of inadequate tissue, malalignment, or abnormal scar placement. If the vermilion alone is inadequate and is restricted by a mucous membrane scar, a V-Y advancement of the vermilion helps (see Fig. 32–6). If there is inadequate bulk for tubercle projection, muscle advancement is necessary. However, the pars marginalis alone should be advanced. If excess bulk is placed beneath the distal philtrum, an unaesthetic fullness will result. Advancement of the pars marginalis alone allows dynamic augmentation of the tubercle yet preserves the philtral dimple (see Fig. 32–12).

If the central vermilion is intrinsically inadequate, a shaved Abbe flap (Fig. 32–10) or composite graft should be used.

Skin Deformities

Secondary scar deformities are common and may involve the entire lip or only a portion of the lip.
White Roll Irregularities. Interruption of a normal white line, if isolated, has many simple solutions. Scar revision with careful approximation of the white roll margins or Z-plasty is often useful and simple. Millard has proposed a small, white roll graft as an effective alternative.[46] Use of a color-simulated tattoo technique at the vermilion-cutaneous junction is effective and can be carried out as an office procedure (Fig. 32–11).[47]
Wide or Irregular Scars. Wide or irregular scars of the skin can generally be managed with excision and precise reapproximation of the skin with careful identification of the white roll and philtral landmarks. In the unilateral cleft lip, if a minor linear discrepancy exists between the normal and cleft sides, an eccentric Z-plasty may be useful. Anizuka et al.[24] have reported success with multiple Z-plasties and camouflaging of a variety of skin deformities in the secondary bilateral cleft lip. The judicious use of Z-plasty in cleft lip scar revision is often helpful. It may, however, produce distortions of the philtral line and upper lip dimple. Dermabrasion techniques are useful when surface irregularities are the dominant problem and the scars are not particularly wide. When the philtral skin is badly scarred, however, total resurfacing with a full-thickness graft may be indicated, as reported by Broadbent[48] and others.

Muscle Deformities

Randall and his associates[43] have emphasized the importance of muscle reconstruction in both primary and secondary lip repair. This emphasis has been reinforced by Kapetansky,[49] Pucket et al.,[45] and others.

The primary release of the orbicularis oris from the maxilla and proper alignment can prevent many secondary muscle deformities.[43] This is particularly true of the pars marginalis. Secondary repair of an inadequate tubercle and correction of a whistle deformity have previously been discussed in the section on vermilion deformities.
Lateral Muscle Bulge. A common secondary deformity is the lateral muscle bulge (Fig. 32–12). This results from inadequate primary muscle release or secondary disruption, and it creates a significant deformity. When this occurs in isolation, careful dissection and muscle readvancement together with adequate maxillary release are indicated. Skin adjustment independent of the muscle is generally indicated because skin elevation may be associated with the scar secondary to hematoma.
Inadequate Muscle. Abnormal indentations may occur as a result of inadequate muscle placement. This often is observed in the nasal sill area but may be associated with a caudal portion of the septum deviating away from the cleft as a result of an imbalance in muscle pull (Fig. 32–12). The indentations can be corrected surgically by secondary muscle advancement and precise approximation.

Bone Deformity

Alveolar and Maxillary Deformities. Management of bone deformities is beyond the scope of this chapter

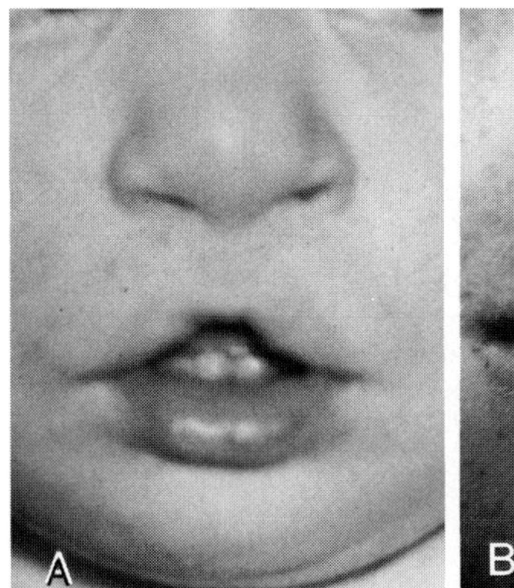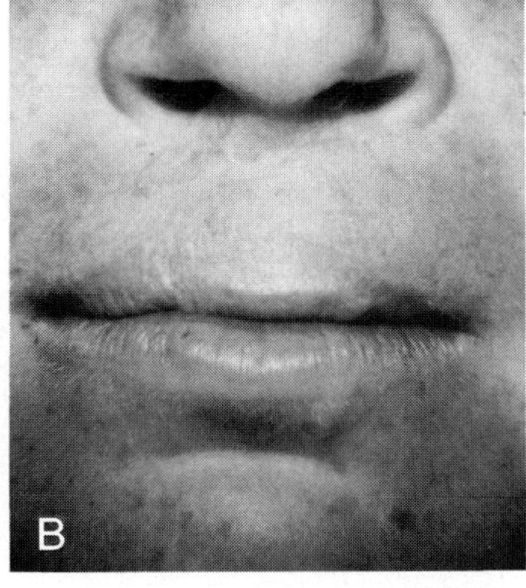

Figure 32–10 Use of a "shaved" Abbe flap for a tubercle deficiency. *A,* Central vermilion deficiency in a 6-year-old with a bilateral cleft lip. *B,* Lip 4 years after Abbe reconstruction.

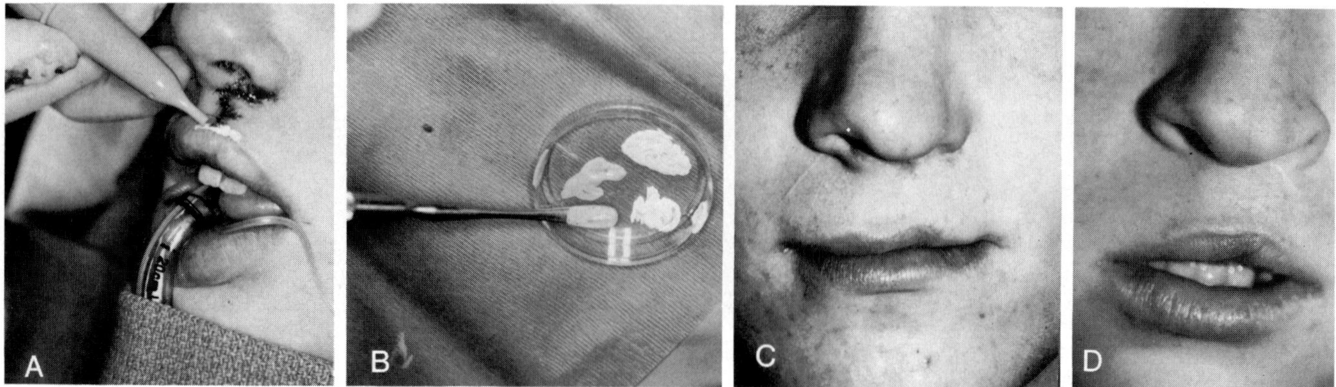

Figure 32–11 *A–D,* Use of a color-matched tattoo technique for establishment of a white roll to frame the upper lip at the suture line.

and is specifically addressed elsewhere (Chaps. 62, 63, 64, and 65). However, bony deficiencies significantly influence secondary lip deformities. Orthodontic treatment and alveolar bone grafting are significant components that influence the timing and correction of secondary lip and nasal sill deformities. Early attention to bony and dental alignment is important to carry out alveolar grafting during mixed dentition as proposed by Bergland et al.[50] Midfacial growth and normal occlusal relationships affect lip function and aesthetics; thus orthognathic evaluation and correction must be considered part of secondary lip repair (see Fig. 32–5).

Premaxillary Deformities. Management of the protruded premaxilla in the bilateral cleft is an essential antecedent to final secondary lip repair. Eppley and his associates have outlined effective surgical principles in premaxillary management.[51] These include:

1. Adequate evaluation of the deformity, including cephalometric studies and occlusal radiology, dental models, and standard photographs.
2. Presurgical dental orthopedic alignment with lateral segment expansion.
3. Delayed surgical repositioning to at least age 8.
4. Concurrent bone grafting and postoperative retention.
5. Concurrent closure of the oronasal fistula.
6. Soft tissue procedures to create an adequate vestibule.
7. Correction of orthognathic deformity at least 1 year following bone grafting.

Attention to these principles assists in the timing of secondary lip repair in the bilateral cleft patient who has an unstable, protruded premaxilla.

Dental Deformities

Concurrent integration of treatment of dental deformities by sequential dental orthopedic, prosthodontic, and fixed orthodontic care is essential for adequate secondary cleft lip repair. Surgical isolation from dental

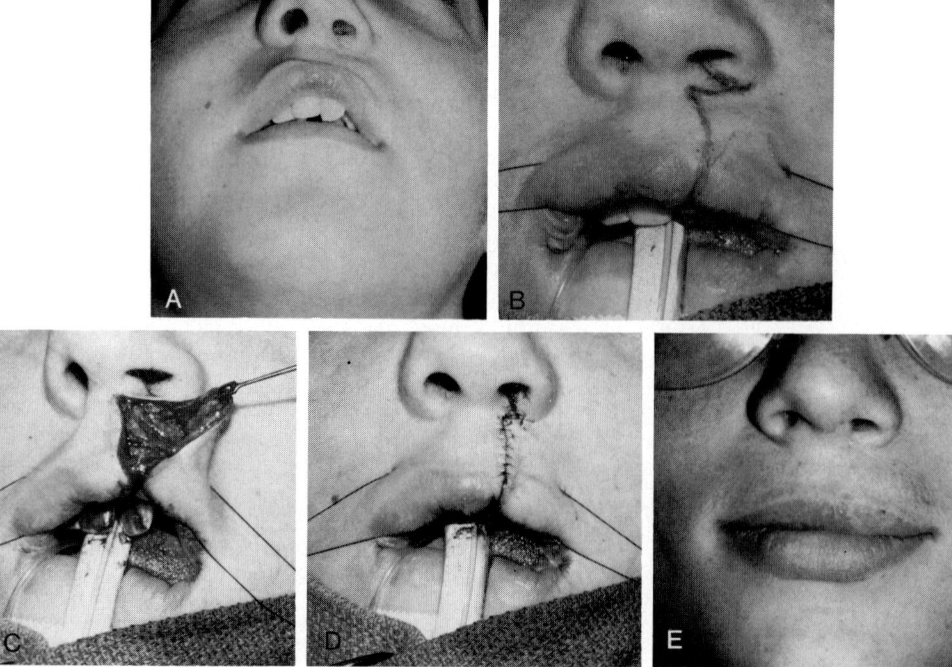

Figure 32–12 A 13-year-old white girl with muscle asymmetry. *A,* Laterally bunched muscle with inadequate soft tissue in the nasal sill and upper lip adjacent to the philtrum. *B–D,* Horizontal cutting of the orbicularis oris with vertical distraction to achieve increased vertical muscle length and reattachment of the muscle. *E,* One year after surgery.

factors generally produces inferior results and may only lead to an indication for further surgical revisions.

Conclusion

Secondary lip revision that is well planned, integrated, and executed can be gratifying for the patient and the surgeon. However, injudicious or poorly timed or executed revisions will produce disappointing results and may forever doom the correction of the deformity.

References

1. Steffensen WH: Further experience with the rectangular flap operation for cleft lip repair. Plast Reconstr Surg 11:49, 1953.
2. Farkas LG, Lindsay WK: Morphology of the adult face following repair of unilateral cleft lip and palate in childhood. Plast Reconstr Surg 52:652, 1973.
3. Amaratunga ND: A comparison of Millard and Le Mesurier's methods of repair of the complete unilateral cleft lip using a new symmetry index. J Oral Maxillofac Surg 46:353, 1988.
4. Musgrave RH: General aspects of the unilateral cleft lip repair. In Grabb WC, Rosenstein SW, Bzoch KR (eds): Cleft Lip and Palate. Boston: Little, Brown, 1971.
5. Terman LM, Merrill MA: Stanford-Binet Intelligence Scale. Boston: Houghton Mifflin, 1960.
6. Tobiasen J, Hiebert J: Children's judgments of facial disfigurement: Stigma or aesthetic? In press, 1988.
7. Tobiasen J, Hiebert J: Psychosocial adjustment to craniofacial surgery. In press, 1988.
8. Hiebert JM, Tobiasen JT: Preoperative counselling: An important adjunct in surgery for facial deformities. In preparation, 1989.
9. Trier WC: Repair of bilateral cleft lip: Millard's technique. Clin Plast Surg 12:605, 1985.
10. Thomson HG: Quadrilateral flap in the repair of unilateral cleft lip. In Grabb WC, Rosenstein SW, Bzoch KR (eds): Cleft Lip and Palate. Boston: Little, Brown, 1971.
11. Millard DR, Jr: A radical rotation in single harelip. Am J Surg 95:318, 1958.
12. Millard DR, Jr: Rotation-advancement advocated. In Cleft Craft. Vol. I. The Unilateral Deformity. Boston: Little, Brown, 1976.
13. Millard DR, Jr: Long upper lip. In Cleft Craft. Vol. II. Bilateral and Rare Deformities. Boston: Little, Brown, 1977.
14. Teale TP: On plastic operations for the restoration of the upper lip. Med Times 35:561, 1887.
15. Erich JB: Secondary deformities of the cleft lip. In Converse JM (ed): Reconstructive Plastic Surgery. Philadelphia: Saunders, 1964.
16. Vaughan HS: The importance of the premaxilla and the philtrum in bilateral cleft lip. Plast Reconstr Surg 1:240, 1946.
17. Holdsworth WG: Later treatment of complete double clefts. Br J Plast Surg 21:127, 1963.
18. Austin HW: The lip lift. Plast Reconstr Surg 77:990, 1986.
19. Gillies HD, Kilner TP: Hare-Lip: Operation for the correction of secondary deformities. Lancet 223:1369, 1932.
20. Harding RL: Secondary repair of bilateral cleft lips. In Grabb WC, Rosenstein SW, Bzoch KR (eds): Cleft Lip and Palate. Boston: Little, Brown, 1971.
21. Peterson R, Ellenberg A, Carroll D: Vermilion flap reconstruction of bilateral cleft lip deformities. Plast Reconstr Surg 38:109, 1966.
22. O'Malley J: The vermilion lip roll for bilateral cleft lip revision. Southeastern Plast Reconstr Surg Newsletter, June, 1973.
23. Millard DR, Jr: A switch then a fork. In Cleft Craft. Vol. II. Bilateral and Rare Deformities. Boston: Little, Brown, 1977.
24. Anizuka J, Hesoka L, Sumiyo N: Aesthetic camouflage of bilateral cleft lip scars. Aesth Plast Surg 11:241, 1987.
25. Wynn SK: Correction of the secondary cleft lip and nasal deformities. In Georgiade NG, Hagerty RF (eds): Symposium on Management of Cleft Lip and Palate and Associated Deformities. St. Louis: Mosby, 1974.
26. Webster JP: Crecentric peri-alar cheek excision for upper lip flap advancement with a short history of upper lip repair. Plast Reconstr Surg 16:434, 1955.
27. Kai S, Ohishi M: Secondary correction of the cleft lip and nose deformity: A new technique for revision of whistling deformity. Cleft Palate J 22:290, 1985.
28. Gillies HD, Millard DR, Jr: The Principles and Art of Plastic Surgery. Boston: Little, Brown, 1957.
29. Abbe R: A new plastic operation for the relief of deformity due to double harelip. Med Rec 53:477, 1898.
30. Sabattini P: Cenno Storics Dell'Origine e Progressa della Rinoplastica e cheiloplastica Sequinto dalla Descrizione de Queste Operazioni Sopra un Solo Individuo. Bologna: Bell'Arti, 1838.
31. Stein SAY: Laebedannelse (cheiloplasty) udfort paa en ny methode. Hospitals-meddelelser 1:212, 1848.
32. Estlander JA: En ny Operation Metod att Alerslalla en Forstand lapp Ellerkind. Fenska Lak Handl 14:1, 1872.
33. Smith JW: The anatomic and physiologic acclimatization of tissue transplanted by the lip switch technique. Plast Reconstr Surg 26:40, 1960.
34. McGregor IA: The Abbe flap: Its use in single and double lip clefts. Br J Plast Surg 16:46, 1963.
35. Peet EW, Patterson TJS: The Essentials of Plastic Surgery. Oxford: Blackwell, 1963.
36. Cannon B, Murray J: Further observations on the use of the split vermilion border flap. Plast Reconstr Surg 11:497, 1953.
37. Esser JFS: Studies in plastic surgery of the face. Plastic operations about the mouth. The epidermis enlay. Ann Surg 65:297, 1917.
38. Cosman B, Crikelair GF: Release of the prolabium in the bilateral cleft lip. Cleft Palate J 3:122, 1966.
39. von Reilen AW: Some aspects in the secondary repair of cleft lip, palate and nasal deformities with case report. Plast Reconstr Surg 10:460, 1952.
40. Falcone AE: Release of adherent prolabium and deepening of labial sulcus in the secondary repair of bilateral cleft lips. Plast Reconstr Surg 38:42, 1966.
41. Horton CE, Adamson JE, Mladick RA, et al: The upper lip sulcus in cleft lips. Plast Reconstr Surg 45:31, 1970.
42. Duffey MM: Restoration of the orbicularis oris muscle continuity in the repair of the bilateral cleft lip. Br J Plat Surg 24:48, 1970.
43. Randall P, Whitaker LA, LaRossa D: The importance of muscle reconstruction in primary and secondary cleft lip repair. Plast Reconstr Surg 54:316, 1974.
44. Robinson DW, Ketchum LD, Masters FW: Double V-Y procedure for whistling deformity in repaired cleft. Plast Reconstr Surg 46:241, 1970.
45. Pucket RL, Reinisch JF, Weiner RS: Late correction of orbicularis discontinuity in bilateral clefts of the lip. Cleft Palate J 17:1, 1980.
46. Millard DR, Jr: White roll free grafts. In Cleft Craft. Vol. I. The Unilateral Deformity. Boston: Little, Brown, 1976.
47. Hiebert JM, Canady J: Tattoo correction of the discontinuous white roll deformity in secondary cleft lip. In press, 1989.
48. Broadbent TR: The badly scarred bilateral cleft lip: Total resurfacing. Plast Reconstr Surg 20:485, 1957.
49. Kapetansky DI: Animation and cosmetic balance in repair of bilateral cleft lip: A modified technique. Cleft Palate J 11:219, 1974.
50. Bergland O, Semb G, et al: Secondary bone grafting and orthodontic treatment in patients with bilateral complete clefts of the lip and palate. Ann Plast Surg 17:460, 1986.
51. Eppley BL, Sclaroff A, Delfino JJ: Secondary management of the premaxilla in bilateral cleft lip and palate patients. J Oral Maxillofac Surg 44:987, 1986.

CHAPTER 33

Correction of Secondary Unilateral and Bilateral Nasal Deformities: Cronin Technique

Thomas D. Cronin, Keith A. Denkler, and Ernest D. Cronin

Anatomy

Although the degree of nasal deformity associated with cleft lip is variable, it is always present. The major deformity consists of a malposition of the lower lateral cartilage on the cleft side. The cartilage on the other side is usually normal. The involved cartilage is displaced posteriorly, laterally, and inferiorly (Fig. 33–1A). The nose is longer on the affected side, and the caudal septum is tilted toward the normal side. The lateral crus on the affected side is flattened or buckled. The alar base is attached too far laterally but also may be too high or too low. There may be a deficiency in the maxilla as evidenced by a depression of the alar base.

Timing of Correction

In our opinion, the optimal time for correction of the cleft lip nasal deformity is the teenage period when the cartilages have developed and are more easily and safely molded during surgery.[1–22] When the nasal deformity has been especially severe, the senior author has carried out corrective surgery as early as 4 to 10 years of age, but the surgery is more difficult because the cartilages are more pliable.[23–26] Although some authors advocate repair of the nose at the time of lip repair, we do not recommend this because of the small and delicate nature of the infant's cartilage.[27–37]

Treatment

In our opinion, the logical treatment is to restore the involved lower lateral cartilage to its normal position in relation to the opposite lower lateral cartilage. This can best be done by an open operation with adequate exposure of the domes.[38]

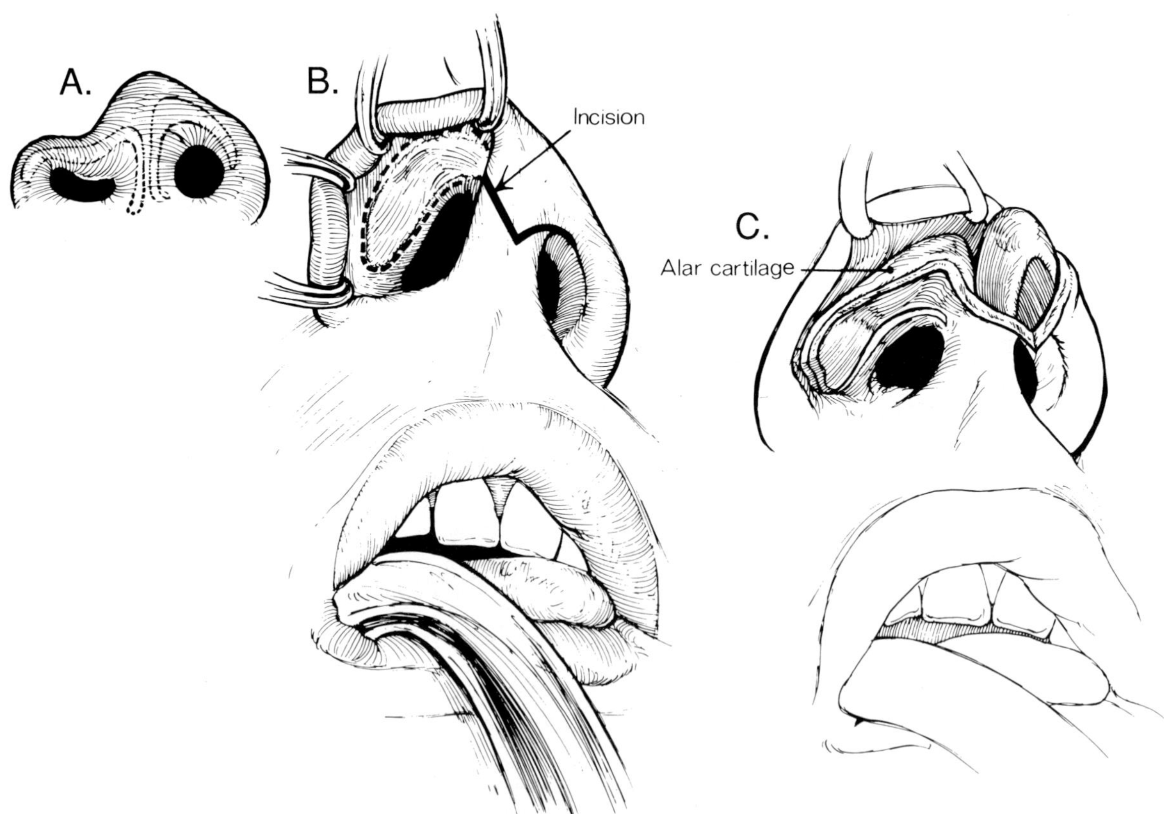

Figure 33–1 *A,* A phantom view of the lower lateral cartilages showing displacement posteriorly, laterally, and inferiorly with flattening of the ala. *B,* The flying-bird incision. The V skin incision should be made in the midcolumella. On the normal side the incision continues just inside the vestibulum sufficiently to elevate the skin over the tip. On the cleft side the ala is everted with a double hook, and the vestibular incision closely follows completely around the margin of the lower lateral cartilage, leaving the mucosa lining attached to it.

C, The skin flap over the tip is turned back, exposing the alar domes. The loose fat and connective tissue is trimmed off the domes. The lower lateral cartilage is dissected up completely to its junction with the medial crus.

Technique

A so-called transcolumella, "flying-bird" incision (Fig. 33–1*B*), or perhaps taking up the entire length of the columella (Fig. 33–2) as a skin flap, gives excellent exposure.[39] The incisions are continued as vestibular incisions just inside the nostril margins to permit the skin to be dissected over the tip, exposing the domes of the cartilages. The loose fat and connective tissue are cleared off the domes (Fig. 33–1*C*). Then the alar margin on the cleft side is everted with a double hook, and the vestibular incision is continued laterally along the border of the lower lateral cartilage, which is easily visible (Fig. 33–1*B*). This incision is continued all the way around the entire length of the cartilage and then up between the lower and upper lateral cartilages, staying close to the lower cartilage. The mucosal lining is left attached to the cartilage as it is dissected free of the overlying skin up to the tip, thereby saving time and the blood supply and ensuring the safety of the cartilage in case cross-hatching should be required.

The cartilage can now be lifted outward, with hooks or forceps, and folded on itself to form a new dome at a more forward position, slightly overcorrecting the deformity. Partial-thickness cross-hatches (Fig. 33–1*E* and *F*) are made if necessary to better shape the new dome. The two domes are sutured together with 5–0 nonabsorbable suture (Fig. 33–1*F*). Great care should be taken to see that this new position of the cartilages provides the proper correction when the skin is replaced over the tip. If they are not properly positioned, the sutures should be removed and replaced (Fig. 33–3).

To correct the excessive length of the nose on the affected side, trimming of the cephalad edge of the

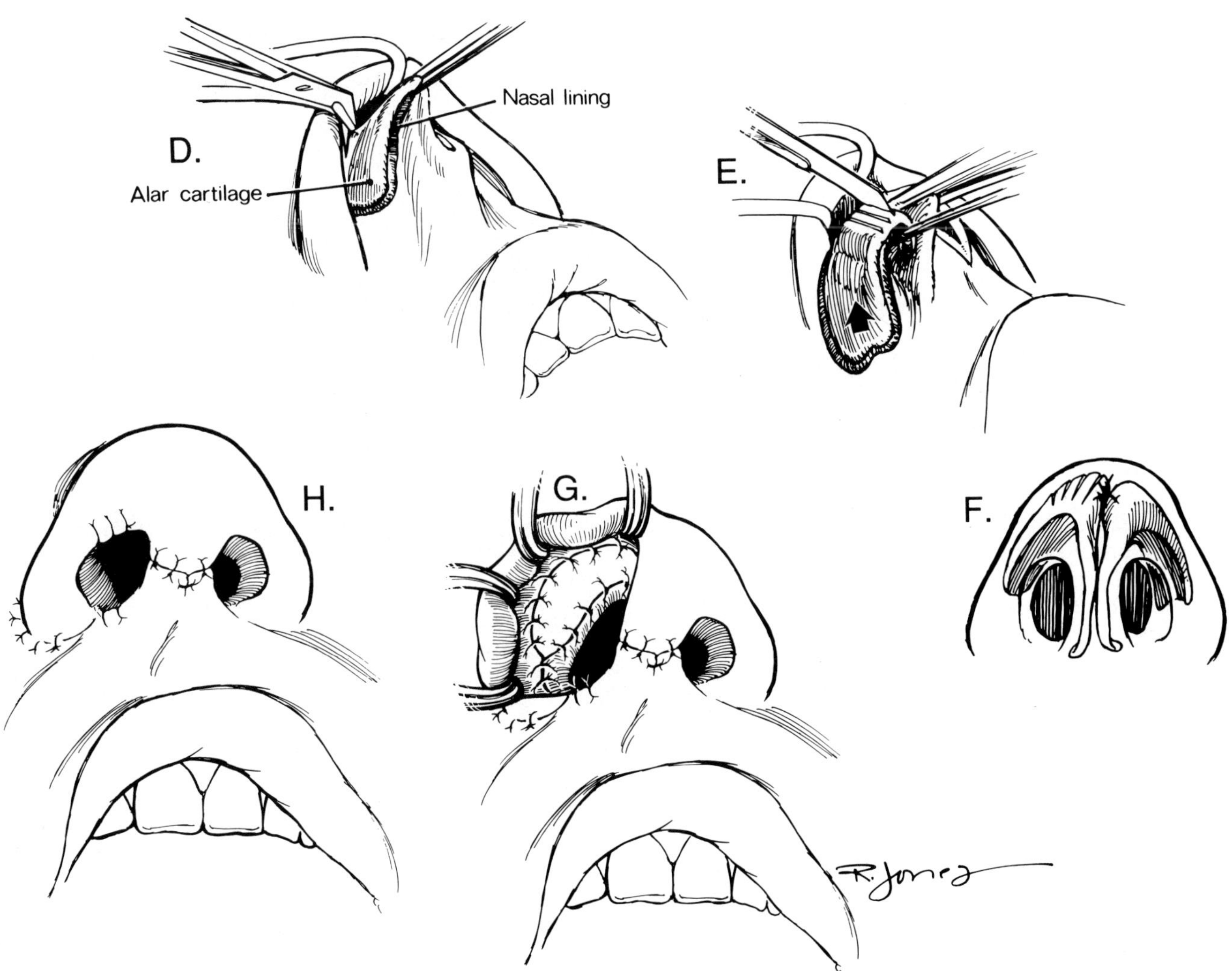

Figure 33–1 *Continued D*, The lower lateral cartilage can now be lifted and folded on itself, forming a new dome in a slightly overcorrected position adjacent to the normal dome. *E*, Several partial-thickness crosshatch incisions are made to facilitate a gentle flexing of the cartilage to form a natural dome. *F*, The lateral crus has been advanced in slight overcorrection and sutured to the adjacent cartilages. The medial crus is lengthened by the advancement.

G, V-Y closure of the defect left in the mucosa after advancement of the lateral crus. Note that the V-columellar incision has been closed with a small V-Y advancement. Also note the sutures of the alar base, indicating that an adjustment has been made here. *H*, Excess tissue has been trimmed from the nostril. The position of the alar base has been improved. (*A–H* from Cronin TD, Denkler K: Correction of the unilateral cleft lip nose. Plast Reconstr Surg 82(3):419–432, 1988. With permission.)

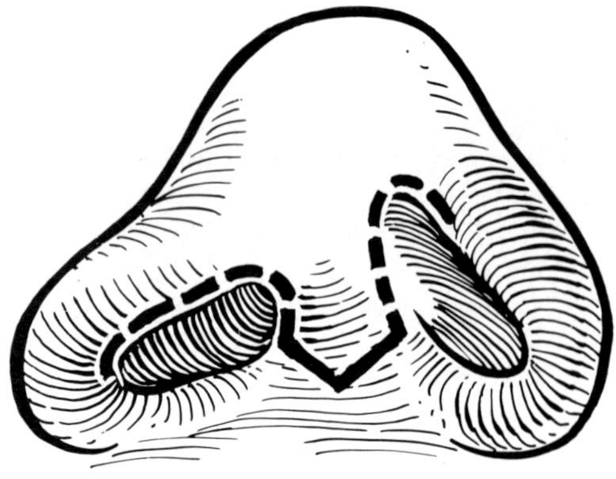

Figure 33–2 Potter (1954) turned up the entire length of the columella to give extensive exposure of the nasal tip.

lower lateral cartilage is done as needed. Any excess skin over the nostril margin also may be trimmed. Advancement of the lower lateral cartilage usually corrects the tip very well in about 80% of cases. The other 20% of patients may need a slight build-up with a cartilage graft. This may be done primarily or it may be done secondarily if the need arises, using septum or contralateral alar cartilage.

Closure of the mucosal defect left by advancement of the lower lateral crus is accomplished by a **V-Y** plasty of the mucosa (Fig. 33–1G) using 4–0 plain catgut, but fine silk is used on the exposed skin. Skin grafts are not needed because there is plenty of mucosa for closure.

Other rhinoplastic procedures, including septoplasty, osteotomies, hump removal, and trimming of the lower lateral cartilages are done as needed.

A small **V-Y** advancement may be gained in the columella (Fig. 33–1G). Frequently the alar base is moved to match the other side (Fig. 33–1H). If the alar base is depressed owing to deficiency of the maxillary segment, the area may be built up with bone, cartilage, or Proplast.

An unsightly scar of the lip requires revision also.

Results

The charts of 53 unilateral cleft lip nasal repairs performed by the senior author since 1950 using this technique were reviewed. Forty-five patients required only one operation to correct their cleft lip nose. Eight patients required a revision of the tip with placement of a cartilage graft over the cleft lateral crus. The opposite lower lateral cartilage or septum served as the donor site. Of these 53 patients, 42 required adjustment of the alar base position. When the alar base was depressed owing to deficiency of the maxillary bone, the area was augmented with cartilage in five patients, bone in three patients, and Proplast in two patients. A Le Fort I advancement procedure corrected the defi-

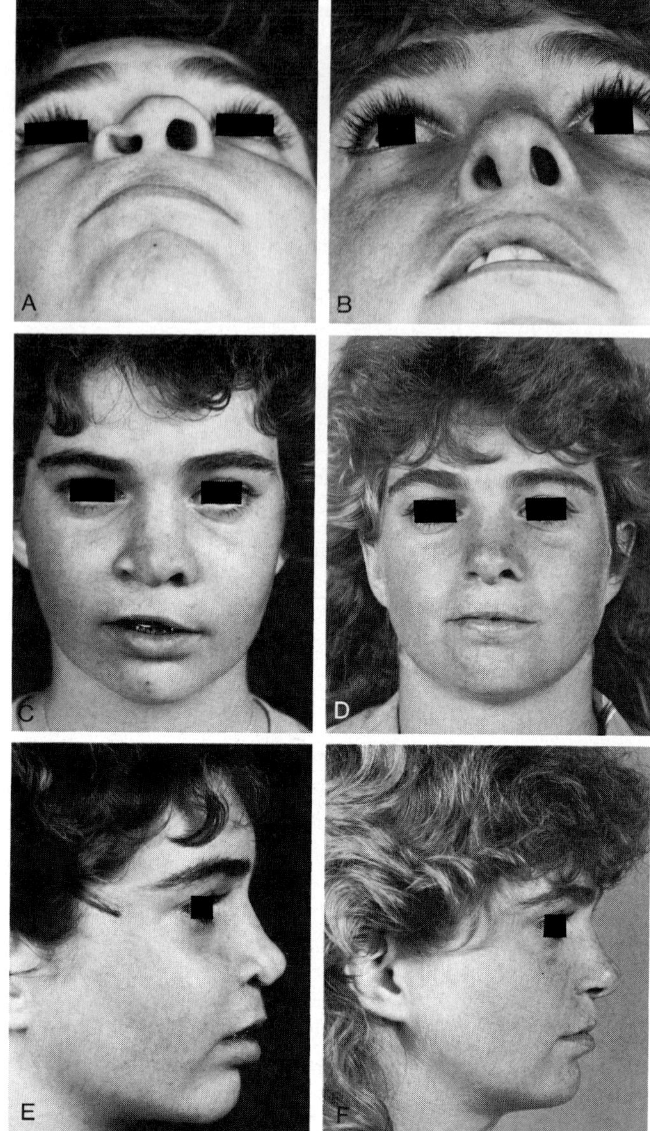

Figure 33–3 This 16-year-old was born with a wide unilateral cleft lip and palate. The lip was repaired at age 2 months. A pushback palate repair was done at the age of 21 months. The patient showed retrusion of the maxilla. A Le Fort I procedure was done at age 16 years. This actually made the nasal deformity worse.

A, The marked flattening of the right ala is apparent. *B,* Correction is obtained by advancing the lower lateral alar cartilage to the tip of the nose and suturing it to the opposite dome. *C* and *E,* Front and lateral views showing the depressed right ala. *D* and *F,* The correction 5½ years after surgery. (*A–F* from Cronin TD, Denkler K: Correction of the unilateral cleft lip nose. Plast Reconstr Surg 82(3):419–432, 1988. With permission.)

ciency in four patients. Twenty-eight patients required a submucous resection or septoplasty.

The results in all teenage or older patients were considered satisfactory, as demonstrated by the before and after pictures. When the cleft lip nasal deformity is photographed, at least three views are required, the most important being the view showing the head tilted back. Next is the lateral view of the affected side and then the front view (Figs. 33–4 and 33–5).

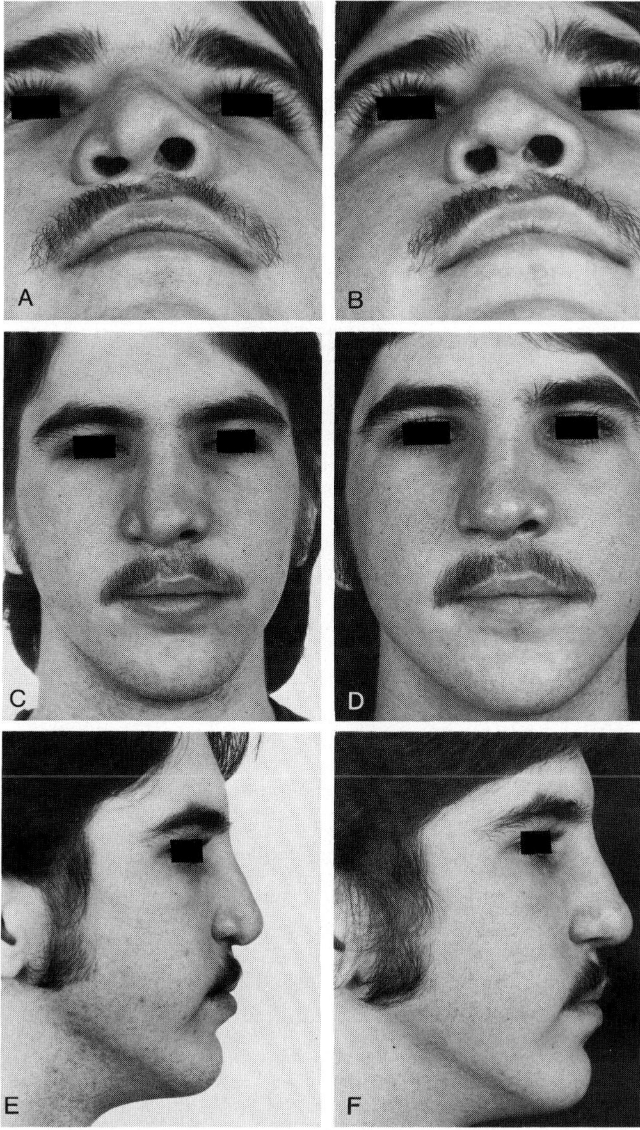

Figure 33–4 *A,* A 16-year-old boy with a typical unilateral cleft lip nasal deformity. *B,* Appearance 6 weeks after correction. *C,* Front view showing the flattened ala and increased length of nose on the right side. *D,* The improved appearance after surgery. *E,* The short ala and flattened tip are visible from the side. *F,* The improved appearance after surgery. (*A–F* from Cronin TD, Denkler K: Correction of the unilateral cleft lip nose. Plast Reconstr Surg 82(3):419–432, 1988. With permission.)

Cronin Bilateral Technique

Timing and Anatomy

We believe that the surgeon should not attempt to correct the nasal deformity of a short columella during the initial repair of the lip because of the small and delicate nature of the alar cartilages and in spite of reports of success with primary repair.[40, 41] We prefer to lengthen the columella when the child is about school age or even later, after the nose has further grown and developed. However, in the initial primary repair of the bilateral cleft lip, one should preserve as much colu-

mellar skin as possible. The nasal floor should be left somewhat wide and no excess tissue discarded because this will later be used in columellar lengthening.

The underlying anatomic problems in a patient with a secondary bilateral cleft lip nose include a short columella, depressed nasal tip, bilateral dislocation of the alar cartilages off the crest of the septum, an obtuse mediolateral crural angle, and a flatness of the nasal tip with a web of skin at the alar rim.[42]

Technique

A peaked incision is made with its apex at a point just above the columellar base (Fig. 33–6*A* and *B*). From there, the incision sweeps down on each side between

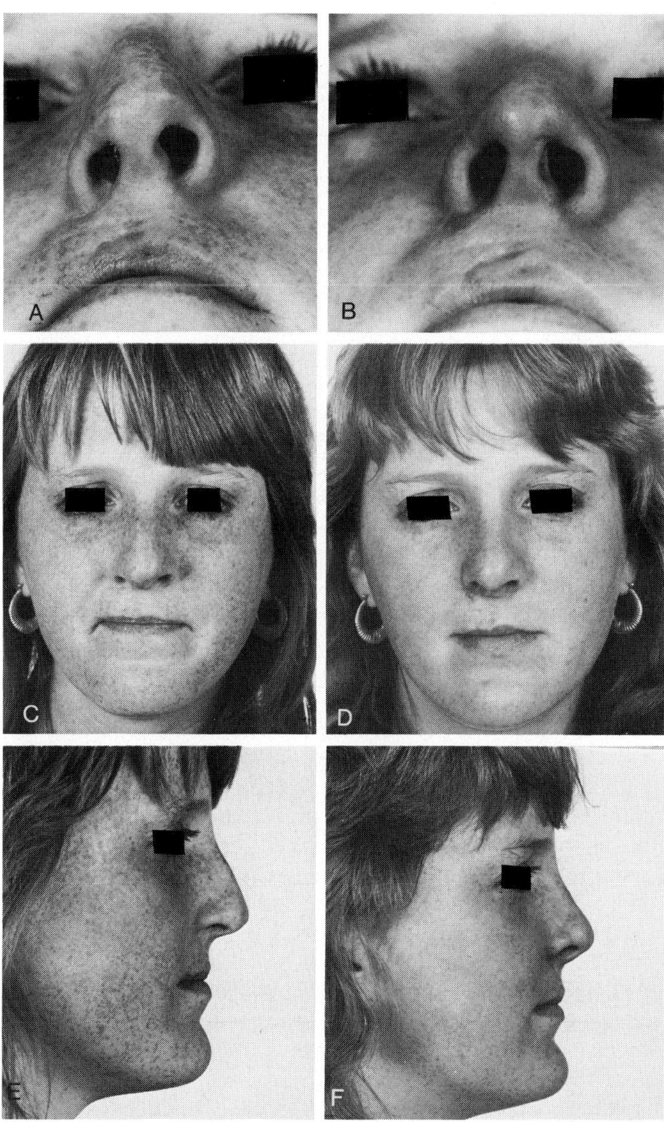

Figure 33–5 *A,* A 16-year-old girl with a unilateral cleft lip nasal deformity. *B,* Note the improved symmetry 10 weeks post surgery. *C,* Mild deformity as viewed from the front. *D,* Appearance after surgery. *E,* Preoperative appearance. *F,* Note that a bone hump was removed in addition to correction of the cleft deformity. (*A–F* from Cronin TD, Denkler K: Correction of the unilateral cleft lip nose. Plast Reconstr Surg 82(3):419–432, 1988. With permission.)

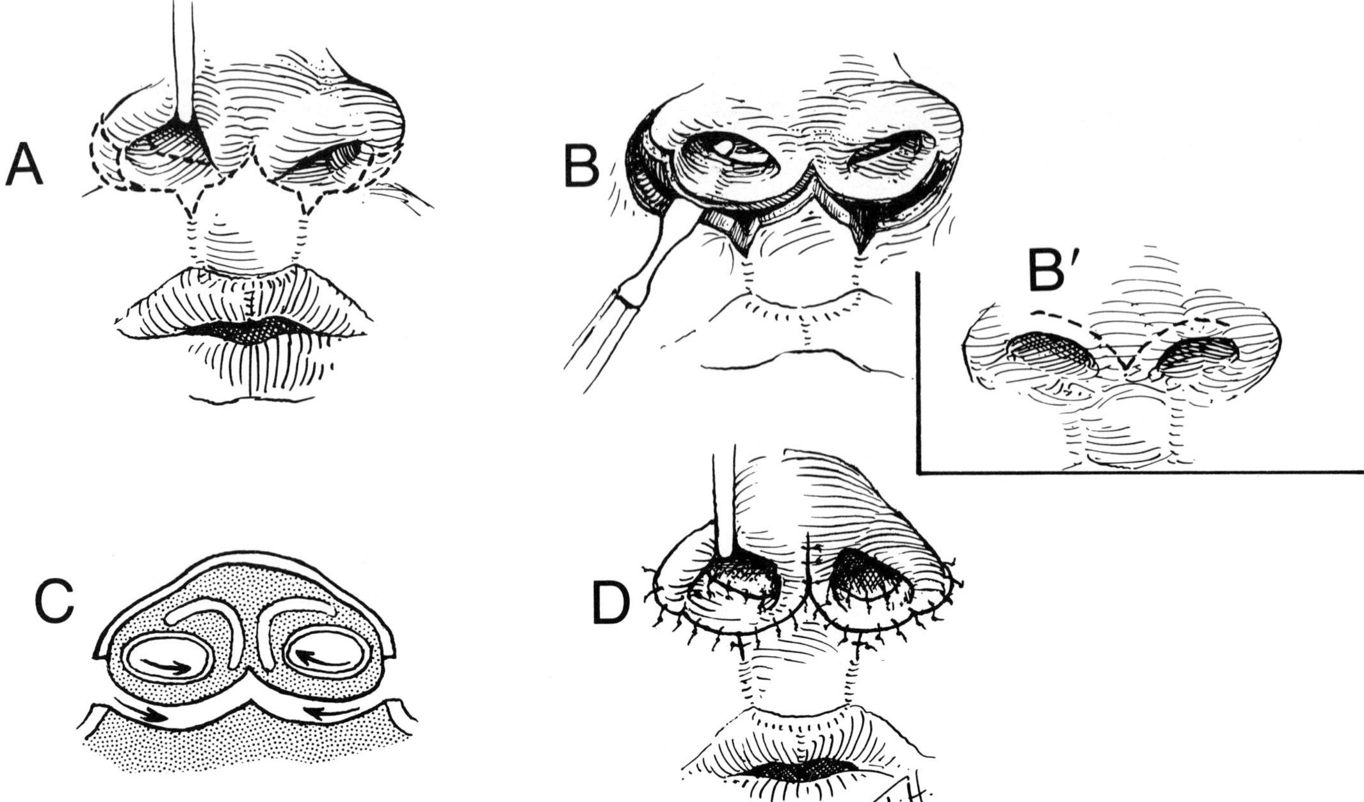

Figure 33–6 Cronin method of columellar lengthening. *A*, Incisions create the bipedicle flaps and half-thickness alar wedge excisions and V excisions in scars of the upper lip. *B*, The flap in the vestibular floor is undermined down to the nasal spine medially. *C*, Cross section of flaps. Arrows indicate the direction of the rotation toward the nasal tip. *D*, After advancement and closure. *A flying-bird incision may be added (B′) for better exposure to suture alar cartilages together.* (*A–D from Cronin TD, Upton J: Lengthening of the short columella associated with bilateral cleft lip. Ann Plast Surg 1(1):75, 1978. With permission.*)

the nasal floor and the lip around the base of the ala. An excessively long alar length may be taken up by removing a half-thickness wedge of their width at the base of the ala (Fig. 33–6A–D). This also gives further columellar advancement. Another incision is made inside the nose, freeing the columella from the septum to produce bipedicle flaps that are somewhat wider laterally than medially (Fig. 33–6B). This makes the base of the lengthened columella pyramidal and prevents a retracted appearance, which might result from narrow flaps. The flaps should contain sufficient subcutaneous tissue to ensure good circulation and bulk to form the columella. When the flaps have been freely mobilized (Fig. 33–6C and D), the tip of the nose is lifted forward with a double skin hook placed in the apices of each nostril. If any tightness remains, the flaps are undermined further laterally. The flaps are sutured together in the midline for a sufficient distance to give the desired increase in length (Fig. 33–6D).

If the tip is too broad, a flying-bird incision may be made to expose the domes (Fig. 33–7). The alar cartilages with their mucosal lining attached are freed up slightly and sutured together at their domes (Fig. 33–7D). Extensive freeing up of the alar cartilages with a V-Y plasty, as in the unilateral deformity, is not needed. Occasionally, a conchal cartilage graft acting as a strut

is required to provide additional projection, but a cartilage graft over the lateral crus, which is sometimes required in the unilateral deformity, is not needed (Fig. 33–8).

The problem of the wide, thick, and flared ala may be solved by several methods. Often the excess width of the alar base is corrected through advancement of the columella. Excess skin of the lip may be taken up by careful skin closure. If not, a small triangle may be excised in conjunction with the lip scars (Fig. 33–7A). An excessively long alar length may be taken up by removal of a half-thickness wedge of their width at the base of the ala, as described earlier (Fig. 33–6A–D). The senior author has described a Z-plasty technique, one arm being the ala and the other the floor of the nostril (Fig. 33–8A–C). This permits narrowing of the alar base without disturbing the lip if the scars do not need revision. This can be done only as a secondary procedure to columellar advancement, because otherwise the bipedicle flap would be cut. Occasionally the columella may require the additional support of conchal ear cartilage struts (Fig. 33–8B,D,E).[43–45]

Lesser variations in the overall technique may be used. In some instances, the inner incision detaching the columella from the septum may not be necessary. When the lip is unduly long vertically, the lip may be

Text continued on page 273

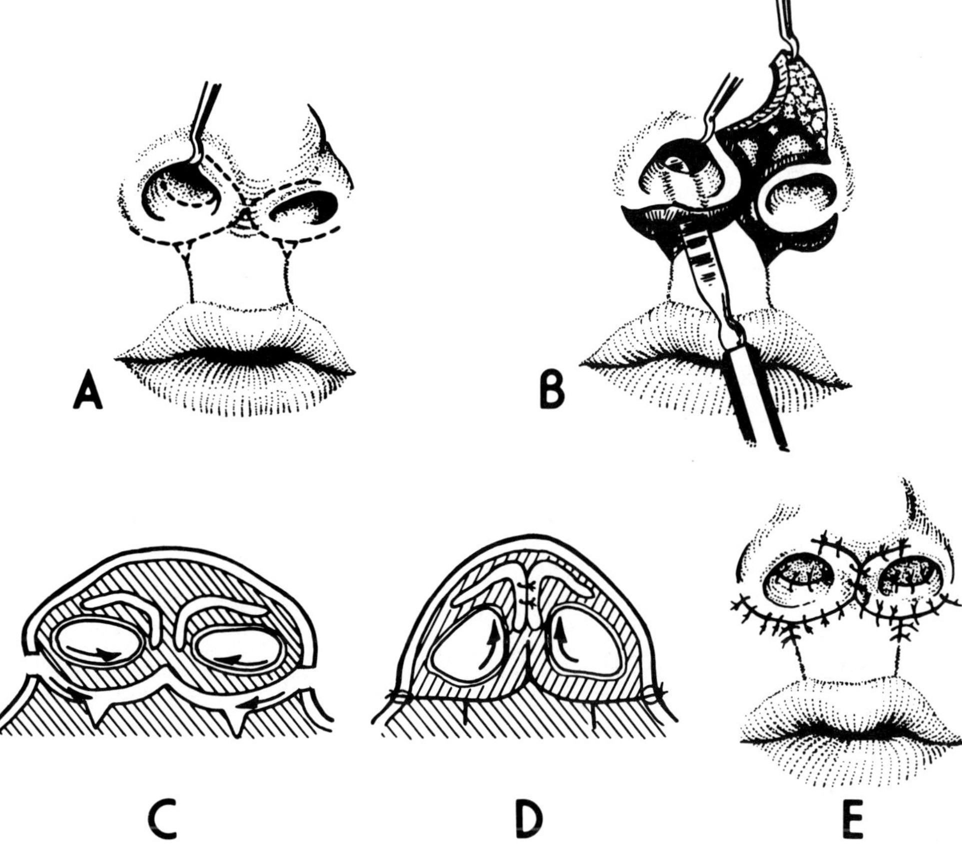

Figure 33–7 Technique of lengthening the short columella associated with bilateral cleft lip. *A*, Outline of incisions. Alar wedges may be excised to narrow the nose. The ala is elevated to show the incision, which separates the columella from the lower edge of the septum. It extends posterolaterally across the nasal floor and facilitates alar rotation. *B*, Elevation of bipedicle flap in the nasal floor. The alar domes have been exposed to allow suturing together. *C* and *D*, Cross section of nose, which illustrates alar rotation to lengthen columella. Half-wedge alar base resections are pictured. *E*, The operation completed. (*A–E* from Cronin TD: Management of the bilateral cleft lip and palate and nose. In Brent B (ed): The Artistry of Reconstructive Surgery. St. Louis: CV Mosby, 1987. With permission.)

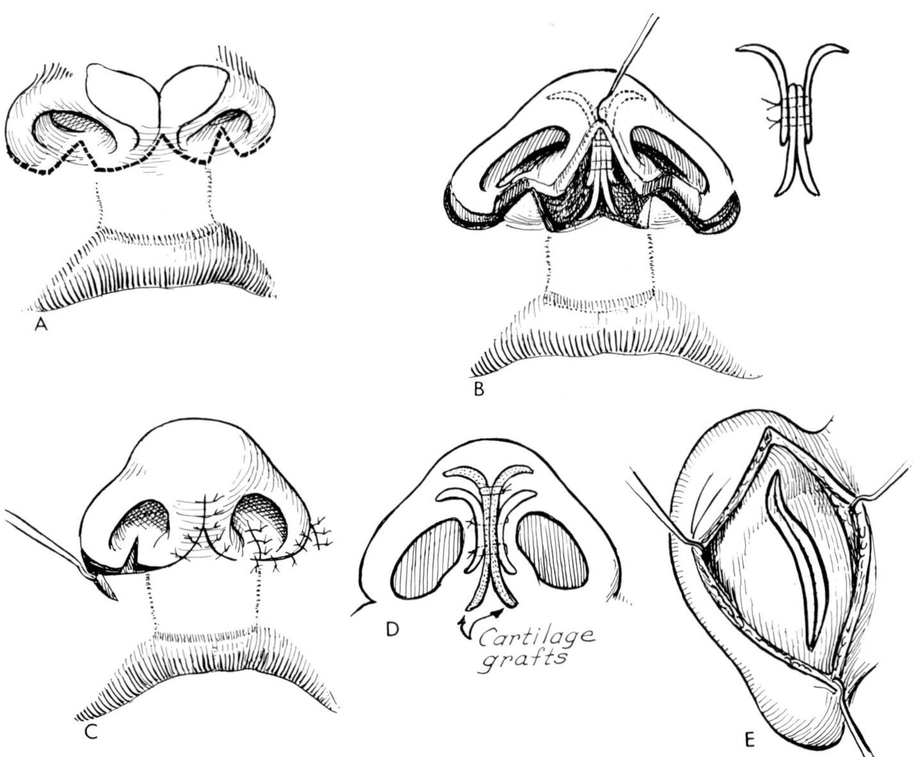

Figure 33–8 Variations of technique in columellar lengthening (Cronin). *A*, A Z-plasty, one arm being the ala and the other the floor of the nostril, permits narrowing of the alar base without disturbing the lip, if the scars do not need revision. *B*, Two pieces of ear cartilage sutured back to back to lengthen the medial crura. *C*, Closure of the wound and completion of the Z-plasty. *D*, Use of a longer piece of ear cartilage when the alar cartilages are delicate and more support is required for the tip. *E*, Technique of removal of an elliptical piece of cartilage from the concha of the ear. Septal cartilage may be used in preference to the ear cartilage. It is a little stiffer. (*A–E* from Cronin TD: The bilateral cleft lip with bilateral cleft of the primary palate. In Converse JM (ed): Reconstructive Plastic Surgery. The Head and Neck. Philadelphia: WB Saunders, 1977. With permission.)

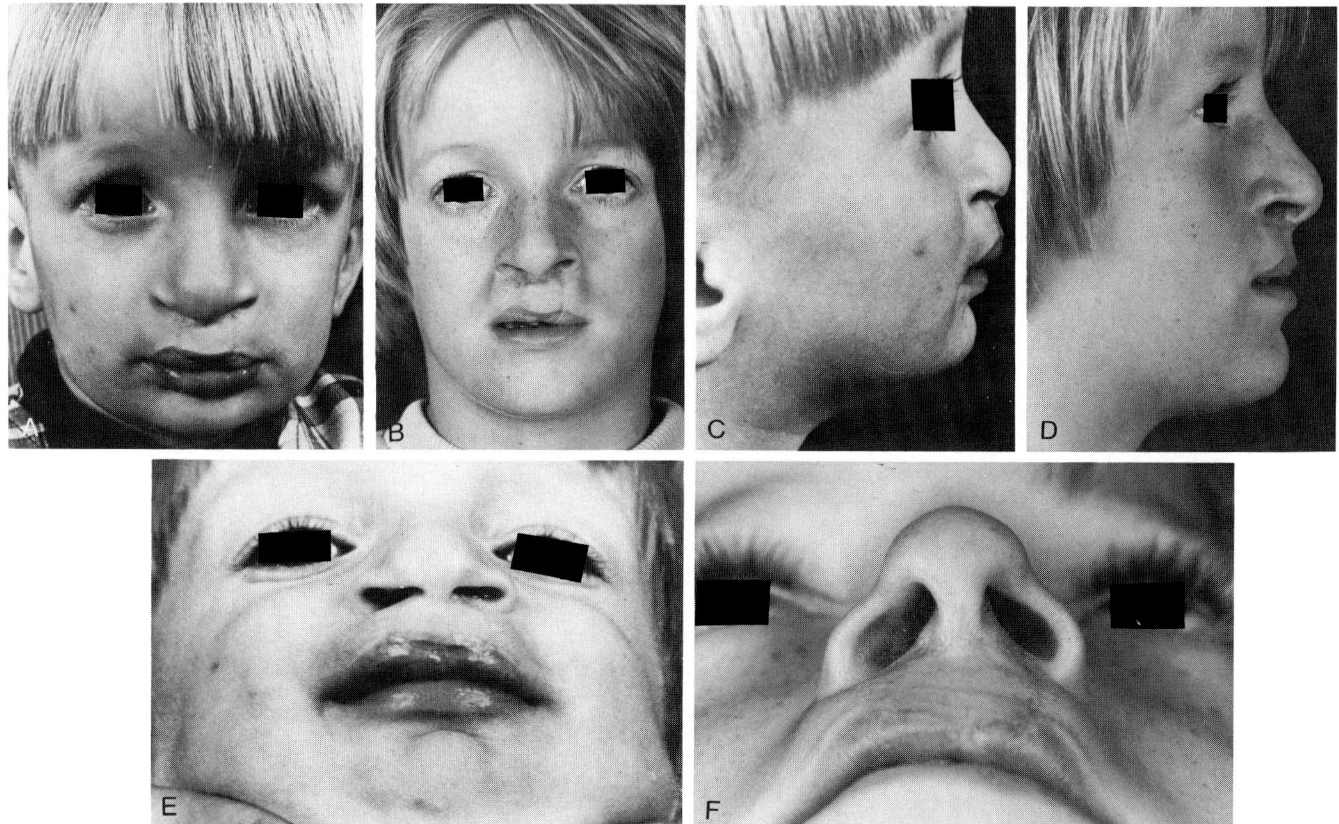

Figure 33–9 *A, C, E,* A 2-year-old boy after repair of cleft of the lip and palate. He demonstrates the typical short columella. *B, D, F,* Patient is shown at age 9, 1 year after columella was lengthened. In addition to the procedure described in the text, the cephalic portion of the alar cartilage was excised and then sutured on top of the remaining cartilage of the dome for additional projection of the tip. The domes were sutured together also.

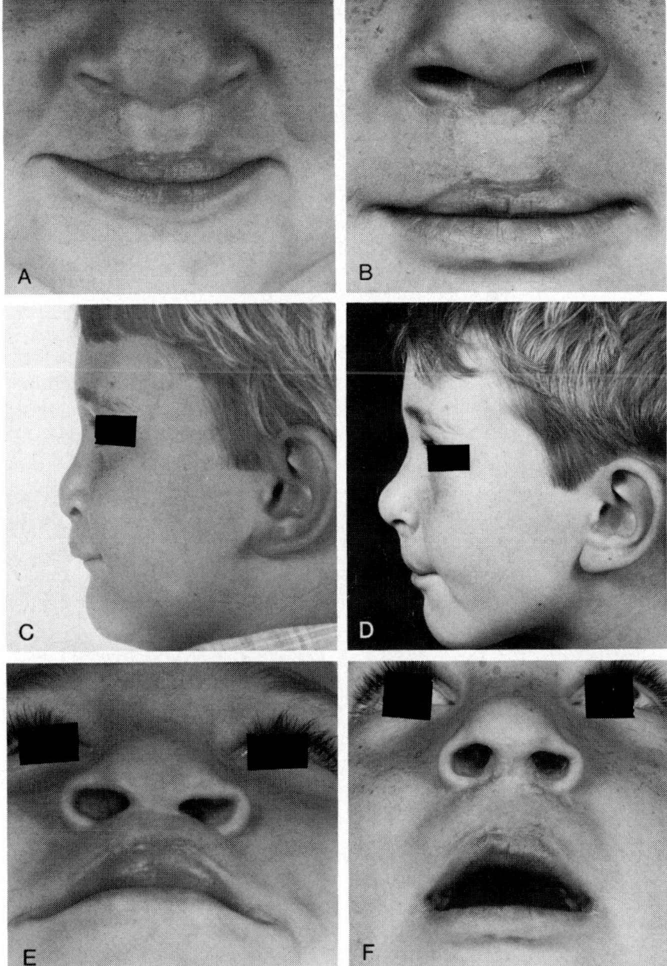

Figure 33–10 *A, C, E,* Preoperative condition at 3 years of age after repair of complete bilateral cleft of the lip and palate. Columella lengthening was done at age 4½. *B, D, F,* Patient is shown 2 years after the columella lengthening procedure combined with suturing of the domes in the midline.

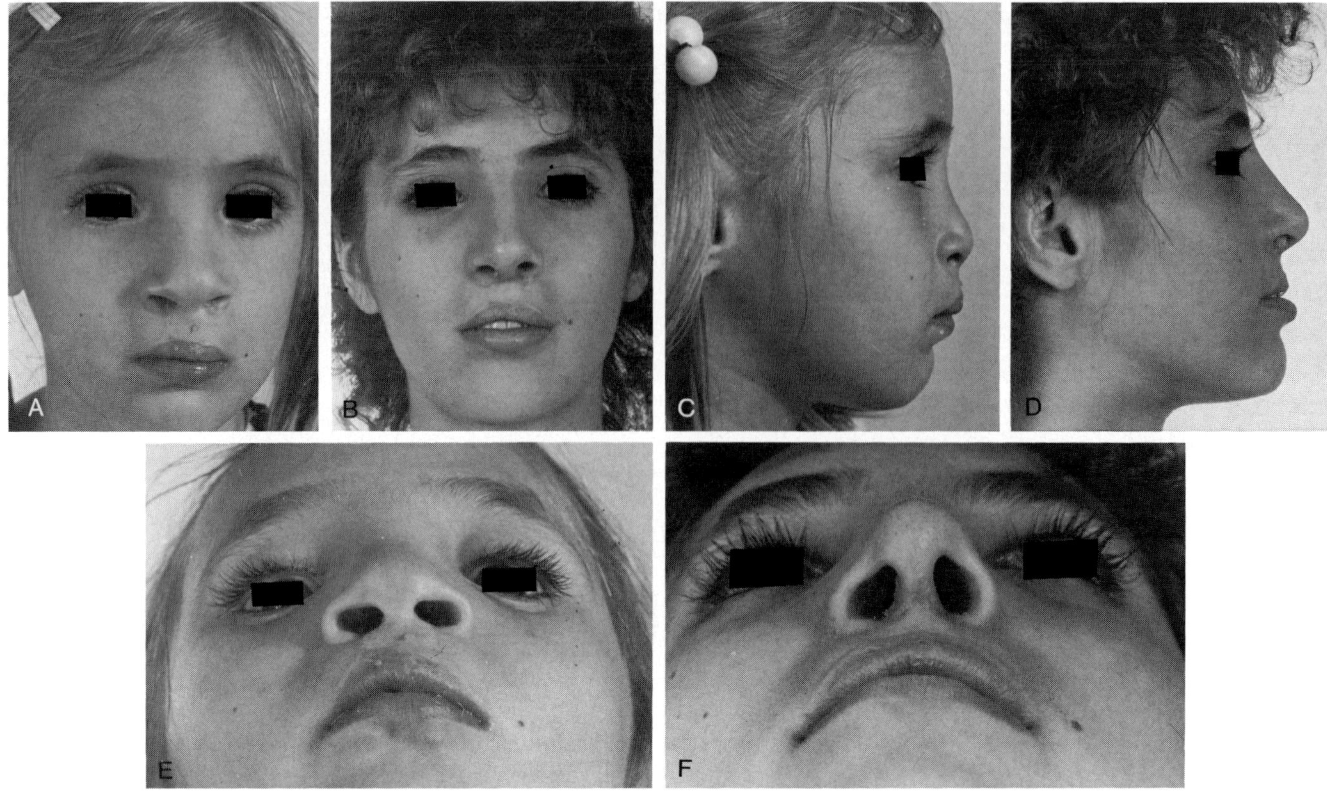

Figure 33–11 *A, C, E,* Four-year-old girl with repaired bilateral cleft of the lip and palate. *B, D, F,* The Cronin columella lengthening procedure was done at age 4, and the alar cartilages were sutured in the midline to obtain greater projection and narrowing of the tip. Also a rhinoplasty was done at age 16, which included a septal cartilage graft placed in a subcutaneous pocket at the nasal tip. The patient is shown at age 16.

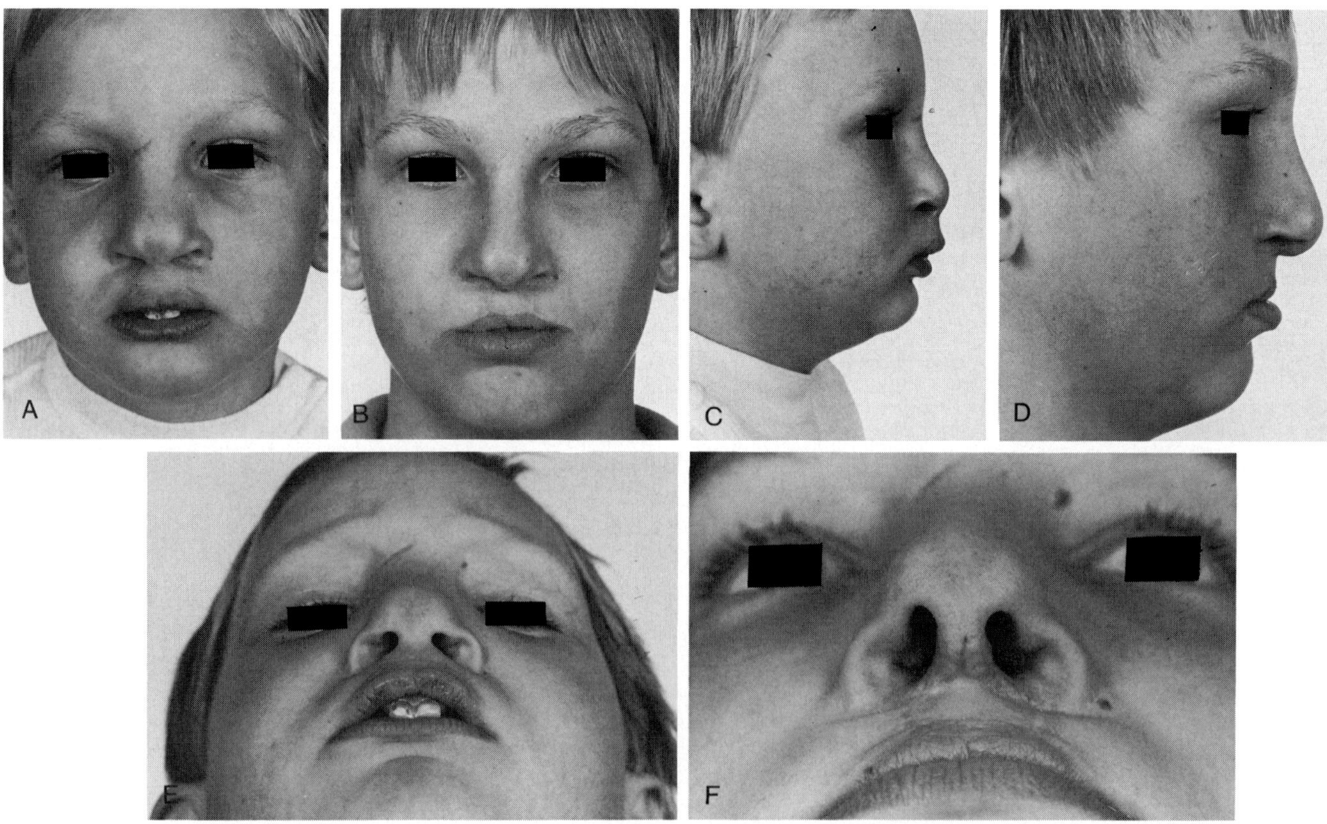

Figure 33–12 *A, C, E,* Preoperative condition after repair of complete bilateral cleft of the lip and palate. The boy had the columella lengthening procedure at age 3½. The alar bases were sutured to the periosteum of the piriform aperture. *B, D, F,* Patient is shown at age 14, 10 years postoperatively. He later had an Abbe flap procedure because of discrepancy between the upper and lower lip.

shortened by taking horizontal flaps from immediately below the nostril (rather than from the nostril floor) and advancing this tissue to lengthen the columella. Maxillary advancement (Le Fort I) or grafts of bone, cartilage, Proplast, or hydroxyapatite may be necessary to achieve more forward projection of the nose and lip.

Results

Approximately 100 patients have undergone this technique since 1950. Most have required only one procedure, but 10% to 15% have needed further columellar lengthening. This technique may be repeated once or, rarely, twice. The technique of Brauer and Forrester as a secondary procedure complements the Cronin columellar advancement, especially if there is excess skin in the area of the domes.[46] However, their technique may tend to produce a hanging columella, which may need revision at a later date.

Overall results with our technique have been good, and several sample patients are shown (Figs. 33–9 to 33–12).[47]

References

1. Gillies HD, Kilner TP: Harelip: Operation for the correction of secondary deformities. Lancet 2:1369, 1932.
2. Figi FA: The repair of secondary cleft lip and nasal deformity. J Int Coll Surg 17:297, 1952.
3. McIndoe AH, Rees T: Synchronous repair of secondary deformities in cleft lip and nose. Plast Reconstr Surg 24:150, 1959.
4. Musgrave R: Surgery of nasal deformities associated with cleft lip. Plast Reconstr Surg 28:261, 1961.
5. Stenstrom SJ, Oberg TRH: The nasal deformity in unilateral cleft lip. Plast Reconstr Surg 28:295, 1961.
6. Merville L: Asymetrie narinaire du bec-de-lievre unilateral. Rev Stomatol 63:392, 1962.
7. Farrior RT: The problem of the unilateral cleft lip-nose. A composite operation for revision of the secondary deformity. Laryngoscope 72:289, 1962.
8. Marcks KM, Trevaskis AE, Berg EM, et al: Nasal defects associated with cleft lip deformity. Plast Reconstr Surg 34:176, 1964.
9. Rees TD, Guy CL, Converse JM: Repair of the cleft lip nose: Addendum to the synchronous technique with full-thickness skin grafting of the nasal vestibule. Plast Reconstr Surg 37:47, 1966.
10. Stenstrom SJ: The alar cartilage and the nasal deformity in unilateral cleft lip. Plast Reconstr Surg 38:223, 1966.
11. Spina V: Repair of unilateral cleft lip-nose. Cleft Palate J 5:356, 1968.
12. Matthews D: The nose tip. Br J Plast Surg 21:153, 1968.
13. Spira M, Hardy SB, Gerow FJ: Correction of nasal deformities accompanying unilateral cleft lip. Cleft Palate J 7:112, 1970.
14. Hogan VM, Converse JM: Secondary deformities of unilateral cleft lip and nose. In Grabb WC, Rosenstein SW, Bzoch KR (eds): Cleft Lip and Palate. Boston: Little, Brown, 1971, p 345.
15. Stenstrom SJ: Alar cartilage and nasal deformity in unilateral cleft lip (follow-up clinic). Plast Reconstr Surg 5(3):359, 1975.
16. Stenstrom SJ: Correction of cleft lip nasal deformity: A refinement of an older method. Plast Reconstr Surg 59:675, 1977.
17. Converse JM, Hogan VM, Barton FE: Secondary deformities of cleft lip, cleft lip and nose, and cleft palate. In Converse JM (ed): Reconstructive Plastic Surgery. 2nd ed, Vol. 4. Philadelphia: Saunders, 1977, p 2165.
18. Ogino Y, Ishida H: Secondary repair of the cleft lip nose. Ann Plast Surg 4:469, 1980.
19. Goodman W, Zorn M: The unilateral cleft lip nose. J Otolaryngol 11(3):198, 1982.
20. Tessier P, Tulasne JF: Secondary repair of cleft lip deformity. Symposium on lip surgery. Clin Plast Surg 12(4):719, 1985.
21. Wilson LF: Correction of residual deformities of the lip and nose in repaired clefts of the primary palate (lip and alveolus). Clin Plast Surg 12(4):719, 1985.
22. Gorney MK. Cleft lip and nose (Part 3). In Stark RB (ed): Plastic Surgery of the Head and Neck. Vol. 1. New York: Churchill Livingstone, 1987, p 568.
23. Ortiz-Monasterio F, Olmedo A: Corrective rhinoplasty before puberty: A long-term follow-up. Plast Reconstr Surg 68:381, 1981.
24. Millard DR, Jr: Earlier correction of the unilateral cleft lip nose. Plast Reconstr Surg 70:64, 1982.
25. Thompson M: The residual unilateral cleft lip nasal deformity: A three-phase correction technique. Plast Reconstr Surg 76(1):36, 1983.
26. Talmant JC: Guidelines for the repair of unilateral cleft lip nose. Ann Chir Plast Esthet 29:123, 1984.
27. McIndoe AH: Correction of alar deformity in cleft lip. Lancet 1:607, 1938.
28. Berkeley WT: The cleft lip nose. Plast Reconstr Surg 223:567, 1959.
29. Berkeley WT: Correction of the unilateral cleft lip nasal deformity. In Grabb SW, Rosenstein SW, Bzoch KR (eds): Cleft Lip and Palate. Boston: Little, Brown, 1971, p 227.
30. McComb H: Treatment of the unilateral cleft lip nose. Plast Reconstr Surg 55:596d, 1975.
31. Kernahan DA, Bauer BS, Harris GD: Experience with the Tajima procedure in primary and secondary repair in unilateral cleft lip nasal deformity. Plast Reconstr Surg 66(1):46, 1980.
32. Broadbent TB, Woolf, RM: Cleft lip nasal deformity. Ann Plast Surg 12:216, 1984.
33. McComb H: Primary correction of unilateral cleft lip nasal deformity: A 10-year review. Plast Reconstr Surg 75:791, 1985.
34. Anderl H: Simultaneous repair of lip and nose in the unilateral cleft (a long-term report). In Jackson IT, Sommerlad BC (eds): Recent Advances in Plastic Surgery. Vol. 1. Edinburgh: Churchill Livingstone, 1985, p 1.
35. Salyer K: Primary correction of the unilateral cleft lip nose: A 15-year experience. Plast Reconstr Surg 77(4):558, 1986.
36. Kapetansky D: Techniques in Cleft Lip, Nose and Palate Reconstruction. Philadelphia: Lippincott, 1987, p 7.
37. Boo-Chai K: Primary repair of the unilateral cleft lip nose in the Oriental: A 20-year follow-up. Plast Reconstr Surg 78:185, 1987.
38. Cronin TD, Denkler KA: Correction of the unilateral cleft lip nose. Plast Reconstr Surg 82(3), 419–432, 1988.
39. Potter J: Some nasal tip deformities due to alar cartilage abnormalities. Plast Reconstr Surg 13:358, 1954.
40. McComb H: Primary repair of the bilateral cleft lip nose: A 10-year review. Le fascicule 4 est managuant. Plast Reconstr Surg 77:701, 1986.
41. Kobus K: Early columella elongation. Ann Plast Surg 18(6):470, 1987.
42. Millard DR: The anatomy of the secondary bilateral nasal deformity. In Cleft Craft. Vol. II, Bilateral and Rare Deformities. Boston: Little, Brown, 1977, p 477.
43. Cronin TD: Lengthening columella by use of skin from nasal floor and ala. Plast Reconstr Surg 21(6):417, 1958.
44. Cronin TD, Upton J: Lengthening of the short columella associated with bilateral cleft lip. Ann Plast Surg 1(1):75, 1978.
45. Cronin TD: The bilateral cleft lip with bilateral cleft of the primary palate. In Converse JM (ed): Reconstructive Plastic Surgery. The Head and Neck, Philadelphia: Saunders, 1977, Ch. 44, p 2048.
46. Brauer RO, Forrester DW: Another method to lengthen the columella in the double cleft patient. Plast Reconstr Surg 38(1):27, 1966.
47. Cronin TD: Management of the bilateral cleft lip and palate and nose in Brent B (ed): The Artistry of Reconstructive Surgery. St. Louis: Mosby, 1987, Ch. 32.

CHAPTER 34

Secondary Correction of the Unilateral and Bilateral Cleft Lip Nasal Deformity: Bardach Technique

Janusz Bardach

Currently, three major approaches are used in the treatment of the nasal deformities associated with unilateral or bilateral clefts, each differing from the other in terms of timing and surgical technique. The newest and most radical approach was designed by Anderl[1, 2] and is strongly advocated by McComb[3] and Salyer.[4, 5] These surgeons emphasize that early correction of the nasal deformity, performed simultaneously with primary cleft lip repair, may ensure the normal, or close to normal, growth and development of nasal structures. Early correction of the nasal deformity alleviates the need for secondary corrections, which are usually performed when the child is 7 to 12 years of age or older. In the surgical procedures for unilateral cleft lip/nose described by the previously mentioned authors, an aggressive and radical approach to the lower lateral cartilage is taken. This involves dissection from the skin and nasal mucosa, repositioning according to the shape of the normal site, and stabilization with sutures in a position symmetric to the normal side. In bilateral clefts, repositioning of both lower lateral cartilages is necessary, creating a new dome and simultaneously lengthening the columella.

This approach is gaining popularity. According to Anderl, McComb, and Salyer, this treatment strategy may be the final correction, precluding the need for additional surgery at a later age. In most patients there is marked improvement; however, a slight deformity may persist, and further surgery may be indicated. The idea of early radical correction undoubtedly is very attractive; however, caution should be used when dealing with the lower lateral cartilages at an early age. More late results need to be analyzed before definite conclusions can be drawn. It would be interesting to know the number of secondary corrections required at a later age subsequent to primary correction of the nasal deformity performed at the time of primary lip repair. Also, it would be very important to know what kind of secondary deformities occur and how they are related to the primary early intervention on the lower lateral cartilages. Furthermore, it would be interesting to know if growth inhibition was observed in the long-term results. This information may not be readily available; nevertheless, we should pursue the study of late results

in a controlled manner so that we do not have to rely on trial and error to learn about the benefits and drawbacks of the concept of early correction of nasal deformity. I think the idea of early definitive correction of the nasal deformity is a very important step toward improving our surgical results.

A second, more conservative approach involves limited correction of the nasal deformity at the time of primary cleft lip repair with final correction performed at a later age. This approach, which I have used for many years, differs from the previously described approach of final correction attempted during primary lip repair. This technique for limited correction includes construction of the floor of the nose, placement of the base of the ala in a position that is symmetric to the normal side, and straightening of the columella. Limited correction of the nasal deformity does not involve repositioning the lower lateral cartilage. Therefore, in the majority of patients, secondary correction is necessary. This approach is applicable to patients with both unilateral and bilateral clefts. In children with unilateral clefts, this approach leads to marked improvement and may sometimes result in final correction. When the optimal position of the nasal tip and columella is obtained, creating a symmetric and well-defined shape of the nose, there is no need for further correction. The major problem evolving from this procedure is the lack of consistent results, and this unpredictability is related, in my opinion, to the great variety of cleft forms.

In most cases, limited correction results initially in marked improvement. However, with growth, the shape of the lower lateral cartilage changes, altering the shape of the nasal tip and ala to the degree that further corrective surgery may be necessary. Our long-term experience indicates that these secondary deformities are usually not as severe as the original one, and this facilitates secondary correction.

A third approach limits primary repair to the lip only, leaving correction of the nasal deformity for a later age. This conservative approach creates the most severe secondary nasal deformities, requiring total rearrangement of the lower lateral cartilages, construction of the nasal floor, and closure of the nasolabial fistulas. Since the deformities associated with unilateral and bilateral clefts differ, they must be discussed and analyzed separately, although the philosophy of treatment and the surgical technique are similar in both deformities.

Correction of the Unilateral Nasal Deformity

The unilateral cleft lip nasal deformity presents a more difficult treatment problem than does cleft lip or cleft palate. The challenge arises from the multiplicity of factors causing the deformity. All these factors were described in Chapter 19, in which the anatomy of unilateral and bilateral cleft noses is described. Since one of the major causes of the nasal deformity is the malposition of the lesser maxillary segment, definite improvement in the shape and position of the nasal elements cannot be obtained without correcting the position of the skeletal base. One of the reasons why many surgical techniques designed to correct the nasal deformity are unsuccessful is that no consideration is given to the correction of the existing asymmetry of the skeletal platform. When assessing the existing nasal deformity and the position of the maxillary segments, it is important to realize that treatment strategy is not limited exclusively to surgical intervention. Orthodontic treatment is a very important part of the combined approach and can be very instrumental in establishing symmetry in the skeletal base. When severe hypoplasia in the area of the piriform aperture causes skeletal asymmetry, and subsequently nasal asymmetry, only bone or cartilage implants can assist in restoring the symmetry of the nose.

Correction of the nasal deformity in patients with unilateral clefts, as performed at the Iowa Cleft Palate Center, is divided into two stages, early and late. The first stage, performed simultaneously with primary lip repair, involves limited correction of the nasal deformity. In the second stage, final correction is attempted, sometimes in conjunction with septoplasty.

During the first stage, the cleft lip is repaired using the triangular flap or rotation-advancement technique. The floor of the nose is constructed using a mucoperiosteal flap from the lateral nasal wall and a mucoperichondrial flap from the nasal septum. The base of the ala is repositioned medially so that it is symmetric with the normal side. The columella is straightened as well. At this stage, we are not concerned with the position of the maxillary segments, since we do not use presurgical orthopedic treatment. Our surgical technique of cleft lip repair is designed to create conditions under which the alignment of the maxillary segments will improve without orthopedic treatment. To achieve this goal, no incisions are made in the sulcus, and there is no undermining of the soft tissue. However, special attention is focused on preservation of the fibrous band between the alveolar ridge and the lip on the cleft side. In regard to lip repair, this band facilitates realignment of the lesser maxillary segment into the proper position because it creates a pulling force similar to the function of an orthodontic appliance. Prior to the second stage, which is performed at approximately 7 to 12 years of age, attention is focused on achieving symmetry of the skeletal platform. This symmetry is an important factor in the success of surgical correction of the nasal deformity. In this second stage we attempt to correct all deformed nasal elements in one operation.

Preoperative Assessment

Preoperative analysis of the nasal deformity prior to lip repair must include evaluation of the following:
1. Cleft form (lip only or both lip and palate).
2. Extent of the cleft (partial or complete).
3. Cleft width.
4. Position of the maxillary segments.
5. Presence of Simonart's band.
6. Presence or absence of the nasal floor.
7. Position of the columella.
8. Position of the base of the ala.
9. Size and shape of the nostril.
10. Symmetry of the nasal tip.

Analysis of these factors is important at the time of both primary and secondary correction of the nasal deformity. However, I believe that careful analysis of these factors is more important during secondary correction than primary because it influences decisions about treatment sequence and techniques. The following factors deserve special consideration when planning the correction of the secondary nasal deformity.

Position of the Maxillary Segments. The position of the maxillary segments must be analyzed in terms of symmetry because they form the skeletal base of the nasal pyramid. We attempt to achieve a symmetric skeletal base prior to correction of the nasal deformity. In the majority of patients, such symmetry is achieved with orthodontic treatment, usually maxillary expansion. If there is hypoplasia of the lesser maxillary segment, onlay bone grafting under the base of the ala on the margin of the piriform aperture may be indicated. In the past, I frequently used preserved, homologous cartilage grafts to create symmetry of the alar bases; however, during follow-up examinations, I found that many of the implants had been partially or completely resorbed.

Presence or Absence of the Nasal Floor. When the nasal floor is absent, I construct it in the same manner employed at the time of the primary lip repair, by using mucoperiosteal flaps from the lateral nasal wall and mucoperichondrial flaps from the nasal septum. If reoperation of the lip is indicated, the floor of the nose is constructed with a two-layer closure in its anterior portion. However, when no lip reoperation is indicated, the floor of the nose is created in one layer. In some patients, the nasal floor is lower on the cleft side than on the normal side, and correction is necessary to establish the proper level on the cleft side. The problem is more difficult when the nasal floor on the cleft side is higher than that on the normal side and the nostril is small. Correction of this situation is extremely difficult and will be discussed later.

Position of the Columella. The columella is usually deviated and is in an oblique rather than a vertical position. The anterior nasal spine also may be displaced to the normal side. The columella is shorter on the cleft side and thus, at the time of nasal tip and nostril reconstruction, an additional skin flap from the upper lip may be needed to lengthen it and to obtain symmetry.

Position of the Alar Base. The base of the ala may be malpositioned posteriorly, inferiorly, laterally, or medially. Repositioning the base of the ala, in many secondary operations, represents a very important step leading to symmetry of the nostrils. As mentioned above, repositioning of the base of the ala may be improved by realigning the lesser maxillary segment or bone grafting alone.

Size and Shape of the Nostril. At the time of primary lip repair, regardless of the severity of the nasal deformity, our action is limited to constructing the nasal floor and positioning the alar base symmetric to the normal side. We are extremely careful to prevent creation of a nostril that is too small. This complication frequently occurs in correction of wide unilateral clefts in which the Millard[6] repair is utilized. Correction of a small nostril is one of the most difficult problems in cleft surgery, and no successful corrective technique has so far been described for this problem. We prefer to deal with a nostril that remains larger than that on the normal side. Correction of the small nostril is still an unsolved problem because the skin envelope on the cleft side is deficient. In this situation, repositioning of the lower lateral cartilage may not create the expected symmetry of the nasal tip and nostrils.

Symmetry of the Nasal Tip. Because asymmetry of the nasal tip is caused by the malpositioned lower lateral cartilage on the cleft side, rearrangement of this cartilage and creation of a new dome are necessary to obtain symmetry of the nasal tip. Following the first stage of limited correction of the secondary nasal deformity, the deformity usually is less severe, and thus its correction may be successfully performed using an external approach, which will be described later in this chapter.

Timing of Correction

As mentioned previously, primary correction of the nasal deformity associated with unilateral cleft lip is always performed at the time of primary cleft lip repair at approximately 3 months of age. The timing of the secondary correction is not as well defined because it depends on the growth and development of the individual, the facial and nasal structures, and particularly, the status of the lower lateral cartilages. Because, in our technique for correction of the secondary nasal deformity, the lower lateral cartilages are rearranged, reshaped, and placed in a new position, they must be strong enough to support the newly formed nasal tip, nostrils, and columella before further procedures are performed. Experience indicates that at 7 to 8 years of age or older, the cartilages are usually well developed and strong.

Corrective rhinoplasty is usually performed at 7 to 12 years of age, depending on the growth and development of the facial structures. At this age, necessary limited septoplasty can be performed as well, especially if it involves straightening of the deflected lower edge of the cartilaginous septum. Prior to correction of the secondary nasal deformity in patients with unilateral clefts, we have to ascertain that both maxillary segments are well aligned, creating an alveolar arch of normal shape. The symmetry of the skeletal base is extremely important for successful nasal construction. In many patients, orthodontic treatment is combined with alveolar bone grafting and onlay bone grafting to establish better symmetry of the skeletal base, a major factor to be considered when planning the secondary correction of the nasal deformity. On rare occasions, when osteotomy is indicated in conjunction with remodeling of the lower lateral cartilage and lengthening of the columella, the corrective operation can be performed at 14 years of age or later.

Surgical Technique for the Primary Cleft Lip Nasal Deformity

Technically, limited correction involves construction of the floor of the nose. Over the years, this has become an integral part of our approach to cleft lip nose repair at 3 months of age. Following the usual preparation for lip repair—that is, making measurements and designing the incision lines—the intranasal incisions are marked to create flaps for reconstruction of the nasal floor. On the lateral nasal wall, the incision is carried to just above the palatal shelf below the lower turbinate. From this incision, the mucoperiosteal flap is raised. Attention is focused on keeping this flap below the lower turbinate, allowing space between the lower turbinate and the reconstructed nasal floor. On the medial side, a mucoperichondrial flap from the nasal septum is raised from the incision parallel to the lower edge of the vomer and 2 to 3 mm above it. The incision in the nasal cavity varies in length depending on the accessibility and width of the cleft (Figs. 34–1 and 34–2).

Both incisions on the lateral nasal wall and septum are extended into the lip according to the marked design and follow the vermilion-cutaneous junction. This allows two flaps to be elevated on each side of the cleft. On the lateral side, these are two mucoperiosteal flaps, one directed upward and the other downward; on the medial side, a mucoperichondrial flap is turned upward and a mucoperiosteal flap is turned downward. Since the incision in the nasal cavity is extended 2 to 3 cm posteriorly, only flaps raised in the nasal cavity will be used to construct the floor of the nose. The mucoperiosteal flaps raised on the maxillary segments allow closure of the raw surface of the flaps lying above, but at the anterior portion of the floor of the nose, a raw area is left at the back. In this manner, the nasal floor is constructed with a double-layer closure anteriorly and a single-layer closure posteriorly.

This technique allows successful closure of the nasolabial fistula. However, depending on the position of the maxillary segments at the time of cleft lip repair and following orthodontic treatment, particularly maxillary expansion, the nasolabial fistula may reappear at a later age and will then require secondary closure. When constructing the nasal floor, we always use periosteal flaps, which are no different from the periosteal flaps described by Skoog.[7] Thus, it can be expected that some new bone formation will occur in the cleft area. Currently, we are not able to indicate the frequency, volume, or quality of new bone formation in the cleft following use of periosteal flaps for reconstruction of the nasal floor. However, in many secondary procedures, we have observed that new bone formation has occurred in the cleft area. We are currently conducting studies to explain this further.

Following creation of the nasal floor, we attempt to place the alar base in a position that is symmetric with the normal side. When the skeletal base is symmetric,

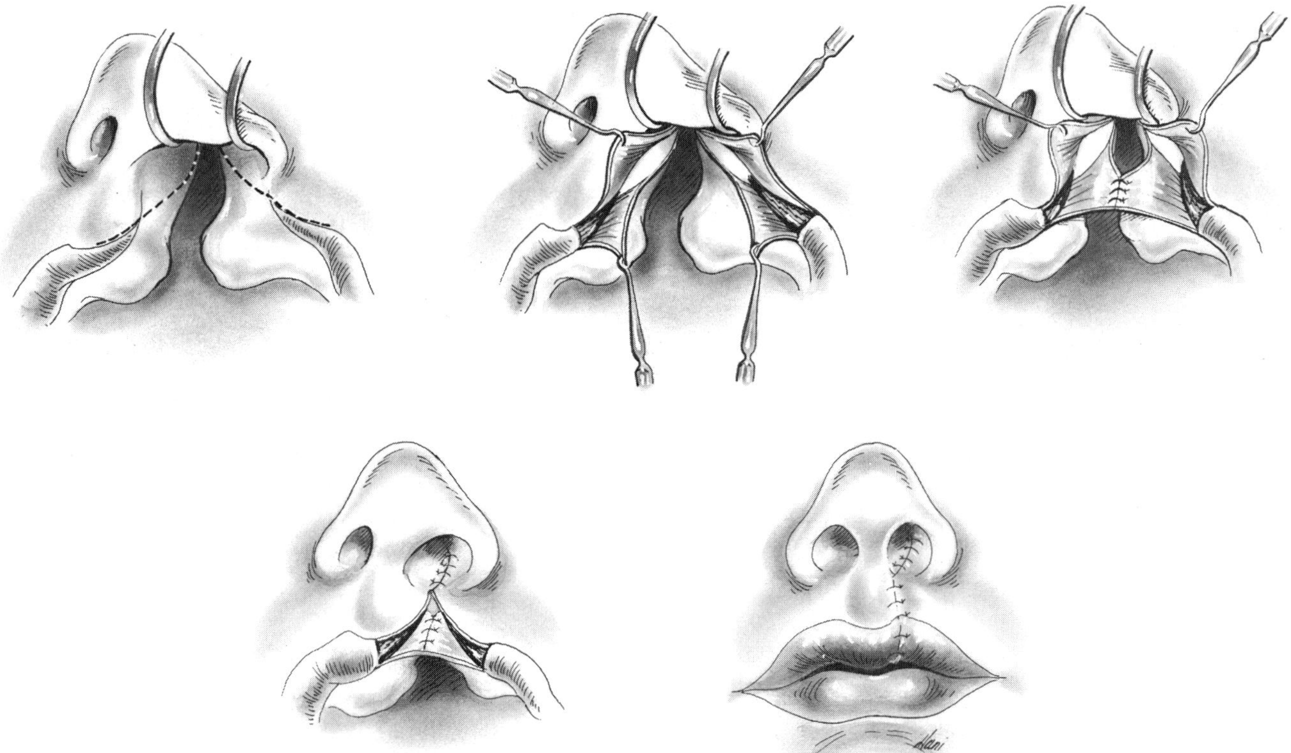

Figure 34–1 Construction of the nasal floor, using mucoperichondrial and mucoperiosteal flaps from the nasal septum, lateral nasal wall, and maxillary segments. Two-layer closure is achieved anteriorly, whereas only a one-layer closure can be achieved posteriorly.

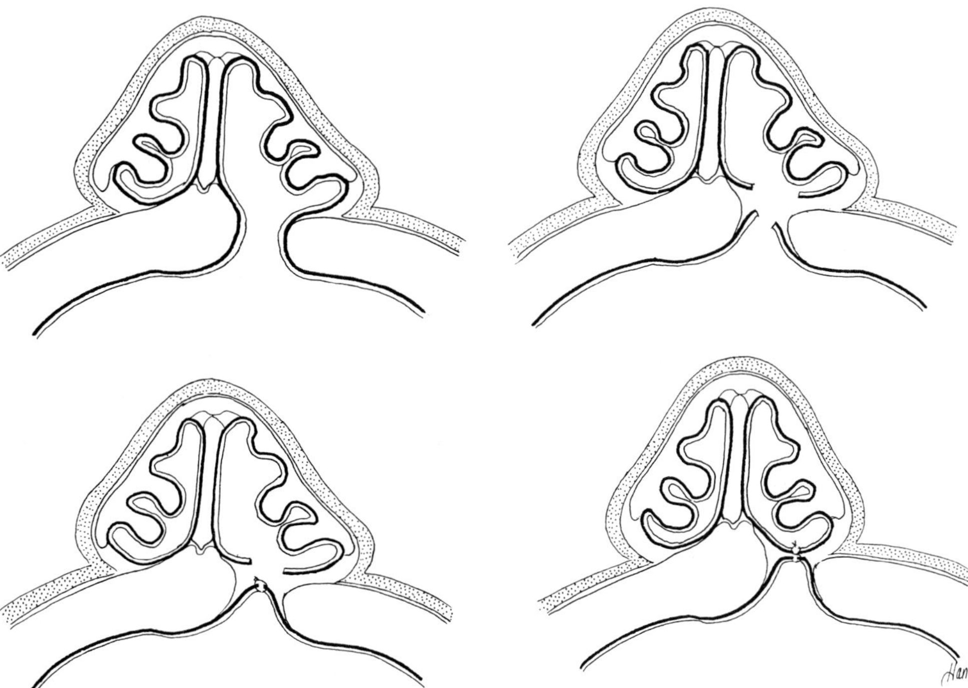

Figure 34–2 Schematic drawing of closure of the nasal floor in the unilateral cleft. Note two-layer closure of mucoperiosteum in the area of the alveolar cleft, which precludes nasolabial fistulas.

this is simple and merely requires adjustment of the distance between the columella and alar base to match that of the opposite side. To achieve this symmetry, some adjustment of skin flaps in the area of the nasal sill may be necessary. A major problem exists when the lesser maxillary segment is collapsed and the skeletal base is asymmetric. In this case, the nasal pyramid is presented as a tilted triangle, and achieving symmetry of the nostrils in this situation is extremely difficult. To create better symmetry of the skeletal base, bone grafting has been used with onlay grafts under the alar base at the edge of the piriform aperture.

When the skeletal asymmetry, which may be caused by collapse of the maxillary segment or hypoplasia, persists despite orthodontic treatment, alveolar bone grafting combined with onlay bone grafting underneath the alar base is performed at approximately 9 years of age. At this age, bone grafting may be helpful in two respects. On the one hand, alveolar bone grafting allows tooth eruption into the cleft area; on the other, it creates symmetry of the skeletal platform for the base of the ala.

Secondary Surgical Correction of the Cleft Lip Nasal Deformity

Secondary correction of the nasal deformity, as indicated previously, is usually performed when the child is between 7 and 12 years of age. This operation, which I described in 1967[8] and elaborated further in 1987,[5] was designed to eliminate all the existing deformities in a one-stage procedure in patients with asymmetry of the skeletal base. This operation was designed to correct asymmetry of the nostrils, deformity of the ala, displacement of the alar base, asymmetry of the nasal tip and columella, absence of the nasal floor, nasolabial fistula, and septal deviation. Correction of septal deviation is not always included in secondary correction. If there is a caudal deviation only, straightening can be performed at any age; however, major septal deviation corrections are delayed until the patient is at least 14 years old.

The approach used for this operation is determined by the existing nasal deformity. The exception is nasal deformity with a small nostril, for which correction presents an extremely difficult and sometimes insoluble problem. Since the main goal is to reconstruct a symmetric nose and since the deformity mostly affects the lower portion of the nose with the lower lateral cartilage as the basic component, we use an external approach with full exposure of the lower lateral cartilages on both sides. The medial crus on the cleft side is shorter than that on the normal side, whereas the cleft-side lateral crus is elongated, displaced caudally, and often S-shaped. To eliminate the asymmetry in the area of the nasal tip and nostrils and malpositioning of the lower lateral cartilage on the cleft side, it is necessary to lengthen the medial crus to the same height as that on the normal side, create a new dome, and reposition and reshape the cartilage on both sides. To achieve this goal, both lateral crura of the lower lateral cartilage are separated completely from the overlying skin and underlying mucous membrane.

This separation is a most important step in the operation and must be performed with extreme caution to avoid tearing the nasal lining. Extensive damage to the nasal lining may be very difficult to correct because there is insufficient tissue to cover the exposed lower lateral cartilage. To avoid this complication, it is helpful to place the index finger in the nostril to support the lower lateral cartilage from below when dissecting the lateral crus. Dissection is easily achieved using sharp scissors and a Freer knife. When both lateral crura have been completely dissected from the skin and mucosa, they are rearranged in a symmetric fashion by reducing excessive cartilage on the cleft side. Sometimes, at the cephalic end, reduction on both sides may be indicated (Figs. 34–3 and 34–4).

Following this step, a 6–0 nylon mattress suture is placed to join both cartilages at the desired height of the dome (as on the normal side), creating symmetric support for the nasal tip. Usually a second suture is placed to ensure that the dome will be stabilized in the desired position. With this maneuver, the medial crus on the cleft side is lengthened and the lateral crus is rearranged to match that of the normal side. As a result, we anticipate that the rearranged nasal tip and nostrils will be symmetric.

Since the lower lateral cartilages were rearranged to lengthen the medial crus on the cleft side, the columella also must be lengthened on that side. This fact was taken into account in planning the initial incisions to raise the skin to expose the lower lateral cartilages. Depending on the existing asymmetry of the columella, we design the incision on the lip, where the additional unequal triangular flap was created at the base of the columella. Attached to it is the elevated remaining skin of the nose. This additional flap from the upper lip is used to lengthen the columella on the cleft side, creating symmetry. It is important to elevate the entire skin of the nose because, following rearrangement of the lower lateral cartilages, redraping the entire skin allows better redistribution and smoother contours of the reconstructed nose. Closure of the defect on the upper lip after the columella has been corrected may have the additional benefit of slightly sliding the midportion of the lip downward, which helps to produce a better contour of the Cupid's bow (Figs. 34–5 through 34–7).

The final step in this operation is placement of the alar base so that it is symmetric to the normal side. This is easily achieved with V-Y advancement. A V-shaped defect is created, and the alar base and nasal sill are moved into the triangular defect. To achieve a stable result, an incision around the alar base may be needed to prevent drawing of the base into its previous position.

As previously mentioned, caudal deviation of the nasal septum can be corrected at any age using an external approach. After completing the operation, nasal packing consisting of gauze treated with antibiotic ointment is inserted. This packing supports the modeling dressing, which remains in place for 7 to 10 days. Serious attention should be given to the postoperative dressing to ensure that the desired configuration of the nose is retained. After insertion of the packing into both nasal passages, the initial modeling is done with paper tape, stabilizing

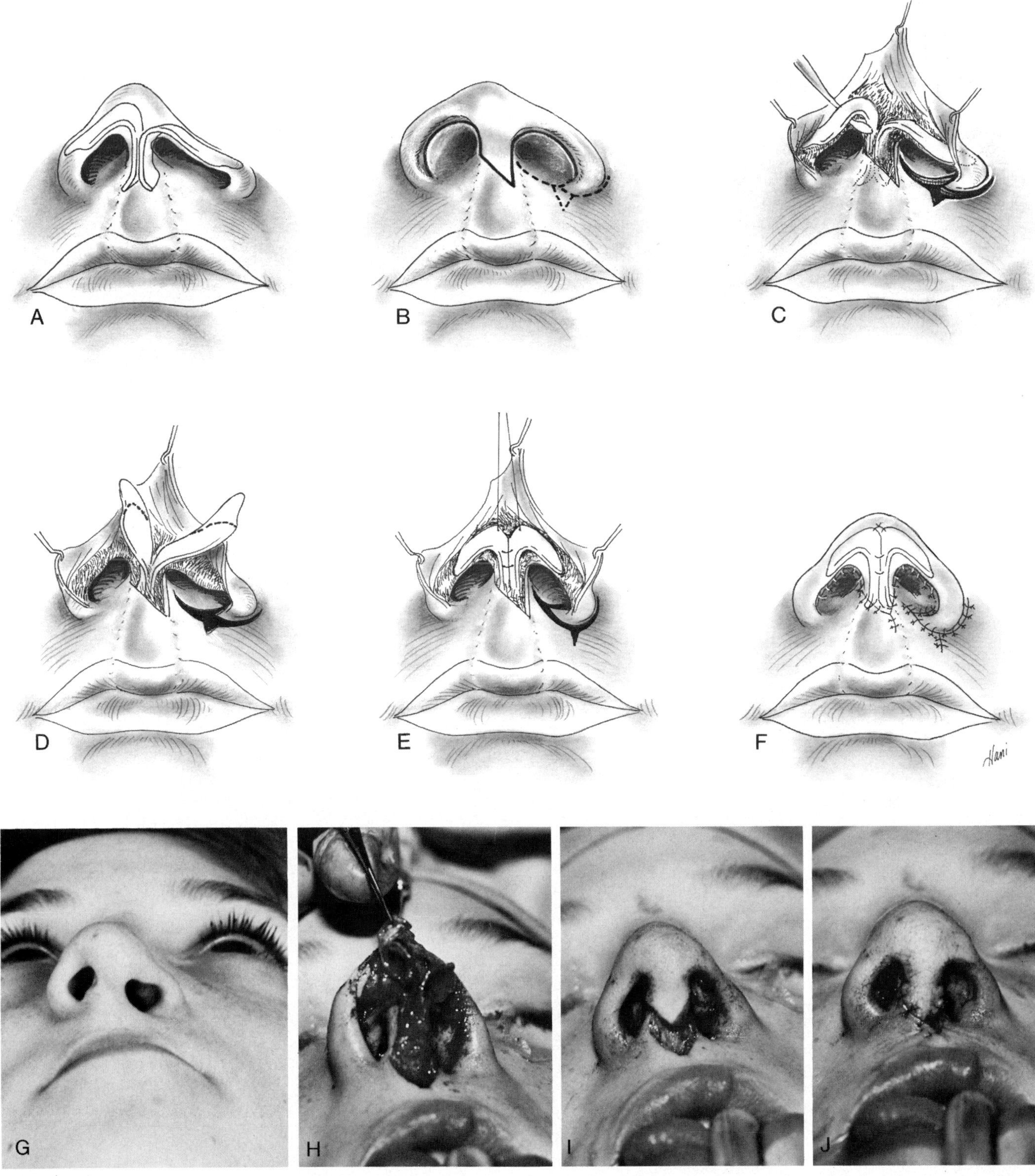

Figure 34–3 Bardach's technique for correction of the secondary cleft lip nasal deformity. *A*, Note the deformity of the lower lateral cartilage, nostril, nasal tip, and alar base. *B*, Design of incisions. The triangular flap in the area of the philtrum is designed to lengthen the columella on the cleft side. *C*, Exposure of both lower lateral cartilages and dissection from the skin and nasal mucosa. *D*, Both lateral crura are completely dissected and elevated. Note the difference in shape and size of the lateral crura. *E*, The reshaped cartilages are sutured in place. *F*, The defect on the upper lip is closed, and sutures are placed in the nasal vestibule. *G*, Typical nasal deformity following unilateral cleft lip nasal repair using the triangular flap technique. *H*, The skin has been raised and both lateral crura have been dissected. *I*, After creating new domes and suturing them together, the change in shape and appearance of the nostrils and nasal tip is evident. *J*, After the columella is sutured in place. Note the symmetry of the nostrils and the change in shape of the nasal tip and the ala.

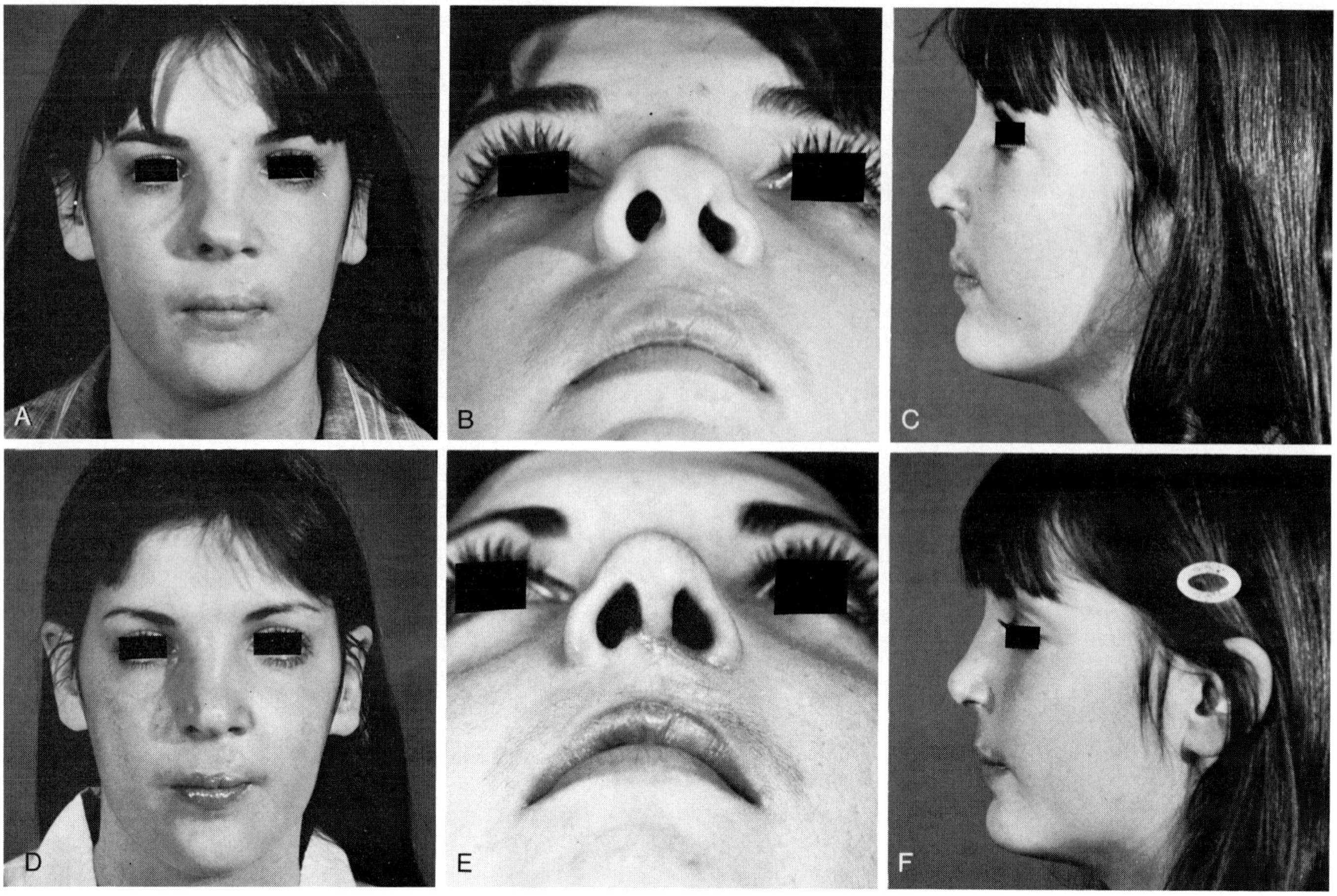

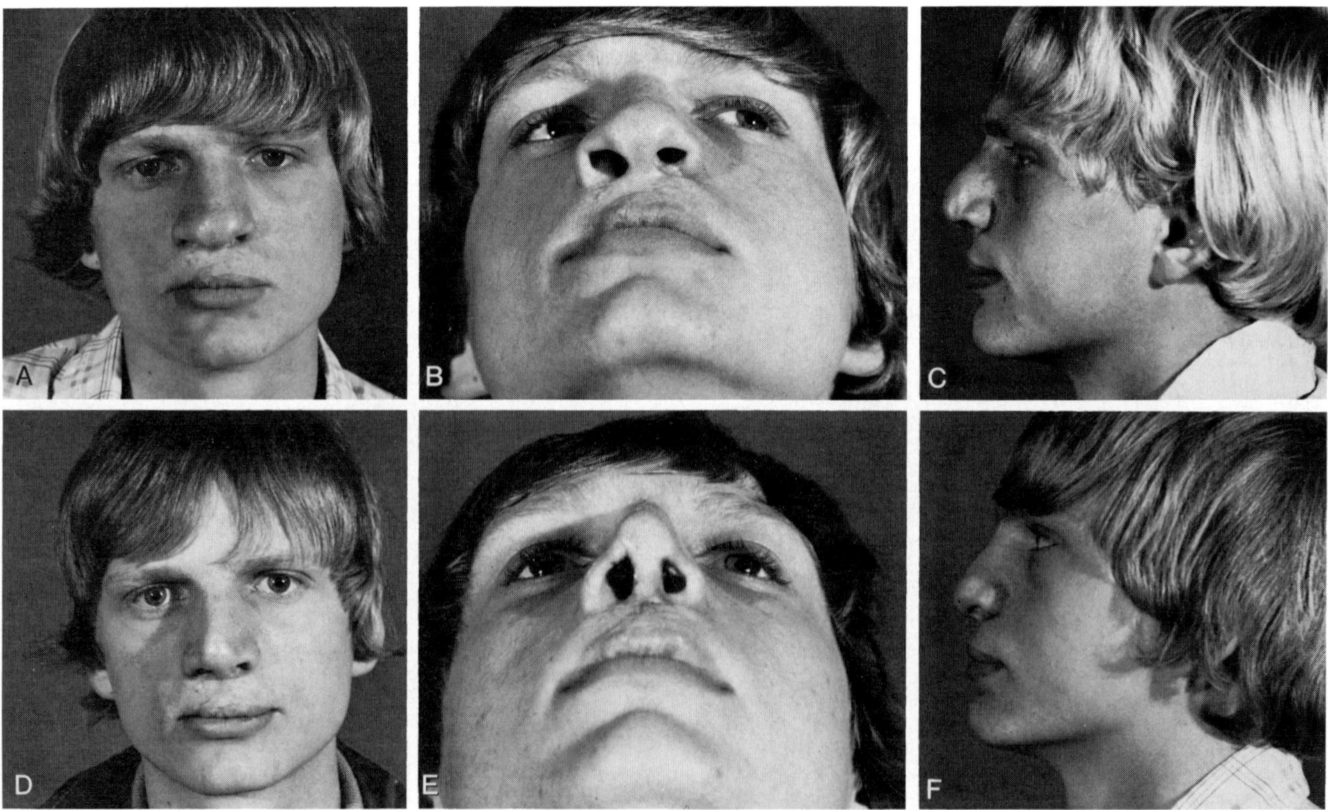

Figure 34–4 *A–C*, Patient with unilateral cleft lip, alveolus, and palate after primary cleft lip repair and primary correction of the nasal deformity. Lip repair was performed using the triangular flap technique. Note nasal deformity in *B* and *C*. *D–F*, The same patient following correction of the secondary nasal deformity using the technique mentioned earlier.

Figure 34–5 *A–C*, Patient with secondary nasal deformity. *D–F*, The same patient after surgery using the previously described surgical technique.

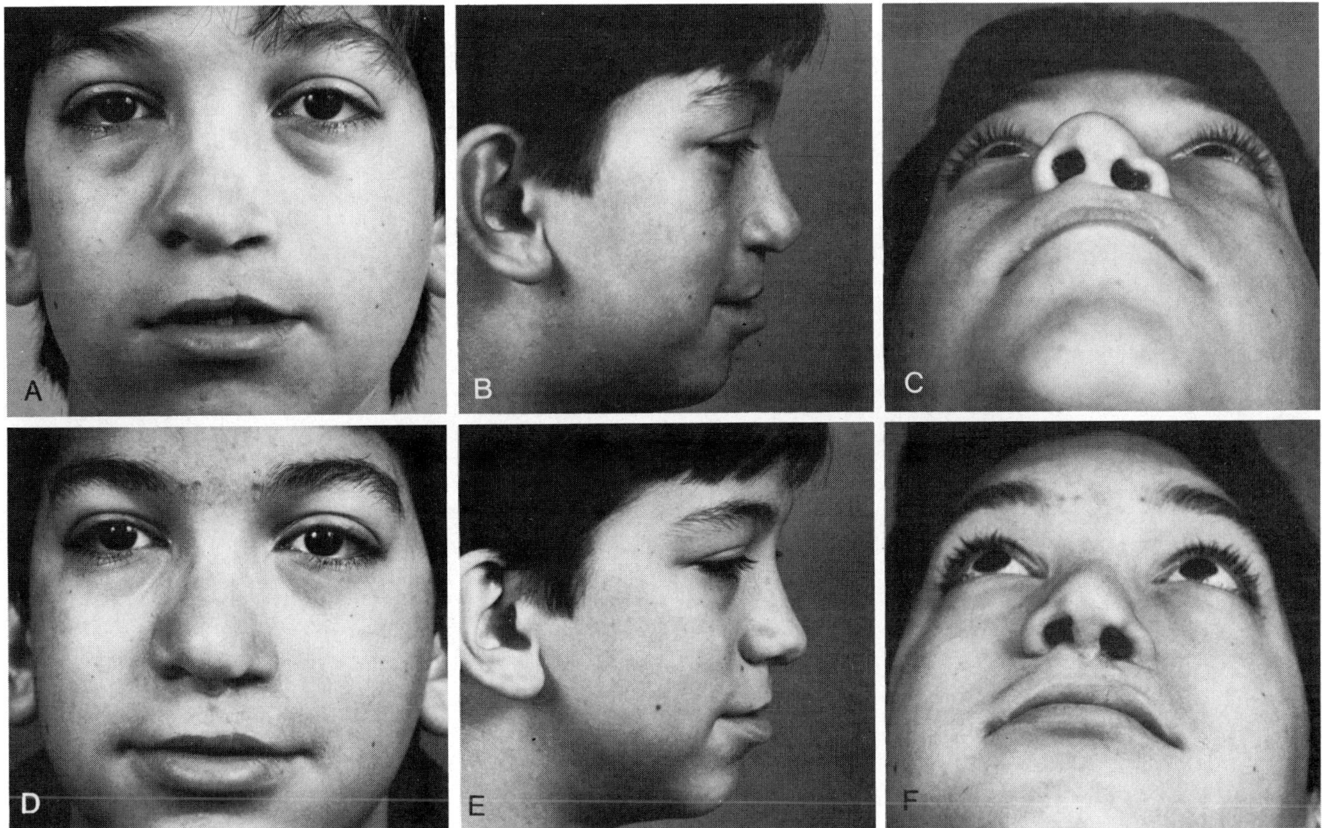

Figure 34–6 *A–C,* Patient with secondary nasal deformity following cleft lip and palate repair on the left side. *D–F,* The same patient after the operation.

the shape and symmetry of the tip and nostrils. This is followed by a dressing of a plaster cast, creating a rigid form. The nasal packing is removed after 48 hours and the nasal dressing after 7 to 10 days. The patient is advised to avoid trauma to the nose for a period of 3 months.

Correction of the Bilateral Nasal Deformity

The anatomy of the bilateral cleft lip nasal deformity differs significantly from that of the unilateral deformity.

Figure 34–7 *A* and *B,* Base view before and after correction of the secondary deformity using the technique described in this chapter.

The differences are related to the initial deformities, which vary substantially.

The cleft form, the extent of the cleft, and the position, size, and shape of the premaxilla and prolabium reflect substantially the severity of the nasal deformity. In partial bilateral clefts, the growth of the nose and other anatomy may be undisturbed, whereas in complete bilateral clefts with a protruding premaxilla, the columella may be extremely short or nonexistent and the prolabium may be attached to the nasal tip. In asymmetric bilateral clefts, the initial and secondary nasal deformities resemble those observed in unilateral clefts.

Preoperative Assessment

In patients with bilateral clefts, our basic approach follows the same principles as those described for unilateral clefts. At the time of primary lip repair, performed in one or two stages depending on the severity of the cleft, limited correction of the nasal deformity is attempted as well. The initial cleft deformity allows us to predict the severity of the secondary nasal deformities. Since we do not rearrange the lower lateral cartilages and lengthen the columella at the time of primary lip repair, we limit our correction of the nose to construction of the floor of the nose and symmetric positioning of the alar bases. Construction of the nasal floor is performed in the same manner as that used for unilateral clefts. However, in patients with a protruding

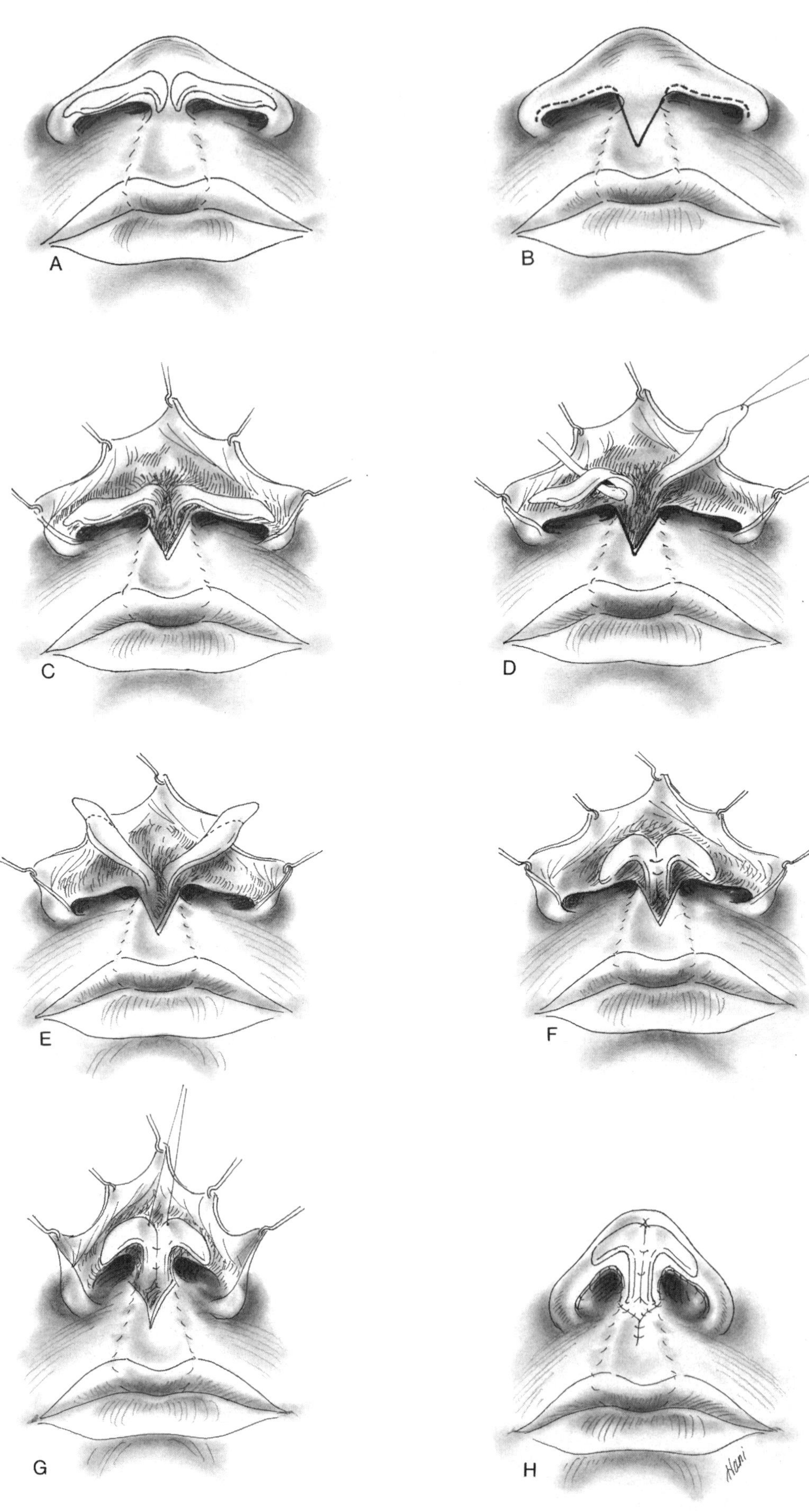

Figure 34–8 Bardach's technique for correction of the secondary deformity associated with bilateral cleft lip repair. *A,* Typical nasal deformity following lip repair in bilateral cleft lip. *B,* Design of the incisions, including creation of the skin flap in the area of the philtrum. *C,* Elevation of the skin. *D,* Dissection of the lateral crura. *E,* Both lateral crura elevated. *F,* Medial crura lengthened. Lateral crura shortened and rearranged. *G,* Suturing the domes. *H,* Final closure.

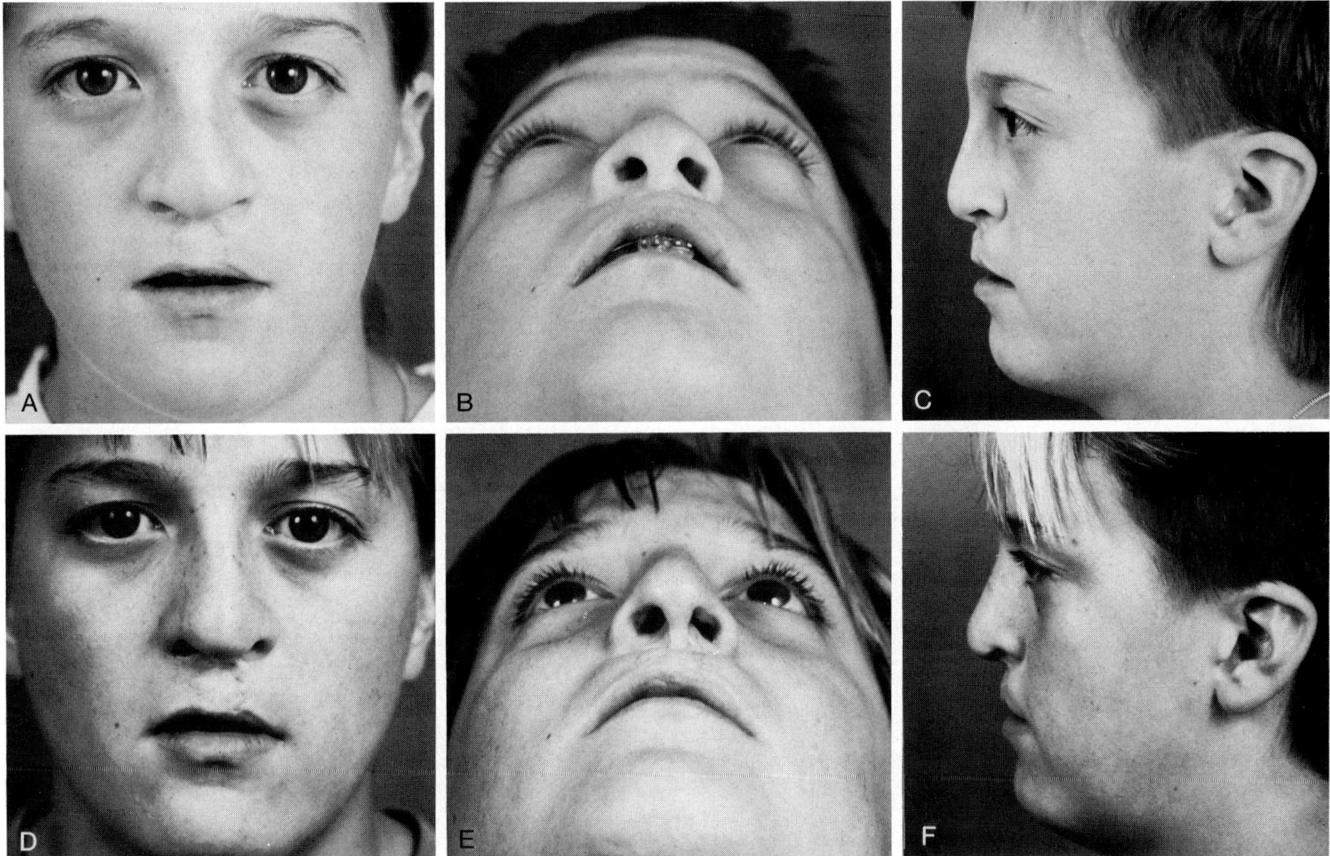

Figure 34–9 *A–C*, Patient with bilateral cleft lip, alveolus, and palate and protruding premaxilla after cleft lip and palate repair and retropositioning of the premaxilla with bilateral bone grafting prior to correction of the secondary nasal deformity. *D–F*, The same patient after the operation.

premaxilla, wide nasolabial and oronasal fistulas remain. These are closed at the time of premaxillary retropositioning combined with bilateral bone grafting, as described in Chapter 69.

The features of the bilateral cleft lip nasal deformity primarily involve the columella, the nostrils, the lower lateral cartilages, the nasal tip, and the bases of the alae. Analysis of the existing secondary nasal deformity helps determine the plan for correction. In my technique, all existing deformities are corrected in a single-stage procedure.[8] These deformities usually include the following:

1. Short columella.
2. Flat, broad nasal tip.
3. Flat nasal alae.
4. Horizontal orientation of the nostrils.
5. Absence of the nasal floor.
6. Lateral displacement of the alar bases.
7. Deformity of the lower lateral cartilages including:
   a. Excessively short medial crura, widely separated at the nasal tip.
   b. Elongated lateral crura.
   c. Obtuse nasal domes.

Timing of Correction and Surgical Techniques

Primary correction of the nasal deformity in the bilateral cleft is done during primary lip repair. At this time, construction of the nasal floor and repositioning of the bases of the alae are performed; however, no attempt is made to rearrange the lower lateral cartilages or to lengthen the columella. This limited correction of the nasal deformity usually does not prevent secondary deformities, and surgical intervention is required at a later age.

Correction of the secondary deformity is usually delayed until the patient is 7 to 12 years old, depending on the growth and development of the nasal and facial structures and the position of the maxillary segments. An important factor to be considered prior to the operation is the status of the lower lateral cartilages, since they must be strong enough to support the rearranged shape of the nasal tip and nostrils. When the premaxilla protrudes, cleft rhinoplasty is delayed until the retropositioning of the premaxilla is completed. In asymmetric bilateral clefts, alignment of the maxillary segments must be considered prior to surgery because the symmetry of the skeletal base plays a major role in achieving successful results in correction of the nasal deformity.

The operation is designed to correct all existing deformities in a single surgical procedure (Fig. 34–8). This may include the following: lengthening of the columella; creation of a projected, refined nasal tip; repositioning of the nostrils from horizontal to oblique; narrowing of the alar bases; repositioning of the lateral

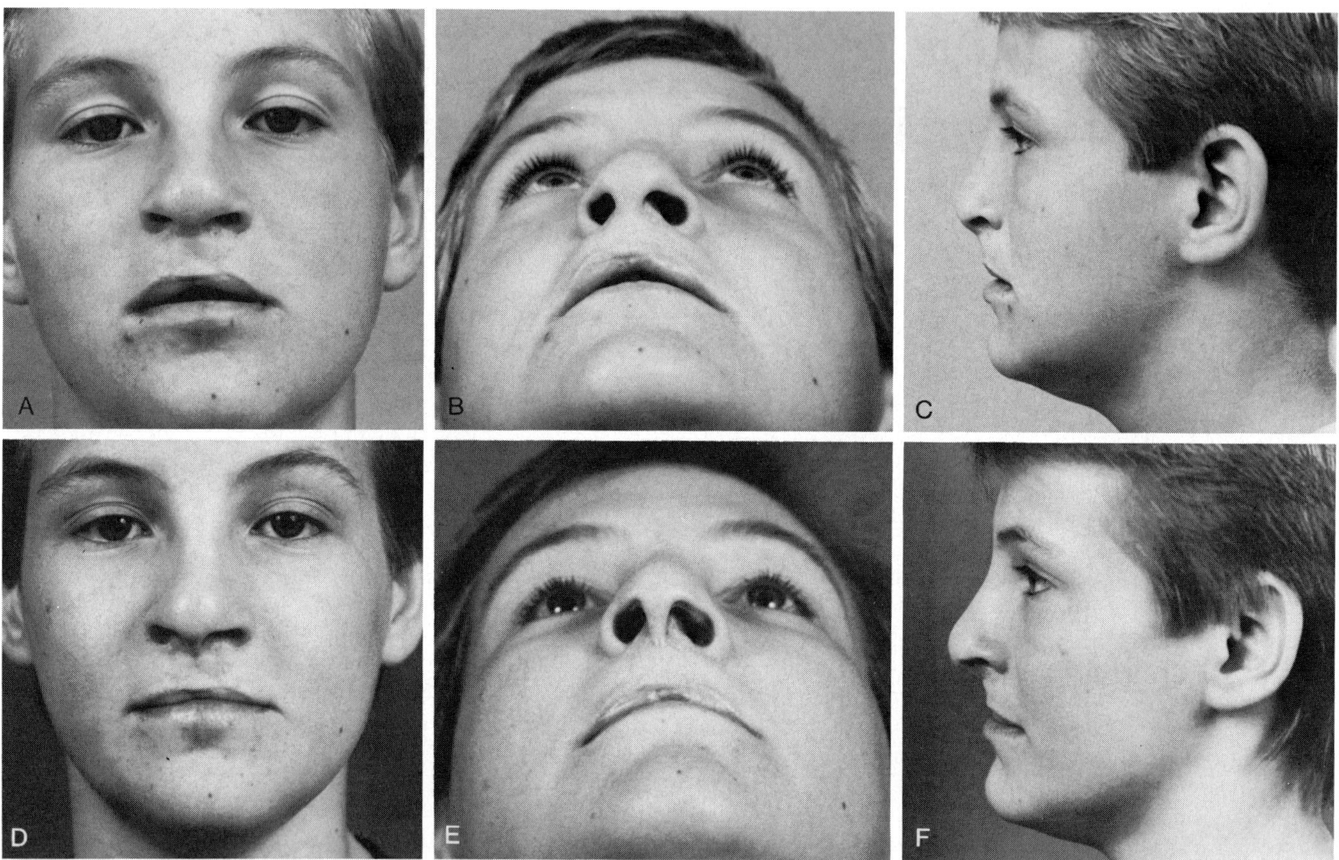

Figure 34–10 *A–C*, Patient with bilateral cleft lip, alveolus, and palate and protruding premaxilla after cleft lip and palate repair and retro-positioning of the premaxilla with bilateral bone grafting prior to correction of the secondary nasal deformity. *D–F*, The same patient after the operation.

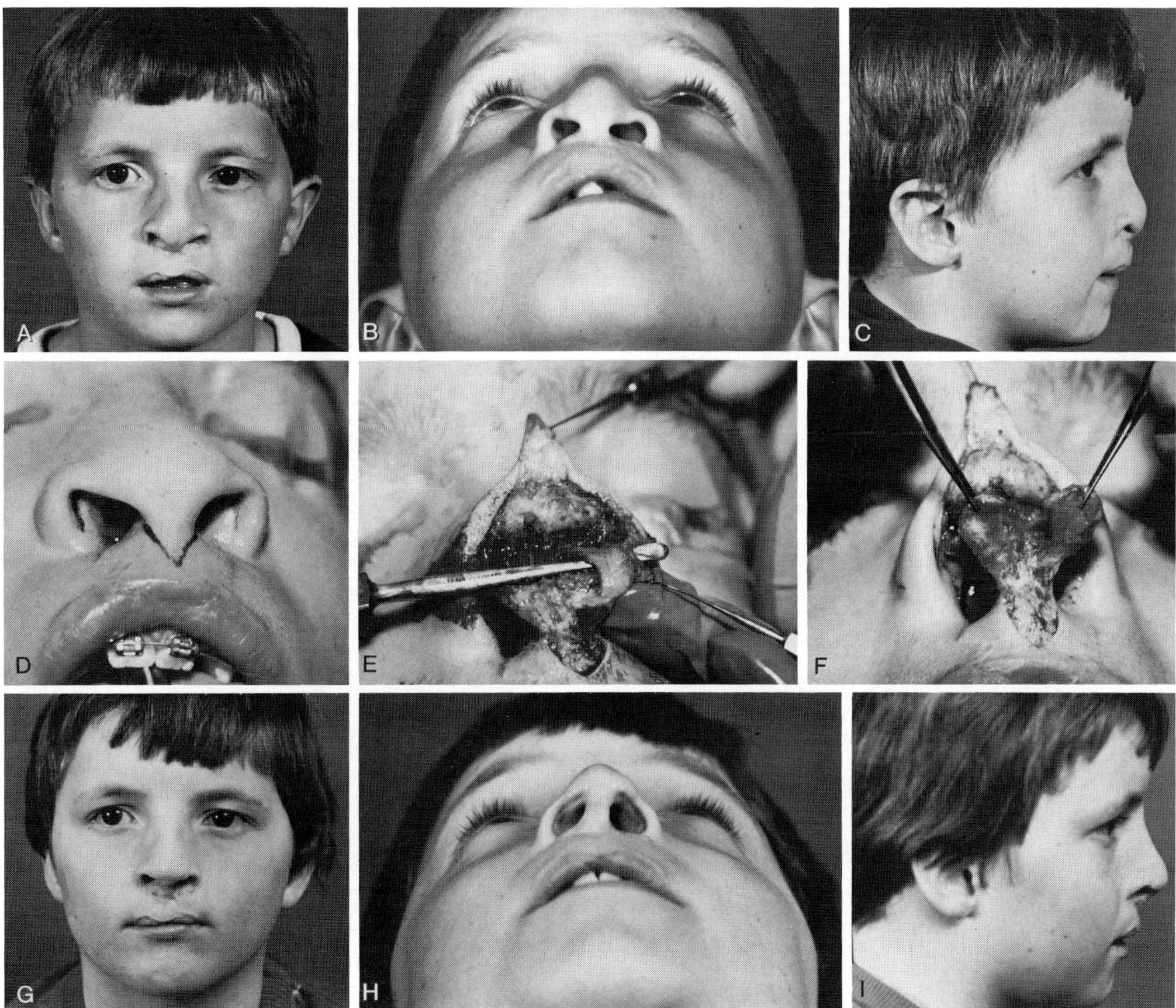

Figure 34–11 *A–C*, Secondary nasal deformity associated with bilateral cleft lip. *D*, Design of the incisions to elevate the skin flap. *E*, Skin flap raised. Dissection of the lateral crus of the lower lateral cartilage. *F*, Both lateral crura dissected and raised prior to rearrangement and suturing at the new lengths to create the nasal tip. *G,H,I*, The same patient 5 years after correction of the nasal deformity.

crura, creation of the domes; and joining of both cartilages at an appropriate height to establish a projected nasal tip. To accomplish these goals in a single surgical procedure, the external approach has been found to be highly advantageous. Columellar lengthening is achieved by using a triangular skin flap attached to the base of the columella to create its extension. This skin flap is designed in the midportion of the lip. It is not unusual to find that the length of the columella must be doubled to achieve a harmonious configuration with the nostrils and nasal tip. When skin is raised, careful dissection of both lateral crura must be completed, freeing them from both skin and nasal mucosa. The only attachment of the lower lateral cartilages remains at the columella by the medial crura, which are usually shorter than normal.

At this point, we rearrange the lower lateral cartilages by lengthening the medial crura, shortening the lateral crura, and establishing the domes in a new position. Joining the domes at the appropriate heights where we expect to have the nasal tip changes the orientation of the nostrils from horizontal to oblique. The reorientation of the shape of the nostrils also is enhanced by medial placement of the base of the ala on both sides, narrowing the nostrils. This can be achieved by reducing the skin between the base of the ala and the columella; however, it may require detachment of the base of the ala with an incision around it. Closure of the medial lip defect plays an important role in narrowing the alar bases, thus improving the shape and appearance of the nose, and in sliding the midportion of the lip inferiorly, creating a better-shaped Cupid's bow (Figs. 34–9 to 34–11).

Postoperative dressings and care are the same as those described for unilateral clefts.

References

1. Anderl H: Extensive primary nose repair in unilateral cleft lip. In Abstracts of the Third International Congress on Cleft Palate and Related Craniofacial Anomalies, Toronto, No. 150, 1977.
2. Anderl H: Simultaneous repair of lip and nose in the unilateral cleft (a long-term report). In Jackson IT, Sommerlad BC (eds): Recent Advances in Plastic Surgery. London: Churchill Livingstone, 1985.
3. McComb H: Primary correction of unilateral cleft lip nasal deformity. A ten year review. Plast Reconstr Surg 75:791, 1985.
4. Salyer K: Primary correction of the unilateral cleft lip nose. A 15 year experience. Plast Reconstr Surg 77:556, 1986.
5. Bardach J, Salyer KE: Surgical Techniques in Cleft Lip and Palate. Chicago: Year Book, 1987.
6. Millard DR, Jr: The unilateral cleft lip nose. Plast Reconstr Surg 34:169, 1964.
7. Skoog T: Repair of the unilateral cleft lip deformity: Maxilla, nose, and lip. Scand J Plast Reconstr Surg 3:109, 1969.
8. Bardach J: Rozszczepy Wargi Gornej i Podniebienia. Warszawa: Panstwowy Zaklad Wydawnictw Lekarskich, 1967.

Primary Surgical Treatment of Cleft Palate

CHAPTER 35

Anatomy of the Cleft Palate

Otto Kriens

Honor those who go first
even if those who came later go further.
SIR SYDNEY SUNDERLAND

The phylogenetic secondary palate is an evolutionary, recently acquired, anatomic entity of mammalianlike reptiles and of mammals. In the posterior region of the bony roof of this "new" oral cavity, the phylogenetic reduction has predominantly affected the pterygoid and has even led to the loss of the epipterygoid, which changed its function to form the alisphenoid (the later middle cranial fossa, anterior to the otic capsule). During the development of the skull, the pterygoid thus became the buttress of the midfacial skeleton against the cranial base (Fig. 35–1).

The branchial system, which is derived from the mesenchyme of the splanchnopleura and not from somites, also has been considerably reduced and/or modified during its development from ancient vertebrates to mammals. Muscles of the first and second branchial arch still disclose their phylogenetic origin and borders by their innervation and adjacent fascias.

As early as 1717, Valsalva had referred to the velum as belonging to the pharynx: "Est re vera pars pharyngis." This idea has recently been substantiated by James Bosma, who named the hard and soft palates the *oral* and *pharyngeal* palates, respectively, and rightfully gave the velum more than an oronasal dimension.[1] The junction of the two is at the spheno-occipital synchondrosis. The borderline further down runs between the first (fifth cranial nerve) and second branchial arch (ninth and tenth cranial nerves). The salpingopharyngeal fascia (von Tröltsch) with its levator palati muscle separates the pharynx from the phylogenetic masticatory region. The tubal cartilage is looked on as an interposition between the internal and external layers of the buccopharyngeal fascia.[2]

Von Luschka's monograph of 1868, *The Pharyngeal Head in the Human*, is a highlight among many anatomic studies on the muscles of the normal mesopharynx and epipharynx, including the pharyngeal palate.[3] Studies on the cleft velar anatomy have been few and have almost exclusively concentrated on muscles.[2, 4–7] Prior to dissections of the cleft palate,[8] which led to the concept of intravelar repair,[9] the main functional-anatomic interest had been concentrated on the palatoglossus and palatopharyngeus muscles, which support the palatopharyngeal sphincter of Whillis.[10] Veau, who also published photographs of cleft bony palates, based his findings of the cleft velar musculature on what he could observe during surgery.[11] Unfortunately, the extensive investigations into the normal fascial apparatus related to the pharyngeal palate have not been expanded to the cleft palate.[12–16] Although recent anatomic descriptions of clinical and autopsy studies have increased our detailed anatomic knowledge, some misconceptions have prevailed—for instance, those concerning the aponeurosis, the hamular fracture, and the palatoglossus muscle.

Cleft Palate Skeleton

There are few publications with a substantial number of illustrations of cleft bony palates.[4, 5, 11, 17] The scarceness of anatomic specimens has barred assessments of the bony cleft palate. Ashley-Montagu[18] and Sillman,[19] however, published data on dissections of infant maxillary gum pads confirming the existence of skeletal points that are applicable to measurements of plaster casts. Methodically, this has paved the way for computer three-dimensional measurements, e.g., with the reflex microscope. Palate topography has still not been investigated with these extremely accurate machines. Measurement of the palate with computed automatic registrations is presented to elucidate the morphology of the infant cleft bony palate.

Width of Palate

The morphology of the cleft bony palate is influenced by primary and secondary changes of intrauterine and postpartum origin. The infant cleft palate is dealt with to illustrate the cardinal morphologic findings in palatal clefts (Fig. 35–2).

Post-tuberosity Width (P–P1)

In noncleft fetuses at term, the hamulus is a distinct bone, demarcated by a suture from the medial pterygoid lamina.[1] In infants, the distance from the hamular base

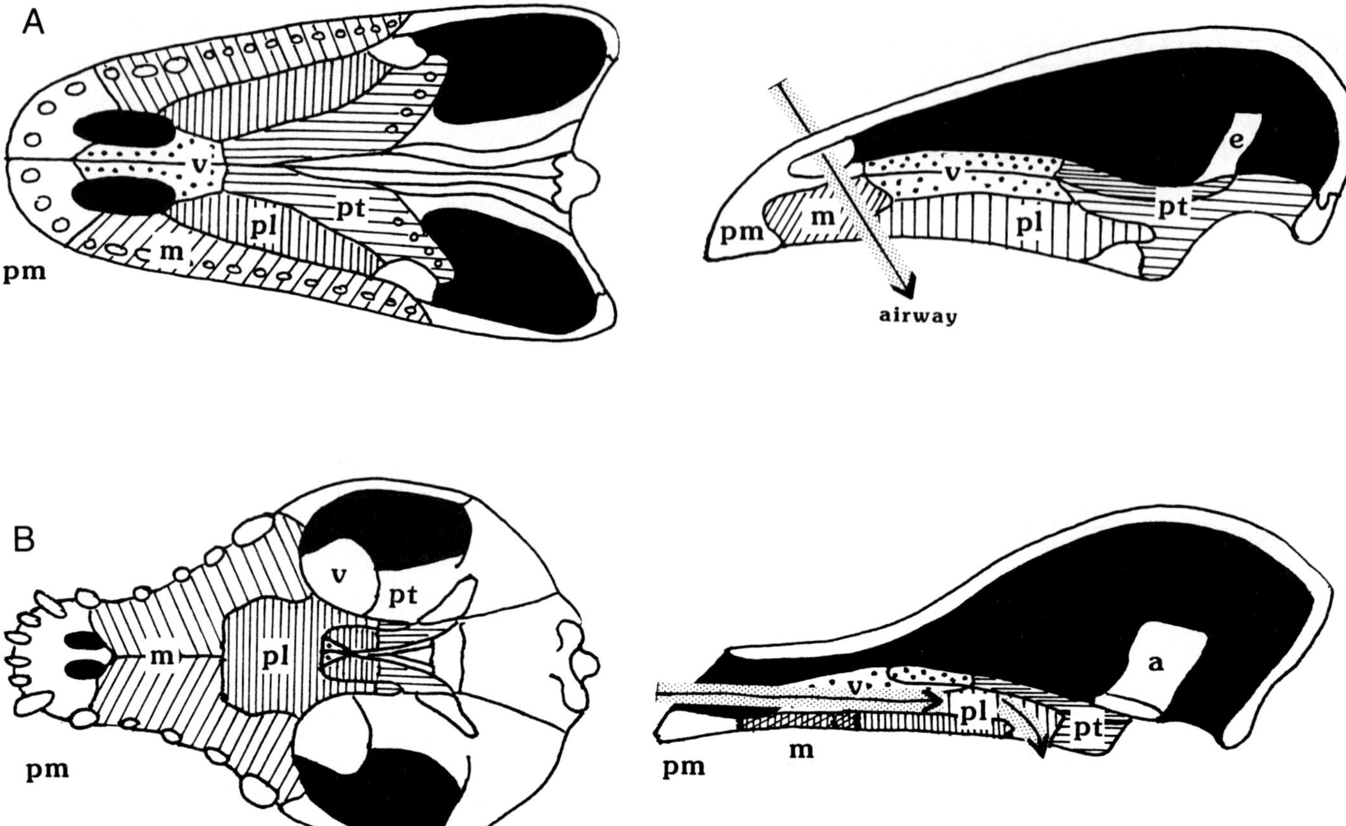

Figure 35–1 Schematic illustrations of the phylogeny of the secondary bony palate. Ventral and lateral aspects of the palatal skelelton are shown in *(A)* a primitive mammalianlike reptile, which existed during the carbon and perm, and *(B)* a dog (after Romer[37]). Coincidental with the reduction of the posterior portion of the bony roof of the mouth there ensued a decrease in the number of teeth and the loss of pterygoid teeth. Bones (maxilla, lateral portions of the palatine), which had been oriented predominantly vertically in the oral cavity of the primary palate, developed considerable horizontal portions, whereas other bones (vomer, pterygoid, and the cranial portions of the palatine) with predominantly horizontal extensions changed into more vertical ones. A simplified summary would be that (1) the bony roof of the primary palate (vomer and pterygoid) posterior to the intermaxillary bone became located at or in the median portion of the cranial base; and (2) the maxilla and palatine form a "new" bony roof of the oral cavity below the recent airways. (pm = premaxilla, v = vomer, pl = palatine, pt = pterygoid, e = epipterygoid, a = alisphenoid.)

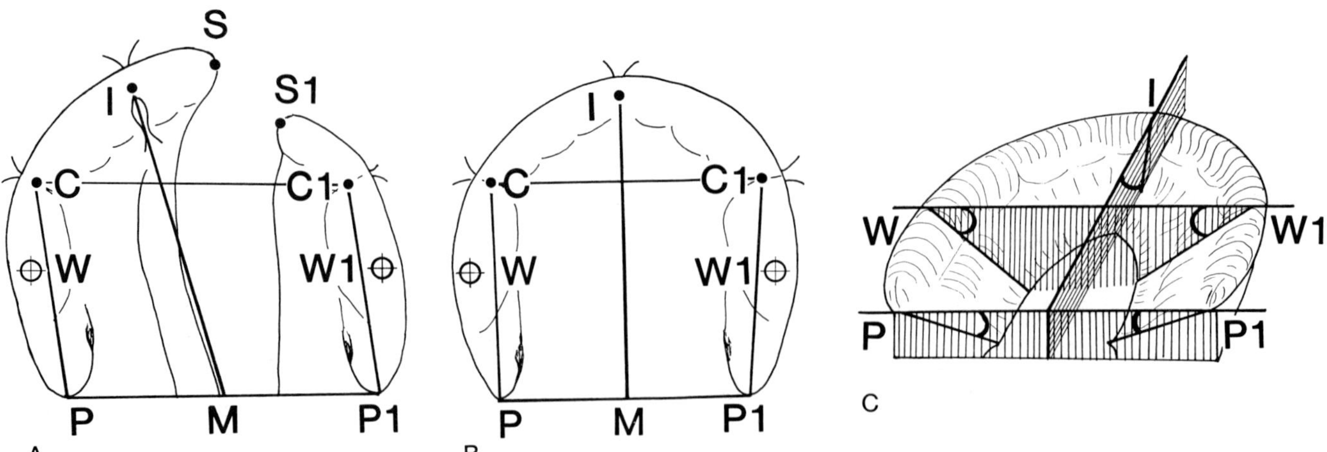

Figure 35–2 Points, distances, and angle used for assessment of the infant palate. *A,* Unilateral cleft lip, alveolus, and palate (UCLP). *B,* Cleft palate (CP). *C,* Vertical angles of the palatal slope at I, W, and P. P–P1 = post-tuberosity points; W–W1 = midalveolar points at maximal transverses arch diameter; C–C1 = transverse distance between canine points; I = interincisor point; M = median point of P–P1; S–S1 = points limiting the clinical cleft width.

to the auditory tube is only 4 to 5 mm, but its length is usually much greater than the 4 mm stated.[6] Although the long infant hamulus is readily palpable, it cannot serve as a reference because it is subject to considerable reduction with age. The post-tuberosity plane P–P1, however, is most constant in the cleft maxillary complex (Fig. 35–3). Because of phylogenetic, ontogenetic, and functional considerations, the P–P1 distance has been suggested as a reference for maxillary assessment.[20]

The post-tuberosity distance increases with the degree of clefting (Table 35–1). The tongue and the enlarged P–P1 distance in clefts affects the shape of the palate and the displacement of the large segment in unilateral cleft lip and palate as well.

A consistent finding in complete infant unilateral cleft lip, alveolus, and palate (UCLP) is a mean deviation to the noncleft side of 15 degrees of the midalveolar point measured from the midsagittal plane through the post-tuberosity distance (Fig. 35–2). Since the mean angles at P and P1 differ considerably (93.6 vs 81.9 degrees), the displacement has been attributed to the interplay of lingual and facial tissue pressure during fetal development.[20] Such interplay is substantiated by the fact that the tongue can be distinctly recognized in fetuses prior to the development of the primordial cartilage in the head. The fetal tongue is dislocated from its median position posteriorly into the cleft palate (CP) or laterally into a UCLP, which results in an opposing medial pressure. Evaluation of the clinical cleft (S–S1) of the alveolus in UCLPs proved that its width is caused by segmental displacements rather than by a defect (Fig. 35–2).

In 91 infants (mean age, 19 days) C–I equals I–S plus the cleft (S–S1) plus S1–C1. According to this equation

(14.2 mm = 7.3 mm + S–S1 + 8.56 mm), the actual cleft width is 14.2 mm − 15.95 mm = − 1.75 mm. The excess tissue, indicated by the minus sign, may be attributed to a possible supernumerary tooth (bud) and to measuring the soft tissue at both ends of the cleft stumps, that is, twice. Although the mean value of the clinical cleft width is 11.5 mm, there is no tissue defect for the mean values of the alveolar cleft.

Intercanine Width (C–C1)

The intercanine distance depends on the number and size of the tooth buds or teeth and the shape of the arch. In the normal infant, C–C1 is 27.2 mm (100%), but this distance decreases considerably in velar (− 19.1%) and complete palate clefts (− 19.4%). In patients with complete UCLP, the diminution is only 11%, and in UCLP patients with a partial cleft lip it is merely 9%. This confirms cineradiographic findings that the infant tongue slips through a cleft into the epipharynx or nasal cavity. In UCLP, the tongue is displaced anterolaterally into the nose and even into the alveolar cleft. Thus, it causes considerably less narrowing of the

Table 35–1. P–P1 Measurement of Infant Hard Palates

Diagnosis	No.	P–P1 (mm)	SD	Correlation Coefficient
No cleft	30	29.5	1.76	0.99
Velar cleft	30	30.0	2.11	0.97
Complete cleft palate	30	31.8	2.24	0.98
Unilateral cleft lip and palate	92	32.2	2.73	0.906

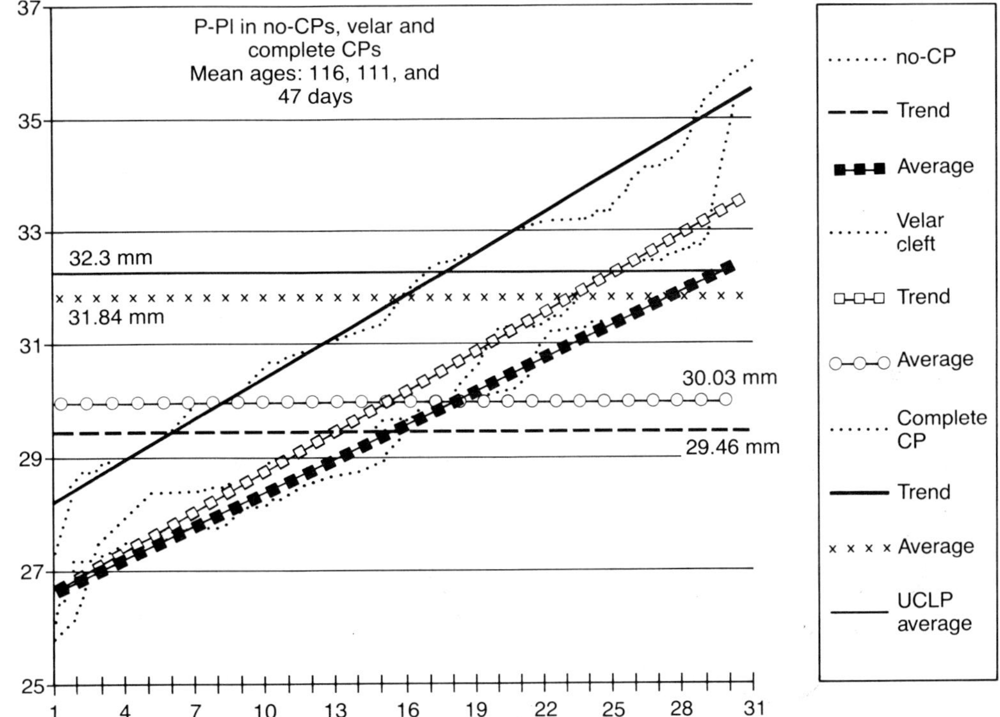

Figure 35–3 Post-tuberosity width (P–P1) in infants with noncleft maxilla, velar cleft, and complete cleft palate. The average values of P–P1 of the normal palate and the velar cleft on the one hand, and of the complete palate cleft and the UCLP on the other, show the similarity of P–P1 values (i.e., 29.5 to 30 mm and 31.8 to 32.2 mm with a gap of 1.8 mm between the two groups).

canine regions. These values correlate with those of the post-tuberosity distances.

Midsagittal Dimensions

The midsagittal dimension (M–I) of the infant hard palate decreases with increasing severity of the palatal cleft and greater post-tuberosity width (P–P1) (Table 35–2). The cleft bony palate is hypoplastic in both the transverse and sagittal dimensions.[6]

Inclinations of Shelves

Shelf inclination is an important morphologic characteristic of the bony palate. It is measured transversely from the occlusal plane. Any point may be chosen, but the best overall information has been found at W (widest transverse diameter of the arch), I, and P (Fig. 35–4).

Table 35–2. Midsagittal Infant Palatal Length Relative to Post-tuberosity Width

Diagnosis	M–I (mm)	P–P1 (mm)
No cleft	28.9	27.2
Velar cleft	26.7	29.1
Complete cleft palate	23.1	30.5

In cleft palates, the intact alveolar arch surrounds the tongue so that the palatal vault can reflect the size and tonus of the tongue. The inclinations of the shelves vary considerably with the size of the cleft and the posterior displacement of the tongue. In patients with UCLP the transverse palatal slope at W and the difference between the angles at W and P differ considerably from comparable measurements in patients with cleft palate only (Table 35–3).

PALATAL INCLINATIONS
Normal infant palate

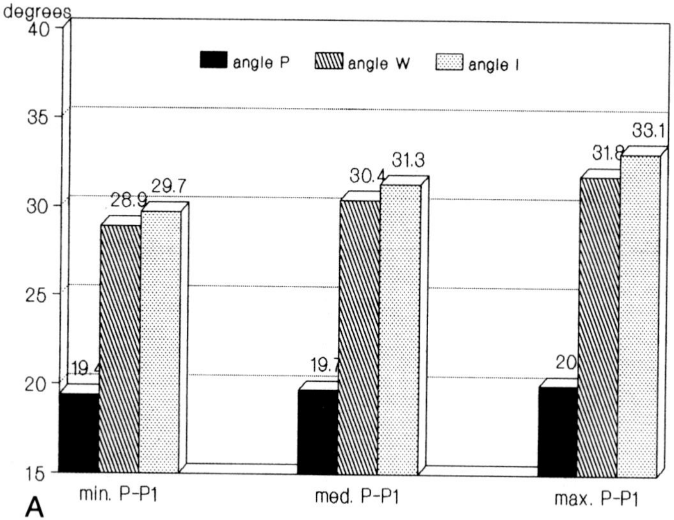

Figure 35–4 Palatal inclinations at P, W, and I in infants with *A*, normal palate, *B*, velar cleft, and *C*, complete palate cleft. With median P–P1 values the transverse palatal slopes at W–W1 are 30 degrees in the noncleft palate, 31.7 degrees in the velar, and 32 degrees in the complete palate cleft. There is hardly any difference between the two latter cleft forms in this respect. The palatal inclinations in the post-tuberosity plane (P–P1) in the normal palate (19 degrees) differ again considerably from those in velar (27 degrees) and complete palate cleft (28 degrees). The inclination at P decreases remarkably in complete palatal cleft with increasing P–P1 values (32 to 26 degrees). The effect of the tongue tonus is reflected by increasing palatal slopes at W and I with wider P–P1 distances in the normal infant palate, whereas there is a reduction of the slope at these points if the tongue is displaced posteriorly through the velar cleft. (Normal palate, velar, and complete cleft groups: n = 30 infants each.)

Infant velar cleft

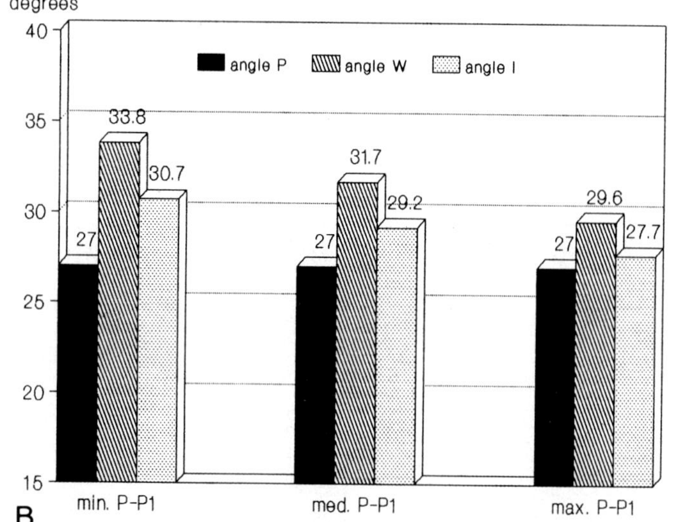

Complete infant cleft palate

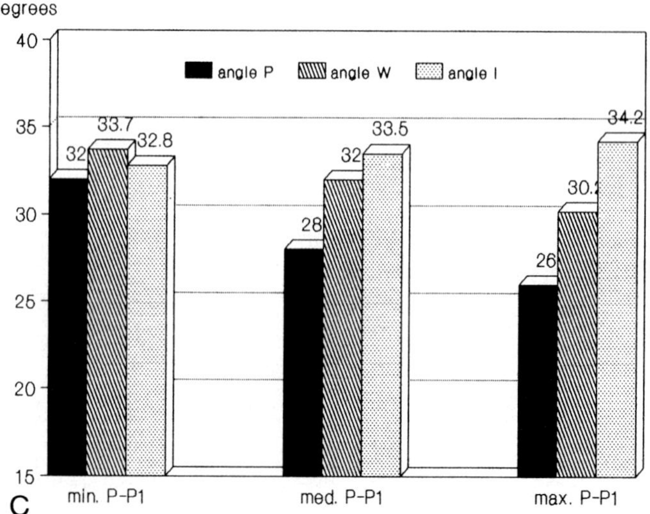

Table 35–3. Palatal Inclinations (Mean Values)

Diagnosis	At W	At P	Difference
Noncleft palate	29.9°	19.7°	10.2°
Velar cleft	31.7°	26.9°	4.8°
Complete cleft palate	32.0°	29.0°	3.0°
UCLP noncleft side	45.2°	29.0°	16.2°
UCLP cleft side	47.7°	31.3°	16.4°

The maximum and minimum trend values of the palatal inclinations elucidate the effects of the tongue in shaping the palatal vault (Figs. 35–4 and 35–5). The mean range of the normal palate inclinations is small: P, 19.4 to 20.1 degrees; W, 28.9 to 31.8 degrees; and I, 29.7 to 33.1 degrees (Fig. 35–4A). These values reflect the formative effect of different sized tongues (Fig. 35–4A) influencing shelf inclination and post-tuberosity distance.

In the infant velar cleft, the slope at P–P1 measures 27 degrees, and this 40% increase against the minimal values in the noncleft palate is present in the entire range of P–P1. The slope at W–W1, however, decreases from 33.8 degrees (minimal P–P1) to 29.6 degrees (maximal P–P1). There is a decline of the midsagittal inclination from 30.7 to 27.7 degrees also. These findings are in accord with clinical observations that the tongue slips through the velar cleft into the epipharynx and therefore is unable to reach forward to the normal extent. Thus, the tongue occupies less space in the palatal vault with increasing P–P1 dimensions (Fig. 35–4B). In complete palate clefts the transverse palatal inclinations reflect the more anterior position of the tongue between the cleft edges. The slope at P (32.1 degrees) is by far the steepest in the minimal P–P1 value group but decreases toward maximal P–P1 values to 26 degrees. The anterior position of the tongue is also reflected by the overall high midsagittal slope measurements at I (32.8 to 34.2 degrees) (Fig. 35–4C).

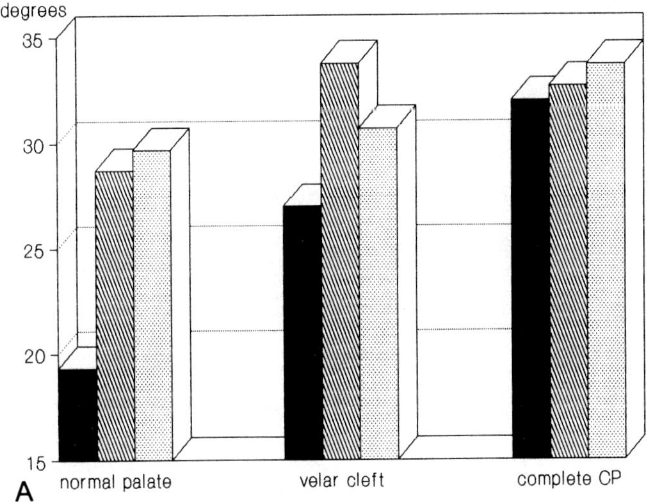

Figure 35–5 Minimal (*A*), median (*B*) and maximal (*C*) trend values of the palatal shelf inclination at P, W, and I are given for normal palates, velar clefts, and complete palatal clefts in infants (models sorted on values of P). In the normal infant palate (left group of columns) the palatal inclination at P stays the same for *A*, *B*, and *C* with a constant increase of the slopes at I and W for models with wider interpterygoid distances (P–P1). In velar clefts the inclination at P is steeper than in the normal palate and stays the same. The inclinations at W and I decrease from the smallest interpterygoid distances to the maximal ones. In complete palatal clefts there is a noteworthy decrease of the palatal shelf inclination at P with greater distances P–P1, while the angle I stays about the same.

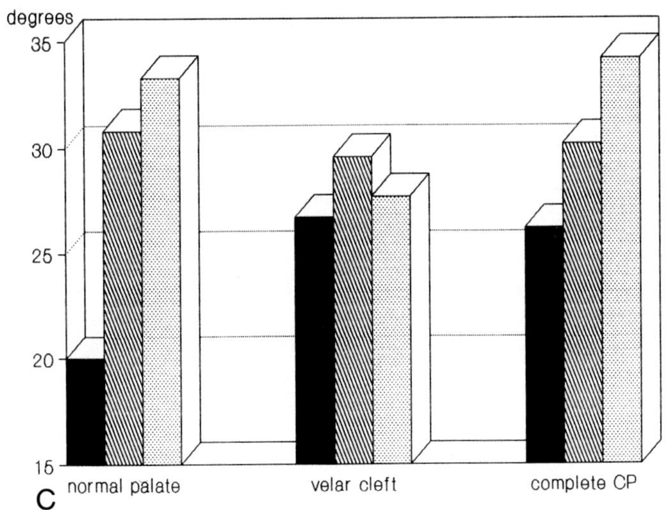

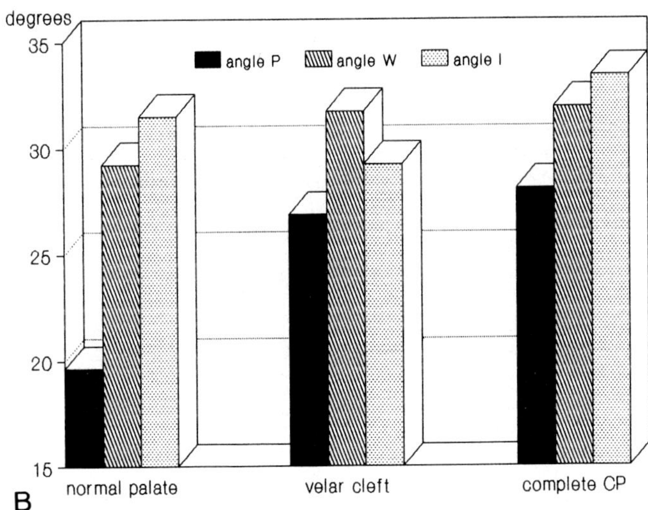

Morphologic Epitomes of Hard Palate

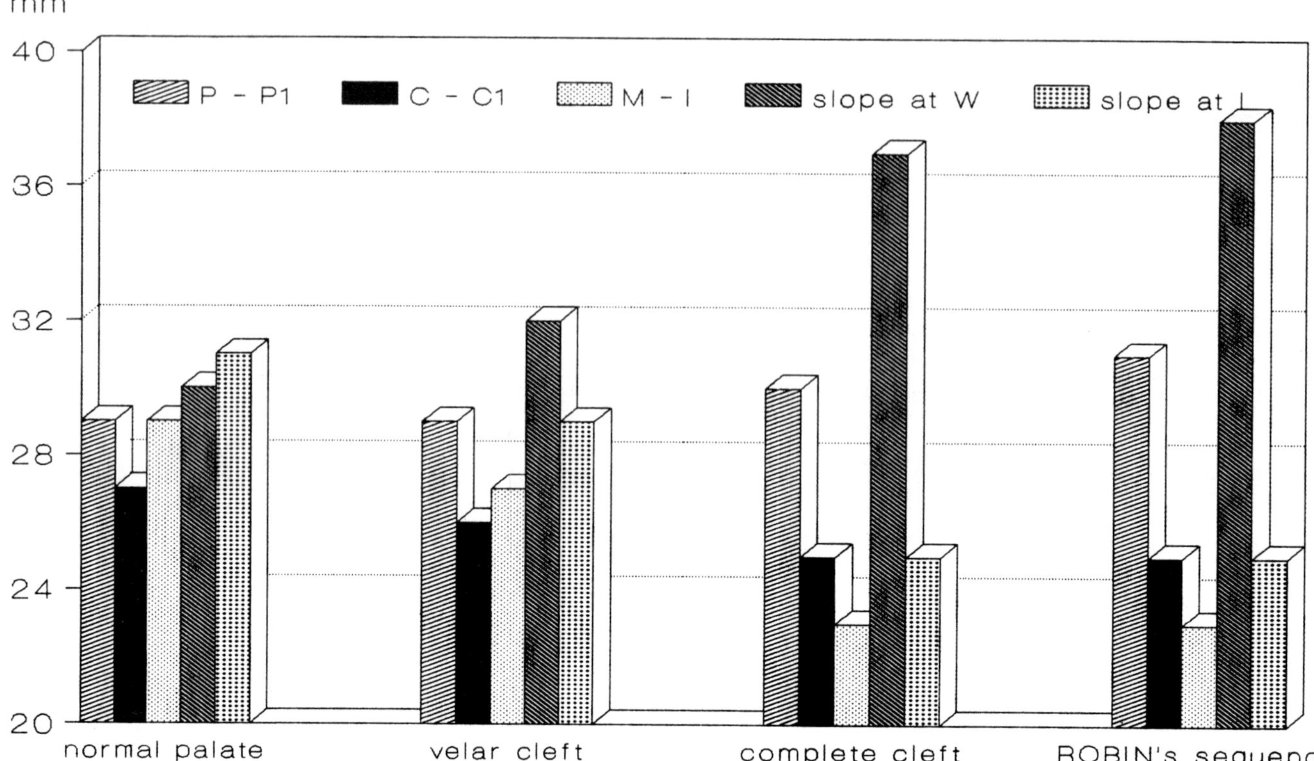

Figure 35–6 Morphologic epitomes of the infant palate. The mean values of five measurements (P–P1, C–C1, M–I, slope at W, and slope at I) characterize the severity of the cleft. The most striking changes are seen in the palatal slopes. The transverse palatal inclination at W–W1 shows an increase of 22.5%, whereas the midsagittal slope at I decreases 17%. Although there is only a slight increase in the distance P–P1, the values of C–C1 and M–I decrease 7.5% and 21%, respectively.

Synopsis

The ratios of distances and palatal slopes support the morphologic description of cleft palates in that the severity of the cleft is indicated by greater quotients (Table 35–4). Five measurements of the infant palate help to comprehend and specify the morphology of the bony palate (Table 35–5). Intrinsic (dental anlagen) and extrinsic factors (the formative dynamics of the tongue and facial tissues) are contained in these descriptive epitomes (Fig. 35–6). Most striking are the reduction of the M–I dimension (from 28.9 to 23 mm) and the considerably increased slope at W (29 to 37.3 degrees) versus the reduction of the midsaggital inclination M–I (31.7 to 24.7 degrees). These noticeable differences may be reproduced in schematic illustrations, morphologic epitomes, which characterize particular types of palate clefts.

The morphologic palate epitomes disclose that Robin's sequence is not a specific morphologic entity but a severe form of the complete cleft of the bony palate. A more severe palate cleft causes a greater shortening of M–I and C–C1 as well as an increase in P–P1. Clefting causes the anteromedial attachment of the velar aponeurosis, to the rudiments of which the cleft velar muscles affix. Secondarily, this anomaly leads to steep palatal inclination measurements and a reduction in the sagittal dimension of both the oral and the pharyngeal palates.

Fascial Apparatus

Fascias are products of muscles such as tendons and aponeuroses and are not merely covers or sheaths.[12, 13] Another characteristic of fascias is their tendency to merge and interlock with one another.[14] They form a network or supportive infrastructure. Finally, fascias are also morphologic, histologic, and even phylogenetic connections between muscle and bone. Outstanding investigations into the nasopharyngeal fascias of the normal nasopharyngeal region were performed more than a hundred years ago.[11, 14, 16]

Velar Aponeurosis

Phylogeny. Phylogenetically, the aponeurosis is derived from the primitive palatopharyngeus muscle.[11] Fibrous

Table 35–4. Ratios of P–P1/M–I and of Slopes at W/I

Diagnosis	P–P1/M–I	W/I
Noncleft palate	29/29 = 1	1
Velar cleft	29/27 = 1.07	32/29 = 1.1
Complete cleft palate	30/23 = 1.3	37/25 = 1.5

Table 35–5. Mean Configuration of Various Forms of the Infant Hard Palate

Diagnoses	P–P1	C–C1	M–I	Slope at W	Slope at I
No cleft	28.7	27	28.9	29	31.7
Velar cleft	29.1	26	26.9	37.7	25.6
Complete cleft palate	30.5	24.5	23	37.1	25.6
Robin's sequence	31.2	24.6	23	37.3	24.7

Note: Three transverse measurements (P–P1, C–C1, slope at W) and two midsagittal evaluations (M–I, slope at I) help to characterize the infant hard palate.

tissues, like fascias, attaching to the aponeurosis have been regarded as substitutes for muscles.[10, 14] They help us to understand the phylogeny of the region. The pathologic findings in velar cleft patients demonstrate that the velar aponeurosis consists of the pharyngeal fascia, which merges with the horizontal tensor tendon and the velar muscles (Fig. 35–7).

The velar aponeurosis constitutes the phylogenetic border between the masticatory region (cranial nerve V) and the velopharynx (cranial nerve IX and X). The aponeurosis belongs to the pharyngeal palate and should therefore be named *velar* rather than *palatal* aponeurosis (Fig. 35–8).

The normal velar aponeurosis serves two functions:

1. In the sagittal direction, it is a junction between the rigid palatine bone and the mobile velopharyngeal muscles.[21] Veau, following this idea, wrote: "The muscles pull the palate long," that is, via their attachments to the velar aponeurosis.[11]
2. In the normal velum, the aponeurosis extends in the transverse direction between the auditory tubes and the fascias, ligaments, and muscles of the lateral oropharyngeal wall. The horizontal tensor tendon

passes around the hamulus into the velar aponeurosis, and its vertical tendon inserts into the pterygomandibular ligament (buccopharyngeal fascia). During deglutition, yawning, and speech, the tensor muscle pulls the lateral edge of the tubal cartilage isometrically downward. At the same time, its horizontal tendon most likely transmits the "pull" from the velar aponeurosis in the transverse direction. Obviously, this connection assists in the coordination of muscle actions in the velopharyngeal region, perhaps by transmitting proprioceptive reflexes.[14]

Whillis supported the erroneous idea that the velar aponeurosis is formed by the expanded tensor muscle tendon.[10] He reported "a split of the aponeurosis near the middle line to enclose the musculus uvulae," a finding that has not been confirmed. Dickson's[22] statements that von Luschka[3] wrote the first description of cleft musculature and detected the lack of the palatal aponeurosis is as false as his assumption that hamular fracture does not affect eustachian tube function on account of the "inferior (tensor) tendon passing around the hamulus and its attachments to the entire length of the posterior rim of the hard palate." Students of velar anatomy are advised to scrutinize von Luschka's monograph on the normal "pharyngeal head" and the extensive anatomic research into the fascial structures of the nasopharyngeal cavity (Fig. 35–9).[14–16]

The rudimentary aponeurosis of the cleft palate dis-

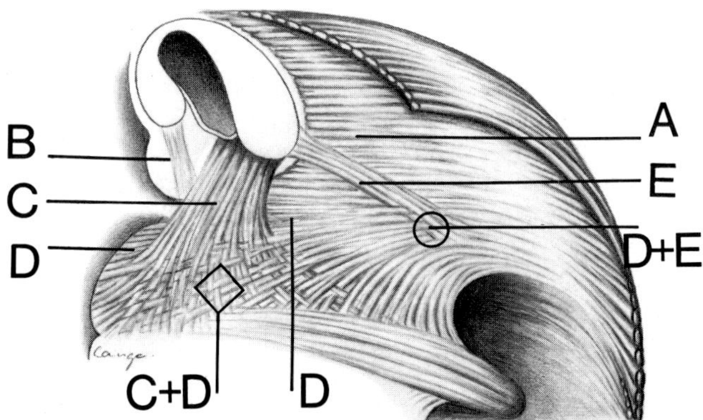

Figure 35–7 Fascias of the normal infant epipharynx. The most important buccopharyngeal fascia (A) forms a coalescent layer around the fibers of the constrictor pharyngis muscle, bordering the sinus of Winslow (W). It attaches strongly at A1 and along the hamulus (pointer). Another portion (A2) enters the anterior portion of the velum to join fibers of the horizontal tensor tendon in the formation of the velar aponeurosis. The tensor tendon (B) swings around the hamulus from a lateral direction into the velar aponeurosis (B1). The tendon has a distinct posterior border over the inferior aspect of the hamulus and can be traced into the velum (B2). Fascial structures from around the levator muscle and ligaments from underneath the membranous portion of the tube also extend into the velar aponeurosis.

Figure 35–8 Muscles in the normal infant epipharynx. A, superior constrictor pharyngis; B, portion of the tensor muscle; C, levator veli palatini muscle; D, palatopharyngeus muscle fibers inserting at the hamulus and passing laterally underneath the levator muscle. Most fibers of the palatopharyngeus and levator veli palatini muscles intermingle in the velum (C + D). D + E represents the area of intertwining muscle fibers of the palatopharyngeus and salpingopharyngeus muscles. The third area of interweaving fibers of the horizontal and longitudinal portions of the palatopharyngeus muscle is not shown.

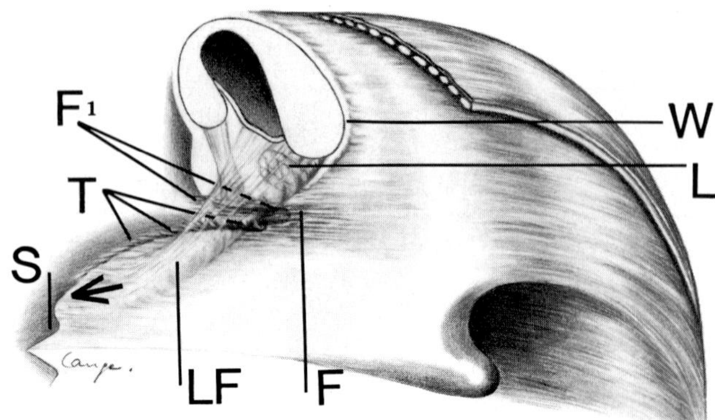

Figure 35–9 Fascias of the cleft velum. The buccopharyngeal fascia borders the sinus of Winslow inferoposterior of the medial tubal edge and affixes to the hamulus. Both portions run forward (F1) as an almost vertical fascia at the inner aspect of the hamulus. The horizontal tensor tendon (T) passes around the hamulus and attaches to the velopharyngeal fascia as a strong transverse bundle with a distinct posterior border. The rudiment of the aponeurosis is but a small strip of fascia, almost vertical and attenuating anteriorly. The anterior fibers of the tensor tendon (T) fan out anteriorly along the posterior edge of the bony palate. The fascia of the levator muscle (LF) and velosalpingeal ligaments enter the velum from a laterocranial position in a forward direction (see Figs. 35–12 and 35–13). W = sinus of Winslow, L = levator muscle, LF = fascia of the levator muscle, F = buccopharyngeal fascia, S = posterior nasal spine.

closes the fundamental nature of velar cleft morphology. Only on first sight does the median nonunion of the main velar muscle slings (palatopharyngeus, levator) seem to be of primary importance. Yet the velar aponeurosis is the prerequisite for the attachment of velar muscles (Fig. 35–10). The missed median union of the velar aponeurosis is the prime morphologic characteristic of the velar cleft, which was recognized as such by Dorrance as early as 1930.[5]

The rudiment of the aponeurosis in the velar cleft reveals its components: the abnormal anterior extension into the velum of the buccopharyngeal fascia and the horizontal tensor tendon. Cleft velar surgery should not be confined only to rearranging muscle fibers within the muscle compartment medial to the pharyngeal fascia.[23–25] These fascial structures are readily and necessarily exposed. Cutting the tensor tendon over the hamulus frees the main pathologic lateral tether of the cleft velar muscle compartment (Fig. 35–11).

In the cleft velum, the horizontal tensor tendon is visualized after the mucosa of the intermaxillary fold is incised and the underlying delicate inner sheath of the buccopharyngeal fascia is separated by blunt dissection. Diligent preparation is guided by the thin fascia. A perforation will result in entering the masticatory region along the lateral pterygoid muscle (Fig. 35–12).

Two landmarks help to identify the rudimentary tensor tendon during surgery: (1) its synovial sheath ("bourse sereuse"[11]) just lateral of the hamulus, and (2) its posterior edge. Passing around the hamulus, the fibers of the tendon fan out anteromedially. They form a thin shiny layer and attach to the velopharyngeal fascia of the velar cleft. This attachment area is the rudiment of the aponeurosis. It reaches from the medial side of the hamulus to the posterior rim of the palatine bone in an almost vertical position (Figs. 35–10 and 35–13).

The posterior border of the tensor tendon is easily visualized just anterior to the tip of the hamulus. Seen from the oral approach, the tensor tendon covers a gliding space lateral to the pharyngeal fascia (Fig. 35–11). The rudiment of the velar aponeurosis becomes visible with a wider anteromedial exposure and after cutting the horizontal tensor tendon over the hamulus. Although the normal velar aponeurosis extends horizontally between the hamular processes, its narrow rudiment is almost vertical. The cleft velar muscles follow their cleft aponeurosis along the inner aspect of the hamulus. This muscle compartment attenuates anteromedially and so does the aponeurotic rudiment (Figs. 35–9 and 35–10).

During the past two decades, the muscular pathology of the cleft velum and its reconstruction have rightfully been emphasized. However, attention has been distracted from the fascial apparatus of the cleft velum. The essence of the velar cleft is not the anterolateral displacement of Veau's "cleft muscle" but rather the lateralization of the aponeurotic rudiments (Fig. 35–13).

The failure to form an aponeurosis not only prevents median muscular union but also contributes to the sagittal reduction and steeper slope of the palatal shelves. It also causes the abnormal displacement of the velopharyngeal fascia medially along the hamulus into the anterior portion of the cleft velum. Although not specifically mentioned, these anatomic relations have been excellently depicted in a reconstruction of serial sections made through the velopharyngeal region of a cleft lip and palate infant by Latham and co-workers.[26] The anatomic locations, direction, and course of the aponeurotic rudiment are especially well outlined in Figures 2 and 3 of their article.

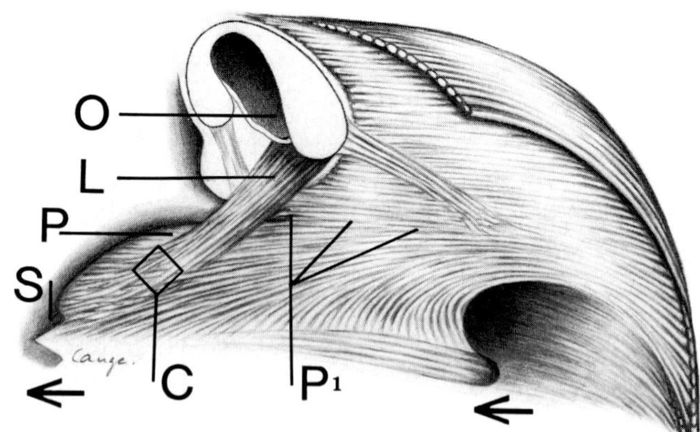

Figure 35–10 Velopharyngeal muscles in the cleft infant velum (right side). The levator muscle (L) has a pathologic posteroinferior convexity and a more anterolateral position below the tubal orifice, which is more inferior in cleft palates. The levator fibers intertwine anteriorly with fibers of the palatopharyngeus muscle to form Veau's "cleft muscle" (rectangle C): Thus Veau's "muscle de la fente" is not one muscle but the anterior portion of two. Fibers of the horizontal portion of the palatopharyngeus muscle pass inferolaterally of the levator muscle (P). Fibers of the palatopharyngeus muscle (P1) inserting at the hamulus or near it belong to the Passavant's portion. The shortening of the cleft palate, indicated by two arrows, can only secondarily be attributed to the muscular displacement, the primary reason being the displacement of the facial apparatus (see Fig. 35–9).

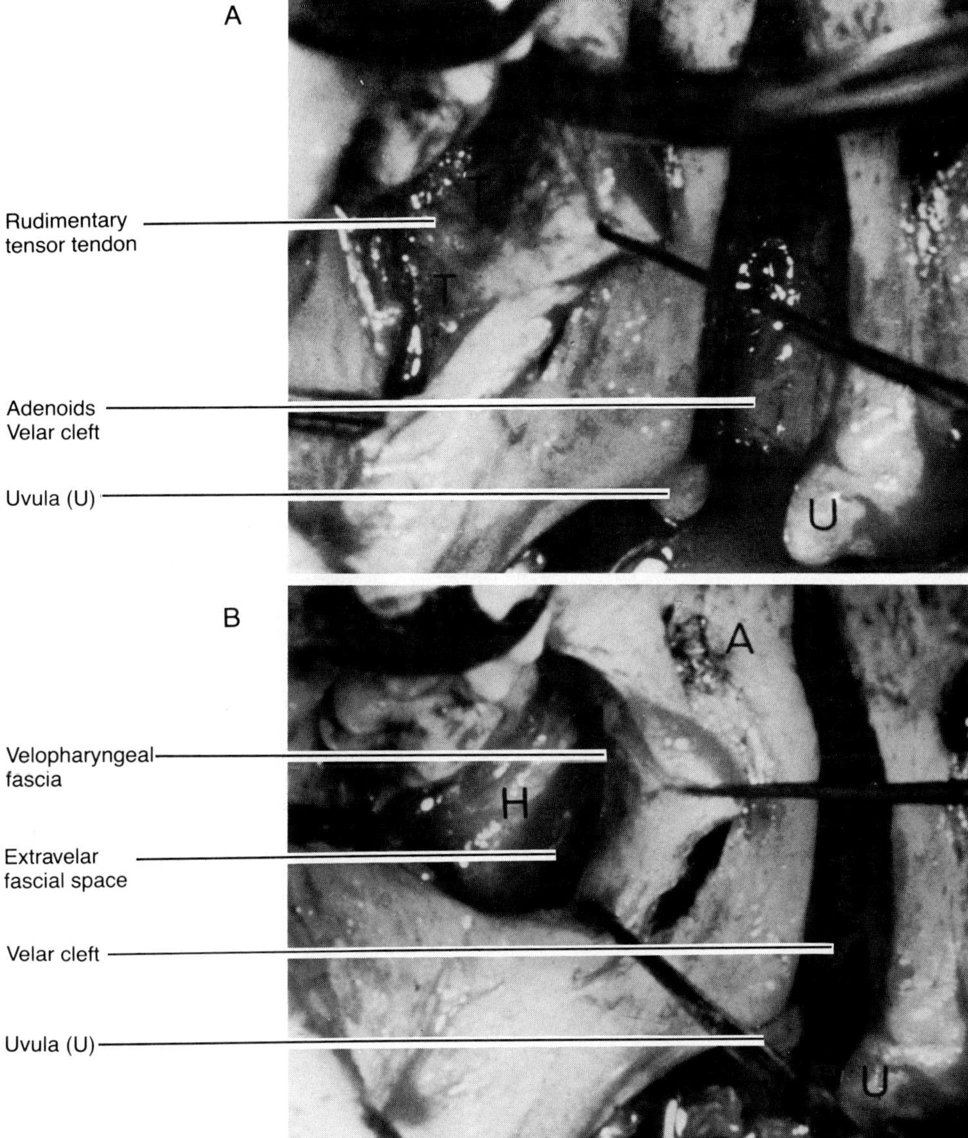

Figure 35–11 Topographic anatomy of the lateral border of the right velum (oral aspect). *A,* The post-tuberosity incision exposes the rudimentary tensor tendon, which enters the cleft velum from around the hamulus and attaches at the velopharyngeal fascia. *B,* Cutting of this tendon exposes the extravelar fascial space, which is bordered medially by the almost vertically oriented fascia. After the tendon has been severed, the traction of the hook can substantially move the velar half medially.

Most anatomic drawings of cleft velar anatomy either lack tendinous structures or show incorrect findings. Some researchers believe they have observed a horizontal velar aponeurosis or at least a portion of it. In Figure 4 of his article, Ruding had the artist show the tensor tendon attached to a velar aponeurosis in the anterior portion of a velar cleft.[6] Such findings would not even be correct for a submucous velar cleft. There are also insertions of sagittal muscle fibers to this "aponeurosis" near the anterior cleft region. In Figure 3 of their article, Fára and Dvorak show the dissection of "a large anastomosis of the tensor tendon with the front bundles of the levator," although in neither the normal nor the cleft velum does the levator muscle attach to the tensor muscle or tendon.[27] Apparently they missed the rudiment of the aponeurosis and failed to dissect the extension of the pharyngeal fascia into the anterior third of the cleft velum of their specimens. Many other researchers and surgeons have erroneously taken for granted the

existence of a horizontal palatal aponeurosis in the cleft palate.[28–32] Illustrations showing a palatal aponeurosis in velar clefts should be revised. The tendinous attachments of the "cleft muscle" to the tunica propria of the mucosa may have been misinterpreted as extending to the velar aponeurosis.

The aponeurosis is seldom correctly understood as an organ of the velar muscles. The velar aponeurosis is generally misinterpreted as a fibrous sheath originating from the tendon of the tensor veli muscle only, "very firmly attached to the mucosa," and giving "the impression of a scar."[6]

Fascias

Embryology. The most important structures develop from "the lateral membranous wall," a remarkably thick, fibrous area adjacent to the membranous portion of the tube between the tensor and levator muscles.[32] It can

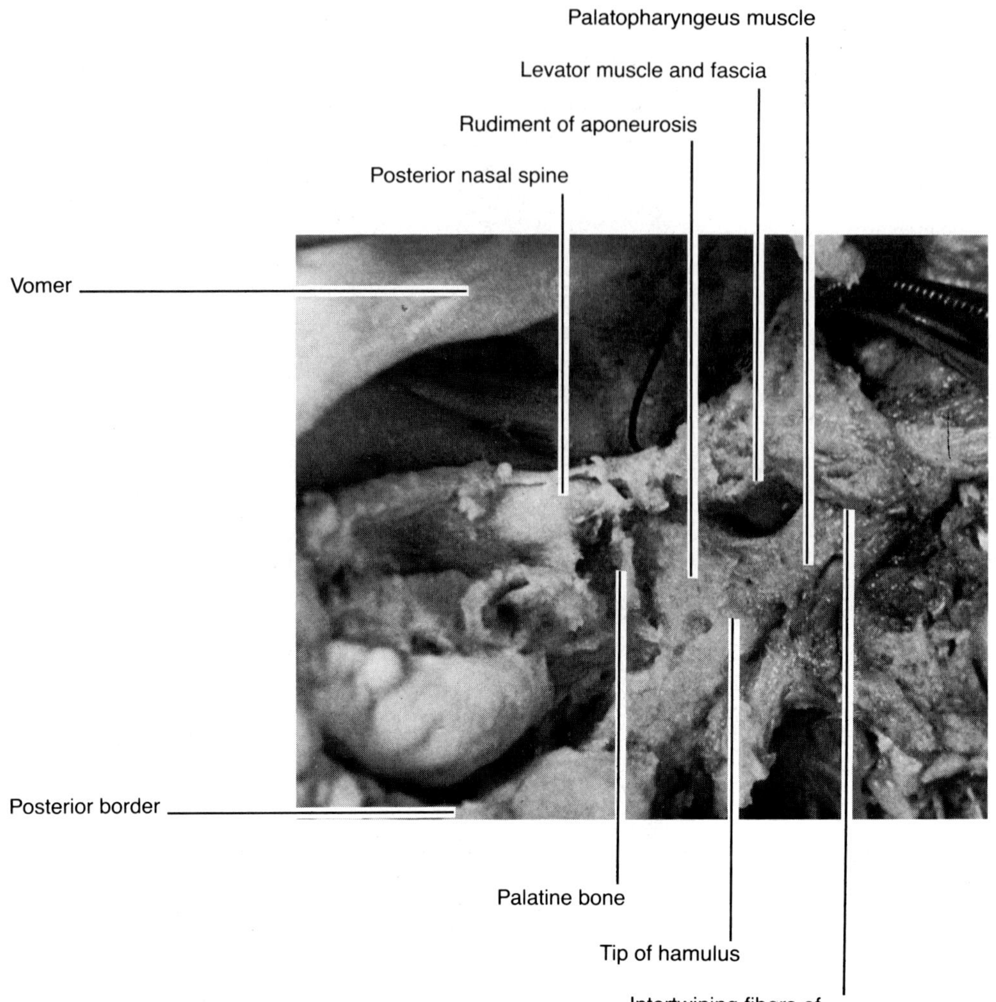

Figure 35–12 Topographic anatomy of the right cleft velar half (oral aspect seen from a medial position). Anterior to the tip of the hamulus the opening of the tensor tendon sheath can be seen, just lateroinferior of the hamulus. The extravelar space has been exposed by posteromedial traction at the anterior portion of the palatopharyngeus muscle (clamp). The rudimentary aponeurosis is dissected medial of the hamulus (near the orifice of the tensor tendon sheath). Fibers of the horizontal portion of the palatopharyngeus muscle pass lateral of the levator muscle. Cutting of the rudimentary tensor tendon at the hamulus would expose the extravelar fascial space as shown in Figure 35–11. The horizontal portion of the palatopharyngeus muscle, which helps to form Passavant's ridge, interweaves with the longitudinal portion in the palatopharyngeal fold.

be identified as early as age 10 weeks, that is, prior to tubal cartilage formation. The "lateral membranous wall" is not dealt with in detail but the phylogenetic borderline between the first and second branchial arch can be clearly seen in the illustrations of a 12-week-old fetus.[33] At this age the tubal length is about 1.5 mm. In a 28-week-old individual with a total tubal length of just under 10 mm there are already structures resembling Ostmann's fat body and the salpingopharyngeal fascia of von Tröltsch.

Buccopharyngeal Fascia. The buccopharyngeal fascia is the mother fascia of the nasopharyngeal cavity and supports the pharynx.[34] It joins the pharyngobasilar fascia cranial to the superior constrictor pharyngis muscle and passes downward and forward around the epipharynx and mesopharynx (sinus of Winslow). It attaches to the hamulus, to the inner margins of the auditory tube fascias, and to the pterygomandibular ligament. An extension continues anteromedially into the cleft velum (see next paragraph on velopharyngeal fascia). The buccopharyngeal fascia is connected by a loose connective tissue layer to the medial cervical fascia (Sappey), which helps to form the carotid and jugular fascial sheath.

Velopharyngeal Fascia. The velopharyngeal fascia is the fascia proper of the cleft palate and can be found only in the cleft velum. It is confined to the area medial of the hamular process and it is derived from the buccopharyngeal fascia. In the normal pharyngeal palate, the fascia is integrated in the velar aponeurosis. In the cleft velum, the velopharyngeal fascia contributes to the rudiment of the aponeurosis. It constitutes the lateral border of the cleft velar muscle compartment.

A striking finding during autopsy dissection of the cleft pharyngeal palate has been the "gliding spaces" lateral to the velopharyngeal fascia.[8] Cutting the tensor tendon opens this layer of loose connective tissue. It serves small vessels. This space is closed cranially by firm fibrous structures at and lateral to the hamulus.

Salpingopharyngeal (von Tröltsch) Fascia. The salpingopharyngeal fascia originates from the entire length of the tubal membrane and attaches to the hamulus. At this location it has connections with the portion of the superior constrictor, which affixes at the pterygoid lamina (musculus pterygopharyngeus Santorini), so that actions of this portion without tensor contractions are likely to affect the tubal membrane. One portion of the buccopharyngeal fascia extends between the entire

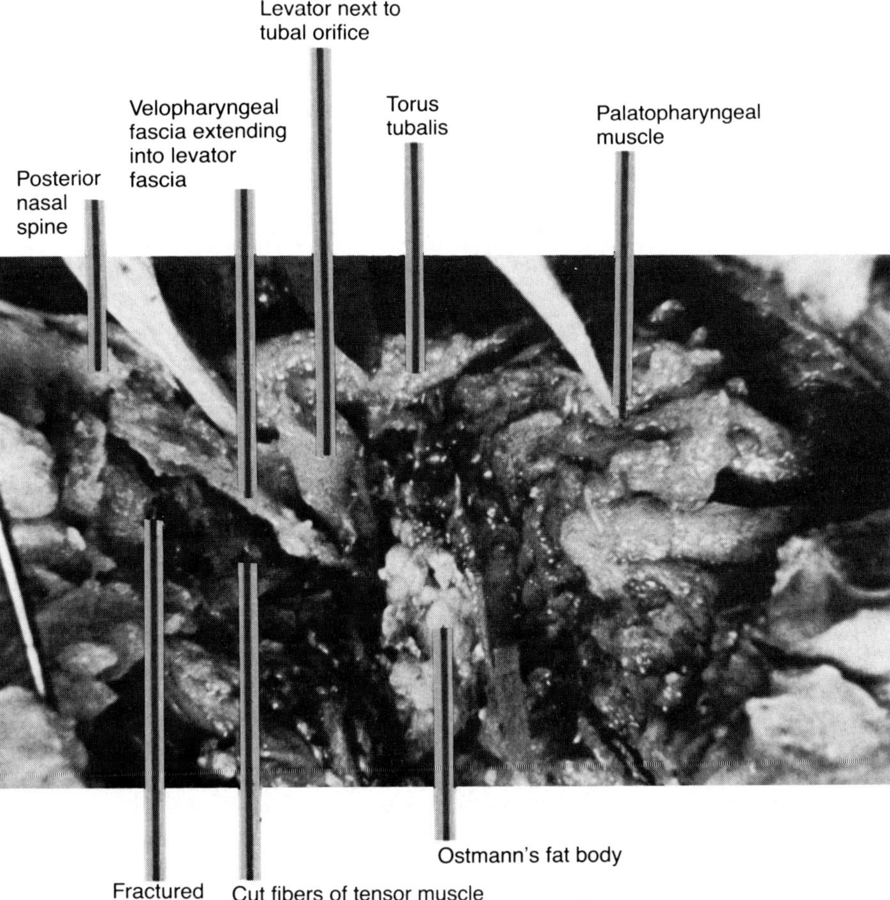

Figure 35–13 Topographic anatomy of right velar half. Oral aspect of horizontal section cranial of the hamular plane. The velopharyngeal fascia extends in a near vertical position to just lateral of the cleft posterior nasal spine (left upper corner). This fascia is continuous with the membranous floor of the auditory tube and von Tröltsch's fascia around the levator muscle. The left wooden pointer rests in the tubal orifice, the right pointer indicates intermingling fibers of the horizontal and downward running portions of the palatopharyngeus muscle.

length of the tubal membrane and the hamulus. From there, it connects with the buccopharyngeal fascia lateral to the superior constrictor. In 1868 von Tröltsch named this fascia, which had already been described by Tourtual, and explained its function. It separates the first from the second branchial arch region—that is, the tensor from the levator muscle.

In a study of the paratubal musculature in a 1-month-old cleft palate infant, the derivatives of the thick "lateral membranous wall" appeared to be squeezed between the levator and the tensor muscles.[35] Because the cleft levator muscle is abnormally positioned lateral to the medial edge of the tubal cartilage and beneath the tubal lumen, the lack of loose connective and fat tissue may be secondary in nature. Two striking findings are the laterocranial position (in relation to the median tubal edge) of at least one portion of the levator muscle and the steep inclination of von Tröltsch's fascia near the tubal orifice, which is positioned more inferiorly than normal. The lumen is completely drawn out in this direction or appears as a recess in an area that shows undulation of the epithelium of the membranous portion of the tube, suggesting elasticity. Perhaps the compression of the tubal lumen by the levator muscle is a result both of the malposition of the levator muscle and the distortion of the salpingopharyngeal fascia.

These findings can also be detected on coronal sections in the study by Latham et al.[26] These authors are concerned with the abnormal pattern of the velar muscles. However, their reconstructions clearly show that the laterocranial displacement of the levator muscle results in an almost direct contact with the tensor muscle. There does not seem to be a significant gliding space (fascias, fat). Furthermore, the membranous portion of the tubal lumen is displaced in the almost vertical direction characteristic of von Tröltsch's fascia in the cleft palate infant.

Salpingopterygopharyngeal (Weber-Liel) Fascia. The fascia of Weber-Liel[16] "covers" the anterolateral aspect of the tensor muscle and separates it from the internal pterygoid muscle. It also is believed to derive from the buccopharyngeal fascia. It is attached skeletally to the pterygoid crest and sphenoid spine.

Ligaments

Salpingopharyngeal (Zuckerkandl) Ligament

The pharyngotubal ligament of Zuckerkandl[36] has been observed when the salpingopharyngeal muscle was not in close contact with the palatopharyngeal muscle, from which it derives.[34] The ligament is believed to be a substitute for muscle fibers, which had been interwoven with it. Thus, the salpingopharyngeal ligament serves as a reinforcement for the same muscle. It attaches to the medial edge of the tubal cartilage near the orifice.

Since the function of the pharyngeal muscles (deglutition, yawning) is grossly synchronous, the contracting salpingopharyngeal muscle and ligament are elevated by the stronger levator muscle in a synergistic opening of the eustachian tube.

Velosalpingeal Ligaments

Up to three bundles have been described passing from the membranous portion of the auditory tube to the nasal side of the velar aponeurosis.[11] They are believed to be fibroelastic reinforcements of the fascial extensions from the velar aponeurosis into the auditory tube. If ligaments are understood as derivatives of muscles, the muscle pertained to here is the levator veli palatini.

Pterygomandibular Ligament

The pterygomandibular ligament originates from the tip of the pterygoid hamulus and runs downward to the retromolar area of the mandible and its mylohyoid line. The pterygomandibular ligament accepts the vertical tendon of the tensor muscle and plays an important role in stabilizing the position of the hamulus. The ligament serves as an attachment for the superior pharyngeal constrictor muscle and the buccinator (ligament bucco-pharyngicium).

Careful parahamular dissection during intravelar veloplasty shows a dense fibrous plane just cranial to the hamulus. It serves as an attachment for von Tröltsch's and Weber-Liel's fascias, a finding that prohibits hamular fracture as well. In the normal palate the medial ends of the tubal fascias terminate at the tip of the hamulus as cleft palates.[3,15] Strong fibers from the membranous portion of the tube (anterior and medial salpingopalatine ligaments) pass transversely into the velar aponeurosis.[14] The pterygomandibular ligament and fibers of the superior constrictor muscle affix to the tip of the hamulus as well. Although the position of the hamulus is likely to be more lateral in the cleft velum, a fracture of the hamulus disrupts its topographic and functional equilibrium within this complex myofascial apparatus (Fig. 35–10).

Cleft Velar Muscles

Developmental Aspects

Phylogeny. Sharks have a pattern of branchial muscles that can be looked on as the base for the other gnathostomata. The shark maxilla is loosely affixed to the cranial base. The levator palatoquadratei muscles of sharks connect the cranial base with the upper jaw (kinetic cranium). This muscle can be compared with the levator muscle of the typical branchial arches in mammals. With the bony union of upper jaw and cranial base, the levator muscle attenuated considerably. The mammalian levator muscle does not originate from the cartilaginous

palatoquadrate (as in sharks) or bones replacing it but from the inferior surface of the anlagen of bones forming the phylogenetically recent lateral cranial base. Thus, there is a reduction in size of the muscle and a spreading of its origin.[37]

Phylogenetically, the tensor veli palatini and the tensor tympani derive from the posterior mandibular adductor muscle. The morphologic union in the human was discovered in 1865 and is a well-confirmed finding.[38] **Ontogeny.** The tensor and levator veli palatini muscles are derived from the foregut and from the first and second branchial arches, respectively. With other mesenchymal elements these muscles extend into the pharyngeal palate as it is formed along with the oral palate from symmetric shelves converging from the margins of the foregut and stomodeum.[1]

Topography

It can be assumed that the origins of the cleft velar muscles and related structures are normal.[6] Their medial portions, however, are displaced anterolaterally. This is particularly true for the levator and palatopharyngeus muscles, which intermingle to form Veau's "cleft muscle."[8]

Levator Palati Muscle

SYNONYMS: *m. peristaphylin intern* (Curveilhier), *m. salpingopalatinus* (Santorini), *m. petrosalpingostaphylinus* (Winslow)

The levator palati muscle originates at the petrous portion of the temporal bone[1] and at the tubal cartilage anterior to the carotid orifice.[34] An abnormal origin from the inferior surface of the tube was detected at autopsy of an infant.[35]

The cleft levator palati muscle runs medially in a downward and forward course along with the salpingopharyngeal fascia. Its fibers intermingle with those of the palatopharyngeus muscle to form the "cleft muscle" medial to Winslow's sinus. Baggerman dissected a cleft velum in which the bundles of Veau's muscle were "macroscopically well visualized."[6] In the cleft palate, the insertions of the levator muscle to the rudiment of the aponeurosis extend to the anterior portion of the cleft. The muscle is of course medial to the velopharyngeal fascia as far anterior as the cleft posterior nasal spine and attaches to the periosteum of the cleft edge, the fascial rudiment, but mainly to the tunica propria of the nasal and oral linings near the cleft posterior nasal spine. The insertions can be defined more distinctly than has been depicted in the literature.[24, 31, 39] The insertion to the tunica propria can be detected on clinical examination as a small, uneven, nodulated area (palatine fovea) posterior to the cleft posterior nasal spine (Fig. 35–14).

After the attachments of the "cleft muscle" have been dissected from the bony cleft edge and the oral and nasal linings have been dissected immediately posterolateral to the cleft posterior nasal spine, delicate dissection reveals muscle fibers of the levator in a discrete

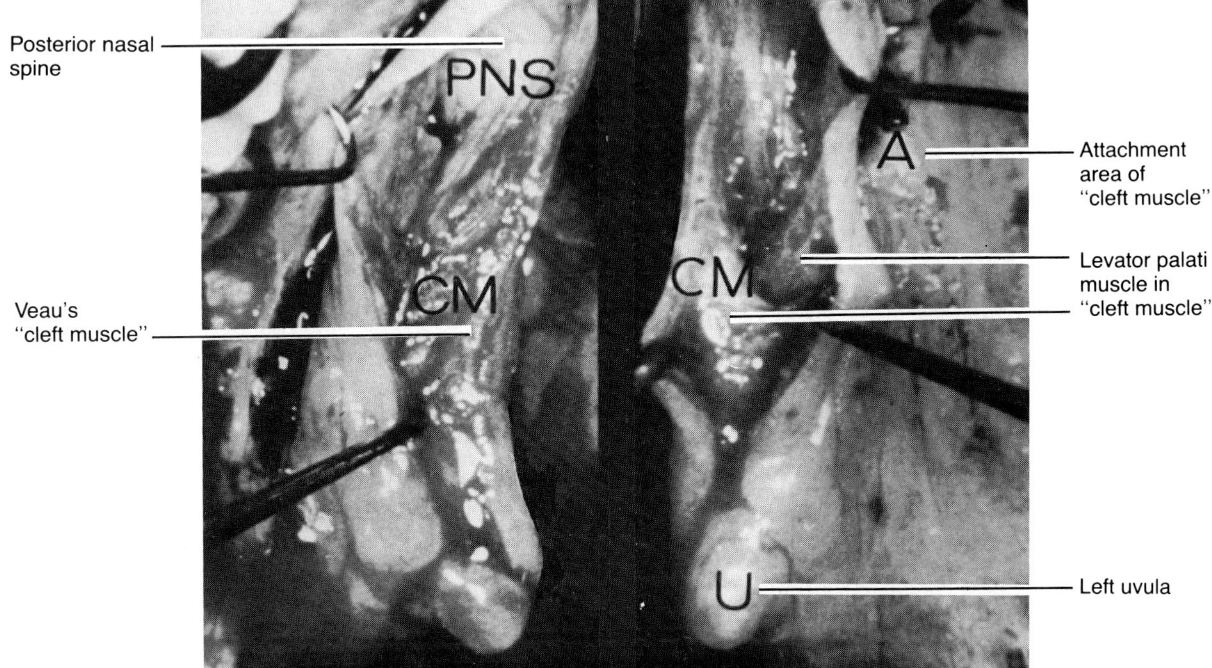

Figure 35–14 Topographic anatomy of the velar cleft edges (oral aspect). Dissection of the right cleft edge and exposure of the cleft posterior nasal spine (PNS) reveals the anteromedial course of the fibers of Veau's "cleft muscle" (CM). Careful further dissection of the left velar half discloses a levator muscle bundle surrounded by the attenuated extensions of von Tröltsch's fascia into the cleft palate (also see Figs. 35–12 and 35–13). On the photograph the attachment area of Veau's cleft muscle at the oral mucosa is exposed at point A and at the posterior nasal spine (PNS) in the other velar half. The attachment area at the nasal lining is not shown. These attachments must be severed for the reconstruction of a levator sling.

fascial compartment within the muscle bulk (Figs. 35–12 and 35–13). They are probably extensions of von Tröltsch's fascia into the cleft velum. They run in a craniolateral direction. Fibers medial and lateral to it belong to the palatopharyngeus muscle, as has been proved by three-dimensional dissection (Fig. 35–9).[26] These muscle fibers are medial to the velopharyngeal fascia, which runs along the inner aspect of the hamulus. During intravelar veloplasty the "cleft muscle"[11] and the pharyngeal fascia are freed from their attachments to allow reconstruction of the muscle sling across the repaired velum.

Freeing the cleft velar muscle from the nasal mucosa is difficult. The anatomic reason for the surgical difficulty is the lack of a layer of submucous salivary glands in the attachment area.[40]

The fibers of the levator that normally turn into the uvula may be neglected in patients with clefts because "they do not exist to all intents and purposes."[6]

In a series of cadaver dissections, the normal levator palati muscle was found to occupy the intermediate 40% of the length of the soft palate. This normal distribution should be the aim in cleft palate repair.[41]

Surgical Anatomy. Ruding made 2- to 3-mm long cuts in the medial border of the nasal mucosa over the "cleft muscle" for a Z-plasty and described the medial border as stiff.[6] A Z-plasty has been advocated to reorient the muscle fibers during cleft palate repair.[23, 25] Walter and Meisel reported about 10 years of experience with a large reversing Z-plasty on the oral and nasal side of each velar half.[25] No attempt was made to dissect the displaced muscular or fascial attachments. A very similar procedure was reported in 1978 and published in 1980.[23]

Difficulties are encountered in dissecting the muscle from the nasal mucosa.[24] It is noted that the "area most likely to have deficiency of tissue is laterally on the nasal side." The anatomic reason for these surgical difficulties is the attachments of the inner layer of the pharyngeal fascia to the nasal lining and the lateral tether of the hamulus by means of the tensor tendon. These surgical interventions are mentioned briefly because no attempt is made to correct the prime anatomic deformity of the cleft velar—that is, the cleft aponeurosis. Surgery is erroneously confined to the cleft velar muscle compartment only.

Tensor Veli Muscle

SYNONYMS: *Peristaphylinus externus* (Riolan 1624), *novus tubae Eustachianiae musculus* (Valsalva 1717), *m. salpingopalatinus* (Santorini 1724), *m. salpingostaphylinus externus* (Winslow 1743), *m. chondrostaphylinus* (Rudinger 1865), *m. dilatator tubae, m. abductor tubae* (von Tröltsch 1864).

The variety of names indicate the uncertainty that existed about the action of the muscle. Still, the present name is a misnomer. As early as 1825 Henle stated that in functional anatomic terms the true stretcher of the palate is the levator not the tensor.[21] Von Tröltsch suggested naming this muscle more correctly the "tensor of the eustachian tube." More recently, others have followed suit.[42–44]

Different portions of the tensor veli muscle originate from normal origins at the scaphoid fossa, the sphenoid spine, and the lateral edge of the eustachian tube. Fibers of its ventral portion originate from Weber-Liel's fascia.[34, 45–47] Except for fibers affixing to the pterygoid and the pterygomandibular ligament, this flat muscle passes medially and downward into a strong horizontal and discrete vertical tendon lateral to the hamulus. This latter medioventral portion attaches to the buccal fascia (pterygomandibular ligament or buccopharyngeal raphe), and the middle portion attaches to the pterygoid.

In the cleft velum, the tensor muscle meets the rudimentary aponeurosis just inferomedial to the hamulus (Fig. 35–10). Unfortunately, the important early investigations into the fascias of the nasopharynx are rarely quoted, yet they hold the key to the understanding of the anatomic essentials of the cleft. It is a false axiom that morphologic changes closer to the cleft margin are more important than those occurring in the cleft velum. The discovery of muscular anomalies in the cleft velum has distracted attention from the fascial apparatus, especially in the hamular region (see earlier section, Fascias).

Superior Constrictor Muscle

The superior constrictor muscle forms the "pharyngeal head"[3] from its attachment at the pharyngeal tubercle down to the pterygomandibular raphe. Its superior fibers pass below and posteriorly around to the levator muscle (sinus of Winslow) and attach to the hamulus. During swallowing, the levator and superior constrictors move cranially to elevate the medial edge of the eustachian tube. Both muscles are the strongest components of the muscular suspensory system of the epipharynx.

Palatopharyngeal Muscle

In the normal velum this muscle originates from the entire width of the velar aponeurosis. In the cleft velum, however, the greater portion of the muscle intermingles with the cleft levator palati muscle to form Veau's "cleft muscle," whereas smaller bundles pass Veau's muscle medially and laterally to affix at the aponeurotic rudiment (Fig. 35–9).[26] Von Kostanecki's concept of the velopharyngeal apparatus as one functional myofacial organ is supported by the fact that the fibers of the palatopharyngeal muscle mingle with those of the superior constrictor in the lateral pharyngeal wall as well as with fibers of the stylopharyngeal muscle in the pharyngopalatine arch.[14]

Passavant's Ridge

Fibers of the palatopharyngeal muscle attach to the tubal cartilage.[14, 21] They may occur separately as the salpingopharyngeal muscle. The more horizontal fibers pass onto the pterygomandibular ligament and help to form Passavant's ridge along with fibers of the superior constrictor.[48]

In 1893, autopsy findings of the velopharyngeal region of an adult male with cleft palate revealed that the palatopharyngeal muscle was remarkably more developed than in normals.[49] Clinically, this compensatory hypertrophy had been noticed by Passavant in 1869.[48] He described a ridge located 3 mm above to 7 mm below the tubercle of the arch of the atlas. Later, there was uncertainty about which muscle formed this ridge. Fergusson,[7] Passavant,[48] Dorrance,[5] Veau,[11] and many more have expressed the opinion that the ridge contains fibers of the superior constrictor. Others claimed that fibers of the palatopharyngeal muscle produced this "bar."[3, 10] Because there are, however, "consistent interconnections" and "hopelessly entangled fibers of both muscles," it seems impossible to differentiate the two in the ridge.[50]

Salpingopharyngeal Muscle

The salpingopharyngeal muscle derives from the lateral portion of the palatopharyngeal muscle. The fibers may intermingle.[34] If they run independently, the intermuscular space contains the pharyngotubal ligament of Zuckerkandl.[36] Only in the noncleft velum does the muscle assist the action of the levator muscle during their combined contraction because the cleft levator muscle moves laterally instead of dorsally.

Palatoglossal Muscle

The palatoglossal muscle is a small bundle in the anterior palatal arch,[34] narrower in the middle of the normal palate than at either end. These findings correlate well with findings of distinct extrinsic glossal muscles in the normal infant. However, the direct muscular relation of the palatoglossal muscle to the soft palate is minor.[1] In the normal velum the palatopharyngeal and palatoglossal muscle loops were found to insert into the anterior part of the aponeurosis.[6]

Fára and Dvorak, in a gross anatomic dissection of a compact "cleft muscle," found almost as strong a bundle of muscle fibers medially along the cleft margin, which they attributed to the palatoglossal muscle.[27] Neither the amount of muscle nor its far anteriorly reaching course correlate with findings produced in a three-dimensional anatomic reconstruction.[26] These fibers apparently belong to the palatopharyngeal muscle. However, the palatoglossal muscle forms a very thin, superficial, and discrete layer of fibers in the anterior palatal arch, hardly visible during surgery.

Uvular Muscle

SYNONYMS: *m. medialis veli, m. azygos, m. levator uvulae, m. palatostaphylinus.*

Comparative Anatomy. This muscle is present in *Cercopithecus* (tail-bearing monkey), the gorilla, and man.[51] However, animals without a uvula, for example, the dog, may have a sagittal palatine muscle. The uvular muscle of man and the palatine muscle of domesticated animals are homologous.[47] In carnivores and the horse, the muscle occurs in pairs, and its fibers unite with those of the palatopharyngeal muscle. This has been rarely observed in primates and not at all in man, in whom the uvular muscle terminates in the uvula.

Microscopic Anatomy. The characteristic findings of the uvular muscle are ringbindings and lateral and terminal buds of the myofibrils.[52] The ringbindings have been found to increase in number with age and are consistently present at the age of 20 years,[53] a finding that should be mentioned in conjunction with the fact that "the uvula develops long after the other muscles have obtained their definite shape."[6] However, in one of the first examinations of an infantile uvula in 1898, practically normal tissue was found.[54] A uvular muscle biopsy of a 6-month-old cleft infant revealed hypolemmal ringbindings and lateral sarcolemmal buds but no Conheim's striation.[7]

There is a single report of a median split of the aponeurosis in the normal velum that accepted the uvular muscle.[10] Although this statement has never been confirmed, it might substantiate the findings of Voth that the uvular muscle is located in its own fascial compartment in the normal palate.[11] In a three-dimensional reconstruction of a cleft palate, the cleft uvular muscle was located at the medioventral aspect of Veau's "cleft muscle."[26]

Function of Velar Muscles

In 1923 the palatoglossus was believed to be the second most important muscle in the velum after the tensor muscle.[4] Its functional importance has been over-rated for a few decades, ever since Whillis in 1932 suggested that the nasopharyngeal isthmus be named the *palatopharyngeal sphincter*, often called the *sphincter of Whillis*.[10] Still, in 1964 it was stressed that the tongue and the palatopharyngeal and palatoglossal muscle loops form the oropharyngeal sphincter.[6] Apparently this notion prevailed until the intravelar reconstruction of the levator muscle sling was described in 1970.[9]

It has been pointed out that the cleft levator veli muscle has two ipsilateral attachments.[7, 9] While the normal levator sling runs in the forward and downward direction, the cleft levator muscle has a posterior convexity. The pathologic course results in a pathologic action. Although the normal levator sling contracts *isotonically* in an upward and backward direction, there is only a limited period of isotonic contraction during the lateral and upward movement of the cleft levator. It terminates in an *isometric* contraction between the two ipsilateral attachments of the cleft levator. Enforced isometric action of an isotonically working muscle results in muscular atrophy. In fact, in a series of 18 autopsies of stillborn cleft infants considerable hypoplasia (some 50% of the norm) was found.[27] Recently, the pathologic action of the cleft levator muscle has been shown on nasendoscopic videofilm. On contraction it occluded the orifice of the eustachian tube.[55]

In the normal infant the portion of the levator adjacent to the auditory tube is a compact, rounded column of muscle enclosed by fascia. The muscle becomes broader as it enters the palate,[11] and the cleft levator muscle has a more anterolateral location under the medial portion of the tube, even compressing the lumen.[35] This finding would correlate with the pathologic course mentioned above. In an autopsy specimen, the levator muscle was found to be made up of two abnormally separated bundles, occupying the space underneath the medial edge of the tubal cartilage and the floor of the lumen, respectively.[35] However, this solitary finding seems to be rather normal because the origin of a smaller second portion of the muscle[3, 15] and two insertions have been reported as "regular" ones.[21]

The dimpling during phonation observed in many normal and cleft palate subjects has been reproduced in cadavers by levator palati traction. On serial histologic sections, these dimplings corresponded to levator insertion. Retropositioning of the levator in palate repairs has resulted in improved speech.[41]

It is wrong to state that after the luxation of the hamulus, the tensor function is taken over by the "cooperating" palatoglossal and palatopharyngeal muscles (see earlier section Pterygomandibular Ligament).[6]

Innervation

The tensor muscle is supplied by a branch of the third division of the trigeminal nerve, which innervates the medial pterygoid muscle also.[56] In the cat, the rostral two-thirds of the medioventral division of the trigeminal motoneuron has been determined to supply the tensor muscle.[57]

It is generally accepted that the remaining velar musculature, specifically the levator veli muscle, is innervated by the ninth cranial nerve, the pharyngeal plexus of the tenth cranial nerve, and the superficial petrous branch of the eighth nerve via the sphenopalatine ganglion, but this branch has not yet been unanimously defined.[58–61] Again in the cat, the related motoneurons within the nucleus ambiguus (i.e., possibly cranial nerve IX or X) have been established.[57] The course of the nerve branches follows that of the stylopharyngeus muscle. The branches that supply the superior constrictor and the levator muscle pass medial to the stylopharyngeus muscle and ascend to the sinus of Winslow, quite similar to the course of the velar arteries. These branches are predominantly vagal, whereas the more rostral branches, which innervate the palatoglossal and palatopharyngeal muscles, pass laterally over the stylopharyngeal muscle and ascend into the soft palate.[56]

Blood Supply

The main blood supply for the velar muscles arrives through the branches of the ascending palatine artery from the facial artery. From outside of the superior constrictor muscle, the vessels enter the soft palate via Winslow's sinus in an anterocaudal direction. They run along the pharyngeal side of the border between the first and second branchial arches, that is, at or through the levator muscle, and supply the central portion of the velar musculature.

The greater palatine artery, which mainly supplies the hard palate, sends only a few small branches posteriorly into the velum. From the same palatine foramen, the lesser palatine artery turns posteriorly and provides blood for the anterior oral side of the soft palate. Branches of the tonsillar artery enter the velum along the palatoglossal muscle and provide blood for the lateral velar portions. Branches of the ascending pharyngeal artery reach their peripheral velar supply zone by perforating the palatopharyngeal muscle.[56] The examination of the arterial supply of the bony cleft palate region in three fetuses has revealed considerable variation.[62]

ACKNOWLEDGMENT. The author gratefully acknowledges the generous support provided by the Wolfgang Ritter Foundation, Bremen.

References

1. Bosma JF: Anatomy of the Infant Head. Baltimore: Johns Hopkins University Press, 1986.
2. Kostanecki von K: Zur Morphologie der Tubengaumenmusculatur und ihrer Fascien. Arch Mikroskop Anat 32:479, 1888.
3. Luschka von H: Der Schlundkopf des Menschen. Tubingen: H. Laupp, 1868.
4. Brophy TW: Cleft Lip and Palate. Philadelphia: Blakiston, 1923.
5. Dorrance GM: Congenital insufficiency of the palate. Arch Surg 21:185, 1930.
6. Ruding R: Cleft palate: Anatomic and surgical considerations. Plast Reconstr Surg 33:132, 1964.
7. Kriens O: Anatomy of the velopharyngeal area in cleft palate. Clin Plast Surg 2:261, 1975.
8. Kriens O: Anatomische Untersuchungen am gespaltenen weichen Gaumen. Chir Plast Reconstr (Springer) 4:14, 1967.
9. Kriens O: Fundamental anatomic findings for an intravelar veloplasty. Cleft Palate J 7:27, 1970.
10. Whillis J: A note on the muscles of the palate and the superior constrictor. J Anat 65:92, 1931.
11. Veau V, Borel S: Division Palatine, Anatomie, Chirurgie, Phonetique. Paris: Masson, 1931.
12. Bardeleben K: Fascien und Fascienspanner. Jenaische Ztschr Naturwiss 12:94, 1878.
13. Bardeleben K: Muskeln und Fascien. Jenaische Ztschr Naturwiss 14:339, 1882.
14. Kostanecki von K: Zur Morphologie der Tubengaumenmusculatur und ihrer Fascien. Arch Mikroskop Anat 32:479, 1888.
15. Tröltsch von NN: Beitrager zur anatomischen und physiologische Wurdigung der Tube- und Gaumenmuskulatur. Arch Ohrenheilkd 1:15, 1864.
16. Weber-Liel FE: Über die Beziehung des M. levator veli zur Tuba eustachii. Monatschr Ohrenheilkd 5:81, 1871.
17. Leukart FS: Untersuchungen über das Zwischenkieferbein des Menschen in seiner und abnormen Metamorphonse. Stuttgart: Schweizbart, 1840.
18. Ashley-Montagu MF: The form and dimension of the palate in the newborn. Int J Orthod Dent Child 694, 1934.
19. Sillman JH: Dimensional changes of the dental arch: Longitudinal studies from birth to 25 years. Am J Orthod 50:11, 1964.
20. Kriens O: Three-dimensional model analyses of infant maxillary plaster models with the reflex microscope. In Kriens O (ed): The Untreated Cleft Lip and Palate. A Multidisciplinary Update. Stuttgart: G. Thieme, 1989, p. 135.
21. Henle J: Schlundmuskeln, Gaumenmuskeln. In Handbuch Systematischer Anatomie des Menschen. Vol. 2. Braunschweig: F. Vieweg & Sohn, 1866, p. 104.
22. Dickson DR: Normal and cleft palate. Cleft Palate J 9:280, 1972.
23. Furlow IT: Double reversing Z-plasty for cleft palate. In Millard DR (ed): Cleft Craft. Vol. 3. Alveolar and Palatal Deformities. Boston: Little, Brown, 1980, p. 519.
24. Randall P, LaRossa D, Solomon M, et al: Experience with the Furlow double-reversing Z-plasty for cleft palate repair. Plast Reconstr Surg 77:569, 1986.
25. Walter C, Meisel HH: A new method for the closure of a cleft palate. J Maxillofac Surg 6:222, 1978.
26. Latham RA, Long RE, Latham EA: Cleft palate velopharyngeal musculature in a five-month-old infant: A three dimensional histological reconstruction. Cleft Palate J 17:1, 1980.
27. Fára M, Dvorak J: Abnormal anatomy of the muscles of the palatopharyngeal closure in cleft palates. Plast Reconstr Surg 46:488, 1970.
28. Brown AS, Cohen MA, Randall P: Levator muscle reconstruction: Does it make a difference? Plast Reconstr Surg 72:1, 1983.
29. Maue-Dickson D, Dickson DR: Anatomy and physiology related to cleft palate: Current research and clinical implications. Plast Reconstr Surg 65:83, 1980.
30. Millard RD: Cleft Craft. Vol. 3. Alveolar and Palatal Deformities. Boston: Little, Brown, 1980, p. 36.
31. Randall P: The cleft palate. In Grabb WC, Smith JW (eds): Plastic Surgery, 3rd ed. Boston: Little, Brown, 1979.
32. Trier WC: Velopharyngeal incompetency in the absence of overt cleft palate: Anatomic and surgical considerations. Cleft Palate J 20:209, 1983.
33. Swarts JD, Rood SR, Doyle WJ: Fetal development of the auditory tube and paratubal structures. Cleft Palate J 23:289, 1986.
34. Proctor B: Anatomy of the eustachian tube. Arch Otolaryngol 97:2, 1973.
35. Doyle WJ, Kitajiri M, Sando I: The anatomy of the auditory tube and paratubal musculature in a one month old cleft palate infant. Cleft Palate J 20:218, 1983.
36. Zuckerkandl E: Beitrag zur Anatomie des Gehororgans. Monatschr Ohrenheilkd 18:201, 1884.
37. Romer AS: The Vertebrate Body, 4th ed. Philadelphia: Saunders, 1970.
38. Rudinger NN: Ein Beitrag zur Anatomie und Histologie der Eustachischen Röhre. Ärztl Intelligenzbl (München) 37:511, 1865.
39. Coston GN, Hagerty RF, Jannarone RJ, et al: Levator muscle reconstruction: Resulting velopharyngeal competence, a preliminary report. Plast Reconstr Surg 77:911, 1986.
40. Voth D: Zur funktionellen Morphologie des menschlichen Gaumens. Anat Anz 110:2, 1961.
41. Boorman JG, Sommerlad BC: Levator palati and palatal dimples: Their anatomy, relationship and clinical significance. Br J Plast Surg 38:326, 1985.
42. Honjo I, Okazari N, Kumazawa T: Experimental study of the eustachian tube function with regard to its related muscles. Acta Otolaryngol 87:84, 1979.
43. Honjo I, Okazaki N, Nozoe T: Role of the tensor veli palatini muscle in movement of the soft palate. Acta Otolaryngol 88:137, 1979.
44. Rich AR: A physiological study of the eustachian tube and its related muscles. Johns Hopkins Hosp Bull 352:206, 1920.
45. Himmelreich HA: M. tensor veli palatini der Saugetiere unter Beruchsichtigung seines Aufbaus, seiner Funktion und seiner Entwicklungsgeschichte. Anat Anz 115:1, 1964.
46. Korner F: Die Muskeln tensor und levator veli palatini. Ztschr Anat Entwicklgesch 111:508, 1942.
47. Kunzel E, Luckhaus G, Scholz P: Vergleichend-anato-mische Untersuchungen der Gaumenmuskulatur. Zeitschr Anat Entwicklgesch 125:276, 1966.
48. Passavant G: Ueber die Verschliessung des Schlundes beim Sprechen. Arch Pathol Anat Physiol Klin Med 64:1, 1869.
49. Röse C: Ueber die Wirkung der Muskulatur bei angeborener Gaumenspalte. Centralbl Allg Pathol Anat 4:64, 1893.
50. Townshend RH: On the formation of Passavant's bar. J Laryngol 60:154, 1940.
51. Lubosch W: Muskeln des Kopfes, viscerale Muskulatur. In Lubosch W (ed): Handbuch vergl. Anat. Wirbeltiere. Vol. 5. Berlin: Urban & Schwarzenberg, 1938.
52. Graf P: Eigenartige Strukturverhaltnisse in der Muskulatur der menschlichen Uvula. Ztschr Anat 114:399, 1949.
53. Wohlfahrt G: Quergestreifte Ringbinden in normalen Augenmuskeln. Anat Anz 74:228, 1932.
54. Hoen AG: On a form of degeneration of striated muscle met with in the uvula. J Exp Med 3:550, 1898.
55. Godbersen GS: Endoscopy in cleft lip and palate patients. The mechanical obstruction of the eustachian tube preoperatively. In Kriens O (ed): The Untreated Cleft Lip and Palate. A Multidisciplinary Up-date. Stuttgart: G. Thieme, 1989, p 99.
56. Broomhead IW: The nerve supply of the muscles of the soft palate. Br J Plast Surg 4:1, 1951.
57. Keller JT, Saunders MC, van Loveren H, et al: Neuroanatomical Considerations of Palatal Muscles: Tensor and levator veli palatini. Cleft Palate J 21:70, 1984.
58. Moritz W: Über die Funktion und Innervation der Muskulatur des weichen Gaumens. Ztschr Anat 109:197, 1939.
59. Nickl VE: Über die Innervation des M. levator veli palatini durch den N. fascialis. Arch Psychiatr Nervenkr 184:117, 1950.
60. Nishio J, Matsuya T, Machida J, et al: The motor nerve supply of the velopharyngeal muscles. Cleft Palate J 13:20, 1976.
61. Rich AR: The innervation of the tensor veli palatini and levator veli muscles. Johns Hopkins Hosp Bull 31:305, 1920.
62. Maher WP: Distribution of palatal and other arteries in cleft and non-cleft human palates. Cleft Palate J 14:1, 1977.

CHAPTER 36

Cleft Palate Repair: Von Langenbeck Technique

William K. Lindsay and Mary Anne Witzel

In 1861, Bernard von Langenbeck, a German surgeon from Berlin, described a new method of palatoplasty or uranoplasty using mucoperiosteal flaps for the repair of the hard palate portion of the defect (Fig. 36–1).[1] This was a great step forward because prior to this time only mucous membrane flaps had been attempted, and these frequently became necrotic. Von Langenbeck's name has been associated with the surgical repair of cleft palate more than that of any other surgeon. The merits and shortcomings of his technique have been debated more than those of any other cleft palate operation.

There has been a reasonable degree of controversy over who should be given credit for devising the mucoperiosteal flap method. Grey Turner considered that Sir William Ferguson deserved the credit, but he could produce no published proof.[2] Wardill, during a Hunterian lecture in 1933, referred to the Langenbeck-Ferguson method, recognizing this controversy.[3] However, in 1873, Ferguson remarked that "in the so-called Langenbeck operation—that is, where mucoperiosteal flaps are taken from the roof of the mouth and drawn toward the middle line—the proceeding is often unsuccessful from the fact that, after some time, the granulations which are thrown out on the upper surfaces of the displaced flaps contract and separate the union that may have taken place between the paired edges of the flaps."[1] One can conclude from this that Ferguson himself gave due credit for the mucoperiosteal flap procedure to von Langenbeck. Other authors seek to give credit for this method both to Johann Dieffenbach (1792–1847) of Germany and to Jonathan Mason Warren (1811–1847) of the United States.[4, 5] Lateral relaxing incisions were the only common factor in the methods of the three surgeons described. Dieffenbach and Warren gave their names to a bone flap method of repairing a cleft palate, whereas von Langenbeck described a method that utilized mucoperiosteal flaps.[6] These developments are all beautifully summarized by Millard.[7]

Von Langenbeck stated, in his article entitled Uranoplasty by Detaching the Mucoperiosteal Lining of the Hard Palate, that "the uranoplasty [repair of the hard palate] consists of the following stages whether staphylorrhaphy [repair of the soft palate] is done at the same time or not: (I) incising the edges of the cleft, (II) division of a palatine musculature, (III) lateral incision, (IV) detaching the mucoperiosteal flaps of the palate, (V) application of sutures."[8]

Von Langenbeck proceeded to describe these five stages in such detail and clarity in his 1861 manuscript that many surgeons performing this procedure today carry out what are essentially the same steps. The description, to follow later in this chapter and illustrated in Figure 36–2, is very similar to von Langenbeck's classic description and is frequently referred to as the modern Langenbeck palatoplasty. I (W.L.) sometimes refer to it as the simple closure palatoplasty because it is the simplest of the palate operations with the possible exception of the bone flap procedures described by Warren,[15] Dieffenbach,[4] and Wise.

Von Langenbeck retained an anterior attachment for the flaps and avoided the ligation of the palatine neurovascular bundles. In effect, a double-based flap was developed on each side of the midline. He also denuded the free border of the nasal septum to allow attachment of the palatal flaps.

The Langenbeck method became very popular in Great Britain and Europe and to a lesser degree in the United States. By the early 1920s, the Langenbeck and

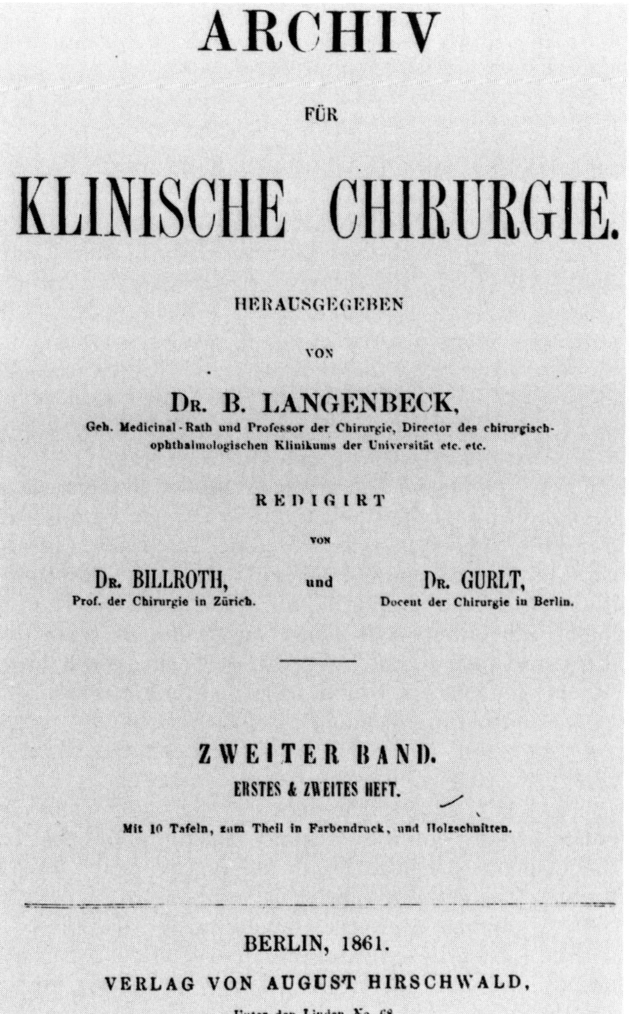

Figure 36–1 The front of the monograph or journal in which Bernard von Langenbeck published the details of his operation for the repair of both the hard and soft palates and the use of mucoperiosteal flaps.

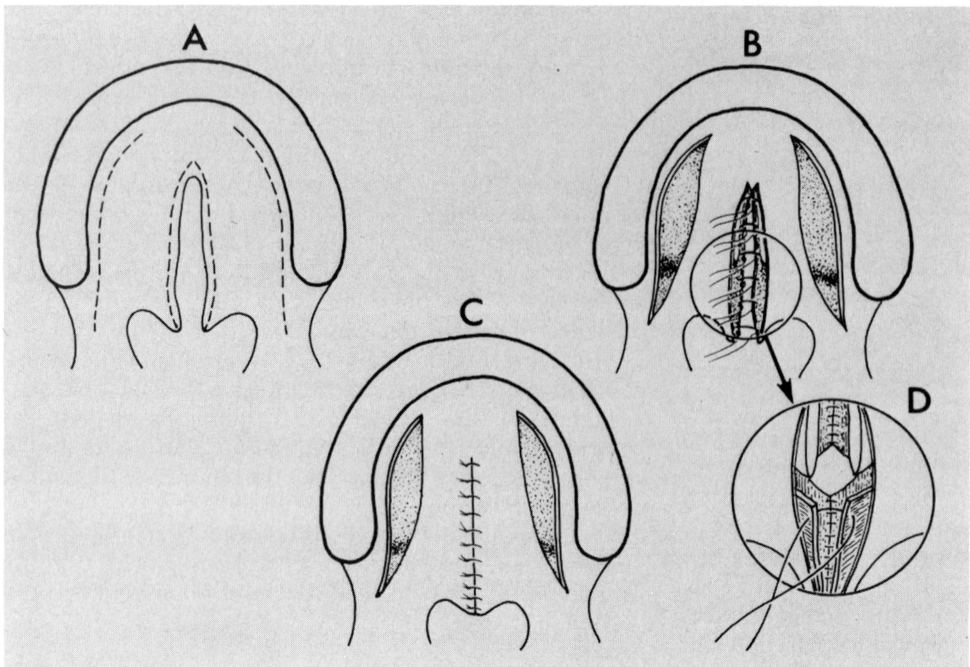

Figure 36–2 Von Langenbeck (simple closure) palatoplasty for isolated cleft palate. *A*, The incision lines for the margins of the soft and hard palate lateral release incisions. *B*, Closure of the nasal mucosa. In this case, direct closure, leaving the nasal mucosa intact, is shown. This is possible only in narrower and less extensive clefts. Not shown is the fact that the hamuli have been infractured; the mucoperiosteal flaps have been elevated, leaving the posterior palatine artery intact but freeing it from its foramen; and some tenuous fibers running from the region of the maxillary tuberosity to the vicinity of the posterior palatine artery have been cut. *C*, Closure of the oral mucosa. Note that the anterior mucoperiosteum is still intact and there is a bipedicled mucoperiosteal flap on either side. The opportunities for pushback are not as great. The lateral open areas are not as large as those shown in the other operations. *D*, An enlarged drawing of the circled area illustrating one of the controversial concepts. The nasal mucosa is transected and allowed to drop back with the soft palate, leaving a controversial raw nasal area. The tensor and levator muscle mass is shown, already dissected from the posterior nasal spine and the palatal aponeurosis. These muscles are directly sutured to each other.

the flap method of Arbuthnot Lane were the two procedures in vogue in Great Britain, whereas the Langenbeck and Dieffenbach-Warren-Davis bone flap techniques were the leading methods in the United States.[9] By 1927, Victor Veau, of Paris, began a scathing attack, in lectures and articles, on the Langenbeck method: "Langenbeck's method results in short, immobile palates due to sclerosis caused by cicatrization of a large bleeding surface of the nasal aspect of the palate which in turn is related to the wide undermining necessary to lower the flaps."[9] It is interesting to note that the technique Veau recommended was based on the Lane flap method plus the use of mucous membrane from the vomer as a flap. By the late 1920s, interest was shifting to push-back or palatal lengthening procedures, led by Sir Harold Gillies and Kelsey Fry. A major objection to the von Langenbeck repair was expressed by Ivy and Curtis in 1934 when they wrote, "Even if complete union occurs, there is much scar tissue contracture which pulls forward the soft palate, creating insufficiency there and preventing velopharyngeal closure so necessary for good speech."[10] Lewin, who in 1964 surveyed methods of management of cleft palate in the United States and Canada, found that half the surgeons participating in the survey used a form of the von Langenbeck repair.[11]

It is obvious that the Langenbeck palatoplasty is worthy of continued in-depth investigation because of its popularity in this era of palatal lengthening surgery and the concerns about velopharyngeal inadequacy. This operation serves also as a baseline for comparison with innovative techniques such as the Furlow procedure.[12]

Objectives of a Cleft Palate Operation

The major objectives of a cleft palate operation can be stated under three headings, none of which is independent:
1. To produce normal speech.
2. To produce anatomic closure.
3. To minimize maxillary growth inhibition and dentoalveolar deformities.

The advantages and disadvantages of a Langenbeck palatoplasty have been debated under these same headings.

Normal Speech

It is agreed by all that velopharyngeal closure is the prime essential for normal speech and that this is dependent on palatal length and mobility together with other velopharyngeal and neuromotor coordination factors. The relative importance of each factor is open to question. It is generally agreed, although it has not been proved, that the Langenbeck operation does not produce as long a palate as the modern push-back procedures but perhaps produces a more mobile palate.

Anatomic Closure

Complete anatomic closure of the palate, separating the nasal cavity from the oral cavity, has a lesser although still significant relationship to speech. Complete physical closure is also attempted to prevent the nasal escape of food and air. The Langenbeck procedure does not offer the surgical satisfaction of attempting to close the extreme anterior end of the hard palate and alveolar regions when the cleft is wide. The mucoperiosteum is not undermined or dissected in this region. Fistulas or residual defects of the anterior portion of the hard palate remain after the Langenbeck operation unless secondary procedures are done.

Dentoalveolar Development and Maxillary Growth

The role of surgery in retarding anteroposterior, lateral, and vertical maxillary growth has been debated since 1949.[13] Both the timing and the type of surgery have been considered. The evidence tends to incriminate the sequelae of surgery as the major factors producing impaired maxillary growth and dentoalveolar deformities. If surgery is a factor, it should be possible to determine which types of surgery are less inhibiting to maxillary growth. The Langenbeck procedure involves less dissection and detachment of tissues from the anterior portions of the hard palate and the alveolus. It was reasoned that this operation might produce less interference with blood supply and involve less fibrous tissue for contraction, thereby causing fewer maxillary growth aberrations. Not operating in the vicinity of the tooth buds probably produces less dentoalveolar deformity.

Operative Technique for the Langenbeck Palatoplasty

This operation is shown in simple diagrammatic form for the isolated cleft palate (Fig. 36–2), unilateral cleft lip and palate (Fig. 36–3), and bilateral cleft lip and palate deformities (Fig. 36–5). The two-flap palatoplasty is illustrated for comparative purposes (Fig. 36–4).

Dissecting the Soft Palate

The marginal soft palate tissues are incised and dissected to create three layers: oral mucosa and submucosa, muscle, and nasal mucosa and submucosa. The lateral borders of the soft palate are incised to produce lateral soft palate release. This includes an atraumatic infracturing of the pterygoid hamulus on both sides. It is impossible to tell from the translations of Bernard von Langenbeck's original article whether he included this in his original operation. This can be a traumatic procedure if the correct plane lateral to the hamulus and immediately medial to the pterygomandibular raphe is not entered properly at the first attempt.

Dissecting the Hard Palate

The medial margins of the hard palate portion of the cleft are next incised to the bone using an incision that is continuous with the soft palate incision. One side is incised at a time to decrease blood loss.

The lateral margins of the hard palate are incised, commencing in the groove medial to the maxillary tuberosity and proceeding forward in the line between the smooth gingivoalveolar mucous membrane and the rugose palatal mucoperiosteum. This incision continues forward to the canine bicuspid region. Mucoperiosteal flaps are elevated by blunt dissection. The posterior palatine arteries are teased from their foramina to allow medial shifting of the mucoperiosteum without tension.

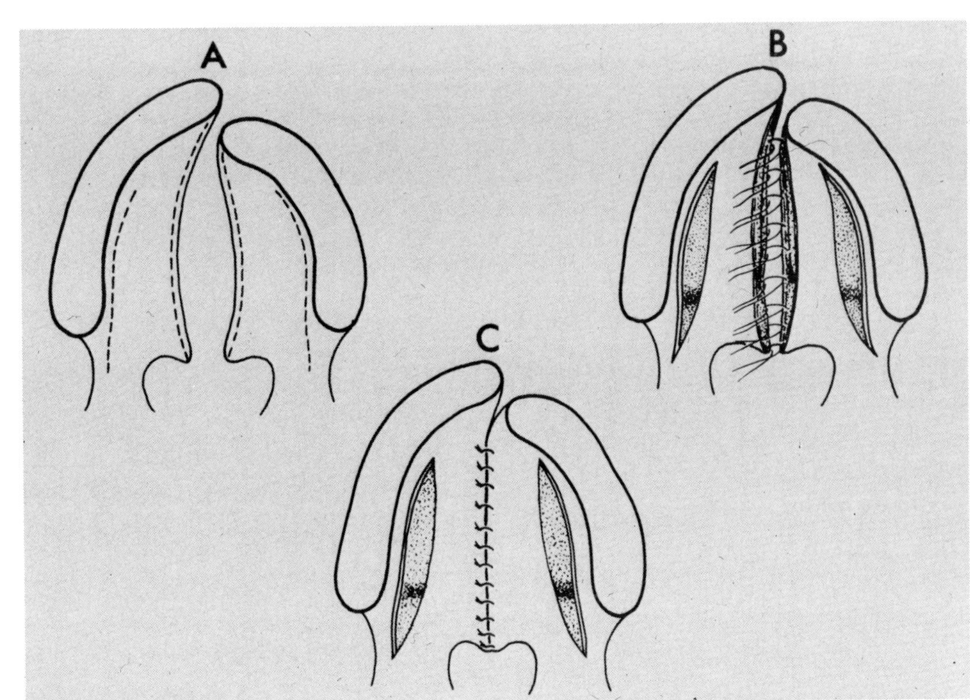

Figure 36–3 Von Langenbeck (simple closure) palatoplasty for complete unilateral cleft lip and palate. *A*, The incision lines. *B*, Mucoperiosteal flaps have been elevated, although they are not well shown in this diagram. The nasal mucosa is closed. In this anomaly, the nasal mucosa on the noncleft or medial side is continuous with the septum and the vomer. More tissue is available to be manipulated and was dealt with as described in Figure 36–2. *C*, Oral mucosal closure. Note that it is impossible to obtain a two-layer closure of the alveolar portion of the cleft with this operation. Pushback is less. Lateral raw areas are smaller because the mucoperiosteum is not detached anteriorly.

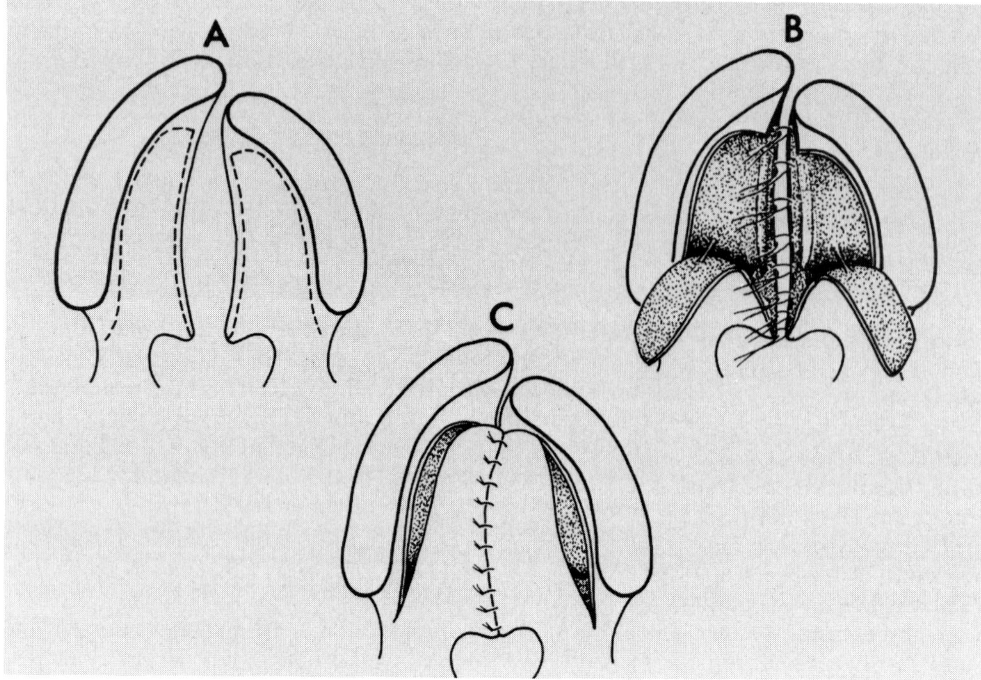

Figure 36–4 Two-flap pushback palatoplasty for complete unilateral cleft of the primary and secondary palates. *A,* The incision lines are joined anteriorly by a line placed obliquely to allow maximum V-Y retrodisplacement of the mucoperiosteum. *B,* Mucoperiosteal flaps have been elevated with posterior palatine arteries intact but teased out of their foramina. Soft palate lateral release incisions have been made. The hamuli are infractured. The nasal mucosa and muscle are closed as in Figure 36–2. *C,* The oral mucosa is closed using the V-Y shift anteriorly, which shifts not only the mucoperiosteum but also the entire palate posteriorly.

The Nasal Mucosa

The nasal mucosa is transected (Fig. 36–2*D*), commencing at its medial portion at a point anterior to the posterior nasal spine and proceeding laterally. This transection is performed after the region of the palatine aponeurosis with its muscle attachments has been detached from the posterior border of the hard palate by blunt dissection and dropped back. This procedure does leave the controversial raw area that has been subjected to so much criticism over the years.

Closure

The nasal mucosa is sutured with interrupted 4–0 polyglycolic sutures (Fig. 36–2). The tensor palatini and levator palatini muscles are each approximated with similar sutures in their new positions. The oral mucosa is closed with 5–0 sutures of the surgeon's choice.

The only difference between this and von Langenbeck's original description is the infracture of the hamulus, which was added to this procedure by Billroth in 1868.[14]

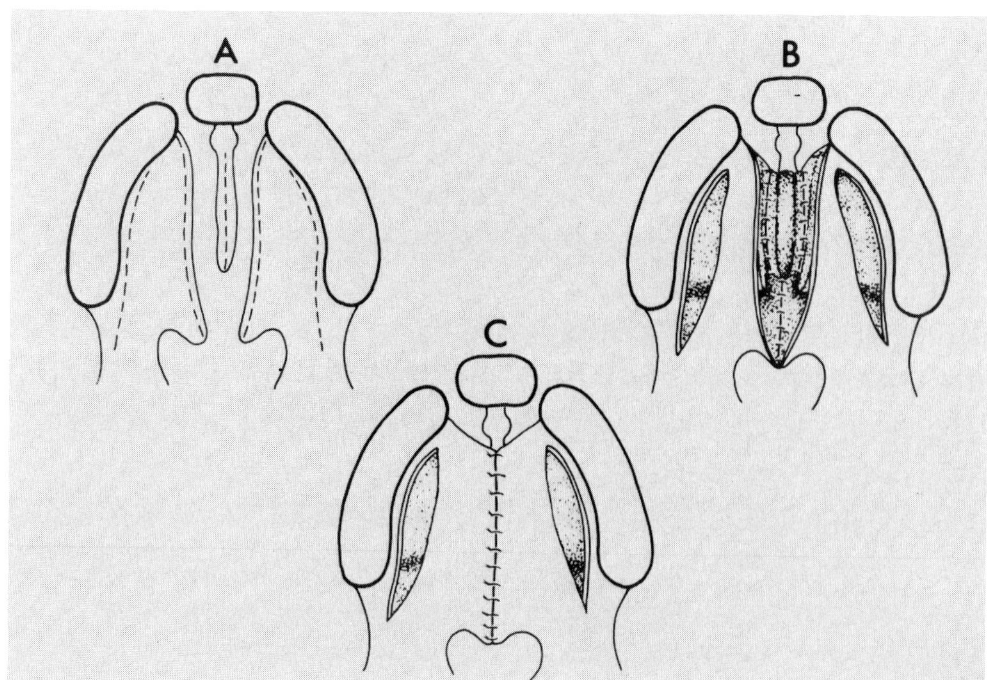

Figure 36–5 Von Langenbeck (simple closure) palatoplasty for bilateral complete cleft lip and palate. The configuration of this deformity varies tremendously, and line drawings can be misleading. *A,* The incision lines. The inferior border of the vomer is incised, and the mucous membrane is elevated from both sides of it. *B,* Mucoperiosteal flaps are elevated without anterior detachment, keeping the posterior palatine arteries intact. Extensive dissection is frequently necessary in the lateral release incision area for this anomaly. The cleft is usually wide, and there is usually considerable hypoplasia. The nasal mucosa is closed. Two suture lines are necessary anteriorly because of the two vomer flaps. *C,* Oral mucosal closure. It is impossible to close the anterior portions of the cleft with this operation. The amount of palatal bone denuded is less, however.

Speech Results

The success of palatoplasty techniques are often judged by speech outcome, particularly nasal resonance and velopharyngeal competence. The current methods of making these judgments are not completely reliable because speech pathologists are not in agreement on what constitutes normal speech or what the criteria for velopharyngeal competence should be. There is no common agreement on the indications for the recommendation of a pharyngoplasty. Imaging techniques such as videofluoroscopy and nasopharyngoscopy should permit more accurate and complete descriptions of velopharyngeal function in cleft palate patients. Morris, in 1973, reviewed the literature on speech results after cleft palate repair and estimated that a 75% success rate of velopharyngeal competence was common regardless of the primary palatoplasty technique used.[15]

The results of most speech outcome studies have favored palatal lengthening techniques over the von Langenbeck technique. However, the controversy continues because of variations in research design, study sample, and surgical techniques, and, in most cases, because of the nonspecific descriptions of the technique. These studies often contain inadequate controls for cleft type and severity, associated anomalies, age at surgery, surgeon's experience, age at evaluation, hearing acuity, intelligence, and methods and standards of assessing speech and velopharyngeal closure.

In a study of speech results in patients with an isolated cleft of the hard and soft palates treated at The Hospital for Sick Children, we attempted to control many of these variables to provide information on velopharyngeal closure and conversational speech.[16] The patients had undergone either the von Langenbeck (modified by Lindsay) or modified Dorrance push-back technique. No significant differences were found between the two groups.

More recently, we reviewed the medical records of all patients with cleft palate born between 1970 and 1979 who had undergone von Langenbeck palate repair by Lindsay.[17] The patients in the study sample had had surgery before 24 months of age (mean 18.62 months, range 15 to 24 months) and no patient had (1) additional cleft palate surgery by any other surgeon, (2) severe hearing, neuromuscular, or intellectual impairment, or (3) submucous cleft palate. Patients also were excluded if they were lost to follow-up. The youngest child was 7 years old at the time of the study. The study sample consisted of 185 patients. Sixty-six had a unilateral cleft lip and palate, 40 had bilateral cleft lip and palate, and 79 had an isolated cleft palate.

The incidence of fistulas was low. There was one fistula of the soft palate. This was repaired at the time of pharyngoplasty at age 6. Four patients had a fistula at the junction of the hard and soft palates and eight patients had a fistula of the posterior hard palate. Most of these patients had isolated cleft palate, and repair was necessary in two and five cases, respectively.

The von Langenbeck technique naturally leaves residual defects of the anterior portion of the hard palate in patients with complete cleft palate. There were 11 fistulas of the anterior hard palate; five patients underwent repair because the fistulas caused symptomatic speech defects. Fifteen of eighty-four patients with complete clefts had an obvious or symptomatic alveolar residual defect.

Adequacy of velopharyngeal function was determined between the ages of 4 and 7 years. Multiview videofluoroscopy and, in more recent cases, nasopharyngoscopy were undertaken if hypernasal resonance and nasal air emission were noted in the child's speech. When these tests confirmed velopharyngeal insufficiency and the parents expressed concern about the child's speech, a pharyngoplasty was recommended. If the child also had a palatal fistula or compensatory articulation, care was taken to occlude the fistula or to establish correct articulatory placement during the assessment to eliminate incorrect judgments of velopharyngeal function. The incidence of velopharyngeal incompetence treated by pharyngoplasty was 25.9% (48 patients). There was no significant difference in the cleft type for those having pharyngoplasty.

Maxillary Growth and Dentoalveolar Development

Rapid changes occur in facial morphology following surgery. The degree to which cleft palate repair inhibits anteroposterior, lateral, and vertical maxillary growth is uncertain, although the timing, type of operation, and individual surgeon are important.[18]

The specialists at the orthodontic division of the Craniofacial Treatment and Research Center of The Hospital for Sick Children, Toronto, have studied the maxilla, alveolus, and dentition of the patients in its von Langenbeck case load on at least two occasions over the years. In a 1969 study, the incidence of anterior crossbite was 12% for the von Langenbeck operation and 62% for a push-back operation.[19] A more recent and international study included both von Langenbeck and push-back cases operated on by the senior author (W.K.L.). The overall maxillary growth did not appear to be different in both groups. However, the inclination of the anterior maxillary incisors was more favorable in the von Langenbeck group.[20]

The Future

The influence of speech pathology on our cleft palate patient population has changed greatly during my generation (W.K.L.). The number of speech pathologists, their training, and their relationship with patients has increased tremendously. The standards of speech expected by speech pathologists have increased proportionately. The emphasis on velopharyngeal function and the speech pathologist's techniques of assessment are much more sophisticated. What surgeons call acceptable speech is no longer acceptable speech to speech pathologists, to parents, to school teachers, and to society in general. The criteria for what we loosely referred to as "cleft palate stigmatization" have become much more sophisticated. Lay assessors have always given lower speech ratings to our postoperative cleft palate population than have the involved professionals, including speech pathologists and plastic surgeons. The increase in the pharyngoplasty rate is not an indication that the speech results of our standard von Langenbeck procedure are becoming worse. Rather, it is an indication that what we formerly considered acceptable speech is no longer acceptable when judged by speech pathologists, parents, school teachers, and society.

The von Langenbeck, or simple closure, primary palate operation is a good but not perfect operation. It produces reasonably acceptable speech, but the criteria for acceptable speech are rising and vary from center to center. Approximately 25% of cleft palate deformities are probably intrinsically hypoplastic and require some form of augmentation. The von Langenbeck operation is a good operation with respect to maxillary, alveolar, and dental development because it can be less traumatic, particularly in the tooth-bearing regions. The region involved is probably inherently hypoplastic in 25% of patients, and approximately 25% of cleft lip and/or palate patients will require orthognathic surgery.

References

1. Ferguson W: Observations on hare lip and cleft palate. Br Med J 1:403, 1874. Month Rev Dent Surg 2:481, 1873.
2. Turner GG: Discussion on the treatment of cleft palate by operation. Proc R Soc Med 20:1891, 1927.
3. Wardill WEM: Cleft palate (Hunterian lecture). Br J Surg 21:347, 1933.
4. Dieffenbach JF: Beitrage zur Gaumennoth. Litt Ann Heilk 6:305, 1826. Cited by Dorrance GM: The Operative Story of Cleft Palate. Philadelphia: Saunders, 1933.
5. Dorrance GM: Operative Story of Cleft Palate. Philadelphia: Saunders, 1933.
6. Peer IA, Walker JC, Meiger R: The Dieffenbach bone-flap method of cleft palate repair. Plast Reconstr Surg 34:472, 1964.
7. Millard DR: Cleft Craft—The Evolution of Its Surgery. III. Alveolar and Palatal Deformities. Boston: Little, Brown, 1980.
8. Von Langenbeck B: Die uranoplastik mittels Ablosung des mukos-periostalen Gaumenuberzuges. Arch Klin Chir 2:205, 1861.
9. Berry J: Discussion on the treatment of cleft palate operation. Proc R Soc Med 20:1887, 1927.
10. Ivy RH, Curtis L: Procedures in cleft palate surgery. Ann Surg 100:502, 1934.
11. Lewin MI: Management of cleft lip and palate in the United States and Canada. Plast Reconstr Surg 33:383, 1964.
12. Furlow LT, Jr: Cleft palate repair by double opposing Z-plasty. Plast Reconstr Surg 78:724, 1986.
13. Graber TM: Craniofacial morphology in cleft palate and cleft lip deformities. Surg Gynec Obstet 88:359, 1949.
14. Billroth T: Über osteoplastische Operationen. Wien Med Wschr 9:1057, 1868.
15. Morris H: Velopharyngeal competence in primary cleft palate surgery, 1961–1970: A critical review. Cleft Palate Rev 10:62, 1973.
16. Witzel MA, Clarke J, Lindsay WK, Thomson HG. Comparison of results of pushback or von Langenbeck repair of isolated cleft of the hard and soft palates. Plast Reconstr Surg 64:347, 1979.
17. Hart N, Witzel MA, Lindsay WK: Unpublished data. The Hospital for Sick Children, Toronto, 1987.
18. Ross RB, Johnston MC: Cleft Lip and Palate. Baltimore: Williams & Wilkins, 1972, p 159.
19. Palmer CR, Hamlen M, Ross RB, et al: Cleft Palate Repair—Comparison of the Results of Two Surgical Techniques. Can J Surg 12:32, 1969.
20. Ross RB: Treatment variables affecting facial growth in complete unilateral cleft lip and palate. Cleft Palate J 24:5, 1987.

CHAPTER 37

Cleft Palate Repair: The Von Langenbeck Technique

*Paul H. M. Spauwen,
Siena M. Goorhuis-Brouwer,
and Harm K. Schutte*

The von Langenbeck palatoplasty is the oldest known successful technique for repair of palatal clefts aiming at a functional separation between the oral and nasal cavities. Von Langenbeck realized that following paring of the cleft edges, extensive lateral relaxing incisions from outside the pterygoid hamuli posterior to the canine region in front were necessary because the bilateral mucoperiosteal flaps were incapable of being stretched to the midline.[1] Good results in relation to closure of the cleft and a low rate of fistula occurrence followed wide adoption of the von Langenbeck procedure. However, dissatisfaction with the functional results led to many modifications of the original operation with the purpose of constructing an active muscle sling for velopharyngeal closure and appropriate functioning of the eustachian tube.

Based on suggestions from Veau and Borel,[2] Podvinec,[3] Ruding,[4] Braithwaite,[5] and Kriens,[6] the need for reconstruction of the displaced halves of the levator veli palatini muscle became apparent. Consequently, levator muscle sling reconstruction was frequently combined with the von Langenbeck operation. Due to these modifications, the classic von Langenbeck technique has been practically abandoned. We will discuss the value of our policy in regard to a modified von Langenbeck technique and question whether there is a need for changing this policy in light of the functional speech results.

At the Cleft Palate Center in Groningen, primary cleft palate repair follows a two-stage regimen. The soft palate is closed at the age of 10 months using a straight-line closure according to the von Langenbeck principle. This procedure includes relocation of the levator muscle insertion but omits fracture of the pterygoid hamuli. The hard palate is closed between 18 and 24 months of age using bipedical mucoperiosteal flaps.

From a surgical point of view, we are satisfied with this procedure, in which safe closure of the cleft edges and a very low fistula rate are predictable and reproducible. However, the early results of the speech outcome, particularly functional velopharyngeal closure and articulatory abilities, are less predictable. Nevertheless, regular and careful follow-up of patients combined with thorough diagnostic methods and adequate treatment may yield satisfying speech abilities.

To demonstrate this, the speech results of our patient group were studied. In the Groningen Cleft Palate Clinic the same type of primary treatment, embedded in a stable, interdisciplinary team organization, has been used for many years, making a coherent patient group available for evaluation.

Patients and Methods

From 1970 to 1985, 733 patients entered the cleft palate treatment program (Table 37–1). The ratio of patients with cleft lip and palate, cleft lip alone, and cleft palate alone is similar to that recorded in the data mentioned by other authors, and the ratio of unilateral to bilateral cases (2:1) is also in accordance with data from the literature.[7] For the purpose of this study, the speech results of a subgroup of patients with any form of cleft palate who had primary treatment between 1971 and 1975 were evaluated.

These 101 patients, who had had their first speech examination before the age of 6 years, were followed to the age of 12 years or earlier if a pharyngoplasty had been performed. Forty-two patients had a unilateral cleft lip and palate and 21 had a bilateral cleft lip and palate. Thirty-eight patients had a cleft palate only.

Speech examinations were carried out at the ages of 4, 6, 8, and 12 years and were performed independently by two qualified speech pathologists, one from the medical and one from the psychology discipline. Velopharyngeal function was diagnosed using listener judgments, the mirror test during sustained vowel production, and stethoscope tubing. Speech was recorded on tape. Velopharyngeal incompetence (VPI), related to a specific degree of hypernasality and nasal escape, was graded using a four-point scale (absent, mild, moderate, or severe). The presence or absence and type of articulatory disorders during spontaneous speech and special test sentences were classified according to a three-point

scale (absent, sufficient, or insufficient). Articulation was graded as good if all the speech sounds normal for the age level of the child were present. Articulation was sufficient if two or three speech sounds were incorrect or absent according to age level. If more speech sounds were incorrect or absent, articulation was graded as insufficient. The results of articulation tests were always placed within the context of the total language and nonverbal development of the child.

Results

Incidence and Type of Speech Problems

At the first speech examination, 66 of 101 children were judged to have velopharyngeal incompetence: the disorder in 30 patients was graded mild, in 21 patients moderate, and in 15 patients severe. Articulatory abilities were good in 26 patients, whereas 37 patients showed sufficient and 38 patients insufficient articulation. In regard to the type of articulatory disorders, weaker articulation of the plosive consonants /p/, /t/, and /k/ and the fricatives /s/ and /f/ was most obvious. When /s/ was affected, marked nasal escape surrounding /s/ was persistently present.

In this group, no significant correlation between velopharyngeal incompetence and the presence or absence of articulatory disorders was found. Thus, velopharyngeal incompetence and articulation are independent variables. The existence and severity of velopharyngeal incompetence do not presuppose articulatory disabilities. In addition, articulatory deficits may exist without any form of velopharyngeal incompetence and may be due to other factors such as lip stiffness or dental arch defects.

Relationship Between Speech Problems and Type of Cleft

The incidence and degree of velopharyngeal incompetence were not related to the type of cleft. However, articulatory disorders were significantly more frequent and severe in children with bilateral cleft lip and palate followed by those with unilateral cleft lip and palate, and were least in cleft palate patients (X^2 test: p < 0.001).

Treatment of Speech Problems

Treatment of velopharyngeal incompetence and/or articulatory disorders consisted of an inferiorly based pharyngoplasty, articulation therapy, or a combination of both. Seventy-two of 101 patients needed additional treatment to improve their speech abilities. Articulation therapy only was given to 37 patients. Articulation therapy followed by an inferiorly based pharyngoplasty was performed in 19 patients, and pharyngoplasty alone was performed in 16 patients. This means that 56 patients received only articulation therapy, whereas 35 patients required a pharyngoplasty.

Table 37–1. The Distribution of Cleft Palate Patients Treated by the Cleft Palate Team, Groningen (1970–1985)

Type of Cleft		Number of Patients
CLP		312
	UCLP	206
	BCLP	106
CLA		231
	UCLA	215
	BCLA	16
CP		190
Total		733

CLP = Cleft lip and palate; CLA = cleft lip and alveolus; CP = cleft palate; UCLP = unilateral cleft lip and palate; BCLP = bilateral cleft lip and palate; UCLA = unilateral cleft lip and alveolus; BCLA = bilateral cleft lip and alveolus.

Speech Performance at the End of the Follow-up Period

Twenty-nine patients did not receive any additional treatment after the primary operation. Of these 29, 28 patients were judged to have good speech. One patient still exhibited mild velopharyngeal incompetence.

Seventy-two patients received additional treatment. Of 37 patients who received articulation therapy only, 22 had good speech ability. Seven patients had mild velopharyngeal incompetence, and eight patients had mild articulatory disorders. All 35 patients who had undergone a pharyngoplasty following articulation therapy or who received a pharyngoplasty alone were judged to have good speech ability.

Overall, at the age of 12 years, 85 patients had good speech, eight patients continued to have mild velopharyngeal incompetence, and eight patients had mild articulatory disorders (Table 37–2).

Discussion

In evaluating and comparing results after surgical treatment of cleft palate, many variables play a part. In particular, speech results should be related to the age at which palatoplasty has been performed, and strict definitions of the technique applied should be reported. Also, surgeon-independent observers, using standardized examination protocols, should clarify the real extent of successes and failures.

In the literature, "success" rates of speech outcome related to the von Langenbeck procedure ranged from 51% to 73%.[8, 9] In our series, following examination before the age of 6 years, the occurrence of both velopharyngeal incompetence and articulatory disorders appears to be rather high.

At first sight, these results may be discouraging. However, after follow-up and treatment to 12 years of age, the speech results are satisfactory. Of 101 patients, 85 achieved a good speech outcome. Thus, the later encouraging results demonstrate that the goals of treatment can be reached, requiring only time.

In our philosophy, these data constitute a challenge to carry out regular diagnostic examinations from an early age, following them with adequate therapeutic measures. It is important to decide beforehand which management strategy should be followed: The four basic options we consider are:
1. Wait for spontaneous development.
2. Perform surgical intervention.
3. Provide specific articulation therapy.
4. Provide both surgical intervention and speech therapy.

In our experience, using these procedures, the speech of most patients appears to improve. For this reason, we continue to use a protocol in which primary surgery is only one part of a comprehensive program.

Table 37–2. Speech Outcome at 12 Years of Age

Procedure	No.	Good	VPI (Mild)	Articulatory Disorders (Mild)
No treatment	29	28	1	0
Speech education	37	22	7	8
Speech education + pharyngoplasty	19	19	0	0
Pharyngoplasty only	16	16	0	0
Total	101	85	8	8

VPI = Velopharyngeal insufficiency

In addition, unfavorable early results after a specific surgical procedure for cleft closure should urge us to scrutinize the timing and technique of the primary operation. Although switching to another technique often seems rational on the basis of logical anatomic-functional principles, actual results lead to reticence. For example, the results of the levator sling reconstruction merely show a trend to improved speech performance but no significant differences compared with techniques that do not involve reconstructing a muscle sling.[10,11] Also, comparison of the push-back with the von Langenbeck technique yields less convincing differences than one would expect.[12] Future prospective studies on comparisons between existing and newly developed techniques may provide more clarity. Recently, in the Groningen Cleft Palate Clinic, a prospective study has been initiated to investigate the effects on speech outcome of a palatoplasty using double opposing Z-plasties according to Furlow compared with the von Langenbeck technique.

References

1. Langenbeck von B: Operation der angeborenen totalen Spalten des harten Gaumens nach einer neuen Methode. Deutsch Klin 8:231, 1861.
2. Veau V, Borel S: Division Palatine: Anatomie, Chirurgie, Phonetique. Paris: Masson, 1931.
3. Podvinec S: Physiology and pathology of the soft palate. J Laryngol 66:452, 1952.
4. Ruding R: Cleft palate: Anatomical and surgical considerations. Plast Reconstr Surg 33:133, 1964.
5. Braithwaite F: Cleft palate repair. In Gibson T: Modern Trends in Plastic Surgery. London: Butterworth, 1964, p 30.
6. Kriens OB: An anatomical approach to veloplasty. Plast Reconstr Surg 43:29, 1969.
7. Gabka J: Hasenscharten und Wolfsrachen. Entstehung, Behandlung und Operationsverfahren. Berlin: Walter de Gruyter, 1967.
8. Blocksma R, Leuz CA, Mellerstig KE: A conservative program for managing cleft palates without the use of mucoperiosteal flaps. Plast Reconstr Surg 55:160, 1975.
9. Musgrave RH, McWilliams BJ, Matthews HP: A review of the results of two different surgical procedures for the repair of clefts of the soft palate only. Cleft Palate J 12:281, 1975.
10. Coston GN, Hagerty RF, Jannarone RJ, et al: Levator muscle reconstruction: Resulting velopharyngeal competence—a preliminary report. Plast Reconstr Surg 77:911, 1986.
11. Brown AS, Cohen MA, Randall P: Levator muscle reconstruction: Does it make a difference? Plast Reconstr Surg 72:1, 1983.
12. Witzel MA, Clarke JA, Lindsay WK, et al: Comparison of results of pushback or von Langenbeck repair of isolated clefts of the hard and soft palate. Plast Reconstr Surg 64:347, 1979.

CHAPTER 38

Two-Stage Palatoplasty

Milivoj Perko

Concerning cleft palate closure, there is little agreement on the proper timing, on whether it should be a one-stage or two-stage repair, or even on whether the hard or soft palate should be closed first, simultaneously with lip repair, or later on. The matter is further complicated by considerable differences between the surgical techniques applied and their various approaches. Reconstruction of the levator muscle, for example, is performed in many different ways[1-4] or not at all.[5] The influence of specific procedures on facial growth and on speech development is still a controversial issue. On the one hand, observation of individuals with unrepaired cleft lip and palate demonstrated practically normal facial growth.[6-9] On the other hand, many authors, among them Millard, found that too radical and too early surgery was responsible for more or less severe maxillary growth disturbance as well as alveolar and dental disorders.[10]

In Zurich 20 years ago palatal closure was routinely performed at 2 years of age by a Veau–von Langenbeck technique modified by Grob.[11] At age 15, maxillary hypoplasia was found in more than 50% of patients with unilateral and bilateral complete cleft lip and palate, and speech results were often far from satisfactory.[12] Maxillary osteotomies for correction of sagittal skeletal disharmony ultimately proved necessary in about 80% of these patients.

To minimize growth impediments and improve speech proficiency, a change in the entire therapeutic approach was deemed imperative in Zurich in the mid-1960s. Based on the current literature of that time and on an extensive quest for treatment alternatives by Dr. Margaret Hotz, a new sequence of surgical intervention as well as new techniques were introduced. Two-stage palate repair, a basic concept introduced in the United States by Slaughter and Brodie[13] and in Europe by Schweckendiek[14] was adopted, based on the observation of Gillies and Fry that leaving the hard palate open led to fewer growth disturbances in cleft patients.[15] The advantage of delayed hard palate closure for facial growth was later confirmed by Schweckendiek's son on publishing his father's long-term results.[16, 17]

In the 1960s and 1970s, two-stage palatal surgery became rather popular with many surgeons.[18-24] However, poor speech results following the use of Schweckendiek's surgical procedure for soft palate repair soon caused many teams to abandon the two-stage approach.[25-28] Discussions at various conferences on speech problems resulting from the original Schweckendiek technique also prompted our team to try a one-stage repair combining a modification of Widmaier's soft palate closure[29] with a Campbell[30] or Pichler[31] vomer flap in the hard palate area. The aim was to avoid the sequelae of denudation of the palatal shelves brought about by raising mucoperiosteal flaps.[32] However, this specific one-stage repair often resulted in residual palatal fistulas in the anterior third of the palate or a gradually deepening groove in the vomer flap area and in subsequent speech disturbances. The transverse position of the lesser maxillary segment was often far from ideal in those patients. Another attempt at closing the entire palate without raising the periosteum from the palatal shelves and using purely mucosal flaps[33] was soon abandoned as being too risky because of the danger of flap necrosis.[3] On the basis of this experience, the Zurich team finally opted for a two-stage palatal closure that differs considerably from the Schweckendiek approach in both timing and technique.

The Zurich Approach

With minor changes in timing, the current therapeutic approach to cleft lip and palate in Zurich has been in use since 1969. It is based on close cooperation between maxillary orthopedic treatment and surgery. Orthopedic guidance is initiated at birth and continued until the child is about 16 months of age.[34] Its main objectives are to keep the tongue out of the cleft, normalize feeding, and allow spontaneous narrowing of the cleft, thus facilitating subsequent soft palate closure and providing more tissue for achieving adequate velar length (Chap. 71). Closure of all complete palatal clefts is performed in two stages, the soft palate around 18 months of age and the hard palate when the child is between 4 and 5 years old. Individual timing depends on developmental factors, particularly speech.

Closure of the Soft Palate

For closure and elongation of the soft palate our modification[3] of Widmaier's technique[29] is as follows (Fig. 38–1):

1. Dissection of two supraperiosteal mucosal flaps in the area of the posterior third of the hard palate, *without any denuding of the palatal shelves.*
2. Sparing mobilization of the nasal mucosa in the same area *without* breaking the hamulus or mobilizing the pterygoid muscles.
3. Dissection of the anterior attachment of the levator palatini muscle and of the muscle fibers on the posterior border of the hard palate.
4. Mobilization of the velar muscular complex on both sides; reconstruction and retropositioning of a transverse muscle sling.
5. Elongation of the nasal mucosa by Z-plasty.
6. Union of the residual musculature in the posterior third of the soft palate.
7. Union and elongation of the oral mucosa by V–Y plasty.

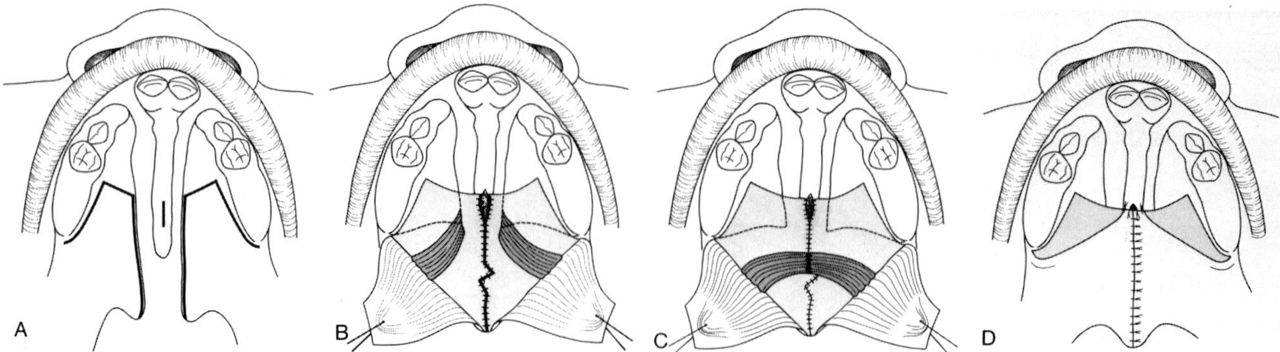

Figure 38–1 Surgical technique for soft palate closure in bilateral cleft lip and palate. *A,* Incision lines; note the short incision of the vomerine mucosa which is performed in bilateral cleft lip and palate cases only. *B,* Oral *mucosal flaps* elevated and held by threads; nasal mucosa elongated by Z-plasty and ventrally sutured to the split vomerine mucosa. Velar musculature exposed but still adherent to its aberrant insertion on the dorsal end of the hard palate. Periosteum on the oral surface of the palatal shelves remains untouched. *C,* Velar musculature detached from its insertion and sutured in the midline. Spontaneous relocation of the muscle sling to its correct anatomical position. *D,* Oral mucosal flaps sutured and retropositioned according to the V–Y principle; ventral end of the flaps sutured to the vomerine mucosa. Triangular raw areas on both sides to be dressed with a compressive pad for a few days. (*A–D* from Hotz M, et al: The Zurich approach, 1964 to 1984. In Hotz M, et al: Early Treatment of Cleft Lip and Palate. Bern. Huber, 1986. With permission.)

Closure of the Hard Palate

Subsequent to soft palate repair, the hard palate cleft narrows spontaneously. There is evidence of growth of the palatal shelves, and in 80% of our unilateral complete cleft patients, the width of the anterior palate cleft is less than 5 mm at the time of hard palate closure (Chap. 71). It is thus possible to close the hard palate area with a minimum of tissue mobilization (Figs. 38–2 and 38–3).[35] In patients with unilateral clefts, only a single mucoperiosteal flap raised from the nonaffected side of the palate is necessary for closure. The lateral incision can be performed well away from the area of the attached gingiva. According to animal experiments by Kremenak et al., this placement of the incision is an additional precaution against maxillary growth disturbance.[32] The palatal mucoperiosteum of the cleft side is not detached at all. Hard palate surgery is performed when the child is 4 to 5 years old, that is, when the anterior maxillary arch has attained about five-sixths of its adult size,[36] or when the speech clinician calls for it. For the Zurich team, the active involvement of speech specialists in decision making as postulated by Witzel[37] has been a matter of course since 1965. One speech specialist (H. Nussbaumer) has followed all patients from the speech clinician's point of view during the past 23 years. Other speech clinicians have assisted her for periods of 5 to 20 years each.

In the period between 1971 and 1987, 233 children with cleft palate were operated on, using the two-stage method described above, and were regularly followed by the surgeon, speech clinician, and orthodontist (Table 38–1). Results are reported below.

Results

Facial Growth

Results of the Zurich approach on facial growth in the 10-year age group were published earlier (see Chap.

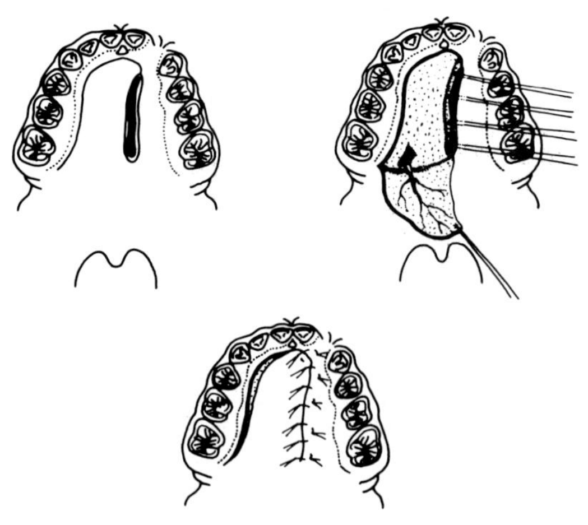

Figure 38–2 Drawing of hard palate closure. (From Perko M: Closure of the hard palate in unilateral cleft palate cases, following previous closure of the soft palate according to the Widmaier-Perko technique. Chir Testa Collo 1:9, 1984. With permission.)

Table 38–1. Sample Size for Two-Stage Palatoplasty

Type of Cleft	Total Patients	Patients with Hard Palate Closed (1987)
Unilateral		
Complete	86	66
Incomplete	15	10
Bilateral		
Complete	54	38
Incomplete	35	28
Palate only		
Complete	10	9
Incomplete	8	5
Total	233	180

Note: The patients in this sample had a two-stage palatoplasty with soft palate repair by Perko's modification of the Widmaier technique.[3, 35] All patients were operated on by the same surgeon (M.P.).

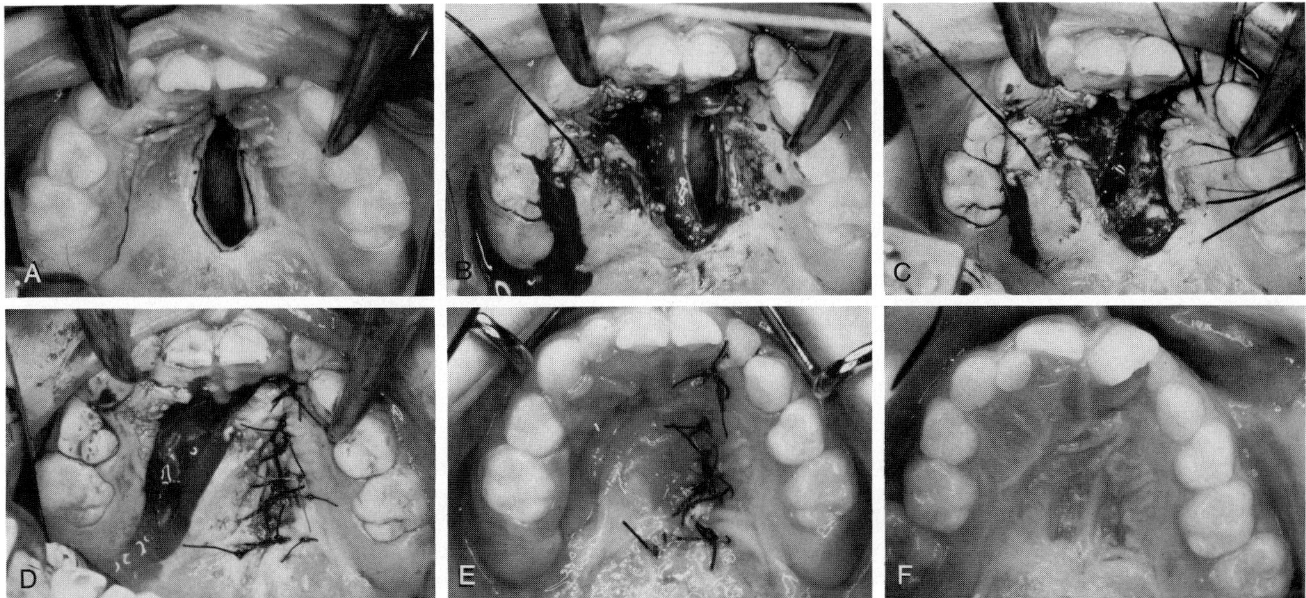

Figure 38–3 Surgical technique of hard palate closure. *A*, The incision line is drawn; *B*, the palatal flap from the nonaffected side is raised; *C*, the vomer flap is mobilized and fitted with sutures under the palatal mucosa of the opposite side; *D*, the mucoperiosteal flap is rotated and sutured; *E*, one week after the intervention, sutures to be removed; *F*, Situation at age 8, 3 years after the intervention. (From Perko M: Closure of the hard palate in unilateral cleft palate cases following previous closure of the soft palate according to the Widmaier-Perko technique. Chir Testa Collo 1:9, 1984. With permission.)

71),[38] and a preliminary study was published for the small sample already available at the 15-year age level.[39]

Speech Results

To evaluate the results of the Zurich two-stage approach on an internationally accepted level, a joint study with Prof. D. R. Van Demark from The University of Iowa was undertaken in December 1986. The random sample comprised 37 subjects with complete unilateral cleft lip and palate, ranging in age from 6 to 16 years. This corresponds to 80.8% of all German-speaking patients with complete unilateral cleft lip and palate in the respective age range treated by the approach described. Reasons beyond the team's influence precluded 11 patients from participation.

The purpose of the study was to describe perceptually the speech articulation, voice quality, and velopharyngeal competence resulting from the Zurich approach. A full report was published by Van Demark et al.[40] In summary, testing consisted of guided conversation with a Swiss speech clinician, repetition of standard sentences, and administration of the Swiss Pressure Articulation Test (SPAT) of 90 consonant elements in 54 items patterned after the Iowa Pressure Articulation Test (IPAT)[41] and partially modified with regard to specific Swiss German phonemes.

Severity Ratings of Articulation Defectiveness and Hypernasality

Ratings were made perceptually on seven-point scales (1 = normal, 7 = severely defective or severely hypernasal). The mean rating of articulation defectiveness was 2.89, and the mean rating of nasality was 2.65. No subject was rated as having severely defective articulation or severe hypernasality.

Articulation Testing

The average number of correct items on the SPAT was 37.89 (range 4 to 54, SD 11.68). Oral distortions occurred on an average of 9.92 items, nasal distortions 4.03 items, pharyngeal substitutions 0.35 items, and glottals 0.24 items. Of the nearly 2000 items produced, 70% were correct, 18% orally distorted, and 7.5% nasally distorted. Glottal-stop and pharyngeal errors occurred only 1.1% of the time.

Velopharyngeal Competence

Perceptually, the majority of the subjects exhibited velopharyngeal competence (40.5%) or marginal velopharyngeal competence (54%). One subject was rated as incompetent. Another subject received secondary lengthening of the palate plus a Teflon implant and was therefore also considered as primarily incompetent. In total, only 5.4% of the sample showed velopharyngeal incompetence and were considered by the American examiner to be in need of secondary management.

Discussion

The Zurich two-stage approach as used for unilateral cases since 1969 and for all complete clefts since 1972 has repeatedly been questioned, based on experience with the Schweckendiek technique, from which it differs

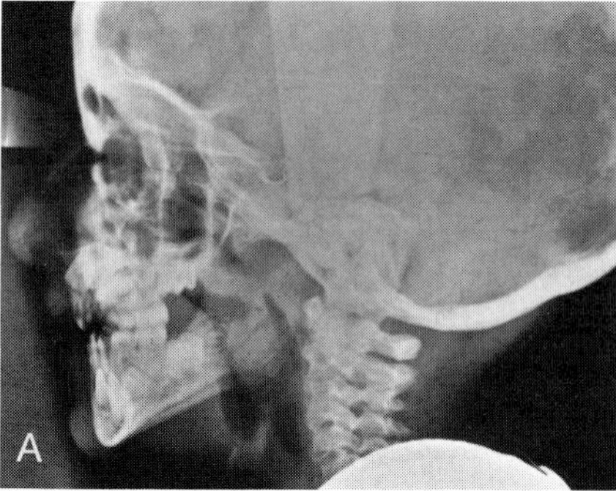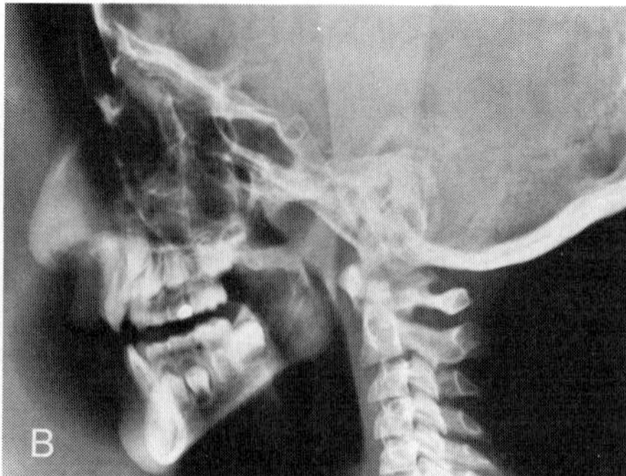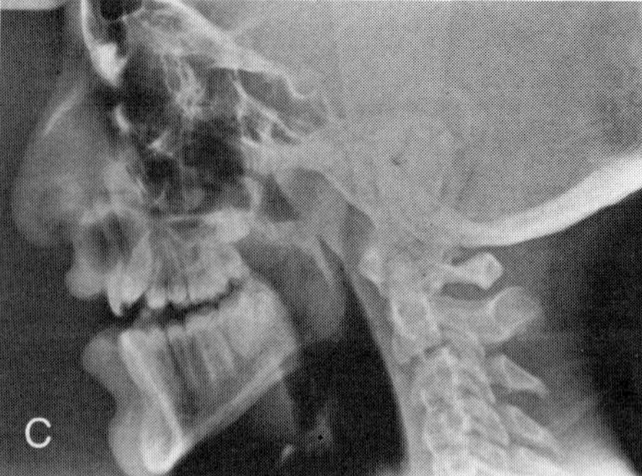

Figure 38–4 Still x-rays on phonation of /e/; functional adaptation of the soft palate through development: *(A)* at age 5 years; *(B)* at age 10 years; *(C)* at age 15 years.

a great deal, or on limited experience with partly modified approaches. The main difference between the Zurich procedure and the Schweckendiek method must be stated clearly: Although avoiding early denudation of the palatal shelves, the Perko technique additionally provides lengthening of the soft palate with a Z-plasty of the nasal layer and detailed anatomic reconstruction of the levator muscle.[3, 35] Consequently, it provides near-normal muscle function. Velopharyngeal competence is established at an early age, and velar function adapts to the gradual deepening of the pharyngeal space through pubertal growth (Fig. 38–4). This could be the reason for Van Demark's observation that the majority of the subjects did *not* exhibit the compensatory articulation errors of glottal stops or pharyngeal fricatives that are commonly attributed to two-stage procedures with delayed hard palate closure.[40] The anatomic repair of the soft palate plus the lengthening provided by the Z-plasty in the nasal layer also may explain the low rate (5.4%) of patients in the Zurich sample who exhibited velopharyngeal incompetence[40] compared with an incompetence rate of 56.4% in Schweckendiek's own cases.[42]

Limited experience and a lack of team cooperation seem to be the reasons for other criticisms such as Montoya's qualifying our procedure as "an elegant solution . . . with limitations: It is rather difficult to perform on wide clefts, abstention from tissue mobilization in the tuberosity area often gives rise to tension on the repaired soft palate, the percentage of heavy scarring and fistulae is rather high."[43] For our approach, maybe more than for others, excellent cooperation between the various specialists on the team is a prerequisite. The preparatory use of infant orthopedic plates[34] contributes a great deal because by the time of soft palate closure the mean posterior cleft width measured on the casts is only 7.7 mm, or about 50% of the initial width (see Chap. 71). Thus, tension is no problem. Soft tissue mobilization is less extensive and traumatic, and as a consequence, bone apposition in the maxillary tuberosity area is less liable to be disturbed by scarring because relaxing incisions around the tuberosities are avoided. As for the problems of fistulas and scarring, no fistulas ever occurred in our two-stage sample of unilateral cleft lip and palate or bilateral cleft lip and palate. Bulky transverse scars were a problem in 20% of our

early patients born between 1969 and 1972, whereas patients born between 1973 and 1979 demonstrate the result of the surgeon's increasing skill and experience in showing a ratio of only 7% bulky scars and 29% slightly prominent scars; 64% have a smooth palate.

The surgical technique for raising purely mucosal flaps and for dissecting the levator muscle bundle on velar closure admittedly is more demanding in skill and experience than the preparation of mucoperiosteal flaps in one-stage procedures. Only experience of long standing will enable clinicians to fully exploit the potential of such an approach. The results of other teams who have tried to adopt our method in the past 15 years have made it evident that local conditions can play a great role in success or failure and that a transfer of approaches is not feasible in all conditions.

References

1. Braithwaite F, Maurice JG: The importance of the levator palati muscle in cleft palate closure. Br J Plast Surg 21:60, 1968.
2. Kriens OB: An anatomical approach to veloplasty. Plast Reconstr Surg 43:29, 1969.
3. Perko M: Two-stage closure of cleft palate. J Maxillofac Surg 7:76, 1979.
4. Furlow LT: Cleft palate repair by double opposing Z-plasty. Plast Reconstr Surg 78:724, 1986.
5. Marsh JL: Palatoplasty. ACPA Symposium on Velopharyngeal Incompetence, Williamsburg, VA, April 24–25, 1988.
6. Ortiz-Monasterio F, Rebeil AS, Valderrama M, et al: Cephalometric measurements on adult patients with nonoperated cleft palates. Plast Reconstr Surg 24:53, 1959.
7. Ortiz-Monasterio F, Serrano A, Barrera G, et al: A study of untreated adult cleft palate patients. Plast Reconstr Surg 38:36, 1966.
8. De Jesus JA: Comparative cephalometric analysis of nonoperated cleft palate adults and normal adults. Am J Orthod 45:61, 1959.
9. Mestre JC, De Jesus J, Subtelny JD: Unoperated oral clefts at maturation. Angle Orthod 30:78, 1960.
10. Millard DR, Jr: Cleft Craft: The Evolution of Its Surgery. Vol. 3. Alveolar and Palatal Deformities. Boston: Little, Brown, 1980, p 58.
11. Grob M: Lehrbuch der Kinderchirurgie. Stuttgart: G. Thieme, 1957, p 90.
12. Gnoinski WM: Early maxillary orthopaedics as a supplement to conventional primary surgery in complete cleft lip and palate cases—Long-term results. J Maxillofac Surg 10:165, 1982.
13. Slaughter WB, Brodie AG: Facial clefts and their surgical management. Plast Reconstr Surg 4:311, 1949.
14. Schweckendiek H: Zur Frage der Fruh- und Spatoperationen der angeborenen Lippen-Kiefer-Gaumenspalten (mit Demonstrationen). Z Laryngol Rhinol Otol 30:51, 1951.
15. Gillies HG, Fry WK: A new principle in the surgical treatment of "congenital cleft palate" and its mechanical counterpart. Br Med J 1:335, 1921.
16. Schweckendiek W: Die zweizeitige Gaumenplastik, Vorzuge-Mangel-Ergebnisse. Fortschr Kiefer-Gesichtschir 16/17:140, 1973.
17. Schweckendiek W: Primary veloplasty: Long-term results without maxillary deformity. A twenty-five year report. Cleft Palate J 15:268, 1978.
18. Herfert O: Two-stage operation for cleft palate. Br J Plast Surg 16:37, 1963.
19. Gabka J: Hasenscharten und Wolfsrachen. In Entstehung, Behandlung und Operationsverfahren. Berlin: De Gruyter, 1964, p 134.

20. Walker DH: Minimal closure in cleft lip and palate surgery. J South Afr Logoped Soc 13:44, 1966.
21. Dingman RO, O'Connor JE: A conservative program of surgical management of the cleft lip and cleft palate patient. Presented at the Second International Congress on Cleft Palate, 1973. (Abstract, p 262.)
22. Blocksma R, Leuz CA, Mellerstig KE: A conservative program for managing cleft palates without the use of mucoperiosteal flaps. Plast Reconstr Surg 55:160, 1975.
23. Friede H, Lilja J, Johanson B: Cleft lip and palate treatment with delayed closure of the hard palate. Scand J Plast Reconstr Surg 14:49, 1980.
24. Malek R, Psaume J: Nouvelle conception de la chronologie et de la technique chirurgicale du traitement des fentes palatines. Resultats sur 20 cas. Ann Chir Plast Esthet 28:237, 1983.
25. Cosman B, Falk AS: Delayed hard palate repair and speech deficiencies: A cautionary report. Cleft Palate J 17:27, 1980.
26. Jackson IT, McLellan G, Scheker LR: Primary veloplasty or primary palatoplasty: Some preliminary findings. Plast Reconstr Surg 72:153, 1983.
27. Robertson NRE, Jolleys A: A further look at the effects of delaying repair of the hard palate. Craniofacial Society of Great Britain, 1st International Meeting, Birmingham 1983. In press, 1989.
28. Poupard B, Coornaert H, Ribiere H, et al: Early bone grafting versus delay of procedures interfering with maxillary bone—twenty year's experience. In Hotz M, et al (eds): Early Treatment of Cleft Lip and Palate. Bern: Hans Huber, 1986, p 95.
29. Widmaier W: Ein eigenes Verfahren zum Verschluss der Gaumenspalte. Chirurgie 30:274, 1959.
30. Campbell A: The closure of congenital clefts and hard palate. Br J Surg 13:715, 1926.
31. Pichler H: Ueber Lippen- und Gaumenspalten. Wien Klin Wschr 3:70, 1934.
32. Kremenak CR, Jr, Huffman W, Olin WH: Growth of maxillae in dogs after palatal surgery. I. Cleft Palate J 4:6, 1967.
33. Perko M: Primary closure of the cleft palate using a palatal mucosal flap: An attempt to prevent growth impairment. J Maxillofac Surg 2:40, 1974.
34. Hotz M, Gnoinski W: Comprehensive care of cleft lip and palate children at Zurich University: A preliminary report. Am J Orthod 70:481, 1976.
35. Perko M: Closure of the hard palate in unilateral cleft palate cases, following previous closure of the soft palate according to the Widmaier-Perko technique. Chir Testa e Collo 1:9, 1984.
36. Brash JC: The Genesis and Growth of Deformed Jaws and Palates. London: Dental Board of the United Kingdom, 1924.
37. Witzel MA, Salyer KE, Ross RB: Delayed hard palate closure: The philosophy revisited. Cleft Palate J 21:263, 1984.
38. Hotz M, Gnoinski W, Perko M, et al: The Zurich approach, 1964 to 1984. In Hotz M, et al (eds): Early Treatment of Cleft Lip and Palate. Bern: Hans Huber, 1986, p 42.
39. Gnoinski WM: Orofacial development up to age 15 in UCLP cases treated according to the current Zürich approach. In Pfeifer G. (ed): Craniofacial Anomalies of Lip, Alveolus and Palate. Principles of Treatment, Long-Term Results. Fourth International Hamburg Symposium. Stuttgart, G. Thieme, 1989.
40. Van Demark DR, Gnoinski W, Hotz M, et al: Speech results of the Zurich approach in treatment of unilateral cleft lip and palate. Plast Reconstr Surg 83:605–613, 1989.
41. Morris HL, Spriestersbach DC, Darley FL: An articulation test for assessing the competency of velopharyngeal closure. J Speech Hear Res 4:48, 1961.
42. Bardach J, Morris H, Olin W: Late results of primary veloplasty: The Marburg Project. Plast Reconstr Surg 73:207, 1984.
43. Montoya P, Martinez Y: Traitement primaire des fentes du palais secondaire. Chir Pediatr 24:337, 1983.

CHAPTER 39

Two-Stage Palatoplasty: Schweckendiek Technique

Wolfram Schweckendiek and Eberhard Kruse

After early complete closure of the palatal cleft, extensive growth aberrations of the maxillary complex may occur. Following these observations, my father, Hermann Schweckendiek, developed the idea of a primary veloplasty. The goals were to preclude severe disturbances of maxillary growth, ensure proper development of speech, and decrease the size of the cleft in the hard palate to facilitate its closure.

Technique of Primary Veloplasty

Improvements in surgical technique since the 1920s have not greatly diminished the incidence of postoperative maxillary deformities in patients with cleft palate. Ritter[1] and Rosenthal[2] drew attention to subsequent midfacial malformations resulting from early palate repair. Studies of patients with cleft palate who had had no early surgery indicated that severe deformities of the maxilla had not occurred.

Herfert, in his experimental studies, revealed that early operations on the hard palate almost always inhibited maxillary growth.[3, 4] Extensive scarring following cleft palate repair also influenced secondary maxillofacial deformities. These findings have been confirmed by experimental studies carried out by Lynch and Peil[5] and by Kremenak and co-workers.[6]

In our opinion, the growth of the maxillary complex is normal when the soft palate is closed during infancy by means of primary veloplasty. The residual cleft in the hard palate becomes narrower with growth of the palate over the years without causing secondary maxillofacial deformities.

The surgical technique is illustrated in Figure 39–1. The edges of the cleft of the soft palate are dissected into three layers, and lateral incisions 1 cm in length are made on both sides along the pterygomandibular raphe. Through medial and lateral incisions, a rubber band is inserted using a special needle, and small foam rubber sponges are inserted on the bands. The cleft is then repaired, suturing each layer separately: nasal mucosa, muscles, and oral mucosa. At the end of the operation, the tension of the rubber band is appropriately adjusted, and the ends of the rubber band are connected to a thread. The rubber band is removed after 7 days. In patients with a narrow cleft (less than 8 mm in diameter), a rubber band is not necessary.

My father started to perform primary veloplasty operations in 1944 with the objective of creating a soft palate that could function normally. He assumed that speech would develop early and that growth and development of the maxilla would not be disturbed. He published this method in 1951 and 1955.[7, 8] The same idea was presented by Slaughter and Pruzansky in 1954.[9]

At present, we perform primary veloplasty on patients between 6 and 8 months of age who weigh an average

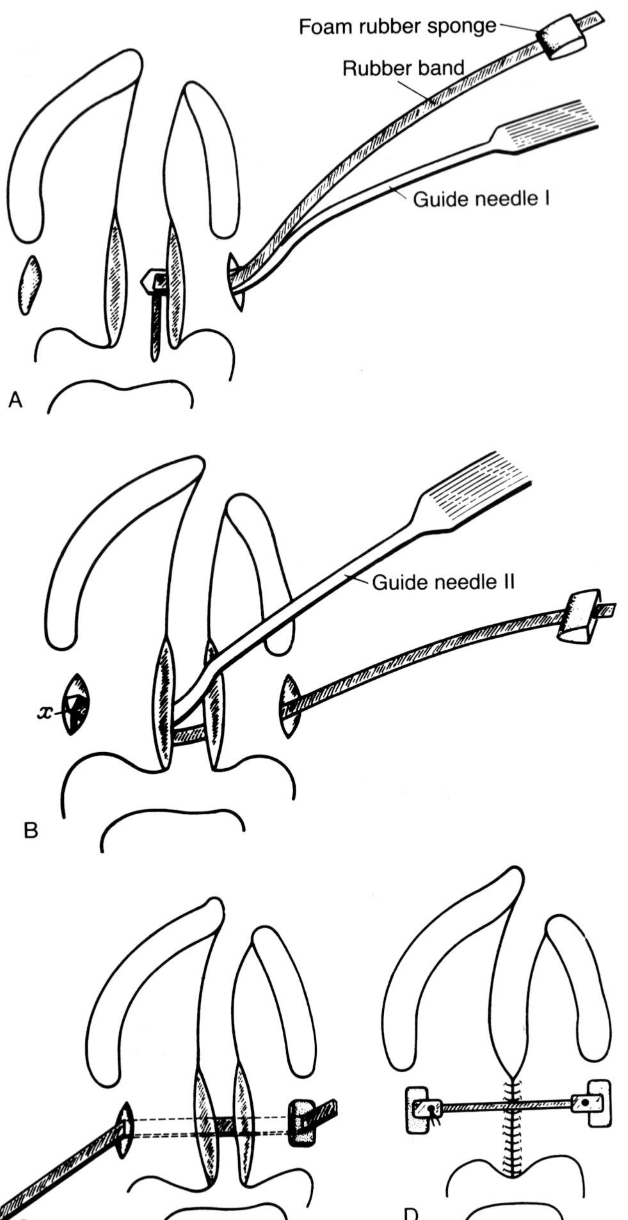

Figure 39–1 *A*, The cleft is dissected in layers in the area of the soft palate, and lateral incisions are made on both sides. *B*, Through these incisions a rubber band is introduced with special needles. The lateral incisions are filled with small foam rubber sponges. *C* and *D*, The cleft is sutured in three layers. At the end of the operation, the tension of the rubber band is adjusted, and the oral ends are joined by a thread.

of 7 to 8 kg. Risk is minor, and postoperative complications are rare. Failures are very uncommon. It should be emphasized that during the primary operation, we mobilize the soft palate at the posterior edge of the hard palate by means of lateral incisions to bring together the muscles of the palate along the midline without tension. We also endeavor at this stage to lengthen the palate by including the pharyngopalatine arch (Table 39–1).[10, 11]

In patients with complete unilateral clefts, we operate on the soft palate first. Three weeks later we perform cleft lip repair. For complete bilateral clefts, we first close one side of the cleft lip and perform primary veloplasty 3 weeks later. Three weeks after that, we close the other side of the lip and the alveolar cleft. This operative sequence is followed because surgery may be carried out on the lip shortly after the primary operation. At the time of the veloplasty, the oral cleft

Table 39–1. Timing of Primary Veloplasty

Age	CLCP Unilateral	CLCP Bilateral	CP Soft and Hard	Total Number
Under 1 year	175	67	102	344
Over 1 year	38	14	59	111
Total Number	213	81	161	455

CLCP = Complete cleft lip and palate

is wide open, facilitating surgery. We postpone the repair of the hard palate.[12] Because surgical intervention is limited to the soft tissue, the bony maxilla has unrestricted growth (Fig. 39–2). On follow-up, minor difficulties were found to occur in only 3% of the patients. However, a number of children required temporary prostheses to cover the cleft so that the spontaneous growth of the upper jaw might continue undisturbed for as long as possible.

Closure of the residual cleft in the hard palate is generally postponed until the patient reaches the age of 11 to 13 years. At that time, normal growth of the maxilla is virtually complete. If for any reason the residual cleft has to be closed at an earlier age—for instance, at 6 to 8 years—the maxilla must be kept under constant orthodontic supervision to prevent subsequent collapse or compression. Serious articulation problems can generally be avoided, that is, sibilants and plosives can be produced almost normally (Fig. 39–3).

In all patients with clefts, final assessment of clinical treatment is possible only after the patients have reached adolescence. During recent years, we have published various preliminary reports on the effects of primary veloplasty on jaw formation and speech. We now have final results for 455 patients in whom surgical closure of the residual cleft was performed. On the average, this cleft became at least 60% to 70% narrower between the primary veloplasty and final closure of the hard palate. In more than 95% of all patients, the edges of the alveolar cleft were in close juxtaposition prior to surgical closure.

We also assessed the growth of the jaws by means of clinical observations and use of plaster dental models for measurement purposes.[13, 14] We have demonstrated that development of the maxilla following primary veloplasty proceeds in an undisturbed manner. The values for the width of the palatine arch, length of the maxilla, and the base of the skull are nearly the same as those for normal adults.

Facial Growth and Orthodontic Results

As we stated previously, we currently have final results on 455 patients with different forms of clefts in whom surgical closure of the residual cleft was performed (Table 39–2). As indicated, narrowing of the residual cleft facilitates surgery of the hard palate. During the period between primary veloplasty and repair of the hard palate, growth and development

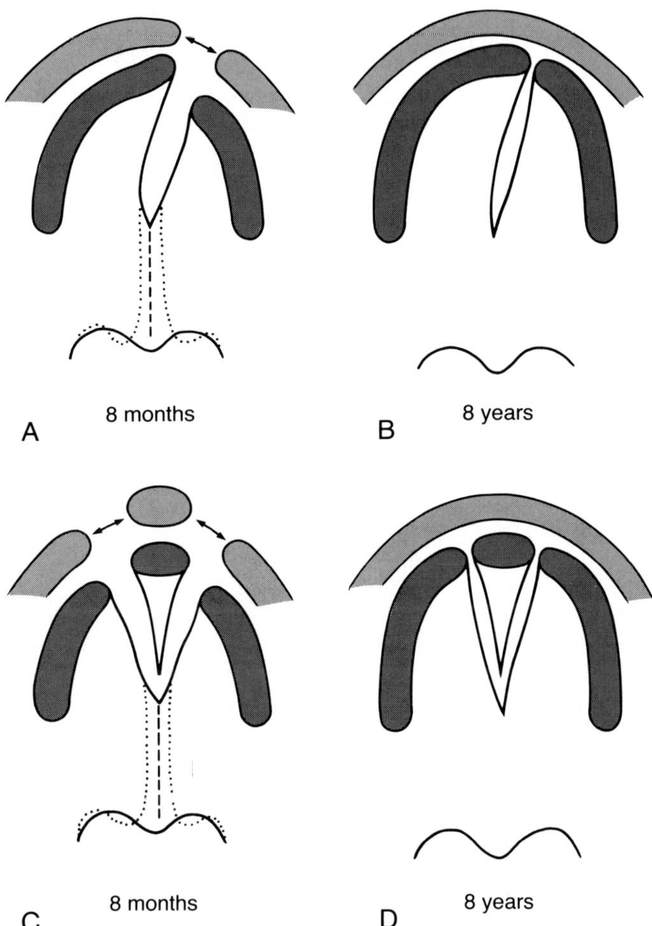

Figure 39–2 Development of the cleft maxilla after primary veloplasty and repair of the cleft lip. *A* and *B*, Model of primary veloplasty at 8 months of age and 8 years in complete unilateral cleft lip and palate. Undisturbed development of the maxilla. *C* and *D*, The same model in complete bilateral cleft lip and palate.

continue. By the time of hard palate repair, the palate is well developed, and closure is easily achieved. This growth has been documented by dental models and photographs.

In complete cleft lip and palate patients, the muscles of the face and of the soft palate form a ring around the maxilla that has a functional influence on growth. Its normal development and function inhibit growth disturbances of the maxillary complex. Consequently, facial growth and development are normal in most patients, a fact that has been documented with frontal and lateral photographs.

Table 39–2. Timing of Uranoplasty

Age	CLCP Unilateral	CLCP Bilateral	CP Soft and Hard	Total Number
Under 12 years	7	2	25	34
12–14 years	150	55	88	293
14–16 years	33	15	24	72
Over 16 years	23	9	24	56
Total Number	213	81	161	455

CLCP = Complete cleft lip and palate

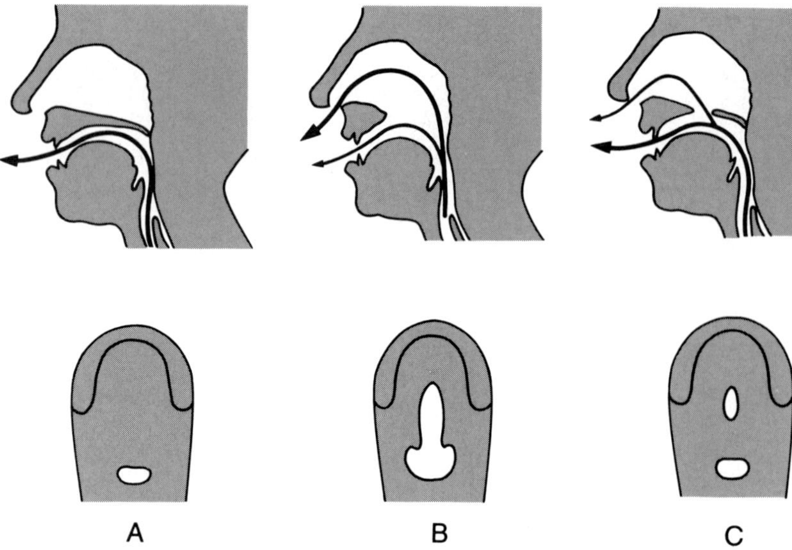

Figure 39–3 *A*, Normal palate. *B*, Unoperated cleft palate; most of the air escapes through the nose. *C*, After primary veloplasty the airflow through the nose is decreased.

With cephalometric measurements it is possible to study the growth of the maxilla. Our patients were examined with this technique by Haakonson-Kuhn,[15] Bardach et al,[16] and Ross.[17] These measurements demonstrated nearly normal maxillofacial growth following primary veloplasty and delayed closure of the hard palate. According to Bardach et al, acceptable results of facial growth were found in 88% of the patients.[16]

In a study by Ross, the results of primary veloplasty from 14 different cleft palate centers and from normal control patients were analyzed and compared.[17] Ross indicated that "the best faces (that is, close to noncleft) were from Marburg with their virtually unoperated palates. The evidence for further growth after palate repair could not be obtained from the radiographs available, but at the late age repair was done, it would be surprising if growth would be greatly affected."

In cleft palate patients certain anomalies in the position and number of the teeth are present. In our patients, some abnormalities of occlusion required orthodontic therapy. Orthodontic treatment of the maxilla is possible in spite of a residual cleft in the hard palate. Treatment is necessary in patients who have positional abnormalities of the teeth adjacent to the cleft (Fig. 39–4).

Orthodontic treatment was influenced by the amount of scarring that existed following cleft palate repair. Treatment in patients with little scarring was achieved easily. However, in patients with severe scarring, orthodontic treatment was very difficult to complete.

After primary veloplasty in patients with Pierre-Robin syndrome the tongue is prevented from falling backward, a fact that favors diminution of the microgenia. The facial profile becomes almost normal in these patients.

Otolaryngologic Results

The influence of the primary veloplasty on the function of the eustachian tube is very positive. We found that the incidence of ear disease diminished after pri-

mary veloplasty, and this also has been confirmed by others.[18, 19] In 202 patients who had primary veloplasty, Grebe found hearing loss and middle ear problems in 25% compared with 57% in other surgical procedures.[21] Bottcher[8] observed slight hearing loss in only 183 of 755 children after primary veloplasty (24.3%), while a review of the literature shows a higher percentage in cleft palate patients. Kittel confirmed these findings in his own investigations.[20]

Speech Results

As far as speech development is concerned, we have found that between 2 and 5 years of age, children with residual clefts of the hard palate have greater difficulties. Children and parents have to spend more time with speech training than is normally necessary. From 3 years of age, speech control by a phoniatrist and speech therapy are often necessary. In spite of the remaining

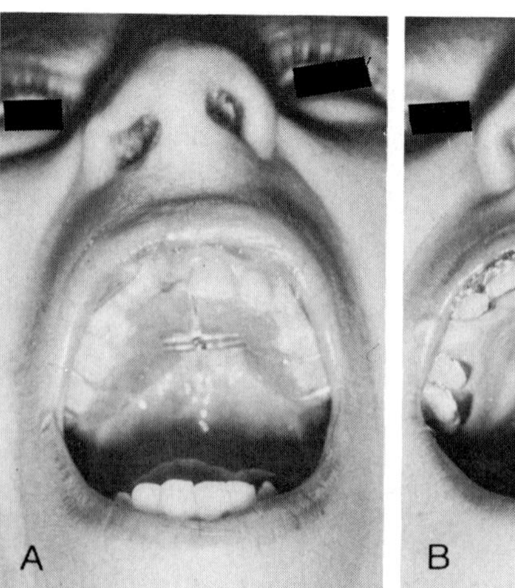
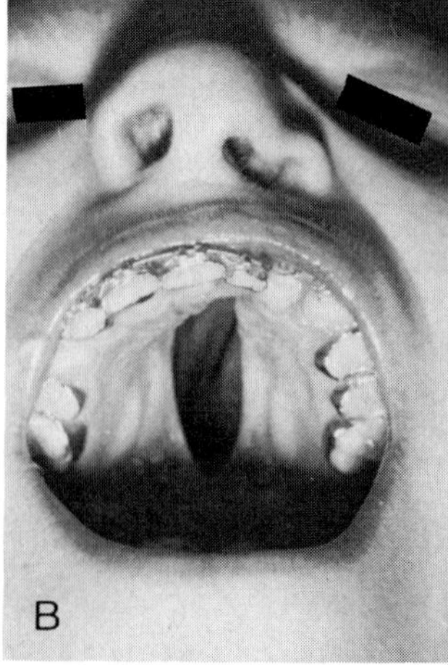

Figure 39–4 Orthodontic treatment is not hindered by the residual cleft in the hard palate. *A*, Palatal plate with an expansion screw. *B*, Treatment using braces.

Table 39–3. Long-Term Results of Primary Veloplasty: Speech Results

Speech Group	CLCP Unilateral	CLCP Bilateral	CP Soft and Hard	Total Number	Percentage
I: Normal	102	34	81	217	47.7
II: Intelligible	90	38	66	194	42.7
III: Moderate	20	9	13	42	9.2
IV: Poor	1	0	1	2	0.4
	213	81	161	455	100.00

CLCP = Complete cleft lip and palate

cleft of the hard palate, many patients speak almost normally. In other patients, we find rhinolalia and articulation errors. These patients need systematic speech therapy. In some cases, we can help them with a plate that covers the residual cleft in the hard palate (Fig. 39–5).

Speech results primarily depend on the adequate function of a long, mobile velum. Therefore, we try to lengthen the soft palate by mobilizing the velar muscles from the posterior edge of the hard palate, restoring the levator muscle sling, and including the pharyngopalatine arch in the veloplasty. Unfortunately, we do not reach our goal in all patients, and in some (about 10%), secondary surgery, for instance by a pharyngeal flap procedure, is necessary later on (Table 39–3).

In our opinion, the best time for closing the residual hard palate cleft is 12 years of age or later. In the past, many patients desired closure of the hard palate later (at the age of 16 years) because they did not have any trouble with the remaining cleft or had not experienced speech difficulties. Occasionally we close the hard palate earlier, when the speech pathologist recommends it or when the patient or his parents press for surgery (Fig. 39–6). In these patients, orthodontic control and treatment are necessary. The speech treatment is provided by our phoniatrist, Dr. Kruse, from the otolaryngology clinic of the University of Marburg.

In our opinion, the main problem in speech rehabilitation is not the residual cleft of the hard palate and its size but the competence of the velopharyngeal mechanism. The earlier velopharyngeal closure is trained by the function of the muscles of the pharynx and the mouth, the better are the speech results. We attempt to create a long mobile velum to avoid the need for secondary surgery to correct velopharyngeal incompetence using pharyngeal flaps.

However, a long mobile velum is not always created. Factors such as hypoplasia of the soft palate or the size of the cleft may result in a short velum. The speech pathologist advocates surgery of the soft palate as early as possible. Presently, many cleft palate centers are in favor of this. We believe that the optimal time for veloplasty is 6 months of age. At the time of primary

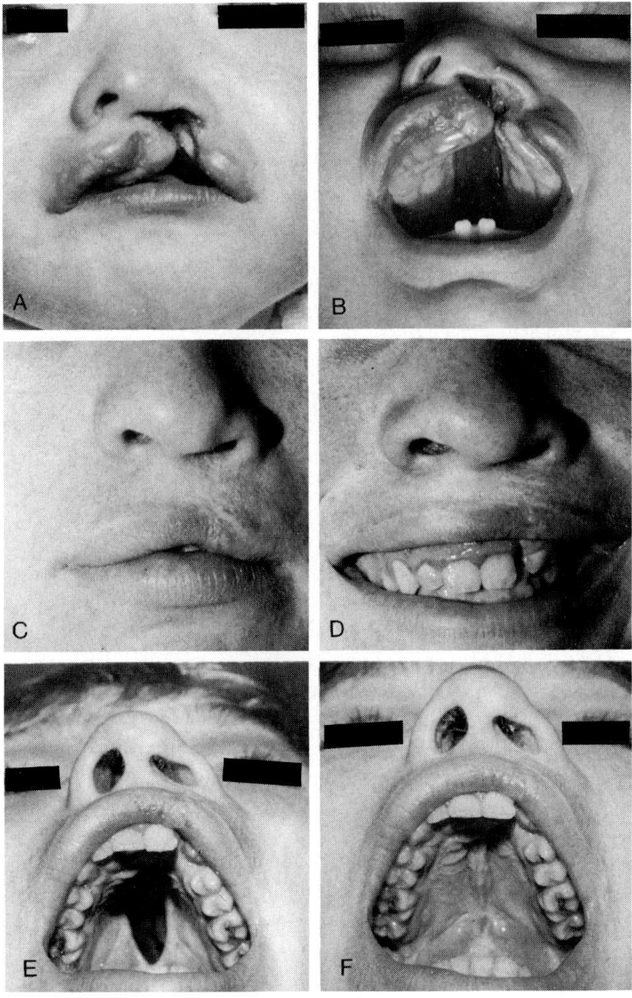

Figure 39–6 A patient with unilateral cleft lip and palate. *A* and *B,* Before primary veloplasty and lip repair. *C* and *D* At 14 years of age, good appearance and normal occlusion. *E,* At 14 years, residual cleft of the hard palate. *F,* At 15 years, 6 months after hard palate repair.

Figure 39–5 *A,* A patient at 6 years of age with a residual cleft of the hard palate. *B,* The residual cleft is temporarily closed with a plate.

veloplasty, special attention is directed to constructing the levator sling. Veloplasty performed at a later age prevents the advantageous influence of the muscles of the mouth and pharynx during early speech development. We advocate early speech treatment and development of the preverbal muscular movements. In this way, we hope to influence the later motor control of the articulation patterns.

Conclusions

In planning and assessing the results of hard palate repair, one must consider the growth of the maxilla and the entire midface. Severe secondary deformities may also have a detrimental effect on speech. Facial aesthetics, occlusion, and mastication are affected. Therefore, hard palate repair is postponed until facial growth is completed. Good collaboration with the orthodontist is essential to ensure proper occlusal relationships and maxillofacial growth. These findings are based on our evaluations published in 1982[21] and on the study of patients in our clinic by Bardach et al.[16] Even the Swiss team (Hotz and Gnoinski) has not observed disadvantages in the two-stage surgery of the palate.[22]

With regard to undisturbed growth of the midface and early development of speech we recommend the following timing of surgical procedures in patients with complete clefts of the lip and palate:

1. Veloplasty is done 3 weeks prior to cleft lip repair. Cleft lip surgery (in patients with unilateral cleft) is done at about 6 months of age.
2. In patients with bilateral clefts, the first side of the cleft lip is repaired at 6 months of age. Veloplasty is done 3 weeks later, and the other side of the lip is closed 3 weeks later.
3. Cleft palate repair is performed at 12 years. Presurgical orthopedic treatment has not been used.

The early veloplasty introduced by my father, Hermann Schweckendiek, forms a muscular ring around the growing maxilla. The residual cleft in the hard palate then becomes narrower without causing deformity of the maxillary complex. Early speech development is possible when the velum has been repaired, and some patients have achieved normal speech even with a residual cleft of the hard palate. Others need speech training for rhinolalia or articulation errors. In some patients, the cleft was closed by a temporary speech plate.

We try to lengthen the velum and create a muscle sling during the primary operation. Unfortunately, this goal is not reached in all patients. Therefore, some patients require secondary surgery with a pharyngeal flap. We think the best time for closing the residual cleft of the hard palate is the age of 12 years or later. Occasionally we close the hard palate earlier if the speech pathologist recommends it or if the patient presses for surgery.

Orthodontic treatment is often necessary in the permanent dentition. Most problems can be easily corrected with routine orthodontic treatment.

Osteoplasty is used in only a few patients. If necessary, we perform a secondary osteoplasty after 12 years of age. Most of these patients had bilateral clefts with a mobile premaxilla. Secondary surgery, such as corrective rhinoplasy, lip revisions, or veloplasties, is usually postponed until adolescence. The late results, in our opinion, can be judged objectively by 17 years of age.[23-27]

References

1. Ritter R: Die Nachteile der Frühoperation bei Lippen-, Kiefer- und Gaumenspalten. Stoma Konstanz 1:10, 1948.
2. Rosenthal W: Die postoperative Kieferverkruppelung nach Lippen- und Gaumenspaltoperationen. Chirurgie 22:483, 1951.
3. Herfert O: Der optimale Zeitpunkt für die Operation der Gaumenspalten. Dtsch Zahn-Mund-Kieferhk 17:265, 1953.
4. Herfert O: Fundamental investigations into problems related to cleft palate surgery. Br J Plast Surg 11:97, 1958.
5. Lynch JB, Peil R: Retarded maxillary growth in experimental cleft palates. Am Surg 32:507, 1966.
6. Kremenak CR, Huffman WC, Olin WH: Growth of the maxillae in dogs after palatal surgery, I. Cleft Palate J 4:6, 1967.
7. Schweckendiek H: Zur Frage der Früh- und Spaltoperationen der angeborenen Lippen-Kiefer-Gaumenspalten. Z Laryngol Rhinol 30:51, 1951.
8. Schweckendiek H: Zur zweiphasigen Gaumenspaltenoperation bei primärem Velumverschluss. In Schuchardt K, Wassmund M (eds): Fortschritte Kiefer- und Gesichtschirurgie. Jb Bd I. Stuttgart: G. Thieme, 1955, p. 73.
9. Slaughter WB, Pruzansky S: The rationale for velar closure as a primary procedure in the repair of cleft palate defects. Plast Reconstr Surg 13:341, 1954.
10. Schweckendiek W: Die Technik der primaren Veloplastik. Chirurgie 34:277, 1963.
11. Schweckendiek W: Primary veloplasty. In Schuchardt K (ed): Treatment of Patients with Clefts of Lip, Alveolus and Palate. Stuttgart: G. Thieme, 1966.
12. Ullik R: Der Zeitpunkt der Lippenplastik. In Schuchardt K, Wassmund M (eds): Fortschritte Kiefer- und Gesichtschirurgie. Jb Bd I. Stuttgart: Thieme, 1955, p 25.
13. Hinuber E, Schweckendiek W: Einfluss der primaren Veloplastik auf die Oberkieferentwicklung bei einseitigen Lippen-Kiefer-Gaumenspalten. In Schuchardt K (ed): Fortschritte der Kiefer- und Gesichtschirurgie. Bd. 16/17. Stuttgart: G. Thieme, 1973, p 169.
14. Edeling C: Spatergebnisse der Kieferform und Okklusion bei Gaumenspaltoperationen nach Schweckendiek. Dissertation. Marburg, 1983.
15. Haakonson-Kuhn M: Lippen-Kiefer-Gaumenspalten im lateralen Fernrontgenbild. Fortschr Kieferorthop 30:311, 1969.
16. Bardach J, Morris HL, Olin WH: Late results of primary veloplasty: The Marburg project. Plast Reconstr Surg 73:207, 1984.
17. Ross RB: Treatment variables affecting facial growth in complete unilateral cleft lip and palate. Cleft Palate J 24:5, 1987.
18. Bottcher R, Schweckendiek W: Hals-, nasen-, ohrenarztliche Gesichtspunkte beim Spaltrager. In Schuchardt K (ed): Fortschritte Kiefer- und Gesichtschirurgie. Jb Bd 16/17. Stuttgart: G. Thieme, 1973, p 218.
19. Grebe G: Die Erkrankungen des Ohres bei Patienten mit Lippen-Kiefer-Gaumenspalten. Dissertation. Marburg, 1966.
20. Kittel G: Discussion. Arch Otorhinolaryngol 216:501, 1977.
21. Kruse E: Langzeitergebnisse der primaren Veloplastik unter phoniatrischen und logopadischen Aspekten. In Pfeifer G (ed): Lippen-Kiefer-Gaumenspalten. Third International Symposium, Hamburg 1979. Stuttgart: G. Thieme, 1982, p 168.
22. Hotz MM, Gnoinski WM: Effects of early maxillary orthopaedics in coordination with delayed surgery for cleft lip and palate. J Maxillofac Surg 7:201, 1979.
23. Schweckendiek W: Primary veloplasty: Long term results without maxillary deformity. Cleft Palate J 15:268, 1979.
24. Schweckendiek W: Two-stage closure of cleft palate: Rationale for its use. In Kehrer B, et al (ed): Long Term Treatment in Cleft Lip and Palate. Bern: Hans Huber, 1981, p 254.
25. Schweckendiek W: Speech development after two-stage closure of cleft palate. In Kehrer B, et al (ed): Long Term Treatment in Cleft Lip and Palate. Bern: Hans Huber, 1981, p 307.
26. Schweckendiek W: Spatergebnisse der Kiefer- und Gaumenform nach primaren Lippen- und Velumplastik und offen gelassener Skelettspalte. In Pfeifer G (ed): Lippen-Kiefer-Gaumenspalten. Third International Symposium, Hamburg 1979. Stuttgart: G. Thieme, 1982, p 69.
27. Schweckendiek W: Langzeitergebnisse der primaren Veloplastik unter hals-, nasen-, ohrenarztlichen, phoniatrischen und logopadischen Aspekten. In Pfeifer G (ed): Lippen-Kiefer-Gaumenspalten. Third International Symposium, Hamburg 1979. Stuttgart: G. Thieme, 1982, p 166.

CHAPTER 40

Two-Stage Palatoplasty and Evaluation of Speech Results

Robby Meijer and Shirley Cohen

Historical Development

Since about 1969 at our Center, complete clefts of the palate have been closed with a two-stage procedure. The decision to follow this route was a direct result of an evolution in the concept of the surgical management of the complete cleft lip. Since 1964, the so-called lip adhesion or preliminary lip repair has been the treatment of choice in all cases of complete clefts, unilateral as well as bilateral.[1] This approach is based on the philosophy that extended surgery—that is, wide undermining—may be detrimental to the growth and development of the maxilla. Two-stage palate repair has been advocated by Schweckendiek,[2] the results of which have been controversial. It was our feeling at that time, however, that if the operation were performed earlier, the reported negative aspects of the two-stage closure might be avoided.

Slaughter and Pruzansky, as early as 1954, studied the results of muscular forces acting in the area of the cleft and recommended that repair of the velum be done without fracturing the bone, undue introduction of scar tissue, or severence of the blood supply.[3] We generally agree with these principles. Their time of closure depended on clinical evaluation and ranged, in the reported cases, from 11 months to 4½ years of age, with the anterior palate subsequently closed later at variable time intervals. Unfortunately, no speech results were reported.

Fára reported his experiences with early (before 8 months) soft palate closure combined with delayed (after 6 years) hard palate closure.[4] Seventy children were studied. To approximate the mobilized muscles in the velum, lateral incisions in the cleft were necessary if the cleft was wider than 12 mm at the junction of the hard and soft palates. Initially, no relaxing incisions were made, but now these incisions are used whenever it seems necessary. Fára found that the anterior clefts were spontaneously reduced by an average of 4 mm in width. However, velopharyngeal function was poor.

In 1979, Herfert reported his results with the Schweckendiek method. He performed most velar closures after the patients were 1 year of age.[5] He found that after 3 to 4 years the anterior palatal cleft had narrowed so much that closure was greatly simplified and facilitated. He stated that normal speech was "encouraged" by the "early" velar closure but did not publish the results.

A reevaluation of the delayed hard palate closure was done by Witzel et al in 1984.[6] They concluded that although delaying the hard palate repair past the age of 12 years produced excellent skeletal relationships, the speech results reported when the procedure was delayed until age 4 to 8 were contradictory. It was also their contention that severe speech problems dominated. Also in 1984, Bardach et al reported on their study of 45 randomly selected patients operated on by Wolfram Schweckendiek.[7] In contrast to the highly acceptable facial growth of these patients, there was an unusually high incidence of velopharyngeal incompetence (estimated success rate only 48.8%). In addition, they reported a high incidence of glottal stops and pharyngeal fricatives, two speech production patterns that can be regarded as compensatory. This was not unexpected because these patients had open hard palate clefts until the age of 13 years.

The purpose of this chapter is to provide additional information about the speech results associated with the primary veloplasty procedure.

Timing and Technique

Soft palate closure is done at approximately 3 to 6 months of age. In patients with complete clefts of the primary and secondary palates, this operation coincides with definitive lip repair. Initially, no relaxing incisions were made, nor were the muscles dissected. The cleft edges were merely freshened as far forward as the palatal shelves could be approximated without undue tension (Fig. 40–1). At times the repair can be somewhat precarious. Dehiscence has occurred at a rate of approximately 40% for partial dehiscences of varying degrees and 5% for complete dehiscence. Partial dehiscence, however, does not seem to influence the presumed effect of the veloplasty on the anterior bony portion of the cleft. In most instances, narrowing of the anterior cleft occurs (Figs. 40–2 and 40–3) with only a few exceptions in the isolated cleft palate category (Fig. 40–4). Under the influence of Kriens in early 1970,[8] the velar closure was modified, and attempts were made to reconstruct the muscular sling, which often necessitates placement of relaxing incisions laterally as well as incisions at or just beyond the bony junction (Fig. 40–5).

Following suitable induction of anesthesia with intubation, a Dingman mouth gag is placed to ensure continuous good exposure. A solution of lidocaine, 0.5%, with epinephrine, 1:200,000, is used to infiltrate the incision sites. Using an angulated Beaver blade, the soft palate edge is split from the uvula to just anterior to the posterior edge of the bony palate. Whenever feasible, the levator muscle is identified and sharply freed from the bone. This may be sufficient to join the muscle from each side in the midline; however, more often than not, small relaxing incisions are necessary around the tuberosity, after which the submucosal structures are bluntly pushed medially to make approximation possible. Submucoperiosteal dissection of the oral as well as nasal mucosae at the bony junction aids in the closure of both mucosal layers. In the very wide cleft,

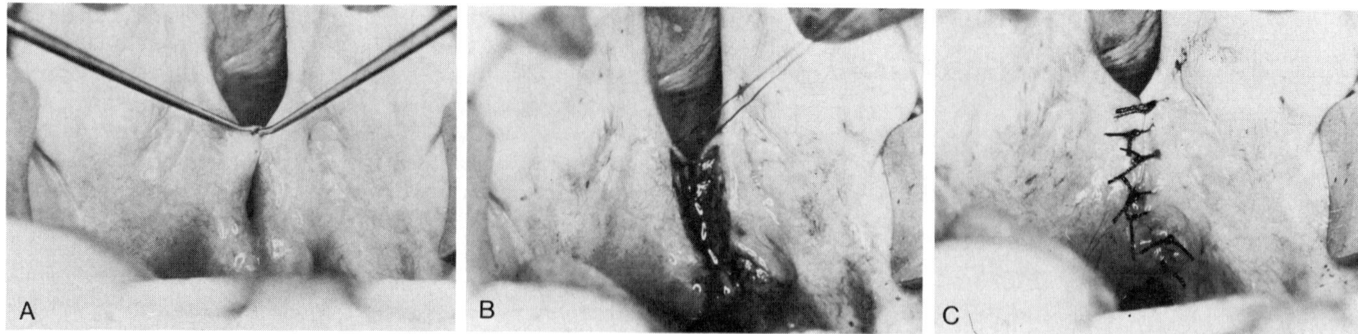

Figure 40–1 *A*, Estimation of extent of velar closure without lateral relaxing incisions. *B*, Nasal side of a three-layer closure without muscle reconstruction. *C*, End of repair.

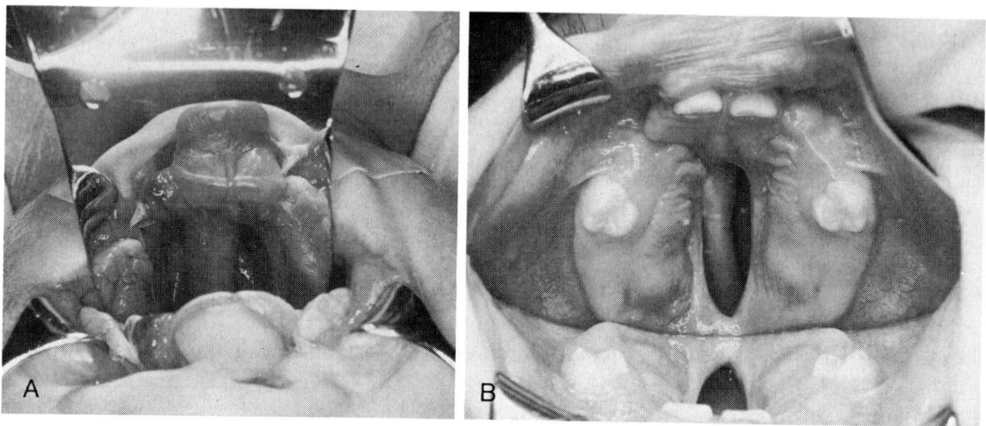

Figure 40–2 *A*, Wide bilateral cleft palate. *B*, Anterior palate development following velar closure.

Figure 40–3 *A*, Isolated cleft palate. *B*, Considerable development of the anterior palatal shelves following velar closure without lateral relaxing incisions.

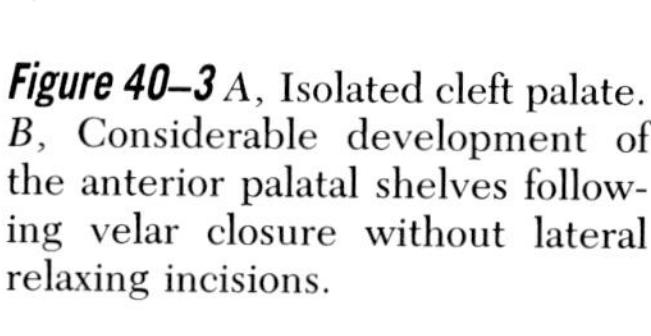

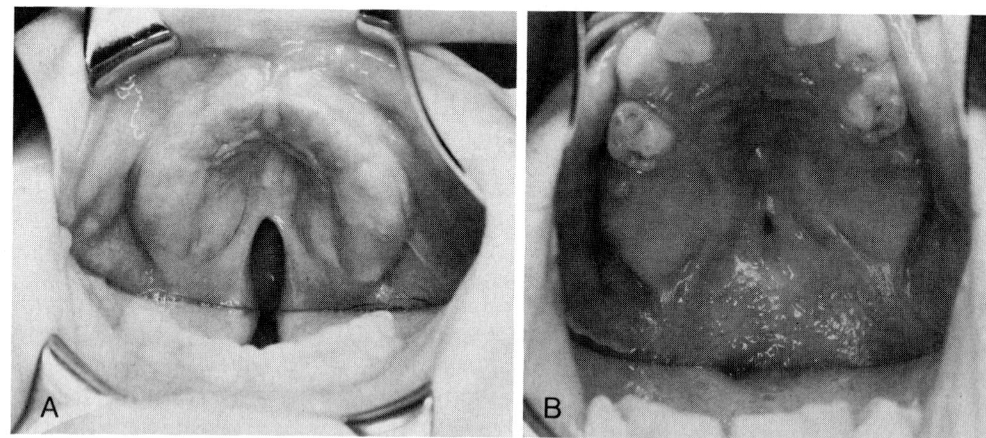

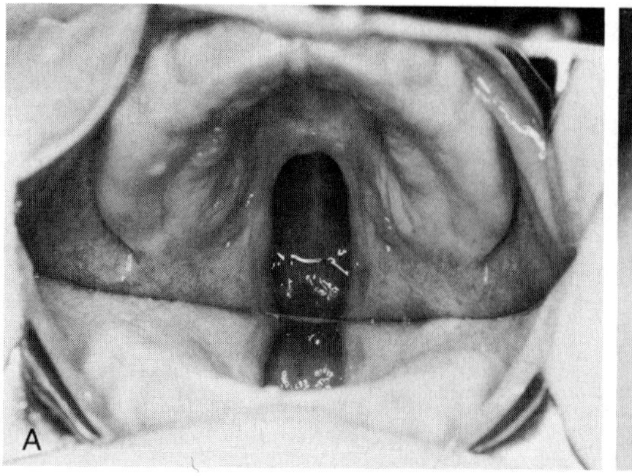

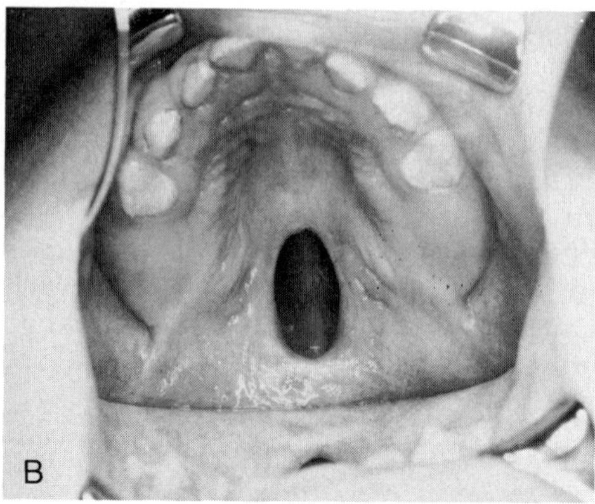

Figure 40–4 *A*, Isolated cleft palate. *B*, Little effect on palatal shelves following velar closure.

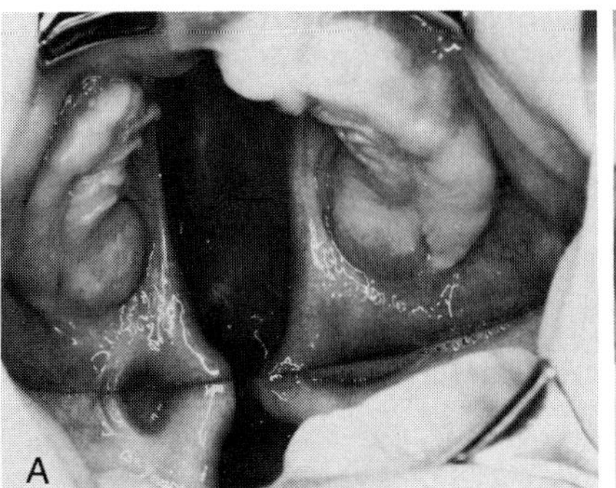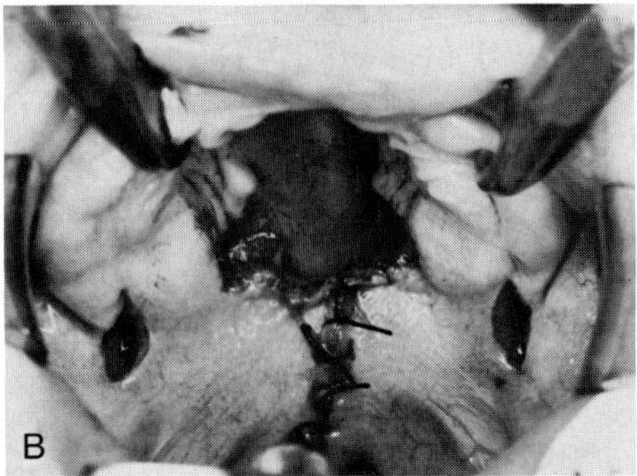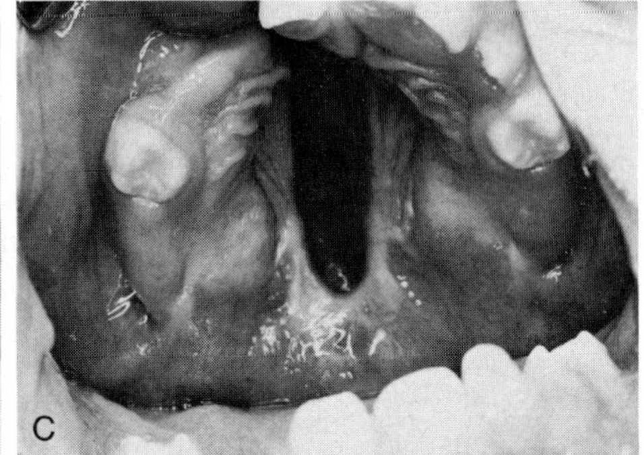

Figure 40–5 *A,* Complete wide unilateral cleft. *B,* Velar closure and muscle reconstruction using lateral and anterior relaxing incisions. *C,* Subsequent effect on anterior palate with little trace of relaxing incisions.

incising these structures may be necessary (Figs. 40–5 and 40–6). The soft palate is then closed in three layers using 4–0 chromic catgut for the nasal mucosa and muscular sling reconstruction and 4–0 black silk sutures for the oral mucosa. Silk leaves a cleaner oral wound and does not have to be removed. In the most anterior portion of the velum, where closure cannot be done, the nasal and oral mucosae are sutured to one another to ensure a closed wound. After approximately 3 months, neither the relaxing incisions nor the incisions at the junction of the soft and hard palates are discernible (Fig. 40–5).

Also, unlike the Schweckendiek method, closure of the remainder of the palate is not delayed longer than 12 to 22 months, avoiding the need for obturators. Hard palate closure is done using either the von Langenbeck technique with or without the use of a vomer flap for a two-layer closure, or occasionally by a modified Widmaier technique (one-layer vomer flap closure). The latter technique is used only when the palatal shelves have progressed medially until only a very narrow space remains.

The remaining anterior cleft is closed as follows. The oral mucoperiosteal flaps are elevated. The width of the cleft dictates whether this is done completely or whether an anterior attachment is maintained. The base of the vomer is incised over its entire length, and a flap is raised to serve as the nasal lining. This flap either is directly sutured to the elevated edge of the nasal mucoperiosteum on the cleft side or, using mattress sutures of 3–0 chromic catgut, is drawn underneath the raised oral mucoperiosteal flap (Fig. 40–7), or a combination of both. These sutures are tied at the end of the closure, ensuring reduction of the potential dead space between the oral and nasal layers. Closure is attempted up to but not including the alveolar portion of the cleft.

An orthodontic evaluation of the maxillary growth of the two-stage palatal closure, as outlined above, has been given at the Third International Symposium for Early Treatment of Cleft Lip and Cleft Palate in Zurich, Switzerland,[9] in 1984. Eighty percent of all unilateral clefts showed favorable results, with absence of or only slight crossbite. In patients with bilateral clefts this figure was 76%. The alveolar portion of the cleft is closed with a bone graft at the mixed dentition stage.

Evaluation of Speech Results

Three previous reports have been made about the speech results from the series of 114 cleft lip and palate and cleft palate patients treated with primary veloplasty during a 16-year period. The first two reports, by Meijer et al[10] (1984) and Cohen et al[11] in 1985, dealt with patients who had good speech results following primary repair. The third report, by Cohen et al[12] in 1986, studied patients who subsequently required a pharyngeal flap.

In the present work, previous reports will be sum-

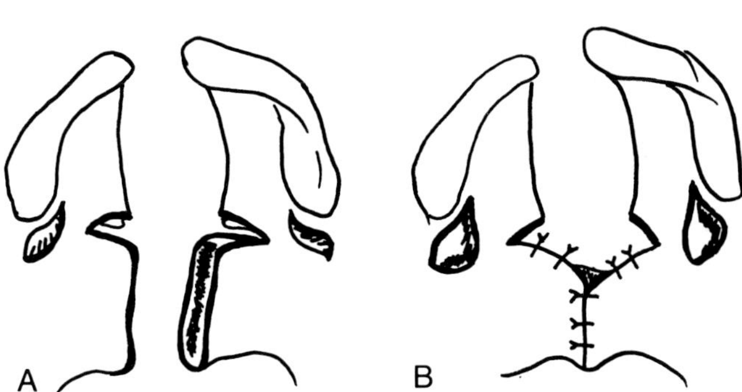

Figure 40–6 *A,* Incisions at bony junction for very wide clefts. *B,* Closure of incisions.

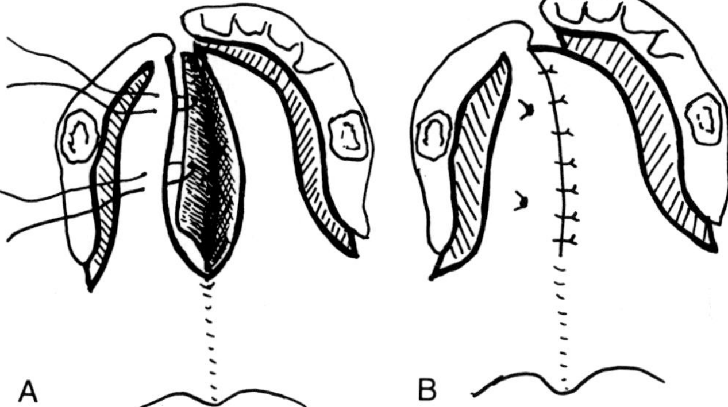

Figure 40–7 *A,* Use of sutures to draw vomer flap laterally. *B,* Final closure with mattress sutures tied, obliterating dead space.

marized and additional data will be presented. The studies included 71 males and 43 females. No patients were eliminated because of mental retardation, hearing loss, or other significant medical diagnosis. Surgery was performed by plastic surgeons belonging to the cleft palate team. Sixty-four percent of patients (or 73) had good speech results following primary repair (by a two-stage procedure). Twenty-nine percent showed good results following pharyngeal flap surgery; 7% continued to have poor speech even after pharyngoplasty. Since these results were reported, data from two additional patients have been added to our series. Both had achieved good speech following primary repair. Therefore, the speech results for the series changed as follows: Of 116 patients, 75 (65%) had good speech results following primary repair, 33 (28%) showed good results following pharyngeal flap surgery, and 8 (7%) continued to have poor speech even after a pharyngeal flap procedure.

Good speech was defined as speech that did not call attention to itself because of hypernasality and/or nasal emission. The evaluation system duplicated as closely as possible the speech pathology protocol developed and used first by Morris[13] and then in several subsequent studies by The University of Iowa Cleft Palate Center.[7, 14]

In the discussion to follow and in Tables 40–1 to 40–5, the abbreviations PP and PF refer to patients who received primary two-stage palate surgery and those who also required pharyngeal flap surgery, respectively. The data for the PF group was taken before the pharyngeal flap procedure was done. Descriptive information about the 116 patients is summarized in Table 40–1. Data about the two additional patients are not incorporated unless indicated by the phrase *116 series*. In the PP group (116 series) 22 (or 29%) of 75 patients did not receive speech therapy.

Speech evaluations used in both studies were those that resulted in the recommendation to consider or not consider palatopharyngoplasty to improve speech. The mean age at evaluation in the PP group was 7 years 1 month and in the PF group, 6 years 5 months. For the two groups (116 series) judgments of speech capability were made by plastic surgeons for ten patients. Data were obtained for the remaining 106 patients by five speech pathologists who were experienced in working with cleft palate patients.

The Iowa protocol and summation of the findings of the two studies follow:

1. *Articulation using Iowa Pressure Articulation Test (IPAT)*. In the PP group (59 patients) 34% received high scores of 36 or more (43 is the perfect score).

Table 40–1. Descriptive Information of 116 Patients Under Study[a]

Description	PP	PF
Age at study		
Range	2½ yr to 21 yr 8 mo	4 yr 5 mo to 21 yr
Mean	7 yr 1 mo	12 yr 5 mo
Sex distribution		
Male	44	27
Female	31	14
Age at surgery		
Average age at velar closure	6 mo	12 mo
Average age at hard palate closure	20 mo	24 mo

PP = Primary palatoplasty; PF = pharyngeal flap surgery
[a]Of 116 patients, 75 had primary surgery only; 41 had pharyngeal flap surgery also.

Sixty-three percent received moderate scores (16 to 35), 3% scored low (11 to 15), and none scored below 10. Seventeen percent made nasal emission errors, 61% made oral distortion errors, and one glottal stop was noted. In the PF group (30 patients) 80% missed more than half the test items. One hundred percent made nasal emission errors, 30% made oral distortion errors, and 16% made glottal errors.

2. *Stimulability to produce /p/ and /s/ phonemes*. In the PP group 96% could produce the phonemes. In the PF group 76% could not produce the phonemes.

3. *Grimacing*. Grimacing was observed in the PP group in 13% and in the PF group in 32%.

4. *Articulation rating*. In the PP group 90% rated in the normal to mildly defective range (on a five-point scale), and 10% scored in the moderately defective range. Of interest is the fact that 63% of the patients were under 7 years of age, the period of time in which articulatory errors are common. In the PF group 76% rated in the moderate to severely defective range.

5. *Nasality rating*. In the PP group 95% rated in the normal to very mild, intermittent hypernasality range (on a seven-point scale). In the PF group 76% rated in the moderate to severe hypernasality range.

6. *Corroborative studies*. Panendoscopy, cinefluoroscopy, videofluoroscopy, and nasendoscopy were used to provide physiologic assessment of velopharyngeal function when velopharyngeal incompetence was suspected. One or more of these tests was used for 26 PF patients. Of these, 92% rated in the velopharyngeal incompetent range and 8% in the marginally incompetent range by the different physiologic studies, which agreed with listener judgment of degree of velopharyngeal incompetence in 25 of 26 cases.

Table 40–2. Post Hoc Velopharyngeal Status of 69 Cases—Iowa Protocol 1984 (116 Series)

Rating	Operative Status	No.	%
Competent	Post primary palatoplasty	58	84
Marginal	Post primary palatoplasty	3	4
Incompetent	Post primary palatoplasty	—	—
	Subtotal	61	12
Not classifiable		8	—
	Total	69	100

Table 40–3. Speech Results in 116 Cases by Cleft Type—116 Series

		Good Postoperative Primary Lip and Palate Repair		Good Postoperative PF		Poor Postoperative PF		
Description	No.	No.	%	No.	%	No.	%	Total %
Incomplete unilateral CL/P	14	7	50	5	36	2	14	100
Complete unilateral CL/P	36	28	78	7	19	1	3	100
Incomplete bilateral CL/P	12	10	83	1	8	1	9	100
Complete bilateral CL/P	24	14	58	9	38	1	4	100
Incomplete CP	16	10	63	5	31	1	6	100
Complete CP	14	6	43	6	43	2	14	100
Total	116	75		33		8		

CL/P = Cleft lip and palate; CP = cleft palate; PF = pharyngeal flap

Utilizing the Iowa protocol, three clinical judgments were made about the causes of speech defects, as follows (116 series):

1. Dental, occlusal, fistula factors (fistula factors were not a part of the Iowa protocol). In the PP group (69 patients) possible or probable adverse effects were noted in 19 patients (28%). No effect was noted in 50 patients (72%). In the PF group (36 patients) possible or probable adverse effects occurred in 13 patients (36%). No effect was seen in 23 patients (64%).

2. Learning factors. In the PP group (69 patients) possible or probable effects occurred in 19 patients or 28%. In the PF group (36 patients) possible or probable effects occurred in 13 patients or 36%.

3. Velopharyngeal functioning. In the PP group (69 patients) 53 patients (77%) rated as competent and 16 patients (23%) as marginally competent. In the PF group (37 patients) 36 patients (97%) rated as incompetent and 1 patient (3%) as marginally competent.

Using predetermined criteria in the Iowa protocol, post hoc ratings of velopharyngeal competence were made to check the clinical judgments made of the PP group as shown in Table 40–2. In this PP group (116 series) of 69 patients, 61 (88%) could be classified, excluding corroborative data, and rated as competent or marginally competent, which agreed with the Saint Barnabas Medical Center rating. The eight who could not be classified had a nasality rating from Saint Barnabas Medical Center of 0 (normal) or +1 (nearly normal). Of the eight, five exhibited a nasal grimace, and two could not produce a good /s/ sound but otherwise were rated as velopharyngeal competent. The corroborative information and clinical judgment differed for one patient, and therefore that patient could not be classified.

In the PF group (37 patients) prior to the pharyngeal flap procedure, post hoc ratings of velopharyngeal competence also were made to check clinical judgments. Twenty-six, or 70%, could be classified. Eight (21%) were rated as having marginal competence and 18 (49%) as having velopharyngeal incompetence. Eleven patients (30%) were not classifiable, seven because they did not have IPAT scores and four because they did not fit the rating criteria exactly.

The number and percentage of good speech results following two-stage primary palatoplasty were tabulated by cleft type (116 series) as shown in Table 40–3. By cleft type, those with incomplete bilateral cleft lip and palate and complete unilateral cleft lip and palate showed the highest percentage of good speech results, and those with complete cleft palate showed the lowest.

Additional information related to dental, occlusal, and fistula factors, as listed in Table 40–4 by cleft type for the PP group (116 series), was obtained. More than half of the factors were found to be present in the bilateral cleft group. Thirteen (65%) of all factors were attributed to occlusion and resulted in distortion of fricative sounds, especially /s/, /z/, and /s/, and affricate sounds, /tʃ/ and /dʒ/. The presence of a hard palatal fistula resulted in two patients in a rating of +1 (very mild)

Table 40–4. Dental, Occlusal, Fistula Factors in 69 Patients by Cleft Type—PP Group (116 Series)

		Dental		Occlusal		Fistula		Total	
Description	No.	Poss	Prob	Poss	Prob	Poss	Prob	Poss	Prob
Incomplete unilateral CL/P	7	1[a]		1[a]				2	
Complete unilateral CL/P	28			1	1	1	1	2	2
Incomplete bilateral CL/P	10			1		1		2	
Complete bilateral CL/P	13	1		3	5		2	4	7
Incomplete CP	5				1				1
Complete CP	6								
Total	69	2		6	7	2	3	10	10

Poss = possible; Prob = probable; PP = primary surgery; CL/P = cleft lip and palate; CP = cleft palate
[a]One patient had two types of errors.

Table 40–5. Dental, Occlusal, Fistula Factors in 36 Patients by Cleft Type—PF Group

Description	No.	Dental		Occlusal		Fistula		Total	
		Poss	*Prob*	*Poss*	*Prob*	*Poss*	*Prob*	*Poss*	*Prob*
Incomplete unilateral CL/P	6	1			1		1	1	2
Complete unilateral CL/P	7			1		1		2	
Incomplete bilateral CL/P	1			1				1	
Complete bilateral CL/P	8		1	2		1		3	1
Incomplete CP	6					1		1	
Complete CP	8			1		1		2	
Total	36	1	1	5	1	4	1	10	3

PF = pharyngeal flap surgery; Poss = possible; prob = probable; CL/P = cleft lip and palate; CP = cleft palate

intermittent degree of hypernasality; in the others it was responsible for possible or probable oral distortion and/or substitution of sounds.

Shelton and Blank[15] cited a number of reports that indicated that oronasal fistulas may have harmful effects on speech. Isberg and Henningsson[16] studied velopharyngeal function using cineradiography in ten patients with hard palate fistulas and velopharyngeal incompetence and found that complete velopharyngeal closure was obtained in some of their patients by occluding the fistula. In our study, the least number of factors was attributed to dentition. In one patient, a malpositioned tooth near the midline in the hard palate was thought to be a possible causative factor in oral distortion.

Dental, occlusal, and fistula factors thought to have a deleterious effect on speech for the PF group are listed in Table 40–5. An equal number of factors was found in the unilateral and bilateral cleft lip and palate groups. The greater number of factors was attributed to occlusion. Occlusal factors in two patients were attributed possibly to an open bite. In two studies of normals, as reported by Starr,[17] open bite occlusion was thought to contribute to defective speech. In our PF series, one fistula, when occluded with a prosthesis, eliminated hypernasal speech.

The number of patients for whom dental, occlusal, and fistula factors were available in the PP and PF groups in the 116 series totaled 105. In 73 (70%) of these patients, no effect on speech relating to these factors was registered. One author (S.C.) has seen patients in which compensatory use of the speech mechanism produced good speech despite the presence of dental, occlusal, or fistula abnormalities.

Studies about the speech results of a particular surgical procedure are enhanced if a tentative conclusion can be presented regarding the probable factors contributing to failure to achieve nasal resonance in the range of normal. The following information, known about five patients who were rated as having poor speech after primary repair and who later underwent a pharyngeal flap procedure, may prove useful in this regard. Learning factors were considered to have a probable effect on these patients as follows. One patient with complete unilateral cleft lip and palate and hemifacial microsomia had maximum conductive hearing loss requiring use of a hearing aid. A second patient with complete bilateral cleft lip and palate had a moderate learning disability, a receptive language delay greater than 3 years, and he came from a non-English speaking home and community. These patients appeared to be at risk for failing to achieve good speech results following palatal repair because of impaired learning.

The average age at velar closure was 6 months later in the PF group than in the PP group, which raises speculation about whether or not the delayed closure was related to the need for the pharyngeal flap procedure. Additional information about the timing of surgery for the two groups does not offer strong evidence to support such a relationship. Sixty-five percent of the PP group had received velar closure by the end of the sixth month, and all had received this procedure before 29 months. In the PF group, 60% had achieved velar closure by the end of the sixth month, and all but five had achieved it before 29 months. Age of closure for the five patients ranged from 3 years to 6 years 3 months. Of these five patients, three retained poor speech following the pharyngeal flap procedure and are among the group mentioned in the preceding paragraph who were thought to have a poor response to surgical intervention because of impaired learning ability.

Discussion

Studies were conducted on the speech of 116 patients who had undergone two-stage palatoplasty. For patients with good speech results the average age at velar closure was 6 months, with hard palate closure at 20 months. In those who required a pharyngeal flap procedure velar closure was achieved at 12 months and hard palatal closure at 24 months.

The later average age at velar closure in the pharyngeal flap group was largely due to the late age at surgery in five patients (ranging from 3 years to 6 years 3 months). Three of these five patients were considered to have poor speech results following pharyngeal flap surgery. They were thought to be at risk for failing to develop good speech following surgical intervention because of impaired learning skills. With our series, there does not appear to be supporting evidence that delayed closure results in the need for pharyngeal flap.

The two studies suggest that two-stage palatoplasty, as performed at our center, yields a satisfactory percentage of good speech results because overall, 65% of the cleft lip and palate and cleft palate patients obtained good speech. By cleft type, the best results were seen in those with complete unilateral cleft lip and palate (78%) and in those with incomplete bilateral cleft lip and palate (83%); the poorest results occurred in those with incomplete unilateral cleft lip and palate and complete cleft palate. Morris[18] estimated the success rate of primary surgery as 75% and as 60% to 70% in a personal communication with one of the authors (S.C.).[19]

The studies suggest that our surgical approach tends to provide an intraoral environment that is conducive to the development of good articulation. For 73 patients with good speech results following primary repair, 90% rated in the normal to mildly defective range in articulation skill. Of interest is the fact that 63% of these patients were under 7 years of age, a period of time in which misarticulation is common. Iowa Pressure Articulation Test scores were available for 59 of these patients. Thirty-four percent received high scores of 36 or more (of a possible 43), only 3% had low scores of between 11 and 15; none scored below 10, and only one glottal error was noted. Data were extrapolated from both studies regarding the possible or probable adverse effects of dental, occlusal, and fistula factors on articulation. In the PP (primary palatoplasty) group, no effect was noted in 50 (72%) of 69 patients, and in the PF (pharyngeal flap) group, no effect was noted in 23 (65%) of 36 patients. When results from both groups were combined, 70% of the 105 patients showed no effect. In each group, occlusal factors were more common than dental or fistula factors.

Our studies provided evidence that factors other than timing and method of palatal repair appeared to affect speech outcome for some of the patients. Five of the 116 patients were judged to be poor surgical candidates due to impaired learning ability. Palatal surgery can be successful only to the extent that the individual can learn how to use the speech mechanism. The Iowa Protocol was used to report and evaluate speech results for the patients in our studies. It was convenient to use and proved to be cost-effective because the research design was already in place.

References

1. Walker JC, Jr, Collito MB, Mancusi-Ungaro A, et al: Physiologic considerations in cleft lip closure: The C. W. technique. Plast Reconstr Surg 37:552, 1966.
2. Schweckendiek W: Zur Frage der Früh- und Spatoperation der angeborenen Lippen-Kiefer-Gaumenspalten. Z Laryngol Rhinol 30:51, 1951.
3. Slaughter WB, Pruzansky S: The rationale for velar closure as a primary procedure in the repair of cleft palate defects. Plast Reconstr Surg 13–14:341, 1954.
4. Fára M, Brousilova M: Experiences with early closure of velum and later closure of hard palate. Plast Reconstr Surg 44:134, 1969.
5. Herfert O: Two-stage operation for cleft palate. Br J Plast Surg 16:37, 1979.
6. Witzel MA, Salyer KE, Ross RB: Delayed hard palate closure: The philosophy revisited. Cleft Palate J 21:263, 1984.
7. Bardach J, Morris HL, Olin WH: Late results of primary veloplasty: The Marburg project. Plast Reconstr Surg 73:207, 1984.
8. Kriens O: An anatomical approach to veloplasty. Plast Reconstr Surg 43:29, 1969.
9. Meijer R, Greenlee R, Cohen SW: The lip adhesion as a base for the early treatment of complete clefts of the lip and palate. In Hotz M, Gnoinski W, Perko M, et al (eds): Early Treatment of Cleft Lip and Palate. Bern: Hans Huber, 1986, p 49.
10. Meijer R, Greenlee R, Cohen SW: Speech results following primary palatoplasty—a partial report. Third International Symposium on Early Treatment of Cleft Lip and Palate, Zurich, 1984, unpublished.
11. Cohen SW, Meijer R, Ciacca K, et al: Speech results following primary palatoplasty. Presented at the Fifth International Congress of Cleft Palate and Related Craniofacial Anomalies, Monte Carlo, 1985.
12. Cohen SW, Meijer R, Winarksy S: Speech results for cases requiring pharyngeal flap. Presented at the Forty-third Annual Meeting of the American Cleft Palate Association, New York, 1986, unpublished.
13. Morris HL: Velopharyngeal competence and the Demjen W/V-Y technique. In Morris HL (ed): The Bratislava Project: Some Cleft Palate Surgical Results. Iowa City: University of Iowa Press, 1978, Chap. 4.
14. Bardach J, Morris H, Olin W, et al: Late results of multidisciplinary management of unilateral cleft lip and palate. Ann Plast Surg 12:235, 1984.
15. Shelton RL, Blank JL: Oronasal fistulas, intraoral air pressure and nasal air flow during speech. Cleft Palate J 21:91, 1984.
16. Isberg A, Henningsson G: Influence of palatal fistulas on velopharyngeal movements: A cineradiographic study. Plast Reconstr Surg 79:530, 1987.
17. Starr DC: Dental and occlusal hazards to normal speech production. In Grabb WD, Rosenstein SW, Bzoch KR (eds): Cleft Lip and Palate. Boston: Little, Brown, 1971, p 672.
18. Morris, HL: Velopharyngeal competence and primary cleft palate surgery. 1960–1971: A critical review. Cleft Palate J 10:62, 1973.
19. Morris HL: Personal communication, September 11, 1984.

CHAPTER 41

Evaluation of Late Results of Cleft Palate Repair

Libby Wilson

In 1971 the cleft palate clinic at Rancho Los Amigos began to perform two-stage cleft palate repair. We were encouraged by reports of favorable influences on facial growth resulting from this surgical procedure.[1-3] At that time we were not yet aware of any reports suggesting potential problems with speech production.

Materials and Methods

Within the first days of life, our patients were fitted with a palatal appliance to facilitate feeding. Soft palate repair was carried out at the same time as lip repair at 3 months of age or later, depending on the age of the patient at the time of his or her first visit to the clinic. As part of the surgical procedure, the muscles were reoriented and approximated as advocated by Randall.[4] Oral mucosal flaps were brought together in the midline, posterior to the greater palatine vessels. We obturated the defect left by the unrepaired hard palate with an acrylic appliance.

We repaired the hard palate when arch expansion and stabilization could be accomplished using the second deciduous molars for appliance retention. Hard palate closure was performed using turnover flaps based on the vomer. The maxillary arch shape was maintained with appliances through completion of orthodontic treatment. When family compliance was good, resulting speech production was only minimally distorted, and maxillary arch form was generally satisfactory.

Unfortunately, we found that the obturating appliances were discarded at a high rate by families. After lip and soft palate repair was carried out, patients frequently did not return. If they did return for follow-up, compensatory articulatory patterns were noted, which we attributed to the open defect in the hard palate.

Results

We carried out two-stage palate repair from 1971 through 1981. For the first 7 years, anterior palatal oral mucosal island flaps were utilized to achieve palatal lengthening. Rather than confusing interpretation of speech results with this additional variable, these patients were excluded from this report.

Between January of 1978 and November of 1981, 36 patients with unilateral clefts of the lip and palate were repaired in two stages. The distribution of sex and side of cleft in our patients is reported in Table 41–1.

Table 41–1. Distribution of the Study Patients in Regard to Side of Cleft and Sex

	L	R	Total
Male	18	9	27
Female	5	4	9
Total	23	13	36

Most soft palate repairs were carried out when the patients were between 2 and 8 months of age. One patient underwent soft palate repair at 1 month and one at 11 months of age. Surgical repair of the hard palate was performed in most patients between 2.5 and 4 years of age. One patient underwent repair at 1 year and another at 6 years of age.

Eight of the 36 patients (22%) did not return for repair of the hard palate. One of these patients has recently returned with a residual cleft of the hard palate at 9 years of age. She demonstrated nasal emission and distorted articulation. Three patients did not return after palate repair. Therefore, no speech information is available. These 11 patients represent 30% of the group

Table 41–2. Summary of Evaluation of Our 36 Study Patients

Initials	Date of Birth	Side of Cleft	Velum	Hard Palate Surgery	Nasal Emission	Articulatory Distortions	Comments
C.M.	9/26/77	L	3½ mo	3 yr + 4 mo	0	All sibilant sounds	
W.B.	6/9/77	R	8 mo	2½ yr	+/−	—	10/79 Lost to follow-up
M.T.	1/20/78	R	4 mo	2 yr	0	0	
C.A.	1/9/78	R	2½ mo	4 yr − 2 mo	0	0	
O.S.	3/3/78	L	4 mo	4 yr	0	S	
M.R.	3/7/78	L	5 mo	3 yr + 7 mo	0	+	10/83 Last visit
B.G.	12/10/77	L	6 mo	0		—	1978 Lost to follow-up
J.B.	4/28/78	L	3 mo	0		—	10/80 Lost to follow-up
E.Q.	4/1/78	L	3 mo	3 yr + 1 mo	+	0	Push-back at 9½ yr
N.N.	7/7/78	L	2½ mo	0	+	+	
M.J.M.	10/20/78	L	3 mo	6 yr	0	/f/, /s/, /ch/, /z/, /j/, /r/	
B.E.	10/24/78	L	8 mo	3 yr		Developmental errors	4/83 Last visit
L.M.	1/3/79	L	4½ mo	3 yr + 4 mo	0	Slight /s/	
J.R.	2/4/79	L	3 mo	0		—	Lost to follow-up
D.W.	5/29/79	R	3½ mo	0		—	Lost to follow-up
R.L.	6/5/79	L	3½ mo	0		—	Lost to follow-up
H.A.	8/2/79	R	7½ mo	2 yr + 9 mo	0	Minimum /s/	
T.A.	8/19/79	L	2½ mo	0		—	Lost to follow-up
C.H.	8/19/79	L	8 mo	0		—	Lost to follow-up
M.R.	9/17/79	R	4½ mo	—	0	0	Age of closure of hard palate not documented
E.A.	2/6/80	L	5½ mo	3 yr + 4 mo	0	Phoneme specific	
J.E.	4/17/80	R	6 mo	2½ yr	+	—	Lost to follow-up
A.B.	4/4/80	R	11 mo	3 yr + 4 mo	0	All sibilant sounds	
J.M.	5/11/80	L	5½ mo	2 yr + 8 mo	+/−	/s/, /sh/, /f/	
R.P.	5/16/80	L	3 mo	6 yr + 3 mo		—	No evaluation available
E.G.	6/2/80	L	7 mo	2 yr + 8 mo	0	/s/, /h/, /r/	
R.G.	6/6/80	L	5 mo	2 yr	0	/r/, /s/, /th/, /l/	
C.R.	7/31/80	L	5½ mo	2½ yr	0	Omits /g/ and /k/	
S.F.	9/2/80	R	2 mo	2 yr + 9 mo	+/−	/s/	
A.P.	11/5/80	R	3½ mo	3 yr + 2 mo	0	/s/	
G.Y.	12/20/80	R	6 mo	3 yr + 4 mo	0	—	No evaluation available
M.M.	1/9/81	L	5 mo	2 yr + 9 mo	+/−	Present	
J.N.	1/31/81	R	5 mo	3 yr + 1 mo	0	/s/, /s/ blends	
R.V.	5/18/81	L	2½ mo	3 yr − 2 mo	0	/s/, /th/, /ch/	
P.P.	6/2/81	R	1 mo	3 yr − 2 mo	0	/s/, /sh/	
J.P.	6/20/81	L	5 mo	1 yr	+	0	Push-back at 5½ yr

of 36. Twenty-five patients, or 70%, of the study group, continue to receive care at Rancho Los Amigos and have had recent speech evaluation by the Rancho team speech pathologist.

Of this group, 20 patients (80%) have no evidence of nasal emission. Three (15%) of the 20 have no articulatory defects. Seventeen of the 20 (85%) have articulatory defects involving the phonemes /s/, /sh/, /th/, /ch/, /z/, /f/, and /r/.

Of the five patients in the group of 25 who were considered to have nasal emission, two were judged to be free of articulatory defects. Videofluoroscopy in these two patients demonstrated small velopharyngeal defects, described as touch closure. Both of these patients have had secondary palatal surgery consisting of palatal push-back or lengthening using a cheek mucosal flap to line the nasal mucosal defect, as described by Kaplan.[5] These patients no longer have nasal emission. Judgment of speech results was made by our team speech pathologist and a consultant who visits monthly. The other three patients had equivocal nasal emission on clinical examination. Articulatory defects involving the phonemes listed previously were present in all three. Videofluoroscopic studies of these patients demonstrated good velopharyngeal function but aberrant tongue function. They are receiving speech therapy and will continue to be reevaluated. A summary of our individual patient results is presented in Table 41–2.

Discussion

It is not the purpose of this chapter to discuss the effect of an unrepaired hard palate on speech production. However, it is worthwhile to consider the findings of Isberg and Henningsson,[6] who described the damping effect of an anterior palatal fistula on the function of the velopharyngeal mechanism prior to proceeding with secondary palatal surgery.

In addition, this chapter emphasizes the importance of considering all factors that contribute to successful completion of a course of treatment. Before committing patients and staff to a treatment protocol requiring a 15- to 18-year period of consistent care, one should be aware of the patient population. In Los Angeles, it is estimated that 25% of the Hispanic population returns to Mexico annually. This percentage agrees closely with the 30% of our study population that was lost to follow-up. Approximately 85% of our patients have Hispanic surnames. With this information, modification of the proposed plan of treatment is necessary.

Our recommendations are as follows.

1. Before embarking on a long-term program, attempt to determine if families will be able to comply with long-term commitments required by multistage treatment.
2. Repair the hard palate before compensatory articulatory patterns develop.
3. Utilize surgical techniques that create the least amount of raw surface, for example, turnover or bookflaps.
4. Finally, if a patient is seen with an unrepaired hard palate and nasal emission, repair the hard palate. Then reexamine the speech production in 6 months using endoscopy and fluoroscopy. Do not carry out secondary surgical procedures, such as pharyngeal flaps, before closing significant residual defects in the hard palate.

References

1. Slaughter WB, Pruzansky S: The rationale for velar closure as a primary procedure in the repair of cleft palate defects. Plast Reconstr Surg 13:341, 1954.
2. Schweckendiek W: Die Technik der primaren Veloplastik. Chirurg 34:277, 1963.
3. Schweckendiek W: Primary veloplasty. In Schuchardt K (ed): Treatment of Patients with Clefts of the Lip, Alveolus and Palate. Stuttgart: G. Thieme, 1966.
4. Randall P: A triangular flap operation for the primary repair of unilateral clefts of the lip. Plast Reconstr Surg 23:331, 1959.
5. Kaplan EN: Soft palate repair by levator muscle reconstruction and a buccal mucosal flap. Plast Reconstr Surg 5:129, 1975.
6. Isberg A, Henningsson G: Influence of palatal fistulae on velopharyngeal movements. A cineradiographic study. Plast Reconstr Surg 79:525, 1987.

CHAPTER 42

Intravelar Veloplasty: A Prospective Study

Jeffrey L. Marsh, Lynn Marty Grames, and Barbel Holtman

The goal of surgical repair for cleft palate is restoration of the static and dynamic anatomic integrity of the palate for normal deglutition and speech without impairment of the subsequent growth of the maxilla. Proponents of various methods of palatoplasty claim either that improved speech intelligibility or less impairment of maxillary growth results from usage of their procedure compared with those of others. Prospective controlled comparative studies of palatoplasty techniques are reported infrequently, however. When comparisons are made, they usually refer to historical data, which makes interpretation of the findings difficult. Surgical restoration of the levator veli palatini musculo-aponeurotic sling (intravelar veloplasty [IVV]) has been advocated since the 1960s as a means of improving velopharyngeal function for speech in patients with cleft palates.[1, 2] However, neither the initial anatomic reports of the operation[1–8] nor the subsequent historical comparative control studies[9, 10] have clearly established the efficacy of intravelar veloplasty. Because of the sound anatomic basis of the hypothesis that underlies intravelar veloplasty—namely, that restoration of the levator sling will improve velopharyngeal function—we initiated a prospective, alternative, single-institution study to test this hypothesis. Analysis of our first consecutive 121 patients is reported.

Methods of Study

Intravelar Veloplasty

The two surgeons agreed to initiate the study in 1982. They standardized the palatoplasty procedures by observing each other operate and then defining the non-IVV and IVV operations. One surgeon (B.H.) ceased operating after performing the sixty-eighth palatoplasty in this series; all subsequent palatoplasties were performed by the remaining surgeon (J.L.M.). Some palatoplasties were performed by resident surgeons. When this was the case, one of the two senior surgeons was present from the beginning to the end of the operation.

All patients received the non-IVV palatoplasty. The non-IVV palatoplasty consisted of mobilization of oral unipedicle mucoperiosteal flaps with skeletonization of the greater palatine neurovascular bundles; mobilization of nasal mucoperiosteal flaps from the posterior and cleft edges of the hard palate; and linear midline repair of each layer independently. The following procedures were not performed: mobilization of vomer flaps; division of the nasal mucoperiosteum or mucosa; fracture of the hamulus; and palatal push-back.

Those patients assigned to the IVV group also received an intravelar veloplasty in addition to the non-IVV palatoplasty. The intravelar veloplasty consisted of dissection of the levator fibers from the overlying and underlying oral and nasal mucosae; sharp separation of the fibers from their insertion on the posterior edge of the hard palate shelves; retroposition of the muscle bundles to the junction of the mid and posterior thirds of the velum; and plication of the muscle bundles across the midline between the oral and nasal mucosal repairs. In actual sequencing, the palatal mucosal and levator bundle dissections were performed first, the nasal mucosal repair second, the IVV third, and the oral mucosal repair last.

Patient Population

All patients presenting with clefts of the secondary palate with or without clefts of the primary palate for multidisciplinary evaluation by the cleft palate team of the Cleft Palate and Craniofacial Deformities Institute, St. Louis Children's Hospital, St. Louis, Missouri, were entered in the study. The infants were alternately assigned, independently for each surgeon, to either the non-IVV or the IVV group. Palatoplasty was performed as soon after each infant's first year birthday as feasible. The first patient in this study underwent palatoplasty on May 13, 1982. To date, 167 patients have been entered in the study, and enrollment continues. Of these, 121 are at least 3 years of age, the minimum age for speech evaluation in this study.

Of the 121 patients potentially available for evaluation, 49 have been eliminated from this study. Of those

eliminated, 15 were lost to follow-up; 14 were operated on by surgeons other than the two who standardized their procedures; nine had chronologically delayed palatoplasties; four had surgical complications that could be expected to affect velopharyngeal function (fistula or dehiscence); and seven had additional anomalies that might have adversely influenced sampling. This left 34 non-IVV and 38 IVV patients available for analysis.

Cleft Type

All patients with overt clefts of the secondary palate with or without clefts of the primary palate were enrolled in the study. Patients with submucous cleft palate were not entered in the study. There was a complete spectrum of palatal clefts ranging from incomplete clefts of the velum through complete bilateral cleft lip and palate (Fig. 42–1). The distribution of cleft types was similar between the non-IVV and the IVV groups except that there was a larger number of bilateral cleft lip and palate patients in the IVV group. The non-IVV group included six patients with Robin sequence; there were four Robin patients in the IVV group.

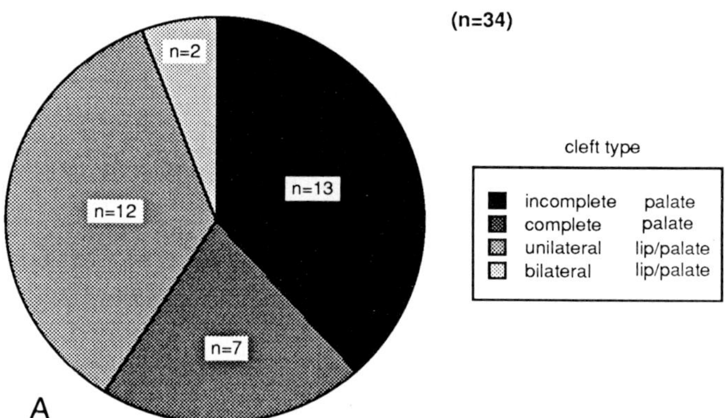

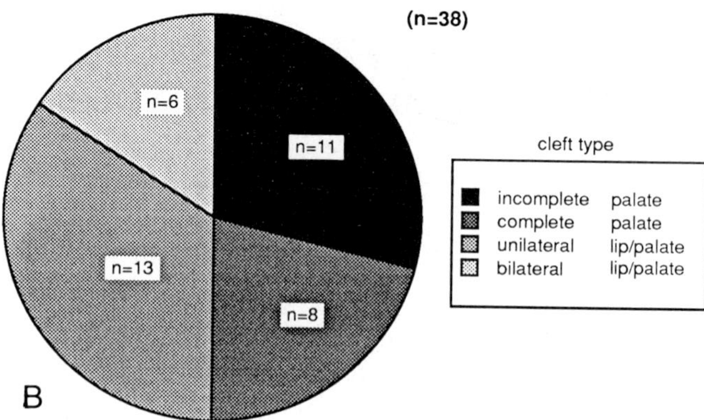

Figure 42–1 Distribution of cleft type: "incomplete palate" = isolated incomplete clefts of the secondary palate; "complete palate" = isolated complete clefts of the secondary palate; "unilateral lip/palate" = unilateral incomplete and complete clefts of the primary and secondary palates; "bilateral lip/palate" = bilateral incomplete and complete clefts of the primary and secondary palates. *A*, Non-intravelar veloplasty (IVV) patients. *B*, IVV patients.

Age at Palatoplasty

Palatoplasty was performed between 12 and 18 months of age for the patients in this study. The mean age for the non-IVV group was 15.3 ± 1.4 months; the mean age for the IVV group was 14.6 ± 1.7 months. There was no statistically significant difference between these mean values.

Technique of Palatoplasty

All patients received a standard palatoplasty. After the introduction of general endotracheal anesthesia, the patient's head was prepared and draped and slid into the surgeon's lap in the Trendelenburg position. A Dingman mouth gag was inserted. The tissues of the velum and the mucoperiosteum of the hard palate were infiltrated with 1:200,000 epinephrine solution. During a wait of 5 minutes for vasoconstriction to develop, bilateral unipedical mucoperiosteal flaps were marked (Fig. 42–2A). The cleft edge of each hemivelum was incised with a No. 12 blade, keeping the incision on the oral side of the hemivelum with a 2-mm cuff of oral mucosa. Using a No. 11 blade, the palatal mucoperiosteum was incised along the lingual aspect of the alveolar ridge from a point posterior of the maxillary tuberosity to the mesial aspect of the palatal shelf. The incision was continued posteriorly toward the velar incision with the No. 11 blade. Care was taken to preserve a 2-mm cuff of oral mucoperiosteum with the nasal mucosal flap to facilitate suturing and avoid vomer dissection.

On connection of the palatal and velar incisions, each mucoperiosteal flap was raised from the osseous palatal shelf using a Joseph elevator. The greater palatine neurovascular bundles were skeletonized using a Joseph elevator and Thackery palatal rasps. The preserved cuff of oral mucoperiosteum, along the hard palate cleft edge, was mobilized off the palatal shelf in continuity with the contiguous nasal mucosa using Joseph and Cronin elevators. The nasal mucosa was closed in straight-line fashion, from ventral to dorsal, using simple interrupted sutures of 4–0 polyglycolic acid on a palatal J needle (Fig. 42–2B). In patients with a bilateral cleft palate, each nasal floor was closed independently using a small, 2- to 3-mm flap of vomer mucosa reflected right and left from a midline incision.

Once the nasal mucosa was repaired, the two operations, intravelar veloplasty and non–intravelar veloplasty, diverged. When intravelar veloplasty was performed, the fibers of the levator were separated superiorly from the nasal mucosa of the velum using Joseph and Cronin elevators. The oral velar mucosa was separated from the levator fibers using Metzenbaum scissors (Fig. 42–2C). Once the levator fibers were

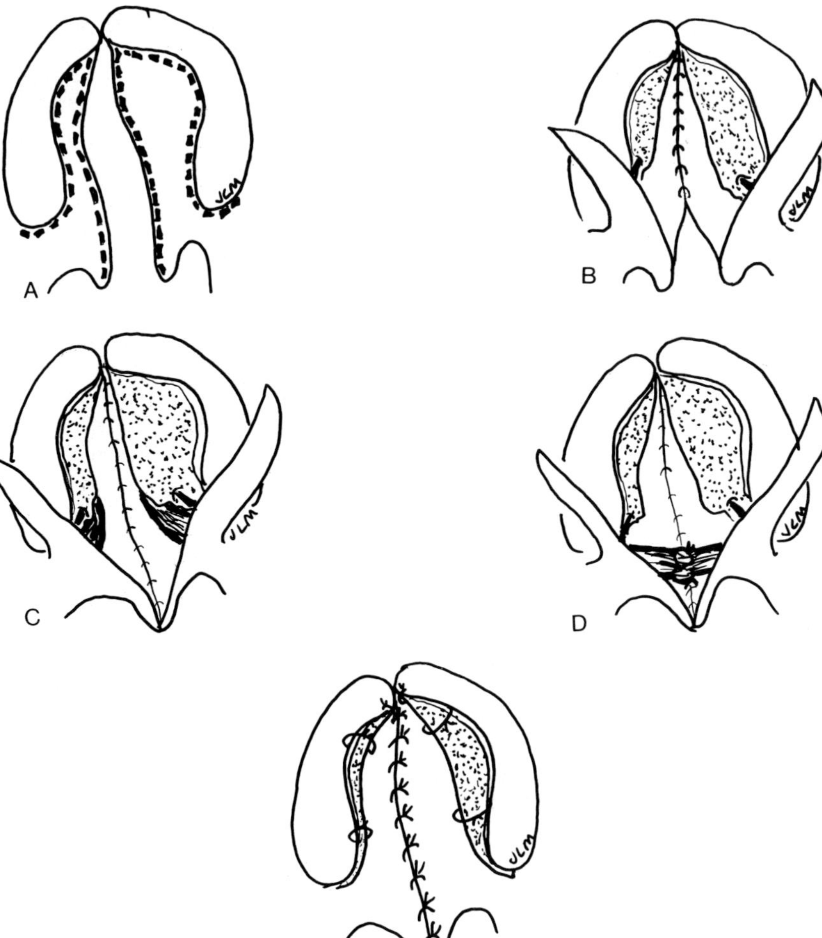

Figure 42–2 Schematic of the operations performed. *A,* The dotted lines indicate the incisions for both the non-IVV and IVV groups. *B,* The nasal mucosa is closed from ventral to dorsal for both groups. *C,* For those patients receiving intravelar veloplasty, the levator veli palatini bundles are skeletonized from the oral and nasal mucosae. The levators are shown still attached to the edge of the osseous palatal shelves. *D,* For those patients receiving IVV, the levators are cut from their osseous insertion. The muscles are retropositioned and plicated across the repaired velar nasal mucosa. *E,* The oral mucoperiosteum is closed in straight-line fashion, and the tips of the flaps are fixed to the alveolar mucosa for both the non-IVV and IVV groups.

skeletonized at their attachment to the posterior edge of the palatal shelf, they were cut free from the bone at their insertion. The closure of the nasal mucosa was then completed. The freed insertions of the levator bundles were then retropositioned and plicated, using horizontal mattress sutures of 4–0 polyglycolic acid, across the repaired nasal mucosa of the velum (Fig. 42–2D).

At this point both operations were completed similarly. The uvula and oral mucosa of the velum were repaired in straight-line fashion using simple interrupted sutures of 4–0 polyglycolic acid. Repair of the palatal oral mucoperiosteum was continued in straight-line fashion with simple interrupted sutures. When tension on the closure at the junction of the hard and soft palates seemed excessive, relaxing incisions were cut into the mucosa posterior to the maxillary tuberosities. There was no dissection of the lateral pharyngeal walls, nor were the hamuli fractured. The tips of the palatal mucoperiosteal flaps were fixed to the alveolar mucosa with simple interrupted sutures of 4–0 polyglycolic acid. Two simple sutures were placed between the lateral edge of the palatal mucoperiosteal flaps and the alveolar mucosa to minimize flap movement until the fibrin clot set (Fig. 42–2E). An orogastric tube was passed, the gastric contents emptied, and the tube removed. The Dingman gag was removed, and the patient was returned to the supine position and extubated. The patient was sent to the postanesthetic recovery room in the lateral decubitus position with elbow splints in place.

Postoperative management was the same for both groups. The child was allowed to drink full liquids as soon after emergence from anesthesia as was safe. The intravenous line was discontinued when the child consistently took oral liquids. A "cleft palate" (nonchew) diet was begun the day after surgery. The child was discharged home when he or she was taking fluids well orally. This time period ranged from the first to the fifth postoperative day, with most children going home on the third postoperative day. A nonchew diet and elbow splints were maintained for 3 weeks after palatoplasty. The child was evaluated in the surgeon's office at that time, and diet and activity were then liberalized.

Speech Evaluation

Perceptual speech and language evaluations were performed at 3, 4, and 6 years of age for the study population (Fig. 42–3). The most recent evaluation has been used for the data presented. The majority of patients (65% for the non-IVV and 71% for the IVV groups) were at least 4 years of age at the time of the speech evaluation used to compile this report. Of those patients evaluated only at the age 3 to 4 years, 12 were in the non-IVV group and 11 were in the IVV group. Of those evaluated between the ages of 4 and 6 years, 17 were in the non-IVV group and 22 were in the IVV group. Of those evaluated at 6 years of age, there were five each in the non-IVV and IVV groups.

All children were evaluated by the same speech pathologist, who was experienced in assessment and

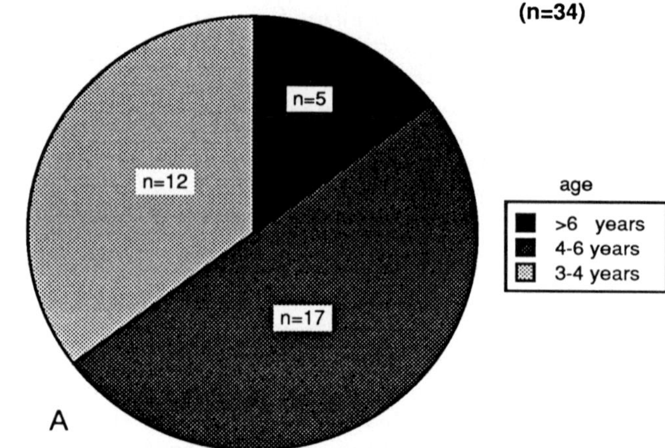

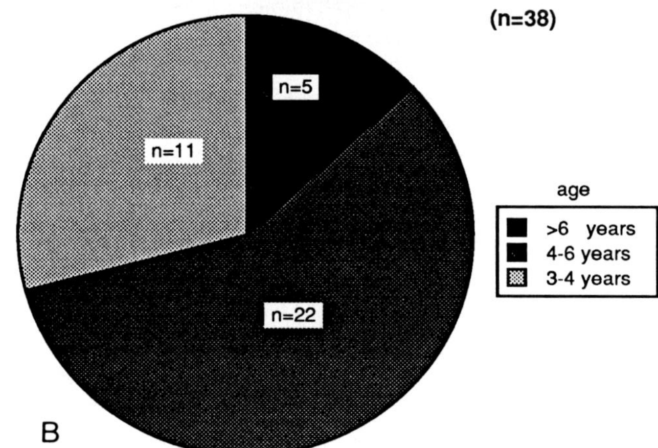

Figure 42–3 Distribution of age at the most recent speech evaluation was used for this study. *A,* Non-IVV patients. *B,* IVV patients.

therapy of cleft palate children. The evaluator was unaware of the patient's veloplasty group at the time of the evaluation. The same test protocol was used for all evaluations. The assessment was heavily weighted toward articulation, phonology, and resonance with additional screens for oral motor skills, language, and voice. Oral peripheral examinations, parent reports, therapeutic histories, and spontaneous language samples also were obtained. Stimulability screens were conducted on those children demonstrating symptoms of velopharyngeal dysfunction.

Treatment recommendations were made on the basis of this evaluation and with consideration of other cleft team members' findings. All patients referred for speech therapy or secondary palatal management had at least one additional speech and language evaluation by an independent speech pathologist. These evaluations all concurred with those of the team speech pathologist. In addition, all patients considered for secondary palatal management underwent nasopharyngoscopic evaluation of the velopharynx by a team consisting of a speech pathologist, pediatric otolaryngologist, plastic surgeon, and prosthodontist.

Table 42–1. Classification System for Velopharyngeal Dysfunction

WNL (within normal limits):   No symptoms of velopharyngeal dysfunction detected.

I: Psychosocially insignificant velopharyngeal dysfunction symptoms; no treatment indicated.

II: Velopharyngeal dysfunction symptoms that warrant a trial period of speech therapy.

III: Velopharyngeal dysfunction symptoms that warrant surgical or prosthetic palatal management.

Classification of Velopharyngeal Status

A four-part rating scale was established to classify the velopharyngeal function for speech of the patients in this study (Table 42–1). Children without any evidence of velopharyngeal dysfunction were classified as within normal limits (WNL). Type I dysfunction included mild, infrequent nasal turbulence or mild, fleeting hypernasality. These children were not referred for speech therapy because the need did not seem to justify the expense, and the outcome could not be assuredly different from the presenting behavior. Type II dysfunction included velopharyngeal dysfunction symptoms that were psychosocially significant but stimulable for change or mild to moderate in character. These patients were referred for a trial of speech therapy followed by re-evaluation. Type III dysfunction included symptoms of velopharyngeal dysfunction that was severe enough to warrant surgical or prosthetic secondary palatal management. All of these patients had received appropriate speech therapy that failed to produce sufficient change in velopharyngeal function to preclude secondary palatal management.

Audiograms

Because hearing is essential to the development of normal speech, the audiograms for the patients in the study were reviewed. The audiograms were obtained at 12 months and 3 years of age. They were rated as within normal limits, abnormal (loss of greater than 10 dB in at least one frequency), or unable to test. Most 12-month audiograms were acquired via sound field testing, were not ear specific, and did not include all frequencies. The 3-year audiograms were ear specific and included all of the usual frequencies. All children with abnormal results on audiograms and/or otologic examinations received otologic management according to their needs both prior to and following the audiographic testing.

Results

Velopharyngeal Status

There was no statistically significant difference between the non-IVV and IVV groups with respect to the distribution of velopharyngeal dysfunction classes (X^2 p = 0.406) (Fig. 42–4). In the non-IVV group, the distribution was WNL = 24%; type I = 29%; type II = 29%; type III = 18%. In the IVV group, the distribution

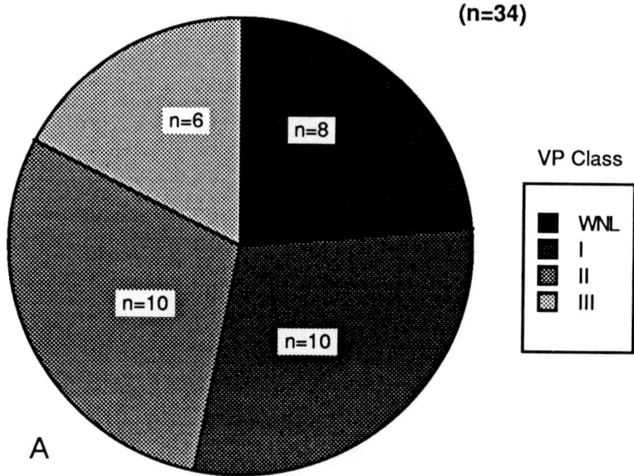

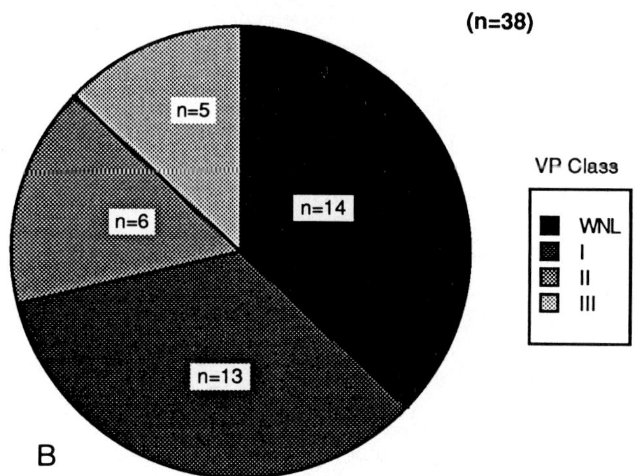

Figure 42–4 Distribution of velopharyngeal status using classification system of Table 42–1 above. *A*, Non-IVV patients. *B*, IVV patients.

was WNL = 37%; type I = 34%; type II = 16%; type III = 13%.

Consolidation of the data according to the need for therapeutic intervention, speech therapy, or secondary palatal management does suggest that there is less velopharyngeal dysfunction among patients who received intravelar veloplasty than among those who did not (Fig. 42–5). In the non-IVV group, 53% did not exhibit dysfunction requiring management whereas 47% did. In contrast, in the IVV group, 71% did not require management whereas only 29% did. These differences, however, were not statistically significant (Fisher's exact test p = 1.000).

An additional interpretation of the data results from analysis of the mean velopharyngeal status as a function of the age of the patient at the time of speech evaluation used in this study (Fig. 42–6). The velopharyngeal dysfunction classes were assigned numerical values to obtain mean scores for each age group: WNL = 0; I = 1; II = 2; III = 3. Whereas the IVV group had

Velopharyngeal Status - Non-IVV Patients

(n=34)

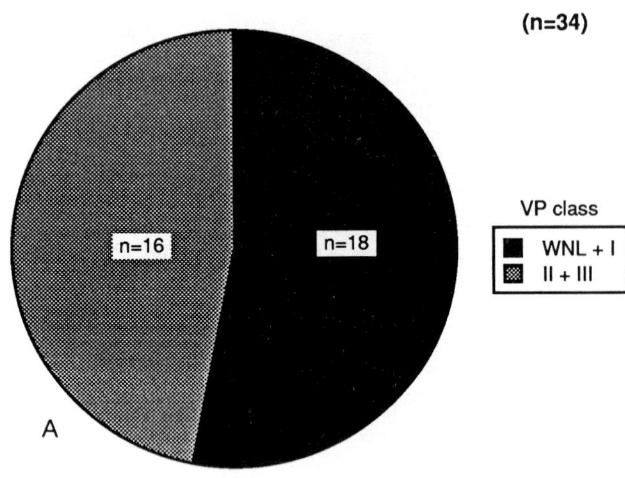

Figure 42–5 Distribution of velopharyngeal status with consolidation of data into those patients not requiring intervention (WNL + I) and those requiring either speech therapy or palatal management (II + III). *A*, Non-IVV patients. *B*, IVV patients.

Velopharyngeal Status - IVV Patients

(n=38)

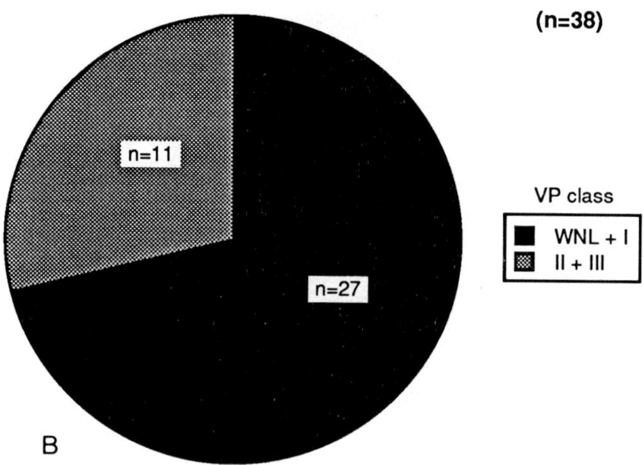

Velopharyngeal Status vs. Age of Speech Evaluation

Figure 42–6 Mean velopharyngeal status classification as a function of the patient's age in years at the time of the speech evaluation used for this study. The probability (Mann-Whitney U test) of the distribution of the paired non-IVV and IVV date for each age being due to chance is indicated.

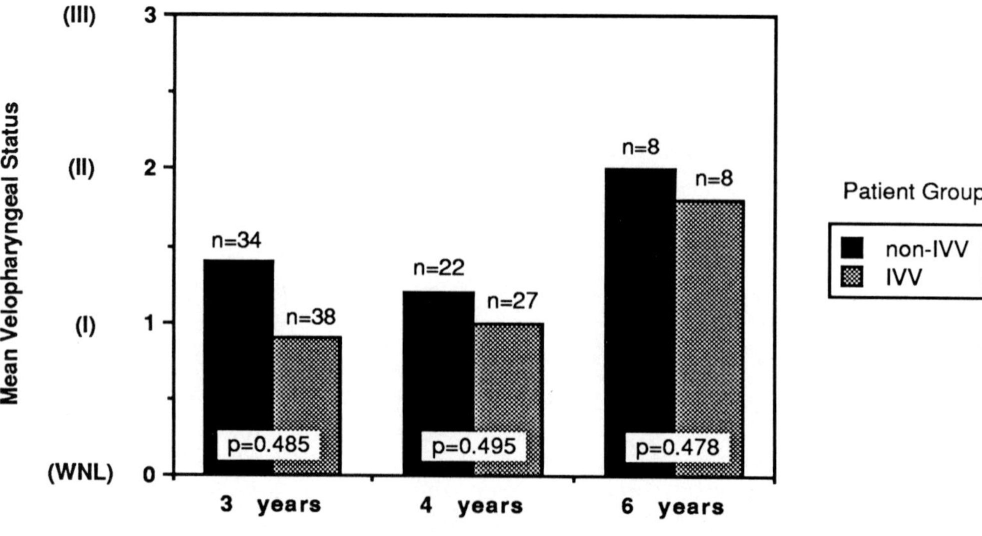

significantly less velopharyngeal dysfunction (mean, 0.9) than the non-IVV group (mean, 1.4) in children evaluated between 3 and 4 years of age (Student's *t* test p = 0.037), the statistical test may be invalid due to the non-normal distribution of the non-IVV data. Use of a more appropriate statistic, the Mann-Whitney U test, could not demonstrate statistical significance (p = 0.485). No statistically significant difference, using the Mann-Whitney U test, could be demonstrated between either the 4- to 6-year groups (IVV mean, 1.0, non-IVV mean, 1.2; p = 0.658) or the 6-year groups (IVV mean, 1.8, non-IVV mean, 2.0; p = 0.705).

Audiograms

Hearing abnormalities were characterized in both groups by mild conductive hearing losses with low static admittance in one or both ears. No sensorineural hearing loss was documented among either the 12-month or the 3-year audiograms. None of the hearing losses at either age were significant enough to require amplification. There was no statistically significant difference at either 12 months (Fig. 42–7) or 3 years (Fig. 42–8) of age between the non-IVV and IVV groups (Fisher's exact test p = 1.000 and p = 0.227, respectively; the "unable to test" data were not included in the statistical analysis).

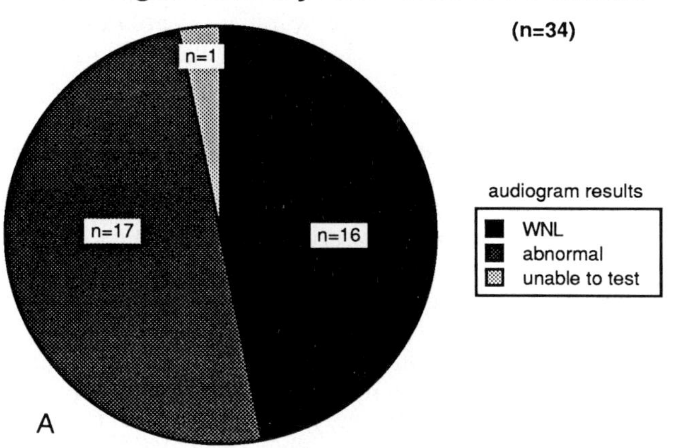

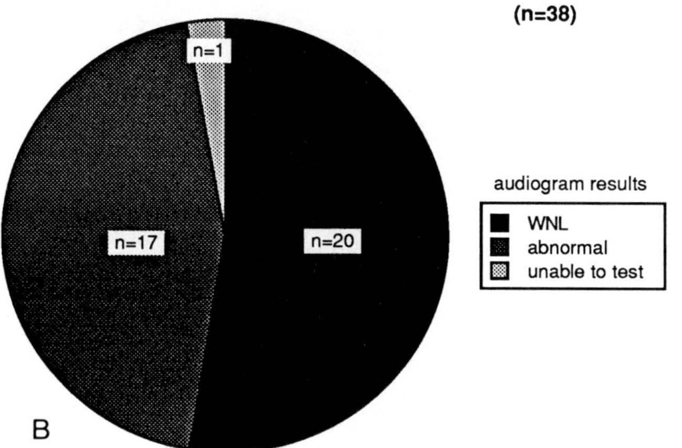

Figure 42–7 Distribution of results of single sample audiogram at 12 months of age. *A*, Non-IVV patients. *B*, IVV patients.

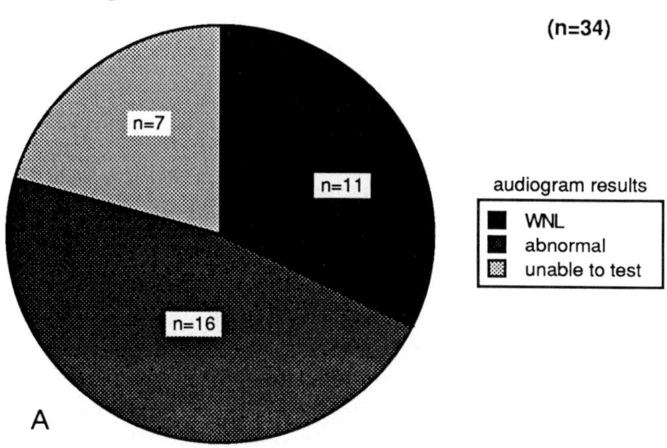

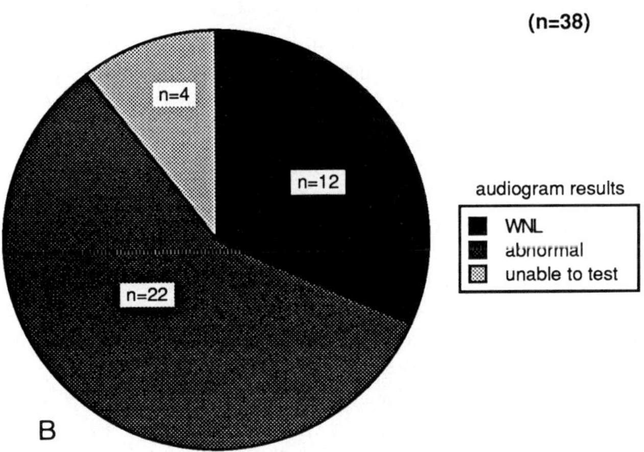

Figure 42–8 Distribution of results of single sample audiogram at 3 years of age. *A*, Non-IVV patients. *B*, IVV patients.

Surgical Morbidity

There were no deaths in either group. Two patients developed postoperative fistulas. One of these had an intravelar veloplasty, the other did not. Both fistulas were pinpoint in size and did not affect speech or deglutition. Patients with asymptomatic fistulas were retained within the study population. Four patients had sufficient dehiscence of the palatoplasty to require secondary palatal management. These patients were eliminated from the study population. One of these had an intravelar veloplasty, the other three did not.

Surgical Costs

Surgical time and costs were evaluated in 1986 for the first 51 patients (26 IVV, 25 non-IVV) reported above.[11] Intravelar veloplasty extended the operative time an average of 12 minutes for one surgeon and 33 minutes for the other. This additional time in the operating room increased the charges both from the hospital, for the operating room, and from the anesthesiology department. There was no surcharge in the professional fee for the additional procedure of intravelar veloplasty. In 1986 dollars, intravelar veloplasty increased the operative costs an average of $400 for surgeon A's patients and $707 for those of surgeon B.

Discussion

This study was undertaken to examine the efficacy of intravelar veloplasty in a prospective controlled manner. One of the surgeons "believed" in the procedure, the other did not. Neither the believer nor the doubter was able to substantiate his or her opinion by reference to the literature. The initial anatomic reports that documented the absence of the levator sling in cleft palate patients either lacked clinical results or presented results from a minority of their study population without specific speech information or control data.[1, 2, 4, 6] Studies published subsequent to the initiation of our investigation in 1982 have presented data that purport to validate the hypothesis that intravelar veloplasty does decrease the incidence of velopharyngeal dysfunction in patients who have had palatoplasty for cleft palate.[9, 10, 12] These studies have been compromised by one or more of the following: their retrospective nature, use of historical controls, participation of multiple surgeons without intersurgeon standardization, participation of multiple institutions, and choice of a basic palatoplasty procedure known to affect velopharyngeal function adversely.

The ideal study would be conducted prospectively and randomized in a single institution. All surgery would be performed by one surgeon. The perceptual speech evaluations would be performed blindly and independently by a series of speech pathologists with cleft expertise. Velopharyngeal function would be documented instrumentally using several modalities, e.g. nasopharyngoscopy, videofluoroscopy, and aerodynamics. Unfortunately, no institution seems to have the control over personnel and the abundance of resources to conduct such a study.

The design of our investigation is an attempt to find the middle ground between laboratory purity and clinical reality. It provides the following features:

1. A prospective study with alternate patient group entry conducted within a single institution.
2. Standardized operative procedures performed by two surgeons experienced in cleft surgery.
3. Perceptual speech evaluation blinded to the operative procedure conducted by the same experienced speech pathologist.
4. Independent additional blinded perceptual speech evaluations for all patients referred for speech therapy or secondary palatal management.
5. Instrumental (nasopharyngoscopy, at least) evaluation of all patients referred for secondary palatal management.

Our findings, taken from a sample of 72 patients with cleft palate, showed no statistically significant difference with respect to velopharyngeal dysfunction between patients who had had intravelar veloplasty and those who had not. This does not necessarily mean that intravelar veloplasty is an ineffective procedure. Rather, the statistical analysis stated that the results collected could be due either to chance—i.e., IVV is ineffective—

or to the positive effect of IVV on a small percentage of patients that cannot be discerned clearly from the current sample size. Furthermore, our combined analysis of all cleft types, which was chosen to obtain a sample size of some statistical validity, could obscure a positive effect of IVV on a specific anatomic subpopulation of patients with cleft palate. Continuing the study to increase the sample size may resolve these issues.

Conclusions

A prospective, alternate study is being conducted to test the hypothesis that intravelar veloplasty favorably affects velopharyngeal function following repair of a cleft palate. Of 167 patients enrolled in the study to date, 121 are at least 3 years of age and therefore suitable for perceptual evaluation of velopharyngeal function. Of these 121, 72 were recoverable for inclusion in this report: 34 underwent palatoplasty without intravelar veloplasty; 38 underwent palatoplasty with intravelar veloplasty. The two surgical groups were similar with respect to the distribution of cleft type, the mean age at time of palatoplasty, and the incidence of abnormal results of audiograms obtained at both 12 months and 3 years of age.

The findings to date are that surgical retropositioning and approximation of the levator veli palatini muscles (intravelar veloplasty) during initial palatoplasty, compared with palatoplasty without intravelar veloplasty:

1. Does not demonstrably affect the incidence of postpalatoplasty auditory perceptual symptoms of velopharyngeal dysfunction.
2. Does not have greater morbidity.
3. Requires a longer operating time.
4. Is costlier because the operating room and anesthesia charges are temporally rated.

These findings suggest that either there is no beneficial effect of intravelar veloplasty on velopharyngeal function or that the effect, if present, is of small magnitude. It is hoped that sequential reports of forthcoming data will clarify these alternatives.

References

1. Ruding R: Cleft palate. Anatomic and surgical considerations. Plast Reconstr Surg 33:132, 1964.
2. Braithwaite F: Cleft lip and palate. In Rob C, Smith R (eds): Clinical Surgery. London: Butterworth, 1966.
3. Braithwaite F: The importance of the levator muscle in cleft palate closure. Br J Plast Surg 21:60, 1968.
4. Kriens O: An anatomical approach to veloplasty. Plast Reconstr Surg 43:29, 1969.
5. Dellon AL, Edgerton MT: Correction of velopharyngeal incompetence by retrodisplacement of the levator veli palatini muscle insertion. Surg Forum 20:510, 1969.
6. Fára M, Dvorak J: Abnormal anatomy of muscles of palatopharyngeal closure in cleft palate. Plast Reconstr Surg 46:488, 1970.
7. Millard DR, Batstone JHF, Heycock MH, et al: Ten years with the palatal island flap. Plast Reconstr Surg 46:540, 1970.
8. Kaplan EN: Soft palate repair by levator muscle reconstruction and a buccal mucosal flap. Plast Reconstr Surg 56:129, 1975.
9. Brown AS, Cohen MA, Randall P: Levator muscle reconstruction: Does it make a difference? Plast Reconstr Surg 72:1, 1983.
10. Dreyer TW, Trier WC: A comparison of palatoplasty techniques. Cleft Palate J 21:251, 1984.
11. Marsh JL, Grames LM, Holtman B: Intravelar veloplasty: A prospective study. Cleft Palate J 26:46, 1989.
12. Coston GN, et al: Levator muscle reconstruction resulting in velopharyngeal competence—a preliminary report. Plast Reconstr Surg 77:911, 1986.

CHAPTER 43

The Furlow Double Reversing Z-Plasty for Cleft Palate Repair: The First Ten Years of Experience

Don La Rossa, Peter Randall, Marilyn Cohen, and Steven Cohen

Review of the Literature

The earliest methods of cleft palate repair sought to achieve surgical closure of the palate with minimum risk to life from hemorrhage and loss of airway.[1–4] Once this was accomplished, efforts were directed at reducing the risk of dehiscence through the introduction of relaxing incisions by Dieffenbach and the multilayered closure by von Langenbeck.[5, 6] The emphasis, however, remained on achieving reliable surgical closure of the palatal defect. Attention to palate function had to be deferred until these basic principles had been established.

The next step in the evolution of palatoplasty was marked by the development of methods to lengthen the palate in an attempt to improve speech results. The efforts of Veau, Dorrance, Kilner, and Wardill culminated in the "push-back" procedures that dominated cleft palate surgery until the late 1960s.[7–12] Refinements were added in an attempt to reduce the potential deleterious effects of denuded bone on facial growth. Nasal lining flaps were devised by Cronin, buccal mucosal flaps by Kaplan, and skin grafts by Dorrance.[8, 13–18] Amidst this focus on achieving increased palatal length, Veau and others were unraveling the details of cleft anatomy that would form the underpinnings of the next generation of cleft palate operations, those that would try to recreate a more normal anatomy and function. In this work, Veau described what is now called the "cleft muscle," a confluence of fibers of the levator and tensor palati muscles, the palatopharyngeus muscle, and the rudimentary palatal aponeurosis.[7]

Fára in 1968 and Kriens in 1969 published their landmark papers on the altered cleft palate muscular anatomy. They reemphasized that the confluence of muscles paralleled the cleft margin to insert on the posterior edge of the hard palate. The muscles were thus oriented in an anterior-posterior direction rather than in the normal transverse direction.[19–24] Kriens recommended dissecting the muscles from their mucosal mantel within the soft palate and redirecting them into a transverse position to recreate the levator sling. His procedure, the intravelar veloplasty, has had a signifi-

cant impact on palatal surgery through the 1970s and 1980s.

His concepts have been embraced to some degree by virtually all cleft palate surgeons. Some reproduced his operation as he described it, with wide dissection of muscle bundles and overlapping of the fibers.[25–29] Others modified it by detaching the muscle insertion from the hard palate but dissecting only enough muscle to sew it end to end.[30] Magnification was used by others to help identify the muscle and reduce trauma to it.[31] It is even possible to use Kriens' concepts to explain why the results from the push-back procedures were improved over those of earlier repairs, because inherent in these operations was a release of the muscle insertion from bone, and the muscle's natural tendency was to become transversely oriented when released.[32]

When one evaluates the results from incorporation of the intravelar veloplasty into palate repairs, they indeed seem improved compared with earlier repair techniques, though not to the degree that one might expect from an operation that seems so anatomically correct and logical. In retrospective series by Trier and Dreyer and by Brown et al., only a 10% improvement in speech results was noted.[33, 34] An ongoing prospective study by Marsh et al. showed similar results.[35] Have we reached the point of diminishing returns, or are there other factors? A critical factor in any study has been the problem of what operation is actually being done both within series and between several series. Only Marsh and co-workers' prospective randomized series has adjusted for this factor by standardizing the operation between surgeons in their study.

Technical expertise may play a significant role in results obtained. Most surgeons will agree that full dissection of the muscle as described by Kriens is difficult to do without traumatizing the muscle. Given the vagaries of wound healing, it is hard not to implicate the potential impact of technique on results. This could, in fact, be the most important factor.

Furlow Technique

In 1978, Furlow introduced an elegant solution to the problem of muscle disorientation. He described his double reversing Z-plasty method of soft palate repair at the Southeastern Society of Plastic Surgeons in Boca Raton, Florida. It was later briefly described, and the original diagrams reproduced, in Millard's *Cleft Craft* and was described in great detail in Furlow's landmark paper in 1986.[36, 37] In the audience was Peter Randall, who brought the idea back to Philadelphia, where we began using it in 1978 and have used it almost exclusively since 1981.[38] Dr. Furlow's concept was simple. Design an operation that will lengthen the palate while simultaneously reorienting the palate muscles to recreate a muscular sling. Combine this with minimal undermining of the hard palate mucoperiosteum, reducing the potential for deleterious effects on facial growth. He has done this operation without relaxing incisions, taking advantage of the arched configuration of the palatal shelves. By undermining the medial edges of the hard palate mucoperiosteum, the mucosal roof is lowered out of the palatal vault, permitting a tension-free closure. A dead space is left between the mucoperiosteum and the bone, but this does not seem to be of consequence.

Surgical Technique

As with all operations, each surgeon modifies the procedure incorporating his or her own ideas and nuances. The following is a description of the technique as it has evolved at the Children's Hospital of Philadelphia.

The principal objective of this procedure involves the management of the soft palate and its musculature. Two opposing Z-plasties are used to reorient the muscles and simultaneously lengthen the soft palate (Fig. 43–1). On the oral side, the posteriorly based flap is composed of mucosa with attached underlying muscle, whereas the anteriorly based flap is mucosa alone. The oral musculomucosal flap is designed on the patient's left side because this seems to be an easier dissection for a right-handed surgeon to perform. On the nasal side, the same situation is created, although the direction of the flaps is reversed, with the posteriorly based, muscle-containing flap on the side opposite the oral musculomucosal flap. The limb of the Z is directed toward the pterygoid hamulus. The angle of the musculomucosal flaps is usually about 60 degrees. The angles of the oral and nasal mucosal flaps vary with the width of the cleft. In narrow clefts the angles approach 60 degrees. In wide clefts with significant tissue deficiency the angles become more obtuse, approaching 80 to 90 degrees.

The flaps are elevated with either a scapel or scissors after paring the medial cleft margin. The nasal mucosa is tough and resilient, permitting scalpel dissection of the oral musculomucosal flap. The incision of the oral mucosal flap is performed with a scalpel until the muscle is identified. The dissection then proceeds anteriorly, preserving the muscle, which lies deep against the nasal mucosa and becomes attenuated as one approaches the hard palate.

The nasal mucosa is carefully dissected from the palatal shelves to permit a midline membranous closure. When necessary, a nasal relaxing incision is made at the junction of the lateral nasal wall and the palatal shelves with a nasal knife introduced through the nostril.

The nasal mucosal and musculomucosal flaps are now cut. The incision follows the reflection of the oral flaps and ends near the eustachian tube orifice. Care must be taken to avoid injury to the orifice with scalpel or suture in this operation. The oral mucoperiosteum is elevated in a medial to lateral direction until sufficient release has been achieved to permit a tension-free midline closure. We use relaxing incisions of the von Langenbeck type when needed. In complete clefts of the palate, a vomer flap is used to close the hard palate, minimizing the need for extensive elevation of mucoperiosteal flaps and achieving a two-layer closure.[39]

The closure is done with 4–0 chromic catgut or 5–0 Vicryl. When closing a cleft of the secondary palate only, the anteriormost portion of the nasal hard palate mucosa is closed first for a short distance because it is a difficult spot to reach. Likewise, when closing a complete cleft, the vomer flap closure is done first. The nasal musculomucosal flap is inset next, followed by closure back to the uvula. The nasal mucosal flap is next inset and the nasal closure completed. The oral soft palate closure is done next, beginning with inset of the musculomucosal flap and finishing with reconstruction of the uvula. The remainder of the hard palate mucoperiosteum is then closed, ending with inset of the oral mucosal flap. Postoperatively, a tongue suture or nasopharyngeal airway (or both) is used for safety. The palatal

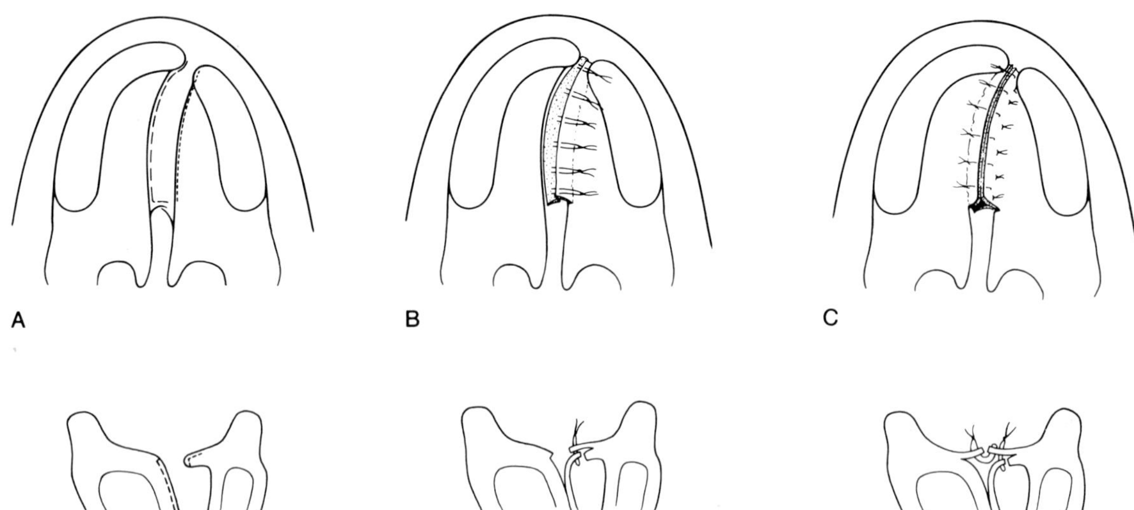

Figure 43–1 *A,* Incision design for the oral mucosal, musculomucosal flaps, relaxing incisions, and vomer flap for repair of a complete unilateral cleft of the palate. *B,* Following elevation of the oral flaps demonstrating design of the nasal mucosal (R) and musculomucosal (L) flaps. The hard palate has been closed with a vomer flap. *C,* Following interdigitation of the nasal mucosal and musculomucosal flaps. Completed closure following interdigitation of the oral mucosal and musculomucosal flaps. (*A–C* From LaRossa D: Cleft palate. In McCarthy JG, ed: Plastic Surgery, 3rd ed, 8 vols. Philadelphia: WB Saunders, 1989. With permission.)

and gingival mucosac are carefully injected with 0.25% bupivacaine for long-term pain relief.

Since 1981, we have used the Furlow operation on all clefts in which improved speech was our primary goal rather than the prevention of regurgitation as in neurologically impaired children. As of May 1988, 166 clefts have been closed.

The potential advantages of the Furlow procedure are the following:

1. Lengthening of the soft palate without hard palate mucoperiosteal lengthening flaps.
2. Reduced dissection and trauma to the palatal muscles by maintaining their attachment to the mucosa on at least one surface.
3. Reorientation of the palatal musculature to a more anatomically correct position, thereby reconstructing the "levator sling."
4. Closure of the soft palate without a straight midline scar.
5. No increased incidence of fistula.
6. Improved speech results.

The potential disadvantages are as follows:

1. Probable increased operative time (not measured).
2. Possible increase in scarring.
3. Possible increased incidence of posterior crossbite.

Clinical Evaluation and Results

As of March 1988, 36 children who underwent the Furlow procedure were at least 6 years post operation and were available for evaluation. Twelve were excluded from the study: Six of these patients had primary pharyngeal flaps; four had known mental retardation, other neurological impairment, or craniofacial syndromes other than cleft lip and palate; and two were older than 19 months of age at the time of closure. Twenty-four children were therefore suitable for evaluation. The distribution of cleft types is shown in Table 43–1. The mean age at closure was 9 months (Table 43–2).

All patients were evaluated by the same speech pathologist for speech and language development. Evaluations consisted of an informal assessment of language development, articulation testing, and a qualitative analysis of vocal quality. The results of the speech analyses were recorded on The Weighted Values for Speech Symptoms Associated with Velopharyngeal Incompetence Form used at the University of Pittsburgh. Patients with weighted scores higher than 2, indicating

Table 43–1. Distribution of Cleft Types According to Veau's Classification

	Cleft Classification			
Procedure	*I*	*II*	*III*	*IV*
Furlow	1/24 (4%)	10/24 (42%)	5/24 (21%)	8/24 (33%)
IVVP	1/19 (5%)	6/19 (32%)	9/19 (47%)	3/19 (16%)
Non-IVVP	2/30 (7%)	12/30 (40%)	11/30 (37%)	5/30 (17%)

IVVP = Intravelar veloplasty

inconsistent or significant velopharyngeal incompetence, were referred for either videofluoroscopy, nasendoscopy, or lateral still x-rays of the soft palate. Patients with subsequent objective evidence of velopharyngeal incompetence were referred for secondary posterior pharyngeal flap (PFF) surgery.

Three "outcome of procedure" variables were considered. The first was whether a second procedure was required (PPF). The second was the speech indicator, which was treated as an ordinal variable with values of 1 to 4 (taken from the Pittsburgh form). The third indicator, nasality, was treated in the same way as the speech indicator. Statistical tests for group differences were obtained using chi-square analysis.

Six of twenty-four (25%) of the children who had Furlow procedures required a posterior pharyngeal flap compared with 57% (17 of 30) who did not have intravelar veloplasty and 68% (13 of 19) who had intravelar veloplasty as the initial procedure (p < 0.01) (Table 43–2). The relative risk of a second procedure was 0.44 (95% confidence interval = 0.22 to 0.88) for the Furlow procedure compared with the nonintravelar veloplasty (p < 0.02), and 0.37 (95% confidence interval = 0.17 to 0.78) for the Furlow procedure compared with the intravelar veloplasty procedure (p < 0.01).

The speech outcome following primary surgery was compared between the Furlow group and those patients who had had palatoplasties with and without intravelar veloplasty (Table 43–3).

The incidence of fistula occurrence was 17% (Table 43–2). The children were not old enough to assess the possible effect of the operation on facial growth. Since the Z-plasty produced increased length at the expense of width, tightness was produced just posterior to the maxillary tuberosities. One might therefore anticipate an increased incidence of posterior crossbite. Whether this will have secondary effects on other aspects of the facial skeleton, such as bizygomatic breadth, remains to

Table 43–2. Summary of Secondary Surgery Required, Occurrence of Fistulas, Mean Age of Primary Palate Repair, and Follow-Up for the Three Groups of Patients

Procedure	Secondary PPF (%)	Fistula (%)	Mean Age at Closure (mo)	Age (yr)	Follow-Up Range (yr)
Furlow (N = 24)	25	17	9	7	5.9–10.1
Non-IVVP (N = 30)	57	20	12	9	4.11–15.10
IVVP (N = 19)	68	63	14	9	5.10–12.6

IVVP = Intravelar veloplasty; PPF = posterior pharyngeal flap

Table 43–3. Results of Speech Outcome Following Primary Palate Repair in the Three Groups of Patients Studied

Type of Procedure	1	2	3	4	Totals
Nasality[a]					
Furlow	15 (65%)	5 (22%)	3 (13%)	0 (0%)	23 (100%)
Non-IVVP	12 (43%)	4 (14%)	9 (32%)	3 (11%)	28 (100%)
IVVP	5 (28%)	1 (6%)	10 (56%)	2 (11%)	18 (100%)
$p < 0.01$					
Speech Indicators[b]					
Furlow	11 (48%)	4 (17%)	8 (35%)	0 (0%)	23 (100%)
Non-IVVP	4 (14%)	7 (25%)	11 (39%)	6 (21%)	28 (100%)
IVVP	5 (28%)	1 (6%)	10 (56%)	2 (11%)	18 (100%)
$p < 0.02$					

IVVP = Intravelar veloplasty

[a]1 = normal; 2 = mild hypernasality; 3 = moderate hypernasality; 4 = severe hypernasality.

[b]1 = competent velopharyngeal mechanism; 2 = competent to borderline competent; 3 = borderline to borderline incompetent; 4 = incompetent velopharyngeal mechanism.

be seen. No negative effect on middle ear disease was observed, nor was any serious morbidity or mortality encountered.

Conclusion

What is the explanation for the improved speech results? Perhaps the lengthening of the soft palate is beneficial; however, palatal length is an inconsistent determinant of speech performance. Muscular reorientation and levator sling reconstruction should have a positive effect on speech production. Leaving the muscle attached to mucosa on one surface facilitates dissection and should reduce trauma and subsequent scarring, perhaps explaining the improved results compared with the intravelar veloplasty. It is possible that the conventional midline scar in the soft palate acts to tether the soft palate's motion as a midline velar incision across a finger joint limits finger extension. The zigzag incision in the soft palate may be as important as it is in the finger. Another possibility is that the technique reduces the caliber of the nasal airway because Z-plasties create length at the expense of width. A pharyngoplasty effect may be created by this narrowing, accounting for better speech performance.

It is probable that a combination of several of these factors occurs and will be defined by future investigators. Regardless of the reasons, the speech results seem significantly better at this point in time. Long-term follow-up and confirmation by others are needed.

References

1. Von Graefe CF: Neue Wege des plastischen Verschlusses von Gaumendefekten. Berl Klin Wochenschr 54:209, 1917.
2. Roux PJ: Observation sur une division congenitale du voile du palais et de la luette, guevie au moyen d'une operation analogue a celle du bec-de-lievre. J Univ Sci Med 15:356, 1918.
3. Roux PJ: Memoire sur la staphylorrhaphie, ou suture du voile du palais. Arch Gén De Méd Par, 1825; J. S. Chaude, 1925.
4. Warren JC: On an operation for the cure of natural fissure of the soft palate. Am J Med Sci 1:1, 1928.
5. Dieffenbach JF: Beitrage zur Gaumennath. Litt Ann Heilk 11:322, 1828.
6. von Langenbeck B: Operation der angeborenen totalen Spaltung des harten Gaumens nach einer neuer Methode. Gösch Deutsche Klin 13:231, 1861.
7. Veau V: Division Palatine. Paris: Masson, 1931.
8. Dorrance GM: The Operative Story of Cleft Palate. Philadelphia: Saunders, 1933, p 3.
9. Dorrance GM, Bransfeld JW: The pushback operation for repair of cleft palate. Plast Reconstr Surg 1:145, 1946.
10. Wardill WEM: Techniques of operation for cleft palate. Br J Surg 25:117, 1937.
11. Kilner TP: Cleft lip and palate repair technique. St Thomas Hosp Rep 2:127, 1937.
12. Converse JM: Victor Veau (1871–1949): The contribution of a pioneer. Plast Reconstr Surg 30:225, 1962.
13. Cronin TD: Method of preventing raw areas on the nasal surface of soft palate in push-back surgery. Plast Reconstr Surg 20:474, 1957.
14. Stark RB: Nasal lining in partial cleft palate repair. Plast Reconstr Surg 32:75, 1963.
15. Stark RB: Cleft palate. In Stark RB (ed): Plastic Surgery. New York. Hoeber Medical Division, Harper & Row, 1962.
16. Mukherji MM: Cheek flap for short palates. Cleft Palate J 6:415, 1969.
17. Kaplan EN: Soft palate repair by levator muscle reconstruction and a buccal mucosal flap. Plast Reconstr Surg 5:129, 1975.
18. Horton CE, Irish TJ, Adamson JE, et al: The use of vomerine flaps to cover the raw area on the nasal surface in cleft palate repair. Cleft Palate J 15:30, 1978.
19. Fára M, Dvorak J: Abnormal anatomy of the muscles of the palatopharyngeal closure in cleft palate. Plast Reconstr Surg 46:44, 1970.
20. Kriens OB: An anatomical approach to veloplasty. Plast Reconstr Surg 43:29, 1969.
21. Kriens OB: Fundamental anatomic findings for an intravelar veloplasty. Cleft Palate J 7:27, 1970.
22. Kriens OB: Anatomy of the velopharyngeal area of cleft palate. Clin Plast Surg 2:261, 1975.
23. Dickson DR, Dickson WM: Velopharyngeal anatomy. J Speech Hear Res 15:372, 1972.
24. Latham RA, Long RE, Latham EA: Cleft palate velopharyngeal musculature in a 5-month-old infant: A three-dimensional histological reconstruction. Cleft Palate J 17:1, 1980.
25. Randall P: The cleft palate in operative plastic and reconstructive surgery. In Barron JN, Saan MN (eds): Operative Plastic and Reconstructive Surgery. London: Churchill Livingstone, 1980.
26. Randall P: Cleft of the alveolus and palate. In Serafin D, Georgiade NG (eds): Pediatric Plastic Surgery. St. Louis: Mosby, 1984.
27. Trier WC, Dreyer TM: Primary von Langenbeck palatoplasty with levator reconstruction: Rationale and technique. Cleft Palate J 21:254, 1984.
28. Trier WC: Primary palatoplasty. Clin Plast Surg 12:4, 1985.
29. Trier WC: Surgery for congenital cleft palate. In Habal MB, Morain WC, Lewin ML, et al (eds): Plastic and Reconstructive Surgery. Vol. 2. Chicago: Year Book, 1986.
30. Edgerton MT, Dellon AL: Surgical retrodisplacement of the levator veli palatini muscle. Plast Reconstr Surg 47:154, 1971.
31. Fisher J: Personal communication, 1988.
32. Lewin M: Personal communication, 1988.
33. Brown AS, Cohen MA, Randall P: Levator muscle reconstruction: Does it make a difference? Plast Reconstr Surg 72:1, 1983.
34. Dreyer TM, Trier WC: A comparison of palatoplasty techniques. Cleft Palate J 21:251, 1984.
35. Marsh J: Presentation of speech results from palatoplasties with and without intravelar veloplasty. Presented at the Velopharyngeal Incompetence Symposium, Williamsburg, VA, 1988.
36. Furlow LT: Double reversing Z-plasty for cleft palate. In Millard DR (ed): Cleft Craft. Vol. 3. Alveolar and Palatal Deformities. Boston: Little, Brown, 1980, p 519.
37. Furlow L, Jr: Cleft palate repair by double reversing Z-plasty. Plast Reconstr Surg 78:724, 1986.
38. Randall P, LaRossa D, Solomon M, et al: Experience with the Furlow double reversing Z-plasty for cleft palate repair. Plast Reconstr Surg 77:569, 1986.
39. Dunn FS: Results of the vomer flap technique used in surgery of the cleft palate during the past eleven years. Am J Surg 92:852, 1956.

CHAPTER 44

Early Cleft Palate Repair and Speech Outcome: A Ten-Year Experience

Debra Susan Dorf and John W. Curtin

Speech problems associated with cleft palate include hypernasality (a resonance problem resulting from abnormal coupling of the oral and nasal cavities that affects vowel production) and highly unusual misarticulation of consonants known as compensatory articulations. These problems significantly impair the unique human characteristic most of us take for granted, intelligible speech. Although the problem of hypernasality of vowels and nasal air emission on consonants may be surgically corrected by means of pharyngoplasty, the misarticulation of consonants associated with a cleft palate can require years of intensive speech therapy.

The primary purpose of cleft palate repair is to provide an intact mechanism for normal speech production. This requires an intact palate of adequate length and appropriate mobility, normal pharyngeal configuration, and muscular integrity. Surgical repair is most often recommended between 18 and 24 months of age[1] despite developmental research showing that consonant-vowel sequences emerge between 6 and 9 months of age in noncleft infants.[2] It is not surprising that the compensatory articulations observed in youngsters and adults with repaired palatal clefts can be traced to the chronology of cleft palate treatment. Although early vocalizations of all babies include some productions of the classically described compensatory articulations, noncleft babies produce these sounds with decreasing frequency toward the end of the first year of life, whereas in babies with unrepaired palatal clefts the frequency of these unusual productions increases during the same period of time. For American English-speaking, noncleft babies, the high pressure consonants that form the essential elements of their language begin to emerge in the first year of life, whereas babies with cleft palate do not develop these essential elements of speech. The continuation and predominance of compensatory articulations have been documented prior to surgical reconstruction and persist postoperatively.[3] Although there has been speculation that earlier palatal reconstruction might reduce these articulatory abnormalities,[4–6] systematic study of this proposal was not reported until recently.[7]

The effect of cleft palate repair on maxillary growth has been influential in determining the protocol for treatment. Ross and Johnston's review of facial growth in surgically repaired cleft lip and palate indicates that this topic remains controversial because of the great number of variables that may affect midfacial growth.[8] Such variables include surgical technique or modification of a specific technique, the number of surgical procedures performed on the hard palate, the surgeon involved, and the inherent facial morphology. Although some evidence suggests that surgical repair of the hard palate results in midfacial growth deficiency, other studies report that surgical repair that does not utilize primary bone grafting does not interfere with growth.[9, 10] Criteria for determining the optimal age for surgery to minimize growth problems still have not been established.

When considering the impact of surgical repair of cleft palate on the development of communication skills, we are reminded that speech production begins with the infant's first cries announcing his or her entrance into the world and develops through predictable stages of phonologic, morphemic, syntactic, and semantic levels during the first year of life. The young infant's vocalizations are characterized by a variety of sound productions, some of which are phonemic (or meaningful) in his or her native language environment and some of which are nonphonemic (or nonmeaningful) in the child's future language system. Toward the end of the first year, nonphonemic productions drop out of the infant's vocal play, and the phonemic sound units become the components of the child's first intelligible utterances. Within the first 6 to 14 months of life, the infant begins to reduce his or her sound production repertoire to the phonemic units of American English. These serve as the basic components of the English language system. During the first year of life, this selection process is characterized by the distinction of three classes of sound production: vowels, nasal consonants (/n/, /m/, /ŋ/), and oral consonants.

Structural and functional adequacy of the speech mechanism is required for this developmental sequence to proceed smoothly. Normal speech is characterized by intraoral pressure build-up and release of an oral air stream for production of the various phonemes, including high pressure consonants (/p/, /b/, /t/, /d/, /k/, /g/, /f/, /v/, /s/, /z/, /ʃ/, /ʒ/, /tʃ/, /dʒ/, /θ/, /ð/) and for production of acceptable oral/nasal resonance balance on vowels and vocalic consonants (/w/, /r/, /l/, /j/). All these sounds are produced normally in the highlighted area of the vocal tract (Fig. 44–1). Three articulatory valves are necessary, oral, velopharyngeal, and laryngeal, to provide constrictions along this vocal tract to produce the various phonemes. These are identified as places of sound production. Velopharyngeal valving occurs simultaneously with other oral constrictions in the production of all speech sounds except the three nasal consonants. Inadequate velopharyngeal closure results in distortion of almost all speech sounds produced in English.

Unrepaired clefts of the palate represent the major type of structural problem that results in velopharyngeal insufficiency. Although all articulation errors represent errors in valving accuracy, specific disorders can be distinguished in patients with structural deficiencies.[11] Such errors in youngsters with a congenital structural

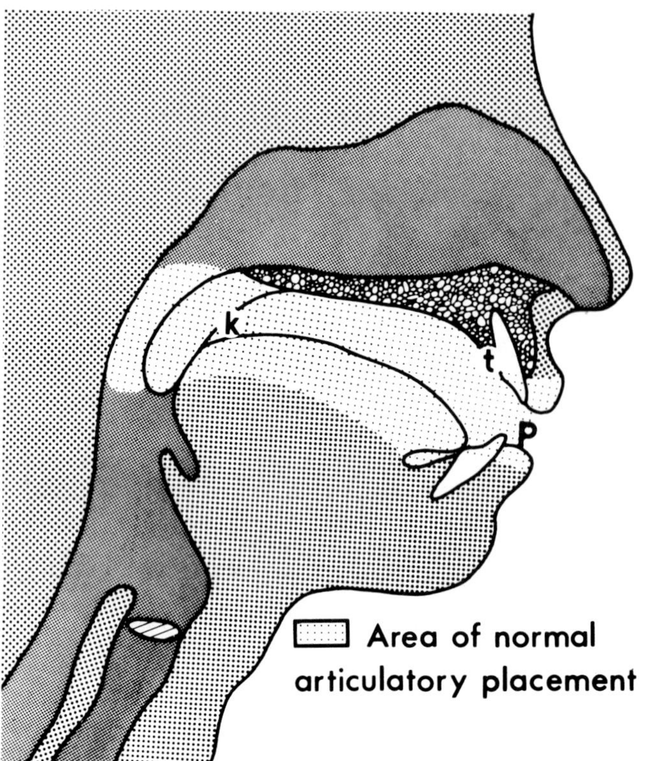

Figure 44–1 Constrictions occur within the highlighted area for articulation of normal speech sounds. Examples of high-pressure consonants are located at places of production. (From Dorf DS, Curtin JW:
Early cleft palate repair and speech outcome. Plast Reconstr Surg
70:1, 77, 1982. With permission.)

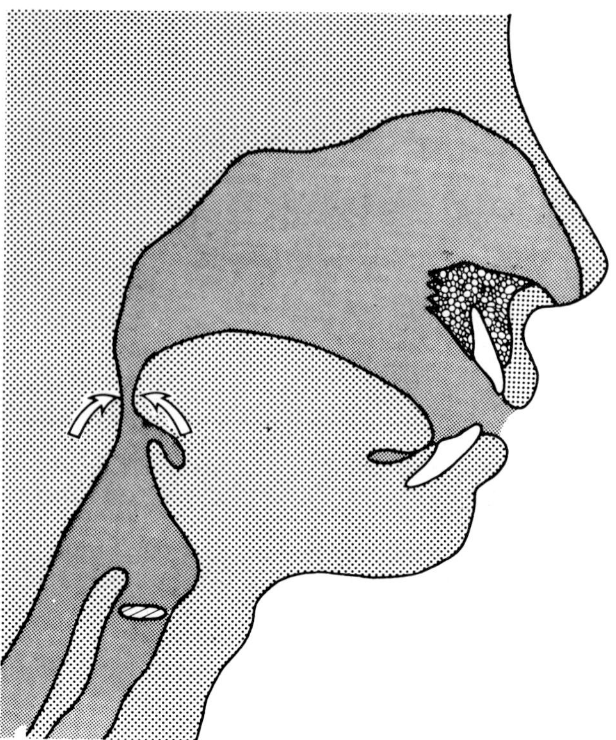

Figure 44–2 Schematic of structurally deficient speech mechanism.
Arrows indicate linguapharyngeal constriction for production of the
compensatory articulation identified as "pharyngeal fricative." Oral
posture was traced from cephalometric radiographs. (From Dorf DS,
Curtin JW: Early cleft palate repair and speech outcome. Plast
Reconstr Surg 70:1, 77, 1982. With permission.)

deficiency, such as unrepaired cleft palate, are predominantly errors in place of production. These are distinguishable from hypernasality and nasal air emission.
Certain types of articulatory compensations result when
there is abnormal coupling of the oral and nasal cavities.
The place of these productions is posterior and inferior
to the velopharyngeal defect. Figure 44–2 shows the
abnormal use of the tongue and pharynx in speech
production. Such compensatory articulations have been
observed even in individuals whose speech mechanisms
have been satisfactorily reconstructed.[11] It has been
speculated that compensatory articulations persist after
velopharyngeal adequacy has been restored because the
abnormal speech production motor patterns have become well established prior to reconstruction.[4] Despite
extensive speech therapy, these early-developing problems have been observed to continue into adolescence
and adulthood.

The development of such abnormal motor speech
patterns has been traced to its origins in infant vocal
play. In 1965, Olson compared the phonologic development of normal infants with that of infants with
unrepaired cleft palate.[3] He reported that infants with
unrepaired cleft palate produced compensatory articulations with increasing frequency from 5 to 30 months
of age, whereas normal infants reduced or eliminated
such productions during the first year of life and utilized
more "normal" American English phonemes.

Although the speech production of cleft palate infants

deviates from the norm, physical management of cleft
palate has frequently been delayed until the second or
third year of life. This places the child with a cleft at
high risk for development of speech and language problems. Although the outcome of speech after reconstruction has frequently been attributed to a specific surgical
technique, the age of the patient at surgery has not
been a well-controlled variable in any of those investigations. This is not to say that surgeons and speech
pathologists have not been concerned about the optimal
age for palate closure. To the contrary, the dilemma has
been how to obtain maximal and early communicative
adequacy without sacrificing orofacial growth components. The present study was undertaken to investigate
these problems.

Materials and Methods

Speech development in 131 cleft palate children from
the Center for Craniofacial Anomalies, University of
Illinois, Chicago, was assessed for the presence or
absence of six perceptually distinguishable compensatory articulations. To control for the variety of factors
that may affect speech and language development, no
child was included who had any of the following conditions:
1. Any known syndrome.
2. Submucous cleft or any other variety of velopharyngeal impairment in the absence of overt cleft.

3. Known moderate, severe, or profound hearing loss.
4. Partially repaired cleft or residual palatal fistula.
5. Significant psychomotor delay, including expressive language delay (characterized by one or more years' delay during the first 3 years of life or known mental retardation).
6. Palatal repair that incorporated a pharyngeal flap.

All patients were evaluated by the first author (D.D.). Speech evaluations began at 6 months of age or earlier if palate closure was to be carried out prior to 6 months of age. An informal play environment was utilized to elicit vocal and verbal responses. Narrow phonetic transcriptions utilizing modifications by Trost for recording compensatory articulations were used in data collection.[11] Speech and language evaluations were routinely repeated at 3-month intervals for all patients. When the child's level of cooperation was such that formal articulation testing could be carried out, between 18 and 30 months of age, standard articulation testing was done using the same modifications of narrow phonetic transcription for data collection.

Perceptual identification of six compensatory articulations (mid-dorsum palatal stops, posterior nasal fricatives, velar fricatives, pharyngeal stops, pharyngeal fricatives, and glottal stops) has been established in a study by Trost.[11] The first author of this paper (D.D.) served as a listener-judge in that perceptual study, in which a level of 93% accuracy for identification of compensatory articulations was established, with 100% accuracy for intrajudge reliability.

The age of 12 months was arbitrarily chosen in this study as the dividing point between early and late palatal closure. This yielded a distribution of the 131 children into two groups: (1) forty-nine children whose palates were repaired between 5 months 15 days of age and 12 months 15 days of age comprised the "early" closure group; (2) eighty-two children whose palates were repaired between 12 months 16 days of age and 27 months of age comprised the "late" closure group.

The age at palatal closure was determined from the operative reports for the 131 children. The greater majority of the cleft palate patients in this series were carefully screened and surgically closed by means of a Wardill-Kilner V-Y retropositioning procedure.[12] When the width of the cleft was minimal, some clefts were closed using a von Langenbeck repair. This latter group included only a very small number of patients. No primary bone grafting, multiple-stage palatal repairs, or any primary pharyngeal flap procedures were included. In this study no attempt was made to relate the type of surgical procedure to (later) speech adequacy for two reasons: (1) A small percentage of the operative reports were unclear about the specific surgical procedure utilized; and (2) more than one surgeon was involved in this study, although the same techniques were utilized. A review of the available operative reports did not suggest a correlation between type of surgical procedure and speech results.

Surgical Technique

After the patient is anesthetized, an intravenous line ensured, and an oral Rae endotracheal tube placed, a 3–0 horizontal silk suture is placed in the tongue as a safety measure until the following morning. A Dingman mouth gag is inserted with a properly fitting tongue blade attachment so that there is no undue pressure on the structures it touches. At this time communication between the surgeon and anesthesiologist is essential to ensure an open airway and no crimping of the endotracheal tube by the tongue blade.

Two to four ml of 1% lidocaine (Xylocaine) with 1:100,000 epinephrine is injected beneath the mucoperiosteum of the hard palate on each side as well as into the soft palate. Enough time should elapse to allow the epinephrine to maximize hemostasis. A small, wet gauze pack is placed in the pharynx to prevent blood from running back into the stomach or trachea and to give a better seal around the endotracheal tube.

If the cleft is isolated to the entire soft palate and one-fourth to one-half of the hard palate, a three-flap procedure is planned (Fig. 44–3). If the cleft is complete and extends through the alveolar process on one or both sides, a four-flap V-Y push-back procedure is anticipated. To minimize bleeding, one side of the procedure is completed from front to back before incisions on the other side are undertaken.

In either the isolated cleft of the secondary palate or the complete cleft of both the primary and secondary palates, the incision begins in the anterior part of the

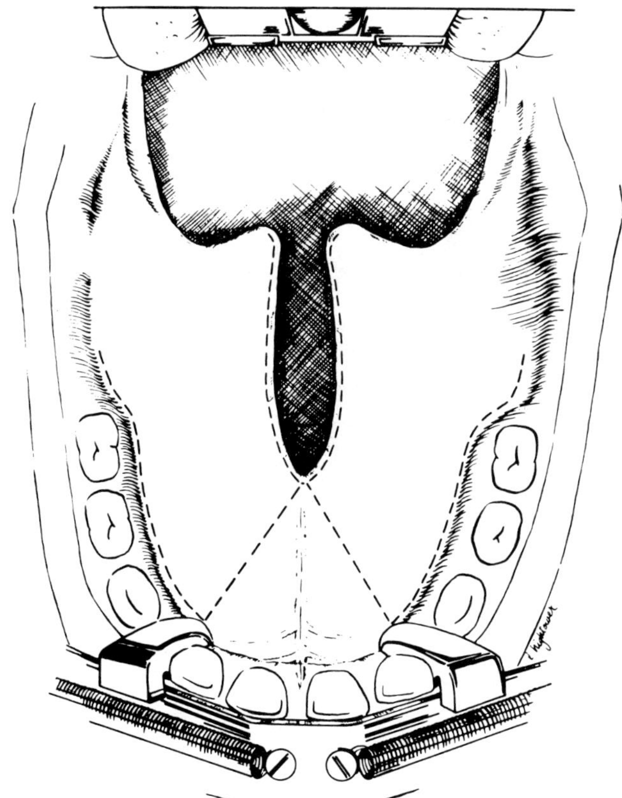

Figure 44–3 Basic design of the mucosal incisions used for the Wardill-Kilner V-Y cleft palate repair. (From Masters F, Levin J: Surgical management of the bilateral cleft palate by V-Y technique (Wardill-Kilner repair). In Symposium on Management of Cleft Lip and Palate and Associated Deformities. Vol. 8. St. Louis: C. V. Mosby, 1974. With permission.)

hard palate, undermining and raising a single or double V-shaped mucoperiosteal flap with a Joseph or Freer elevator. The medial edge of the soft palate and remaining hard palate cleft is freshened by removing a very thin strip of mucosa with either a No. 11 or No. 15 scalpel blade (Fig. 44–4). Next, an incision is started at the anterior and most lateral part of the mucoperiosteal flap, proceeding posteriorly along the highest lateral part of the palatal vault. When the area of the maxillary tuberosity is reached, the scalpel incision curves outward or laterally posterior to the tuberosity and then proceeds further toward the pharynx in the buccal mucosa. Once in awhile, the fat pads of Bouchut will prolapse and have to be sectioned and coagulated.

Blunt dissection of the musculature is carried out to allow for eventual mesial movement of the musculature of the soft palate. This dissection should allow for palpation and later visualization of the hamular process with the tendon of the tensor palati passing over it (Fig. 44–5). This process is very easily fractured and pushed medially in the young infant under 1 year of age. The hamulus should be completely detached to release this part of the tendon of the tensor palati muscle and produce a surgical closure of the soft palate with minimal tension. Wardill stated, "The importance of division of the hamulus process cannot be overestimated, since by its destruction the tensors of the palate are released and one of the greatest obstacles to easy suturing and free mobility is removed."[13]

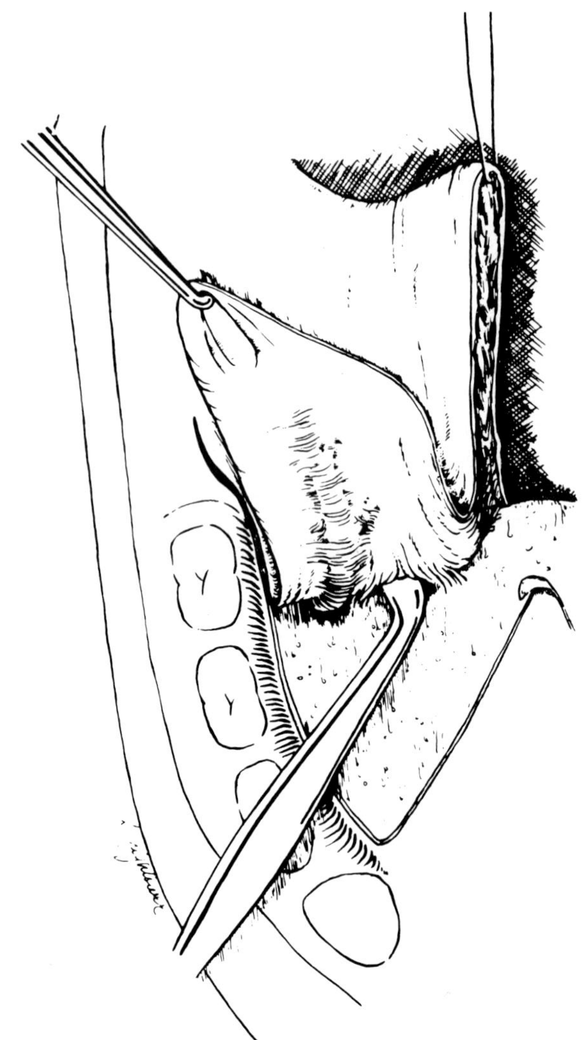

Figure 44–5 The elevation of the tensor veli palatini muscle from the hamular process will aid in relaxing the midline closure. (From Masters F, Levin J: Surgical management of the bilateral cleft palate by V-Y technique (Wardill-Kilner repair). In Symposium on Management of Cleft Lip and Palate and Associated Deformities. Vol. 8. St. Louis: C. V. Mosby, 1974. With permission.)

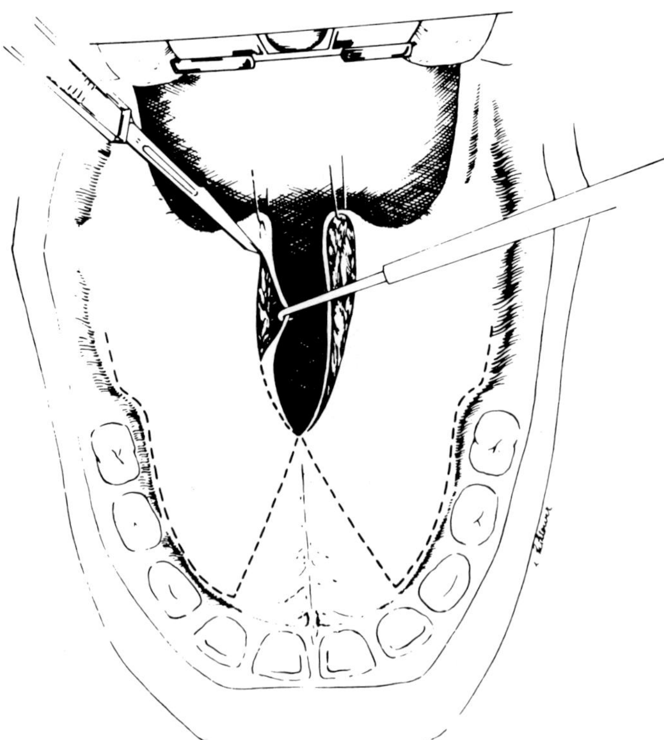

Figure 44–4 The cleft margin is gently pared to create a raw surface for ultimate closure. (From Masters F, Levin J: Surgical management of the bilateral cleft palate by V-Y technique Wardill-Kilner repair). In Symposium on Management of Cleft Lip and Palate and Associated Deformities. Vol. 8. St. Louis: C. V. Mosby, 1974. With permission.)

We return to the most anterior point of the lateral mucoperiosteal flap of the hard palate. Using a Joseph elevator, the most anterior part is gently stripped from the hard palatal bone and reflected (Fig. 44–6). Extreme care must be exercised as one nears the posterior edge of the hard palate on the medial side. Here the mucoperiosteum is very thin, and a horizontal tear could take place. As the lateral area of the mucoperiosteal flap is reflected, one encounters the neurovascular bundle protruding through the posterior palatine foramen. By now this dissection has exposed the palatine aponeurosis, which is attached to the posterior border of the hard palate. It is here that the surgeon has a decision to make. He may detach this aponeurosis from the bone without detaching or injuring the nasal mucosa, or he can simply detach by sharp dissection both the aponeurosis and the attached mucosa in one scissor cut as far laterally as allowed (Fig. 44–7).

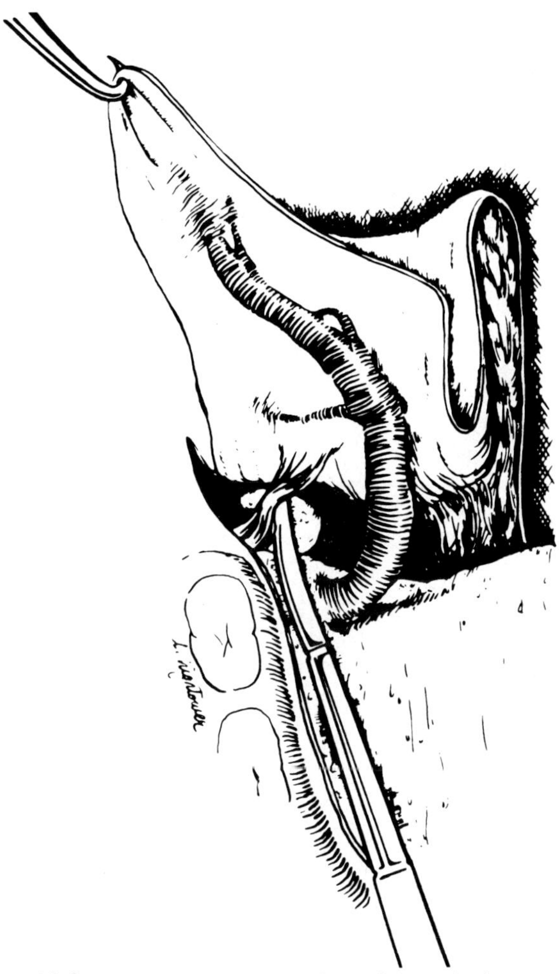

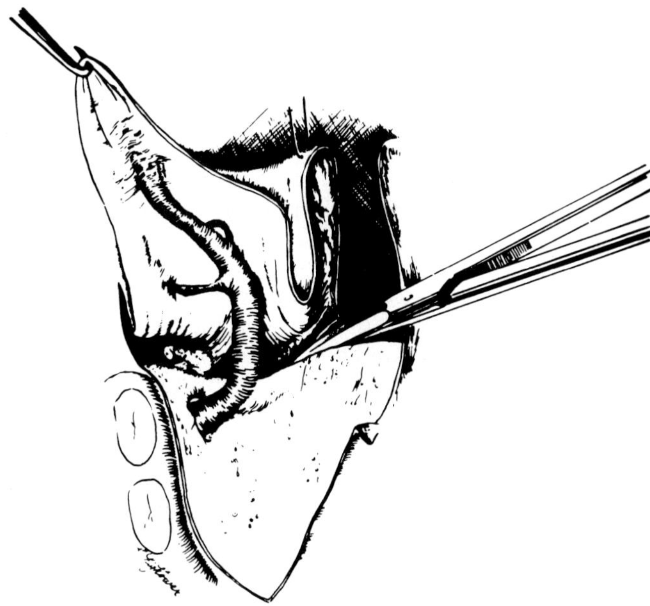

Figure 44–7 The nasal mucosa is divided behind the free margin of the bony margin. (From Masters F, Levin J: Surgical management of the bilateral cleft palate by V-Y technique (Wardill-Kilner repair). In Symposium on Management of Cleft Lip and Palate and Associated Deformities. Vol. 8. St. Louis: C. V. Mosby, 1974. With permission.)

Figure 44–6 The posterior flaps are elevated from the bony surface. (From Masters F, Levin J: Surgical management of the bilateral cleft palate by V-Y technique (Wardill-Kilner repair). In Symposium on Management of Cleft Lip and Palate and Associated Deformities. Vol. 8. St. Louis: C. V. Mosby, 1974. With permission.)

The neurovascular bundle is visible at all times and can be avoided. We prefer to maintain the continuity of the neurovascular bundle always. Immediate and spontaneous retropositioning of the hard and soft palate takes place. Next, with the neurovascular bundle retracted, we remove with a chisel and hammer the posterior wall of the palatine canal and gently push the palate and attached neurovascular bundle backward and medially (Fig. 44–8). This maneuver further enhances relaxation of all palatal tissues.

The complete separation of the palatine process laterally allows considerable mesial movement and retropositioning. It is this surgeon's (J.C.) firm belief that all of these incisions and maneuvers make for a more successful palatal closure with less immediate or subsequent tension than with the von Langenbeck and other palatal closure procedures. In other words, the push-back method (without closure of the nasal mucosa) derives its value from release of the abnormally attached levator and palatopharyngeal muscles, not from an actual increase in length of the palate.[12, 14]

When all of the necessary operative steps are performed on one side of the hard and soft palates, the

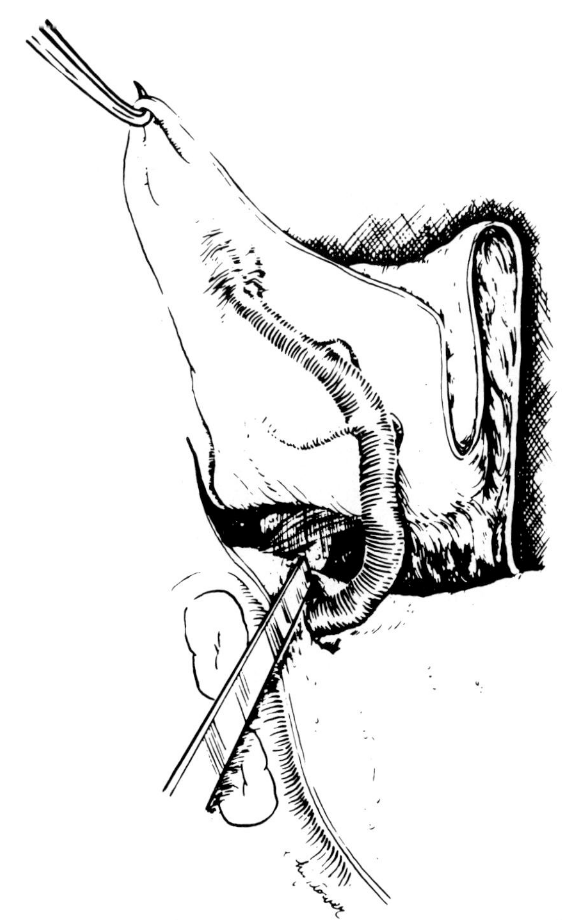

Figure 44–8 The posterior flap also may be lengthened by resection of the posterior aspect of the greater palatine foramen. (From Masters F, Levin J: Surgical management of the bilateral cleft palate by V-Y technique (Wardill-Kilner repair). In Symposium on Management of Cleft Lip and Palate and Associated Deformities. Vol. 8. St. Louis: C. V. Mosby, 1974. With permission.)

reflected mucoperiosteal flap is returned to its original site to lie limply against the palatal bone again; it is allowed to "breathe" for awhile. The dissection of the opposite side of the palate can now be undertaken.

When the aforementioned operative maneuvers have been completed on both sides, a thorough search for bleeding points is carried out. Occasionally, if oozing continues in the lateral recesses following blunt undermining, a Gelfoam pack can be inserted, to be removed at the end of the operation.

A layer-by-layer closure of the medial edges of the hard and soft palates can begin, using 5–0 Vicryl absorbable sutures (Fig. 44–9). Closure begins at the anterior part by approximating the single triangular mucoperiosteal flap and proceeds to the most anterior part of the two lateral flaps that have been retropositioned by all of the previous maneuvers. Horizontal mattress sutures are used for eversion, and occasionally an additional stitch is used for reinforcement because only a one-layer closure is possible in this technique. If the cleft extends through the alveolus and a four-flap closure is necessary, the two anteriorly attached trian-

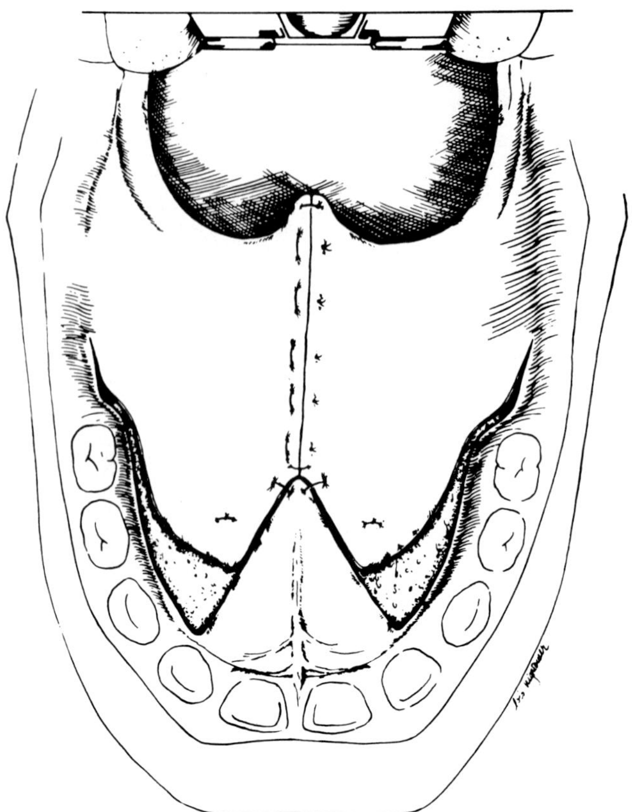

Figure 44–10 The appearance of the repaired palate at termination of the procedure. (From Masters F, Levin J: Surgical management of the bilateral cleft palate by V-Y technique (Wardill-Kilner repair). In Symposium on Management of Cleft Lip and Palate and Associated Deformities. Vol. 8. St. Louis: C. V. Mosby, 1974. With permission.)

gular flaps are first sutured to each other in the midline. The nasal mucosal layer of the soft palate is approximated to include the uvula. Suture knots are placed on the nasal side.

The levator musculature is next joined by deep-seated, horizontal mattress sutures throughout the entire musculature of the soft palate. We use a slightly heavier suture at the forepart of the musculature because the greatest amount of the tension is present at this area. It may be possible to put two layers of buried sutures in the muscle closure. Again, these buried sutures are placed with their knots tied on the nasal side. Finally, the mucosa on the oral side of the cleft is sutured with horizontal mattress sutures of 5–0 Vicryl (Fig. 44–10). Ruding has very succinctly said that the surgical closure of the musculature should imitate normal embryologic development as much as possible because the cleft is closed in utero in an anteroposterior direction, causing the palatal musculature to move posteriorly also.[15]

In wider clefts extending into the hard palate with a bony defect, an opening into the nasal chamber may be detected at one or both lateral edges of the mucoperiosteal flaps. This opening should be obliterated by placing sutures from the raw edge of the flap to the periosteum on the nasal side of the hard palatal bone. If periosteum cannot be found, a small drill hole can be

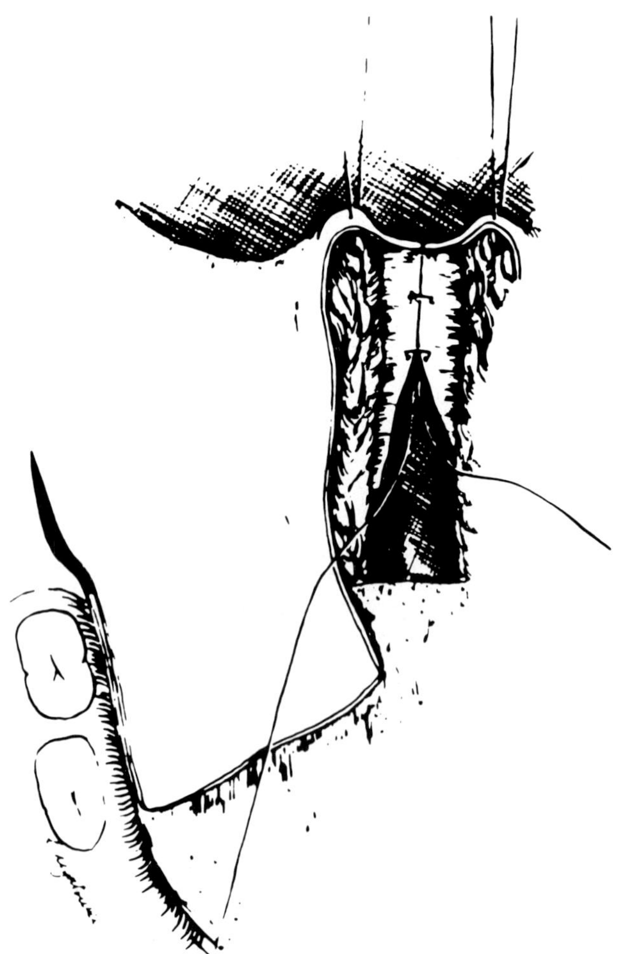

Figure 44–9 The nasal mucosa is closed with interrupted absorbable sutures. (From Masters F, Levin J: Surgical management of the bilateral cleft palate by V-Y technique (Wardill-Kilner repair). In Symposium on Management of Cleft Lip and Palate and Associated Deformities. Vol. 8. St. Louis: C. V. Mosby, 1974. With permission.)

placed in the hard palate. The suture is directed through this hole, and the flap is cinched to close the opening.

Finally, the pharyngeal pack is removed, and the oral cavity and pharynx are suctioned. Surveillance of the entire operative field is completed to detect any bleeding. No packs or Gelfoam are used in the lateral recesses of the palatal vault. The assistant surgeon must stand by until the patient is extubated and must ensure that the airway is satisfactory. Arm restraints are immediately applied and are to be worn for 2 weeks postoperatively.

Within an hour or two following completion of surgery, some persistent bloody discharge will ooze from the exposed areas of the hard and soft palates. This is coincident with the diminution of the epinephrine effect. The infant's condition should be periodically checked by the resident staff in the recovery room and when the child returns to the pediatric floor. Prophylactic antibiotics as a rule are not given.

Results

Chi-square analysis was used to compare the two subject groups on the single dependent variable of presence or absence of compensatory articulations. Pooling the data for all cleft types, a significant difference (p <0.0001) was found between the early closure and late closure groups. In other words, as seen in Figure 44–11, compensatory articulations developed less frequently in children whose palatal repair occurred prior to 12 months 15 days of age. Of the 82 subjects composing the late closure group, nearly 90% developed compensatory articulations. Among the 49 early closure subjects, fewer than 5% developed compensatory articulations, and more than 95% developed normal articulation skills.

These findings were consistent regardless of cleft type (Fig. 44–12). Unilateral cleft lip and palate, isolated cleft palate, and bilateral cleft lip and palate yielded similar statistical findings. These findings suggest that more normal speech development occurs when palatal reconstruction is completed prior to the traditionally suggested age of 18 to 24 months.

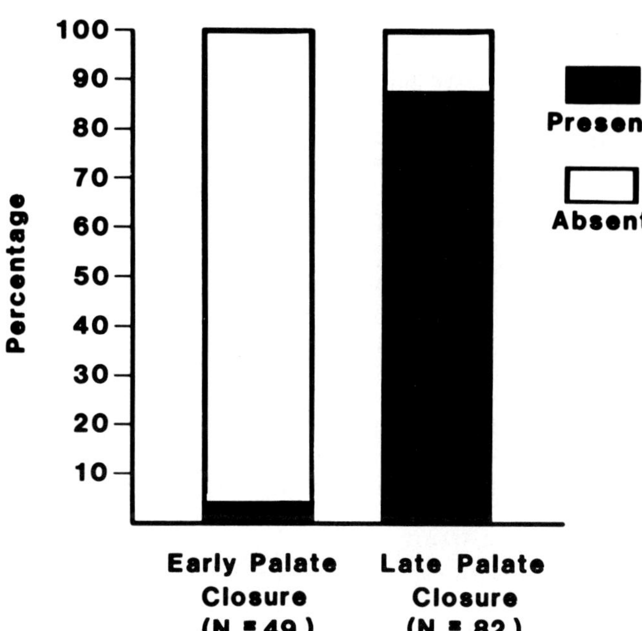

Figure 44–11 Bar graph indicates higher incidence of normal articulation in group with early palate closure.

Discussion

Although the design of this study utilized age as the factor dividing subjects into two groups, analysis of subject performance revealed that chronologic age was not the key factor in the development of long-term articulatory abnormalities. Rather, the child's stage of phonemic development, or articulation age, at the time of palatal reconstruction appeared to have determined the articulatory patterns that were observed postoperatively. Individual analysis of the speech development of the two early closure subjects who did develop compen-

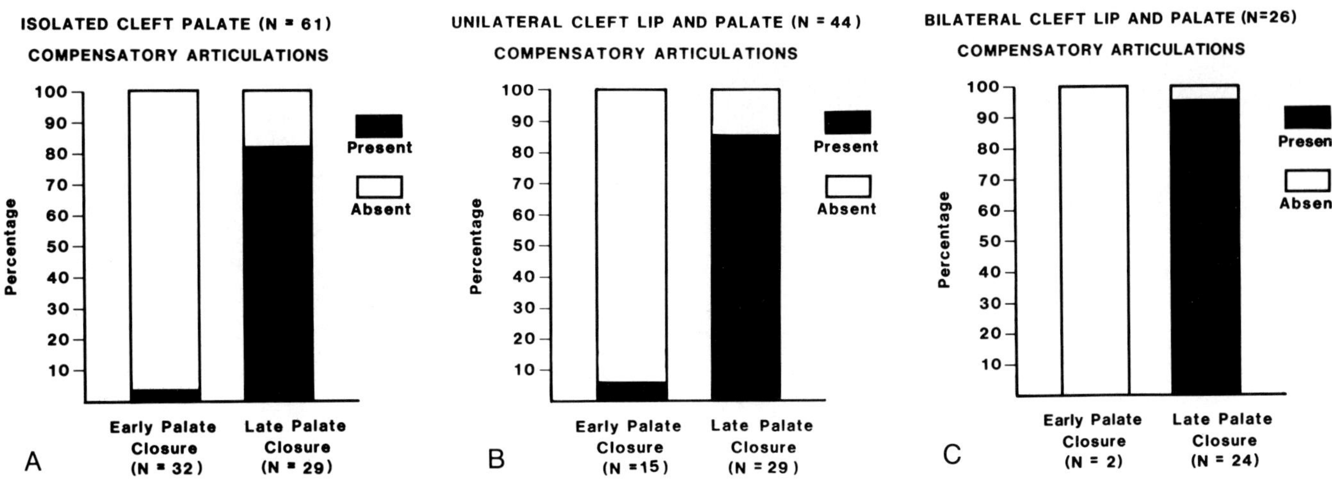

Figure 44–12 A–C, Bar graphs indicate higher incidence of normal articulation in early palate closure group when analyzed by cleft type.

satory articulations supported this concept of early onset of phonemic development. In these two children, compensatory articulations had already been established prior to surgery and continued postoperatively.

Along the same line of thought, subjects in the late closure group who did not develop compensatory articulations demonstrated a slightly later than normal onset of phonemic development. This slight lag in verbal development may in fact have worked to their advantage to prevent the preoperative establishment of compensatory articulations. Thus, from the standpoint of speech, *articulation age* rather than chronologic age appeared to be the key factor in the timing of palatal surgery. When the palate can be closed prior to the onset of phonemic development, it may be possible to minimize abnormal speech patterns. This brings the child with a cleft palate one step closer to normalcy.

No attempt was made to correlate the presence or absence of compensatory articulations with the severity of the cleft for two reasons. First, in a study by Bishara and colleagues on isolated cleft palate, the measured width of the cleft was, in fact, inversely correlated with the severity of the speech defect.[16] Second, studies that have attempted to correlate severity of cleft with severity of speech defect have looked only at the type of cleft, not the configuration or width of the cleft. The results of these studies have been inconsistent. More severely defective speech has been reported by some in isolated cleft palate and by others in bilateral cleft lip and palate.[17]

Rather than using chronologic age alone as the deciding factor in determining timing of the initial palate repair, the stage of each child's phonemic development should be considered if maximum speech potential is to be achieved and if speech development is to parallel that of the child's normal peers. Determining this stage of development through early speech and language evaluations, beginning at 6 months of age, thus becomes an essential component in the habilitation of children with cleft palate.

Continued research is needed to ensure that specialists do not place disproportionate emphasis on the achievement of normal speech compared with craniofacial growth considerations. Preliminary studies have shown no significant difference in the facial growth patterns of the early closure group compared with those of the late closure group.[18] Continued cooperative research between surgeons and speech pathologists is imperative to base these important decisions on substantiated findings.

ACKNOWLEDGMENT. The authors wish to acknowledge Joanne Darrow for her patience and careful preparation of the manuscript.

References

1. Lewis GK: Recent trends in surgical treatment of the cleft palate. J Int Coll Surg 56:478, 1956.
2. Smith BL, Oller DK: A comparative study of pre-meaningful vocalizations produced by normally developing and Down's syndrome infants. J Speech Hear Dis 46:46, 1981.
3. Olson D: A Descriptive Study of the Speech Development of a Group of Infants with Unoperated Cleft Palate. Dissertation. Chicago: Northwestern University, 1965.
4. Schultz LW: Correct time and sequence for closure of cleft lip and palate. Am J Surg 87:651, 1954.
5. Veau VE: Division Palatine. Paris: Masson, 1931.
6. Metzger JT: Consideration of factors in determining age for closure of congenital palatal clefts. Cleft Pal Bull 7:7, 1957.
7. Dorf DS, Curtin JW: Early cleft palate repair and speech outcome. Plast Reconstr Surg 70:1, 74–79, 1982.
8. Ross RB, Johnston MC: Facial growth in surgically repaired cleft lip and palate. In Cleft Lip and Palate. New York: Kreiger, 1978.
9. Aduss H: Craniofacial growth in complete unilateral cleft lip and palate. Angle Orthod 41:202, 1971.
10. Friede H, Pruzansky S: Longitudinal study of growth in bilateral cleft lip and palate from infancy to adolescence. Plast Reconstr Surg 49:392, 1972.
11. Trost JE: Articulatory additions to the classical description of the speech of persons with cleft palate. Cleft Pal J 18:193, 1981.
12. Curtin JW, Pruzansky S: Cephalometric evaluation of the Wardill pushback procedure in cleft palate repair. Bull Cleft Palate Rehab, July 1960.
13. Wardill WEM: The technique for operation for cleft palate. Br J Surg 25:119, 1937.
14. Kaplan EN: Cleft palate repair at three months? Ann Plast Surg 7:185, 1981.
15. Ruding R: Cleft palate—anatomic and surgical considerations. Plast Reconstr Surg 33:132–147, 1964.
16. Bishara SE, VanDemark DR, Henderson WG: Relation between speech production and oro-facial structures in individuals with isolated clefts of the palate. Cleft Pal J 12:452, 1975.
17. Spriestersbach D, Sherman D (eds): Cleft Palate and Communication. New York: Academic Press, 1968.
18. Ziesemer R: A Longitudinal Roentgenocephalometric Study of Facial Growth in Patients with Cleft Palate Following Early and Late Complete Closure of the Palate. Thesis. Chicago: University of Illinois, 1987.

CHAPTER 45

Two-Stage Palatoplasty

K. K. H. Gundlach

Cleft lip and palate surgery did not exist in Central Europe until the beginning of the nineteenth century. Von Grafe reported that in 1816 he had successfully operated on a cleft of the soft palate.[1] The subsequent 100 years were named "the century of surgeons" because of the enormous progress that was made. This was the time when, among others, Bernhard von Langenbeck, Professor at the University of Berlin and the first president of the German Surgical Society, developed new surgical techniques for clefts of the lip and palate.[2] Even today, many surgeons close the hard palate according to von Langenbeck's technique and use lateral incisions to shift the palatal mucoperiosteum toward the midline. In 1928 Georg Axhausen became director of the Berlin Maxillofacial Clinic. His best known operation is the palatoplasty, which combined elements of the different methods developed by von Langenbeck, Ernst, and Veau.[3] It has been performed at our hospital for many years with great success, and it still is within our repertoire today.

Karl Schuchardt, a disciple of Axhausen, took over direction of the Northwest German Maxillofacial Clinic in 1945. In 1954 he invited the most prominent European cleft surgeons to the First International Symposium in Hamburg. On that occasion, Hermann Schweckendiek's paper evoked a lively discussion. Since 1944 he had been closing the velar cleft first, postponing closure of the hard palate until the patient was 5 to 6 years of age. Later, he realized that malocclusion still occurred; thus he waited until the patient was 12 to 14 years old and all permanent teeth had erupted before closing the hard palate.[4, 5]

At Nordwestdeutsche Kieferklinik in Hamburg, we adopted a modified regime of two-stage palatoplasty in the early 1970s. In our opinion, early closure of the velum allows normal speech development and physiologic function of the eustachian tube. By postponing closure of the hard palate, compression of the upper dental arch and maxillary collapse are avoided.

In an earlier study, we realized that we gradually have reduced the age of patients at the time of veloplasty.[6] The median age has decreased from 5 years of age in 1960 to 2 years of age currently. Like colleagues in other medical specialties,[7] we had a problem in admitting children younger than 2½ years, because infants 18 to 30 months of age often experience severe anxiety and pain of separation in the hospital. However, we overcame this problem by allowing mothers to share the same room.

Materials and Methods

Patient and Methods

In May 1987, the Iowa Cleft Palate Team and the team from Hamburg started a joint research project (patients from both centers were evaluated by teams of specialists from both centers). In Hamburg, patients of Nordwestdeutsche Kieferklinik who had been selected by age and by diagnosis were invited to participate. Among these were 40 children who had been treated for complete unilateral clefts of the lip, alveolus, and palate; 23 of these accepted the invitation. Two-stage palatoplasty had been performed in 18 patients: seven were between 15 and 17 years of age, and 11 were either 8 or 9 years old. All patients were evaluated by two surgeons, two otolaryngologists, two orthodontists, a speech therapist, and a speech pathologist. Photographs, radiographs, and dental impressions of the upper and lower arches were taken. Rhinomanometry also was carried out. In October 1987, the Hamburg team visited and evaluated the Iowa Cleft Palate Center patients.

Surgical Timing and Techniques

All of the *older* patients had been operated on three to five times. On the average, lip repair was performed at 6 months. In one patient, an early primary osteoplasty had been performed; in three others a late primary osteoplasty had been done at age 14 years. In all seven patients the palate was closed in a two-stage procedure: soft palate at age 5 months to 4 years, hard palate at age 3 to 11 years. Only two patients had a pharyngoplasty as a secondary procedure.

Patients in the *younger* age group had been operated on two to four times. Primary lip repair was performed at 6 months of age. In five patients a late primary bone graft had been done at age 8 years. Palate repair was carried out using a two-stage procedure: the soft palate was closed at ages ranging from 2 years 3 months to 3 years 6 months, and the hard palate was closed at 4 to 8 years of age.

Patients in both age groups underwent the same surgical techniques for a two-stage palate repair. The soft palate was repaired first by performing intravelar veloplasty with two bipedicle flaps according to the von Langenbeck-Ernst-Veau technique (Fig. 45–1). The hard palate was repaired using local flaps without any type of push-back. Pharyngoplasties were performed rarely.

Criteria for Speech Evaluation

When evaluating speech, one is working with "soft data." There is no way to find a yardstick for measuring speech and for obtaining hard data on
1. Pitch and quality of the voice (nasal or denasal).
2. Velopharyngeal closure and articulation.

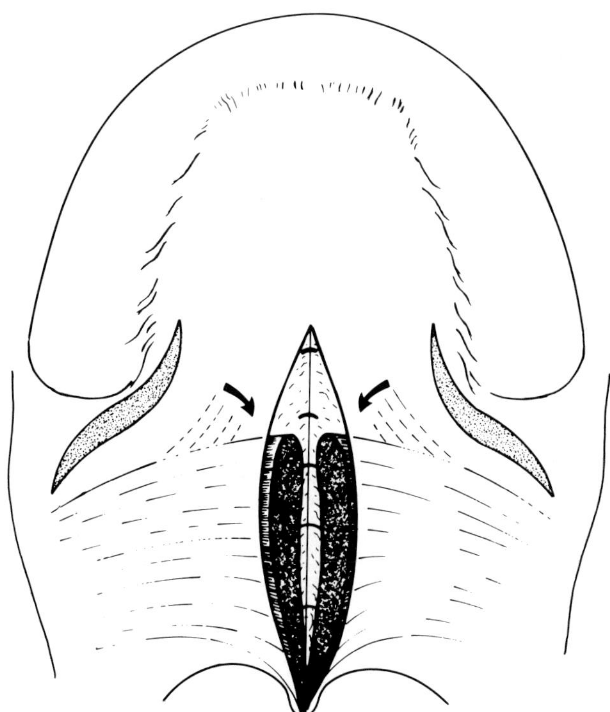

Figure 45–1 Intravelar veloplasty using two bipedicle flaps according to von Langenbeck, Ernst, and Veau.

3. Compensatory articulation (specifically, glottal stops and pharyngeal fricatives).
4. Intelligibility of speech.
5. Facial grimacing during speech production.

In Hamburg the following three grades were used to evaluate speech:

1. Perfect articulation. Inconspicuous voice, inconspicuous flow of speech. Speech may vary with local dialect, but person cannot be identified as a cleft palate patient.
2. Intelligible speech. Average or good voice may exhibit some nasality and/or a few pharyngeal fricatives, e.g., /th/ may be substituted for /s/ or /z/.
3. Major articulation faults: i.e., difficult to understand, or major faults in voice and articulation, especially hypernasality or use of glottal stops and pharyngeal fricatives.

Orthodontic Treatment

Most patients have had orthodontic treatment. Dental impressions were taken to determine which deviations of the palatal dimensions were due to surgery. Therefore, when evaluating the dental casts, we included only those patients who did not have any orthodontic treatment whatsoever up to the age of 8 years. Twelve patients fit these criteria. Eight of these were 8 years old, and four were 16 years old but had not had orthodontic therapy at age 8 years. Therefore, the casts taken at age 8 years could be evaluated.

Results

Maxillofacial Growth or Occlusion

In unilateral clefts of lip, alveolus, and palate the *maxillary arch* is asymmetric. Typically, the arch collapses. We followed this event in our patients. Results indicated that the canine on the cleft side was displaced medially at the time of evaluation. The distance between the cleft side canine and the normal first molar was 40.6 mm on the average. This distance was smaller than that between the normal canine and the cleft side first molar (43.8 mm). It also was smaller than the corresponding distance in the normal control group (44.9 mm).

The arch collapse was even more severe in terms of the occlusion. The incidence of crossbite in patients with clefts (9 of 22 maxillary segments) was very high at the level of the canine. It was still high at the level of the molars (5 of 24) (see Table 45–1).

We also measured the three dimensions of the palate and compared these measurements with the same measurements from the control group. Transversely, we measured with calipers the upper arch width between the first molars (44.3 mm). This measurement did not differ significantly from that in the control group (44.9 mm). However, there was a difference in the measurement of the width between the canines (27.2 mm in the cleft group compared with 31.7 mm in the control group) (Table 45–2).

Table 45–1. Transverse Measurements in Palates of 8-Year-Old Patients with Unilateral Clefts of Lips, Alveolus, and Palate

	8-Year-Old Patients, No Orthodontic Treatment	
	Cleft	*Control*
Distance (mm)		
C3–H6	40.6	45.0
H3–C6	43.8	44.8
Crossbite		
Canine	9 of 22	3 of 28
First molar	5 of 24	3 of 25

C3 = canine on cleft side; C6 = first molar on cleft side; H3 = canine on healthy side; H6 = first molar on healthy side

Concerning the deviations of the sagittal plane, the dental arch length (32.0 mm) showed only a slight deviation from that of the control group (33.9 mm). In the vertical dimension, palatal height measured at the level of the first molars varied significantly between the cleft group (13.7 mm) and the control group (17.2 mm; Table 45–2).

Speech

For the evaluation of *speech* we used three grades, as described previously. In both cleft lip and palate groups the result of speech testing was good, with an average grade of 1.2 in the younger group (8- or 9-year-olds). In the older patient group (15 to 16 years) we found an average grade of 1.1 (Table 45–3).

We used seven grades to evaluate *nasality*: grade 1, no nasality noted; grade 1.5, very slight degree of nasality; grade 2 or 3, minor nasality; Grade 4, 5, 6, or 7, various degrees of major nasality. In both groups there was only slight nasality. However, the younger patients (grade 1.7 on the average) scored better than the older ones (grade 1.9; Table 45–3).

Otolaryngology

Hearing evaluation revealed that most patients had no significant conductive loss. Twenty-five percent of patients had mild losses (less than 30 dB). None of the patients had moderate (30 to 40 dB) or severe (greater than 40 dB) conductive losses. Patients in the older group scored better than the younger ones.

Table 45–2. Three-Dimensional Evaluations of Maxilla in 8-Year-Old Children with Unilateral Clefts of the Lip, Alveolus, and Palate

	8-Year-Old Patients, No Orthodontic Treatment	
	Cleft	*Control*
Upper Arch Width		
6–6 mm	44.3	44.9
3–3 mm	27.2	31.7
Upper arch length	32.0	33.9
Palatal height	13.7	17.2

Table 45–3. Evaluation of Speech and Nasality (Average Grades) in Patients with Unilateral Clefts of Lip, Alveolus, and Palate

	Grades (Arithmetic Means)	
	Speech	*Nasality*
8- to 9-year-old patients	1.2	1.7
15- to 16-year-old patients	1.1	1.9

Discussion

Many surgeons today feel that a cleft of the lip, alveolus, and palate should be closed completely within the first months of life. We do not believe in this and prefer the two-stage palatoplasty. Nevertheless, we have altered the timing of palatal closure during the last 25 years so that patients now are considerably younger at the time of veloplasty than in the 1960s. In this study we found that in patients who had been operated on in the 1970s, the function of the velum with regard to speech, nasality, and hearing (that is, the function of the eustachian tube) was close to normal. The Hamburg speech therapist and the Iowa speech pathologist have come to the same conclusion: Near-normal results were due to the technique of soft palate closure, which included reconstruction of the cleft muscle.

Many cleft teams today advocate repairing the palate earlier than we did in these patients. On the one hand, speech pathologists reason that normal velopharyngeal anatomy is necessary for learning to speak.[8] On the other hand, otolaryngologists stress that a mucoserotympanum is less likely to develop if ventilation of the tympanum is improved.[9] Although we understand this reasoning and follow these recommendations, our data suggest that there is no need to close the velum as early as age 6 months in all patients.[6] To individualize the timing for closure of the palate seems to be more valuable than closing the entire cleft as early as possible.[10] Therefore, we feel that *small* velar clefts (up to 5 mm wide) should be closed early (at the time of labioplasty at 4 to 6 months of age). *Wide* velar clefts, however, should be closed later (at approximately age 1.6 to 2.6 years), because denuding the bony palate too early must interfere with growth and development of the maxillary arch.

It is especially important that timing and surgical techniques of palatoplasty *also* not interfere much with the normal growth of the hard palate. Here we follow Schweckendiek's idea to a certain extent: Once the velar part of the cleft is closed, the anterior part of the palatal cleft becomes smaller automatically. Children wear a plate to cover the gap between the shelves. We try to repair the hard palate before the child enters school. By following this schedule, physiologic development of the maxillary arch is not hindered.

We know that orthodontists can repair almost everything, but it is much better if a surgeon produces palates that need not be repaired to begin with. Ross evaluated several variables affecting facial growth in patients with cleft lip and palate from several cleft centers.[11] He did not include data from the Hamburg patients but had evaluated the Marburg patients that Schweckendiek himself had treated. Ross stated, "The best faces (that is, close to noncleft in appearance) were from Marburg with their unoperated palates." In 1987, Ross even pooled the Marburg data with the sample that had had no surgery owing to their excellent maxillary growth and development.[12]

On the occasion of the Third International Symposium on Early Treatment of Cleft Lip and Palate held in September 1984 in Zurich, nobody presented speech results based on patients with delayed hard palate closure. At the State-of-the-Art Conference in Iowa in 1987 we were able to do so. I believe our results were by all means at least as good as the data obtained from patients with one-stage closure.

References

1. Grafe von C: Die Gaumennaht. J Chirurgie Augen-Heilk 1:1–54, 1820.
2. Schober KL: Die deutsche Gesellschaft für Chirurgie—ihre Grunder und deren Ziele. In Schreiber HW, Carstensen G (eds): Chirurgie im Wandel der Zeit 1945–1983. Berlin: Springer, 1983, pp 1–10.
3. Axhausen G: Technik und Ergebnisse der Spaltplastiken. Munchen: Hanser, 1952.
4. Eckstein A: Ruckblick auf das Erste Internationale Hamburger Symposium über Lippen-Kiefer-Gaumenspalten 1954. In Pfeifer G (ed): Lippen-Kiefer-Gaumenspalten. Stuttgart: G. Thieme, 1982, pp 4–9.
5. Schweckendiek W: Vierzig Jahre primare Veloplastik. In Lippen-Kiefer-Gaumenspalten, Zweites Rostocker Expertensymposium, April 24–27, 1985. Wilhelm-Pieck-Universitat Rostock, Sektion Stomatologie, 1985, pp 35–36.
6. Gundlach KKH, Maerker R: Differenzierte Behandlung bei unterschiedlichen Formen von Gaumenspalten und Sprechergebnisse. In Lippen-Kiefer-Gaumenspalten, Zweites Rostocker Expertensymposium, April 24–27, 1985. Wilhelm-Pieck-Universitat Rostock, Sektion Stomatologie, 1985, pp 49–52.
7. King LR: Optimal treatment of children with undescended testes. J Urol 131:734–735, 1984.
8. Eggeling V: Sprachheilpadagogische Überlegungen zum Zeitpunkt des Gaumenverschlusses bei Spalttragern. Dtsch Z Mund-Kiefer-Gesichts-Chir 5:179–182, 1981.
9. Herberhold C: Zur Problematik des Mucoserotympanon. In Pfeifer G (ed): Lippen-Kiefer-Gaumenspalten. Stuttgart: G. Thieme, 1982, pp 184–185.
10. Pfeifer G: Die Gaumenplastik in Abhangigkeit von Art, Ausdehnung und Umgebung der Spalten. In Pfeifer G (ed): Lippen-Kiefer-Gaumenspalten. Stuttgart: G. Thieme, 1982, pp 197–203.
11. Ross RB: Variables affecting facial growth in cleft lip and palate—an international study. In Hotz M, Gnoinski W, Perko M, et al (eds): Early Treatment of Cleft Lip and Palate. Toronto: Hans Huber, 1986, pp 238–246.
12. Ross RB: Treatment variables affecting growth in unilateral cleft lip and palate. Part 5: Timing of palate repair. Cleft Palate J 24:54–63, 1987.

CHAPTER 46

Cleft Palate Repair: Two-Flap Palatoplasty. Research, Philosophy, Technique, and Results

Janusz Bardach

There are many more controversies and misconceptions related to palatoplasty than to cleft lip repair. The main reason for this is that palate repair has been considered the primary cause of maxillofacial growth aberrations for almost 40 years. Many clinical and experimental studies have been conducted on the relationships between palatoplasty, maxillofacial growth, and speech. Lip repair, on the other hand, has only recently become the focus of interest, and few studies have been performed to assess its role in facial growth. Palatoplasty remains an area in which many questions are unanswered and many problems misunderstood.

When discussing palatoplasty, it is important to differentiate between misconceptions and controversies. Some misconceptions that have been widely accepted for many years without being challenged have led to the belief that no further investigation is necessary because the issues have been "well documented" or proved. The common belief that palatoplasty is deleterious to maxillofacial growth has been expressed in the very general statement that cleft palate repair is the main cause of maxillofacial growth aberrations. Given this degree of generalization, any attempt to question the basic findings leading to this hypothesis is precluded. Furthermore, the solidly established "dogma" is no longer challenged. The idea that palatoplasty is harmful to facial growth was proposed about 40 years ago. Since that time, little has been done to confirm or negate this notion.

Many years of clinical observation as well as numerous clinical and experimental studies have led me to question the idea that palatoplasty is detrimental to maxillofacial growth. Many new surgical procedures have been developed, so this hypothesis may not apply in all cases. Also, the team approach toward treatment of cleft patients has become established in many centers, further weakening the "validity" of this concept. The misconception that I intend to challenge in this chapter is thus: Cleft palate repair has a deleterious effect on maxillofacial growth.

This general misconception is usually elaborated as follows:

1. Interference with palatal bone and periosteum by undermining mucoperiosteal flaps affects facial growth and results in aberrations of various degrees of severity.
2. Each surgical technique results in some exposure of bare palatal bone. Healing of these bare areas through secondary intention leads to scarring and consequently to maxillofacial growth aberrations.

Misconceptions of the cause-and-effect relationships in palatoplasty exist because on the one hand, lip repair has not been considered a possible cause of growth aberrations. On the other hand, there have been only a few well-designed clinical and experimental studies that have provided any information on the influence of palate repair on facial growth. There are even fewer studies that provide verified data on how the timing of palate repair, the sequence of surgical procedures, and various surgical techniques influence maxillofacial growth and speech production. As a result, many controversies remain regarding the timing of the operation, the sequence of procedures, and the surgical techniques. Despite the fact that a great deal of information on palatoplasty is available, the information we have is not sufficient to allow definite conclusions to be drawn in regard to the aforementioned controversies. We know next to nothing about the role of the individual surgeon in the results of palatoplasty, although there is no doubt that an experienced surgeon using a precise technique and a gentle touch is able to perform palatoplasty with a higher rate of success than a surgeon with little experience whose surgical skills and choice of techniques leave much to be desired.

The concept that cleft palate repair is detrimental to facial growth has been widely accepted despite the fact that to date there is no adequate substantiation of this concept from clinical or experimental studies. Also, some practitioners are still of the opinion that palatoplasty is the major factor in maxillofacial growth aberrations. To understand why these concepts have been so readily accepted, we must examine the state of the art in cleft management approximately 40 years ago.

At that time, treatment of cleft deformities was limited to surgical intervention. Orthodontists and speech pathologists did not routinely participate in cleft treatment. Even during the early 1950s, when the team approach had already been accepted in the United States, treatment of cleft patients in Europe typically continued to be managed by surgeons alone. According to the information presented in this book, even at present, treatment of clefts is limited to surgery, with occasional help from orthodontists or speech pathologists, in some developing cleft centers.

Forty years ago, surgical techniques differed from those used today. For example, cleft lip repair was usually performed according to the Mirault and Veau techniques. In both techniques and their modifications, lip repair was performed under excessive tension. Cleft palate repair was carried out using the von Langenbeck and Veau techniques. Palatal closure obtained with the von Langenbeck technique was performed under excessive tension, typically resulting in oronasal fistulas in the anterior palate and at the border of the hard and soft palates. Veau's concept of closing the anterior palate at the time of primary lip repair contributed greatly to anteroposterior growth inhibition of the midface. At that time, more advanced techniques (like the Le Mesurier cleft lip repair and Wardill-Kilner cleft palate repair) were only beginning to gain popularity. Surgical techniques used 40 years ago led frequently to multiple lip and palate operations, which, combined with insufficient (and sometimes absent) orthodontic treatment, led to a high incidence of secondary maxillofacial deformities caused by midfacial growth inhibition.

The majority of surgeons had only a vague understanding of the factors contributing to maxillofacial growth inhibition, and there were no reliable studies that indicated which procedures in the sequence of cleft lip and palate treatment were detrimental to maxillofacial growth. Surgeons, frustrated by a high incidence of severe secondary maxillofacial deformities, delayed cleft lip and palate repair. I was trained to perform lip closure when the patient was 1 to 2 years old and cleft palate repair at 6 to 8 years of age at the earliest. Under these circumstances, the suggestions by Graber and Herfert that cleft palate repair was the primary cause of maxillofacial growth aberrations, were readily acknowledged.[1-7] Finally, surgeons could blame the procedures rather than themselves. However, critical analysis of the publications by Graber and Herfert indicates that the data they presented were not adequate to support the hypothesis that palatoplasty had a detrimental effect on maxillofacial growth.

Review of Experimental and Clinical Studies

The concept that cleft palate repair was detrimental to facial growth was formulated in the late 1940s and early 1950s by Graber[1-4] in the United States and Herfert[5-7] in Germany. Graber evaluated growth and development of patients operated on by a plastic surgeon in Chicago who used a radical approach for cleft palate repair. Cephalometric studies revealed a high incidence of maxillofacial growth inhibition. Graber also found that the earlier surgery was performed, the more severe the growth inhibition. Any interpretation of Graber's results is questionable because he did not specifically describe the surgical technique used for palate repair. As far as I know (based on my knowledge of this surgical technique), the procedure used would be detrimental to facial growth regardless of the patient's age at the time of surgery.

Graber's results must be interpreted with caution. His data were based on a very specific group of patients who underwent a given surgical procedure that resulted in a very poor clinical outcome. Unfortunately, the results of Graber's studies often are generalized to apply to surgical techniques that have not been analyzed to support the assumption that palate repair is detrimental to facial growth. If no objective analysis of other surgical techniques has been performed, it cannot be assumed that all techniques used in palatoplasty represent a major contributing factor in maxillofacial growth aberrations.

Herfert[5-7] based his conclusions on clinical and experimental observations. He reported that all of his patients who were operated on between 2 and 5 years of age exhibited a severe degree of maxillofacial growth inhibition. He was the first to suggest that the very nature of palatoplasty, which includes raising mucoperiosteal flaps, affects the growth centers in the bony palate, leading to aberrations of facial growth. Herfert also stressed the relationship between age and the severity of growth impairments. That is, the earlier palatoplasty was performed, the greater the resulting growth aberrations.

In an attempt to support his clinical observations with experimental data, Herfert designed a study using a dog model. His first experiment involved elevation of a mucoperiosteal flap on one side of the palate with ligation of the posterior palatine artery and removal of a narrow strip of mucoperiosteum from the lateral edge of the raised flap. The flap was then returned to its bed and sutured. A narrow strip of denuded bone was exposed next to the alveolar ridge. After sacrificing the dogs, the skulls were directly measured. Asymmetry of the palate was found, the side operated on being narrower than the side that had not been operated on.

In a second study, Herfert used a similar design; however, ligation of the palatine artery was not performed. The results still showed palatal asymmetry but to a less severe extent than that seen in his first study. On the basis of his clinical observations and experimental studies, Herfert concluded that palatoplasty—specifically, the raising of mucoperiosteal flaps and leaving denuded bone exposed—resulted in maxillary growth impairment that led to secondary maxillofacial deformities.

It is interesting that in all the literature devoted to experimental research in cleft palate, no critical assessment of the first study by Herfert is to be found. His study was conducted on only five dogs, of which one died immediately after surgery and another was considered an unoperated control. The remaining three constituted the "experimental group."

The small number of subjects in his experimental studies, the lack of homogeneity, and the fact that no statistical analyses were performed make Herfert's conclusions much weaker than they appear. Furthermore, the unoperated side of the palate was used as a control, which makes the experimental design questionable. Growth aberrations on the operated side may have influenced the unoperated side. Additionally, in his clinical observations he neglected to take into account the effects of lip repair, the type of cleft, cleft width, and dysmorphogenesis—all factors that should be considered in the evaluation of clinical results.

Critical analysis of Herfert's findings shows that the studies were inconclusive because of the flaws in his experimental design. Graber's results were biased because the surgical technique used was a radical approach and resulted in severe maxillofacial deformities. Despite the questionable scientific merit of these early studies, these experiments stimulated further investigation into the influence of palatoplasty on facial growth.

Kremenak and colleagues[8] followed Herfert's design and repeated his experimental study by removing a strip of mucoperiosteum adjacent to the alveolar ridge. They found that denudation of the bone resulted in significant maxillofacial growth inhibition, especially in the transverse dimension. Unfortunately, Kremenak and his associates also used the unoperated side of the palate as a control, making interpretation of the results difficult. The findings of this study were similar to those of Herfert. However, in both studies the same design weaknesses also applied to interpretation of the results.

In all subsequent studies, Kremenak assumed that palatoplasty resulted in some denudation of the bony palate. Based on this unproved assumption, Kremenak conducted further studies that indicated that denudation of the palatal shelf adjacent to the alveolar ridge was the cause of maxillofacial growth disturbances. Also, he reported that the temporary elevation of the mucoperiosteum and the severing of the major palatine artery were not relevant factors in growth aberrations. It was concluded that wound contracture must be prevented to preclude growth impairment in experimental animals following partial denudation of the bony palate. This hypothesis led to a study designed by Kremenak's associate Koopman,[9] who found that grafting of the denuded bone with buccal mucosa prevented maxillofacial growth inhibition.

These findings were supported by Jonsson and Strenstrom[10] and Jonsson and Hallmans,[11] who examined maxillary growth after unilateral closure of a surgically induced defect in the hard palate of beagle puppies. The hard palate, together with all of the mucoperiosteum, was removed except for a 4-mm strip of bone in the midline. On one side, the nasal mucoperiosteum was covered with a full-thickness free skin graft; on the other, the raw surface was left for secondary epithelialization. Findings revealed no difference in total maxillary length between the two sides of the maxilla. However, the overall difference in growth aberrations of the maxilla indicated that reducing the amount of scar tissue by covering the raw surface with the free skin graft resulted in reduction of maxillary growth impairment following palatal surgery.

Further studies by Dabelsteen and Kremenak[12] and Squier and Kremenak[13, 14] focused on the role of myofibroblasts in the healing of palatal wounds in beagles. It was suggested that fibroblasts, with actin filaments found in granulation tissue, were the main cause of scar contraction leading to convergence of the wound margins and interference with the normal growth of the underlying bony structures. Quantitative study of the healing palatal mucoperiosteal wound in beagles revealed that complete repair and remodeling of the tissue was likely to take longer than 18 days. The authors, on the basis of experimental studies and infrastructural observations, emphasized that myofibroblasts, with their contractile properties, may be responsible for the contraction of the healing palatal wound and subsequent growth aberrations. As a logical consequence, Kremenak and associates[15] suggested minimizing contraction of surgical wounds in the hard palate by using various topical pharmacologic agents. Kremenak and co-workers[16] simulated V–Y palatoplasty in beagles. They concluded that this procedure caused restriction of maxillary width but did not affect maxillary length.

Studies by Kremenak and his associates contributed interesting information about the influence of various surgical procedures on maxillofacial growth. However, these results should be discussed within the limitations of their particular experimental design. Although these studies used a better design than Herfert's and included appropriate statistical analyses, they were conducted on the basis of the following erroneous assumption: Cleft palate repair always results in partial denudation of the bony palate. Another factor should be taken into consideration. Like Herfert, Kremenak and his colleagues used one side of the palate as a control. This factor again neglects the interdependency of growth processes and does not take into account the fact that the control side could have been affected by the effects of the operated side on the growth of the entire maxillofacial complex.

Sarnat[17] presented experimental studies suggesting that cleft palate repair was not detrimental to facial growth. His study in macaque rhesus monkeys (*Macaca mulatta*) revealed that unilateral elevation and partial removal of mucoperiosteum, with the severing of the palatine artery and partial resection of the hard palate and adjacent sutures, did not produce grossly apparent growth arrest in either the face or the palate. Lynch and Peil[18] found that creation of palatal clefts in puppies resulted in no significant changes in growth patterns compared to the control group. The palatal cleft was created by resection of the medial palatal suture and partial resection of the vomer. In the group in which the cleft palate was closed using mucoperiosteal flaps, a significant decrease in transverse palatal growth was demonstrated. It was suggested that the binding effect of the scar tissue following palatoplasty caused inhibition in the transverse dimension.

Studies on dogs by Meijer and Prahl[19] employed two different surgical procedures for cleft palate closure: the Dieffenbach and the von Langenbeck techniques. Both were evaluated for their possible influence on facial growth and occlusion. The results indicated that Dieffenbach's bone flap operation had a more detrimental effect on the maxillary complex and occlusion than did the von Langenbeck technique. The authors' conclusion that lateral relaxing incisions for repair of palatal clefts should be used with great prudence and avoided whenever possible seems stronger than warranted by the evidence presented in their study.

Studies by Verwoerd-Verhoef[20] indicated that interruption of the orbicularis oris muscle interferes minimally with facial growth but that creation of a bony defect in the alveolus and palate results in growth aberrations and inhibiton, primarily in the anteroposterior dimension. These studies describe a useful and replicable animal model for testing the effects of various surgical techniques for closure of surgically created defects. They also demonstrate that the rabbit model can be successfully employed in experimental studies of cleft lip and palate.

A series of experimental studies by Freng[21–23] and

Freng and Voss[24] explored the role of the periosteum in surgically induced palatal clefts. The reparative potential of single- and double-layered mucoperiosteum was examined in surgically induced palatal clefts in cats. At 2 months of age, the entire midpalatal suture and adjoining bone were resected, creating a bony defect 4 mm wide. The nasal mucoperiosteum was left intact. A flap of oral mucoperiosteum was then used to cover the bony defect, creating complete coverage by undisrupted mucoperiosteum on the oral and nasal sides. At 13 months of age, all the animals were sacrificed. It was found that the entire palatal defect was filled with new bone. In 5 of the 15 animals, a normal-looking midpalatal suture had been reestablished. The author indicated that new bone formation in the palatal defect may lead to maxillary growth arrest; however, this conclusion was not based on cephalometric measurements.

In another study, Freng[21] used single-layer periosteoplasty in midpalatal clefts. The results seemed to indicate that one-layer closure of the midpalatal suture in cats resulted in reduction of transverse maxillary growth by up to 50%. Freng's[23] experimental studies on the growth of the middle face, particularly early bony fusion in the different palatal and maxillary sutural systems, indicated that the midpalatal suture was essential for growth and development of the maxillary complex in the transverse dimension. No inhibition of facial growth in the anteroposterior or vertical dimension was observed. Freng explored the restorative potential of the mucoperiosteum and provided more information about new bone formation in surgically induced palatal clefts.

Some surgeons have reported observations indicating that palatoplasty performed at an early age does interfere with facial growth, causing secondary maxillofacial deformities.[25, 26] Bernstein[27] advocated a delay of palatoplasty until the age of 36 months or later. In his opinion, cleft palate repair performed before all deciduous molars were in proper occlusion resulted in midfacial growth inhibition. Wada and Miyazaki[28] found that palate repair at 2 years of age resulted in restriction of anteroposterior and transverse maxillary growth. Abe and colleagues[29] found that, following lip repair at 3 months of age and palatoplasty at 14 months, growth inhibition was apparent in the anteroposterior and transverse dimensions of the maxillary complex. To minimize interference with the bony palate at the time of cleft palate repair and to avoid denudation of the palatal shelves, Perko[30] introduced a surgical technique that made use of mucosal flaps instead of mucoperiosteal flaps for closure of the cleft.

Not all specialists involved in the management of cleft lip and palate considered early palatoplasty detrimental to normal facial growth. Bill and associates[31] did not observe alteration in facial growth after early surgery (before 2 years of age). Ross and Lindsay[32] found that the best facial-skeletal relationships occurred in patients who had palate repair before 18 months of age using the von Langenbeck technique. In addition, these authors emphasized that significant differences in skeletal relations occurred depending on the surgeon's proficiency.

Robertson and Jolleys[33] presented the results of a well-designed clinical study in two groups with complete unilateral cleft lip and palate. Forty infants were randomly assigned to two groups. Patients from both groups underwent lip and soft palate repair at 3 months of age using the same surgical techniques. In one group the hard palate was repaired at 12 months of age, and in the other the hard palate was repaired at 4.5 to 5 years of age. Examination at 4.5 and 7 years revealed no significant difference in occlusion between the two groups. The authors concluded that early hard palate repair did not affect facial growth. Mapes and colleagues[34] and Robertson and Fish[35] indicated that conservative, nontraumatic palatoplasty stimulated acceleration of the maxillary growth rate and that more normal dimensions were achieved in the following years.

A longitudinal cephalometric study by Krogman and colleagues[36] of the craniofacial growth patterns in children with clefts from birth to 6 years of age was one of the most impressive studies in this area. Two types of clefts were studied: (1) unilateral cleft lip, alveolus, and palate; and (2) cleft palate only. A general postoperative "catch-up" growth was observed in both groups, but more growth occurred in the cleft palate only group. These authors concluded that conservative palatoplasty stimulated rather than inhibited growth in both the maxillofacial skeletal complex and the soft tissues of the labial complex. This study supports the hypothesis that palatoplasty performed with minimal trauma facilitates maxillofacial growth and an acceptable, normal, craniofacial dental growth pattern.

Results of cephalometric studies by Bishara[37–39] indicated that when a Wardill-Kilner palatoplasty was performed on a patient with cleft of the palate only, anteroposterior and vertical skeletal and facial relationships were not affected. Bishara stressed that cleft populations and normal populations represent two distinct groups with different craniofacial characteristics.

Strong evidence that palatoplasty has no detrimental effect on maxillofacial growth was stressed by Aduss: ". . . orthodontists, acting as roentgenocephalometricians, documented craniofacial growth for these patients and revealed that iatrogenic aberrations of craniofacial growth were no longer a consequence of palatal surgery." He also emphasized that these findings may be due in part to the fact that surgeons have modified their techniques, the timing of surgery, and the number of surgeries performed on the palate. On the other hand, Aduss stressed that, by working with a cleft team, the orthodontist can integrate his goals more efficiently with those of the other specialists in treatment of the cleft patient.

The belief that palatoplasty has deleterious effects on facial growth stimulated some surgeons to design new procedures that involved neither the raising of mucoperiosteal flaps nor closure of the hard palate at an early age. A classic example of these procedures was the concept that offered a compromise solution to the demands of both speech pathologists (who advocated early palatoplasty) and orthodontists (who favored late palatoplasty).

Such a concept was initiated by Herman Schweckendiek[40, 41] and further developed by his son Wolfram.[42] The soft palate was repaired at an early age (about 6 months), and the hard palate was left unrepaired until approximately 12 to 16 years of age. The premises were that primary veloplasty created a functioning velopharyngeal mechanism for early speech development, while the unrepaired hard palate allowed unrestricted facial growth. Slaughter and Pruzansky[43] also formulated a rationale for velar closure as a primary procedure. Unfortunately, no follow-up was presented by these latter authors.

To learn more about this concept, the cleft palate team from the Iowa Cleft Palate Center evaluated 45 patients with unilateral cleft lip, alveolus, and palate. All were operated on by Wolfram Schweckendiek. Examination revealed a high incidence of short palates with poor mobility and velopharyngeal incompetence. However, facial growth was highly acceptable in the majority of patients. The Marburg experience,[44] combined with our series of primary veloplasty patients, demonstrated that two-stage palatoplasty was not the best solution for cleft palate repair.

Another surgical technique, in which the primary goal was to avoid undermining of the mucoperiosteum, was described by Perko,[30] who developed use of mucosal flaps for closure of the palatal defect. Some surgeons use vomer flap mucoperiosteum or mucosa for closure of the hard palate cleft in a two-stage sequence for palatoplasty. Others use a vomer flap and a free skin graft (see Chap. 3). All these procedures were designed to minimize the negative effect of palatoplasty on maxillofacial growth because these surgeons expressed strong convictions that palate repair was the primary cause of growth aberrations. None of them ever questioned the validity of this concept.

Critical review of the literature indicates that there is little evidence (clinical or experimental) to suggest that cleft palate surgery is a primary cause of maxillary growth impairment. Because palatoplasty is closely related to maxillofacial growth and speech production, there is a definite need for further well-designed studies that use standardized criteria and a uniform protocol to generate a reliable data base. There is also a need to answer the question of whether techniques for palatoplasty that do not involve raising mucoperiosteal flaps or exposure of bare bone differ in results from palatoplasty techniques that do involve raising mucoperiosteal flaps or exposure of bare bone. Such issues must be investigated as we attempt to define the role of orthodontics and its importance in the treatment of cleft patients. Experimental and clinical studies present good arguments for and against the hypothesis that palatoplasty is the major cause of facial growth aberrations. However, the results must be interpreted within the limits of the various study designs. Continuous disagreement about the influence of palate repair on facial growth is probably the result of the various experimental models and designs used to study this problem. Thus, the evidence generated so far should be regarded as inconclusive.

Experimental Studies at the Iowa Cleft Palate Center

Our challenge of the hypothesis that palatoplasty is the main cause of maxillofacial growth aberrations is based on long-term clinical experience and observations, clinical studies, and experimental research. It is our opinion that:

1. Cleft palate repair is not the major or only cause of maxillofacial growth aberrations.
2. Interference with the periosteum and bony palate does not negatively affect facial growth.
3. Cleft palate repair does not necessarily result in exposure of bare palatal bone.

Some of the above mentioned hypotheses have been substantiated by our experimental and clinical studies. Others require further investigation.

One of the major factors that stimulated my interest in exploring the influence of cleft lip and/or palate repair on facial growth was the clinical observation of adolescents and adults with cleft lip and palate whose lips had been repaired but in whom no palatal surgery was done. Many of these patients exhibited midfacial growth inhibition and subsequent maxillofacial deformities identical to those observed in patients who had had cleft lip and palate repair. Those observations, made in different countries (U.S.S.R., Poland, Bulgaria, Turkey, and China), led to the hypothesis that lip repair may be an important factor in facial growth aberrations.

Clinical observations led to the assumption that the sequence of surgical procedures is relevant when analyzing the causal agents interfering with facial growth. In the past, there was a period of 2 to 8 years between cleft lip and palate repair. Presently, this period is shorter; however, we still have an approximate 12-month interval between cleft lip repair (usually performed at 3 months of age) and palate repair (12 to 24 months of age). This sequence of two major surgical procedures indicates that at the time period between the two operations, the probable cause of maxillofacial growth aberrations is limited to lip repair exclusively.

Facial growth aberrations do not develop immediately following lip or palate surgery. The evidence of secondary maxillofacial deformities may appear after several years, when it is impossible to distinguish which surgical procedure, cleft lip or palate repair, was the main cause of growth disturbances.

Another clinical observation raised my doubts about the widely accepted hypothesis that palate repair is the primary cause of facial growth aberrations. When I changed my choice of surgical technique of palatoplasty from the method of Veau and Wardill-Kilner to two-flap palatoplasty, it became evident that the frequency and severity of growth aberrations markedly decreased. In using the Veau and Wardill-Kilner palatoplasty techniques, large areas of denuded bone were exposed, and the subsequent healing process, followed by scar contracture, appeared to result in growth disturbances. On the contrary, the use of two-flap palatoplasty and the attempt to leave minimal or no bare bone exposed apparently prevented serious growth aberrations.

Two other factors must be considered when discussing facial growth in individuals with clefts: congenital dysmorphogenesis and proficiency of the surgeon. Congenital dysmorphogenesis, which is expressed in the initial deformity by a variety of characteristics (cleft form, severity of the cleft, cleft width, hypoplasia of the soft and bony tissue, positioning of the maxillary segments, tissue deficiency, nasal deformity, and so on) may affect facial growth despite adequate surgical and orthodontic treatment. Some factors related to congenital dysmorphogenesis can be measured and studied; however, some of them, in particular hypoplasia, cannot be studied clinically because there is no technique available to measure the amount of hypoplasia that exists or to assess its influence on subsequent growth.

Another problem that must be considered when reviewing the factors that may influence maxillofacial growth is the surgeon's proficiency. It is obvious that cleft lip or palate repair performed with a rough technique and under great tension will probably have a more detrimental effect on facial growth than the same operation performed in a gentle manner and with minimal tension. It is my strong conviction that the surgeon rather than the surgical technique is the important variable that ensures the successful and beneficial outcome of the operation. There is no question that a specific surgical procedure does not work the same way in every surgeon's hands. The surgical technique is good only when the surgeon is good. At the same time, if a particular surgical technique proves to be efficient in the hands of many surgeons, this fact is an indication of its high validity. For all these reasons, the role of a surgeon in any clinical study cannot be overlooked.

To distinguish between the influence of cleft lip repair and cleft palate repair on maxillofacial growth, experimental studies with animal models are necessary. It is impossible in human populations, for ethical reasons, to design study groups in which various treatment protocols may be applied; there is a possibility that one of the proposed protocols may not be considered by the author of the study to be an optimal treatment. Research using animal models allows investigation of factors that cannot be readily studied in humans, and for this reason, animal models will always be of value. When using animal models, investigators must not only be aware of the limitations of such models but must also recognize that the choice of animal may have a pronounced effect on the findings.

In our laboratory experiments, research was initially conducted using a rabbit model and then was changed to a beagle model. The change of model was in part brought about by the criticism of Sarnat,[45] who indicated that lagomorphs are not the best animals for experimental research on craniofacial growth. In a literature search, we found that a great variety of animals (rats, cats, rabbits, dogs, and primates) have been used to study craniofacial growth. Since we could not find a study that compared animal models, we elected to work with the beagle model, being well aware of the limitations of this model. In 1988, we published a comparative study of the role of animal models in experimental studies of craniofacial growth following cleft lip and palate repair.[46] In this study, we found that in some respects both animal models (rabbits and beagles) yielded similar results, whereas in other respects the results differed significantly. The results obtained did not allow us to draw strong conclusions about which animal model might be more appropriate.

In several experimental studies, we tested the hypothesis that cleft lip repair is a major factor in midfacial growth aberrations,[47–56] and in several other studies, we explored the hypothesis that cleft palate repair is an important factor in facial growth aberrations.[44, 57–60] In both rabbits and beagles, a single design was used to assess the effects of cleft lip or palate repair independently of surgical creation of the cleft lip, alveolus, and palate. To eliminate the effect of surgical creation on the cleft, two control groups were used in each study: unoperated controls and animals with surgically created clefts of the lip, alveolus, and palate that were left unrepaired. It was established that lip repair is an important factor influencing maxillofacial growth. In both animal models, the pressure of the repaired lip affected maxillary length most severely. In beagles, maxillary widths and posterior facial lengths were also inhibited.[47–51, 57]

The results of our studies investigating the influence of cleft lip repair on maxillofacial growth stimulated us to extend our research into the role of palate repair, because this was considered to be a prime cause of growth inhibition and aberrations. The varying opinions expressed about the influence of palatoplasty on facial growth are probably the result of the multiplicity of surgical techniques, experimental models, and designs used to study the problem. We performed studies investigating the role of palatoplasty on craniofacial growth in rabbits and beagles, using a design identical to that used in our previous studies on the influence of cleft lip repair. We also explored how exposure of bare bone following palatoplasty influenced craniofacial growth. The defects of the lip, alveolus, and palate were surgically created as in our previous studies. The palatal defect was closed using two-flap palatoplasty in which two mucoperiosteal flaps were raised and approximated in the midline and sutured to each other and to the nasal mucosa.

In our experiments with rabbits,[58] we found that two-flap palatoplasty resulted in asymmetric maxillary and mandibular growth. We interpreted this to mean that palatal repair may simultaneously inhibit growth in some dimensions and enhance growth in others. In both rabbits and beagles, two-flap palatoplasty did not slow overall facial growth. In beagles, facial growth following two-flap palatoplasty was indistinguishable from that seen in normal unoperated animals. Maxillary length was found to be within normal limits, whereas maxillary width was substantially increased compared with that found in nonrepaired animals.[59] These findings are in contrast to those reported by Kremenak[8, 16]; however, it is possible that the differences may be attributed to variations in experimental design.

Our findings stimulated us to design a new study to

assess the effects of palatoplasty in which bare bone was exposed lateral to the mucoperiosteal flaps. Sixty-six beagle puppies were divided into four groups: two control and two experimental groups. The first control group consisted of normal unoperated beagles, and the second control group consisted of animals with surgically created palatal defects simulating unrepaired palatal clefts. The experimental groups consisted of animals with surgically created defects. In the first group, the palatal defects were closed using two-flap palatoplasty, leaving a strip of exposed bare bone 1 to 2.5 mm wide lateral to both mucoperiosteal flaps. In the second experimental group, the defects were closed using a single mucoperiosteal flap to increase the area of exposed bare bone on one side to 7 to 8 mm.

Direct cephalometric measurements on the skull following sacrifice after 28 weeks of age included 34 craniofacial variables. The most severe craniofacial growth aberrations occurred in animals whose palatal defects were closed using a single mucoperiosteal flap, exposing a very wide area of bare bone on one side. In animals in which the palatal defect was closed using two-flap palatoplasty to minimize the area of exposed bone, the growth aberrations were insignificant. These findings suggest a relationship between the area of exposed bare bone and the degree of craniofacial growth aberrations. The smaller the area of exposed bone, the less severe the growth aberrations.

Evidence was found that two-flap palatoplasty stimulates new bone formation in surgically created palatal defects. In animals in which two-flap palatoplasty was performed, a large area of the surgically created palatal defect (62.2%) had been replaced with new bone, the structure of which was indistinguishable from that of a normal palate. In animals with surgically created clefts that were left unrepaired, a significantly smaller area was replaced with new bone (40.48%). These findings suggest that two-flap palatoplasty with mucoperiosteal flaps stimulates new bone formation and bone remodeling, which may be responsible for enhanced anteroposterior and transverse growth. In bone remodeling following two-flap palatoplasty in the beagle model, new bone formation led in some cases to complete closure of the surgically induced defect.

In humans, there is no clinical evidence that two-flap palatoplasty stimulates new bone formation within the cleft defect. However, it might be expected that by approximating two layers of periosteum, one from the oral side and one from the nasal side, new bone formation might occur.

New bone formation within the palatal cleft does not seem as important as solid two-layer closure of the entire hard palate. When the entire palate is closed with two layers, it does not make any difference whether or not there is a bony bridge between the two palatal shelves. Therefore, attempts to insert cartilage or bone implants into the palatal cleft are totally unneeded and unjustified.

Our experimental findings differ substantially from those of Herfert and Kremenak.[5–8] We understand that the results of each study must be interpreted within the limitations of the experimental design. The results of our studies led us to conclude that some existing concepts and hypotheses need to be studied more carefully. There is no question that further experimental studies using a uniform protocol and animal model should be conducted in various centers so that we may compare and arrive at verifiable conclusions.

Clinical Studies at the Iowa Cleft Palate Center

Our observations of adolescents and adults who underwent lip repair but not palate repair demonstrated that these patients showed the same anteroposterior growth inhibition as that observed in patients who had had both lip and palate repair. Based on this observation, we questioned which operation, lip repair or palate repair, or both, was responsible for subsequent growth disturbances. These observations gave further support to the idea that palate repair is neither the major nor the only cause of maxillofacial growth aberrations.

Clinical observations and comments in the literature suggest that lip repair is probably one of the important variables modulating craniofacial growth. To verify this hypothesis, we initiated a series of experimental and clinical studies.[52, 60] Postoperative increases in lip pressure in animal models were found to be significantly correlated with various craniofacial growth aberrations. The experimental findings led us to hypothesize that lip repair in infants with complete unilateral cleft lip, alveolus, and palate results in increased lip tension, which is transferred as pressure to the maxillary segments and may contribute to subsequent craniofacial growth aberrations. Forty-four infants with complete unilateral cleft lip, alveolus, and palate and 148 normal control infants were followed until 2 years of age.[52] Lip pressure measurements in the infants who had had lip repair were found to be significantly higher than those in normal infants. Also, lip pressure in the cleft infants remained significantly higher than that in the normal control children for the entire 2-year duration of the study. Thus, increased lip pressure, when the palate is unrepaired, should be considered a factor modulating subsequent craniofacial growth.

Two studies were conducted by speech pathologists at the Iowa Cleft Palate Center to evaluate the efficacy of two-flap palatoplasty with regard to speech production. In the first study, 45 children with unilateral cleft lip and palate who underwent two-flap palatoplasty (as described by Bardach) were examined primarily for speech patterns, using a previously designed protocol.[61] The findings from this investigation indicate that as a primary palatoplasty technique, the two-flap method can be expected to produce a velopharyngeal mechanism that is appropriate for normal oral speech in four out of five patients. This success rate of 80% compares quite favorably with rates reported for other methods (about 70%).[62, 63] In addition, this surgical technique can be expected to yield no postoperative palatal fistulas. However, more than half of the patients needed further dental treatment (62%) or speech therapy (51%) before normal speech production was achieved. These findings indicate that the two-flap method is highly satisfactory in the correction of cleft palate.

Results similar to those above were found in another study conducted in 1987 in cooperation with a team of specialists from the Hamburg Cleft Palate Center (see Chap. 12). In this study, 58 patients, all treated by the Iowa cleft palate team and all operated on by one surgeon (J.B.), were evaluated by specialists from the Iowa and Hamburg teams. The results were found to be successful in 80% to 85% of the patients. Maxillofacial growth was evaluated by two orthodontists. Cephalometric findings revealed slight underdevelopment of the midface and the mandible, which resulted in a favorable maxillomandibular relationship in the majority of the patients. Of 56 patients, only 3 (5.3%) required, in all probability, orthognathic surgery at a later age. All patients exhibited facial growth that was judged to be acceptable with regard to facial proportion and appearance.

Geometric Analysis of Two-Flap Palatoplasty

The concept that cleft palate repair is detrimental to facial growth is based on the assumptions that palatoplasty results in partial exposure of bare bone adjacent to the alveolar ridge and lateral to the mucoperiosteal flaps, and that this denudation of the bone leads to maxillary growth aberrations.[6–8] The assumption that palatoplasty results in exposure of bare bone adjacent to the alveolar ridge is true when applied to the four-flap palatoplasty technique in which posterior transposition of the mucoperiosteal flaps intentionally exposes bare bone on each palatal shelf. It is also true for the von Langenbeck palatoplasty, in which bare bone is left exposed lateral to the mucoperiosteal flaps. The same assumption cannot be applied to other surgical techniques for palate repair. Specifically, it does not apply to the two-flap palatoplasty described and used by Salyer and me. Two-flap palatoplasty does not require posterior transposition of the mucoperiosteal flaps to achieve complete closure. Closure of the palatal cleft is achieved by downward rotation of the mucoperiosteal flaps.

In 1967, I reported that most palatal clefts could be closed without exposing bare bone by using the two-flap palatoplasty technique.[64] I hypothesized that this was true because of the various angulations of the palatal shelves and the downward rotation of the mucoperiosteal flaps during closure. To test this hypothesis, a geometric analysis was performed by Bardach and Nosal in 1985.[65] Geometric analysis is a useful tool for investigating the actual transposition of the mucoperiosteal flaps because it demonstrates that some assumptions applied to two-flap palatoplasty, widely believed to be true, are actually false.

The two assumptions that were analyzed were:

1. The amount of bone exposed lateral to the mucoperiosteal flaps must be equal to or greater than the width of the palatal cleft to achieve tension-free closure.

2. Closure of the palatal cleft can be achieved only when the sum of the widths of the palatal shelves is greater than the width of the palatal cleft.

We want to emphasize that geometry is only one factor that contributes to effective closure of a palatal cleft. Other factors, for example, tissue elasticity and the stretch-relaxation phenomenon, play an important role in palatoplasty and allow closure of cleft defects that are even wider than those predicted on a geometric basis alone.

Two main factors must be considered in the analysis of the geometry of two-flap palatoplasty. The first is the discrepancy between the actual and apparent width of the palatal shelves. The second factor is the downward rotation of the mucoperiosteal flaps from their actual slopes into the horizontal plane of closure. Downward rotation allows the surgeon to use the actual total widths of both mucoperiosteal flaps. The role of both factors increases as the slopes increase. The magnitude of the angle of rotation determines the amount of additional closure that can be achieved by rotation. The initial slope, angle of rotation, cleft width, and widths of the palatal shelves are geometric factors that allow analysis and prediction of palatal closure (Figs. 46–1 and 46–2). The equations described by Nosal can be helpful when actual values are used in place of the variables. These also explain the principle of downward rotation of the mucoperiosteal flaps and closure of the cleft with no tension or exposure of bare bone. According to one

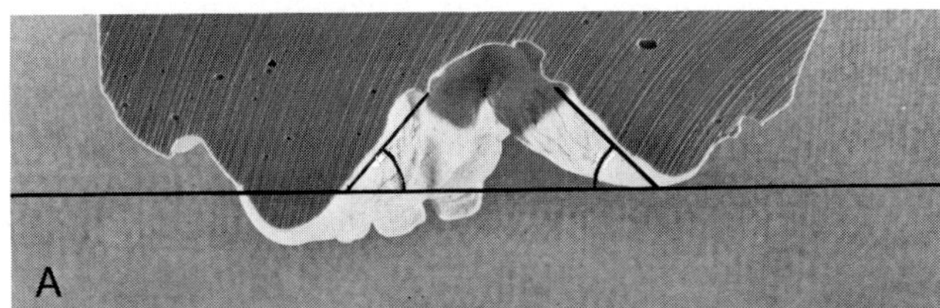

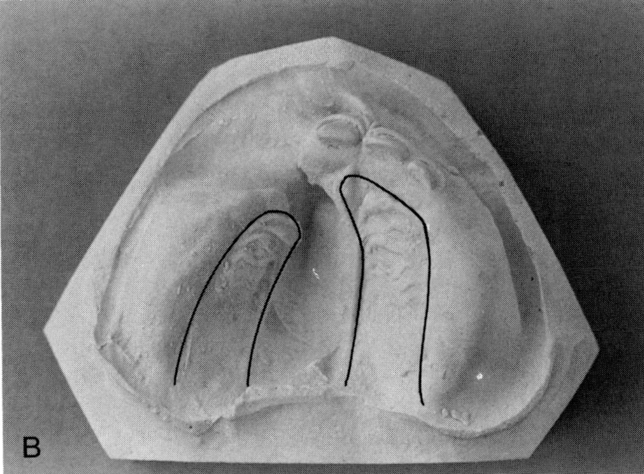

Figure 46–1 Wide unilateral cleft of the palate. *A,* The actual width of the palatal shelves and the angulation at × degrees. *B,* The projected widths of the palatal shelves. The projected widths are approximately one-third shorter than the actual widths of the palatal shelves. The difference depends on the slope of the palatal shelves.

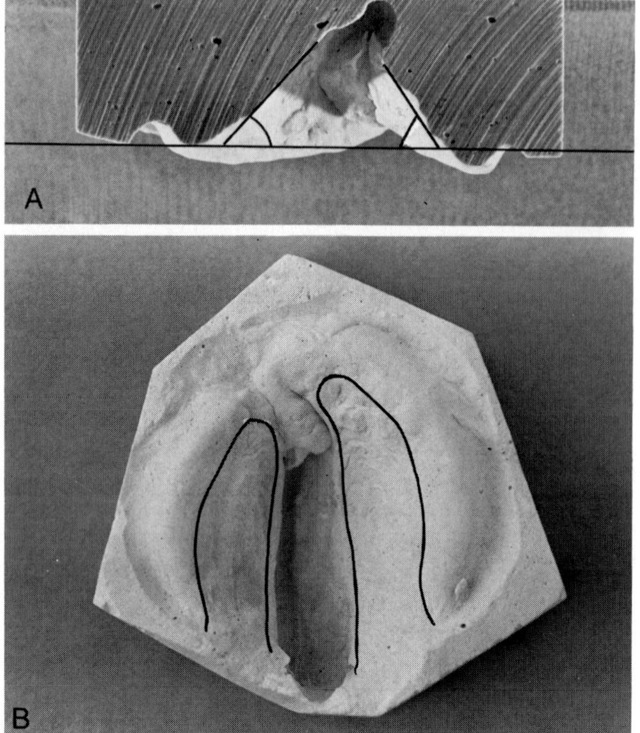

Figure 46–2 *A,* Palatal cleft with steep slopes and angulation of × degrees. *B,* The projected widths of the palatal shelves, which are shorter than the actual widths.

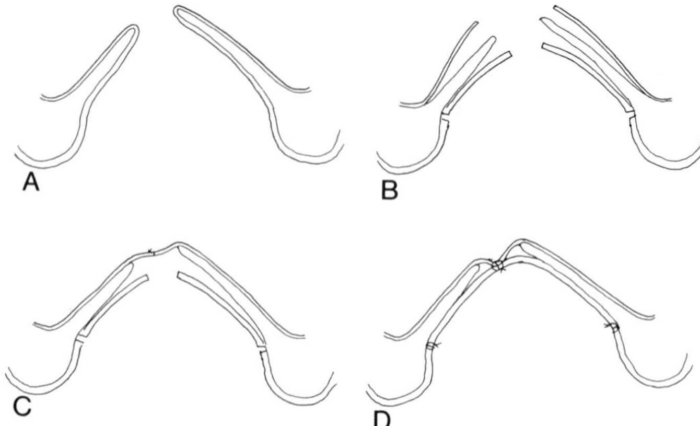

Figure 46–3 *A,* Schematic view of the unilateral palatal cleft. *B,* The mucoperiosteal flaps are undermined. *C,* The mucoperiosteal flaps on the nasal side are sutured together. *D,* The mucoperiosteal flaps on the oral side are attached with mattress sutures to the mucoperiosteum on the nasal side. Note the complete closure of the defects lateral to the mucoperiosteal flaps.

equation, when the palatal cleft is 10 mm wide and both palatal shelves are 10 mm in actual width and are positioned at an angle of 60 degrees with respect to the horizontal plane of closure, the cleft can be closed without tension or exposure of the bare bone. The same equation indicates that all parameters play important roles in our ability to predict the amount of closure of the palatal cleft that can be achieved without tension and exposed bare bone. The equation and the parameters are as follows:

$$C = A \times [1 - \cos(X)] + B \times [1 - \cos(Y)]$$

Where
C = Width of the cleft to be closed without tension or exposed bare bone
A = Actual width of the palatal shelf on the cleft side
X = Angle between the palatal shelf and the horizontal closure plane on the cleft side
B = Actual width of the palatal shelf on the noncleft side
Y = Angle on the noncleft side

The second assumption that was geometrically analyzed by Nosal implied (fallaciously) that closure of the palatal cleft can be achieved only when the sum of the widths of the palatal shelves is greater than the widths of the palatal cleft. This assumption is false because the usual measurements indicate the apparent, not the actual, widths of the palatal shelves. The importance of this second equation becomes apparent when the values of the apparent widths of the palatal shelves and the angles of the shelves are substituted. Then we can

derive a measurement of the actual amount of tissue available for closure of the cleft (Figs. 46–3 and 46–4).

Geometric analysis of two-flap palatoplasty, as described by Nosal, is presented in more detail in *Surgical Techniques in Cleft Lip and Palate.*[66] This analysis creates a theoretical base for the practical use of two-flap palatoplasty in which closure of the palatal cleft, with simultaneous closure of the lateral defects, is performed without leaving bare bone exposed. According to our experience, such closure can be achieved in the majority of patients with unilateral clefts and clefts of the palate only. It is difficult to achieve the same closure in patients with bilateral clefts (Figs. 46–5 through 46–8).

Surgical Technique

The main objective of cleft palate repair is to close the palatal defect completely and create an adequately

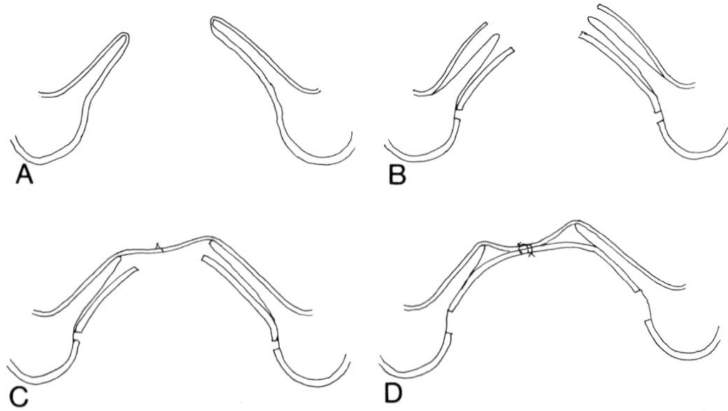

Figure 46–4 *A,* A wide unilateral cleft of the palate. *B,* Undermining of the mucoperiosteal flaps on the oral and nasal sides. *C,* Closure of the mucoperiosteal flaps on the nasal side. *D,* The oral mucoperiosteal flaps are sutured together and attached to the nasal mucoperiosteum. Note the exposure of bare bone lateral to the mucoperiosteal flaps on the oral side.

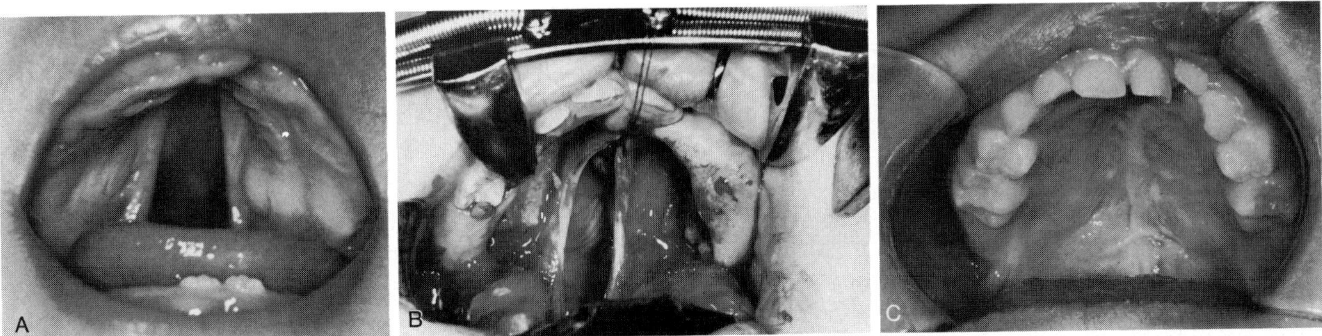

Figure 46–5 *A*, A wide unilateral cleft of the palate. *B*, The initial stage of closure of the nasal layers. *C*, Eight years after two-flap palatoplasty.

Figure 46–6 *A*, A bilateral cleft of the lip, alveolus, and palate. *B*, Following two-flap palatoplasty with no bare bone exposed laterally to the mucoperiosteal flaps.

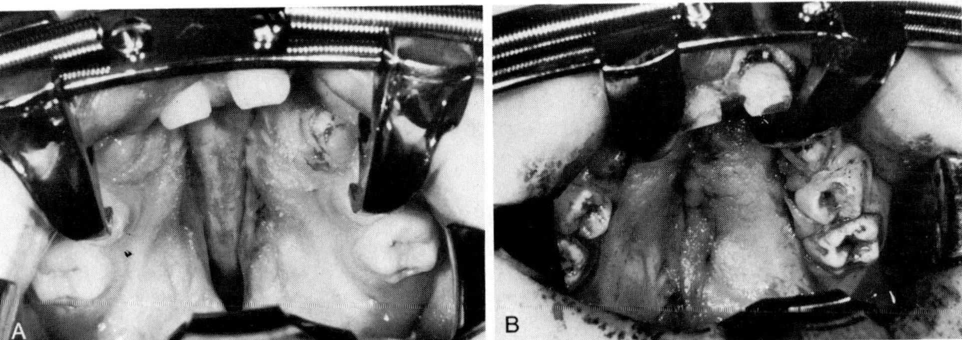

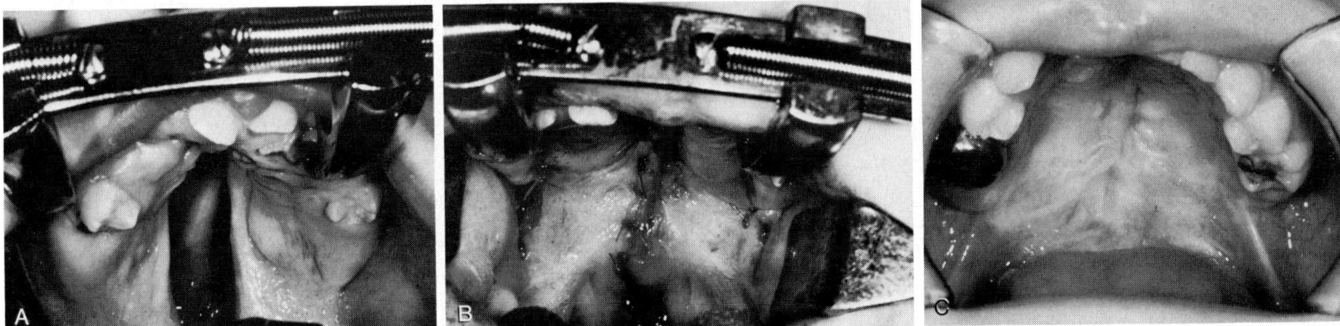

Figure 46–7 *A*, A unilateral cleft of the lip and alveolus and bilateral cleft of the palate. *B*, Closure of the palatal cleft without exposure of bare bone. *C*, The palate several years later.

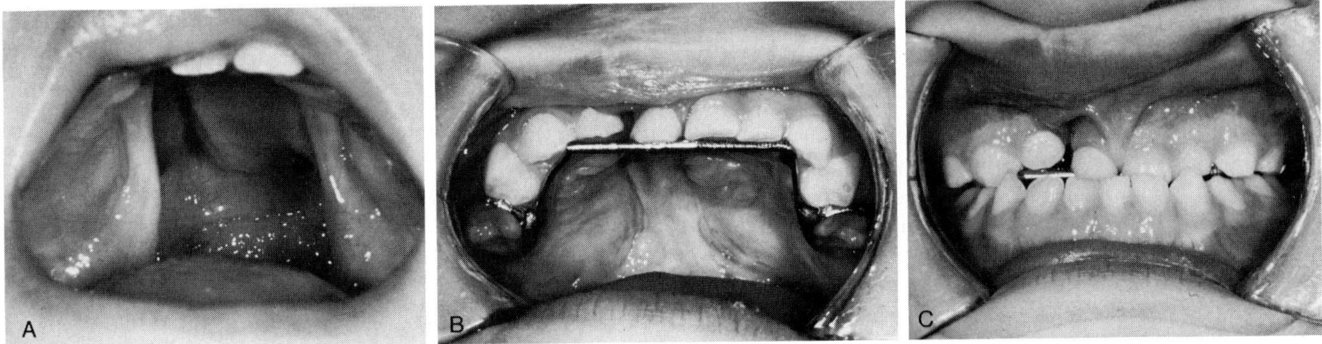

Figure 46–8 *A*, An extremely wide cleft of the palate. *B*, After two-flap palatoplasty at the time of maxillary expansion. *C*, Anterior crossbite.

functioning velopharyngeal mechanism for normal speech production. Thus, the main criteria for determining the success of palatoplasty are subsequent speech production and reconstruction of the palate without residual fistulas. In our opinion, which is supported by experimental research[59] and long-term clinical observations,[44, 64, 66–68] the two-flap palatoplasty performed according to our principles and techniques has minimal adverse effects on craniofacial growth. The concept that cleft palate repair is detrimental to facial growth is based on the assumption that this procedure always results in exposure of bone adjacent to the alveolar ridge.[5–8, 25] This assumption is true for the Wardill-Kilner-Peet four-flap palatoplasty (Oxford technique), which has been used extensively. In this technique, posterior transposition of the mucoperiosteal flaps intentionally exposes a relatively large area of bare bone on each side of the hard palate. Bare bone exposure also occurs with the von Langenbeck technique. This technique is not used as frequently now as in the past. Palatal bone exposure in these techniques results in scarring of those areas and leads to growth aberrations of various degrees of severity.

The two-flap palatoplasty does not require posterior transposition of the mucoperiosteal flaps and allows complete closure of the palatal cleft with minimal or no areas of denuded bone exposed in most patients. Thus, the concept and surgical technique of two-flap palatoplasty are totally different from the concepts and techniques in the operations mentioned previously.

Two-flap palatoplasty, which has been used at our center since 1972, was described initially by me in 1967[64] and elaborated by me in 1984.[67] Most recently, the technique has been decribed by Salyer and me in 1987.[66] Two-flap palatoplasty combines certain elements of other operations with some innovative details. In 1967 I formulated the hypothesis that in the majority of cases, two-flap palatoplasty allowed closure of the palatal cleft with minimal or no exposure of the bare bone adjacent to the alveolar ridge and lateral to the mucoperiosteal flaps. I reasoned that downward rotation of the mucoperiosteal flaps from their slanted position at various angles to a more horizontal position resulted in a gain in the horizontal dimension, allowing closure of the cleft with little or no exposure of bare bone.

Three major elements determine the possibility of closure of the palatal cleft without exposure of bare bone: (1) width of the palatal cleft, (2) width of the palatal shelves, and (3) angulation of the palatal shelves.

In the course of geometric analysis (described earlier), equations were designed that are used to predict the closure of the palatal cleft with or without bare bone exposure. This analysis disproved the assumption that the amount of bare bone exposed lateral to the mucoperiosteal flaps in two-flap palatoplasty must be greater than or equal to the width of the palatal cleft to achieve tension-free closure. It should be noted that geometry presents only one factor that contributes to effective closure of the palatal cleft. Other factors such as tissue elasticity and the stretch-relaxation phenomenon should be considered in any surgical technique.

Evaluation of patients prior to cleft palate repair should include assessment of the following factors:
1. Type of cleft
2. Width of cleft
3. Shape of cleft
4. Distance between the maxillary segments
5. Position of the maxillary segments
6. Presence of the vomer in the midline of the cleft
7. Attachment of the lower edge of the vomer to the palatal shelf on the noncleft side
8. Widths of the palatal shelves
9. Inclination of the palatal shelves
10. Position and mobility of the premaxilla
11. Length, symmetry, and mobility of the soft palate
12. Degree of motion of the lateral pharyngeal walls
13. Presence and quality of dentition
14. Distance between the posterior edge of the soft palate and pharyngeal walls
15. Presence of Passavant's pad
16. Presence and amount of adenoid tissue
17. Size and status of the tonsils

In our center, palatoplasty is usually performed at 9 to 18 months of age to create an adequate mechanism for early speech development. The type and severity of the palatal cleft assist in determining the best time for surgery. Two-flap palatoplasty, as previously described, incorporates several elements from other operations as well as some new features. The design and rationale of

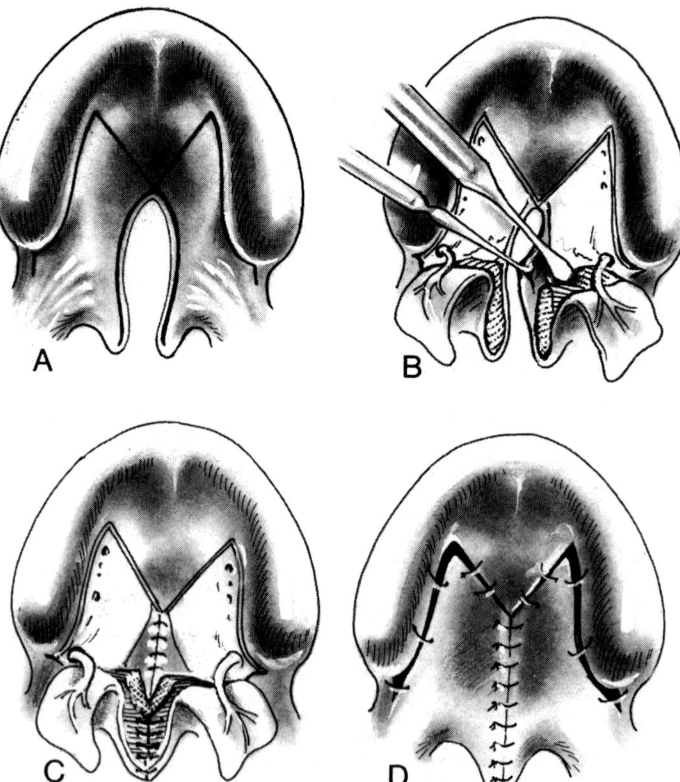

Figure 46–9 Two-flap palatoplasty for cleft palate only. *A*, The design of the incisions. *B*, Dissection of the nasal layer and dissection of the muscles of the soft palate from the edge of the hard palate and nasal periosteum. *C*, Closure of the nasal layer and the muscles of the soft palate. *D*, The mucoperiosteal flaps are closed with 4–0 chromic catgut.

each step in the two-flap palatoplasty allows this surgical technique to be considered a unique procedure, despite the fact that it represents a compilation of various surgical techniques modified by original maneuvers. The idea of raising two mucoperiosteal flaps was adopted from von Langenbeck's technique. However, in von Langenbeck's procedure, the flaps remain attached anteriorly, limiting their mobility and sometimes preventing closure of the anterior palate next to the alveolar ridge.

Special attention is given to complete closure of the entire palatal cleft with emphasis on closure of the anterior palate to prevent oronasal fistulas in this area. Mucoperiosteal flaps, based on the posterior palatine arteries, are raised and approximated at the midline, creating an oral layer. Lateral incisions follow along the pterygomandibular raphe; however, we do not attempt to enter the space of Ernst or fracture the hamulus. The neurovascular bundles are identified and preserved. Depending on the width of the cleft, the neurovascular bundles may be dissected from the mucoperiosteal flaps to increase the mobility of the flaps and lessen tension when suturing them at the midline.

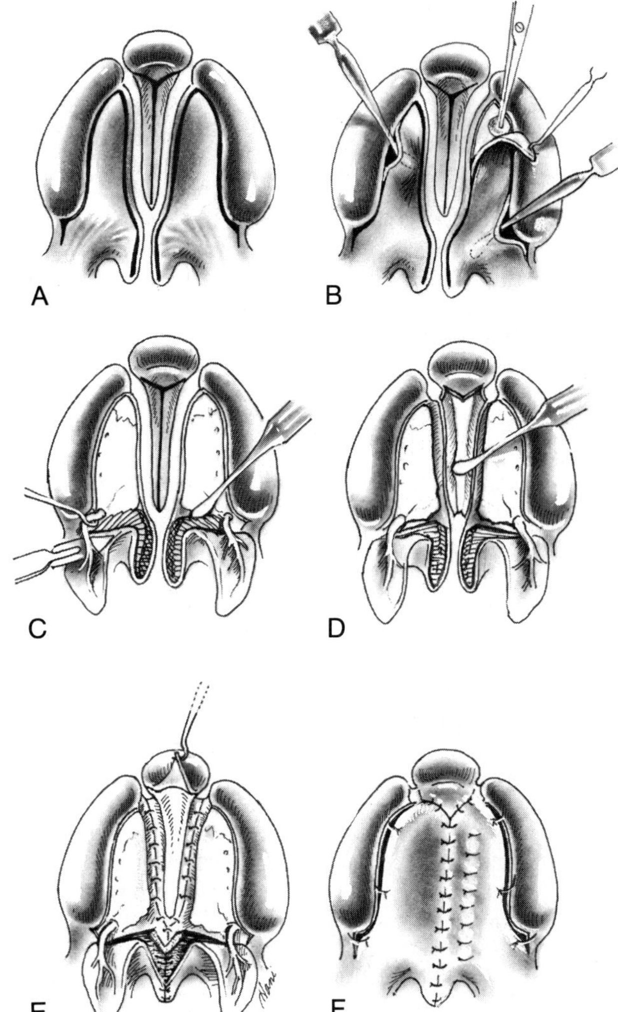

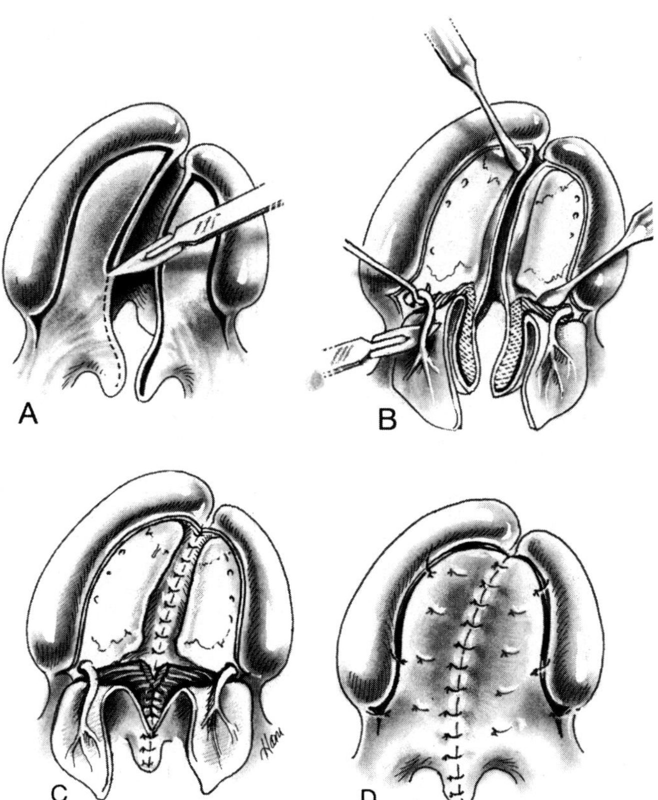

Figure 46–10 Two-flap palatoplasty for repair of the unilateral cleft palate. *A*, The design of the incisions on the hard and soft palates. Note the narrow strip of mucoperiosteum left at the medial edge of the palatal shelf in the area of the hard palate to increase the widths of the mucoperiosteal flaps for the nasal layer. *B*, The mucoperiosteal flaps on the oral side are raised. The neurovascular bundle is lengthened by dissection of the pedicle from the mucoperiosteal flap at the desired length. The muscles of the soft palate are detached from the posterior edge of the bony palate and from the nasal mucoperiosteum. *C*, The nasal layer and muscle of the soft palate are sutured with 4–0 chromic catgut. *D*, The mucoperiosteal flaps are sutured together and attached in the area of the hard palate to the nasal layer. The lateral incisions are closed if possible.

Figure 46–11 Two-flap palatoplasty for repair of bilateral cleft of the palate. *A*, The design of the incisions. *B*, The undermining of the mucoperiosteal flaps. *C*, The dissection of the muscles of the soft palate from the posterior edge of the bony palate and lengthening of the neurovascular bundles. *D*, Raising the mucoperiosteal flaps from the vomer for closure of the nasal layer. *E*, The nasal layer and muscles of the soft palate are sutured. *F*, The mucoperiosteal flaps are sutured using vertical mattress sutures. The lateral incisions are closed if possible. The mucoperiosteal flap from the premaxilla is joined with the mucoperiosteal flaps of the hard palate.

Incisions on the medial margins of the cleft are designed to create an adequate amount of mucoperiosteum for the nasal layer to be sutured free of tension. Depending on the width of the cleft, the width of the strip of mucoperiosteum on the oral side is determined. This serves as a nasal layer after it is dissected, elevated, and turned over facing the nasal cavity. It is important to estimate carefully how much tissue will be needed to close the nasal layer (Figs. 46–9 through 46–11).

The hard palate is always closed in two layers. The nasal mucoperiosteum is widely undermined and mobilized on both sides of the cleft and then approximated at the midline to create the nasal layer. Mucoperiosteal flaps are also approximated at the midline to create an oral layer. An important innovation in this operation is the close approximation of the oral and nasal layers in the area of the hard palate, thereby not only eliminating the dead space between the two layers but also stabilizing the mucoperiosteal flaps in the desired position. This is done by using vertical mattress sutures, a technique that has proved to be highly effective in almost totally eliminating fistulas in the area of the anterior palate. In some cases, lengthening of the neurovascular bundles by dissection from the mucoperiosteal flaps facilitates tension-free closure of wide clefts.

Creation of the muscle sling starts with careful dissection of the muscles of the soft palate from the posterior edge of the hard palate and the nasal mucoperiosteum. The muscles should be freed from both the hard palate and the nasal mucoperiosteum to create a functional muscle sling. This procedure also contributes to some lengthening of the soft palate.

Closure of both layers, nasal and oral, should be done under no tension. Closure of the nasal layer starts at the alveolar ridge and proceeds toward the uvula. The muscles of the soft palate and the oral mucoperiosteum are sutured from the uvula toward the alveolar ridge.

Following complete closure of the cleft, we attempt to close the area of exposed bone lateral to the mucoperiosteal flaps. If complete closure is impossible due to excessive tension, reduction of the exposed bone is recommended as well as covering the bare bone with (Avetine) microfibrillar collagen hemostat or oxidized cellulose (Oxycel) to stimulate healing of the denuded area.

We definitely prefer one-stage total closure of the palatal cleft to two-stage palatoplasty as described by Veau or Schweckendiek.[42, 69] The residual cleft, whether in the soft or hard palate, negatively affects speech production. Thus, the two-stage palate closure cannot be considered beneficial.

References

1. Graber TM: A cephalometric analysis of the developmental pattern and facial morphology in cleft palate. Angle Orthod 19:91, 1949.
2. Graber TM: Craniofacial morphology in cleft palate and cleft lip deformities. Surg Gynecol Obstet 88:359, 1949.
3. Graber TM: Changing philosophies in cleft palate management. J Pediat 37:400, 1950.
4. Graber TM: The congenital cleft palate deformity. J Am Dent Assoc 48:375, 1954.
5. Herfert O: Experimenteller Beitrag zur Frage der Schadigung des Oberkiefer-Wachstums durch vorzeitige Gaumenspaltoperation. Dtsch Zahn-Mund-Kieferheilk 20:369, 1954.
6. Herfert O: Tierexperimentelle Untersuchungen über die biologische Wertigkeit von Bruckenlappen (Axhausen) und Stiellappen (Palatinalappen) bei der Gaumenplastik. Dtsch Zahn-Mund-Kieferheilk 24:112, 1956.
7. Herfert O: Fundamental investigations into the problems related to cleft palate surgery. Br J Plast Surg 11:97, 1958.
8. Kremenak CR, Huffman WC, Olin W, Jr: Growth of maxillae in dogs after palatal surgery. I. Cleft Palate J 4:6, 1967.
9. Koopman CF, Jr: The effects of autogenous free intraoral grafting on maxillary growth after mucoperiosteal denudation of palatal shelf bone in young beagles. Thesis, University of Iowa, 1975.
10. Jonsson G, Stenstrom S: Maxillary growth after palatal surgery: An experimental study on dogs. Scand J Plast Reconstr Surg 12:131, 1978.
11. Jonsson G, Hallmans G: Healing of palatal defects with and without skin grafts: An intraindividual experimental study on dogs. Internat J Oral Surg 9:128, 1980.
12. Dabelsteen E, Kremenak CR: Demonstration of actin in the fibroblasts of healing palatal wounds. Plast Reconstr Surg 62:429, 1978.
13. Squier CA, Kremenak CR: Myofibroblasts in healing palatal wounds of the beagle dog. J Anat 130:585, 1980.
14. Squier CA, Kremenak CR: Quantitation of the healing palatal mucoperiosteal wound in the beagle dog. Br J Exp Pathol 63:573, 1982.
15. Kremenak CR, Searls J, Barrett R, et al: Inhibition of palatal postsurgical wound contraction; effects of pharmacologic agents (abstract). J Dent Res 55B:297, 1976.
16. Kremenak CR, Wada T, Seydel S, et al: Effects of VY palatoplasty simulations on maxillary growth in beagles (abstract). J Dent Res 57A:94, 1978.
17. Sarnat BG: Palatal and facial growth in macaca rhesus monkeys with surgically produced palatal clefts. Plast Reconstr Surg 22:29, 1958.
18. Lynch JB, Peil R: Retarded maxillary growth in experimental cleft palates: Mechanical binding of scar tissue in puppies. Am Surg 32:507, 1966.
19. Meijer R, Prahl B: Influences of different surgical procedures on growth of dentomaxillary complex in dogs with artificially created cleft palate. Ann Plast Surg 1:460, 1978.
20. Verwoerd-Verhoef H: Schedelgroei onder Invloed van aangezichts Spleten. Drukkerij Van Gerwen, Den Dunen, 1974.
21. Freng A: Single layered periosteoplasty in experimental mid-palatal clefts: A histological study in the cat. Scand J Plast Reconstr Surg 13:401, 1979a.
22. Freng A: The restorative potential of double layered mucoperiosteum: A study on experimental mid-palatal clefts in the cat. Scand J Plast Reconstr Surg 13:313, 1979b.
23. Freng A: Growth of the middle face in experimental early bony fusion of the vomeropremaxillary, vomeromaxillary and mid-palatal sutural system: A roentgencephalometric study in the domestic cat. Scand J Plast Reconstr Surg 15:117, 1981.
24. Freng A, Voss R: Bony or connective tissue union of operated experimental palatal clefts: Implications on growth of the dentomaxillary complex; a biometrical study in the domestic cat. Scand J Plast Reconstr Surg 16:233, 1982.
25. Blocksma R, Leuz CA, Beernink JH: A study of deformity following cleft palate repair in patients with normal lip and alveolus. Cleft Palate J 12:390, 1975.
26. Blocksma R, Leuz CA, Mellerstig KE: A conservative program for managing cleft palates without the use of mucoperiosteal flaps. Plast Reconstr Surg 55:160, 1975.
27. Bernstein L: The effect of timing of cleft palate operations on subsequent growth of the maxilla. Laryngoscope 78:1510, 1968.
28. Wada T, Miyazaki T: Growth and changes in maxillary arch form in complete unilateral cleft lip and cleft palate children. Cleft Palate J 12:115, 1975.
29. Abe M, Tatematsu M, Kato T, et al: A longitudinal study of postoperative changes of arch form and dimensions in complete unilateral cleft-lip and palate from birth to 3 years (abstract). Cleft Palate J 14:343, 1977.
30. Perko M: The closure of cleft palate using a mucosal flap. In Marchac D (ed): Transactions of the Sixth International Congress of Plastic and Reconstructive Surgery. Paris: Masson, 1976, pp 241.
31. Bill AH Jr, Moore AW, Coe HE: The time of choice for repair of cleft palate in relation to the type of surgical repair and its effect on bony growth of the face. Plast Reconstr Surg 18:469, 1956.
32. Ross RB, Lindsay WK: Surgical variables affecting facial growth in complete unilateral cleft lip and palate (abstract). Presented at the Fourth International Congress on Cleft Palate and Related Craniofacial Anomalies, Acapulco, Mexico, 1981.
33. Robertson NRE, Jolleys A: The timing of hard palate repair (Abstract). Cleft Palate J 14:346, 1977.
34. Mapes AH, Mazaheri M, Harding RL, et al: A longitudinal analysis of the maxillary growth increments of cleft lip and palate patients (CLP). Cleft Palate J 11:450, 1974.
35. Robertson NRE, Fish J: Early dimensional changes in the arches of cleft palate children. Am J Orthod 67:290, 1975.
36. Krogman WM, Mazaheri M, Harding RL, et al: A longitudinal study of the craniofacial growth pattern in children with clefts as compared to normal, birth to six years. Cleft Palate J 12:59, 1975.
37. Bishara SE: Cephalometric evaluation of facial growth in operated and nonoperated individuals with isolated clefts of the palate. Cleft Palate J 10:239, 1973.
38. Bishara SE: Comparisons of the effect of two palatoplasties on facial and dental relations. Cleft Palate J 11:261, 1974.
39. Bishara SE: Effects of the Wardill-Kilner (V/W-Y) palatoplasty on facial growth. Angle Orthod 45:55, 1975.
40. Schweckendiek H: Zur zweiphasigen Gaumenspalten-operation bei primarem Velumverschug. Fortschr Kiefer Gesichtschir I, 1944.
41. Schweckendiek H: Zur Frage der Frish- und Spatoperation der angeborenen Lippen-Kiefer-Gaumenspalten. Z Laryngol 30:51, 1951.
42. Schweckendiek W: Primary veloplasty: Long-term results without maxillary deformity. A twenty-five year report. Cleft Palate J 15:268, 1978.
43. Slaughter WB, Pruzansky S: The rationale for velar closure as a primary procedure in the repair of cleft palate defects. Plast Reconstr Surg 13:341, 1954.
44. Bardach J, Morris HL, Olin WN: Late results of primary veloplasty: The Marburg Project. Plast Reconstr Surg 73:207, 1984.
45. Sarnat BG: Discussion of "A comparative study of facial growth following cleft lip repair with or without soft-tissue undermining: An experimental

study in rabbits," by Bardach J, Mooney M, and Giedrojc-Juraha ZL. Plast Reconstr Surg 69:754, 1982.

46. Bardach J, Kelly KM: Role of animal models in experimental studies of craniofacial growth following cleft lip and palate repair. Cleft Palate J 25:103, 1988.

47. Bardach J, Klausner EC, Eisbach KJ: The relationship between lip pressure and facial growth after cleft lip repair: An experimental study. Cleft Palate J 16:137, 1979.

48. Bardach J, Eisbach KJ: The influence of primary unilateral cleft lip repair on facial growth. Cleft Palate J 14:88, 1977.

49. Bardach J, Robert DM, Yale J, et al: The influence of simultaneous cleft lip and palate repair on facial growth in rabbits. Cleft Palate J 17:309, 1980.

50. Bardach J, Mooney M, Giedrojc-Juraha ZL: A comparative study of facial growth following cleft lip repair with or without soft-tissue undermining: An experimental study in rabbits. Plast Reconstr Surg 69:745, 1982.

51. Bardach J, Kelly KM: The influence of lip repair with and without soft tissue undermining on facial growth in beagles. Plast Reconstr Surg 82:747, 1988.

52. Bardach J, Bakowska J, McDurmott-Murray J, et al: Lip pressure changes following lip repair in infants with unilateral clefts of the lip and palate. Plast Reconstr Surg 74:476, 1984.

53. Eisbach K, Bardach J, Klausner E: The influence of primary unilateral cleft lip repair on facial growth, Part II: Direct cephalometry of the skull. Cleft Palate J 15:109, 1978.

54. Bardach J, Mooney MP: The relationship between lip pressure following lip repair and craniofacial growth: An experimental study in beagles. Plast Reconstr Surg 73:544, 1984.

55. Bardach J: Facial growth following cleft lip and palate repair: Experimental studies in rabbits and beagles. In Jackson IT, Sommerland B (eds): Recent Advances in Plastic Surgery. Edinburgh: Churchill Livingstone, 1984.

56. Bardach J, Mooney M, Bakowska J: The influence of lip repair on facial growth: A comparative study in rabbits, beagles and humans. In Williams HB (ed): Transactions of the Eighth International Congress of Plastic and Reconstructive Surgery. Montreal: R.B.T. Printing, 1983.

57. Bardach J, Kelly KM, Jakobsen JR: Simultaneous cleft lip and palate repair: An experimental study in beagles. Plast Reconstr Surg 82:31, 1988.

58. Bardach J, Roberts DM, Klausner EC: Influence of two-flap palatoplasty on facial growth in rabbits. Cleft Palate J 16:402, 1979.

59. Bardach J, Mooney M, Bardach E: The influence of two flap palatoplasty on facial growth in beagles. Plast Reconstr Surg 69:927, 1982.

60. Bardach J, Martin R, Mooney M, et al: Bone formation in the canine palate following partial resection. In Dixon AD, Saruat BG (eds): Normal and Abnormal Bone Growth: Basic and Clinical. New York: Alan R. Liss, 1985.

61. Morris HL, Bardach J, VanDemark DR, et al: Results of two-flap palatoplasty with regard to speech production. Eur J Plast Surg 12:16, 1989.

62. McWilliams BJ, Morris HL, Shelton RL (eds): Cleft Palate Speech. Toronto: Brian C. Decker, Mosby, 1988.

63. Morris HL: Velopharyngeal competence and primary cleft palate surgery, 1960–1971: A critical review. Cleft Palate J 10:62, 1973.

64. Bardach J: Rozszczepy Wargi Gornej i Podniebienia. Warsaw, Panstwowy Zaklad Wydawnietw Lekarskich, 1967.

65. Bardach J, Nosal P: Geometry of the two-flap palatoplasty. Unpublished manuscript.

66. Bardach J, Salyer KE: Surgical Techniques in Cleft Lip and Palate. Chicago: Year Book, 1987.

67. Bardach J: Unilateral cleft palate repair. In Gates GA (ed): Current Therapy in Otolaryngology–Head and Neck Surgery. Philadelphia: Brian C. Decker, 1984.

68. Bardach J, Morris HL, Olin W, et al: Late results of multidisciplinary management of unilateral cleft lip and palate. Ann Plast Surg 12:235, 1984.

69. Veau V: Division Palatine. Paris: Masson, 1931.

Secondary Surgical Treatment of Cleft Palate

CHAPTER 47

Anatomy and Physiology of the Velopharynx

Martin D. Cassell, Jerald B. Moon, and Hani Elkadi

Modern anatomic textbooks generally give only a cursory treatment of velopharyngeal anatomy and an even more casual treatment of velopharyngeal physiology. It is rare even to find the term *velopharynx* applied to the soft palate and superior pharynx. Much of this deficiency can be attributed to a failure to recognize the highly detailed studies of the early anatomists and the important contributions available in the clinical literature. Although an exhaustive and detailed description of the anatomy and physiology of the velopharynx is beyond the scope of this chapter, we have attempted to provide a broad overview of its current status. In this, we hope to provide the clinician with basic information concerning the normal velopharynx and to highlight some of the many deficiencies in our knowledge and understanding.

The Velopharynx

The velopharynx is a musculomembranous valve extending from the caudal margins of the oral cavity to the posterior pharynx (Fig. 47–1). The anterior opening of the velopharynx, the oropharyngeal isthmus, is bounded on either side by the palatoglossal arches and inferiorly by the dorsum of the tongue. The anterosuperior limit of the velopharynx is the line of attachment of the soft palate along the posterior margin of the palatine bones. The notion of the soft palate as forming the true roof of the pharynx is best appreciated if the soft palate is considered in its elevated position.[1] In this position, the oral surface of the soft palate is continuous with the posterior and lateral walls of the pharynx. The superior limit of the velopharynx thus becomes defined as the line of apposition of the soft palate with the posterior pharyngeal wall. Cineradiographic studies in-

dicate that the level of velar apposition with the posterior pharyngeal wall lies about 1 cm above the level of the atlas, very close to the plane of the pharyngeal tubercle on the basilar part of the occipital bone (Fig. 47–2).[2]

In its relaxed position, the posterior border of the soft palate defines the anterior limits of a large aperture in the velopharynx, the nasopharyngeal isthmus or hiatus nasopharyngeus.[1] The lateral borders of the nasopharyngeal isthmus are defined by the ridge produced by the palatopharyngeus muscle proper (the so-called *palatopharyngeal sphincter*, see below) and posteriorly by the pharynx above the pharyngeal ridge (of Passavant). Jones[1] suggested that the ridge of Passavant itself was the true posterior limit of the nasopharyngeal isthmus, although studies in living subjects indicate that the line of apposition of the soft palate is normally above the ridge.[2] This superior limit approximates the level of the tori tubarii and thus includes the "true" pharyngeal part of the nasopharynx in the velopharynx.[3]

Identification of the soft palate with the roof of the pharynx excludes the space behind the choanae traditionally referred to as the *nasopharynx*. Various terms have been suggested for this region, including *epipharynx*,[4] although that suggested by Negus—*posterior nasal cavity*—seems most appropriate.[5]

Basic Structure of the Velopharynx

Excluding the vascular and nerve plexus, the pharyngeal part of the velopharynx consists of four layers: an internal layer of mucous membrane, an internal fibrous layer, a muscular layer, and an external fibrous layer. The internal fibrous layer is continuous superiorly with the pharyngobasilar fascia, whereas the external fibrous layer is usually termed the *buccopharyngeal fascia*. The internal and external fibrous layers represent the epimysial coverings of the pharyngeal muscles. This basic scheme of organization is continued in the soft palate with some modification because both surfaces of the soft palate are covered with mucous membrane.

Mucous Membrane

The velopharyngeal mucous membrane is typical oral mucosa consisting of nonkeratinizing, stratified squamous epithelium, with a well-developed lamina propria. Anterolaterally, the velopharyngeal mucosa is continuous with the oral mucosa over the palatoglossal arches. Inferiorly, the velopharyngeal mucosa is reflected over

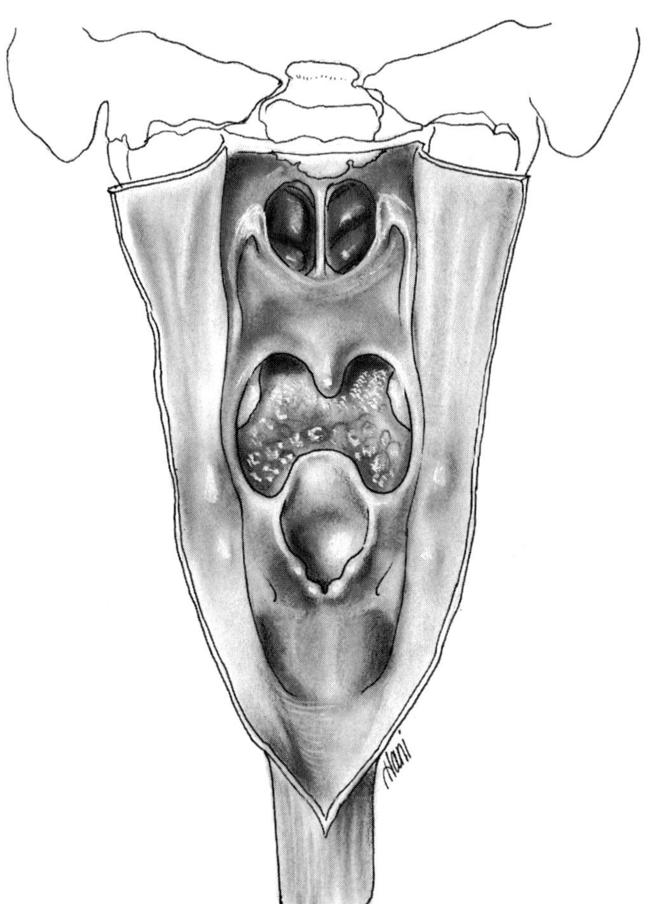

Figure 47–1 Posterior view of the velopharynx, pharynx, and larynx. The posterior wall of the pharynx has been opened by a longitudinal incision and its walls reflected laterally.

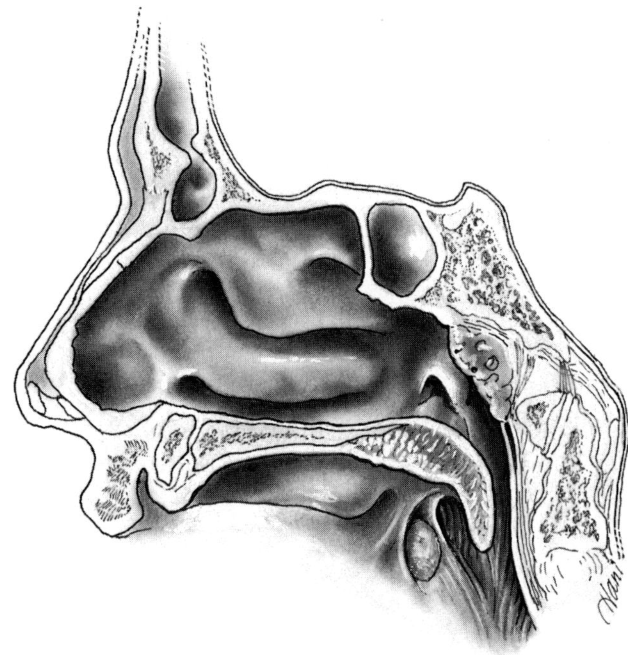

Figure 47–2 Lateral view of the nasal cavity and velopharynx.

the palatine tonsils to become continuous with the nonpapillate mucosa over the postsulcal part of the tongue and the epiglottic folds. Anterosuperiorly, the mucosa on the oral surface of the soft palate is continuous with the keratinized mucosa of the hard palate. Along the border of the nasopharyngeal isthmus, there is a transition from the typical stratified squamous epithelium of the velopharynx to the respiratory type of ciliated, columnar epithelium (Fig. 47–3). Anteriorly, the transition between the nasal mucosa at the inferior border of the choanae and the mucosa of the soft palate is abrupt.[6] Over the lateral and posterior surfaces of the pharynx a band of transitional epithelium is interposed between the stratified squamous epithelium of the velopharynx and the ciliated epithelium (Fig. 47–3). This transitional band, which is composed of patches of stratified and ciliated epithelium as well as true transitional epithelium, overlies the tori tubarii and the pharyngeal recesses (fossae of Rosenmueller) and continues into the mucosa overlying the basilar part of the occipital bone.[6] Inferiorly, the velopharyngeal mucosa is continuous with the mucosa of the remainder of the pharynx and esophagus (Fig. 47–1).

Grossly, the velopharyngeal mucosa appears smooth and continuous except where it is thrown into folds by underlying structures (Figs. 47–1 to 47–3). The most prominent of these folds are the palatoglossal and palatopharyngeal arches (anterior and posterior pillars of the fauces). The palatoglossal arch contains the palatoglossus muscles and associated connective tissue. The palatopharyngeal arch contains connective tissue and vertically running muscle fibers traditionally referred to as part of the palatopharyngeus muscle. As will be described in the section on velopharyngeal musculature, we have designated these fibers as a distinct muscle, the *palatothyroideus*. On the posterior wall of the pharynx, a horizontal ridge (the ridge of Passavant) can be observed in some living subjects. This ridge may be produced by fibers running horizontally from the palate to the superior pharynx, which we refer to as part of the true

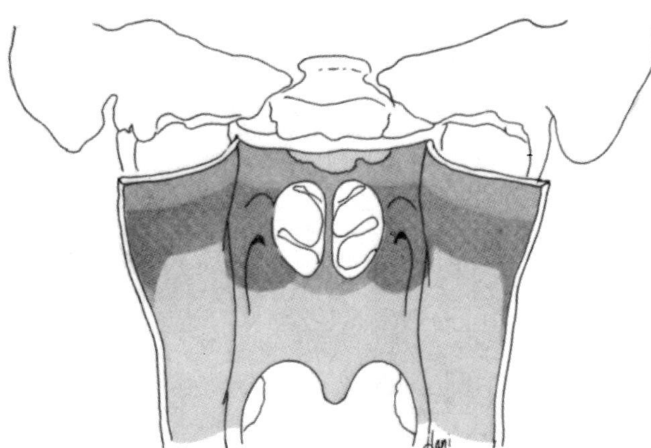

Figure 47–3 Semidiagrammatic representation of the velopharynx similar to that depicted in Figure 47–1 showing the distributions of the respiratory epithelium (midgray area), transitional epithelium (dark gray area), and stratified squamous epithelium (light gray area).

palatopharyngeus muscle.[1] In the region of the torus tubarius, three ridges are usually apparent (Fig. 47–3). Running almost anteriorly from the lateral ledge of the torus is the small salpingopalatal fold. From below the opening of the auditory tube, a ridge formed by the levator palati muscle (the torus levatorius) runs anteromedially into the soft palate. Also, from the opening of the auditory tube medial to the torus levatorius, the salpingopharyngeal fold runs almost vertically downward (Fig. 47–1 to 47–3).

Internal and External Fibrous Layers of the Velopharynx

The internal and external fibrous layers of the velopharynx, though generally thin, constitute a supporting framework for the velopharynx (Fig. 47–4A). Superiorly, the internal fibrous layer extends beyond the superior border of the superior constrictor muscle and is considerably thickened. This thick layer, generally termed the *pharyngobasilar fascia*, is firmly attached to the basilar part of the occipital bone, the pterygoid tubercle, and the adjacent surface of the petrous part of the temporal bone. The pharyngobasilar fascia sweeps under the auditory tube and is attached to the processus tubarius and the posterior border of the medial pterygoid plate (Fig. 47–4 and 47–5). The pharyngobasilar fascia also is continuous with the thinner epimysium of the levator palati, which passes onto the nasal surface of the soft palate (Fig. 47–4A).

The internal fibrous layer is thin over the constrictor muscles, particularly over the inferior constrictor, and its extent is difficult to discern in gross dissection. Below the pterygoid hamulus, the fibrous layer appears to be continuous with the fibrous layer over the palatal arches and is reportedly attached to the pterygomandibular raphe.[7] Along the posterior surface of the pharynx,

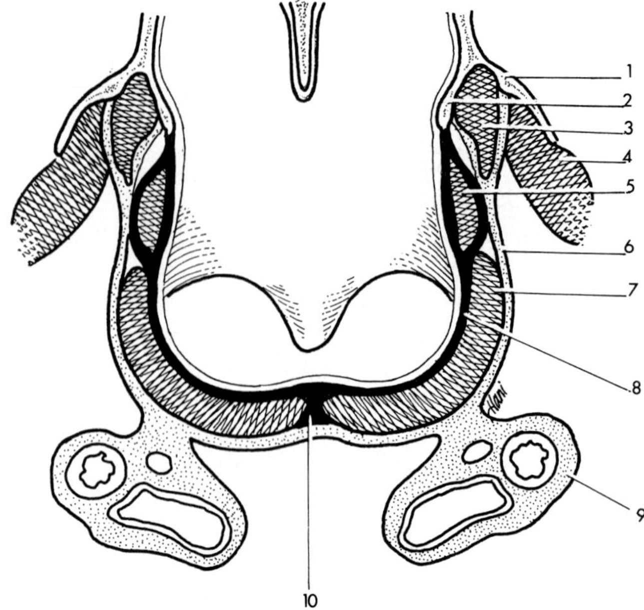

Figure 47–4 Schematic representation of a horizontal section through the superior pharynx just below the level of the auditory tube, depicting the relationships and attachments of the velopharyngeal fascia. (1) Lateral pterygoid plate; (2) medial pterygoid plate; (3) tensor palati; (4) medial pterygoid; (5) levator palati; (6) buccopharyngeal fascia (external fibrous layer); (7) superior constrictor; (8) pharyngobasilar fascia (internal fibrous layer); (9) carotid sheath; (10) pharyngeal raphe.

however, the internal fibrous layer is greatly thickened to form the median pharyngeal raphe (Fig. 47–4A). Superiorly, the raphe expands and is attached to the pharyngeal tubercle on the occipital bone. The pharyngeal raphe provides not only a suspensory mechanism for the posterior pharynx but also the insertion for the

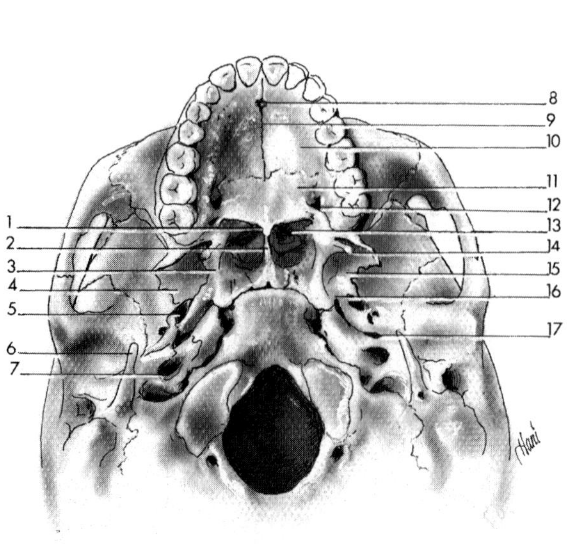

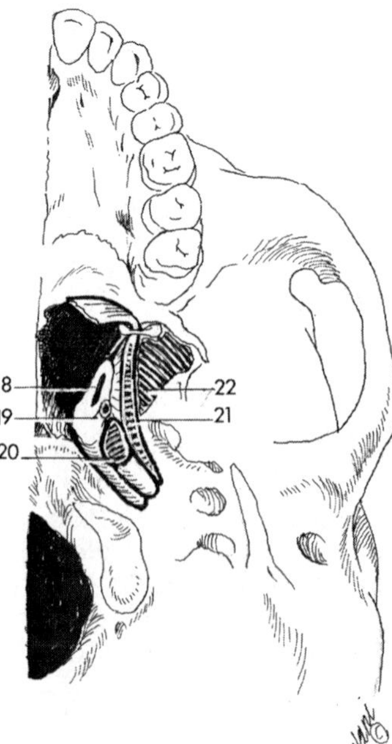

Figure 47–5 External surface of the base of the skull (left) and diagrammatic representation showing the origins of velopharyngeal muscles (right). (1) Posterior nasal spine; (2) vomer; (3) medial pterygoid plate; (4) lateral pterygoid plate; (5) foramen ovale; (6) styloid process; (7) carotid canal; (8) incisive fossa; (9) intermaxillary suture; (10) palatine process of maxilla; (11) horizontal plate of palatine bone; (12) greater palatine foramen; (13) left posterior nasal aperture; (14) pterygoid hamulus; (15) pterygoid fossa; (16) scaphoid fossa; (17) opening of auditory tube; (18) tubal cartilage; (19) salpingopharyngeus; (20) levator palati; (21) tensor palati; (22) medial pterygoid.

pharyngeal constrictors. A recent examination of 18 cadavers (M. D. Cassell, unpublished observations, 1988) revealed that in 16 cases the superior constrictor was completely inserted into the raphe; in only two specimens could muscle fibers be found inserting into the basilar part of the occipital bone.

The palatine, or velar, aponeurosis is a sheet of fibrous connective tissue extending to about 1 cm posterior from the posterior border of the hard palate (Fig. 47–4B). Generally, its posterior limit lies along a line joining the hamuli, but medially its fibers thin out gradually and pass more posteriorly than this limit. Although commonly referred to as the aponeurosis of the tensor palati, the palatine aponeurosis receives contributions from the epimysial coverings of the velar musculature and the salpingopharyngeal fascia. On the evidence of earlier studies, Kriens described the palatine aponeurosis as a direct continuation of the velopharygeal fascia.[8] A detailed description of the continuity between the palatine aponeurosis and the velopharyngeal fascia will not be made here. It is evident, however, that the fascia running between the soft palate and the tubal cartilage (the so-called salpingopalatine ligaments) and the membranous part of the auditory tube (the fascia of Tröltsch) is retained in the cleft palate, even in the absence of a palatine aponeurosis.[8]

The external fibrous layer, or buccopharyngeal fascia (Fig. 47–4A), is thinner than the internal fibrous layer, and its precise extent is difficult to discern. Superiorly, it merges with the pharyngobasilar fascia and laterally with the carotid sheath and fascia overlying the buccinator muscle (Fig. 47–4A).

Velopharyngeal Musculature

In the broadest terms, the musculature of the velopharynx consists of four U-shaped muscular slings that converge on the soft palate (the levatores palati, the palatoglossi, the palatothyroidei, and the palatopharyngei), and a paired muscle mass (the musculi uvulae) lying on the soft palate. Associated with these muscles are paired longitudinal muscles running from the auditory tube (the salpingopharyngei), a U-shaped muscle sheet forming the superior pharynx (the superior constrictors), and a pair of L-shaped muscles contributing to the palatine aponeurosis, the tensores palati (Figs. 47–5 and 47–6).

Palatoglossus. The palatoglossus muscle runs from the soft palate to the laterodorsal surface of the tongue (Fig. 47–7). In its midportion, the fibers of the palatoglossus form a narrow fasciculus, approximately 5 mm in diameter, which fans out on approaching its attachments to the tongue and soft palate (Fig. 47–7).[9] The attachment of the palatoglossus to the laterodorsal surface of the tongue appears to be along a continuation of the fascial sheath of the muscle itself. There appears to be little evidence to support the common assertion that the fibers of the palatoglossus merge with the transverse musculature of the tongue. The palatal attachment of the palatoglossus is more complex (Fig. 47–7B). Kuehn and Azzam reported that the fascicles at the superior

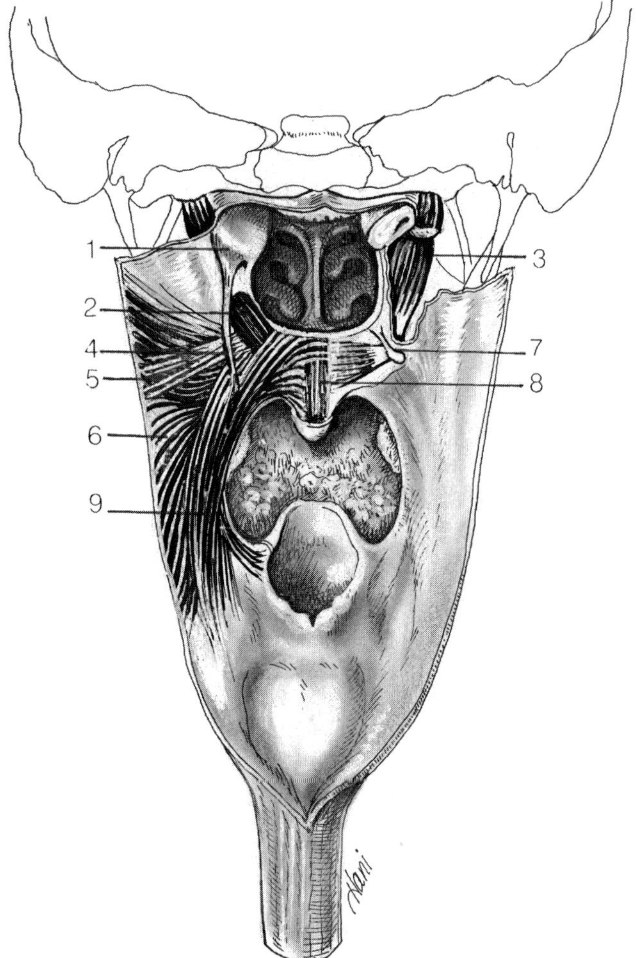

Figure 47–6 Posterior view of the velopharynx. The mucosa on the left side has been removed to show the musculature of the velopharynx. (1) Tubal cartilage; (2) levator palati; (3) tensor palati; (4) salpingopharyngeus; (5) palatopharyngeus; (6) superior constrictor; (7) pterygoid hamulus; (8) musculi uvulae; (9) palatothyroideus.

end of the palatoglossus fan out and intermingle with the mucous glands and connective tissue lying beneath the mucosa on the oral surface of the palate.[9] Others report that the upper fascicles of the palatoglossus split into superior and inferior bundles on entering the palate.[10] The inferior bundle runs toward the midline beneath the palatal mucosa. Contrary to the information in many texts, these muscle fibers stop short of the midline and do not interdigitate with fascicles from the contralateral muscle (Fig. 47–7B). The superior bundle of palatoglossal fibers pierces the palatal mass of the levator palati to end in connective tissue lateral to the musculi uvulae.[10]

In the parasagittal plane, the oblique course of the palatoglossus muscle is generally in line with the oblique course of the levator palati in the same plane (Fig. 47–8). The two muscles are thus commonly considered antagonistic.[9] In an oblique coronal plane, however, the levatores palati are directed toward the midline, whereas the palatoglossi curve laterally away from the midline (Figure 47–8A). These differences in direction

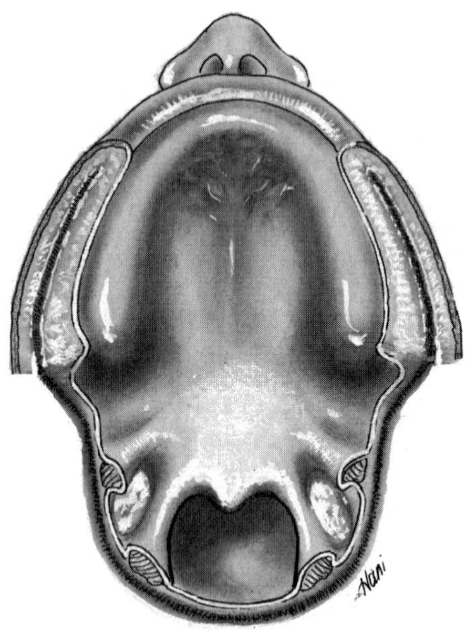
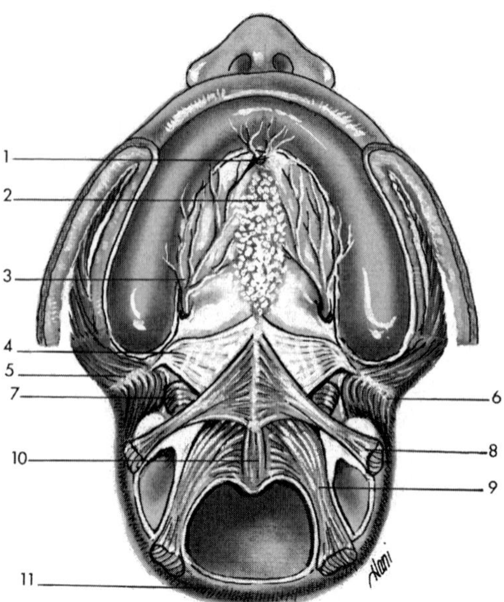

Figure 47–7 Ventral view of the velopharynx in a horizontal section at the level of the oral fissure. (1) Incisive fossa; (2) palatine mucous glands; (3) greater palatine nerves and vessels; (4) pterygoid hamulus and tensor palati; (5) buccinator; (6) pterygomandibular raphe and superior constrictor; (7) levator palati; (8) palatoglossus; (9) palatothyroideus; (10) musculus uvulae; (11) superior constrictor.

should be considered when referring to the levator palati and palatoglossus as antagonistic.

The anterior fauces (palatoglossal arch) contain a sheet of elastic fibers extending from the soft palate to the tongue. Fibers of the palatoglossus muscle insert into perpendicularly oriented elastic fibers.[9] The elastic fibers of the palatoglossal arch may assist in restoring the soft palate to its rest position.

Palatothyroideus and Palatopharyngeus. Many of the earliest descriptions of the velopharyngeal musculature recognized a clear distinction between the vertical muscle fibers running from the soft palate to the larynx and inferolateral pharynx, and the horizontal muscle fibers running from the soft palate laterally and posteriorly into the superior pharynx.[11] In consequence, the vertically running fibers were designated *m. thyrostaphylini* or *m. thyropalatinus*, whereas the horizontal fibers were termed *m. pharyngostaphylini* or *m. pharyngopalatinus*.[11–13] This scheme not only defines two distinct velopharyngeal muscles but also brings the description of these muscles in man in line with the situation in other mammals.[1, 14] Despite the clarity of the earlier descriptions and the exhortations of Jones,[1] modern anatomic texts use the term *palatopharyngeus* to describe the vertical muscle running in the posterior fauces and largely ignore the horizontal fibers that represent the "true" palatopharyngeus.

The present description has therefore sought to revise the nomenclature of these velopharyngeal muscles by restoring the term *palatothyroideus* to the muscle fibers running vertically from the soft palate to the larynx and inferior pharynx (Figs. 47–6 and 47–9). Aside from purely anatomic and comparative evidence, the most compelling reason for distinguishing these two muscles is their clear functional differences. The vertically running fibers of the palatothyroideus are in a position to act as a depressor of the soft palate, a suggestion consistent with the results of electromyographic studies (see Physiology of Velopharynx section below). On the

other hand, the horizontal fibers of the palatopharyngeus may play a role in closing the nasopharyngeal isthmus through movement of the pharyngeal walls.[15]

The palatothyroideus muscle is a thick fasciculus of muscle fibers running within the posterior fauces from the soft palate to the thyroid cartilage and inferior pharynx (Figs. 47–6 and 47–9). The palatal attachment of the palatothyroideus consists of two fasciculi that pass either side of the levator palati (Fig. 47–9). The anterolateral fasciculus, which lies between the levator palati and the tensor palati, is attached to the posterior border of the hard palate and to the palatine aponeurosis at and behind the posterior nasal spine.[7, 16] Some fibers reportedly join in the median plane with fibers from the contralateral muscle.[17] The posteromedial fasciculus, located behind the levator palati, is attached to the palatine aponeurosis and is joined by fibers from the opposite muscle near the midline. Some fibers of the palatothyroideus appear to be attached to the palatine raphe, whereas other fibers reportedly pass over the musculi uvulae.[18] The two fasciculi merge at the posterolateral border of the palate and descend in the posterior fauces behind the tonsil. The inferior attachments of the palatothyroideus have not been studied in any detail, and there are conflicting descriptions in the anatomic literature. According to most texts,[7] the fibers of the palatothyroideus pass posteromedial to the fibers of the stylopharyngeus and, with fibers from that muscle, attach to the superior horn and posterior border of the thyroid cartilage (Fig. 47–6). These descriptions usually note a few fibers passing posteromedially in the pharynx to attach to the internal fibrous layer. Other texts[16] describe three groups of fasciculi in the inferior part of the palatothyroideus: an anterior fasciculus that attaches to the thyroid cartilage, a lateral fasciculus that runs into the internal fibrous layer, and a posterior fasciculus that attaches to the pharyngeal raphe, with a few fibers crossing the midline to decussate with the fibers of the opposite muscle. Clearly, a more detailed

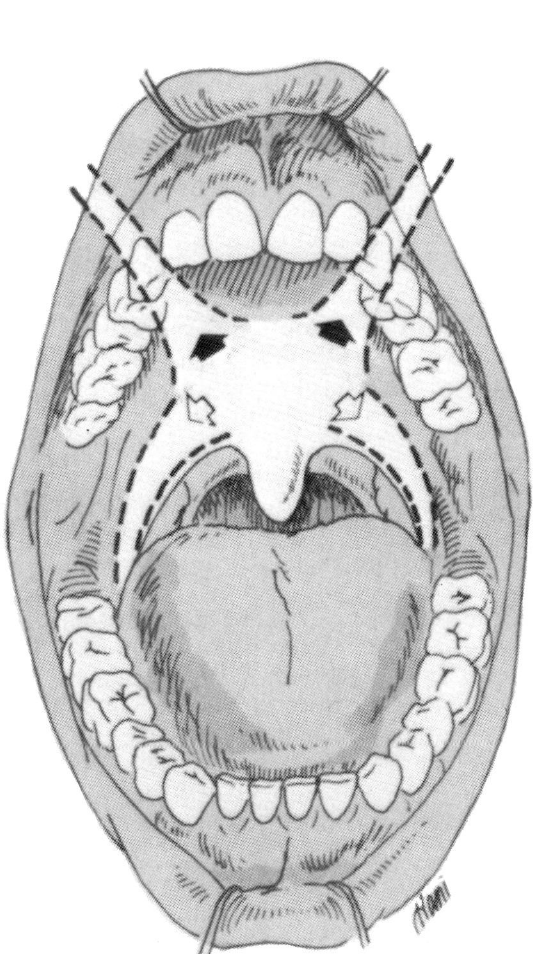

Figure 47-8 Semidiagrammatic representation of the relative orientation of the palatoglossi and levatores palati when viewed from the front.

Figure 47-9 Muscles of the velopharynx, viewed from behind. (1) Levator palati; (2) palatothyroideus; (3) musculi uvulae; (4) palatopharyngeus; (5) torus tubarius; (6) salpingopalatine fold; (7) salpingopharyngeus; (8) pharyngobasilar fascia; (9) nasal conchae.

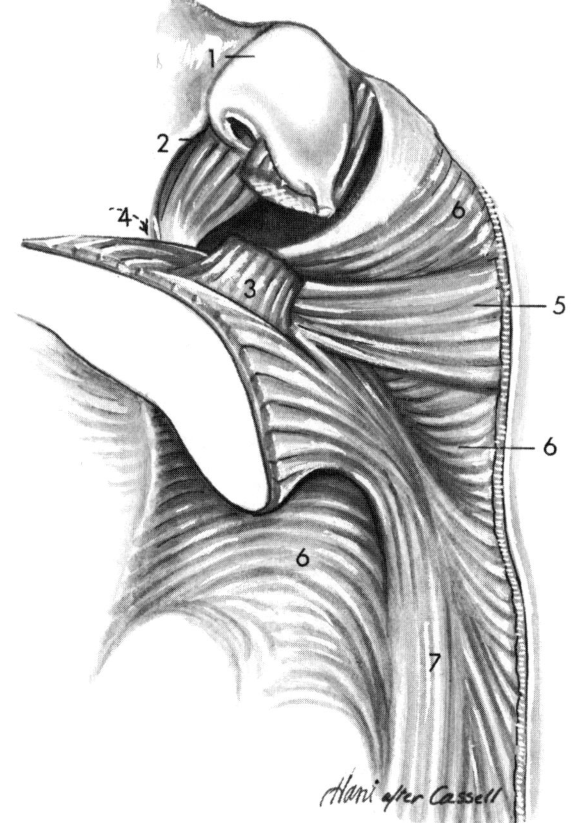

Figure 47-10 Oblique view of the velopharyngeal musculature in the region of the auditory tube. (1) Auditory tube; (2) tensor palati; (3) levator palati; (4) pterygoid hamulus; (5) palatopharyngeus; (6) superior constrictor; (7) palatothyroideus.

study of the inferior attachments of the palatothyroideus is warranted.

The best modern descriptions of the palatopharyngeus muscle are those given by Whillis,[17] Harrington,[19] and Dickson and Dickson.[20] The palatopharyngeus is a thin triangular lamina of muscle fibers running horizontally from the posterolateral surface of the palate to the pharyngeal raphe (Fig. 47–10). Laterally, the palatopharyngeus is related to the medial pterygoid plate anteriorly and to the pterygoid hamulus, the pharyngobasilar fascia, and the internal fibrous layer overlying the superior constrictor. Medially, the palatopharyngeus is related to the salpingopharyngeus, the anterolateral fasciculus of the palatothyroideus and the levator palati (Fig. 47–10). The palatal attachment of the palatopharyngeus extends to the superior surface of the palatine aponeurosis,[17] although the position of this attachment varies.[20] In six dissections of fetal heads, Dickson and Dickson reported that the palatopharyngeus was attached posterior to the levator palati (one case), anterolateral to the levator palati (three cases), and to both sides of the levator palati (two cases).[20] Some of the fibers of the palatopharyngeus appear to penetrate the insertion of the levator palati.

The posterior attachments of the palatopharyngeus were not described in detail by either Whillis,[17] Harrington,[19] or Dickson and Dickson.[20] Presumably, the posterior fibers of this muscle eventually attach to the pharyngeal raphe, as is the case in other mammals.[1, 14] It should be noted, however, that both Whillis and Dickson and Dickson consider the palatopharyngeal fibers that they describe to be part of the superior constrictor, and Harrington considers them part of his "m. pterygopharyngeus." This is despite the fact that both the palatopharyngeus and the superior constrictor are separated by the pharyngobasilar fascia and a branch of the ascending palatine artery and despite the statement by Whillis that the palatopharyngeal fibers are "on the same plane relative to the pharyngeal constrictors as the pharyngopalatinus (i.e., palatothyroideus)".[17]

The palatopharyngeus muscles are reportedly responsible for the production of the pharyngeal ridge (of Passavant) in the pharyngeal mucosa.[17, 20]

Salpingopharyngeus. The salpingopharyngeus is a variable fasciculus of muscle fibers running from the posterior surface of the cartilage of the auditory tube to the larynx and inferior pharynx (Fig. 47–11). When present, the salpingopharyngeus consists of between one and five fascicles covered by connective and glandular tissue.[20–22] This connective and glandular tissue appears to form the bulk of the salpingopharyngeal fold.[20] According to Bosma,[22] the salpingopharyngeus has a fan-shaped attachment to the length of the posterior lamina of the tubal cartilage, including the torus tubarius (Fig. 47–11). Both McMyn[21] and Harrington[19] report a variety of contributions from the palatopharyngeus and palatothyroideus. The fasciculi of the salpingopharyngeus descend

on the lateral wall of the pharynx, blending with the fibers of the palatothyroideus and stylopharyngeus to attach to the larynx and pharynx. Dickson and Dickson[20] make the interesting assertion that the muscle fibers of the salpingopharyngeus "arise" from the palatothyroideus muscle.

Musculi Uvulae. The musculi uvulae are two muscle masses on either side of the midline of the soft palate running in an anteroposterior direction. Although the old description of these muscles as a single muscle (that is, azygos musculus uvulae) is not generally accepted,[23] it appears in the adult that little if any nonmuscular tissue separates the muscles on either side.[18] The musculi uvulae follow a flattened S-shaped course over the nasal surface of the soft palate (Fig. 47–12). The "bellies" of the muscles overlie the muscular sling of the levator palati.[18, 23, 24] Anteriorly, the musculi uvulae originate from the palatine aponeurosis behind the posterior border of the hard palate but not from the hard palate itself.[18] There appears to be no evidence for the common assertion that the musculi uvulae arise from the posterior nasal spine (Fig. 47–12).[7] Anteriorly, the palatine aponeurosis, with some fibers of the palatothyroideus, overlies the musculi uvulae, and some muscle fibers of the musculi uvulae originate from the inferior surface of the palatine aponeurosis. Langdon and Klueber reported the variable appearance of transversely running muscle fibers in the anterior soft palate that turn posteriorly to join the musculi uvulae.[18] These authors also reported a "recurrent" bundle of muscle fibers that arise from the underside of the palatine aponeurosis, pass inferiorly, and curve up to enter the ventral (oral) surface of the musculi uvulae. The musculi uvulae pass over the levator sling but are separated from that muscle mass by a plane of connective tissue.[24] The musculi uvulae taper as they enter the uvula to terminate among palatal glandular tissue and fibers of the palatine raphe.[18] In its posterior part, muscle fibers of the palatoglossus

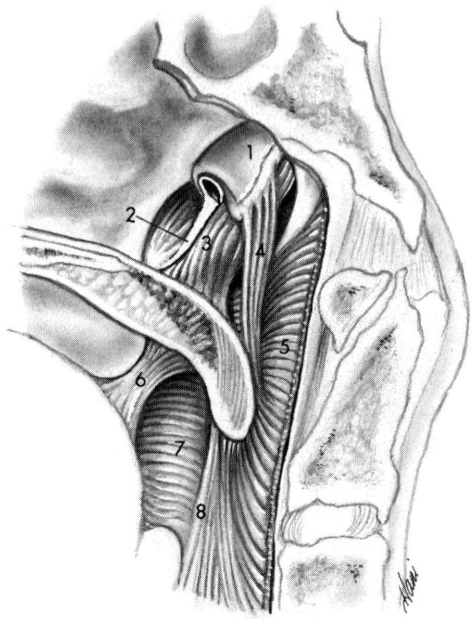

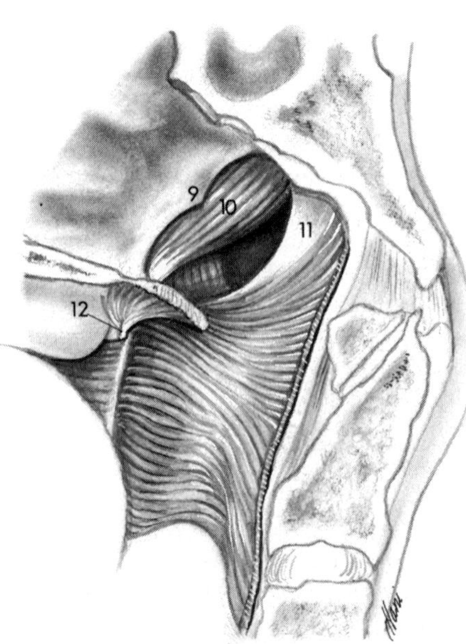

Figure 47–11 Lateral view of velopharyngeal musculature showing the origin and relationships of the salpingopharyngeus. On the right, the auditory tube and most of the velopharyngeal musculature have been removed to expose the tensor palati. (1) Tubal cartilage; (2) salpingopharyngeal fascia (of Troltsch); (3) levator palati; (4) salpingopharyngeus; (5) palatopharyngeus; (6) palatoglossus; (7) superior constrictor; (8) palatothyroideus; (9) processus tubarius on medial pterygoid plate; (10) tensor palati; (11) pharyngobasilar fascia; (12) pterygoid hamulus.

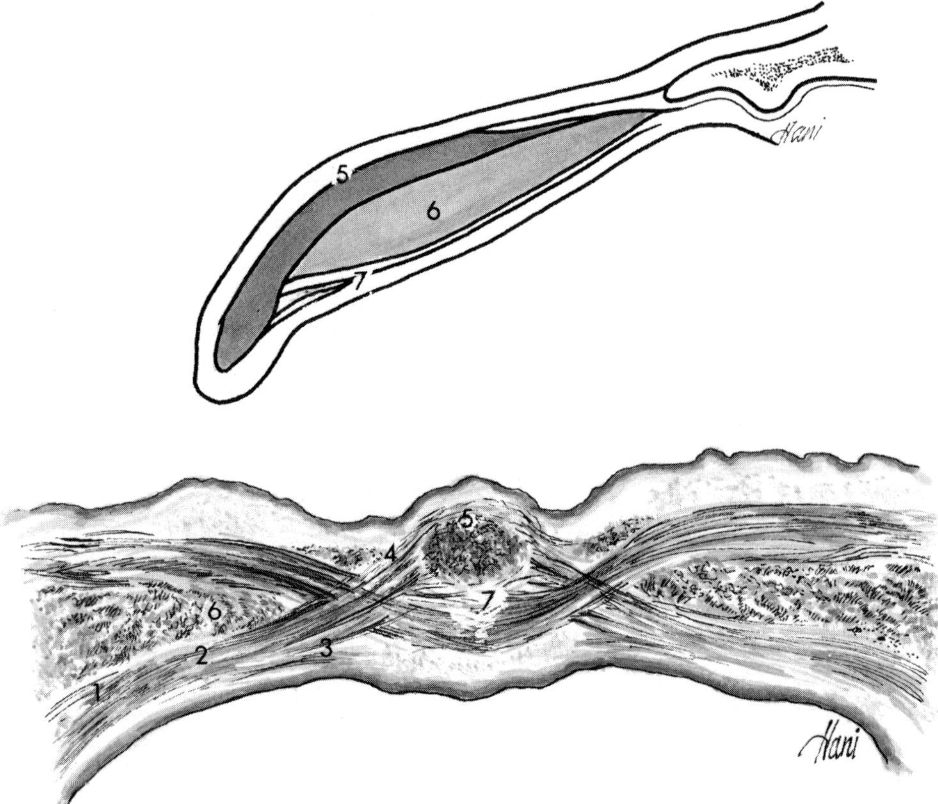

Figure 47–12 Longitudinal (schematic) and coronal sections through the soft palate showing the course and relationships of the musculi uvulae. (1) Palatoglossus; (2) fibers of palatoglossus entering transverse musculature of soft palate; (3) inferior bundle of palatoglossus; (4) superior bundle of palatoglossus; (5) musculi uvulae; (6) transverse musculature (levator palati) of soft palate; (7) palatine raphe.

and palatothyroideus pass over and into the musculi uvulae.[18] These fibers may be important in attaching the musculi uvulae to the more flexible posterior part of the soft palate.[25]

Superior Constrictor. The superior constrictor muscle has been included here although its role in velopharyngeal physiology is debatable. The superior constrictor arises from a series of bony and fibrous attachments extending from the pterygoid hamulus to the posterior tongue (Fig. 47–13). Superiorly, the superior constrictor arises from the lateral surface of the pterygoid hamulus (Fig. 47–5) and rarely, the adjacent part of the medial pterygoid plate.[19] Below the hamulus, the fibers of the superior constrictor intermingle and are continuous with the whole posterior margin of the buccinator down to the retromolar trigone. However, the existence of a

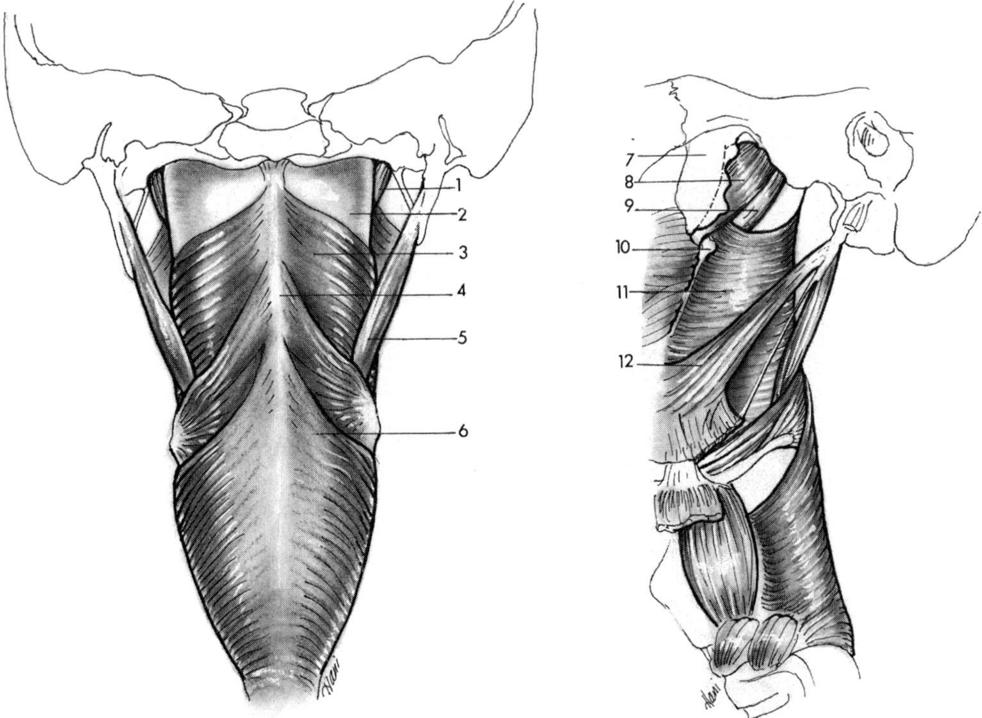

Figure 47–13 Posterior (left) and lateral (right) views of the pharyngeal constrictors and associated muscles. (1) Levator palati; (2) pharyngobasilar fascia; (3) superior constrictor; (4) insertion of middle constrictor on pharyngeal raphe; (5) stylopharyngeus; (6) inferior constrictor; (7) lateral pterygoid plate; (8) tensor palati; (9) levator palati; (10) pterygoid hamulus; (11) superior constrictor; (12) styloglossus.

grossly identifiable, tendinous intersection between the buccinator and the superior constrictor—the pterygomandibular raphe—has been categorically denied.[26] Inferiorly, the superior constrictor is attached to the posterior end of the mylohyoid line and to fibrous tissue on the posterolateral aspect of the tongue.[19] The fibers of the superior constrictor pass upward and posteriorly to insert into the pharyngeal raphe (Fig. 47–13). Rarely, the upper fibers of the superior constrictor attach to the basilar part of the occipital bone (M. D. Cassell, unpublished observations, 1988). Externally, the lower half to two-thirds of the superior constrictor is overlapped by fibers of the middle constrictor (Fig. 47–13).

Levator Palati (Levator Veli Palatini). The levatores palati muscles descend from the base of the skull to insert into the nasal surface of the soft palate (Figs. 47–9 and 47–14). The origin of the levator palati appears to be only slightly variable, even in persons with cleft palate.[8] The levator palati arises by a small tendon from the inferior surface of the petrous part of the temporal bone, anterior to the entrance to the carotid canal (Fig. 47–5), from the fascia forming the upper part of the carotid sheath, and by a few fascicles arising from the inferior surface of the adjacent tubal cartilage.[21, 27] The fibers of the levator palati pass downward, forward, and medially along the inferior border of the tubal cartilage. The salpingopharyngeal fascia (fascia of Tröltsch) that forms a section of the membranous part of the auditory tube (Fig. 47–11) and continues onto the soft palate reportedly forms a "gliding plane" between the tubal cartilage and the levator palati.[8]

The insertion of the levatores palati into the palate is complex and may relate to the different orientation of fiber groups within the muscles themselves.[27, 28] According to Ruding's illustrations, the anterior fibers of the levator palati insert into the palatine aponeurosis on its oral surface.[28] Consistent with this, a recent report denied the existence of *any* muscular insertions into the nasal surface of the aponeurosis.[29] Kriens, quoting earlier reports, referred to a small anterior bundle of levator fibers arising from the tubal cartilage and inserting into the palatine aponeurosis.[8] The bulk of the posteromedial fibers of the levator palati pass medially beneath the musculi uvulae to merge with the fibers of the contralateral muscle. The resulting "levator sling" occupies the intermediate 40% of the soft palate.[29] The muscle fibers of the levator palati intermingle with fibers of the palatopharyngeus, palatothyroideus, and palatoglossus. Posterior to the main mass of the "sling," the intermingling of the levator and palatopharyngeus fibers is related to the palatal "dimple."[29] Some posterior fibers of the levator palati reportedly pass into the uvula,[28] although this has been denied.[29]

Tensor Palati (Tensor Veli Palatini) and the Palatine Aponeurosis. Recent studies indicate that the tensor palati acts largely in association with the tensor tympani in facilitating aeration of the middle ear.[30, 31] Although the involvement of the tensor palati in velopharyngeal function is probably minimal, its contribution to the palatine aponeurosis and proximity to the velopharyngeal musculature justifies a description here.

Superiorly, the bony attachments of the tensor palati include the lateral part of the medial pterygoid plate, the roof of the pterygoid fossa, the scaphoid fossa, and the spine of the sphenoid (Fig. 47–5). The bulk of the muscle (75% to 80%) is attached to the lateral hook of the tubal cartilage and the fibrous tissue forming the membranous portion of the auditory tube.[32] The fibers of the tensor palati pass vertically or obliquely downward (Fig. 47–14), depending on their origin, converging into a broad, flat tendon that passes around the pterygoid hamulus. Most anatomic texts refer to the presence of a bursa between the tendon of the tensor palati and the hamulus. However, Ross failed to find a bursa in 32 gross dissections or in microscopic examination of eight hamuli.[32]

The attachments of the tensor palati tendon to the palate and adjacent structures are complex. The anterolateral fibers of the tendon attach continuously to the tuberosity and alveolar process of the maxilla and the posterior border of the hard palate as far anteriorly as the palatine crest and as far medially as the posterior nasal spine.[8, 21, 28, 32] An attachment to the pterygoid hamulus, which is present consistently in most mammals,[33] is found inconsistently in man,[21, 32] and is considered to be of little functional importance.[32] A "vertical" aponeurosis, arising from the tubal fibers of the tensor palati *before* they pass around the hamulus, has been reported to insert into the buccopharyngeal fascia overlying the buccinator.[8] The majority of the fibers of the tensor palati tendon attach to the palatine aponeurosis, merging with fibers of the contralateral muscle (Fig. 47–14). Ross reports that the outer fibers of the tensor palati give rise to fibers that pass into the superficial fascia on the oral surface of the soft palate.[32] This observation may account for some statements that the palatine aponeurosis "splits" into two laminae that surround the musculi uvulae.[17]

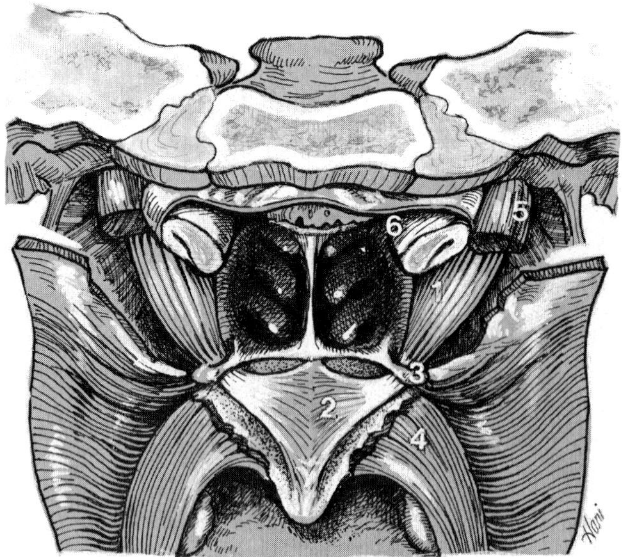

Figure 47–14 Posterior view of velopharyngeal musculature following removal of levator palati and musculi uvulae. (1) Tensor palati; (2) tensor aponeurosis; (3) pterygoid hamulus; (4) palatothyroideus; (5) levator palati (cut); (6) tubal cartilage and pharyngobasilar fascia.

Physiology of the Velopharynx

Primary velopharyngeal movements can be divided roughly into two groups: (1) movements of the velum toward the posterior pharyngeal wall, and (2) mesial movements of the lateral pharyngeal walls. Anterior movements of the posterior pharyngeal wall and bulging of the nasal surface of the velum are also often considered when discussing velopharyngeal function. Numerous techniques, including ultrasound, cineradiography, endoscopy, and observation of anatomic relationships have been employed to study the contributions of velopharyngeal muscles to these movements.[34] However, the majority of these reports utilized electromyography (EMG) to relate muscle activity to velopharyngeal movement patterns. Although it might seem intuitively attractive to relate muscle activity directly to movement of structures, interpretation of such data must be made with some caution. Although a discussion of EMG methodology is beyond the scope of this chaper, the reader is referred to Kuehn et al for an excellent review.[35]

Velar Elevation

During breathing at rest and nasal sound production, the velum is maintained in a lower position to allow for the movement of air between the oral and nasal cavities. During attempts to produce oral speech sounds, the normally functioning velum moves posteriorly and superiorly to contact the posterior pharyngeal wall. The elevated velum is typically highest at its middle segment, whereas contact against the posterior pharyngeal wall is accomplished in its third quadrant.[36] Velar height and displacement will, of course, vary during connected speech as a function of phonetic context.

It is generally well accepted that the muscle primarily responsible for velar elevation is the levator palati (Fig. 47–9). Recording speech from 26 subjects, Fritzell observed a close relationship between levator muscle activity and the production of oral speech sounds.[37, 38] Specifically, contraction of this muscle moved the midportion of the velum upward and backward. These observations have been supported by numerous investigators.[20, 39–41]

An additional observation made by Fritzell[37, 38] and Bell-Berti[40] was a positive relationship between the extent of velar elevation and the magnitude of levator EMG activity. However, correlations reported by Fritzell[37] ranged from 0.46 to 0.94. He suggested that the superior constrictor, palatopharyngeus (palatothyroideus), and palatoglossus muscles may influence velar elevation in some subjects. The suggestion was supported and expanded on by Kuehn et al.[35] These investigators recorded EMG activity from the levator palati, palatoglossus, palatopharyngeus (palatothyroideus), and superior constrictor muscles and related measured activity to velar position as observed on lateral x-rays. In contrast to previous reports, they found that "levels of levator muscle activity independent of other muscle activity were not directly related to velar position."[35]

Kuehn et al did find a systematic interaction among levator palati, palatoglossus, and palatopharyngeus muscle activity. They posited that a trading relationship exists among these three muscles in positioning the velum. That is, velar elevation resulting from levator muscle activity could be offset or attenuated by activity in the palatoglossus or palatopharyngeus. Therefore, various combinations of activity in these three muscles may give rise to the same velar position. Superior constrictor muscle activity was recorded for each speech sound measured in the Kuehn et al study, although inconsistently. They concluded that its participation in velar elevation was questionable.[35]

Velar Lowering

Given that levator muscle activity results in movement of the velum toward a closed position, it would seem logical to assume that velar lowering would involve a cessation, or at least a reduced level, of levator muscle activity. This pattern has, in fact, been observed by all investigators studying velar movement.[37–40] There is, however, some disagreement about the precise mechanism involved in lowering the velum. In her study of three subjects, Bell-Berti suggested that in addition to cessation of levator activity, velar lowering was accomplished by "the natural tendency of tissue to return to its rest position, and not from increased activity in any muscle."[40] This possibility is supported by the observation of elastic fibers in the anterior faucial pillars.[9]

An alternative explanation for velar lowering involves muscle activity. Historically, increased activity in two muscles has been associated with velar lowering. Westlake and Rutherford suggested that the tensor palati (Fig. 47–14) is favorably situated to pull the palate down and forward.[42] More recent study, however, has cast doubt on the role of the tensor palati during speech production. Fritzell found that the tensor was consistently active during swallowing and chewing only.[37] During speech, the muscle was typically inactive, and when active it bore no relationship to speech. Tensor palati activity does appear to be related to respiration. Hairston and Sauerland found that the tensor was activated during the inspiratory phase, tensing the palate and providing an unimpeded airway.[43]

The second muscle thought by some to contribute to velar lowering is the palatoglossus (Fig. 47–8). Anatomically, the palatoglossus is in a position to lower the palate.[9] Fritzell[37] and Lubker et al[39] found the palatoglossus to be active during palate lowering. Fritzell asserted that opening involves more than simple gravitational forces following cessation of levator palati activity. He suggested that the palatoglossus pulls the palate down for nasal sound production and at the end of phonation. Fritzell also noted a small amount of activity at the onset of phonation, presumably as a part of some preparatory soft palate positioning movement. In contrast, Bell-Berti found that the palatoglossus was active for tongue movement and palatal narrowing but not for palatal lowering.[40] She did, however, report that an additional subject not included in the original report showed palatoglossus activity during the production of nasal consonants. On the basis of anatomic evidence, Kuehn and Azzam supported the role of the palatoglossus in palate lowering.[9] Following dissection of 25 cadaver heads, Kuehn and Azzam suggested that the palatoglossus had a favorable mechanical ability to lower the velum. This view of palatoglossus function fits the concept of coordinated or interrelated palatoglossus, palatopharyngeus, and levator activity proposed by Kuehn et al and reviewed earlier.[35]

Lateral Pharyngeal Walls

It is well established that mesial movement of the lateral pharyngeal walls contributes to velopharyngeal closure. Much less established is a description of how this is accomplished. Early reports attributed lateral pharyngeal wall movement to the salpingopharyngeus muscle.[44] However, its contribution to such movement has since been discounted.[20] Current explanations for lateral pharyngeal wall movement center on two muscles, the levator palati and the superior constrictor.

On the basis of anatomic dissection, Dickson and Dickson proposed that lateral pharyngeal wall movement consisted of inward deflection of the torus tubarius.[20] Given the relative positions of the levator palati and the torus tubarius (Figs. 47–9 and 47–11), they concluded that levator muscle activity was responsible for both velar and lateral pharyngeal wall movement. Support for this theory was provided by Honjo et al,[45] Niimi et al,[34] and Isshiki et al.[46] Honjo et al observed three adult patients with facial defects that allowed direct visualization of their velopharyngeal mechanism.[45] Three major observations were made from these views and additional radiographic and anatomic investigations. First, lateral pharyngeal wall movement appeared to occur most prominently at the torus tubarius. Second, lateral pharyngeal wall motion coincided well with soft palate motion, implying that the same muscle was involved in both movements. Further, they suggested that the amount of lateral pharyngeal wall movement was directly related to the extent of velar elevation. Finally, the relationship of the levator musculature to the torus tubarius placed it in a favorable position to draw the torus inward during contraction. Niimi et al recorded EMG information from the levator and superior constrictor musculature and concluded that the levator was responsible for lateral pharyngeal wall motion.[34] Isshiki et al anesthetized the levator musculature unilaterally and observed the consequences on velar and lateral pharyngeal wall movement.[46] On the anesthetized side, velar elevation was insufficient compared to the control side. Further, lateral pharyngeal wall motion was nonevident on the anesthetized side. Although cautioning that they could not confirm the injected site of the anesthesia, Isshiki et al did conclude that the levator was most likely responsible for mesial movement of the lateral pharyngeal wall.[46]

An alternative explanation is that the superior constrictor muscle (Fig. 47–12) is responsible for lateral pharyngeal wall motion. Using videofluoroscopy, Skolnick,[47, 48] Skolnick et al,[49] and Shprintzen et al[50] observed

that maximal mesial movements of the lateral pharyngeal wall occurred well below the velar eminence. These findings were supported by Iglesias et al,[51] who observed maximal excursions at or just below the level of the hard palate. These data conflict with the notion proposed by Honjo et al[45] and Dickson and Dickson[20] that maximal excursions occurred at the torus tubarius. Iglesias et al suggest that methodological problems with the Honjo et al study might have led to misinterpretation of their radiographic images.[51]

Skolnick et al suggested that the levator cannot be involved because maximal lateral pharyngeal wall movement occurs below the level of the torus tubarius.[49] Conversely, proponents of the levator muscle argue that the superior constrictor cannot be involved because lateral pharyngeal wall movement occurs too high in the pharynx. Dickson and Dickson argued that there are no superior constrictor fibers above the level of the hard palate.[20] However, the role of the horizontal fibers of the palatopharyngeus (Fig. 47–10) in lateral pharyngeal movement has not been addressed in the current literature. It is evident that a firm understanding of the relative contributions of the levator palati and superior constrictor muscles to movement of the lateral pharyngeal walls does not yet exist.

Posterior Pharyngeal Wall

In the mid-1800s, Passavant described a bulging forward of the posterior pharyngeal wall in a cleft palate subject.[13] Passavant's ridge has since been reported in normal subjects as well.[15, 52] Delineation of the exact mechanism by which this ridge is formed is not clear. Glasner postulated that some active process may increase tension on the musculature comprising Passavant's ridge, causing the ridge to appear.[53] Dickson and Dickson[20] and McWilliams et al[54] suggested that the superior constrictor may contribute to the ridge, although the horizontal fibers of the palatopharyngeus have also been implicated.[17] McWilliams et al suggested that Passavant's ridge does contribute to velopharyngeal closure in some patients who demonstrated the ridge.[54] This is especially true in patients with repaired palatal clefts. However, others have concluded that in normal speakers the observed magnitude of anterior movements of the posterior pharyngeal wall is probably not significant in the production of speech.[55, 56]

Velar Bulging

Until recently, much less attention has been focused on the musculi uvulae relative to the other velopharyngeal muscles. Kuehn et al referred to historical notions that contraction of the musculi uvulae (Figs. 47–4, 47–6, and 47–13) shortens the velum, an action that might oppose velopharyngeal closing movements.[57] Azzam and Kuehn proposed that the musculi uvulae contribute to the convexity of the nasal surface of the soft palate.[23] They concluded that the primary role of these muscles was to "add bulk to the dorsal surface of the soft palate, which would aid in occlusion of the velopharyngeal port during speech and deglutition." In contrast, Boorman and Sommerlad suggested that musculi uvulae activity is not essential for normal speech produced by noncleft speakers.[24] Their conclusions were based on two observations. In fresh cadavers, traction applied bilaterally to the levator palati muscles with no manipulation of the musculi uvulae produced the nasal convexity of the soft palate. Second, anesthesia of the musculi uvulae produced no visible alteration in the nasal convexity or ridging of the palate and no perceptive changes in speech output.

In an attempt to elucidate further a possible role for the musculi uvulae during speech production, Kuehn et al recorded EMG data from the levator palati and musculi uvulae during a series of speech and nonspeech tasks.[57] Two possible roles for the musculi uvulae were proposed: a stiffness-modifying mechanism and a velar extensor mechanism.

As a stiffness-modifying mechanism, the musculi uvulae would act to control the velar-distorting forces of the levator palati muscle. That is, levator contraction in association with compliant musculi uvulae might result in distortion of the velum by stretching the top layer upward instead of moving the entire velum. The velum must be stiff enough to avoid such distortion but at the same time have enough compliance to allow it to stretch in reaching the posterior pharyngeal wall.

As a velar extensor, the musculi uvulae might act as either a flexible beam or a pulling force about a boundary. The curved beam model is based on the fact that the musculi uvulae lie in the top half of the curved velum and are attached anteriorly to the palatal aponeurosis (Figs. 47–4 and 47–13). On contraction, a compressional force is exerted along the nasal side of the velum. Because the oral side of the velum is relatively compliant, the compressional force would act to straighten the curved velum and extend it posteriorly. The pulling force model is based on the fact that the musculi uvulae extend across the dorsal aspect of the "levator sling." The sling acts as a boundary around which the musculi uvulae can exert a force, thereby extending the velum posteriorly.

Conclusion

In the present chapter we have attempted to provide a broad overview of the normal anatomy and physiology of the velopharynx. In doing so, we have gone against the trend seen in most modern anatomy texts by not treating the soft palate and superior pharynx as separate, distinct structures. This approach is embodied in our use of the term *velopharynx,* a term rarely used in anatomy texts. It is evident, however, that much remains to be learned concerning the normal velopharynx. It is a pity that the challenges put foward by Dickson and Dickson[20] in their earlier review of velopharyngeal anatomy and physiology remain largely unanswered.

References

1. Jones FW: The nature of the soft palate. J Anat 74:147, 1940.
2. Calnan J: Movements of the soft palate. Br J Plast Surg 5:286, 1955.
3. Leela K, Kanagasuntheram R, Khoo FY: Morphology of the primate nasopharynx. J Anat 117:333, 1974.
4. Cave AJE: The epipharynx. J Laryngol Otol 74:713, 1960.
5. Negus VE: Comments on the term epipharynx. J Laryngol Otol 75:828, 1961.
6. Ali MY: Histology of the human nasopharyngeal mucosa. J Anat 99:657, 1965.
7. Warwick R, Williams PL (eds): Gray's Anatomy, 36th ed. Philadelphia: Saunders, 1975.
8. Kriens O: Anatomy of the velopharyngeal area in cleft palate. Clin Plast Surg 2:261, 1975.
9. Kuehn D, Azzam N: Anatomical characteristics of palatoglossus and the anterior faucial pillar. Cleft Palate J 15:349, 1978.
10. Langdon HL, Klueber KM, Barnwell YM: The morphology of m. palatoglossus in the 15-week human foetus. Anat Anz 146:12, 1979.
11. Winslow JB: Anatomical Exposition of the Structure of the Human Body. Philadelphia: 1733.
12. Luschka HV: Der schlund Kopf des Menschen. Tübingen: M. Lauppische Buchhandlung, 1868.
13. Passavant G: Ueber die Verschliessung des Schlundes beim Sprechen. Virchow's Archiv Path Anat Physiol Klin Med 46:1, 1869.
14. Ruckert J: Der Pharynx als Sprache- und Schluckapparat. Munich: Th. Riedel, 1882.
15. Calnan J: Modern views on Passavant's ridge. Br J Plast Surg 10:89, 1957.
16. Sicher H: Oral Anatomy. St. Louis: C V Mosby, 1975.
17. Whillis J: A note on the muscles of the palate and superior constrictor. J Anat 65:92, 1930.
18. Langdon HL, Klueber DM: The longitudinal fibromuscular component of the soft palate in the 15-week human foetus; musculus uvulae and palatine raphe. Cleft Palate J 14:337, 1978.
19. Harrington R: M. pterygopharyngeus and its relation to m. palatopharyngeus. Laryngoscope 55:499, 1945.
20. Dickson D, Dickson W: Velopharyngeal anatomy. J Speech Hear Res 15:372, 1972.
21. McMyn JK: The anatomy of the salpingopharyngeus muscle. J Laryngol Otol 55:1, 1940.
22. Bosma JF: A correlated study of the anatomy and motor activity of the upper pharynx by cadaver dissection and by cinematic study of patients after maxillo-facial surgery. Ann Otol 62:51, 1953.
23. Azzam N, Kuehn D: The morphology of musculus uvulae. Cleft Palate J 14:78, 1977.
24. Boorman J, Sommerlad B: Musculus uvulae and levator palatini: Theoretical, anatomical and functional relationship in velopharyngeal closure. Br J Plast Surg 38:33, 1985.
25. Voth D: Zur functionellen Morphologie des Menschlichen Gaumens. Anat Anz 110:165, 1961.
26. Gaughran GRL: The pterygomandibular raphe—anatomical artifact. Anat Rec 184:410a, 1976.
27. Rohan RF, Turner L: The levator palati muscle. J Anat 90:153, 1956.
28. Ruding R: Cleft palate. Anatomic and surgical considerations. Plast Reconstr Surg 33:132, 1964.
29. Boorman JG, Sommerlad BC: Levator palati and palatal dimples: Their anatomy, relationship and clinical significance. Br J Plast Surg 38:326, 1985.
30. Kamerer DB, Rood SR: The tensor tympani, stapedius and tensor veli palatini muscles—an electromyographic study. Otorhinolaryngol 86:416, 1979.
31. Doyle WJ, Rood SR: Comparison of the anatomy of the Eustachian tube in the rhesus monkey (*Macaca mulatta*) and man: Implications for physiological modeling. Ann Otol 89:49, 1980.
32. Ross MA: Functional anatomy of the tensor palati. Arch Otolaryngol 93:1, 1971.
33. Himmerleich HA: M. tensor veli palatini der Saugeteire unter Berucksichtigung seines Aufbas, seiner Funktion und seiner Entstehungsgeschichte. Anat Anz 115:1, 1964.
34. Niimi S, Bell-Berti F, Harris K: Dynamic aspects of velopharyngeal closure. Folia Phoniat 34:246, 1982.
35. Kuehn D, Folkins J, Cutting C: Relationships between muscle activity and velar position. Cleft Palate J 19:25, 1982.
36. Bzoch K, Graber T, Aoba T: A study of normal velopharyngeal valving for speech. Cleft Palate Bull 9:3, 1959.
37. Fritzell B: The velopharyngeal muscles in speech. Acta Otolaryngol, Suppl 250, 1969.
38. Fritzell B: Electromyography in the study of the velopharyngeal function—a review. Folia Phoniat 31:93, 1979.
39. Lubker J, Fritzell B, Lindqvist J: Velopharyngeal function: An electromyographic study. Q Prog Stat Resp-Speech Trans Lab (Stockholm) 4:9, 1970.
40. Bell-Berti F: An electromyographic study of velopharyngeal function in speech. J Speech Hear Res 19:225, 1976.
41. Kuehn D: Velopharyngeal anatomy and physiology. Ear Nose Throat J 58:316, 1979.
42. Westlake H, Rutherford D: Cleft Palate. Englewood Cliffs: Prentice-Hall, 1966.
43. Hairston L, Sauerland E: Electromyography of the human palate: Discharge patterns of the levator and tensor veli palatini. Electromyog Clin Neurophysiol 21:287, 1981.
44. Harrington R: A study of the mechanism of velopharyngeal closure. J Speech Hear Dis 9:325, 1944.

45. Honjo I, Harada H, Kumazasa T: Role of the levator veli palatini muscle in movement of the lateral pharyngeal wall. Arch Oto Rhinol Laryngol 212:93, 1976.
46. Isshiki N, Harita Y, Kawano M: What muscle is responsible for lateral pharyngeal wall movement? Ann Plast Surg 14:224, 1985.
47. Skolnick L: Video velopharyngography in patients with nasal speech, with emphasis on lateral pharyngeal motion in velopharyngeal closure. Radiology 93:747, 1969.
48. Skolnick L: Videofluoroscopic examination of the velopharyngeal portal during phonation in lateral and base projections—a new technique for studying the mechanics of closure. Cleft Palate J 7:803, 1970.
49. Skolnick L, McCall G, Barnes M: The sphincteric mechanism of velopharyngeal closure. Cleft Palate J 7:803, 1970.
50. Shprintzen R, McCall G, Skolnick L, et al: Selective movement of the lateral aspects of the pharyngeal walls during velopharyngeal closure for speech, blowing and whistling in normals. Cleft Palate J 12:51, 1975.
51. Iglesias A, Kuehn D, Morris H: Simultaneous assessment of pharyngeal wall and velar displacement for selected speech sounds. J Speech Hear Res 23:429, 1980.
52. Fletcher S: A cinefluoroscopic study of the posterior wall of the pharynx during speech and deglutition. Masters thesis, University of Utah, Salt Lake City, 1957.
53. Glasner E, Skolnick L, McWilliams B, et al: The dynamics of Passavant's ridge in subjects with and without velopharyngeal insufficiency— a multiview videofluoroscopic study. Cleft Palate J 16:24, 1979.
54. McWilliams B, Morris H, Shelton R: Cleft Palate Speech. Philadelphia: B. C. Decker, 1984.
55. Hagerty R, Hill M, Pettit H, et al: Posterior pharyngeal wall movement in normals. J Speech Hear Res 1:203, 1958.
56. Hagerty R, Hill M: Pharyngeal wall and palatal movement in postoperative cleft palates and normal palates. J Speech Hear Res 3:59, 1960.
57. Kuehn D, Folkins J, Linville R: An electromyographic study of the musculus uvulae. Cleft Palate J 25:348, 1988.

CHAPTER 48

The Dynamic Muscle Sphincter of the Pharynx

Miguel Orticochea

Program of Surgical Treatment for the Cleft Patient

In our program of surgical treatment for children with cleft lip and palate, three basic procedures are planned.
1. The lip cleft is repaired at 3 months of age.[1]
2. The hard and soft palates are closed at the age of 2 years by means of a minimal palatorrhaphy to allow maximum mobility of the repaired soft palate. We never lengthen or push back the soft palate.
3. The velopharyngeal incompetence that remains in the great majority of patients after this minimal palatorrhaphy is corrected 6 months later at the age of 2½ years by construction of a dynamic muscle sphincter in the oral pharynx behind and below the palate.[2, 3]

When properly constructed in a child of 2½ to 5 years of age, the sphincter closes to a pinpoint by simultaneous contractions of its four walls: the soft palate moves upward and backward, the lateral walls formed by the palatopharyngeus muscles move toward the midline, and the circular or angular posterior border formed by the union of the posterior tonsillar pillars with the posterior pharyngeal flap moves upward and slightly forward (Fig. 48–1). There is no loss of the contractile activity of the pharyngeal muscles, and the sphincter regulates the amount of air that passes into the nasopharynx and nasal cavities during speech in a reflexive or automatic manner.

In older patients, particularly those with a fibrous, rigid short palate secondary to traumatic cleft palate surgery, the sphincter is triangular in shape, the walls are less flexible (particularly the anterior and posterior walls), and closure occurs only through approximation of the transplanted posterior pillars. The triangular-shaped lumen of the sphincter becomes an anteroposterior slit (Fig. 48–2).

Whatever the sphincter's mechanism for closure, its muscular contraction exerts a recurrent centripetal force toward the midline on the oral and nasal mucosa of the transplanted posterior pillars and on the scar tissue that occludes the lateral oronasal passages. This force gradually stretches these structures and increases their size until they become a *true membrane or diaphragm with a central sphincteric orifice* (Figs. 48–3 and 48–4). This is a new anatomic structure that is totally different from the three original passages or orifices created by the surgeon during the operation (Fig. 48–5).

All patients born with a cleft palate undergo an operation to create a dynamic muscle sphincter of the pharynx at the age of 2½. Fig. 48–6 shows that velopharyngeal incompetence at that age is minimal. It is my opinion that it is preferable to create the dynamic muscle sphincter of the pharynx at an early age in an operation that lasts only 20 minutes than to wait until the patient is older and has gone through years of speech therapy and sometimes even psychiatric treatment.

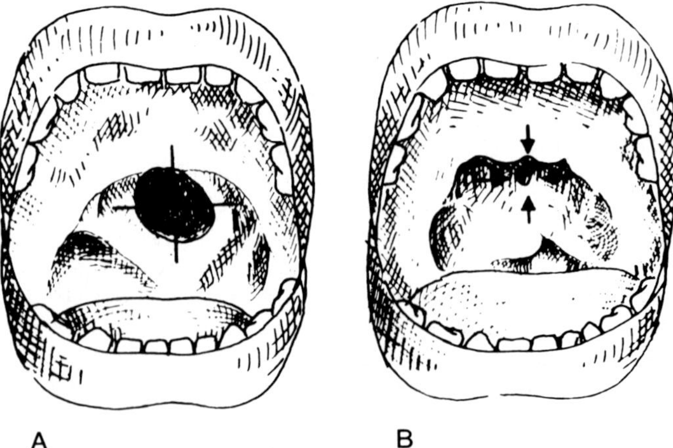

A   B

Figure 48–1 *A*, Open sphincter. *B*, Closed sphincter. The four walls of the sphincter contract concentrically. (From Orticochea M: A review of 236 cleft palate patients treated with dynamic muscle sphincter. Plast Reconstr Surg 71:183, 1983. With permission.)

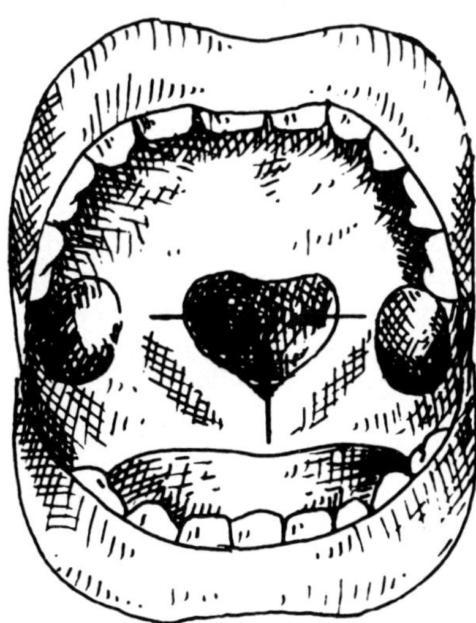

Figure 48–2 The dynamic muscle sphincter closes by contraction of the posterior pillars and the superior constrictor. The soft palate does not contract owing to previous traumatic palatorrhaphy. In these patients, the sphincter closes completely without velopharyngeal incompetence. (From Orticochea M: A review of 236 cleft palate patients treated with dynamic muscle sphincter. Plast Reconstr Surg 71:183, 1983. With permission.)

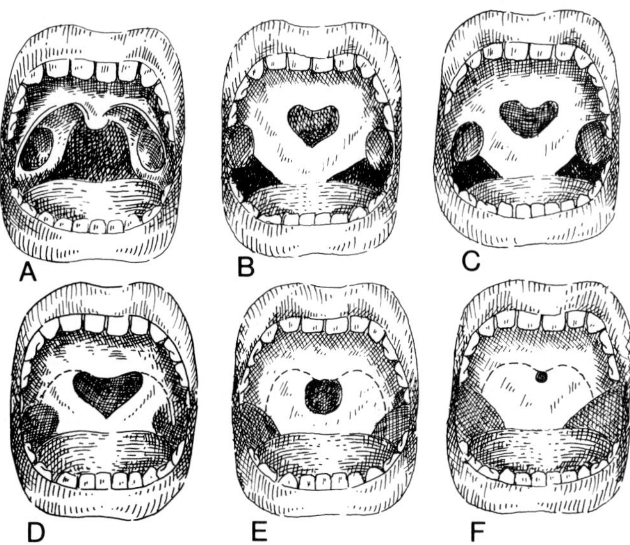

Figure 48–4 A–C, Evolution of surgical technique. D–F, Closure of the oronasal pharyngeal sphincter during production of certain sounds. (From Orticochea M: Construction of a dynamic muscle sphincter in cleft palates. Plast Reconstr Surg 41:324, 1968. With permission.)

Velopharyngeal Incompetence

A dynamic oronasal muscle sphincter should be created in patients who have velopharyngeal incompetence with good muscular function of the palate, for example, patients with (1) a congenital short palate, (2) a submucous cleft palate, (3) a repaired cleft palate with inadequate velopharyngeal closure, and (4) a short, fibrous, rigid palate subsequent to traumatic cleft palate surgery.

Velopharyngeal incompetence in the cleft palate patient is an evolving, progressive, nonregressive condition that shows no spontaneous improvement. First, the lesion occurs in the palate—a short cleft palate. This lesion appears from birth to 2½ years of age. In the second stage of the sequence, the lesion appears in the pharynx (at approximately 2½ to 4 years of age). As the pharynx begins to grow, the first symptoms of velopharyngeal incompetence begin to appear (Fig. 48–6). The early symptoms of velopharyngeal incompetence continue to increase. Once velopharyngeal insufficiency has been diagnosed, the patient requires surgical treatment.

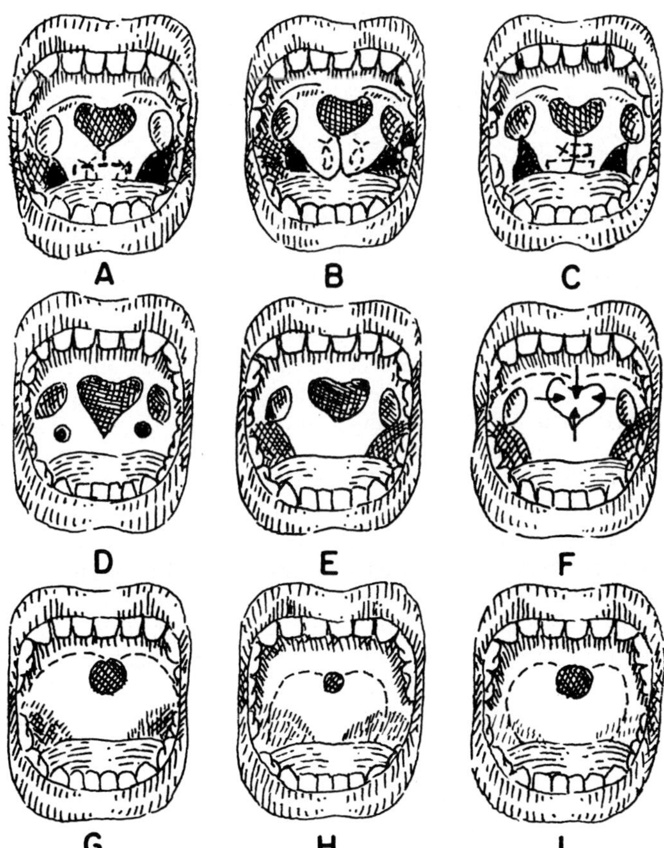

Figure 48–3 A, The flaps sutured with U sutures of multifilament 4–0 nylon. B–F, Evolution of the sphincter during the first 2 postoperative weeks. The lateral openings with their raw surfaces gradually stenose and heal. G, There is a new anatomic entity. A muscular membrane with an active rounded central sphincter links the soft palate to the posterior pharyngeal wall. H, The sphincter closes when saying "a-a-a." I, The sphincter at rest. (From Orticochea M: Results of the dynamic muscle sphincter operation in cleft palates. Br J Plast Surg 23:109, 1970. With permission.)

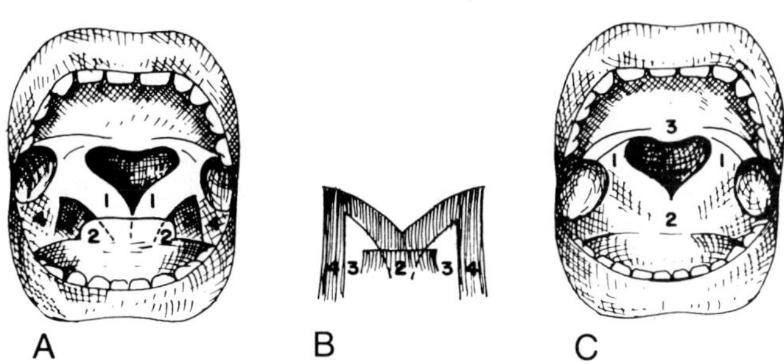

Figure 48–5 A, Schematic representation of the dynamic muscle sphincter. B, Schematic representation of the raw surfaces on the lateral and posterior walls when the surgery is over. C, The sphincter 4 weeks after surgery, showing the posterior pillars (1) with the palatopharyngeus muscles, joining of the posterior pillars to the superior constrictor muscle (2), and the soft palate (3). (From Orticochea M: A review of 236 cleft palate patients treated with dynamic muscle sphincter. Plast Reconstr Surg 71:181, 1983. With permission.)

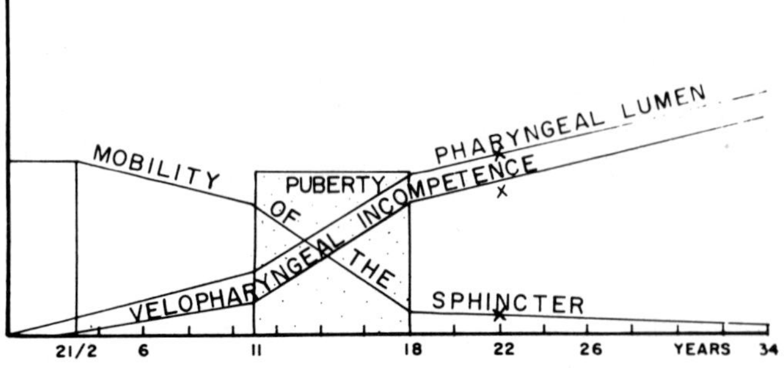

Figure 48–6 Velopharyngeal incompetence increases with age, especially during puberty. The impairment of velopharyngeal incompetence parallels growth of the pharyngeal lumen. Mobility of the sphincter decreases with age, especially during puberty. (From Riski JE, Riefkohl R, Georgiade S, Georgiade NG: A rationale for modifying the site of insertion of the Orticochea pharyngoplasty. Plast Reconstr Surg 73:893, 1984. With permission.)

Next, the lesion occurs in both the pharynx and brain (at 4 or more years of age) and becomes a cerebral lesion with continued phonic patterns that, once established, are very difficult to correct. Velopharyngeal incompetence worsens with age in relation to growth of the pharynx (Fig. 48–7).

Increase in the size of the pharyngeal lumen continues throughout life. The pharynx grows slowly from birth to puberty. It dramatically expands in width during puberty and grows slowly in adulthood. In old age, the size of the pharynx again enlarges as a result of atrophy of the pharyngeal mucous membrane (Fig. 48–6). The phoniatric problem of the cleft patient lies primarily in the palate but is subsequently located in the pharynx, where the dynamic muscle sphincter is built.

The Passavant Sphincter

The nasopharyngeal sphincter is created by the harmonious contraction of various muscles: (1) the superior constrictor muscles at the level of the nasopharynx that move the posterior wall forward and inward in a semicircle; (2) the levator veli palatini muscles, which raise

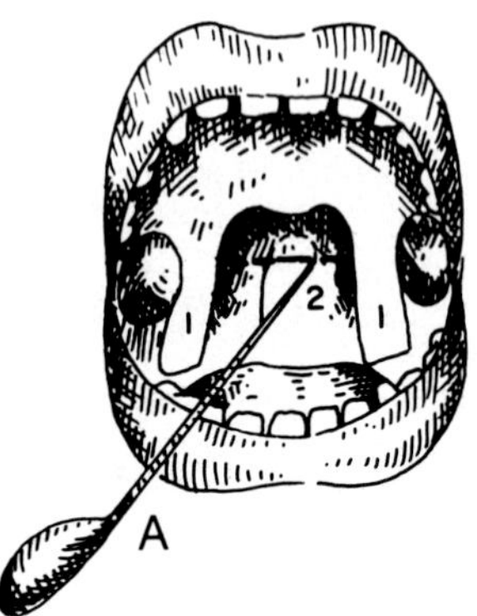
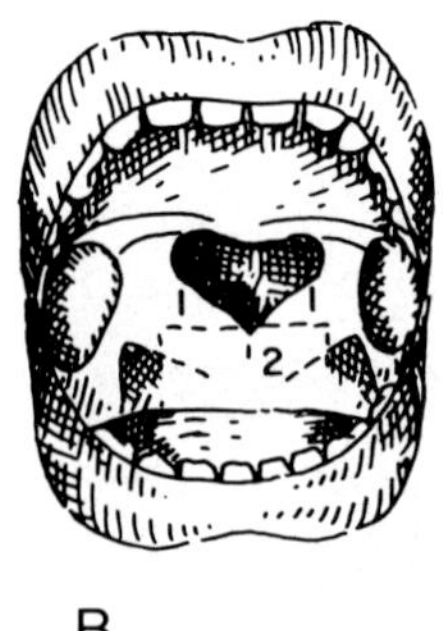

Figure 48–7 Schematic representation of the dynamic muscle sphincter. *A,* The pharyngeal flap is raised. It is preferable to place it high rather than low. *B,* Sphincter after surgery. The posterior pillars (1 and 1) and inferiorly based pharyngeal flap (2) should be created with little undermining. (From Riski JE, Riefkohl R, Georgiade S, Georgiade NG: A rationale for modifying the site of insertion of the Orticochea pharyngoplasty. Plast Reconstr Surg 73:893, 1984. With permission.)

and retract the soft palate toward the Passavant pad; and (3) the palatopharyngeus muscles, which complete the closure between the oral pharynx and the nasal pharynx by contraction, moving the lateral pharynx walls toward the midline.

The sphincter described by Passavant[4, 5] contracts dozens of times a minute during conversation, regulates the column of air that emerges from the lungs, and vibrates in the larynx. As the air stream reaches the oral pharynx, it takes one of two paths, depending on the phoneme being produced: (1) emerging partly or totally through the nasal cavity, or (2) emerging partly or totally through the oral cavity.

I do not know how Passavant discovered the nasopharyngeal sphincter.[6] I have seen it two or three times in patients with eye tumors who have had an orbital exenteration with complete removal of the bony walls of the orbital cavity. In these patients the nasal pharynx can be seen through the orbital cavity, and Passavant's nasopharyngeal sphincter and its great mobility can be observed as well. Currently, the same observations are possible with nasendoscopy.

The Dynamic Muscle Sphincter of the Pharynx

Many years ago I treated a patient with complete unilateral cleft lip, alveolus, and palate who underwent surgery in the interior of Colombia. The palate was short, and the patient had severe velopharyngeal incompetence. Through observation of this patient I concluded that the muscles acting during the gag reflex could be engaged for speech production; thus, the idea for a dynamic muscle sphincter was born. The gag reflex involves contraction of the posterior pillars of the tonsils, which contain the palatopharyngeus muscles. These muscles have the same cerebral representation as the other muscles—the levator veli palatini and the superior constrictor—of Passavant's sphincter.

Based on this observation, a surgical procedure was designed to change the lower insertion of the posterior pillars from the lateral walls to the posterior wall of the pharynx. Thus, a dynamic muscle sphincter of the pharynx was created that can open and close dozens of times a minute. Furthermore, this sphincter has the same cerebrocortical role as the nasopharyngeal sphincter described by Passavant[5] because the palatopharyngeus and superior constrictor muscles that are a part of the Passavant nasopharyngeal sphincter are used in its construction.

Reconstruction of the Muscle Sphincter

Surgeons are familiar with the diverse types of sphincters such as, for example, the pyloric, ileocecal, and vesical sphincters. These sphincters are resected by the surgeon if a tumor exists but normally are not reconstructed. The method of creating a dynamic muscle sphincter of the pharynx marked the beginning of a new era of operative technique. In the near future when there is a need to remove a sphincter, a new sphincter will be reconstructed to replace the removed or malfunctioning one.

Preoperative Physical Examination of the Pharynx

Prior to surgical intervention, the surgeon should first conduct the physical examination. The following items are observed: (1) the mobility of the soft palate, (2) the distance in millimeters between the posterior border of the soft palate and the posterior pharyngeal wall (for this measurement a wooden tongue depressor is used), (3) the development and mobility of the posterior pillars, (4) the size of the tonsils, which may help or interfere with the surgery of the dynamic muscle sphincter and its subsequent functioning.

Surgical Technique

The surgical technique is illustrated in Figs. 48–8 to 48–10. The description of the technique used at present is the same as that published in 1968 and 1979 with no modifications.[2, 3]

The following are some of the details of this surgery. The flap based on the posterior oropharyngeal wall should be brought to the height of the posterior pillars, but it is preferable to bring it to a high rather than a low level (Fig. 48–7). The nearer the superior constrictor muscle is to the Passavant pad, the more constricting force it will exert. I believe that it is preferable to make the flap high, not low. Conservative surgery with limited raising of the flaps will result in less postoperative

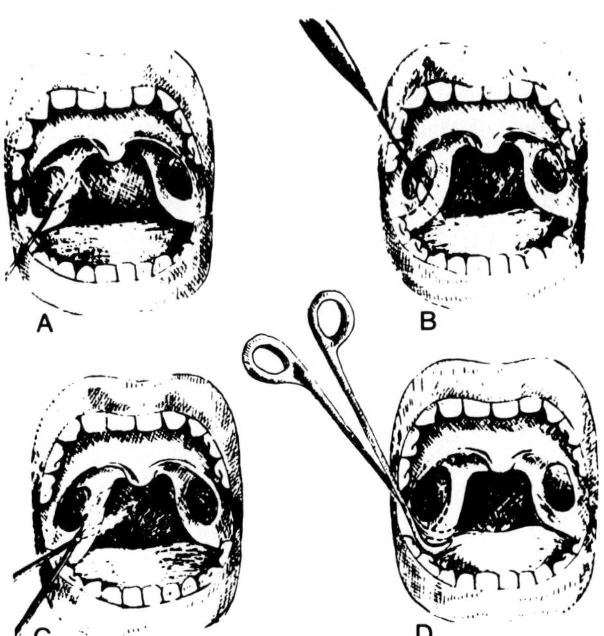

Figure 48–8 Patient in the Rose position. *A* and *B,* A vertical incision is made in the mucosa of the posterior pillar of the pharynx along the groove which separates it from the tonsil; the incision extends to the lower tonsillar pole. *C,* With spreading movements of Steven's scissors, the fibers of the palatopharyngeus muscle are separated from the superior constrictor. When the whole mass of the palatopharyngeus is free, it is retracted medially, and the mucosa on the posterior aspect of the posterior pillar is incised in the same line. *D,* The inferior insertion of the posterior pillar is sectioned with enucleation scissors underneath the lower pole of the tonsil. (From Orticochea M: Results of the dynamic muscle sphincter operation in cleft palates. Br J Plast Surg 23:109, 1970. With permission.)

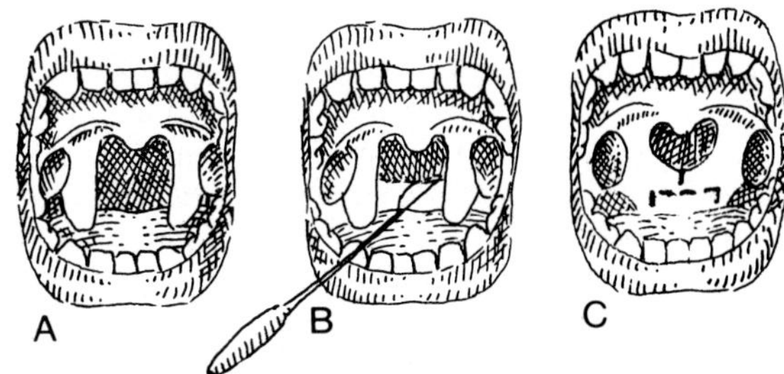

Figure 48–9 *A,* The posterior pillars containing the entire palatopharyngeus are separated from the tonsils and the lateral pharyngeal walls. Its lower third remains attached at the upper poles through which their innervation passes. *B,* An inferiorly based flap, 5 mm high by 2 cm wide, is prepared on the posterior pharyngeal wall projecting at the level of the superior third of the tonsil. The flap includes the superior constrictor muscle and is raised. *C,* The pharyngeal flap turned down and the lateral flaps in position for suturing. (From Orticochea M: Results of the dynamic muscle sphincter operation in cleft palates. Br J Plast Surg 23:109, 1970. With permission.)

scarring, better mobility of the transposed muscles, and consequently, better speech.

Closing the cleft by means of a conservative palatoplasty, without lengthening the anteroposterior dimension of the palate, preserves maximum mobility and voluntary contractile capacity of the soft palate. The space created between the posterior edge of the soft palate and the posterior pharyngeal wall is left open. Later, at approximately 2½ years of age, a contractile muscular sphincter is constructed by transplanting the posterior tonsillar pillars from the lateral walls to the posterior pharyngeal wall (Fig. 48–4).

The vagus nerve enters the upper part of the palatopharyngeus muscles at the level of the soft palate, innervating these muscles. Its integrity must be preserved during the muscular transplant. The construction of a dynamic oronasal pharyngeal sphincter enables the surgeon and the speech therapist to dispense with the tonsils as organs for obstructing the space between the soft palate and the posterior pharyngeal wall.

In adults or in patients with very short palates in whom there is a greater risk of dehiscence, only one of the palatopharyngeus muscles is transplanted. Three months later, in a second operation, the sphincter is completed by transplanting the second palatopharyngeus muscle.

The sphincter is created by transposing the posterior tonsillar pillars with the enclosed palatopharyngeus

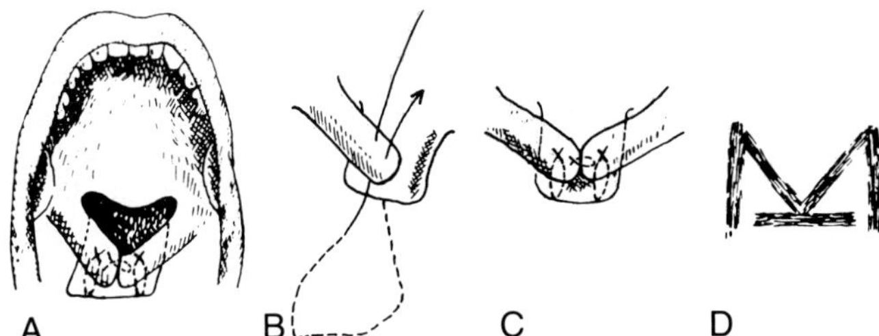

Figure 48–10 *A–D,* Technique for suturing the posterior pillars to the inferiorly based flap in the posterior pharyngeal wall. A U stitch is used with monofilament 4–0 nylon, joining both posterior pillars to prevent their dehiscence. (From Orticochea M: Construction of a dynamic muscle sphincter in cleft palates. Plast Reconstr Surg 41:326, 1968. With permission.)

muscles from the lateral pharyngeal walls to the mid-section of the posterior pharyngeal wall (Fig. 48–3). The pillars must be inserted with no tension to avoid dehiscence in the postoperative period. It is imperative that the posterior pillars be sutured together at the midline next to the posterior pharyngeal wall. Leaving a separation between the pillars allows air to escape from the oral to the nasal pharynx (Fig. 48–10).

Once both posterior pillars have been sutured, the sphincter is formed, concluding the surgical operation. Three openings or passages conduct air between the oral and nasal pharynges. All three have different walls and different anatomic characteristics, and all follow a different course of evolution (Figs. 48–3 and 48–5).[8, 9]

In the central opening, the oronasal pharyngeal sphincter, the borders are formed by the mobile edge of the soft palate and the two posterior pillars covered with mucosa. There is no raw surface around the circumference. Accordingly, its shape and width remain unchanged postoperatively, with no reduction of the lumen. The posterior pillars contain the palatopharyngeus muscle covered with mucosa on three sides: the nasal, oral, and inner aspects. The posterior vertex of the sphincter is placed above the pharyngeal flap in front of the posterior wall of the pharynx. This flap is designed to create a bed in which the transposed posterior pillars are sutured into the posterior pharyngeal wall.

The two lateral openings on both sides of the transposed posterior pillars have broad, raw surfaces on the walls and undergo gradual stenosis as they heal during the first weeks of the postoperative period. Eventually, their lumen disappears completely. The raw surfaces in the pharynx are outlined in Figures 48–3, 48–4, and 48–5. Contrary to the sequence of events in palatal "pushback" procedures or in pharyngeal flaps, which reduce the anteroposterior dimension, the lumen of the pharynx is narrowed in the transverse diameter with no adverse effect on the mobility of the soft palate (Figs. 48–1, 48–3 and 48–4).

The operation usually results in minimal bleeding. Local anesthesia with vasoconstrictive agents should not be used because it could result in necrosis of the flaps. When raising the flap on the posterior pharyngeal wall, two small veins that descend vertically are visible behind the superior constrictor in the retropharyngeal region. Transection of these veins should be avoided. The veins should be tied off with catgut.

The inferiorly based pharyngeal flap on the posterior pharyngeal wall should be 5 mm high and have a variable width depending on the size of the pharynx. However, laterally this flap should never reach the raw surface that is left after raising the posterior pillars (Figs. 48–5 and 48–7). A portion of mucosa (see 3 and 3 in Fig. 48–5) should be left to divide the raw surface on the posterior pharyngeal wall and the two lateral raw surfaces that remain after raising the lower ends of the posterior pillars. By not joining these three surfaces, creation of a large scar is prevented that would impair the movements of the sphincter in the postoperative stage.

At what level should the flap of the posterior pharyn-

geal wall be outlined? The flaps formed by the posterior pillars (No. 1 in Fig. 48–7) should be raised first. Only after this should the posterior pharyngeal wall flap be outlined at a level easily reached by the posterior pillars. Consequently, the suture is left free of tension (Figs. 48–7 and 48–10).

Anatomy of the Muscle Sphincter

The dynamic muscle sphincter is made up of four musculomucosal walls (Figs. 48–1 and 48–5C). The lateral walls are formed by the posterior tonsillar pillars, which contain the palatopharyngeus muscles. The posterior pillars of the lateral pharyngeal wall are detached from and along the lower third of the tonsils and remain joined to the lateral pharyngeal wall in front of the medial and upper thirds of the tonsils, through which they are innervated. Thus, the mobility of the palatopharyngeus muscles is maintained. The posterior inferior wall, formed by the superior constrictor muscle, moves upward when the sphincter is closed. The anterior superior wall, formed by the free border of the soft palate, has variable mobility depending on the results of the previous palatoplasty. If this was traumatic, the free border of the palate becomes fibrous and rigid. If it has neither mobility nor the ability to contract, it does not contribute to the closing of the sphincter (Fig. 48–2).

At our surgery department, where the dynamic pharyngeal sphincter muscle is made, it has proved very useful to add a medical history sheet with two diagrams to the surgical notes (Figs. 48–6 and 48–11). Thus, in accordance with the pharyngeal symptomatology and the age and sex of the patient, a prognosis is given of the quality of phonation.

Pathological Anatomy in the Adolescent and Adult with Velopharyngeal Incompetence

Construction of the dynamic muscle sphincter in the adolescent or adult involves dealing with the following anatomic and physiologic conditions:

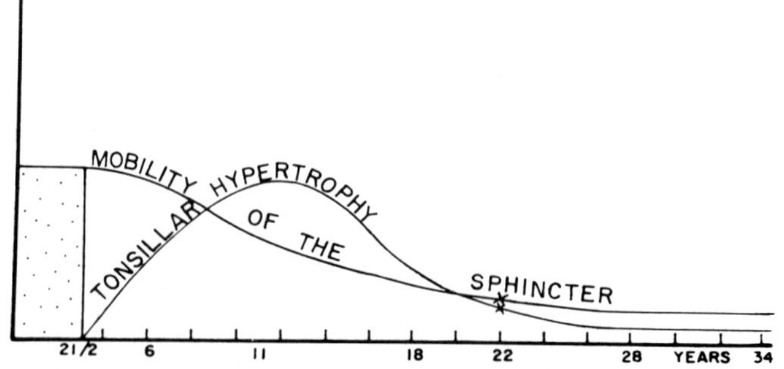

Figure 48–11 Mobility of the sphincter decreases with age. Usually the tonsillar hypertrophy increases during the first years of life and decreases from the age of 14 years on. For this reason, the dynamic muscle sphincter should be constructed at 2½ years of age, before tonsillar hypertrophy occurs. (From Riski JE, Serafin D, Riefkohl R, Georgiade GS, Georgiade NG: A rationale for modifying the site of insertion of the Orticochea pharyngoplasty. Plast Reconstr Surg 73:893, 1984. With permission.)

1. Considerable development of the pharynx, formed by a cavity (lumen) of large anteroposterior, transverse, and vertical dimensions (Fig. 48–6).
2. Lack of development of the posterior pillars of the tonsils in relation to the size of the pharynx. When the posterior pillars are moved, they may be too small and too short to reach the posterior wall of the pharynx.

These anatomic features make construction of the sphincter more difficult in an adult than in a child. As a consequence, we advise that the sphincter in an adult be made in two stages: (1) The larger posterior pillar is transposed to the posterior wall of the pharynx, and (2) 3 months later, the remaining posterior pillar is transposed. This sequence prevents tension of the flap and postoperative dehiscence. The dynamic muscle sphincter created in an adolescent or an adult has a larger diameter and lesser contractile capacity than that in a young child (Figs. 48–6 and 48–11).

Marked velopharyngeal incompetence in the adolescent and adult improves with construction of the sphincter, and the voice quality becomes less nasal (Fig. 48–6). However, this surgery in adults does not provide the same benefit as it does a preschool age child because by this age a cerebral phonic pattern is solidly established.

When a dynamic muscle sphincter in an adolescent or adult is insufficient owing to a lack of contractile

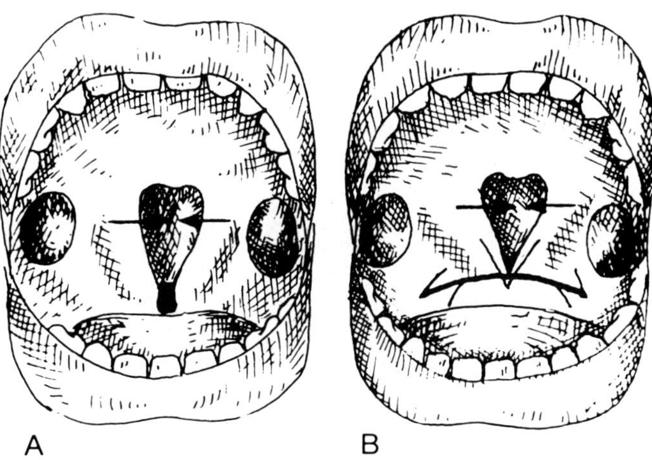

Figure 48–13 *A*, The posterior pillars are attached to a scar on the posterior pharyngeal wall (dotted line) and do not reach the midline. The sphincter will not close completely. Its function will be greatly diminished. Consequently, there is some velopharyngeal incompetence. This is due to the fact that the tension produced by the muscular tonus and by the contraction of the palatopharyngeus muscles has raised the superiorly based flap constructed on the posterior pharyngeal wall. A large raw surface is left on the posterior pharyngeal wall, producing a large scar later on (dotted line). *B*, The posterior pillars are fixed to a transverse scar, which should be removed, and two lateral Z-plasties should be performed on the posterior pharyngeal wall. Insertion of the posterior pillars is raised by means of a V-Y plasty. (From Orticochea M: A review of 236 cleft palate patients treated with dynamic muscle sphincter. Plast Reconstr Surg 71:184, 1983. With permission.)

capacity or too large a diameter, the residual velopharyngeal incompetence may be improved by reducing the size of the sphincter (Fig. 48–12).

Secondary Surgery of the Dynamic Muscle Sphincter of the Pharynx

In my experience, the most common causes of poor concentric closure of the sphincter are as follows:

1. *Attachment of the posterior pillars to the posterior pharyngeal wall, impairing the elevation of the superior constrictor muscles (Fig. 48–13A, B).* This condition may result from a surgical procedure that leaves a large raw surface on the posterior pharyngeal wall. A similar large raw surface may be observed subsequent to creation of a superiorly based pharyngeal flap or following adenoidectomy or tonsillectomy. Following construction of a dynamic muscle sphincter, two types of scars may be observed on the posterior pharyngeal wall: fibrous nodular scars and transverse and concave downward scars. Fibrous nodular scars must be removed and repaired by means of a V-Y plasty (Fig. 48–13*A*). Transverse and concave downward scars must be removed, and two lateral Z-plasties must be performed on the posterior pharyngeal wall. The insertion of the posterior pillars is raised by a V-Y plasty (Fig. 48–13*B*).
2. *Lack of union of the posterior pillars in the midline of the posterior pharyngeal wall.* This condition may result from inappropriate primary surgery in which the lower edges of the posterior pillars were not

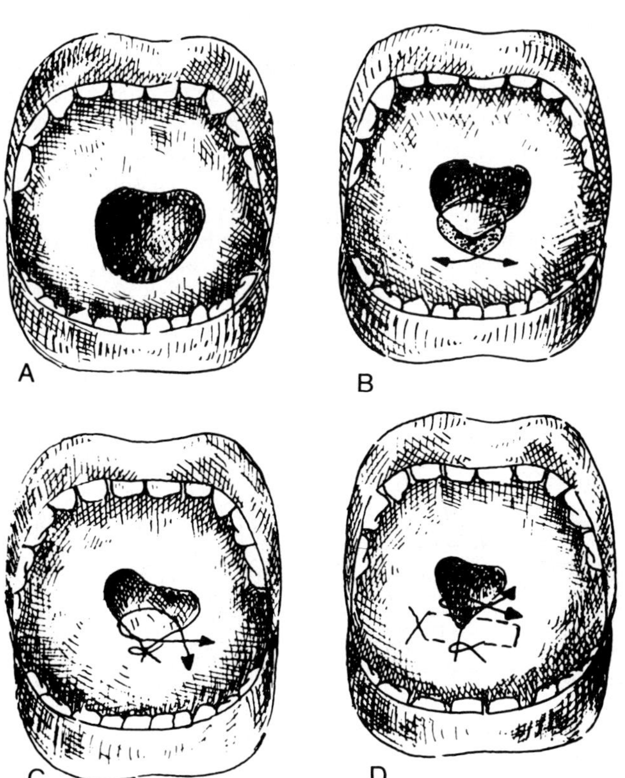

Figure 48–12 *A*, Large sphincter with velopharyngeal incompetence. *B*, The mucosa of the lower vertex of the sphincter should be removed. *C* and *D*, Both palatopharyngeus muscles are sutured together with nonabsorbable material. (From Orticochea M: A review of 236 cleft palate patients treated with dynamic muscle sphincter. Plast Reconstr Surg 71:185, 1983. With permission.)

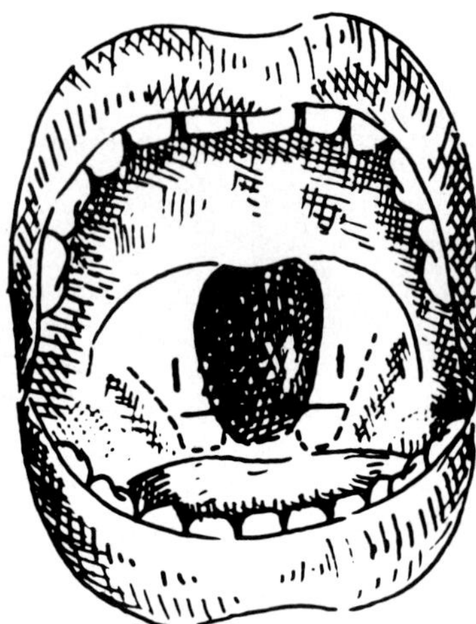

Figure 48–14 The inferior poles of the posterior pillars are dissected and sutured in the midline. (From Orticochea M: A review of 236 cleft palate patients treated with dynamic muscle sphincter. Plast Reconstr Surg 71:186, 1983. With permission.)

sutured together at midline. Another cause is partial dehiscence of the flaps postoperatively. If the separation of the posterior pillars is slight, the mucosa of the lower vertex of the sphincter should be removed and both palatopharyngeus muscles sutured together with nonabsorbable sutures (Fig. 48–12). If there is a wide separation, the lower poles of the posterior pillars should be detached, sutured again in the midline, and then joined together (Fig. 48–14).

3. *Sphincter with large lumen not closing completely during contraction.* This condition results most frequently from transposition of the posterior pillars with little muscular tissue and without including the entire muscular mass. The lower end of the palatopharyngeus muscles must be dissected and the posterior pillars sutured together in the midline (Fig. 48–14).

Treatment of Hypertrophied Tonsils and Adenoids in Cleft Palate Patients Previously Operated on for Dynamic Muscle Sphincter of the Pharynx

A preschool-age patient who has been operated on for cleft palate and has undergone a dynamic muscle sphincter procedure has the same chances of tonsil and adenoid hypertrophy as a normal person. The patient whose cleft palate has been closed without creation of a dynamic muscle sphincter of the pharynx will have a greater likelihood of hypertrophy of the tonsils and pharyngeal adenoids than a normal person. This predilection may be caused by velopharyngeal incompetence with excessive ventilation—a great deal of hot air exits from the lungs and a great deal of cold air enters from the outside. This hyperventilation originates an inflammatory and infectious process of the nasopharyngeal and oral mucosa followed by hypertrophy of the Waldeyer tonsillar ring.

Among these patients, as in normal persons, a small percentage will have tonsil and adenoid hypertrophy calling for surgery. When it is medically indicated to operate on hypertrophied tonsils and adenoids (for example, in patients with rheumatoid arthritis, heart lesions, or acute nephritis), the removal of the tonsils is performed without any consequences to the patient's phonation.

A patient with a cleft palate that is closed at the age of 2 years who undergoes a dynamic muscle sphincter procedure at the age of 2½ years will have no velopharyngeal incompetence and no hyperventilation of the pharynx. This is one of the great advantages of the dynamic muscle sphincter in patients with a cleft palate as well as one of the great differences between this technique and others, in which resection of the tonsils produces serious phonation disorders.[7]

Surgical Technique

The surgical procedure for hypertrophied tonsils and adenoids in a patient with dynamic muscle sphincter is based on the following principles:

1. The removal of hypertrophied tonsils is simple because they are in front of the sphincter and its muscle-mucous membrane. The tonsils are visible and accessible during the operation (Fig. 48–15A).
2. The hypertrophied tonsils are removed leaving a maximum amount of mucosa, so that there is a small raw surface. The fibers of the palatopharyngeal muscle should not be injured.
3. Any raw surface vessels that may bleed are compressed downward with forceps rather than sideways (Fig. 48–15B). If they were compressed sideways with hemostatic forceps, the sphincter would be widened laterally, and its transverse diameter would be increased. The vessels are tied with catgut.
4. To resect the nasopharyngeal adenoids, the sphincter is dilated gently, the adenotome being inserted to remove the adenoids. The adenoids are removed by

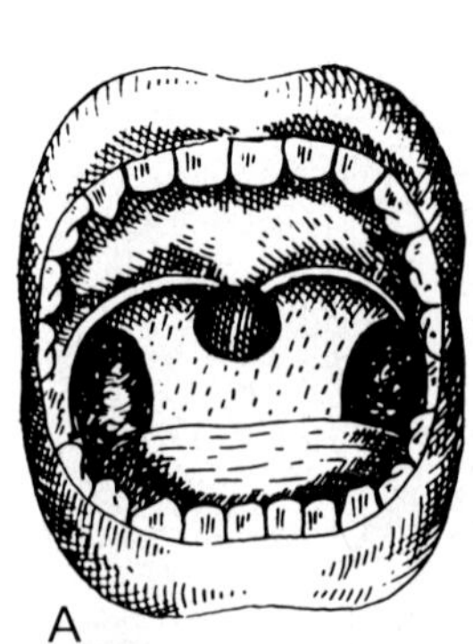
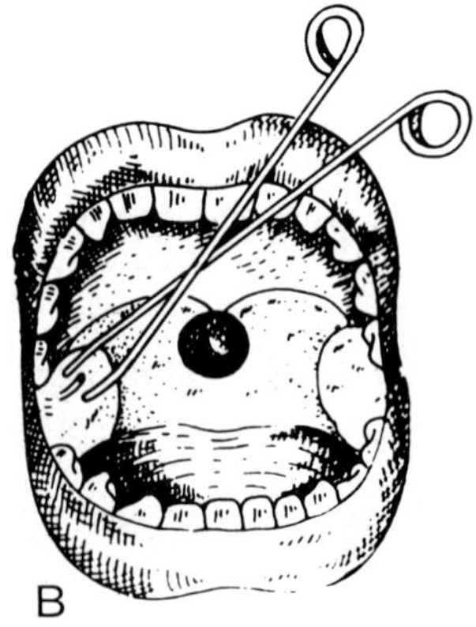

Figure 48–15 *A*, Hypertrophic tonsils in a patient with a dynamic muscle sphincter. *B*, Removal of the tonsil, leaving as much mucosa as possible. The bleeding vessels of the raw surface are clamped from above downward. (From Orticochea M: Traitement des amygdales et des adenoides hypertrophiques chez le malade opere de division palatine avec sphincter musculaire. Ann Chir Plast Esthet 1:81–83, 1977. With permission.)

gentle handling of the adenotome, taking care not to injure the posterior wall of the nasal pharynx. The tissue of the adenoids, once detached, is aspirated by a cannula through the sphincter.

Discussion

Two main conclusions may be drawn. First, the morphology and activity of the sphincter are independent of the type of cleft that preceded the origin of velopharyngeal incompetence, and second, the muscular membrane, with the sphincter in its center, develops better and acquires better anatomic and physiologic properties the earlier the surgery is performed (Fig. 48–6).[10]

Effect of the Sphincter on Speech

The dynamic function of the sphincter that controls the exact amount of air passing into the nasopharyngeal cavity and from there to the nasal cavity is an automatic and reflex action. When the operation is carried out at the age of approximately 2½ years, before the patient has acquired bad speech habits, and provided that the anatomic components of the oronasal cavity that take an active part in the emission of sounds are intact or reconstructed, normal speech without hypernasality is obtained, and speech therapy is necessary only for voice training (Fig. 48–6). On the other hand, in pubertal children or adults with velopharyngeal incompetence, the reconstructed sphincter evolves differently from its behavior in the small child, and it will have neither the speed of movement, the elasticity, nor the ability to close that are seen in young children. In such patients the anatomic and physiologic structures have a set pattern of adaptation during speech, and this tends to persist as before with only partial improvement after the operation. These patients need prolonged speech therapy to overcome their longstanding patterns. Nevertheless, all patients who had hypernasality before surgery improved to some degree after construction of the sphincter (Fig. 48–6).

Effects of the Sphincter on Growth of the Pharynx

During puberty, especially in males, there is extensive development of the pharynx, and the severity of velopharyngeal incompetence increases in the cleft palate patient. The posterior pillars do not increase proportionately in size, remaining small in relation to the degree of velopharyngeal incompetence and the distance separating them from the posterior wall of the pharynx. On the other hand, the capacity of fibroblasts to heal, which is so important in this technique, decreases as the years pass. These three factors—the growth of the pharynx, the limited development of the posterior pillars, and the decrease in fibroblastic ability to heal—make construction of the sphincter and its later contractile capacity much more difficult and less effective in adults, especially men, than in children of preschool age (Fig. 48–6).

In adulthood as well as in puberty, women possess a smaller pharynx and better anatomic conditions for constructing the sphincter than men. Therefore, in women, too, the sphincter is morphologically superior and has greater contractile capacity than in men.

Effect of the Sphincter on Swallowing

When swallowing, the sphincter closes during the passage of food from the oral to oropharyngeal cavity, preventing it from entering the nose.

The Sphincter and the Tonsils and Adenoids

The tonsils are located in front of the pharyngeal diaphragm and the adenoids lie behind it. They no longer contribute to the closure of the velopharynx, and their management should be the same as that in the normal patient. Any patient who has had a dynamic sphincter repair should be seen regularly by an otorhinolaryngologist. Patients who have velopharyngeal incompetence associated with hypertrophy of the tonsils pose a problem for the surgeon: which to do first, the sphincter or the tonsillectomy? To try to construct a sphincter with enlarged, hypertrophied tonsils that hide the posterior pillars is a difficult and time consuming surgical technique. To construct a sphincter a few months after a tonsillectomy is equally difficult and time consuming because the scar, which occupies the tonsil bed, hides the posterior pillars and the palatopharyngeal muscle. Under such circumstances, it is difficult to construct a strong, powerful sphincter by transplanting the whole muscular mass. I perform the tonsillectomy and the dynamic sphincter construction in one stage, but this leaves too much raw surface exposed.

ACKNOWLEDGMENTS. I dedicate this study to Von Passavant, who in 1862 described the sphincter named for him, and to Enrique Apolo, who took the knowledge on cleft lip and palate patients from Europe to Uruguay.

References

1. Orticochea M: A new method for repair of total or partial cleft lips. Transactions of the Fourth International Congress of Plastic and Reconstructive Surgery. Amsterdam, Excerpta Medica, 1969, p 337.
2. Orticochea M: Construction of a dynamic muscle sphincter in cleft palate. Plast Reconstr Surg 41:323, 1968.
3. Orticochea M: Results of the dynamic muscle sphincter operation in cleft palates. Br J Plast Surg 23:108, 1970.
4. Passavant G: Über die Operation der angeborenen Spalten des harten Gaumens und der damit Complicierten. Hasenscharten Arch Ohr Nas Kehlkopfheilk 3:193, 1892.
5. Passavant G: Über die Beseitigung der naselnden Sprache bei angeborenen Spalten des harten und weichen Gaumens (Gaumensegel, Schulundnaht und Rucklagerung des Gaumensegels). Arch Klin Chir 6:33, 1865.
6. Passavant G: Über die Verbesserung der Sprache nach der Vranoplastik. Dtsch Gesellschaft Chir 7:128, 1878.
7. Orticochea M: Traitement des amygdales et des adenoides hypertrophiques chez le malade opere de division palatine avec sphincter musculaire dynamique du pharynx. Ann Chir Plast 22:81, 1977.
8. Orticochea M: Indications et opportunite chirurgicale du sphincter musculaire dynamique du pharynx. Ann Chir Plast 19:5, 1974.
9. Orticochea M: Discussion. A rationale for modifying the site of insertion of the Orticochea pharyngoplasty. Plast Reconstr Surg 73:892, 1984.
10. Lendrum J: The Orticochea dynamic pharyngoplasty. Br J Plast Surg 37:160, 1984.

CHAPTER 49

Pharyngoplasty: Jackson Technique

Ian T. Jackson

Before considering palatal rehabilitation, it is relevant to examine the presently accepted philosophy of rehabilitation of the unsatisfactory lip repair. Correction of the secondary deformity of the cleft lip and nose has led to the development of many techniques; there is no single one that applies to all lip problems. Everyone would now agree that a careful assessment should be made of the aesthetic and functional aspects of the deformity. The lip height is assessed with regard to the balance of the lip and also the transverse tightness. Just as important is the observation of the position of the orbicularis oris and its function. According to the surgeon's analysis of the situation, the method of correction is established and executed, frequently converting the previous repair to a rotation-advancement type of flap with accurate reconstruction of the orbicularis oris muscle. On rare occasions in which oversacrifice of lip tissue has occurred, an Abbe flap is employed.

It is strange that, in light of this very well reasoned and logical approach to lip and nose deformity, in the case of the cleft palate patient with velopharyngeal incompetence after the initial repair there exists what can only be described as a "blunderbuss" approach. It seems that in the mind of most surgeons, "velopharyngeal incompetence" equals "pharyngeal flap," the only anatomic and physiologic change made over the years being conversion from the inferiorly based Rosenthal[1] procedure to the superiorly based technique of Sanvanero-Rosselli[2]—at least a step in the right direction! Where is the careful analysis on which to base a procedure that is so characteristic of reconstructive surgery of the lip? In one's own experience and that of others, it seems unlikely that such an illogical attitude is justifiable. This reasoning has led to a careful assessment of the anatomic cause of velopharyngeal incompetence and formulation of an operative procedure based on the finding of that investigation.

Preoperative Assessment

The presence and degree of velopharyngeal incompetence, together with any coexisting articulation defects, are comprehensively assessed and established by the speech pathologist and the plastic surgeon.[3] If at all possible, nasendoscopy, usually with the flexible endoscope, is performed. In children under the age of 4 to 6 years, it is unusual to be able to carry out this investigation because of lack of patient cooperation. The information obtained from endoscopy can be summarized as the extent and type of movement of the soft palate, any palate deformation occurring with movement, movement of the posterior and lateral pharyngeal walls, and the size and shape of the velopharyngeal defect. The presence of bubbling of saliva also can be a significant finding because it indicates escape of air from the oral to the nasal cavity. In the noncleft patient, any incoordination around the velopharyngeal sphincter may be highly significant. An adjunctive and most helpful investigation is videofluoroscopy, as described by Skolnick[4]; it is important to understand the information gained from each particular view. This information will augment the evidence for or against a particular procedure.

Videofluoroscopy

Lateral View. This view shows the functional height of the palate, where the knee of maximum palatal muscular contraction occurs, the movement of the posterior pharyngeal wall and where it occurs (Passavant's ridge), and the velopharyngeal gap on non-nasal sounds. In addition to these findings, the speed of palatal movement is noted. In many individuals with velopharyngeal incompetence it is significant that the speed of palatal movement is considerably reduced. The thickness of the palate, particularly posteriorly, gives an indication of muscle bulk.

Anterior View. This view allows assessment of the degree and speed of movement of the lateral pharyngeal walls.

Basal View. This view is rather like the view obtained by endoscopy and shows the movement of the soft palate and the lateral and posterior pharyngeal walls. With good technique, the shape of the soft palate can be examined and the size and shape of the velopharyngeal defect noted. It must be said, however, that this is an extremely difficult view to obtain and on many occasions is not produced in a fashion that makes meaningful diagnosis possible.

Treatment Strategy

From an educated assessment of the investigations mentioned above, a clear idea of the cause of the velopharyngeal incompetence can be obtained in almost all patients. It seems reasonable to suggest that the method of surgical rehabilitation be chosen according to the established cause. The methods of palatal reconstruction that are available are

1. Re-repair of the palate with reconstruction of the palatal muscular mechanism
2. Superior pharyngeal flap
3. Sphincter pharyngoplasty.

Re-repair of the Palate

Intraoral Examination. Good palatal movement is seen, but it occurs too far forward. The muscular contraction from ridges is causing a V-shaped formation from front to back. The central V-shaped structure is virtually devoid of muscle activity.

Nasendoscopy. There is a typical V-shaped appearance with muscles running anteroposteriorly rather than transversely, indicating a lack of proper muscle reconstruction at the time of the original repair. The maximum palatal movement is too far forward. There is good posterior and lateral pharyngeal wall movement.

Videofluoroscopy. Lateral view reveals that the knee of muscular movement is too far forward. The palate is thin posteriorly, indicating lack of muscle bulk. There is good posterior wall movement with a marked Passavant's ridge. On anterior and basal views, there is good lateral and posterior wall movement.

Pharyngeal Flap Procedure

Intraoral Examination. Little or no palatal movement is observed.

Nasendoscopy. Little or no palatal movement is seen. Good lateral wall movement occurs.

Videofluoroscopy. Lateral view shows little or no palatal movement. There may be good posterior pharyngeal wall movement, but there is no velopharyngeal closure. Palatal thickness is of no importance. Anterior and basal views show good lateral wall movement with or without good posterior pharyngeal wall movement.

Sphincter Pharyngoplasty

Intraoral Examination. Good palatal movement is observed, and the muscles appear to be in a good position.

Nasendoscopy. There is good palatal movement far back on the soft palate. Little or no lateral wall movement is seen with or without good posterior pharyngeal wall movement.

Videofluoroscopy. From the lateral perspective the palate appears short, but there is good muscular thickness with the muscular knee in a good position. There may or may not be good posterior pharyngeal wall movement. Anterior and basal views show poor lateral pharyngeal wall movement, with or without good posterior pharyngeal wall movement.

Another group of patients in whom the sphincter pharyngoplasty could be considered is the group in whom there is generally poor function in all areas making up the velopharyngeal sphincter mechanism. The remainder of this chapter is dedicated to the sphincter pharyngoplasty, and therefore only this rehabilitative technique will be considered.[3, 5]

Sphincter Pharyngoplasty: Operative Technique

Having used the available evidence to decide which procedure is indicated to deal with the functional anomaly resulting in velopharyngeal incompetence, management proceeds without delay. As Orticochea has stated, "Velopharyngeal incompetence is like cancer. There is nothing to be gained by waiting to see what will happen."[6] The outcome is already known; significant improvement never occurs without surgical treatment.

The operation is carried out under general anesthesia using an oral endotracheal airway. The operating position is obviously a personal perference. The most effective position for the surgeon is probably seated with the feet firmly placed on a small stool to prevent the legs from becoming fatigued and the patient's head brought to the surgeons lap; this results in extension of the patient's neck. A Dott or Dingman mouth gag is inserted. It is most satisfactory to have a degree of hypotension in these patients, but this can be difficult owing to the head position. The posterior pharyngeal wall and the posterior pillars of the fauces are infiltrated with 0.5% lidocaine (Xylocaine) and 1:400,000 epinephrine (Adrenalin). It is advisable to wait a minimum of 5 minutes, preferably somewhat longer, to allow the pharmacologic effect of this injection to take place. Illumination is difficult in this procedure, and one has to opt for someone standing behind the surgeon and manipulating operating lights as necessary, wearing a head light, or having an assistant wearing a head light. Unfortunately, most head lights tend to get in the way of the assistants in this confined space, but again the decision to use one or not is often a personal preference. It is best to consider this procedure a "one man" operation (Fig. 49–1). The operation itself is divided into three stages: (1) raising the faucial flaps, (2) incising the posterior pharyngeal wall, and (3) insetting the flaps.

Raising the Faucial Flaps

Before the flaps are raised, it is wise to observe and carefully palpate the posterior and lateral pharyngeal

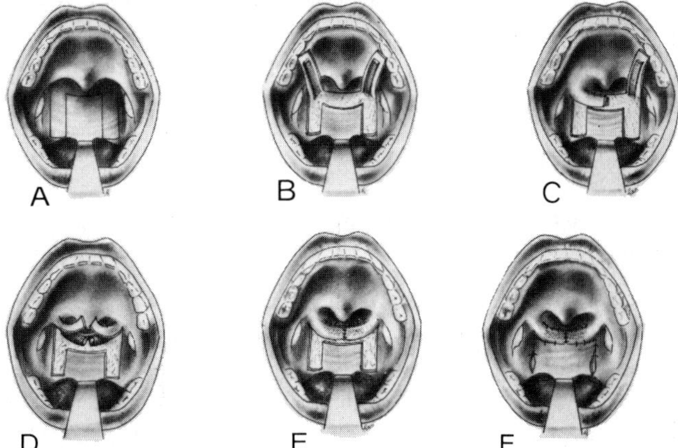

Figure 49–1 Pharyngoplasty: Jackson approach. *A,* Pharyngoplasty drawn on the posterior pharyngeal wall. Illustration shows the transverse incision on the posterior pharyngeal wall and the lateral pharyngeal flaps, consisting of the posterior tonsillar pillars. *B,* The flaps have been elevated together with the palatopharyngeus muscles. A transverse incision has been made on the posterior pharyngeal wall. Because of tension, the posterior pharyngeal wall opens widely. *C,* The medial edge of the tonsillar pillar flap is sutured to the superior edge of the transverse pharyngeal incision. *D,* After the superior edges of the posterior tonsillar pillar flaps have been sutured to the superior edge of the posterior pharyngeal wall incision, the palatopharyngeus muscles are sutured end to end. *E,* The distal ends of the tonsillar pillar flaps are sutured together end to end. *F,* The lateral edges of the tonsillar pillars are sutured to the inferior margin of the transverse pharyngeal incision. The lateral defects are closed directly. (From Bardach J, Salyer K: Surgical Techniques in Cleft Lip and Palate. Chicago: Year Book, 1987.)

walls. On one occasion, a previously undiagnosed arteriovenous malformation was encountered with interesting consequences that will be described later under complications. A recent article relating to pharyngeal flaps suggests that anomalous branches of the carotid or the internal carotid itself may occasionally lie on the posterior pharyngeal wall.[7] Should either of these situations be suspected, it would probably be wise to postpone the operation and investigate the patient with carotid angiography before continuing any surgical procedure. A large tonsil may also be a problem, and it is possible to find oneself cutting through tonsillar tissue. If this is the case, it is sometimes wise to remove the tonsils, conserving the mucosa, before proceeding with the pharyngoplasty.

If there are no contraindications, an incision is made anterior to the posterior pillar of the fauces through the mucosa to expose the palatopharyngeus muscle and is continued as far down the lateral pharyngeal wall as is necessary to lift the total extent of the posterior pillar. Using a small dissector (each surgeon has his particular favorite), the muscle fibers are separated vertically, and the dissector is introduced behind them, working medially onto the posterior pharyngeal wall. In this way, a large portion of the palatopharyngeus is elevated with the posterior faucial pillar. A vertical incision is then made in the posterior pharyngeal wall to form a flap that is approximately 1 to 1.5 cm in width. The faucial pillar flap is totally mobilized over its whole length. A further check is made to ensure that no large vessels are included in the flap. The inferior border of the flap is divided using straight scissors. The flap is then lifted, based cranially, and any bleeding vessels are coagulated. It is usually possible to close the pillar defect with a few interrupted 4–0 catgut sutures. A similar procedure is then carried out on the contralateral side, and that defect is also closed.

Incising the Posterior Pharyngeal Wall

If it has not been done before, the uvula is now pulled as far forward on the soft palate as possible and is maintained there with a suture taken on the soft palate. This exposes the velopharyngeal area very adequately. A transverse incison is made at the top of the tonsillar fossa at the cranial extent of the incision for the medial edge of the faucial flap. This incision is taken from one tonsillar area to the other, connecting the most cranial parts of the vertical posterior pharyngeal wall incisions. The mucosa of the posterior pharyngeal wall springs apart, opening a gap about 0.5 cm wide. Bleeding points are coagulated.

Suturing the Flaps

The faucial flaps are rotated medially, and the *medial edges* of the flaps are sutured to the *cranial edge* of the incison on the posterior pharyngeal wall. In the midline, the flaps lie at right angles to their original position, and their caudal ends are sutured together. Further narrowing of the pharyngeal sphincter can be controlled very accurately by beginning to suture the *lateral edges* of the flaps together in the midline. Like all other pharyngoplasties, exact measurements in millimeters tend to be ridiculous because of the biology of the healing process. Therefore, it is enough to say that a sphincter mechanism of somewhere between 8 and 10 mm in diameter (the end of a pencil) is aimed for. Actually, one can never forecast what the eventual diameter of this orifice will be owing to the inconsistency of intraoral healing. This suturing establishes a transverse shelf high up on the posterior pharyngeal wall with the mucosa of the flaps now facing cranially. The palatopharyngeus muscles can be picked up bilaterally and sutured in the midline with interrupted sutures of absorbable material, the choice being decided by the surgeon's preference. The anterior edge of the mucosal shelf is actually the lateral margin of the faucial flaps. This latter edge is pulled caudally and sutured to the caudal free edge of the transverse posterior pharyngeal wall incision. In this way, the muscle reconstruction is covered, and there are no residual raw areas.

If the patient has been operated on under hypotensive anesthesia, normal tension is established, and bleeding is watched for. Should this be of any consequence, it must be stopped at this time. The patient is taken to the recovery room after extubation and observed carefully to rule out any airway problems. Observation following this period is done either in the intensive care area or the intensive nursing area overnight. The patient is usually discharged after 24 to 48 hours.

Postoperative Progress

Ideally, there should be hyponasality lasting for 2 to 3 months. Following this period, there should be a gradual transition to normal or near-normal speech. Speech therapy is indicated only for articulation errors. If the patient has residual hypernasality or becomes hyponasal, further adjustment of the velopharyngeal aperture will be necessary.

Hypernasality

Treatment of hypernasality consists of reexploration with elevation, mobilization, and advancement of the faucial flaps to further narrow the velopharyngeal opening. The medial edges of the flaps are sutured together so that the sphincter is reduced in diameter. Often the method chosen varies with the local findings.

Hyponasality

The velopharyngeal mechanism is carefully examined under anesthesia, and the sphincter area is enlarged either by moving the flaps apart or carrying out a midline Z-plasty when there is a tight band in the midline. In both hyponasality and hypernasality the sphincter diameter aimed for is about the size of a pencil. This measurement has been arrived at solely by experience.

Complications of Sphincter Pharyngoplasty

Intraoperatively, there may be bleeding, but this is usually fairly easily identified and coagulated. It is important, however, to study the position of the carotid vessels prior to carrying out this procedure. On the occasion described earlier when an arteriovenous malformation was encountered, the bleeding was uncontrollable by conventional measures, and it was necessary to suture a large pressure pack into the raw area to stop the bleeding. A tracheostomy was carried out, and pharyngoplasty was completed. Ten days later, the patient was brought back to the operating room, and the pack was gently removed. There was no evidence of further bleeding. The patient achieved an excellent result from the pharyngoplasty.

Postoperatively, it is conceivable (as with all posterior pharyngeal procedures) that airway problems might develop, and the same careful postoperative observation is advocated as that advised for palate repairs and pharyngeal flaps. There may be some neck pain and stiffness, but this seems to be less of a problem than it is with posterior pharyngeal flaps.

Hypernasality has been improved but not totally corrected in 10% of cases, and hyponasality has occurred in 2% of cases. These problems can be corrected or improved as discussed above. As with pharyngeal flaps, there is considerable concern in the patients with hyponasality that they may also have some degree of sleep apnea. If this is suspected when the patient is assessed by the craniofacial team, an assessment is performed at the Sleep Disorders Center. Sleep apnea has been definitely confirmed in one patient with Treacher-Collins syndrome, a repaired cleft, and pharyngeal flap. It has not been demonstrated in any cases of sphincter pharyngoplasty, although postoperative snoring occurs in almost all patients—the price that has to be paid for speech improvement. There has been a concern about development of middle ear infection as a result of this procedure, but all patients have been carefully assessed by the otorhinolaryngologist on the team without establishing any relationship between the two entities.

Why Sphincter Pharyngoplasty?

As stated earlier, it was felt that the procedure carried out for secondary reconstruction of the palate in patients with velopharyngeal incompetence needed to be very closely tailored to the causal elements of the condition. One must be careful not to fall into the trap of attempting to develop a universal cure for a problem that is multifaceted. That philosophy is best summed up by the statement, "When the only tool you have is a hammer, the whole world begins to look like a nail." It seems logical that when the soft palate is functioning adequately but is too short and there is no viable way to make the palate longer, then the answer is to maintain the good palatal function and reduce the dimensions of the velopharyngeal sphincter mechanism, particularly when lateral pharyngeal wall movement is less than optimal. It would be ideal, of course, if the reconstructed sphincter always functioned actively. Although this does happen, it does not occur in every case (Fig. 49–2). Fortunately, due to the upward movement of the soft palate, the lateral walls of the velopharyngeal aperture are pulled forward and tend to close together, unlike the mechanism that closes the vocal cords.

If the muscles of the palate are positioned wrongly, an initial reconstruction of the soft palate levator mechanism should be performed. A proportion of these patients will do very well and will not require any further surgery. Many will achieve a good mobile soft palate but will still have some degree of velopharyngeal incompetence. This latter group comprises patients who can be very well rehabilitated with sphincter pharyngoplasty. Although this approach involves two operations, it is certainly more anatomically and physiologically sound than opting immediately for a pharyngeal flap.

Although healing around the orifice of the velopharyngeal sphincter is not totally controllable following

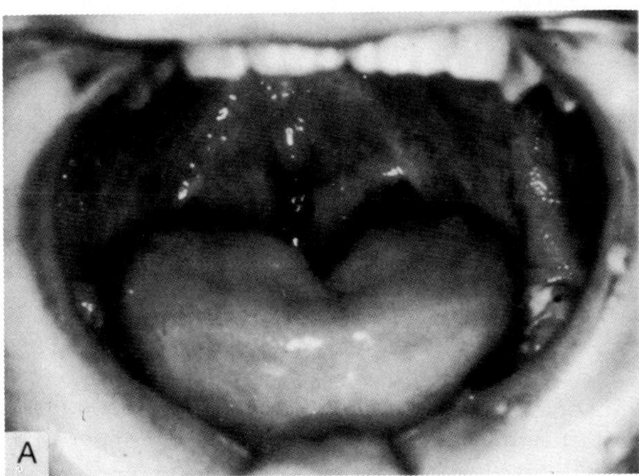
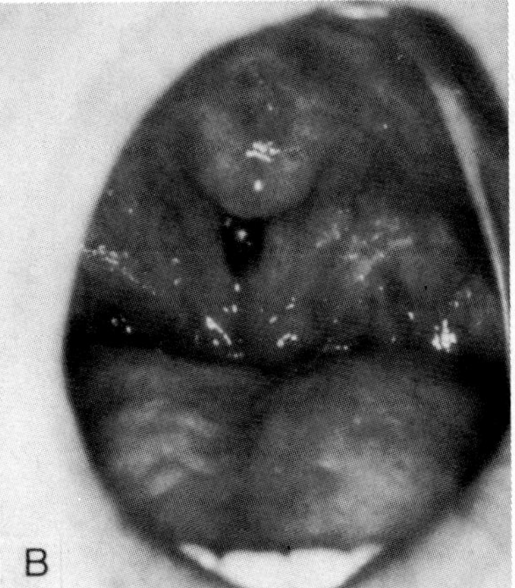
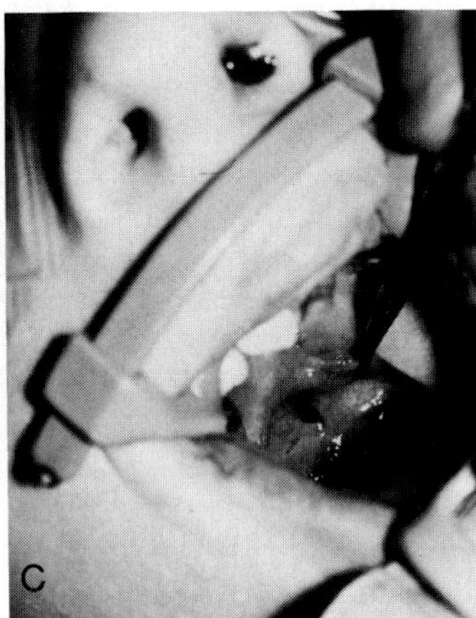
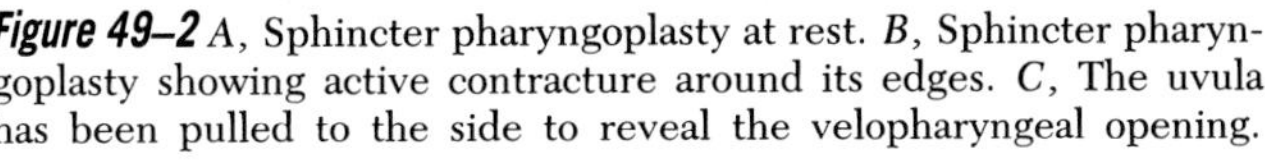

Figure 49–2 A, Sphincter pharyngoplasty at rest. *B*, Sphincter pharyngoplasty showing active contracture around its edges. *C*, The uvula has been pulled to the side to reveal the velopharyngeal opening. The mucomuscular shelf on the posterior pharyngeal wall formed by the drawing in of the posterior pillars of the fauces can be easily seen.

sphincter pharyngoplasty, it is much more so than healing around the lateral ports of the pharyngeal flap. Only one posterior vertical suture line is incorporated in the recreated sphincter; therefore, contracture of the sphincter due to scarring is unlikely to occur. The sphincter may be pulled backward and downward by posterior scarring, thus reducing it to a slit rather than a circle. This result contrasts very favorably with the ports of the pharyngeal flap, which have the capacity to contract rather dramatically. Several patients seen on referral after the so-called "controlled port" operation have had total closure of the velopharyngeal area. In contrast, the opposite problem of pharyngeal flap shrinkage may also occur.

Should persistent hypernasality occur or should hyponasality develop, the sphincter can be further modified. Perhaps one of the most significant advantages of the sphincter pharyngoplasty is the ability to use it when a pharyngeal flap has failed. Satisfactory speech results can be obtained after this procedure (see earlier under Postoperative Progress). As yet, although there have been cases of hyponasality and snoring at night (the latter being a common sequel to operations that narrow the velopharyngeal opening), no cases of true sleep apnea have occurred with the sphincter technique. The operation itself, once the technique is understood, is very easy to do. It also is very quick. There are no residual raw areas and few postoperative symptoms. *It must be stressed, however, that this is not the operation for all patients with velopharyngeal incompetence. It is used only when indicated by careful preoperative assessment.*

In a previous publication, satisfactory results were reported in an independent review of 100 patients with a follow-up of 1 year or longer. Since then, the technique has been modified considerably. The patients are younger, and the results have consequently improved. Sphincter pharyngoplasty was performed in patients with velopharyngeal incompetence, who are considered the ideal candidates for this procedure. The average follow-up was 5.3 years. Of the 46 patients, 42 (91%) were judged to have satisfactory results not requiring any further rehabilitative surgery. Of the four failures, one underwent a Le Fort I maxillary advancement procedure after the pharyngoplasty, and another had his tonsils and adenoids removed. The condition of both these patients had been satisfactory prior to these surgical events. One patient had persistent hypernasality, and the fourth developed hyponasality. These patients responded satisfactorily, although it must be said that speech in the fourth patient continues to be slightly hyponasal.

In a series of 50 patients with pharyngeal flaps that were performed with the customary lack of definite indications for doing the procedure and followed for 8 years, seven required revision, division, or conversion to sphincter pharyngoplasty. Thus, the success rate was 86%; however, in the failures, there were no mitigating circumstances as in the two patients with failure of the sphincter pharyngoplasty. When the pharyngeal flap procedure is chosen for the correct indications, the results seem better, but the clinical sample is too small to make any definite statements. A review of pharyngeal flaps performed for the correct indications has not been reported.

Use of Sphincter Pharyngoplasty in Noncleft Patients

Sphincter pharyngoplasty has previously been reported using the original sphincter operation[8] in 20 noncleft patients, of whom 19 obtained acceptable speech results. In these patients a mixture of trauma, tonsillectomy, and neurologic problems resulted in velopharyngeal incompetence.[9] A further study has been undertaken using the pharyngoplasty procedure described in this chapter with the following results.

Results

This study comprised 12 patients who had velopharyngeal incompetence without clefting and were treated with sphincter pharyngoplasty. Two patients were excluded—one had a congenital absence of the palate, and the other had a palate defect due to carcinoma resection. They both had excellent results following sphincter pharyngoplasty, but it was judged to be incorrect to include them with the study group. Of the remaining ten patients, seven had neurologic deficits (myotonia, one; spastic paralysis, one; hemiplegia, two; palatal paresis, three). One patient had neurofibromatosis, another had just had tonsils and adenoids removed, and in the last patient there was no known cause. In nine patients, there was enough improvement that no further surgery was required. In one patient, a child aged 6 with velocardiofacial syndrome and mental subnormality, there was no change in the speech pattern. Based on results of the previous study and this one, sphincter pharyngoplasty appears to be a useful therapeutic measure in these difficult patients.

Sphincter Pharyngoplasty Following Failed Pharyngeal Flap Surgery

In the past, when a pharyngeal flap failed to control velopharyngeal insufficiency, this was the "end of the road" for the patient. The sphincter pharyngoplasty has changed this outlook. The old flap is divided at the posterior pharyngeal wall and becomes an extension of the soft palate. A standard sphincter pharyngoplasty is then performed to reduce the velopharyngeal aperture.

Results

The patients in this study were mostly referred from other institutions. In eight patients with hyponasality following superiorly based pharyngeal flap surgery the pharyngeal flap was converted to a sphincter pharyngoplasty. Seven required no further surgery, and one was improved but may require further correction. Sixteen patients with hypernasality after pharyngeal flap surgery underwent sphincter pharyngoplasties. Fourteen required no further surgery, and in two the condition is unchanged and further correction is required.

Revision of Sphincter Pharyngoplasties

As stated earlier, four patients required revision in a series of 46. Two had hypernasality due to secondary procedures, maxillary osteotomy, or tonsillectomy. These two and another with hypernasality required no further surgery after revision. The remaining patient with hyponasality improved after revision, although the problem was not entirely eliminated.

Discussion

The sphincter pharyngoplasty described here is a variation of older concepts. The Hynes procedure has some similarities, but such well-defined flaps of mucosa and muscle were not transferred.[10] Moore described a similar technique using the salpingopharyngeus.[11] Orticochea was the true originator of the present-day sphincter concept, but he placed his flaps on an inferiorly based pharyngeal flap.[12–15] This procedure was found to be unsuitable for Caucasians and thus was modified so that the flaps were placed on a superiorly based pharyngeal flap.[16] However, as has been described earlier, it is unnecessary to raise any flaps on the posterior pharyngeal wall. This procedure has produced a velopharyngeal orifice that is more stable and is placed higher in position, which is probably significant from a functional point of view.[3, 16] Reichert described a somewhat similar operation but the flaps were smaller and contained no muscle.[17] This procedure has been used occasionally in very mild cases of velopharyngeal incompetence. Pigott, noting the similarity between the Hynes and Orticochea procedures, has coined the term *Hynacochea*.[18]

Many others have now begun to use the sphincter technique and have reported on their good results.[19, 20] Others have expressed their satisfaction in discussion either privately or openly at meetings. Frequently, when the technique is presented, it is seen by proponents of pharyngeal flaps as a direct attack on this procedure. This attitude shows a lack of appreciation that the technique is a refinement that has only become possible because of the newer techniques of investigation. It is performed when it is indicated, as is a pharyngeal flap, although it has to be said that as one becomes experienced and comfortable with this procedure, it is the most common rehabilitative measure employed. This is as it should be because today all palates should have good mobility, and therefore one shrinks from placing anything in the soft palate that might in any way interfere with this much valued movement. The fact that the velopharyngeal aperture does not retract because of the lack of raw areas and circumferential incisions is significant.

We have seen no cases of sleep apnea. This is due to the fact that the aperture can only increase in size. It will never *decrease* because scarring is minimal and occurs in a vertical rather than a horizontal direction. Thus, the disastrous total closure of the velopharyngeal area, which occurs occasionally with pharyngeal flaps, has not been seen. Hyponasality or hypernasality tends to exist for 3 months after surgery when the local reaction has settled; there is little change in the speech pattern established after this.[8] Revision of the velopharyngeal opening is possible, and the procedure can be used to rehabilitate the patient who has a failed pharyngeal flap. In patients requiring Le Fort I or Le Fort II advancement, the sphincter pharyngoplasty has never caused any obstruction to advancement, a problem that has occurred on several occasions with pharyngeal flaps, which, when tight and scarred, have required division. In all of these cases, rehabilitation has been performed using sphincter pharyngoplasty 6 months after the maxillary advancement. The availability of this procedure has allowed treatment of velopharyngeal incompetence to be eminently more logical, and, it is hoped, has produced consistently better results in the cases in which it is indicated.

References

1. Rosenthal W: Zur Frage der Gaumenplastic. Zentralbl Cir 51:1621, 1924.
2. Sanvanero-Rosselli G: Divisione palatine e sua cura chirurgica. Atti Con Int Stomatol 36:391, 1935.
3. Jackson IT: Sphincter pharyngoplasty. Clin Plast Surg 12:711, 1985.
4. Skolnick ML: Video velopharyngography in patients with nasal speech with emphasis on lateral pharyngeal motion in velopharyngeal closure. Radiology 93:747, 1969.
5. Bardach J, Salyer K: Surgical Techniques in Cleft Lip and Palate. Chicago: Year Book, 1987.
6. Orticochea M: Personal communication, 1978.
7. MacKenzie-Stepner K, Stringer DA, Lindsay WK, et al: Abnormal carotid arteries in the velocardiofacial syndrome: A report of three cases. Plast Reconstr Surg 80:347, 1987.
8. Jackson IT, Silverton JS: Sphincter pharyngoplasty as a secondary procedure in cleft palate. Plast Reconstr Surg 59:518, 1977.
9. Jackson IT, McGlynn M, Huskie CF: Velopharyngeal incompetence in the absence of cleft palate. Results of treatment in 20 cases. Plast Reconstr Surg 66:211, 1980.
10. Hynes W: Pharyngoplasty by muscle transplantation. Br J Plast Surg 3:138, 1950.
11. Moore FT: A new operation to cure nasopharyngeal incompetence. Br J Surg 47:424, 1960.
12. Orticochea M: Construction of a dynamic muscle sphincter in cleft palates. Plast Reconstr Surg 41:323, 1968.
13. Orticochea M: Results of the dynamic muscle sphincter operation. Br J Plast Surg 23:108, 1970.
14. Orticochea M: Indications et opportunité chirurgicale du sphincter musculaire dynamique du pharynx. Ann Chir Plast 19:5, 1974.
15. Orticochea M: A review of 236 cleft palate patients treated with dynamic muscle sphincter. Plast Reconstr Surg 71:180, 1983.
16. Jackson IT: A review of 236 cleft palate patients treated with dynamic muscle sphincter. Plast Reconstr Surg 71:187, 1983.
17. Reichert H: The lateral velopharyngoplasty: A new method for the correction of open nasality. J Maxillofac Surg 2:95, 1974.
18. Pigott RW: Personal communication, 1984.
19. Stratoudakis AC, Bambace C: Sphincter pharyngoplasty for correction of velopharyngeal incompetence. Ann Plast Surg 12:243, 1984.
20. Riski JE, Serafin D, Riefkohl R, et al: A rationale for modifying the site of insertion of the Orticochea pharyngoplasty. Plast Reconstr Surg 73:882, 1984.

CHAPTER 50

Bilateral Transverse Pharyngeal Flaps for Hypernasal Speech

Donald I. Kapetansky

Designing a surgical procedure to assist with palatal function requires many considerations. The basic problem usually is inadequate flow resistance control by the combined motion of the palate with the posterior and lateral pharyngeal walls.[1, 2] Adequacy of the nasal passages is essential for the nonturbulent flow of air for normal resonance in speech production. Healing in the nasopharynx after any surgical procedure must permit normal airflow through the nose so that normal nasal physiologic processes can continue to function.

Airflow through the nose is necessary for drainage of the nasal sinuses and function of the middle ear through the eustachian tube. Nasal obstruction also can cause difficulty with chewing and swallowing. In addition, pleasurable kissing is very difficult if the nose is obstructed.

The surgical procedure required to correct a hypernasal speech problem must be designed so that adequate air passes from the mouth and nose.[3–14] The mechanism allowing passage of air must be constructed to permit control of the amount of air needed or closed off completely depending on the particular phoneme. We have been disappointed with the long-term results of vertical pharyngeal flaps because the lateral apertures produced may vary in size with progression of healing. Often the central obturation gradually diminishes, the pharyngeal flap "tubes" being due to the remaining raw surface.

Owsley demonstrated in dogs that vertical incisions on the posterior pharyngeal wall through the constrictor muscles cause loss of motor innervation.[15] We performed biopsies on 23 vertical pharyngeal flap samples and consistently demonstrated loss of striated muscle fibers under microscopic examination.[16] Clinically, this results in further shrinking of the tissue and can lead to total detachment of the flap after a long period of time. Therefore, we felt that the design of the surgical procedure should preserve the motor innervation, in this case, branches of the ninth and tenth cranial nerves, to the constrictor muscles so that the obturator effect would be maintained. Additionally, continuity of the lateral wall muscle fibers with the muscle bundles extending into the pharyngeal flap tissue could have the potential to further stimulate lateral wall motion.[17]

Design of the New Variable Air Resistor

We designed our first new procedure to see if the muscle component of the pharyngeal flap construction could be modified to allow maintenance of the mass of the healed tissue.[18, 19] Our observations revealed a great tendency for healed vertical pharyngeal flaps to shrink. In some patients merely the size of the pedicle diminished, but in others the flap continued to shrink and progressed to detachment of the flap in 2 to 5 years. Many patients initially had good early speech results with elimination of hypernasality; however, due to the changes in the pharyngeal flap, hypernasality gradually returned.

When constructing a vertical flap, surgeons expect some narrowing of the healed tissues owing to a tubing effect unless the raw surface of the flap is covered with a mucosal flap. A serious disadvantage of the vertical pharyngeal flap is that vertical incisions denervate the constrictor muscles enclosed in the flap tissue because the ninth and tenth cranial nerves (motor) are severed during these procedures.

Therefore, to maintain the mass of the constructed pharyngeal flap, the muscles and ninth and tenth cranial nerves must be dissected as a unit (unless neoneurotization can be anticipated, as in the Abbe flap correction for the lip). A series of 23 vertical pharyngeal flap samples were subjected to biopsy for microscopic examination of the muscles. No striated muscle bundles were present in any of these specimens.

The first procedure required is removal of the tonsils and adenoids, usually 1 or 2 months prior to the flap surgery. If the tonsils are not removed, they obturate the small lateral ports, which must remain open for breathing and speech. The adenoids are removed to prevent bleeding that may occur during surgery and would be difficult to control. In three patients, normal speech occurred after tonsillectomy.[20, 21]

Speech assessment can be done as early as 2.5 to 3 years of age. Hypernasality varies in grade of intensity. Speech therapy is given a 6-month trial in some borderline cases. We feel that early speech or surgical intervention is indicated once a positive diagnosis of hypernasality is made. The longer a child substitutes or omits sounds, the more difficult it may become to correct speech with therapy. Moreover, the psychological frustration of the child is usually manifested in overt antisocial behavior. After all, if a child cannot communicate verbally, he may often resort to a form of antisocial behavior to gain attention to his needs.

Our observation of the remarkable change in behavior of these children following surgery has enlightened us to the severe stress to which the speech-impaired child can be subjected. The behavior is manifest as body language because the child's attempt to communicate before surgery is expressed with very physical mannerisms. This behavior contrasts with the more docile postoperative state when speech communication is effective and the smile of the joy of human expression pervades. Many of these children have been placed on medication used for "overactive" and "difficult" children and are able to discontinue the medication when normal speech communication is effective. Grandparents routinely note the ability to communicate by telephone after surgery, an ability that is lacking before surgery, probably owing to the lack of visual cues when using a telephone for conversation.

Our preference is to admit the child to the hospital on the morning of surgery. Most patients are observed in the hospital for one night following surgery. Surgery is performed using general, oral, endotracheal anesthesia. The Dingman mouth gag or similar device greatly aids in the exposure of this difficult surgical area. The soft palate and posterior pharyngeal wall are infiltrated with a long-acting local anesthetic. We now use 0.25% lidocaine with 0.125% bupivacaine and 1:300,000 epinephrine. This has three important effects; the lidocaine acts quickly and the bupivacaine lasts more than 10 hours, giving the anesthesia personnel an opportunity to carry the patient under a lighter general anesthesia; wake-up time is shorter, and spontaneous respirations are more easily maintained during surgery. Finally, not only does the adrenalin assist in prolonging the local anesthetic effect but the minimal bleeding also is a great help for providing clarity of the surgical field and for allowing accuracy of dissection and ease of suture placement.[22, 23] The use of local anesthesia does not affect the ability to swallow or breathe after surgery.

To save anesthesia time, we usually inject the local anesthetic solution prior to draping the patient and adjusting the table, lights, and instruments. Five minutes after the local anesthetic has been injected, the surgery begins. The full thickness of the entire uvula is split with a midline incision (Fig. 50–1A). The levator muscle is not incised. The hemiuvulae are retracted with sutures (we prefer 5–0 polyglycolic acid suture material). A No. 15 scalpel is used to start the first oblique incision. Usually one can start higher on the left side and extend the incision obliquely across the posterior pharynx to the right side, almost at a transverse level. The incision is usually 3 to 4 cm in length (Fig. 50–1B).

The second incision starts at least 2 cm lower on the left and ends at a point more than 1 cm lower on the right and crosses the posterior pharyngeal wall almost

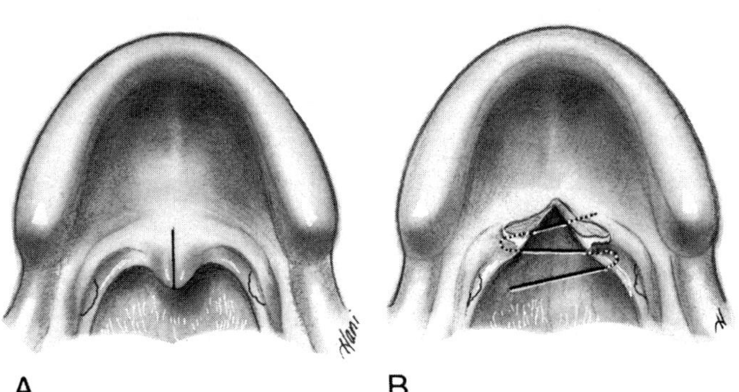

A   B

Figure 50–1 *A*, The uvula is split, and the S-shaped incision is outlined on the posterior pharyngeal wall. *B*, The two pharyngeal flaps are elevated and retracted, and the donor site is partially repaired.

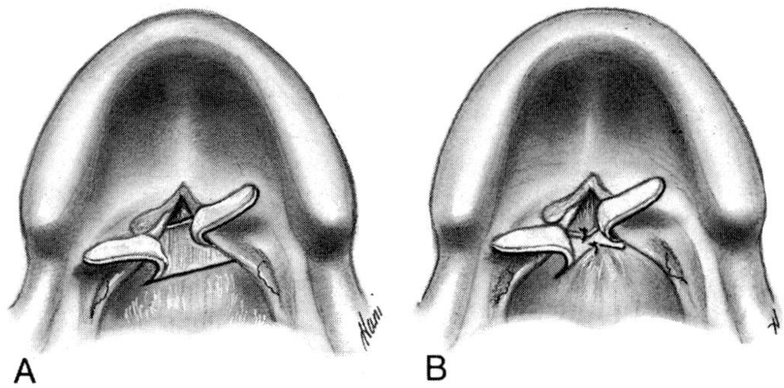

A   B

Figure 50–2 *A*, The S-shaped incision is cut and elevated. *B*, The donor site is repaired.

transversely. The third incision starts from a point at least 1 cm lower on the left and extends to a point more than 2 cm lower on the right in an oblique direction. The constrictor muscle fibers are bluntly dissected in the planes of each of these three incisions down to the prevertebral fascia. Tunneling at this deep level under the three incisions connects the dissection at this level of the tissue plane in the prevertebral fascia. The first two incisions are connected at the far right by a semicircular incision, defining the first pedicle. The second and third incisions are similarly connected at the left side, defining the second pedicle. Sutures are placed through the tip of each flap for retraction (Fig. 50–2A). Important branches of the carotid arteries, such as the ascending pharyngeal arteries, must be avoided during surgery. This artery was frequently seen in our series of patients, but injury of these vessels was consistently avoided.

The donor site was left unrepaired in a small series of patients. Although minimal bleeding during surgery was observed from the open wound of the posterior pharynx, occasional postoperative bleeding was more troublesome. Closure of the wound on the posterior pharyngeal wall occludes the bleeding source. One patient in this series of 800 had a severe bleeding problem and required a blood transfusion and revision of the wound. In all the remaining patients the donor site was repaired with no further bleeding problems. The repair places tension along the wound margins, aiding blood vessel retraction and coagulation. The first polyglycolic suture is carried through the midline of the prevertebral fascia and the left inferior wound edge of musculomucosal tissues (Fig. 50–2B). This suture is tied with some tension, but not too tightly. The second suture also extends from the prevertebral fascia to the right superior musculomucosal tissues.

Following closure of the donor area, we proceed with the definitive placement of the two transverse pharyngeal flaps. The left and more superiorly based pedicle is turned on its long axis (Fig. 50–3A) and sutured into the nasal aspect of the uvula and soft palate defect. The first suture extends from the cephalad edge of the flap to the right hemiuvula, defining the left aperture. The next sutures advance the flap in the nasal aspect of the dissection. Although the soft palate incision opens the soft palate, the levator muscles are usually anterior to the repair and are not divided.

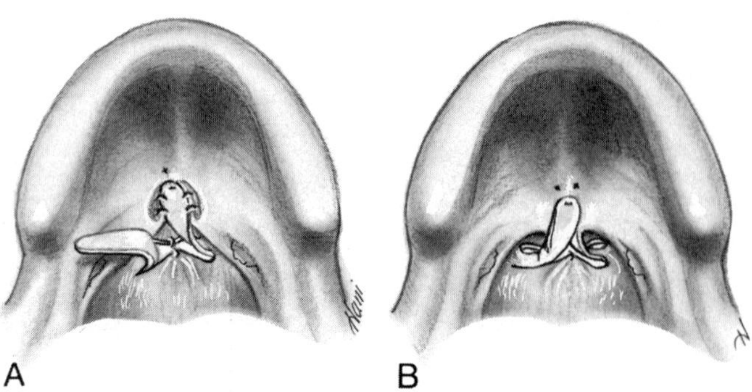

Figure 50–3 *A,* Suture in numbered order for the cranial (left) flap. *B,* The caudal (right) flap is cut and inset into the oral side of the palate by the suture numbers.

The tip of the pedicle is maintained in the crotch of the incision by using a retraction suture and converting it to a horizontal mattress suture. The nasal side of the repair is completed with sutures from the right side of the uvula to the caudal side of the pedicle. Finally, the right and more caudally based flap is brought into the oral side of the palate and directly sutured to the uvula halves with interrupted sutures (Fig. 50–3*B*). A horizontal mattress suture takes up the tension in the tip, using a converted retraction suture. No bleeding should be apparent. Levin's tube is used to suction the stomach. Hexadrol is given parenterally during the procedure, usually 2 mg intramuscularly and 2 mg intravenously, to minimize postoperative airway problems. Thus, the use of the steam tent is obviated.

Postoperative Management

Intravenous hydration during and following surgery is extremely important because dehydration produces an increased amount of postoperative discomfort for the patient. We find it extremely important to try to discuss the postoperative management with the patient prior to surgery. A child as young as 3 years of age is able to cooperate in his or her postoperative care. Simple preoperative discussion with the patient that drinking after surgery will make him or her feel better and will ease any discomfort is all that is necessary. The word *pain* is not used; *discomfort* is used instead. Patients are advised that they will be given sips of water or apple juice, soda pop that has gone "flat," or anything else they would like to drink. It is emphasized that the more they drink, the less discomfort they will experience. This preoperative training has been very successful in getting the youngsters to drink after surgery.

Postoperatively, fluids must be offered about every 20 minutes after the anesthetic effects wear off and the tendency for emesis is no longer a factor. This maintains hydration and minimizes pain. Usually room temperature fluids are preferred by the patient. Apple juice is better than citrus juice, which can sting the raw tissues. Colas and soda pop can be used if the carbonation is allowed to dissolve into the air. Flavored ices on a stick are preferred by some of our patients. If hydration is thus maintained, the temperature of the patient will remain near normal. Usually, the patients drink satis-

factorily within 3 hours after surgery, and they can be released from the hospital on the morning after surgery.

Fortunately, the use of local anesthesia during the operation greatly assists in carrying the patient in a lighter plane of general anesthesia, which also permits more rapid recovery.

Pain is controlled with elixir of Tylenol 60 mg per year of age up to 600 mg, and codeine 1 mg per 4 lb up to 30 mg, given every 4 hours as needed for pain. Plain Tylenol elixir also is very effective.

Some stiffness of the neck may be apparent for 3 to 7 days following surgery, usually concerning the family more than the patient. Many of the patients do not ingest food in the first week after surgery and will often lose a small amount of weight. It has been our experience that this weight is replaced rapidly in the second and third weeks following the surgical procedure. Therefore, we concentrate mostly on maintaining adequate hydration until the appetite returns. As would be expected, there is a great amount of variation in this, and some youngsters go back to eating quite satisfactorily within 1 or 2 days after the surgical procedure.

The pyramidal raw surface between the two flaps and the posterior pharyngeal wall are used for a nasal respiratory passage after surgery. As this closes down with healing, this "planned" scar formation will open the two lateral ports for breathing and speech. Speech therapy usually begins about 1 month after surgery, and rapid improvement in the degree of hypernasality is usually seen.

Fine-Tuning Procedure

Failure to obtain optimal speech results usually means that the lateral ports are not the ideal size for the patient. In about 5% of patients further reduction in size of the ports is needed; in about 1%, the ports need further enlargement. An adjustment procedure has been designed to correct these problems. This procedure is performed on an outpatient basis, requires less than 30 minutes of operative time, and usually involves minimal postoperative pain. General anesthesia is used in most cases. The same local anesthetic solution as used in the primary procedure is infiltrated; bleeding is then of little consequence, facilitating visualization for the placement of sutures. To reduce the size of the apertures, a flap of mucosa and submucosa is raised on the oral surface of the posterior border of the soft palate, with an incision along a line about 6 mm from the posterior border of the soft palate (Fig. 50–4). The flap is carefully elevated (Fig. 50–5) and sutured (Fig. 50–6) into an incised pocket along the side of the constructed pharyngeal pedicle. With variation in the placement of these incisions, the aperture can be reduced to one-half or one-third of its size. The design of these two flaps can be reversed, incising the midline of the pharyngeal pedicle (Fig. 50–7). This flap is brought laterally (Fig. 50–8) after raising a flap from the nasal aspect of the soft palate (Fig. 50–9).

In the small group of patients in whom denasality results as healing progresses, the apertures can be

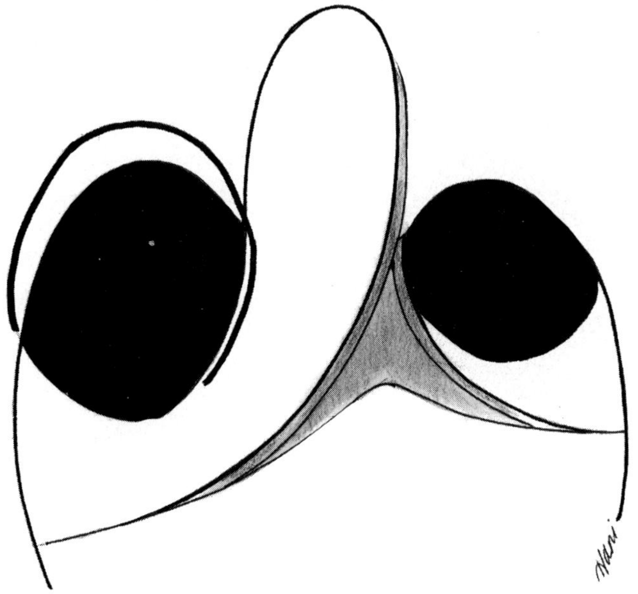

Figure 50–4 Reduction of the portal with incision along the side of the pharyngeal obturator extending onto the oral surface of the soft palate.

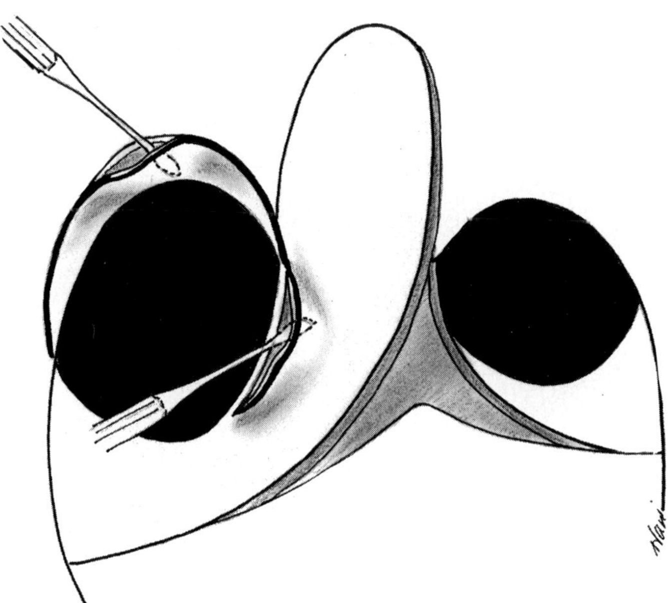

Figure 50–5 Blunt dissection of the tissue.

Figure 50–6 Interdigitation of the two flaps.

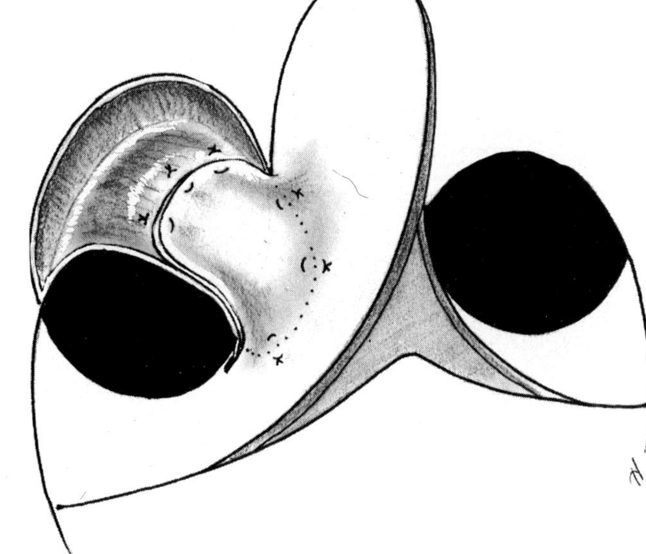

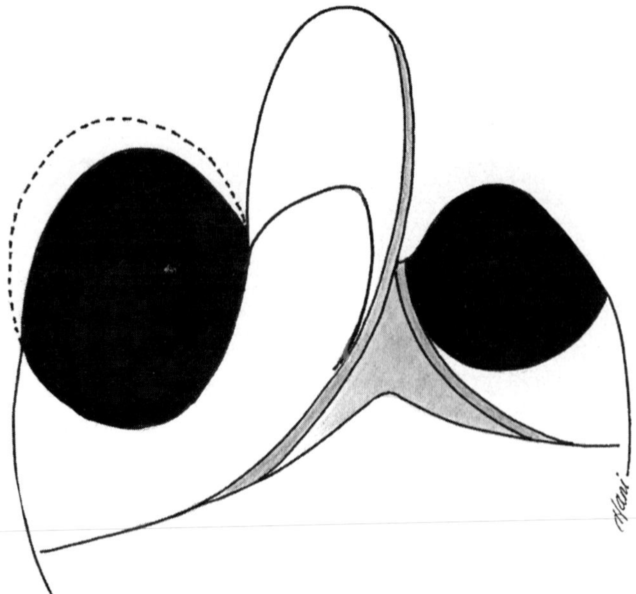

Figure 50–7 Alternate portal reduction by inverted V-incision of the pharyngeal obturator, continuing onto the nasal aspect of the soft palate.

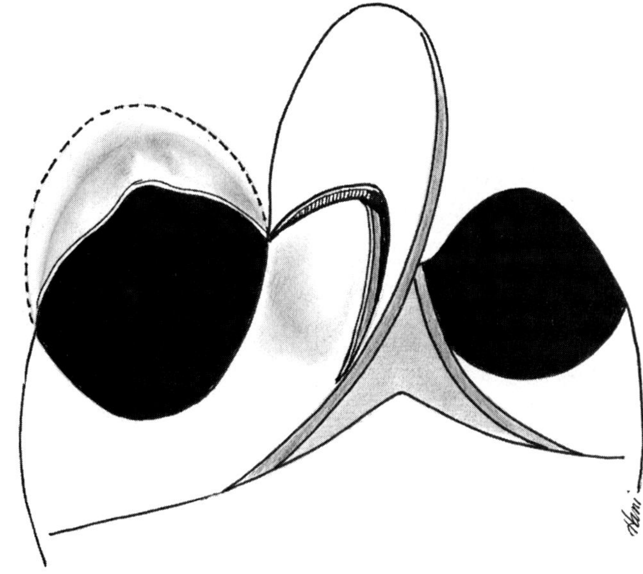

Figure 50–8 Elevation of the flaps.

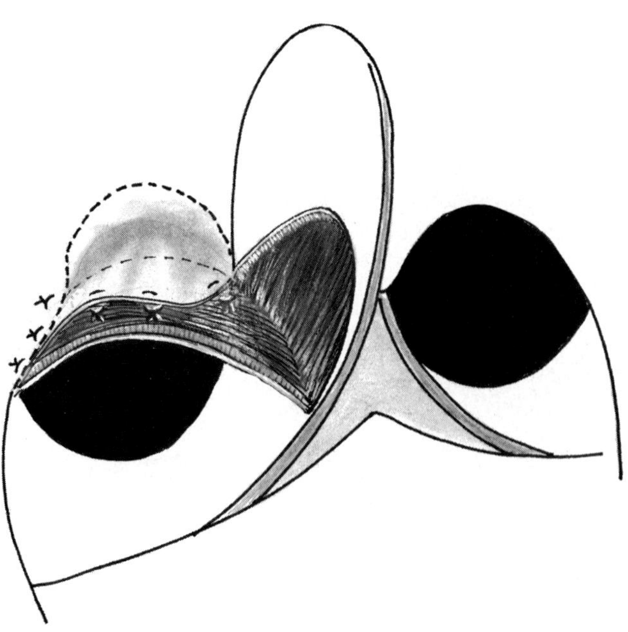

Figure 50–9 Interdigitation of the two flaps.

opened by the use of a **Y-V** advancement flap at the perimeter or a **Z**-plasty along the aperture margin.

The New Modified Procedure

Improvement of the transverse pharyngeal flap procedure was developed for patients who had a very short soft palate. Instead of placing the two pharyngeal flaps at the midline, each flap was inserted into overlapping portions of the breadth of the posterior border of the soft palate (Fig. 50–6). This configuration was so successful that we have used this as our procedure of choice except for patients with submucous cleft palate. Most patients with submucous cleft palate have a sufficient amount of soft palate tissue, and the clinical results in this group of patients were rarely disappointing following use of our original primary procedure. Our group of submucous cleft palate patients numbers 272 of the 800 cases reviewed for this report.

Our revised primary procedure also requires preliminary removal of tonsils and adenoids, with a check on the need for pressure equalization tubes, usually 6 to 8 weeks prior to this pharyngeal flap procedure. We prefer a 2-week period of normal respiratory health if the patient develops an upper respiratory infection. General anesthesia is controlled with an oral endotracheal tube system. Both general and local anesthesia are used as previously described.

The posterior portion of the soft palate and the posterior pharyngeal wall are infiltrated with a local anesthetic solution of 0.25% lidocaine, 0.125% bupivacaine, and 1:300,000 epinephrine. The lidocaine gives rapid onset of local anesthesia, the bupivacaine gives prolonged anesthesia, and the adrenalin permits a drier field for ease of identification of the surgical anatomy. The use of local anesthesia also permits a lighter general anesthetic and a more rapid recovery postoperatively.

The first incision is made in a lazy-**S** shape, extending across the posterior border of the soft palate (Fig. 50–10A). It crosses the midline at the center of the posterior edge of the palate and extends on each side along a line 5 or 6 mm anterior to the posterior border. On the right half the incision is on the oral aspect, and on the left side the incision runs on the nasal aspect of the palate. Both arms of this incision are carried laterally to the full extent of the soft palate. Submucosal mobilization (Fig. 50–10B) is done carefully to avoid entering the muscles of the soft palate. Retraction sutures of polyglycolic acid on noncutting needles through these dissected palatal flaps can be used to expose the posterior pharyngeal wall.

The three incisions on the posterior pharyngeal wall are planned (Fig. 50–10A). The first incision begins high on the left side, as high as the constrictor muscles extend. It extends slightly obliquely from left to right and ends somewhat lower on the right side than on the left side. The second incision begins at least 2 cm lower on the left side and extends to a minimum of 1 cm lower on the right side and is almost horizontal. The third incision begins at least 1 cm lower on the left side

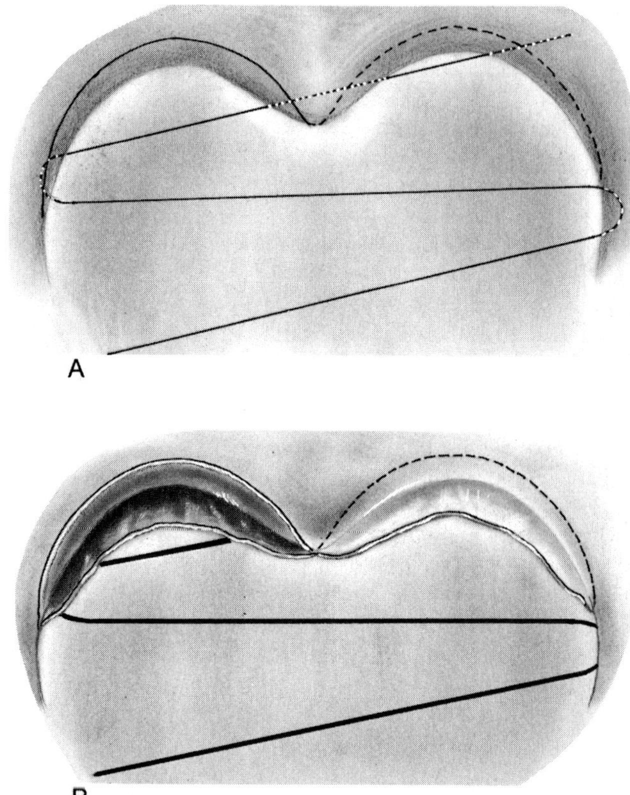

Figure 50–10 *A*, Long S-shaped incision along the posterior border of the soft palate, and wide S-shaped incision of the posterior pharyngeal wall. *B*, Opened posterior soft palate.

and extends to a point minimally 2 cm lower on the right side.

By blunt dissection the three incisions are carried perpendicularly down to the prevertebral fascia, being careful to preserve the innervation for the ninth and tenth cranial nerves on the deep aspect of the constrictor muscle fibers. The two flaps are elevated at the level of the prevertebral fascia by blunt dissection, preserving the innervation. When this is completed, the tips of the two flaps are cut in a semicircle. The cranial flap is based on the left side, and the caudal flap is based on the right side. The tips of these flaps are held with 5–0 polyglycolic acid sutures for retraction. At this point there is a minimal amount of bleeding, and control of bleeding is accomplished using a 3–0 polyglycolic acid suture from the midline prevertebral fascia to the left inferior musculomucosal tissues (Fig. 50–12A). Occasionally, a second suture is used to help bring this tissue up under some tension but not excessively tight because the donor site does not need to be completely closed. The purpose of these sutures is to create tension along the incision lines so that there will be minimal risk of postoperative bleeding. A second suture or two also is placed from the midline prevertebral fascia upward to the right superior musculomucosal incision. These sutures also are tied with some tension for control of bleeding on the wound margin. Once these sutures are tied, bleeding is usually no problem, and only rarely is electrocoagulation required to assist with any further bleeding sites.

The actual attachment of the pharyngeal pedicles occurs at this point in the procedure. The left, cranial-based flap is brought into the posterior border of the soft palate and rotated on its long axis so that its caudal border is first sutured to the nasal mucosa with interrupted 5–0 polyglycolic acid sutures (Figs. 50–11A and 50–12A). The repair continues along the left posterior palatal border on the nasal aspect with interrupted sutures. Small bites of the pedicle tissue are taken to avoid impairment of the circulation of the pedicle for healing. At the midline the retraction suture that had been placed in the pedicle is used for a mattress suture and is brought to the right of the midline and oriented to bring the cranial pharyngeal pedicle into the nasal aspect (Fig. 50–12A). This mattress suture releases the tension on the repair. Usually a single suture is used to bring the mucosal tissue from the right side of the soft palate over to the left transverse pedicle to open the tissues on the posterior border of the soft palate (Fig. 50–12A). This also creates an additional margin for adhesion of the first pedicle to the nasal aspect of the soft palate and helps to lengthen the palate border, which is especially useful in the patient with severe shortening of the soft palate.

When this process has been completed, the surgery proceeds by bringing the right pharyngeal flap up into the oral aspect of the soft palate (Figs. 50–11B and 50–12B). The first suture is taken at the extreme right side

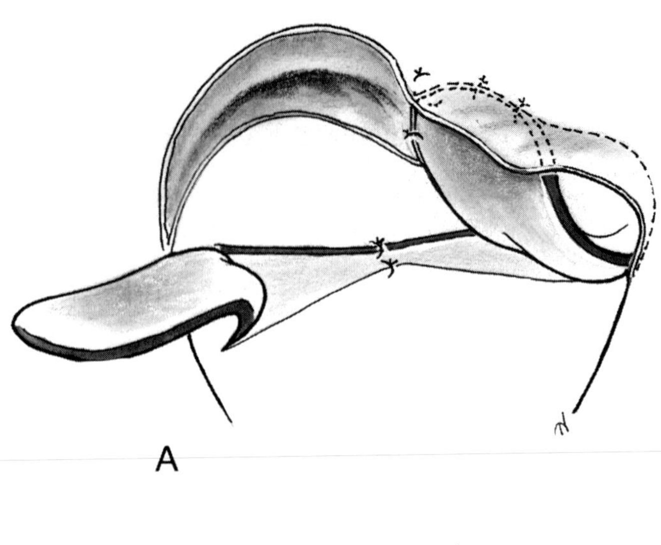

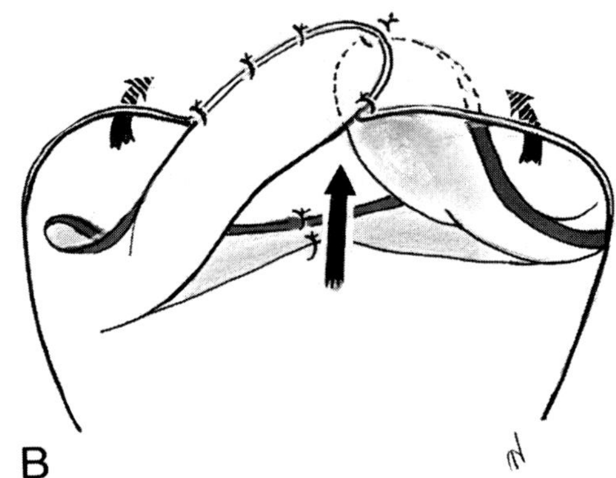

A

B

Figure 50–12 *A*, Partial closure of donor site; rotation and insertion of flap into the soft palate. *B*, Advancement onto oral surface of soft palate with lateral portals indicated.

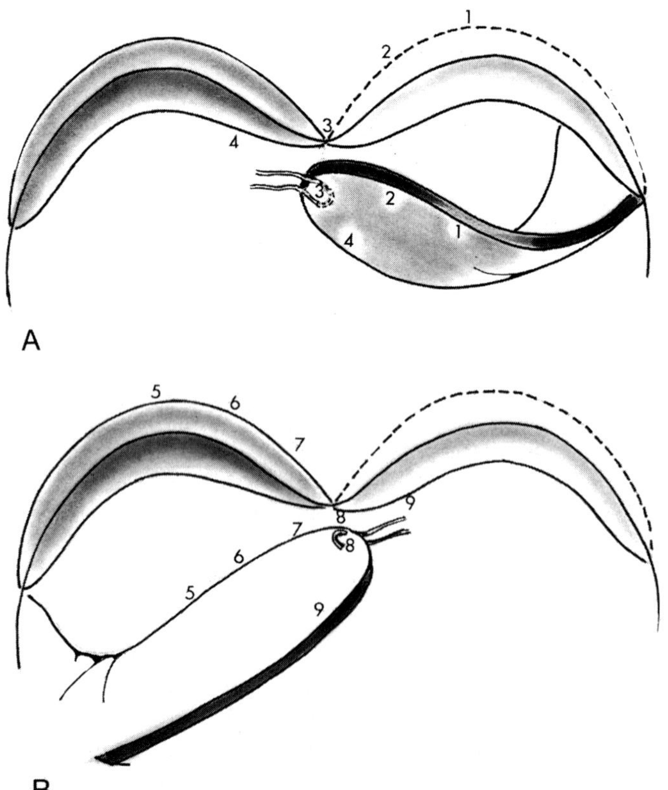

A

B

Figure 50–11 *A*, Suture order of cranial (left) flap. *B*, Suture order of caudal (right) flap.

of the soft palate to a position near the base of the pedicle. Again, these sutures take a small bite on the pedicle side. The circulation should not be impaired by placement of these sutures. A row of sutures is continued along the posterior border of the soft palate (usually two or three more sutures are needed), bringing the tip of the flap into the center of the soft palate. Here the center of the palate is fixed to the pedicle using the previously placed tip traction suture to form a mattress suture. This suture releases the tension caused by placement of this pedicle. The final suture or two is placed on the left side of this pedicle to bring some of the left-sided soft palate tissues over to give a broader area of adhesion. The end result of this repair is the placement of as much tissue as possible from the soft palate into contact with the two pharyngeal flaps. Thus healing can progress over as wide an area as possible, maximizing the area of the soft palate. The postoperative protocol followed is the same as that described for the previous procedure, the new variable air resistor.

Observation of healing has shown that the tissues do not tend to shrink but instead maintain or enlarge the tissue apparent in this area. The tissue in an extremely small soft palate can be augmented in this fashion, and if necessary a second small operation consisting of turnover flaps can be used to further increase the size of the apparent tissue in the soft palate area and decrease the size of the two ports used for speech, breathing, and swallowing.

Speech therapy is usually started or restarted approximately 1 month after the surgical procedure. If hypernasality does not decrease, the secondary procedure of turnover flaps is used because we have found that less satisfactory results occur in patients in whom the lateral ports have healed with an unusually large aperture on one or both sides. Younger patients seem to improve extremely rapidly, perhaps because they have had less time to try to compensate for the speech difficulties usually encountered with hypernasality.

Evaluation of Results

One of our earliest studies was an attempt to see if the constrictor muscles and their innervation by the ninth and tenth cranial nerves were able to survive and function after the transfer procedure. Patients were evaluated 6 months after the pharyngeal flap procedure. In a study designed by McClung using bipolar electrodes, the muscle activity in the pharyngeal flap was analyzed. The bipolar leads were brought out to a Honeywell standard recording device. The leads were set to record during speech and swallowing. The results showed consistent electric potentials during muscle activity.

A second study was carried out with standard speech recordings before and after surgery. These recordings were mixed into a master tape using a standard series of random numbers. The tapes were than played for a group of untrained listeners to rate intelligibility on a numbered scale from zero to five. The results were analyzed for matching preoperative and postoperative tapes. The difference in speech assessment was significant at the p = .05 level. The entire study was supervised by the professor of speech pathology at Wayne State University, Mervyn Falk.

A third study was carried out to examine a random group of patients by nasendoscopy. This study was done under the experienced supervision of Dr. Robert Shprintzen. The results of this evaluation showed lateral wall motion in all of the patients. In a separate group of 1000 subjects, Shprintzen was able to demonstrate good lateral wall motion in only one-third of the patients.

Summary

Eight hundred patients have now undergone the transverse pharyngeal flap procedure in the past 16 years. In contrast with the reports in the literature,[24] we have had no mortality. Long-term follow-up has brought some problems to our attention as well as valuable conclusions. The patient with a submucous cleft responds extremely well to the midline attachment of the paired pharyngeal flaps. We had 272 patients in this subgroup. Only on rare occasions was a second procedure required to adjust the twin portals.

Patients with repaired cleft palates with residual hypernasality do better with the modified attachment of the twin pharyngeal flaps to the entire posterior border of the soft palate. Indeed, the hypoplastic soft palate can be variably augmented with this design. A second procedure is needed in about 5% of cases to further reduce the lateral ports: in about 1% of cases these twin ports need to be enlarged for ideal speech control.

Objective data on speech results are elusive, and it is difficult to compare one group of treated patients with another group undergoing a standardized method of therapy in a different locality. Observation revealed that prior to surgery 90% of our patients could not be understood in telephone conversation by a family member, and the remaining 10% had great difficulty with this form of communication. Following this procedure, almost all of our patients were easily understood over the telephone.

References

1. Dalston RM, Warren DW: Comparison of Tonar II, pressure-flow and listener judgments of hypernasality in the assessment of velopharyngeal function. Cleft Palate J 23:108, 1986.
2. Redenbaugh MA, Reich AR: Correspondence between an accelerometric nasal/voice amplitude ratio and listeners' direct magnitude estimations of hypernasality. J Speech Hear Res 28:273, 1985.
3. Skoog T: The pharyngeal flap operation in cleft palate. A clinical study of eighty-two cases. Br J Plast Surg 18:265, 1965.
4. Brondsted K, Liisberg WB, Orsted A, et al: Surgical and speech results following palatopharyngoplasty operations in Denmark 1959–1977. Cleft Palate J 21:170, 1984.
5. Stueber K, Wilhelmsen HR: Use of the pharyngeal flap in the treatment of congenital velopharyngeal incompetence. Plast Reconstr Surg 73:219, 1984.
6. Younger R, Dickson RI: Adult pharyngoplasty for velopharyngeal insufficiency. J Otolaryngol 14:158, 1985.
7. Longacre JJ, DeStefano GA: The role of the posterior pharyngeal flap in rehabilitation of the patient with cleft palate. Am J Surg 94:882, 1957.
8. Owsley JQ, Blackfield HM: The technique and complications of pharyngeal flap surgery. Plast Reconstr Surg 35:531, 1965.
9. Trigos I, Ysunza A, Gonzalez A, et al: Surgical treatment of borderline velopharyngeal insufficiency using homologous cartilage implantation with videonasopharyngoscopic monitoring. Cleft Palate J 25:167, 1988.
10. Coston GN, Hagerty RF, Jannarone RJ, et al: Levator muscle reconstruction: Resulting velopharyngeal competence—a preliminary report. Plast Reconstr Surg 77:911, 1986.
11. Orticochea M: Indications and the convenient moment for surgery of the dynamic muscle sphincter of the pharynx. Ann Chir Plast 19:5, 1974.
12. Orticochea M: A review of 236 cleft palate patients treated with dynamic muscle sphincter. Plast Reconstr Surg 71:180, 1983.
13. Orticochea M: Treatment of hypertrophic tonsils and adenoids in the patient operated on for cleft palate with dynamic muscular sphincter of the pharynx. Ann Chir Plast 22:81, 1977.
14. Furlow LT, Jr, Williams WN, Eisenbach CR, 2nd, et al: A long-term study on treating velopharyngeal insufficiency by Teflon injection. Cleft Palate J 19:47, 1982.
15. Owsley JQ, Creech BJ, Dedo H: Poor speech following the pharyngeal flap operation: Etiology and treatment. Cleft Palate J 9:312, 1972.
16. Kapetansky DI: Techniques in Cleft Lip, Nose and Palate Reconstruction. Philadelphia: Lippincott, 1987.
17. Shprintzen RJ, McCall GN, Skolnick ML: The effect of pharyngeal flap surgery on the movements of the lateral pharyngeal walls. Plast Reconstr Surg 66:570, 1980.
18. Kapetansky DI: Bilateral transverse pharyngeal flaps for repair of cleft palate. Plast Reconstr Surg 52:52, 1973.
19. Kapetansky DI: Transverse pharyngeal flaps: A dynamic repair for velopharyngeal insufficiency. Cleft Palate J 12:44, 1975.
20. MacKenzie-Stepner K, Witzel MA, Stringer DA, et al: Velopharyngeal insufficiency due to hypertrophic tonsils. A report of two cases. Int J Pediatr Otorhinolaryngol 14:57, 1987.
21. Shprintzen RJ, Sher AE, Croft CB: Hypernasal speech caused by tonsillar hypertrophy. Int J Pediatr Otorhinolaryngol 14:45, 1987.
22. Klingenstrom P, Westermark L: Local effects of adrenaline and phenylalanine-lysyl-vasopressin in local anesthesia. Acta Anaesth Scand 7:131, 1963.
23. Klingenstrom P, Westermark L: Local tissue oxygen-tension after adrenaline, noradrenaline and Octapressin in local anaesthesia. Acta Anaesth Scand 8:261, 1964.
24. Musgrave RH, Bremner JC: Complications of cleft palate surgery. Plast Reconstr Surg 26:180, 1960.

CHAPTER 51

Pharyngoplasty

William C. Trier

Competent velopharyngeal mechanisms exist in 70% to 90% of patients undergoing palatoplasty in centers treating patients with cleft lip and palate.[1-8] Reasons for these improved results appear to be better surgical techniques and the use of intravelar veloplasty as part of the palate repair procedure. Fistulas,[9] excessive tightness, shortness, and immobility of the palate due to excessive scarring can be prevented by precise surgery to allow approximation of the mucoperiosteal flaps without tension. In addition, careful preservation of the greater palatine arteries and suturing of the palate by everting vertical mattress sutures to provide a broad apposition of the edges of the flaps are more likely to ensure uncomplicated healing.[10-12]

Although there has been some controversy about the value of intravelar veloplasty, the majority of reports indicate an improvement in the rate of velopharyngeal competence when this procedure is used.[1, 13-20] According to our data, pharyngoplasty has been more frequently performed for clefts of the palate only and submucous cleft palate (overt or occult), and for a relatively small number of patients with congenital palatal incompetence. Of the 129 patients studied who have had adequate follow-up, only 22 had unilateral clefts of the lip and palate.

In my opinion, primary pharyngoplasty may be indicated at the time of primary palatoplasty in older patients with unrepaired clefts or in patients with very wide clefts who required a pharyngeal flap for initial repair in early childhood (12 to 16 months). Primary pharyngoplasty does not seem warranted as a routine primary procedure.[21]

Moran has reported that Trendelenburg conceived the operation of the pharyngeal flap and performed it in animals,[22] but it was Schoenborn who reported the first pharyngeal flap operation in a human.[23] The first flap was inferiorly based, but Schoenborn later reported performing a superiorly based flap. Padgett was the first to report pharyngeal flap surgery in the United States in seven patients,[24] and Moran carried out pharyngeal flap surgery in 35 patients.[22]

Anatomy and Physiology

Speech in cleft patients who cannot close the velopharyngeal orifice is characterized by hypernasality and nasal emission in all vowel and all consonant sounds with the exception of the nasals. The presence of an unrepaired alveolar cleft in a patient with a unilateral or bilateral cleft lip ordinarily does not cause hypernasality or nasal emission. Defects of the hard or soft palate, and particularly failure to achieve posterior closure of the palatopharyngeal mechanism, results in the typical stigmatized speech of the patient with a cleft. It is important to plug an alveolar cleft or an anterior fistula posterior to the alveolar cleft with dental wax during evaluation to be certain that it is not contributing to abnormal speech.

Velopharygneal closure depends on the levator veli palatini muscles contracting as a sphincter in conjunction with the superior pharyngeal constrictor muscle. Dickson et al[25, 26] and Maue-Dickson,[27, 28] Kuehn,[29] and Honjo et al[30-32] believe that the levator muscle alone is responsible for velopharyngeal closure. Latham et al have demonstrated in anatomic studies that the palatopharyngeus joins with the levator muscle to close the velopharynx.[33] Pigott[34] and Croft et al[35] have ascribed a significant role for the uvular muscle in velopharyngeal closure. However, recent studies by Boorman and Sommerlad cast doubt on this latter hypothesis.[13]

The levator veli palatini muscles elevate the soft palate and draw it posteriorly. They also produce medial movement of the pharyngeal walls during phonation as they pass on the lateral pharyngeal walls lateral to the torus tubarius of the eustachian tube.[36] Innervation of the soft palate musculature, with the exception of the tensor muscle, is by way of the pharyngeal plexus and consists of the ninth, tenth, and eleventh cranial nerves. The bulbar portion of the eleventh cranial nerve, the pharyngeal branch of the vagus nerve, provides motor innervation. The lesser palatine nerve (ninth cranial nerve) provides sensory innervation.

Indications for Pharyngoplasty

Patients who fail to achieve velopharyngeal closure typically develop compensatory articulation patterns in the effort to make sounds correctly.[37, 38] Glottal stops, pharyngeal fricatives, abnormal positioning of the tongue, and other means may be used in the attempt to produce intelligible vowels and consonants. This frequently results in increased *un*intelligibility. Absence of an adequate physical mechanism for speech requires, therefore, a physical means of altering the abnormal structures.

This can be accomplished by the use of a speech appliance, an obturator or speech bulb that occludes the velopharyngeal orifice sufficiently to produce speech. Speech appliances are not well tolerated by many patients; they require expert fitting and fabrication, frequently need modification, and may in the long run be as expensive as a surgical means of providing an adequate mechanism. An advantage of the speech appliance is that it can be removed when the patient sleeps or is engaged in strenuous physical activity, ensuring an adequate nasal airway. The appliance, can, of course, be decreased in size if it provides excessive nasal airway obstruction or denasality in speech.

Surgical modification of the velopharyngeal mechanism can be carried out by augmentation of the posterior pharyngeal wall using cartilage,[39] silicone,[40, 41] Teflon,[42–47] or injectable collagen.[48] Gersuny initially used paraffin for pharyngeal wall augmentation.[49] Pharyngoplasty is most commonly performed by constructing a pharyngeal flap that is inserted into the soft palate. Hynes,[50] Orticochea,[51] and Sullivan[52] have all reported various types of pharyngoplasty using musculomucosal flaps of palatopharyngeal muscle with or without a posterior pharyngeal flap.

Diagnosis of Velopharyngeal Inadequacy

The diagnosis of velopharyngeal inadequacy—either incompetence due to the physiologic abnormality or insufficiency due to an inadequate anatomic structure or structures—requires the diagnostic skills of an experienced speech pathologist using test phonemes, as in the Iowa Pressure Articulation Tests or the Templin-Darley Test. Evaluation of continuous and spontaneous speech is particularly important because the eliciting of specific phonemes may not always disclose abnormal velopharyngeal closure.

In addition to trained-listener observation, aerodynamic studies of the palatopharyngeal mechanism,[53, 54] nasopharyngoscopy, and videofluoroscopy are frequently used measures. The author has relied particularly on pressure-flow studies as the most objective means for determining the extent of the ability to achieve closure of the velopharyngeal orifice both preoperatively and postoperatively. Nasopharyngoscopy and videofluoroscopy disclose the type of closure, the contribution of lateral pharyngeal wall movement, the contribution of the soft palate, and the level of closure in estimating the likely effects of operation.[34, 55, 56]

Pharyngoplasty

There is a considerable difference of opinion about the type of pharyngoplasty that should be performed. One argument concerns the use of superiorly based or inferiorly based pharyngeal flaps. Inferiorly based flaps are certainly more easily and more rapidly performed. A study by Whitaker and coauthors has shown no significant difference beween the results following superiorly based pharyngeal flaps and inferiorly based flaps in conditions in which either flap could be used.[57] Graham and his colleagues, in reporting complications of pharyngeal flap surgery, noted ten cases of complete flap separation and eight cases of partial flap separation, suggesting that the flaps, which were inferiorly based, had simply been of inadequate length and had been sutured into the palate under tension.[58]

This author uses a superiorly based pharyngeal flap because, within reason, there is no limit to the length that can be provided. Furthermore, the site from which the flap has been raised can be visualized readily in the event of postoperative bleeding that might require reoperation. An inferiorly based flap completely ob-

scures the underlying donor site. In addition, an inferiorly based flap has the theoretical disadvantage of tethering the soft palate in an inferior direction. Finally, because the nasopharynx narrows in a cephalad direction, better obturation is obtained from the superiorly based flap.

Another controversy concerns whether the flap should be dynamic or adynamic. Kapetansky[59] and McCoy[60] have advocated laterally based flaps that will retain their nerve supply, allowing them to contract and provide closure of the velopharyngeal orifice although they are smaller. A midline vertical pharyngeal flap requires the division of the lateral nerve supply to the pharyngeal muscles. Biopsies of midline vertical pharyngeal flaps have revealed only scar tissue without viable muscle tissue, so the flap is not contractile.[61] As noted earlier, however, because velopharyngeal closure depends primarily on the levator muscles and because they are responsible for lateral pharyngeal wall motion, the velopharyngeal mechanism is dynamic regardless of which flap is used and whether or not the flap itself is dynamic.

Finally, one should note that the epithelial surface of wounds should be kept as intact as possible to prevent unwanted wound contraction. Specifically, unlined pharyngeal flaps or unlined flaps of any sort tend to "tube" as they heal. A flap that had comprised the entire posterior pharyngeal wall may tube into a narrow midline structure that provides inadequate obturation. Lining the pharyngeal flap with flaps of nasal mucous membrane retains the width of the flap and provides a broad, raw defect into which the flap can be sutured.

The High-Attached, Superiorly Based, Lined Pharyngeal Flap

The technique of pharyngeal flap surgery used by the author was described by Owsley and coauthors in 1966.[62] Since 1976, however, the author has added intravelar veloplasty to the pharyngeal flap operation, as will be discussed later.[63]

Selection of Patients

Patients for whom a diagnosis of velopharyngeal inadequacy has been made should undergo modification of the velopharyngeal mechanism as soon as possible to prevent the development of compensatory articulation patterns.[37, 38] Patients are followed at 6-month intervals to be certain that adequacy of velopharyngeal closure is maintained. When it becomes apparent, however, that the velopharyngeal mechanism is inadequate, correction is carried out as soon as possible. Speech therapy may be effective in correcting articulation errors, but in the presence of velopharyngeal inadequacy normal speech cannot be achieved and continued therapy may only frustrate the patient.

Anesthesia

Anesthesia is administered through an oral endotracheal tube. Although the author prefers the use of a guarded tube, the choice of the tube is left to the anesthesiologist; however, it must be made clear that the Dingman mouth gag can significantly compress the unguarded tube. Ethrane is preferred as an anesthetic agent, and therefore an adequate amount of epinephrine solution in lidocaine can be used for its hemostatic effect. A dilution of 1:200,000 epinephrine is quite adequate.

Position of the Patient

The patient is placed in the supine position with the top of the head level with the top of the operating table. A folded towel is placed beneath the scapulae to provide some extension of the head and neck to permit better access to the posterior oral pharynx. Shot-filled bags, sandbags, or a foam plastic ring is used to maintain the head in the face-up position. The hard and soft palates are infiltrated with the lidocaine and epinephrine solution in an amount not to exceed 3 μg per kg. A 7-minute wait allows the epinephrine solution to produce an adequate hemostatic effect.

Surgical Technique

The soft palate is split through the uvula and down the central raphe or central scar of the palate to a point just posterior to the hard palate (Fig. 51–1). In the patient who has had palatoplasty and intravelar veloplasty, the intact levator sling is exposed and left in continuity. Depending on review of the patient's previous operative reports (when obtainable) or when the patient has a submucous cleft and it is likely that the levator muscles are inserted abnormally into the hard palate, the anatomy of the soft palate is observed as the soft palate is split. Because the oral incision extends farther anteriorly than the nasal mucous membrane incision, the pharyngeal flap can be easily sutured to the anterior end of the nasal mucous membrane defect. This extent of dissection allows the posterior pharyngeal wall to be visible well above the tubercle of the atlas.

Marking for Flap. After the soft palate has been split, malleable retractors are inserted, and the lateral borders of the proposed pharyngeal flap are marked with puncture marks of indelible marking solution (Fig. 51–1). The lateral borders of the flap lie at the lateral border of the posterior pharyngeal wall just before it curves onto the lateral pharyngeal wall. Placement of the tip of the proposed pharyngeal flap is estimated, and puncture marks are made transversely so that the flap will be long enough to reach without tension to the anterior end of the nasal mucous membrane defect in the palate. The posterior pharyngeal wall is infiltrated with lidocaine and epinephrine solution.

Muscle Dissection and Preparation of Turnback Flaps. As noted, an intact levator mechanism is preserved. If intravelar veloplasty has not been carried out previously, the levator muscles are identified and dissected from the overlying and underlying mucous membrane, the point of insertion is divided, and the muscles are dissected medially until they can be made to lie trans-

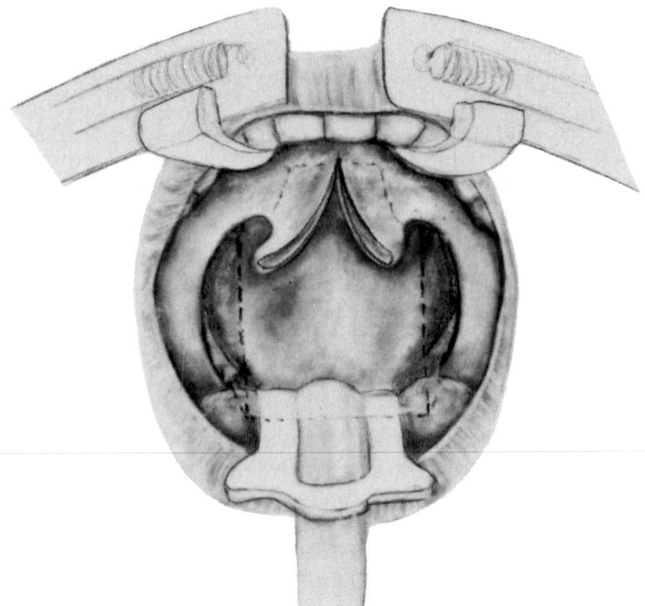

Figure 51–1 Soft palate is divided in the midline. Incision on oral side reaches posterior edge of hard palate. On nasal surface, incision ends about 1 cm short of hard palate to leave an adequate cuff of mucous membrane to which anterior end of pharyngeal flap is sutured. Proposed pharyngeal flap (dotted lines) is outlined on posterior pharyngeal wall with puncture marks of marking solution. The width of the flap may include the entire width of the posterior pharyngeal wall, or it may be narrower depending on the degree of the patient's velopharyngeal incompetence. The length of the flap extends from above the tubercle of the atlas to its distal end so that the flap is long enough to reach the anterior end of the palate defect without tension but at the same time is not redundant and hangs against the posterior pharyngeal wall.

versely without tension (Fig. 51–2). The nasal mucous membrane turnback flaps are then raised by making a lateral incision just posterior to the farthest anterior extent of the nasal mucous membrane incision and carried posteriorly, parallel to the midline incision and approximately a centimeter or so in width back to the posterior border of the soft palate. The flaps are raised from the muscle (Fig. 51–3).

Elevation of Pharyngeal Flap. A silk suture is inserted through the tip of the proposed pharyngeal flap as a traction suture. Incisions are made along the lines for incision that have been marked laterally on either side of the flap just through the mucous membrane. A transverse incision is made at the site marked at the distal end of the flap (Fig. 51–4A). Using retraction provided by the malleable retractor, scissor dissection provided by Metzenbaum scissors, and the traction suture, the transverse and lateral incisions are joined and the flap is dissected from the prevertebral fascia of the posterior pharyngeal wall by dissecting first on one side and then on the other until the flap is raised to a point above the level of the tubercle of the atlas (Fig. 51–4B).

As Owsley has pointed out, failure to elevate the flap above the tubercle of the atlas is probably responsible for failure of the pharyngeal flap to correct velopharyngeal inadequacy.[62] Bleeding in the donor site usually

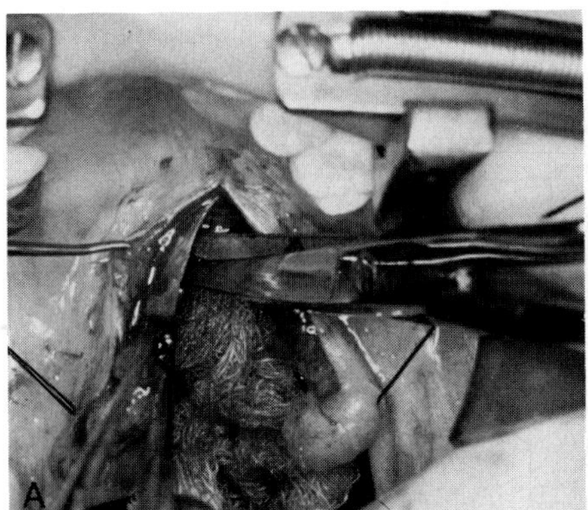 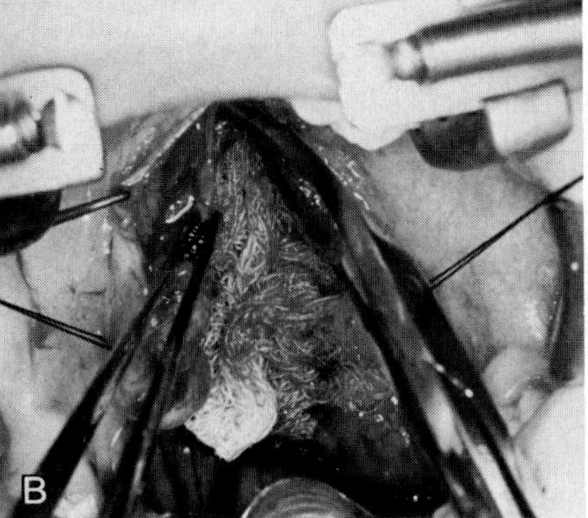 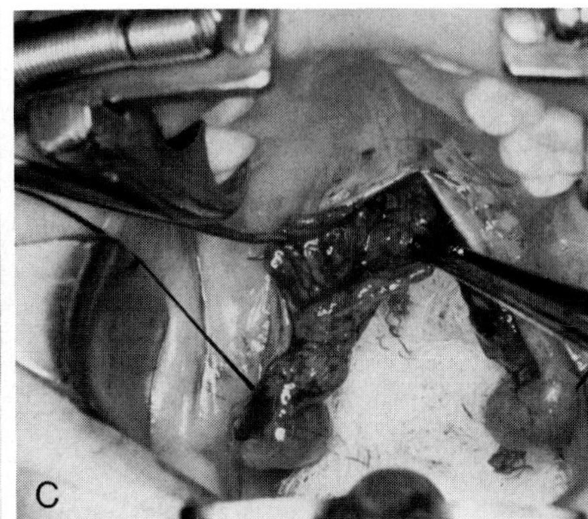

Figure 51–2 *A*, Shows dissection around patient's right levator muscle with the scissors dissecting between nasal mucous membrane and the muscle. *B*, The muscle divided at its insertion into the hard palate. *C*, Muscle being drawn medially and posteriorly.

ceases spontaneously. Occasionally a few bleeding vessels require electrocoagulation. The flap should now reach, without tension, to the anterior end of the midline palatal incision.

Posterior Pharyngeal Wall Closure. I believe it is preferable to close the posterior wall because patients appear to be more comfortable when it is closed. Closure is ordinarily readily accomplished by means of interrupted sutures of chromic catgut, beginning at the center of the defect and closing the defect in a caudal

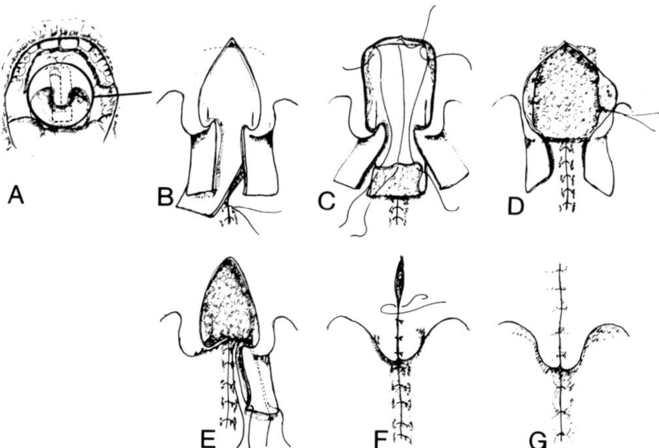

Figure 51–3 *A*, Outline of the proposed flap on the posterior pharyngeal wall. The three parallel dotted lines indicate the outline of the nasal mucous membrane turnback flaps outlined on the nasal surface of the soft palate. These are divided anteriorly about 1 cm posterior to the posterior edge of the hard palate and are dissected off the muscle. *B*, Pharyngeal flap has been raised with closure of the posterior pharyngeal wall. The two turnback flaps have been elevated from the muscle and lie on either side of the pharyngeal flap. *C*, Sutures are placed between the flap and the nasal mucous membrane at the posterior edge of the hard palate and along the lateral borders of the nasal surface of the soft palate. Sutures are actually inserted so that when tied, the knots will be on the nasal mucosal surface rather than as shown (incorrectly) in the drawing. *D*, Flap is sutured in place on the nasal surface of the soft palate with its raw undersurface facing downward into the oral cavity. The flap is sutured at the lateral sides until a lateral port of appropriate size exists on each side. *E*, Sutures of catgut catch the tip of the turnback flaps, which are sutured to the lateral edges and the center of the pharyngeal flap. *F* and *G*, Suturing of the nasal surface of the soft palate, uvula, and oral surface of the soft palate.

direction and then closing the cephalad portion of the donor defect to just beneath the base of the pharyngeal flap (Fig. 51–5).

Inset of Flap. Two retention sutures of chromic catgut are inserted as mattress sutures, each catching one corner of the end of the pharyngeal flap and drawing the raw surface of the flap against the nasal surface (Fig. 51–3C). These mattress sutures are left untied until complete closure of the oral mucous membrane is accomplished. A suture of chromic catgut is then inserted between the center of the end of the pharyngeal flap and the nasal surface of the anterior end of the midline palatal incision, inverting the suture so that the knot is placed on the nasal surface. Closure is then carried out with similar sutures, first on one side and then on the other, working in an anterior to posterior direction until the lumen of the lateral port between the lateral pharyngeal wall and the border of pharyngeal flap appears to be small enough to provide closure on phonation but large enough to permit an adequate airway on expiration and inspiration (Fig. 51–3D).

Although Hogan has reported the use of lateral port control using a 14F catheter as a template on each side,[64, 65] this author has merely used a right-angle hemostat as a guide (Fig. 51–6). If the lateral port remains too large after suturing the flap to the nasal mucous membrane of the palate on each side, additional decrease in port size can be achieved by splitting the edge of the posterior pillar and suturing the flap to its posterior edge.

Turnback Flaps. The turnback flaps are sutured to the raw undersurface of the pharyngeal flap by catgut sutures placed at each lateral corner of the two turnback flaps. These flaps are sutured to the edges of the pharyngeal flap at its base. A third suture fixes the medial corner of each turnback flap to the center of the base of the pharyngeal flap, so that when the three sutures are tied they will pull the lining flaps down to the base of the pharyngeal flap and toward each other (Fig. 51–3E). A suture of polydiaxanone is then inserted through the tip of the uvula. Sutures of chromic catgut are used to close the nasal surface of the uvula, and closure is carried posteriorly between the two turnback flaps, suturing them together to line the raw surface of

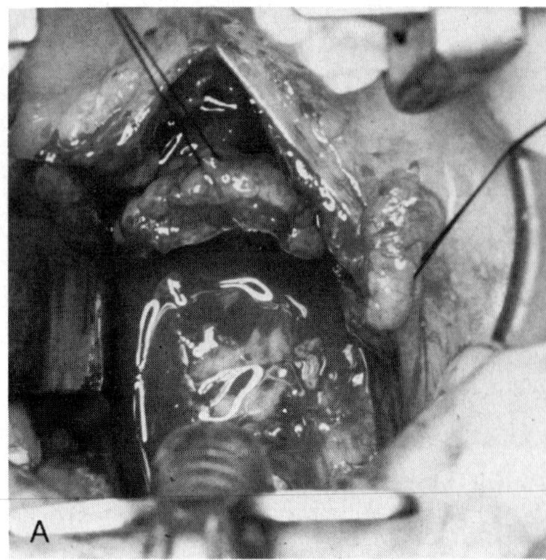
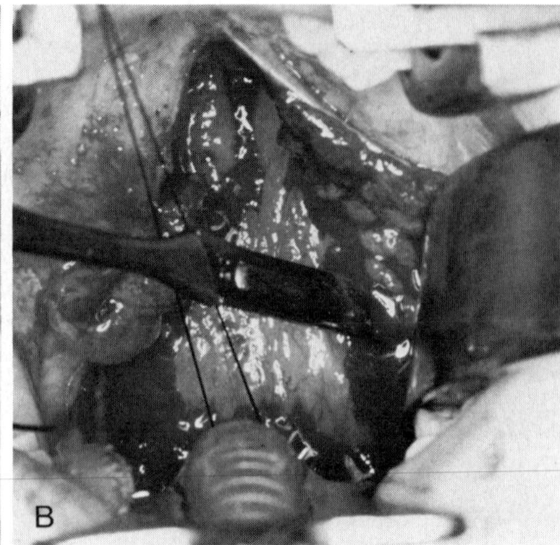

Figure 51–4 *A,* Lateral incisions made along the border of the pharyngeal flap. The suture is made through the tip of the flap. A malleable retractor provides exposure on the patient's left side. *B,* Elevated flap above the level of the tubercle of the atlas.

the pharyngeal flap more securely (Fig. 51–3*F* and *G*).
Levator Muscle Suture. If an adequate muscle sling has not been identified, the retropositioned levator muscles are overlapped in the midline by inserting two mattress sutures, one from each side, through the mucous membrane of the oral surface of the palate and catching the levator muscle on the opposite side (Fig. 51–7*D*). These sutures, along with the anterior retention sutures, are left untied until complete closure of the oral mucous membrane is accomplished. Attempts to suture one levator muscle directly to the other are likely to result in tearing of the frequently very delicate muscle. Overlapping of the muscles shortens the muscle sling, increasing its efficiency, and also provides a broad apposition of muscle to muscle.

Oral Mucous Membrane Closure. The oral mucous membrane is then closed using vertical mattress sutures of 4–0 polydiaxanone, along with some additional simple interrupted sutures. The two retention sutures and two muscle sutures are tied (Fig. 51–8). The operative areas are carefully inspected to be sure that there is no bleeding. Blood and mucus are aspirated from the oral cavity. A heavy silk suture is inserted as a tongue suture for small children if there is any question of the adequacy of the airway in the postoperative period. The tongue suture is removed 12 to 24 hours postoperatively.

Postoperative Care

Patients are started on clear liquids as soon as they can tolerate them postoperatively. Antibiotics are not administered. Intravenous fluids are given until oral intake is adequate, and patients are discharged from the

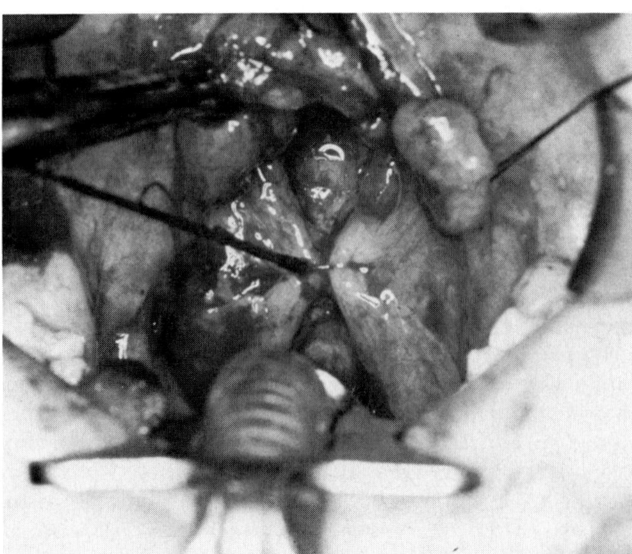

Figure 51–5 The first catgut suture approximating the posterior pharyngeal wall mucous membrane has been tied. Closure caudally and in a cephalad direction is then carried out so that the entire posterior pharyngeal wall is sutured except for a small portion just beneath the flap and at the caudal end.

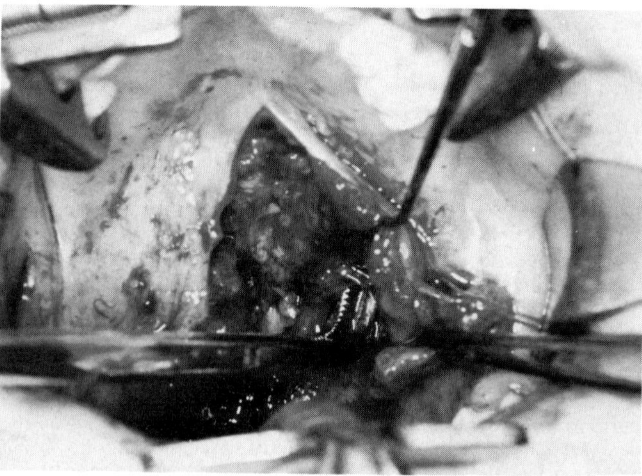

Figure 51–6 A right angle clamp is shown with its tip in the lateral port on the left side. The dimensions of the lateral port can be estimated in this fashion and, depending on the degree of velopharyngeal incompetence of the patient, the size of the lateral port can be adjusted.

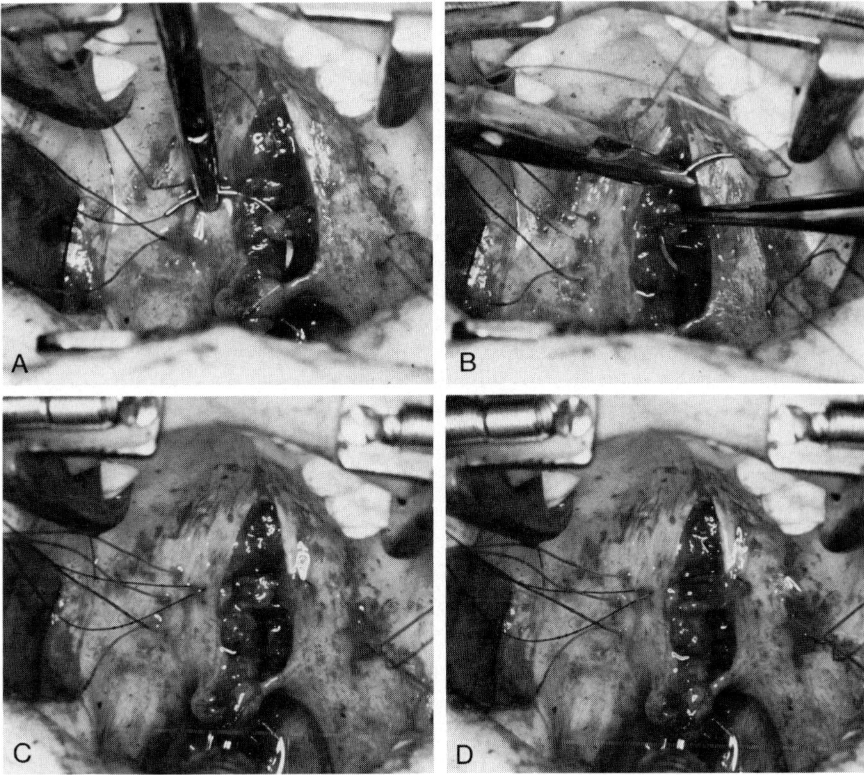

Figure 51–7 A, Left levator muscle is transfixed with a mattress suture that has been inserted on the patient's right side through the oral mucous membrane. *B*, Right levator muscle is transfixed with a similar mattress suture. *C*, Both muscle sutures inserted, each transfixing the opposite levator muscle. The levator muscle is shown between the two incised borders of the soft palate. *D*, Muscles are overlapped by traction on the muscle suture.

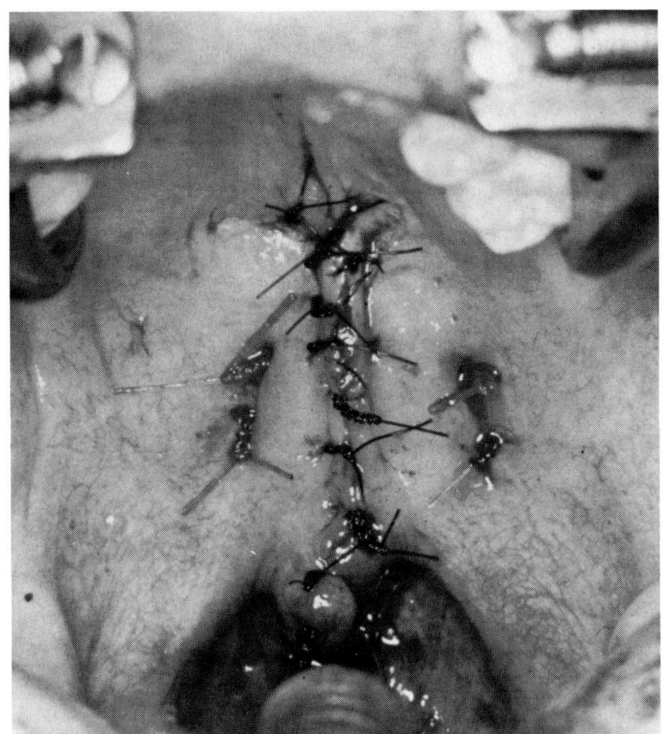

Figure 51–8 Completed pharyngoplasty with both the retention sutures and the muscle sutures tied and the soft palate reapproximated in the midline with vertical mattress sutures and simple sutures.

hospital on full liquids and a soft diet. They are instructed not to eat food that requires chewing for at least 4 weeks following the operation. Also, strenuous physical exercise or athletics are prohibited for 4 weeks after the operation. Patients are instructed not to use straws.

Follow-up Examination

Following discharge, patients are seen 1 week following the operation and return for follow-up examination at 1 month. Although a dramatic change in the degree of velopharyngeal competence is usually seen immediately after the operation, a reasonable estimate of the correction achieved cannot be made until at least 6 months after surgery, when healing is complete, edema has subsided, and the patient is able to use the velopharyngeal mechanism freely.

Results

The author has been able to study three groups of patients for whom follow-up information is available.[66] The first group consisted of 21 patients operated on between July of 1967 and July of 1969 at the University of North Carolina, although adequate data are available on only 13 patients. Two of these patients had a repaired unilateral cleft lip and palate, four had a submucous cleft palate, three had a bilateral cleft lip and palate, and four had a cleft of the secondary palate alone.

The second group consisted of 29 patients treated at the University of Arizona between 1971 and 1975 with data available on 25. Five of these patients had a repaired unilateral cleft lip and palate, 11 had a submucous cleft palate, five had a cleft of the secondary palate, six had congenital palatal incompetence, one had a partially paralyzed palate secondary to an acoustic neuroma, and one had a primary pharyngoplasty at the time of palatoplasty.

The third group consisted of 113 patients operated on between 1976 and 1983 at the University of North Carolina, of whom 91 presented adequate follow-up information. Fifteen of these patients had a repaired unilateral cleft lip and palate, 32 had a submucous cleft palate, 8 had congenital palatal incompetence, 16 had a repaired bilateral cleft lip and palate, and 20 had an isolated cleft of the secondary palate only.

Since 1976, intravelar veloplasty has been added to our pharyngoplasty technique with the expectation of improving velopharyngeal closure. This expectation was based on three hypotheses: first, that closure of the lateral port on either side of the flap depended on adequate lateral pharyngeal wall motion medially;[30] second, that the levator muscle was primarily responsible for a lateral pharyngeal wall motion;[31] and third, that levator function was significantly improved by detaching the levator muscle from the hard palate during intravelar veloplasty.[32]

Speech evaluation in a total of 38 patients who had pharyngeal flap surgery without intravelar veloplasty

Table 51–1. Postoperative Speech Evaluations in 38 Patients (Without Intravelar Veloplasty)

	No. Patients	Percent
Normal	22	57.9
Mild hyponasality	1	2.6
Mild-moderate hyponasality	1	2.6
Moderate-severe hyponasality	4	10.5
Mild hypernasality/nasal emission	6	15.8
Mild-moderate hypernasality/nasal emission	2	5.3
Moderate-severe hypernasality/nasal emission	2	5.3

revealed that 89.4% achieved velopharyngeal adequacy (Table 51–1). Limited pressure-flow data in six patients revealed adequate velopharyngeal closure in five and borderline closure in one patient.

Results in 91 patients who had undergone intravelar veloplasty at the time of pharyngoplasty and for whom data are available are shown in Table 51–2. Again, 89% of the patients achieved velopharyngeal adequacy. Pressure-flow data in 72 of these 91 patients revealed adequate velopharyngeal closure in 93%. In the group of patients without intravelar veloplasty, 10.5% had moderate hyponasality. In the group with intravelar veloplasty, 7.7% had moderate to severe hyponasality.

Nasal obstruction was severe enough in three patients in the group without intravelar veloplasty that secondary surgical revision or division of the flap had to be performed. In the group of patients who had pharyngoplasty with intravelar veloplasty, secondary revision was not necessary. The incidence of hyponasal speech and nasal obstruction is disturbing and has been noted by a number of other authors.[67–69] It may be desirable to increase the size of the lateral port, with the expectation that intravelar veloplasty might then be effective in closing the larger lateral ports.

Conclusion

Pharyngoplasty by means of a high-attached, lined, superiorly based pharyngeal flap has provided velopharyngeal adequacy in over 89% of patients. Intravelar veloplasty, although theoretically an attractive adjunct to pharyngoplasty, has not been demonstrated to improve the results of pharyngoplasty. It is possible that intravelar veloplasty at the time of pharyngoplasty may

Table 51–2. Postoperative Speech Evaluations in 91 Patients (With Intravelar Veloplasty)

	No. Patients	Percent
Normal	22	24.2
Mild hyponasality	10	11.0
Mild-moderate hyponasality	10	11.0
Moderate-severe hyponasality	7	7.7
Mild hypernasality/nasal emission	24	26.4
Mild-moderate hypernasality/nasal emission	8	8.8
Moderate-severe hypernasality/nasal emission	10	11.0

provide better dynamic closure of lateral ports, permitting the construction of larger ports that would still close adequately on phonation.

References

1. Dreyer TM, Trier WC: A comparison of palatoplasty techniques. Cleft Palate J 21:251, 1984.
2. Holtmann B, Wray RC, Weeks, PM: A comparison of three techniques of palatorrhaphy: Early speech results. Ann Plast Surg 12:514, 1984.
3. Kaplan I, Labandter H, Ben-Bassat M, et al: A long-term follow-up of clefts of the secondary palate repaired by von Langenbeck's method. Br J Plast Surg 31:353, 1978.
4. Krause CJ, Tharp RE, Morris HL: A comparative study of the results of the von Langenbeck and the V–Y pushback palatoplasties. Cleft Palate J 13:11, 1976.
5. Lindsay WK: Von Langenbeck palatorrhaphy. In Grabb WC, Rosenstein SW, Bzoch K (eds): Cleft Lip and Palate: Surgical, Dental and Speech Aspects. Boston: Little, Brown, 1971, p. 393.
6. Musgrave RH, McWilliams BJ, Matthews HP: A review of two different surgical procedures for the repair of clefts of the soft palate only. Cleft Palate J 12:281, 1975.
7. Reidy JP: The other 20 percent: Failure of cleft palate repair. Br J Plast Surg 15:261, 1962.
8. Ross RB, Johnston MC: Cleft Lip and Palate. Baltimore: Williams & Wilkins, 1972.
9. Oneal RM: Oronasal Fistulas. In Grabb WC, Rosenstein SW, Bzoch KR (eds): Cleft Lip and Palate: Surgical, Dental and Speech Aspects. Boston: Little, Brown, 1971.
10. Byars LT: Personal communication, 1956.
11. Musgrave RH, Bremmer JC: Complications of cleft palate surgery. Plast Reconstr Surg 26:180, 1960.
12. Trier WC, Dreyer TM: Primary von Langenbeck palatoplasty with levator reconstruction: Rationale and technique. Cleft Palate J 21:254, 1984.
13. Boorman JG, Sommerlad BC: Muscular uvulae and levator palate: Their anatomical and functional relationship in velopharyngeal closure. Br J Plast Surg 38:333, 1985.
14. Brown AS, Cohen MA, Randall P: Levator muscle reconstruction: Does it make a difference? Plast Reconstr Surg 72:1, 1983.
15. Dellon AL, Edgerton MT: Correction of velopharyngeal incompetence by retrodisplacement of the levator veli palatini muscle insertion. Surg Forum 20:510, 1969.
16. Edgerton MT, Dellon AL: Surgical retrodisplacement of the levator veli palatini muscle. Plast Reconstr Surg 47:154, 1971.
17. Fara M, Dvorak J: Abnormal anatomy of the muscles and palatopharyngeal closure in cleft palates. Plast Reconstr Surg 46:488, 1970.
18. Kriens OB: An anatomical approach to veloplasty. Plast Reconstr Surg 43:290, 1969.
19. Kriens OB: Fundamental anatomic findings for an intravelar veloplasty. Cleft Palate J 7:27, 1970.
20. Kriens O: Anatomy of the velopharyngeal area in cleft palate. Clin Plast Surg 2:261, 1975.
21. Stark RB, Frileck: Primary pharyngeal flap and palatorrhaphy. In Grabb WC, Rosenstein SW, Bzoch KR (ed): Cleft Lip and Palate: Surgical, Dental and Speech Aspects. Boston: Little, Brown, 1971, p. 407.
22. Moran RE: The pharyngeal flap operation as a speech aid. Plast Reconstr Surg 7:202, 1951.
23. Schoenborn K: Über eine neue Methode der Staphylorrhaphie. Arch Klin Chir 19:527, 1876.
24. Padgett EC: The repair of cleft palates after unsuccessful operation. Arch Surg 20:453, 1930.
25. Dickson DR: Normal and cleft palate anatomy. Cleft Palate J 9:288, 1972.
26. Dickson DR, Grant JCB, Sicher H, et al: Status of research in cleft palate anatomy and physiology, July 1973—Part I. Cleft Palate J 11:471, 1974.
27. Maue-Dickson W: Section II—Anatomy and physiology, 3. The velopharyngeal mechanism. Cleft Palate J 14:270, 1977.
28. Maue-Dickson W: The craniofacial complex in cleft palate: An updated review of anatomy and function. Cleft Palate J 16:291, 1979.
29. Kuehn DP: Velopharyngeal anatomy and physiology. Ear Nose Throat J 58:316, 1979.
30. Honjo I, Harada H, Kumajawa I: Role of the levator veli palatini muscle in movement of the lateral pharyngeal wall. Arch Otol Rhinol Laryngol 212:93, 1970.
31. Honjo I, Okazaki N, Nozoe T: Role of the tensor veli palatini muscle in movement of the soft palate. Acta Otolaryngol 88:137, 1979.
32. Honjo I, Harada H, Okazaki N: Significance of levator muscle sling formation in cleft palate surgery: Evaluation by electrical stimulation. Plast Reconstr Surg 65:443, 1980.
33. Latham RA, Long RE, Latham EA: Cleft palate velopharyngeal musculature in a five-month-old infant: A three-dimensional histological reconstruction. Cleft Palate J 17:1, 1980.
34. Pigott RW: The nasendoscope appearance of the normal palatopharyngeal valve. Plast Reconstr Surg 43:19, 1969.
35. Croft CD, Shprintzen RJ, Daniller A, et al: The occult submucous cleft palate and the musculus uvulae. Cleft Palate J 15:50, 1978.
36. Argamaso RV, Shprintzen RJ, Strauch B, et al: The role of lateral pharyngeal wall movement in pharyngeal flap surgery. Plast Reconstr Surg 66:214, 1980.
37. Dorf DS, Curtin JW: Early cleft palate repair and speech outcome. Plast Reconstr Surg 70:74, 1982.
38. Trost JE: Compensatory articulation: Errors, types, patterns and treatment approaches. Presented at the Annual Meeting of the American Cleft Palate Association, Seattle, Washington, May 23, 1984.
39. Hagerty RF, Hill MJ: Cartilage pharyngoplasty in cleft palate patients. Surg Gynecol Obstet 112:350, 1961.
40. Blocksma R: Correction of velopharyngeal insufficiency by Silastic pharyngeal implant. Plast Reconstr Surg 31:268, 1963.
41. Brauer RI: Retropharyngeal implantation of silicone gel pillows for velopharyngeal incompetence. Plast Reconstr Surg 51:254, 1973.
42. Furlow LT, Williams WN, Eisenbach CR, et al: A long-term study on treating velopharyngeal insufficiency by Teflon injection. Cleft Palate J 19:47, 1982.
43. Kuehn DP, VanDemark DR: Assessment of velopharyngeal competency following Teflon pharyngoplasty. Cleft Palate J 15:145, 1978.
44. Lewy R, Cole R, Wepman J: Teflon injection in the correction of velopharyngeal insufficiency. Ann Otol Rhinol Laryngol 74:874, 1965.
45. Smith JK, McCabe BF: Teflon injection in the nasopharynx to improve velopharyngeal closure. Ann Otol 86:559, 1977.
46. Sturim HS, Jacob CT: Teflon pharyngoplasty. Plast Reconstr Surg 49:180, 1972.
47. Ward PH, Stoudt R, Goldman R: Improvement of velopharyngeal insufficiency by Teflon injection. Tri Am Acad Ophthalmol Otol 71:923, 1967.
48. Trier WC: Unpublished information.
49. Gersuny R: Über eine subcutane Prosthese. Heilkunst 21:199, 1900.
50. Hynes W: Pharyngoplasty by muscle transplantation. Br J Plast Surg 3:128, 1950.
51. Orticochea M: Construction of a dynamic muscle sphincter in cleft palates. Plast Reconstr Surg 41:323, 1968.
52. Sullivan DE: Bilateral pharyngoplasty as an aid to velopharyngeal closure. Plast Reconstr Surg 27:31, 1961.
53. Warren DW, DuBois AB: A pressure-flow technique for measuring velopharyngeal orifice area during continuous speech. Cleft Palate J 1:52, 1964.
54. Warren DW: Velopharyngeal orifice size and upper pharyngeal pressure-flow patterns in normal speech. Plast Reconstr Surg 33:148, 1964.
55. Skolnick ML: Videofluoroscopic examination of the velopharyngeal portal during phonation in lateral and base projections—a new technique for studying the mechanics of closure. Cleft Palate J 7:803, 1970.
56. Skolnick JL, McCall GN: Velopharyngeal competence and incompetence following pharyngeal flap surgery: Video-fluoroscopic study in multiple projections. Cleft Palate J 9:1, 1972.
57. Whitaker LA, Randall P, Graham WP, et al: A prospective and randomized series comparing superiorly and inferiorly based posterior pharyngeal flaps. Cleft Palate J 9:304, 1972.
58. Graham WP, Hamilton R, Randall P, et al: Complications following posterior pharyngeal flap surgery. Cleft Palate J 10:176, 1973.
59. Kapetansky DI: Bilateral transverse pharyngeal flaps for repair of cleft palate. Plast Reconstr Surg 52:52, 1973.
60. McCoy FJ, Zahorsky CL: A new approach to the elusive dynamic pharyngeal flap. Plast Reconstr Surg 49:160, 1972.
61. Owsley JQ, Creech BJ, Dedo HH: Poor speech following the pharyngeal flap operation: Etiology and treatment. Cleft Palate J 9:312, 1972.
62. Owsley JQ, Lawson LI, Miller ER, et al: Experience with the high attached pharyngeal flap. Plast Reconstr Surg 38:232, 1966.
63. Trier WC: The pharyngeal flap operation. Clin Plast Surg 22:697, 1985.
64. Hogan VM: A clarification of the surgical goals in cleft palate speech and the introduction of the lateral port control (LPC) pharyngeal flap. Cleft Palate J 10:331, 1973.
65. Hogan VM, Schwartz MF: Velopharyngeal incompetence. In Converse JM, McCarthy JG (eds): Reconstructive Plastic Surgery. Philadelphia: Saunders, 1977.
66. Jarvis BL, Trier WC: The effect of intravelar veloplasty on velopharyngeal competence following pharyngeal flap surgery. Cleft Palate J 25:389, 1988.
67. Smith BE, Skef Z, Cohen M, et al: Aerodynamic assessment of the results of pharyngeal flap surgery: A preliminary investigation. Plast Reconstr Surg 76:402, 1985.
68. Thurston JB, Larson DL, Shanks JC, et al: Nasal obstruction as a complication of pharyngeal flap surgery. Cleft Palate J 17:148, 1980.
69. VanDemark DR, Hardin MA: Longitudinal evaluation of articulation and velopharyngeal competence of patients with pharyngeal flaps. Cleft Palate J 22:163, 1985.

CHAPTER 52

Augmentation of the Posterior Pharyngeal Wall

Raymond O. Brauer, Donna R. Fox, and David Humphreys

Surgery for the patient with a cleft has advanced considerably in the past 30 to 40 years. We can now operate on unilateral clefts so successfully that the Cupid's bow shows minimal scarring, and the nose has a nearly normal appearance. Advances in palate repair have not really kept pace; we still see patients after primary palatoplasty who have nasal speech. The most neglected patient is the one with an immobile but short palate who has had years of unsuccessful speech therapy because of velopharyngeal dysfunction. This problem is anatomic.

Evaluation of the patient with nasal speech is based on clinical impressions, multiplanar videofluoroscopy, and a variety of other methods including nasendoscopy. We have chosen to use videofluoroscopy because we can observe the length and thickness of the palate, the width of contact between the palate and pharyngeal wall, the distance between the soft palate and the pharyngeal wall, and the timing of the palate and pharyngeal movement as well as the approximate contact point on the pharyngeal wall. This modality provides the best visualization not only of the anatomy but also of the physiologic aspects of speech.

When the videofluoroscopic record shows a gap between the palate and the pharyngeal wall the surgeon can choose one of three possible methods of improving or achieving normal speech. First, push-back repair can be considered if none has been performed; such a repair may suffice if it is carried out before the age of 4 or 5 years. After the age of 4, additional procedures are usually needed. The second procedure commonly used is a pharyngeal flap. This is not a normal anatomic procedure and should be reserved for the patient with a gap greater than 6 mm or for the paralyzed palate. In our opinion, the flap is the court of last appeal.

The third choice is augmentation of the posterior pharyngeal wall. This is a logical solution because it addresses the problem where the need is greatest. This procedure moves the posterior pharyngeal wall forward so that the active palate can make contact with the pharyngeal wall, thus directing the airflow out of the mouth and preventing its escape into the nose (Figs. 52–1 and 52–2). The real problem with this technique has been in finding the optimal material to use for augmentation. At present we use a Dacron-wrapped silicone gel implant, which is tolerated well by most patients.

Definition of Speech

Normal speech can be defined as normal resonance, normal articulation, and normal language. Normal velopharyngeal closure is necessary to achieve normal oral resonance. Without normal closure, abnormal nasal resonance and articulation will occur. Normal articulation is influenced by proper dentition and tongue movement as well as by velopharyngeal closure. Normal language depends on the integrity of sensory, motor, perceptual, and cognitive abilities. Without normal resonance, normal speech cannot be achieved; normal resonance depends on structures acting together to produce velopharyngeal closure.

Velopharyngeal closure is the result of the combined movements of several structures: the superior and posterior movements of the soft palate, the medial movement of the lateral walls of the pharynx, and possibly, to a limited extent, the anterior movement of the posterior pharyngeal wall. In some instances a deficiency in the soft palate movement is compensated by the medial movement of the lateral pharyngeal wall and may be further compensated by the presence of large tonsils and adenoids.

Nasal speech with nasal emission of sounds can be heard in the patient with a repaired cleft or congenitally short palate and in those who have limited or no movement of the soft palate. It is also heard in the patient with a palate of normal length and function who has an excessively deep nasopharynx. Nasal speech may occur after adenotonsillectomy in a patient with a short soft palate or when a deep nasopharynx is revealed for the first time.

Velopharyngoplasty or a pharyngeal flap procedure is indicated when little or no palatal motion is present or when a gross deficiency exists in the velopharyngeal structures. These procedures appear to be less suitable for minor deficiencies. Augmentation of the posterior pharyngeal wall is a relatively simple procedure that can be used to produce velopharyngeal closure in the patient who has minimal or borderline velopharyngeal competence.

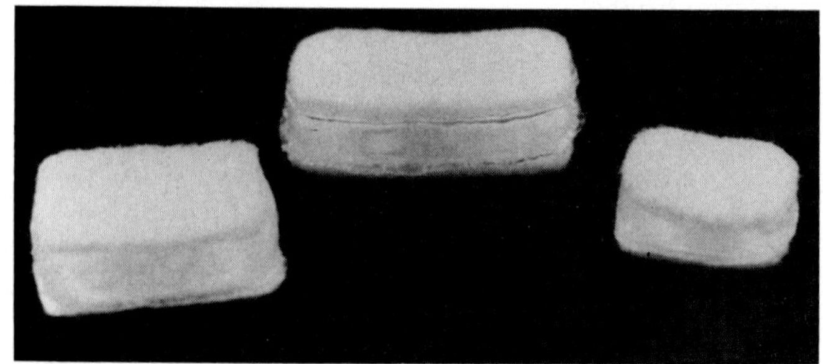

Figure 52–1 These are the three implants with different widths but the same 9-mm thickness.

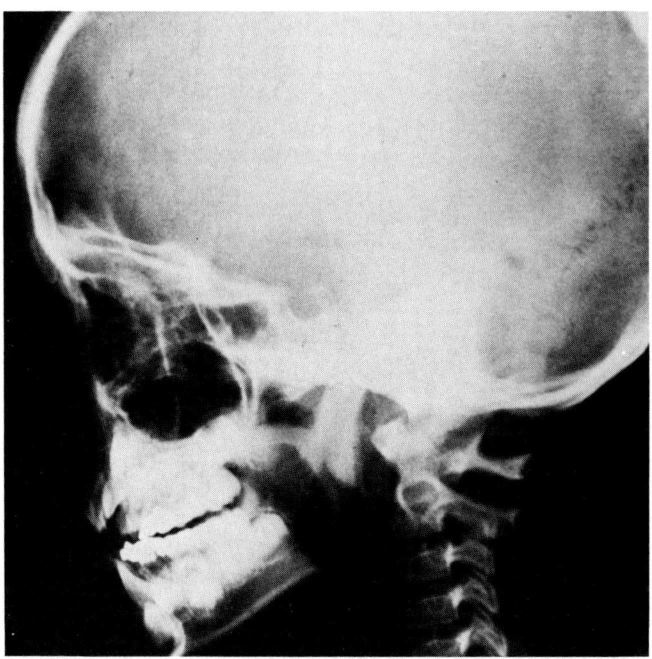

Figure 52–2 The knee formation of the soft palate, showing excellent closure against the posterior pharyngeal wall that is pushed away by the implant. This is the same patient seen in Figure 52–7.

History of Augmentation Procedures

Earliest use of a procedure to build up the posterior pharyngeal wall may have occurred in 1900 when Gersuny injected Vaseline into several patients.[1] He did not report any complications, but Eckstein in 1904 reported that one of Gersuny's patients had died of a fatal lung embolism.[2] Others suffered unilateral blindness. Eckstein injected paraffin and reported no complications.

In 1912 Hollweg and Perthes[3] inserted autogenous cartilage through an external approach. Lando[4] inserted homogeneous cartilage grafts using a transoral approach in 1950. Hynes[5, 6] reported use of mucosal and muscle flaps to build up the posterior pharyngeal wall in 1950 and 1953. In 1951 Vinas and Jager[7] first started using autogenous cartilage; later they tried homogeneous cartilage and other implants.

Early American reports on augmentation of the posterior pharyngeal wall were made by Hagerty and associates in the 1960s.[8, 9] They used homogeneous cartilage inserted through a transverse incision in the posterior pharyngeal wall and reported no extrusions, but there was an expected rate of absorption of 2% to 3% each year. They reported an improvement in speech intelligibility and articulation with less nasal emission and less nasal sound. The speech results were better in patients under 10 years of age.

Calnan reported his experience with autogenous cartilage and its attached perichondrium, introduced through an intraoral route, in patients who had nasal speech after adenoidectomy.[10] He reported subsequent normal speech in all patients.

Blocksma reported his experiences with solid Silastic, medium X30146; solid Silastic, soft shredded, S60508; sponge Silastic, coarse; and RTV fluid Silastic with stannous octoate catalyst, S5392.[11] Of the four materials reported, the RTV fluid Silastic proved somewhat successful, and in 1964 Blocksma described the techniques he used to instill the RTV.[12] He noted speech improvement in 23 of 27 patients; however, he advised against the routine use of Silastic in the posterior pharynx as a corrective procedure for velopharyngeal incompetence.

Lewy et al reported a single patient in whom 3 to 5 ml of Teflon in glycerine was injected into Passavant's line; speech improvement resulted.[13] In 1968, Bluestone et al reported their experiences with 12 patients in whom Teflon paste was injected into the posterior pharyngeal wall.[14, 15] Five of these patients had speech that was judged to be very close to normal. All experienced some improvement, and there were no serious complications. Sturim and Jacob reported their experiences with the injection of Teflon in glycerine in 23 patients.[16] Their results showed 12 patients with good speech and 10 with improved speech. Calnan implanted Teflon felt and solid plastics, but all these materials extruded, and their use was discontinued.[17]

Ousterhout et al presented a case report on pharyngeal bursa associated with velopharyngeal incompetence.[18] Benson described a roentgenographic cephalometric study of palatopharyngeal closure in normal adults during vowel phonation in 1974.[19] Altermatt et al reported the histopathologic findings after Teflon injection in 1985.[20] Furlow et al reported obstructive sleep apnea following treatment of velopharyngeal incompetence by Teflon injection.[21]

Personal Surgical Experience

In 1954 I (R.O.B.) inserted homogeneous cartilage using an intraoral approach, with disappointing speech results. In 1963 carved, solid Silastic implants were used in a number of patients. Most of these implants were extruded, but in one patient the speech changed from markedly nasal to normal. Later, we placed room temperature vulcanizing silicone (RTV) in a prepared pocket in the posterior pharyngeal wall. This, too, eroded through the overlying muscle and mucosa, and its use was discontinued. I also made my own "pillow" implants from soft silicone rubber provided by the Dow Corning Company to which Dacron wool was fixed with glue. A number of these implants extruded, necessitating removal, and they are no longer used. The ideal material for implantation is one that is readily available, easy to use, well tolerated by the body, not absorbed, and will not drift or disappear. In 1968 the Dow Corning Company provided me with some small silicone bags filled with silicone gel. In an effort to prevent gradual erosion of the overlying soft tissue, I wrapped the Silastic bags in Dacron wool, sutured with 5–0 Dacron. These implants were inserted into a prepared pocket in the posterior pharyngeal wall in several patients and have not extruded.

Based on this experience Dow Corning then prepared a special implant or "pillow" with Dacron wool glued to silicone gel bags. These have been made in three sizes: 28 x 15 x 9 mm, 20 x 15 x 9 mm, and 15 x 10 x 9 mm (see Fig. 52–1). These are the implants that we have used quite successfully during the past 20 years.

Preoperative Management

Physical examination centers on the soft palate as a search is made for a bifid uvula, submucous cleft, short soft palate, or deep nasopharynx, but most important, the presence of palatal motion. Although the physical examination is helpful, the most reliable information is provided by a videofluoroscopic study of the palate.

The second author (D.R.F.) has found that in some instances it is necessary to fatigue the patient before the extent of the deficiency is revealed in the study. The case history usually indicates the presence of intermittent nasality (see Fig. 52–2). The extent of the space or gap between the flexed soft palate and the posterior pharyngeal wall is measured from the lateral film. Almost all of the patients in the series demonstrated active soft palate motion and had a gap of 6 mm or less.

The patient is examined 2 days before surgery to rule out any upper respiratory infection and is placed on oral antibiotics to reduce the chance of infection of the implant. An intravenous bolus of antibiotic is used during surgery. It is better to perform this surgery during late spring, summer, or fall when the chances of an upper respiratory infection are decreased.

Operative Technique

The surgery is performed under endotracheal anesthesia supplemented by 1% lidocaine with 1:1000 epinephrine injected along both sides of the posterior pharyngeal wall and in the planned midline incision for hemostasis. A delay of 5 minutes is recommended before making the incision.

The upper end of the vertical midline incision is placed 1 cm below the adenoid area so that it will not overlay the implant (Fig. 52–3). A transverse incision is contraindicated in the event a later pharyngeal flap should be required.

The 1- to 1¼-inch incision extends through the muscle to expose the white, shiny prevertebral fascia. The soft palate is retracted to visualize the dissection as it extends beneath the muscle and adenoid area to the base of the skull (Figs. 52–3 and 52–4). The many fibrous septa are cut with either a right-angled Beaver knife or a right-angled scissors. The pocket is made almost the full width of the posterior pharyngeal wall, taking care to avoid injury to the lateral ascending arterial vessels. The posterior pharyngeal wall is measured transversely to determine the size of the implant to be used. The implant is soaked in 1,000,000 units of aqueous penicillin solution, and the same penicillin solution is instilled into the dissected pocket and the

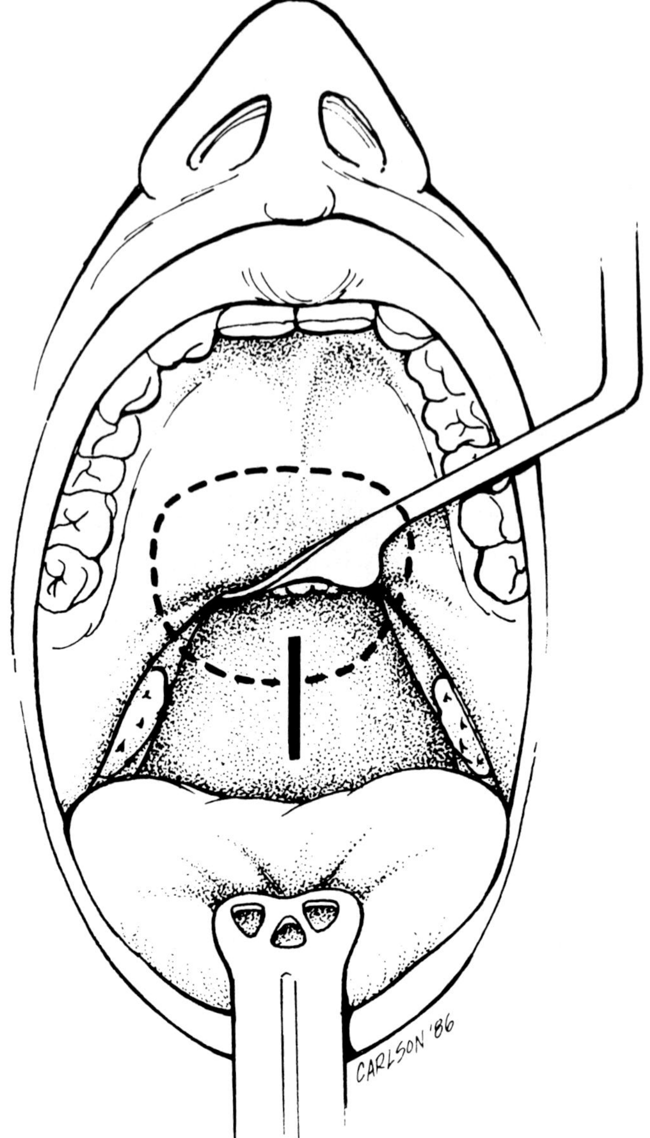

Figure 52–3 The heavy line is the 1¼-inch incision below or distal to the adenoid area. The palate is retracted to reveal the area of planned pocket dissection illustrated by the dotted lines.

surrounding areas to reduce the amount of contamination of the implant. Bleeding is controlled by inserting cottonoids into the dissected pocket. This also helps to determine the extent of the dissection.

The implant is then inserted in a transverse position and is pushed superiorly as far as possible (Figs. 52–5, 52–6, and 52–7). Ideally, none of the implant is visible below the upper margin of the incision. If it is visible, it should be removed and the pocket enlarged before replacing the implant. The incision is closed in two layers with interrupted 5–0 Vicryl starting at the superior end of the incision and closing the muscle layer first and the mucosa last. When the second muscle suture is placed, I often fix it to the posterior pharyngeal wall to help close any dead space. Figure 52–8 shows the bulge of one of the early round implants. Figure

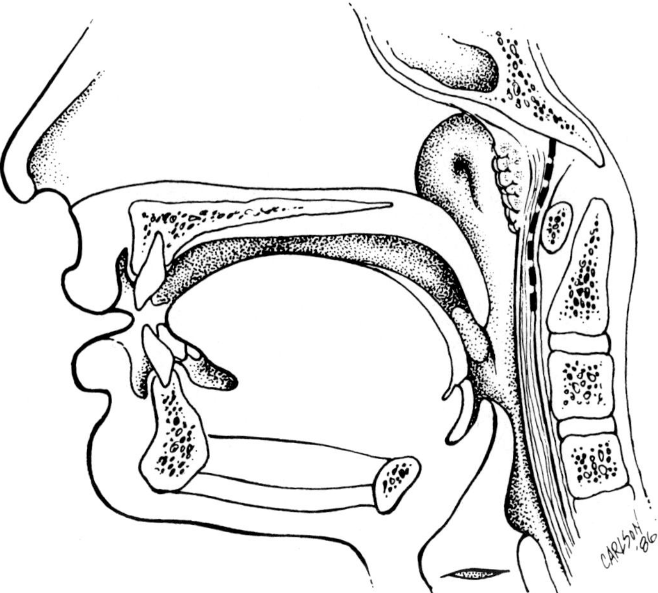

Figure 52–4 The dotted line shows the vertical extent of the dissection.

52–7 is a videofluroscopic study of a palate at rest, and Figure 52–1 shows the closure of this palate on phonation with an implant in place.

Postoperative Care

Postoperative care is simple. The patient is often discharged on the day of surgery but is kept on a soft diet for 4 or 5 days. It is expected that he or she will have a sore throat or a stiff neck for several days postoperatively. Oral antibiotics are continued for 4

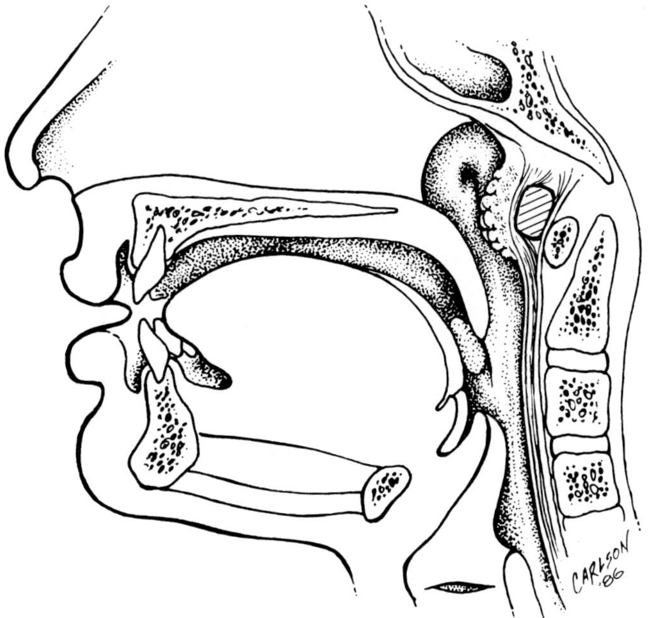

Figure 52–5 The implant is placed deep to the adenoid mass as high as possible.

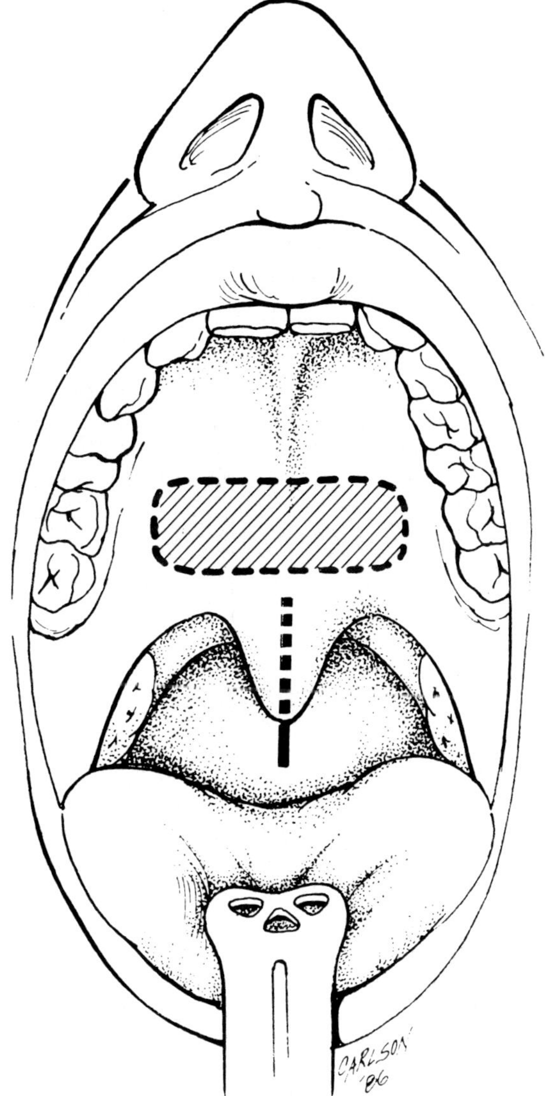

Figure 52–6 This photograph shows the final positioning of the implant. It actually ends beneath the midportion of the soft palate.

days postoperatively. I often see the patient at weekly intervals for about 3 weeks and then again after a month.

Visual evidence of infection of the implant is a small, raised, grapelike process in the posterior pharyngeal wall, usually slightly below the site of placement of the implant, indicating need for further treatment with antibiotics. There also may or may not be a sore throat. If the infection persists, the implant must be removed. Removal is performed in the operating room, with special attention to removal of all of the Dacron velour. After a period of 6 to 12 months, another implant can be inserted. Late exposure of the implant is accompanied by repeated sore throat attacks and bad breath.

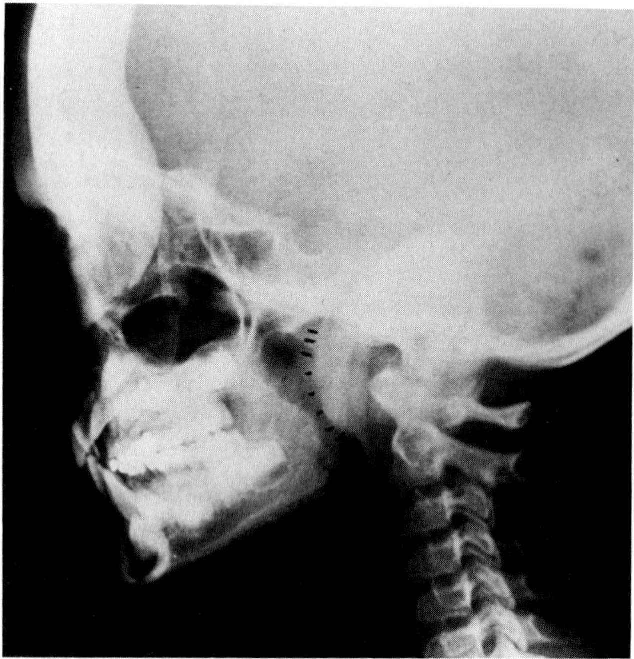

Figure 52–7 A radiograph of the soft palate at rest with the margin of the posterior pharyngeal wall outlined by the dotted lines and pushed forward by an implant.

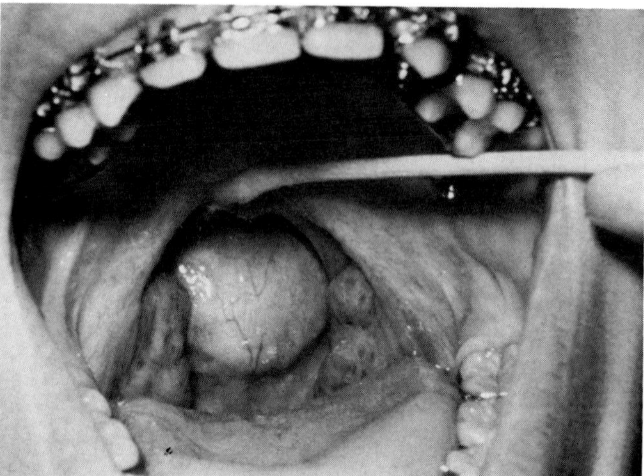

Figure 52–8 Photograph of one of the round implants that has been in place for several years. Patient had normal resonance and speech.

Complications

The major complication has been loss of the implant. Such loss occurred in 9 of the 70 patients in the series. In seven of these nine patients, evidence of exposure was found within 2½ to 4 months after the operation. However, in two patients the implant became exposed as late as 3 and 5 years after surgery. Exposure of the implant in the early time period probably means that there was sufficient contamination at the time of insertion to produce subsequent infection. Long-term loss of the implant suggests that the patient had a systemic infection as a reaction to other types of foreign bodies.

In four of the nine patients a gel implant was successfully replaced after a delay of 6 months to several years. Successful replacement probably could have been accomplished in the other five patients, but they failed to return for surgery.

Another possible cause of infection and loss of the implant occurs in the patient with deep adenoid crypts. These crypts need to be gently probed or explored either before or after dissection. If the crypt extends into the dissected pocket, placement of the implant should be delayed and the crypt excised and closed. This occurred in 1 of the 70 patients.

Speech Results

This 20-year series consisted of 70 patients who had implants inserted in the posterior pharyngeal wall (Table 52–1). Preoperatively, all patients had mild to severe nasal speech. Most were referred by speech pathologists or other physicians, or they were self-referred. Careful preoperative speech evaluation was not done on all patients because speech was obviously nasal.

A preoperative fluoroscopic study was done in all patients who demonstrated a gap of 6 mm or less. The degree of nasality was usually related to the extent of the gap; however, nasal speech also occurred with intermittent or weak closure. Many of these patients with intermittent closure had normal speech much of the time, but speech deteriorated with fatigue (end of day) or when the patient was excited or angry. A common complaint of these patients was that they could not be understood on the telephone, a real handicap in today's world.

There were 70 patients in the study, but only 65 had successful implants; seven of these were lost to follow-up when the families moved away from Houston. (Patients are quick to relate to the primary surgeon in the event of complications, which leads me to believe that

Table 52–1. Augmentation of Posterior Pharyngeal Wall: Summary of Results

Type of Implant
Dacron-wrapped gel pillow—64
Dacron-wrapped silicon block—6

Age at Surgery
Average 10.66 yr
Range 3–26 yr

Length of Follow-Up
Average 40.8 mo
Range 1 wk–15 yr
7 patients were lost to follow-up

Speech Results–58 Patients
Normal resonance 44/58 (75.8%)
Normal resonance and articulation 33/58 (61%)
Slight nasality 14/58 (24.1%)

Loss of Implant–9 Patients
Successful reaugmentation 4/9 (45%)
Unsuccessful reaugmentation 1/9 (11%)
Did not return for augmentation 4/9 (45%)
Implant removal 1.5–66 months postoperatively
Lost within 4 months 7/9 (78%)

they also had a successful result from the surgery.) (Fig. 52–1).

The remaining 58 patients underwent postoperative speech evaluation. The two senior authors (R.O.B. and D.R.F.) examined 30 of these patients independently and were in agreement 95% of the time. R.O.B. rated 21 to have normal resonance, D.R.F. rated 22 to have normal resonance. R.O.B. rated six as nasal, and D.R.F. rated eight as nasal. The remaining 28 postoperative speech evaluations were performed by R.O.B. or other speech pathologists.

Forty-four (75%) of the 58 patients had normal resonance. Thirty-five of these also had normal articulation, whereas the remaining nine had normal resonance with articulation defects.

There were 14 patients (24.1%) with persistent nasal speech after surgery. All patients but one showed marked improvement. They were rated as nasal although the nasality was often perceptible only to the trained ear. Postoperative videofluoroscopic studies were not performed in 20 patients; however, 18 of these had normal resonance. In the presence of normal resonance, postoperative fluoroscopic studies were probably not needed. Five of the 14 patients had nasal speech postoperatively when videofluoroscopy showed velopharyngeal closure. Another five had normal resonance even though a small gap was revealed; apparently the anteroposterior deficit was compensated for by exceptional lateral wall movement.

Some Special Cases

Four patients received surgery even though they did not fit the preoperative protocol. The first patient had a 15-mm gap on fluoroscopy with hypernasality; after surgery the gap was reduced to 5 mm, and the nasality was significantly improved. A second implant was advised but was never carried out. A second patient had a 15-mm gap; in this patient a simultaneous push-back repair and implant was carried out. After surgery, even though the patient's speech was still nasal, she could be understood on the telephone for the first time in her life.

Surgery was performed early in the series on the third patient, who had a 7-mm gap preoperatively. Her speech was extremely nasal, and two pillows were inserted but resulted in little improvement in her speech. Five months later, a third pillow was inserted beneath the first two, reducing the gap on the fluoroscopic study to 1 mm. Her speech remained quite nasal, and a pharyngeal flap was performed without removal of the pillows. Little improvement in speech was obtained even after the pharyngeal flap was performed.

The fourth exceptional patient was a 23-year-old patient with mild Crouzon's disease. She, too, had nasal speech with poor palatal movement and a 5-mm gap on the videofluoroscopic study. However, she had excep-

tionally active lateral walls preoperatively. It was thought that if a medium-sized implant was inserted without disturbing the lateral wall musculature, speech could be improved. This proved to be a surgical triumph because postoperatively she had normal resonance, and closure was evident on fluoroscopy.

Conclusions

Augmentation of the posterior pharyngeal wall is a logical approach to the correction of an anatomic deficit. It offers the patient a chance to overcome a significant speech problem with a relatively short operative procedure. The improvement is immediate and the implants are well tolerated. This procedure is far more logical than a pharyngeal flap. Augmentation of the posterior pharyngeal wall is definitely a procedure whose time has come. Every surgeon who performs surgery on the cleft patient should become familiar with this procedure so that it can be offered to patients. Adherence to the criteria of good palatal movement and a gap of 6 mm or less should maximize the chance of normal resonance after augmentation.

References

1. Gersuny R: About a subcutaneous prosthesis. Zschr Heilk 21:199, 1900.
2. Eckstein H: Demonstration of a paraffin prosthesis in defects of the face and palate. Dermatologica 11:772, 1904.
3. Hollweg E, Perthes G: Treatment of Cleft Palates. Tübingen: Franz Pietzcher, 1912.
4. Lando RL: Transplant of cadaveric cartilage into the posterior pharyngeal wall in treatment of cleft palate. Stomatologia 4:38, 1950.
5. Hynes W: Pharyngoplasty by muscle transplantation. Br J Plast Surg 3:128, 1950.
6. Hynes W: The results of pharyngoplasty by muscle transplantation in "failed cleft palate" cases. Ann R Coll Surg Engl 13:17, 1953.
7. Vinas JC, Jager E: The "Push Forward" in Velopharyngeal Incompetence. Transactions of Fifth International Congress of Plastic Surgery, Melbourne, 1951.
8. Hagerty RF, Hill MJ: Cartilage pharyngoplasty in cleft palate patients. Surg Gynecol Obstet 112:350, 1961.
9. Hagerty RF, Mylin WK, Hess DA: Augmentation pharyngoplasty. Plast Reconstr Surg 44:353, 1969.
10. Calnan JS: Permanent nasal escape in speech after adenoidectomy. Br J Plast Surg 24:197, 1971.
11. Blocksma R: Correction of velopharyngeal insufficiency by Silastic pharyngeal implant. Plast Reconstr Surg 31:268, 1963.
12. Blocksma R: Silicone implants for velopharyngeal incompetence: a progress report. Cleft Palate J 1:72, 1964.
13. Lewy R, et al: Teflon injection in the correction of velopharyngeal insufficiency. Ann Otol Rhinol Laryngol 74:874, 1965.
14. Bluestone CD, et al: Teflon injection pharyngoplasty. Cleft Palate J 5:19, 1968.
15. Bluestone CD, et al: Teflon injection pharyngoplasty status 1968. Laryngoscope 78:558, 1968.
16. Sturim HS, Jacob CT, Jr: Teflon pharyngoplasty. Plast Reconstr Surg 49:180, 1972.
17. Calnan JS: Congenital large pharynx. Br J Plast Surg 24:263, 1971.
18. Ousterhout DK, Jobe RP: Pharyngeal bursa associated with velopharyngeal incompetence—case report. Plast Reconstr Surg 47:187, 1971.
19. Benson D: Roentgenographic cephalometric study of palato-pharyngeal closure of normal adults during vowel phonation. Cleft Palate J 9:43, 1972.
20. Altermatt HJ, Gebbers JO, Sommerhalder A, et al: Histopathologic findings in the posterior pharyngeal wall 8 years after treatment of velar insufficiency with Teflon injection. Laryngol-Rhinol-Otol 64:582, 1985.
21. Furlow LT, Jr, Block AJ, Williams WN: Obstructive sleep apnea following treatment of velopharyngeal incompetence by Teflon injection. Cleft Palate J 23:153, 1986.

CHAPTER 53

The Influence of Pharyngeal Flap on Facial Growth

*Gunvor Semb
and William Shaw*

Approximately 20% to 30% of patients who have undergone palatoplasty, regardless of the technique, still have poor speech. A substantial proportion of these may be considered to be in need of some form of secondary surgery.[1] One of the most common procedures is the attachment of a superiorly based pharyngeal flap to the posterior edge of the soft palate (Fig. 53–1), more accurately described as palatopharyngoplasty.[2] As with all secondary procedures, the desirability of additional surgery is not always clear-cut, and the benefits and risks must be carefully weighed in each case.

Factors Affecting Facial Development

Facial growth is known to be highly vulnerable to surgical insult, and it is not inconceivable that the growth disturbances associated with primary repair may be accentuated by pharyngoplasty, especially when it is performed on a young child. Indeed, current theories of facial growth suggest that pharyngoplasty may adversely affect subsequent development in two ways:
1. By inducing functional adaptations in facial form secondary to increased airway resistance.
2. By inhibiting anteroposterior maxillary growth.

Airway Resistance

A long-suspected association between nasal airway resistance and facial form has been substantiated in recent years because definite changes in facial development have been identified in children who have excessive adenoid tissue in the nasopharynx. In these children there is an increase in anterior facial height, and both the maxilla and mandible are retrusive.[3] The mandibular ramus is positioned vertically in relation to the nasal floor, and the gonial angle is obtuse.[4] The adaptive nature of these characteristics is highlighted by the small but significant "normalization" that follows adenoidectomy.[5] The causal mechanism for these adaptations is improperly understood, but part of the explanation may lie in the alterations of head posture that are necessary to facilitate breathing and the muscular and facial tension that ensues. Thus the head, extended in relation to the cervical column, is associated with an increased anterior facial height, small anteroposterior dimensions, and retrognathism.[6]

Nasal airway resistance is reported to be high in the cleft population.[7] Secondary restorative procedures such as pharyngeal flaps significantly reduce the nasopharyngeal airspace further and have an especially adverse effect on upper airway breathing in children.[8–10]

Facial form in individuals with repaired clefts of the lip and palate has many of the characteristics of the "adenoidal facies," and it would not be unreasonable to suppose that the occlusion of the nasopharynx sought by pharyngoplasty together with other preexisting influences such as tongue displacement might further accentuate these adaptations.[11, 12]

Maxillary Restraint

The second way in which pharyngoplasty may disturb facial development is by restraining the normal forward growth of the maxilla. In patients with repaired clefts of the palate, the maxilla is already retruded to some degree, mainly as a result of the binding effect of residual scar tissue in the retromaxillary region.[13] The extent to which the presence of a pharyngeal flap is likely to be a significant additional factor is difficult to estimate. On the one hand, the pharyngeal flap is intended to be dynamic, and electromyographic activity has been found in superiorly based flaps.[14] As such, there is some similarity to the growth-restraining forces mediated by the orthodontist's use of headgear in the treatment of maxillary protrusion. On the other hand, resting levels of force in a pharyngeal flap are unlikely

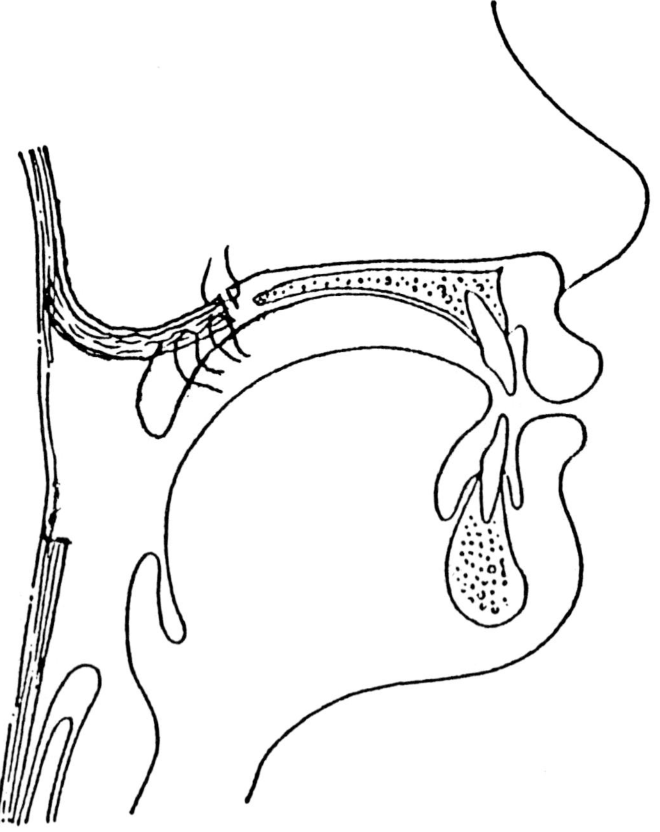

Figure 53–1 Palatopharyngoplasty.

to be of sufficient magnitude to inhibit growth (forces of 250 to 500 gm per side are required for effective headgear wear), and the duration of higher levels of force reached during speech and swallowing is arguably too brief to be a significant restraint.

Previous Studies

Only a minority of children with repaired cleft palate receive pharyngeal flap surgery and it is perhaps not surprising that studies dedicated to the subsequent impact of this procedure on facial growth are sparse. One study reported by Subtelny and Pineda-Nieto included 24 patients who had undergone pharyngeal flap surgery between the ages of 7 and 11 years.[15] Of these, 19 subjects had repaired palatal clefts, and five had congenital palatal insufficiency. Group comparisons were made with 18 individuals with repaired palatal clefts but no pharyngeal flaps and with a reference group of 28 noncleft individuals. The number of subjects in the cleft palate group with unilateral or bilateral clefts of the lip and alveolus was not specified. In two different statistical analyses, the available postoperative cephalometric records were matched according to age. Preoperative records were not included.

The authors reported one major difference between the groups: the anterior prominence of the maxilla was reduced (that is, was restrained) to a greater extent in the pharyngeal flap group. However, their published tables contradict this finding. Maxillary prominence (SNA) in the pharyngoplasty cleft palate group was reduced by only 4.42 degrees during the period of observation compared with a reduction of 6.61 degrees in the nonpharyngoplasty cleft group. Apart from the lack of preoperative records, further doubt about the reliability of these findings is raised by the remarkably high SNA value of 87.75 degrees reported for the nonpharyngoplasty cleft group at baseline (the range for noncleft normal values being 80 to 82 degrees), suggesting that this group contained a significant proportion of subjects with bilateral clefts of the lip and palate and associated premaxillary protrusion.

Long and McNamara examined the effects of pharyngoplasty on facial growth in 17 patients (nine with cleft palate only, eight with unilateral cleft lip and palate).[16] Each patient was matched with a control of the same cleft type, sex, presurgical mandibular growth direction (facial axis angle), and cranial base size. Pharyngeal flap surgery was performed in patients between 5 and 7 years of age, and annual cephalometric records were available for 3 years before and 3 years after surgery. Although matched for mandibular growth direction, presurgical differences between the flap and control groups emerged for some other variables. Patients who later received a pharyngoplasty had a greater upper anterior facial height and a more retrusive maxilla and mandible. Following surgery, increased vertical growth of the mandible was evident, implying a functional adaptation to increased airway resistance similar to that found in adenoidal noncleft children.

Pearl and Kaplan obtained cephalometric records of 25 patients, of whom 12 had a repaired cleft involving the palate and 13 had noncleft palatopharyngeal incompetence.[17] Each child had undergone a pharyngeal flap *and palatal push-back* operation 3 to 10 years previously. No control patients were included, but the cephalometric measurements of the patients, confined to anteroposterior relationships, were compared with published norms for noncleft children. The authors found a degree of maxillary and mandibular retrusion that they considered to be no more than that which would be anticipated in any cleft population. They concluded that the combined push-back and pharyngeal flap was not deleterious to growth.

Present Study

Purpose

The present study addresses two questions:
1. Does the skeletal pattern of children with cleft lip and palate diagnosed as requiring a pharyngeal flap for correction of palatopharyngeal incompetence differ from that of cleft lip and palate children with competent palatopharyngeal function?
2. Following a pharyngeal flap operation, is the pattern of skeletal development altered?

Sample

Records of 257 consecutive patients with complete unilateral cleft lip and palate were abstracted from the Oslo Cleft Lip and Palate Growth Archive. Patients with a soft tissue (but not bony) bridge across the cleft were also included. All had had surgery performed at the Department of Plastic Surgery, University Hospital in Oslo and had had regular follow-up examinations by the Oslo Cleft Palate Team. The approach to primary surgical management in Oslo has been relatively consistent since 1954, only minor modifications having been made (see Chap. 4).[18, 19] Among the 257 patients, 52 (20%) had undergone palatopharyngoplasty with a superiorly based pharyngeal flap (Fig. 53–1). Of these, 33 were male and 19 were female.

Cephalometry

All patients were represented by serial cephalometric records obtained under standardized conditions and for which extensive digitization had been performed. For the present report, the reference points and planes considered are shown in Figure 53–2. Definition of the landmarks is in accordance with the description by Bjork.[20] In addition, an ss′ point was used, defined as the projection of ss on the NL line. All digitizing was performed by the same individual (G.S.).

Analysis of Prepharyngoplasty Skeletal Form

Each of the 52 patients who underwent pharyngoplasty was matched with a control from the remainder

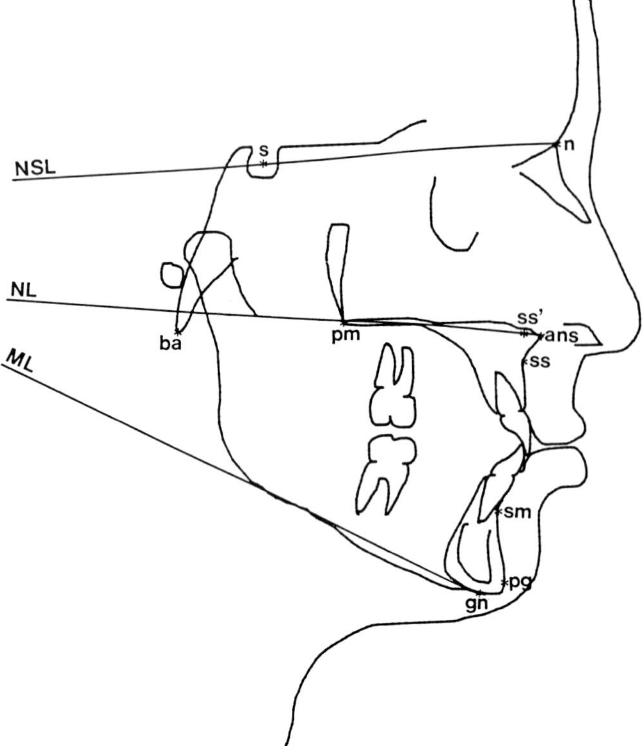

Figure 53–2 Reference points and planes. Cephalometric landmarks and planes. s, sella; n, nasion; ba, basion; pm, pterygomaxillare; ans, anterior nasal spine; ss, subspinale (A point); ss', intercept of ss perpendicular on nasal line; sm, submandibulare (B point); pg, pogonion; gn, gnathion; NSL, nasion-sella line; NL, nasal line; ML, mandibular line.

of the sample. Each matched pair had had a lateral cephalometric film taken at the same age (within 12 months). In the pharyngoplasty group, the record used was always taken before the operation; in patients in whom the operation had not been performed until the teens, a record obtained before the child had reached age 12 was used. Pairs also were matched for sex and for presence or absence of a soft tissue bridge. Details of the distribution of age at the time of pharyngoplasty and the ages of controls are presented in Table 53–1.

Mean values for the 52 pharyngoplasty patients and their matched pairs were compared by a paired t test (Table 53–2). Major differences between the pharyngoplasty patients and controls were not evident; however, some minor differences did emerge. Although anterior maxillary protrusion was the same in both groups (s–n–ss), maxillary length (ss'–pm) was 1.5 mm shorter on average in the pharyngoplasty group (p = 0.043), and upper facial height (n–ss') was 1.4 mm less on average (p = 0.007). Lower facial height (ss'–gn) was also slightly less (mean difference 1.7 mm, p = 0.043), and the mandible was slightly more protrusive in the pharyngoplasty group (s–n–pg, mean difference 1.3 mm, p = 0.029).

The maxillary shortness combined with a normal maxillary protrusion in the pharyngoplasty group is consistent with a predisposition toward palatopharyngeal incompetence and the need for pharyngoplasty. The

Table 53–1. Age of Records Used for Prepharyngoplasty Controlled Comparison (52 Matched Pairs)

Age When Record Obtained (years)	Pharyngoplasty Group	Control Group
4	10	10
5	13	13
6	14	14
7	7	6
8	3	4
9	2	3
10	1	2
11	2	0

reduction in anterior facial height is less readily explained, but the reduced lower facial height and concomitant mandibular protrusion is broadly in keeping with current functional adaptation therapy: that is, if airway obstruction is associated with increased facial height and mandibular retrusion, then lack of obstruction (palatopharyngeal incompetence) might be expected to produce the opposite effect. In the context of facial development in a cleft population, this would mean a lesser expression of the characteristics of adenoidal facies.

Analysis of the Influence of Pharyngoplasty

To study the possible growth interference caused by childhood pharyngoplasty, this part of the study was confined to those patients in whom pharyngoplasty was performed at age 12 or younger and for whom 5-year (minimum) postoperative records were available. This yielded 29 pharyngoplasty patients, 17 males and 12 females. Each patient was matched with a control case of the same sex and the presence or absence of soft-tissue bridging. Comparison of the mean change in facial dimensions occurring during the period of observation for the 29 pharyngoplasty patients and their controls was performed by a paired t test (Table 53–3).

Table 53–2. Prepharyngoplasty Controlled Comparison (52 Matched Pairs)

	Pharyngoplasty Group $\bar{x}$	Control Group $\bar{x}$	Probability
Anteroposterior relationships			
s–n–ss	79.00	78.70	0.683
s–n–pg	75.12	73.85	0.029
ss–n–sm	4.16	5.13	0.156
n–ss–pg	172.68	170.50	0.136
ss'–pm	43.91	45.43	0.043
Vertical relationships			
NSL–NL	8.45	9.62	0.074
NSL–ML	35.79	37.19	0.093
NL–ML	27.34	27.58	0.786
n–ss'	41.44	42.82	0.007
ss'–gn	58.63	60.29	0.043
Cranial base angulation			
n–s–ba	130.92	131.79	0.324

Table 53–3. Controlled Comparison of Amount of Change Occurring in the Pharyngoplasty Group between Preoperative and Follow-up Registration (29 Matched Pairs)

	Pharyngoplasty Group $\bar{x}$	Control Group $\bar{x}$	Probability
Anteroposterior relationships			
s–n–ss	−3.86	−3.43	0.568
s–n–pg	3.18	3.17	0.991
ss–n–sm	−5.37	−4.81	0.525
n–ss–pg	13.90	13.27	0.739
ss′–pm	0.88	1.13	0.747
Vertical relationships			
NSL–NL	−1.34	−1.67	0.714
NSL–ML	−1.63	−1.81	0.873
NL–ML	−0.29	−0.14	0.912
n–ss′	9.89	9.02	0.100
ss–gn	14.50	13.08	0.142
Cranial base angulation			
n–s–ba	−1.51	−1.08	0.592

The overall impression is one of similar growth in the pharyngoplasty and control groups, with slightly greater increases in the previously shorter upper and lower anterior facial heights of the pharyngoplasty group (nonsignificant trends, p = 0.1 and 0.14 respectively). This might be interpreted as weak evidence of a functional adaptation to the increased airway resistance produced by the pharyngeal flap.

A repeated measures analysis of variance was performed as a final exploration of difference between the pharyngoplasty group and their pair-wise matched controls.[21] For this analysis, each pair was considered as an experimental unit with two factors: treatment group (pharyngoplasty/no pharyngoplasty), and time (presurgery/follow-up). In this analysis a group effect would suggest that there were intrinsic differences between the pharyngoplasty and control patients not attributable to the operation and a time effect would imply growth changes independent of the operation. Of particular interest, a significant interaction would imply differential development of the two groups, suggesting a surgical interference with growth.

The results of the repeated measures analysis of variance confirm the earlier analyses. Significant growth changes attributable to the passage of time were identified for all variables except maxillomandibular planes angle (NL–ML). Significant group differences confirmed the pharyngoplasty group's intrinsically shorter maxillary length (ss′–pm, p = 0.004) and smaller upper facial height (n–ss, p = 0.02); NSL–NL, p = 0.025). No effects attributable to receipt of a pharyngoplasty were identified apart from weak trends suggesting "catch-up" changes in the pharyngoplasty group for upper and lower facial height (n–ss, p = 0.1; ss′–gn, p = 0.14).

Discussion

The general uniformity of the program of surgical care at Oslo, the standardization of records, and the relatively large sample of documented cases of a particular cleft subtype (complete unilateral cleft lip and palate), offer a reasonable opportunity to study the influence of pharyngoplasty on facial growth.

The importance of including preoperative measures in studies of surgical intervention are highlighted in this investigation because certain preexisting differences were apparent between the group who had been diagnosed as requiring a pharyngeal flap and the controls, who did not. In the pharyngoplasty group, maxillary length and upper and lower facial height were shorter, and the mandible was slightly more protrusive. On the average, these differences were not large and would not appear to offer particularly useful diagnostic guidelines for identifying patients who might require pharyngoplasty. The reduced maxillary depth is certainly in keeping with the excessive size of the palatopharyngeal port, which might contribute to the nasality in speech identified by the speech pathologist and, in turn, the selection of pharyngoplasty as the treatment of choice following clinical examination.

The other minor differences in mandibular position are generally compatible with the current theory of functional adaptation to nasal airway obstruction or, in the case of the palatopharyngeal incompetence group, the lack of it. Similarly, the weak trends identifying an assimilation of anterior facial height following pharyngoplasty conform conveniently to theoretical expectations. However, the modest nature of observed changes fails to contribute substantially to the current debate on the adaptability of facial form to airway resistance. Pharyngoplasty cannot be regarded as an equivalent (but opposite) effect to adenoidectomy. Above all, the important conclusion of this study is that performing a superiorly based pharyngeal flap operation does not appear to carry a risk of adversely affecting subsequent facial growth in either the anteroposterior or the vertical dimension.

References

1. Spriestersbach DC, Dickson DR, Fraser FC, et al: Clinical research in cleft lip and cleft palate: The state of the art. Cleft Palate J 10:113, 1973.
2. Lindsay WK: Surgery. In Ross RB, Johnston MC (eds): Cleft Lip and Palate. Baltimore: Williams & Wilkins, 1972, p. 155.
3. Linder-Aronson S: Adenoids—their effect on mode of breathing and nasal airflow and their relationship to characteristics of the facial skeleton and the dentition. Acta Oto-Laryngologica (Suppl) 265, 1970.
4. Koski K, Lahdemaki P: Adaptation of the mandible in children with adenoids. Am J Orthod 68:660, 1975.
5. Linder-Aronson S: Effects of adenoidectomy on dentition and nasopharynx. Am J Orthod 65:1, 1974.
6. Solow B, Tallgren A: Head posture and craniofacial morphology. Am J Phys Anthropol 44:417, 1976.
7. Warren DW, Duany LF, Fischer ND: Nasal pathway resistance in normal and cleft lip and palate subjects. Cleft Palate J 6:134, 1969.
8. Warren DW, Trier WC, Bevin AG: Effect of restorative procedures on the nasopharyngeal airway in cleft palate. Cleft Palate J 11:367, 1974.
9. Guilleminault C, Eldridge FL, Tilkian A, et al: Sleep apnea syndrome due to upper airway obstruction: A review of 25 cases. Arch Intern Med 137:296, 1977.
10. Kravath RE, Pollak CP, Borowiecki B, et al: Obstructive sleep apnea and death associated with surgical correction of velopharyngeal incompetence. Pediatrics 96:645, 1980.
11. Harvold EP: The role of function in the etiology and treatment of malocclusion. Am J Orthod 54:883, 1968.
12. McKee TL: A cephalometric radiographic study of tongue position in individuals with cleft palate deformity. Angle Orthod 26:99, 1956.

13. Ross RB: Treatment variables affecting growth in cleft lip and palate. Part 6. Techniques of palate repair. Cleft Palate J 24:64, 1987.
14. Broadbent TR, Swinyard CA: The dynamic pharyngeal flap: Its selective use and electromyographic evaluation. Plast Reconstr Surg 23:301, 1959.
15. Subtelny JD, Pineda-Nieto: A longitudinal study of maxillary growth following pharyngeal flap surgery. Cleft Palate J 15:118, 1978.
16. Long RE, Jr., McNamara JA, Jr: Facial growth following pharyngeal flap surgery: Skeletal assessment on serial lateral cephalometric radiographs. Am J Orthod 87:187, 1985.
17. Pearl RM, Kaplan EN: Cephalometric study of facial growth in children after combined pushback and pharyngeal flap operations. Plast Reconstr Surg 57:480, 1976.
18. Abyholm FE, Borchgrevink HC, Eskeland G: Cleft lip and palate in Norway. III. Surgical treatment of CLP-patients in Oslo 1954–75. Scand J Plast Reconstr Surg 15:15, 1981.
19. Borchgrevink HC: Cleft palate repair. In Muir IFK (ed): Current Operative Surgery—Plastic and Reconstruction Surgery. London: Bailliere Tindall, 1986.
20. Bjork A: Kaebernes relation til det ovrige kranium. In Lundstrom A (ed): Nordisk Larobok i Ortodonti, Suppl 4. Stockholm: Sveriges Tandlakarforbunds Forlagsforening, 1975.
21. Winer BJ: Statistical Principles in Experimental Design, 2nd ed. New York: McGraw Hill, 1971.

CHAPTER 54

Airway Obstruction and Apnea in Cleft Palate Patients

Steven Gray

Symptoms of airway obstruction have been recognized for many years. It has only been in the last decade, however, that the consequences of partial airway obstruction and apnea have been identified and treated. The consequences of acute airway obstruction or prolonged apnea resulting in respiratory arrest or death are not infrequently addressed by any surgeon who performs surgery that may alter or affect the airway. Cleft patients are at risk for partial airway obstruction and apnea. Frequently the cleft may be associated with other craniofacial anomalies that are predisposed to airway compromise such as the Robin anomaly. Hypertrophy of the tonsils and adenoids may lead to partial airway obstruction similar to that seen in noncleft children. Subglottic stenosis, laryngomalacia, and poor swallowing coordination (due to nervous system immaturity) are among several other causes of airway difficulty that may affect the infant airway, including those with clefts.

Probably the most common cause of airway obstruction in cleft patients occurs in those who have received a pharyngeal flap. Although the incidence of pathologic airway obstruction in these patients is not known, nearly all cleft surgeons are aware of patients who have suffered from losing their nasal airway. It is likely that partial airway obstruction and apnea is under-recognized and undertreated because the emphasis in treatment of clefts has historically been on correction of speech, often at the expense of the airway.

It was not until the late 1960s and early 1970s, through reports by Ainger,[1] Bland,[2] Cronje,[3] and Gerald,[4] that it was realized that chronic hypoxia due to partial airway obstruction could lead to serious cardiopulmonary disorders. Gerald et al[4] described cor pulmonale and pulmonary edema in patients with chronic upper airway obstruction, and Bland et al[2] described pulmonary hypertension and congestive heart failure in children with similar symptoms. Since then, upper airway obstruction causing hypoventilation and cor pulmonale has become known as cardiopulmonary syndrome. As the people who suffered from chronic hypoxia were better studied, it became apparent that many of them also experienced other symptoms of this disease such as failure to thrive, chronic fatigue, tiredness, inattentiveness, and irritability. The results of pharyngeal flap surgery are now scrutinized more carefully with respect to both speech and airway patency. Because of this attention, it is likely that revision surgery will focus on obtaining the best speech and airway function.

Pharyngeal Flap

The placement of the pharyngeal flap requires special consideration and carries with it the unique risk of creating obstructive sleep apnea.[5] This may occur as acute obstruction in the immediate postoperative period or may occur as chronic airway obstruction manifested by obstructive sleep apnea accompanied by mouth breathing. Orr et al reported acute postoperative death resulting from airway obstruction.[6] It is now well recognized that patients receiving pharyngeal flaps are at risk for acute airway obstruction in the postoperative period.[7] Most of these cleft patients have had excellent nasal breathing since birth. Placement of the pharyngeal flap and the presence of pharyngeal edema in the postoperative phase requires these patients to adapt suddenly to oral breathing during the sleep phase. Orr et al showed that the majority of postoperative pharyngeal flap patients experienced some obstructive sleep apnea during the early postoperative period.[6] When retested after 3 months, only 10% had abnormal results on sleep studies. This report attests to the difficulty experienced by a pediatric patient in suddenly changing from nasal breathing to oral breathing during the sleep period. This difficulty can be compounded by the effects of anesthesia postoperatively or any postoperative sedation.

The surgeon must be aware that resolution of apneic events does not occur in all patients and that it is possible for apnea to reappear following scar contracture of the pharyngeal ports. The presence of apneic symptoms demands evaluation to determine the severity of the apneic events (the symptoms of apnea and the work-up are discussed in the next section). If apnea does exist, the surgeon must decide, generally in consultation with other specialists who deal with obstructive sleep apnea, such as otolaryngologists, pulmonologists, or neurologists, whether or not the apnea is severe enough to warrant a revision procedure on the pharyngeal flap. The surgeon should avoid considering the development of sleep apnea in the pharyngeal flap patient as a surgical failure because this attitude may prevent him from diagnosing the existence of this condition in his patients. It must be remembered that the surgery is performed to obturate the velopharyngeal port; sleep apnea should be considered as a possible consequence, not a complication, of the procedure.

The ability to control the size of the pharyngeal ports at the time of the placement of the pharyngeal flap is also controversial. The development of sleep apnea in patients undergoing pharyngeal flap surgery, regardless of technique or procedure, points out the difficulty of controlling the scar contracture around the velopharyngeal ports that exist postoperatively. To further compound this problem, the pharyngeal flaps have a tendency to curl or tube (Fig. 54–1), thus shrinking the width of the flaps. Other tendencies of the pharyngeal flaps due to scarring are contraction and subsequently tethering of the palate. If scarring and consequent contraction of the pharyngeal flap pull the palate inferiorly, two other conditions occur:

1. The velopharyngeal ports may be displaced inferiorly in the pharynx, positioning the ports below the area of maximal velopharyngeal movement (this does not maximize the patient's own ability to close the ports).
2. Infiltration of scar tissue around the velopharyngeal ports may further reduce their capacity for lateral and medial wall motion.

This independent variable of scar contracture is probably the most significant factor in determining the final size of the ports. This factor may overshadow our attempts to try to tailor pharyngeal flaps and control port size.

When reconstructed nasopharyngeal ports are too large, velopharyngeal incompetence persists. When ports are too small, hyponasality and, more important, snoring and nasal obstruction (associated at times with sleep apnea) can occur. Bjork in 1961 reported that 20 mm^2 is the maximal amount the velopharyngeal port may be open and still allow clinically normal speech.[8] Since that report, many surgeons have used that measurement to determine the port size during reconstruction. Ports this small provide good pharyngeal competence but are accompanied by a high rate of significant nasal obstruction. Furthermore, if there is good pharyngeal wall motion so that the ports are dynamic, they can be larger than 20 mm^2 and still provide good speech.

Despite the concept of tailoring pharyngeal flaps, the velopharyngeal surgeon not infrequently encounters patients with ports that are either too large or too small.

Ports That Are Too Large

Patients who have velopharyngeal ports that are too large have significant hypernasality. Generally, there are no nasal breathing complaints. In these patients the ports need to be narrowed. Patience should be used prior to revision because a port may continue to contract postoperatively. Revision should be delayed for 6 months after the original pharyngoplasty procedure. The method used for revision depends partly on the degree of port narrowing that must be achieved. If, for instance, flap contracture or necrosis has resulted in very large ports and a very thin, narrow, or nonexistent pharyngeal flap, it is best to repeat the pharyngeal flap procedure. This usually necessitates taking down whatever remnant of the flap is present and then raising another pharyngeal flap. Despite the fact that the superior constrictor has already been raised from the donor site, there is enough tissue to create a second flap if the revision procedure is done after the donor site is well healed. An alternative

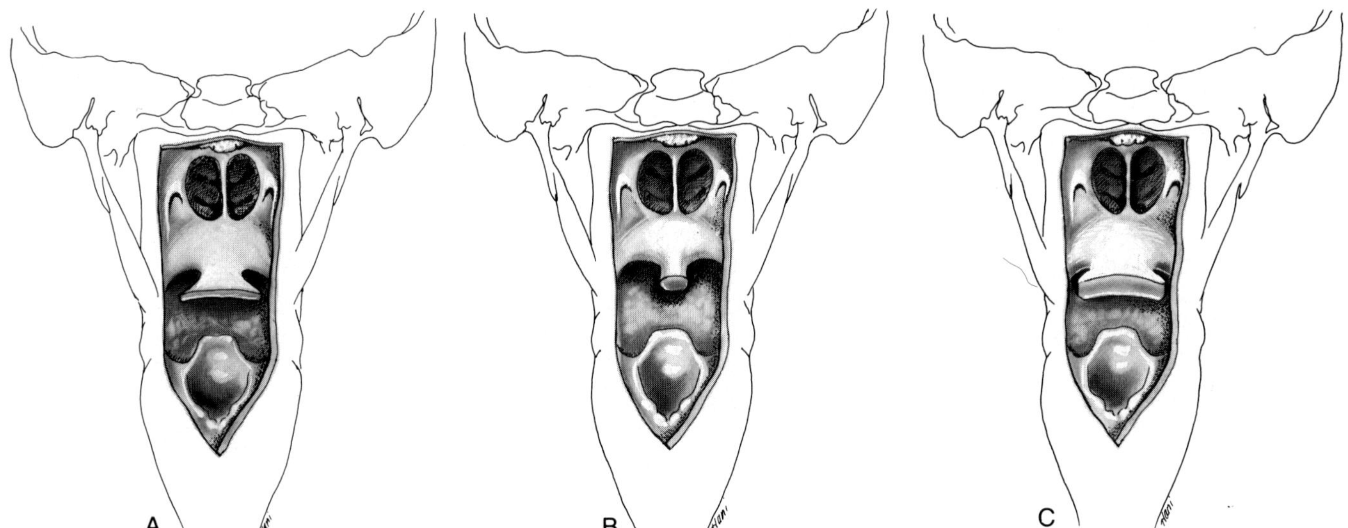

Figure 54–1 View of pharyngeal flap with posterior wall removed. *A,* Normal flap (superiorly based). *B,* Small pharyngeal flap as a result of flap contracture, tubing, or intentional "tailoring" by surgeon to correct a specific velopharyngeal defect in closure. Note large ports. *C,* Large pharyngeal flap with pharyngeal ports nearly obstructed or too small. Thick flaps may lead to port collapse and closure during exhalation.

to this procedure is to perform a pharyngeal flap that does not use the same donor site such as a transverse pharyngeal flap or a sphincter pharyngoplasty. Kapetansky has reported good success in using a transverse pharyngeal flap following failure of a superiorly or inferiorly based pharyngeal flap.[9]

If there is no need to redo the entire pharyngeal flap, port narrowing may be accomplished using one of three techniques. The first is Teflon injection into the port. This is accomplished by injecting a small amount of Teflon into the port area and is best suited for minor corrections. The site of injection should be away from any large vessels and in areas that are less dynamic in port closure. This site is best assessed by nasendoscopy. The best site is usually the posterior, medial aspect of the velopharyngeal port.[10] Although Teflon is approved for human use, it is not approved by the Food and Drug Administration (FDA) for nasopharyngeal injection. Therefore, Teflon use in this way requires appropriate informed consent. The second method uses a scarification technique. Essentially this technique induces further scar contracture of the port, thus narrowing it. This may be done with cautery or a knife, and again is best done away from vessels and away from the more dynamic areas of "port closure." The areas that generally seem to be most dynamic in port closure are the lateral walls in a superiorly or inferiorly based pharyngeal flap. The third technique is that of portal tissue excision from the port. In this technique a wedge-shaped piece of tissue can be excised from the port, thus narrowing it.

Ports That Are Too Narrow

If ports are too narrow, the patient will present with some of the following characteristics: hyponasality, snoring, obstructed nasal breathing, and sleep apnea. Speech in these patients is generally good even with hyponasality. If the patient reports considerable snoring and obstructed nasal breathing, or if any doubt exists about possible apnea, a sleep study should be obtained. If nasal obstruction or sleep apnea is present, the nasopharynx and oropharynx should be thoroughly ex-

amined. We have encountered a few cases in which adenoids that were not removed preoperatively became obstructive and inhibited nasal breathing despite adequately sized ports. We have also seen documented sleep apnea due to hypertrophic tonsils that obstructed the nasopharyngeal ports. After examination, if it appears that the problem is indeed the size of the ports, port enlargement must be considered. Ports can be enlarged in four general ways. If the scar tissue surrounding the port is relatively immature, then ports may be dilated. Some surgeons feel that injection of the port with steroids or placement of a long-term stent is helpful. Although the authors know of successful results through the use of nasopharyngeal port dilation, steroid injection of the ports, and placement of nasopharyngeal stents for up to 3 months, the results are not predictable, and these methods seem to delay but not prevent the ports from becoming too small.

A second method consists of transferring tissue to the ports with local flaps created from the pharyngeal walls. The port is incised, and a local flap is moved into the port at the area of incision, thus expanding it. A stent may be needed to hold the flap in place until adequate healing has occurred.

The third method, which carries a much higher success rate but may result in velopharyngeal incompetence, consists of taking down the pharyngeal flap (Fig. 54–2). In this procedure, the flap is sectioned so that again the soft palate is free from the nasopharynx. The flap should be detached so that a moderate ridge of tissue remains on the posterior wall to help provide obturation. The ridge should be located in the same area as Passavant's ridge. The surgically exposed ridge of tissue should be covered with mucosa as much as possible, avoiding extensive surgical dissection. If this procedure is done in a child, velopharyngeal incompetence may return. However, this procedure has been very successful in the teenager or adult who has had a pharyngeal flap placed as a child. These older patients rarely exhibit velopharyngeal incompetence following pharyngeal flap release.

Selection criteria for pharyngeal flap release include (1) total or near total nasal obstruction; (2) no current

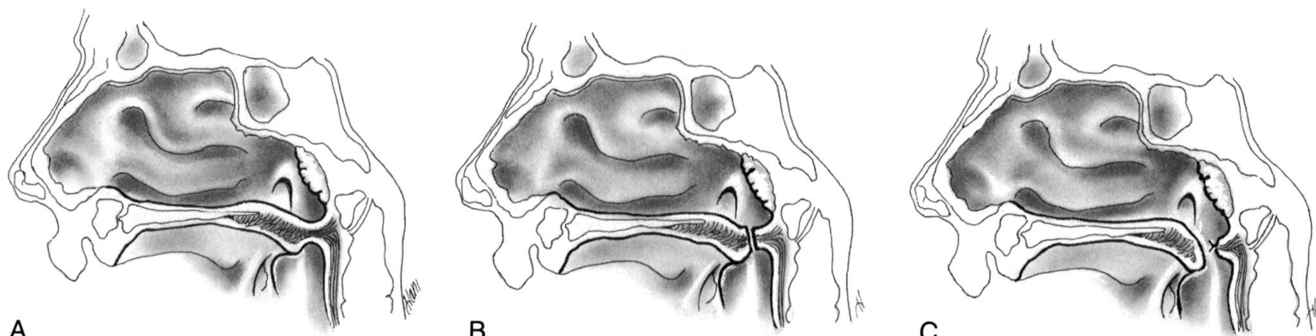

Figure 54–2 Pharyngeal flap release. *A*, Position of flap connecting palate to posterior pharyngeal wall at desired level, just inferior to adenoid pad. *B*, Pharyngeal flap is sectioned so that a small to moderate ridge of tissue is left on the posterior pharyngeal wall. This aids in continued obturation of the velopharyngeal opening after flap release. *C*, Posterior wall ridge is covered with mucosa as much as possible.

velopharyngeal insufficiency; (3) a palate that is severely scarred and tethered to the posterior pharyngeal wall so that the entire posterior edge of the soft palate is closely approximated to the posterior pharyngeal wall. Following flap release, the velopharyngeal gap is not large.

The fourth method, trimming the flap to enlarge the ports, is simple and occasionally successful. Unless mucosal coverage of the trimmed area is performed, the port will again contract. Trimming of the flap alone will often provide only temporary improvement.

Adhesions tethering the flap may alter the position of the newly created ports and may also decrease the dynamic motion of the ports. In those instances, lysis of adhesions may be needed.

We have experienced good success with a method of port enlargement that is derived from the concept of the uvulopalatopharyngoplasty used by otolaryngologists to correct obstructive sleep apnea (Fig. 54–3). This procedure is combined with a tonsillectomy and involves closure of the tonsillar fossa by suturing the posterior tonsillar pillar to the anterior tonsillar pillar. Incision of the junction of the anterior soft palatal portion with the medial wall of the flap leads to anterior advancement of the lateral and anterior ports as the tonsillar fossa is closed. If more port enlargement is needed, partial resection of the soft palatal portion of the port can be performed. If partial resection of the palate is necessary, the incision should be beveled so that mucosa can be preserved and complete mucosal coverage can be provided.

Adenoidectomy and Tonsillectomy

Controversy exists about whether or not a patient should have a prepharyngeal flap adenoidectomy. The arguments for doing a prepharyngeal flap adenoidectomy are as follows:

1. Removal of adenoid tissue may improve the nasopharyngeal airway following placement of the pharyngeal flap. Although adenoid tissue can assist in velopharyngeal closure by providing more nasopharyngeal tissue, the same tissue can become quite obstructive to a nasopharyngeal port following placement of the pharyngeal flap. Removal of adenoid tissue is very difficult after a pharyngeal flap has been placed. Generally, it is not possible to work through the nasopharyngeal ports to remove the adenoid tissue. Thus the adenoid tissue has to be removed transnasally with electrocautery and sinus endoscopic equipment.
2. There is some concern, although it is not proved, that resolution of the adenoid tissue due to growth and maturity will change velopharyngeal closure. This resolution of adenoid tissue will cause the pharyngeal ports to become too open, and the patient will again develop velopharyngeal incompetence.
3. Gates et al demonstrated that adenoidectomy is effective in reducing persistent middle ear effusions in noncleft patients.[11] Severeid et al, in assessing the efficacy of adenoidectomy in cleft patients, performed

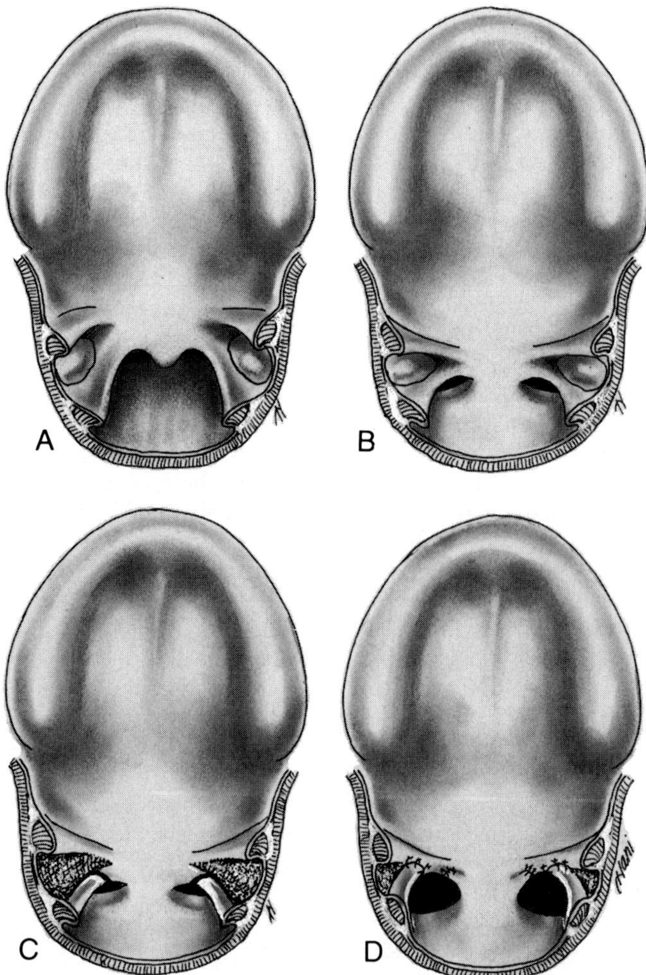

Figure 54–3 Port enlargement method. *A*, Normal oropharyngeal anatomy before pharyngeal flap. Note position of tonsillar pillars. *B*, Oropharyngeal anatomy following pharyngeal flap. Tonsillar pillars are oriented more posteriorly, and posterior tonsillar pillar constitutes the anterior portion of the velopharyngeal port. Note space occupied by tonsil. *C*, Tonsillectomy performed with tonsillar fossa bare, anterior tonsillar pillar to anterior border of velopharyngeal port. Releasing incision is performed through anterior port as shown. *D*, Posterior tonsillar pillar sutured to anterior tonsillar pillar with closure of tonsillar fossa. Port mucosa should not be injured except by releasing incision. This avoids further scar contracture. Scar contracture of port is opposed by anterior tonsillar pillar, which has already been displaced posteriorly from original pharyngeal flap. Compare positions in *A*, *B*, and *C*. Absorbable sutures are used.

a retrospective study and concluded that age rather than adenoidectomy was the major factor resulting in resolution of ear disease.[12] The efficacy of adenoidectomy in cleft patients has not been proved, although, as mentioned previously, it appears that adenoidectomy is beneficial in noncleft patients suffering from persistent middle ear effusions. Because of the risk of causing velopharyngeal incompetence, it is difficult to design a study to assess the efficacy of adenoidectomy in the cleft patient. Some otolaryngologists point out that since adenoidectomy may be beneficial in treating ear disease, it should be performed in those patients who have already developed velopharyngeal incompetence and who will require placement of a pharyngeal flap.

The arguments against a prepharyngeal flap adenoidectomy are:

1. The procedure may leave scarring in the selected surgical site for the pharyngeal flap. This scarring may make the procedure more difficult or may impair the blood supply to the flap. Neither of these effects has been proved.
2. The procedure may be unnecessary. There are patients with minimal to nonexistent adenoid tissue in whom the routine removal of adenoid tissue before pharyngeal flap placement would be superfluous.
3. The effect of adenoidectomy in cleft patients for improvement of ear disease has not been proved.

At the Iowa City Cleft Palate Center, we perform prepharyngeal flap adenoidectomy in patients who have demonstrated severe ear disease or have so much adenoid tissue that we feel that partial obstruction of the pharyngeal ports may possibly develop. This prepharyngeal flap adenoidectomy is generally performed at least 8 weeks prior to the pharyngeal flap procedure. Parents need to be warned that velopharyngeal incompetence will be more obvious following adenoidectomy and prior to placement of the pharyngeal flap.

Another indication for adenoidectomy, as recommended by the American Academy of Otolaryngology—Head and Neck Surgery, is chronic and recurrent purulent nasal pharyngitis despite adequate medical or immunotherapy. Because of the risk of developing velopharyngeal incompetence in cleft patients, adenoidectomy for recurrent purulent nasal pharyngitis should be avoided. If adenoidectomy is necessary, a partial adenoidectomy may be considered.

Tonsillectomy and adenoidectomy are indicated when obstruction of the airway occurs and is related to sleep apnea, cor pulmonale, or failure to thrive. Obligate mouth breathing, not solely attributed to other causes, is occasionally an indication. Although mouth breathing has not been proved to be deleterious, it may indicate that sleep apnea is occurring at night. Therefore, patients that are obligate mouth breathers should be evaluated for sleep apnea. There is concern that obligate mouth breathing may lead to orofacial growth and orthodontic abnormalities. A discussion of that topic is beyond the scope of this chapter. Tonsillectomy and adenoidectomy in these patients usually will improve the airway but may not change the orofacial growth and orthodontic problems. When performing tonsil and adenoid surgery in cleft patients, one must weigh carefully the risks of possibly increasing velopharyngeal dysfunction compared with the benefits of an improved upper airway.

Tonsillectomy without adenoidectomy appears to carry no higher risk in the cleft patient than in the normal population. Tonsillectomy is recommended when:

1. Tonsils are causing occlusion of pharyngeal flap ports or occlusion of the oropharyngeal airway.
2. Tonsils are so large that they cause difficulty with eating and swallowing.
3. Recurrent tonsillitis occurs despite adequate medical therapy. Recurrent tonsillitis may be complicated by peritonsillar abscess, abscessed cervical nodes, acute airway obstruction, febrile seizures, cardiac valvular disease with recurrent streptococcal tonsillitis, and recurrent otitis media. Indications for tonsillectomy in this group are stronger.

Apnea

Apnea is defined as a cessation of respiratory airflow. The respiratory pause may be central, obstructive, or mixed. Central apnea occurs when no respiratory effort by the muscles of respiration is made. Obstructive apnea occurs when respiratory effort is made but no airflow occurs owing to obstruction of the upper airway. Short episodes of apnea (less than 10 to 15 seconds in duration) can be normal at all ages. Apnea becomes pathologic when it is associated with cardiopulmonary symptoms such as cyanosis, pallor, hypotonia, or arrhythmias. Chronic mild to moderate apnea may become pathologic when symptoms of sleep deprivation (daytime somnolence, inattentiveness, fatigue) or failure to thrive occur.

Although the type of apnea experienced by cleft patients is usually due to obstruction, it behooves the surgeon to be aware of other factors influencing breathing that may affect the occurrence of apnea in the patient. Short episodes of obstructive apnea may occur in healthy infants[13] with crying, feeding, defecation, and Valsalva maneuvers. Rest or bottle feeding causes an early termination of inspiration. Nevertheless, most term infants can feed without significant alteration of minute ventilation. Some infants have a 40% to 50% drop in minute ventilation and a 10% to 13% drop in pO_2 during continuous feeding. This may explain why infants suffering from mild to moderate apnea become symptomatic during feeding. Additionally, in some apnea-prone preterm infants, milk regurgitation appears to trigger laryngeal and esophageal reflexes that may precipitate episodes of obstructive or mixed apnea. Chronic partial airway obstruction leads to hypoxia and hypercapnia. As the pCO_2 continues to increase, the respiratory center in the brain becomes insensitive to carbon dioxide.[2, 14] It has been well described that many patients suffering from mild to severe sleep apnea of an obstructive nature frequently develop central apnea. Consequently, many patients with obstructive apnea initially may actually have mixed apnea. Resolution of the obstructive apnea may not lead to a rapid clinical improvement because of the component of central apnea. In most cases, the central apnea will slowly correct itself following resolution of the obstructive component.

Symptoms and Signs

A history and physical examination are usually adequate to alert the physician that partial airway obstruction is present. Snoring, noisy breathing, and stridor are hallmark findings indicating that partial airway obstruction is present. Frequently the parents will volunteer information indicating that the noisy breathing is interrupted by silence, which indicates that an obstructive apneic event is occurring. Occasionally the parents will indicate that the child struggles for breath and sleeps restlessly. In a study of 81 patients with documented cardiopulmonary syndrome, Yonkers and Spaur found that snoring or stridor was the most common symptom.[15] Lethargy, frequent upper respiratory tract infection, and failure to thrive were common symptoms.

In the majority of patients partial airway obstruction becomes worse during sleep because the pharyngeal musculature is relaxed as a child enters stage II or rapid eye movement (REM) sleep. With relaxation of the pharyngeal musculature, the partially obstructed airway is further compromised. It is normal for children to have nasal breathing during sleep. Those children who depend on an oral airway can develop significant sleep apnea. Patients with pharyngeal flaps may exhibit nocturnal oral breathing and sleep apnea. These children may have poor sleep habits, nightmares, enuresis, and the characteristics of people who are sleep deprived such as irritability, daytime somnolence, and inattentiveness.

Physical examination should focus on the respiratory rate, blood pressure, and signs indicating the presence of partial airway obstruction and increased respiratory effort. Because the airway starts with the nose and ends with the pulmonary alveoli, a thorough examination should include the nasal, nasopharyngeal, oral, oropharyngeal, and laryngeal structures. Obstructions of the airway should be carefully sought, with the realization that some obstructions that are dynamic may be recognizable only during sleep (such as pharyngeal wall collapse) or feeding (double aortic arch). If a complete examination of the upper airway reveals no obstruction in the awake child, yet noisy breathing persists, examination of the trachea, bronchi, and distal airway is warranted. This is best done with a chest x-ray followed by a bronchoscopic examination.

Other signs of partial airway obstruction include mouth breathing, chest wall retractions, poor growth, large tonsils or adenoids, and cardiovascular signs indicating cor pulmonale. A differential diagnosis for nasal obstruction includes alar collapse (valving); deviated nasal septum; polyps, nasal masses, or tumors such as an encephalocele, dermoid, or hemangioma; choanal stenosis; and atresia. If the internasal anatomy is normal, one must consider whether there is hypertrophy of the turbinates or if they are chronically congested, thus interfering with nasal breathing. The nasopharynx should be examined for obstructive adenoids and for other nasopharyngeal masses, such as angiofibroma, which usually occurs in the male adolescent population. Pharyngeal flaps are frequently the cause of nasal obstructions, and nasendoscopy should be performed to evaluate the obstruction. Oral and oropharyngeal obstructions can include the tonsils, macroglossia, and micrognathia, and occasionally redundant or excessive pharyngeal tissue such as occurs in children with Hunter's syndrome or in patients with poor neuromuscular control (as with cerebral palsy).

Laryngeal examination should include a dynamic examination for evaluation of the vocal cords to reassure the physician that the cords demonstrate normal inspiratory and expiratory motion. Vocal cord paresis or paralysis may be the first sign of a velopharyngeal shunt dysfunction and will cause the patient to breathe increasingly noisily. Laryngomalacia is a common cause of noisy breathing and partial obstruction in infants. By 18 months, this obstruction has usually resolved in the normal child. However, severe laryngomalacia may persist for many years, especially in children with craniofacial syndromes such as Goldenhar's syndrome. Laryngomalacia may develop in patients who have a progressive neuromuscular disease that decreases the tone of the laryngeal and pharyngeal muscles. When laryngomalacia is severe enough, treatment may include a tracheostomy or an epiglottoplasty.[17] If this examination does not reveal the cause of the airway obstruction, a further work-up is indicated. Most often this includes either a flexible or rigid bronchoscopic examination. Subglottal stenosis is occasionally present in patients with craniofacial disorders, either as part of their initial syndrome or because of previous intubation. Tracheomalacia or vascular compression of the trachea, generally due to abnormal anatomy of the cardiovascular system, may be the cause of partial obstruction of the trachea. Tracheal compression due to pectus excavatum and scoliosis may be a factor in some of these patients.

Although in most cases sleep apnea or partial airway obstruction may be diagnosed from the history and physical examination, a formal sleep study can help determine the severity of the disease. This is helpful if correction of the cause of sleep apnea may require surgery more involved than a tonsillectomy or adenoidectomy (such as takedown or revision of pharyngeal flap) or may carry with it significant risks (tracheostomy). A sleep study (polysomnogram) provides documentation of the disorder and gives the physician quantified data that can help to determine whether intervention is needed and whether improvement is achieved postoperatively. Although the effects of moderate to severe obstructive apnea are well known in the cardiopulmonary syndrome, the effects of minimal to mild sleep apnea are not well documented. If a sleep study shows moderate to severe obstructive apnea, intervention is performed. If minimal to mild obstructive apnea is found but is asymptomatic (not pathologic as described earlier), a case can be made for adopting a wait-and-see approach. If the causative factor of the apnea is expected to improve (such as laryngomalacia), one may wish to wait before intervening surgically. If mild apnea is pathologic or symptomatic or if the causative factor is not expected to improve (such as a pharyngeal flap with small ports), intervention to correct the apnea is warranted. Because the long-term effects of mild apnea are not known, close follow-up is essential if a wait-and-see approach is taken to watch for the development of sleep apnea symptoms and signs as described above.

A sleep study also can be of value in diagnosing patients in whom the history is hard to obtain or is mildly suggestive of a sleep disorder. Our policy has been to obtain a sleep study if we are the least bit suspicious of a sleep disorder or if correction of the sleep disorder will require major intervention. We do not obtain sleep studies if we feel that the obstruction is due to tonsil or adenoid hypertrophy and a tonsillectomy or adenoidectomy will suffice. A cassette audio recording performed by the parents at home of the child during sleep may be very helpful in determining if sleep apnea is present. A recent radiologic modality, cinecomputed tomography, can be helpful in evaluating dynamic airway collapse and in determining the site of obstruction. At present, this technique has some limitations in determining the cause of the collapse, particularly at the glottic level. It does offer a tremendous advantage in that it is capable of evaluating both the airway and the cardiovascular system simultaneously.

Sudden Infant Death Syndrome

Sudden infant death syndrome is defined as the sudden death of an infant or young child that is unexplained by the history and in which postmortem examination fails to demonstrate the cause of death. At this time there is no evidence that suggests that sleep apnea is a risk factor for sudden infant death syndrome.[17]

Micrognathia and Macroglossia

Pediatric patients with craniofacial disorders frequently exhibit micrognathia and relative macroglossia. Although these terms may be imprecise in describing the etiology of the mandibular and tongue defect, they do cause the clinician to consider the likelihood of airway obstruction. Since Pierre Robin described the association of micrognathia with upper airway obstruction, clinicians have associated these clinical findings with the term *Pierre Robin syndrome*.[18] The Robin malformation is not a syndrome with a single pathogenesis and may be associated with many other syndromes encountered by the craniofacial surgeon.[19-21] Regardless of the etiology, these patients do suffer from airway obstruction. This obstruction usually becomes manifest at, or shortly after, birth. Some patients with the Robin malformation may have an adequate airway until major craniofacial surgery is performed. Following surgery, the alterations of the structural airway support and accompanying edema may necessitate a tracheostomy.

Many clinicians label the region of obstruction in the Robin malformation as pharyngeal, and no further work-up for a more precise localization of the obstructed area is performed. Shprintzen and Sher et al categorized oral pharyngeal obstruction into four types.[21, 22] Type one occurs if the base of the tongue contacts the posterior pharyngeal wall, thus occluding the upper airway. Type two obstruction occurs when the tongue contacts the velum, which in turn contacts the posterior pharyngeal wall, causing an airway obstruction due to the tongue, velum, and posterior wall. A type three obstruction results when the lateral pharyngeal walls collapse medially, obstructing the oral pharynx. Type four obstruction represents collapse of the pharynx in a sphincteric manner. In a retrospective review of the endoscopic findings of 60 patients with the Robin triad of micro-

gnathia, U-shaped palatal cleft, and upper airway obstruction, it was found that the type of obstruction was never homogeneous within a certain diagnostic syndrome. A clinician must guard against assuming that the region of obstruction in these patients is pharyngeal. A proper evaluation of these patients includes an adequate nasal, nasopharyngeal, oropharyngeal, and laryngeal examination. A work-up similar to that described previously in the apnea section on airway obstruction should be performed. At the Iowa Cleft Palate Center, we have encountered choanal stenosis and atresia, laryngomalacia, subglottic stenosis, and pathologically obstructing tonsils and adenoids in patients with micrognathia and airway obstruction.

Other conditions may produce symptoms of airway obstruction similar to those encountered in the micrognathic patient. The Beckwith-Wiedemann syndrome, which is associated with macroglossia, or the pharyngeal hypotonia encountered in patients with velocardiofacial syndrome are examples of oral or oropharyngeal airway obstruction. Treatment for patients with oropharyngeal airway obstruction after appropriate diagnostic work-up and assessment of the entire airway is aimed at correcting the obstruction or bypassing it. Indications for surgical intervention are similar to those described above for the treatment of patients with obstructive apnea. In the neonate, infant, or toddler, it is usually most effective to bypass the airway obstruction when it is due to micrognathia. This is accomplished with a tracheostomy. Many other procedures have been proposed to correct the glossoptosis that can occur in these patients. Glossopexy is popular in some centers, although it is looked on with disfavor in others. Sher et al have reported that glossopexy has been performed with success in their institution for patients suffering from a type one obstruction.[22] Hyoid suspension has been proposed with some success. Our experience with glossopexy has not been favorable, and hyoid suspension has produced mixed results. For patients with serious airway obstruction, placement of a tracheostomy tube is the tried and true treatment. In patients with laxity of the pharyngeal tissue or with pharyngeal hypotonia, a uvulopalatopharyngoplasty may be indicated. We have performed uvulopalatopharyngoplasty successfully for treatment of airway obstruction due to pharyngeal hypotonia in patients with neuromuscular disease.

With growth, the airway obstruction due to micrognathia may resolve. This result depends partially on mandibular growth, which in turn depends on the initial etiology of the micrognathia. Shprintzen has reported that fewer than 20% of all patients with Robin malformation exhibit true catch-up growth.[21] Nevertheless, many patients may be decannulated from a tracheostomy without surgical correction despite lagging mandibular growth. Decannulation of the tracheostomy should be a controlled process, and proper monitoring of adequate ventilation should be accomplished during and after decannulation. Failure of decannulation may not necessarily be due to micrognathia even though that was the initial reason for the airway obstruction and the need for tracheostomy. Thus, an examination of the entire airway should again be performed prior to an attempt at decannulation, and failure of decannulation should raise concern that other factors may be responsible for airway obstruction, as the following report demonstrates.

This case concerns a child who required a tracheostomy 1 month after birth for isolated severe micrognathia and airway obstruction. He was the product of twin gestation, and although full-term, he had a birth weight of 1900 gm. At 1 month, he was evaluated at The University of Iowa for failure to thrive and hypotonia. Further evaluation revealed severe partial airway obstruction and prolonged obstructive apneic spells, which were felt to be due to his severe micrognathia. Following tracheostomy, he showed remarkable growth and development. At 8 months, he was brought in for decannulation, which was performed successfully. Two nights of postdecannulation monitoring showed normal oxygen saturations and carbon dioxide levels. Eight weeks later, he was readmitted for failure to thrive and sleep apnea symptoms. A sleep study showed that oxygen saturation dropped into the 40s to 60s with mild carbon dioxide retention. Airway examination revealed a moderate adenoid pad and oropharyngeal collapse. A tonsillectomy and adenoidectomy was performed, suturing the posterior tonsillar pillar forward to the anterior tonsillar pillars, which caused further tightening of the pharyngeal walls as occurs in a uvulopalatopharyngoplasty. Five days later, the patient had normal results on a sleep study and has had no further trouble in follow-up.

References

1. Ainger LE: Large tonsils and adenoids in small children with cor pulmonale. Br Heart J 30:356, 1968.
2. Bland JW Jr, Edwards FK, Brinsfield D: Pulmonary hypertension and congestive heart failure in children with chronic upper airway obstruction. New concepts of etiologic factors. Am J Cardiol 23:830, 1969.
3. Cronje RE, Human GP, Simson IW: Hypoxaemic pulmonary hypertension in children. Afr Med J 40:2, 1966.
4. Gerald B, Dungan WT: Cor pulmonale and pulmonary edema in children secondary to chronic upper airway obstruction. Radiology 90:679, 1968.
5. Shprintzen RJ: Pharyngeal flap surgery and the pediatric upper airway. Int Anesthesiol Clin 26:79, 1988.
6. Orr WC, Levine NS, Buchanan RT: Effect of cleft palate repair and pharyngeal flap surgery on upper airway obstruction during sleep. Plast Reconstr Surg 80:226, 1987.
7. Kravath RE, Pollack C, Borowiecki B, et al: Obstructive sleep apnea and death associated with surgical correction of velopharyngeal incompetence. J Pediatr 96:645, 1980.
8. Bjork L: Velopharyngeal function in connected speech. Acta Radiol, Suppl 202, 1961.
9. Kapetansky D: Transverse pharyngeal flaps: A dynamic repair for velopharyngeal insufficiency. Cleft Palate J 12:44, 1975.
10. Smith JK, McCabe BF: Teflon injection in the nasopharynx to improve velopharyngeal closure. Ann Otol Rhinol Laryngol 86:559, 1977.
11. Gates GA, Avery CA, Prihoda TJ: Effect of adenoidectomy upon children with chronic otitis-media effusion. Laryngoscope 98:58, 1988.
12. Severeid LR: Development of cholesteotoma in children with cleft palate: A longitudinal study. In McCabe BF, Sade J, Abramson M (eds): Cholesteotoma. First International Conference, Iowa City, IA. Birmingham, AL: Aesculapius Publishing, 1977.
13. von Someren V, Stothers JK: A critical dissection of obstructive apnea in the human infant. Pediatrics 71:721, 1983.
14. Talbot AR, Robertson LW: Cardiac failure with tonsil and adenoid hypertrophy. Arch Otolaryngol 98:277, 1973.
15. Yonkers AJ, Spaur CR: Upper airway obstruction and the pharyngeal lymphoid tissue. Otolaryngol Clin North Am 20:235, 1987.
16. ZalZal GH, Anon JB, Cotton RT: Epiglottoplasty for the treatment of laryngomalacia. Ann Otol Rhinol Laryngol 96:72, 1987.
17. Southall DP, Talbert DG, Johnson P, et al: Prolonged expiratory apnea and hypoxaemia. Lancet 2:1125, 1985.
18. Robin P: Glossoptosis due to atresia and hypotrophy of the mandible. Am J Dis Child 48:541, 1934.
19. Hanson JW, Smith DW: U-shaped palatal defect in the Robin anomalad: Developmental and clinical relevance. J Pediatr 87:30, 1975.
20. Cohen MM, Jr: The Robin anomalad: Its nonspecificity and associated syndromes. J Oral Surg 34:587, 1976.
21. Shprintzen RJ: Palatal and pharyngeal anomalies in craniofacial syndromes. Birth Defects Original Article Series 18(1):53, 1982.
22. Sher AE, Shprintzen RJ, Thorpy MJ: Endoscopic observations of obstructive sleep apnea in children with anomalous upper airways: Predictive and therapeutic value. Int J Pediatr Otorhinolaryngol 11:135, 1986.

CHAPTER 55

Oronasal and Nasolabial Fistulas

Craig R. Dufresne

The primary goals of palatal surgery are the closure of the cleft between the oropharynx and the nasal passages and the construction of a functional velum that allows for good speech production. The art and science of palatal surgery have evolved through the years so that the results now yield fewer complications and greater success in regard to speech, dental occlusion, and facial morphology. Although a single operation and primary healing of the palate are often the desired goal in palatal surgery, failures can occur, and oronasal or nasolabial fistulas can develop subsequently.[1–3] These secondary fistulas can occur in the palate anywhere along the site of the original cleft.[4, 5] They represent either a failure of technique or the healing process itself. Often their presence is heralded by the escape of air during speech or of liquid or food while eating.[1]

The incidence varies greatly between surgeons and cleft centers. The usual incidence reported in the world literature varies from 5% to 29%.[2, 5–7] At the Facial Rehabilitation Center at the Johns Hopkins Hospital an active roster of 330 patients with clefts is seen each year, and an additional 100 new patients are seen and evaluated. The incidence of fistulas varies with surgeons and the techniques they employ. In the author's experience, it is maintained at around 7% per year (4 of 55 patients, 1987). Successful correction of the various secondary fistulas encountered approaches 85% per year (4/28, 1987).

The location of the fistulas is most often in the anterior palate. Few of these, however, are symptomatic.[5,7] Fistulas in the middle or posterior palate are much less frequent but are more often symptomatic. Lindsay noted, after careful evaluation of his patient population, that in 1962, among 612 patients, 20% had fistulas or residual defects located in the perialveolar area, 11% of lesions were found in the hard palate, and 1% were noted in the soft palate.[5] A second review carried out in 1969 revealed that 31% of 111 patients had residual defects in the perialveolar area.[5] No other regions appeared to have any significant residual defects. Part of the reason behind these findings lay in the fact that there was no attempt to close the perialveolar area completely at the time of the primary surgery. Lindsay considered it preferable to avoid extensive surgery and therefore scarring in this region.[5] The von Langenbeck, or four-flap push-back procedure, does not allow complete closure of the anterior palate and therefore results in a higher incidence of fistulas.[2, 5] In our experience, there is a much higher incidence of fistula formation in patients who have had island flap palatoplasties or push-back palatoplasties with retrodisplacement of the levator palatini muscles.[8, 9]

Historical Overview

Historically, many attempts and various techniques have been employed to bring more tissue into the palatal region to make up for what nature failed to provide. At the turn of the twentieth century some gallant if not extreme efforts were carried out to bring healthy tissue into the oropharynx.[1] One surgeon sacrificed a patient's fifth digit when he used it as a pedicled flap to close a palatal cleft and help with the reconstruction of the nose and premaxilla. The blood supply was gradually reduced under tourniquet, and the digit was finally detached.[2]

More often, however, surgeons relied on tubed pedicles from the neck, chest, or inner upper arm to reconstruct large defects in the palate.[1-3, 5] These tubed pedicles were rotated into place, often employing ingenious designs in fixation in combination with other procedures such as pharyngeal flaps for reconstruction. Other surgeons successfully used forehead, nasolabial, or cheek flaps to reconstruct defects of any large magnitude.[12]

Today these techniques are used in ablative tumor surgery more than in palatal surgery. In wide clefts or large fistulas with a paucity of local palatal tissue, lining tissue can be obtained from several sources:

1. The nasal cavity. Septal and turbinate flaps from this region have been used but can result in significant growth disturbances if flaps are large or if the craniofacial sutures or growth centers are disturbed.
2. Local tissue adjacent to the defect. Turnover flaps and adjacent transposition flaps can be used.
3. Local buccal, vestibular, or facial regions.
4. Distant areas. Tissue from distant sites can be brought into the region; microvascular techniques can be employed in extreme instances.[1-5, 8, 10-12]

Our Center has reserved most of these techniques for patients with extensive craniofacial cleft syndromes.

Flaps from the anterior, lateral, or dorsal portion of the tongue still enjoy some degree of favor in our Center because of the high degree of success associated with them. Again, they are reserved for recurrent, recalcitrant fistulas in which extensive scar tissue is present. Caution has to be exercised not to sacrifice too much tissue for the sake of closing the fistula, thereby jeopardizing intelligent speech.[2, 13]

Some nonsurgical techniques have been employed to close fistulas with some success. Tincture of cantharides has been used as a cauterizing agent to help heal palatal fistulas in the immediate postoperative period. Others have used palatal appliances or splints until the fistulas closed or narrowed by themselves with vascularized tissues.[2, 14, 15] Our experience has shown that palatal appliances are useful in hyperactive children or in those in whom it is difficult to maintain protection of the suture line.

Today we agree with practitioners at several other Centers who believe that the most effective and most popular methods of closure are flaps utilizing a combination of local palatal, lip, or mucosal tissues.[2, 4, 14-17] The fistulas are then closed in a two-layer fashion without tension and with vascularized tissues. Bone grafts are often incorporated into the procedure to reconstruct the bony defects and to add to the aesthetic appearance of the final result.[18-23] This type of reconstruction, when it is necessary, in essence results in a three-layer closure.[10]

Nasolabial Fistulas

By definition, a nasolabial fistula is a defect on the labial side of the alveolus that often involves the alveolar bone and communicates with the nasal cavity.[4] An opening between the oral and nasal cavities is present in each patient with a complete unilateral cleft lip, alveolus, and palate. During primary lip repair this opening is closed as the floor of the nose is closed, and a normal sulcus is created. In most cases, the primary repair remains intact; however, a nasolabial fistula can recur. A nasolabial fistula may result from inadequate closure, excessive tension, or infection during the primary lip repair, or it may appear later, when the maxillary segments are expanded during orthodontic treatment.[1, 2, 4-6, 10, 14, 15]

The location of a nasolabial fistula may vary from high in the sulcus to close to the alveolar ridge.[4, 5, 24] Sometimes it extends through the entire height of the alveolus. A nasolabial fistula may be symptomatic, allowing air and fluids to pass through the nose. A very small and superiorly located nasolabial fistula may remain asymptomatic and may be visible only when the lip is pulled upward.[2, 4, 5, 7]

If it is determined that closure of a nasolabial fistula is necessary, the timing of the operation then depends on the orthodontic treatment (Fig. 55–1). When maxillary expansion is planned, closure is delayed until expansion is complete. Bone grafting is often carried out at this time.[1, 4, 15] Closure of a nasolabial fistula prior to expansion may be successful, but the fistula may reopen. In combination with cancellous bone grafting, the success rate is very high with the additional advantage of stabilization of the maxillary arch (Figs. 55–2 and 55–3).[1-5, 10, 14, 15, 25-27]

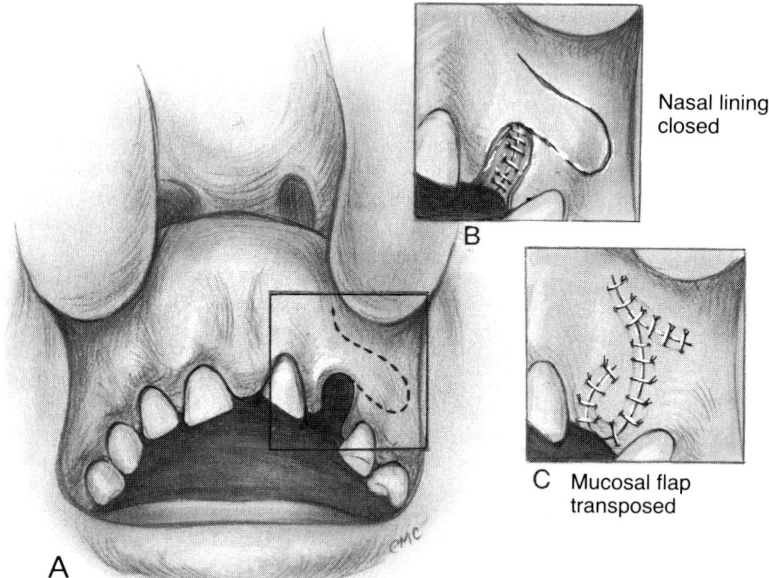

Figure 55–1 Two-layer closure of a small anterior naso-labial fistula that can communicate into the anterior nasal floor. *A,* Design of the labial mucosal flap. *B,* Closure of the palatal side with local flaps. *C,* Mucosal flap transposed.

When there is a large bony defect in combination with the nasolabial fistula, closure is carried out with bone grafting.[4, 28, 29] This operation is often done at the time of eruption of the dentition. A two-layer closure has been found by most authors to achieve the most successful results.[4, 15, 28] Mucoperiosteal flaps raised on both margins of the fistula on the alveolar side are turned over and sutured together, the raw surface being turned toward the sulcus (Fig. 55–4). A mucosal or mucoperiosteal flap from the surrounding tissue is used as the outer layer in closure. Advancement, rotation-advancement, or transposition flaps from the buccal mucosa or palate are used, depending on the size and location of the defect, to ensure a tension-free closure (Figs. 55–5 and 55–6).[1, 2, 4, 5]

Some authors feel that another advantage of bone grafting in this region is an improvement in the tone of the voice. They feel that completion of the bony arch improves resonance and reduces the nasal tones noted with both large and small fistulas.[28] These fistulas are difficult to obturate, enabling air to be expelled into the nose whenever the lips lose contact with the prosthesis. Therefore, a solid repair is recommended for the best results.[2, 14, 15, 28]

Oronasal Fistulas

Oronasal fistulas occur most frequently in the anterior portion of the palate, at the junction of the hard and soft palates, and in the soft palate. These fistulas tend to occur following palatoplasty for treatment of unilateral and bilateral complete clefts of the lip, alveolus, and palate and for treatment of cleft palate only.[1–5]

Oronasal fistulas may have many causes. The most common are hematomas between the oral and nasal layers, wound dehiscence due to excessive tension, partial necrosis of the mucoperiosteal flaps, insufficient attachment of the oral layer in the area of the hard palate, inadequate closure anteriorly of the nasal and oral layers, and postoperative traumatic manipulation.[2, 4, 5] Incomplete closure of the palate results in the passing of air, fluids, and food from the oral into the nasal cavity. Depending on their size, shape, and location, these fistulas may result in functional problems and adversely affect speech production.[2, 4]

Oronasal Fistulas in the Hard Palate

Fistulas in the hard palate can take on various configurations depending on the original clefting deformity. A narrow crevicelike fistula can occur in the oronasal area along the line of the original repair of the cleft palate. The best results have been obtained when the repair is performed in two layers with a tension-free suture line that completely closes the fistula.[24] The incisions are made along the medial edges of the fistula so that two flaps can be rotated to form the nasal layer. On the noncleft side, a mucoperiosteal flap is raised and mobilized toward the cleft side, creating the second layer of closure on the oral side. Vertical mattress sutures or simple sutures are used to ensure proper positioning of the mucoperiosteal flaps and to close each layer of tissue (Figs. 55–7 and 55–8).[1–5, 14, 15, 30, 31]

It is of paramount importance that each nasal and mucoperiosteal flap be adequately undermined and mobilized so that it can be secured in its new position without tension.[4] In most cases, transposition of a single mucoperiosteal flap is sufficient for complete closure of the fistula.[2, 4]

When the fistula is wide and long, a re-creation of the original repair is carried out in the hard palate to achieve complete closure. In secondary defects of the hard palate, a total secondary palatoplasty with two-layer closure and mobilization of one or both mucoperiosteal flaps results in a more successful repair than

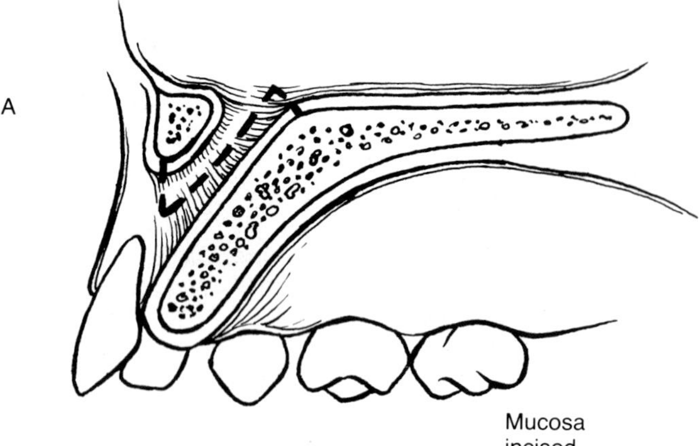

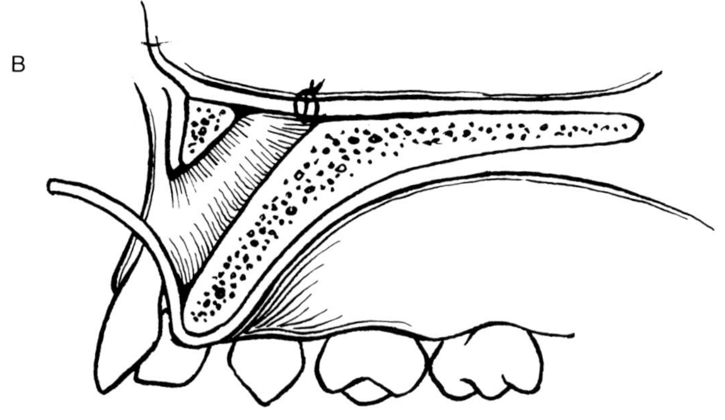

Figure 55–2 Schematic drawings of the two-layer closure of the nasolabial fistula with a large bony deficiency. *A,* Musocal flaps are designed to close the defect. *B,* Flaps are elevated and the nasal side closed. *C,* Bone graft is added to the bony defect, and the labial side is closed.

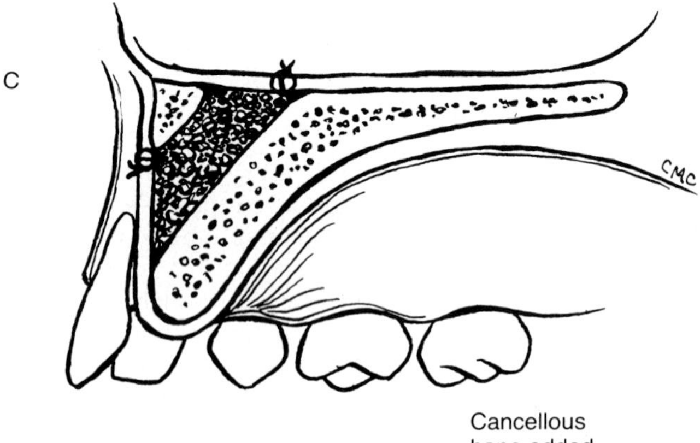

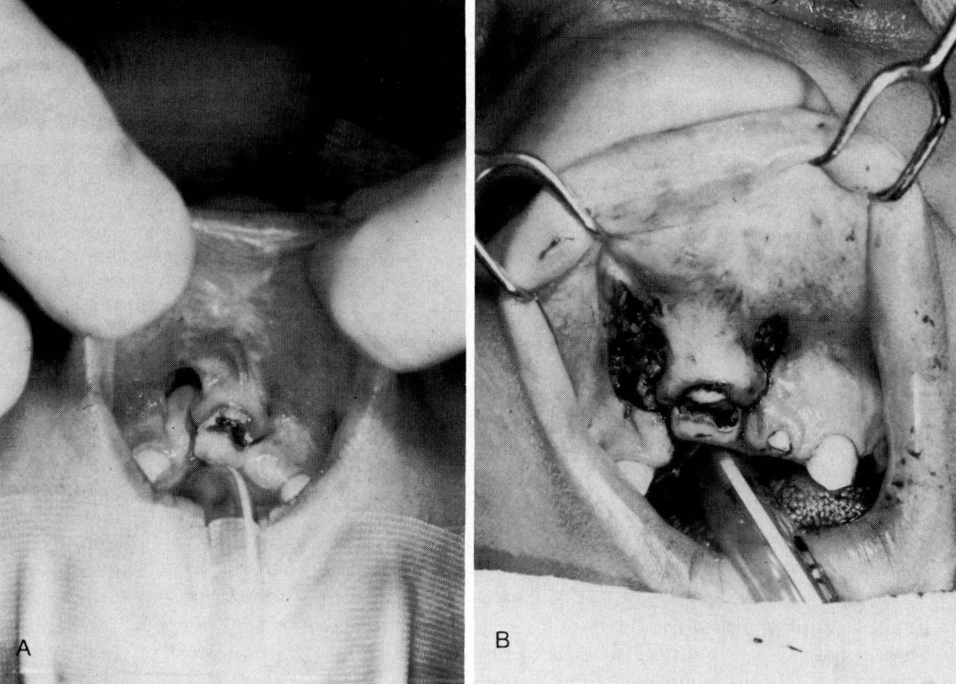

Figure 55–3 Young patient with a symptomatic nasolabial fistula on both sides of the premaxilla, with a single badly decayed central incisor. *A*, Appearance at the time of surgery. *B*, Mucosal flaps elevated and the nasal sides closed; bone graft was added subsequently, and anterior closure was achieved by labial mucosal flaps.

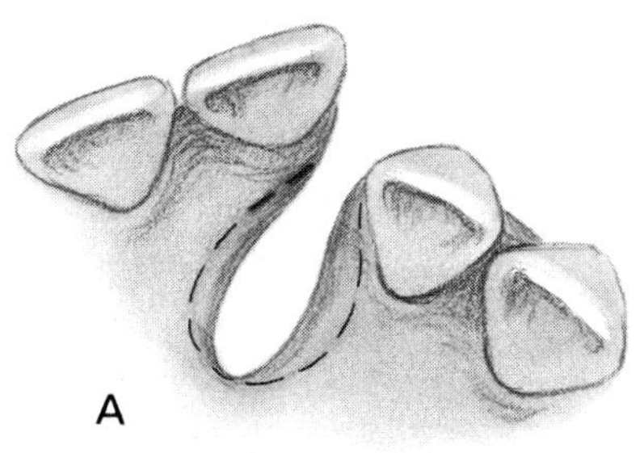

A

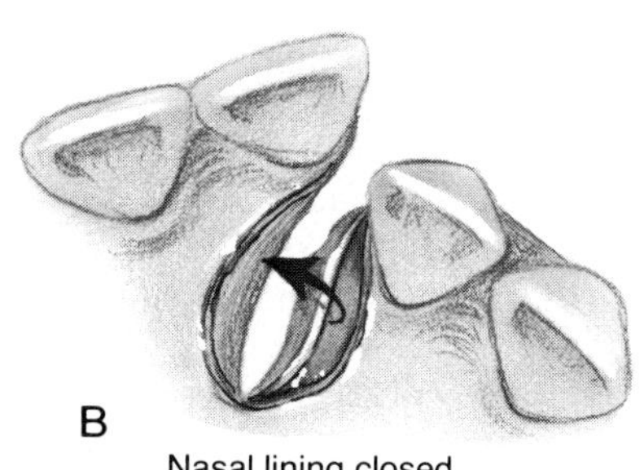

B

Nasal lining closed

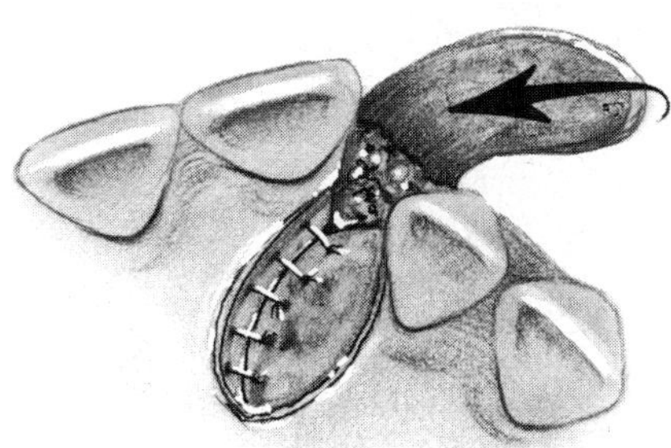

C Mucosal flap elevated and bone added

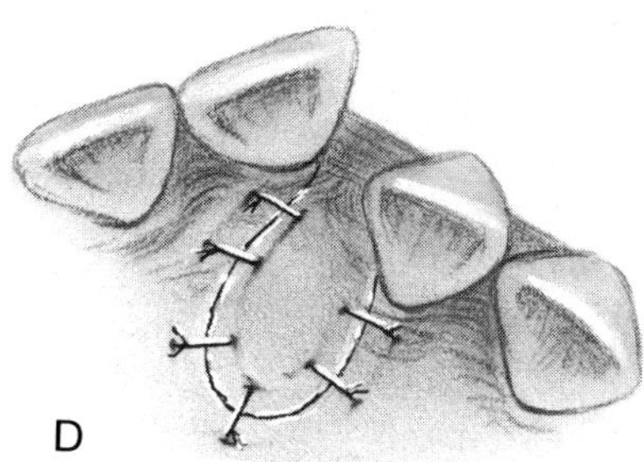

D Mucosal flap sutured

Figure 55–4 Palatal view of oronasal fistula with bony deficiency. *A*, Palatal incisions are designed for a two-layer closure. *B*, Nasal floor closed. *C*, Bone graft added to alveolar surface. *D*, Mucosal flap placed in position for final closure of the palatal side.

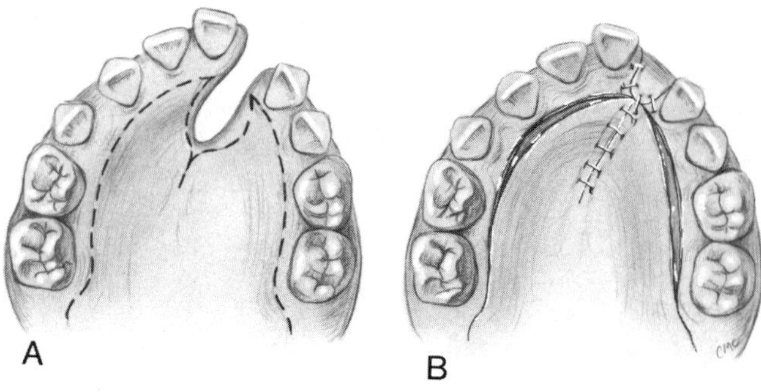

Figure 55–5 Two-layer closure of an oronasal fistula in the anterior palate and alveolus following a unilateral cleft palate repair. *A,* The fistula with the design of the incisions for a two-layer closure. *B,* Closure of the fistula with an inner nasal layer, mucoperiosteal flaps transposed, and a mucosal flap from the sulcus.

attempts to use small local flaps without careful closure of the nasal layer.[1–5]

When a round fistula is present, closure can be achieved by a different technique. On one side of the oronasal fistula, a semicircular flap is based on the edge of the fistula. This is then raised and turned over so that the mucosa faces the nasal cavity. This flap is then sutured to the freshened edges of the fistula to form the nasal layer. The transposition flap from the oral muco-periosteum is raised on the opposite side of the fistula and is used for the oral layer, resulting in complete closure of the palatal fistula.[2, 4, 15]

Oronasal fistulas in the anterior area of the hard palate may result from wide bilateral clefts or excision of the premaxilla. The resultant defect within the alveolar arch and anterior palate can be quite large. A double-layer closure of this defect can be performed using a muco-periosteal flap from the hard palate as a turnover flap to form the nasal layer and a mucosal flap from the buccal or labial region as the oral layer. A shallow sulcus and a secondary upper lip deformity may result from this procedure. However, in many cases this technique may be the only way to obtain successful closure of the defect. Bone grafts have been helpful in increasing the rate of success and improving the aesthetic results (Figs. 55–9 to 55–12).[2, 4, 5, 14, 15]

A much more difficult situation arises when there is a large defect in the anterior hard palate. Mucosal flaps often do not reach into the deep palatal regions. A

tongue flap should be reserved for large defects of the hard palate, especially when multiple operations have been performed on the palate and many scars jeopardize flap survival.[1, 2, 13] When oronasal fistulas in the area of the hard palate are surrounded by dense scar tissue, any secondary procedure can fail. Careful preoperative evaluation and planning are necessary for each patient, particularly for those with secondary fistulas. If the success of a surgical closure is questionable, a prosthesis can be recommended, although these are usually reserved for patients who are not good surgical candidates or in whom multiple attempts at correction have failed.[2, 4, 14, 15]

Oronasal Fistulas of the Soft Palate

Oronasal fistulas of the soft palate require correction if there is loss of intraoral pressure during speech. If there is adequate function of the soft palate and good speech production, correction is not necessary. Moderate to large oronasal fistulas of the soft palate are repaired using a two-layer closure and relaxing incisions in the lateral soft palate tissue.[2, 4]

The goal of correction of fistulas in the soft palate is not only to close the defects but also to create a functional soft palate that has adequate velopharyngeal closure (Fig. 55–12).[1, 2, 4] Because these lesions are often due to scarring, a total reoperation and complete two-flap palatoplasty (with all the previously described steps)

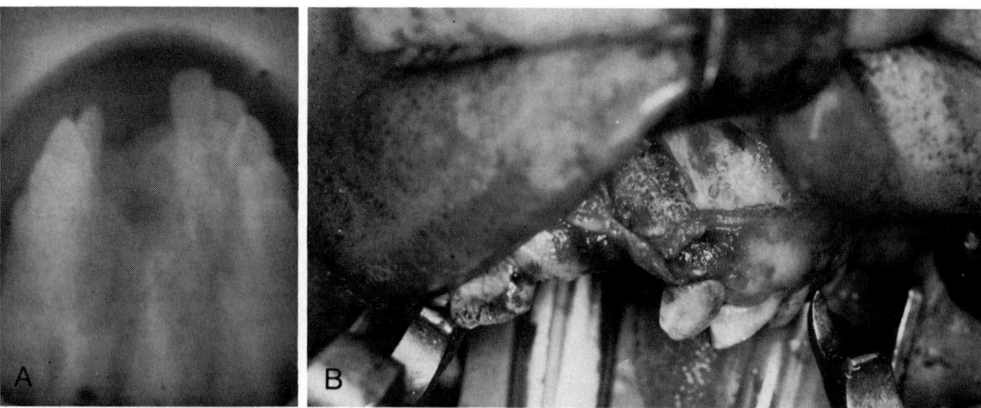

Figure 55–6 A clinical example of a 25-year-old patient with a moderate sized symptomatic anterior alveolar, nasolabial fistula. *A,* X-ray of the alveolar defect. *B,* An example of the technique used to pack the bony defect with the cancellous bone from the iliac crest after freshening the edges of the bony cleft. The final closure is then carried out with labial mucosal flaps in the manner demonstrated.

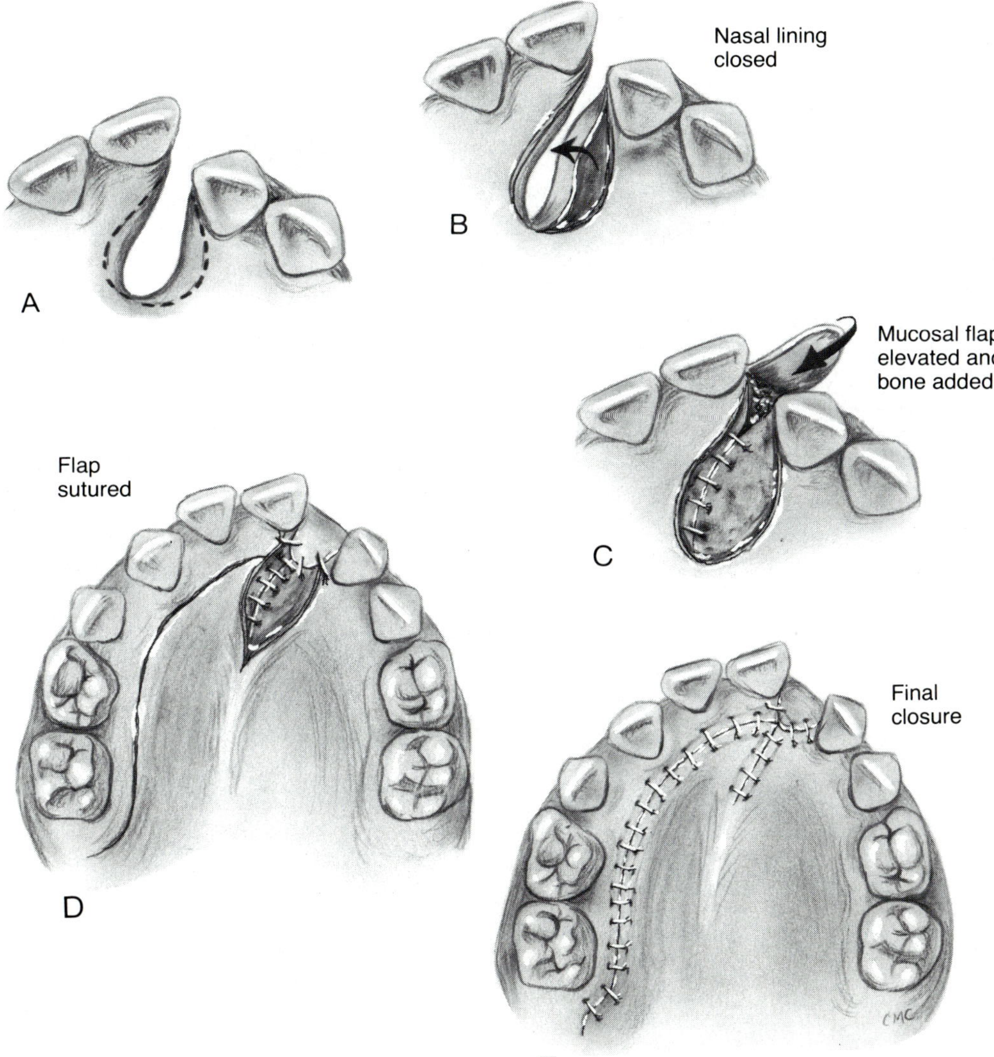

Figure 55–7 Two-layer closure of an anterior oronasal fistula. *A*, Nasal lining is designed from tissue around the fistula. *B*, Careful undermining with turnover flaps aligned in place. *C*, Closure of the nasal lining is achieved with cancellous bone grafts added when there is significant bony deficiency and then closed anteriorly with a sulcus mucosal flap. *D*, The labial flap is secured in place and a large mucoperiosteal flap is mobilized. *E*, The final appearance of the closure.

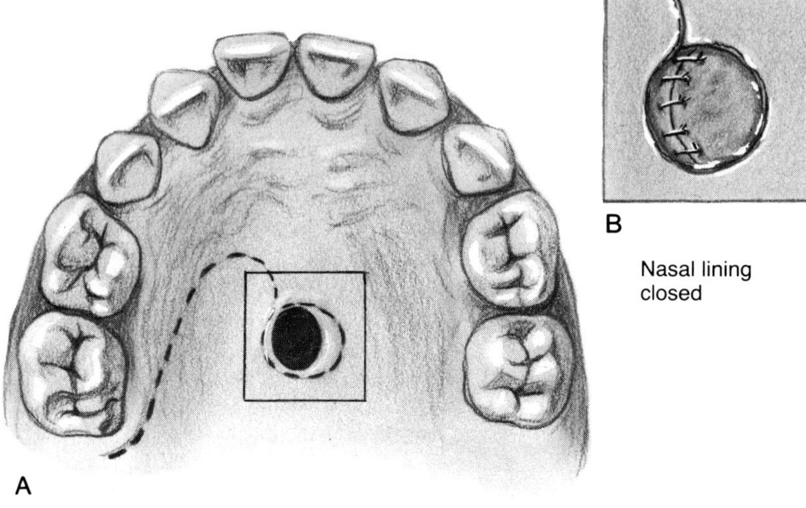

A

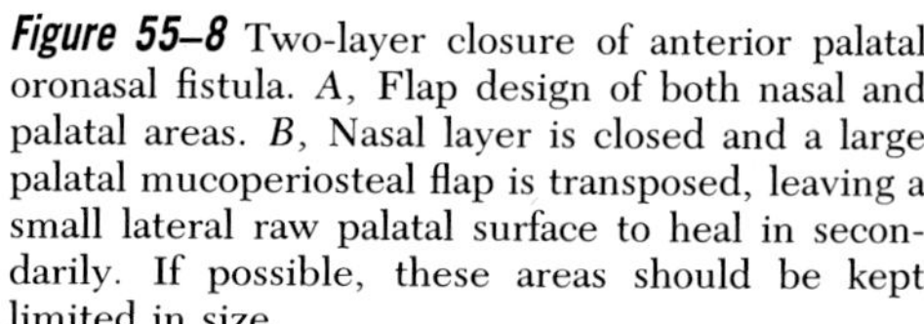

B

Nasal lining
closed

Figure 55–8 Two-layer closure of anterior palatal oronasal fistula. *A,* Flap design of both nasal and palatal areas. *B,* Nasal layer is closed and a large palatal mucoperiosteal flap is transposed, leaving a small lateral raw palatal surface to heal in secondarily. If possible, these areas should be kept limited in size.

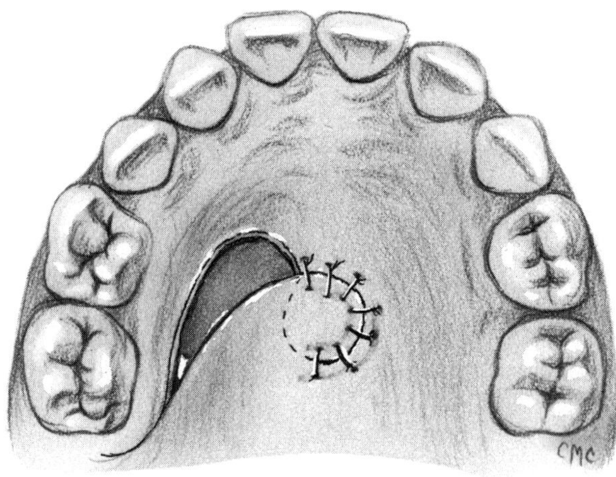

C   Flap transposed

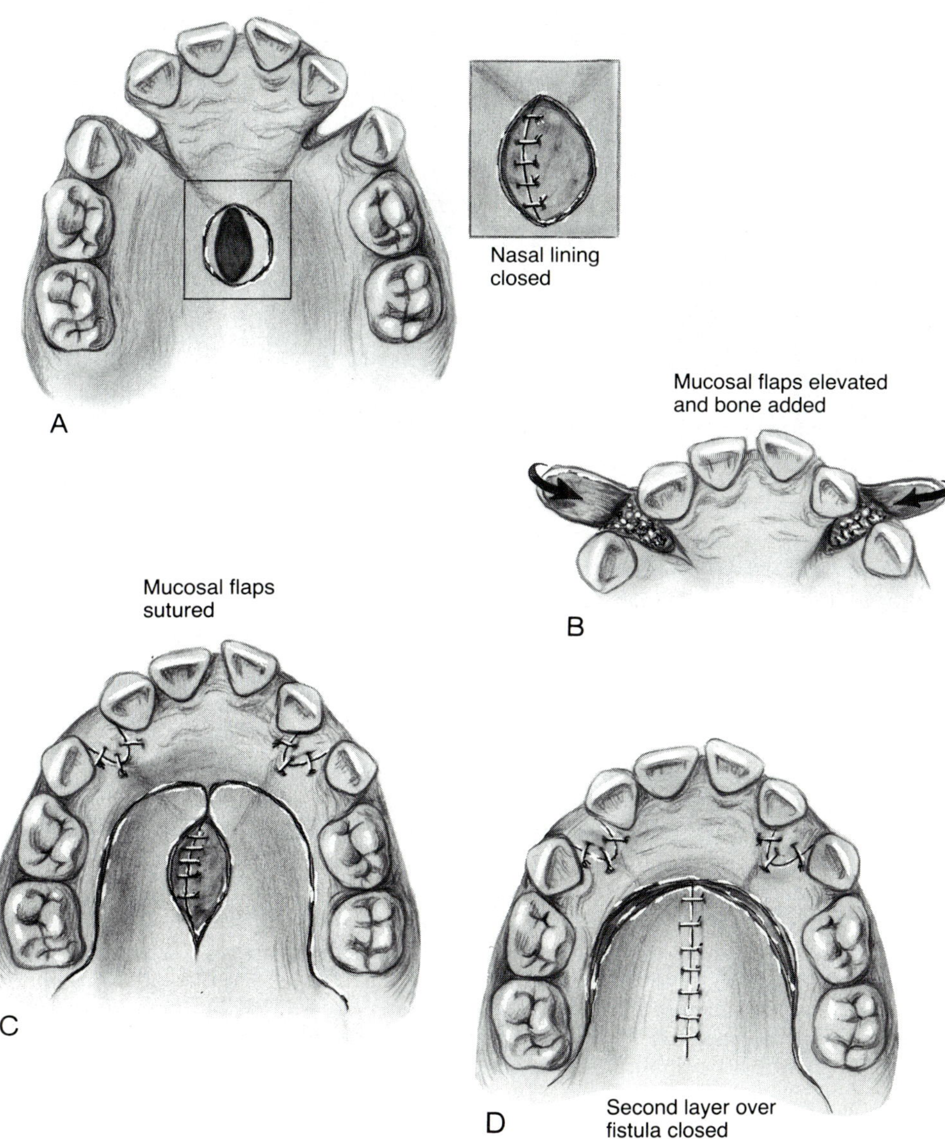

Figure 55–9 Two-layer closure of an oronasal fistula in the anterior palate following a bilateral cleft palatoplasty. *A,* Design of the incisions around the fistula with closure of the nasal side. *B,* Mucosal flaps from the buccal sulcus raised to close the alveolar clefts after bone graft has been added. *C,* Closure of the alveolar areas and raising of mucoperiosteal flaps. *D,* The final reconstruction and closure of the palatal side.

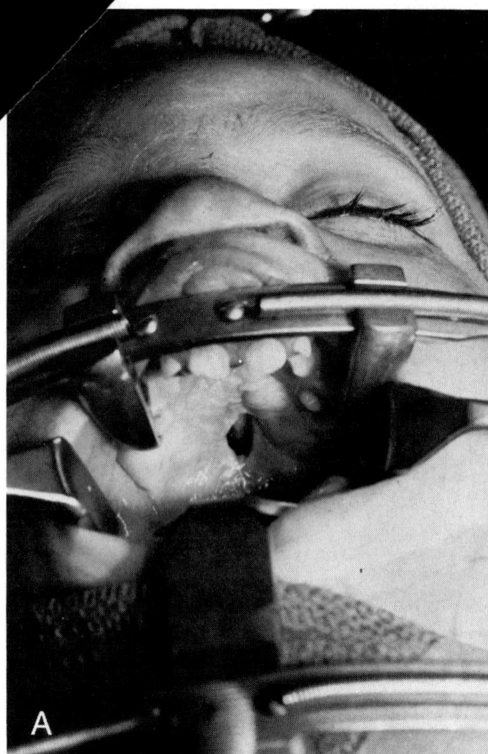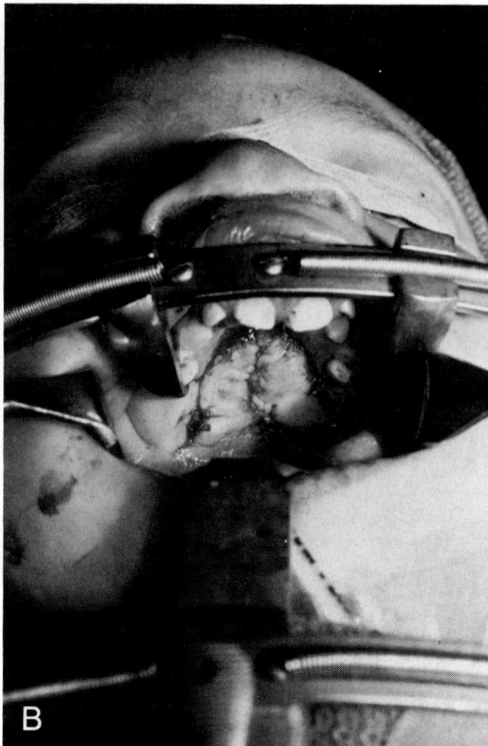

Figure 55–10 Clinical example of a palatal oronasal fistula following a bilateral cleft palatoplasty. *A,* Appearance at the time of surgery. *B,* After final reconstruction using the two-layer mucoperiosteal flap closure.

is the recommended procedure. In the majority of cases, reconstruction of the soft palate by means of a total secondary palatoplasty not only eliminates the fistulas but also improves the function of the velopharyngeal mechanism for speech production.[1,4]

Small oronasal fistulas at the border between the hard and soft palates are treated in the same fashion as small rounded oronasal fistulas in the region of the hard palate.[4] Larger fistulas in this area may require total reoperation and reconstruction with elevation and mobilization of both mucoperiosteal flaps. Careful mobilization in the area of the maxillary tuberosity, lengthening of the neurovascular bundle, and wide undermining of the nasal mucosa should be carried out. The muscles of the soft palate must be totally detached from the posterior edge of the hard palate so that areas of tension are totally eliminated.[1–5, 14, 15] If these maneuvers are still not sufficient, incorporation of tissue from other sources is necessary. In these cases, pharyngeal flaps are readily available and very successful. The sources of the tissue should be carefully selected to avoid compromising speech or facial growth.[1,5]

Any secondary operation on the palate is inherently more difficult in terms of undermining the mucoperiosteal flaps and mobilizing the entire palate because of the scarring that has resulted from the primary operation.[4] Experience has shown, however, that the closure of large oronasal fistulas is most successful when a total reoperation is performed.[2,4] These secondary palatoplasty procedures may improve the function of the soft palate, providing more efficient velopharyngeal closure for speech purposes.[4, 5, 7]

Complications can also arise from any of these sec-ondary procedures on the palate. Necrosis of a portion of the flap or the whole mucoperiosteal flap occurs if the flaps are not attached to the nasal layer or if there is dead space between the mucoperiosteal flaps, palatal shelves, and nasal layers. Sutures themselves, if tied too tightly, can result in necrosis along the incision line. The suture material should be absorbable and secured tightly enough to approximate the flap edges only.[3]

The hard palate has a remarkable propensity to regenerate and thus the raw surface that remains is quick to heal. In the past, infections used to play a greater role in palate surgery, particularly hemolytic streptococcus infections.[2, 3] Today the practice at the Facial Rehabilitation Center is to cancel operation of any patient with a history of upper respiratory infection within 2 weeks of any upcoming surgery and to place those with chronic ear infections on the appropriate antibiotics several days prior to surgery. All patients receive prophylatic cephalosporin antibiotic coverage if they are not allergic to it. Any complication of primary or secondary palate surgery can result in problems with speech production or subsequent facial deformity.[2, 3, 5] Careful reexamination and reassessment should be carried out before the next step is planned.[1–5, 14, 15, 24]

Conclusions

The incidence and character of oronasal and nasolabial fistulas following cleft palate surgery appear to be changing.[2, 3, 5, 7] As techniques have improved and as multi-specialty collaboration has enhanced the delivery of care, understanding of the long-term effects of surgery

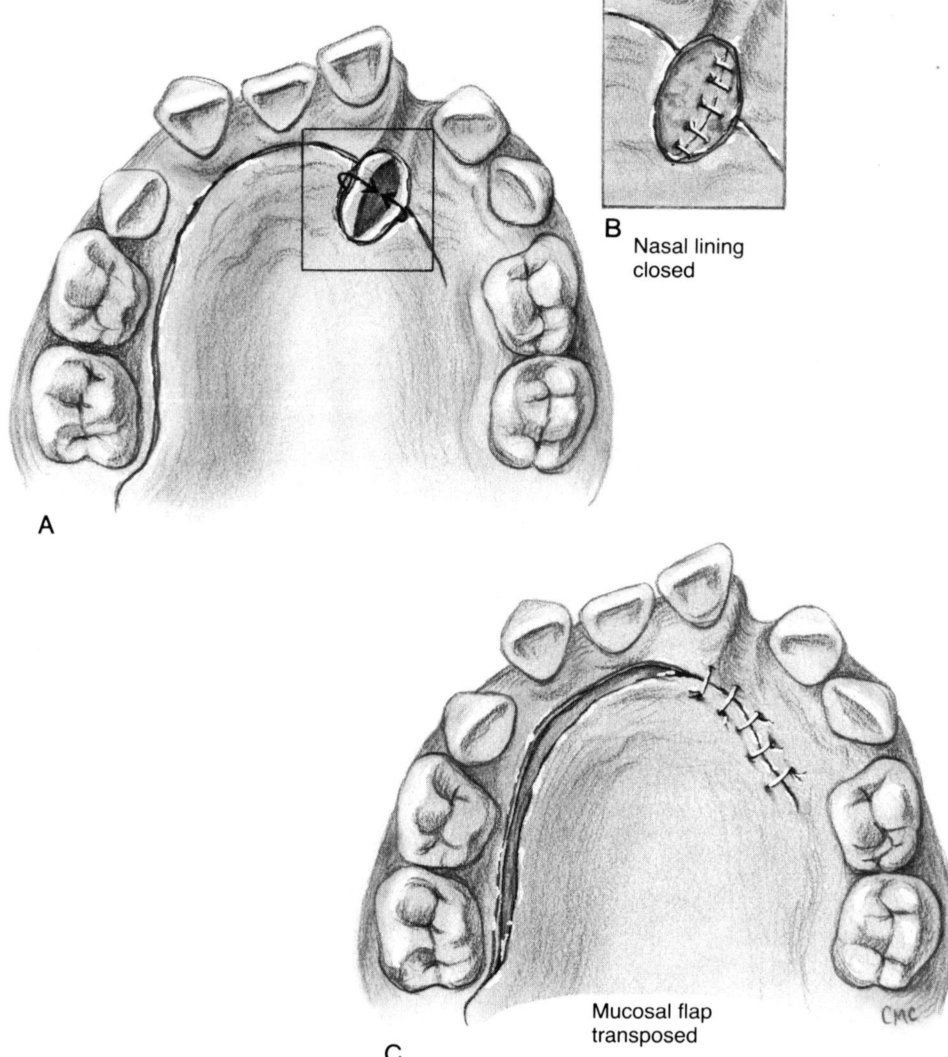

Figure 55–11 Two-layer closure of an oronasal fistula at the junction of the hard and soft palates. *A,* The closure is designed to create a turnover palatal flap for the (*B*) nasal closure. *C,* A palatal mucoperiosteal flap is transposed over the fistula to close the defect. This technique leaves a raw surface to heal secondarily.

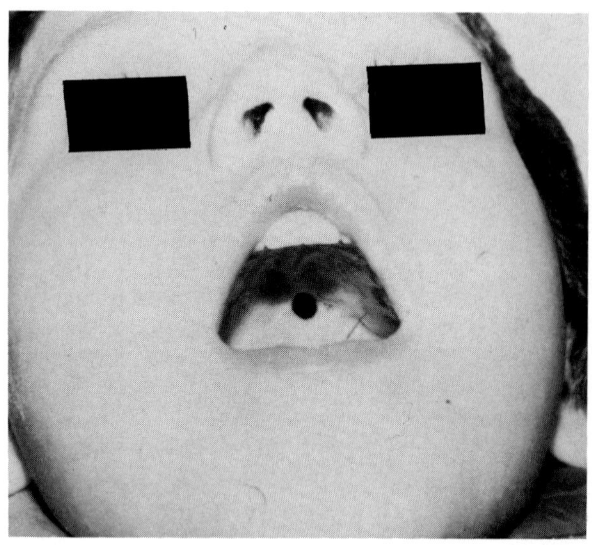

Figure 55–12 Clinical example of an oronasal fistula at the junction of the hard and soft palates.

and its complications has been achieved.[2–5, 16, 17] Today more thoughtful and concise approaches can be used to respond to the daily challenges offered by cleft lip and palate surgery, yielding more functional and predictable results.

References

1. Converse JM: Palatal defects: Oronasal fistulas. In Converse JM (ed): Reconstructive Plastic Surgery. Vol. 4. Philadelphia: Saunders, 1977, pp 2198–2201.
2. Millard RD, Jr: Cleft Craft: The Evolution of Its Surgery. Vol. III: Alveolar and Palatal Deformities. Boston: Little, Brown, 1980.
3. Randall P: Surgery for cleft palate. In Goldwyn RM (ed): The Unfavorable Result in Plastic Surgery. Boston: Little, Brown, 1985, pp 277–286.
4. Bardach J, Salyer K: Surgical Techniques in Cleft Lip and Palate. Chicago: Year Book, 1987, pp 215–223.
5. Lindsay WK: The end results of cleft palate surgery and management. In Goldwyn RM (ed): Long Term Results in Plastic and Reconstructive Surgery. Boston: Little, Brown, 1980, pp 62–67.
6. Cambell Reid DA: Fistulas in the hard palate following cleft palate surgery. Br J Plast Surg 15:377, 1962.
7. Lindsay WK, LeMesurier AB, Farmer AW: A study of the speech results of a large series of cleft palate patients. Plast Reconstr Surg 29:273, 1962.
8. Luce EA, McClinton M, Hoopes JE: Long-term results of the island flap palatal push-back. Plast Reconstr Surg 58:332, 1976.
9. Millard DR Jr, Batstone JHF, Heycock MH, et al: Ten years with the palatal island flap. Plast Reconstr Surg 46:540, 1970.
10. Bell WH: Surgical Correction of Dentofacial Deformities. Vol. III. Philadelphia: Saunders, 1985, pp 574–591.
11. Edgerton M, DeVito F: Closure of palatal defects by means of hinged nasal septal flap. Plast Reconstr Surg 31:537, 1963.
12. McWilliams BJ: Cleft palate management in England. Speech Pathol Ther 3:3, 1960.
13. Jackson I: Use of tongue flaps to resurface lip defects and close palatal fistulas in children. Plast Reconstr Surg 49:537, 1972.
14. Salyer K: Cleft and velopharyngeal function. In Selected Readings in Plastic Surgery. Dallas. University of Texas Health Science Center, Dallas, Vol. 3(23), 1983.
15. Salyer K: Cleft and velopharyngeal function. In Selected Readings in Plastic Surgery. Dallas. University of Texas Health Science Center, Dallas, Vol. 3(23), 1985.
16. Bardach J, Roberts DM, Klausner EC: Influence of two-flap palatoplasty on facial growth in rabbits. Cleft Palate J 16:402, 1979.
17. Bardach J, Mooney M, Bardach E: The influence of two-flap palatoplasty on facial growth in beagles. Plast Reconstr Surg 69:927, 1982.
18. Freng A: Growth of the middle face in experimental early bony fusion of the vomeropremaxillary, vomeromaxillary and midpalatal sutural system: A roentgencephalometric study in the domestic cat. Scand J Plast Surg 15:117, 1981.
19. Freng A, Voss R: Bony or connective tissue union of operated experimental palatal clefts: Implications on growth of the dentomaxillary complex. A biometric study in the domestic cat. Scand J Plast Reconstr Surg 16:233, 1982.
20. Georgiade NC, Pickrell KL, Quinn GW: Varying concepts in bone grafting of alveolar palatal defects. Cleft Palate J 1:43, 1964.
21. Koberg WR: Present view on bone grafting in cleft palate (a review of the literature). J Maxillofac Surg 1:185, 1973.
22. Rehzmann AH, Koberg WR, Koch H: Long-term post-operative results of primary and secondary bone grafting in complete clefts of the lip and palate. Cleft Palate J 7:206, 1970.
23. Robertson NRE, Jolleys A: Effects of early bone grafting in complete clefts of lip and palate. Plast Reconstr Surg 42:414, 1968.
24. Musgrave RH, Bremner JC: Complications of cleft palate surgery. Plast Reconstr Surg 26:180, 1960.
25. Bill AH Jr, Moore AW, Coe HE: The time of choice for repair of cleft palate in relation to the type of surgical repair and its effect on bony growth of the face. Plast Reconstr Surg 18:469, 1956.
26. Lindsay WK: Von Langenbeck palatoplasty. In Grabb WC, Rosenstein SW, Bzoch KR (eds): Cleft Lip and Palate: Surgical, Dental and Speech Aspects. Boston: Little, Brown, 1971.
27. Witzel M, Salyer KE, Ross B: Delayed hard palate closure: The philosophy revisited. Cleft Palate J 21:4, 1984.
28. Jackson M, Jackson I, Christie F: Improvement in speech following closure of anterior palatal fistulas with bone grafts. Br J Plast Surg 29:295, 1976.
29. Jackson I, McLennan G, Scheker L: Primary veloplasty or primary palatoplasty: Some preliminary findings. Plast Reconstr Surg 72:153, 1983.
30. Wynn SK: Long-term results after cleft palate closure by bilateral osteotomy technique. Plast Reconstr Surg 58:71, 1976.
31. Wynn SK: Influence of cleft palate closure by osteotomy technique on growth of the dentomaxillary complex in human beings. Ann Plast Surg 3:129, 1979.

CHAPTER 56

Scientific Evaluation of Facial Surfaces in Craniofacial Malformations Using Computer Graphics Methods

Court B. Cutting

Much of the plastic surgery research done in cleft lip and palate and other craniofacial anomalies has been based on clinical impressions. Unfortunately, the clinical impressions of experts are often diametrically opposed to one another. *Quantitative* evaluation of facial form following different types of treatment provides the only hope of raising this research out of the quagmire of personal opinion. This chapter describes the direction of the research in progress in our center to achieve the goal of comprehensive, quantitative measurement and evaluation of facial form.

If measurement of facial form is to be comprehensive, landmark points will not be an adequate data set. Although point distances and angles will continue to be an essential part of cephalometrics, attention must be directed to the shapes of the curving surfaces between these landmark points. I feel that this is the reason why most plastic surgeons do not spend much time making point measurements of facial form in a case involving soft tissue reconstruction. The eye of the plastic surgeon takes in all of the surface data rather than just the landmark points. This is a far richer data set than that provided by anthropometry. The surgeon then uses his own intuitive computer, that is, his brain, to process all the data and arrive at a surgical plan. Our measurement and analysis methods must take in and process the same rich surface data seen by the human eye. Newer data sources such as computed tomography (CT) and magnetic resonance imaging (MRI) allow us to peer deeper into the object of study than is possible with the human eye. Thus, volumes as well as surfaces will have to be measured and evaluated.

Comprehensive measurement and evaluation of facial form requires computer methods. Traditional two-dimensional cephalometrics and anthropometry can be handled without a computer because only relatively short lists of data measurements are dealt with. As we reach for a well-sampled measurement of the facial surface, this traditional approach quickly breaks down. We are swamped with data. Computers provide the only reasonable way to handle it all.

This chapter describes the tools that will be available to the student of craniofacial anomalies in the not-too-distant future. The researcher will examine craniofacial anomalies on a computer graphics work station using "user friendly" software that will not require extensive knowledge of computers to operate. The researcher in craniofacial anomalies usually has spent most of his or her life studying biochemistry, dentistry, surgery, and so on. It is not reasonable to expect this individual to know a great deal about computer science. This chapter outlines the general design of these tools from the clinical user's point of view. To allow this material to reach as broad an audience as possible, the clinical reader will occasionally find digressions into mathematics or computer science. These sections can be safely skipped by the nontechnical reader unless the text specifically directs the clinical reader not to miss a certain concept.

Data Sources

This section describes the sources of input of biologic data into a computer-based environment. Many of these data sources are well known to clinicians and are described only briefly. Other, less well known data sources are described in more detail.

Cephalometric x-rays will continue to be an important source of data in the study of craniofacial anomalies for the foreseeable future.[1–5] There are now large libraries of cephalometric data from patients with craniofacial anomalies. The value of these records should not be underestimated. They are often the only quantifiable data source from such patients during the past several decades. It is essential that as much information be gleaned from them as possible. However, the two-dimensional nature of those x-rays and the landmark point–based methods of analysis have appeared to be quite limiting in recent years.

Recently, we have described a method for extracting magnification-free, three-dimensional landmark information from these data.[6, 7] This approach has led to important new insights in treatment planning for patients with hemifacial microsomia. Work is also in progress on methods of extracting the ridge curves of the skull (e.g., orbital rims, mandibular border, opening of the piriform aperture, petrous ridge, etc.) from cephalograms. The algorithm needed to accomplish this is a straightforward extension of that described by Dr. Grayson (Chap. 57). Syndromologic insights have also increased by an order of magnitude. The three-dimensional cephalogram is described more fully in this volume in Chapter 57.

Three-dimensional cephalometric data have also provided exciting new insights into treatment planning and syndromology of bilaterally symmetric anomalies. We have recently described the three-dimensional bone fragment movements required to normalize the facial skeleton in Crouzon's disease that are not appreciated from either the posteroanterior or lateral cephalogram. Although the human face and the canine face are both bilaterally symmetric, there are no series of osteotomies that can be appreciated from the lateral view that will carry the canine face into a human shape. To do this requires three-dimensional osteotomies and three-dimensional freedom of movement. On a smaller scale the same situation appears to be true for the patient with Crouzon's disease.

The cephalogram will continue to be used in the near future for several reasons. The cephalostat is relatively inexpensive and takes up little room in a clinical environment involved with craniofacial anomalies. The radiation dose is low, and sedation of the patient is not required. Eventually small CT or MRI scanners that will replace the cephalostat may become available, but this is many generations of scanners in the future. It seems to us that the cephalogram will continue to be the dominant tool in the longitudinal study of postoperative facial bone growth.

Computed tomography and magnetic resonance imaging have shown themselves to be rich data sources for the study of craniofacial anomalies. A number of authors have demonstrated that these data can be used in three dimensions to create synthetic images of the facial skeleton.[8–14] We are very enthusiastic about the future of three-dimensional CT and MRI scanning. The experience in our unit during the past 6 years has tempered this enthusiasm with the realities of using these modalities. The principal problem has been cost (approximately $800 for a three-dimensional CT study, not including the three-dimensional processing). Such studies also require about an hour of time in the scanner. This requirement makes the studies difficult to schedule and requires sedation for infants. The radiation dose for a three-dimensional CT scan is not negligible. The realities of three-dimensional CT scanning have forced us to realize that we will usually get one preoperative three-dimensional CT study per patient and, if there is a clinical problem following surgery, an occasional postoperative study. This modality will certainly not be used for routine postoperative follow-up. Cephalograms and facial-light scans are far more likely candidates for use in longitudinal data collection.

Anthropometry will continue to be a useful source of data in the near future. Anthropometry involves measuring distances and angles directly from the surface of the face.[15, 26] Unfortunately, it is a landmark-based system. Comprehensive input from the surface of the face is not possible with anthropometry. The amount of time spent per patient with anthropometry is considerable. We feel that traditional anthropometry will eventually be replaced by automatic facial surface scanners used in conjunction with three-dimensional cephalometric data.

Stereophotogrammetric and moire topographic studies will continue to be useful in collecting facial surface data.[17–19] Moire topographic studies use interference fringes of light to code depth in a two-dimensional photograph. By this means a three-dimensional topologic map of the face is generated, although the resolution of the system is low. Stereophotogrammetric studies use trigonometric match-up of points seen from two separate views at an angle to one another to code for depth. Berkowitz and Cuzzi[20] and Savara et al[21] have applied stereophotogrammetry to the study of the facial surface in craniofacial anomalies. Although the biologic data-gathering equipment needed for stereophotogrammetric studies is simple and inexpensive, the per patient cost of processing the data at a commercial cartographic laboratory may approach that of a three-dimensional CT study. One major advantage of stereophotogrammetric studies compared with automatic facial light scanning is that stereophotogrammetric data gathering is done in an instant with a simultaneous pair of flash pictures. The automatic light scanners require several seconds. An infant with cleft lip and palate would have to be asleep for performance of an automated scan. Stereophotogrammetric studies do not suffer from this limitation. Baumrind et al[22, 23] and others are doing their own three-dimensional processing of stereophotograms, which markedly decreases the cost. Examples of stereophotograms of patients with craniofacial anomalies appear in Figures 56–1 and 56–2.

Automatic light scanners are an excellent source of facial surface data for the study of craniofacial anomalies, particularly cleft lip and palate. What follows is a description of one such device, the Echo scanner from Cyberware Laboratories,[24] although several different designs currently exist.[25, 26] A line of laser light is projected vertically on the surface of the face. A laser is used to keep the beam from spreading. A video camera views this line from an angle (Fig. 56–3A) and sweeps out 480 horizontal scan lines to read the entire video frame (Fig. 56–3B). A clocked digital counter is started at the beginning of the horizontal scan sweep. The counter is stopped when the laser light is detected. The count obtained is proportional to the distance of the facial surface at that point from the center of the axis of rotation of the device. In this way, each complete video frame provides 480 radius measurements. If the whole device is rotated about the subject's face, many contour lines can be collected in a short time (Fig. 56–3C and D). Berkowitz et al have described a scanner for dental models that operates on a similar principle.[27] Arridge et

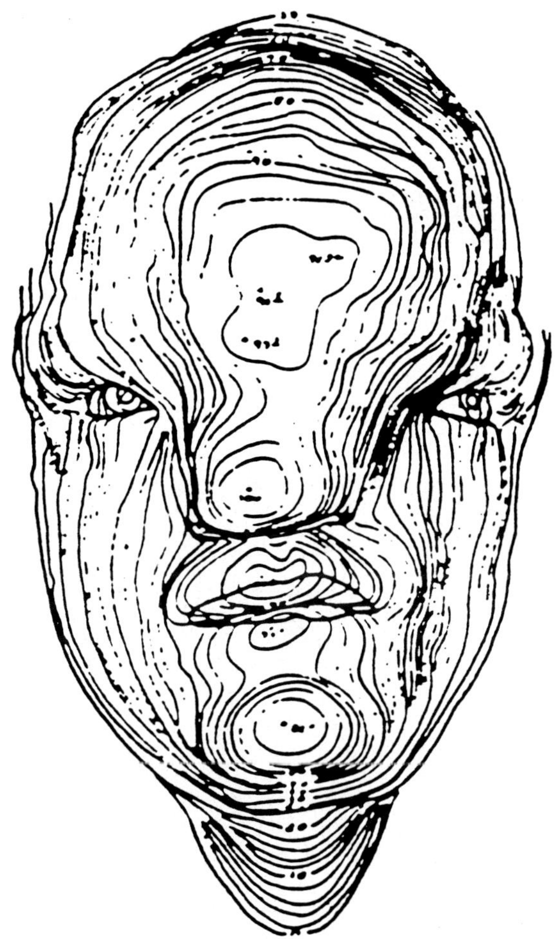

Figure 56–1 Stereophotogram of a patient with hypertelorism. (From Berkowitz S, Cuzzi J: Biostereometric analysis of surgically corrected abnormal faces. Am J Orthod 72:526, 1977. Used with permission.)

seconds. Although the initial start-up cost is relatively high, the per patient processing cost is very low (literally, the cost of the magnetic media used to store the data). In contrast, in stereophotogrammetric studies the start-up cost is relatively low, but the per patient cost is quite high. Another advantage over stereophotogrammetric studies is that the data are immediately available in digital form. This allows the data to be postprocessed on a work station that will be described later. Figures 56–4 and 56–5 show use of the scanner to study the lip-nose complex of patients with clefts of the lip and palate. Figure 56–6 is a full facial scan of a patient with Apert's syndrome.

Casts and moulages continue to be an excellent source of three-dimensional surface data.[28, 29] The moulages can be scanned by a laser scanner at a later time for digital manipulation of the data.[24, 27] Figure 56–7 illustrates the collection of data on a complete unilateral cleft lip and nose by cast-moulage methods kept in three-dimensional registration with the skull base by means of face bow transfer. I would like to encourage workers doing research on cleft lip and palate to collect pre- and postoperative moulages on their patients at regular intervals. Even if the researcher is not yet able to invest in a scanner, in several years scanners will become much less expensive, and the software to process the data will be readily accessible. Moulages are an inexpensive, easily accessible way to save important research records of children with craniofacial anomalies.

Serial histologic sections are another important source of three-dimensional volume data for the study of craniofacial anomalies. If each serial slice is digitized with a two-dimensional video scanner, the data are not much different than those obtained by CT or MRI. To the computer programs that process the data and create three-dimensional images, these data are simply another three-dimensional stack of slices. Histologic sections are used principally in embryologic research and in the study of anatomic specimens. King and associates created three-dimensional images of normal and bilateral cleft lip specimens by performing three-dimensional reconstructions from serial sections by hand (Fig. 56–8).[30]

al have described a laser scanner that works on a slightly different principle.[25]

Automatic light scanners have numerous advantages. The most obvious is that no ionizing radiation is required. Also, a scan can be performed in only a few

Figure 56–2 Stereophotogram of a patient with Treacher Collins syndrome. (From Savara B, Miller S, Demuth R, et al: Biostereometrics and computer graphics for patients with craniofacial malformations: Diagnosis and treatment planning. Plast Reconstr Surg 75:495, 1985. Used with permission.)

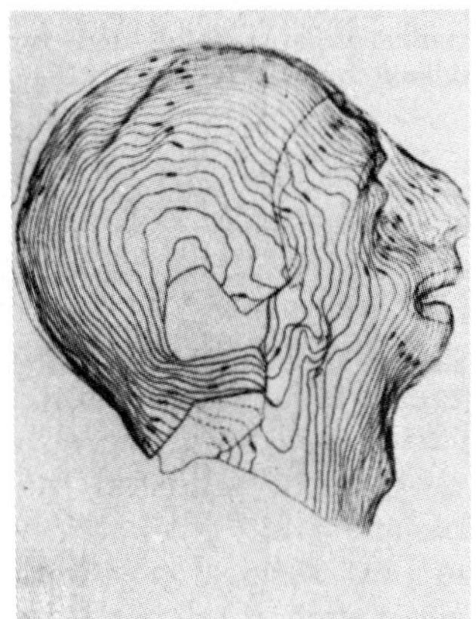 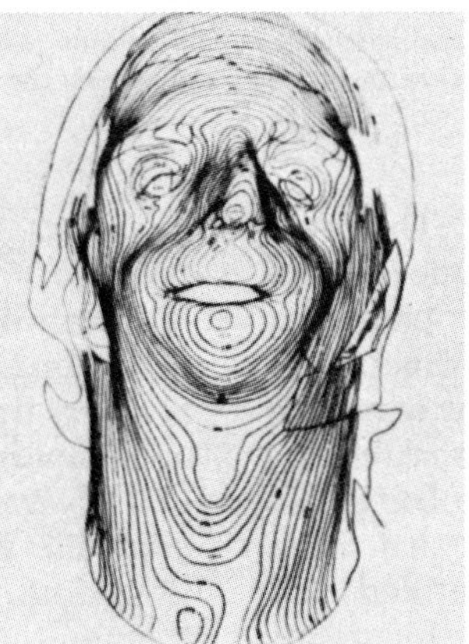 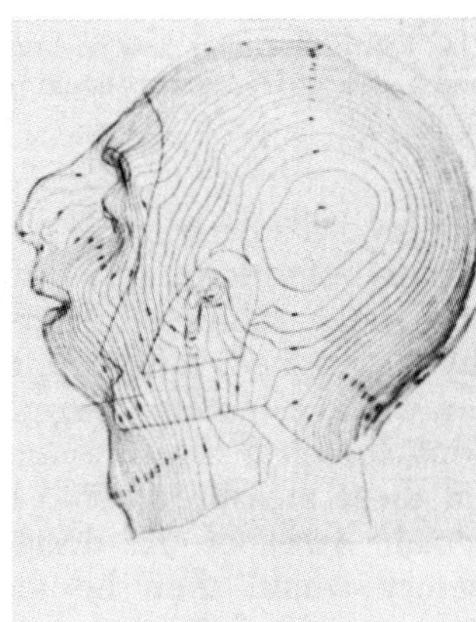

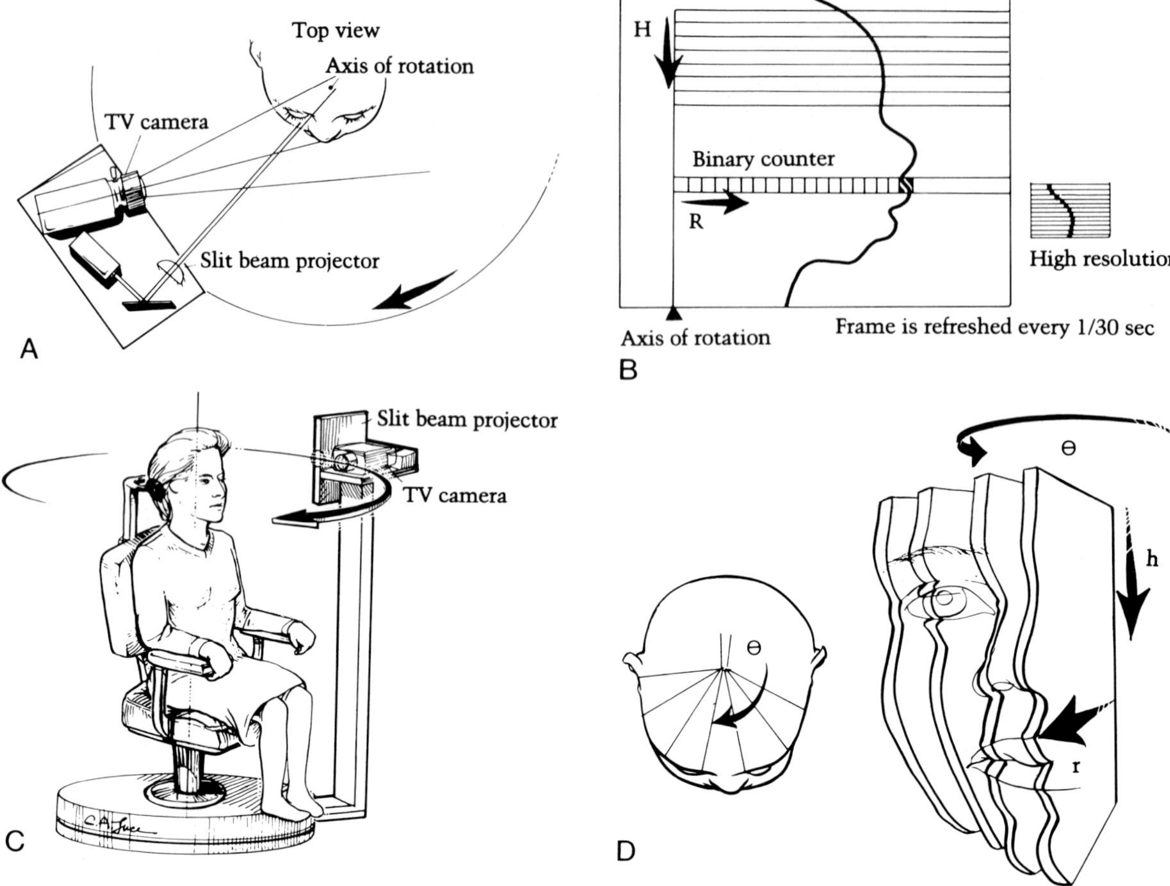

Figure 56–3 *A*, Top view of laser scanner. A line of laser light is projected on the surface of the face. A video camera views this line at a known angle. *B*, A counter is started at the beginning of each video scan line. The counter is stopped when the laser light is detected. This count is proportional to the radius from the center of the axis of rotation of the device to the surface of the face. In this way, an entire contour line is measured with each video frame. *C*, The entire device is rotated at a constant rate about the subject's face. *D*, This results in a series of contours that represents the entire surface.

Ultrasound remains a promising but as yet untapped source of three-dimensional data from craniofacial patients in utero. Although other modalities are preferable in the postnatal period, ultrasound is unsurpassed for prenatal diagnosis. The current use of ultrasound involves the examination of two-dimensional slices of fetal anatomy using a linear array of ultrasonic transducers. This situation is analogous to two-dimensional CT prior to the era of three-dimensional reconstruction. Severe problems, however, must be solved before three-di-

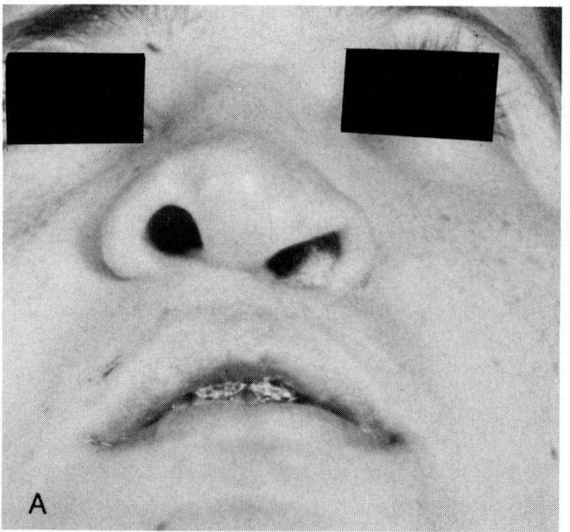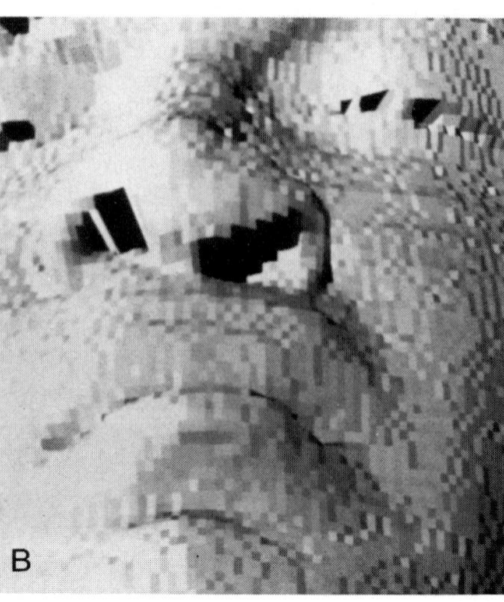

Figure 56–4 Photograph (*A*) and scan (*B*) of a patient with a unilateral cleft lip nose deformity.

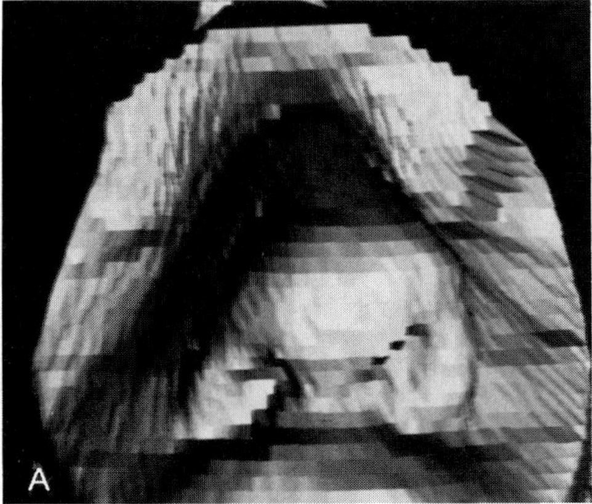
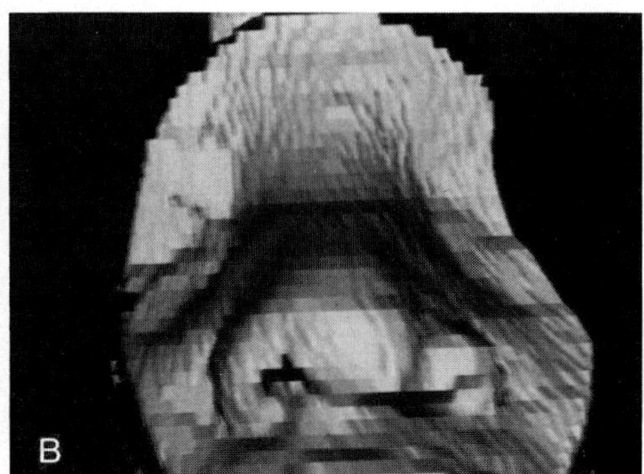

Figure 56–5 *A* and *B*, Laser scans of moulages of the nose in patients following cleft lip repair in which there had been no primary nasal correction except for repair of the floor of the nose.

mensional reconstructions of fetuses suspected of having a craniofacial malformation based on ultrasound data become a reality. Either a two-dimensional array of transducers will have to be constructed or a mechanism for uniformly sweeping the uterus with a linear array will have to be devised. Much fetal motion artifact will be present if scan time is not kept short. Finally, ultrasound images have a great deal of noise in them. Image processing methods will be required to extract the real biological signal.

Software for the Analysis of Craniofacial Malformations

Raw Data Input and Query Programs

On entry into the craniofacial anomalies software structure, the clinician first will be asked to identify a data source that he or she wishes to work on. This may be any of the patient data sources described elsewhere in this chapter. This data will have been abstracted into the closed polyhedral surface format also described elsewhere in this chapter. It will then be presented to the clinician as a solid model of the object on the computer screen. Because the work station is displaying only surfaces at this time, modeling and editing of solids can be done in real time. Utilities will be provided to allow the clinician to section the object in any arbitrary plane. If the data are in the form of a CT or MRI scan, the original data will then be queried, and this new reformatted "slice" will be displayed. Utilities also will be provided to allow the clinician to cut the solid into pieces. Translucent views of the original data that fall on the newly cut surface can be displayed. This will appear to the user as if he or she is truly cutting all of the original data, whereas really only the surfaces are displayed. In the case of CT or MRI scans, it can be seen that the quality of the program that finds closed polyhedra around surfaces of a volume-sampled solid is of paramount importance. Utilities also must be present to allow the clinician to change the gray scale over which the radiolucency data are projected, perform histograms, take distance and angle measures, and so on. These are functions currently provided on commercially available CT and MRI scan viewing stations and will not be discussed here.

Surgical Simulation

Surgical simulation is a relatively straightforward extension of the solids editing program mentioned above.

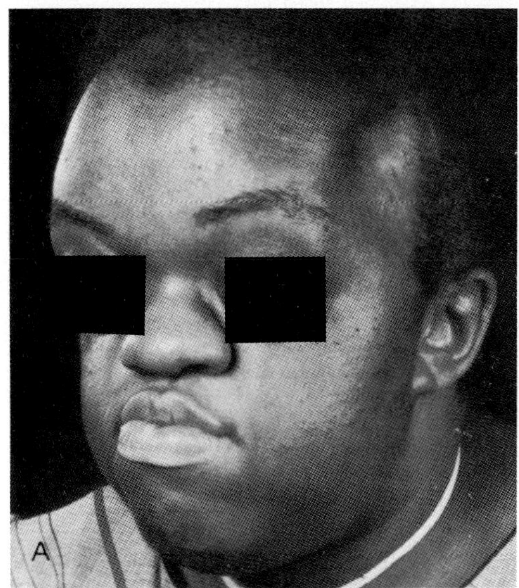
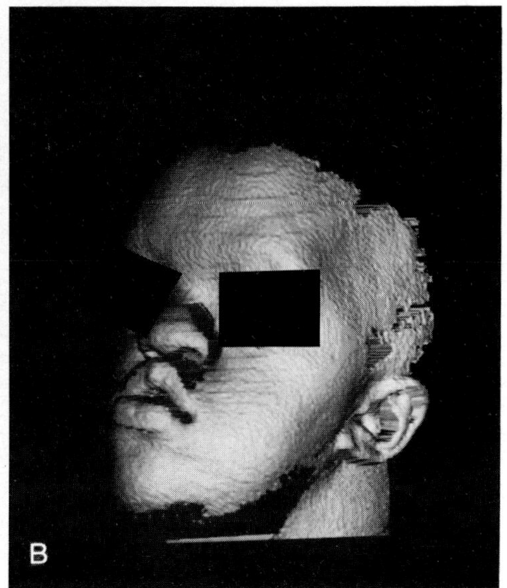

Figure 56–6 Photograph *(A)* and laser scan *(B)* of a patient with Apert's syndrome prior to Le Fort III advancement of the midface. (From Cutting C, McCarthy JG, Karron D: Three-dimensional input of body surface data using a laser light scanner. Ann Plast Surg 21:38, 1988.)

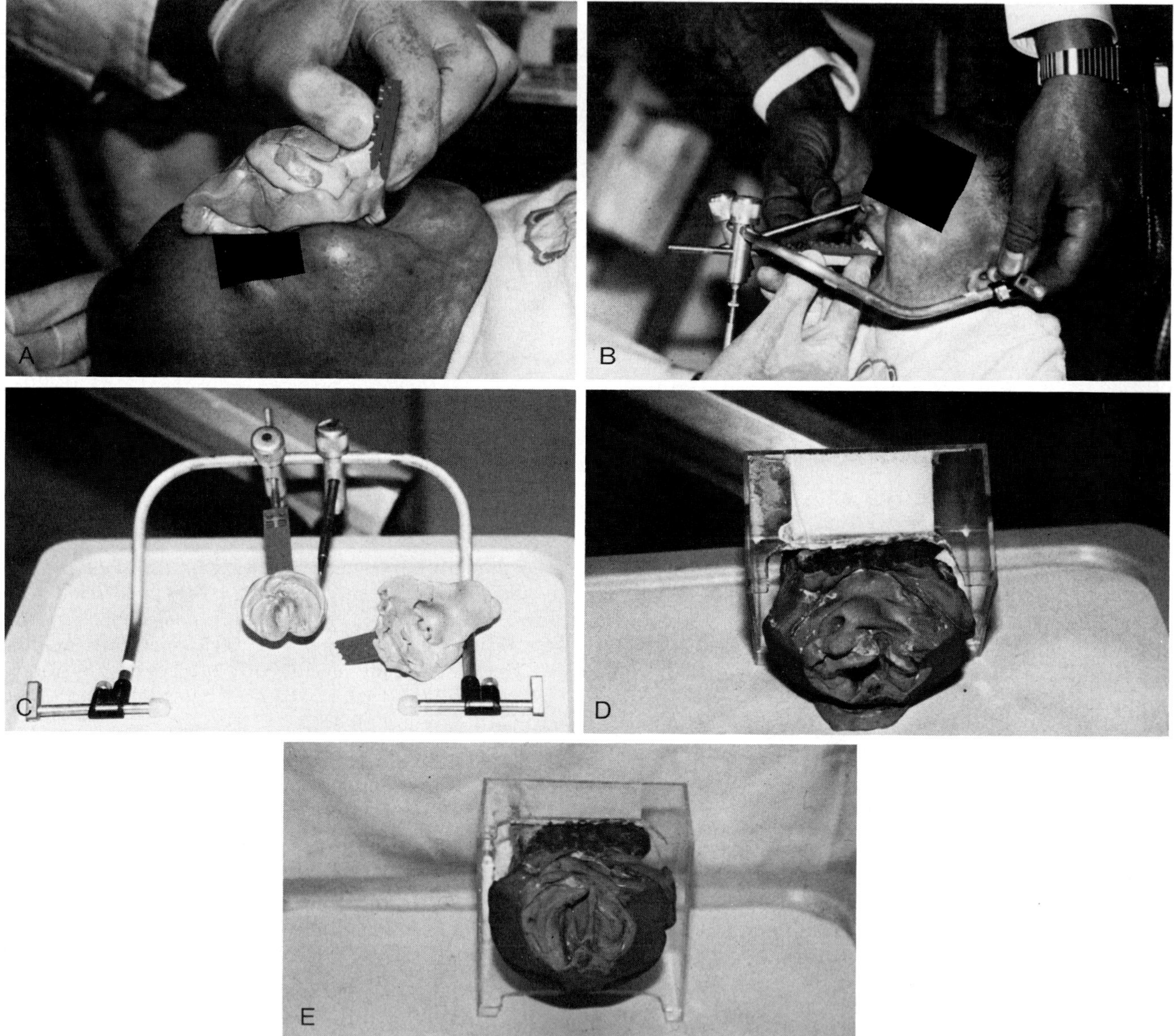

Figure 56–7 Method of collecting a three-dimensional moulage referenced to the skull base in an awake infant with cleft lip, alveolus, and palate. *A*, After a dental impression has been made, a nasal impression is taken in three-dimensional registration with the dental impression. *B*, The nasal impression is removed, and the dental impression is taken in registration with the skull base using a head frame. *C*, The apparatus. *D*, The nasal aspect of the moulage mounted in a three-dimensional reference box. *E*, The dental aspect of the impression. (From Petrover J et al: New method for taking a moulage of the lip-nose-palate complex in infants with cleft lip and palate. In preparation. Used with permission.)

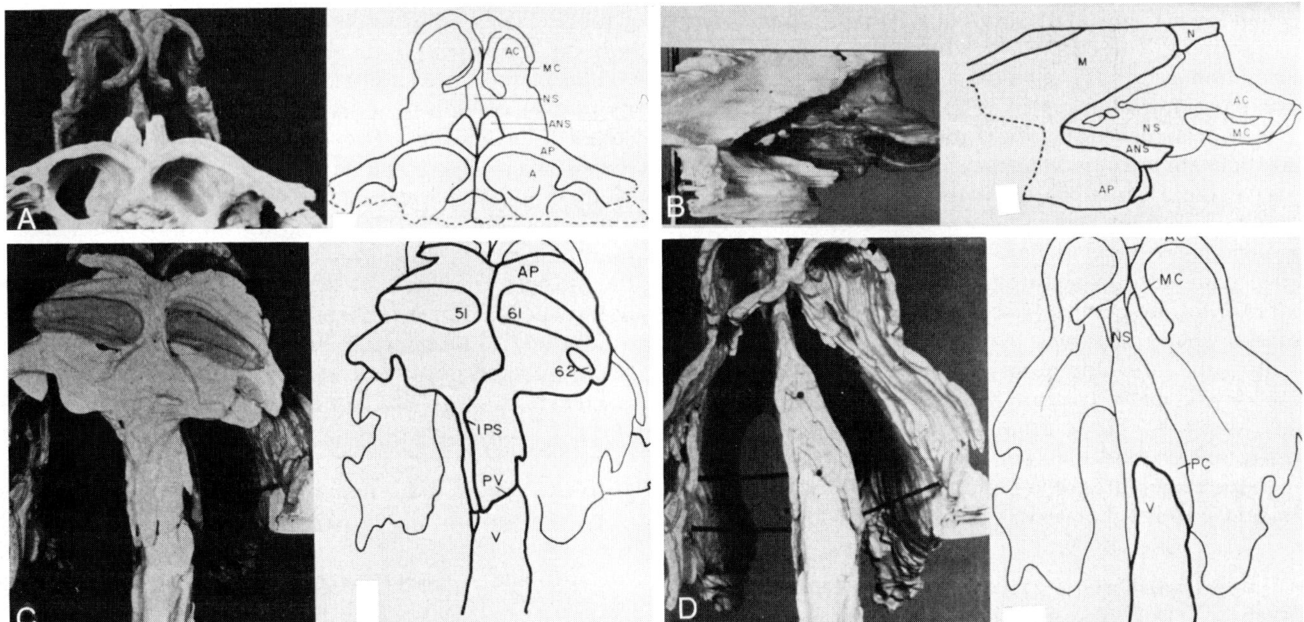

Figure 56–8 Three-dimensional reconstructions made by hand from serial sections from a normal fetus *(A and B)* and a fetus with bilateral cleft lip, alveolus, and palate *(C and D)*. (From King B, Workman C, Latham R: An anatomic study of the columella and the protruding premaxillae in a bilateral cleft lip and palate infant. Cleft Palate J 16:223, 1979. Used with permission.)

Surgical simulation has been described previously in the literature.[6, 7, 31–34] Movement of the solid pieces created by the osteotomy simulation is well known in computer graphics.[36] Recently, in a paper written by the author and his colleagues, the notion of optimization of bone fragment positioning was introduced.[6, 7, 32, 36, 37] As a first pass, the computer is allowed to position the bone fragments based on a best fit to normal landmark position. The clinician then refines these movements to correct for biologic factors. This work is described in a separate chapter in this book (Chap. 62).

The future of surgical simulation lies in soft tissue modeling, growth prediction, and the development of a more comprehensive cephalometric system. All of the surgical simulation work done thus far has been directed at the facial skeleton. In the end, it is only the skin surface that concerns the patient aesthetically.[38] Soft tissue has been avoided by computer modelers thus far owing to its elasticity. There is an area of engineering known as finite element modeling that represents an elastic structure as a composite of a number of discrete "finite elements."[39–42] The deformation characteristics of the element are known. If the elements are then combined and subjected to a mechanical load, the deformation of the composite object can be calculated. The skin surface result of movements of osteotomy fragments under a soft tissue envelope can best be predicted in this way.

Growth prediction is an essential component in the future of surgical simulation. The craniofacial anomalies community has become very aware of the serious psychosocial consequences of not correcting these major facial malformations early enough. From a purely surgical point of view, it would be better to allow these children to become full grown prior to surgery. The program would then be a three-dimensional one without the need to be concerned with growth. Results with this approach have revealed that the psychosocial consequences of such a course can be devastating. To avoid these problems, most centers have moved toward correcting the problems at an early age. Surgical planning has, of necessity, become a four-dimensional problem. The empiric approach is crucial to the success of this venture. Longitudinal studies of facial growth of patients following surgery at an early age are vital. This growth data must be fed back into surgical planning programs for the next generation of patients. Optimization routines for automatic osteotomy fragment positioning must include growth changes as a variable.

The last major improvement in surgical planning rests on the development of a new and comprehensive cephalometric system. Currently, cephalometrics involves the study of landmark points. This is an inadequate data set for accurate surgical planning. The surface points on the bone and skin also must be taken into account to plan surgery accurately. The new cephalometric system will be discussed in detail in the sections that follow.

Syndromology

The specific study of craniofacial syndromes will be greatly facilitated by using a quantitative morphometric approach. Although the actual software structure will be described in the sections that follow, it is appropriate to comment on how syndrome identification, classification, and an understanding of their pathomechanics are facilitated by this approach. Although autopsy studies are sometimes possible, they are rare. For this reason, the "in vivo" dissection capabilities provided by this software are invaluable for an understanding of pathomechanics. CT and MRI scans of growing patients may be examined, sometimes longitudinally, for anatomic information that may elucidate the pathogenesis of a particular syndrome.

A comprehensive statistical method is also of importance here. Syndrome identification also is accomplished better using a statistical approach. Recently, I thought a newborn patient had Pfeiffer's syndrome. The three-dimensional pattern recognition capabilities of our pediatric geneticist (Marcia Wishnick) suggested Antley-Bixler syndrome instead based on a perceived difference in facial shape that was somehow hard to describe. Ideally, the development of a new cephalometric method will allow pattern recognition to be quantitatively defined. Three-dimensional imaging based on prenatal ultrasound data should soon become a reality. The benefits of this development on prenatal genetic counseling to families at risk could be considerable.

New Cephalometric System Based on Geometric Hierarchy

Our current research will develop an entirely new and comprehensive cephalometric system. The need for this has arisen from the rich new data sets that have become available from clinical work with patients with craniofacial anomalies. The older cephalometric systems involve analysis of points identified from two-dimensional x-rays. In this volume, Grayson has described our recent three-dimensional extrapolation of this approach (Chap. 57). In either version, landmark points are the only data of interest. Distances and angles are calculated (often by hand) to perform syndrome analysis and surgical planning. Most workers in the field now use electronic point digitizer pads and personal computers for this task.[1, 3, 4, 31] The three-dimensional cephalogram really requires that the data be examined with the aid of three-dimensional computer graphics. Landmark points will continue to be the most useful cardinal geometric elements in the study of the human face.

Unfortunately, too much information is omitted if we rely on landmark points alone.

The new cephalometrics system will be built on a hierarchy of points, curving lines, surfaces, and the solids they enclose. The key concept is that of a *geometric hierarchy*. The idea springs from the author's view of human pattern recognition. We start identifying a sampled object by first locating the most outstanding points in its structure, move to the prominent ridges on the surface, and last, look at the shape of the surfaces in between. After establishing this geometric hierarchy, the pattern is recognized and the object identified. The software to be described will proceed in this same way.

The first step up from landmark points is ridge curves.[59] Examples of ridge curves are the orbital rims, mandibular border, temporal line, piriform aperture, posterior edge of the lesser wing of the sphenoid, and so on. A drawing of the major ridge curves of the skull appears in Figure 56–9. Most of the landmarks of conventional cephalometrics can be found on ridge curves. After finding the ridge curves of the skull, new landmark points may be found as curvature and torsion maxima on the ridge curves (these will be explained later). By connecting landmarks across ridge curves with geodesic lines, the surface regions will have been demarcated (Fig. 56–10). Following this logic a step further, the surface regions on either side of a solid can be connected to subdivide a sampled solid into standard homologous solid regions for analysis. The way in which a clinician will be able to establish this *geometric hierarchy* and the theoretic basis for it follows.

The theoretic basis for this project derives directly from differential geometry.[43–47] To use the software, the clinician must learn a little about the geometry of curving lines and surfaces. An essential concept is that of curvature at a point (Fig. 56–11). At any point on a curving line it is possible to fit the perimeter of a circle to the point and its immediate neighbors. The inverse of the radius of this circle is called the *curvature of a point*. If the circle lies on one side of the line, the

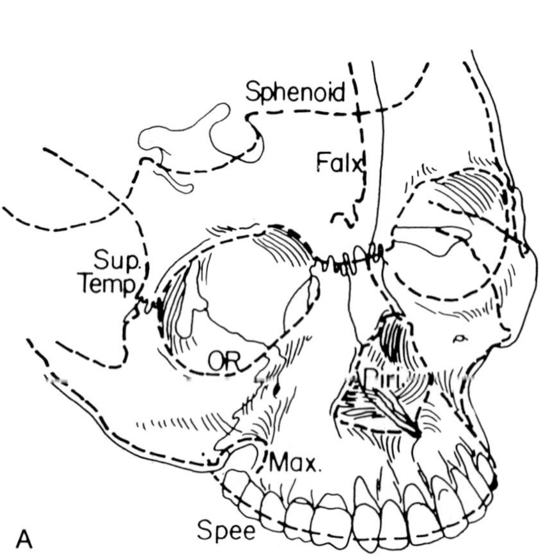

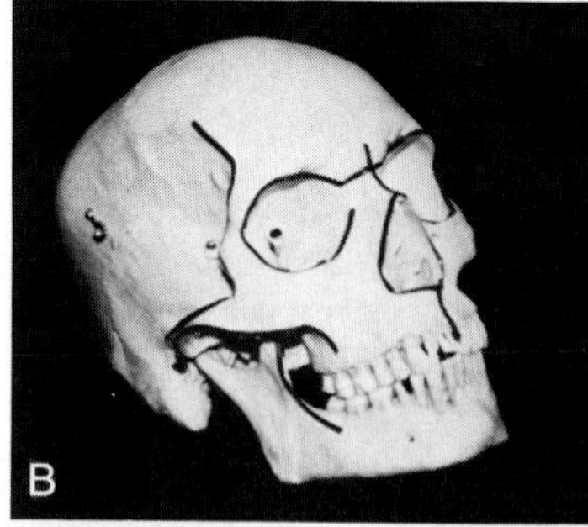

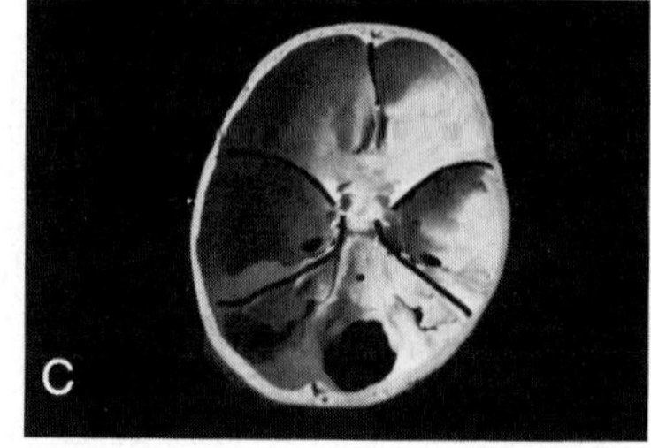

Figure 56–9 Ridge curves of the skull. *A,* A line drawing of some of the ridge curves of the maxilla and cranial base. *B* and *C,* A photograph of the same curves outlined on a skull from *(B)* the outside and *(C)* the inside. (From Bookstein FL, Cutting C: A proposal for the apprehension of curving craniofacial form in three dimensions. In Vig K, Burdi A (eds): Craniofacial Morphogenesis and Dysmorphogenesis. Monograph, Craniofacial Growth Series, Ann Arbor: Center for Human Growth and Development, University of Michigan, 1988, pp 127–140. Used with permission.)

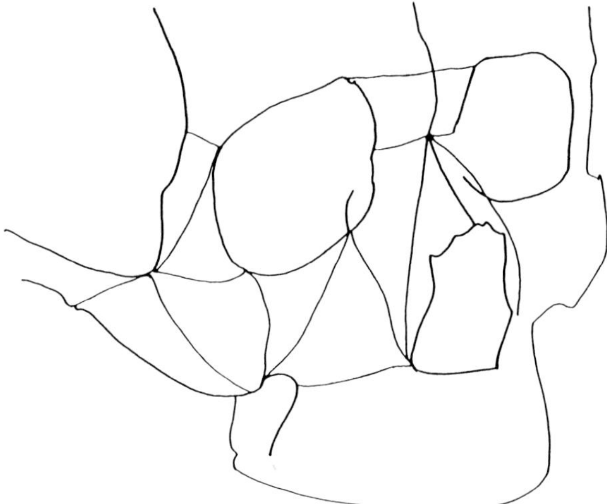

Figure 56–10 Homologous surface regions of the midface. Ridge curves are extracted first and then local curvature maxima on them are used as landmarks. Geodesic lines across the surface are used to connect landmark points to break the surface of the midface into standard regions.

curvature is positive; if on the other side, the curvature is negative. For a curving line in a plane, the curvature varies as a function of arc length along the curve. Furthermore, if the curvature as a function of arc length is known, the shape of the line is completely described.

For a three-dimensional line that twists through space we will need another concept called *torsion*. Torsion is the amount by which the line "twists" out of the plane along the axis of a line. Torsion also varies as a function

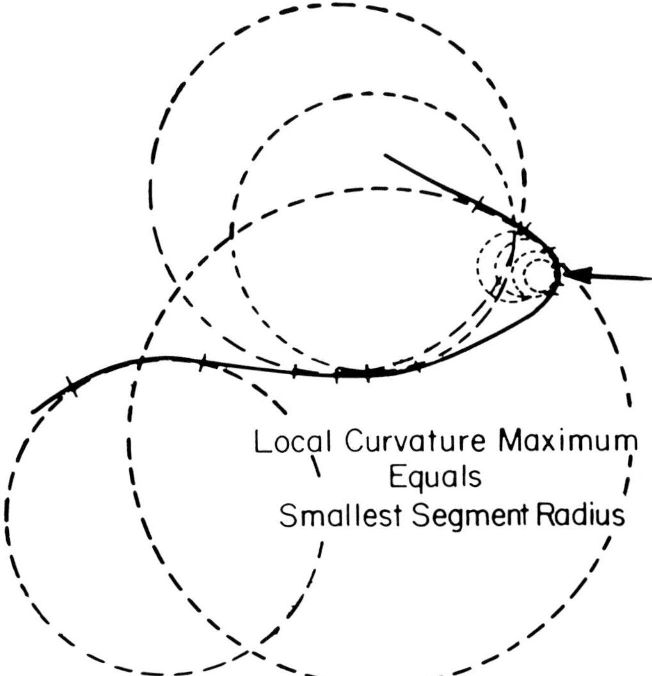

Figure 56–11 Concept of curvature on a plane curve. For any point on the curve, there is a circle that best fits the point and its nearest neighbors. The inverse of the radius of this circle is the curvature at any point. The curvature varies along the curve as a function of arc length.

of arc length. In three dimensions, if curvature and torsion are known as functions of arc length, the shape of the space curve is uniquely defined.

The concept of curvature as it applies to surfaces also must be understood. The great nineteenth century mathematician Gauss said that any point on a smoothly curving surface could be viewed as having two curvatures associated with it at right angles to one another (Fig. 56–12). Furthermore, there are only three kinds of points: parabolic, hyperbolic, and cylindric. A parabolic point has both of its centers of curvature on the same side of the surface (Fig. 56–12A). A hyperbolic point (e.g., a saddle point) has its centers of curvature on opposite sides of the surface (Fig. 56–12C). A cylindric point has one of its principal curvatures as zero (Fig. 56–12B). Gaussian curvature at a point is simply the result of multiplying these two principal curvatures together. Parabolic points have a positive Gaussian curvature because both curvature values have the same sign. Hyperbolic points have a negative Gaussian curvature because the two curvatures always have opposite signs. Cylindric points have a Gaussian curvature of zero.

Now let us put these previously unfamiliar geometric ideas into a familiar cephalometric context. When viewed as three-dimensional surface points, examples of parabolic points might be the gonion, pogonion, and anterior nasal spine. Furthermore, these points are "more parabolic" than any of the points on the surface in the neighborhood of the point. By *more parabolic* we mean that the Gaussian curvature is greater at the landmark point than it is at any of the neighboring points. Examples of hyperbolic points might be A point, B point, and nasion. At the nasion, we have a classic saddle-shaped surface. The nasion point is "more hyperbolic" than any of its neighboring points. This is equivalent to saying that its Gaussian curvature is smaller than any of the nearby points. A computer might find a hyperbolic landmark by searching the surface for a local Gaussian curvature minimum. Similarly, a parabolic landmark might be found by a computer as a local Gaussian curvature maximum.

Cylindric points are found on ridges on the surface such as at the orbital rims or the lower mandibular border. "Very cylindric points" might be found by searching a local surface region for a point where the absolute value of one of the principal curvatures was very large while the other principal curvature approached zero. Once this starting point on the ridge curve is found, the rest of the ridge curve can be found by moving out in opposite directions from the starting point, looking for neighboring points where the absolute value of one of the principal curvatures is a local maximum.

With this background, we can discuss how the new cephalometric program might look to the clinician. First, a rotating surface representation of the facial bones (CT or MRI scan) or skin surface (light scanner) is examined by the clinician. A set of three utility functions is presented as a menu to help the clinician find all of the standard landmark points. PARABOLIC POINT FINDER and HYPERBOLIC POINT FINDER start

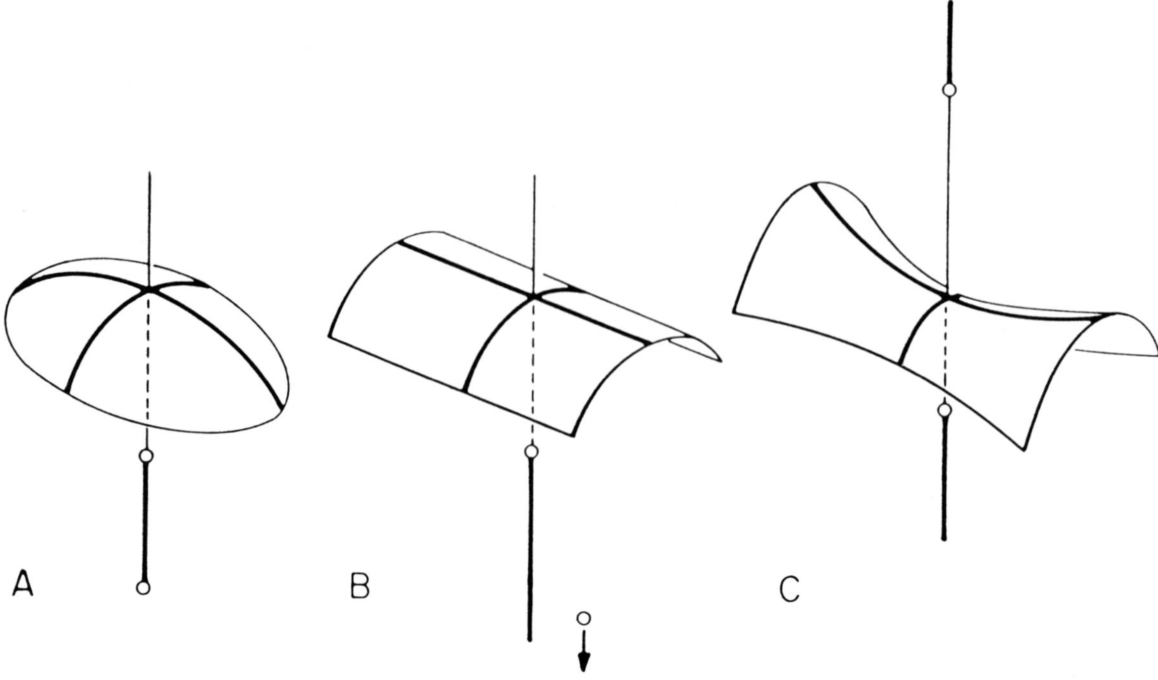

Figure 56–12 Concept of curvature as it applies to a surface point. According to Gauss, any surface point can be viewed as having a maximum and a minimum curvature value at right angles to one another. *A,* On a parabolic point both axes of curvature are on the same side of the surface. *B,* In a cylindric point one of the curvature values is zero (i.e., flat). *C,* In a hyperbolic point the axes of curvature are on opposite sides of the surface. (From Bookstein FL, Cutting C: A proposal for the apprehension of curving craniofacial form in three dimensions. In Vig K, Burdi A (eds): Craniofacial Morphogenesis and Dysmorphogenesis. Monograph, Craniofacial Growth Series. Ann Arbor: Center for Human Growth and Development, University of Michigan, 1988, pp 127–140. Used with permission.)

when the clinician points near the landmark in question. The computer then searches the neighboring points and quickly finds the desired point. The third function is a MANUAL POINT FINDER. After the point is found the landmark name may be typed in. Alternatively, the clinician or cephalometric technician may follow a programmed protocol that asks the user to find points in a specific order with the program filling in the landmark names automatically.

There are also three line-finder routines. RIDGE CURVE FINDER starts with the clinician selecting a point near the desired ridge curve. The computer then searches the neighboring surface for the ridge curve starting point and traces it in both directions until the clinician specifies that the end has been found. MANUAL CURVE FINDER also may be used to identify a ridge curve by hand. GEODESIC CURVE FINDER is the last routine that finds a curving line across a surface. A geodesic line is the shortest line traveling along the surface between two points on a surface. The clinician gives the computer two landmark points, and the machine finds the geodesic line across the surface that lies between them. Because the landmarks have been located previously by the clinician, it is unlikely that the clinician will use the GEODESIC CURVE FINDER directly. It is more likely that the program will automatically find the requisite geodesic lines. The established lines are labeled with an identifier manually or, in a programmed series, as for the landmark points.

A new set of landmark points will arise from the automatic analysis of ridge curves. Local curvature and torsion maxima and minima of the points on the ridge curve may be used to identify some landmark points. The menton and gonions, for example, are local curvature maxima on the curve that is the inferior mandibular border. Some new landmarks, such as the "corners" of the orbits, are also expected to be found in this way.

At this point, the heuristic part of the cephalometric identification procedure is over, and the computer does the rest. By use of the point and ridge finder utilities the clinician will have generated a "map" of the facial surface much like that seen in Figure 56–10. The computer then sets about the task of HOMOLOGY MAPPING. This is the second key concept in the development of this new cephalometric system. Up to this point, we have been discussing the means by which man and machine together go about establishing a GEOMETRIC HIERARCHY through volume-sampled data. This was the first key concept. Now the abstracted points, lines, surface regions, and solids must be homologously mapped into a standard schema.

Much of this work has already been done by the clinician as just described. For example, after the anterior nasal spine landmark on a patient has been found and labeled, it is mapped to other homologous landmarks obtained from various patients and a normal sample. In this way, we can compare the anterior nasal spine landmark of patients with the normal form. This idea is deeply rooted in the cephalometric tradition.[2, 5] By comparing homologous anatomic landmarks of patients and normal subjects it is possible both to study quantitatively the facial deformity of a syndrome as a group and to study individual patients for the purposes of surgical treatment planning.

The concept of HOMOLOGY MAPPING must now be extended beyond landmarks into ridge curves, surface regions, and solid regions.[48–51] To do this requires use of the concept of parametric representation. A single quantitative parameter may be mapped onto a curving line segment in a three-dimensional space. It is customary to assign the parameter a value of 0.0 at the beginning of the line segment and a value of 1.0 at the end of the segment. Parameter values in the middle of the line segment are usually defined as a proportion of the total length of the segment. For example, the point midway between the menton and the gonion on the inferior mandibular border would be assigned a parametric value of 0.5 of that line segment.

This parameter may be used to map homologous points on curving line segments between different individuals. In the example just given, comparing points with the same parameter value of 0.5 between different individuals means that the midpoints between their mentons and gonions on the line of the inferior mandibular border will be grouped together for statistical purposes. Using the parametric concept, points on a smoothly curving three-dimensional line may be compared in much the same way as landmarks.

Points on a surface region require two parameters to describe a location uniquely. The best example is the latitude-longitude system for describing a location on the surface of the earth. It takes two parametric numbers (in this case latitude and longitude) to identify a unique location on a smoothly curving surface in three dimensions. In Figure 56–10 it is possible to break down the facial surface into regions that are bounded on four sides by lines. Each of these lines has its own single valued parametric representation. By pairing the parameters on opposite borders of the region, it becomes possible to identify any point on the surface with just two parametric numbers. This process is similar to looking at a sheet of ruled graph paper. The paper has four border lines, the top and bottom lines sharing the same "right-left" parameter and the right and left border lines sharing the same "top-bottom" parameter. A point in the middle of the paper would have a parametric value

of 0.5 in the right-left parameter and 0.5 in the top-bottom parameter.

This same two-parameter schema may be used to identify a point on a smoothly curving surface that is bounded by three or four line segments (Fig. 56–13). The mathematics of parametric surface representation have been well developed in the computer-aided design literature.[35, 52, 53] Fortunately for the clinician, all of this parametric mapping of homologous surface points may be done entirely by computer once the corner landmarks and border curves have been found.

Parametric mapping of solid regions requires three parameters. When the earth is viewed as a solid, a latitude and longitude define only a surface point. If we add a third parameter—namely, distance from the center of the earth—we know exactly where we are within the solid. In the case of Figure 56–10, each surface region might be matched with a landmark on the opposite side of the solid. Parametric distance between this point and the surface above provides the necessary third parameter for assignment of solid homology.

Statistics in the New Cephalometric System

The concept of the abstraction of a volume sample into a progressively simpler GEOMETRIC HIERARCHY followed by heuristic landmark point identification and then progressively more complex parametric HOMOLOGY MAPPING of the volume sample has many important applications, not the least of which is the development of a new cephalometric method. It becomes possible to perform statistical operations on lines, surfaces, and volumes.

The simple ability to average surfaces would lift the comparison of surgical treatment methods in craniofacial anomalies out of the quagmire of anecdotal reporting. Surgeons are currently given to reporting the efficacy of a new treatment procedure with photographs of their best results. In any other field of medicine, this manner of reporting would be totally unacceptable. In introducing a new chemotherapeutic drug at a cancer symposium, if the presenter tried to attest to its efficacy by presenting one or two long-term survivors, he would be a laughingstock. Yet this continues to be the manner of

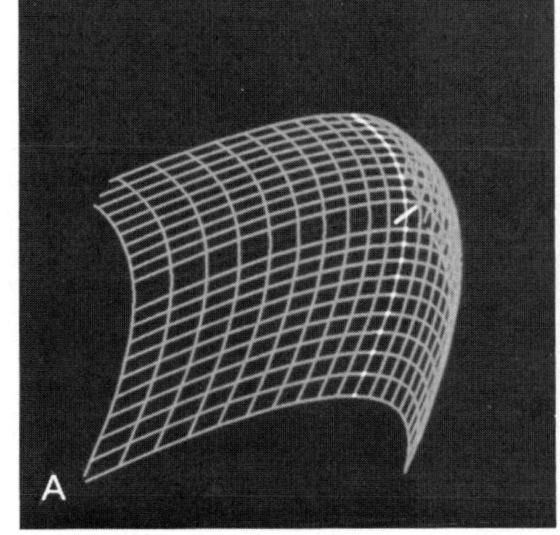
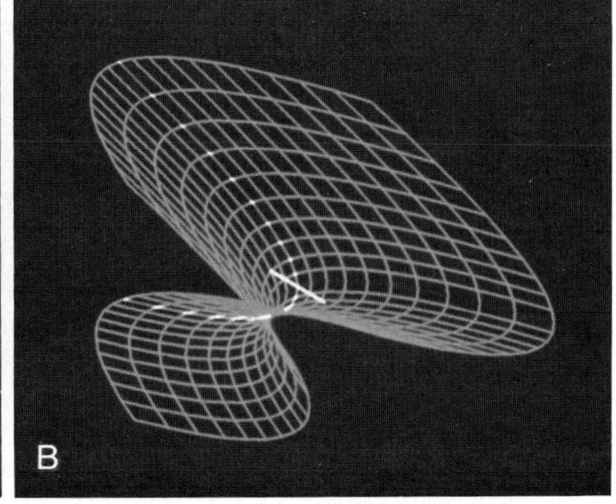

Figure 56–13 Two parameters are required to identify a point uniquely on a surface. A parabolic surface *(A)* and a hyperbolic surface *(B)* are shown with their lines of equal parametric value ruled on the surface.

presentation of surgical results. Chemotherapists would demand to know the mean survival with this new drug and whether the outcome was statistically significantly better than the current treatment method. Workers in the field of craniofacial anomalies should strive to achieve the same high standards. In chemotherapy, results can be reported with a single number, that is, survival. Craniofacial surgery results are multidimensional, making numerical reporting more difficult. We feel that three-dimensional computer graphics makes this difficult problem tractable.

Color-coded three-dimensional computer graphics will be the most likely way to present the results of multidimensional statistical comparisons of the human face to the clinician. Reporting comparisons using huge lists of numbers will not be very useful. Color will be used to represent the statistical dimension. For example, probabilities of a difference from normal could be projected onto a color range from red to blue with white in the middle. If a point on the surface of an average face in a patient with Crouzon's disease were the same as normal it would be colored in a simple black-to-white gray scale. If it were three or more standard deviations too large in some measure, it would be colored with a blue intensity scale. Three or more standard deviations too small would result in red scale coloration. Intermediate scales would represent intermediate deviations. In this way a single, color-coded, three-dimensional computer graphic could present the results of many thousands of statistical computations to the clinician in an easily understood format. Touching the surface with a cursor could be made to present the actual quantitative result in a region of the image. It should be stressed that the study of craniofacial anomalies is a four-dimensional problem: the study of the change in three-dimensional shape over time.

If color is used to report the statistical dimension, then time must be used to report growth. The appropriate intuitive report format to the clinician might be color-coded, three-dimensional animations of the change in facial shape over time. Appreciation of such a "film loop" repeated over time would allow the clinician to grasp intuitively statistical comparisons of the growing three-dimensional form of patients with craniofacial anomalies. I fear at this point that the means of presenting statistical results of comparisons between groups of surfaces will be more easily developed than the methods of performing the statistical comparisons. This challenge should provide suitable fodder for geometrically inclined statisticians in the years to come.[48-50]

The Craniofacial Anomalies Work Station

The hardware required to produce a craniofacial anomalies work station is rapidly becoming more accessible. When the author began this work, the hardware cost six times that of the hardware currently in use and was two hundred times less powerful. During the next few years, the kind of computer graphics power, memory size, and central processing power required to fulfill the needs of this application will be available on a personal computer. The student of craniofacial anomalies will study his data using "user friendly" programs that are no more difficult to use than those of a word processor.

This section will describe the specific hardware requirements of such a work station. The following paragraphs may be skipped by the nontechnical reader. The principal problem to be handled by the hardware involves the management of very large volumes of data. A single CT or MRI scan can occupy more than 20 megabytes, even when maximally packed. To deal with data interactively requires large amounts of disk and random access memory (RAM). Magnetic disks will soon be replaced by optical disks for the storage of medical data. Write-once-read-many (WORM) disk storage is ideal for medical data. The usual objection to the WORM disk is that the laser writes the data on the disk permanently so that the optical disk cannot be erased and rewritten. This is not a problem for medical data because once the study is performed, the original data should never be altered anyway. Optical WORM disk storage is also very high density, storing a gigabyte or more on a single removable disk.

Graphics functions implemented in hardware are essential. The three-dimensional, CT-based, surgical simulation program currently in use by the author models the skull as approximately 600,000 polygons, which must be rendered in as close to real time as possible. Volume-rendered translucent views of CT or MRI data become tractable only with the use of dedicated graphics hardware. Fortunately, this kind of high-performance graphics hardware is becoming more powerful and less expensive.

High-speed data communications hardware also is essential. Data from the various scanners should be capable of being transmitted directly to the work station without the need for intermediate transfer on magnetic media. Direct connection to the department of radiology for the acquisition of CT and MRI scans is highly desirable. A high central processing speed also is essential for the efficient handling of data. Increasing use of parallel processing and reduced instruction set (RISC) central processing units currently hold the greatest promise in this regard.

From a technical viewpoint, the software used to process data on craniofacial anomalies must have three ingredients. The first is a common database format for the storage of points, lines, surfaces, and volumes. The second is isolation of graphics functions into a common subroutine library. The last is a modular program structure. These three essential factors will be described below.

The database structure for surfaces and volumes is of paramount importance. If multiple utility programs are used to examine a source of medical data, a robust and efficient common data storage format is essential. For the storage of surface data we have adopted a modification of Baumgart's winged-edge data structure.[54] These data are stored as lists of vertices, edges, and faces.[55] The surfaces of all solids are stored as closed polyhedra. It should be noted that this is a solids modeling approach. To those already doing research in this area, it may seem unnecessary to insist on a connected surface around solids. This is done so that the CT and MRI data that generated these surfaces in the first place can be back-referenced as enclosed, edited solids. This editing can be most easily done using a simplified surface extraction procedure from the original CT or MRI data. This step also is very helpful in distilling the geometric hierarchies from within the data that will be used for pattern recognition and quantitative analysis.

A database must be capable of storing any kind of information in its structure. The Baumgart data structure just described stores only the topologic data of the objects. We feel that this is the reason why no general purpose subroutine library has ever emerged from Baumgart's original dissertation. To this end, Betsy Haddad and Kenneth Perlin of our group have written an "extension" system to Baumgart's library. This allows the user to attach any kind of information he or she wishes to any of the vertices, faces, edges, or objects.

Storage of the basic CT or MRI data is currently being accomplished using QSH, a program-subroutine library written by Gerald Maguire and Marilyn Noz.[56–58] At its foundation, QSH has a common data storage format for volume-sampled data. Programs that read CT and MRI scan tapes from most commercially available scanners exist and put the data into QSH format. There are a number of display, reformat, and image-processing programs that allow the data to be rapidly accessed, processed in a variety of ways, and viewed.

It is essential to be able to go back and forth easily between volume and surface databases. Mr. Alan Kalvin, under the direction of Robert Hummel and Marilyn Noz, has written a program that finds a closed polyhedron around a solid detected in a CT or MRI scan. This program uses a three-dimensional extrapolation of two-dimensional image-processing algorithms to find the surface. This solid surface is then put into the surface database structure just described. In this way the surface around bone or soft tissue can be found and converted to the surface storage format. A program will soon be written that partitions a complete CT or MRI study into a smaller unit by "cutting" it with a closed polyhedron. By narrowing the region of interest, the scan may be examined much more quickly. In this way, solids can be efficiently edited and processed using the surface data format, and the result of the editing can be applied to the original CT or MRI data.

It also is essential that the graphics elements of the software structure be isolated from the rest of the software. At this point in the development of computer graphics hardware, no standard set of capabilities exists. For this reason, each work station manufacturer has written its own system graphics software that uses only the facilities provided by its hardware. At the system level there is no uniformity of graphics subroutine calls. The graphics kernel system (GKS) addresses this problem for two-dimensional graphics but is woefully inadequate for high-performance three-dimensional graphics requirements. PHIGS plus is coming closer to meeting the needs of this application but has not yet gained widespread acceptance in the graphics hardware community. For the purposes of this project, all of the utility programs use a high-level graphics subroutine library that consists of less than 20 subroutines. This subroutine library must be created for each machine that is to run the craniofacial anomalies surgical simulation and analysis program.

This project was constructed using multiple small general-purpose programs linked together by an executive program superstructure. This is in keeping with the UNIX philosophy. UNIX is an operating system that has become dominant in the scientific and engineering community. This program is being written in the C programming language under the UNIX operating system, which is the most portable software environment currently available. For this reason, it is anticipated that the software that results from this project will attain widespread distribution and run on a large number of different machines.

ACKNOWLEDGMENTS. Work in progress reported in this chapter is supported by a grant from the National Institute of Dental Research No. DE03568—12.

The author wishes to acknowledge and thank his coworkers on this project: Fred L. Bookstein of the University of Michigan provided mathematical guidance in carrying out this software development and developed all of the relevant statistics. Barry Grayson, Joseph G. McCarthy, and Hiechun Kim of the Craniofacial Anomalies Unit of the Institute of Reconstructive Plastic Surgery at New York University helped to develop the clinical direction of this project. Gerald Maguire of Columbia University and Marilyn Noz of New York University joined the project and brought their QSH software with them. Robert Hummel, Kenneth Perlin, Jack Schwartz, and Paul Wright of New York University provided the computer science faculty support for this project. And last, but by no means least, I would like to thank the computer science graduate students Alan Kalvin, Betsy Haddad, Pat Bedard, and Dan Karron, without whom this project would not have been possible.

References

1. Baumrind S, Miller D: Computer-aided head film analysis: The University of California San Francisco Method. Am J Orthod 78:41, 1980.
2. Broadbent BH, Golden W: Bolton Standards of Developmental Growth. St. Louis: C. V. Mosby, 1975.
3. Ricketts R, Bench R, Hilgers J, et al: An overview of computerized cephalometrics. Am J Orthod 61:1, 1972.
4. Ricketts R: Divine proportion in facial esthetics. Clin Plast Surg 9:401, 1982.
5. Riolo ML, Moyers RE, McNamara JS, et al: An Atlas of Craniofacial Growth. Monograph No. 2, Craniofacial Growth Series. Ann Arbor: Center for Human Growth and Development, University of Michigan, 1974.
6. Cutting C, Bookstein F, Grayson B, et al: Three-dimensional computer assisted design of craniofacial surgical procedures: Optimization and interaction with cephalometric and CT-based models. Plast Reconstr Surg 77:877, 1986.
7. Cutting C, Grayson B, Bookstein F, et al: Computer-aided planning and evaluation of facial and orthognathic surgery. Clin Plast Surg 13:449, 1986.
8. Cook L, Dwyer S, Batnitzky S, et al: A three-dimensional display system for diagnostic imaging applications. IEEE Comput Graphics Appl 3:13, 1983.
9. Herman G, Liu H: Display of three-dimensional information in computed tomography. J Comput Assist Tomogr 1:155, 1977.
10. Herman G, Liu H: Three-dimensional display of human organs from computed tomograms. Comput Graphics Image Proc 9:1, 1979.
11. Marsh J, Vannier M: The "third" dimension in craniofacial surgery. Plast Reconstr Surg 71:759, 1983.

12. Merz P: Computer guides facial reconstruction. JAMA 249:1409, March 18, 1983.
13. Udupa J, Herman G, Margasahayam P, et al: A turnkey system for the display and analysis of 3D medical objects. Proc SPIE 671:154, 1986.
14. Vannier M, Marsh J, Warren J: Three-dimensional CT reconstruction images for craniofacial surgical planning and evaluation. Radiology 150:179, 1984.
15. Farkas L, Ross RB, James J: Anthropometry of the face in lateral facial dysplasia: The bilateral form. Cleft Palate J 14:41, 1977.
16. Farkas L: Anthropometry of the Head and Face in Medicine. New York: Elsevier North-Holland, 1981.
17. Coblentz A, Herron R (eds): Applications of Human Biostereometrics. Proc SPIE 166, 1978.
18. Frobin W, Hierholzer E: Analysis of human back shape using surface curvatures. J Biomech 15:379, 1982.
19. Herron R (ed): Biostereometrics '82. Proc Soc Photo-Opt Instru Engl 361, 1982.
20. Berkowitz S, Cuzzi J: Biostereometric analysis of surgically corrected abnormal faces. Am J Orthod 72:526, 1977.
21. Savara B, Miller S, Demuth R, et al: Biostereometrics and computer graphics for patients with craniofacial malformations: Diagnosis and treatment planning. Plast Reconstr Surg 75:495, 1985.
22. Baumrind S, Moffit F, Curry S: Three-dimensional x-ray stereometry from paired coplanar images: A progress report. Am J Orthod 84:292, 1983.
23. Baumrind S, Moffit F, Curry S: The geometry of three-dimensional measurement from paired coplanar x-ray images. Am J Orthod 84:313, 1983.
24. Cutting C, McCarthy JG, Karron D: Three-dimensional input of body surface data using a laser light scanner. Ann Plast Surg 21:38, 1988.
25. Arridge S, Moss J, Linney A, et al: Three-dimensional digitization of the face and skull. J Maxillofac Surg 13:136, 1985.
26. Moss J, Linney A, Grinrod S, et al: Three-dimensional visualization of the face and skull using computerized tomography and laser scanning techniques. Eur J Orthod 9:247, 1987.
27. Berkowitz S: Automatic laser scanning of dental models. Read before the American Cleft Palate Association, San Antonio, TX, 1987.
28. Wada T, Miyazaki T: Growth and changes in maxillary arch form in complete unilateral cleft lip and palate children. Cleft Palate J 12:115, 1975.
29. Wada T, Mizokawa N, Miyazaki T, et al: Maxillary dental arch growth in different types of cleft. Cleft Palate J 21:180, 1984.
30. King B, Workman C, Latham R: An anatomic study of the columella and the protruding premaxillae in a bilateral cleft lip and palate infant. Cleft Palate J 16:223, 1979.
31. Bhatia S, Sowray J: A computer aided design for orthognathic surgery. Br J Oral Maxillofac Surg 22:237, 1984.
32. Cutting C, Bookstein F, Grayson B, et al: Computer aided planning of orthognathic surgery. Read before the Plastic Surgery Research Council Meeting, Detroit, MI, April 1–4, 1984.
33. Marsh J, Vannier M, Stevens WG, et al: Computerized imaging for soft tissue and osseous reconstruction in the head and neck. Clin Plast Surg 12:279, 1985.
34. Udupa J: Computerized surgical planning: Current capabilities and medical needs. Proc Soc Photo-Opt Instru Engl 626, 474, 1986.
35. Foley J, van Dam A: Fundamentals of Interactive Computer Graphics. Reading, MA: Addison-Wesley, 1982.
36. Caceci M, Cacheris W: Fitting curves to data. Byte 9:340, 1984.
37. Luenberger D: Linear and Non-linear Programming. London: Addison-Wesley, 1973.
38. Willmott DR: Soft tissue profile changes following correction of class III malocclusions by mandibular surgery. Br J Orthodont 8:175, 1981.
39. Gallagher R, Simon B, Johnson P, et al: Finite Elements in Biomechanics. New York: Wiley, 1982.
40. Rice J: Finite element methods. In Numerical Methods, Software, and Analysis: IMSL Reference Edition. New York: McGraw-Hill, 1983, pp 320–324.
41. Rockey K, Evans H, Griffiths D, et al: The Finite Element Method. New York: Wiley, 1983.
42. Zienkeiwicz O: The Finite Element Method. New York: McGraw-Hill, 1977.
43. Borisenko A, Tarapov I: Vector and Tensor Analysis with Applications, Silverman R (trans). New York: Dover, 1968, pp 45–47.
44. Guggenheimer H: Differential Geometry. New York: Dover, 1977.
45. Hilbert D, Cohn-Vossen S: Geometry and the Imagination. New York: Chelsea, 1952.
46. Kreyszig E: Introduction to Differential Geometry and Riemannian Geometry. Toronto: University of Toronto Press, 1968.
47. Lipshutz M: Differential Geometry. New York: McGraw-Hill, 1969.
48. Bookstein FL: The Measurement of Biological Shape and Shape Change. Lecture Notes in Biomathematics. Vol. 24. New York: Springer, 1978.
49. Bookstein FL: Tensor biometrics for changes in cranial shape. Ann Hum Biol 1413:437, 1984.
50. Bookstein FL: A statistical method for biological shape comparisons. J Theoret Biol 107:475, 1984.
51. Thompson D: On the theory of transformations or the comparison of related forms. In Bonner JT (ed): On Growth and Form. Cambridge: Cambridge University Press, 1961, pp 325–368.
52. Gordon W, Risenfeld R: B-spline curves and surfaces. In Barnhill R, Riesenfeld R (eds): Computer Aided Geometric Design. New York: Academic Press, 1974, pp 95–126.
53. Rogers D, Adams J: Mathematical Elements for Computer Graphics. New York: McGraw-Hill, 1976.
54. Baumgart BG: Geometric Modeling for Computer Vision. Thesis (Ph.D.). Stanford: Stanford University, 1974.
55. Preparata F, Shamos MI: Computational Geometry. New York: Springer, 1985.
56. Maguire G, Noz M: Standardizing the raster display for medial images using a fixed set of frame buffer primitives. J Med Sys 10:209, 1986.
57. Maguire G, Jaeger J, Farde L, et al: Use of graphic techniques for error evaluation. J Med Sys 11:277, 1987.
58. Noz M, Maguire G: QSH: A minimal but highly portable image display and handling tool kit. Comput Meth Prog Biomed (in press, 1988).
59. Bookstein FL, Cutting C: A proposal for the apprehension of curving craniofacial form in three dimensions. In Vig K, Burdi A (eds): Craniofacial Morphogenesis and Dysmorphogenesis. Monograph, Craniofacial Growth Series. Ann Arbor: Center for Human Growth and Development, University of Michigan, 1988, pp 127–140.

CHAPTER 57

Tensor and Three-Dimensional Cephalometric Method of Anthropometric Analysis

Barry H. Grayson

Conventional cephalometric analysis defines craniofacial morphology in terms of the two-dimensional locations of points (landmarks), the lengths of lines, and the angles between pairs of lines. These representations have been of considerable clinical use in comparing individuals to population norms and in planning and assessing the progress of orthodontic treatment.[1]

Traditional methods of cephalometric analysis significantly limit our ability to describe craniofacial form.[2] Many measurements describe structures by their relations to other structures. For instance, maxillary A–point and mandibular B–point may be measured by the angle they make with the "normally positioned" cranial base, the line S–N. We have thereby inadvertently presumed that those landmarks are both normally positioned in the form under study, an assumption that goes unverified.

A second limitation of the conventional cephalometric method is its representation of a three-dimensional object by compressing it into a two-dimensional cephalogram. This introduces artifacts such as perspective distortion, radiographic enlargement, and foreshortening.

A third limitation of conventional cephalometric methods, which we will concentrate on in this chapter, is the routine reduction of all cephalograms to "analyses" using fixed sets of variables. The usual study of deformity proceeds in two steps—first, selection of an arbitrary set of measurement variables, and then clinical or statistical summaries of those variables. The alternative we recommend, tensor analysis, reverses the order of these steps. First, a biologic effect of interest is selected, and second, measurements of those effects are provided. For instance, we may study a population of special interest, perhaps one with a specific craniofacial syndrome. We then consider, by a variety of concealed algebraic maneuvers, all possible measures of a set of landmarks and determine which of all the possible distances or proportions best express the particular abnormality under investigation. That is to say, the tensor method of cephalometric analysis makes possible a rigorous statistical analysis of landmark data without requiring the specification of particular shape measures in advance. The technique extracts the particular shape measures that are most clearly diagnostic of the form or syndrome under study.

The statistical details of the tensor analysis have been presented elsewhere.[3] In this short chapter we can only illustrate the logic of these studies. We start out by grouping conventional cephalometric landmarks in sets of three, forming triangles. For the diagnosis of a deformity, these triangles are compared to the triangles of the same landmarks encountered in an age- and sex-matched normative population (Figure 57–1) in a manner that is independent of preexisting measurement schemes. In Fig. 57–2, the triangles on the left (ABC) could represent any three conventional cephalometric landmarks in their typical locations in a mean normal film. On the right, triangles A'B'C' show their locations in the patient or syndrome. We interpret the comparison as a deformation of this triangle for a single case or a mean in a specific study population.

The deformation can be mathematically described by its effect on the shape of a circle. A uniform deformation transforms the circle into an ellipse. The ellipse has two perpendicular axes. The circle, it can be shown, has two perpendicular diameters that correspond to the axes of the ellipse undergoing the transformation. When the lengths of the axes of the circle and the ellipse are compared to one another, one shows the greatest ratio of change between the forms, and one the least. This pair of changes in length of the axes, together with their orientation on the form, exhaust the geometric descrip-

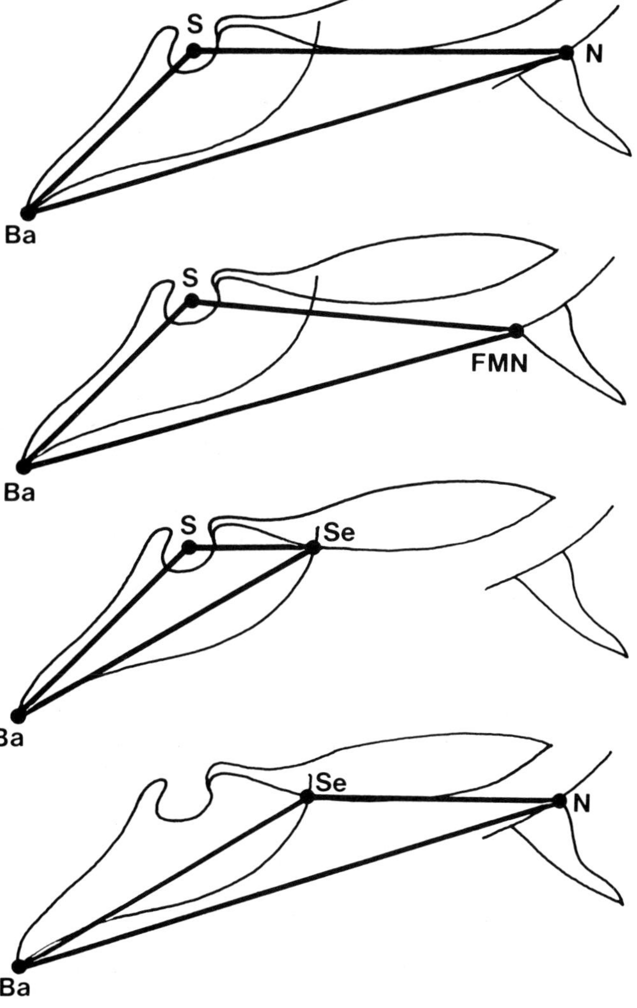

Figure 57–1 Cephalometric landmarks linked together in sets forming triangles. Quantitative comparison of these triangles can be made between the normal and study populations. Ba = basion, S = sella turcica, N = nasion, FMN = frontomaxillary nasal suture, and SE = sphenoethmoidal intersect.

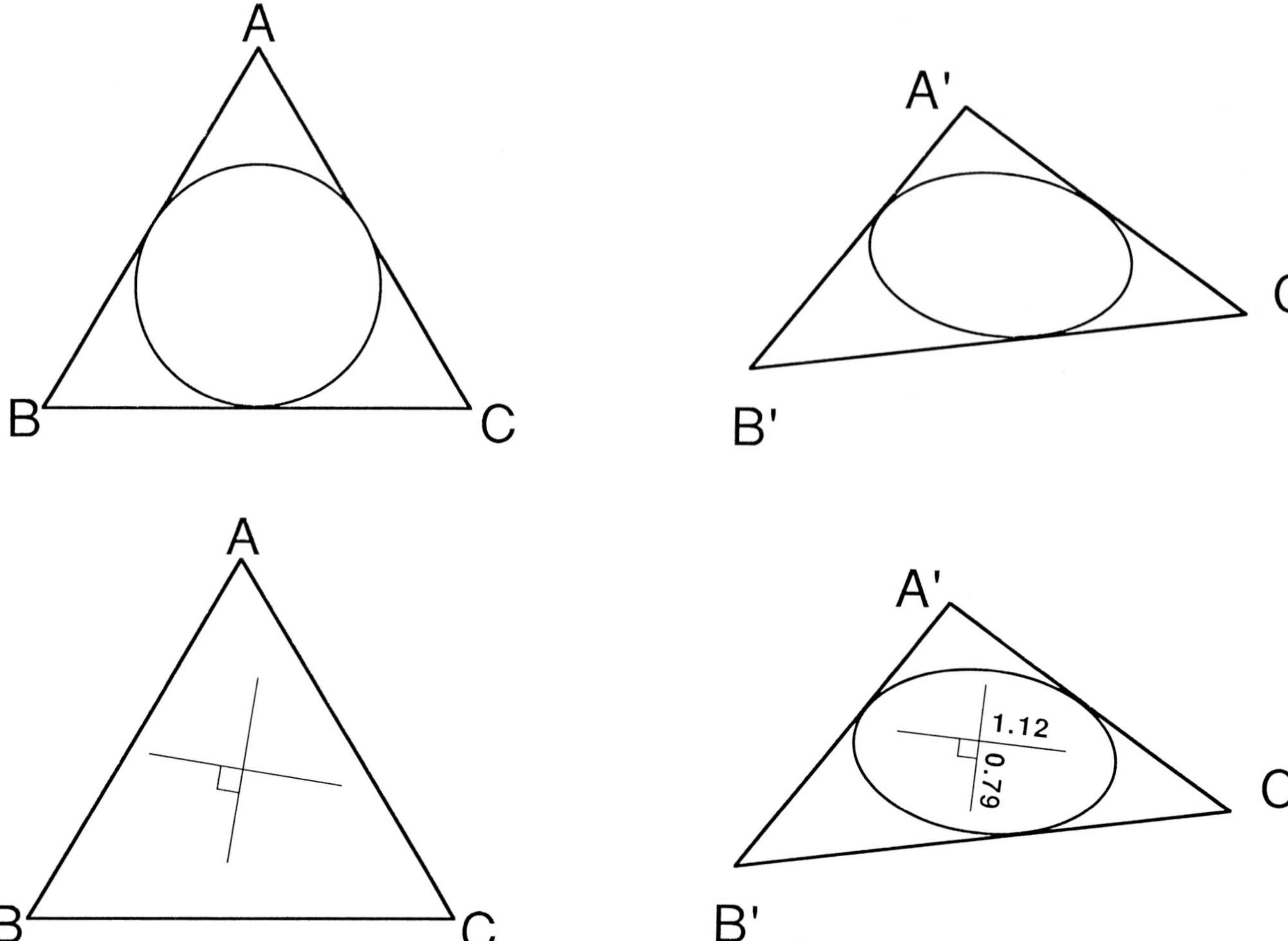

Figure 57–2 Triangles on the left (ABC) are composed of any three conventional cephalometric landmarks. On the right (triangles A'B'C') is a deformation of these triangles that may represent the mean deformation for a triangle in a specific study population. Change in shape of the triangles results in transformation of a circle into an ellipse. Perpendicular axes of the circle and ellipse are compared. Change in length of each axis provides a geometric description or summary of the overall change in shape of the triangles. In this example there is a reduction of 21% in a nearly vertical direction and an increase of 12% in a nearly horizontal direction. Perpendicular axes are pictures of tensors, which are coordinate-free representations of geometric change.

tion of the change in shape of the triangles. In this example we see a reduction, or a shrinkage, of 21% in an approximately vertical direction and a lengthening, or stretch, of 12% in an approximately horizontal direction. Neither in this case nor in general do these axes align with conventional measures of the landmarks ABC. Consequently, changes that are not usually considered are recorded.

The crossing lines displayed in these triangles are pictures of the axes in the description of change. This is a tensor description, a coordinate-free representation, or a geometric shape change.

Following is an example of the use of these descriptions in syndromology. Figure 57–3 shows the findings of a study[4] dealing with the effects of unilateral cleft lip and palate on facial height. The distance from nasion to pogonion—"net facial height"—is 5% short of normal in the typical patient of the sample. This is the least abnormal dimension in any of the large facial triangles. However, the upper component of this measurement, the distance from cranial base to ANS, is 7% short of normal. Note that the direction of greatest reduction in

length does not, in this population, align along axes that pass through conventional cephalometric landmarks. With the assistance of a computer, one can consider, triangle by triangle, an entire set of cephalometric landmarks. The computer then determines which of the triangles most significantly differ from those found in a matched normative population and sketches the orientation of these discrepancies. Thus, the analysis finds the particular shape measures most clearly manifesting the individual or group difference, indicating both the direction(s) and the magnitude(s) of deformation.

Three-Dimensional Cephalometrics

At the very beginning of the cephalometric method, Broadbent and Bolton[5] stressed the importance of coordinating the lateral (LAT) with the posteroanterior (PA) cephalogram to arrive at a distortion-free definition of craniofacial form. Because the LAT and PA films occupy positions at 90 degrees to each other, with their use one can reconstruct much of the three-dimensional

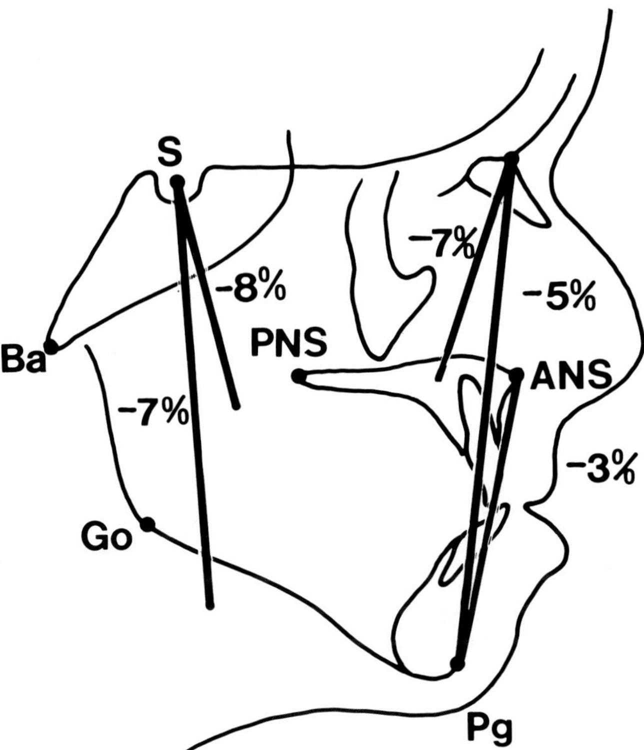

Figure 57–3 Directions and magnitudes of reduction in mean face height observed in a population of cleft lip and palate patients. Note that the direction of greatest reduction in length does not always align along axes that pass through conventional cephalometric landmarks. Ba = basion, S = sella turcica, Go = gonion, PNS = posterior nasal spine, ANS = anterior nasal spine, Pg = pogonion.

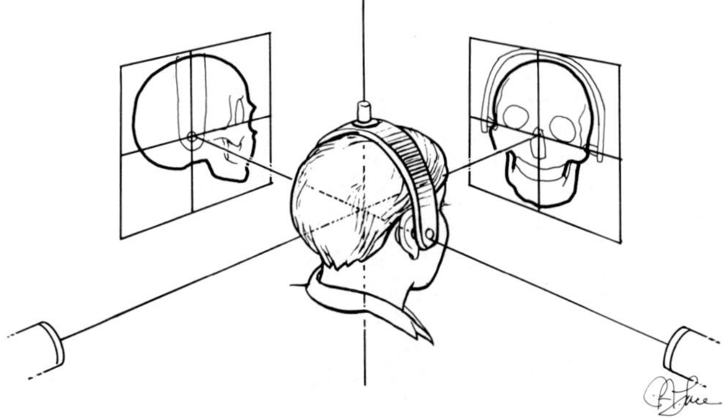

Figure 57–4 Knowing the three-dimensional locations of the point source of an x-ray beam and the shadow of an anatomic landmark on the cephalometric film allows determination of a line in three dimensions. Given lines from both the posteroanterior and the lateral cephalograms, the three-dimensional position of the landmark in question can be determined.

data describing the original craniofacial form in space (Figure 57–4).

A point on the x-ray film represents a line in space—that is, the three-dimensional locations of the point source of an x-ray beam and the shadow of an anatomic landmark on the cephalometric film together specify a line in three dimensions (Figure 57–4). From the two lines representing the two landmarks in both the posteroanterior and lateral cephalograms, the three-dimensional position of the landmark in question can be determined.[6] Collecting three-dimensional landmark points in this manner yields a constellation of landmarks for the face that is visualized most easily by connecting the points with lines (Figure 57–5).

The three-dimensional cephalometric landmark definition is subject to some sources of error and definitional instabilities. Aside from the usual cephalometric sources of error, the principal problem is that a number of these three-dimensional landmarks do not actually lie on the skeleton. A case in point is the angle of the mandible (that is, gonion). The gonion seen on the posteroanterior cephalogram is lateral to the gonion seen on the lateral view. The three-dimensional intersection of a vertical plane through the posteroanterior gonion and a line through the gonion seen on the lateral x-ray yields a three-dimensional intercept that does not actually lie on the skeleton. It should be noted that use of intercepts rather than points actually on the skeleton is well established in conventional cephalometric usage (e.g.,

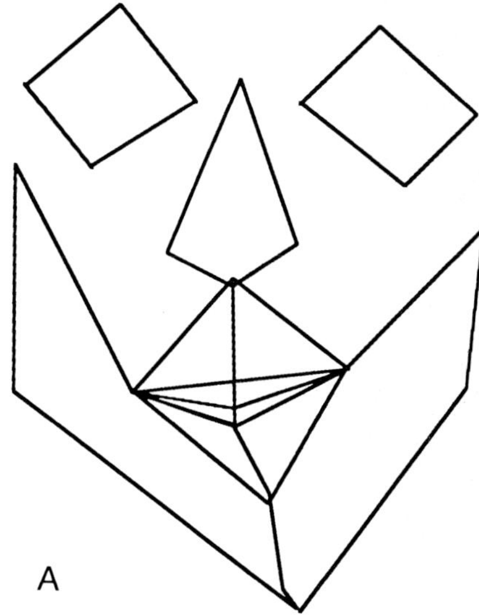

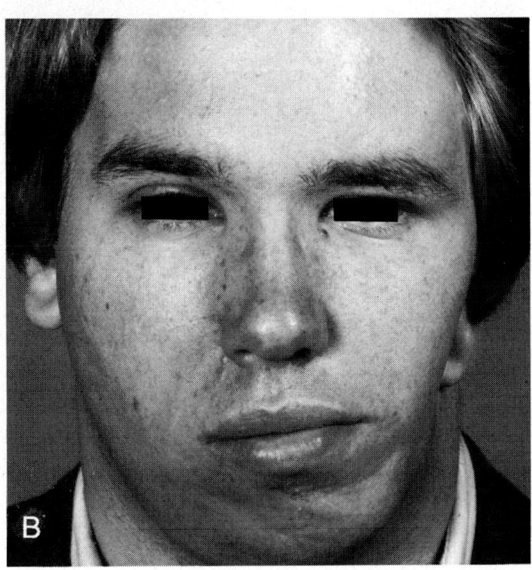

A   B

Figure 57–5 *A,* Three-dimensional cephalometric landmark points connected by straight lines, illustrating the asymmetric craniofacial morphology of a patient with hemifacial microsomia. *B,* Frontal photograph of the same patient with hemifacial microsomia.

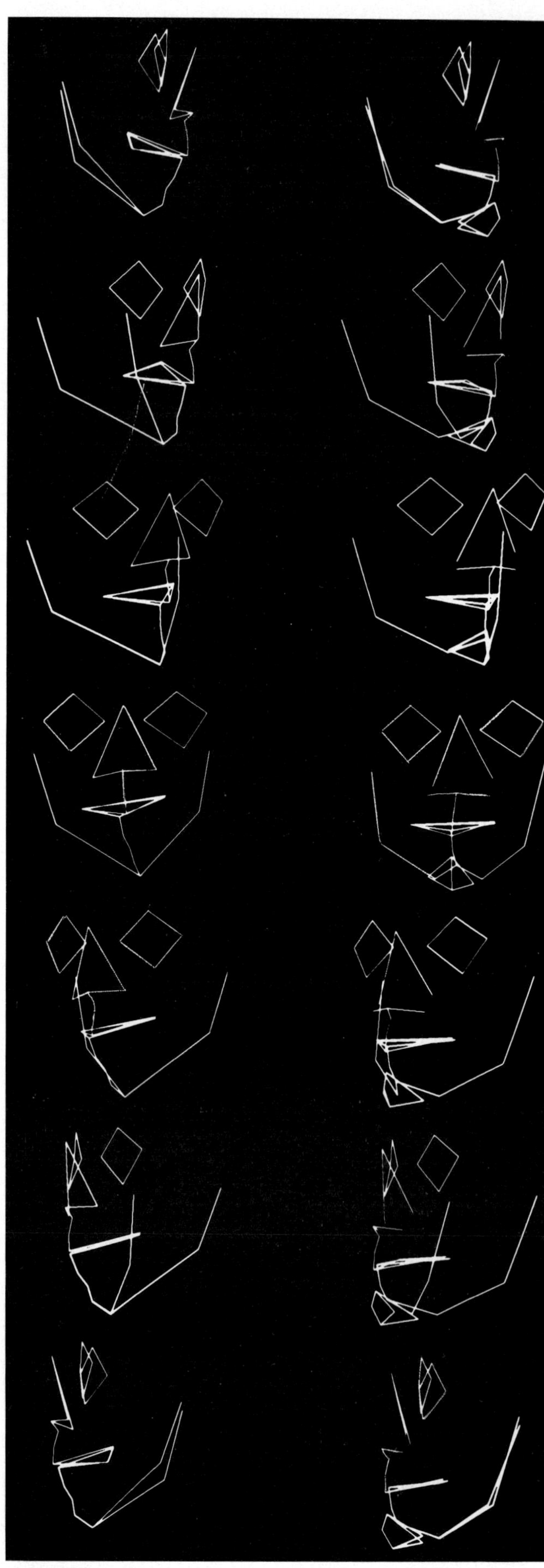

Figure 57-6 Preoperative and computer-optimized, postsimulation, three-dimensional line drawing of a patient with hemifacial microsomia. Three-dimensional landmark point locations were obtained by the method illustrated in Figure 57–4. Simulation involves a sagittal split of the mandible, Le Fort I procedure, and genioplasty. The preoperative animation sequence appears in the left column, and the postsimulation sequence appears on the right. As you move down the columns, the heads turn from one side to the other.

GoI [gonial intercept]). As long as these intercepts are consistently defined, they may be used for any conventional purpose for which landmarks are used, such as the tensor descriptions of anomaly we described above.

In particular, the three-dimensional landmark constellations that result may be used for optimal surgical planning, as is done frequently for two-dimensional data (mock surgery on cephalometric tracings). Figure 57–6 shows a stick-figure representation of a patient with hemifacial microsomia and a three-dimensional surgical plan. The surgical simulation indicates the extent of three osteotomies, Le Fort I, sagittal split, and genioplasty, computed to create a normal form "most closely." Such computations must be adjusted in the light of a great many clinical factors.

Three-dimensional cephalometric technique requires considerable care in the identification of bilateral, cephalometric landmarks, especially orbital or dental landmarks. When executed accurately, the technique has several advantages compared with the three-dimensional CT scan in the study of craniofacial form.

1. Normative data exist for the three-dimensional cephalogram. (Our studies borrow usage of the Broadbent-Bolton PA and LAT cephalometric templates.)[7] It is unlikely that normative data exist for the more extensive visualization of the CT scan.

2. A pair of cephalograms involves approximately a 26-mrad skin dose to the subject. By comparison, a closely spaced series of CT slices totals about 6.5 rad. Hence, it is much more practical to use a three-dimensional cephalogram in the anticipation that it will be repeated, as for longitudinal studies of growth and relapse following surgery.

3. The cost of a pair of cephalograms is a negligible fraction of the cost of a CT scan.

4. The young patient does not need to be sedated in the course of this procedure.

5. Archives of cephalogram pairs have been collected through decades of orthodontic treatment and research. Using these data, one could proceed immediately with three-dimensional study of large populations of treated cases. Morphometric methods already exist for analysis of three-dimensional landmark data, whereas they are emerging only very slowly for analyses of comparable CT data.

Changes in the geometry of the face may not be well detected in projected images; three-dimensionalization improves the precision of cephalometric analysis in the study of craniofacial treatment. Mock surgery, originally introduced as a two-dimensional technique, gains in accuracy when it has access to the three-dimensional cephalometric record, just as it is enhanced when the corresponding computation is carried out using data from the CT scan. Because of the existence of normative data, a first step in surgical planning using the three-dimensional cephalogram can be computed automatically. The three-dimensional cephalogram serves as the link between the CT scan and the norms for this computation.[8] In all these applications, three-dimensional cephalometric data may be recorded and manipulated using equipment no more sophisticated than the now ubiquitous personal computer. Only simple algebra and simple graphics are required.

ACKNOWLEDGMENTS. The author wishes to acknowledge the use of material in this chapter borrowed from papers co-authored with Drs. F. L. Bookstein, C.B. Cutting, J. G. McCarthy, and Mr. H. Kim.

References

1. Steiner CC: Cephalometrics in clinical practices. Angle Orthod 29:8, 1959.
2. Moyers RE: Handbook of Orthodontics, 4th ed. Chicago: Year Book, 1988.
3. Bookstein FL: Size and shape spaces for landmark data in two dimensions. Stat Sci 1:181–242, 1986.
4. Grayson BH, Bookstein FL, McCarthy JG, et al: Mean tensor cephalometric analysis of a patient population with clefts of the palate and lip. Cleft Palate J 24:267, 1987.
5. Broadbent BH, Sr: A new x-ray technique and its application to orthodontia. Angle Orthod 1:45–66, 1931.
6. Cutting CB, Bookstein FL, Grayson BH, et al: Three-dimensional computer-assisted design of craniofacial surgical procedures: Optimization and interaction with cephalometric and CT based models. Plast Reconstr Surg 77:877, 1986.
7. Bolton BH, Sr, Broadbent BH, Jr, Golden WH: Bolton Standards of Dentofacial Development Growth. St. Louis: C.V. Mosby, 1975.
8. Grayson BH, Cutting CB, Bookstein FL, et al: The three-dimensional cephalogram: Theory, technique and clinical application. Am J Orthod Dentofac Orthop 94:327–337, 1988.

CHAPTER 58

The Complete Unilateral Cleft Lip and Palate: Serial Three-Dimensional Studies of Excellent Palatal Growth

Samuel Berkowitz

When to close the palatal cleft should not be the dilemma many surgeons seem to find it to be. Treatment priorities for most surgeons include intelligible speech first followed by normal palatal and facial development and dental occlusion. In some instances, such a priority system has justified poor reconstructive surgery that has created midfacial deformities with the excuse that the patient can at least speak well. Sufficient evidence is now available to support the views that good palatal and facial development, dental occlusion, and intelligible speech are not mutually exclusive and that all treatment goals are attainable if the surgeon tailors the reconstructive procedures to the individual anatomic changes of the cleft palate. A treatment plan based on the patient's age alone disregards the benefits that can be derived from reconstruction and the possibility of attaining normal palatal anatomy and function.

The unsettling experience of performing the same surgical procedure on similar cleft types with different and often growth-inhibiting consequences has led to futile attempts to develop new and untested techniques. The history of cleft palate surgery is replete with such hit-or-miss approaches to find a surgical solution to very complex biologic problems. However, it has been only in the last 40 years since the introduction of roentgenocephalography and the collection of serial dental casts starting at the newborn period that clinical research has begun to focus on examination of the developing affected face and palate to exploit the many cause-and-effect relationships that might exist between palatal surgery and subsequent facial development. These studies highlighted the facts that the success of treatment depended on many factors over which the surgeon had little or no control and that surgical solutions lay in developing individual treatment plans rather than fitting each patient's treatment to a fixed formula.

Unfortunately, there are still no complete answers to basic questions about whether the cleft palate represents a nonunion of parts that are intrinsically adequate, inadequate, or even in excess. The nature of the distortion and derangement of the skeletal components seen at birth and the effects of surgery and growth on the palatal segments have been studied only in part. This deficiency in our understanding of palatal development, which is essential to further refine and improve rehabilitative procedures, is due somewhat to the lack of an appropriate measuring instrument. With the development of new biometric techniques, a multiphased, three-dimensional growth study of serial palatal casts has been designed to expose new information that formerly went unnoticed or unappreciated. An intensive quantitative and qualitative assessment of the changing cleft palate of patients with different cleft types who have undergone various treatment procedures has been planned to answer the following questions:

1. Are the rates and extent of growth of normal palates different from those of cleft palates?
2. What ages show the most rapid growth, and how is such growth expressed?
3. What is the effect of surgical trauma and scarring on palatal size and form?
   a. Does the growth rate accelerate or decelerate after surgical closure?
   b. How can physiologic surgery be defined as it relates to palatal changes? By physiologic surgery, we mean cleft palate repair that does not interfere with maxillofacial growth.
   c. Which part of the dental arch is influenced more by surgical correction?
   d. Is the magnitude of the palatal scarring influenced by the width and length of the cleft palate relative to the amount of available soft tissue?

The answers to these questions are expected to supply objective criteria for surgical treatment planning by showing that the morphologic and spatial relationships of the palatal segments may be the prime determinant of the ultimate occlusion and arch form.

Growth Studies to Be Performed

Geometric Study of the Complete Unilateral Cleft Lip and Palate Compared with the Noncleft Palate

Serial studies of 16 complete unilateral cleft lip and palate patients from birth to 6 years of age who showed good speech and palate development were selected for a spatial-temporal analysis. Ten patients with clefts limited to either the lip and alveolus or to the soft palate were used as the control group (normal palate). As a result of the limited sampling population, sophisticated statistical tests were postponed until more of these cases are analyzed. This preliminary report will be limited to the reporting of (1) trends in palatal growth between the cleft and noncleft cleft segments (comparison will be made with the noncleft palate group); (2) linear dimensions that describe the palate's changing size and form; and (3) graphic displays of the changing shape of the palatal vault.

Future phased studies will include patients with all cleft types who have had both successful and unsuccessful surgical treatment. A consortium of cleft palate research centers will be established to compare the various treatment philosophies on palatal growth and development.

Surgical Treatment. Ralph Millard Jr. performed all of the surgery. Lip adhesion was done before 2 months of age followed by definitive lip surgery at approximately 3 to 6 months of age. The hard and soft palates were repaired between 12 and 30 months of age using either a (1) simple mucoperiosteum approximation, (2) von Langenbeck plus vomer flap, or (3) vomer flap procedure. The choice of surgical procedure depended on the size and shape of the cleft space relative to the available palatal mucosal tissue and the desire to limit palatal scarring.

Orthodontic Treatment. A crossbite of either the deciduous canine or deciduous canine and first and second deciduous molars was corrected after 4 years of age using a fixed palatal expander. The corrections were completed within 3 to 6 months and were retained with a fixed transpalatal arch. None of the patients had had neonatal maxillary orthopedic treatment or primary bone grafting. Secondary bone grafts were performed when the patients were between 8 and 10 years of age. Cranial bone grafts were used in the majority of patients.

Method. An electromechanical digitizer (The Preceptor, manufactured by Micro Control Systems, Inc.) was used to extrapolate spatial three-dimensional data from serial cleft palate casts (Fig. 58–1). The data are stored in digital form and are amenable to computer manipulation, storage, and analysis. This allows later inspection and analysis of details that are found to be more important than was first thought and is of major importance for this project. Palatal landmarks are listed (Fig. 58–2).

Measurements. The first phase of this three-dimensional study describes the changes in the size of the palate's surface area, cleft space, and various dental and anthropometric linear dimensions. Changes in the palate slopes reflect the force systems that influence its geometric form.

Palatal Surface. The palatal surface to be measured is limited anterolaterally by the alveolar crest and posteriorly by a line connecting points P and P' (right and left postgingivale, which is comparable to the pterygomaxillary fissure [Ptm]). These points are also the posterior extent of the alveolar crest. The palatal surface area lateral to the alveolar crest (and anterior to the premaxillary crest) was not evaluated because its boundary, which is dependent on impression technique, is highly variable.

Cleft Space. The cleft space is viewed as a changing, two-dimensional, irregular plane bounded laterally by the medial border of the hard palate. In unilateral clefts the anterior limits are bounded by a line drawn between the anterior ends of the alveolar crests, Ac and Ac', and posteriorly by line PC to PC', which is drawn between the posterior medial limits of the palatal segment at the clefts, points PC and PC'. In isolated cleft palates this is the posterior limit of the cleft space as well. The cleft anterior point (CAP) of the palatal cleft is defined either when the palatal segments are in contact or when the cleft is limited to the hard palate. Cleft posterior point (CPP) is the posterior point of the cleft space within the hard palate. In patients with bilateral clefts the cleft space has anterior and posterior divisions separated by

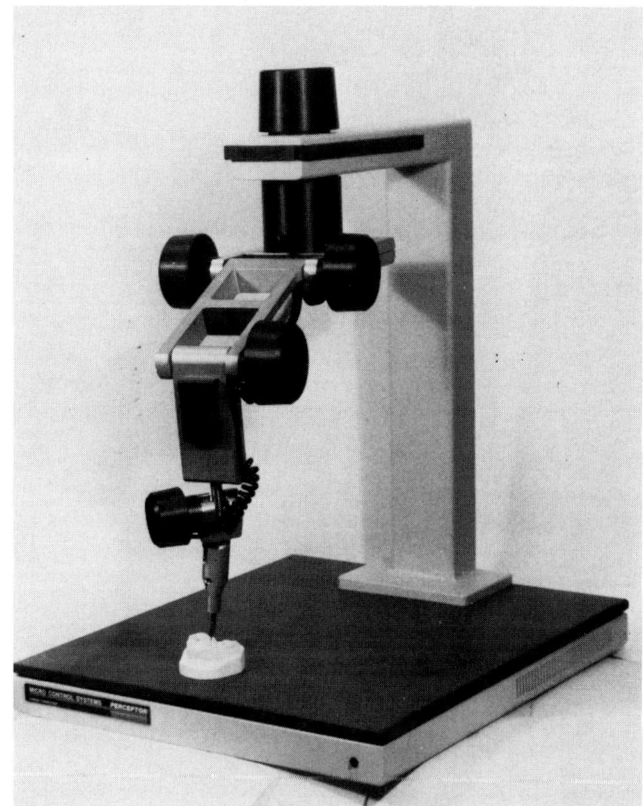

Figure 58–1 Perceptor—an electromechanical hand-held digitizer manufactured by Micro Control Systems.

a line drawn between the anterior limits of the palatal crests (AC points). The anterior cleft space is bounded laterally by a line drawn from the lateral extent of the premaxillary crests to the respective AC points.

Slopes. The first slope (1) is the angle of the palatal vault on the P-P' line—for example, P–PC, P'–PC'. Slope 2 is the slope at the middle of each palatal segment tangent to the crest (A) and at the levels of the first and second deciduous molars.

Linear Divisions. Linear divisions are two- and three-dimensional. The distance between the teeth on opposing arches and the right and left postgingival (P and P') was utilized to measure arch widths. The anteroposterior dimension is measured from the incisal papilla to the postgingival line.

Tooth Location. The height of the teeth is reduced to the alveolar crest and therefore tooth size does not influence the vault space dimensions. Various interarch dimensions using the central fossa of the teeth were recorded. Special attention was given to increases in vertical alveolar height in orthodontically treated and nontreated cases using the palatal rugae as a reference system for measuring the effects of growth and surgery.

Using the Palatal Rugae As a Reference System for Measuring the Effects of Growth and Treatment

The palatal rugae are easily identifiable palatal landmarks. They are distant from active growth sites and have been demonstrated by Lebret to be excellent

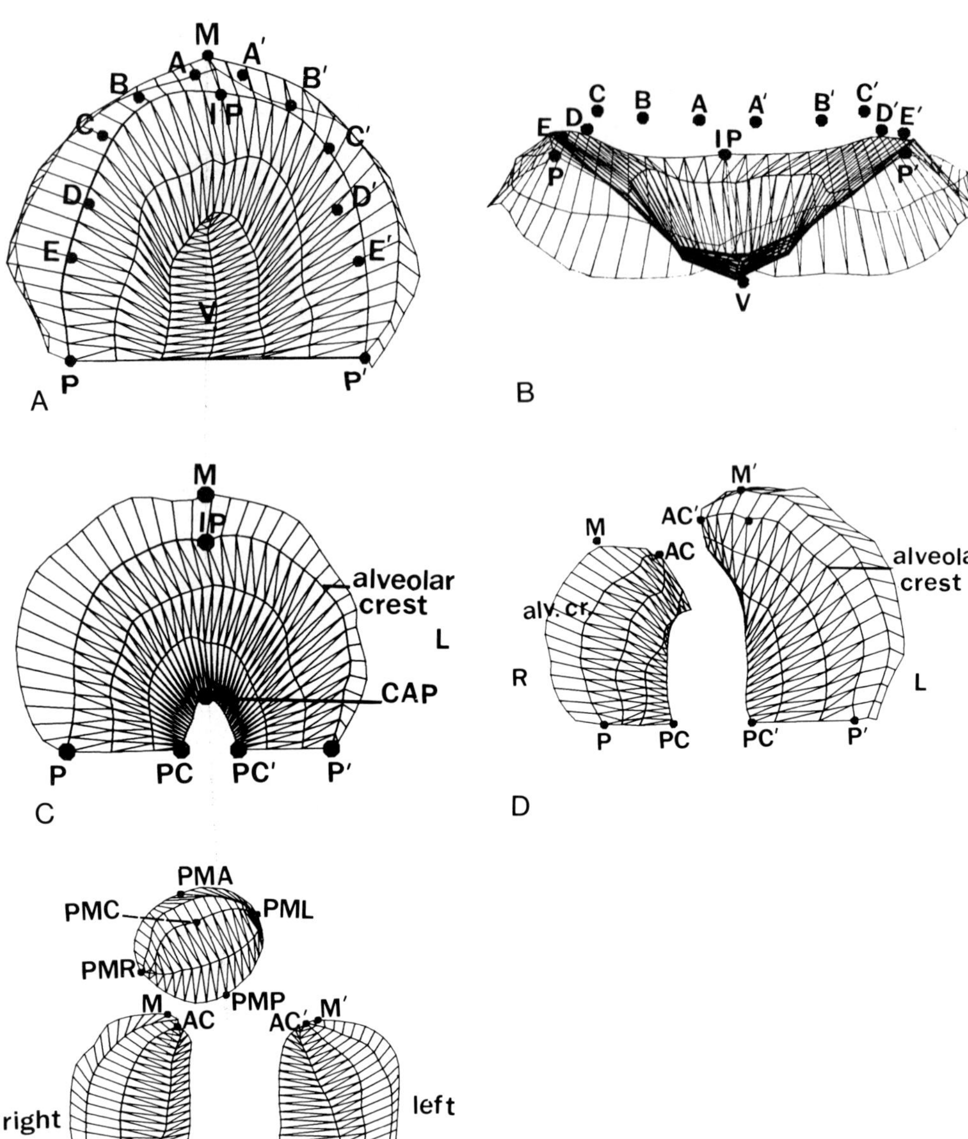

Figure 58–2 Landmarks utilized in geometric study of the various palates. Key: M—anteriormost extent of palate; IP—incisal papilla; A—central incisor; B—lateral incisor; C—cuspid; D—first molar; E—second molar; P—postgingival; V—highest vault point. CAP—cleft anterior palate; PC—cleft point on PP^1 line (CPP—not shown—is the posterior extent of a palatal cleft within the palate); AC—anteriormost point of the crest at the cleft.

Premaxilla landmarks: PMA—anterior extent; PMC—center of crest; PML—left extent of crest; PMR—right extent of crest; PMP—posteriormost point.

The *anterior cleft area* is bounded by the premaxilla lines drawn from PMR to AC and PML to AC' and from AC to AC'. The *posterior cleft area* is lines AC to AC', PC to PC', AC to PC, and AC' to PC'.

reference points for palatal growth studies.[1] Using a Korkhaus symmetrograph,[2] he demonstrated that the median palatal contour remains stable and is largely unaffected by growth changes. The position of the rugae relative to the median raphe and to the teeth remains almost constant. The boundary between palate and alveolar bone at the level of the molars is located approximately 3.33 mm in vertical height from the apex of the vault. Since Korkhaus lists the mean palatal height with standard deviations at 5 and 18 years of age, comparison with the cleft population is possible.[2]

In the cleft palate population, palatal rugae, in combination with other landmarks such as the vomer, can be used in the following ways: (1) Prior to lip surgery they show the location and extent of appositional bone growth and the effect of orthopedic devices. (2) After the molding of palatal segments the change in rugae position depicts the change in the palate's geometric orientation. (3) After the palatal segments have been stabilized and prior to and after palatal closure, they can be used to study, respectively, growth, degree of mucosal displacement due to surgery, and growth changes after surgery. Because the size and relationship between the rugae change with growth, the centroid of the rugae (or the most anterior rugae on each side) and various teeth are used for purposes of superimposition in serial images to demonstrate palatal growth changes. (4) The rugae are also used to study the effects of orthodontic treatment on palatal form.

The geometric alignment of the palatal rugae is very irregular and forms unique relationships that can be identified at various ages. When the palatal cleft space is open, points on the crest of the vomer are utilized for reference as well. The anterior rugae (sometimes centroid) points are superimposed or are placed in the same anteroposterior position when the palatal segments are displaced. The distance between rugae on the same side increases with palatal growth, the greater change occurring between the most posterior rugae points.

An example of using the palatal rugae as reference points in a serial study of a complete unilateral cleft lip and palate is shown in Figs. 58–3 and 58–4. Serial outlines of the palate are drawn, and three rugae points in each lateral palatal segment and the edge of the vomer (V) are identified. After the palatal segments or mucoperiosteum is displaced, other landmark points such as P and P′ can be substituted but are kept at the same anteroposterior position. Afterward, the new rugae points plus tooth landmarks then become the reference points for later superimposition.

This serial study demonstrates that palatal changes are accurately represented in the superimposed drawings when using the vomer, rugae, and tooth landmarks as reference points. Major palatal growth occurs at the posterior border, with some appositional growth changes occurring at the lateral surface and anterior poles of the arch.

Results

STUDY I. Investigate Surface Area and Dimensional Changes in 16 Patients with Complete Unilateral Cleft Lip and Palate from Birth Through 6 Years of Age

Palatal Surface Area (Fig. 58–5). Twenty percent of the patients showed a marked increase in growth rate during the first 12 months. Fifty percent demonstrated a rapid increase until 20 months of age. Eighty percent showed the greatest rate of growth between 12 and 20 months of age (prior to the age when most had palatal surgery).

In almost all patients the increase in palatal growth leveled off between 20 and 28 months of age. Afterward, growth continued until 10 years of age but at a lesser rate. In 50% of patients there was a second period of growth that leveled off between 4 years 4 months of age and 4 years 8 months of age. These cases demonstrated an increase in size but at a slower growth rate. In 80% of the patients a slight acceleration in growth rate appears from 2 years 4 months to 6 years of age. This study clearly demonstrates that extreme care needs to be exerted when interpreting serial group data to avoid missing or misinterpreting meaningful growth dynamics of some cases. Therefore, each case will be analyzed in great detail to identify all the possible growth variations that may occur.

STUDY II. Comparison of Palatal Changes in Patients Who Had Intact Palates with Those Who Had Complete Unilateral Clefts of the Lip and Palate

Since a normal palate series of casts was not available for study, patients with either a cleft of the lip and alveolus or those with a cleft of the soft palate or of the uvula only were selected to be a control "normal" population.

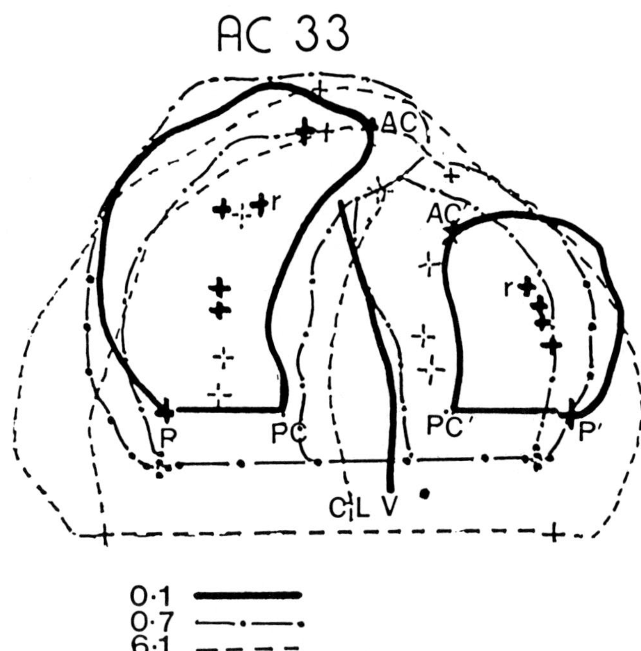

Figure 58–3 AC33 superimposed images of palatal casts at 1 month, 7 months, and 6 years 1 month of age. Casts were superimposed on the vomer edge (V) while the most anterior rugae were placed at the same anteroposterior level and near each other. This technique shows medial movement of the lesser palatal segment after lip adhesion and medial posterior movement of the premaxillary portion of the lesser segment. The cleft line (CL) is closer to the larger segment. Rugae on the larger segment are at the same transverse position but are located more posteriorly. Most of the palatal growth in length and width occurred at the posterior border.

Fifty percent of the noncleft palate patients showed less growth acceleration than 50% of those with complete unilateral cleft lip and palate (Fig. 58–5). Fifty percent of both groups showed growth leveling off between 20 and 24 months of age; however, the noncleft palate patients showed a growth spurt until 32 months of age. Palatal growth in the cleft group occurs at a slower rate until approximately 5 years 6 months of age. It must be emphasized that increases in alveolar development associated with tooth eruption account for much of the increase after 3 years of age.

STUDY III. Growth Rates in Smaller (Cleft) Segments Versus Those in Larger Segments

The chart in Figure 58–6 shows that in more than 50% of patients the smaller (cleft) segment is growing more rapidly than the larger segment until 6 years of age. Caution needs to be exerted in making comparisons between the smaller and larger segments after surgery because it is hard to differentiate the two segments from each other.

STUDY IV

Patient A. This patient had a complete unilateral cleft lip and palate (Figs. 58–7 and 58–8).
History. The lip was united at 2 months of age, and the
Text continued on page 465

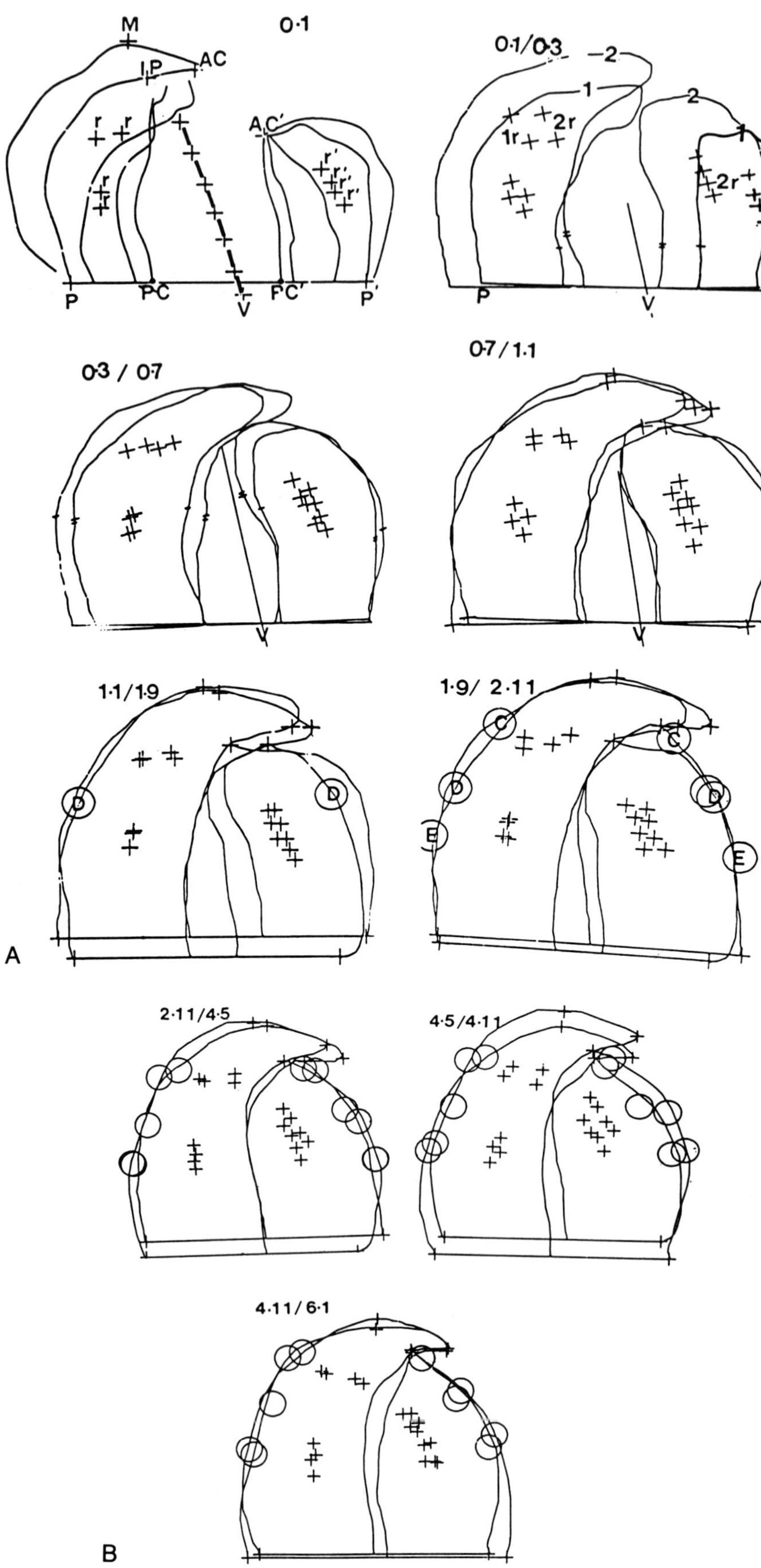

Figure 58–4 Graphic display of palatal geometric and growth changes. 0.1: Newborn cast r and r' rugae points on the right and left palatal segments, respectively. PP' = line connecting postgingival points that designate the posterior limits of the hard palate. PC and PC' = the points on PP' line at the cleft space, V = vomer point on the PP' line.

Superimposition technique: *A,* To determine geometric palatal changes, the lines P-P' are superimposed and the vomer point (V) is used for registration. This technique demonstrates changes in palatal relationships and the amount of palatal growth to each segment in two dimensions but does not reveal where growth occurs. Casts 0.1, 1.3, 1.7, and 1.1. *B,* To determine where palatal growth is taking place, internal landmarks, such as the rugae, must be utilized for superimposition purposes (see Fig. 58–3). When palatal surgery displaces the rugae points, new ones need to be selected. The changing location of rugae points describes the degree of mucosal displacement. The following serial casts (0.1, 0.3, 0.7, and 1.1) are superimposed on the PP' line using the V point for registration to demonstrate changes in palatal relationships brought on by surgery. The casts (1.9, 2.11, 4.5, 4.11, and 6.1) show changes to palatal size brought on by growth. The circles represent the deciduous cuspids, first deciduous molars, and second deciduous molars.

Results: Anteroposterior palatal growth is continuous in order to accommodate the permanent molars, most of it occurring at the posterior border. The palatal width also increased between 4.11 and 6.1, even though the width between the teeth shows no change. Quantitative measures will be reviewed in another study using a larger sample of similar cases.

Figure 58–5 Changes in palatal surface area (between the alveolar ridges and the posterior edge of the hard palate) in the 16 complete unilateral cleft lip and palate cases are compared with the same area in 10 noncleft cases. In the normal population, the average growth increments from birth to 1½ years are rapid and steady. From 1¾ years to 2 years of age, the growth acceleration decreases. A second growth spurt occurs between 2 and 3 years of age. Palatal growth slows down for a short period of time but then accelerates until 5 years of age, when it decelerates again. Palatal growth changes in the unilateral cleft population are highly variable. Twenty percent of the cases show a very rapid period of growth from 3 to 6 months of age, then a slowdown for 3 months with a second growth spurt between 1 and 1½ years of age. No additional growth occurs between 1 year 9 months and 3 years 3 months of age, but a second growth spurt then follows and lasts until 6 years of age. Fifty percent of the cases show steady growth acceleration until 1 year 9 months of age. This is followed by a temporary slowdown for 3 months and then a second period of growth acceleration until 4½ years of age. Eighty percent of the cases show a slow rate of growth until 1 year of age, followed by a rapid period of acceleration until 1½ years of age. Growth acceleration is much slower thereafter. Comments: The greatest period of growth acceleration in the cleft and noncleft populations occurs between 1 and 1½ years of age. Therefore, it would be advisable not to perform any growth-inhibiting surgery prior to this important growth period. Early palatal growth is more rapid in the cleft series than in the normal population.

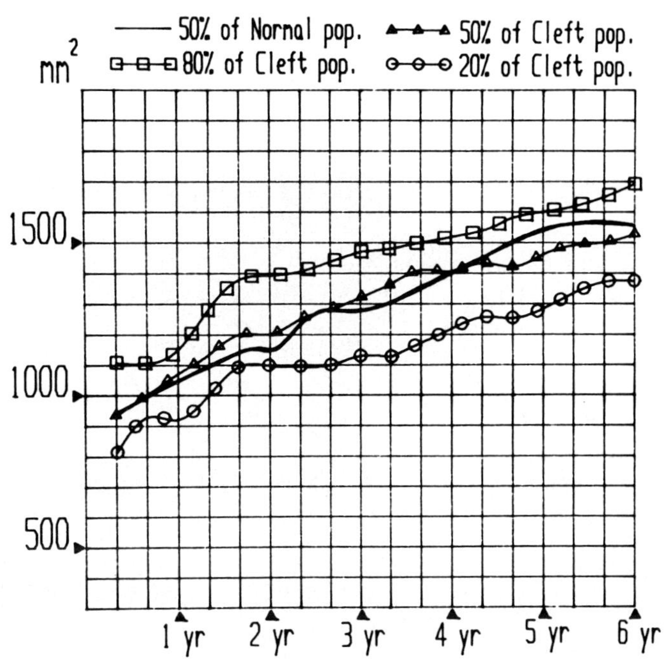

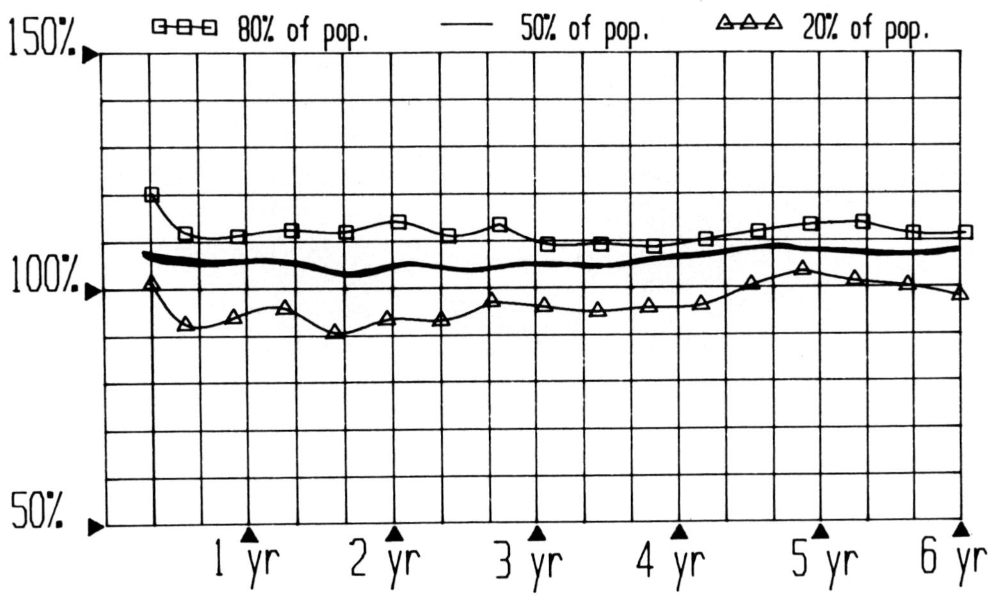

Figure 58–6 Complete unilateral cleft of the lip and palate. The ratio of the growth of the smaller to the larger palatal segment. At all ages the smaller cleft palatal segment, in most instances, is growing more rapidly than the noncleft segment. This conclusion supports the existence of the phenomenon of "catch-up growth."

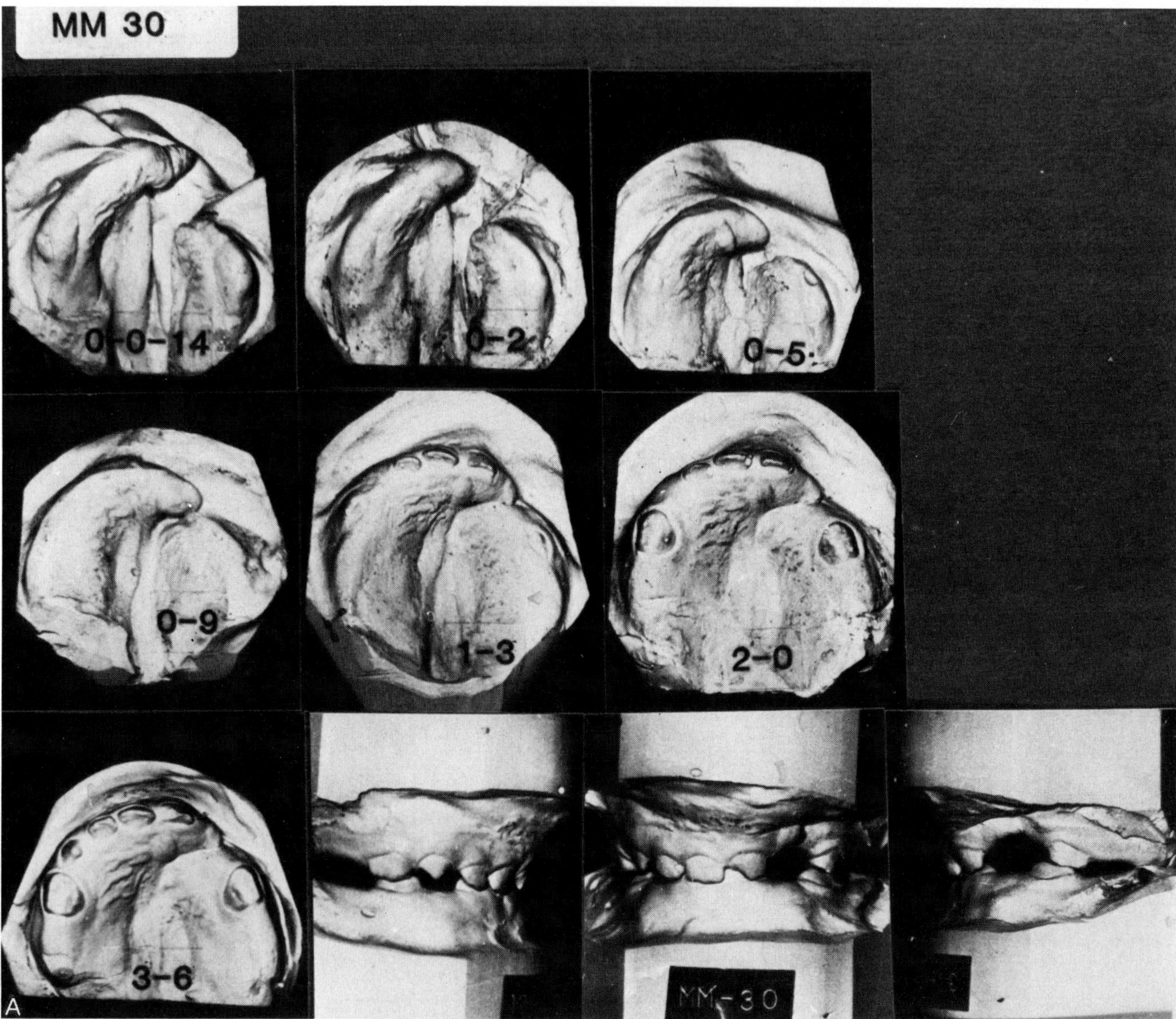

Figure 58–7 *A* and *B*, Case MM-30: serial palatal photographs at each age. *C*, Casts from 9 years 9 months to 12 years 8 months of age. These casts were not subjected to three-dimensional analysis. Left deciduous cuspid was still in crossbite at 9 years of age. Rotated permanent central and lateral incisors were orthodontically corrected. Alveolar bone graft (using cranial bone) performed at 10 years of age permitted the left lateral incisor to be brought into ideal position. Excellence in occlusion reflects normal midfacial and palatal growth. *D*, Case MM-30: complete unilateral cleft of the lip and palate. Good speech and palatal development are evident. Upper left, newborn period; upper right, lip adhesion; lower left, excellent palatal size and form. Left deciduous lateral incisor is in the line of the cleft. It will be removed within a year. Lower middle, the deciduous cuspid on the lesser palatal segment is in crossbite due to mediopalatal rotation. Lower right, excellent fascial aesthetics. Comments: The palatal cleft was closed at 16 months of age with a conservative von Langenbeck procedure leaving very little denuded bone. Palatal development has followed normal growth gradients.

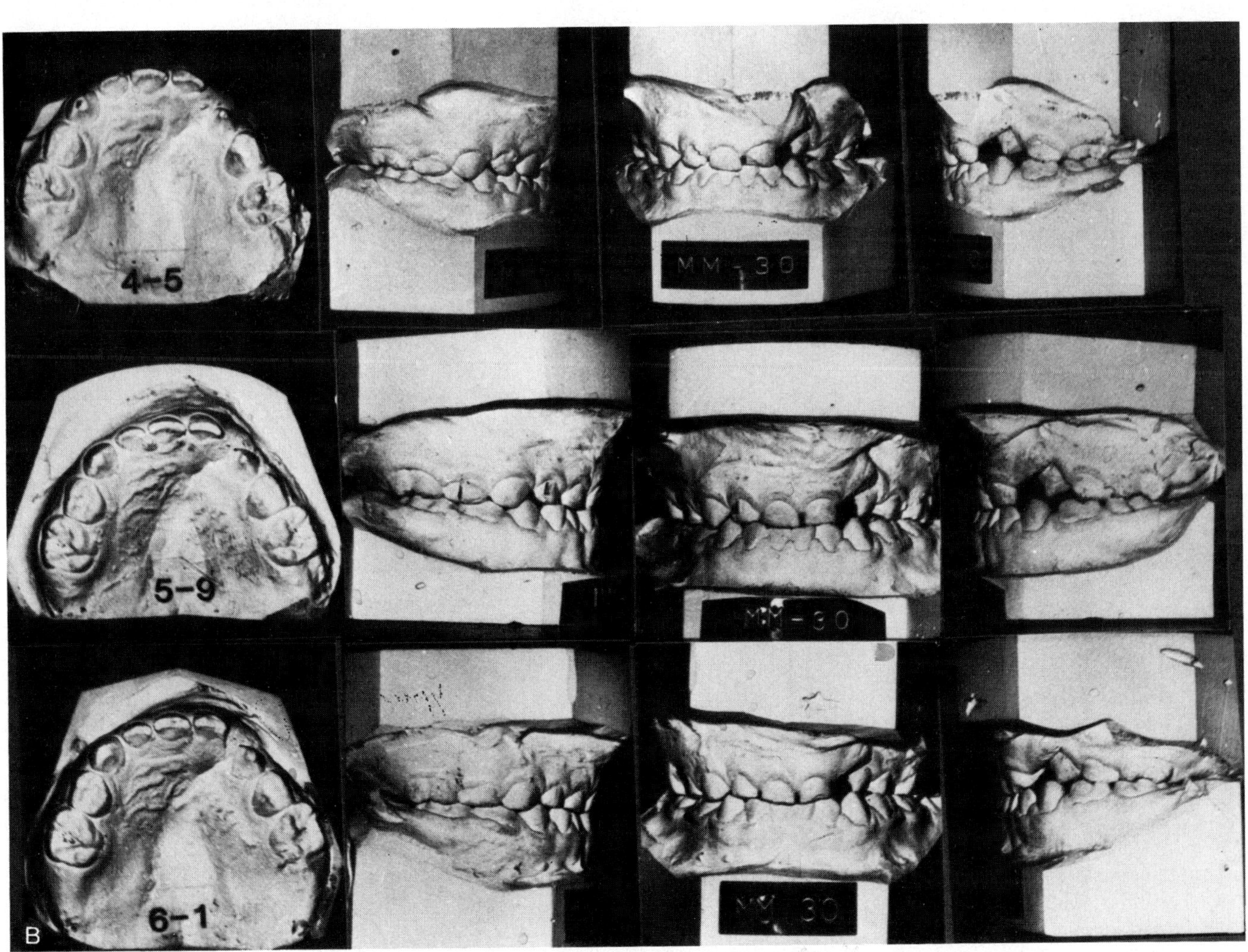

Figure 58–7 Continued

Illustration continued on following page

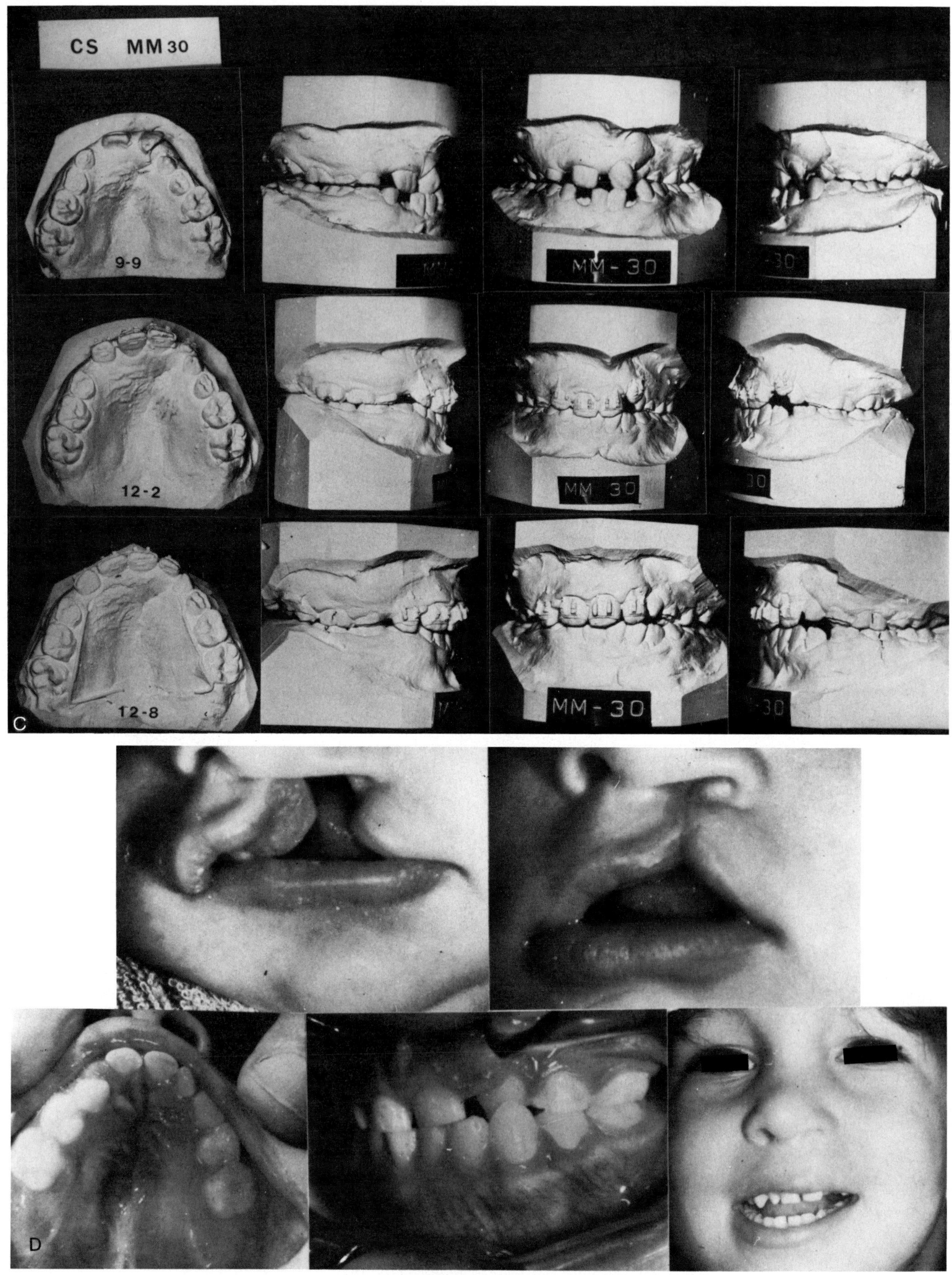

Figure 58–7 Continued

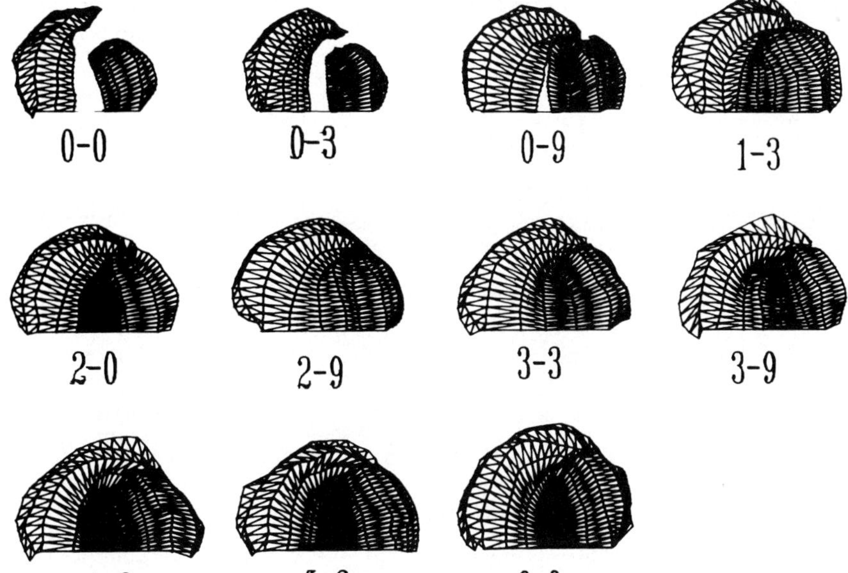

Figure 58–8 Case MM-30. Serial palatal growth and cleft space changes at each age (years/months). All images are drawn to the same scale.

hard and soft palatal cleft was closed at 16 months of age using a von Langenbeck procedure. No orthodontic treatment was performed. An alveolar bone graft was performed at 10 years of age.

One of the 16 patients with complete unilateral cleft of the lip and palate was selected to demonstrate the time sequence analysis of the changing geometric form and surface area measurements (Figs. 58–9, 58–10, and 58–11, and Table 58–1).

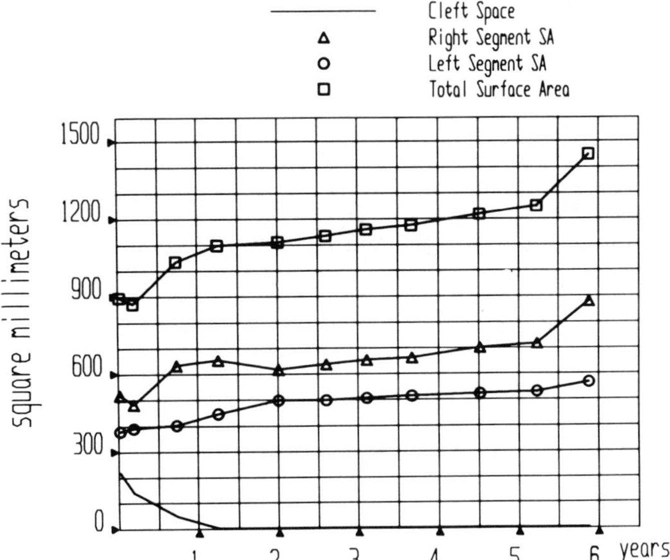

Figure 58–9 Case MM-30. Time sequence analysis of palatal surface area and cleft space size. The graph shows two periods of palatal growth acceleration: one from 3 to 6 months of age and the other at 5 years 6 months of age. The growth of the noncleft segment accelerates earlier than that of the cleft segment. Cleft segment between 9 months and 2 years of age grows more rapidly until 5 years of age. A second period of growth acceleration occurs at 5 years 3 months of age.

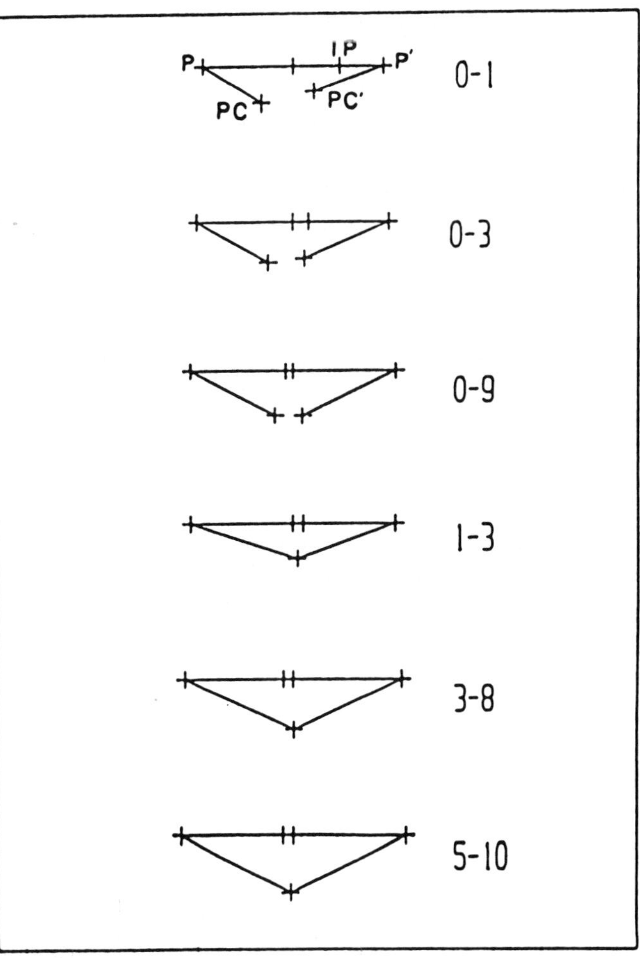

Figure 58–10 Vault angulation at the P-P′ line. In Case MM-30 the cleft palatal segment is steeper than the noncleft segment at birth. Within the first year the slopes of the two segments are similar, with the vault space becoming progressively flatter.

MM30: VAULT CONTOUR

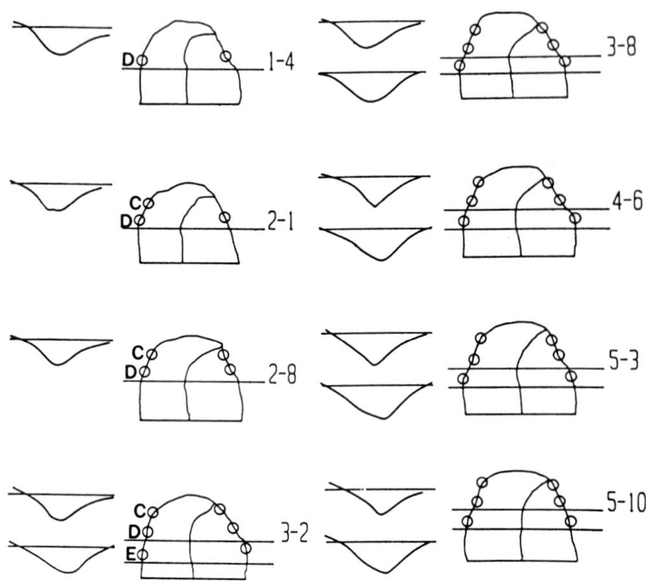

Figure 58–11 Vault contour (1 year 4 months to 5 years 10 months) cross sections were made at the level of the first and second deciduous molars. After 1 year 4 months of age the vault contour at the level of the second deciduous molar is more ovoid and deeper than that at a more anterior location.

Findings: Serial Palatal Growth and Cleft Space Changes. The computer-drawn surface of each cast is drawn to scale, demonstrating the size and shape changes occurring under the influence of growth and surgery. An extension of the premaxillary portion of the larger segment was due to the presence of an underlying ectopically positioned malformed tooth. When it was removed at 3 months of age, the surface area diminished. The premaxillary portion rotated posteromedially, and the lesser palatal segment moved medially, narrowing the posterior palatal width. With removal of the projecting unerupted malformed tooth, the surface area of the larger segment was reduced by 6.8%. The

palatal cleft was closed at 16 months of age. Between 3 and 9 months of age the larger palatal segment increased 31.6% while the smaller segment increased only 3.17%. Afterward, the lesser segment increased 11.2%, which was 5 times more rapid than the larger segment's change in surface area. For the next 9 months the lesser segment increased by another 11.26%. At 5 years 3 months of age, the larger segment's surface area increased an additional 15.76% while the lesser segment's surface arch increased only 6.68%. The second growth rate acceleration in palatal growth occurred between 5 years 3 months and 5 years 10 months of age.

Comments. A temporary reduction in three-dimensional surface area is not an unusual finding immediately after palatal surgery has been performed. In some instances it may be due to the undermining of the palatal mucoperiosteum and the fact that it was moved medially to cover the cleft space; the vault height is reduced as well. The cleft surface area at the time of surgery was only 46 mm^2 and represented 4.47% of the total palatal surface area.

The time sequence analysis shows that the smaller segment increased at a more rapid rate and to a greater degree than the larger segment. Although there is an early period of growth deceleration, the potential does exist for the growth rate to undergo a second period of growth acceleration. After 2 years of age, the increase in palatal surface area is generally associated with an increase in alveolar height.

Palatal Vault Angulation. At the newborn state the palatal vault slope at the postgingivale (P–P′) line of the larger segment is more acute than that of the cleft segment (Fig. 58–10 and Table 58–2). Notice that the incisal papilla point (IP) is located closer to P′. After lip repair, the larger segment angle becomes more obtuse, and the IP point approaches the midline. After the palatal cleft is surgically closed by bringing the undermined palatal mucoperiosteum together at the midline, the vault height is slightly decreased. However, the palatal vault height increases with the growth of the alveolar arch relative to the height of point P and P′.

Measurements of Palatal Widths. Interdeciduous canine (C–C), first interdeciduous molars (D–D), and second interdeciduous molar widths (E–E) did not increase after they erupted (Table 58–3). This finding is similar to that reported by Barrow and White from a normal population.[3] The posterior palatal width as measured by the distance between points P and P′ increased steadily

Table 58–1. Measurements of Interdental Two-Dimensional Complete Unilateral Cleft of Lip and Palate (Case MM-30)

Age	C–C (mm)	D–D (mm)	E–E (mm)	VHD (mm)	VHE (mm)	Angle E (degrees)
1–4	—	32	—	11	—	—
2–1	—	32	—	11	—	—
2–8	27	32	—	10	—	—
3–2	26	33	40	10	10	27
3–8	25	32	39	10	11	30
4–6	26	33	41	11	12	29
5–3	26	32	42	12	13	30
5–10	27	31	42	10	12	29

C–C = Interdeciduous canine; D–D = first interdeciduous molars; E–E = second interdeciduous molars; VHD = vault height at the level of the first deciduous molar; VHE = vault height at the level of the second deciduous molar.

Two-dimensional distance between the teeth on the right and left side of the arch show very little change from 1 year 4 months to 5 years 10 months of age. Vault height is also stable and greater at the posterior one-third of the arch.

Table 58–2. Vault Angles in a Complete Unilateral Cleft (Case MM-30)

Age	RS	Change	LS	Change
0–0	21.7		33.9	
0–3	25.3	17%	31.6	−7%
0–9	28.4	12%	30.5	−3%
1–3	21.1	−26%	10.3	37%
3–8	26.7	27%	26.2	36%
5–10	28.0	5%	29.0	11%

Note: All measurements are in degrees of rotation. Vault angulation at the level of the posterior edge of the palate is not stable prior to palatal closure. After cleft closure it appears to become flatter.

RS = right palatal segment; LS = left palatal segment.

Table 58–3. Measurements of Palatal Widths (Case MM-30)

	Distances			
Age	P–P'	P–PC	PC–PC'	PC'–P'
0–1	32.75	13.44	9.83	12.87
0–3	34.83	16.91	6.61	15.22
0–9	37.26	19.19	5.04	17.79
1–3	37.15	18.97	0.00	20.60
2–0	37.74	18.68	0.00	23.12
2–7	38.65	20.56	0.00	21.47
3–2	40.04	21.59	0.00	22.11
3–8	39.45	21.85	0.00	22.20
4–6	41.50	23.96	0.00	23.00
5–3	41.19	24.01	0.00	22.75
5–10	41.03	20.92	0.00	20.12

Posterior palatal width became wider with time, increasing by almost 30%. Transverse palatal growth at 9 months of age (P-PC and PC'-P') shows a 43% increase. The initial medial movement of the cleft segment immediately after lip or soft palate repair usually reduces the posterior palatal width.

between 1 month and 5 years 10 months of age. This finding was unique in that the overexpansion seen in the newborn cast did not change because of compressive lip forces owing to the fact that the inferior turbinate of the left cleft side had already made contact with the vomer at the newborn stage.

Comment. Mandibular arch dimensions showed the same consistency in width as judged by the constancy of the buccal occlusion.

Patient B. This patient had complete unilateral cleft of the lip and palate (Figs. 58–12A and B, 58–13, 58–14, and Tables 58–4 and 58–5).

History. Lip adhesion was performed at 2 months of age, definitive lip surgery at 6 months of age, and hard and soft palate repair at 24 months of age. A class I occlusion developed with the left deciduous cuspid erupting in crossbite owing to mesioangular rotation of the left palatal segment. No orthodontic treatment was performed.

Graphic Representation of Palatal Growth Changes (Fig. 58–4). Casts 0.1, 0.3, 0.7, and 1.1 were superimposed on the vomer edge with the P–P' line registered.

Casts 1.9, 2.11, 4.5, 4.11, and 6.1 were superimposed on the right first deciduous molar with the P–P' line paralleled.

Findings. Lip adhesion reversed the muscular force fields operating on the detached palatal segment, causing the left palatal segment to move bodily medially. The premaxillary portion of the larger segment had rotated medioinferiorly, making contact with the lesser segment at points AC. From birth to 7 months of age the surface area of the larger palatal segment increased by 24%, whereas the surface area of the smaller cleft segment showed a more rapid growth and increased by 39%. Within 4 months the total surface area increased by 36% while the cleft space decreased by 54%. Between 7 months and 6 years 1 month of age the total surface area increased by 41%. The growth rate decreased steadily to 1 year 1 month of age. A rapid period of growth acceleration occurred between 4 years 6 months and 5 years of age. From 7 months to 6 years of age the posterior width of the palatal segment increased by 19%, and the anteroposterior length increased by 20%. During this same period there was no significant increase in intercuspid first interdeciduous molar or second interdeciduous molar width. The palatal vault became progressively flatter at the P–P' line, but at the line between the first deciduous molars it became steeper.

Comments. Good palatal growth and development as determined by the developing occlusion can be characterized by (1) early acclerated growth of the lesser palatal segment compared with the larger noncleft segment, (2) an increase in growth of the palatal surface area to approximately 3 years of age, at which time it appears to level off, and (3) a second period of growth acceleration after physiologic surgery, occurring between 4 years 6 months and 6 years of age.

Graphic presentation of early palatal segmental relationships prior to palatal cleft closure can be shown using the vomer line coupled with the P–P' line. The location of palatal growth can be shown when the teeth and rugae are utilized for purposes of registration.

Table 58–4. Complete Unilateral Cleft Lip and Palate—Measurements Between Landmarks (Case AC-33)

	Distances						
Age	P–P'	P–PC	PC–PC'	PC'–P'	C–C	D–D	E–E
0–0	36.78	12.88	14.46	13.84	0.00	0.00	0.00
0–3	36.99	18.88	8.08	14.61	0.00	0.00	0.00
0–7	33.52	15.40	10.12	13.08	0.00	0.00	0.00
1–1	34.65	14.62	7.01	13.02	0.00	0.00	0.00
1–8	35.59	17.47	5.80	16.97	0.00	31.08	0.00
2–11	33.51	20.51	0.00	17.65	22.09	29.26	37.47
3–4	35.90	20.99	0.00	18.67	22.88	30.17	37.45
3–10	36.01	21.61	0.00	19.50	21.63	30.03	36.69
4–6	36.23	21.74	0.00	19.82	22.28	29.01	37.44
5–0	35.42	21.14	0.00	19.81	22.94	30.54	37.32
5–7	36.82	21.38	0.00	20.31	22.85	30.97	38.28
6–4	41.51	24.07	0.00	22.05	21.98	31.09	38.01

Posterior palatal width decreased after lip adhesion, then progressively increased by 24% at 6 years 4 months of age. Distance between teeth on opposite sides of the arch remained constant.

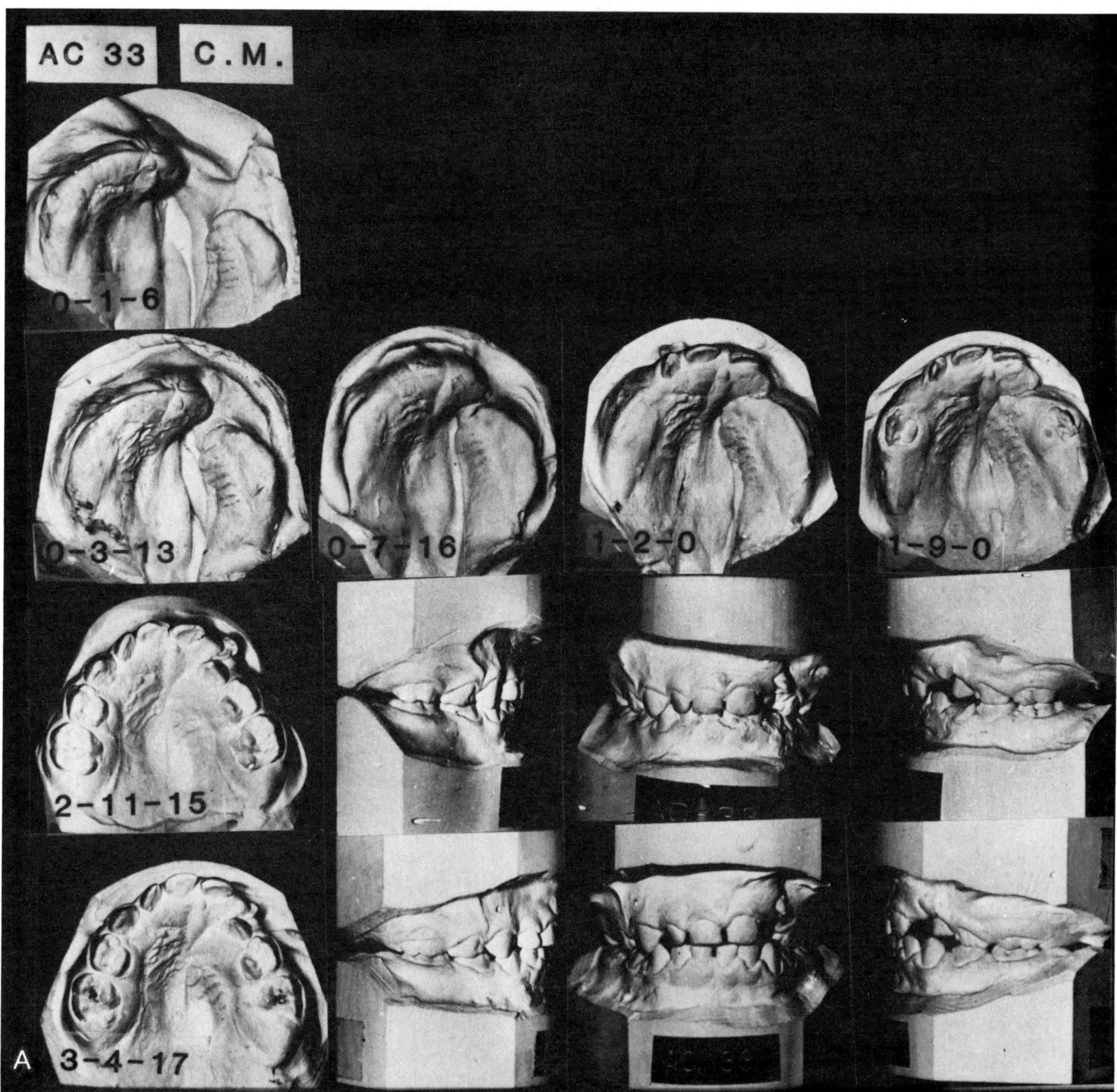

Figure 58–12 A and B, Case AC-33. Complete unilateral cleft lip and palate. Serial palate photographs.

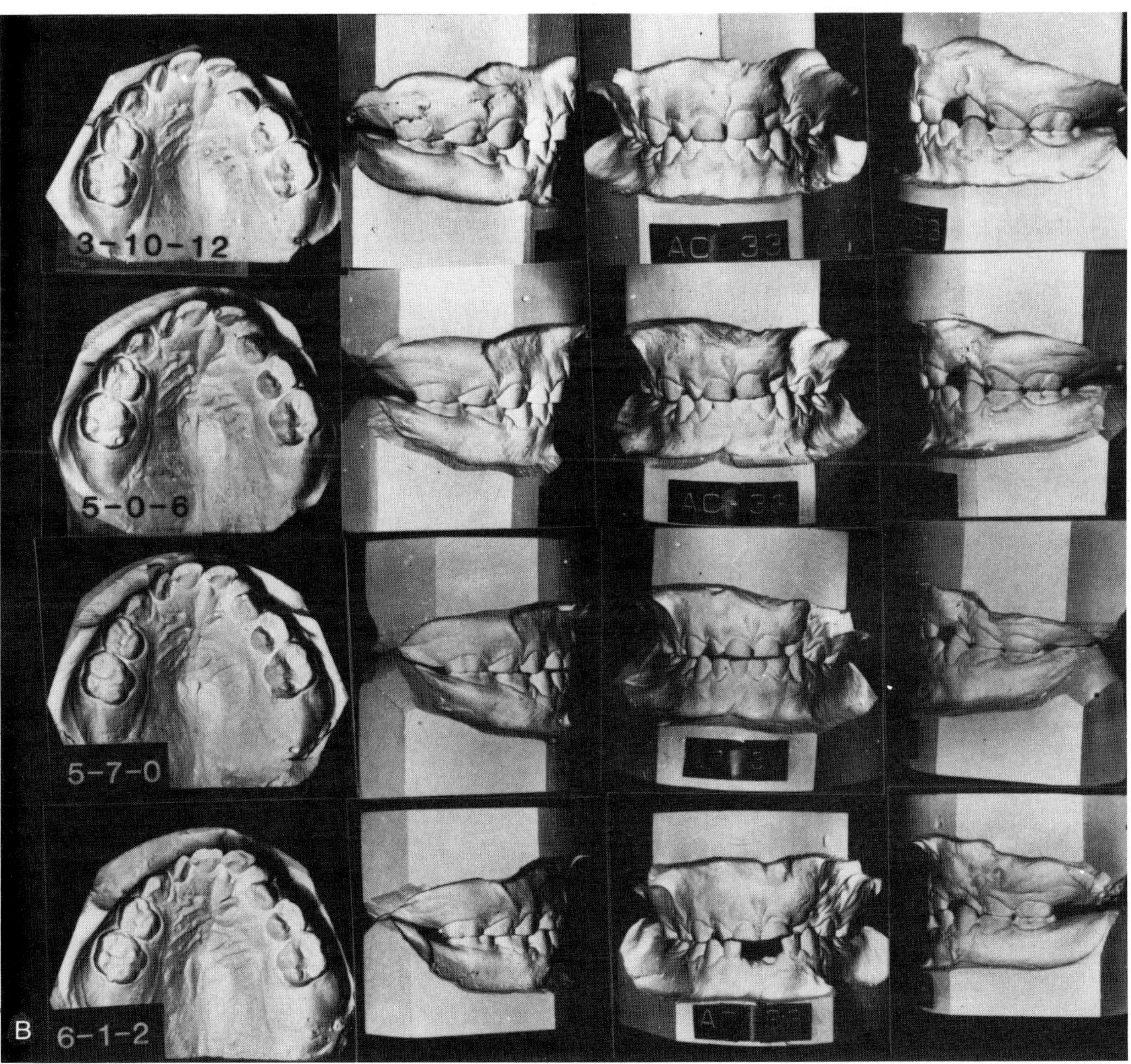

Figure 58–12 Continued

Table 58–5. Complete Unilateral Cleft Lip and Palate—Measurements Between Landmarks (Case AC-33)

Age	Distances				Arc Distance			Angles	
	AC–AC′	ACx	ACy	Md	P–AC	P–IP	P′–P-IP	P–PC	P′–PC′
0–0	12.13	5.73	8.40	27.76	50.47	35.89	29.98	31.73	34.52
0–3	7.11	−2.15	5.99	31.20	53.03	39.17	39.09	29.34	29.55
0–7	5.36	−4.88	1.92	31.85	56.85	46.28	38.63	33.38	36.16
1–1	9.03	−8.72	1.71	29.84	59.21	44.17	35.33	0.93	0.05
1–8	6.30	−5.36	2.80	35.46	64.81	46.21	37.55	29.19	31.06
2–11	8.30	−7.42	3.02	36.74	65.49	50.86	36.91	26.35	31.05
3–4	10.89	−9.87	1.46	35.78	64.70	45.77	35.67	23.62	26.77
3–10	6.89	−6.38	1.86	36.93	62.65	47.82	37.48	27.29	30.53
4–6	6.86	−6.66	0.80	34.81	64.09	49.89	36.76	27.88	30.85
5–0	6.67	−6.38	1.29	37.89	66.02	51.73	39.57	29.05	31.21
5–7	5.35	−5.26	0.52	37.54	64.61	50.28	40.05	27.21	28.77
6–4	5.49	−5.14	1.72	37.78	62.71	50.45	40.97	24.64	27.09

Note: All distances are given in millimeters, angles are given in degrees. Anteroposterior dimensions increased by 43% as measured between the incisal papilla (IP) to the P–P′ line. Three-dimensional distance along the alveolar crest of the larger segment increased by 24%, whereas on the lesser segment it increased by 38%. This clearly demonstrates the greater growth potential of the lesser palatal segment to increase in size and "catch up" with the larger segment. Relationship of the AC points to each other is highly variable. They will be analyzed in greater detail in another study.

Studies on maxillary arch width in normal palates by Barrow and White[3] showed that there was very little increase in intercanine width between 3 and 5 years of age; however, between 5 and 9 years of age it increased by approximately 4 mm. The second interdeciduous molar distance increased by only 1.5 mm between 5 and 10 years of age. Bjork and Skieller[4] concluded that the increase in the posterior width of the maxillary arch at Ptm (P point) is greater than at the canines during this same period.

Measurements of the noncleft palates showed that (1) the distance between the canines, first deciduous molars, and second deciduous molars does not increase between 3 and 5 years of age; and (2) the vault height increased by approximately 10%, and the vault form at the posterior third of the palate became flatter with time.

Discussion

Presently there is much controversy about which surgical procedure should be utilized to close the palatal cleft, when the procedure should be done, and whether neonatal maxillary orthopedic treatment has any long-term utility. Although the results of treatment have greatly improved in the last 25 years, there is still much that needs to be done to improve differential diagnosis and treatment planning.

The history of cleft palate surgery reveals that poorly conceived, badly executed, and ill-timed operations performed at birth are to blame for poor surgical results in many cases.[5, 6] When these findings were reported in the 1950s, a movement to delay surgical treatment until school age developed to minimize the deleterious effects of surgery on palatal and facial growth.[7–9] These advo-

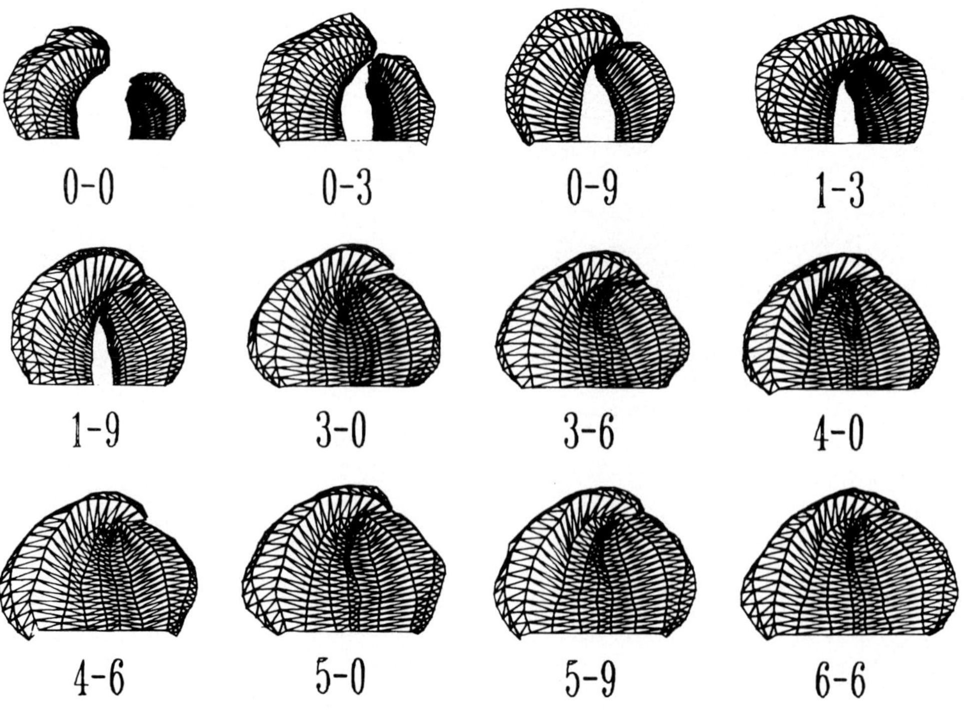

Figure 58–13 Computer-generated images of each cast drawn to scale.

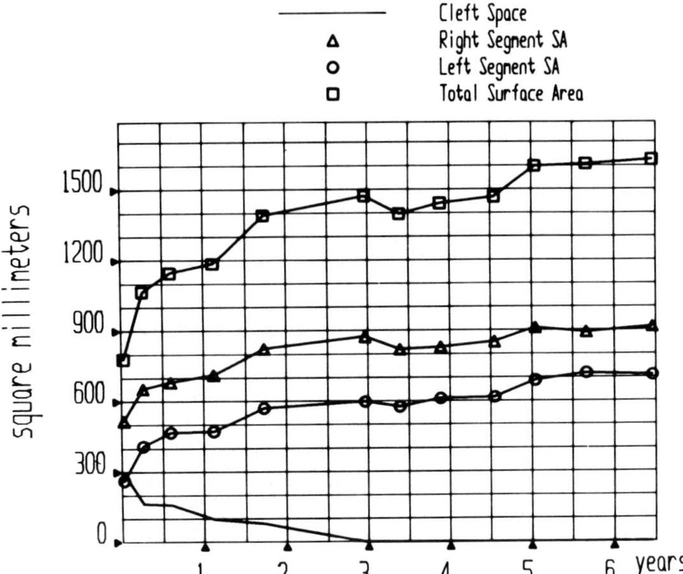

Figure 58–14 Case AC-33. Time sequence analysis of palatal growth in a case of complete unilateral cleft lip and palate. Smaller cleft segment grows more rapidly during the first 6 months of age and then tapers off but begins to accelerate after 4 years 6 months of age.

cates recommended use of obturators while waiting for the palate to mature. Presumably, proponents of this school of thought assumed that all operations on the palate posed a definite impediment to the natural maxillary growth process. Those who believed in a contrary concept of treatment advocated surgical repair of the cleft palate before 1 year of age to avoid perverted patterns of speech that would require prolonged and difficult reduction at a later age.[10–13] This group gave priority to speech development over palatal and facial development. Still others took a middle-of-the-road view and advocated performance of palatal surgery between 12 and 24 months of age.[14–19] Even among this group there was much variation in treatment sequence—that is, whether to unite the soft palate prior to or simultaneously with closure of the hard palate. The literature is full of conflicting reports on the "best" age and the "best" surgical technique to be utilized. The majority of these cross-sectional studies have limited significance because the investigators used inadequate case samples. By lumping the various cleft types together and not considering the age at surgery in relation to the techniques utilized, they failed to expose the significant factors that determined the final result.[20, 21]

The questions remain: Were the different outcomes due to the types of surgery utilized? Was the skill of the operator the relevant factor, or were there significant diagnostic differences within each cleft type? How important were some or all of these factors? Serial palatal growth studies starting at the newborn period have shown that too many variants were operating in these studies to permit the formulation of simple and all-inclusive rules, such as fixing the age at which *all* clefts of the palate should be repaired. They demonstrated that biologic variations, such as the extent of the palatal cleft in relation to the amount of surrounding available

mucoperiosteum, were beyond the control of the surgeon and that these factors could spell the difference between therapeutic success and failure.

Pruzansky frequently stated that his most important contribution to the cleft palate literature was the conclusion that "cleft lip and palate do not represent a single fixed entity subject to generalizations of description and classification and least of all to rigid therapeutic formulas."[22] An anatomic classification system based on the location and completeness of the cleft does not reveal sufficient information about the ultimate effect of surgery and fails to highlight the remarkable range of geometric variation existing within each cleft category. For example, some unilateral clefts exhibit wide separation of the palatal shelves. Others are less separated, and in some, actual overlap of the palatal segments occurs, even prior to surgical closure of the lip. The cleft palatal segments are tilted to various degrees medially and superiorly. Even though they are similarly classified, various degrees of incompleteness of the cleft in the lip and palate may exist in combinations too numerous to describe conveniently.

The bilateral cleft lip and palate and isolated cleft palate also show a high degree of geometric variation. Bilateral clefts of the lip and palate may be complete or incomplete. The premaxilla may be of varying size, depending on the number of tooth buds, and may be symmetric or asymmetric. In isolated cleft palates, the cleft may extend forward from the uvula in varying degrees; in extreme cases it reaches the nasopalatine foramen. The outline of the cleft may be wide or narrow, piriform or V-shaped. The significance of the anatomic variation within each cleft type in predicting the final palatal form and occlusion is still unknown, but one can suspect that the geometric parameters, taken in combination, may be important in predicting the final outcome.

Early Growth Studies on the Natural History of Cleft Palate Are in Conflict

Some studies of clefts that were not operated on have produced conflicting results with regard to the effects of a cleft on jaw growth. Peyton concluded that cleft palate consists of normal tissues that are abnormally displaced.[23, 24] Mestre et al and Ortiz-Monasterio et al[25–27] have shown that clefting has no effect on palatal or facial growth. Slaughter et al first recognized the great anatomic variation even within similarly classified clefts.[28] They suggested that there *are* great differences in the amount and quality of palatal tissue among the several cleft types and even among the same types. The amount of palatal tissue relative to cleft size increases with growth, but the timing of growth varies. In some patients, the greatest proportional changes occur earlier than in others, so that cleft space closure may have to be delayed to avoid producing growth-inhibiting scar tissue. These findings were later verified by Pruzansky, Pruzansky and Lis, Pruzansky and Aduss, Slaughter et al, Pruzansky et al, Lis et al, and Krogman et al, who stated that growth of both hard and soft tissue increases at a rapid rate.[29–36] They observed postoperative "catch-up growth" in almost every case. At the age of 6 years the maxillary complex is usually acceptably normal. They further reported that after palate surgery there may be a growth lag of 14 to 20 months, but after the "shock" pause the processes of orderly development take over and may even accelerate. Berkowitz et al and Mapes et al stated that the maxillary growth rate lags temporarily following surgery but then accelerates to achieve normal length.[37, 38] Robertson and Fish showed that the final results depend not only on the procedures employed but also on the type and degree of deformity seen at birth.[39] Gnoinski's 15-year study highlighted the interference in facial growth by some types of surgical operations.[40]

On the other hand, others believe that skeletal deficiency is characteristic of the cleft population.[41–44] Huddart et al and Boo-Chai concluded that mesodermal deficiency associated with the cleft led to growth deficiency.[45, 46] Scott hypothesized that cleft palates were underdeveloped at birth because the cleft palatal segments in complete clefts were detached from the downward- and forward-growing nasal septum and therefore did not receive its growth impetus.[47, 48] He believed that deficient palates could be stimulated to further growth by functional orthopedic devices. McNeil and Burston accepted Scott's message and led a movement that advocated the use of neonatal maxillary orthopedic treatment to stimulate palatal development.[49–51] A decade later a state-of-the-art report by an international committee concluded that neonatal maxillary orthopedic treatment with or without primary bone grafting had no long-term utility.[52]

Although the mechanism of growth at the midpalatal suture is very dissimilar to that occurring at the cleft space, the two phenomena are comparable in that they stimulate strong dissenting opinions. Scott concluded that all sutural growth ends by 1 year of age, whereas Latham stated that it lasts until 3 years of age.[47, 53] Persson and Thilander claim that it continues until 13 years of age.[54] Bjork and Bjork and Skieller demonstrated that palatal appositional growth continues until 13 to 14 years of age and anteroposterior length increases until 16 to 18 years of age.[4, 55] They stressed that growth was an intermittent process with various periods of rest. Sutural growth continues in girls up to 16 years and in boys up to 18 years of age. Freng was unable to judge whether sutural growth was passive or active, but it continues past puberty and occurs in spurts.[56] As to growth at the cleft space, Berkowitz has shown that appositional bone growth at the cleft border is responsible for increased cleft closure after molding action is complete.[57, 58] This growth is highly variable, and in rare instances, even with additional palatal and facial growth, the cleft width can actually increase. Berkowitz suggested that the surgeon needs to consider the possibility that spontaneous growth at the cleft border can reduce cleft space size, thus influencing the choice of surgical procedures.[19] Therefore, timing of palatal surgery should not be based on age alone. In some instances, when the cleft space is narrow, it can be closed early; however, when the cleft space is very wide, it is wiser to wait for additional growth to occur. In the very rare instances

when it does not occur, one should utilize an obturator. Those who favor late palatal closure seem to favor this treatment approach.

Need for Improved Measuring Techniques

Xerographic studies of casts were an advance over previous measuring systems because they permitted a more accurate description of dimensional and surface area changes. Huddart concluded from these measurements that in patients with complete unilateral cleft lip and palate, the palatal mucosa is deficient by 16 years of age compared to a normal population of the same age. He even mentioned that presurgical orthopedic treatment may hinder palatal growth.[59–61]

In 1971, Mazaheri and coworkers reported on changes in arch form and dimensions in unilateral cleft lip (UCLP) and palate and cleft palate only.[62] They reported the existence of a significant pattern of anteroposterior and lateral growth retardation immediately after surgical treatment. By 4 years of age the arch lengths were of more normal size, whereas arch widths were smaller and remained smaller. Mapes et al reported on the results of a longitudinal study of UCLP. There appeared to be asymmetric growth of the palatal segment with the affected palatal segment showing a greater growth rate.[38] Unfortunately, these studies still did not answer questions relating to the relationship between palatal growth rates and the timing of surgical procedures, nor did they recognize the large range of growth variation that exists within each cleft type.

Stockli was very critical of his own research and reported that there are great limitations to the use of xerography for the study of cleft palate casts.[63] He emphasized that *arch form* needs to be considered in the treatment of an infant with complete cleft of the lip and palate and recognized that *three-dimensional measurements* would be more appropriate for longitudinal and comparative palatal growth studies. The ideal measuring system would express in numerical terms the spatial relationship of the two maxillary segments in the frontal and sagittal planes, particularly in the region of the alveolar cleft. He called for more extensive three-dimensional analyses of casts using more exacting measuring techniques.

Conclusion

The geometric three-dimensional analysis of serial palatal casts has exposed important information about the palate's physical changes that occur under the influence of growth and surgery. A longitudinal analysis of complete unilateral cleft lip and palate patients has verified the existence of catch-up growth during the first 2 years of life. It appears that the lesser cleft segment has the potential to grow more rapidly than the noncleft segment. A second period of accelerated growth is possible after physiologic (nonscarring) surgery is utilized to close the palatal cleft. A study of vault contours and palatal growth demonstrates that physiologic surgery does (1) allow normal palatal height to exist within 1 year after surgery; (2) permit medially positioned palatal segments to be moved into normal alignment; and (3) permit normal transverse and antero-posterior palatal growth and vertical alveolar development.

In the presence of extremely wide cleft spaces that do not decrease spontaneously, a von Langenbeck procedure would leave wide lateral areas of denuded bone, causing severe scarring and palatal growth inhibition. In this circumstance, it is better to use a vomer flap with or without a von Langenbeck procedure to avoid the consequences of excessive palatal scarring. There are instances when the cleft space is so large (due to osteogenic deficiency) that the treatment of choice is use of an obturator rather than a surgical solution.

References

1. Lebret L: Growth changes of the palate. J Dent Res 41:1391, 1962.
2. Korkhaus GA: A new orthodontic symmetrograph. Int J Orthod 16:665, 1930.
3. Barrow GV, White JR: Development changes of the maxillary and mandibular dental arches. Am J Orthod 22:41–46, 1952.
4. Bjork A, Skieller V: Growth in width of the maxilla studied by the implant method. Scand J Plast Reconstr Surg 8:26, 1974.
5. Graber TM: Craniofacial morphology in cleft palate and cleft lip deformities. Surg Gynecol Obstet 88:359, 1949.
6. Graber TM: The congenital cleft palate deformity. J Am Dent Assoc 48:375, 1954.
7. Schweckendiek W: Primary veloplasty: Long term results without maxillary deformity. A twenty-five year report. Cleft Palate J 15:268, 1978.
8. Hotz R: The indications for preoperative and postoperative orthopedic treatment of cleft lip and palate. In Hotz R, et al (eds): Early Treatment of Cleft Lip and Palate. Bern: Hans Huber, 1964, p 78
9. Hotz M, Gnoinski W, Perko M, et al: The Zurich approach, 1964 to 1984. In Hotz M, et al (eds): Early Treatment of Cleft Lip and Palate. Toronto: Hans Huber, 1984.
10. Holdsworth WG: Early treatment of cleft lip and cleft palate. Br Med J 1:304, 1954.
11. Jolleys A: A review of the results of operations on cleft palates with references to maxillary growth and speech function. Br J Plast Surg 7:229, 1954.
12. Robertson NRE, Jolleys A: The timing of hard palate repair. Scand J Plast Reconstr Surg 8:49, 1974.
13. Dorf DS, Curtin JW: Early cleft palate repair and speech outcome. Plast Reconstr Surg 70:74, 1982.
14. Slaughter W, Pruzansky S: The rationale for velar closure as a primary procedure in the repair of cleft palate defects. Plast Reconstr Surg 13:341, 1954.
15. Slaughter W, Pruzansky S, Harris HL, et al: A new surgical concept for repair of congenital clefts of lip and palate. Surg Clin North Am 38(4):945, 1958.
16. Blocksma R, Leuz CA, Mellerstag K: A constructive program for managing cleft palates without the use of mucoperiosteal flaps. Plast Reconstr Surg 55:160, 1975.
17. Dingman RO, Grabb WC: A rational program for surgical management of bilateral cleft lip and palate. Plast Reconstr Surg 46:239, 1971.
18. Dingman RO, O'Connor JE: A conservative program of surgical management of the cleft lip and cleft palate patient. Presented at The Second International Congress on Cleft Palates, Copenhagen, 1973 (Abstract 262).
19. Berkowitz S: Timing cleft palate closure—age should not be the sole determinant. In Cohen M, Rollnick BR (eds): Craniofacial Dysmorphology: Studies in Honor of Samuel Pruzansky. New York: Alan R. Liss, 1985.
20. Koberg W, Koblin I: Speech development and maxillary growth in relation to technique and timing of palatoplasty. J Maxillofac Surg 1:44, 1973.
21. Robertson NRE, Jolleys A: The timing of hard palate repair. Scand J Plast Reconstr Surg 8:49, 1974.
22. Pruzansky S: Description classification and analysis of unoperated clefts of the lip and palate. Am J Orthod 39:590, 1953.
23. Peyton WT: The dimensions and growth of the palate in normal infants and in the infant with gross mal-development of the upper lip and palate. Arch Surg 22:704, 1931.
24. Peyton WT: Dimensions and growth of the palate in infants with gross maldevelopment of the upper lip and palate. Am J Dis Child 47:1265, 1934.
25. Mestre JC, DeJesus J, Subtelny JD: Unoperated oral clefts at maturation. Angle Orthod 30:78, 1960.
26. Ortiz-Monasterio F, Rebeil AS, Valderrama M, et al: Cephalometric measurements on adult patients with unoperated cleft palates. Plast Reconstr Surg 24:53, 1959.
27. Ortiz-Monasterio F, Rebeil AS, Barrera G, et al: A study of untreated adult cleft palate patients. Plast Reconstr Surg 38:36, 1966.
28. Slaughter WB, Pruzansky S, Harris HL: Cleft lip and cleft palate, surgical considerations. Pediatr Clin North Am 3:1029, 1956.
29. Pruzansky S: Factors determining arch form in clefts of the lip and palate. Am J Orthod 41:827, 1955.
30. Pruzansky S: The foundation of the cleft palate center and training program at the University of Illinois. Angle Orthod 27:69, 1957.
31. Pruzansky S, Lis EF: Cephalometric roentgenography of infants: Sedation, instrumentation and research. Am J Orthod 44:159, 1958.
32. Pruzansky S, Aduss H: Arch form and the deciduous occlusion in complete unilateral clefts. Cleft Palate J 1:411, 1964.
33. Slaughter WB, Pruzansky S, Harris HL: Cleft lip and cleft palate: Surgical considerations. Pediatr Clin North Am 3:1029, 1969.
34. Pruzansky S, Aduss H, Berkowitz S, et al: Monitoring growth of the infant with cleft lip and palate. Trans Eur Orthod Soc 1973, p 538.
35. Lis E, Pruzansky S, Koepp-Baker H: Cleft lip and cleft palate: Perspectives in management. Pediatr Clin North Am 3:995, 1956.
36. Krogman WM, Mazaheri M, Harding RL: A longitudinal study of craniofacial growth in children with clefts as compared to normal, birth to six years. Cleft Palate J 12:59, 1979.
37. Berkowitz S, Krischer J, Pruzansky S: Quantitative analysis of cleft palate casts. Cleft Palate J 11:134, 1974.
38. Mapes AH, Mazaheri M, Harding RL, et al: A longitudinal analysis of the maxillary growth increments of cleft lip and palate patients (CLP). Cleft Palate J 11:450, 1974.
39. Robertson NRE, Fish J: Early dimensional changes in the arches of cleft palate children. Am J Orthod 67:290, 1975.
40. Gnoinski W: Early maxillary orthopaedics as a supplement to conventional primary surgery in complete unilateral cleft lip and palate cases—long-term results. J Maxillofac Surg 10:165, 1982.
41. Stark RB: Pathogenesis of harelip and cleft palate. Plast Reconstr Surg 13:20, 1954.
42. Coupe TB, Subtelny JD: Cleft palate deficiency or displacement of tissue. Plast Reconstr Surg 26:600, 1960.
43. Innis CO: Some preliminary observations on unrepaired hare-lips and cleft palates in adult members of the Dusau Tribes of North Borneo. Br J Plast Surg 15:173, 1962.
44. Pitanguay MD, Franco T: Non-operated facial fissures in adults. Plast Reconstr Surg 39:569, 1967.
45. Huddart AG, MacCauley FJ, Muriel EH, et al: Maxillary arch dimensions in normal and unilateral cleft palate subjects. Cleft Palate J 6:471, 1969.
46. Boo-Chai K: The unoperated adult bilateral cleft of the lip and palate. Br J Plast Surg 24:250, 1971.
47. Scott JH: Growth of facial sutures. Am J Orthod 42:381, 1956.
48. Scott JH: Further studies on the growth of the human face. Proc R Soc Med 52:263, 1959.
49. McNeil CK: Oral and Facial Deformity. London: Pitman and Sons, 1954.
50. Burston WR: The early orthodontic treatment of cleft palate conditions. Dent Pract 9:41, 1958.
51. Burston WR: The early orthodontic treatment of alveolar clefts. Proc R Soc Med 58:767, 1965.
52. Berkowitz S: Orofacial growth and dentistry. Section III. State of the art report. Cleft Palate J 14:288, 1977.
53. Latham RA: The development, structure and growth pattern of the human mid-palatal suture. J Anat 108:31, 1971.
54. Persson M, Thilander B: Palatal suture closure in man from 15 to 35 years of age. Am J Orthod 72:42, 1977.
55. Bjork A: Facial growth in man studied with the aid of metallic implants. Acta Odontol Scand 13:9, 1955.
56. Freng A: Growth in width of the dental arches after partial extirpation of the mid-palatal suture in man. Scand J Plast Reconstr Surg 12:267, 1978.
57. Berkowitz S: Stereophotogrammetric analysis of casts of normal and abnormal palates. Am J Orthod 60:1, 1971.
58. Berkowitz S, Krischer J, Pruzansky S: Quantative analysis of cleft palate casts. Cleft Palate J 11:134, 1974.
59. Huddart AG: Maxillary arch dimensions in cleft palate cases. In Cole R (ed): Early Treatment of Cleft Lip and Palate. Proceedings of Second International Symposium. Chicago: Northwestern University Cleft Lip and Palate Institute, 1970, p 46.
60. Huddart AG: Maxillary arch dimensions in cleft palate cases. In Cole R (ed): Early Treatment of Cleft Lip and Palate Proceedings of Second International Symposium. Chicago: Northwestern University Cleft Lip and Palate Institute, 1971, p 15.
61. Huddart AG, Huddart AM: An investigation to relate the overall size of the maxillary arch and area of palatal mucosa in cleft lip and palate cases at birth to the overall size of the upper dental arch at 5 years of age. In Cohen M, Rollnick BR (eds): Studies in Honor of Samuel Pruzansky. New York: Alan R. Liss, 1985.
62. Mazaheri M, Harding RL, Cooper JA, et al: Changes in arch form and dimensions of cleft patients. Am J Orthod 60:19, 1971.
63. Stockli PW: Application of a quantitative method of arch form evaluation in complete unilateral cleft lip and palate. Cleft Palate J 8:322, 1971.

CHAPTER 59

Anthropometry of the Face in Cleft Patients

Leslie G. Farkas

The vast number of cleft lip repair methods indicates the existence of numerous variations in the anomaly, each requiring a slightly different approach. The usual classification of clefts into complete or incomplete, and unilateral or bilateral types does not cover all variations. Detailed quantitative analysis of the hard and soft tissues creating the facial defects and disproportions helps the surgeon choose the most appropriate treatment. Furthermore, objective criteria for preoperative, postoperative, and late findings of the cleft lip anomaly permit identification of the most efficient treatment technique within an institution and comparison of treatment effectiveness among several institutions.[1]

Direct anthropometric measurements are used to generate objective data about deformities, dislocations, and the degree of soft-tissue defects in the face. Because the nasolabial complex is aesthetically extremely sensitive,[2] anthropometric measurements must be taken throughout the entire facial framework, even in cases of isolated cleft lip. When the cleft is only one symptom, as in 154 currently recognized facial syndromes,[3] a more detailed anthropometric examination of the face is required.

Use of anthropometric techniques offers the following benefits in clinical study of cleft lip and palate anomalies:
1. Uniformity in judgment of the preoperative and postoperative morphologic changes in the face, based on the sum of quantitative assessment.
2. Creation of a new clinical classification of the anomaly—mild, moderate, and severe—based on quantitative abnormalities in the surface and skeletal anatomy of the face.
3. Detailed data for identifying and delineating facial syndromes.
4. Help in understanding the postoperative development of the face, particularly the cleft nose deformity.

Preoperative Assessment

Seven measurements of the soft nose and seven of the lips (Figs. 59–1 and 59–2) provide valuable information about the location and extent of the soft-tissue defects (abbreviations in general use are listed in Table 59–1). Although some measurements must be obtained while the child is sedated, many nose measurements (e.g., al–al, n–sn, nasal bridge deviation, ac–ac) and all measurements revealing proportions in other craniofacial regions (Fig. 59–3) may be taken without sedation.

Unilateral Cleft Lip

In the nose (Fig. 59–1A), the size of the soft tissue cleft is the difference between the right and left nasal floor widths (sbal–sn' or sbal–sn). The degree of horizontal alar cartilage displacement is shown by the soft nose width (al–al), the distance between the facial insertion points of the ala (ac–ac), and the distance between the alar base insertion points (sbal–sbal). Vertical displacement is demonstrated by the differences between the right and left columellar heights (sn–c', r and l) and the right and left alar lengths (ac–prn, r and l). The direction and extent of the nasal bridge deviation from the medial axis of the face and of the columella from the vertical are also valuable for determining displacement. The nasal index $\dfrac{(al\text{–}al \times 100)}{n\text{–}5n}$, formed by displacement. The nasal index (al–al $\times$ 100), formed by the nose width and height, also should be determined.

In the lips (Fig. 59–1B), the paramedial vertical upper lip heights on the noncleft side (sn'–cph) and close to the cleft (sn'–cph') show the size of the defect in the midportion of the upper lip.[4] The medial height of the upper lip skin (sn–ls) is the distance from the subnasale to the labiale superius. Measurement of the noncleft side (cph–ch) is used to identify the philtral point on the cleft side ("cph").[4] The distance between the two philtral points (cph and cph') yields the size of the cleft in the upper lip (not illustrated). Measurement of the lower lip vermilion height helps in estimating the upper lip vermilion height. Distances between the alar base insertion points and the ipsilateral philtral points (sbal–cph and sbal–"cph") or the labial fissure commissures (sbal–ch, r and l) contribute information about the dislocation of the alar base on the cleft side.

Bilateral Cleft Lip

In the nose (Fig. 59–2A), the sizes of the clefts are identified by the distances between the alar base insertion and the ipsilateral columellar base points (sbal–sn' or sbal–sn, r and l). The horizontal displacement of the alar cartilages is shown by the alar base width (sbal–sbal), the width between the facial insertion points of the alae (ac–ac), the soft nose width (al–al), and the projective alar lengths (ac–prn, r and l). Differences between the paired measurements (sbal–sn, r and l; ac–prn, r and l) reveal asymmetries. The extent of the columellar defect, shown by the columellar lengths (sn'–c', r and l) and the nasal tip protrusion (sn–prn), completes the record of the initial nasal defect. Measurement of the columellar width (the distance between the columellar base points [sn']) frequently indicates an abnormally wide formation. The degree of nasal bridge deviation should be determined if the bilateral cleft lip is asymmetric.

In the lips (Fig. 59–2B), the measurements are con-

Figure 59–1 Preoperative measurements in complete unilateral cleft lip and palate. *A,* Surface measurements of the nose: 1, distance between the alar base (sbal) and the edge of the columella base (sn′), right and left; 2, alar base width (sbal–sbal); 3, alar base facial insertion width (ac–ac); 4, soft nose width (al–al); 5, nasal tip protrusion (sn–prn); 6, columella height (sn–c′), right and left; 7, projective ala length (ac–prn), right and left.

B, Surface measurements of the mouth: 1, distance between the highest point of the Cupid's bow (cph) on the noncleft side and the edge of the columella base (sn′); 2, distance between the lowest point on the Cupid's bow (ls) and the midpoint at the base of the columella (sn); 1/1 distance between the surrogate philtral landmark (cph′) bordering the cleft and the ipsilateral columella base (sn′). The position of the surrogate cph′ point is determined by transferring the philtral landmark (cph–ls) on the noncleft side to the vermilion-cutaneous border of the cleft;[4] 3, distance between the philtral point on the noncleft side (cph) and the ipsilateral commissure (ch) of the labial fissure. The highest point of the Cupid's bow on the cleft side ("cph") is determined by transferring the distance between the philtral point and the labial commissure (cph–ch) from the noncleft side; 4, distance between the highest point of the Cupid's bow (cph or "cph") and the ipsilateral alar base (sbal) on the cleft and noncleft sides; 5, distance between the alar base (sbal) and the ipsilateral commissure (ch) of the labial fissure on both sides of the cleft; 6, midline lower lip vermilion height; 7, labial fissure width ch–ch).

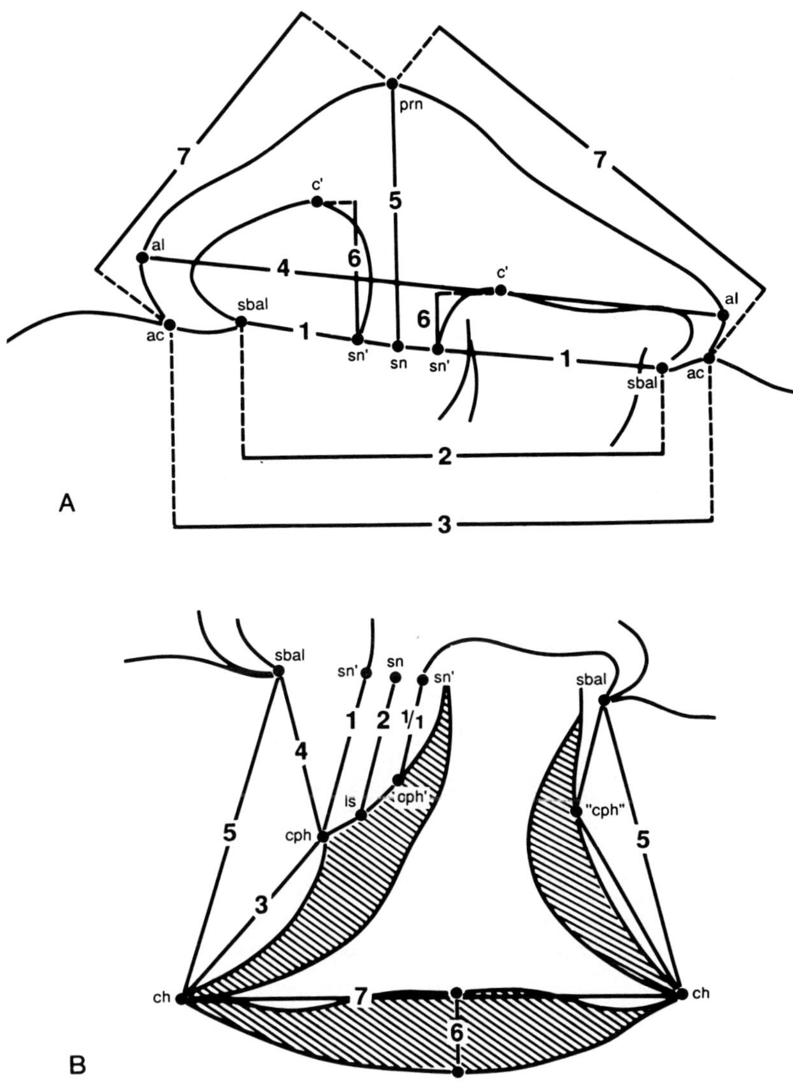

centrated on the central portion—the prolabium. Because the columella may be abnormally wide (sn′–sn′), this measurement cannot always be used for planning the width of the philtrum. Because many surgeons use the prolabium to create the entire central portion of the upper lip,[4–8] precise determination of its size is recommended. The frenulum labii can be used[7] to locate the midaxis of the prolabium, which helps to identify the height of the prolabium (sn–ls) or the height of the middle portion of the upper lip skin. Comparison of the height of the vermilions of the prolabium and the lower lip will help in estimating the ideal vermilion height in the repaired upper lip. The width is measured in the widest portion of the prolabium. The lateral vertical upper lip measurements (sbal–ch, r and l) show the relative positions of the alar bases (sbal, r and l) and the labial fissure commissures (ch, r and l) and tell us the approximate height of the lateral portions of the upper lip.

Other Craniofacial Regions

The basic proportion indices of the head, face, orbits, and ears offer valuable data about the quality of their proportions (Fig. 59–3).[9] The head type is determined by the cephalic index, in which the head width is expressed as a percentage of head length $\frac{(eu-eu \times 100)}{g-op}$. The facial index expresses the relationship of face height and width $\frac{(n-gn \times 100)}{zy-zy}$. The orbital type is given by the intercanthal index $\frac{(en-en \times 100)}{ex-ex}$, which expresses the intercanthal width as a percentage of biocular width. Ear indices (right and left) $\frac{(pra-pa \times 100)}{sa-sba}$ are calculated from the width and height measurements of the ears. The nasal index should be determined. The tissue defect of the upper lip precludes identification of the

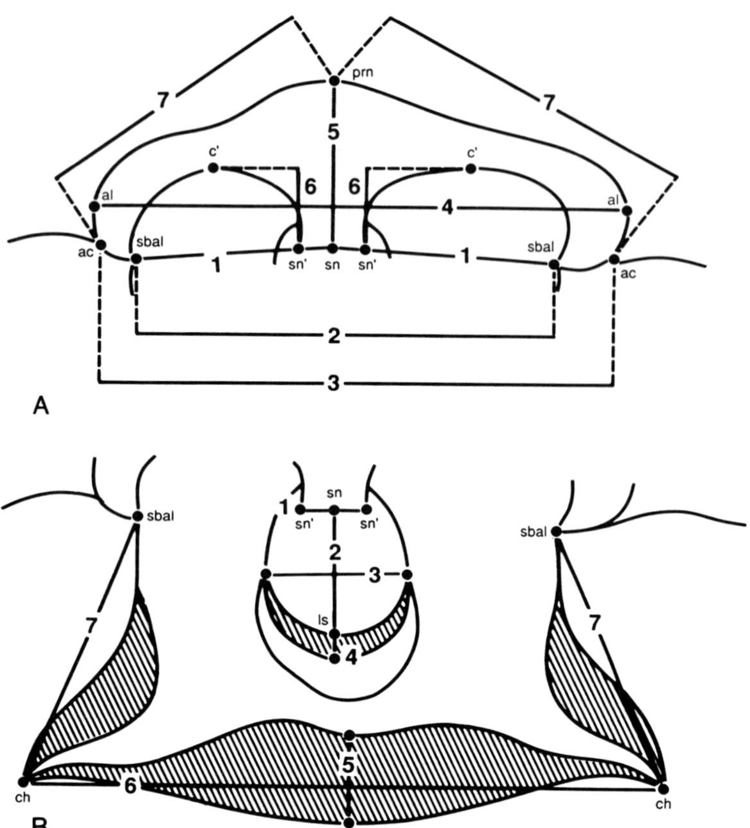

Figure 59–2 Preoperative measurements in complete bilateral cleft lip and palate. *A*, Surface measurements of the nose: 1, distance between the alar base (sbal) and the edge of the columella base (sn′), right and left; 2, alar base width (sbal–sbal); 3, alar base facial insertion width (ac–ac); 4, soft nose width (al–al); 5, nasal tip protrusion (sn–prn); 6, columella height (sn–c′), right and left; 7, projective ala length (ac–prn), right and left.
B, Surface measurements of the lips: 1, columella base width (sn′–sn′); 2, prolabial height (sn–ls); 3, maximal prolabial width; 4, thickness of prolabial mucosa; 5, lower lip vermilion height; 6, labial fissure width (ch–ch); 7, distance between the alar base (sbal) and the ipsilateral commissure of the labial fissure (ch), right and left.

upper lip height–mouth width index $\frac{(sn-sto \times 100)}{ch-ch}$ before the lip repair.

Postoperative Assessments

First Postoperative Examination

The first postoperative examination should take place 1 year after the lip repair or at admission for cleft palate repair. In unilateral clefts, the differences between the noncleft and cleft sides are noted, particularly in the lateral upper lip heights (sbal–ls′, r and l), the nasal floor widths (sbal–sn′ or sbal–sn, r and l), the alar lengths (ac–prn, r and l), the alar base levels (sbal, r and l), and the shape and size of the nostrils.[10, 11] The nasal index, upper lip height–mouth width index, and the more general craniofacial proportions (cephalic, facial, intercanthal, and ear indices) should be repeated.

Second Postoperative Examination

A more detailed examination is recommended at the time of a secondary operation for repair of lip or nasal defects. The measurements taken at the first postoper-

Table 59–1. Abbreviations

ac	= alar curvature point (point of alar base insertion into the face)
al	= alare
c′	= highest point of the columella
ch	= cheilion
cph	= crista philtri landmark preserved on noncleft side
cph′	= crista philtri landmark estimated on noncleft side
"cph"	= crista philtri landmark surrogate on cleft side
en	= endocanthion
eu	= eurion
ex	= exocanthion
g	= glabella
gn	= gnathion
li	= labiale inferius
ls′	= labiale superius below the subalare
ls	= labiale superius
m′	= midpoint of the nasal root at the level of the eye fissure
mf	= maxillofrontale
n	= nasion
op	= opisthocranion
pa	= postaurale
pra	= preaurale
prn	= pronasale
sa	= superaurale
sba	= subaurale
sbal	= subalare
sn	= subnasale (midpoint of the columellar base)
sn′	= edge of the columellar base
sto	= stomion
zy	= zygion

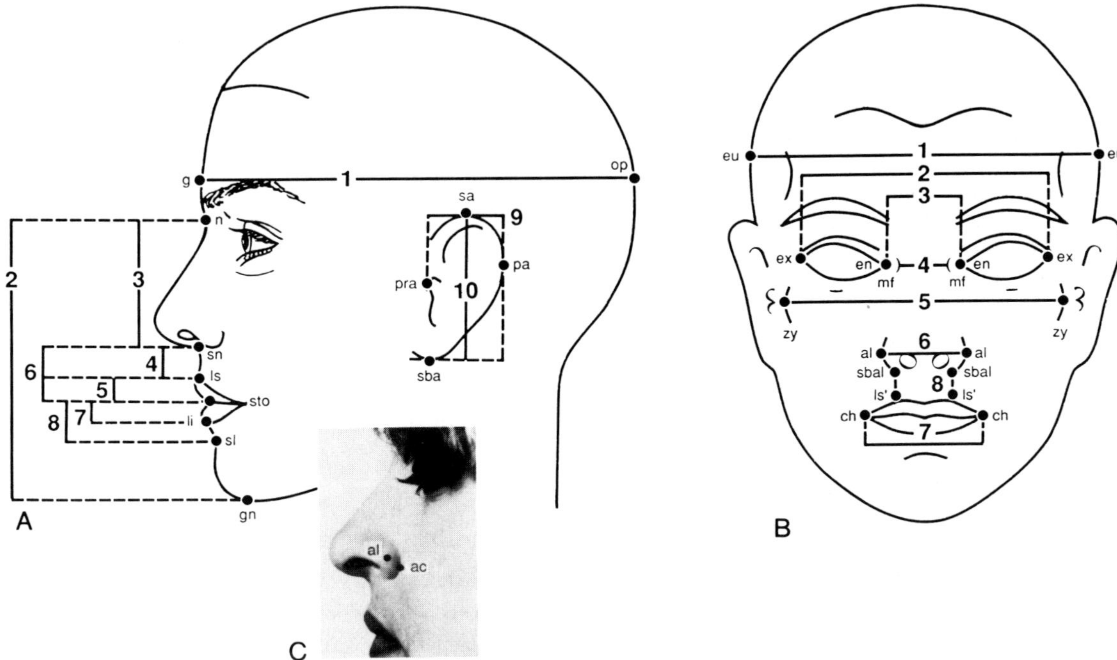

Figure 59–3 Preoperative measurements of the head and face. *A,* Lateral view: 1, head length (g–op); 2, face height (n–gn); 3, nose height (n–sn); 4, upper lip skin height (sn–ls); 5, upper lip vermilion height (ls–sto); 6, upper lip height (sn–sto); 7, lower lip vermilion height (sto–li); 8, lower lip height (sto–sl); 9, ear width (pra–pa); 10, ear height (sa–sba).

B, Frontal view: 1, head width (eu–eu); 2, biocular width (ex–ex); 3, intercanthal width (en–en); 4, nasal root width (mf–mf); 5, face width (zy–zy); 6, nose width (al–al); 7, mouth width (ch–ch); 8, lateral upper lip height (sbal–ls′).
C, Profile view of alar base facial insertion (ac). al = the most lateral point of the ala.

ative examination should be repeated and the columellar height and nasal tip protrusion must also be determined. The nasal tip protrusion–soft nose width proportion index $\dfrac{(\text{sn–prn} \times 100)}{\text{al–al}}$, and the columellar height–tip protrusion index $\dfrac{(\text{sn–c}' \times 100)}{\text{sn–prn}}$ should also be analyzed. The nose–face height index and the nose–face width index indicate any disharmony between the nose and face.[12]

In addition, the aesthetic appearance of the nose depends on the nasal root–nose width index $\dfrac{(\text{mf–mf} \times 100)}{\text{al–al}}$. The inclinations of the nasal bridge, upper face, columella, and upper lip, the nasofrontal and nasolabial angles, and the relationship of the upper and lower lip heights can help to determine the nature and extent of the late deformities.[2, 13]

Third Postoperative Examination

The final examination of the lips and nose of a patient born with cleft lip and palate should be carried out when the face has reached maturity. Table 59–2 shows the mean absolute increases in selected nasal and lip measurements between 6 and 18 years of age for North American Caucasians. At 6 years of age, in both sexes, the medial upper lip height has achieved the highest percentage of its adult value and the columellar height the lowest percentage. The nose height shows the

greatest absolute increase between 6 and 18 years of age.

These data facilitate estimation of the growth that has occurred in the lip and nose of patients who have a

Table 59–2. Age-Related Changes in Major Measurements of the Nose and Upper Lip in North American Caucasians Between 6 and 18 Years of Age

Measurement/Sex	Mean Percentage of Total Growth Achieved at Age 6 Years	Mean Increase Between Ages 6 and 18 Years	
		Percentage of Total Growth	Absolute (mm)
Columellar height (sn–c′)			
Male	71.1	28.9	3.3
Female	70.1	29.9	3.2
Nasal tip protrusion (sn–prn)			
Male	73.3	26.7	5.5
Female	76.7	23.3	4.5
Nose height (n–sn)			
Male	75.6	24.4	12.9
Female	80.4	19.6	19.6
Nose width (al–al)			
Male	82.4	17.6	6.1
Female	88.5	11.5	3.6
Lateral lip height (sbal–ls′)			
Male	88.8	11.2	1.8
Female	92.5	7.5	1.2
Medial lip height (sn–sto)			
Male	91.3	8.7	1.9
Female	95.4	4.6	0.9

repaired cleft lip and can help to clarify differences in growth and late results with different surgical procedures.[14–16]

Detailed nose measurements taken after lip repair can provide clues to its ultimate appearance. An abnormally short and wide columella will remain abnormal. Disproportion between a markedly small nasal tip protrusion and a wide soft nose will not improve with age. Asymmetries in size and shape of the nostrils will not disappear; on the contrary, they may increase with growth. The nasal bridge inclination will be influenced by the upper face inclination (maxilla) and the columellar length.

The form and size of the soft nose and the shape of the nostrils differ between some Caucasian ethnic groups[10] and, more strikingly, between various races. Furthermore, the aesthetic quality of the nose is judged partly by the relationships between the individual nose measurements and partly by the harmony existing between the nose and the face. When the final corrective nose surgery is planned, the following proportion indices may be helpful:[9]

Proportion Indices of the Nose

1. Nasal index: $\dfrac{al-al \times 100}{n-sn}$

2. Nasal root–nose width index: $\dfrac{mf-mf \times 100}{al-al}$

3. Nostril–nose width index: $\dfrac{sbal-sn\ r\ and\ l \times 100}{al-al}$

4. Nasal root depth–width index: $\dfrac{en-m'\ sag \times 100}{mf-mf}$

5. Nasal tip protrusion–width index: $\dfrac{sn-prn \times 100}{al-al}$

6. Nasal root depth–tip protrusion index: $\dfrac{en-m'\ sag \times 100}{sn-prn}$

7. Alar length–nose height index: $\dfrac{ac-prn \times 100}{n-sn}$

8. Columellar length–nasal tip protrusion index: $\dfrac{c'-sn \times 100}{sn-prn}$

Proportion Indices of the Nose and Face

1. Nose–face width index: $\dfrac{al-al \times 100}{zy-zy}$

2. Nose–face height index: $\dfrac{n-sn \times 100}{n-gn}$

3. Nasal root–intercanthal width index: $\dfrac{mf-mf \times 100}{en-en}$

4. Upper lip–nose height index: $\dfrac{sn-sto \times 100}{n-sn}$

The nasofrontal, nasolabial, and nasal tip angles, and the inclination of the columella (from the vertical) provide further data about the aesthetic quality of the nose. However, the nose is only one portion of the facial profile. Its angles and inclinations must form a harmonious unit with the remaining facial profile inclinations: forehead, lower face, mandible, chin, and the general profile line.[2]

Identification and Quantification of Abnormality

The patient's measurements and/or proportions must be compared with normal values taken from a population similar in age, sex, race, and, if possible, ethnic groups. Differences between ethnic groups have been detected in some facial signs within the young adult North American Caucasian population[18] and between North American and European Caucasians (Farkas, unpublished data). Tables 59–3 to 59–8 report the control values (means and standard deviations) of the 26 measurements and eight proportion indices of the head and face described in this chapter. Most of the data for children less than 4 years of age were obtained from a West German population[19] and were adjusted statistically for use in North American Caucasians.[20] Measurements and indices for children aged 4 and 5 years were obtained from a current North American population study (30 subjects of each sex in each age group, Farkas, unpublished data). Most of the upper lip height norms were taken from a Czech population study.[21] The remaining control values have been previously published in monographs describing 112 craniofacial measurements[22] and 155 proportion indices for North American Caucasians aged 6 to 18 years.[9] Normal values for asymmetries of the paired measurements of the nose and upper lip were reported in healthy subjects 6 to 18 years of age[22] and in young adults.[11]

The patient's measurement and/or index is considered abnormal if it does not fall within the range of mean ± 2 SD. The degree of abnormality is determined from the difference between the abnormal value and the closest normal value and is expressed as a percentage of the latter.

The large number of control values for measurements and/or indices facilitates the identification and quantification of the smallest deviation from the normal in North American Caucasian patients between 4 and 18 years old, the time period when corrective procedures are undertaken for patients born with facial clefts.

Conclusion

Quantitative study of facial clefts was first documented more than half a century ago,[23] and uniform assessment

Table 59–3. Normal Values for Head Measurements and Proportion Index in Children Less than 6 Years Old

Measurement/ Proportion and Sex	0–15 days Mean SD	16 days–6 mo Mean SD	6–12 mo Mean SD	1 yr Mean SD	2 yr Mean SD	3 yr Mean SD	4 yr Mean SD	5 yr Mean SD
Measurements								
Head width (eu–eu)								
M	93.7 6.6	100.6 10.1	120.3 7.4	127.3 5.8	132.0 5.8	135.5 5.5	136.4 4.7	138.2 4.0
F	93.7 4.9	97.9 7.0	118.1 6.7	123.7 6.1	128.1 6.7	132.9 3.8	135.8 3.9	135.4 3.8
Head length (g–op)								
M	121.0 7.4	135.6 10.7	153.7 9.0	165.2 6.5	171.6 7.8	176.4 5.8	181.5 6.2	180.5 6.2
F	115.7 2.5	133.2 11.6	149.7 6.4	158.5 9.2	169.6 6.8	171.7 5.3	175.2 5.2	178.8 5.2
Index								
Cephalic $\left(\dfrac{\text{eu–eu} \times 100}{\text{g–op}}\right)$								
M	76.8 3.0	73.7 5.0	78.0 6.6	76.7 4.9	76.6 4.8	76.5 4.1	75.2 3.4	76.7 3.6
F	80.3 4.0	73.3 4.7	78.5 4.5	77.7 5.1	75.1 4.7	77.0 3.2	77.6 3.2	75.8 2.9

All measurements and indices for children aged 0 days to 3 years are taken from the German data[19] adjusted for the North American population.[20] Data for 4- and 5-year-old children are the new North American norms (Farkas).

Table 59–4. Normal Values for Face Measurements and Proportion Index in Children <6 Years Old

Measurement/ Proportion and Sex	0–15 days Mean	SD	16 days–6 mo Mean	SD	6–12 mo Mean	SD	1 yr Mean	SD	2 yr Mean	SD	3 yr Mean	SD	4 yr Mean	SD	5 yr Mean	SD
Measurements																
Face width (zy–zy)																
M	74.8	5.9	83.7	5.9	99.2	5.9	106.2	5.9	107.6	5.9	111.3	5.9	110.2	5.4	111.8	5.1
F	75.8	5.2	81.0	5.2	99.5	5.2	103.7	5.2	105.9	5.2	108.7	5.2	106.8	4.6	109.4	3.6
Face height (n–gn)																
M	52.8	5.8	62.5	5.8	74.1	5.8	80.0	5.8	85.8	5.8	90.1	5.8	96.4	4.3	96.7	3.5
F	54.6	5.1	59.8	5.1	71.3	5.1	76.1	5.1	84.5	5.1	86.6	5.1	92.6	3.5	96.5	4.6
Index																
Facial index $\left(\dfrac{\text{n–gn} \times 100}{\text{zy–zy}}\right)$																
M	68.4	5.1	73.3	5.1	74.0	5.1	75.1	5.1	79.4	5.1	80.8	5.1	87.6	4.2	86.7	3.6
F	70.6	4.7	72.6	4.7	71.6	4.7	73.3	4.7	79.6	4.7	79.4	4.7	86.9	4.9	88.3	4.8

All measurements and indices for children aged 0 days to 3 years are taken from the German data[19] adjusted for the North American population.[20] Data for 4- and 5-year-old children are the new North American norms (Farkas).

Table 59–5. Normal Values for Orbital Measurements and Proportion Index in Children <6 Years Old

Measurement/ Proportion and Sex	0–15 days Mean	SD	16 days–6 mo Mean	SD	6–12 mo Mean	SD	1 yr Mean	SD	2 yr Mean	SD	3 yr Mean	SD	4 yr Mean	SD	5 yr Mean	SD
Measurements																
Intercanthal width (en–en)																
M	23.3	2.6	26.2	2.6	29.2	2.6	29.4	2.6	30.2	2.6	30.2	2.6	30.3	1.9	30.8	2.1
F	23.8	2.3	25.1	2.3	28.4	2.3	29.0	2.3	29.6	2.3	29.3	2.3	29.0	2.0	29.4	2.2
Biocular width (ex–ex)																
M	61.8	6.2	64.9	5.7	74.6	6.3	76.0	4.7	76.6	4.5	77.9	3.3	77.2	3.3	78.7	4.2
F	61.7	3.5	62.0	5.9	70.1	5.4	73.9	3.4	74.6	3.6	75.5	3.2	75.3	2.4	76.5	2.5
Index																
Intercanthal index $\left(\dfrac{\text{e–en} \times 100}{\text{ex–ex}}\right)$																
M	37.1	2.3	40.1	2.3	39.5	2.3	39.0	2.3	39.8	2.3	39.3	2.3	39.2	1.6	39.2	2.0
F	37.7	2.2	39.7	2.2	40.5	2.2	39.4	2.2	39.8	2.2	39.2	2.2	38.5	2.2	38.5	2.6

All measurements and indices for children aged 0 days to 3 years are taken from the German data[19] adjusted for the North American population.[20] Data for 4- and 5-year-old children are the new North American norms (Farkas).

Table 59–6. Normal Values for Nose Measurements and Proportion Index in Children < 6 Years Old

Measurement/ Proportion and Sex	0–15 days Mean	SD	16 days– 6 mo Mean	SD	6–12 mo Mean	SD	1 yr Mean	SD	2 yr Mean	SD	3 yr Mean	SD	4 yr Mean	SD	5 yr Mean	SD
Measurements																
Nose width (al–al)																
M	19.4	2.1	22.2	2.1	25.5	2.1	26.3	2.1	26.4	2.1	27.0	2.1	28.4	1.7	28.9	1.5
F	19.9	2.0	20.7	2.0	24.0	2.0	25.5	2.0	25.9	2.0	26.6	2.0	27.8	1.3	28.5	1.5
Nose height (n–sn)																
M	21.7	2.4	25.6	3.4	30.7	2.3	34.4	2.4	35.9	2.9	36.3	2.3	39.5	1.9	38.9	2.7
F	23.2	0.8	24.7	3.5	31.0	2.9	32.0	2.8	34.8	2.4	36.0	2.6	37.8	1.9	39.3	2.1
Tip protrusion (sn–prn)																
M	6.8	0.8	8.0	1.4	9.8	1.6	10.3	1.7	10.8	1.9	11.9	1.4	13.0	1.1	13.3	0.8
F	6.8	1.2	7.4	1.4	8.6	1.3	10.2	1.4	10.8	1.5	11.7	1.3	12.3	1.1	13.1	1.2
Root width (mf–mf)																
M													17.2	1.3	18.0	1.4
F													17.3	0.9	17.4	1.1
Alar base insertion width (ac–ac)																
M													28.3	1.5	28.3	1.4
F													27.7	1.5	28.3	1.3
Alar base width (sbal–sbal)																
M													16.7	1.3	17.4	1.3
F													16.1	1.0	16.8	1.3
Nostril floor width, left (sbal–sn,1)																
M													9.8	1.8	9.3	1.0
F													9.0	1.1	9.2	1.2
Columellar height, left (sn–c′,1)																
M													6.9	0.9	6.7	0.8
F													6.7	0.8	7.1	0.9
Nasal bridge inclination (degrees)																
M													27.6	4.1	28.2	4.5
F													29.0	4.2	28.9	3.1
Nasolabial angle (degrees)																
M													106.0	10.4	104.6	11.9
F													109.2	10.0	108.6	9.2
Indices																
Nasal index $\left(\dfrac{al–al \times 100}{n–sn}\right)$																
M	92.6	5.9	89.5	5.9	84.2	5.9	77.2	5.9	74.3	5.9	75.0	5.9	72.1	5.3	74.7	6.4
F	88.1	6.2	87.2	6.2	78.9	6.2	81.2	6.2	75.2	6.2	74.6	6.2	73.6	4.8	72.6	4.7
Columellar length-nasal tip protrusion index $\left(\dfrac{c^1–sn\ 1 \times 100}{sn–prn}\right)$																
M													53.7	7.1	50.4	6.3
F													54.7	5.2	54.4	7.2

All measurements and indices for children aged 0 days to 3 years are taken from the German data[19] adjusted for the North American population.[20] Data for 4- and 5-year-old children are the new North American norms (Farkas).

Table 59–7. Normal Values for Orolabial Measurements and Proportion Index in Children < 6 Years Old

Measurement/ Proportion and Sex	0–15 days		16 days– 6 mo		6–12 mo		1 yr		2 yr		3 yr		4 yr		5 yr	
	Mean	SD	Mean	SD	Mean	SD	Mean	SD	Mean	SD	Mean	SD	Mean	SD	Mean	SD
Measurements																
Upper lip height (sn–sto)																
M	10.8[a]	14.3	2.5[b]	15.5	3.2[b]	16.7	3.4[b]	18.5	2.1[b]	19.4	2.0[b]	19.4	1.1	19.5	1.4	
F	10.9[a]	13.9	2.2[b]	14.4	2.5[b]	16.1	2.6[b]	18.1	2.4[b]	18.6	1.9[b]	18.7	1.4	18.9	1.3	
Upper lip skin height (sn–ls)																
M													13.8	1.3	13.6	1.1
F													12.6	1.5	13.0	1.7
Lateral lip height, left (sbal–ls′)																
M													14.0	1.3	13.9	1.3
F													13.1	1.2	13.3	1.8
Upper vermilion height (ls–sto)																
M	6.8	1.3	6.6	1.3	7.2	1.3	8.0	1.3	8.1	1.3	8.0	1.3	7.5	1.0	7.6	0.9
F	6.2	1.3	6.5	1.3	6.9	1.3	8.1	1.3	8.1	1.3	7.5	1.3	7.6	1.1	7.5	1.1
Lower vermilion height (sto–li)																
M	5.4	1.6	6.3	1.6	6.8	1.6	8.1	1.6	8.4	1.6	7.8	1.6	7.0	1.3	7.4	1.1
F	6.6	1.6	6.2	1.6	6.8	1.6	7.8	1.6	7.8	1.6	7.2	1.6	6.9	1.3	7.1	1.3
Lower lip height (sto–sl)																
M													15.1	1.5	15.2	1.2
F													14.4	1.3	15.1	1.2
Mouth width (ch–ch)																
M	30.3	4.7	30.7	4.0	35.7	4.7	37.8	3.8	38.7	3.3	39.0	2.9	38.9	2.5	40.7	2.4
F	30.0	3.0	30.5	3.7	35.8	4.1	38.3	4.1	39.2	3.3	39.6	2.9	37.9	2.2	39.5	2.7
Upper lip inclination																
M													10.9	6.1	8.7	7.8
F													12.1	7.0	9.9	8.0
Indices																
Upper lip height-mouth width index $\left(\dfrac{\text{sn–sto} \times 100}{\text{ch–ch}}\right)$																
M	36.6	7.2	43.3	8.5	43.9	10.2	44.8	8.4	45.2	8.5	49.7	6.6	50.2	4.8	48.1	4.3
F	36.8	8.8	40.1	7.6	42.7	8.1	41.4	9.0	46.0	6.3	45.9	8.0	49.4	4.8	48.0	5.0
Lower-upper lip height index $\left(\dfrac{\text{sto–sl} \times 100}{\text{sn–sto}}\right)$																
M													77.4	6.1	78.3	5.9
F													77.7	8.8	80.5	7.3

[a]West German norms.[19]
[b]Czech norms.[21]
Unless otherwise noted, all measurements and indices for children aged 0 days to 3 years are taken from the German data[19] adjusted for the North American population.[20] Data for 4- and 5-year-old children are the new North American norms (Farkas).

Table 59–8. Normal Values for Ear Measurements and Proportion Index in Children < 6 Years Old

Measurement/ Proportion and Sex	0–15 days		16 days– 6 mo		6–12 mo		1 yr		2 yr		3 yr		4 yr		5 yr	
	Mean	SD	Mean	SD	Mean	SD	Mean	SD	Mean	SD	Mean	SD	Mean	SD	Mean	SD
Measurements																
Ear width, left (pra–pa, l)																
M	24.1	2.3	27.2	2.3	29.3	2.3	30.9	2.3	32.1	2.3	32.2	2.3	34.8	2.0	33.9	2.1
F	25.7	2.1	26.7	2.1	29.5	2.1	31.8	2.1	32.1	2.1	31.9	2.1	31.8	1.8	32.7	2.0
Ear length, left (sa–sba, l)																
M	35.4	3.7	40.7	4.5	47.5	3.4	49.8	2.5	52.4	3.1	51.8	3.4	52.9	2.7	53.6	2.8
F	34.8	3.3	37.9	4.2	45.8	3.9	48.7	3.1	51.1	3.0	51.1	2.9	50.1	2.7	51.0	2.6
Index																
Ear index, left $\left(\dfrac{\text{pra–pa} \times 100}{\text{sa–sba}}\right)$																
M	69.2	4.2	68.4	4.2	63.1	4.2	63.6	4.2	62.8	4.2	63.6	4.2	65.8	4.0	63.3	3.1
F	72.4	3.7	69.5	3.7	64.3	3.7	65.3	3.7	62.8	3.7	70.8	3.7	63.5	3.9	64.2	4.5

All measurements and indices for children aged 0 days to 3 years are taken from the German data[19] adjusted for the North American population.[20] Data for 4- and 5-year-old children are the new North American norms (Farkas).

of preoperative and postoperative changes in patients who have cleft lip and palate was first proposed two decades ago.[24, 25] Nevertheless, the present status of cleft lip surgery, and especially the problems connected with the cleft–lip nose, require more detailed studies of both the hard and soft tissues of the face. Uniformity in methods of examination and close cooperation between institutions[8, 26] would be the fastest way to eliminate the remaining problems in cleft lip treatment.

The measurements recommended in this chapter represent the minimal quantitative data that should be available before surgery and they provide the only objective information about the degree of soft tissue damage. They are essential for objective judgment of the postoperative results. The proportion indices are the best indicators of age-related changes in the growing face, revealing harmony, disharmony, or disproportion. Proportion indices examined at the completion of the facial maturation process are the most reliable indicators of the aesthetic quality of the face, a final product of natural forces influenced by surgical interventions.

ACKNOWLEDGMENTS. The development of the craniofacial norms in 4- and 5-year-old children was made possible by a grant from The Easter Seal Research Institute, Toronto. This manuscript was prepared with the assistance of the Medical Publications Department, The Hospital for Sick Children, Toronto.

References

1. Bardach J: Is there a need for clinical cleft lip and palate research? Plast Reconstr Surg 80:825–826, 1987.
2. Farkas LG, Munro IR, Kolar JC: Relationships of profile segment inclinations in the face of North American Caucasians. In Farkas LG, Munro IR (eds): Anthropometric Facial Proportions in Medicine. Springfield, IL: Charles C Thomas, 1987, pp 67–77.
3. Cohen MM, Jr: Syndromes with cleft lip and cleft palate. Cleft Palate J 15:306–328, 1978.
4. Bardach J, Salyer K: Surgical Techniques in Cleft Lip and Palate. Chicago: Year Book, 1987, pp 28–29, 127–128.
5. Stark RB, Ehrmann NA: The development of the center of the face with particular reference to surgical correction of bilateral cleft lip. Plast Reconstr Surg 21:177–192, 1958.
6. Lee ST: A new approach to bilateral cleft lip repair. Ann Acad Med Singapore 12:347–351, 1983.
7. Takahashi H, Maeda K: Reconstruction of the vermilion for bilateral complete cleft lip. Ann Acad Med Singapore 12:352–358, 1983.
8. Noordhoff MS: Standardization of protocols for multi-center research. Abstract Book, The First Asian Pacific Cleft Lip and Palate Conference, Singapore, April 15–19, 1988, p 97.
9. Farkas LG, Munro IR (eds): Anthropometric Facial Proportions in Medicine. Springfield, IL: Charles C Thomas, 1987.
10. Farkas LG, Hreczko TA, Deutsch CK: Objective assessment of standard nostril types—A morphometric study. Ann Plast Surg 11:381–389, 1983.
11. Farkas LG, Deutsch CK, Hreczko TA: Asymmetries in nostrils and the surrounding tissues of the soft nose—A morphometric study. Ann Plast Surg 12:10–15, 1984.
12. Lindsay WK, Farkas LG: The use of anthropometry in assessing the cleft–lip nose. Plast Reconstr Surg 49:286–293, 1972.
13. Farkas LG, Kolar JC, Munro IR: Geography of the nose: A morphometric study. Aesthetic Plast Surg 10:191–223, 1986.
14. Farkas LG, Lindsay WK: The columella in cleft lip and palate anomaly. In Huston JT (ed): Transactions of the Fifth International Congress of Plastic and Reconstructive Surgery, Melbourne, February 22–26, 1971. Melbourne: Butterworths, 1971, pp 373–381.
15. Farkas LG, Lindsay WK: Morphology of the adult face following repair of bilateral cleft lip and palate in childhood. Plast Reconstr Surg 47:25–32, 1971.
16. Farkas LG, Lindsay WK: Morphology of the adult face following repair of unilateral cleft lip and palate in childhood. Plast Reconstr Surg 52:652–655, 1973.
17. Farkas LG, Munro IR, Kolar JC: Linear proportions in above- and below-average women's faces. In Farkas LG, Munro IR (eds): Anthropometric Facial Proportions in Medicine. Springfield, IL: Charles C Thomas, 1987, pp 119–129.
18. Kolar J: Ethnic differences in facial proportions. In Farkas LG, Munro IR (eds): Anthropometric Facial Proportions in Medicine. Springfield, IL: Charles C Thomas, 1987, pp 19–28.
19. Hajnis K: Kopf-, Ohrmuschel- und Handwachstum. (Verwendung bei den Operationen der angeborenen Missbildungen und Unfallsfolgen.) Acta Univ Carol [Biologica] 19:277–294, 1974.
20. Csima A, Szathmáry T: Facial proportion indices in children less than 6 years old. In Farkas LG, Munro IR (eds): Anthropometric facial proportions in medicine. Springfield, IL: Charles C Thomas, 1987, pp 163–165.
21. Figalova P, Smahel Z: The growth of the skull and face in children from 3 months to 6 years of age (in Czech). Burians' Laboratory of Plastic Surgery. Praha (Czechoslovakia): Czechoslovak Academy of Science, 1972.
22. Farkas LG: Anthropometry of the Head and Face in Medicine. New York: Elsevier, 1981.
23. Peyton WT, Ritchie HP: Quantitative studies on congenital clefts of the lip. Arch Surg 33:1046–1053, 1936.
24. Farkas LG, Hajnis K, Kliment L: Coded surgical case history for cleft lip and cleft palate. A draft. Part I. Acta Chir Plast (Prague) 9:109–120, 1967.
25. Hajnis K, Farkas LG: Anthropological record for congenital developmental defects of the face (especially clefts). Acta Chir Plast (Prague) 11:261–267, 1969.
26. Fong PH, Ngim R, Lee ST: Measuring the cleft deformity. Abstract Book, The First Asian Pacific Cleft Lip and Palate Conference, Singapore, April 15–19, 1988, p. 93.

CHAPTER 60

Cleft Lip and Palate Research: Approaches at the Cellular and Molecular Level

Christopher A. Squier
and Kevin M. Kelly

The history of research in almost every scientific discipline has been an account of extending knowledge by explaining phenomena at ever more fundamental levels. Nowhere has this progress been more evident recently than in the biomedical sciences. In almost all areas, advances have been predicated on progress in the methods of investigation.

The development of the microscope in the seventeenth century revealed the structural organization of tissues and organs at a cellular level. This permitted Virchow, in 1858, to put forward the fundamental proposition that cells are also the units of disease.[1] Despite considerable improvements in the design of the light microscope in the eighteenth and nineteenth centuries, it was not until the electron microscope was developed in the middle of the twentieth century that the next significant advances occurred. The greatly improved resolution available through the use of electrons rather than light permitted visualization of structures within the cell. It became apparent that the similar patterns of cell organization in different tissues and organs in the body had a counterpart at the subcellular level. Cells in widely differing tissues had remarkably similar collections of intracellular components—the cell organelles.

Although light and electron microscopy permitted the identification and description of hitherto unrecognized structures, it was soon apparent that the ultimate causal mechanisms in biology resided at the molecular level. Specific molecules, in particular, proteins and nucleic acids, were found to have important functions in information storage and the determination of structure. Methods of examining these molecules have developed rapidly in recent decades, enabling molecules to be separated, characterized, and manipulated. Within the past 10 years, it has become possible to identify the genes and gene sequences responsible for the synthesis and control of many of these molecules. These discoveries have raised exciting possibilities for better understanding of the pathogenesis of various diseases and the ontogenesis of congenital deformities that may lead to prevention and improved treatment.

Our purpose here is to review briefly several of the experimental approaches currently being used to understand cleft lip and palate at the cellular and molecular levels. Consistent with the focus of this book, we offer a perspective for the clinician or scientist who is interested in relating these approaches to the clinical problem.

Approaches to the Diagnosis and Prevention of Clefting

The malformations associated with cleft lip or palate have been well characterized at the clinical and microscopic levels for more than half a century.[2, 3] However, little is known about the causes of clefts or the processes of development that bring about their manifestation. At one level, cleft lip or cleft palate can be thought of merely as the result of a failure of the primary or secondary palate to fuse properly. Although correct, this perspective belies the fact that this common phenotype may be produced by a variety of factors, because it seems reasonably certain that clefting is an etiologically heterogeneous disorder involving the influence of genetic and environmental factors (see Chap. 14). How these factors are related during development is currently an area of extensive investigation because there is only limited understanding of the mechanisms involved in the normal process, not to mention aberrant development. Approaches to the problem of clefting involve unraveling a complex sequence of events extending from the level of the gene to that of the organ. These sequences not only change with time but are also apparently subject to environmental modification.

Perhaps the most exciting new development is the ability to identify the gene or genes that code for the synthesis of growth factors and messengers. If the factors that direct and regulate growth can be identified, it will be possible to develop probes to recognize aberrations early in prenatal development.[4] There is growing evidence that cleft palate susceptibility is genetically based, perhaps involving genes associated with the major histocompatability loci.[5] The use of DNA probes to produce genetic and physical maps of chromosomes will undoubtedly have a profound effect on our understanding of the genetic basis of this congenital malformation. The identification of genes that contribute to cleft susceptibility and the control of normal palatal differentiation will be of enormous importance because these will represent the intersection of pathways of normal and aberrant development and provide a key to the understanding of congenital malformations.

Eventually it may even be possible to prevent a genetic defect by inserting a cloned normal gene into the germ line in place of the defect. However, it is important to recognize that although molecular genetic techniques now make it possible to localize and decode nucleotide base sequences, much work remains to be done to bridge the gap between recognition of the genetic factors associated with clefting and an understanding of the mechanisms leading to the malformation.

To begin unraveling the sequence of events leading to a cleft lip and palate it is necessary to work with an appropriate model. Studies using humans present so many confounding variables that it is extremely difficult if not impossible to assess the contribution of a particular factor to the process under investigation. Moreover, investigators are morally constrained from knowingly withholding optimal treatment from or administering detrimental treatment to patients. Thus, clinical studies create practical and ethical problems that are compounded when the events that are of interest are occurring in utero. Consequently, there has been a tendency to develop animal models that can simulate events in the human. Animals as varied as the alligator, chick, rat, and mouse have been used.[6] In this regard, specific strains of mice have been particularly useful because of the ease with which the normal processes of craniofacial development can be perturbed.

Clefts of the palate in animals can be induced so dependably and reliably with various teratogens administered during development that what was often a random event has become predictable and subject to controlled experimentation. However, as researchers seek to disentangle and analyze smaller and smaller components of the developmental process, it becomes desirable to work with a system less complex than the whole organism. Here, organ and tissue or cell culture can play an important role. The value of in vitro systems lies in the ability to manipulate the development process to identify components that can then be studied at the histologic, cellular, and molecular levels. It is now possible to maintain whole embryos in culture during development,[7] to isolate elements that are of interest (such as the palatal shelves), or simply to grow "sheets" of similar cells. The conditions of culture can be rigorously controlled, and it is possible, by using chemically defined media, to eliminate unknown influences that are introduced by culture fluids containing serum.

Nevertheless, there are many problems to be resolved in the use of culture systems for such purposes. For example, there is a need to distinguish the changes that may represent real developmental aberrations from artifacts due to culture.[8] A marked advantage of culture systems applied to the study of palatal development has been the ability to use human material,[9] but this use is now threatened by current ethical and political controversies.

There are obvious limitations to the use of any model system, whether animal or culture. It is important not only to be able to see the relations between observations at different levels but also to be aware of the limitations and drawbacks when extrapolating results obtained within an individual system. For example, to what extent can observations on the alligator palate in culture be applied to humans? The answer depends in part on the type of question that is being asked and, in particular, on the level at which an answer is expected. Organogenesis in reptiles and birds may not closely resemble that in mammals, but events at a cellular or molecular level can have considerable relevance.

By means of systems such as those previously mentioned, it has been possible to examine normal and abnormal development at increasingly fundamental levels. An example of this is the insight that has been gained into the process of palatal development. Descriptions of events at gross anatomic and histologic levels in humans and animals have been available for almost a century; however, these accounts did not offer mechanistic explanations of development. It was through the use of electron microscopy for examining cellular events that some of the key factors involved in palatal development were identified. Ultrastructural studies revealed the presence of subcellular organelles (lysosomes) in the epithelial lining of the palatal shelves that are able to bring about cellular breakdown.[11] This is a significant event because after contact of the shelves, the loss of epithelial covering at the line of fusion permits mesenchymal continuity across the palate. However, if development is disturbed sufficiently to prevent approximation of the palatal processes (for example, by culturing the palatal shelves singly), the lysosomal enzymes will still bring about epithelial disruption.[12] This is good evidence for the existence of a preexisting developmental "program" at a more fundamental level. An essential part of this program involves interactions between the epithelium and mesenchyme, as shown by Ferguson and Honig.[12] Their studies indicate that interference with epithelial-mesenchymal interactions prevents epithelial cell death. As a result, the palatal shelves fail to fuse, thereby creating a palatal cleft. Thus, the explanation for a developmental anomaly is extended to an even more fundamental level.

The nature of the messengers involved in epithelial-mesenchymal interactions as well as in other developmental interactions remains one of the most important yet elusive questions in biology. Probable messengers include soluble factors such as epidermal growth factor and transforming growth factor, but it is likely that components of the connective tissue matrix and epithelial basement membrane are also involved.[13] Isolation and purification of such factors open up a new level of investigation because it is then possible to produce specific antibodies with which to localize (and visualize) the distribution of these factors in tissues and organs. This may be done either at the light microscope level (immunohistochemistry) or the electron microscope level (immunocytochemistry), as we will illustrate later in this chapter.

Approaches to the Treatment of Clefts

So far, we have concentrated on cellular and molecular approaches toward understanding cleft lip or palate that will enable us to diagnose it prenatally and perhaps eventually to prevent it. Those possibilities are in the future. Meanwhile, much effort is still being directed toward the clinical treatment of the disorder. The major aim in treatment is to restore structure and function to as near normal levels as possible. This inevitably means surgery.

Paradoxically, the rapid growth of knowledge about cellular and molecular processes has created problems for those concerned with research on the treatment and management of disease and abnormal development. The new technology is fashionable, and often the uncritical use of sophisticated methods may disguise an approach that is not suited to the problem. Although the quantity of information obtained may be impressive, frequently the data are only descriptive, and to describe is not to explain or to understand. What is important is to be able to relate this increasingly more basic knowledge in a meaningful way to the original problem—that is, not to miss seeing the forest for the trees.

The manner in which new information is perceived and used depends on the perspective of the viewer. For the surgeon and clinician, an investigation of the clinical problem at the cellular and tissue level represents basic research that may seem to offer them little help in the care and treatment of a patient. For the molecular biologist, events at the level of the organ or organism represent incomprehensible interactions of the fundamental processes concerned. This difference in perspective makes it important to link the various levels of observation and explanation conceptually. Figure 60–1 represents a diagrammatic sequence of the spectrum between a clinical problem such as cleft palate and the different levels of investigation at which it can be approached. This sequence will be explored further in the remaining part of the chapter by discussing examples of experimental approaches to two surgical treatment problems.

Wound Contraction

One of the recognized problems following primary cleft palate surgery is inadequate growth of the midfacial skeleton. Wound healing following surgical closure mimics many of the processes that occur during embryologic development, yet we know very little about the cellular and molecular events of tissue repair and healing. Postnatal events are not always as amenable to study as those of the embryo, and animal models or culture systems that might be suitable for studying development are not always appropriate after differentiation has ceased and distinct species differences have emerged. For these reasons, many of the studies of cleft repair and healing have used mammals and frequently primates. Based on a series of experiments using the beagle, Kremenak and his colleagues postulated a causal relationship between wound contraction in the palatal mucosa following palatoplasty and developmental deformities in the adjacent facial skeleton.[14–17] It is important to understand the mechanism of contraction if we are to control or prevent this process. The section that follows uses this question as an example of applying different levels of investigation to approach a clinical problem.

The process of wound contraction in the oral mucosa has not been described as it has been in skin, where contraction frequently accompanies the healing of excisional wounds. In skin, maximum contraction coincides with the proliferation of fibroblasts and the production of collagen as granulation tissue is formed.[18–20] Contractility is mediated by a population of fibroblasts within the granulation tissue with a characteristic morphology (including the presence of intracellular microfilaments consisting of actin) and intercellular junctions.[21, 22] These are termed *contractile fibroblasts* or *myofibroblasts,* since myosin is also believed to be associated with the contractile process in these cells.[23–27]

Fibroblasts can be identified with the light microscope; however, it is not possible to distinguish the presence of cells containing actin filaments and intercellular junctions because these are only recognizable

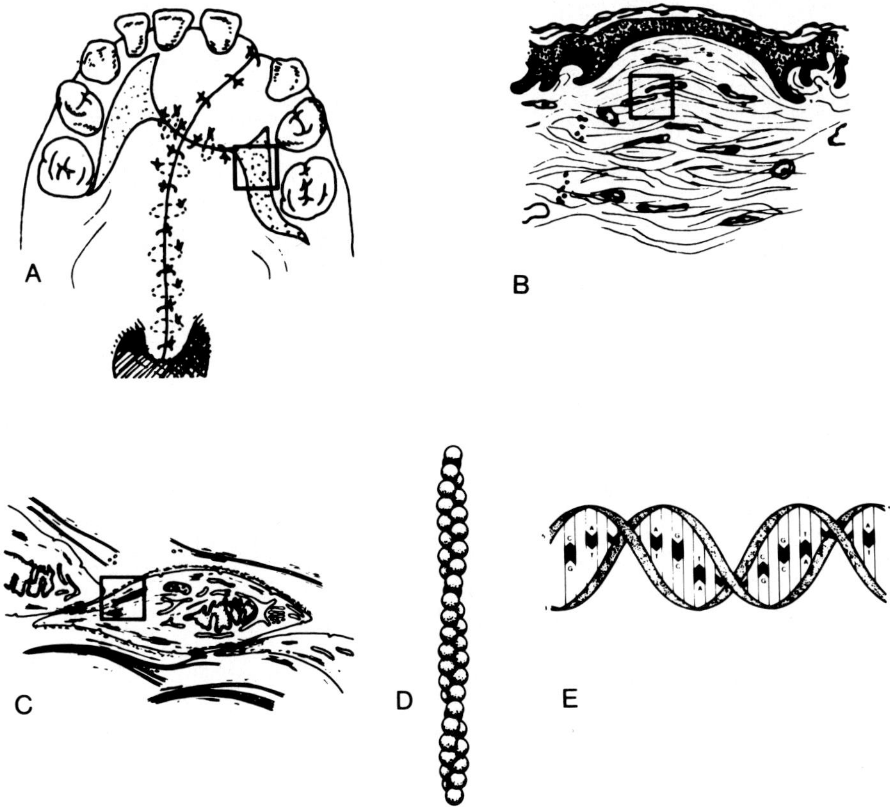

Figure 60–1 Diagram representing increasingly fundamental approaches to a clinical problem. Each boxed-in portion indicates the area illustrated in the next part of this figure. *A,* The repaired cleft (clinical level). *B,* Cell and tissue events in the healing wound (tissue level). *C,* Ultrastructure of cells (contractile fibroblasts) in the wound (cellular level). *D,* The actin molecule present in the contractile fibroblast (molecular level). *E,* DNA sequences that code for a protein such as actin (genetic level).

at the ultrastructural level. In an electron microscopic study of the healing mucoperiosteal wound in the beagle palate, cells with the characteristics of contractile fibroblasts were identified, including bundles of microfilaments and intercellular junctions (Fig. 60–2).[28] Quantification of the numbers of these cells in wounds at different stages of healing indicated that their frequency was related to the period of maximal contraction.[29] Such observations enable a gross phenomenon, wound contraction, to be interpreted in terms of a subcellular component, the intracellular microfilaments. However, precise identification requires the characterization of the microfilaments as the contractile protein actin, which cannot be accomplished by morphologic examination alone (in this case, electron microscopy).

As we have already mentioned, the identification of specific molecules has been greatly facilitated by the application of antibody techniques that permit their visualization. Thus, the presence of cells in the healing wound that stain immunochemically for actin indicates a potential for wound contraction (Fig. 60–3). In a young individual, wound contraction influences subsequent growth and results in morphologic abnormalities of the middle face. It is therefore possible to demonstrate the molecular basis for a process that is evident at a clinical level. Such results alone do not solve the clinical problem, but they do suggest several possibilities for therapy that might improve the outcome. One would be to alter the surgical procedures to avoid large granulating wounds adjacent to the alveolar arches. A possibility

that is being explored in our laboratories is to use cultured tissue grafts derived from the same patient to cover the wounds. Another approach is suggested by our finding that contractile fibroblasts are present in contracting palatal wounds. Contractile fibroblasts are responsive to the action of anticontractile agents such as theophylline and papaverine, which interfere with the actin contraction mechanism in these cells.[26] It is possible that local treatment of the healing wound with such agents could inhibit contraction sufficiently during the critical contractile phase to preclude the undesirable growth sequelae.

Bone Formation

An allied problem of current interest is the need to better understand the biologic conditions necessary to promote bone growth following soft tissue closure of the cleft.[30, 31] The processes by which bone cells lay down mineral in bone has been greatly elucidated by electron microscopic observations. These have demonstrated that small organelles, the matrix vesicles, are budded off by osteoblasts and serve as centers of calcification.[32] The major question that remains concerns the origin of these cells and the factors necessary to induce bone growth.

There have been various attempts to modify surgical procedures to provide conditions conducive to bone regeneration. Many of these procedures focus on providing periosteal continuity as a putative source of osteogenic cells.[33–35] However, the assertion that perios-

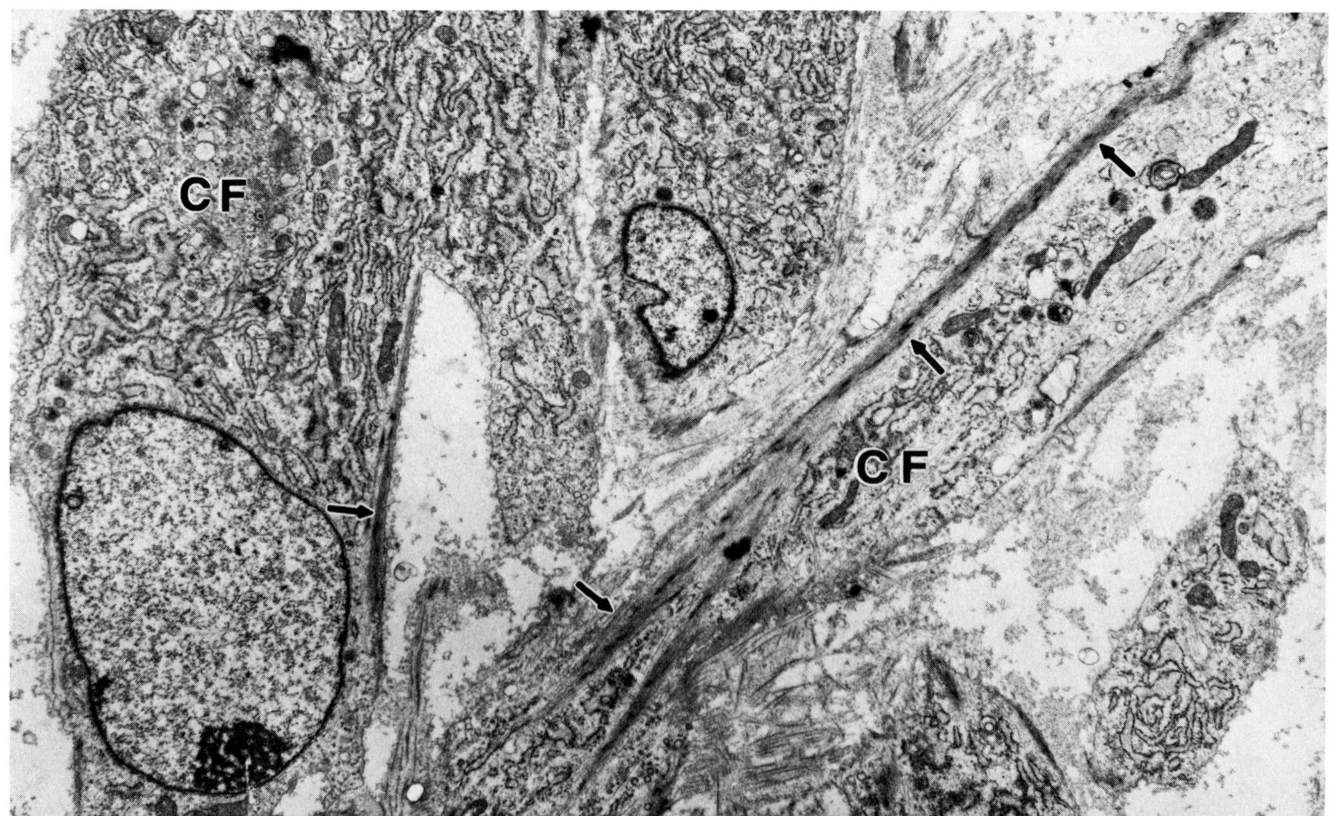

Figure 60–2 Several contractile fibroblasts (CF) in a healing wound at 5 days. Bundles of microfilaments are clearly evident (arrows), and the periodic densities along the filaments probably represent myosin (magnification × 8500).

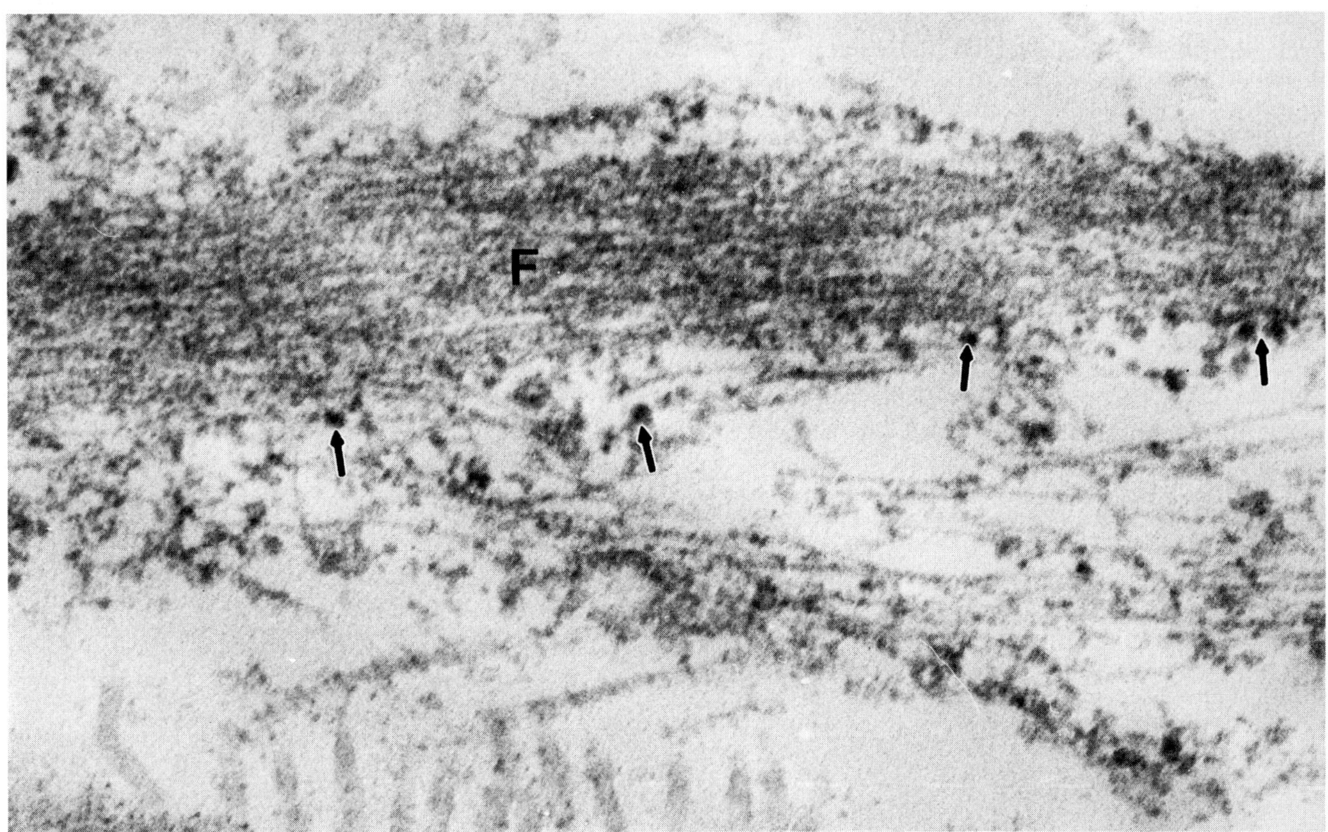

Figure 60–3 A high magnification electron micrograph of part of a contractile fibroblast from a palatal wound showing actin filaments (F), to which are bound particles (arrows) representing anti-actin antibodies (magnification × 160,000).[22]

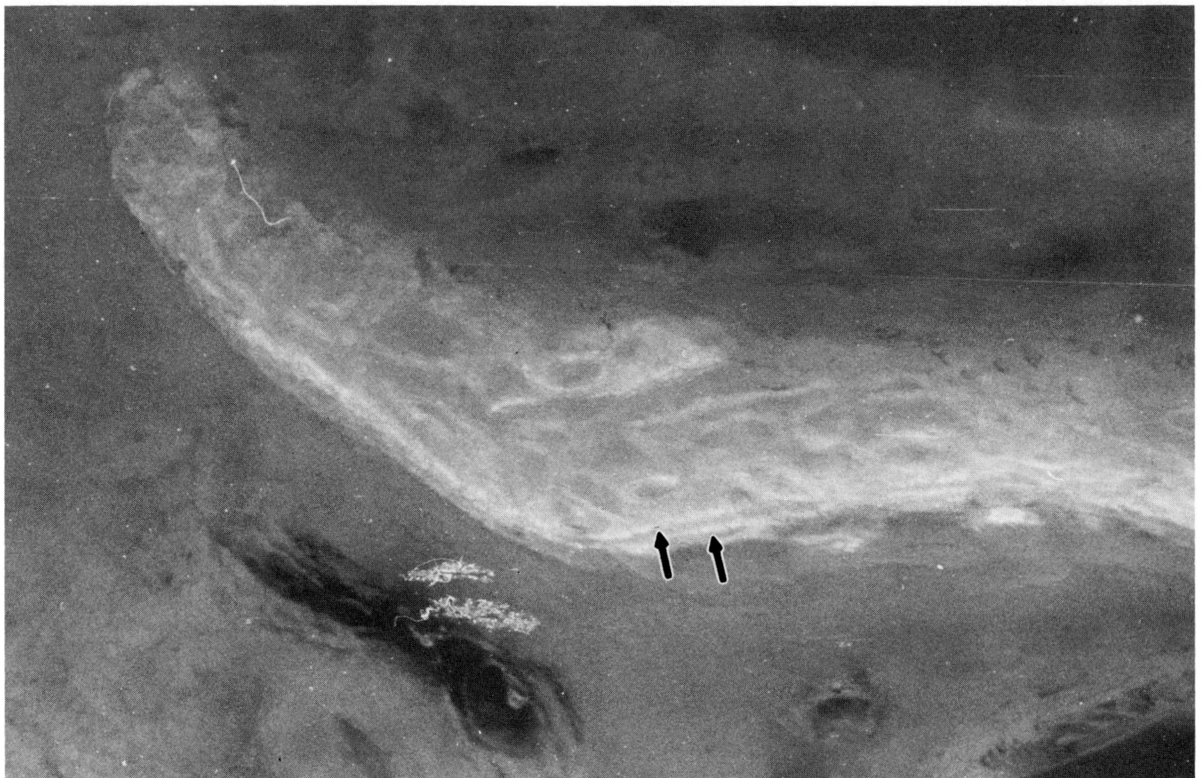

Figure 60–4 Micrograph taken using fluorescent microscope to show the sites of bone formation (arrows) in a healing beagle palate after sequential injection of a marker ("DCAF") (magnification × 25).

teal closure of bony defects is important for bone formation within the palatal cleft is still unproved.

Given the current availability and allure of molecular techniques, it might seem desirable to attempt to search for molecular messengers of the cells in the periosteum to assess their osteogenic potential. Although such studies might lead to a greater understanding of the periosteum, the findings will have limited relevance to surgical treatment unless it can be clearly demonstrated that periosteum does indeed play an essential role in bone growth after cleft repair. In the studies cited above, we have chosen to address this problem by first determining the role of periosteum taken from a variety of skeletal sites in bone growth in the palate.[30, 31] By means of a timed sequence of labeled bone markers, we have been able to obtain a dynamic picture of bone formation in the experimental situation (Fig. 60–4). Cellular events associated with bone growth are being monitored by electron microscopy.

The obvious sequel to such research would be to identify biologic messengers that might promote and direct osteogenic activity to restore structure and function at a clinical level. Unfortunately, there is still limited knowledge about the possible origins of bone cells and the factors necessary to bring about bone formation. Both osteoclasts and osteoblasts may have extraskeletal origins, the former from a monocyte-macrophage cell line, the latter from a local stromal cell, which could be situated in endosteum or periosteum. There also is controversy about the nature of the cytokines that might control bone cell activity and both specific factors, such as osteoclast-activating factor and human skeletal growth factor, and more widespread factors, such as interleukin 1 and tumor necrosis factor, may be involved.[36] The unraveling of the fundamental events controlling bone growth and bone remodeling obviously will have a significant impact on clinical treatment of craniofacial anomalies.

Conclusion

We have reviewed several of the current cellular and molecular approaches to cleft lip and palate research. The knowledge gained from investigations at the cellular and molecular levels will be reflected in a better understanding of developmental aberrations such as cleft lip and palate and subsequently may lead to improved treatment and eventually to prevention. However, the realization of clinical gains from experimental research rarely is immediate and never is guaranteed. The rate of progress is not rapid because the researcher is faced with complex processes that, even when proceeding normally, are as Runner says, ". . . among the best kept secrets in all of biology."[37]

ACKNOWLEDGMENTS. The authors are grateful to Dr. C. R. Kremenak for his critical reading of the manuscript. The work was supported by NIDR Grant No. DE05837–07.

References

1. Virchow R: Die Cellularpathologie. Berlin: Hirschwald, 1858.
2. Pohlmann G: A dissertation on the embryology of the face. Thesis. Leipzig, 1910.
3. Warbrick JG: The development of the nasal cavity and upper lip in the human embryo. J Anat 94:351, 1960.
4. Moore GE, Ivens A, Chambers J, et al: Linkage of an X chromosome cleft palate gene. Nature 326:91, 1987.
5. Goldman AS: Biochemical mechanism of glucocorticoid- and phenytoin-induced cleft palate. In Moscona AA, Monroy A (eds): Current Topics in Developmental Biology. Orlando: Academic Press, 1984.
6. Ferguson MWJ, Honig LS, Slavkin HC: Differentiation of cultured palatal shelves from alligator, chick and mouse embryos. Anat Rec 209:231, 1984.
7. Sadler TW, Horton WE, Hunter ES: Mammalian embryos in culture: A new approach to investigation of normal and abnormal developmental mechanisms. In Lash JW, Saxen L (eds): Developmental Mechanisms: Normal and Abnormal. New York: Alan R. Liss, 1985.
8. Neubert D, Blankenburg G, Lewandowski C, et al: Misinterpretations of results and creation of "artifacts" in studies on developmental toxicity using systems simpler than in vivo systems. In Lash JW, Saxen L (eds): Developmental Mechanisms: Normal and Abnormal. New York: Alan R. Liss, 1985.
9. Yoneda T, Pratt RM: Glucocorticoid receptors in palatal mesenchymal cells from the human embryo: Relevance to human cleft palate formation. J Craniofac Genet Dev Biol 1:411, 1981.
10. Abbott BD, Pratt RM: Human embryonic palatal epithelial differentiation is altered by retinoic acid and epidermal growth factor in organ culture. J Craniofac Genet Dev Biol 7:241, 1987.
11. Mato M, Aikawa E, Katahira M: Appearance of various types of glycosomes in the epithelia covering lateral palatine shelves during a secondary palate formation. Guinea J Med Sci 15:46, 1966.
12. Ferguson MJW, Honig S: Experimental fusion of the naturally cleft embryonic chick palate. J Craniofac Genet Dev Biol Suppl 1:323, 1985.
13. Fyfe D, Ferguson MW, Chiquete R: Tenascin distribution during palate development in mouse and chick embryos. J Dent Res 66:898, 1987.
14. Kremenak CR, Searls JC: Experimental manipulation of midfacial growth: A synthesis of five years of research at the Iowa Maxillofacial Growth Laboratory. J Dent Res 50:1488, 1971.
15. Olin WH, Morris J, Geil J, et al: Contraction of mucoperiosteal wounds after palate surgery in beagle pups. J Dent Res 53:378, 1974.
16. Kremenak CR: Physiological aspects of wound healing: Contraction and growth. Otolaryngol Clin North Am 17:437, 1984.
17. Kremenak CR, Seydel SK, Jakobsen JR: Cleft palate survey and maxillary growth: Methodological considerations in identifying a possible sex difference in treatment effect on beagles. In Burdi AR, Vig K (eds): Craniofacial Morphogenesis and Dysmorphogenesis. Sansibar, MI: Center for Human Growth and Development, 1988.
18. Abercrombie M, Flint MH, James DW: Collagen formation and wound contraction during repair of small excised wounds in the skin of rat. J Embryol Exp Morphol 2:264, 1954.
19. Dunphy JE: Wound Healing. New York: Medcom Press, 1974.
20. Peacock EE, Van Winkle W: Repair of skin wounds. In Peacock EE (ed): Wound Repair, 2nd ed. Philadelphia: Saunders, 1976, pp 54–79.
21. Dabelsteen E, Kremenak CR: Demonstration of actin in the fibroblasts of healing palatal wounds. Plast Reconstr Surg 62:419, 1978.
22. Squier CA, Leranth CS, Ghoneim S, et al: Electron microscopic immunochemical localization of actin in fibroblasts. Histochemistry 78:513, 1983.
23. Majno G, Gabbiani G, Hirschel BJ, et al: Contraction of granulation tissue in vitro: Similarity to smooth muscle. Science 173:548, 1971.
24. Gabbiani G, Majno G, Ryan GB: The fibroblast as a contractile cell: The myo-fibroblast. In Kulonen E, Pikkarainen J (eds): Biology of Fibroblast. New York: Academic Press, 1973, pp. 139–154.
25. Gabbiani G, Ryan GB, Lamelin J-P, et al: Human smooth muscle auto-antibody. Its identification as anti-actin antibody and a study of its binding to nonmuscle cells. Am J Pathol 72:473, 1973.
26. Ryan GB, Cliff WJ, Gabbiani G, et al: Myofibroblasts in human granulation tissue. Human Pathol 5:55, 1974.
27. Montandon D, D'Andiran G, Gabbiani G: The mechanism of wound contraction and epithelialization. Clinical and experimental studies. Clin Plast Surg 4:325, 1977.
28. Squier CA, Kremenak CR: Myofibroblasts in healing palatal wounds of the beagle dog. J Anat 130:585, 1980.
29. Ghoneim S, Squier CA, Slatter SE: Quantitation of contractile fibroblasts in healing palatal wounds. J Dent Res 58:1132, 1979.
30. Bardach J, Martin R, Mooney MP, et al: Bone formation in the canine palate following partial resection. In Dixon AD, Sarnat BG (eds): Normal and Abnormal Bone Growth: Basic and Clinical Research. New York: Alan R. Liss, 1985, pp 365–377, 1985.
31. Bardach J, Squier CA, Kelly KM: The role of periosteum in bone formation in the alveolus and palate following various surgical procedures (in press, 1989).
32. Irving JT: Interrelation of matrix lipids, vesicles and calcification. Fed Proc 35:109, 1976.

33. Skoog T. The use of periosteal flaps in the repair of the primary palate. Cleft Palate J 2:332, 1965.
34. Rintala A, Soivio A, Ranta R, et al: On the bone-forming capacity of periosteal flap in surgery for cleft lip and palate. Scand J Plast Reconstr Surg 8:58, 1974.
35. Azzolini A, Riberti C, Rosselli D, et al: Tibial periosteal graft in repair of cleft lip and palate. Ann Plast Surg 9:105, 1982.
36. Marks SC, Popoff SN: Bone cell biology: The regulation of development, structure and function in the skeleton. Am J Anat 183:1, 1988.
37. Runner MN: Epigenetically regulated genomic expressions for shortened stature and cleft palate are regionally specific in the 11 day mouse embryo. J Craniofac Genet Dev Biol Suppl 2:137, 1986.

CHAPTER 61

Expanding the Perception of Cleft Morphology: Anthropometric Studies of Body Growth, Size, and Form

Kevin M. Kelly

The growth, size, and form of each individual result from interactions between the individual's genetic endowment and the environment, beginning at conception and ending at death. Orofacial clefts are one manifestation of these interactions. Clefting occurs when some factor or factors alter the normal development and growth of the lip, palate, and maxilla. There has been considerable debate in the literature about whether these factors are expressed in other aspects of the growth patterns of affected children. This debate is important because the answer to this question has significant implications on efforts to improve the treatment of patients with clefts and on efforts to understand the etiology of clefting.

A few studies have attempted to determine whether children with clefts exhibit normal growth patterns and, if not, what might be the causes of abnormal growth. For example, there are some indications that growth size is impeded. Because the very nature of the cleft raises apprehensions about feeding difficulties, many studies of physical development in children with clefts address concerns about nutrition therapy rather than etiology.

This chapter is intended to review anthropometric studies of body growth in patients with orofacial clefting. This review recounts the considerable somatic variability that has been observed among patients with clefts and reveals that these observations are a collection of diverse and often contradictory findings. The reasons for this heterogeneity as well as alternate methods for exploring physical development and somatic variability in children with clefts are discussed.

Studies of Body Growth in Individuals with Clefts

Studies of general body growth among individuals with orofacial clefts can be roughly divided into three categories. The first category focuses exclusively on birth weights associated with clefting.[1-8] The articles in this first category are generally the earliest reports. They begin with an article in 1959 by Lutz,[1] although more recent epidemiologic studies also fall into this category.[2, 3] The second category contains studies in which the growth process has been followed from birth into the initial months or years of childhood.[9-13] In these studies, the investigators address a specific clinical concern: the potential necessity for therapeutic intervention. In addition, these studies test the early reports of low birth weights in newborns with clefts.[1, 4-6] The studies in the third category,[14-20] like those of the second, examine physical development following birth. However, they differ from studies in the second group in two important elements: They focus on growth through adolescence to adulthood, and, with the exception of Dahl's 1970 monograph,[14] they address the role of hormonal deficiencies in the etiology of clefting.

In 1959, Lutz published the first documentation of body size associated with clefting.[1] Lutz found that, with the exception of the significantly lower mean birth weight of females with an isolated cleft palate, the birth weights of children with clefts were comparable to those of normals. Similar findings were observed in later surveys by Fraser and Calnan,[4] Drillen et al,[5] and Bonaiti et al.[2] On the other hand, a 1960 report by the Toronto Research Institute of the Hospital for Sick Children[6] and a 1967 study conducted by Rintala and Gylling[7] found lower mean birth weights in infants with cleft lip and/or cleft palate. Other investigators have found no differences in birth weights between children with clefts and normals.[3, 8]

A number of investigators[9-13] have called attention to the need for careful monitoring of physical growth in children with clefts during early childhood. These studies suggest a pattern of impaired growth that begins at birth. Avedian and Ruberg's preliminary study of 37 infants with cleft palate indicates that full recovery of perinatal weight loss occurs by 6 months of age.[9] However, these data are unique in providing this assessment. All other indications are that any recovery occurs during a period of years rather than months.[10, 11, 12]

In response to the birth weight findings in the 1960 Toronto report[6] and those described by Drillen et al,[5] Ranalli and Mazaheri[10] examined the growth of children with clefts in a longitudinal study of the heights and weights of 279 propositi. The data were recorded at 6-month intervals from birth to 6 years of age. These investigators divided the children into four groups: (1) isolated cleft lip (CLO), (2) unilateral cleft lip and palate (uCLP), (3) bilateral cleft lip and palate (bCLP), and (4) isolated cleft palate (CPO). By dividing the patient population into these groups, the authors were able both to assess the effects of the severity of the cleft on growth and to compare the growth differences among different cleft types.

The children with clefts studied by Ranalli and Mazaheri, unlike the affected infants in the Toronto report and the Drillen et al study, were a little longer and heavier at birth than the control group of unaffected children. However, Ranalli and Mazaheri found no significant differences in either height or weight data between the cleft groups and normals from birth to 6 years of age. Nor did they find any differences among cleft types; thus they concluded that the severity of the cleft was not a factor. However, the authors suggest that children with clefts experience a growth lag following birth but that by 3 years of age they have caught up with the norm. Ranalli and Mazaheri attribute this temporary growth lag to "early feeding difficulties, a tendency to frequent upper respiratory infections, and repeated hospitalization for lip and/or palate surgery."[10]

Seth and McWilliams evaluated weight gain from birth to 2 years of age in a longitudinal study of 77 children with at least a cleft palate.[11] In this study, the authors combined data from children with either cleft lip and palate or an isolated cleft palate. Weights were recorded at monthly intervals from birth to 12 months of age and then every other month until age 2. Monthly weights were compared to normative data for each gender. At birth, the mean weight of females with cleft palates did not differ significantly from that of normal females. On the other hand, the males in the Seth and McWilliams cleft palate group were significantly heavier at birth than normals; the authors do not regard this finding as clinically significant because the difference was less than one-quarter of a kilogram. However, in the months following birth, the mean weights of the children with clefts began to lag behind normals to such an extent that "at least 71% of both males and females had lower relative percentile weights at 20 to 24 months than they had at birth."[11]

Jensen and her colleagues[12] presented data on the weights and lengths of 411 male and 267 female Danish children with clefts. The patients were divided into three groups according to cleft type: (1) isolated cleft lip (CLO), (2) combined cleft lip and palate (CLP), and (3) isolated cleft palate (CPO). Within this classification, the patients were further assigned to one of four grades for both cleft lip and cleft palate; these grades described the extent of the cleft. Birth weight and birth length were obtained from the birth registry. Weight and length measurements were made by the authors at 9 weeks and 22 months of age during their examination of the children.

In comparison with normals, only CPO males had significantly lower birth weights, whereas only CPO females exhibited significantly shorter birth lengths. At 9 weeks of age, the CLO females were the only group whose mean weight was not significantly less than that of normals. By 22 months, the mean weight of CLO males was again within normal values, but the mean weights of both males and females with either CLP or CPO remained significantly below normal. The mean length of 9-week-old CLP males was significantly re-

duced compared with that in other subgroups. By 22 months of age, this was also true for both males and females with CLP or CPO. In general, weight and length in CLP and CPO children were lower compared with these parameters in the CLO children. The authors indicate that these growth lags are associated with the severity of the cleft and suggest that they are most plausibly explained by feeding difficulties, recurrent infections, and surgery. They conclude that their "extended method of classification might render possible a selection of high-risk groups and improve differentiation of surgical methods."[12]

In sharp contrast to the findings described above, Felix-Schollaart[13] recently reported finding few significant differences between the lengths and weights of normals and groups of children with isolated cleft lip, combined cleft lip and palate, and isolated cleft palate who were measured at 3-month intervals from birth to 2.5 years of age. The sole indication of impaired growth in this study was the discovery that CLP males were significantly shorter than CLP females and normal males. Furthermore, Felix-Schollaart noted that the occurrence of feeding difficulties, intestinal disorders, and respiratory infections among the cleft groups did not differ significantly from the rates observed among normals.

Dahl's study[14] of 272 Danish adult males with clefts is one of the more comprehensive examinations of the morphologic variation associated with clefting. Although this study focuses on craniofacial morphology, the data are more comprehensive and include direct anthropometric measures of standing height, radius length, tibia length, knee width, and wrist width, as well as radiographic measurements of radius length and width (in addition to standard cephalometric analyses, which will not be discussed here).

Dahl found several significant differences between the anthropometric measurements taken in patients with each cleft type (isolated cleft lip, isolated cleft palate, combined cleft lip and palate) and in normal controls. The mean height, radius length, and knee width in the three cleft types were significantly less than these measurements in unaffected adult males. Among males with isolated cleft lip (N = 62) and those with combined cleft lip and palate (N = 153), height, radius length, and knee width were the only aspects of somatic development significantly different from normals. However, among the 57 males with isolated cleft palate, Dahl found in addition to the differences in height, radius length, and knee width, significant reductions in the length of the tibia. Dahl made no attempt to determine whether these measures differed among the cleft types. In fact, the measurements are mentioned by Dahl only in passing, although they have been placed somewhat in context by Jensen et al.[15] However, the fact remains that the Dahl study has documented a number of differences in cleft morphology that have yet to be examined in other groups.

The timing of height and weight deficits was investigated by Hunter and Dijkman[16] in a cross-sectional study of 45 pairs of 3- to 17-year-old same-gender twins discordant for cleft of the lip and/or palate. They found that between 3 and 10 years of age, the affected twin was not (on average) shorter or lighter than his or her unaffected twin. However, after 10 years of age, both the height and weight of the cleft twin tended to fall below that of the normal twin. The authors conclude that the data are consistent with linkage between "the endocrine controls of maturation at puberty" and the genesis of cleft lip and/or palate.[16] The significance of the Hunter and Dijkman study lies in its documentation of the timing of the deficits. Although Dahl had previously noted significantly reduced adult heights in persons with clefts relative to normals, the Hunter and Dijkman data first suggested that this diminution resulted from events in adolescence and was not the result of feeding difficulties, infections, or surgical interventions experienced in the months immediately following birth.

The prevalence of growth hormone deficiencies among cleft children exhibiting impaired growth was explored by Rudman et al.[17] These investigators measured the heights of 200 children with cleft lip or cleft palate who possessed no other "apparent congenital anomaly." The children ranged in age from 7 to 14 years. Rudman and his colleagues found that the heights of 60% of the 43 children with cleft lip only, 62% of the 114 children with cleft lip and palate, and 56% of the 43 children with isolated cleft palate were below the fiftieth percentile for their age group; 14%, 12%, and 12%, respectively, fell below the third percentile for their age group. After the anthropometric assessment, tests for endogenous growth hormone function were performed on the 25 children falling below the third percentile for height. A small number of children with growth hormone deficiencies were found in each cleft type, but the numbers were insufficient to reach any conclusions about whether one cleft type was more frequently affected than another. However, the data[17] suggest that children with cleft lip or cleft palate are 40 times more likely to experience growth hormone deficiency than noncleft children.

Several recent studies[13, 18–20] have addressed the importance of hormonal deficiencies in the etiology of clefting. Their approach is to elaborate on the growth patterns of children with clefts and assess the likelihood that hormonal deficiencies have produced the observed patterns. Duncan et al[18] observed differences among the growth patterns of 31 children with isolated cleft palate and 34 children with clefts of the lip with or without cleft palate (CL[P]). Sequential height measurements were recorded at varying intervals for a group of patients of both genders who ranged in age from newborn to approximately 20 years old. These investigators found that children with CPO tended to have lower height percentile norms as they got older, whereas CL(P) children had a bimodal pattern that separated them into a short group (below the fiftieth percentile) and a tall group (above the seventieth percentile). No explanation was offered for the CL(P) data except for the suggestion that something has interfered with the "usual genetic determination of height."[18] However, Duncan et al noted that the CPO growth pattern "nearly simulates that of patients with isolated growth hormone deficiency."[18]

Jensen et al concluded that growth delays observed in their semilongitudinal yearly survey of 48 males with combined cleft lip and palate resulted from extrinsic factors (feeding difficulties, infection, surgery), not from growth hormone deficiencies.[13] These investigators analyzed measurements of height, radius length, and skeletal maturity recorded when the subjects were between 6.5 and 19.5 years of age. They found that CLP males continued to be smaller than unaffected males throughout adolescence, although these differences were significant at only three ages: 8.5, 9.5, and 10.5 years. Differences between the radius lengths of their normal controls and the children with clefts were significant at 14.5 and 15.5 years. At each of these ages, the mean radius length of the children with clefts was less than that of the normals. In contrast to the findings of Dahl,[2] radius length was not comparatively small in the "adult" (19.5 years old) portion of the group. The CLP males had a less noticeable growth spurt during puberty. However, their total growth period was longer, and thus they were able to catch up with the normal control group. However, at no time during the growth period did any of the cleft children exhibit an especially low growth rate. Thus the authors conclude that a growth hormone deficiency is not the likely cause of the growth retardation.

Two recent cross-sectional studies conducted by Bowers and her associates[19, 20] attempted to test the hypothesized association of clefting with growth hormone regulation. They considered the degree to which the heights and body mass indices of children with clefts varied from normals as a function of cleft type, gender, and age. The body mass index (BMI), calculated as "weight in kilograms divided by the square of height in meters," was included in their analyses as an economical parameter for relating weights and heights. Height and BMI data were converted to "z scores," which express the values in terms of standard deviations from norms and allow comparisons among children of different ages.

In their initial study,[19] the authors evaluated height and body mass data in 252 children with clefts who ranged in age from 2 to 18 years. Patients with known genetic disorders "that only sometimes include clefts" as well as "patients with diagnosis of stenoses, malignancies or trauma" were excluded from the study. Included among these 252 patients were 43 individuals with Pierre Robin syndrome, Treacher Collins syndrome, hemifacial microsomia, or branchial arch syndrome. Also included were five patients with "other facial clefts." With the exception of ten individuals with Pierre Robin syndrome and isolated cleft palate, the "syndromic" data did not figure into the authors' discussion. Thus, in effect, the study group included 219 children divided according to gender and assigned to one of four cleft types: (1) isolated cleft lip (N = 20), (2) isolated cleft palate (N = 67), (3) unilateral cleft lip and palate (N = 87), and (4) bilateral cleft lip and palate (N = 44).

Bowers et al[19] found that children with unilateral CLP and those with CPO were significantly shorter than the norm. Specifically, males with unilateral CLP as well as those with CPO were significantly shorter and thinner (reduced BMI) than normal, whereas females with CPO differed from normals only in their shorter height. The heights and BMIs of the remaining subgroups were all within normal limits. The authors concluded that the differences in body growth observed among patients with different cleft types suggest that the "congenital metabolic variation contributes to the development of orofacial clefting and influences postnatal development in certain types of clefts."[19]

In the second study[20] Bowers et al expanded on their assessment of growth status by examining age-related differences in height and body mass data among the 144 children identified in the initial study who possessed either an isolated cleft palate or a unilateral cleft lip and palate. In addition to the original categorization by cleft type and gender, the children were divided into three age groups: the first group comprised children aged 2 years 0 months to 7 years 11 months; the second, 8 years 0 months to 13 years 11 months; and the third, 14 years 0 months to 18 years 11 months. The authors chose the time intervals "to approximate the expected times of adrenarche and gonarche."[20]

Although somewhat constrained by the statistical limitations inherent in working with a small number of observations, the authors offer the following interpretations. On average, uCLP males were shorter and thinner in childhood but demonstrated some recovery in adolescence. The average height and body mass of CPO males fell below the male norms as well as the z scores of uCLP males. Furthermore, the authors indicated that adolescent catch-up was less evident in CPO males than in males with uCLP. Similarly, CPO females were shorter than normal and tended, on average, to be shorter than uCLP females. Prior to age 8, the average height of uCLP females did not differ significantly from that of normal females. However, after age 8, the heights of uCLP females tended to decline relative to the female norms. Body mass in CPO and uCLP females was not significantly altered. Based on the findings reported in this and previous studies, Bowers et al reached the not unanticipated conclusion that the "alteration in growth status is associated with age group as well as sex and diagnosis."[20]

Discussion

The preceding review of the literature reveals the diverse and contradictory nature of the morphologic variation observed among patients with clefts. These observations represent the investigative efforts of researchers in the Netherlands, France, Denmark, Great Britain, Canada, and the United States and, as such, attest to the certain though still undefined tendency toward abnormal physical development in children with clefts.

Researchers have tended to conclude that factors such as poor nutrition, increased rates of upper respiratory and middle ear infections, and surgical interventions are the underlying causes of any abnormal growth pattern observed in children with clefts.[10-13, 15] However, some investigators[16-20] see patterns in their data that suggest that there is continued expression of the factors responsible for clefting. Thus, there is general agreement about the need for careful monitoring of the physical development of these children. The groups at risk for impaired physical development and the extent of that risk remain open to debate.

When attempting to explain these diverse and contradictory findings, all factors pertaining to the size, treatment, and ethnicity of the patient samples should be considered. Given the differences in the methodologies of these studies, it is apparent that further generalizations are unwarranted. However, this cursory account of these studies reveals much about the dominant clinically based perception of the morphology of patients with clefts, which may well be the reason for the heterogeneous results presented by these studies.

During the past several decades, researchers have proposed a number of systems for characterizing the morphology of orofacial clefts. Each system has been designed to categorize variability as well as to simplify the recording of the various manifestations of clefting. Although each of the anthropometric studies was in part an attempt to discern the patterns of growth, all of the methodologies employed relied on these clinical characterizations of the cleft to define the groups under study.

Shprintzen et al[21] have raised serious questions about the clinical implications of broad categorical terms such as *cleft palate child*. From a clinical perspective, the cleft classifications address those aspects of morphology that are most important for correcting the anomaly—namely, those features that characterize the structure and anatomy of the face and mouth. However, an appreciation of the underlying etiologies of a disorder is fundamental to proper genetic counseling and proper patient prognosis and treatment (see Chapter 15).[22] Orofacial clefts have long been acknowledged to have a variety of etiologies that exhibit teratogenic as well as genetic components (see Chapter 14). It is extremely important not to confuse "clinically homogeneous groupings" with "etiologically homogeneous groups." The orofacial focus of the classifications ignores other aspects of morphology that—although not directly involved in treatment—represent the products of the same developmental process that resulted in the cleft.

There are good ontogenetic reasons for thinking that at least some children with clefts might be smaller than normal. Recent genetic analyses[23, 24] suggest that more than one-third of the cases of nonsyndromic CL(P) arise from a single major locus. As Wright notes, most genes affect many aspects of the phenotype.[25] This is true for gene products such as the growth factors that have come under increased scrutiny in the search for a genetic basis for clefting[17–20] and whose expression or nonexpression affects general body growth and morphology as well as growth and morphology of the face and head.[26] Thus, the single major locus hypothesis suggests that a substantial proportion of the CL(P) population will share other forms of morphologic variation.

Although clinicians are well aware of how anthropometric measurements can be used to monitor physical development, they are generally unfamiliar with how these data might be applied to partition morphologic variation. When used in combination with multivariate methods of analysis, anthropometric measurements have proved to be an important tool in understanding the etiology and expression of an extensive number of genetic and congenital disorders.[27] Unfortunately, the methodologies applied to the study of body growth and form in cleft populations have, to date, provided investigators with little latitude for new groupings.

Multivariate statistical methods are essential for the identification and characterization of these new taxa. For example, cluster analysis was designed specifically to separate objects into groups (clusters) suggested by the data rather than defined a priori. Given the fact that clefting is etiologically heterogeneous, an empirically derived classification of individuals offers several attractions. On the other hand, discriminant analysis can be used to reveal linear combinations of variables (discriminant functions) that highlight the differences among groups designated by the investigator. These discriminant functions can then be used to classify unknown individuals. Protocols employing these statistical methods would enable researchers to redivide as well as subdivide clinically meaningful and useful taxa in an attempt to identify etiologically homogeneous units.

The recognition that more appropriate methods exist for characterizing the physical development and somatic variability of children with clefts is the starting point for the more difficult task of deciding what type of variability might be important. There is a great need for concentration on these types of studies. Clefting cannot be looked on as an isolated craniofacial anomaly. Investigators must be prepared to assess the symmetry and proportions of the body as well as those of the head and face. Descriptions of standard anthropometric measurements and proper measurement techniques[28, 29] and discussions of appropriate statistical methods[30–34] are readily available. In fact, Meaney and Farrer[27] provide an extensive compilation of anthropometric measurements that have been successfully applied to other genetic and congenital disorders. However, the measurements appropriate for characterizing the somatic variability associated with clefting are currently unknown. Therefore, the success of efforts to expand our perception of cleft morphology will depend on cooperation among physicians, geneticists, epidemiologists, and anthropologists.

References

1. Lutz KR: Birth weights in clefts. Cleft Palate Bull 9:47, 1959.
2. Bonaiti C, Briad ML, Feingold J, et al: An epidemiological and genetic study of facial clefting in France. I. Epidemiology and frequency in relatives. J Med Genet 19:8, 1982.
3. Owens JR, Jones JW, Harris F: Epidemiology of clefting. Arch Dis Child 60:521, 1985.
4. Fraser GR, Calnan JS: Cleft lip and palate: Seasonal incidence, birth weight, birth rank, sex, site, associated malformations and parental age. Arch Dis Child 36:420, 1961.
5. Drillen CM, Ingram TTS, Wilkinson EM: The Causes and Natural History of Cleft Lip and Palate. Baltimore: Williams & Wilkins, 1966.
6. Cox MA (ed): The Cleft Lip and Palate Research Centre: A Five Year Report 1955–1959. Toronto: Hospital for Sick Children, 1960.
7. Rintala AE, Gylling U: Birth weight of infants with cleft lip and palate. Scand J Plast Recontr Surg 1:109, 1967.
8. Ingalls IH, Taube IE, Klingberg MA: Cleft lip and palate: Epidemiologic considerations. Plast Reconstr Surg 34:1, 1964.
9. Avedian L, Ruberg RL: Impaired weight gain in cleft palate infants. Cleft Palate J 17:24, 1980.
10. Ranalli DN, Mazaheri M: Height-weight growth of cleft children, birth to six years. Cleft Palate J 8:400, 1975.
11. Seth AK, McWilliams BJ: Weight gains in children with cleft palate from birth to two years. Cleft Palate J 25:146, 1988.
12. Jensen BL, Kreiborg S, Dahl E, et al: Cleft lip and palate in Denmark, 1976–1981: Epidemiology, variability, and early somatic development. Cleft Palate J 25:258, 1988.
13. Felix-Schollaart B: Solitary, Non-syndromic Cleft Lip and/or Palate. A Comparison Between Cleft Lip, Cleft Lip and Palate and Cleft Palate on Epidemiologic Characteristics and Growth. Amsterdam: Rodopi, 1989.
14. Dahl E: Craniofacial morphology in congenital clefts of the lip and palate. Acta Odontol Scand 28, Suppl 57, 1970.
15. Jensen BL, Dahl E, Kreiborg S: Longitudinal study of body height, radius length and skeletal maturity in Danish boys with cleft lip and palate. Scand J Dent Res 91:473, 1983.
16. Hunter WS, Dijkman DJ: The timing of height and weight deficits in twins discordant for cleft of the lip and/or palate. Cleft Palate J 14:158, 1977.
17. Rudman DR, Davis GI, Priest JH, et al: Prevalence of growth hormone deficiency in children with cleft lip or palate. J Pediatr 93:378, 1978.
18. Duncan PA, Shapiro LR, Soley RL, et al: Linear growth patterns in patients with cleft lip or palate or both. Am J Dis Child 137:159, 1983.
19. Bowers EJ, Rosario FM, Whitaker LA, et al: General body growth in children with clefts of the lip, palate, and craniofacial structure. Scand J Plast Recontr Surg 21:7, 1987.
20. Bowers EJ, Rosario FM, Whitaker LA, et al: General body growth in children with cleft palate and related disorders: Age differences. Am J Phys Anthropol 75:503, 1988.
21. Shprintzen RJ, Siegel-Sadewitz VL, Amato J, et al: Anomalies associated with cleft lip, cleft palate or both. Am J Med Genet 20:585, 1985.
22. Jones MC: Etiology of facial clefts: prospective evaluation of 428 patients. Cleft Palate J 25:16, 1988.
23. Chung CS, Bixler D, Watanabe I, et al: Segregation analysis of cleft lip with or without cleft palate: A comparison of Danish and Japanese data. Am J Hum Genet 39:603, 1986.
24. Marazita ML, Spence MA, Melnick M: Major gene determination of liability to cleft lip with or without cleft palate: A multiracial view. J Craniofac Genet Dev Biol Suppl 2:89, 1986.
25. Wright S: Genic and organismic selection. Evolution 34:825, 1980.
26. Tanner JM: Foetus into Man: Physical Growth from Conception to Maturity. Cambridge: Harvard University Press, 1978.
27. Meaney FJ, Farrer JA: Clinical anthropometry and medical genetics: A compilation of body measurements in genetic and congenital disorders. Am J Med Genet 25:343, 1986.
28. Weiner JS, Lourie JA (eds): Practical Human Biology. New York: Academic Press, 1981.
29. Lohman TG, Roche AF, Martorell R (eds): Anthropometric Standardization Reference Manual. Champaign, IL: Human Kinetics Books, 1988.
30. Seal H: Multivariate Statistical Analysis for Biologists. New York: Wiley, 1964.
31. Sneath PHA, Sokal RR: Numerical Taxonomy. San Francisco: W.H. Freeman, 1973.
32. Van Vark GN, Howells WW (eds): Multivariate Statistical Methods in Physical Anthropology. Dordrecht: D. Reidel, 1984.
33. Preus M, Fraser FC: A methodology for establishing a diagnostic index for syndromes of unknown etiology. Clin Genet 10:249, 1976.
34. Preus M: Numerical classification of syndromes. Hosp Prac 20:111, 1985.

Correction of Skeletal Defects and Deformities Associated with Cleft Lip and Palate

CHAPTER 62

Planning Orthognathic Surgery

Barry H. Grayson

Planning the skeletal, soft tissue, and dental correction of craniofacial deformities requires careful collection of data from various sources including the patient's description or perception of his problem (chief complaint), medical and dental history, clinical examination, analysis of medical photographs, cephalometric analysis, examination of the panoramic or dental radiographs, and evaluation of dental study models.

Chief Complaint

The patient's report of his own problem provides vital information to the clinician. It should direct attention to the patient's perceived needs, which may or may not be those that are most obvious to the clinician. Careful listening during the interview and the ensuing dialogue with the patient helps to assess the patient's motivation and expectations.

Medical and Dental History

Does the patient have medical risk factors that would contraindicate surgical reconstruction? A review of the patient's medical history should alert the clinician to, or rule out, potential medical problems. Does the periodontal and restorative status, past and present, suggest that the patient is a candidate for preoperative orthodontic therapy? Does the patient provide evidence that he is capable of maintaining a level of oral hygiene and health that is acceptable for the postoperative period? Periodontal disease, periapical pathology, and carious lesions must be corrected before combined surgical-orthodontic therapy is begun.

Clinical Examination

The patient should first be examined in a neutral position with the Frankfort horizontal parallel to the floor and with the teeth and condyles in centric occlusion (teeth in maximum intercuspation). The forehead and orbits are examined to rule out eyelid ptosis or any disparity or asymmetry of contour, such as plagiocephaly or orbital dystopia. Any exophthalmos, unilateral or bilateral, must be noted and determined to be attributable to a deficiency of the orbital roof, floor, or both. The interorbital distance is evaluated for signs of hypertelorism or hypotelorism.

At this point the head should be examined from above ("bird's eye" view) and below ("worm's eye" view). Attention also is directed to a sagittal view to assess the transverse dimensions of the midface. In addition, the malar eminences should be evaluated from the frontal, lateral, and submental points of view. Examination of the nose includes evaluation of the dorsum, frontonasal angle, nasolabial angle, and alar base width and symmetry. A similar examination is performed in the subnasal region. Posture and competence of the lips are recorded. The location and density of scar tissue resulting from previous surgery may alter the response of the lip to surgical movement of the maxilla and teeth. The presence of scar tissue in the lip and on the palate may restrict maxillary advancement and increase the tendency for relapse. The interlabial gap should rarely exceed 3.5 mm at rest, and there should not be more than 1 to 2 mm of gingival exposure on smiling. Maxillary incisor show at rest should not exceed 3.5 mm for males or 5.0 mm for females.

An intraoral examination follows, with particular care given to the palatal, tonsillar, and lingual anatomy. Occlusion is studied with respect to its transverse and sagittal relationships. Lateral and protrusive excursions of the mandible as well as the path of the mandible on opening and closing are recorded. The function of the temporomandibular joint is evaluated.

Bilateral flatness or facial concavity is often seen in the canine fossa region but is more severe on the affected side in patients with unilateral cleft lip and palate. This condition sometimes includes bony deficiency up to the inferior orbital rim and along the piriform aperture on the affected side. Consideration may be given to correcting this asymmetric midface deficiency by performing a Le Fort I advancement. Specifically, a Le Fort I osteotomy with a high vertical extension is performed on the affected side, and the maxilla is advanced and if necessary rotated around the vertical axis (y axis) as it is brought forward. The net effect is a greater advancement of the teeth and wall of the anterior maxilla on the affected, more deficient side. The plan for correcting an asymmetric midface deficiency will have an impact on the preoperative orthodontic positioning of the teeth.

It is also wise to examine the ears and neck region for abnormalities associated with congenital syndromes. An evaluation of oral habits, deglutition, and respiration sometimes explains structural abnormalities such as open bite and vertical dysplasia of the facial skeleton.

Evaluation of the Dental Study Model

Evaluation of dental study models may define abnormalities in the arch form, individual tooth position, occlusal planes, and transverse arch width. Presurgical resolution of these problems by orthodontic therapy will facilitate surgery, optimize intermaxillary fixation, and improve postoperative stability. Dental models not only are helpful in establishing the diagnosis or the degree of deformity but are also useful for performing mock surgery.

Execution of mock surgical procedures on the study models permits the clinician to construct an interocclusal acrylic splint for fixation. In addition, model surgery provides an opportunity to evaluate the postoperative occlusion anticipated from performing the surgical treatment plan.

Cephalometric Tracings and Mock Surgery

By tracing the lateral and posteroanterior cephalograms, one can identify objectively the skeletal and soft tissue landmarks that are helpful in evaluating bony and soft tissue morphology and in planning the surgical correction. Figure 62–1 schematically outlines the specific points that are commonly used in evaluating the lateral cephalogram. Use of a computer to digitize the landmark data from a pair of lateral and posteroanterior cephalograms results in a three-dimensional display of cephalometric landmarks. This three-dimensional cephalogram can be subjected to the same range of geometric analyses and comparisons with normative populations that have been traditionally performed on two-dimensional cephalograms (discussed in Chap. 57).

In the lateral cephalogram alone, two-dimensional craniofacial anatomy can be assessed in the vertical and horizontal dimensions and compared with normative data, controlling for age and sex. Several sources of normative data exist for this purpose.[1,2] Equal in importance to controlling for age and sex is scaling the normative data to account for the overall size of the patient. Data from the patient are then compared with

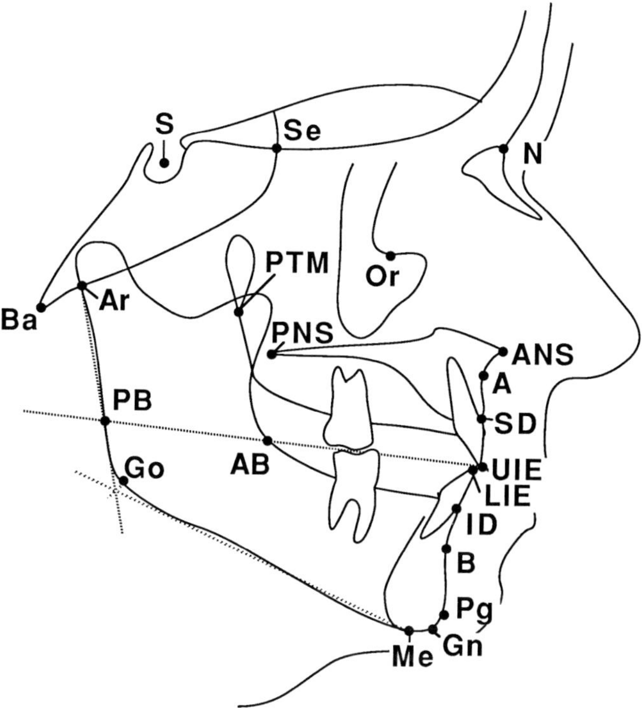

Figure 62–1 Key cephalometric landmarks: N = nasion; S = sella; O = orbitale; ANS = anterior nasal spine; PNS = posterior nasal spine; A = point; SD = supradentale; UIE = upper incisal edge; LIE = lower incisal edge; ID = infradentale; B = point; Pg = pogonion; GN = gnathion; Me = menton; Go = gonion; Se-E = sphenoethmoidal intersect; Ar = articulare; AB = anterior border of mandible; PB = posterior border of mandible; Ba = basion; PTM = pterygomaxillary fissure.

the scaled normal mean data. One can then evaluate the proportionality of various parts of the face. The two-dimensional cephalometric analysis, as performed at the New York University Institute of Reconstructive Surgery, is divided into four parts: (1) vertical facial measurements, (2) horizontal midface measurements, (3) horizontal lower face measurements, and (4) dental measurements. This approach allows the clinician to view and evaluate each component individually and to relate the various components to one another and to the entire craniofacial complex.

Vertical Facial Cephalometric Measurements

The following measurements are helpful in evaluating the face in the vertical dimension (Fig. 62–2).
1. Me-N (anterior total face height, or TFH)
   a. N-ANS (anterior upper face height, or UFH)
   b. ANS-Me (anterior lower face height, or LFH)
2. The ANS-Me measurement can be subdivided into:
   a. ANS-SD (subpiriform maxilla); increased in vertical maxillary excess (long face syndrome) and reduced in short face syndrome following tooth extraction or alveolar remodeling
   b. ANS-UIE (subpiriform maxilla plus height of upper incisal crown); changes with dental extraction, abrasive incisal wear, and inclination of the incisors

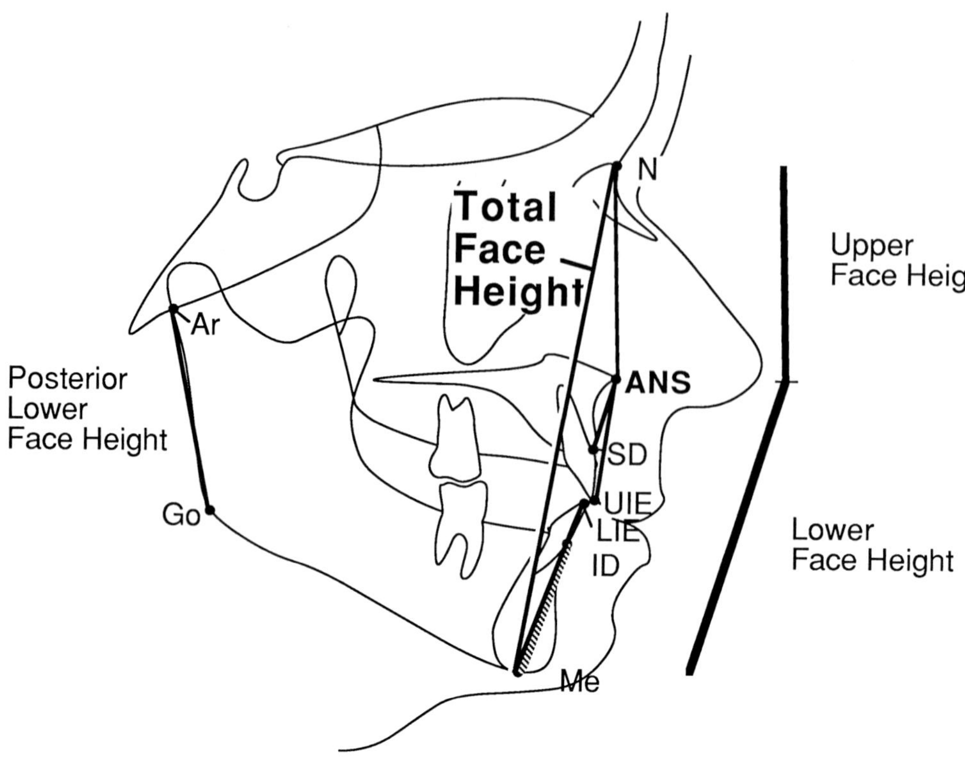

Figure 62–2 Total face height (Me–N) may be divided into upper face height (N–ANS) and lower face height (ANS–Me). Lower face height (LFH) consists of five components: ANS–SD, ANS–UIE, interincisal gap, Me–LIE (lower incisal edge), and Me–ID. Posterior lower face height is defined as Ar–Go.

    c. Me-LIE (height of anterior mandible)
    d. Me-ID (height of anterior mandible, exclusive of teeth); often increased in mandibular deficiency syndromes (dentoalveolar overbite) and reduced following extractions and resultant alveolar crest remodeling
    e. Interincisal relationship
3. Ar-Go (posterior lower face height)
4. SN/MP (angular relationship between the inferior border of the mandible and the anterior cranial base) (Fig. 62–3); often increased in skeletal open bite, micrognathia, and long face syndrome and frequently reduced in mandibular prognathism and short face syndrome
5. Ar-Go-Me (angular relationship of mandibular ramus and body), or gonial angle

Horizontal Midface Measurements

The following measurements are employed to evaluate the midface in a horizontal plane (Fig. 62–4).
1. SN (length of anterior cranial base)
2. SNA (angular measurement defined by sella–nasion and nasion–A lines); generally increased in maxillary hyperplasia and reduced in maxillary hypoplasia

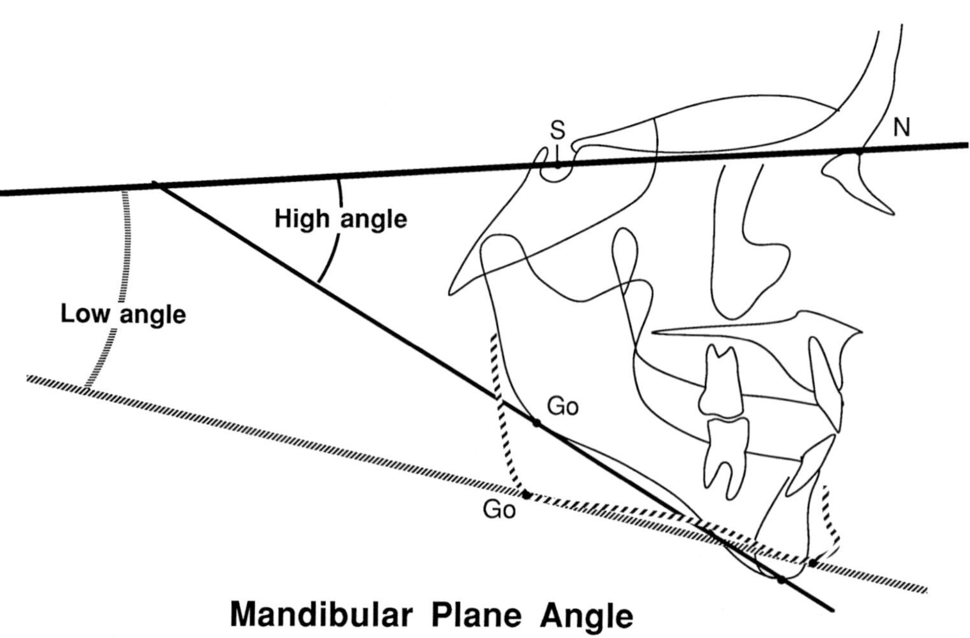

Figure 62–3 Mandibular plane angle. As the mandible rotates clockwise, the angle made by the inferior border with the cranial base (S–N) becomes more obtuse (high angle) as in patients with micrognathia or long face syndrome. In patients with a low angle, the mandible may appear more protrusive.

Mandibular Plane Angle

4. ANB (angular relationship of points A, N, and B); increased in maxillary protrusion or mandibular retrusion and decreased in maxillary retrusion or mandibular protrusion

Dental Measurements

These values are helpful in determining dental stability and orthodontic management.

1. 1̲-SN (the inclination of the maxillary incisor with respect to the anterior cranial base [SN])
2. 1̅-MP (the angle of the lower incisor with respect to the inferior border of the mandible)
3. 1̲ to 1̅ (angular relationships of maxillary and mandibular incisors to one another)

Occlusal stability and periodontal health are related to the position of the dental arches with respect to their bony bases in the craniofacial complex. An optimal relationship between the maxillary and mandibular dentition is also required for postoperative stability and the maintenance of sound periodontal health.

It should be noted that postsurgical skeletal relocation is not necessarily associated with a comparable amount of soft tissue change. Moreover, in the preoperative period one cannot precisely predict the amount of relapse or skeletal regression that may occur during the long term following a surgical advancement or recession procedure. In the growing child, the effects of natural development on the mobilized skeletal segment cannot be accurately predicted prior to surgery.

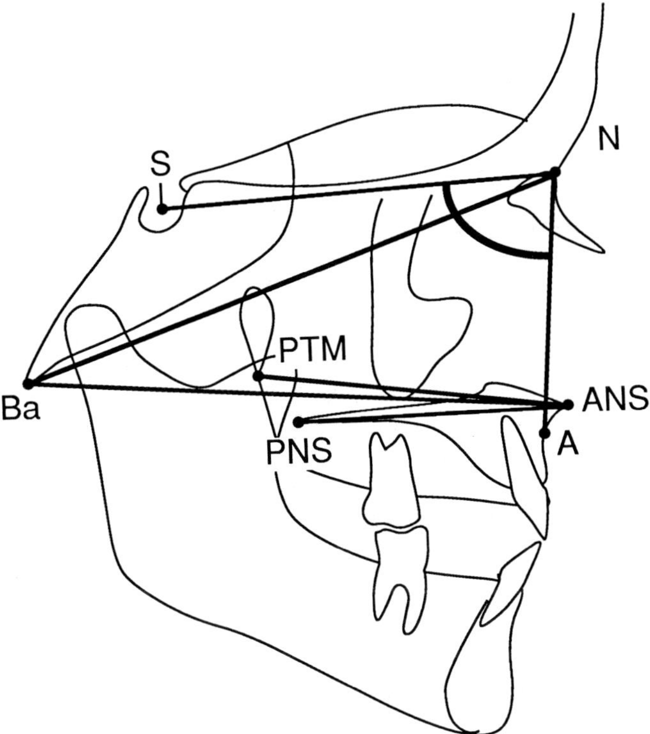

Figure 62–4 Midface horizontal measurement may be divided into cranial base (S–N and Ba–N) and lower midface (Ba–ANS, PTM–ANS, ANS–PNS). The SNA angle defines the position of the maxilla relative to the anterior cranial base. The appraisal of this angle should include the possibility that the cranial base may be tilted.

3. ANS-PNS (anteroposterior depth of maxilla at palatal plane); increased in maxillary hyperplasia and reduced in maxillary hypoplasia
4. Ba-ANS (linear distance from the basion to the anterior nasal spine). This describes the location of the anterior maxilla with respect to the posterior cranial base. A protrusive maxilla will show a larger than normal measurement in this area
5. PTM-ANS (linear distance from the maxillary tuberosity to the anterior nasal spine). This measurement describes the anteroposterior depth of the lower maxilla. It is particularly useful in the presence of clefts of the hard palate when the posterior nasal spine is affected
6. Ba-N (linear distance from the basion to the frontonasal suture on the midsagittal plane). This describes the overall length of the cranial base.

Horizontal Lower Face Measurements

The following areas are of significance in cephalometric assessment of the lower face in the horizontal plane (Fig. 62–5).

1. Ar-Pg (oblique mandibular measurement from the articulare to the pogonian)
2. Go-Pg (linear measurement from the gonion describing mandibular body length to pogonion)
3. SNB (angular relationship of point B to anterior cranial base); increased in mandibular protrusion and reduced in mandibular micrognathia

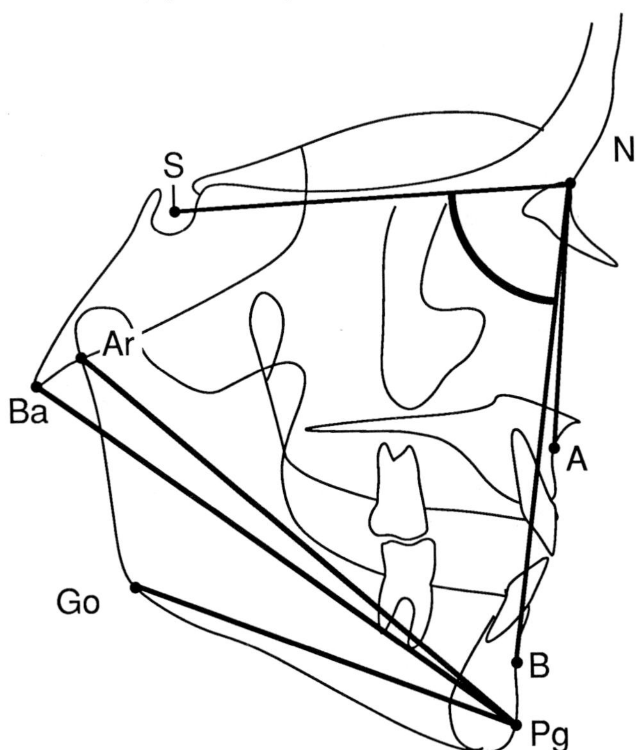

Figure 62–5 Lower face horizontal measurements may be divided into overall oblique mandibular length (Ar–Pg) or mandibular body length (Go–Pg). The downward and forward projection of the body, away from the posterior cranial base, is measured between the basion and pogonion. The SNB angle defines the position of the mandible relative to the anterior cranial base. The anteroposterior position of the mandible relative to the maxilla is described by the ANB angle.

Few studies in the literature deal accurately with this subject. It is known that mandibular advancement procedures associated with closure of a large anterior open bite frequently result in a high degree of postoperative relapse. Similarly, the higher the level of osteotomy in the midface advancement (Le Fort III versus Le Fort I), the greater the degree of relapse. The presence of scar tissue in the lip and palate will contribute to relapse and can to some degree be anticipated by overcorrection in the plan.

The effect of maxillary advancement on the size of the nasolabial angle is variable. Any discussion of change in the nasolabial angle following maxillary advancement must consider the following: the inclination of the incisors, preservation or excision of the anterior nasal spine, size or projection of the anterior nasal spine, height of the osteotomy, and a history of previous lip and nasal surgery.

Mock Surgery on Cephalometric Tracings

The lateral cephalogram is covered with a transparent sheet of matte acetate, on which the principal cephalometric anatomy and landmarks are traced (Fig. 62–6A). Additional acetate sheets are used to trace the bones and associated soft tissues that will be mobilized during surgery (Fig. 62–6B [left]). Illustrated in Figure 62–6B [right] is the composite of a preoperative tracing and a tracing of the mandibular body showing advancement with the resultant profile change. Simulation of the Le Fort I, II, or III procedure and various segmental osteotomies may be evaluated in the same way. The clinician utilizing this method must be acutely aware of the surgical and dental limitations surrounding each procedure. The ability to predict the soft tissue changes resulting from cephalometric mock surgery depends on an understanding of the ratio of change between bone movement, soft tissue movement, and relapse. Three variables that directly influence the ability to predict this ratio are surgical technique, intrinsic quality (quantity, density, presence of previous surgical scars) of the soft tissue, and the direction and magnitude of the skeletal change.

Mock Surgery on Photographic Records

The lateral photograph is enlarged to life size. This is done by including in the photograph a ruler held at the midsagittal plane of the face. When printing the photograph, a ruler is placed on the enlarging table while the image is adjusted in size so that the projected ruler is the same size as the real ruler. The print that is produced shows the ruler and the profile in life size. This image is printed several times for use during mock surgery on the photograph.

A scalpel blade is used to cut the portion of facial anatomy that corresponds to the planned bony surgery. Figure 62–7A is a photograph of a young man with midface hypoplasia secondary to cleft lip and palate. The nasal tip (below the nasal bone) is separated from the philtrum to show the tip elevation that results from maxillary advancement. The nasolabial angle becomes more obtuse owing to the combined effect of maxillary advancement (including the anterior nasal spine) and the resultant elevation of the nasal tip. The inferior border of the chin is cut, repositioned superiorly, and advanced, simulating a vertical reduction genioplasty with advancement (Fig. 62–7B).

A tracing of the profile in the original photo superimposed on the mock surgical photo allows the clinician to measure the direction and the magnitude of the soft tissue change needed to achieve this aesthetic result. The variables affecting the accuracy of this predictive activity are surgical technique, quality of the soft tissue, and the direction and magnitude of bony change. This

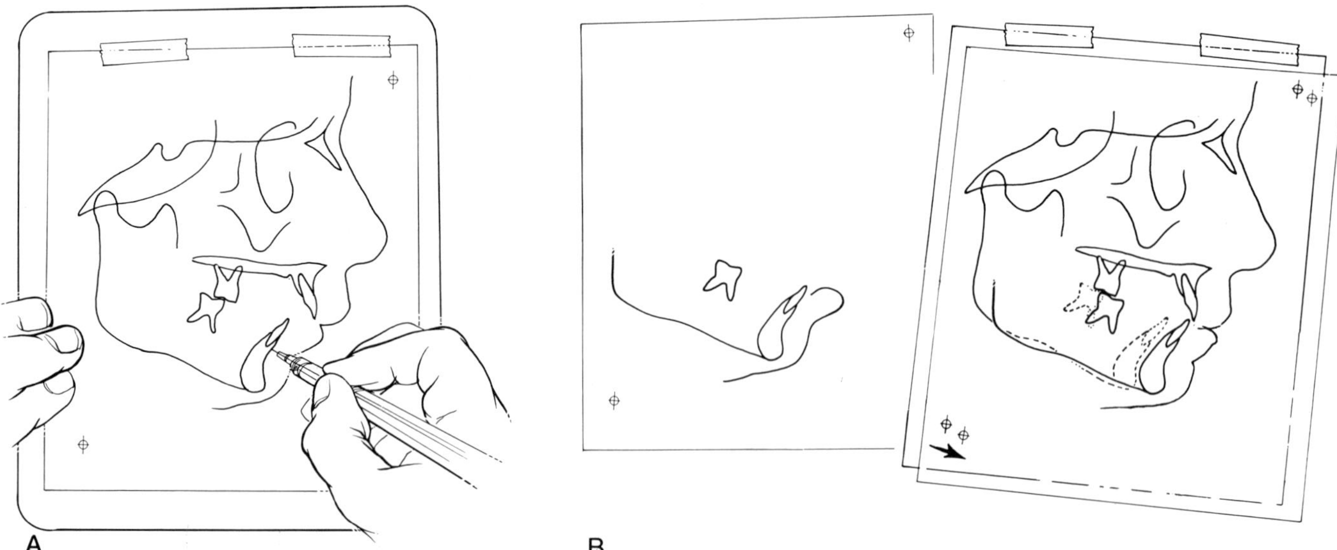

A   B

Figure 62–6 *A* The lateral cephalogram is covered with a transparent sheet of matte acetate, on which the cephalometric anatomy and landmarks are traced. *B,* (Left), An additional acetate sheet is used to trace the bone and associated soft tissue that will be mobilized during surgery. (Right), The composite of a preoperative tracing and a tracing of the mandibular body is illustrated, showing advancement with the resulting profile change.

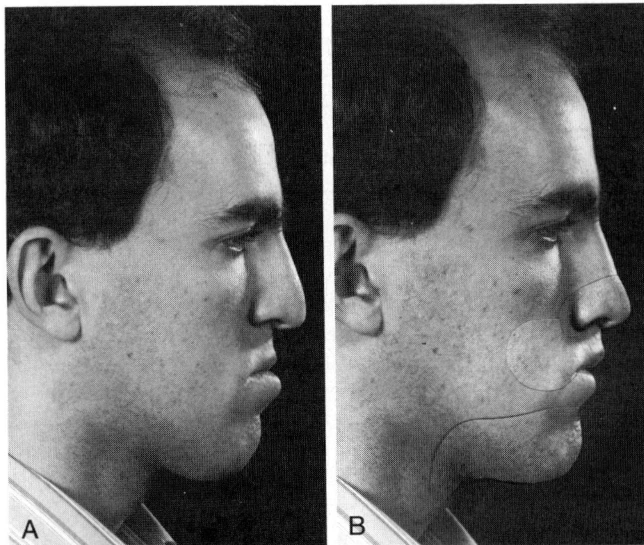

Figure 62–7 *A*, Photograph of an adult male with midface hypoplasia and nasal and lip deformity secondary to cleft lip and palate. The vertical height of the mandibular symphysis is long. *B*, Mock surgery on a life-sized photographic enlargement demonstrating change in profile resulting from simulation of a Le Fort I maxillary advancement and vertical reduction genioplasty. Note nasal tip elevation, advancement of the alar base and paranasal region, and vertical reduction of chin height.

activity allows the surgeon to evaluate the estimated outcome of alternative surgical procedures.

Mock Surgery on Articulated Study Models

A set of dental study models is carefully mounted on an articulator. The articulator, a hinged device which allows the study models to move with the same relative motion as in the patient, enables the clinician to plan the surgical correction and construct an acrylic bite registration (splint) of the desired occlusal and skeletal change. The casts are cut and repositioned to mimic the surgical procedure. The bite splint is fabricated directly

on the occlusal surfaces of the repositioned casts. This "occlusal index" should be thin yet sufficiently strong to tolerate stress. Once the surgical osteotomies are completed, the maxillary and mandibular teeth are keyed into the occlusal splint, establishing the planned change in both dental and skeletal relationships simultaneously.

Three-Dimensional Planning of Orthognathic Surgery

The lateral cephalogram alone is of little value in describing the essential features of asymmetric facial deformity. Two-dimensional cephalometric data may be

Figure 62–8 Three-dimensional CT scan of the craniofacial complex showing separation of frontal bar, Le Fort III, and Le Fort I osteotomy fragments. As in mock surgery on cephalograms, these components can be moved to emulate the proposed surgical plan.

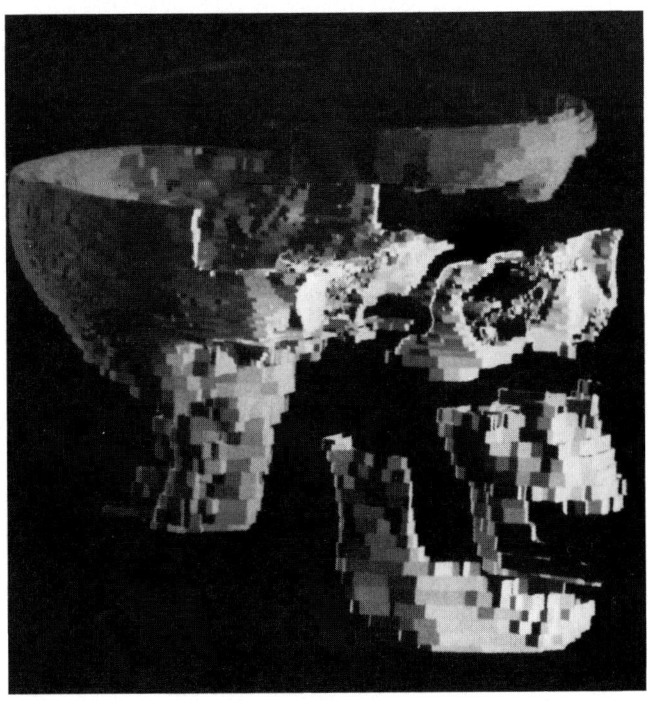

used to create a three-dimensional cephalometric landmark set that permits evaluation of these complex craniofacial deformities and makes possible surgical simulation. This is done by entering into a computer the X, Y, and Z coordinates of cephalometric landmarks seen in both the lateral and posteroanterior cephalograms. They are thus combined to produce a three-dimensional "constellation" of landmarks (Chap. 57). Figure 62–5 is a preoperative computer-optimized, three-dimensional cephalometric illustration of a patient with hemifacial microsomia. Three-dimensional mock surgical simulation involves a sagittal split of the mandible, a Le Fort I procedure, and genioplasty. Mock surgery can be done automatically by having the computer achieve a "best fit" of the patient landmark data to those of an age- and sex-matched normal population. The clinician can then modify the surgical design according to clinical constraints, using interactive computer graphic techniques.

This interactive phase of surgical planning may be performed on three-dimensional computed tomographic (CT) scan reconstructions of the patient's facial skeleton. A program has been developed that allows osteotomy fragments to be created in three dimensions and surgery to be simulated much as it would be in the operating room. An example of this kind of visualization is shown in Figure 62–8. The three-dimensional CT scan visualization can be linked directly with the cephalometric data so that the surgical simulation is done in a conjoined way.

Fusion of the cephalometric and CT-based models gives the user the advantages of both forms of three-dimensional representation.[3] The cephalometric form provides access to a large normative data base necessary for the optimization and measurement operations, whereas the CT-based model provides superior visualization for the interactive surgical simulation. This linking of classic cephalometric analysis with CT will be necessary until a comprehensive, three-dimensional cephalometric representation based on a normative data base of CT scans is developed.

References

1. Bolton BH, Sr, Broadbent BH, Jr, Golden WH: Bolton Standards of Dentofacial Developmental Growth. St. Louis: C. V. Mosby, 1975.
2. Riolo ML, Moyers RE, McNamara JS, et al: An Atlas of Craniofacial Growth. Monograph 2, Craniofacial Growth Series, Center for Human Growth and Development. Ann Arbor: University of Michigan Press, 1974.
3. Cutting CB, Bookstein FL, Grayson BH, et al: Three-dimensional computer-assisted design of craniofacial surgical procedures: Optimization and interaction with cephalometric and CT based models. Plast Reconstr Surg 77:877, 1986.

CHAPTER 63

Orthognathic Surgery for Patients with Cleft Lip and Palate

Ian R. Munro and Kenneth E. Salyer

Orthognathic surgery, which is the restoration of the jaws to their correct position, is part of orthomorphic surgery. The latter, which involves the reconstruction of normal facial contours, includes both soft and hard tissue. In the last 15 years far greater advances have been made in correction of the facial skeleton of cleft patients than in reconstruction of the soft tissue. Ideal facial restoration can be achieved only by a multidisciplinary team, which must include a surgeon experienced in the problems of both the soft tissue and hard tissue that occur in clefts, an orthodontist, speech pathologist, prosthodontist, dental technician, and otolaryngologist. To maintain the necessary expertise, the team should meet on a weekly or biweekly basis and treat at least 30 to 40 new patients a year requiring multidisciplinary cleft management. The complexity of the problems associated with cleft patients is far greater than that of other patients undergoing routine orthognathic surgery.

The Problem and Etiology

All patients with complete unilateral or bilateral clefts will develop malalignment of the teeth and some degree of malocclusion. This includes the failure of dental eruption into the line of the cleft during the mixed dentition stage, which is related to lack of bone in the cleft. Malocclusion can result from malalignment of the teeth and can be corrected by orthodontic treatment at the appropriate time. However, more severe types of malocclusion are due to basal bone disharmony, which is due in all cases, to underdevelopment of the maxilla rather than overgrowth of the mandible and results from a variety of causes.

Repair of the alveolus with bone grafts in infancy almost inevitably has caused retromaxillism. The timing and technique of repair of the hard and soft palates has had variable effects. Ross has found that the surgeon rather than the technique may have the greatest detrimental effect.[1–3] The worst examples of retromaxillism have occurred in patients who have had multiple operations to correct the hard palate, resulting in development of palatal fistulas and subsequent repeated attempts to close these. Because the overall problem in cleft lip and palate patients is one of aesthetics, even when there is a good repair of the lip and nose, midfacial flatness due to retromaxillism produces a most unpleasing appearance.

History

A variety of techniques for orthognathic surgery will be described, but the fundamental technique is that known as the Le Fort I maxillary advancement. This operation was first performed approximately 130 years ago for removal of a nasopharyngeal tumor. The maxilla was split at the level that has become known as the Le Fort I osteotomy.[4, 5] In 1939, Axhausen discussed the total mobilization of the maxilla with anterior repositioning to correct deformities in patients with cleft lip and palate who had hitherto been managed by surgery to set back the mandible.[6] He reported a patient who had had this maxillary advancement procedure in 1941. Schuchardt reported fracturing the junction between the maxillary tuberosity and the pterygoid plates, thus developing the principle of the modern maxillary osteotomy.[7] Gillies and Rowe[8] and Gillies[9] reported in 1947 that they had brought the maxilla into the desired position in a cleft patient by reopening the alveolar and palatal clefts and dividing the bone into two parts. Postoperative immobilization using elastics lasted more than 12 weeks. Subsequently, this timing was shortened by using an iliac bone graft.

In 1951 Dingman and Harding[10] reported their extensive experience with midface osteotomies. Schmidt in 1954 reported dividing the junction between the maxilla and the pterygoid region with a specially designed curved chisel.[11] Obwegeser particularly has promoted the Le Fort I osteotomy and has stressed that the fragments need to be fully mobilized so that they can be brought into the desired position without tissue resistance.[12] He also stressed the use of large bone grafts between the pterygoid plates and the maxillary tuberosity. In 1967 Hogeman and Wilmar[13] reported on the long-term stability of the maxilla in cleft patients undergoing Le Fort I maxillary advancement. The use of screws and miniplates for fixation of the mobilized segments was a further improvement in this surgery.[14, 15]

Orthognathic Surgical Techniques
Bone Grafting of the Alveolus

In cleft patients, there is a dental distortion in the region of the cleft alveolus. There may be either an alveolar fistula or an intact gingiva but no bone in the alveolar cleft. In either situation, teeth can neither erupt nor be moved orthodontically into this area. Closure of the fistula and simultaneous insertion of cancellous bone have allowed effective orthodontic closure of the gap in the dental arch.[16-18] Cancellous rather than cortical bone must be packed into the defect. Cancellous bone can be obtained through a small incision, 2 to 3 cm long, lateral to the iliac crest; the lateral cortical iliac bone is elevated, and cancellous bone is removed with a curette.

Alternatively, a short incision can be made in the hairline in the parietal region, the outer cortex of the skull exposed, and a bur used to remove the outer cortex; cancellous bone is then removed from the diploë to use as a graft.[19] This cranial technique has minimal morbidity for the patient compared to the iliac bone technique, but it is more difficult to harvest a large amount of bone and can be risky if the surgeon is not used to making bur holes in the skull.

Figure 63–1A illustrates a technique for closing a unilateral alveolar fistula. An incision is made around the margins of the fistula, and a buccal sulcus sickle flap (A) is elevated. The nasal lining and oral lining at the margins of the cleft are elevated and turned inward and sutured, as shown in Figure 63–1B. Palatal flaps are created after the technique of Veau, mobilized medially, and sutured (Fig. 63–1C). The gap is then packed with cancellous bone and the buccal flap (A) is placed over this to close the defect (Fig. 63–1D). There may be subsequent orthodontic problems using buccal mucosa in the region of the gingiva, and an alternative technique utilizing mobilization of gingival flaps is shown in Figure 63–2. Figure 63–3 shows a similar technique for closing a bilateral alveolar fistula. Bilateral clefts are much more difficult to close simultaneously because of the problems of elevating the mucoperiosteum off the posterior surface of the premaxilla. It is very important that the premaxilla not be devascularized on its lingual and/or labial surface. Figure 63–4, again, shows a variation using gingival flaps rather than buccal sulcus flaps.

Le Fort I Maxillary Advancement

In adults with a complete cleft lip and palate that has not been operated on, Ortiz-Monasterio has shown that the maxilla and mandible are in a normal relationship.[20, 21] When a class III malocclusion is present, it is always attributed to retromaxillism secondary to the scarring produced by the cleft repair. In the hands of an experienced cleft surgeon, the incidence of patients developing retromaxillism should be as low as 10% to 20%. However, patients who have been treated by an inexperienced surgeon and have undergone several operations to repair the palate are more likely to have significant retromaxillism.

In the past, it was common for the mandible to be set back to produce a normal occlusion with the retropositioned maxilla. This produced a very flat, unaesthetic facial appearance. Currently, the standard treatment is a Le Fort I maxillary advancement. The indications for mandibular surgery will be discussed later. The ideal treatment combines surgery and orthodontic procedures. Orthodontic braces are used to align the teeth in the dental arch in the upright position over the basal bone, but no attempt is made to advance the teeth into correct occlusion. The advancement of the bone is carried out through a maxillary osteotomy.

Figure 63–5 shows the surgical technique for a Le Fort I maxillary advancement in a patient with a unilateral cleft. The technique includes nasotracheal intubation, infiltration of the upper buccal sulcus with 1:200,000 epinephrine (Adrenalin), an incision in the upper buccal sulcus medial to the zygomatic buttress on the noncleft side, a limited incision on the cleft side in the upper buccal sulcus with a short incision anteriorly, and a further incision posteriorly. This is particularly necessary if differential movement of the maxillary segments is desired. A subperiosteal dissection of the maxilla is carried out to the pterygoid plates, and careful dissection of the nasomucoperiosteum is performed,

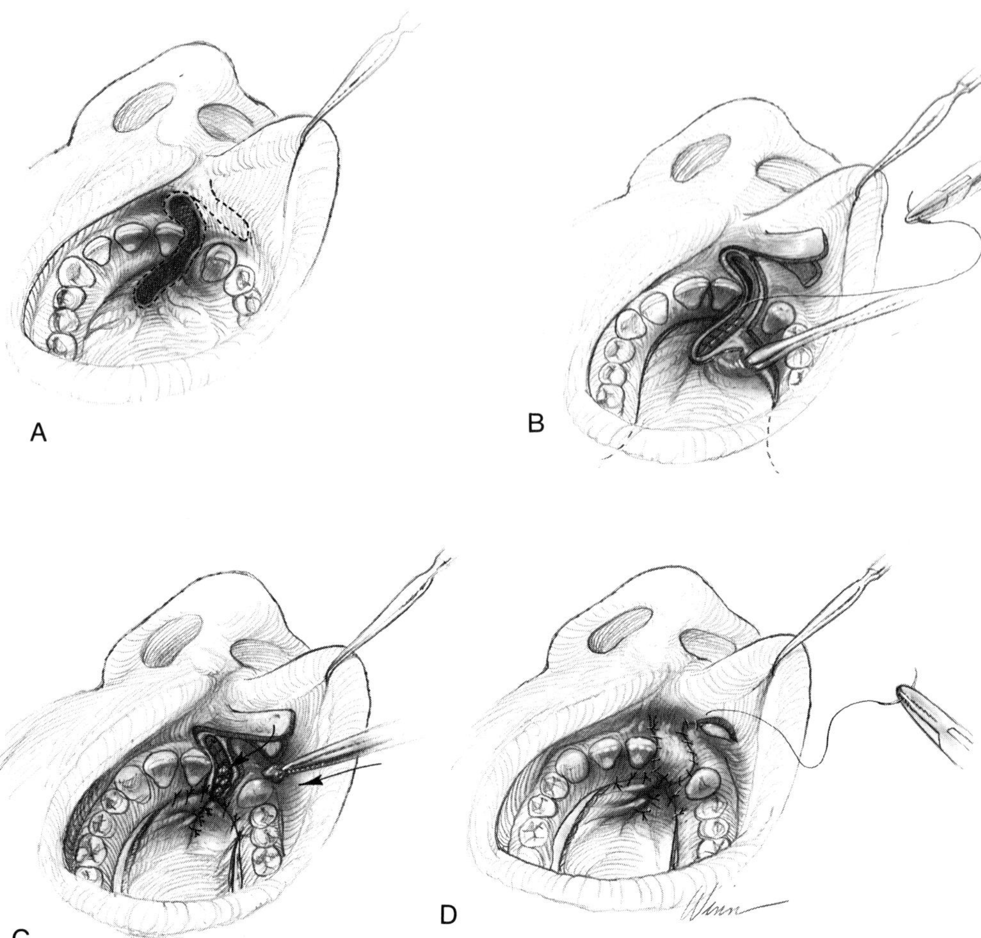

Figure 63–1 *A*, Patient with unilateral alveolar-nasal fistula. Incisions marked at margins of cleft to create a buccal sulcus flap. *B*, The nasal lining is dissected upward and sutured. Lateral palatal mucoperiosteal Veau flaps are elevated. *C*, Cancellous bone is packed into the defect, and the palatal flaps are advanced and sutured anteriorly. Bone may be left exposed posteriorly and laterally. *D*, The buccal sulcus flap is rotated down and sutured at its margins and to the palatal flaps.

Figure 63–2 *A*, Nasal lining is turned inward and sutured. Palatal flaps are advanced and the fistula is packed with cancellous bone as in Figure 63–1. The gingiva and periosteum are elevated, dividing at the papillae. A back cut is made two, three, or four teeth lateral to the cleft. *B*, The gingivoperiosteal flap is advanced to close the labial side of the fistula. If the gap is large, gingival flaps can be elevated from either side of the cleft.

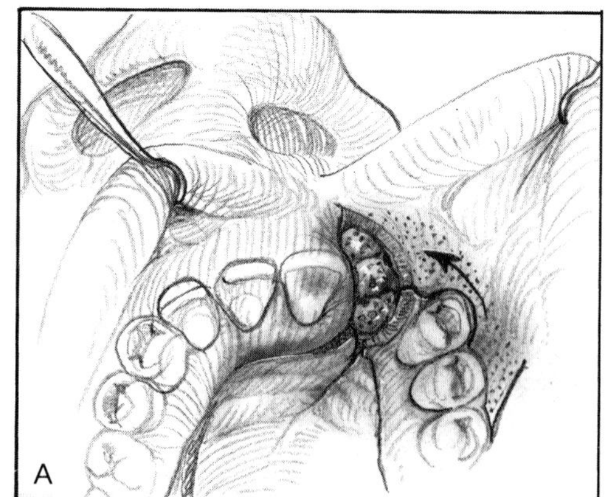
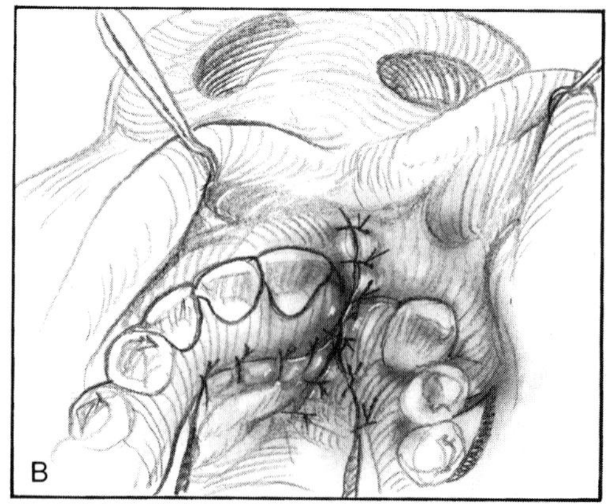

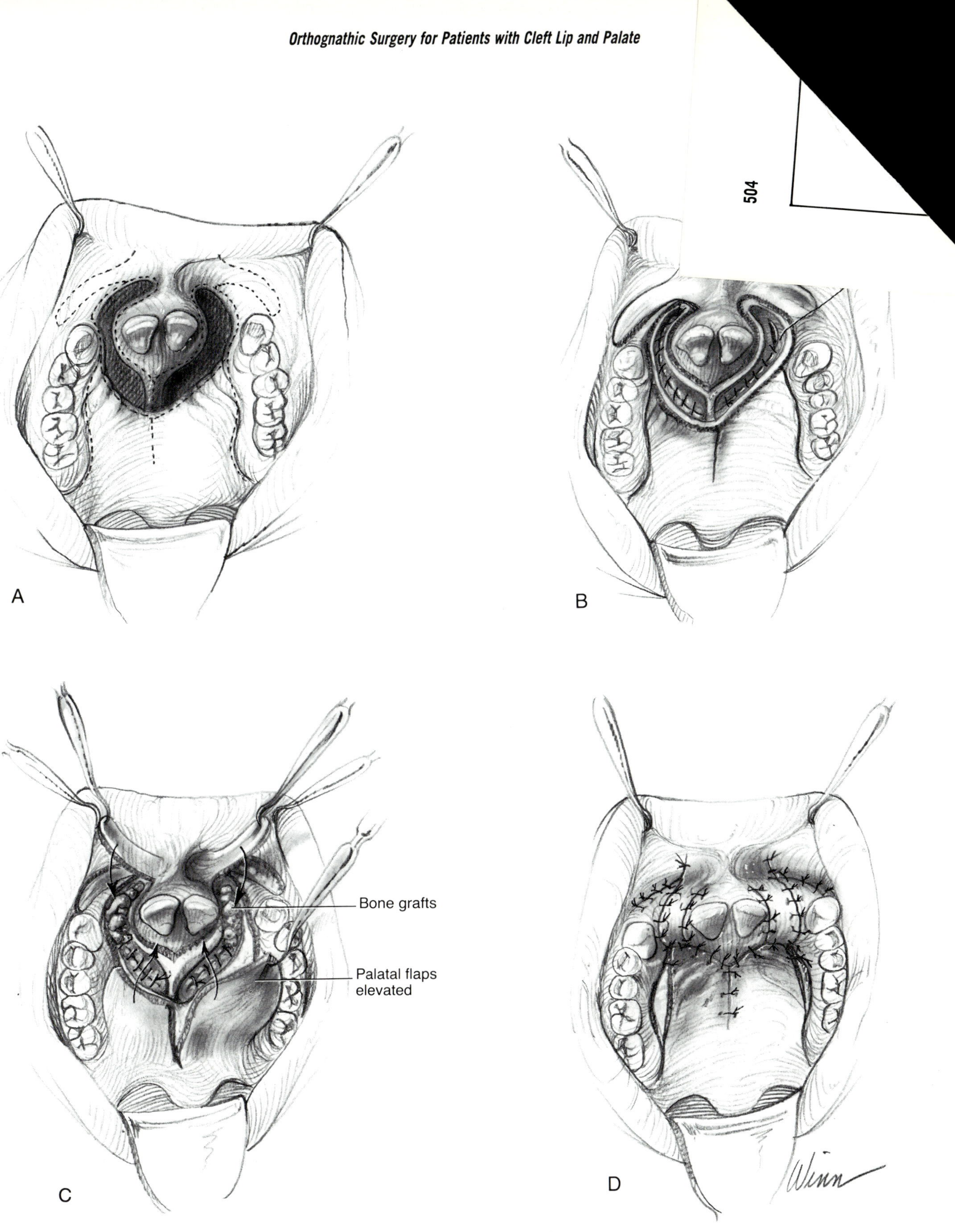

Figure 63–3 *A*, Closure of bilateral alveolar fistulas. Note the incisions around the premaxilla and the midline palatal incisions. Care must be taken not to allow the incisions for these buccal sulcus flaps to encroach on the mucosal blood supply to the premaxilla from its labial surface. *B*, The nasal lining is turned inward and sutured. *C*, The clefts are packed with cancellous bone. *D*, The flaps are sutured together. The most difficult area is at the posterior border of the premaxilla.

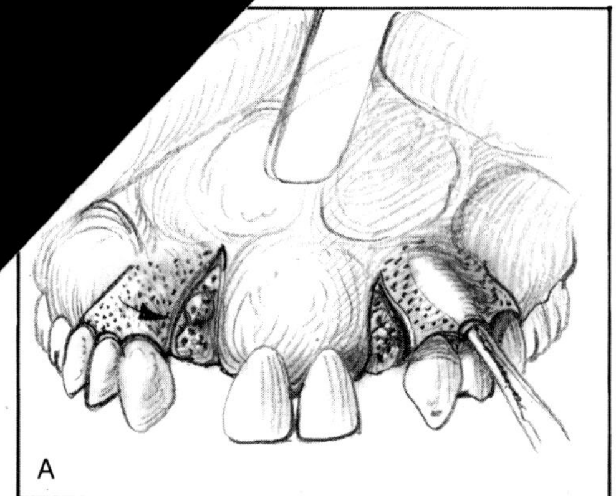

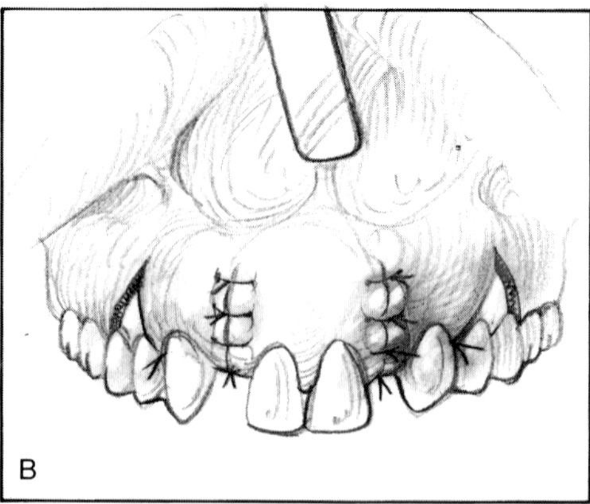

Figure 63–4 *A,* Closure of bilateral alveolar fistula with labial gingivoperiosteal flaps. If the fistula gap is large, the gingival flap should be made larger and should arise from four or even five teeth. *B,* The gingival flaps are advanced and sutured, leaving small defects laterally.

particularly along the margins of the septum (which is usually deviated) and along the nasal floor on the side of the cleft. The maxilla is then cut transversely with a saw from the piriform margin to the maxillary tuberosity. The height of the transverse cut on the piriform margin must be at least above the canine root but can be placed higher on the maxilla as far as the level of the inferior orbital foramen if greater facial convexity is required.

A variety of customized, more complex osteotomies have been described, taking the transverse line even further up to include parts of the inferior orbital rim, but we believe that this is technically too difficult and unnecessary because these areas can be satisfactorily augmented by the addition of onlay split cranial bone grafts. The nasal septum and lateral nasal walls are transected. The pterygomaxillary junction is divided, and the segments can then be down-fractured by finger pressure. Then the segments are moved forward into an acrylic wafer that has been designed for the desired occlusion. The jaws are wired together over the acrylic wafer. Holding the mandible upward and ensuring that the condyle is correctly seated in the temperomandib-

ular fossa, L-shaped or 110-degree–shaped miniplates are applied across the piriform margin and zygomatic buttress (Fig. 63–5B). It is important that these plates be contoured exactly to the shape of the bone. Four self-tapping screws for each plate are inserted, two above and two below the line of the osteotomy.

When the plates are rigidly fixed, the patient is taken out of occlusion, and the mandible is moved passively upward and downward to ensure that it comes back directly into the acrylic wafer. The acrylic wafer should be left attached to the orthodontic bands of the maxilla. Bone grafts may or may not be inserted (as discussed later), and the mucosa is closed. If bone grafts are to be used, it is extremely important to repair the nasal lining completely. This is done when the maxilla has been mobilized completely and is in the down-fractured position.

If the patient has a deviated nasal septum, the mucoperichondrium and mucoperiosteum can be elevated off the septum easily when the maxilla is down-fractured and the septum either straightened or removed, as in a submucous resection. The nasal mucosa from the lateral

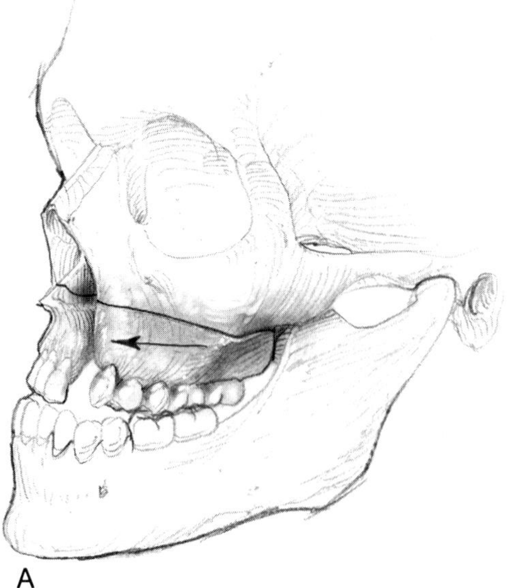

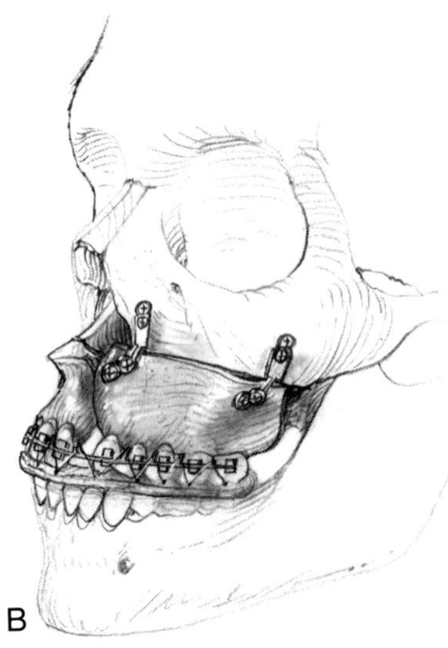

Figure 63–5 *A,* Le Fort I maxillary advancement. The transverse maxillary incisions are made above the level of the nasal floor and above the canine root. *B,* The maxillary segments are mobilized and advanced forward, and are fitted into an acrylic wafer that establishes the desired occlusion with the mandible. Miniplates are then inserted at the piriform margin and zygomatic buttress. The mandible is taken out of the acrylic wafer and passively moved upward and downward to ensure that it returns to the correct occlusion.

nasal wall and the septal floor are sutured to restore the intact nasal lining (Fig. 63–6C, D).

A Le Fort I osteotomy with differential movement may be necessary in those patients with gross hypoplasia of the cleft maxillary segment who have not had orthodontic treatment. The teeth on the cleft side are elevated, and the maxillary segment is contracted medially. More extensive mobilization of the soft tissues is necessary. The lesser segment is advanced forward and moved laterally and inferiorly to produce a normal occlusal plane (Fig. 63–6A–F). The two maxillary segments are fitted into the acrylic splint, the nasal lining is repaired, and a fifth miniplate is used across the

alveolar cleft at the base of the piriform fossa for increased stabilization (Fig. 63–6E and F).

It is common for patients to have an alveolar fistula at the time of the Le Fort I osteotomy. This can be closed at the time of maxillary advancement. In these patients, the buccal sulcus flap technique should be utilized to avoid devascularizing the maxilla (Fig. 63–7). In addition, creation of Veau flaps should be kept to a minimum or avoided, if possible, because they may endanger the blood supply to the maxilla. The Le Fort I osteotomy in a patient with a bilateral cleft is considerably more difficult than that in an individual with a unilateral cleft. This difficulty lies in the increased

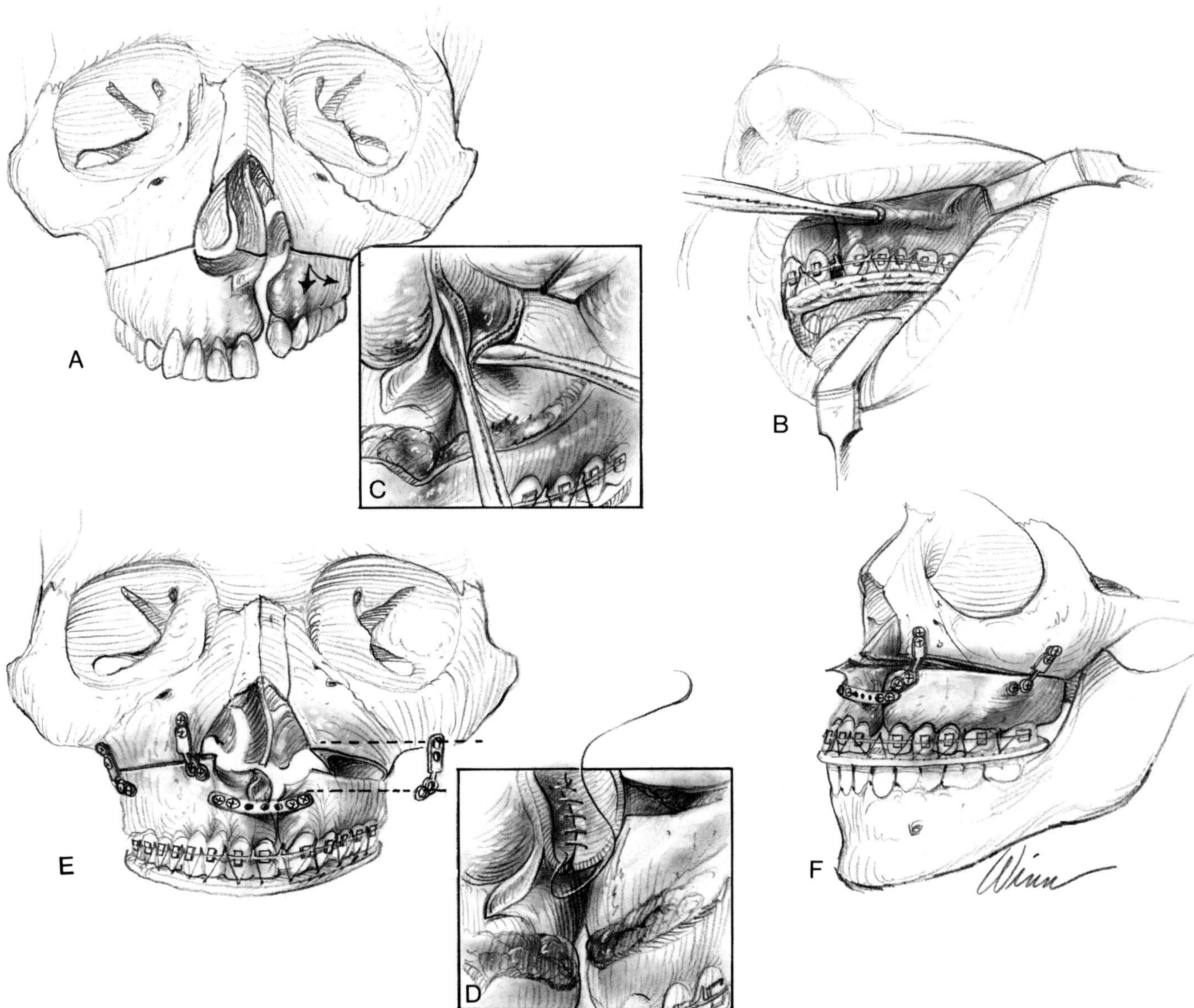

Figure 63–6 *A*, If there has been no orthodontic alignment of the maxillary segments and the lesser segment is collapsed medially and raised upward, it can be mobilized downward and laterally with an osteotomy. *B*, Because of the extensive mobilization of the oromucoperiosteum that will be necessary to allow movement of the maxillary segment forward, laterally, and downward, a more limited mucoperiosteal elevation in the buccal sulcus should be carried out. *C*, The mucosa is elevated off the lateral nasal wall, off its insertion along the repair of the cleft, and off the nasal septum. *D*, The nasal lining is repaired with the maxilla still in the down-fractured position. The deviated nasal septum can be corrected at this time if necessary. *E*, The two maxillary segments are fitted into the acrylic wafer and the desired occlusion with the mandible established. Miniplates are inserted at the piriform margin and zygomatic buttress, and a fifth plate is inserted across the alveolar cleft to further stabilize this segment.

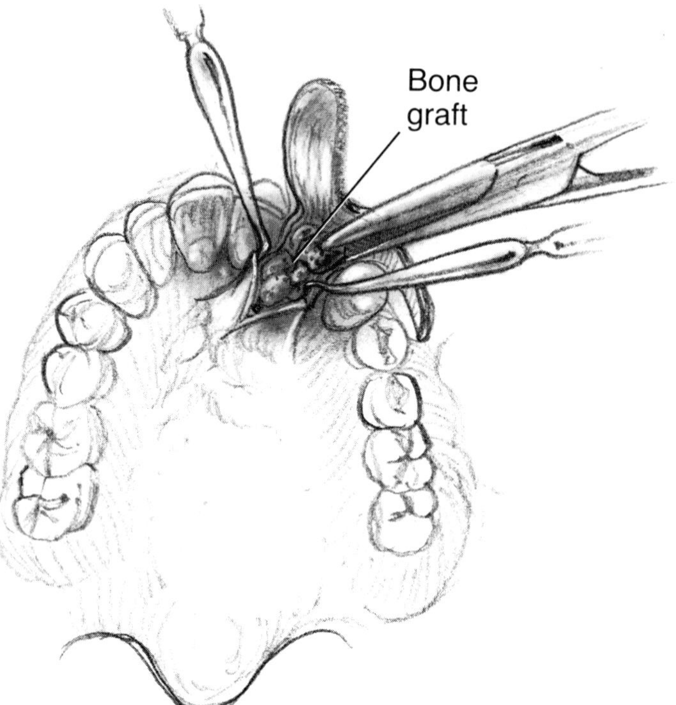

Figure 63–7 An alveolar fistula can be closed at the same time that a Le Fort I osteotomy is performed. A buccal sulcus flap is the best method for closing the gap in the gingiva to avoid further stripping and devascularizing the mobilized maxillary segment.

amount of scarring that occurs in the region of the alveolus as well as the line of the cleft palate repair. It is extremely difficult to mobilize each maxillary segment and the premaxilla to allow advancement, and there is great risk of devascularizing the premaxillary segment. The most ideal form of treatment is orthodontic alignment of the maxillary segments and premaxilla followed by closure of the alveolar fistula with bone grafting performed 6 months to 1 year before the Le Fort I maxillary advancement is done. If this sequence is followed, the stability of the maxillary arch can be reinforced by applying a castcap splint to the entire maxillary dental arch prior to performing the maxillary osteotomy as for a standard Le Fort I maxillary advancement.

In the past, Obwegeser was so concerned about the danger of devascularizing segments that he advocated carrying out a Le Fort I osteotomy in patients with a bilateral cleft and alveolar fistula, moving each segment into the required position but making no attempt to close the alveolar fistula. This was done in a second stage some months later. However, if the upper buccal sulcus incisions over the maxilla are kept to a minimum and tunneling of the mucoperiosteum is carried out sufficiently to allow osteotomy of the anterior maxilla, and if elevation of Veau flaps on the palate is also kept to a minimum and only a stab incision is used over the anterior premaxilla, it is possible to mobilize each maxillary segment (moving each one forward and laterally), reposition the premaxilla, and close the alveolar fistulas at the same time (Fig. 63–8A–F). As in the Le

Fort I procedure in a patient with a unilateral cleft, a fifth miniplate can be applied, extending from one maxilla to the other across the anterior premaxilla, for increased stabilization. Bone grafts can be applied across the anterior maxillary wall and into the pterygoid maxillary junction and the alveolar clefts (Fig. 63–8H).

Postoperative Management

With the current use of miniplates for immediate postoperative intermaxillary fixation, it is now safe to extubate the patient at the end of surgery. Because of scarring, the posterior forces attempting to rotate the advanced maxilla backward are tremendous. Thus it is advisable to keep intermaxillary elastic bands in place, fitting the teeth into an occlusal splint, for a period of time following surgery that may vary from 1 to 5 weeks. However, to ensure a safe airway postoperatively, these elastics should not be applied until the day following extubation.

Use of Bone Grafts

In the past, when the transected segments were held together with wire and patients were placed in intermaxillary fixation for 6 to 8 weeks, bone grafts were considered mandatory. The grafts were placed over the anterior maxilla, across the osteotomy site, and into the pterygomaxillary space. With the use of miniplates, the need for these bone grafts has diminished. We currently use bone grafts across the anterior maxilla when large advancements of at least 8 to 10 mm are performed. Bone grafts also are inserted into the pterygomaxillary junction to help prevent relapse. An alternative use is augmentation of the anterior maxilla, in addition to that achieved by advancement of the teeth into occlusion.

Currently, we prefer split cranial bone grafts because there is far less resorption of cranial bone compared with rib or iliac bone and much less morbidity for the patient. Cranial grafts can be taken through a coronal or hemicoronal incision. An extracranial technique, using a bur to cut through the outer cortex over the lateral parietal region and carefully passing an osteotome through the diploë to remove the outer cortex, is possible. This technique should be used only by a surgeon experienced in it because there is danger of running the osteotome through the inner cortex, cutting the dura mater, and injuring the brain.

Alternatively, and particularly if very large amounts of bone are required, a neurosurgeon can perform a full craniotomy. The bone is removed and split into inner and outer layers, and the inner cortex is then replaced in the skull. The bone graft is cut and shaped as required and placed over the anterior maxilla. It is held in place with one lag screw to prevent any movement and facilitate bone healing (Fig. 63–9).

Mandibular Surgery

Surgery of the mandible is indicated in two situations. If there is true mandibular prognathism, as assessed

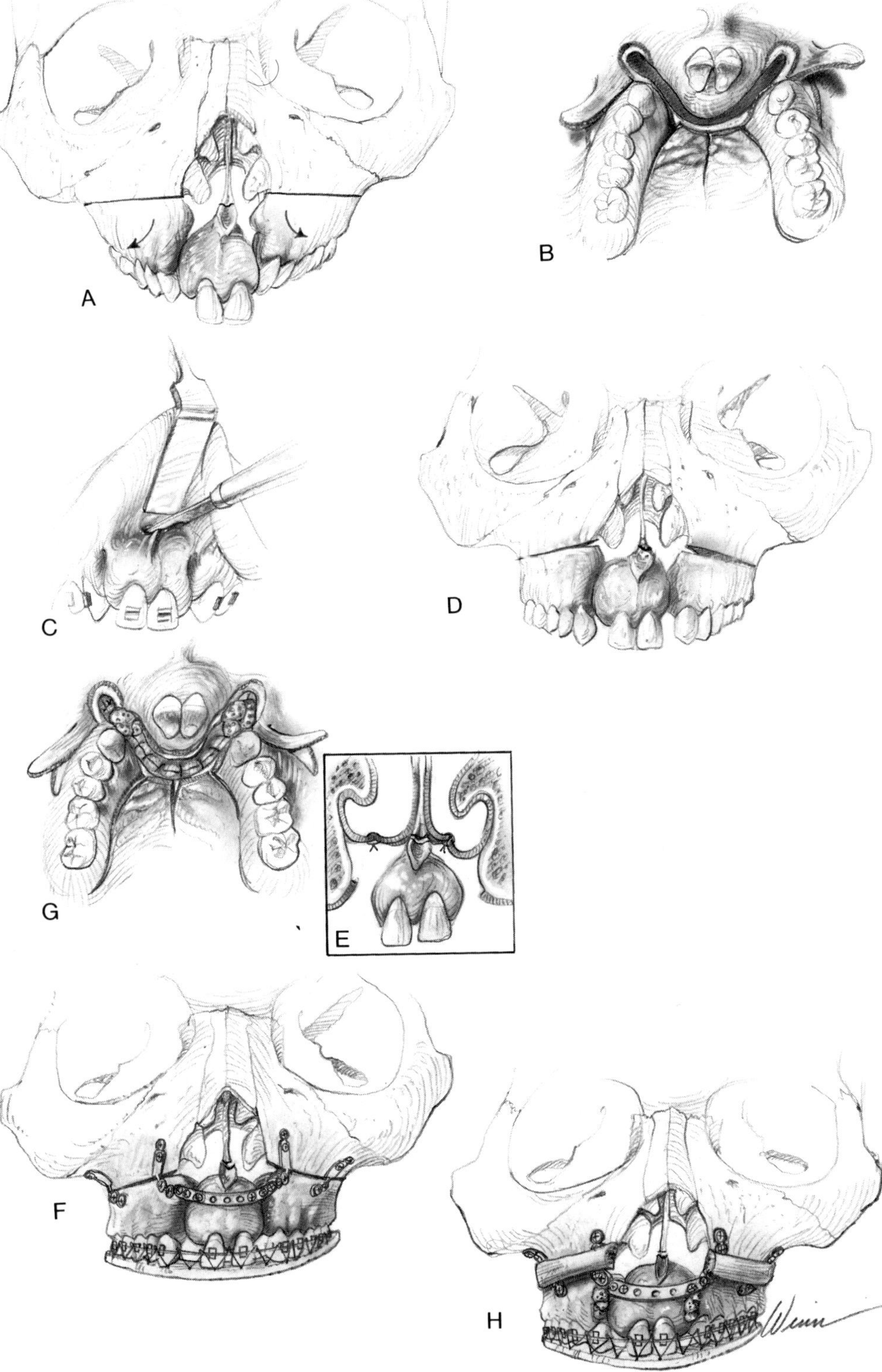

Figure 63–8 A, Osteotomy lines for a bilateral cleft of the maxilla with alveolar fistulas and medial maxillary collapse. *B*, Buccal sulcus flaps are created, and tunneling of the anterior maxilla is carried out through them. Very limited dissection of the Veau flaps should be carried out. *C*, A stab incision is made through the mucosa over the premaxilla to divide the nasal septum. *D*, The maxillary segments and premaxilla are down-fractured and mobilized into the required position. *E*, The nasal lining is sutured from the lateral nasal wall to the mucosa elevated off the side of the nasal septum. *F*, The maxillary segments are stabilized with miniplates, and a fifth plate is inserted from each maxilla across the midline to stabilize the premaxilla. This maneuver is performed by tunneling under the mucosa. *G*, The alveolar fistulas are closed and bone grafts are placed in the usual way. *H*, Additional bone grafts can be inserted over the osteotomy lines and in the region of the pterygomaxillary junction if required.

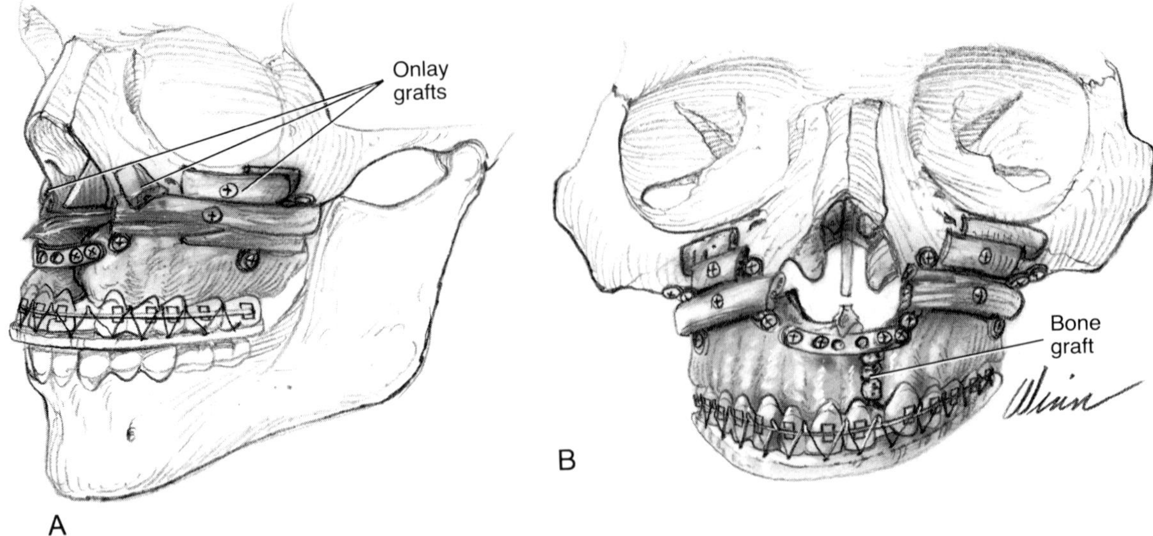

Figure 63–9 *A* and *B,* Split cranial bone grafts are placed over the osteotomy site in large advancements of the maxilla and can be placed further up on the maxilla for increased augmentation of the facial profile. They are held in place with one lag screw.

cephalometrically and aesthetically, the mandible can be set back at the same time the maxilla is advanced. We have found that in very large maxillary advancements, such as those requiring more than a 10-mm advancement, there is a significant degree of relapse of the advancement in spite of the use of miniplates. The amount of relapse is proportional to the increased advancement. Therefore, we feel that maxillary advancement should be limited and combined with a simultaneous mandibular setback.

The techniques we use to set back the mandible are either a subcondylar vertical ramus osteotomy or a sagittal split osteotomy. Surgical exposure for both these techniques is accomplished through the same lower posterior buccal sulcus incision. The lateral ramus of the mandible is exposed and, in the vertical subcondylar osteotomy, a right-angled oscillating saw is used to make a vertical cut from the mandibular notch to the inferior border of the mandible. The mandible is set back, and the posterior segment is placed lateral to the anterior segment. It is usually necessary to wire these segments together, keeping the patient in intermaxillary fixation for 6 to 8 weeks during healing. The advantage of this technique is the very low incidence of damage to the inferior alveolar nerve.

The sagittal split technique entails dividing the medial cortex of the ascending ramus above the lingula with a saw, bringing the saw cut through the cortical bone along the external oblique line, and cutting the lateral cortex approximately opposite the second molar tooth. The mandible is then split sagittally with fine osteotomes to avoid damaging the inferior alveolar nerve. The mandible is placed in occlusion with an acrylic splint. Because the mandible has been set backward, the anterior part of the lateral cortex overlaps the medial part of the mandible, and this should be removed with a saw or bur. Then the sagittal split is rigidly fixed with three lag screws (Fig. 63–10). These can be inserted through the transcutaneous approach utilizing a trocar and cannula, or, alternatively, a right-angled drill and screwdriver can be used to insert the screws with some difficulty intraorally, avoiding the 3- to 4-mm scar beneath the angle of the mandible. Rigid fixation of the mandible eliminates the need for prolonged rigid intermaxillary fixation postoperatively. However, the technique of intermittent usage of dental elastics, as previously explained, should be used.

Genioplasty

If the patient has a small chin or if an extensive setback of the mandible is required, an advancement genioplasty can be performed during the same operation. The amount of advancement of the chin can be calculated in advance from cephalometric tracings and drawings. If the chin is excessively long, it can be reduced in vertical height at the same time. It is best to perform the genioplasty last, after the jaw surgery is complete, to check the aesthetic appearance of the face.

The genioplasty is performed through an anterior lower buccal sulcus incision, stripping the mucoperiosteum off the chin and passing beneath the mental foramen laterally and inferiorly. The mucoperiosteum over the lower border of the chin in the midline should be left attached. A reciprocating saw is used to make a transverse cut across the chin below the level of the mental foramen, extending laterally to the mental nerve.

If the chin height is to be reduced vertically, the lower cut is made first with a saw, and a parallel cut is made the required amount above this, staying below the mental foramen. The middle segment is removed. The inferior segment is then brought upward, advanced forward the necessary measured amount, and held in place with one miniplate, either T-shaped or H-shaped (Fig. 63–10B). The mucoperiosteum over the chin should be closed in two layers, ensuring that the peri-

Figure 63–10 A, In patients requiring extensive maxillary advancement (more than 10 mm) or who have true associated mandibular prognathism, simultaneous two-jaw surgery can be performed using a Le Fort I maxillary advancement combined, usually, with a bilateral sagittal mandibular osteotomy and setback. A compensatory advancement genioplasty may be necessary to maintain a good profile. *B*, The position of the maxilla is established by measurements from the normal bone above; it is fixed in place with miniplates. The mandible is set back and fitted to the maxilla over the predesigned acrylic wafer. The sagittal split is stabilized with three lag screws, and the genioplasty segment is advanced and held with a T-shaped or double-T-shaped miniplate.

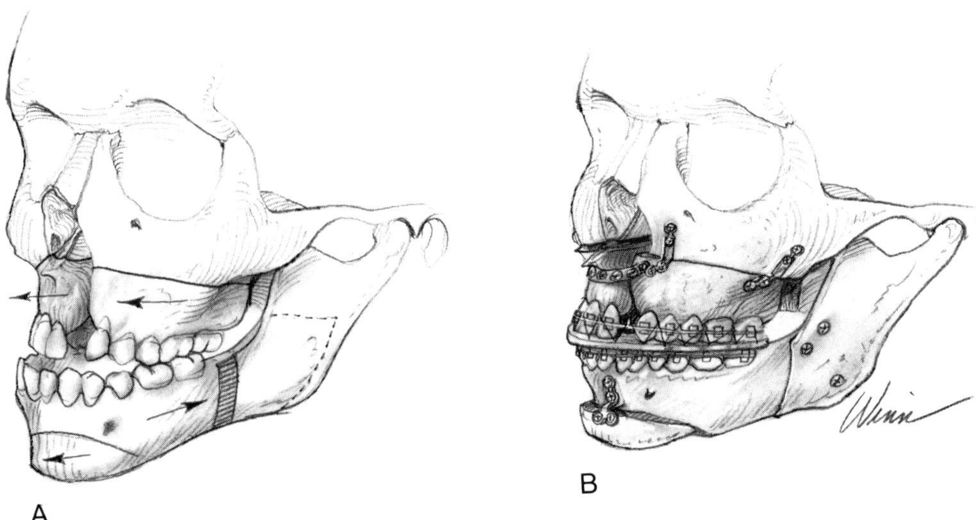

osteum is brought upward and sutured before the mucosa is closed. At the end of the operation, the skin of the chin should be taped upward to prevent prolapse of the lip downward.

Split Lamellar Technique

Salyer has recently described a facial osteotomy technique that, instead of moving the bilamellar maxilla, splits the bone into inner and outer lamellae.[22] This technique maintains the internal lamella in a native position, allowing it to act as a reference point for the bony topography and providing a stable facial framework for rigid fixation. The outer lamella is cut and advanced, allowing aesthetic orthomorphic reconstruction of the malar and paranasal deficiency of the maxilla. Through a transbuccal incision, the entire maxilla, infraorbital nerve, inferior and lateral orbital rims, and the lateral malar zygomatic complex are identified (Fig. 63–11A). An angled retractor is placed in the orbits to protect the globe from below.

Using an oscillating saw, the front of the maxilla is split through the maxillary buttress and the paranasal region in the frontal plane (Fig. 63–11B). Using a right-angled oscillating saw, the malar bone is then cut through at a level that will allow the malar bone to be advanced in continuity with the remaining outer lamella of the maxilla (Fig. 63–11C). This procedure can be performed alone or in combination with screw and miniplate fixation (Fig. 63–11E). It can also be performed in combination with bone grafting or maxillary Le Fort I advancement. This technique also has been used in patients who have previously undergone bone grafting and yet have inadequate projection and contour in the face. The bone graft is left attached to the anterior lamella and is then split in the fashion described (Fig. 63–11).

Split lamellar osteotomy is particularly adaptable, allowing for freedom of reconstruction as sliding and rotational translocations of the maxilla and malar region become possible. This technique provides membranous bone that is thin enough for the surgeon to bend, contour, and curve without fracturing and facilitates improved aesthetic balance in the cleft patient.

Timing of Surgery

Closure of the alveolar fistula with bone grafting is best performed in the period of mixed dentition, just prior to the eruption of the canine teeth. This is usually between 7 and 10 years of age. Once the fistula has been closed and the cancellous bone has healed, solid bony union of the cleft will have been achieved. The canine teeth will tend to erupt spontaneously into this bone and can be guided by the orthodontist into the dental arch. Teeth are then aligned, and orthodontic braces are removed. Orthodontic braces should not be retained for a prolonged period of time.

Ideally, orthognathic surgery is performed when growth of the patient is complete. This usually means around the age of 15 years for girls and 17 to 18 years for boys. Orthodontic bands are applied prior to surgery, and the teeth are aligned within each arch. The bands are left in place to facilitate intermaxillary fixation during surgery and the use of dental elastics postoperatively. In children with gross malocclusion and a severe facial deformity, we have performed maxillary advancements in children as young as the age of 9 or 10 years. In these cases, it is important to perform the osteotomy high on the maxilla to avoid disturbing the unerupted teeth. The operation must be justified for psychosocial reasons. Furthermore, the patient and parents must understand that there is a very strong possibility that a repeat operation may be needed because the maxilla will not grow anteriorly following surgery, although it will grow vertically.[23]

Ideally, we prefer to correct irregularities of cleft lip scarring and the cleft lip nose 6 months after orthognathic surgery. It is extremely difficult to perform

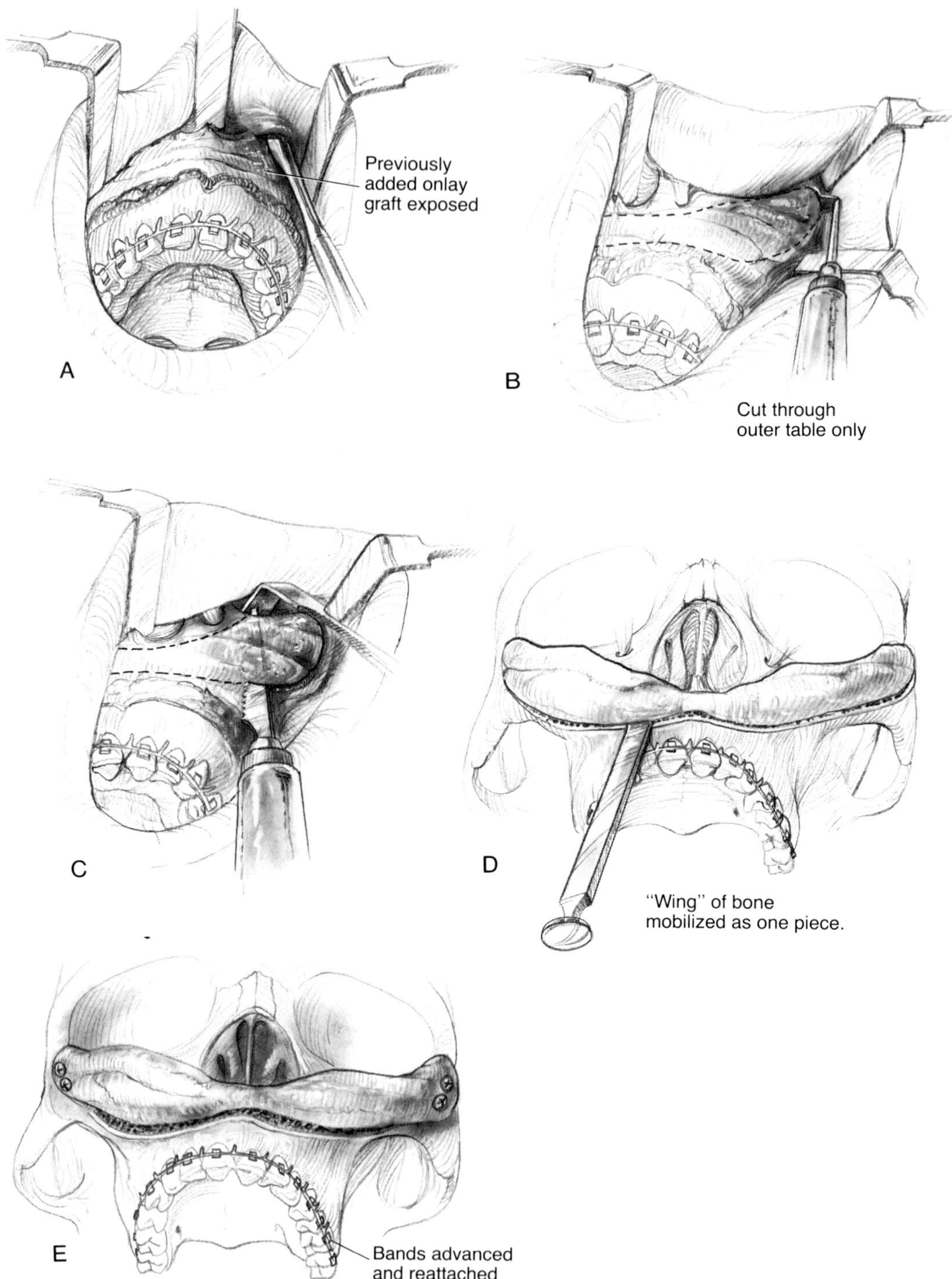

Figure 63–11 *A*, The anterior maxilla is stripped subperiostally up to the inferior orbital rim and over the malar bone. *B*, A maxilla that has had previous onlay bone grafting. An oscillating saw is used to divide this bone up to and including the inferior orbital rim. *C*, The malar bone is cut at a bevel with a right-angle oscillating saw. *D*, The segment is mobilized with an osteotome for advancement. *E*, The segment is held in the advanced position with lag screws.

refined surgery on the soft tissues at the same time as orthognathic surgery. However, this soft tissue surgery can be performed at a younger age without any deleterious effect on maxillary growth. These patients may have retromaxillism and, in particular, severe repositioning of the alar base. To produce the best correction of the nose, it is necessary to mobilize all the soft tissue attachments of the alar base to the bony margins of the piriform fossa and then augment the basal bone with an onlay split cranial graft at the same time. This bone graft will have no adverse effect on subsequent forward maxillary growth but does allow better correction of the nose.

Problems of Speech Related to Clefts

Patients with cleft lip and palate may have speech problems related to malocclusion anteriorly or the velopharyngeal mechanism posteriorly. There may be anterior sibilant distortion related to dentition. This is particularly common in patients who have an alveolar fistula, a gap in the dental arch, or an anterior class III malocclusion. These problems can be corrected by closing the fistula and either bringing a tooth into the dental arch or replacing it with a prosthetic tooth on a dental plate. Occlusion can be corrected by a maxillary osteotomy, which in turn will correct the anterior sibilant distortion.[24]

Some patients who undergo maxillary advancement are at risk of developing worse speech quality than they had before surgery.[25, 26] We believe that all patients undergoing maxillary advancement should have nasendoscopy performed by the speech pathologist and surgeon together. One of three conditions may then be seen. If there is normal velopharyngeal closure, these patients are not at risk of developing worse speech as a result of a maxillary advancement. However, if there is touch closure or even slightly incomplete closure, particularly if there has been a large amount of speech therapy in the past, there is a great risk of developing velopharyngeal insufficiency following maxillary advancement. Third, there is the group of patients who already have velopharyngeal insufficiency, whether or not they have had a previous pharyngeal flap.

Two alternatives are then possible. The patient can be counseled about the likelihood of developing worse speech quality following maxillary advancement. Also, 6 months after maxillary surgery, a pharyngeal flap procedure can be carried out to correct the speech problem. In many centers it has been considered dangerous to perform a pharyngeal flap at the time of maxillary advancement, particularly if the patient is kept in postoperative intermaxillary fixation, because of the hazards to the airway in the immediate postoperative period. However, with a well-organized team and a good intensive care unit, this hazard can be decreased by maintaining postoperative nasotracheal intubation for several days, even with the patient in intermaxillary fixation. Presently, with the use of miniplates and the elimination of postoperative rigid intermaxillary fixation, the hazard has been diminished considerably. Therefore, in the patient who already has velopharyngeal insufficiency or in whom it can be predicted to develop, we now advise a pharyngeal flap procedure at the same time as the maxillary advancement. It is very important to make the pharyngeal flap long and loose so that tension is not created at the time of the maxillary advancement (Fig. 63–12).

There is also a group of patients who already have a pharyngeal flap in place at the time a maxillary advancement procedure is required. These patients may have normal speech, or they may still have incompetent velopharyngeal closure. In either case, maxillary advancement is not possible when a tight pharyngeal flap is present. In these patients, a new superiorly based pharyngeal flap is created and lifted high, which lifts the base of the previous pharyngeal flap, thus lengthening it (Fig. 63–13A). The new flap is inserted into a fresh fish-mouth incision in the soft palate below the previous flap, thus correcting incompetence, lengthening the previous flap, and allowing maxillary advancement (Fig. 63–13B).

Conclusions

In cleft patients who have had good primary surgery with only one operation performed to close the hard and soft palates, the incidence of retromaxillism requiring orthognathic surgery should probably be no higher than 10% to 20% of all cases (Figs. 63–14 to 63–17). Orthognathic surgery in cleft patients is considerably more difficult than a Le Fort I osteotomy in a noncleft patient. The difficulty lies in mobilizing and advancing the segments without jeopardizing the blood supply to the maxilla. In addition, the very large amount of scarring has a tendency to cause relapse of the maxilla, even after the osteotomy site is healed. Therefore, we like to overcorrect the occlusion in these patients by 1 to 2 mm or more if the advancement is extensive.

The use of orthognathic surgery in cleft patients has considerably raised the standard of aesthetic appearance that can be achieved as a final result for cleft patients. Planning of the surgery should be done using a multidisciplinary approach; the fundamental purpose of the surgery is a good aesthetic appearance as well as good occlusion. Determining the required amount of basal bone movement is based initially on an aesthetic judgment of the face, enhanced by cephalometric data and the achievement of normal occlusion. When the amount of advancement required for normal occlusion limits the amount of advancement to the midface needed for a good aesthetic appearance, either the split lamella technique can be utilized or additional split cranial grafts can be layered over the maxilla and zygomas up to the level of the inferior orbital rims, if necessary, to produce the correct convex contours of the face. We strongly believe that these patients should be managed by a multidisciplinary team that is experienced in dealing with a large number of cleft patients from the orthodontic, dental, speech, prosthetic, and plastic surgery points of view.

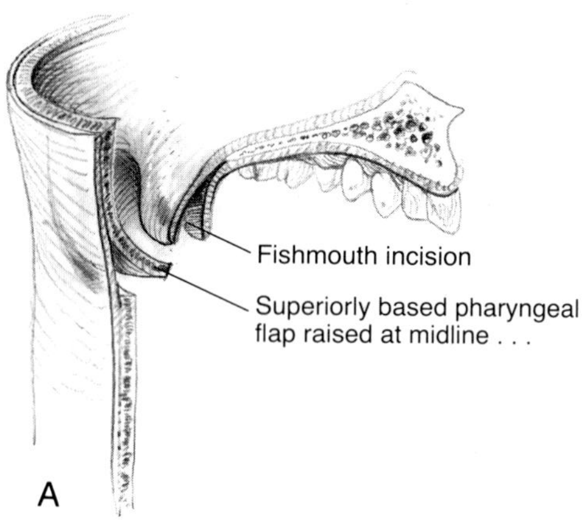

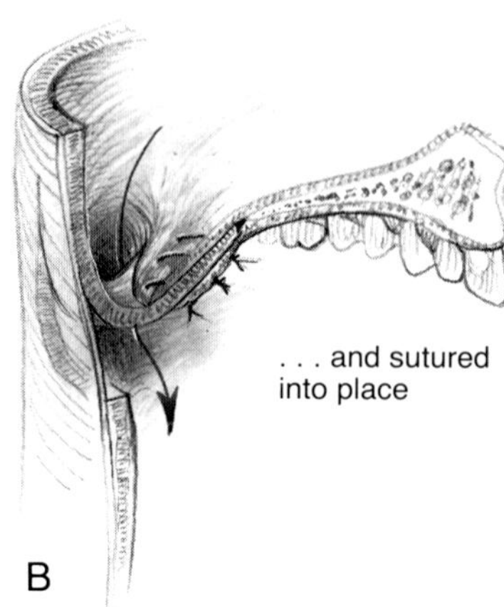

Figure 63–12 *A,* If a pharyngeal flap is necessary at the time of maxillary advancement, a wide superiorly based pharyngeal flap is elevated, and a fishmouth incision is created in the soft palate to divide the oral and nasal layers. *B,* The pharyngeal flap is inserted into the fishmouth incision and sutured, ensuring that the flap is long and loose to allow subsequent maxillary advancement.

Figure 63–13 *A,* In a patient who needs a Le Fort I maxillary advancement but already has a pharyngeal flap in place the flap will need to be lengthened and frequently an additional flap will be needed to help prevent incompetence if it is present. A new superiorly based pharyngeal flap is elevated below the previous flap; as it is dissected upward, it will lengthen the previous flap. *B,* A new fishmouth incision is created in the soft palate beneath the insertion of the previous pharyngeal flap, and then the flap is brought up, creating a double-layered flap, as shown.

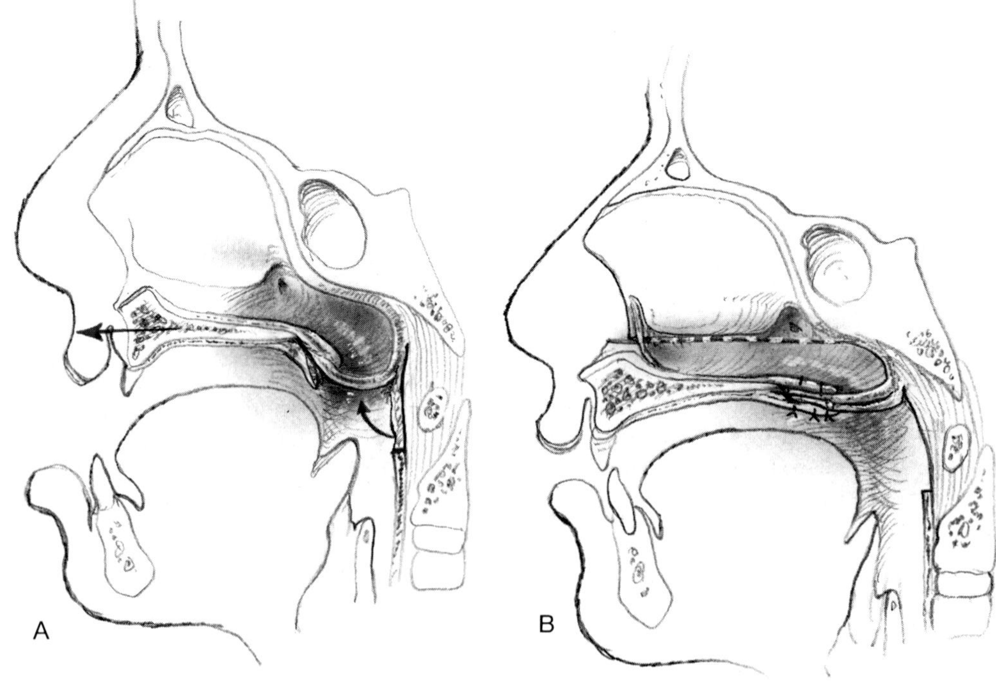

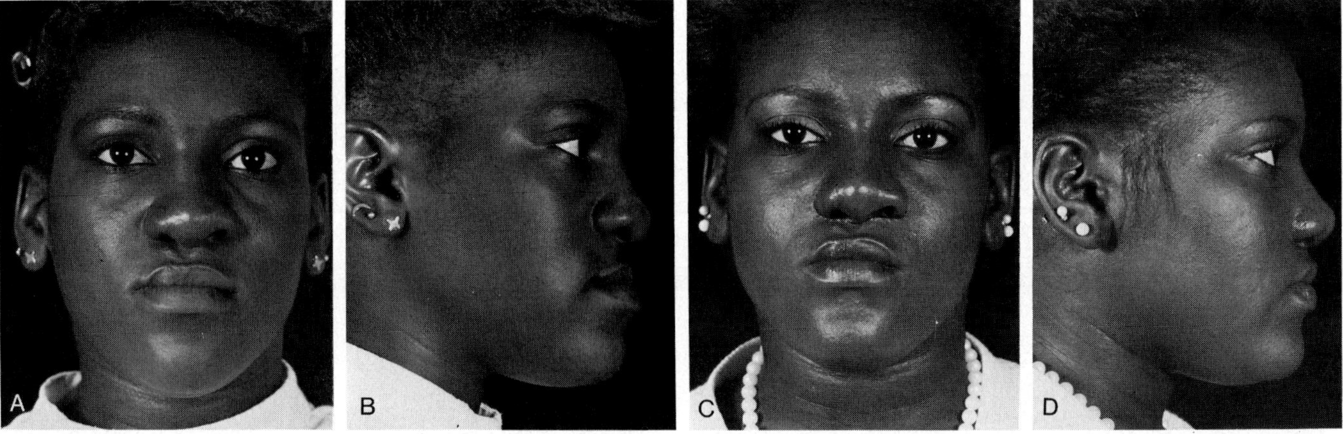

Figure 63–14 *A* and *B*, Preoperative view of a 17-year-old black female with unilateral cleft deformity and retromaxillism. *C* and *D*, Three years following maxillary advancement with onlay grafting to the maxilla and cleft nasal reconstruction.

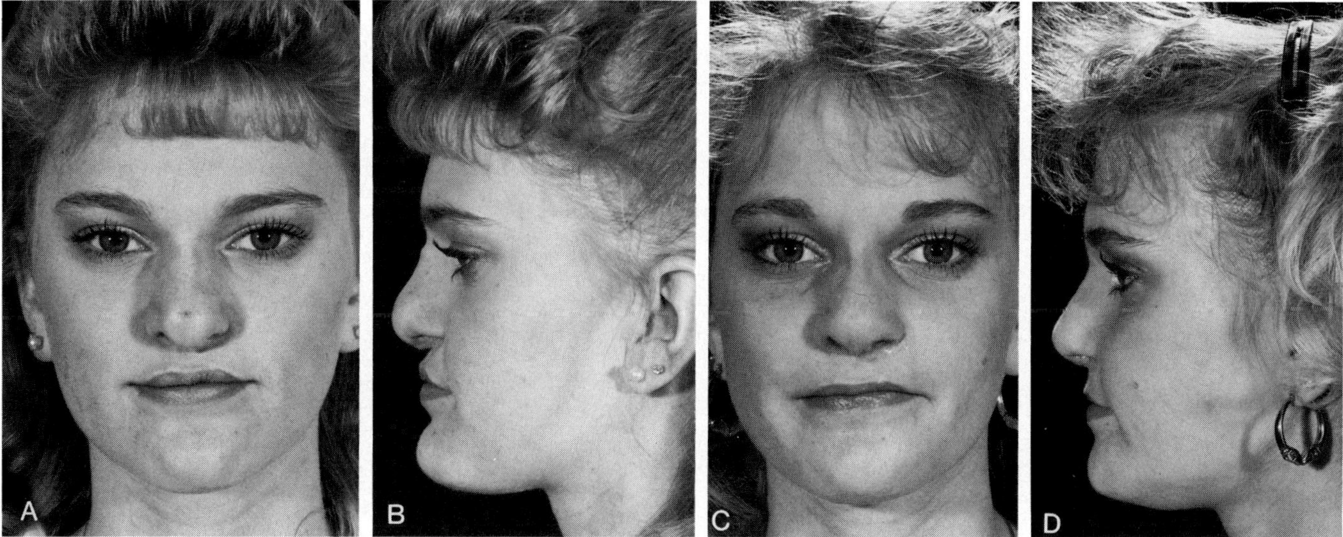

Figure 63–15 *A* and *B*, Female with left unilateral cleft lip and palate, retromaxillism, and severe maxillary hypoplasia. *C* and *D*, Postoperative result following initial onlay bone grafting of the maxilla with cleft nasal reconstruction and a subsequent operation of split lamellar advancement of the previous bone grafts.

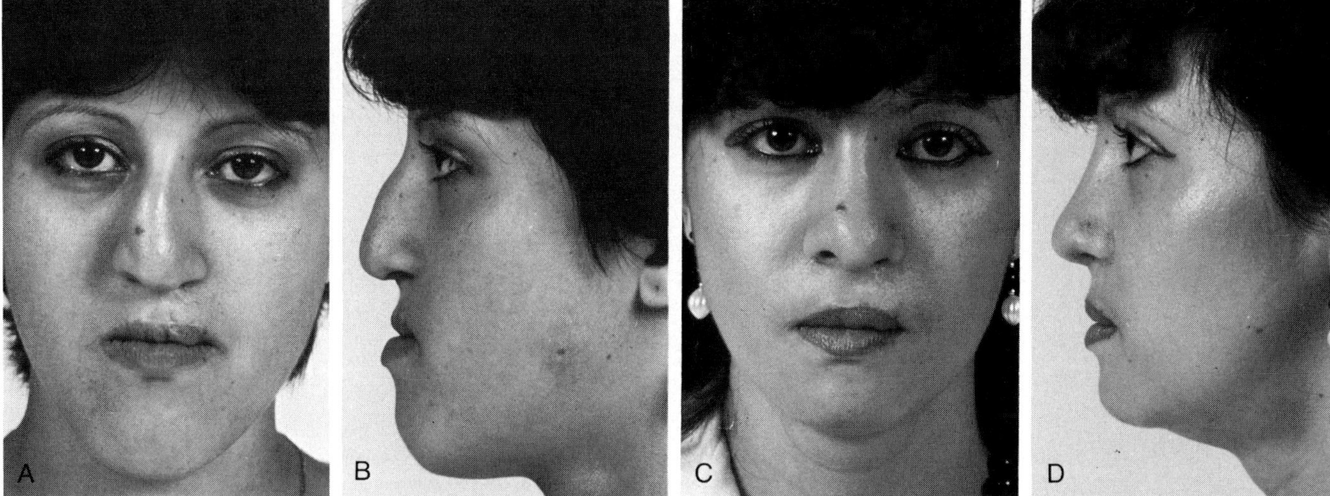

Figure 63–16 *A* and *B*, Seventeen-year-old female with severe retromaxillism, true mandibular prognathism, and a long chin. *C* and *D*, Four years following a Le Fort I maxillary advancement of 9 mm, simultaneous mandibular setback of 10 mm, vertical reduction of the chin by 8 mm with simultaneous advancement of 3 mm, and a superiorly based pharyngeal flap. Two years later reconstruction of the cleft lip and nose was carried out.

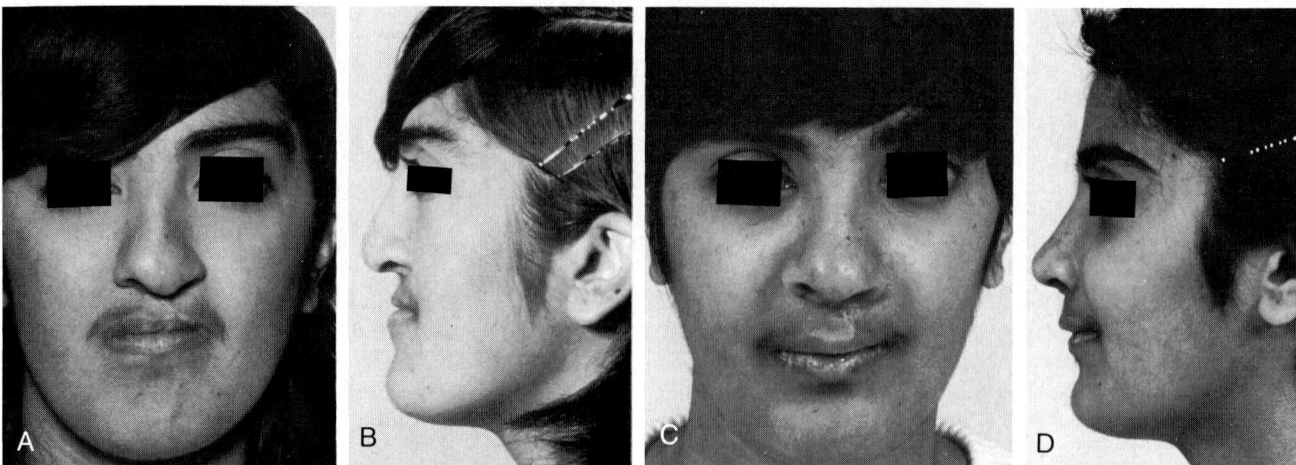

Figure 63–17 *A* and *B*, Nineteen-year-old female with severe retromaxillism and medial collapse of the dental arch. *C* and *D*, Six months following a Le Fort I advancement of 10 mm in two segments with an 18-mm widening of the molar teeth, a simultaneous superiorly based pharyngeal flap, and a subsequent revision of the cleft lip and nose.

References

1. Ross RB: Treatment variables affecting facial growth in complete unilateral cleft lip and palate: Part 5: Timing of palate repair. Cleft Palate J 24:54–63, 1987.
2. Ross RB: Treatment variables affecting facial growth in complete unilateral cleft lip and palate: Part 6: Techniques of palate repair. Cleft Palate J 24:64–70, 1987.
3. Ross RB: Treatment variables affecting facial growth in complete unilateral cleft lip and palate: Part 7: An overview of treatment and facial growth. Cleft Palate J 24:71–77, 1987.
4. Drommer R: The history of the "Le Fort I osteotomy." J Maxillofac Surg 14:119–121, 1986.
5. Langenbeck BV: Beitrage zur Osteoplastik—Die osteoplastische Resektion des Oberkiefers. Goschen, A., Deutsche Klinik. Berlin: Reimer, 1859.
6. Axhausen G: Die operative Orthopadie bei den Fehlbildungen der Kiefer. Dtsch Zach-, Mund- Kieferheilk 6:582, 1939.
7. Schuchardt K: Ein Beitrag zur chirurgischen Kieferorthopadie unter Berucksichtigung ihrer Bedeutung für die Behandlung angeborener und erworbener Kieferdeformitaten bei Soldaten. Dtsch Zahn-, Mund- Kieferheilk 9:73, 1942.
8. Gillies H, Rowe NL: L'osteotomie du maxillaire superieur envisagee essentiellement dans les cas de bec de lievre totale. Rev Stomat 55:545, 1954.
9. Gillies HG: The Principles and Art of Plastic Surgery. London: Butterworth, 1957.
10. Dingman RO, Harding RL: The treatment of malunited fractures of the facial bones. Plast Reconstr Surg 7:505, 1951.
11. Widmaier W: Die chirurgische Behandlung der postoperativen Kieferdeformierungen nach Lippen-Kiefer-Gaumenspalten Operationen. Thesis. Tubingen, 1959.
12. Obwegeser H: Eingriffe am Oberkiefer zur Korrektur des progenen Zustandsbildes. Schweiz Mschr Zahnheilk 75:356, 1965.
13. Hogeman KE, Wilmar K: Die Vorverlagerung des Oberkiefers zur Korrektur von Gebisbanomalien. In Schuchardt K (ed): Fortschr Kiefer- Gesichtschir Hrsg. Stuttgart: G. Thieme, 1967.
14. Beals SP, Munro IR: The use of miniplates in craniomaxillofacial surgery. Plast Reconstr Surg 79:33–38, 1987.
15. Salyer KE: Techniques in Aesthetic Craniofacial Surgery. New York: Gower Publishing, 1988, pp 214–242.
16. Abyholm FE, Borchgrevink HC, Eskeland G: Cleft lip and palate in Norway: III. Surgical treatment of cleft lip and palate patients in Oslo. Scand J Plast Reconstr Surg, Suppl 2, 1981.
17. Abyholm FE, Bergland O, Serub G: Secondary bone grafting of alveolar clefts, Scand J Plast Reconstr Surg, Suppl 2, 1981.
18. Berglund O, Semb G, Abyholm F: Elimination of residual alveolar cleft by secondary bone grafting and subsequent orthodontic treatment. Cleft Palate J 23:175, 1986.
19. Wolfe SA, Berkowitz S: The use of cranial bone grafts in the closure of alveolar and anterior palatal clefts. Plast Reconstr Surg 72:659, 1983.
20. Ortiz-Monasterio F, Rebeil AF, Valderrama M, et al: Cephalometric measurements on adult patients with non-operated cleft palates. Plast Reconstr Surg 24:53, 1959.
21. Ortiz-Monasterio F, Serrano A, Barrera G, et al: A study of untreated adult cleft patients. Plast Reconstr Surg 38:36, 1966.
22. Salyer KE, Hall CD, Bruce DA: Lamellar split osteotomy: A new craniofacial technique. Presented at the 67th meeting of the American Association of Plastic Surgeons, Palm Beach, Florida, May, 1988.
23. Bachmayer DI, Ross RB, Munro IR: Maxillary growth following Le Fort III advancement surgery in Crouzon, Apert and Pfeiffer syndromes. Am J Orthod Dentofac Orthopaed 90(5):420–430, 1986.
24. Witzel MA, Ross RB, Munro IR: Articulation before and after facial osteotomy. J Maxillofac Surg 8:195–202, 1980.
25. Witzel MA, Munro IR: Velopharyngeal insufficiency after maxillary advancement. Cleft Palate J 14:176–180, 1977.
26. McCarthy JC, Coccaro PJ, Schwartz MD: Velopharyngeal function following maxillary advancement. Plast Reconstr Surg 64:180, 1979.

CHAPTER 64

Treatment of Skeletal Deformities in the Cleft Patient

E. Keller and Ian T. Jackson

Without an understanding of the management of the skeletal aspects of the cleft deformity, the possibility of achieving an optimal aesthetic and functional result is considerably reduced. In the child with a unilateral cleft, the maxilla on the cleft side is invariably hypoplastic at birth and remains so;[1] in the bilateral cleft, hypoplasia may be observed on both sides. When there is a soft tissue cleft, no matter how minimal, there is an underlying bony defect; this is most severe in the complete cleft of the primary palate. These skeletal deficiencies lead to a lack of support for the alar base, nostril, sill, and columellar base. There is frequently an anterior crossbite and an absence of a segment of the alveolus that prevents tooth eruption in the affected area. In addition to alveolopalatal and associated hypoplasia, there may be maxillary vertical or anteroposterior deficiency with a class III skeletal malocclusion, which results in a rather typical facial deformity in cleft patients. It is important to address these skeletal-dental aspects of the anomaly in the correct way and at the proper time.

Alveolopalatal Cleft Closure and Bone Grafting

The defect in the alveolus is the first of the skeletal problems to be treated. Since the work of Boyne,[2, 3] Boyne and Sands,[4, 5] and Abyholm et al,[6, 7] it has been accepted that the optimal time for secondary bone grafting of the defect is around 8 to 9 years of age.[8, 9, 10] The orthodontist evaluates the patient's overall dental condition, in particular, the position and developmental stage of the maxillary central incisor, cuspid, and lateral incisor (if present). At this time the orthodontist may opt to perform some alignment of erupted teeth or expansion of the arches prior to beginning bone grafting. In the ideal situation, the incisor roots should be completely formed and the cuspid positioned high in the proximal segment. This condition will help prevent damage to the root of the incisor at the time of surgery and allow bony reconstruction of the cleft. In addition, supernumerary and selected deciduous teeth in the cleft area should be removed prior to bone grafting.

Two aspects of the alveolar bone grafting procedure need to be addressed prior to describing the procedure. The first is the selection of the donor site; the iliac crest is our first choice because of the large amounts of cancellous bone that can be harvested from it.[8, 11, 12, 13, 14] More recently, the use of cranial bone has been described.[15] There are significant objections to the use of cranial bone; for one thing, the harvesting cannot be accomplished simultaneously with the repair, and thus the procedure is prolonged. Also, cranial bone, in contrast to iliac bone, lacks the characteristics of abundant cellular-rich cancellous bone, which can be packed into spaces and molded into shapes. After some experience with cranial bone, we have returned to using cancellous bone from the iliac crest for alveolar bone grafting. It is important to note that in our center bone grafts from the skull are frequently used for reconstruction of the craniofacial skeleton.[16] Surgical morbidity from iliac crest harvesting from the medial ilium is quite low, particularly in the young patient.[12]

The second consideration is closure of the soft tissue defect of the alveolus. Either buccal mucosa or gingiva may be used. Gingiva is a better choice because it provides a more physiologic environment for subsequent tooth eruption and for dental prostheses.[2, 3, 6] On occasion, when the defect is very wide or in selected bilateral cases, the rotation advancement flap of buccal mucosa may be required.[8]

Surgical Techniques

Alveolopalatal Cleft Closure with Bone Grafting and Simultaneous Lip-Nose Reconstruction

In patients with a vertically short lip, unsatisfactory scar, or divided orbicularis oris muscle, a total reoperation of the lip is usually performed. The resulting wide surgical access allows an easier repair of the palatal and labial cleft.[11, 17] The through incision is done with a No. 11 blade, opening the entire lip and extending the incision through the floor of the nose and alveolus. The lip segments are retracted on both sides using silk sutures; a wide view of the alveolar and floor of nose defect is thereby obtained. In most unilateral clefts there is nasal obstruction on the cleft side due to hypertrophy of the lower turbinate, septal deviation, and cranial displacement of the vomerine ridge. To provide a good airway, the turbinate is frequently trimmed. The cartilaginous septum is repositioned and the vomerine ridge is excised. The bony septum (vomer) may have to be repositioned in the same operation. An incision is made vertically on either side of the alveolar cleft, and the mucoperiosteum is elevated from the medial and lateral sides of the cleft as far posteriorly as necessary—i.e., to the posterior extent of the palatal fistula and bony defect. An incision is made anteroposteriorly along the palatal edges of the cleft. This allows elevation of medial and lateral mucoperiosteal flaps that are used for repair of the nasal floor. This repair is made easier by using a specially designed circle needle on 4–0 chromic catgut. To move the alar base into its correct position, the short (hypoplastic) lateral edge should be lengthened. This is accomplished by making an unequal Z-plasty, bringing a larger flap from the medial edge.

Attention is now turned to the palate. If the defect is large, it may be necessary to fashion two mucoperiosteal flaps as designed by Veau. Smaller palatal defects can often be closed with a single flap. When the medial palatal defect is closed, it is usually possible to close, or almost close, the lateral defects to minimize exposure of the bare bone.

At this point, the anterior and alveolar portions of the cleft require oral closure. This closure is achieved by elevating the gingiva from the buccal aspect of the lesser alveolar segment and the anterior face of the maxilla. This is done by introducing the elevator from the edge of the alveolar defect. To mobilize the gingiva, it is incised in the gingival sulcus and then vertically in the bicuspid-molar region. It is usually possible to move the gingival flap medially to close the alveolar defect. If mobility is insufficient, a horizontal incision is made through the periosteum at the superior edge of the anterior flap. Before closure, the bony defect is packed with cancellous iliac bone. In selected patients, a large corticocancellous block of iliac bone is first placed to fill most of the defect. This may be wedged into position to assist skeletal retention of the previously expanded alveolodental segments. The nostril sill area, the nasal spine, and the subalar base region are also grafted. The soft tissue defect is now closed by advancing the gingival flap.

When there is a large defect, or in patients with bilateral clefts, a buccal flap may be necessary to achieve closure,[8] but this should be avoided if at all possible. With nonkeratinized buccal mucosal cover, teeth do not erupt well, and often the bulk of the flap may cause problems with prosthetic reconstruction.

On completion of the cleft closure, the lip-nose repair is performed in standard fashion. The lower lateral cartilage is dissected out, using an intercartilaginous or bucket handle approach, and placed in its correct anatomic position. In the lip, particular attention is paid to reconstruction of the orbicularis oris muscle.

Alveolopalatal Cleft Closure and Bone Grafting with Intact Lip

With the lip retracted using silk sutures, an incision is made around the anterior part of the buccal cleft. The remaining incisions are made as described in the previous section. Again, the mucoperiosteal flaps are elevated up to the level of the nasal floor. To get a safe and secure closure of the nasal floor, a Reverdin needle is used.[8] This instrument carries the suture through the nose and through one of the flaps. The suture is then released. The Reverdin needle is then withdrawn and reloaded with the other end of the suture. It is then introduced through the other flap, released, and withdrawn. The two ends of the suture are pulled out, and the knot is tied on the oral surface with the wound edges everted to the nasal side. The remainder of the closure and bone grafting proceeds as described above.

Onlay Bone Grafting

Onlay bone grafting is indicated when the maxilla is hypoplastic or when the maxillary segments are asymmetric. The potential donor sites for onlay bone grafting are the skull, rib, and iliac crest. Because of the scar and pain at the donor site, the rib is not considered satisfactory for bone grafting. The iliac crest is an easily accessible and good source of cancellous bone. Through a 1- to 1.5-cm incision, a drill hole can be made, and, using a curette, large volumes of cancellous bone can be obtained. This bone can be conveniently packed through a small maxillary buccal sulcus incision into a subperiosteal pocket on the anterior aspect of the maxilla. It is easy to mold, thus establishing the desired contours. The disadvantage of this material, especially in a tight periosteal pocket, is unpredictable resorption. In this situation, cranial bone is more advantageous. The skull is approached through a temporoparietal incision, and skull shavings are taken using a hammer and osteotome. An outer table graft can also be harvested using a contouring bur and osteotome.[16] The shavings can be inserted in layers, or the block can be contoured and inserted. Stabilization is achieved by the confines of the periosteum—e.g., careful preoperative planning and periosteal reflection are mandatory to achieve symmetric aesthetic results. Care is taken not to place the dense cortical cranial bone in the alveolar region where tooth eruption is expected. Occasionally, with the outer table graft a lag screw is used to secure the graft to the piriform aperture rim.

The advantages of skull bone are an inconspicuous and almost painless donor site and a graft that will resorb less than any other because it is composed of very dense cortical membranous bone. One disadvantage of skull bone is the difficulty encountered in contouring particularly dense bone blocks. Also, cranial bone is less resistant to infection than other types of donor bone. Both rib and iliac bone can better resist infection. If graft exposure occurs, complete loss of the cranial cortical grafts is predictable, whereas particulate iliac bone may only be partially lost.

Because of predictable long-term stability, cranial bone, stabilized in a self-contained pocket, is recommended for onlay maxillary bone grafting.

Advantages of Alveolar Bone Grafting

The advantages of alveolar bone grafting (Fig. 64–1) are several. The graft provides bone through which teeth can erupt, and thus dental arch form and aesthetics can be greatly improved. Dental and gingival health is improved because osseous support and keratinized gingiva are provided to the teeth on either side of the cleft. In bilateral clefts, the mobile premaxilla is stabilized. Alveolar bone grafting stabilizes the maxillary segments, which allows the use of a fixed dental prosthesis. The closure of the alveolar cleft provides separation of nasal and oral cavities. Hypernasality may be improved as a result of the anterior cleft closure.[18] The symmetry of the maxilla and nose is improved by the onlay grafting

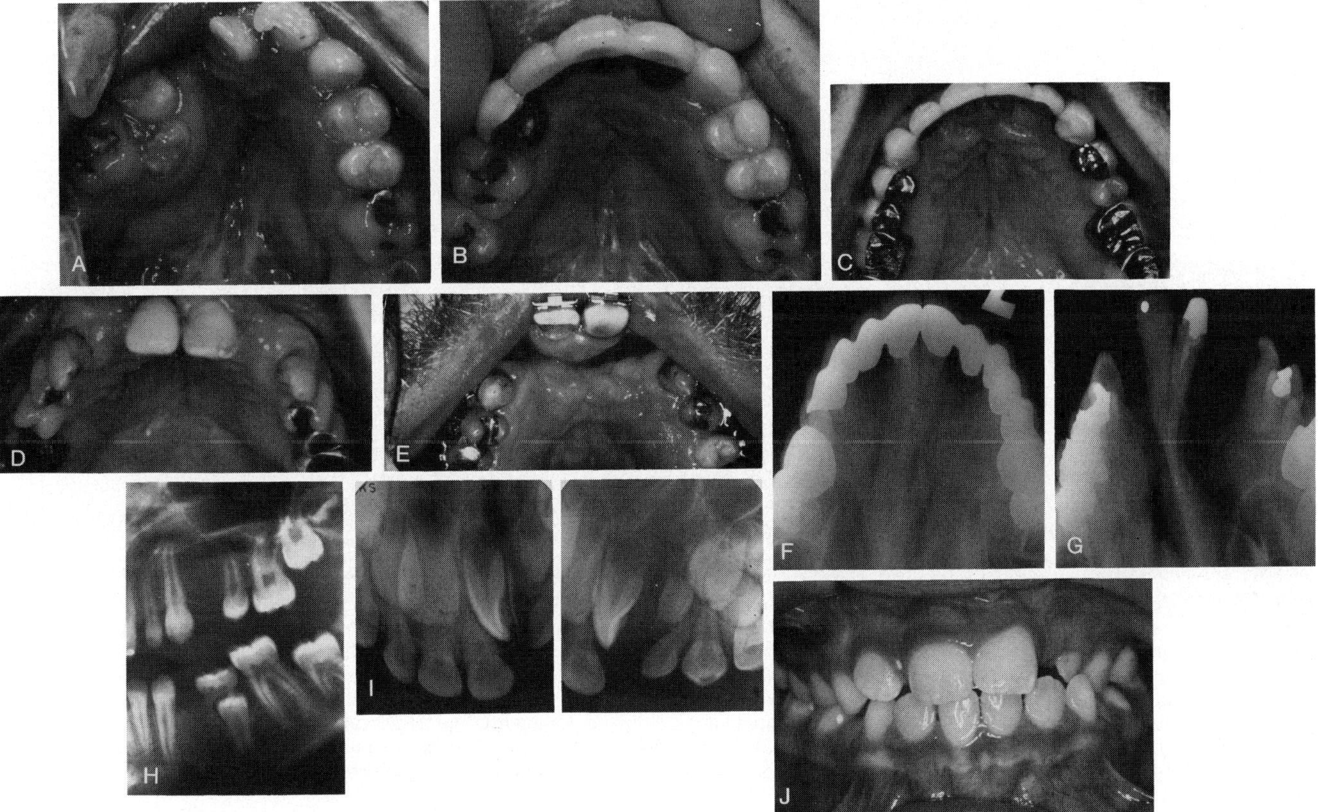

Figure 64–1 Bone grafting of alveolar-palatal cleft. This figure demonstrates the benefits of maxillary palatal-alveolar cleft closure and bone grafting. Arch continuity is established to allow fixed prosthetic reconstruction.

A and *B*. Patient with unilateral cleft before and after bone grafting. Note the improvement in soft tissue inflammation and dental hygiene in B.

C–E. Healthy soft tissue is provided on the alveolus and adjacent dentition. *C* and *D*. Patient with bilateral cleft before and after bone grafting. Note the improvement in soft tissue inflammation and dental hygiene. *E*. A firm anterior segment allows for fixed prosthetic reconstruction.

F and *G*. Osseous tissue is provided to support adjacent dentition. These occlusal radiographs were taken before and after bone grafting in a patient with a bilateral cleft. Note that the nasal floor as well as the alveolus is bone grafted.

H–K. Bone tissue is provided for eruption of permanent dentition in a growing child. *H*. Intraoral radiographs were taken before and after grafting in a 5-year-old unilateral cleft patient. Note the developing permanent lateral incisor and cuspid high in the alveolus. *I*. Six years later the permanent dentition has erupted (lateral incisor and cuspid) into the previous cleft site. *J*. Patient before surgery at age 5.

Illustration continued on following page

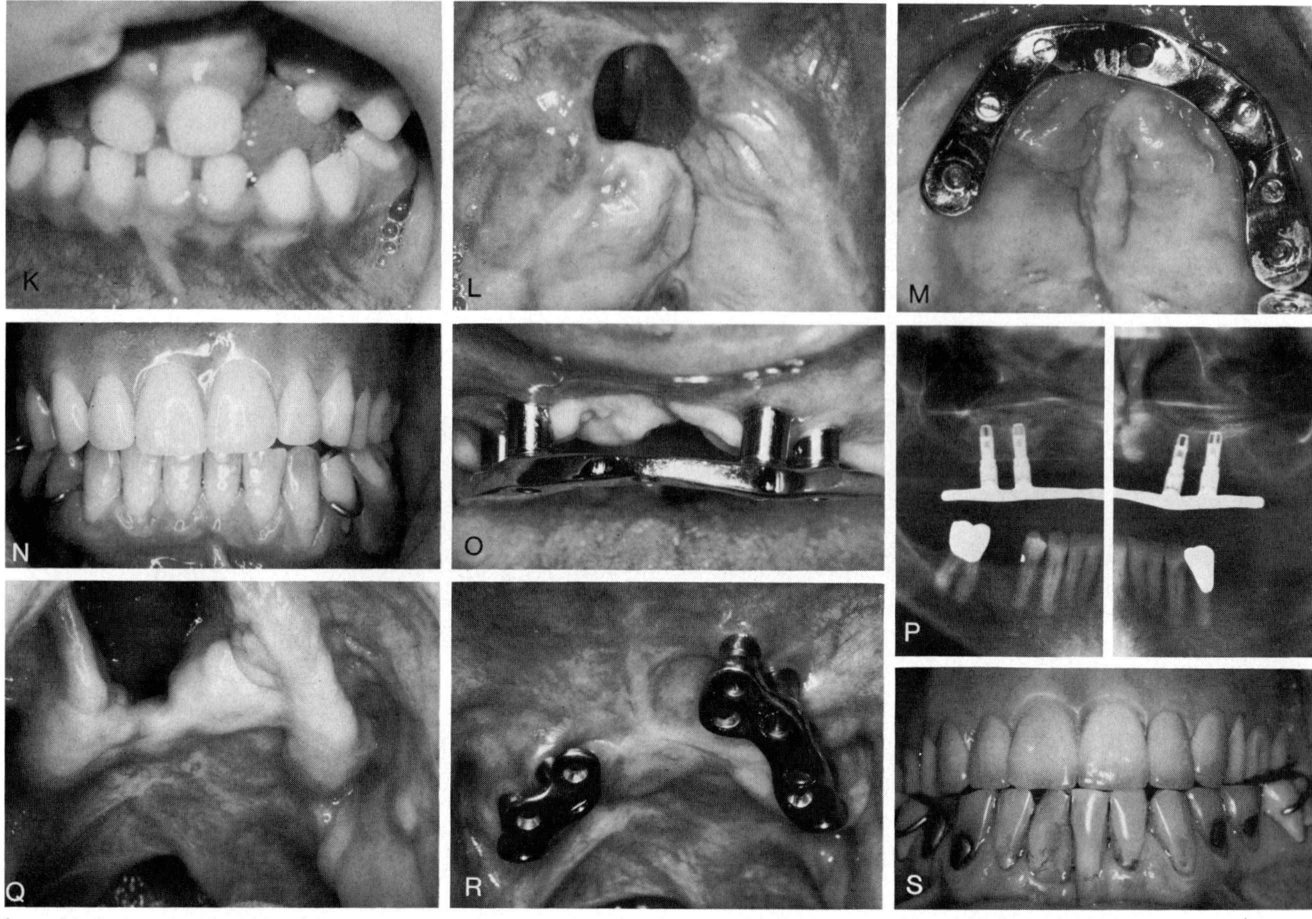

Figure 64–1 *Continued K.* The same patient at age 11. The lateral incisor is deformed and hypoplastic and will require a crown restoration. Bone support is provided for titanium-osseointegrated implants and a fixed osseoprosthesis in the edentulous cleft patient. *L* and *M.* Patient with unilateral edentulous cleft prior to bone grafting and following bone grafting and cleft closure. *N* and *O.* Radiographic and clinical views of the palatal bar attached to titanium endosseous implants. *P.* A fixed-removable (bone-anchored) dental prosthesis is later constructed.

Q–S. Reduction of anterior airflow in large clefts. Cleft closure in this edentulous patient reduced anterior airflow leakage through the large oronasal defect. Following construction of a fixed osseoprosthesis, hypernasality was noticeably reduced. Improvement in speech articulation also occurred owing to the fixed-removable (endosseous implant-supported) prosthesis. *Q* and *R.* Large cleft defect before and after its closure and placement of the titanium endosseous implant. *S.* Fixed-removable osseoprosthesis.

of the maxilla and creation of a nostril sill and nasal spine (see Figs. 64–2, 64–3, and 64–4). Nasal function may be improved by raising the nasal floor until it is equal to that of the noncleft side and placing the septum in its correct anatomic position. Finally, bone grafting of alveolar palatal clefts in edentulous patients allows simultaneous or delayed placement of titanium osseointegrated implants, which initially stabilize the graft and later function as bone anchorage for a dental prosthesis[9, 10] (Fig. 64–1E and F).

Osteotomies in Secondary Cleft Lip and Palate Deformity
(Figs. 64–2 through 64–7)

In the patient with midface retrusion and a class III skeletal malocclusion, a maxillary osteotomy is desirable for functional and aesthetic reasons. However, it is not necessary to perform this until after facial growth is complete (as judged by appropriate maturation indica-

---

Figure 64–2 Quadrangular Le Fort I maxillary osteotomy. Patient with unilateral cleft treated with segmental quadrangular Le Fort I advancement osteotomy with simultaneous iliac bone grafting for stabilization and infraorbital, paranasal, and zygomatic augmentation (an alveolar cleft had been previously closed and grafted). *A.* Diagram illustrating quadrangular Le Fort I osteotomy. *B.* Intraoperative photograph of quadrangular Le Fort I osteotomy in a noncleft patient. *C* and *D.* Patient before and after quadrangular Le Fort I maxillary osteotomy with infraorbital, paranasal, and zygomatic augmentation. *E* and *F.* Same patient before and after surgery.

G and *H.* Lateral cephalograms before and after surgery. Note class

III skeletal open bite malocclusion corrected by maxillary advancement and posterior maxillary impaction. Alveolar-palatal bone grafting was accomplished during a separate surgical procedure.

I and *J.* Maxillary occlusal-palatal photographs taken before and after surgery. Note postsurgical lateral positioning of the lesser segment and eventual eruption of cuspid into the bone-grafted alveolar cleft.

K and *L.* Anterior occlusion before and after surgery. Note correction of class III open bite malocclusion and eruption of the maxillary cuspid. Some relapse of the transverse correction of the lesser segment is noted; there is an end-to-end occlusion posteriorly on the left.

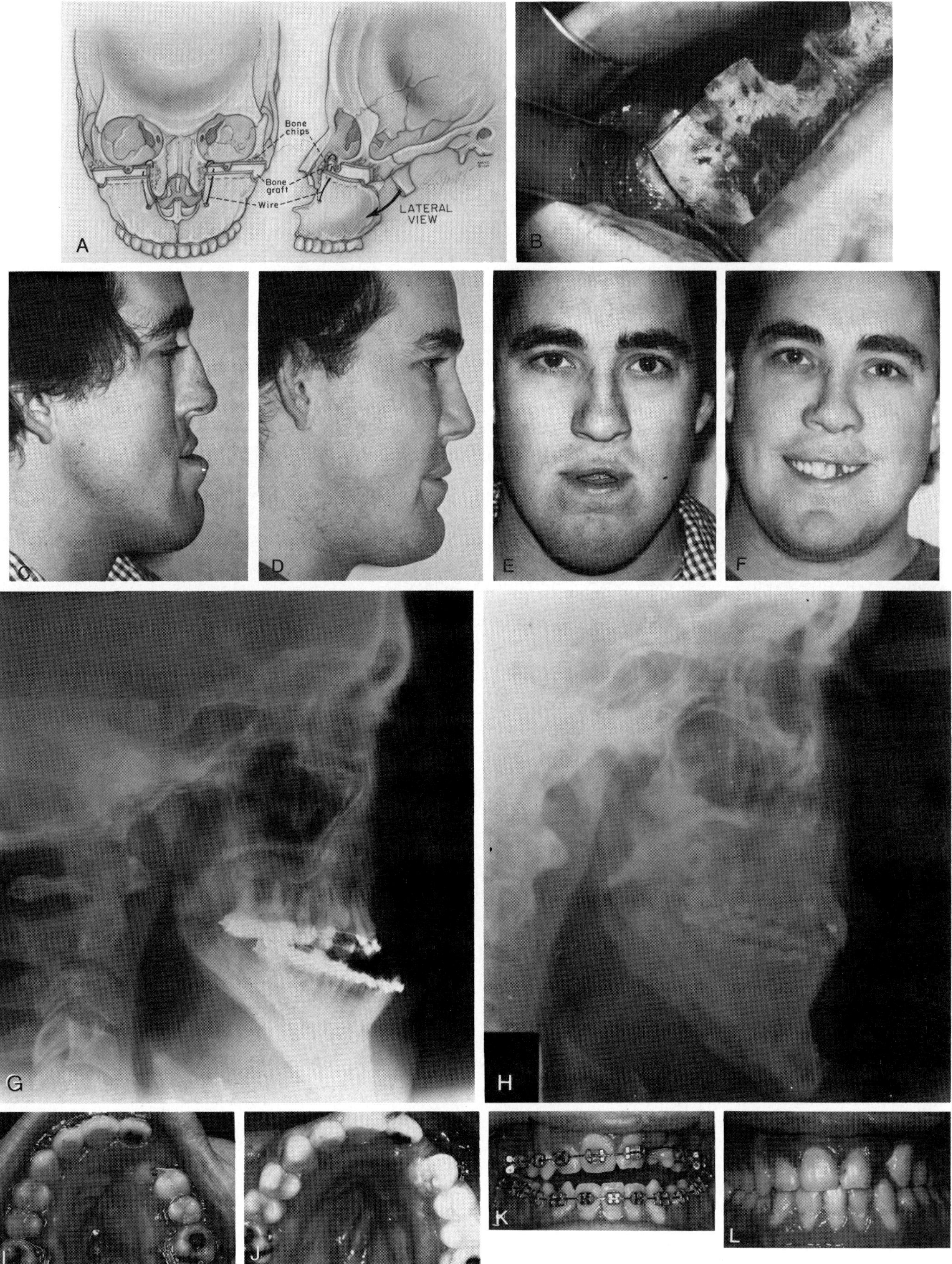

Figure 64–2 See legend on opposite page

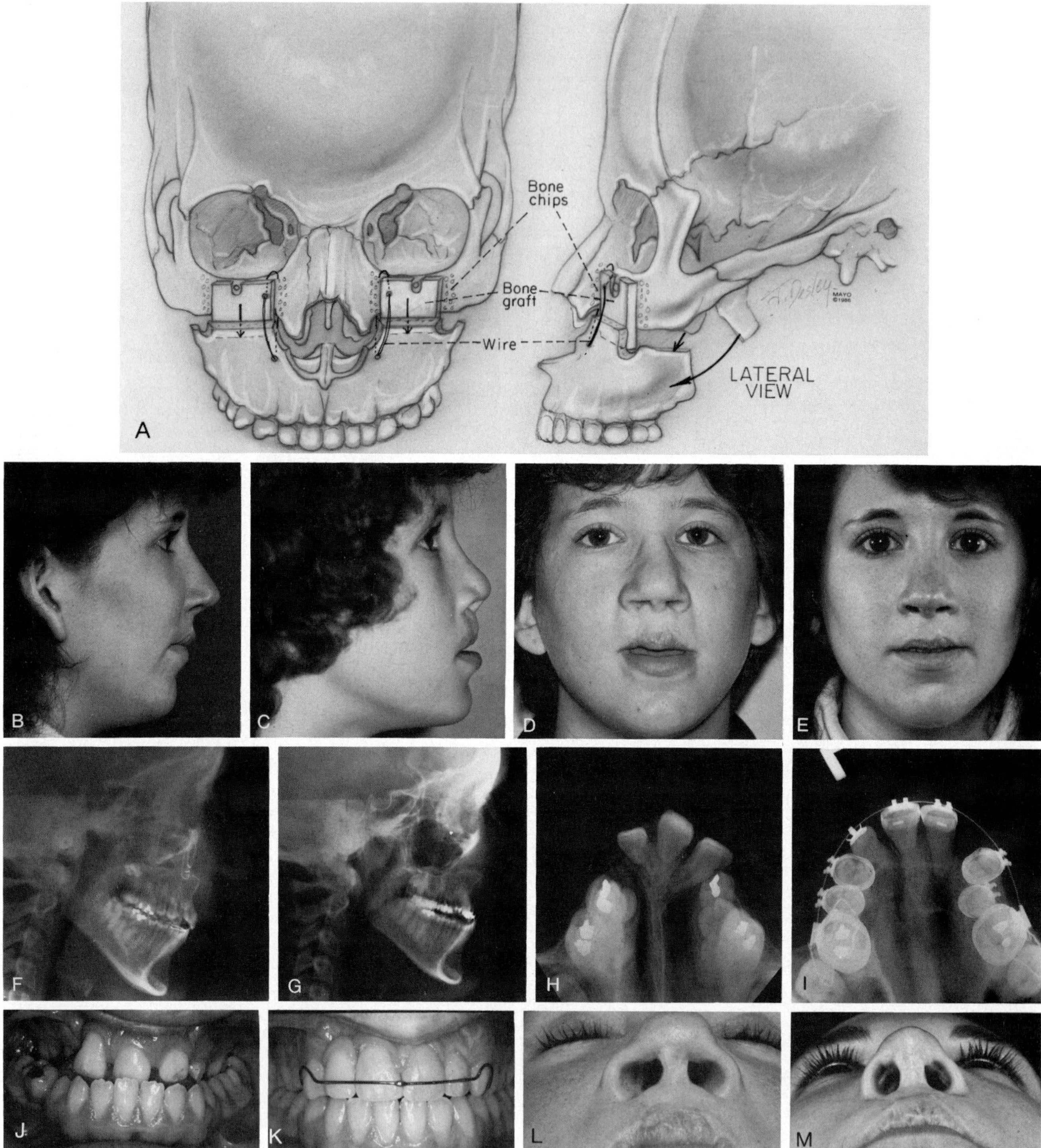

Figure 64–3 Low-level Le Fort I maxillary osteotomy in a patient with a bilateral cleft. Patient with a bilateral cleft of the lip, alveolus, and palate underwent two surgical procedures after the lip and palate were repaired. In the first procedure, bilateral alveolar bone grafting was performed. In the second procedure, a low-level Le Fort I maxillary osteotomy was performed with iliac bone grafts for stabilization and onlay bone grafts in the infraorbital-zygomatic areas for augmentation.

A. Diagram of low-level Le Fort I osteotomy with onlay-inlay infraorbital-zygomatic bone graft augmentation. *B* and *C*. Patient before and after surgery. Note paranasal and infraorbital augmentation.

D and *E*. Same patient before and after Le Fort I maxillary osteotomy. Note alar base support and nasal-lip reconstruction. *F* and *G*. Lateral cephalograms before and after surgery. Note correction of class III skeletal malocclusion. Also note infraorbital onlay bone graft and infraorbital-paranasal transosseous wiring.

H and *I*. Occlusal radiographs before and after osteotomy. Note correction of the palatal width and alveolar-palatal bone graft.

J and *K*. Anterior occlusion before and after surgery. The right lateral incisor has been replaced with a prosthesis.

L and *M*. Before and after correction of the secondary nose-lip deformity, performed 6 months after the osteotomy.

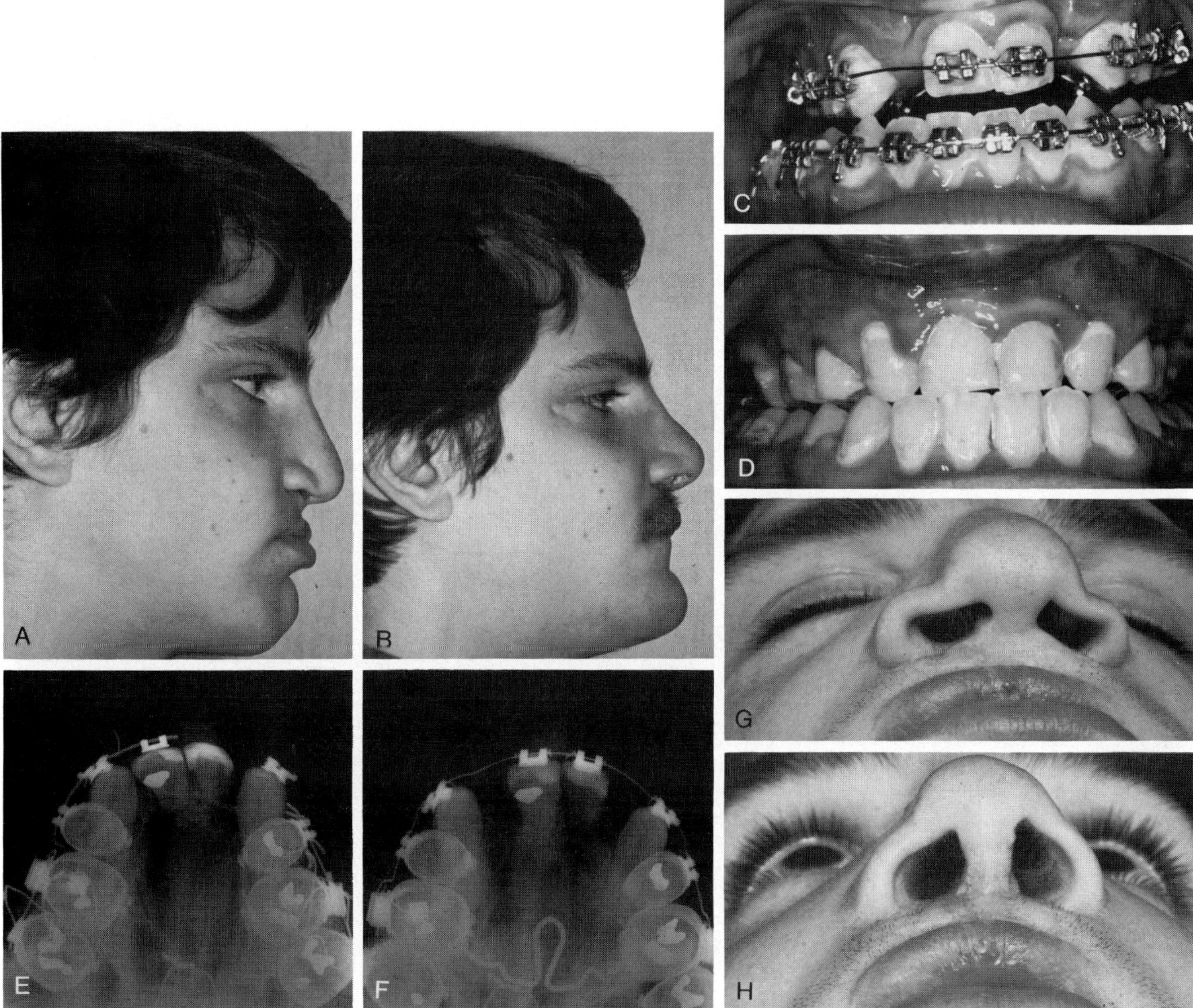

Figure 64–4 Quadrangular Le Fort I maxillary osteotomy (segmental) in bilateral cleft patients. Patient with cleft lip, alveolus, and palate received bilateral alveolar-palatal bone grafts and segmental maxillary Le Fort I advancement osteotomy with iliac bone grafting for stabilization and infraorbital-zygomatic augmentation.

A and *B*. Patient before and after quadrangular Le Fort I maxillary osteotomy with infraorbital and paranasal augmentation. *C* and *D*. Same patient with occlusion before and after surgery. Note closure of lateral incisor space bilaterally, which eliminates the need for prosthetic treatment. *E* and *F*. Occlusal radiographs before and after osteotomy illustrating the differential advancement of the bilateral posterior segments and palatal bone grafting. *G* and *H*. Before and after correction of the secondary nasal deformity, performed 6 months after the osteotomy.

tors and serial cephalometric factors). The reason for this delay is that relapse may result from continued mandibular growth.[19, 20] If the deformity is severe and the child has emotional problems, osteotomy can be advised prior to completion of facial growth provided that it is understood that the osteotomy may have to be repeated at a later date.

Clinical examination includes assessment of facial symmetry, secondary lip or nasal deformities, alveolo-palatal cleft or fistulas, dental occlusion and arch form. A Panorex (orthopantomogram) study illustrates dental factors (unerupted, missing, or supernumerary teeth and the status of erupted teeth) and the alveolopalatal

bone defect. A cephalogram permits an analytic examination of the maxilla and mandible relative to each other and the skull base. Anteroposterior and vertical growth discrepancies in the maxilla or mandible are characterized and quantitated by various cephalometric angular and linear measurements. Dental impressions are taken and study models constructed. These allow further examination of dental occlusion and arch form.

The facial, dental, and radiographic records are analyzed, and an orthodontic and orthognathic surgical treatment plan is formulated. After completion of presurgical orthodontic treatment, additional dental study models are constructed and are utilized for presurgical

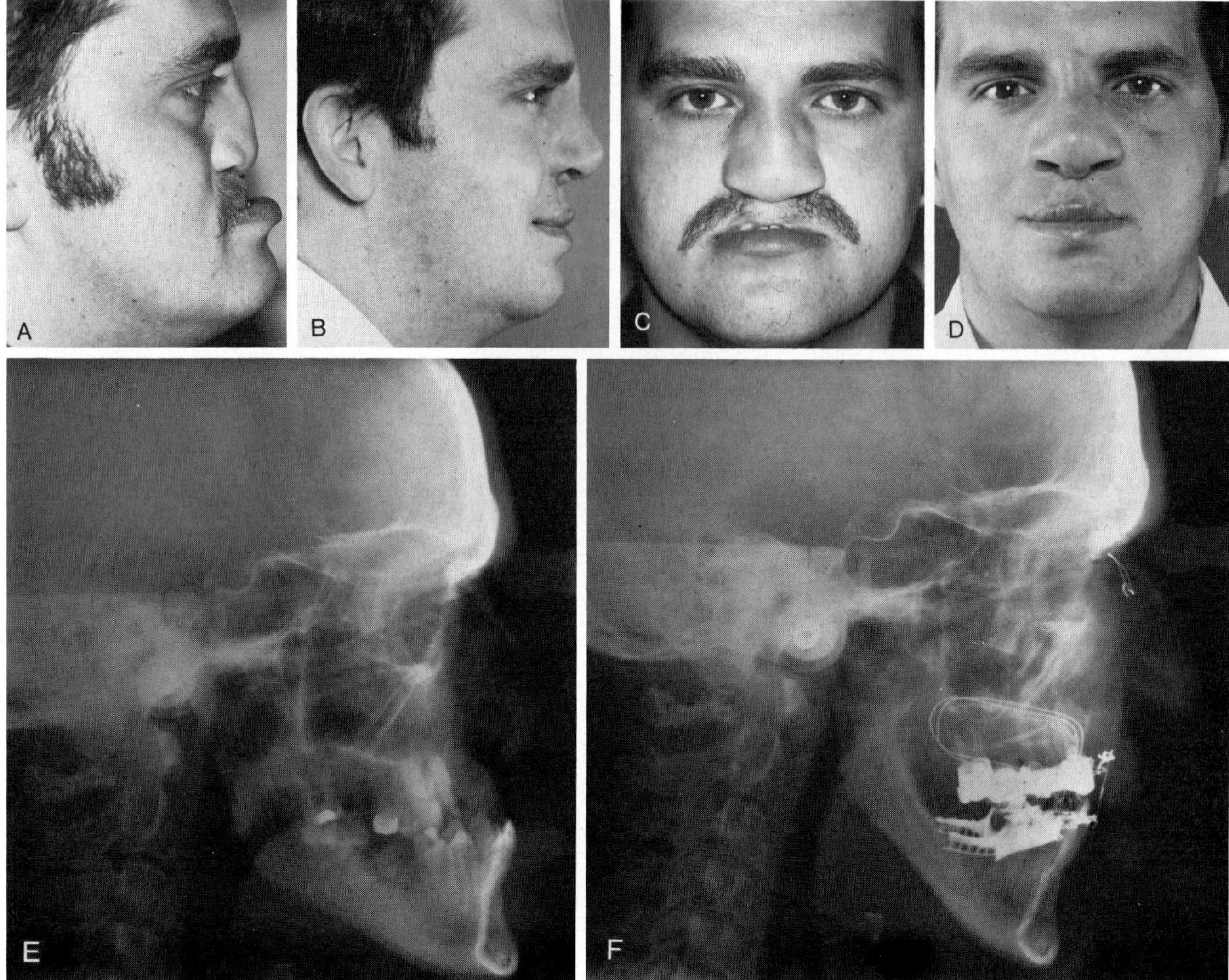

Figure 64–5 Bimaxillary osteotomies for severe maxillary deficiency in bilateral cleft patients. Severe skeletal class III malocclusion in a patient with bilateral cleft of the lip, alveolus, and palate. A vertical mandibular ramus osteotomy for retropositioning of the mandible was performed 3 years prior to the maxillary Le Fort II advancement osteotomy.

A and *B*. Patient before and after Le Fort II advancement osteot-omy. Note correction of the secondary lip-nasal deformity, which was performed 6 months after the maxillary osteotomy. Nasal reconstruction was accomplished in part with a cranial bone graft. *C* and *D*. Same patient before and after surgery. Note reconstruction of the upper lip vermilion with an Abbe flap. *E* and *F*. Lateral cephalograms taken before and after osteotomy. Patient had multiple missing teeth, and reconstruction was achieved with a removable partial denture.

models to determine the feasibility of the surgery and eventually, to aid in construction of surgical splints. The splint is used following segmented osteotomy to establish proper occlusion intraoperatively.

In analyzing the profile of the cleft patient, it is important to note that in most cases there is a retruded maxilla rather than a prognathic mandible. In the past, prior to refinement of maxillary osteotomy procedures, the mandible was frequently repositioned posteriorly in these patients. The facial profile was improved, but the patient was aesthetically and functionally compromised. Midface deficiency persisted, and more important, osteotomy stability was compromised. Tongue function and airway adequacy were adversely affected in patients with moderate to severe skeletal discrepancies, and this contributed to skeletal instability and relapse. Mandib-ular prognathism can occur in conjunction with cleft deformities, but represents a separate familial mandibular deformity.

Maxillary Osteotomy

All levels of maxillary osteotomy (Le Fort I, II, or III) may be indicated in cleft patients with a secondary maxillary deformity. The most common is the Le Fort I procedure, which may be performed at a low or high level and may be segmentalized or nonsegmentalized. The Le Fort II osteotomy or one of its modifications is occasionally indicated. The Le Fort III osteotomy is rarely used unless other coexisting facial deformities are present (e.g., Apert's or Crouzon's deformity). It is unusual to perform separate orbital procedures in patients with simple lip and palatal clefts, but these have been necessary in rare patients with associated facial clefts or craniosynostosis.

Le Fort I Osteotomy Without Lip Revision or Cleft Closure (Figs. 64–2, 64–3, and 64–4)

A Le Fort I procedure can be performed in various ways depending on the dental, skeletal, or aesthetic deficiencies present, as well as the patient's age and health.[21, 22] If the cleft patient has an anterior fistula or bony cleft, the question of whether to repair the soft and hard tissue defect before, during, or after the osteotomy has to be addressed. Although there are occasionally indications for one method or another, the choice is frequently based on the surgeon's preference and experience. If the cleft is large or is associated with extensive scar tissue, separating the two procedures provides a more complete and predictable correction. Ongoing orthodontic treatment may dictate a need to separate the cleft bone grafting and maxillary osteotomy procedures. In addition, if large anteroposterior, transverse, or vertical skeletal movements are required, it is best to separate the soft and hard tissue procedures. If cleft closure is performed separately from the osteotomy skeletal correction, the surgeon has more latitude and can be more versatile in performing the correction and a conventional osteotomy can be performed. The chance of compromised blood supply to the soft tissue flaps and skeletal segments is also reduced.

Surgical Technique

In the ideal situation, the operation should be performed under hypotensive anesthesia with endotracheal intubation. The buccal sulcus and the anterior surface of the maxilla may be infiltrated with 0.5% Xylocaine and 1:100,000 epinephrine. Hyaluronidase can be added to increase dissipation of the anesthetic fluid. A heavy silk suture is placed bilaterally on the upper lip. This is less traumatic than the standard retractor. If the bony cleft is large, it may not be possible or wise to repair it at this time. In this case, closure is performed prior to or following the osteotomy procedure, depending on the type of osteotomy procedure and the amount of skeletal advancement needed.

Frequently, the osteotomy procedure is designed to reduce or significantly eliminate the skeletal cleft defect. This is common in patients with unilateral or bilateral clefts when occlusion will allow advancement of the cuspid into the lateral incisor position. Careful presurgical orthodontic management is crucial in these patients (Figs. 64–3 and 64–4).

Limited incisions (vertical or horizontal, depending on the surgeon's preference) are made in the buccal sulcus (5 mm above the mucogingival junction in the cuspid-bicuspid region) on the lesser segment. The periosteum is elevated posteriorly to the groove between the maxillary tuberosity and the pterygoid plates, anteriorly to the edge of the piriform aperture, and superiorly to the level of the infraorbital rim and fora-

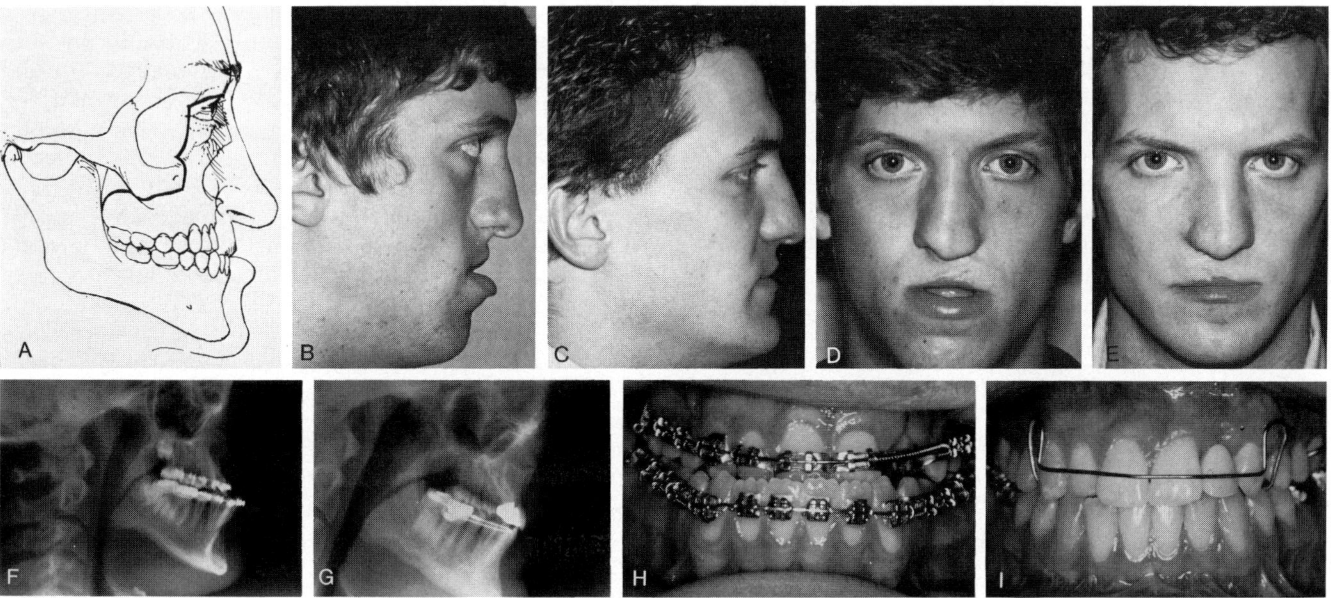

Figure 64–6 Patient with unilateral cleft of the lip, alveolus, and palate. This patient had a piramidal Le Fort II advancement osteotomy with an iliac crest bone graft added for stabilization. An advancement-vertical reduction anterior mandibular horizontal osteotomy was performed as well, along with alveolar-palatal cleft bone grafting. Nasal-lip reconstruction was accomplished 6 months after the osteotomy. *A.* Diagram of pyramidal maxillary Le Fort II osteotomy. *B* and *C.* Patient before and after surgery. Note improvement of the profile due to maxillary and mandibular advancement osteotomies. *D* and *E.* Same patient before and after surgery. *F* and *G.* Lateral cephalograms taken before and after surgery. Note correction of the class III malocclusion. *H* and *I.* Anterior occlusion before and after surgery. Note correction of class III occlusion and alignment of cuspid into the bone-grafted cleft.

men. A buccal sulcus retractor is inserted, and an osteotomy is performed by means of a side-cutting bur or reciprocating saw at the level dictated by the aesthetic requirements of each patient. If significant infraorbital augmentation is desired, a high-level osteotomy (quadrangular Le Fort I) is performed, and interpositional inlay-onlay iliac bone grafting is performed.[22] If significant vertical maxillary positioning is required (either impaction or augmentation) or if segmentalization is required (which is common in the cleft patient), the osteotomy is kept low at the level of the floor of the nose. The osteotomy extends posteriorly to the maxillary tuberosity-pterygoid plate groove. Anteriorly, a retractor is inserted to protect the nasal mucosa, and the incision is carried through the edge of the aperture and extended posteriorly along the lateral nasal wall, just anterior to the palatine vessels. The palatine vessels are frequently cauterized or clipped following the down-fracture maneuver.

Through a horizontal buccal sulcus incision on the greater segment, the periosteum is raised from the anterior maxilla, the lateral wall of the piriform aperture, the floor of the nose, and the vomer. The mucoperiosteum is also raised from the other side of the vomer—i.e., the cleft side. The cartilaginous septum and vomer are separated from the maxillary rostrum using a curette and chisel. The technique of segment osteotomy is similar on each side. A curved pterygoid osteotome is placed in the retrotuberosity groove, and with gentle tapping, the maxilla is separated from the pterygoid plates. These segments can frequently be down-fractured with finger and thumb pressure without first utilizing the curved pterygoid osteotome. Anterior segment mobilization is more difficult than when the noncleft maxilla is intact, and Tessier maxillary mobilizers placed behind the tuberosities can provide additional anterior segmental mobilization. This mobilization should be relatively gentle to preserve as much mucoperiosteum (blood supply) as possible. Often there is considerable postmaxillary fibrous scar tissue, which must be broken down (usually by finger dissection) to allow adequate and effortless maxillary advancement. In patients requiring maxillary advancement of more than 8 mm, it is best, as noted previously, to perform bone grafting 6 months before a conventional Le Fort I osteotomy procedure.

A previously fabricated splint is wired to the mobilized segments using an awl introduced through the palate (circumpalatal wire) or by wiring the orthodontic brackets directly to the splint. The maxilla is advanced and placed into intermaxillary fixation. If a mandibular procedure is also planned, an interim splint is utilized. Any adjustments for facial height problems are made according to the preoperative plan. Miniplates, straight or L-shaped, are applied bilaterally on the zygomaticomaxillary buttress and the piriform aperture margins if adequate bone is available. Transosseous wires to the infraorbital rim may be required in selected patients.[22] This creates a stable maxilla. If inlay or onlay grafts are required, the choice is between iliac and cranial bone. The choice is determined by the preference and experience of the surgeon. If cranial bone is chosen, it should be stabilized with lag screws. The sulcus incisions are then closed with continuous horizontal mattress sutures. The intermaxillary fixation is removed at the termination of the procedure, and jaw stability and condylar position are tested. The splint is maintained in position so that the occlusion can be checked postoperatively and an even occlusal contact can be maintained. If signs of relapse occur, intermaxillary elastics or wires can be reapplied.

Le Fort I Osteotomy with Lip Revision and Alveolopalatal Cleft Closure

In patients with less extensive clefts, bone grafting of the maxillary cleft can be performed in conjunction with the maxillary osteotomy,[21] provided well-vascularized flaps can be designed to allow access for osteotomies and proper coverage of the bone grafts.

Lip revision can be included in the same operation when indicated. When the lip is opened, the extent of the maxillary cleft and the typical nature of the nasal deformity are clearly displayed. At this point, it is necessary to consider the vascular supply of the maxillary segments. Only the buccal or the palatal supply can be compromised, but not both. Otherwise, the segment would become ischemic. In larger clefts, a decision is usually made to move the gingiva from the lesser segment and the mucoperiosteal palatal flap from the greater segment.

A vertical or horizontal incision is made to give access for elevating the mucoperiosteum from the lateral wall of the piriform aperture, the vomerine ridge, and the septum. A horizontal sulcus incision from the right to left bicuspids can also be made through the alveolar cleft to allow access for the osteotomy procedure.

The alar base is separated from the maxilla by subperiosteal dissection, which is continued up to the infraorbital rim and nerve. Medially, the vomerine ridge and the septum are widely displayed. The airway should be considered at this point. The hypertrophied inferior turbinate may be trimmed. The cranially displaced vomerine ridge should be resected, and the septum should be scored to correct the usual deviation onto the cleft side. With these three areas attended to, the airway on the cleft side should now be clear.

At this point, the lower lateral cartilage of the nose is mobilized by means of an intercartilaginous and a rim incision. The cartilage is separated from the skin and is brought out as a "bucket handle." The alar cartilage is dissected from the mucosa up to the medial crus and is repositioned using a 4–0 nylon suture taken from the nasal tip through the cartilage and back again. This will be tied over a gauze pledget later in the procedure.

Closure of the nasal floor is done using unequal Z-plasty in the anterior one-third of the floor. A large mucoperiosteal flap is brought from the medial to the lateral side. This maneuver establishes nasal symmetry. The alveolar defect is closed with a gingival flap. The maxilla is cut with a reciprocating saw or a Lindeman bur. This cut is carried along the lateral wall of the piriform fossa and posteriorly along the anterior surface of the maxilla to the pterygomaxillary groove. A curved osteotome is used to separate the tuberosity from the pterygoid plates. This segment can then be mobilized using finger pressure. Soft tissue behind the tuberosity has to be broken down to allow advancement. On the greater segment, the mucoperiosteum is elevated through a horizontal or vertical sulcus incision from the anterior maxilla, piriform aperture, and nasal spine. This reflection is extended posteriorly to the pterygomaxillary groove. An Obwegeser piriform aperture retractor or curved periosteal elevator is then placed from the vertical incision and is hooked over the edge of the piriform aperture. The anterior portion of the osteotomy can be made in a similar fashion utilizing a closed retractor to protect the soft tissue laterally. The curved osteotome again separates the tuberosity from the pterygoid plates. In the medial area, the mucoperiosteum is elevated from the nasal floor and lateral piriform aperture wall using an Aufricht retractor or a curved periosteal elevator. The lateral nasal wall is exposed and cut with the saw or bur. It is now possible to mobilize the segment in a manner similar to that used for the lesser segment. The palatine arteries may at this point be visible and can be clipped or cauterized.

It is convenient to elevate the Veau flap from the greater segment and suture it to the palatal edge on the lesser segment. The mobilized segments are now placed in a palatal-occlusal splint. Splint stabilization is accomplished with transpalatal wires or wires attached to orthodontic brackets. The maxilla is then placed in its correct anteroposterior position by relating the splint to the mandibular teeth and establishing intermaxillary fixation. On the lesser segment, miniplates are placed on the lateral edge of the piriform aperture and the zygomaticomaxillary buttress. Similarly, miniplates may be placed on the greater segment to give secure skeletal fixation. If there is good anterior soft tissue cover, an anterior miniplate can be placed high on the alveolus between the two segments. Because the segments are at this point stable, the intermaxillary fixation is released, but the splint is retained on the upper dentition. The alveolopalatal defect is filled with block corticocancellous and particulate cancellous iliac bone graft. Bone graft material may also be placed over the osteotomy site and under the alar base of the lesser segment. The gingival flap is advanced and closed in an impermeable, everted manner. All intraoral incisions are closed with horizontal mattress sutures. The lip is reconstructed by repositioning the orbicularis oris muscle. The palatal-interocclusal splint is maintained in position and utilized to access the occlusion continually. If there is a tendency to relapse, intermaxillary fixation can be reestablished using elastics and wires. If the internal skeletal fixation is secure, this is not likely to occur.

Particular Situations

Vertically Short Lesser Segments

In the past, vertical and transverse relapse of the lesser segment was common when the lesser segment

was corrected orthodontically (vertically and transversely) prior to total maxillary advancement and bone grafting. With the advent of miniplate internal skeletal fixation, this multiple procedural approach is no longer necessary, and the length of orthodontic treatment is frequently reduced. The surgical procedure can be done in a single stage with accurate bone grafting and skeletal stabilization of the lesser segment. Vertical and transverse relapse is less likely with this approach.

Maxillary Retrusion in Patients with Bilateral Alveolopalatal Cleft

Because of the concern for viability of the premaxillary segment in patients with bilateral clefts, it is considered safer to perform the correction in two stages (see Fig. 64–3). However, if the premaxilla is in the correct position and both posterior segments require advancement, one can combine the osteotomy and cleft bone grafting procedure (see Fig. 64–4). Because of the extent of the cleft posterior to the premaxilla, it may be necessary to use buccal mucosal flaps to ensure satisfactory oral closure. Six months later a standard Le Fort I osteotomy is performed.

Severe Maxillary Retrusion

When the degree of maxillary retrusion is greater than 1.0 cm (Fig. 64–5), a jaw-sharing procedure may be considered, especially if there is considerable scarring of the palate, the reason being that maxillary relapse is a distinct possibility.

In the planning process, an advancement of less than 1.0 cm can be made in the maxilla, and the remainder of the occlusal correction can be achieved by performing a mandibular setback osteotomy. Miniplate fixation is again advised if there is adequate bony tissue.

Le Fort II Osteotomy

When there is paranasal retrusion extending to the infraorbital rims, regardless of the size of the nose, pyramidal Le Fort II osteotomy (Fig. 64–6) is indicated.[23] An alternative procedure is a high Le Fort I osteotomy with onlay bone grafting.[22] If the osteotomy is not placed high enough or if the onlay-inlay interpositional grafts are not placed and contoured properly, the Le Fort I procedure may give an abnormal relationship between the upper maxilla, orbital rim region, and bony nasal pyramid. Cephalometry is helpful for assessment, but the decision to use the Le Fort II osteotomy is often based exclusively on an aesthetic appreciation of the facial profile and full face appearance. This is particularly true in deciding how far to extend the osteotomy out toward the zygomatic region.

The approach to the upper part of the osteotomy may be made by a coronal flap or by the paranasal incisions originally described.[24] The periosteum is elevated from the nasal bridge and from the medial orbital walls behind the medial canthal ligaments and the lacrimal ducts. This elevation is taken along the floor of the orbit to the point where the infraorbital rim is to be cut. The periosteum is raised from the front of the maxilla as far inferiorly as possible. An osteotomy is made across the bridge using a reciprocating saw. If the paranasal approach is used, the intervening skin is elevated and protected with Aufricht nasal retractor. The orbital contents are protected with malleable retractors, and osteotomies are taken down to and across the orbital floors, over the infraorbital rims, and onto the anterior surface of the maxilla, either medial or lateral to the infraorbital nerve. Some care is taken to ensure that the infraorbital nerve is not damaged as the osteotomy extends across the orbital floor. This portion is frequently performed with fine chisels.

A limited posterior upper buccal sulcus incision is made, taking care not to expose the buccal fat pad. The periosteum is elevated superiorly to the infraorbital rim osteotomy and posteriorly to the pterygotuberosity groove. The osteotomy is continued down the anterior face of the maxilla, across the zygomaticomaxillary buttress, and into the pterygotuberosity groove. Using a curved osteotome, the tuberosity is separated from the pterygoid plates.

To free the maxilla, a curved osteotome is inserted through the transverse nasal cut, and, using a downward and backward movement, the vomer is separated from the skull base. Using Rowe's maxillary disimpaction forceps, Tessier maxillectomy mobilizers, and finger dissection as in the Le Fort I procedure described above, the maxillary segment is completely mobilized and advanced. Fixation is achieved with internal skeletal miniplates in the frontonasal region bilaterally, the infraorbital rim, and occasionally the zygomaticomaxillary buttress. Bone defects from the advancement are grafted with skull bone or with bone from the iliac crest. In selected patients with additional nasal defects, a skull bone graft may be inserted to achieve a satisfactory nasal bridge and good protrusion of the nasal tip (Fig. 64–5). This graft is taken from the temporoparietal region and may be from the outer table or full thickness, depending on the bone thickness required. The graft is stabilized with a wire or two lag screws at the nasofrontal junction; the use of only one screw allows the graft to swing from side to side.

Kufner Osteotomy

Some authorities have felt that a large nose is a contraindication to the Le Fort II procedure. However, for reasons to be discussed later, this objection is probably not valid. In light of this, it is reasonable to consider the Kufner procedure (Fig. 64–7).[25] In this procedure, the vertical cuts are made paranasally through the infraorbital rim down to the lateral rim of the piriform aperture, and the lateral cuts are taken out to the zygoma and through the infraorbital or lateral-orbital rim in this region. The nose is left completely apart from the nasal floor and septum as in the Le Fort I osteotomy. The resulting U-shaped segment of maxilla is mobilized and advanced.

Steinhauser,[26] Souyris,[27] Champy,[28] and Keller and Sather[29] have all described variations and modifications

of the Kufner procedure.[25] This procedure has the following disadvantage: The maxillary segment may break into several pieces when it has a thin piriform rim, and the procedure is contraindicated when this anatomy is encountered on surgical exposure. In these patients, the quadrangular Le Fort I osteotomy procedure is indicated.[22] One should also include as much of the zygomaticomaxillary buttress and the lateral piriform aperture as possible in this procedure to lessen the possibility of fracture. An abnormal relationship between the maxilla and the nose may result, and there may be steps on the infraorbital rim that can be difficult to eliminate. Careful attention to detail when placing the infraorbital grafts medially and laterally will reduce the incidence of this complication.

The presence of a large nose in the cleft deformity can be used to gain an excellent result from a rhinoplasty; one should never hesitate to advance a prominent nose.

If the Kufner Le Fort II osteotomy is to be utilized in the cleft patient, the alveolopalatal defect should be bone grafted at least 6 months prior to the osteotomy procedure. Even with a firm transpalatal splint, segment mobilization of the bilateral segments is extremely difficult.

Comments on Special Situations

When the routine Le Fort II procedure is used in patients with bilateral clefts, there is not the same concern for premaxillary vascularity, and thus in most cases it is permissible to perform simultaneous maxillary advancement and bilateral cleft closure.

If the occlusal discrepancy is large (i.e., more than 1.0 cm), a shared bimaxillary procedure is indicated. In the past, the Le Fort II osteotomy was thought to show less relapse than the Le Fort I and therefore allowed greater advancements. This was never adequately proved. In our experience, a 3- to 4-mm over advancement is routinely performed in anticipation of a predictable relapse with the routine Le Fort II procedure. For this reason, the Kufner (quadrangular) Le Fort II or quadrangular Le Fort I osteotomy with wedging and stabilizing interpositional grafts give noticeably more stable short-term correction.[22, 29] Miniplate fixation has greatly reduced the chances of relapse in the short term. One must remember that rigid internal fixation devices or interpositional bone grafts provide skeletal stability only until the osteotomy sites heal. Afterward, numerous factors affect the stability of skeletal correction.[20]

Special Considerations in Advancement Osteotomies of the Maxillopharyngeal Flaps

On rare occasions, a heavily scarred pharyngeal flap may impede maxillary advancement. When this happens, one should not hesitate to divide the flap. A subsequent sphincter pharyngoplasty can be performed with great ease. Lengthening or repositioning the flap is not advised because this adds to further scarring of the flap and may reduce the chances of obtaining a

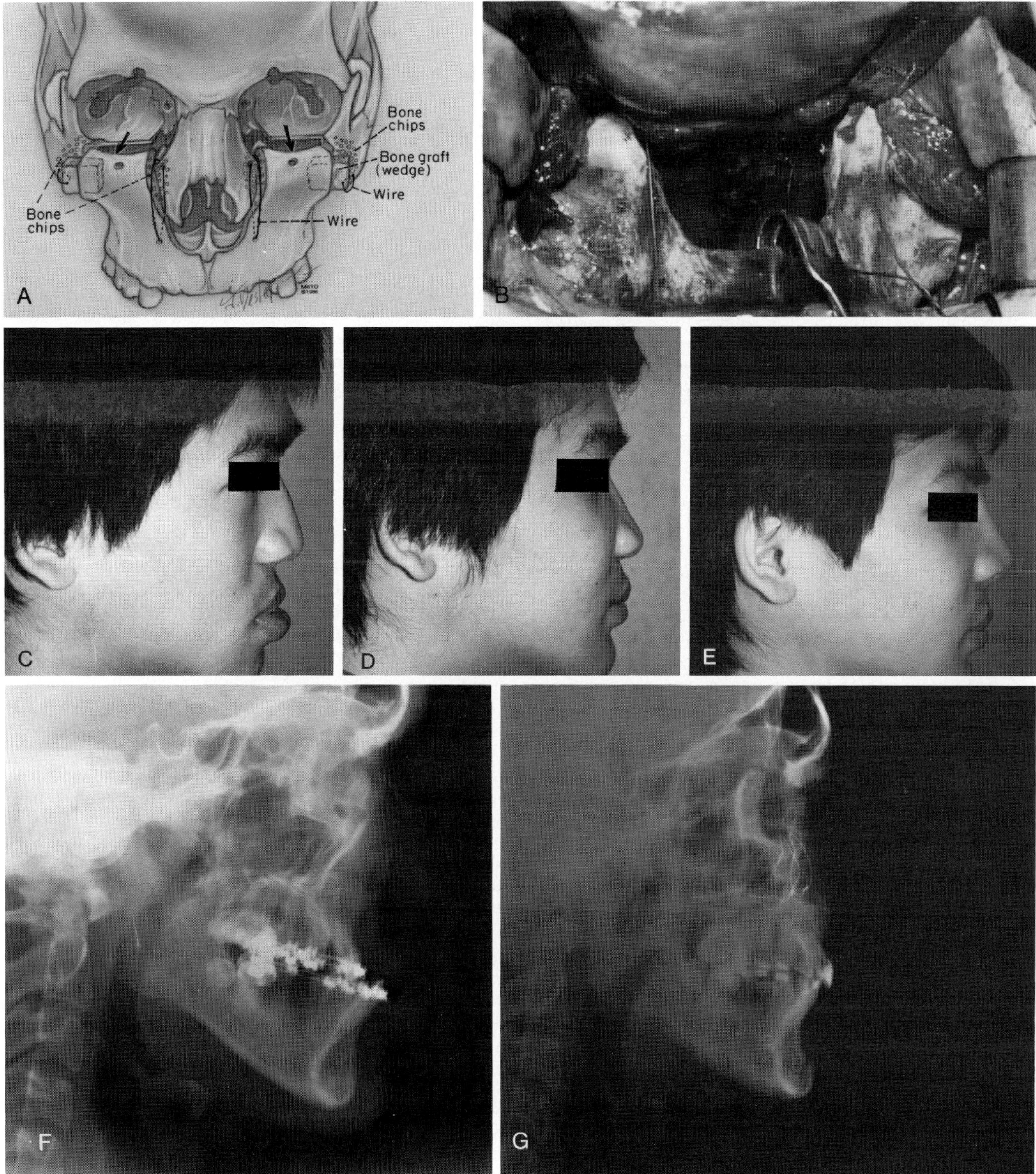

Figure 64–7 Quadrangular Le Fort II maxillary osteotomy in the unilateral cleft patient. Patient with a unilateral cleft treated with quadrangular Le Fort II osteotomy, bilateral mandibular body ostectomy, anterior mandibular segmental osteotomy, and mandibular anterior horizontal osteotomy. Nasal reconstruction with cranial bone graft was performed 6 months after the osteotomy.

A. Diagram of a quadrangular Le Fort II osteotomy showing the osseous cuts, wire fixation, and onlay-inlay bone graft stabilization. *B.* Intraoperative photograph of the mobilized segment (of the quadrangular Le Fort II osteotomy) in a noncleft patient. Alveolar-palatal bone grafting preceded the maxillary osteotomy by 6 months.

C, D, E. Patient before and after maxillary quadrangular Le Fort II osteotomy, multiple mandibular osteotomies, and correction of nasal deformity (6 months after the osteotomies). *F* and *G.* Lateral cephalograms taken before and after surgery.

satisfactory speech result. With proper retrotuberosity and retropalatal soft tissue release, the soft palate is not affected by maxillary advancement.

Velopharyngeal Incompetence

Velopharyngeal incompetence may occur with any maxillary advancement osteotomy, especially when it is present preoperatively. In this situation, the velopharyngeal incompetence becomes worse. However, there have been reports to the contrary.[17, 30, 31, 32] Procedures have been designed in which the hard palate mucosa is elevated posteriorly using an anterior U-shaped incision, and a posterior cut is taken from the tuberosity across the hard palate in front of the greater palatine vessels. In this manner, in theory, the soft palate is left behind when the maxilla moves forward.[33] However, evidence is lacking to suggest that this procedure achieves its goal.

Retrotuberosity Bone Grafting

Retrotuberosity bone grafting was formerly claimed to be an absolute necessity for maxillary stability.[34] In fact, this was not true because the maxilla was frequently unstable and became displaced. We abandoned this procedure in our practice 14 years ago without any significant consequences. Miniplate fixation has further contributed to its demise. When miniplate osteosynthesis is not possible, correct positioning of the interpositional bone grafts (quadrangular Le Fort I or II) anteriorly (paranasal, infraorbital, or zygomatic) provides the necessary skeletal stability and obviates the need for retrotuberosity bone grafting.

Rhinoplasty

In cleft patients, it is strongly advised that only the nasal tip be corrected at the time of the osteotomy—i.e., repositioning the alar base and lower lateral cartilage to achieve symmetry. Experience has shown that the final rehabilitative procedure should be an aesthetic rhinoplasty (Figs. 64–3 to 64–7) that requires a different approach from that of a maxillary osteotomy. If intermaxillary fixation is used at the same time, a rhinoplasty will compromise the airway and there will be a tube in the nose, making fine aesthetic judgment virtually impossible. However, when internal skeletal fixation is provided, intermaxillary fixation may be released, the endotracheal tube may be placed transorally, and selected nasal procedures can be considered.

Fixation

Miniplates may not be available, or the quality of bone or the level of osteotomy may preclude their proper utilization. In these situations, craniomaxillary wiring, direct intraosseous wiring combined with splints, or splints and intermaxillary fixation are quite reliable. Miniplate osteosynthesis is more time-consuming. However, stability is more predictable and the airway is less likely to be compromised if intermaxillary fixation is avoided. The obvious benefits of plates compensate for their expense. When performing the quadrangular Le Fort I or II osteotomy, interpositional onlay-inlay grafts, properly placed and stabilized with wire osteosynthesis, can give skeletal stability that is equal to that achieved with miniplates.

Complications

Airway Compromise

Airway compromise is generally secondary to postoperative edema or continued bleeding. Also, one should never overlook the possibility of a retained foreign body in the upper or lower airway. These complications are less likely with reduced employment of intermaxillary fixation. In addition, reduced operating time, reduced intraoperative bleeding under controlled hypotensive anesthesia, and maximum use of corticosteroids have led to reduced postoperative edema. The use of retained nasotracheal or nasopharyngeal airways is helpful in airway management in the immediate postoperative period. In cases of acute impairment, intermaxillary fixation is released and tracheostomy can be performed on an elective or emergency basis. Management of a marginal nasal airway is a significant clinical challenge. Inspired humidified air, local or systemic decongestants, systemic antihistamines, local nasal toilet, and establishment of an oral airway by various mechanical means in the patient with intermaxillary wiring may be beneficial in selected patients.

Laceration of Lacrimal Duct

Laceration of the lacrimal duct can occur in the Le Fort II procedure and can be carefully repaired with fine suture material and magnification if the duct is small. There is rarely a problem with lacrimal duct blockage because a frequently lacerated duct will spontaneously repair itself or empty into the nose at a high level.

Infection

Infection is rare in Le Fort osteotomy procedures because internal wound drainage into the nose or sinus is adequate. When infection is present, it is usually related to an exposed bone graft, which should be removed. If a wire or a metal plate is responsible, it should be removed.

Loss of Maxilla

Loss of the maxilla is a rare complication that usually involves a portion of one of the segments (anterior segment in a bilateral cleft or the lesser segment in a unilateral cleft). The affected area should be allowed to sequestrate and should then be removed; the overlying mucosa should be preserved. The area should be allowed to heal in a good position. The residual defect may be reconstructed later with bone grafts.[10]

Relapse

If relapse occurs in the early postoperative period, intermaxillary fixation with wires or elastics should be reestablished and the position held for a length of time, depending on the reason for loss of jaw position. An established relapse will require a secondary osteotomy. If a Le Fort II or III osteotomy was performed initially, the relapse frequently occurs at the dental-alveolar level, and a Le Fort I osteotomy may be adequate to re-establish skeletal-dental proportions. Pseudorelapse is occasionally seen and may occur when maxillary advancement is performed prior to completion of facial growth. The mandible continues to grow, and a class III malocclusion subsequently develops. Freihofer[20] found this to be the most common cause of relapse in a large series of patients. Skeletal overcorrection of 2 to 5 mm is included in all maxillary advancement osteotomy procedures. The degree of overcorrection is dictated by the magnitude of advancement, the level of osteotomy, and individual considerations such as the degree of associated lip-nose deformity and occlusion.

Conclusion

An understanding of the disordered skeletal anatomy in the cleft patient is essential. With wide elevation of periosteum, advancement of the periosteal envelope, and fixation of block onlay bone grafts, bone resorption is less frequent or significant. This is especially true when cranial bone is utilized. Additionally, osteotomies become more stable with miniplate fixation and selected use of interpositional stabilizing bone grafts. Decreased operating time, improved anesthetic techniques, improved surgical techniques, and decreased use of intermaxillary fixation have reduced postoperative morbidity following maxillary osteotomy. Skeletal surgery enhances the aesthetic and functional results in cleft patients.

References

1. Dado DV, Kernahan DA: Radiographic analysis of the midface of a stillborn infant with a unilateral cleft lip and palate. Plast Reconstr Surg 78:238, 1986.
2. Boyne PJ: Autogenous cancellous bone and marrow transplants. Clin Orth Rel Res 73:199, 1970.
3. Boyne PJ: Use of marrow-cancellous bone grafts in maxillary alveolar and palatal clefts. J Dental Res 53:821, 1974.
4. Boyne PJ, Sands NR: Secondary bone grafting of residual alveolar and palatal clefts. J Oral Surg 30:87, 1972.
5. Boyne PJ, Sands NR: Combined orthodontic-surgical management of residual palato-alveolar cleft defects. Am J Orthod 70:20, 1976.
6. Abyholm FE, Borchgrevink HC, Eskeland G: Cleft lip and palate in Norway (iii). Clinical treatment of CLP patients in Oslo 1954–1975. Scand J Plast Reconstr Surg 15:15, 1981.
7. Abyholm FE, Berbland O, Semb G: Secondary bone grafting of alveolar clefts. Scand J Plast Surg 15:127, 1981.
8. Jackson IT: Closure of secondary palatal fistulae with intraoral tissue and bone grafting. Br J Plast Surg 25:93, 1972.
9. Keller EE, Van Roekel NB, Desjardins RP, et al: Prosthetic-surgical reconstruction of the severely resorbed maxilla with iliac bone grafting and tissue-integrated prostheses. Int J Oral Maxillofac Implants 2:155, 1987.
10. Tolman DE, Desjardins RP, Keller EE: Surgical-prosthodontic reconstruction of oronasal defects utilizing the tissue-integrated prosthesis. Int J Oral Maxillofac Surg Implants 3:31, 1988.
11. Jackson IT, Vandervord JG, McLennan JG, et al: Bone grafting of the secondary cleft lip and palate deformity. Br J Plast Surg 35:345, 1982.
12. Keller EE, Triplett WW: Iliac bone grafting: review of 160 consecutive cases. J Oral Maxillofac Surg Implants 45:11, 1987.
13. Keller EE, Desjardins RP, Eckert SE, et al: Composite bone grafts and titanium implants in mandibular discontinuity reconstruction. Int J Oral Maxillofac Surg Implants 3:261, 1988.
14. Tidstrom KD, Keller EE: Secondary reconstruction of mandibular discontinuity with composite grafts (iliac bone and titanium mesh tray). Review of 34 consecutive patients. (In press, 1989).
15. Wolfe SA, Berkowitz S: The use of cranial bone grafts in the closure of alveolar and anterior palatal clefts. Plast Reconstr Surg 72:659, 1983.
16. Jackson IT, Pellet C, Smith JM: The skull as a bone graft donor site. Ann Plast Surg 11:533, 1983.
17. Jackson IT: Cleft lip and palate. In Mustarde JC, Jackson IT (eds): Plastic Surgery in Infancy and Childhood. Edinburgh: Churchill Livingstone, 1988.
18. Jackson MS, Jackson IT, Christie FB: Improvements in speech following closure of anterior palatal fistulae with bone grafts. Br J Plast Surg 29:295, 1976.
19. Freihofer IIPM, Jr: Results after midface osteotomies. J Maxillofac Surg 1:30, 1973.
20. Freihofer HPM, Jr: Results of osteotomies of the facial skeleton in adolescence. J Maxillofac Surg 5:267, 1977.
21. Henderson D, Jackson IT: Combined cleft lip revision, anterior fistula closure and maxillary osteotomy: A one-stage procedure. Br J Oral Surg 13:33, 1975.
22. Keller EE, Sather AH: Quadrangular Le Fort I osteotomy (surgical technique and review of 54 consecutive patients). (In press, 1989).
23. Henderson D, Jackson IT: Nasomaxillary hypoplasia: The Le Fort II osteotomy. Br J Plast Surg 11:77, 1973.
24. Witzel MA, Munro IR: Velopharyngeal insufficiency after maxillary advancement. Cleft Palate J 14:176, 1977.
25. Kufner J: Four year experience of major maxillary osteotomies for retrusion. J Oral Surg 29:549, 1971.
26. Steinhauser EW: Variations of Le Fort II osteotomies for correction of midfacial deformities. J Maxillofac Surg 8:258, 1980.
27. Souyris F, Caravel JB, Reynaud JP: Osteotomies "intermediaires" de l'etage moyen de la face. Ann Chir Plast 18:149, 1973.
28. Champy M: Surgical treatment of midface deformities. Head Neck Surg 2:451, 1980.
29. Keller EE, Sather AH: Intraoral quadrangular Le Fort II osteotomy. J Oral Maxillofac Surg 45:223, 1987.
30. Schwarz C, Gruner E: Logopaedic findings following advancement of the maxilla. J Maxillofac Surg 4:40, 1976.
31. McCarthy JC, Coccaro PT, Schwartz MD: Velopharyngeal function following maxillary advancement. Plast Reconstr Surg 64:180, 1979.
32. Schendel SA, Deschraeger M, Wolford LM, et al: Velopharyngeal anatomy and maxillary advancement. J Maxillofac Surg 7:116, 1979.
33. Wake M: Personal communication, 1975.
34. Obwegeser HL: Surgical correction of the small or retrodisplaced maxilla. Plast Reconstr Surg 43:351, 1969.

CHAPTER 65

Management of Jaw Deformities in the Cleft Patient

Jeffrey C. Posnick, Mary Anne Witzel, and Arlene P. Dagys

The satisfactory management of patients with cleft lip and palate presents challenging clinical problems for reconstructive surgeons. Close cooperation is required among a multitude of specialists who wish both to concentrate on one aspect of the patient's care and to integrate their talents for the patient's overall well-being.

Patients with a repaired cleft, skeletal dysplasia, and malocclusion must undergo complete assessment including evaluations of breathing patterns, speech and velopharyngeal function, occlusion, facial soft- and hard-tissue aesthetics, and psychosocial status. At the very least, the assessment team must include the reconstructive surgeon, orthodontist, speech pathologist, and social worker or psychiatrist. Objective measurements and assessments, including computed tomography (CT) scans, cephalometric analysis, anthropometric surface measurements, occlusal analysis, nasendoscopy, videofluoroscopy, and psychological profile analysis, contribute to the surgical planning and the evaluation of surgical outcome. Although the patient may request correction of only a lip scar, nasal deformity, or poor speech, true functional and aesthetic improvement may depend on the establishment of a normal bony architecture. In such cases, there is little room to compromise with simple, soft tissue camouflage procedures.

In general, the central problem for patients with a cleft, skeletal dysplasia, and malocclusion is maxillary hypoplasia resulting from the original birth defect or previous surgical interventions. The usual surgical procedure is the Le Fort I maxillary osteotomy in one or more segments. This procedure originated in Europe. In 1867, Cheever performed a unilateral Le Fort I osteotomy to remove a nasopharyngeal tumor.[1] Later, Wassmund[2] performed an osteotomy of the maxilla according to the fracture lines described by Rene Le Fort[3] in a patient with an open bite deformity.

Schuchardt was the first to separate the Le Fort I osteotomy at the pterygoid plates.[4] Gillies and Rowe first described mobilization of collapsed maxillary segments in a patient with a cleft.[5] Obwegeser showed that the down-fractured maxilla could be moved in any direction either as one unit or in segments.[6–10] Bell, experimenting in dogs, demonstrated the blood supply, revascularization, and bone healing that occurred with this procedure.[11, 12] A more complete history of the Le

Fort I osteotomy can be found in an article by Freihofer.[13]

Well planned and meticulously executed orthognathic surgery can "clean up" many residual problems of clefting: vertical, horizontal, and transverse maxillary hypoplasia; a vertically long, retrognathic chin; a deviated septum and enlarged inferior turbinates; residual oronasal fistulas; cleft defects requiring bone grafting; dental gaps resulting from congenitally absent teeth; anterior speech articulation errors; and, when necessary, mandibular prognathism or retrognathism.

Timing of Maxillofacial Surgery

In general, correction of maxillofacial deformities is planned to take place when the skeleton is mature. Maxillofacial growth is generally complete between the ages of 14 and 16 in females and 16 and 18 in males.[14] Skeletal growth is variable, however, and assessment of each patient must be based on either epiphyseal plate closure, documented on hand radiographs, or cessation of maxillofacial growth, documented on sequential cephalometric radiographs taken at 6-month intervals.

Occasionally, psychosocial considerations will take precedence, and early maxillofacial surgery will be undertaken for the patient's overall benefit, even though revision osteotomy will most likely be required at the time of skeletal maturation. In addition, if mandibular hypoplasia is known to be causing sleep apnea (as occasionally in patients with Pierre Robin syndrome), mandibular advancement may be performed at an early age and revision osteotomy planned for the time of skeletal maturation.[15] Hypoplasia must be confirmed as the cause of the apnea by means of a sleep study demonstrating significant oxygen desaturation of a peripheral rather than central origin. Causes such as large tonsils or an obstructing pharyngeal flap must be ruled out.

Integrated Team Approach

Early identification of abnormal growth patterns of the facial skeleton is critical in patients who have clefts. As soon as a maxillofacial deformity is anticipated or identified, the surgeon and orthodontist must cooperate in assessing the problems and planning treatment. Cephalometric analysis, occlusal analysis, and overall clinical judgment can permit reasonable predictions. Proper planning will avoid years of ineffective orthodontic treatment.

Preoperative speech assessment involving a clinical examination, nasendoscopy, and videofluoroscopy is necessary to characterize both velopharyngeal function and anterior articulation problems resulting in sibilant distortions. Objective preoperative evaluation is important because velopharyngeal function tends to deteriorate after maxillary Le Fort I osteotomy with advancement.[16] Closure that was adequate preoperatively may become borderline postoperatively, whereas closure that was borderline may become inadequate.[17] Articulatory distortions due to malocclusion also are identified and cause-and-effect relationships determined. Intraoperative correction of crossbite, open bite, dental gap, and anterior fistulas can predictably correct the sibilant distortions.[17, 18]

A thorough preorthodontic and preoperative periodontal assessment and oral hygiene regimen must be completed. Dental caries and periodontal disease must be prevented or treated before surgery.

At our institution, all preorthognathic surgical patients undergo neurosensibility facial assessment by a trained occupational therapist. Light touch perception, static and moving two-point discrimination, and vibratory sensation are measured in the infraorbital nerve and inferior alveolar-mental nerve distributions. Postoperative reassessment is done at intervals to identify sensory loss resulting from maxillary, mandibular, or chin surgery.[19–22]

Patients with congenital absence of the lateral incisor tooth on the cleft side of the maxilla require finishing prosthetic treatment if the dental gap has not been closed either orthodontically or surgically. A skilled prosthodontist can construct a permanent functional and aesthetic prosthesis with minimal abutment requirements only if the surgeon has provided a stable bony framework.

Postoperative monitoring of skeletal and dental relapse is critical to achieve desirable facial balance and occlusion. This requires close cooperation between patient, orthodontist, and surgeon. Previous studies have shown that skeletal stability is rarely achieved until 1 year after jaw surgery.[23] During this interval, meticulous monitoring and close scrutiny of the occlusion by both surgeon and orthodontist must continue. Although an understanding of both dynamic and static cephalometric analysis can greatly assist in recognizing skeletal relapse, the orthodontist best understands the physiology and mechanics of tooth movement and can determine when to use elastic traction to limit relapse and maintain good results. However, the orthodontist cannot be expected to appreciate the subtleties of blood supply to the dento-osseousmusculomucosal segments, wound healing, bone graft healing, limitations of bone plating, direct wiring fixation techniques, and sinus or airway management. The surgeon's office, on the other hand, may not be equipped for appropriate postoperative radiographic monitoring.

Diagnosis and Treatment Planning

Facial Aesthetics

A basic appreciation of facial aesthetics and a thorough, systematic approach to the analysis of facial deformities are prerequisites for planning and correction of maxillofacial deformities. Facial proportions, facial symmetry, and the relationship of the maxillary anterior teeth to the upper lip both in smiling and in repose must also be considered.[24] A combination of cephalometric analysis, anthropometric surface measurements,

and CT techniques can supplement but not overshadow the thorough clinical examination.

Since antiquity, man has pursued the elusive embodiment of the concept of beauty. The achievement of an aesthetically pleasing human face is the goal of that enterprise in relation to patients with clefts. Farkas and colleagues found significant differences between the proportions of vertical and horizontal anthropometric measurements in Caucasian faces and the relationships dictated by nine classic Greek canons of facial proportion depicted by Renaissance artists.[25] The head is wider and longer in the neoclassic canon, whereas the modern Caucasian has an elongated lower face and a larger chin. Ricketts suggested that the "golden mean" could be applied to the human face.[26] However, it has long been known that absolute symmetry is uninteresting, monotonous, and boring.[27]

Numerous cephalometric systems have been devised to evaluate the relationships between the cranium, facial bones, and dental structures.[26, 28–30] Every system has attempted to obtain information about jaw-to-jaw, cranial base-to-jaw, and tooth-to-jaw relationships. Cephalometric analysis can be static (comparing the patient at one time with standards derived from age- and sex-matched groups) or dynamic (comparing findings in the patient at various intervals).

The relationship between the upper lip and the maxillary anterior tooth must be considered both in smiling and in repose when assessing a patient with a jaw deformity. Ideally, with the upper lip at rest, about 2 to 3 mm vertical height of the central incisor teeth will be visible. With a broad smile, 1 to 2 mm vertical height of gingiva will show above the central incisor crowns. In patients with a cleft and maxillary hypoplasia, the teeth and gingiva may not show through the upper lip, producing an edentulous appearance. On the other hand, patients with bilateral cleft lip and palate may have an elongated premaxilla, exposing an excessive amount of tooth and gingiva. A congenital cleft lip that has undergone surgical repair and perhaps multiple revisions may vary considerably from the normal; the dynamic range of the upper lip is probably drastically reduced, and the lip is often vertically short and immobile. In such a patient, planning of maxillofacial surgery may necessitate compromise. For overall aesthetic improvement, the upper jaw may have to be placed so that tooth exposure is slightly excessive with the lip at rest and gingival exposure slightly inadequate with the lip in a broad smile.

Ideally, the dental midlines and the midline of the chin should match the facial midline. Aesthetically, perhaps the most important match is the chin to the facial midline, followed by the matching of the maxillary dental midline, and then the mandibular dental midline matched to the facial midline.

Attempts should be made to predict soft tissue response to orthognathic surgery. The ratio of soft to hard tissue change is rarely 1:1. Because ratio tables have been generated that permit a relatively accurate prediction of results, the amount of hard tissue alteration required to achieve the desired soft tissue redraping can be judged to the millimeter.[27, 32–35] However, the response of soft tissue to movement of bone in scarred and tethered cleft lips differs from that of normal lips.

Occlusal Analysis

Occlusion is best analyzed after alginate dental impressions are obtained, cast in stone, and mounted on an articulator with a face bow transfer. Orthodontic treatment and jaw surgery must often be combined to correct occlusal-plane canting, open bite, crossbite, and dental gaps and to position dental midlines on the facial midline.

By "operating on" the dental models preoperatively, the surgeon and orthodontist can plan to the millimeter the anteroposterior, horizontal, and vertical maxillary and mandibular changes required to achieve the ideal facial aesthetic appearance and occlusion. Intraoperatively, it is difficult to judge the facial aesthetics and lip-tooth relationships, and the surgeon must rely on preoperative judgment of desired aesthetic changes and the precise measurements calculated with the orthodontist during the model surgery. A-cut-as-you-go approach in orthognathic surgery is rarely preferred. Greater accuracy is achieved by using a prefabricated acrylic interocclusal final splint in one-jaw surgery and the addition of an intermediate splint in combined maxillary and mandibular (two-jaw) surgery.

Surgical Technique

The surgical techniques used in orthognathic surgery in patients with repaired clefts are unique. Recognition and correction of numerous subtle residual problems present special challenges for the surgeon, demanding variations in technique.

Maxillary Surgery

The central surgical correction of maxillary hypoplasia with vertical, horizontal, or transverse discrepancies is the Le Fort I osteotomy in one or more segments. When the cleft maxilla has not previously received bone grafts, it is segmentally united only by fibrous tissue and is easily released for differential repositioning by down-fracturing. This surgical reorientation is considerably less expensive and less time consuming than preoperative orthodontic reorientation. Setting this as a surgical goal does not obviate orthodontic tooth movement but rather clarifies and separates the surgical and orthodontic goals.

The surgeon must achieve a delicate balance between aggressive soft tissue scar release to permit relocation of the maxilla and meticulous maintenance of blood supply to avoid postoperative avascular necrosis of bone and teeth. When the maxilla is in three segments (that is, when the premaxilla and the left and right lesser segments are separate because of bilateral clefting with no previous bone grafting and fistula closure), the surgeon must preserve the labial mucosal pedicle of the premaxilla to ensure a blood supply to the premaxillary

segment. On completion of the premaxillary osteotomy, this pedicle will provide the only blood supply to the dento-osseousmucosal unit. Use of the circovestibular incision of the standard Le Fort I down-fracture would render the premaxilla avascular, causing it to be lost. When the premaxillary segment requires repositioning, we separate it from the nasal septum using a curved chisel and mallet, approaching from the palatal side. This technique avoids separation of the labial mucosal pedicle from the underlying bone.

Careful application of the viscoelastic, soft tissue properties of Gibson and Kenedi (that is, "creep" and "stress relaxation") permits the surgeon to advance the cleft maxilla 7 to 12 mm with little difficulty.[36] On occasion, we have advanced a cleft maxilla 24 mm horizontally. In most patients, this is the maximum horizontal advancement possible.

Careful attention to placement of the incision not only preserves the maxillary blood supply but also allows oral side wound closure of residual oronasal fistulas. Buccal mucosal flaps and tongue flaps are used only rarely because they do not place "attached gingiva" adjacent to tooth-bearing surfaces. Sliding mucogingival rotation flaps can usually provide attached gingiva where needed.[37]

During the past 2 years, we have performed Le Fort I osteotomy on 45 patients with repaired clefts. Stabilization of osteotomized segments in all patients has been accomplished with bone miniplates and screws. A bone miniplate across the osteotomy is secured, generally with one plate at each zygomatic buttress and one at each nasal aperture. Internal fixation techniques ensure reliable placement of osteotomy segments and may diminish postoperative skeletal relapse. With stable internal fixation, unwiring of the jaws for postoperative airway management is of little concern. However, we believe that postoperative relapse may occur even with the best planning, current surgical techniques, and internal fixation. We feel that this tendency is decreased if intermaxillary fixation is maintained for the initial 6 to 8 weeks postoperatively.

Bilateral interposition of iliac autogenous bone grafts in the osteotomy gap between the zygomatic buttress and the nasal aperture is worthwhile. In addition, the cleft defects are filled with bone grafts. Bone graft placement may be a major factor in preventing relapse.[38, 39]

After achieving the ideal occlusion intraoperatively and releasing the intermaxillary fixation to check the bite, we often leave the jaws unwired for 24 to 48 hours to permit early extubation and recovery. The jaws are then rewired in the orthodontic clinic before the patient is discharged from the hospital.

Mandibular Surgery

In general, the mandible does not require surgical repositioning in patients with clefts except in some patients who have Pierre Robin syndrome. Overall functional and aesthetic needs determine whether mandibular repositioning is indicated. Camouflage procedures consisting of mandibular setback to obviate "maxillary surgery" should be avoided at all costs. In general, any cleft jaw deformity that is present is in the maxilla, not the mandible. Excluding those with Pierre Robin syndrome, less than 15% of our patients who had clefts and required maxillary surgery developed a jaw deformity that required mandibular repositioning. When mandibular repositioning is required, we prefer to use a sagittal split osteotomy technique, which may be more physiologic, allowing better bone-to-bone contact of segments. Stabilization is generally accomplished with two to four bicortical screws at each osteotomy site. Other surgeons prefer placement of bone miniplates or direct interosseous wiring of segments.[40–50] In any case, a basic principle is to ensure that the condyles are well seated in the fossa before the segments are stabilized and immobilized.

Residual, somewhat unpredictable, malocclusion after sagittal split mandibular osteotomies that have been stabilized with internal fixation (miniplates or screws) has led to the development of intricate techniques to maintain the preoperative position of the condyle in the glenoid fossa. The osteotomies are then completed, and the mandible is repositioned and stabilized with bone miniplates or screws. Condylar or proximal segment orientation is maintained before the osteotomy is stabilized. Whether the additional time, dissection, and manipulation required ultimately limit postoperative malocclusion remains to be seen.

When planning surgery, it is important to avoid increasing the posterior facial height through mandibular autorotation. Increases greater than 3 to 5 mm are inherently unstable and tend to relapse.

Sagittal split mandibular osteotomies are said to result in a greater incidence of permanent paresthesias of the inferior alveolar-mental nerve than vertical oblique osteotomies,[19–22, 51–53] but this has not been consistently documented in large series.

Retraction to expose the cortical cuts of the sagittal split osteotomies often requires application of leverage to the maxillary tuberosity region, which may displace a recently stabilized maxilla. Therefore, when two-jaw surgery is undertaken, we prefer to complete all cortical cuts of the sagittal split osteotomies before carrying out maxillary osteotomies and stabilization. Then we complete the mandibular sagittal splits.

The transbuccal trocar system is extremely useful for stabilizing the mandibular segments with bone miniplates or bicortical screws. The trocar system is placed through a 4-mm submandibular incision on each side of the face. A visible scar may occur but rarely causes problems. The more recent introduction of right-angle drills and screwdrivers may allow placement of rigid fixation in the mandible without facial incisions.

Chin Surgery

Frequently, the chin is vertically long and retrognathic. An intraoral vertical reduction and horizontal advancement genioplasty can be safely completed with minimal morbidity if basic principles are adhered to.

The mucosa is incised to the depth of the vestibule to ensure an adequate mucosal cuff at wound closure, which limits wound dehiscence and prevents postoperative problems with the attached gingiva. The blood supply to the chin button should be maintained through a soft tissue attachment along the inferior and lingual aspects of the flap.

The chin and bilateral inferior border of the mandible are exposed through subperiosteal dissection. Dissection superior to the mental nerve is avoided to prevent excessive traction and accidental avulsion of the neurovascular bundle. In the horizontal osteotomy at least 2 mm of bone should be left below the mental foramen to avoid laceration of the nerve in the mandibular canal.

In most cases, chin stabilization with either three transosseous wires or two separate two-screw miniplates is satisfactory. The need for adequate stabilization should not, however, be underestimated.

The posterior extent of the chin osteotomy must be determined during the planning phase. The greater the vertical reduction, the more posteriorly the osteotomy should be extended to avoid a visible "step off" on either side. "Step off" can be reduced through bone burring with a rotary drill but should be managed primarily as part of the genioplasty procedure.

Management of Oronasal Fistulas, Bony Clefts, and Dental Gaps

Not infrequently, the reconstructive surgeon is presented with a skeletally mature patient who has maxillary hypoplasia and malocclusion requiring a Le Fort I osteotomy, closure of a residual oronasal fistula, and grafting of bony clefts, as well as a dental gap caused by congenital absence of a lateral incisor that also requires closure. Simultaneous management of these problems is not only possible but at times may be preferable to staged reconstruction.

Based on a complete understanding of the maxillary segmental blood supply, the surgeon selects the incisions to ensure water-tight, three-layer fistula closure and segmental repositioning. Before closure of the nasal side mucosa, septoplasty consisting of submucous resection of the deviated posterior portion and scoring and repositioning of the anterior cartilaginous septum are performed through the down-fractured maxilla. The inferior turbinate on the cleft side, which may be enlarged or edematous or may even be blocking the true nasal passage, is reduced through the down-fractured maxilla. Once the turbinate has been reduced, water-tight closure of the nasal mucosa is much easier to accomplish. The bony floor of the nose can then be built up with a bone graft to ensure symmetry with the opposite nasal floor.

The residual dental gap, the bony cleft, and the oronasal fistula can be effectively managed through a maxillary segmental osteotomy with differential repositioning. This essentially transfers the dental gap to the posterior region of the dental arch, where a small gap is well tolerated within the bite. This approach obviates "cutting down" the normal tooth structure adjacent to the cleft that would be necessary if a dental bridge were constructed to fill the gap. It also gives a more natural, aesthetically pleasing smile than either fixed bridgework or a removable partial denture. The canine tooth, which now assumes the lateral incisor position, can be shaped slightly so that it looks like an incisor. Perhaps more important, in patients with bilateral cleft lip and palate with a large residual labial and palatal fistula, differential lateral segment advancement may permit closure of a recalcitrant fistula by closing down the anatomic dead space and approximating bony and mucosal edges.

Our most gratifying results in cleft orthognathic surgery have been achieved in patients with the worst preoperative situation: bilateral clefts with collapsed, hypoplastic lesser maxillary segments; vertically long and mobile premaxillas; large residual labial and palatal oronasal fistulas; alveolar, palatal, and nasal floor bony cleft defects; enlarged inferior turbinates; deviated nasal septa; bilateral dental gaps; and a vertically long and retrognathic chin. Proper diagnosis, careful treatment planning, and meticulous technique make it possible to solve these multiple residual problems during one operation.

Management of Velopharyngeal Function

Management of velopharyngeal function in patients with clefts who need maxillary Le Fort I advancement requires preoperative assessment including clinical examination, nasendoscopy, and videofluoroscopy. The ability to obtain velopharyngeal closure tends to deteriorate after advancement of the maxilla, but prospective analysis allows reliable identification of patients at high risk for acquiring or increasing velopharyngeal incompetence (VPI) at surgery.[17, 54, 55]

Various philosophies exist concerning the timing and type of management of velopharyngeal incompetence in patients at high risk. Some patients with cleft palate already have a pharyngeal flap. The flap may be sectioned or lengthened if it limits maxillary advancement during Le Fort I osteotomy; however, we have not found this necessary. In a patient who either has inadequate preoperative velopharyngeal closure or is at high risk for inadequate postoperative closure, a pharyngoplasty can be performed either simultaneously with the maxilllary advancement or 6 to 12 months later.

We prefer to delay pharyngoplasty. Posterior palatal dissection is necessary to inset a pharyngeal flap. This dissection may further compromise the maxillary blood supply, especially when multiple segments or simultaneous dissection of full-thickness palatal flaps for palatal fistula closure are involved. If nasotracheal intubation is used throughout the operation, tube placement can obscure flap dissection and insetting, compromising the result. On the other hand, changing the intubation during the procedure increases anesthetic risk. If a Dingman mouth gag is placed to expose the posterior pharynx after completion of jaw surgery, the traction may slightly dislodge the maxilla. Furthermore, even without intermaxillary fixation, partial blockage of the nose and mouth due to these simultaneous procedures

often prolongs painful and uncomfortable intubation that may increase morbidity. The pharyngoplasty, if later required, can be combined with any secondary rhinoplasty or lip scar revision, avoiding an extra anesthetic.

When surgical correction of velopharyngeal incompetence is delayed or the patient is at high risk for acquiring postoperative velopharyngeal incompetence, the patient and family should be adequately forewarned. Careful preoperative counseling prepares the patient for temporary changes in vocal quality.

Skeletal Stability After Le Fort I Maxillary Advancement

Although the soft tissue changes and the skeletal stability associated with Le Fort I osteotomy have been previously reported,[32, 34, 56–62] most studies concerned with long-term skeletal stability group populations of patients that are quite different and use short follow-up periods or inadequate methods of analysis. Recently, we reported on long-term skeletal stability after Le Fort I maxillary advancement in 30 consecutive patients with unilateral cleft lip and palate.[23] Cephalometric radiographs taken preoperatively, immediately postoperatively, and 6 to 8 weeks, 1 year, and 2 years postoperatively were analyzed. Amount and timing of relapse, correlation between advancement and relapse, effect of performing multiple jaw procedures, and effectiveness of various methods of skeletal fixation were analyzed. The cephalometric tracings of the preoperative and serial postoperative lateral cephalograms were digitized to calculate horizontal and vertical maxillary changes.

We found that skeletal relapse tends to occur in patients with cleft lip and palate who undergo Le Fort I maxillary advancement. The degree of relapse is not necessarily correlated with the amount of advancement. Simultaneous mandibular surgery or genioplasty have no influence on the amount of maxillary skeletal relapse. More than half of the vertical relapse and about half of the horizontal relapse occur during the first 6 to 8 weeks, and vertical and horizontal stability are achieved by 1 year. Skeletal relapse occurs with both miniplate and direct wire fixation after Le Fort I osteotomy, but the use of miniplate fixation techniques allows greater initial and long-term mean effective horizontal maxillary advancement than direct transosseous wire fixation.

Complications

Other than the complications of anesthesia and airway compromise, perhaps the most devastating complication of maxillofacial surgery is the loss of bone segments and teeth secondary to avascular necrosis. This risk is greatest after Le Fort I segmental osteotomy in patients with a bilateral cleft, but when careful surgical technique is used, it should occur rarely if ever.

Residual malocclusion is most commonly the result of poor planning, poor execution of surgery, or skeletal or dental relapse. However, patients of even the most skilled surgeons may experience postoperative malocclusion necessitating a second procedure. Correct diagnosis, meticulous surgical technique including aggressive soft tissue dissection, planned overcorrection in anticipation of relapse, rigid fixation techniques, autogenous bone grafting, postoperative intermaxillary fixation, and class III elastics when indicated can minimize the incidence of this problem. A poor facial aesthetic appearance is generally due to poor recognition and planning preoperatively.

The inferior alveolar-mental nerve, which runs directly through the mandible, may be bruised, producing temporary paresthesias when either ramus osteotomies or genioplasty osteotomies of the mandible are performed. Permanent sensory loss in the lower lip–chin region occurs in at least 10% of patients.[63–65] Injury to the infraorbital nerve with sensory loss in the upper lip distribution may be present after maxillary Le Fort I osteotomy but is rarely permanent. In general, poor objective documentation of neurosensibility changes after osteotomies makes the true incidence of permanent sensory loss and resulting disability difficult to judge.

Residual mobility of maxillary segments is most common after three-part maxillary osteotomies in patients with bilateral cleft lip and palate. The true incidence is unknown but can be minimized through meticulous three-layer fistula closure techniques, autogenous cancellous bone grafting, and rigid fixation combined with prefabricated acrylic splint wiring to the maxilla for at least 6 to 8 weeks postoperatively. A small palatal wound dehiscence may occur in the incisive foramen region with partial graft loss and partial fistula recurrence leading to nonunion of the premaxillary segment. However, this residual fistula is generally considerably smaller than the original, permitting successful secondary regrafting and fistula closure. Recurrent oronasal fistulas should be extremely rare in patients with unilateral clefts.

Laryngeal granuloma secondary to surgical intubation has been seen in two of our patients.[55] Postoperative nasendoscopy is helpful in diagnosing this problem as well as in documenting changes in velopharyngeal function.

Patient Cases

Patient 1—Unilateral Cleft Lip and Palate

A 23-year-old woman had undergone cleft lip and palate repairs at the usual ages. Maxillary hypoplasia, mild mandibular prognathism, and a vertically long chin were diagnosed when she was 20 (Fig. 65–1). Velopharyngeal function was assessed as adequate. A Le Fort I osteotomy with advancement, sagittal split setbacks of the mandible, and vertical reduction genioplasty were performed. The maxilla was stabilized with miniplates, and the mandible and chin with direct wire fixation. Postoperatively, an anterior open bite deformity developed as a result of upper jaw relapse. Two years later the patient was reassessed at our center for revision osteotomy. Additional orthodontic alignment was required before repeat jaw surgery. Model surgery was carried out, and a 5-mm intrusion in the right second molar region and 4 mm in the left second molar region were planned. Horizontal advancement of 12 mm on the right side and 14 mm on the left, and a 5-mm vertical reduction genioplasty also were planned.

Intraoperatively, the maxilla was stabilized with titanium bone miniplates, an interocclusal acrylic splint was wired to the upper jaw, and intermaxillary fixation was applied. The residual left labial and palatal oronasal fistula was closed, and an iliac bone graft was packed into the cleft, the floor of the nose, and the alveolus. An interpositional bone graft also was placed along the lateral maxillary walls. A 5-mm vertical wedge was removed from the chin, and stabilization was achieved with three transosseous wires.

Eighteen months postoperatively, the skeleton was judged to be stable, and a five-unit fixed bridge was constructed to fill the dental gap due to congenital absence of the lateral incisor. Velopharyngeal function remained clinically and nasendoscopically adequate 1 year postoperatively.

Patient 2—Unilateral Cleft Lip and Palate

A 28-year-old woman born with a left cleft lip and palate had undergone 16 cleft repair procedures in Hong Kong, including multiple attempts at oronasal fistula closure, revision pharyngoplasties, and Le Fort I osteotomy. On our examination, her left maxillary central, lateral, and canine teeth were absent, the palate was severely scarred, and residual labial and palatal oronasal fistulas were present (Fig. 65–2). An extremely tight pharyngoplasty was in place, and velopharyngeal incompetence was marked on clinical, nasendoscopic, and videofluoroscopic examination. The maxilla was severely hypoplastic and the mandible prognathic. The chin was vertically long and retrognathic.

Major orthodontic treatment was required in preparation for jaw surgery. At the time of surgery, maxillary Le Fort I osteotomy in two segments was performed, and the residual labial and palatal oronasal fistulas were closed simultaneously, Iliac bone was grafted to the palate, the floor of the nose, and the alveolar cleft, and bilateral sagittal split osteotomies of the mandible with setback, vertical reduction, and advancement genioplasty were performed. The maxilla and chin were stabilized with miniplates, and the mandible was stabilized with bicortical screws in the rami regions. A revision pharyngoplasty was carried out 6 months postoperatively.

Patient 3—Bilateral Cleft Lip and Palate

A skeletally mature 18-year-old male who had been born with a complete bilateral cleft lip and palate presented with maxillary hypoplasia, a mobile premaxilla, residual bilateral labial and palatal oronasal fistulas, residual bony clefts, and dental gaps in the region of the congenitally absent lateral incisors (Fig. 65–3). A vertically long and retrognathic chin and a crooked nose

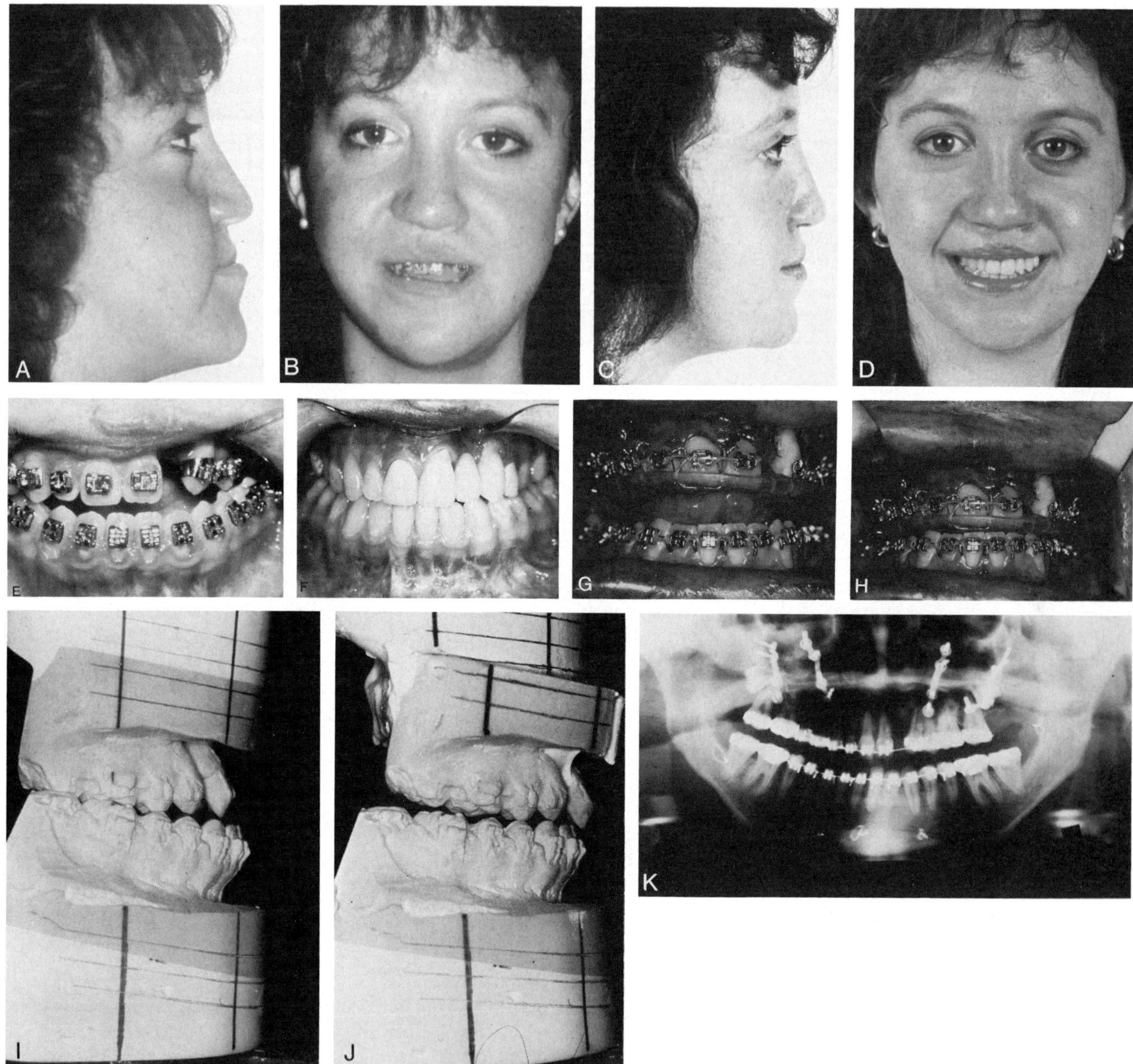

Figure 65–1 A 23-year-old woman with a repaired left cleft lip and palate. *A*, Preoperative profile view. *B*, Preoperative frontal view with smile. *C*, Postoperative profile view. *D*, Postoperative frontal view with smile. *E*, Occlusion before revision osteotomy. *F*, Occlusion after fixed bridge construction. *G*, The maxilla stabilized with an interocclusal acrylic splint wired to it. After the bone miniplates are in place, the intermaxillary fixation is released and occlusion is checked. *H*, Occlusion well interdigitated in the splint after stabilization of the maxillary Le Fort I osteotomy with miniplates. *I*, Alginate impressions cast in stone and mounted on an articulator with a face bow transfer. *J*, Dental models showing the maxilla repositioned for the preferred occlusion. Precise horizontal and vertical measurements are made for use during surgery. An interocclusal acrylic splint is constructed. *K*, Postoperative panoramic radiograph.

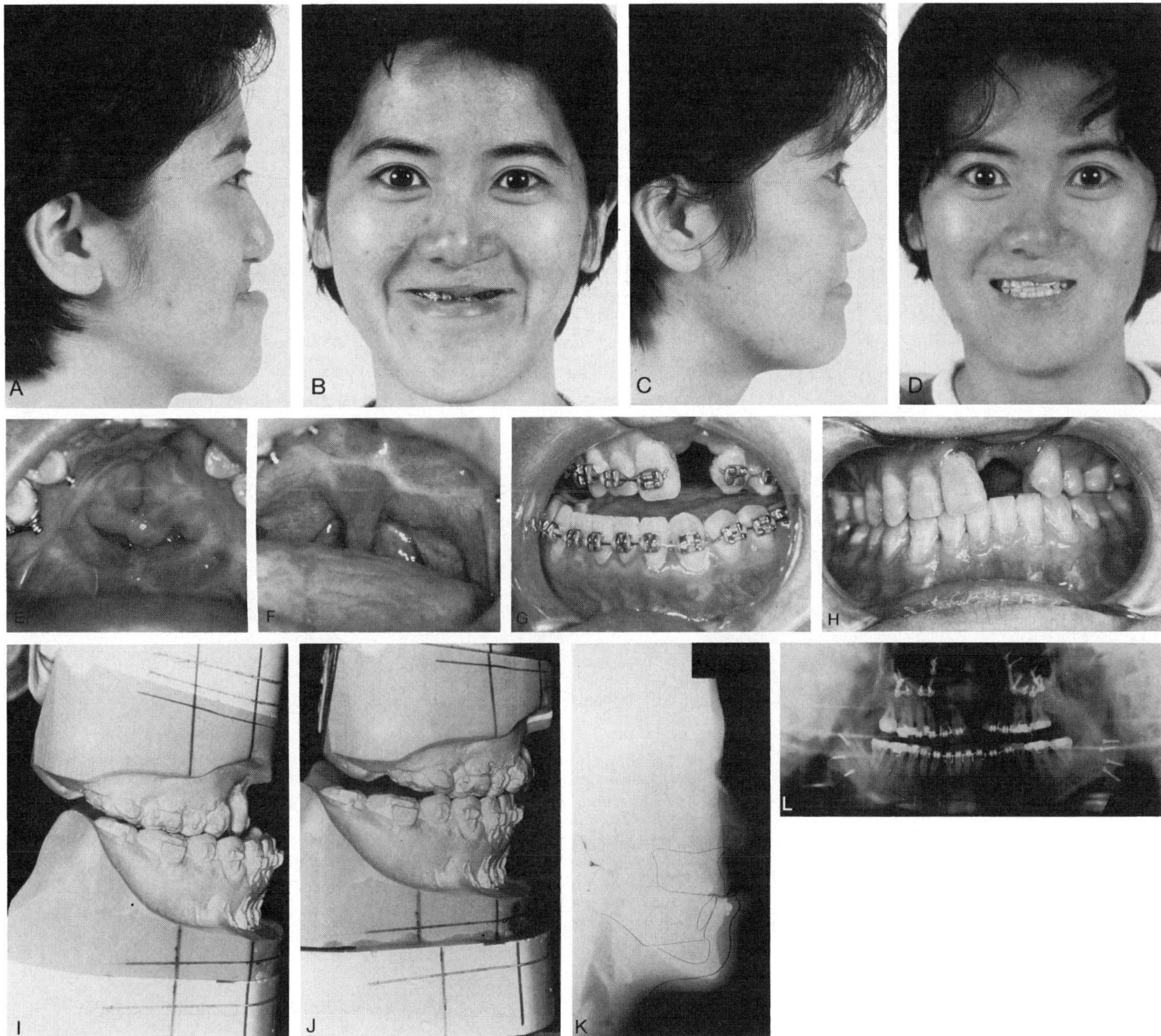

Figure 65–2 A 28-year-old woman with repaired cleft lip and palate. *A*, Preoperative profile view. *B*, Preoperative frontal view with smile. *C*, Postoperative profile view. *D*, Postoperative frontal view with smile. *E*, Preoperative view of the scarred palate demonstrating residual oronasal fistulas. *F*, Preoperative view of the tightly tethered pharyngoplasty. *G*, Preoperative occlusal view showing 12 mm of negative overjet, collapsed maxillary segments, and anterior open bite deformity with full class III malocclusion. *H*, Postoperative and postorthodontic occlusal view. *I*, Articulated dental models marked and ready for planning surgery. *J*, The mandibular dental model is set back for ideal occlusion, and a final acrylic interocclusal splint is constructed to be used at the time of surgery. *K*, Preoperative lateral cephalogram. *L*, Postoperative panoramic radiograph.

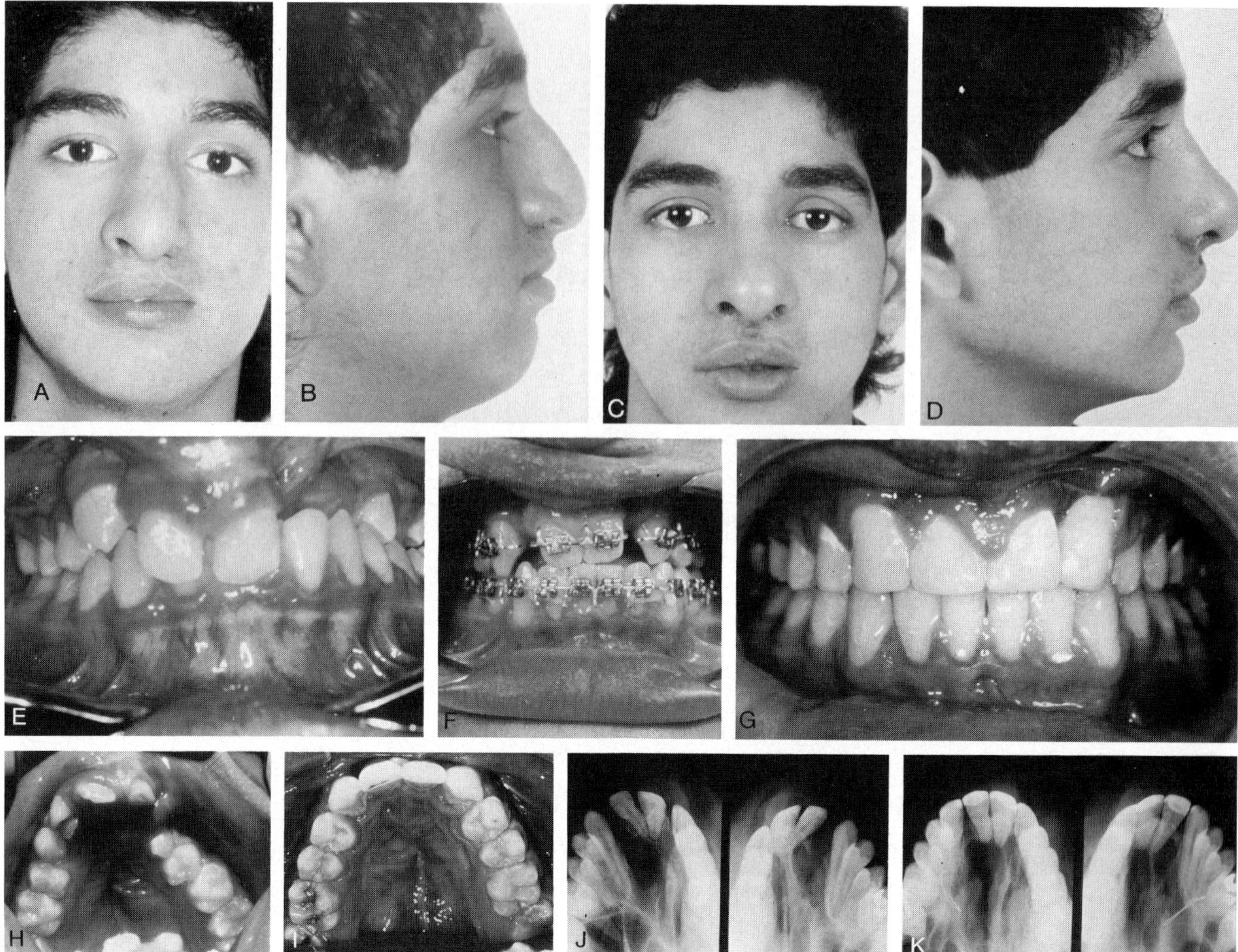

Figure 65–3 A 17-year-old with repaired bilateral cleft lip and palate. *A,* Frontal view. *B,* Lateral view. *C,* Frontal view after maxillary and chin surgery as well as revision rhinoplasty and columella lengthening. *D,* Lateral view after the same procedures. *E,* Occlusal view at 13 years of age. Note that the premaxilla appears to be long vertically. *F,* After preoperative orthodontic treatment in preparation for jaw surgery. *G,* Eighteen months postoperatively after removal of orthodontic bands. *H,* Occlusal view in mixed dentition phase. The cheek rotation flap used to close the palatal fistula has decreased the vestibular depth and placed nonkeratinized mucosa over the tooth-bearing surface. A sliding mucogingival rotation flap would have been preferable. *I,* Maxillary dental arch form after maxillary Le Fort I osteotomy with differential repositioning of segments to close residual fistulas and dental gaps in the region of the congenitally absent lateral incisors. *J,* Occlusal radiographs before Le Fort I osteotomy, fistula closure, and iliac bone grafting, demonstrating lack of continuity of the maxillary arch. *K,* Postoperative occlusal radiographs demonstrating the bony bridge on both sides stabilizing the maxilla into one unit.

with a dropped tip and short columella also were present. The patient underwent 18 months of preoperative orthodontic treatment in preparation for orthognathic surgery.

Surgery included a maxillary Le Fort I osteotomy in three segments with differential repositioning to ensure simultaneous closure of the residual oronasal fistula, iliac bone grafting to the alveolar and palatal bony clefts, and closure of the dental gaps in the region of the congenitally missing lateral incisors. A vertical reduction and advancement genioplasty also was completed. Interpositional iliac grafts were placed along the lateral maxillary walls. The dentition was further restored with composite veneers postorthodontically. Revision rhinoplasty with columella lengthening was carried out 6 months postoperatively.

Patient 4—Bilateral Cleft Lip and Palate

A skeletally mature 16-year-old girl with complete bilateral cleft lip and palate had undergone lip and palate repair at the usual ages but was left with a hypoplastic maxilla, a mobile premaxilla with residual labial and palatal oronasal fistulas, residual palatal and alveolar bony clefts, anterior open bite, vertical maxillary excess, excessive mandibular vertical height with a relatively short upper lip, and a vertically long and retrusive chin (Fig. 65–4). Her nasal septum was badly deviated, and nasal breathing was obstructed. She had a pharyngeal flap in place but with slight hyponasality. Sibilant distortion related to her anterior malocclusion was present.

Major orthdontic treatment was required in prepara-

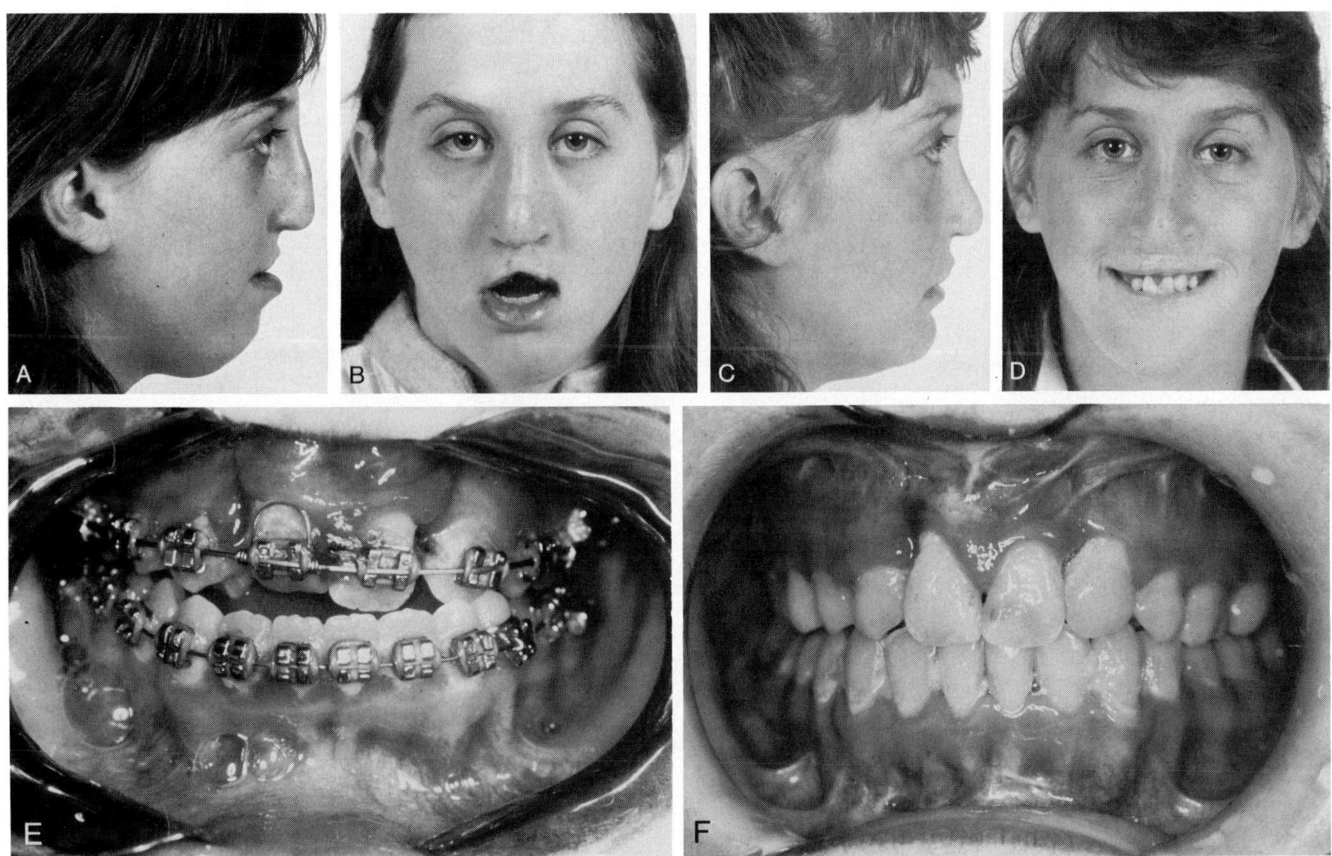

Figure 65–4 A 16-year-old girl with bilateral complete cleft lip and palate. *A*, Lateral preoperative view. *B*, Frontal preoperative view. *C*, Lateral postoperative view. *D*, Smiling frontal postoperative view. *E*, Preoperative occlusion after completion of orthodontic treatment in preparation for jaw surgery. *F*, Occlusion one year postoperatively after removal of orthodontic bands.

tion for jaw surgery. She underwent a maxillary Le Fort I osteotomy in three segments with simultaneous closure of residual labial and palatal oronasal fistulas, iliac bone grafting to the bony clefts, bilateral sagittal split osteotomies with setback, vertical reduction and advancement genioplasty, septoplasty, and reduction of the inferior turbinates. Stabilization was accomplished with titanium bone miniplates in the maxilla and bicortical screws in the mandible. Hyponasality and the sibilant distortion were improved. A revision rhinoplasty was carried out as a secondary procedure.

Patient 5—Isolated Cleft Lip and Palate

A 19-year-old woman with an isolated palatal cleft had undergone palate repair at 18 months of age (Fig. 65–5). No further revisions were required. On examination, she had a marked maxillary hypoplasia with class III malocclusion and a vertically long and retrognathic chin. Preoperatively, nasendoscopy and videofluoroscopy indicated borderline velopharyngeal closure. There was a circular pattern of closure with occasional bubbling of mucus through the velopharyngeal port. Resonance was normal, but nasal air emission was inconsistent. A sibilant distortion was attributed to abnormal tongue placement. This patient was considered at high risk for postoperative velopharyngeal incompetence.

Preoperative orthodontic therapy was arranged, and a maxillary Le Fort I osteotomy with advancement and posterior intrusion was planned. The chin required vertical reduction and advancement. The maxilla was stabilized with titanium bone miniplates and the chin with direct transosseous wires. Velopharyngeal incompetence and hypernasality were noted postoperatively despite the development of a circular closure pattern with a Passavant's ridge. A superiorly based pharyngeal flap was carried out 6 months postoperatively.

ACKNOWLEDGMENTS. The authors would like to thank Drs. R. B. Ross, D. Engel, N. Shapera, M. Taylor, and B. Tompson, our orthodontists in the Craniofacial Treatment Center, Division of Orthodontics, The Hospital for Sick Children, in Toronto, for their help and assistance.

This manuscript was prepared with the assistance of the Medical Publications Service, The Hospital for Sick Children.

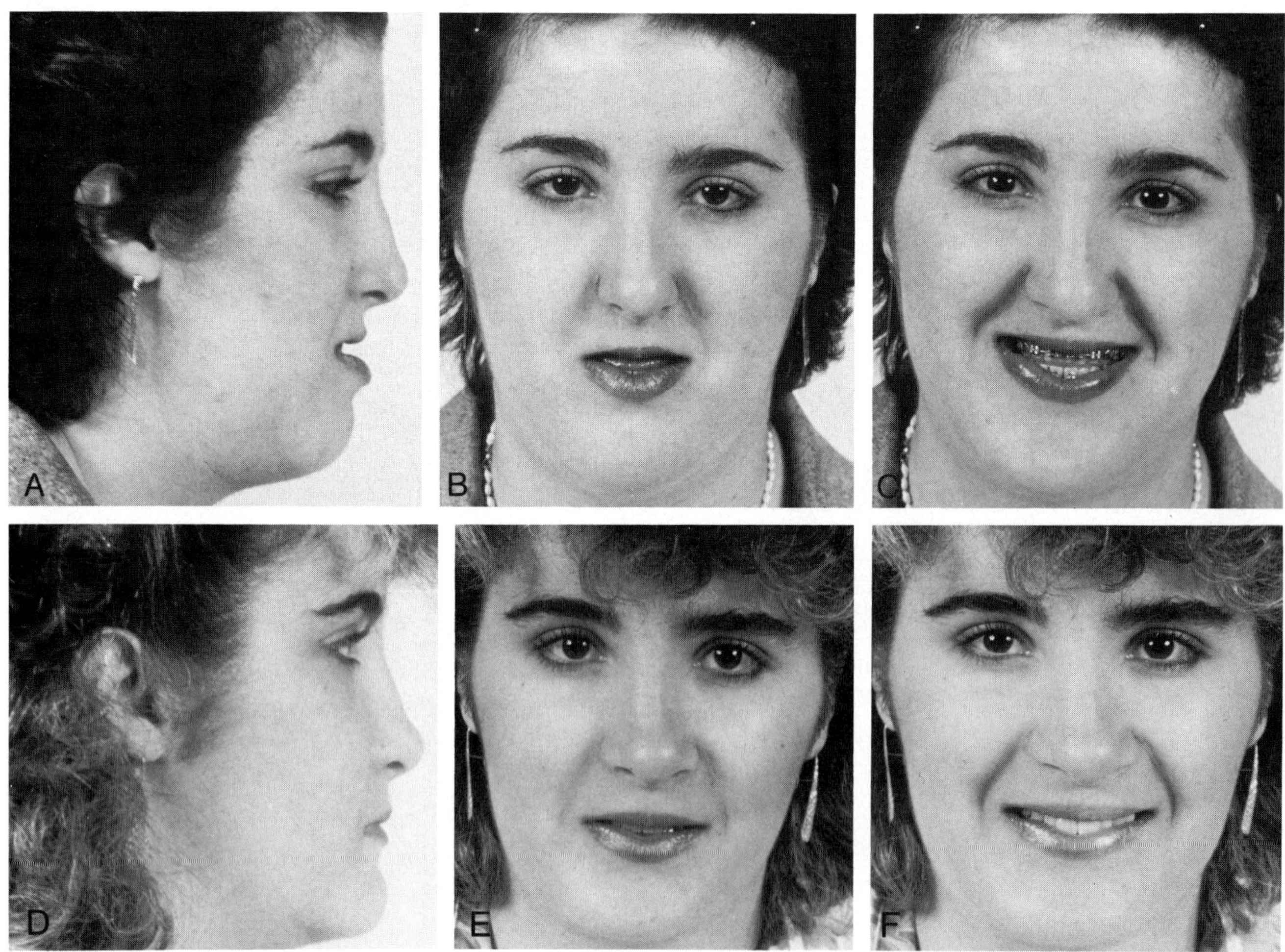

Figure 65–5 A 19-year-old woman with isolated cleft palate. *A,* Lateral preoperative view. *B,* Frontal preoperative view. *C,* Smiling frontal preoperative view. *D,* Lateral postoperative view. *E,* Frontal postoperative view. *F,* Smiling postoperative view.

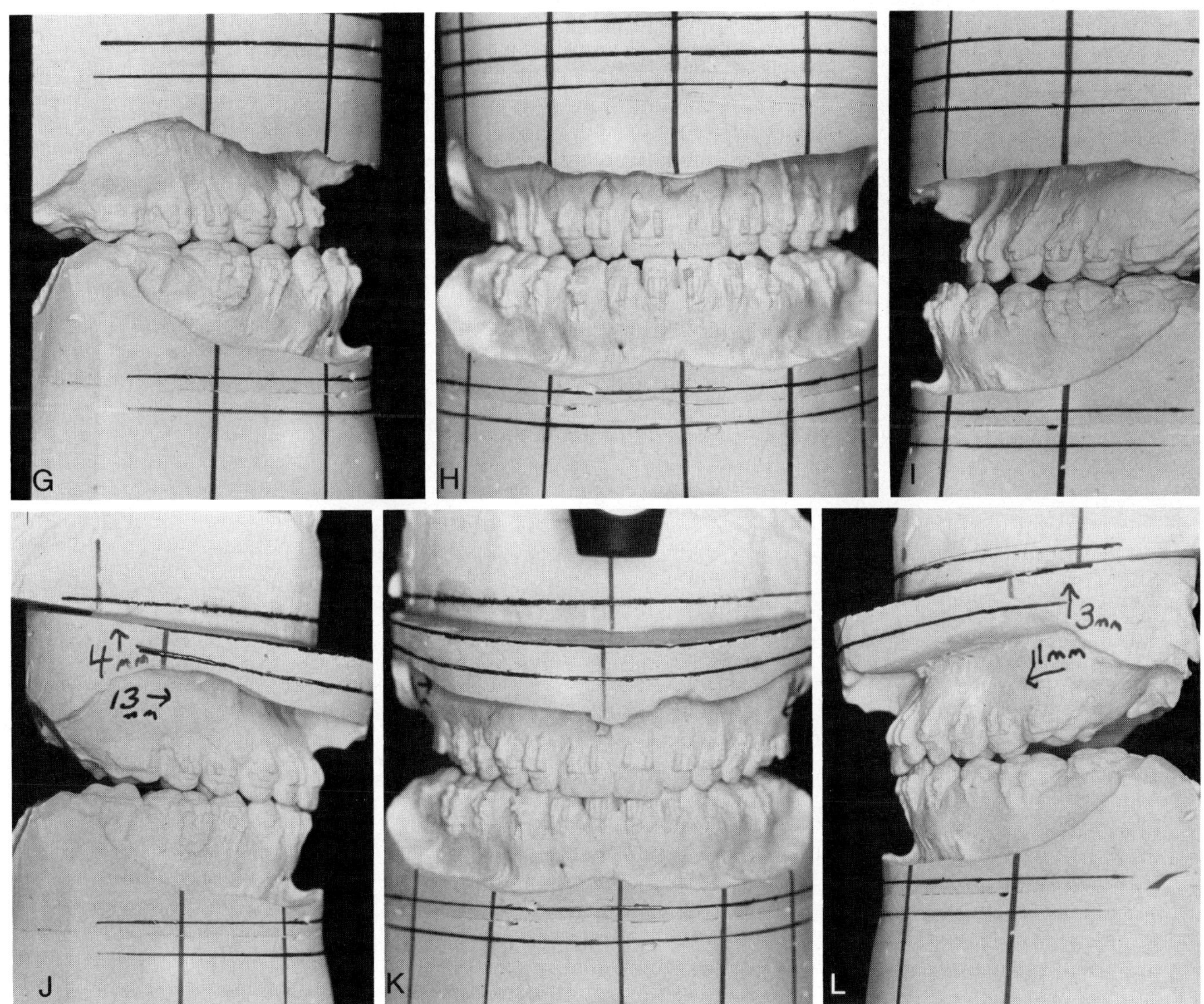

Figure 65–5 *Continued G,* Right lateral view of dental model articulated in preparation for model surgery. *H,* Frontal view. *I,* Left lateral view. *J,* Right lateral view of articulated model repositioned through model surgery. *K,* Frontal view. *L,* Left lateral view demonstrating 11-mm advancement with 3-mm posterior intrusion.

Illustration continued on following page

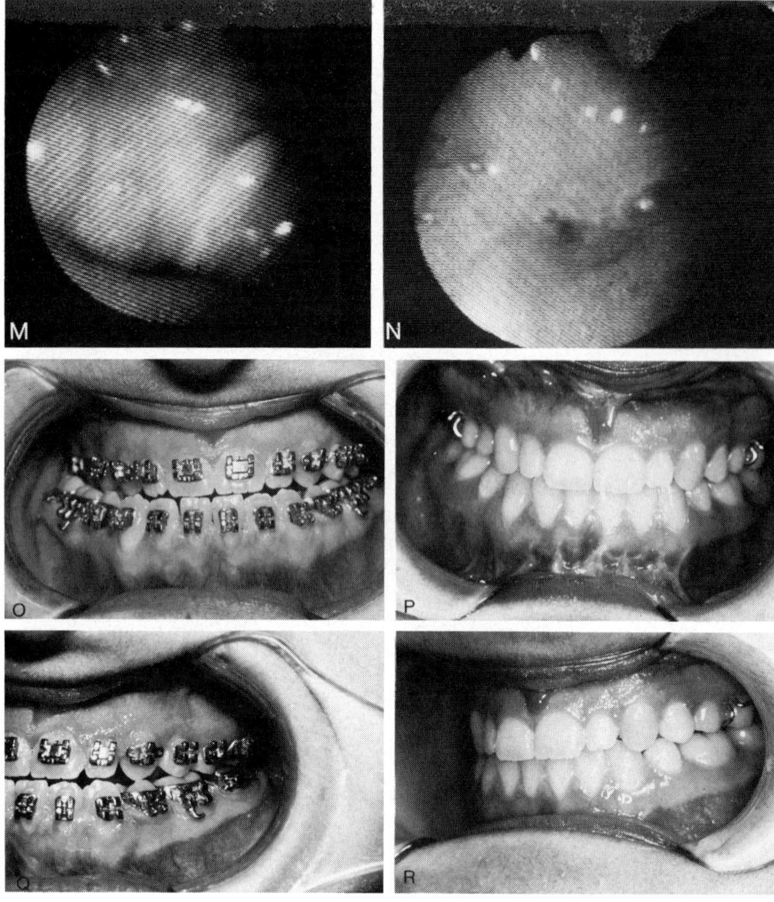

Figure 65–5 *Continued M,* Nasoendoscopic view of velopharyngeal incompetence 1 year after Le Fort I osteotomy. Note the small central defect despite a significant Passavant's ridge. *N,* Nasoendoscopic view of borderline velopharyngeal closure with bubbling of mucus through the velopharyngeal port during speech. *O,* Frontal occlusal view with orthodontic treatment under way. *P,* One year postoperatively after removal of orthodontic bands. *Q,* Left oblique occlusal view with orthodontic bands in place. *R,* One year postoperatively.

References

1. Maloney F, Worthington P: The origin of the Le Fort I maxillary osteotomy: Cheever's operation. J Oral Surg 39:731, 1981.
2. Wassmund M: Praktische Chirurgie des Mundes und der Kiefer. Leipzig; Meusser, 1935.
3. Le Fort R: Experimental study of fractures of the upper jaw: Parts I and II. Rev Chir de Paris 23:208–227, 360–379, 1901.
4. Schuchardt K: Ein Beitrag zur chirurgischen Kieferorthopadie unter Berucksichtigung ihrer Bedeutung für die Behandlung angeborener und erworbener Kieferdeformitaten bei Soldaten. Dtsch Zach-, Mund- Kieferheilk 9:73, 1942.
5. Gillies HD, Rowe NL: L'osteotomie du maxillaire superieur envisagee essentiellement dans les cas de bec de lievre total. Rev Stomat (Paris) 55:545, 1954.
6. Obwegeser H: In Trauner R, Obwegeser H: Zur Operationstechnik bei der Progenie und anderen Unterkieferanomalien. Dtsch Zahn-, Mund- u Kieferheilk 23:1, 1955.
7. Obwegeser H: Cirugia del "mordex apertus." Rev Odont Argentina 50:429, 1962.
8. Obwegeser H: Der offene BiB aus chirurgischer Sicht. Schweiz Mschr Zahnheilk 74:668, 1964.
9. Obwegeser H: Eingriffe am Oberkiefer zur Korrektur des progenen Zustandsbildes. Schweiz Mschr Zahnheilk 75:365, 1965.
10. Obwegeser HL: Surgical correction of small or retrodisplaced maxillae. The "dish-face" deformity. Plast Reconstr Surg 43:351, 1969.
11. Bell WH, Levy BM: Revascularization and bone healing after anterior mandibular osteotomy. J Oral Surg 28:196, 1970.
12. Bell WH: Biological basis for maxillary osteotomies. Am J Phys Anthropol 38:279, 1973.
13. Freihofer HP, Jr; Results of osteotomies of the facial skeleton in adolescence. J Maxillofac Surg 5:267, 1977.
14. Ross RB: Treatment variables affecting facial growth in complete unilateral cleft lip and palate. Cleft Palate J 24:75, 1987.
15. Riley RW, Powell N, Guilleminault C: Current surgical concepts for treating obstructive sleep apnea syndrome. J Oral Maxillofac Surg 45:149, 1987.
16. Witzel MA, Munro IR: Velopharyngeal insufficiency after maxillary advancement. Cleft Palate J 14:176, 1977.
17. Witzel MA: Orthognathic defects and surgical correction: The effects on speech and velopharyngeal function. Thesis. Pittsburgh: University of Pittsburgh, 1981.
18. Witzel MA, Ross RB, Munro IR: Articulation skills before and after facial osteotomies. J Maxillofac Surg 8:195, 1980.
19. Posnick JC, Grossman JAI, Zimbler AG: Normal cutaneous sensibility of the face. Plast Reconstr Surg (in press).
20. Fiamminghi L, Aversa C: Lesions of the inferior alveolar nerve in sagittal osteotomy of the ramus—experimental study. J Maxillofac Surg 7:125, 1979.
21. Brusati R, Fiamminghi L, Sesenna E, et al: Functional disturbances of the inferior alveolar nerve after sagittal osteotomy of the mandibular ramus: Operating technique for prevention. J Maxillofac Surg 9:123, 1981.
22. Nishioka GJ, Zysset MK, Van Sickels JE: Neurosensory disturbance with rigid fixation of the bilateral sagittal split osteotomy. J Oral Maxillofac Surg 45:20, 1987.
23. Posnick JC, Ewing M: Skeletal stability after Le Fort maxillary advancement in patients with unilateral cleft lip and palate. Plast Reconstr Surg (in press).
24. Bell W, Proffitt W, White R: Surgical Correction of Dentofacial Deformities. Vols. 1 and 2. Philadelphia: WB Saunders, 1980.
25. Farkas LG, Hreczko TA, Kolar JC, et al: Vertical and horizontal proportions of the face in young adult North American Caucasians: Revision of neoclassical canons. Plast Reconstr Surg 75:328, 1985.
26. Ricketts RM: Divine proportion in facial esthetics. Clin Plast Surg 9:401, 1982.
27. Byrd HS: Craniofacial anomalies I: Cephalometrics. Selected Readings in Plastic Surgery 4:1, Dallas, TX: Baylor University Medical Center, 1987.
28. Lines PA, Steinhauser EW: Diagnosis and treatment planning in surgical orthodontic therapy. Am J Orthod 66:378, 1974.
29. Baumrind S, Korn EL, Ben-Bassat Y, et al: Quantitation of maxillary remodeling. 2. Masking of remodeling effects when an "anatomical" method of superimposition is used in the absence of metallic implants. Am J Orthod Dentofac Orthop 92:463, 1987.
30. Friede H, Kahnberg KE, Adell R, et al: Accuracy of cephalometric prediction in orthognathic surgery. J Oral Maxillofac Surg 45:754, 1987.
31. Hershey HG, Smith LH: Soft-tissue profile change associated with surgical correction of the prognathic mandible. Am J Orthod 65:483, 1974.
32. Freihofer HP, Jr: The lip profile after correction of retromaxillism in cleft and non-cleft patients. J Maxillofac Surg 4:136, 1976.
33. Suckiel JM, Kohn MW: Soft-tissue changes related to the surgical management of mandibular prognathism. Am J Orthod 73:676, 1978.

34. Bell WH, Scheideman GB: Correction of vertical maxillary deficiency: Stability and soft tissue changes. J Oral Surg 39:666, 1981.

35. Willmot DR: Soft tissue profile changes following correction of class III malocclusions by mandibular surgery. Br J Orthod 8:175, 1981.

36. Gibson T, Kenedi RM: Biomechanical properties of skin. Surg Clin North Am 47:279, 1967.

37. Hall HD, Posnick JC: Early results of secondary bone grafts in 106 alveolar clefts. J Maxillofac Surg 41:289, 1984.

38. Araujo A, Schendel SA, Wolford LM, et al: Total maxillary advancement with and without bone grafting. J Oral Surg 36:849, 1978.

39. Tessier P, Tulasne JF: Secondary repair of cleft lip deformity. Clin Plast Surg 11:747, 1984.

40. Luhr HG: Zur stabilen Osteosynthese bei Unterkieferfrakturen. Dtsch Zahnaerztl Z 23:754, 1968.

41. Luhr HG: Stabile Fixation von Oberkiefer-Mittelgesichtsfrakturen durch Mini-Kompressionsplatten. Dtsch Zahnaerztl 234:851, 1979.

42. Champy M: Surgical treatment of midface deformities. Head Neck Surg 2:451, 1980.

43. Harle F: Le Fort I osteotomy (using mini-plates) for correction of the long face. Int J Oral Surg 9:427, 1980.

44. Horster W: Experience with functionally stable plate osteosynthesis after forward displacement of the upper jaw. J Maxillofac Surg 8:176, 1980.

45. Drommer R, Luhr H: The stabilization of osteotomized maxillary segments with Luhr miniplates in secondary cleft surgery. J Maxillofac Surg 9:166, 1981.

46. Steinhauser EW: Bone screws and plates in orthognathic surgery. Int J Oral Surg 11:209, 1982.

47. Van Sickels JE, Jeter TD, Aragon SB: Rigid fixation of maxillary osteotomies: A preliminary report and technique article. Oral Surg Oral Med Oral Pathol 60:262, 1985.

48. Harsha BC, Terry BC: Stabilization of Le Fort I osteotomies utilizing small bone plates. Int J Adult Orthod Orthognath Surg 1:69, 1986.

49. Rosen HM: Miniplate fixation of Le Fort I osteotomies. Discussion by H G Luhr. Plast Reconstr Surg 78:748, 1986.

50. Beals SP, Munro IR: The use of miniplates in craniomaxillofacial surgery. Plast Reconstr Surg 79:33, 1987.

51. Simpson W: Problems encountered in the sagittal split operation. Int J Oral Surg 10:81, 1981.

52. Martis CS: Complications after mandibular sagittal split osteotomy. J Oral Maxillofac Surg 44:101, 1984.

53. Nishioka GJ, Mason M, Van Sickels JE: Neurosensory disturbance associated with the anterior mandibular horizontal osteotomy. J Oral Maxillofac Surg 46:107, 1988.

54. Swanson E, Witzel MA, Posnick JC: The effect of pharyngeal flap surgery on velopharyngeal closure: Nasendoscopic findings in 40 patients. Plast Surg Forum 11:77, 1988.

55. Sandor GKB, Witzel MA, Posnick JC: The use of nasendoscopy in predicting velopharyngeal function after maxillary advancement. Proceedings, 46th Annual Meeting, The Cleft Palate-Craniofacial Association, April, 1989, p 23.

56. Willmar K: On Le Fort I osteotomy: A follow-up study of 106 operated patients with maxillo-facial deformity. Scand J Plast Reconstr Surg 12:1–68, 1974.

57. Hedemark A, Freihofer HP, Jr: The behavior of the maxilla in vertical movements after Le Fort I osteotomy. J Maxillofac Surg 6:244, 1978.

58. Tideman H, Stoelinga P, Gallia L: Le Fort I advancement with segmental palatal osteotomies in patients with cleft palates. J Oral Surg 38:196, 1980.

59. Braun TW, Stoereanos GC: Long term results with maxillary advancement in cleft palate patients in oral and maxillofacial surgery. Proceedings from the Eighth International Conference on Maxillofacial Surgery, 1982, p 265.

60. Teuscher U, Sailer HF: Stability of Le Fort I osteotomy in class III cases with retropositioned maxillae. J Maxillofac Surg 10:80, 1982.

61. Luyk NH, Ward-Booth RP: The stability of Le Fort I advancement osteotomies using bone plates without bone grafts. J Maxillofac Surg 13:250, 1985.

62. Garrison BT, Lapp TH, Bussard DA: The stability of Le Fort I maxillary osteotomies in patients with simultaneous alveolar cleft bone grafts. J Oral Maxillofac Surg 45:761, 1987.

63. White RP, Peters PB, Costich ER, et al: Evaluation of sagittal split-ramus osteotomy in 17 patients. J Oral Surg 27:851, 1969.

64. Walter JM, Jr, Gregg JM: Analysis of postsurgical neurologic alteration in the trigeminal nerve. J Oral Surg 37:410, 1979.

65. Zaytoun HS, Jr, Phillips C, Terry BC: Long-term neurosensory deficits following transoral vertical ramus and sagittal split osteotomies for mandibular prognathism. J Oral Maxillofac Surg 44:193, 1986.

CHAPTER 66

Bone Grafting of the Cleft Maxilla

Katherine W. L. Vig,
Raymond J. Fonseca,
and Timothy A. Turvey

Delayed or secondary alveolar bone grafting in patients with cleft lip and palate is a well-established method of treatment. Early reports of alveolar bone grafting were described in the German literature by Lexer[1] and Drachter[2] before Axhausen[3] popularized the technique that is now considered the state-of-the-art treatment in many American and European cleft palate centers. Although introduced by surgeons in Europe, Boyne and Sands[4] refined and developed the surgical technique of alveolar bone grafting in the United States. The contemporary surgical management of autogenous bone grafting in the cleft palate patient has been well documented in the literature and is supported with long-term studies.

There are several alternative donor sites from which autologous bone may be harvested. The most widely used donor site is the iliac crest (Figs. 66–1 to 66–4), which provides a source of considerable amounts of cancellous bone. However, the morbidity associated with invasive surgery to the hip has made calvarial bone an attractive alternative.

The first descriptions of utilizing cranial bone as graft material were reported in the German literature by Konig[5] and Muller.[6] Reports of cranial bone for repair of craniofacial defects continued to appear in the literature, but it was not until Smith[7] reported an increase in revascularization and greater volumetric stability of cranial bone grafts in an animal model that this source of bone became well accepted by clinicians. This finding was later supported by Zins and Whitaker.[8] Tessier[9] described the clinical application of cranial bone grafts in surgery on the craniofacial skeleton, and Wolfe and Berkowitz[10] reported use of cranial bone specifically to reconstruct the maxilla and palate in the presence of a cleft. The technique for harvesting bone from the cranium necessitates an increase in operating time. Some clinicians have concerns about whether cranial bone is a viable alternative donor site to the iliac crest.

More recently, allogeneic bone has been suggested as an alternative method of providing bone for grafts in the cleft region by Nique et al[11] (Figs. 66–5 to 66–8). Orthodontic management, including the movement of teeth into the allogeneic grafted area, requires an understanding of the biology of bone formation, osteoinduction, and angiogenesis. Clinical observation and doc-

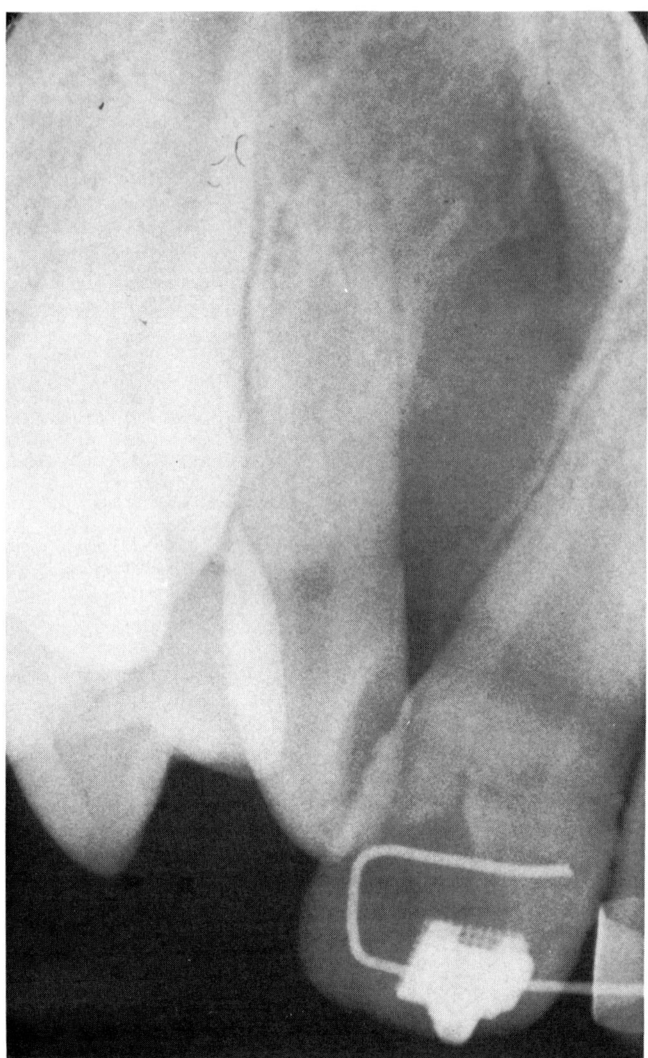

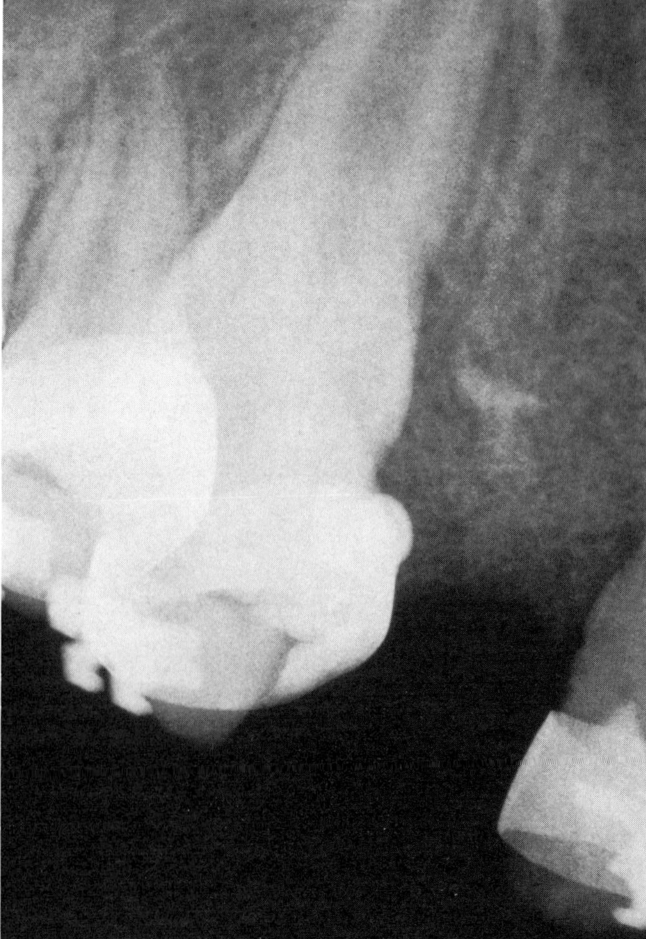

Figure 66–1 Case report of a patient with an autologous bone graft. Periapical radiograph of a 9-year-old boy with a complete right unilateral cleft of the lip and palate. The right permanent canine was unerupted, and the lateral incisor was peg-shaped.

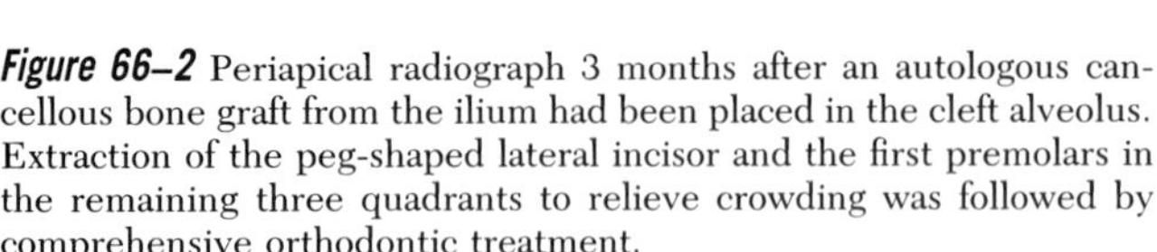

Figure 66–2 Periapical radiograph 3 months after an autologous cancellous bone graft from the ilium had been placed in the cleft alveolus. Extraction of the peg-shaped lateral incisor and the first premolars in the remaining three quadrants to relieve crowding was followed by comprehensive orthodontic treatment.

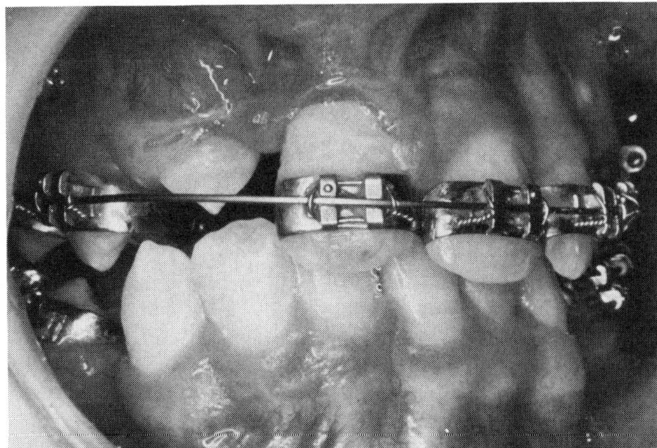

Figure 66–3 Intraoral photograph 1 year after surgery showing the eruption of the maxillary right canine into the bone graft.

umentation indicates that the permanent canine will erupt into allogeneic bone grafts (Fig. 66–6). Freeze-dried cadaver bone eliminates the morbidity associated with a second surgical site, especially the postsurgical discomfort in the hip when the iliac crest is selected as the donor site. The utility of the procedure, in terms of

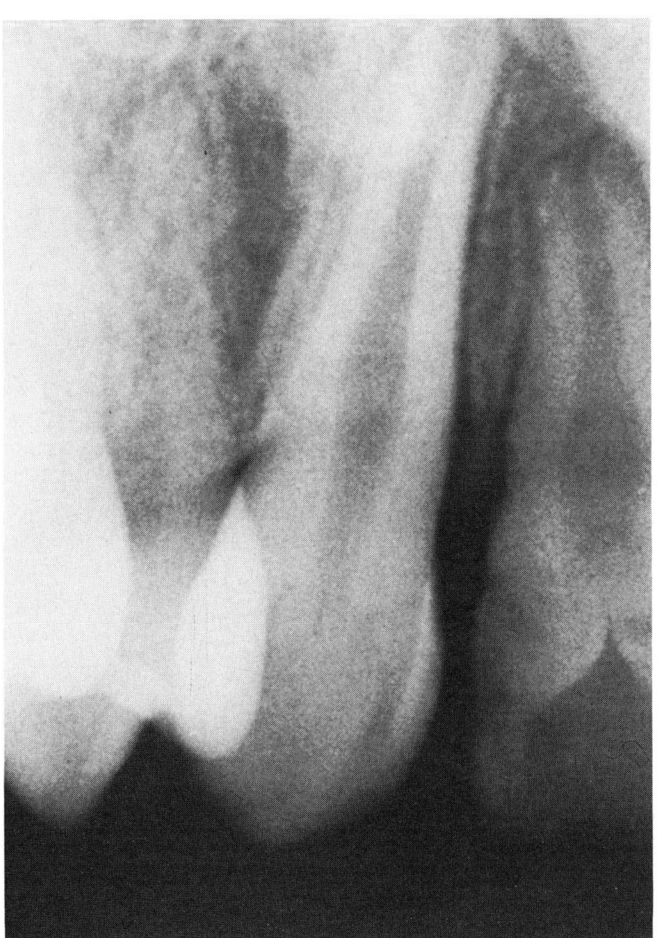

Figure 66–4 Periapical radiograph 4 years after treatment. The maxillary right canine is adjacent to the central incisor, which shows root resorption. The interdental crest bone height between the incisor and canine was satisfactory, with no periodontal defect.

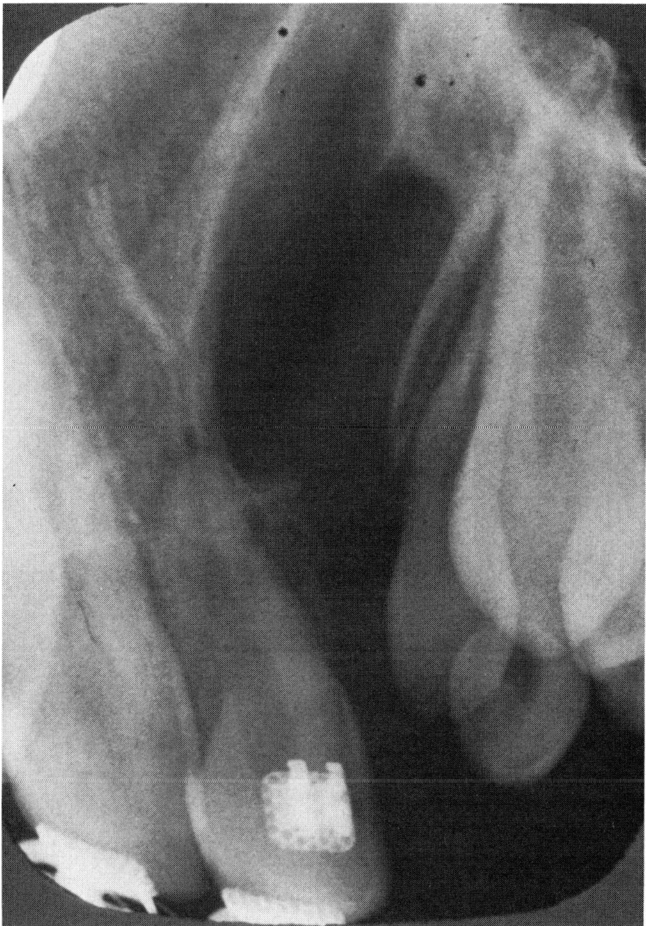

Figure 66–5 Periapical radiograph of a 9-year-old boy with a complete unilateral cleft of the left lip and alveolus.

risk-benefit and efficacy of treatment, may make this the preferred method of obtaining bone for future alveolar bone grafting.

Rationale of Bone Grafting

Clefts of the lip are usually repaired during the first 3 to 6 months after birth, and clefts of the palate are often repaired at 1 to 2 years of age. Early closure of the lip results in establishment of continuity of the perioral musculature, which benefits the infant from both facial aesthetic and functional points of view. Continuity of a functioning soft palate is an important prerequisite for the development of speech. Repair of the palate may be a one- or two-stage procedure and may be performed with or without the provision of an obturator. Continuity of the soft tissues is obtained, but bony defects in the alveolus and hard palate remain. Primary bone grafting in conjunction with primary cleft repair was popular during the 1950s, but long-term evaluation of results indicated that this technique interfered with the normal growth and development of the maxilla.[12–14] This finding resulted in primary alveolar bone grafting being abandoned in children under 2 years of age by many cleft teams and craniofacial centers.

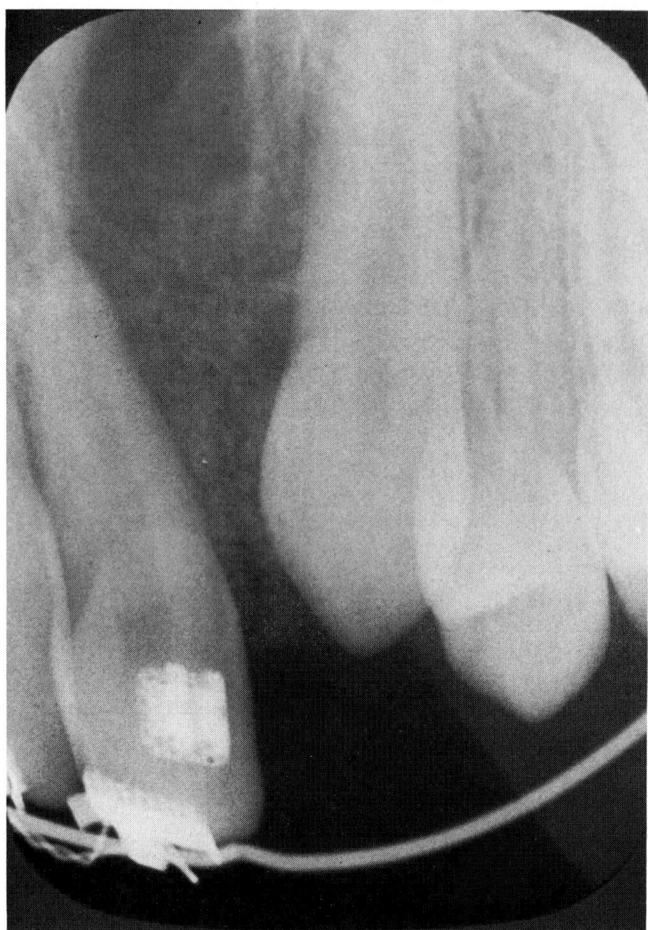

Figure 66–6 Periapical radiograph 6 months after an allogeneic bone graft was placed and the maxillary left lateral incisor extracted. Note eruption of the permanent canine through the freeze-dried bone.

Contemporary repair of the residual alveolar and hard palate cleft supports the concept of secondary bone grafting described by Boyne and Sands.[4]

Primary Bone Grafting

Controversy still exists about primary versus secondary bone grafting of the cleft maxilla and palate. Rosenstein et al[15] have refuted studies that indicate that primary bone grafting has an unfavorable effect on subsequent maxillary growth. Their results indicate that no interference with growth of the maxilla occurs when closure of the hard palate is achieved with rib grafts at the time of primary lip closure provided that there is minimal reflection of the soft tissues, presumably to reduce the amount of scarring. The long-term results indicate an improved arch form with eruption of the permanent dentition into the graft site with bony bridging.

Secondary Bone Grafting

The rationale for secondary bone grafting has focused on the currently accepted view that maxillary growth in the sagittal and transverse dimensions is virtually com-

plete by 9 to 11 years of age, which is considered the optimal age for secondary bone grafting.[16, 17] Additionally, this timing coincides chronologically with the eruption of the permanent cuspids. The placing of an alveolar bone graft provides bone into which the cuspid can erupt and, with the lateral incisor, be moved by orthodontic appliances into the cleft site. In patients with bilateral clefts, the placing of bone grafts stabilizes the premaxilla and promotes eruption of the permanent canines into the dental arch.

Clinical Studies

Indications for alveolar bone grafting include closure of persistent oronasal fistulas, bone support for unerupted and erupted teeth adjacent to the cleft, stabilization of the premaxillary segment in bilateral cases, continuity of the alveolar ridge, and support of the alar base and nasolabial contour. The optimal age recommended for alveolar bone grafts is currently 9 to 11 years of age.[16–18] The rationale for the timing and management of autologous alveolar bone grafts is well documented.[17, 19, 20] Because a reasonable goal of cleft palate rehabilitation

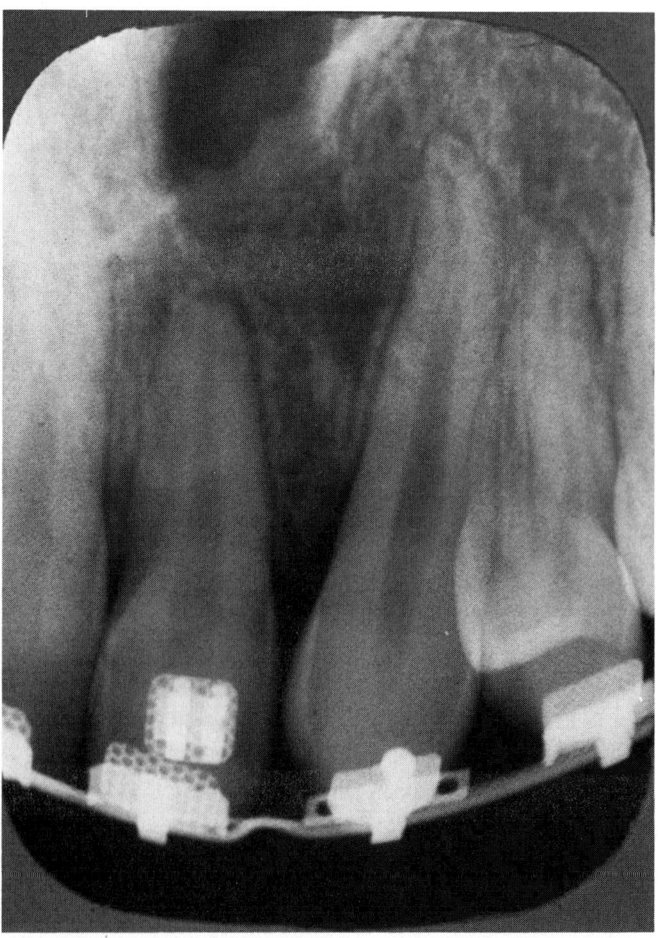

Figure 66–7 Periapical radiograph 3 years after surgery. The maxillary left canine is uprighting itself adjacent to the central incisor. Note the bony bridging and satisfactory height of crestal bone between the canine and the incisor.

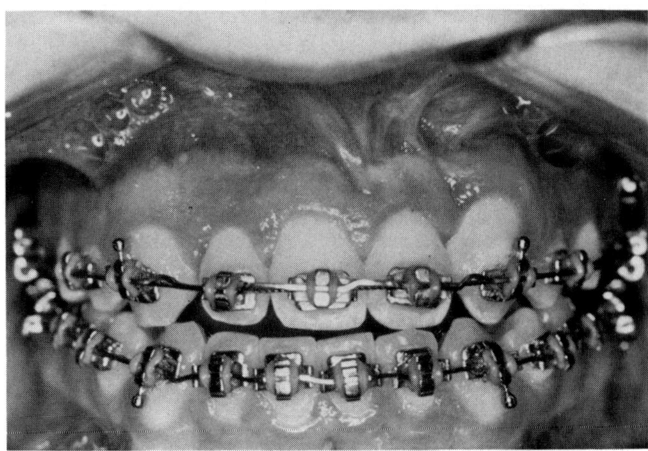

Figure 66–8 Intraoral photograph of the erupted canine with closure of the oronasal fistula. A satisfactory periodontal condition existed, although oral hygiene was poor.

is to eliminate the need for prosthetic replacement of missing teeth, early bone grafting may occasionally be recommended prior to eruption of the incisor adjacent to the cleft. If these teeth are allowed to erupt when there is inadequate bone in the cleft site, they may become periodontally compromised.

With the advent of freeze-dried bone and the use of allogeneic bone in grafting the alveolus, the presence of sequestra during the first 3 months after surgery is to be expected. The biologic response differs between allogeneic bone and autologous bone; therefore it is prudent for the orthodontist to delay moving adjacent teeth into the allogeneic grafted cleft for at least 3 months after surgery.

Autogenous Bone Grafts

Retrospective clinical studies[21, 22] indicate that autogenous bone is clearly the more successful grafting material. The morbidity associated with harvesting cancellous bone from the iliac crest has resulted in the calvarium's becoming an alternative donor site. Caddy and Reid[23] have described a technique by which particulate bone can be obtained using a trephine biopsy method. An interdisciplinary study by Turvey et al[16] reported that patients with both unilateral and bilateral cleft benefited from autogenous alveolar bone grafts. Clinically significant improvements were evaluated by an orthodontist, a periodontist, a prosthodontist, and an oral and maxillofacial surgeon. A long-term comprehensive clinical study by Bergland et al[17] indicates the benefits of secondary bone grafting and subsequent orthodontic treatment. Both these studies used iliac crest donor sites.

Allogeneic Bone Grafts

The morbidity associated with a second operative site needed to provide donor bone for the cleft graft has been a concern of some surgeons. The utilization of allogeneic freeze-dried bone for alveolar bone grafting

as an alternative to autogenous bone was suggested by Backdahl et al.[24] However, satisfactory results were reported in only 40% of cases, whereas the success rate was 100% with autogenous bone grafts, resulting in a reversion to autogenous bone grafts. When Marx et al[25] compared particulate allogeneic and autogenous bone grafts in 22 mongrel dogs, credibility and interest in allogeneic bone for cleft grafting were revived. This study was followed by a study in humans performed by Nique et al,[11] who used particulate allogeneic bone grafting in unilateral cleft palate patients. Although this was a preliminary study in which the patients were not followed for a sufficient period of time to evaluate whether the unerupted canine would erupt through the allogeneic material, a subsequent evaluation by Vig and Fonseca[26] that included some of these former patients indicated that eruption would occur through allogeneic grafts (Figs. 66–5 to 66–8).

The use of banked bone in oral and maxillofacial surgery is not common, although favorable results have been reported in the orthopedic and neurosurgical literature. In a clinical study, Allard et al[27] compared autografts with allografts in patients with unilateral alveolar clefts. They found no difference in clinical behavior between autologous and allogeneic bone grafts.

Surgical Aspects

The technique of alveolar bone grafting in both unilateral and bilateral clefts is described in the literature and is performed under general anesthesia with either oral or nasal endotracheal intubation.[4, 21] The presence of a pharyngeal flap may require an oral anode tube.

Recipient Site Surgery

The preparation of the cleft site to receive either an autologous or allogeneic graft follows the same basic principles. These include careful examination and subsequent closure of the area in which an oronasal fistula has been present to avoid inclusion of an epithelial-lined tract. The nasal soft tissue is repositioned superiorly to form the floor of the nose, and the bone graft is packed into the prepared site. Closure is completed with a four-corner flap over the graft site and multiple simple interrupted sutures to approximate the remainder of the incision. Repair of bilateral alveolar cleft grafts follows a procedure similar to that used for unilateral clefts, both clefts being grafted in one stage. Repositioning of the premaxilla may also be performed if it is necessary. Allogeneic bone is not recommended for grafting in bilateral cases because the vascularity of the soft tissues is often compromised with scarring and dehiscence of bone spicules. This commonly occurs with allogeneic grafts and may increase the chances of infection, ultimately jeopardizing the stability of the premaxilla.

Alveolar bone grafting in both unilateral and bilateral clefts utilizes the four-corner advancement flap technique previously reported by Troxell et al,[21] which has the advantage of bringing the attached gingiva into the operative site. Although unerupted teeth will erupt through mucogingival tissue, it is preferable from a periodontal aspect to promote eruption of the permanent canine through attached gingiva. When the amount of advancement is greater than the available tissue, a finger-flap technique can be utilized for both unilateral and bilateral repair.[4] In this technique, a midline-pedicled horizontal flap is rotated into the area of the labial soft tissue defect to obtain closure. This soft tissue flap is sutured from the crest of the ridge to its base and can be rotated if necessary.

Donor Site Surgery

Iliac Crest. When the ilium is used as a donor source, cancellous bone is harvested through a 3-cm incision placed posterior and parallel to the anterior iliac crest. The incision stops 1 cm before the anterior tip of the spine to prevent injury to the lateral femoral cutaneous nerve. The dissection proceeds to the crest of the ilium, which is cartilaginous in children. Without stripping muscle, the cartilaginous cap is fractured with an osteotome and retracted medially. Through this opening, the cancellous bone is removed with a curette until adequate bone chips have been obtained for the alveolar graft. The pedicled cartilaginous cap is returned to its original position on the ilium and is held in place with several circumferential wire sutures anchored to the muscle and fascia. The wound is then closed in layers and is not drained.

Cranium. The parietal eminence is the usual donor site from which cancellous bone is obtained. A 6-cm long and 0.5-cm wide strip of the scalp is shaved downward from the midline just over the eminence. Drapes are stapled to the scalp, and a sterile adhesive dressing is placed over the surgical area. The incision site is infiltrated with a vasoconstrictor (2% Xylocaine with 1:100,000 epinephrine), and the incision is made through all scalp layers at once. Electrocautery is utilized for hemostasis, and the pericranium is elevated and retracted with the scalp flaps. A drill is then used to score through the outer cortex and several 1- × 4-cm pieces are outlined. The inferior edge of each piece of scored outer cortex is beveled to permit insertion of a spatula osteotome to allow the flexible blade to engage just below the outer cortex. The osteotome is malleted, and the operator observes the leading edge of the osteotome to ensure that it remains just beneath the cortex. The cortex also may be removed by utilizing a pneumatic saw placed in the cancellous bone and cutting just under the plate.

Once several plates have been removed, the cancellous bone may be harvested with curettes, osteotomes, or a pneumatic saw. Vascular channels are sometimes encountered, and hemostasis is achieved with bone wax. The bone plates are replaced and held in place by suturing the scalp layers over them. Drains are usually not placed, and the scalp is closed in two layers. Antibiotic ointment is coated over the wound, and a cellophane-covered dressing is sutured in place over the incision. The cancellous bone harvested from the cranium is more brittle than that harvested from the ilium, probably because of its greater cellular density. This may also explain the rapid revascularization that occurs with calvarial bone.

Orthodontic Aspects

The contemporary management of the alveolar cleft by bone grafting has provided the orthodontist with a continuity of bone in the cleft site into which teeth may erupt or be moved with orthodontic forces. Secondary bone grafting before the eruption of the permanent canine has the advantage of allowing the grafted site to respond to the erupting canine with sufficient alveolar bone to facilitate mesial migration of the canine into the cleft site with closure of the space and uprighting of the canine. The ability of the orthodontist to align teeth in the cleft site has been a significant advance in the management of the cleft maxilla during the past decade (Figs. 66–3 and 66–7).

Long-term studies by Bergland et al[17] have provided convincing evidence that secondary bone grafting followed by orthodontic movement of teeth into the grafted site is a predictable method of eliminating the residual alveolar cleft. The preferred bone in these studies was autologous cancellous iliac chips, and results from a longitudinal study evaluating the effect of secondary alveolar bone grafting on subsequent maxillary growth indicated no interference or disturbance in normal sagittal or vertical growth vectors. This finding is not surprising because the age of 9 to 11 years is optimal for bone grafting, and sagittal and transverse growth of the maxilla is virtually complete at this age.

The orthodontic implications of moving teeth into allogeneic bone is related to the biologic response of the recipient site. Because this type of graft is acellular and avascular, osteoinduction of the surrounding host tissue will have to occur if new bone is to become available for orthodontic tooth movements into the cleft site. Likewise, the eruption of the canine into the grafted area requires the formation of new bone. Although allogeneic bone grafts have been confined to repairs of unilateral clefts, there is growing clinical support for this type of graft material.

Experimental Studies in Bone Grafting

Bone is one of the most frequently transplanted tissues in the body, and tissue banks issue more units of bone than any other tissue.[28] The same genetic principles and immunologic rules governing transplanted bone in other body regions apply to transplanted bone in the oral cavity with the added risk of infection from the wide variety of resident bacteria. Contemporary knowledge of bone graft surgery has involved animal models such as the tibia in mice, maxillary osteotomies in monkeys, and a comparison of particulate allogeneic and autologous bone grafts into the cleft maxillas in dogs.[25]

The value of a bone graft in the oral cavity is the provision of a mechanical scaffold. The viability of the original cell population is unlikely to be a source from which the graft is revascularized or from which osteogenic cells are derived. The bone graft elicits an angiogenic response from the recipient site, and the proliferation and migration of endothelial cells and osteogenic cells are an integral part of the early stages of healing.

There is a difference in the biologic response to allogeneic and autologous bone grafts. An earlier angiogenic response is initiated by autologous bone during the first week after the graft is placed. Survival of some of the transplanted osteoblasts in the autologous graft promotes osteogenesis during the first couple of weeks. Allogeneic bone grafts are characterized by an initial hypervascular response with proliferation of the blood vessels occurring 7 to 14 days later. The invading vasculature is accompanied by osteogenic replacement of the avascular and acellular allogeneic bone graft by a process of osteoinduction at the recipient site, with new bone being laid down at the periphery. Autologous bone grafts have more intracortical bone replacement than allogeneic grafts, and replacement of the graft takes approximately 3 to 6 months in the autologous graft system. In the allogeneic graft system, the hypervascular response gradually disappears, and replacement of the graft is delayed 6 months to 1 year. Histologically, granulation tissue with fibroblastic and vascular response is followed by a proliferation of immature osteoid tissue at the graft periphery. The temporal sequence of this response is delayed in the allogeneic graft, and osteoid is replaced by mature bone with sequestration of spicules of the avascular, acellular freeze-dried bone.

Discussion

The advantage of bone grafting in the cleft maxilla is the provision of stability to the segments, especially the mobile premaxilla in the bilateral cleft patient. Bone in the alveolus eliminates the residual alveolar cleft and promotes eruption of the cuspid into a more favorable position. The subsequent orthodontic movement of teeth adjacent to the cleft is facilitated, and periodontal support of these teeth is improved. The preferred graft material is autologous bone, typically harvested from the ilium. However, many surgeons are avoiding the morbidity associated with the hip as the second surgical site and are obtaining bone from the calvarium. This donor site has gained popularity because it involves less postoperative pain and a shorter hospitalization. The morbidity associated with a second operative site can be avoided if allogeneic bone is substituted. This bone is sterilized and can be preserved to maintain its morphology and inductive properties while possessing minimal antigenicity.

The biologic basis for bony bridging and stabilization of the cleft is fundamental to an understanding of the clinical relevance of the different graft materials. The increased length of time needed for consolidation of allogeneic bone makes it unsuitable for bilateral clefts and also has important orthodontic implications. The movement of teeth into an allogeneic graft should be delayed for at least 3 months after surgery, whereas the orthodontist can confidently move adjacent teeth into an autologous graft a month after surgery.

Although autogenous bone is still considered the most ideal graft material, recent clinical reports and comparative studies in both animal models and humans suggest that allogeneic bone should be investigated as a competing alternative. In terms of morbidity and risk-benefit this graft material may be the preferred bone graft of the future.

Future Perspectives

In clinical fields in which empiricism prevails and criteria for success or failure are based on clinical judgment, the new science of clinimetrics may provide a more objective method for evaluating our treatment results.[29, 30] Decision analytic techniques applied to studies of the efficacy of alternative treatment methods provide the clinician with a method of evaluating the outcomes of treatment quantitatively.[31] The decision to advocate either autogenous or allogeneic bone grafts should be based on clinical judgment quantified in objective terms. Clinicians in the future will need to decide, at least to some extent, the cost-benefit and risk-benefit terms of available options. A second surgical site with its accompanying morbidity is a risk factor in the use of autologous grafts. Only an evaluation of the benefits of the competing graft alternatives can decisively influence the comparison of autologous and allogeneic grafts for the cleft patient.

The need to provide a sound biologic basis for clinical decisions requires the use of appropriate animal models to test questions that cannot be addressed by clinical trials in humans. Animal models are morphologic rather than etiologic to the human situation. This is an inherent limitation of animal studies and must be borne in mind both in terms of the rationale for the experiments and for the inferences that can realistically be made to clinical situations. Bone biology is a rapidly progressing field and at the molecular level technical expertise is required to answer many of the fundamental and clinically pertinent questions it raises. Maintenance of a bridge between the clinician and the basic scientist is essential when much of the fundamental research is laboratory based; otherwise the clinical applications may be jeopardized through a failure of communication between scientist and clinician.

References

1. Lexer E: Die Verwendung der freien Knochenplastik nebst Versuchon über Gelenkverstifung un Gelenktransplantation. Langenbecks Arch Klin Chir 86:939, 1908.
2. Drachter R: Die Gaumenspalte und deren Operative. Behandlung Dtsch Chir 131:1, 1914.
3. Axhausen W: The osteogenic phases of regeneration of bone. J Bone Joint Surg 38:593, 1956.
4. Boyne PJ, Sands NR: Secondary bone grafting of residual alveolar and palatal clefts. J Oral Surg 30:87, 1972.

5. Konig F: Der Knocherne ersatz grosser Shadeldefelente. Zentralbe Chir 17:467, 1890.
6. Muller W: Zur Frage der temporarey Schadelreselstion an Stelle der Trepanation. Zentralbe Chir 17:65, 1890.
7. Smith ID, Abramson M: Membranous versus endochondral bone autografts. Arch Otolaryngol 99:203, 1974.
8. Zins JE, Whitaker LA: Membranous versus endochondral bone autografts: Implications for craniofacial reconstruction. Plast Reconstr Surg 72:778, 1983.
9. Tessier P: Autogenous bone grafts taken from the calvarium for facial and craniofacial applications. Clin Plast Surg 9:531, 1982.
10. Wolfe SA, Berkowitz S: The use of cranial bone grafts in the closure of alveolar and anterior palatal clefts. Plast Reconstr Surg 72:659, 1983.
11. Nique T, Fonseca RJ, Upton LG, et al: Particulate allogenic bone grafts into maxillary alveolar clefts in humans: A preliminary report. J Oral Maxillofac Surg 45:386, 1987.
12. Freide H, Johanson B: A follow-up study of cleft children treated with primary bone grafting. Scand J Plast Reconstr Surg 8:88, 1974.
13. Freide H, Johanson B: Adolescent facial morphology of early bone-grafted cleft-lip and palate patients. Scand J Plast Reconstr Surg 16:41, 1982.
14. Jolleys A, Robertson NRE: A study of the effects of early bone grafting in complete clefts of the lip and palate—five year study. Br J Plast Surg 25:229, 1972.
15. Rosenstein SW, Monroe CW, Kernahan DA, et al: The case for early bone grafting in cleft lip and cleft palate. Plast Reconstr Surg 70:297, 1982.
16. Turvey AT, Vig K, Moriarty J, et al: Delayed bone grafting in the cleft maxilla and palate: A retrospective multidisciplinary analysis. Am J Orthod 86:244, 1984.
17. Bergland O, Semb G, Abyholm FE: Elimination of the residual alveolar cleft by secondary bone grafting and subsequent orthodontic treatment. Cleft Palate J 23:175, 1986.
18. Waite E, Kersten RB: Residual alveolar and palatal clefts. In Bell WH, Proffit WR, White RP (eds): Surgical Correction of Dentofacial Deformities. Philadelphia: WB Saunders, 1980.
19. Boyne PJ, Sands NR: Combined orthodontic-surgical management of residual palato-alveolar cleft defects. Am J Orthod 70:21, 1976.
20. Vig KWL, Turvey TA: Orthodontic–surgical interaction in the management of cleft lip and palate. Clin Plastic Surg 12:735, 1985.
21. Troxell JB, Fonseca RJ, Osbon B: A retrospective study of alveolar cleft grafting. J Oral Maxillofac Surg 40:721, 1982.
22. Witsenburg B: The reconstruction of anterior residual bone defects in patients with cleft lip, alveolus and palate. J Maxillofac Surg 13:1977, 1985.
23. Caddy CM, Reid CD: An atraumatic technique for harvesting cancellous bone for secondary alveolar bone grafting in cleft palate. Br J Plast Surg 38:540, 1985.
24. Backdahl M, Nordin K, Nylen B, et al: Transactions of the International Society of Plastic Surgeons, 3rd Congress. Amsterdam: Excerpta Medica, 1963, p 252.
25. Marx RE, Miller RI, Ehler WJ, et al: A comparison of particulate allogenic and particulate autogenous bone grafts into maxillary alveolar clefts in dogs. J Oral Maxillofac Surg 42:3, 1984.
26. Vig KWL, Fonseca RJ: Allogeneic versus autogenous bone grafts in the cleft maxilla (Abstract). Oxford: Craniofacial Society of Great Britain, 1988.
27. Allard RH, Lekkas C, Swart JG: Autologous versus homologous bone grafting in osteotomies, secondary cleft repairs and ridge augmentations: A clinical study. Oral Surg Oral Med Oral Pathol 64:269, 1987.
28. Feinberg SE, Fonseca RJ: Biological aspects of transplantation of grafts. In Fonseca RJ, Davis WH (eds): Reconstructive Preprosthetic Oral and Maxillofacial Surgery. Philadelphia: WB Saunders, 1986.
29. Feinstein AR: What kind of basic science for clinical medicine? N Engl J Med 283:847, 1970.
30. Feinstein AR: The clinician as scientist. In Vig PS, Ribbens KA: Science and Clinical Judgment in Orthodontics. Monograph 19, Craniofacial Growth Series, Center for Human Growth and Development. Ann Arbor: University of Michigan, 1986.
31. Weinstein MC, Fineberg HB: Clinical Decision Analysis. Philadelphia: WB Saunders, 1980.

CHAPTER 67

Influence of Alveolar Bone Grafting on Facial Growth

Gunvor Semb and William Shaw

When cancellous bone grafting from the iliac crest was introduced in Oslo in 1977, it was soon apparent that dental rehabilitation of the great majority of patients with alveolar clefts could be reliably completed without bridgework (Fig. 67–1). The results and experiences of the first 378 consecutive patients have been presented in detail elsewhere (see Chap. 4).[1, 2]

The substantial and immediate clinical benefits of mixed dentition bone grafting made its inclusion in the program at Oslo routine, and it was offered to every patient in whom the presence of any degree of alveolar clefting precluded full orthodontic alignment of the maxillary dentition. However, just as primary bone grafting was once hailed as an important breakthrough, only to fall later into disrepute because of its deleterious effects on facial growth, it was clear that the long-term effect of mixed dentition bone grafting also should be critically evaluated.[3–5]

Enemark et al presented a follow-up of mixed dentition grafting and reported no impairment of growth in the anteroposterior dimension but a reduction in upper facial height (on linear but not angular measurements).[6] Ross analyzed 28 patients from three different centers who had had grafting performed between 4 and 11 years of age (including 16 boys with unilateral cleft lip and palate from Oslo in whom grafting was done between 9 and 10.9 years) and concluded that "bone grafting in the late mixed dentition adversely affects the vertical dimensions of the anterior maxilla and indirectly the lower face."[7] However, no control material was included. No adverse effects on anteroposterior development following bone grafting at 9 years of age or later were reported. Thus, the purpose of the present report is to make a detailed evaluation of facial growth in patients in whom grafting has been done who have reached 16 years of age.

Materials and Methods

The material for this report is drawn from the records of consecutive cleft lip and palate patients who have had all surgery performed at the Department of Plastic Surgery, University Hospital, Oslo and have had regular follow-up examinations by the Oslo Cleft Palate Team.

Figure 67–2 presents the sequence of primary surgical management in Oslo. This sequence has been relatively consistent since 1953 with only minor modifications (see Chap. 4). The bone grafting procedure (cancellous bone from the iliac crest) and the subsequent orthodontic treatment have been described in detail elsewhere.[1, 2, 8–10]

Bone grafts were initially performed on patients rang-

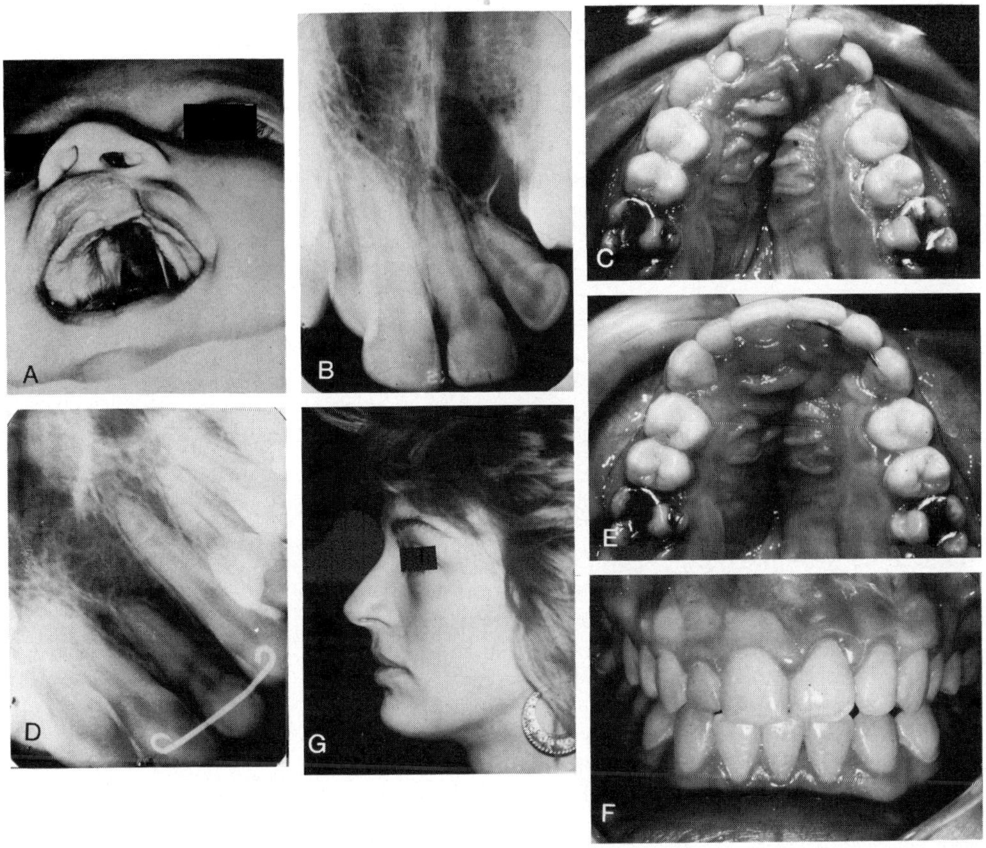

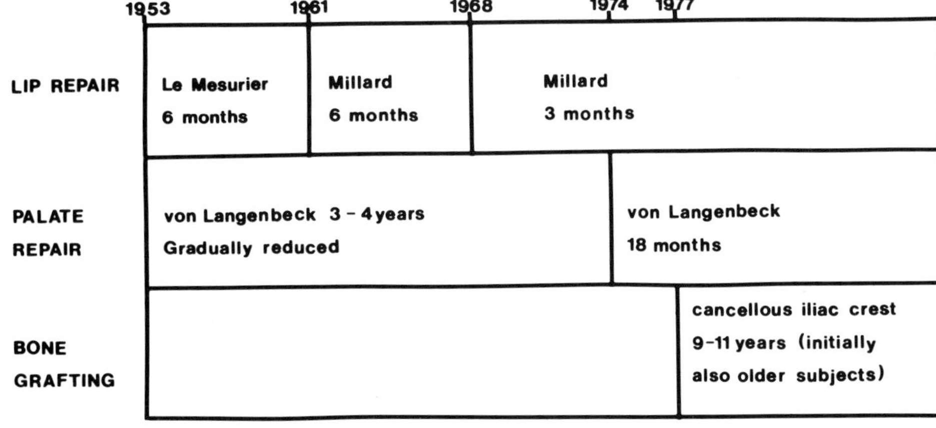

Figure 67–1 *A*, Girl with complete unilateral cleft of the maxilla. *B*, Radiograph of cleft region prior to bone grafting at 11½ years. *C*, Maxillary arch prior to bone grafting. *D*, Radiograph 10 years postoperatively. *E* and *F*, Maxillary arch and occlusion 10 years postoperatively and 6 years after completion of orthodontic treatment. *G*, Profile at age 21.

ing in age from 8 to 18 years. The lower age limit of 8 years was set to avoid interference with subsequent growth, and the upper age limit of 18 years was set because it was not considered economically justifiable to remove a recently inserted bridge to perform bone grafting.

Sample and Records for the Present Study

The present investigation was confined to 70 patients with grafts (49 males, 21 females) born with a complete unilateral cleft of the lip and palate, including those with a soft tissue (but not bony) bridge (Simonart's band) across the cleft (ten males and seven females had a soft tissue bridge). Every patient in this group received a bone graft *between 8 and 15 years of age* and had pregraft and 16-year (±0.75 year) cephalometric records available. Within this group, a subsample of 28 patients who had received a graft by *age 12* was defined (17 males, 11 females; 3 males and 4 females had a soft tissue bridge).

For a control group, reference was made to 30 patients born between 1954 and 1963 because they were considered too old for grafting when the procedure was introduced (24 males, 6 females, 4 males, and 1 female had a soft tissue bridge). Cephalometric records were made in each at 9 years (±0.75 year) and 16 years (±0.75 year).

Figure 67–2 The timetable of surgical management in Oslo since 1954. Bone grafting was introduced in 1977 when rehabilitation in many documented cases was already complete.

	1953	1961	1968	1974 1977
LIP REPAIR	Le Mesurier 6 months	Millard 6 months	Millard 3 months	
PALATE REPAIR	von Langenbeck 3 – 4 years Gradually reduced			von Langenbeck 18 months
BONE GRAFTING				cancellous iliac crest 9–11 years (initially also older subjects)

Cephalometry

The reference points and planes are shown in Figure 67–3. The definition of the landmarks is in accordance with that of Bjork.[11] In addition, ss' point was used, defined as the projection of ss on the NL line. The craniofacial dimensions were computed from lateral skull radiographs obtained under standardized conditions. The measurements were registered twice during the same sitting, and average values were calculated. All digitizing was performed by the same individual (G.S.).

Statistical Analysis

Comparison of mean changes between 9 (± 0.75) and 16 (± 0.75) years in the grafted and control groups using the Student t-test was performed (Table 67–1). This comparison was confined to the subsample of 28 who received their grafts at between 8 and 12 years (all initial films were pregraft).

Stepwise multiple regression also was performed on these groups, taking the cephalometric values at 16 years of age as the dependent variables, and the corresponding cephalometric values at 9 years (always presurgical in the grafted group), sex, presence or absence of a soft tissue bridge, primary surgical management period (as represented by date of birth [Fig. 67–1]), and presence or absence of a bone graft as the independent (predictor) variables. Cephalometric values at 9 years of age were included as a measure of developing facial form independent of later surgical intervention; sex and soft tissue bridging were included to take account of their influence on facial growth,[12] and primary surgical management period (date of birth) was included to allow an appraisal of possible systematic effects over time related to primary surgery.

Various statistics are computed in stepwise multiple

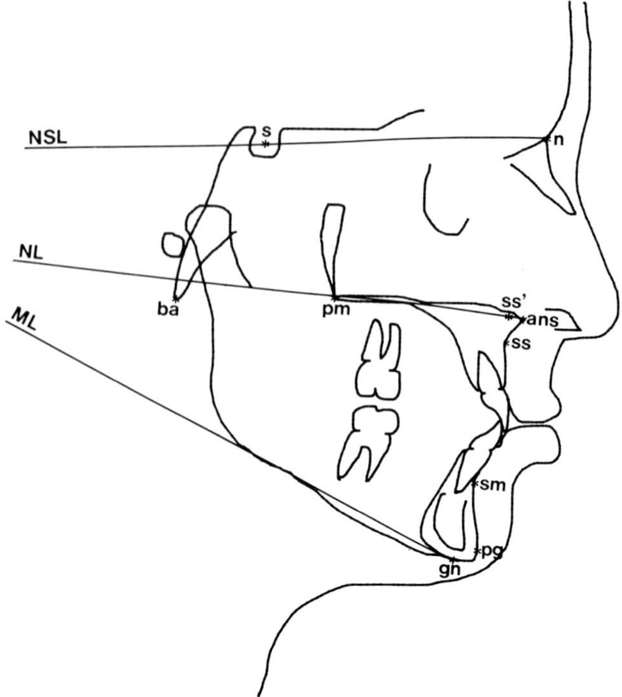

Figure 67–3 Reference points and planes. Cephalometric landmarks and planes. s, sella; n, nasion; ba, basion; pm, pterygomaxillare; ans, anterior nasal spine, ss, subspinale (A point); ss', intercept of ss perpendicular on nasal line; sm, submandibular (B point); pg, pogonion; gn, gnathion; NSL, nasion–sella line; NL, nasal line; ML, mandibular line.

regression analysis, and a summary of the output for each parameter is listed in Table 67–2. The coefficients labeled B are called partial regression coefficients because they are adjusted for other independent variables in the equation; significance levels are listed. The ex-

Table 67–1. Comparisons of Cephalometric Values at 9 Years, 16 Years, and for Changes Between 9 and 16 in Nongraft Versus Grafted Groups

	Comparison of Means at 9 Years					Comparison of Means at 16 Years					Comparison of Mean Change Between 9 and 16 Years				
	Nongraft N = 30 9 ± 0.75 year		*Grafted N = 28 9 ± 0.75 year*			*Nongraft N = 30 16 ± 0.75 year*		*Grafted N = 28 16 ± 0.75 year*			*Nongraft*		*Grafted*		
	x	*SD*	*x*	*SD*	Significance*	*x*	*SD*	*x*	*SD*	Significance*	*x*	*SD*	*x*	*SD*	Significance*
Anteroposterior relationships															
s–n–ss	76.6	3.9	74.6	3.7	NS	74.5	4.1	72.9	3.8	NS	−2.1	1.5	−1.7	1.8	NS
s–n–pg	74.9	3.3	74.5	3.4	NS	77.0	3.7	76.3	3.9	NS	2.1	1.9	1.8	2.4	NS
ss–n–sm	2.7	3.0	1.2	3.3	NS	−0.6	3.0	−1.4	2.9	NS	−3.3	1.7	−2.6	2.2	NS
n–ss–pg	176.6	6.7	179.8	7.6	NS	185.2	7.0	186.9	8.0	NS	8.6	3.8	7.1	4.8	NS
ss'–pm	44.3	2.7	43.9	2.7	NS	46.3	3.2	44.9	2.9	NS	2.0	1.9	1.0	1.7	NS
Vertical relationships															
NSL–NL	10.3	3.7	9.3	3.4	NS	9.5	3.5	8.1	3.9	NS	−0.8	2.3	−1.1	2.5	NS
NSL–ML	37.7	4.9	37.1	4.6	NS	35.5	4.8	36.3	5.9	NS	−2.3	3.2	−0.8	3.4	NS
NL–ML	27.4	6.2	27.8	4.8	NS	25.9	5.6	28.2	5.8	NS	−1.6	4.1	0.4	3.7	p < 0.05
n–ss'	45.9	2.6	45.8	3.6	NS	53.1	3.0	52.1	3.9	NS	7.2	1.6	6.4	2.1	NS
ss'–gn	63.0	3.6	62.1	4.3	NS	72.0	4.0	72.4	6.0	NS	9.0	3.5	10.3	2.9	p < 0.05
Cranial base angulation															
n–s–ba	131.7	4.1	132.9	4.1	NS	131.1	4.9	132.3	4.9	NS	−0.6	2.2	−0.6	2.1	NS

*NS = not significant.

Table 67–2. Selected Statistics from Stepwise Multiple Regression Including Presence or Absence of a Bone Graft (N = 58)

Dependent Variables at 16 Years	Independent Variables (Significant Partial Regression Coefficients)			Explanatory Value (R^2 change as %)
	Variable	*Partial Regression Coefficient (B)*	*Significance*	
Anteroposterior relationships				
s–n–ss	s–n–ss at 9	0.96	<0.001	84
s–n–pg	s–n–pg at 9	0.93	<0.001	68
ss–n–sm	ss–n–sm at 9	0.73	<0.001	65
n–ss–pg	n–ss–pg at 9	0.85	<0.001	69
ss'–pm	ss'–pm at 9	0.91	<0.001	65
Vertical relationships				
NSL–NL	NSL–NL at 9	0.81	<0.001	63
NSL–ML	NSL–ML at 9	0.88	<0.001	62
	Sex	−2.04	<0.05	2
NL–ML	NL–ML at 9	0.77	<0.001	58
	Sex	−2.31	<0.05	3
n–ss'	n–ss' at 9	0.89	<0.001	71
	Sex	−1.97	<0.001	6
	Date of birth	−0.39	<0.01	1
	Bone grafting	2.81	<0.05	1
ss'–gn	ss'–gn at 9	0.97	<0.001	66
	Sex	−3.05	<0.001	6
Cranial base angulation				
n–s–ba	n–s–ba at 9	1.00	<0.001	81

planatory value (R^2 change) gives an indication of the relative importance of each individual independent value. Thus in Table 67–2 the relative values of measurements at points s–n–ss at 9 years of age are seen to be good predictors of values measured at s–n–ss at 16 years, and 84% (R^2 = 0.84) of the observed variability at 16 years is explained by the corresponding value at 9 years.

A further stepwise multiple regression analysis was performed on the 16 (±0.75)-year cephalometric values of the larger group of 70 subjects, *all of whom* had received a bone graft between the ages of 8 and 15 years. This regression model tested the hypothesis that *if* bone grafting were harmful, subjects receiving the graft *early* should demonstrate greater maxillary growth impairment. The same independent variables were included, but interest in bone grafting was focused on the child's age at grafting.

Results

The t-test did not reveal any statistically significant differences at the 5% level between the control and the grafted group, either at 9 or at 16 years of age (Table 67–2). The extent of change in cephalometric values between 9 and 16 years was similar in both the grafted and nongrafted groups. Only two parameters, NL–ML (lower face angulation) and ss'–gn (lower face height), showed statistically significant differences at the 5% level, the grafted group showing a tendency toward a slightly greater increase in lower facial height.

In the first regression model (Table 67–2) the strong predictive value of the 9-year-old craniofacial dimensions was revealed. For example, at age 16, 84% of the variability in maxillary protrusion (s–n–ss) and 65% of the variability in maxillary length (ss'–pm) was explained by the corresponding value at 9 years. For only one parameter, however, did the presence or absence of a bone graft emerge as a minor although significant predictor of facial form at 16 years. The presence of a bone graft was associated with a slightly greater increase in upper facial height (n–ss'), explaining an additional 1% of this parameter's variation at 16 years of age.

A number of sex differences between 9 and 16 years emerged. Sex explained an additional 6% of the variation in both upper and lower facial height (n–ss', ss'–gn) and accounted for somewhat less variation in upper and lower facial angulation (NSL–NL, NL–ML), these values being larger in males. The cranial base angle (n–s–ba) was smaller in males, and there was a tendency for a smaller upper facial height (n–ss') in patients with more recent birth dates.

In the second regression model (Table 67–3), the dimensions recorded in the preoperative radiograph again proved to be the most accurate predictors of facial form at 16 years of age. For example, the preoperative values of s–n–ss accounted for 78% of the variability in this dimension at 16 years. The variable of interest here, age at which grafting was performed, emerged only twice as a minor though statistically significant partial regression coefficient. For maxillary protrusion (s–n–ss) there was an inverse correlation with age at grafting— that is, there was a tendency toward greater protrusion with earlier grafting. There was also a tendency for a minor increase in cranial base angulation (n–s–ba) with later grafting.

For several parameters, sex and the primary surgical management period (birth date) again emerged as minor significant predictors of facial form at 16 years of age, with a tendency toward smaller values for maxillary length, upper and lower facial height, and more obtuse

Table 67–3. Selected Statistics from Stepwise Multiple Regression, Including Age at Bone Grafting (N = 70)

| Dependent Variables at 16 Years | Independent Variables (Significant Partial Regression Coefficients) | | | Explanatory Value (R^2 change as %) |
	Variable	Partial Regression Coefficient (B)	Significance	
Anteroposterior relationships				
s–n–ss	Preoperative s–n–ss	0.89	<0.001	78
	Date of birth	−0.64	<0.01	1
	Age at grafting	−0.56	<0.05	1
s–n–pg	Preoperative s–n–pg	0.95	<0.001	70
ss–n–sm	Preoperative ss–n–sm	0.83	<0.001	70
n–ss–pg	Preoperative n–ss–pg	0.88	<0.001	69
ss′–pm	Preoperative ss′–pm	1.01	<0.001	71
	Sex	−1.01	<0.05	2
	Soft tissue bridge	1.01	<0.05	1
Vertical relationships				
NSL–NL	Preoperative NSL–NL	0.80	<0.001	59
NSL–ML	Preoperative NSL–ML	0.98	<0.001	68
NL–ML	Preoperative NL–ML	0.88	<0.001	67
n–ss′	Preoperative n–ss′	0.79	<0.001	50
	Sex	−2.56	<0.001	12
ss′–gn	Preoperative ss′–gn	0.92	<0.001	66
	Sex	−4.31	<0.001	11
Cranial base angulation				
n–s–ba	Preoperative n–s–ba	0.93	<0.001	84
	Sex	1.44	<0.01	1

cranial base angulation in females. Later primary surgical management dates were associated with reduced maxillary protrusion and more obtuse cranial base angulation. Finally, the presence of a soft tissue bridge was positively correlated with maxillary length.

Discussion

The principal finding is the lack of evidence of any anteroposterior or vertical maxillary growth disturbance in grafted subjects. On the contrary, bone grafting was associated with increased upper facial height and, when performed early, with slightly greater maxillary protrusion (Tables 67–2 and 67–3). The suggestion of increased lower facial height associated with grafting from the direct comparison of mean change (Table 67–1) was not confirmed by regression analysis, indicating that this trend occurred independent of bone grafting.

After the corresponding values at 9 years have been considered, it should be noted that inclusion of the bone graft variables adds little to the prediction of the craniofacial dimensions at 16 years of age (approximate explanatory value of 1%). Thus, there is no evidence that bone grafting alters the individual's pattern of facial growth established by 9 years of age to any clinically significant extent, either favorably or unfavorably.

Clinical Implications

It has long been generally accepted that reconstructive cleft surgery can inhibit maxillary growth.[13, 14] Major controversies under discussion involve the optimal timing for surgery and techniques that minimize these growth disturbances. By exposing children with clefts to the additional surgical procedure of mixed dentition bone grafting, the risk of further interference with growth cannot be disregarded, and the apparent safety of the procedure applied to this sample may reflect certain specific details:

Age at Grafting. The principal mode of growth of the maxilla has been discussed elsewhere.[1, 2, 8] The available evidence from noncleft subjects indicates that growth in width and length of the anterior maxilla has almost ceased by 8 years of age and should not be subject to interference by surgery performed after this age.[15–18]

In addition to the downward and forward translation of the maxilla that characterizes midfacial growth, accretion of bone on the occlusal aspects of the alveolar process makes a substantial contribution to the increase in upper facial height. It is therefore essential that the bone graft can accommodate the eruption of teeth through the transplanted area and also participate in subsequent growth. Nine years' clinical experience indicates that the vertical development of the alveolar process does continue undisturbed following the insertion of a bone graft. The quality of the result is certainly improved when grafting is carried out prior to the eruption of the permanent maxillary canine.

Flap Design. The management of mucoperiosteal flaps, especially in the palate, is also regarded as a significant factor in maxillary growth inhibition.[19] The palatal mucoperiosteal flaps raised during bone grafting in Oslo are small compared to those raised with other techniques;[20, 21] they are not displaced, and bone is not denuded on the palatal aspect. On the buccal side, the lateral mucoperiosteal flap is advanced to cover the cleft and sutured to the smaller medial flap. Thus, only a small area of denuded bone buccal to the second deciduous molar may occasionally be left for secondary epithelialization, and it seems unlikely that this could have any inhibiting effect on subsequent growth.

Conclusion

The present study suggests that maxillary growth is not affected by placement of a cancellous alveolar bone graft after 8 years of age. These findings confirm the clinical experience gained from a relatively large number of cleft individuals with grafts whose orthodontic treatment is now complete.

References

1. Bergland O, Semb G, Abyholm FE: Elimination of the residual alveolar cleft by secondary bone grafting and subsequent orthodontic treatment. Cleft Palate J 23:175, 1986.
2. Bergland O, Semb G, Abyholm F, et al: Secondary bone grafting and orthodontic treatment in patients with bilateral complete clefts of the lip and palate. Ann Plast Surg 17:460, 1986.
3. Rehrmann AH, Koberg WR, Koch H: Long-term postoperative results after primary and secondary bone grafting in complete clefts of lip and palate. Cleft Palate J 7:206, 1970.
4. Rehrmann AH: The effect of early bone grafting on the growth of upper jaw in cleft lip and palate children. A computer evaluation. Minerva Chir 26:874, 1971.
5. Friede H, Johanson B: A follow-up study of cleft children treated with primary bone grafting I. Orthodontic aspects. Scand J Plast Reconstr Surg 8:88, 1974.
6. Enemark H, Sindet-Pederson S, Bundgaard M: Long-term results after secondary bone grafting of alveolar clefts. J Oral Maxillofac Surg 45:913, 1987.
7. Ross RB: Treatment variables affecting facial growth in complete unilateral cleft lip and palate. Part 3: Alveolus repair and bone grafting. Cleft Palate J 24:33, 1987.
8. Abyholm FE, Bergland O, Semb G: Secondary bone grafting of alveolar clefts. Scand J Plast Reconstr Surg 15:127, 1981.
9. Abyholm FE, Borchgrevink HC, Eskeland G: Cleft lip and palate in Norway. III. Surgical treatment of CLP patients in Oslo 1954–1975. Scand J Plast Reconstr Surg 15:15, 1981.
10. Eskeland G, Bergland O, Borchgrevink H, et al: Management of the cleft alveolar arch. In Jackson JT, Sommerland BC (eds): Recent Advances in Plastic Surgery. No. 3. London: Churchill Livingstone, 1985.
11. Bjork A: Kaebernes relation til det ovrige kranium. In Lundstrom A (ed): Nordisk Larobok i Orthodonti. 4 uppl. Stockholm: Sveriges Tandlakarforbunds Forlagsforening, 1975.
12. Semb G, Bergland O, Shaw WC: The effect of a soft tissue bridge (Simonart's band) on facial growth in complete unilateral clefts. Paper presented to the European Association of Cranio-Maxillo-Facial Surgery, Bremen, 1987.
13. Graber TM: A cephalometric analysis of the development pattern and facial morphology in cleft palate. Angle Orthod 19:91, 1949.
14. Slaughter WB, Brodie AG: Facial clefts and their management in view of recent research. Plast Reconstr Surg 4:203, 1949.
15. Sillman MA: Dimensional changes of the dental arches: Longitudinal study from birth to 25 years. Am J Orthod 50:824, 1964.
16. Bjork A, Skieller V: Growth in width of the maxilla studied by the implant method. Scand J Plast Reconstr Surg 8:26, 1974.
17. Bjork A, Skieller V: Postnatal growth and development of the maxillary complex. In McNamara JA, Jr (ed): Factors Affecting the Growth of the Midface. Ann Arbor: The University of Michigan, Center for Human Growth and Development, 1976.
18. Bjork A, Skieller V: Growth of the maxilla in three dimensions as revealed radiographically by the implant method. Br J Orthod 4:53, 1977.
19. Kremenak CR: Physiological aspects of wound healing: Contraction and growth. Otolaryngol Clin North Am 17:437, 1984.
20. Boyne PJ, Sands NR: Secondary bone grafting of residual alveolar and palatal clefts. J Oral Surg 30:87, 1972.
21. Krantz-Simonsen E: Secondary bone grafting for repair of residual cleft defects in the alveolar process and hard palate. Int J Oral Maxillofac Surg 15:1, 1986.

CHAPTER 68

Twenty-Five Years of Experience with Primary Bone Grafting

Heinz Reichert and Karin Manzari

Operating on a young child born with a cleft lip, alveolus, and palate is certainly one of the most exciting and rewarding tasks for the plastic surgeon, but it also may present a long-term, complex treatment endeavor. Although the results of most surgical interventions can be judged after the first few months, patients with cleft lip, alveolus, and palate need follow-up observation for many years until they are fully grown. Only then can one really learn whether the timing of surgical procedures, surgical techniques, orthodontic treatment, and speech therapy have led to a satisfactory aesthetic and functional result.

Rationale for Primary Bone Grafting

Eduard Schmid introduced primary bone grafting into cleft surgery in the early 1950s.[1, 2] The idea soon spread all over the world because it seemed so logical that one should not only unite the soft components of lip, alveolus, and palate but, to prevent collapse of the maxillary segments, fill the bony defect with an autogenous bone graft (Fig. 68–1).

Many surgeons visited our department in Stuttgart in the 1950s to learn the new technique of primary bone grafting. In the following years, in many cleft centers, especially in Europe, primary bone grafting was introduced as a routine method of surgical treatment of clefts. The most startling finding following bone grafting was that teeth were erupting through this transplanted bone.

Our initial enthusiasm for primary bone grafting seemed to be justified by one of Schmid's first cases, a male infant with a wide bilateral cleft of the lip, alveolus, and palate. Bone grafting performed on this patient was helpful in moving the premaxilla in line with the lateral maxillary segments, preventing their collapse behind the premaxilla.

Application and Evaluation

We remained convinced that primary alveolar bone grafting is beneficial for growth and development of the maxilla. Therefore, we decided to widen the application of this technique and started to utilize bone grafting at the time of closure of the palatal defect.[3–5] This was done on the assumption that the bony structure in the hard palate would keep the soft palate in its pushed-back position. We also thought that at a later age, when dentures might be needed, they would be held better by suction on a hard palate in which the cleft defect was filled with new bone. Speech results and the shape

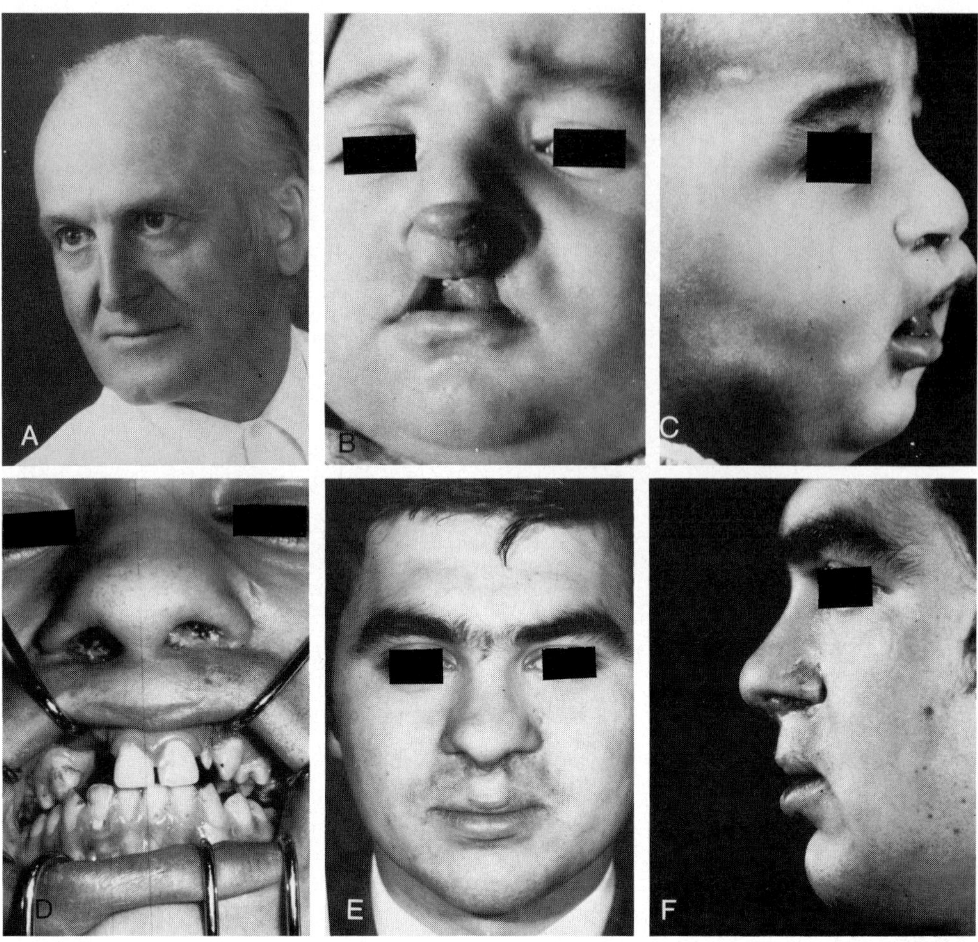

Figure 68–1 A, Eduard Schmid of Stuttgart introduced primary bone grafting into cleft surgery in the early 1950s.[1, 2] *B,* One of Schmid's first cases for primary bone grafting in whom the implant stabilized the protruding premaxilla. *C,* Under the influence of the united muscle ring, the premaxilla lined up with the lateral segments. *D,* Almost normal occlusion at the age of 14 years. *E* and *F,* Front and profile views of the adult patient.

of the upper dental arch at the time of secondary dentition seemed to prove that this procedure was successful.

Despite our initial fascination with primary bone grafting, we became aware of many critical voices raised in many cleft centers in Europe and the United States. Because our own team also became reluctant to use this technique, we decided to reexamine 43 patients with complete clefts of the lip, alveolus, and palate who had been operated on between 1964 and 1968 using the primary bone grafting technique. We found that the results of the lip repair were aesthetically and functionally satisfactory. Most of the lip repairs had been performed using the Millard technique[6, 7] and in selected cases Reichert's modification.[8]

Examination of the alveolar arch showed that bone grafting was effective in preventing maxillary collapse except in two patients. However, in examining the occlusion, we found hypoplasia in the area of the cleft and an open bite in 25 of the 43 patients. The orthopedic correction of this deformity was extremely difficult and time consuming. In several patients it was necessary to perform an osteotomy to achieve normal occlusion. These findings stimulated us to change our entire approach to treatment of patients with cleft lip, alveolus, and palate. Our new approach, begun in 1982, was greatly influenced by the cleft palate team from Zurich (Hotz, Gnoinski, Perko).[9, 10]

Currently we use presurgical orthopedic treatment. Applying this treatment in the first days of life, we not only achieve good shape of the alveolar arches but also stimulate the growth of the maxillary segments toward the cleft, so that the gap between the segments becomes smaller without causing collapse of the lesser maxillary segment.

Following presurgical orthopedic treatment, we perform cleft lip repair at 4 to 6 months of age. For wide clefts, we use the Millard technique.[6, 7] For narrow and incomplete clefts, we use the wave-line technique introduced by Pfeiffer in 1970.[11–13] For very wide clefts and also for bilateral clefts, the technique of Celesnik (first closing only the upper portion of the cleft lip, thus transforming the cleft into an incomplete one)[14] has made it possible to avoid extensive mobilization of the soft tissue and seems to stimulate growth potential in the maxilla as well as the prolabium (Fig. 68–2).

In 1982 we also changed our approach to treatment of the palatal cleft (Fig. 68–3). We now use primary veloplasty combined with Widmaier's technique for closure of the entire palatal cleft.[15] Creation of the muscle sling as advocated by Kriens is beneficial for the speech results associated with it[16] (Fig. 68–4). We agree with the basic philosophy of Schweckendiek that early closure of the soft palate enhances normal speech production[17] (Figs. 68–5, 68–6, and 68–7). Therefore, veloplasty is performed at approximately 12 months of

Text continued on page 563

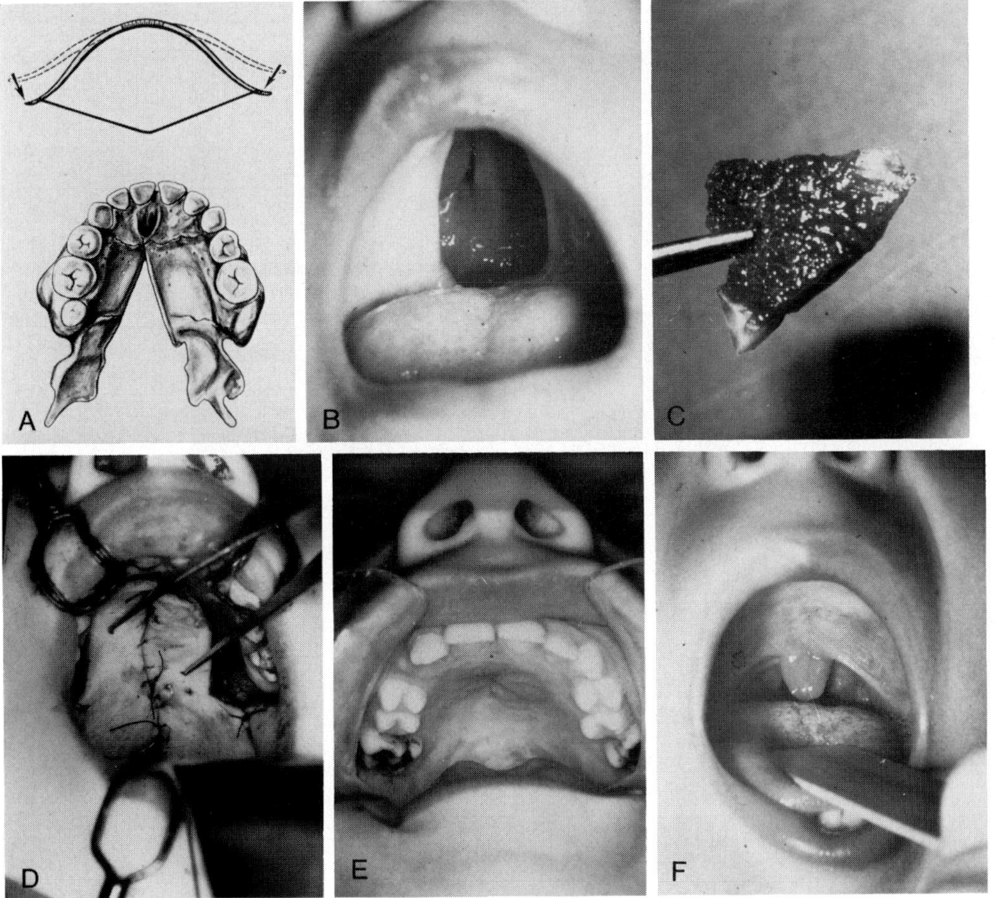

Figure 68–2 A, Widmaier's technique, used since 1959, of closing the velum with two triangular flaps mobilized above the palatine arteries, leaving the blood supply of the growing frontal jaw intact.[15] *B,* Alveolus and hard palate closed by a vomerine flap covering the bone implant. Schematic of closing the velum cleft. *C,* The two flaps united and pushed back. *D,* Very long soft palate with good speech result but deep impression in the area of the anterior hard palate and alveolus.

Figure 68–3 A, Drawing by Reichert explaining his idea of bridging very wide clefts in the hard palate with a bone graft to prevent compression in the molar region.[3–5] *B,* Wide palatal cleft. *C,* Triangular-shaped bone graft from hip. *D,* Palate closed according to Veau with bone graft between the nasal and oral layers. *E* and *F,* Well-rounded dental arch; long, mobile soft palate.

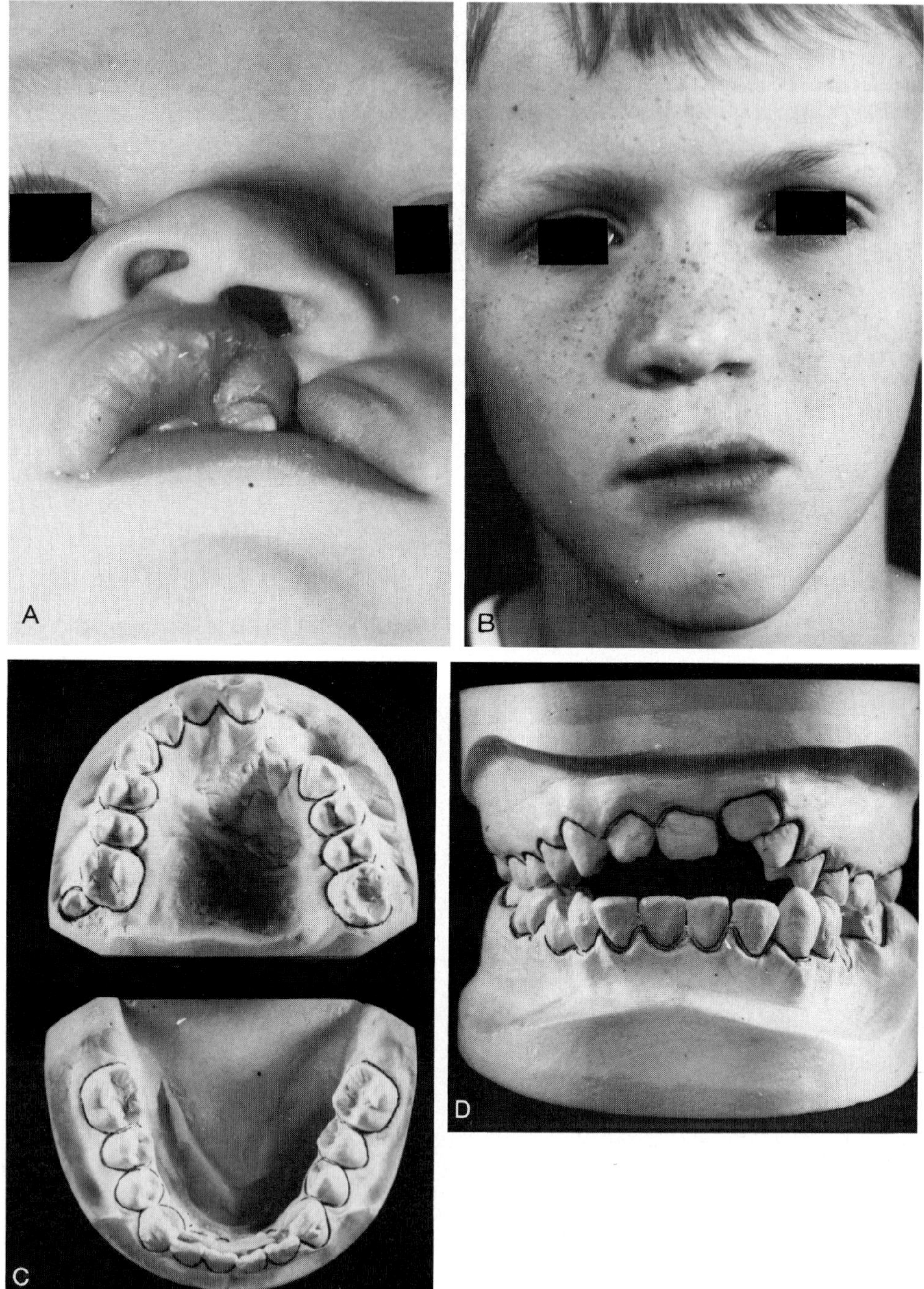

Figure 68–4 *A*, Six-month-old before lip closure combined with primary bone grafting. *B*, Appearance at the age of 10 years. Lip closed according to Reichert and Millard techniques.[6, 7] *C*, Seemingly well-rounded upper dental arch with a primary bone graft in the dental region. *D*, Very marked vertical growth deficiency in the cleft region.

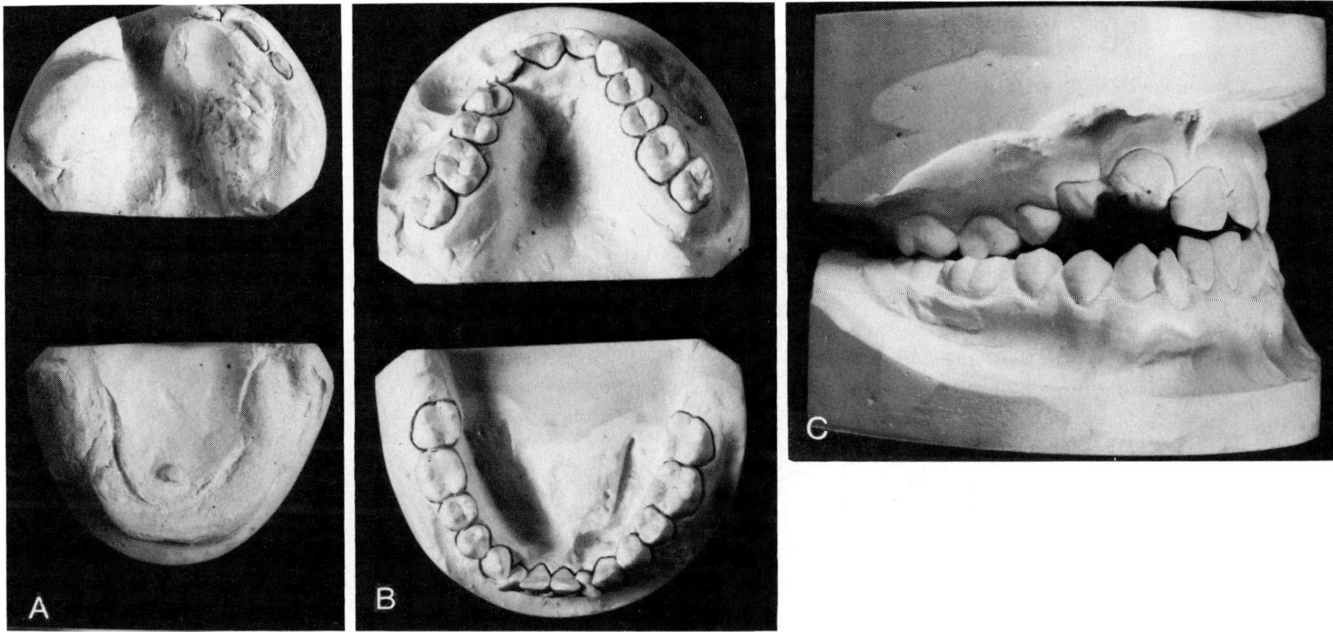

Figure 68–5 *A*, Wide unilateral cleft of the lip and palate before primary bone grafting. *B*, Only slight compression during second dentition. *C*, Very marked hypoplasia in the cleft region.

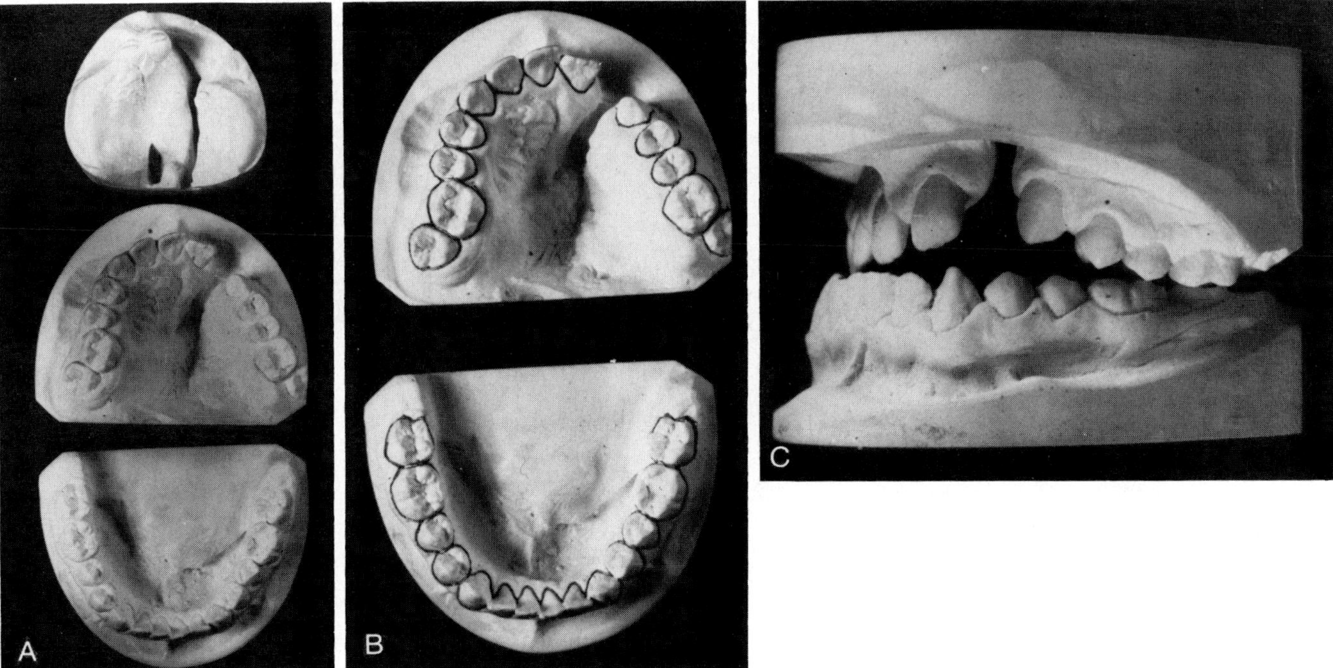

Figure 68–6 *A–C*, Same findings as those seen in Figures 68–4 and 68–5 and in more than 50% of the reexamined patients with primary bone grafting. Primary bone grafting was stopped in 1981.

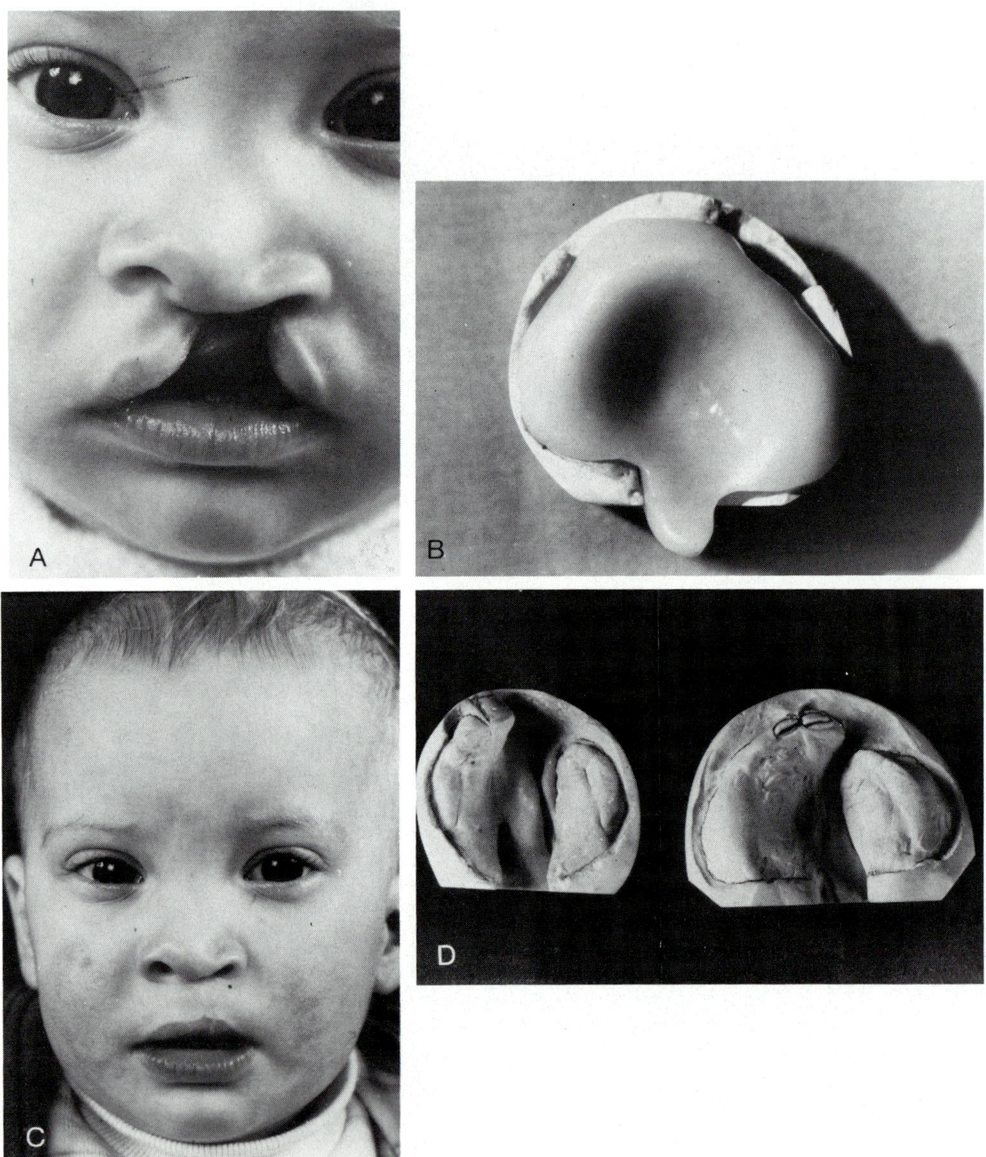

Figure 68–7 *A*, Wide unilateral cleft lip and palate. *B*, Orthopedic plate as described by Hotz.[9] *C*, After lip closure at the age of 7 months. *D*, Strong growth potential has narrowed the bony cleft without compressing the upper jaw.

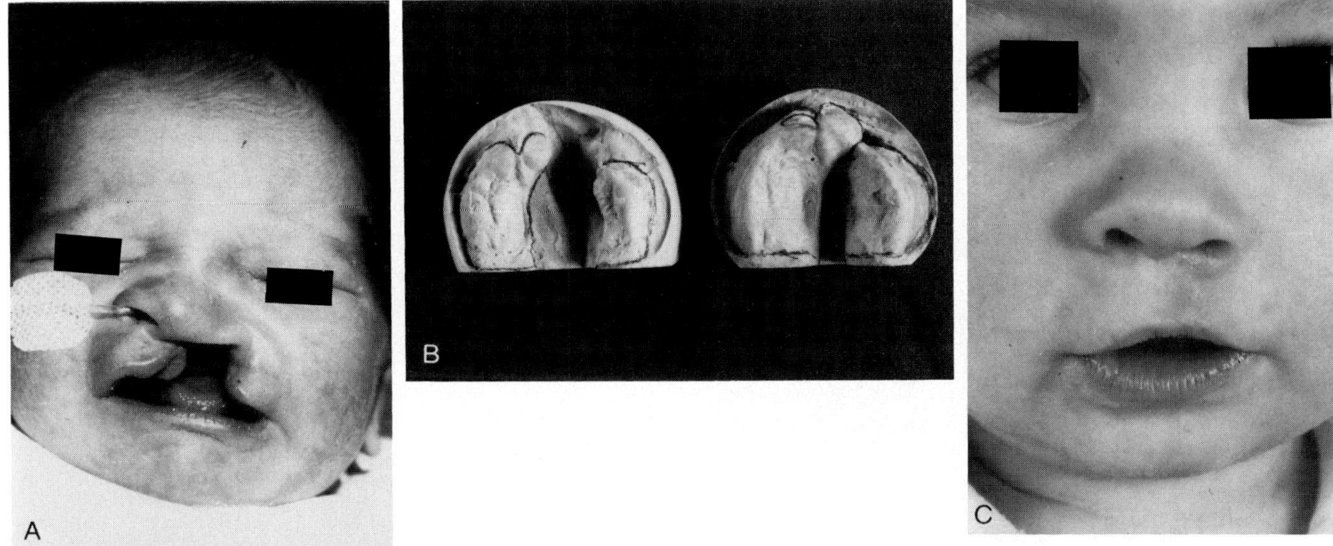

Figure 68–8 *A,* Wide cleft lip and palate. *B,* Plaster models demonstrating extensive growth, especially of the premaxilla and right maxillary fragment under the influence of the orthopedic plate. *C,* At 1 year of age.

Figure 68–9 *A,* Newborn child with wide complete unilateral cleft lip and palate. *B,* Models showing favorable influence of orthopedic plate and marked narrowing of bony gap without compression of upper jaw. *C,* Six months after lip closure using the Millard technique.[6, 7]

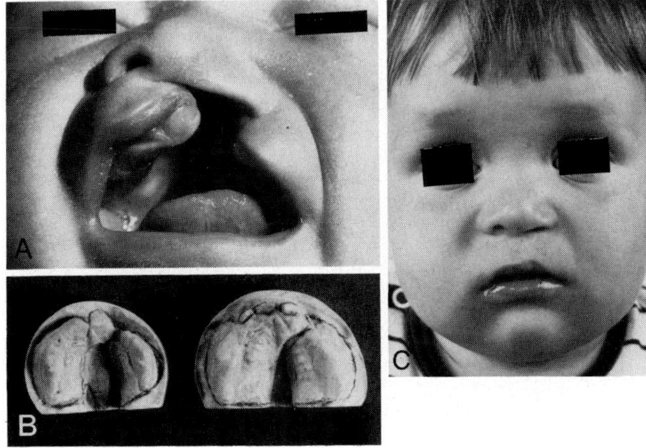

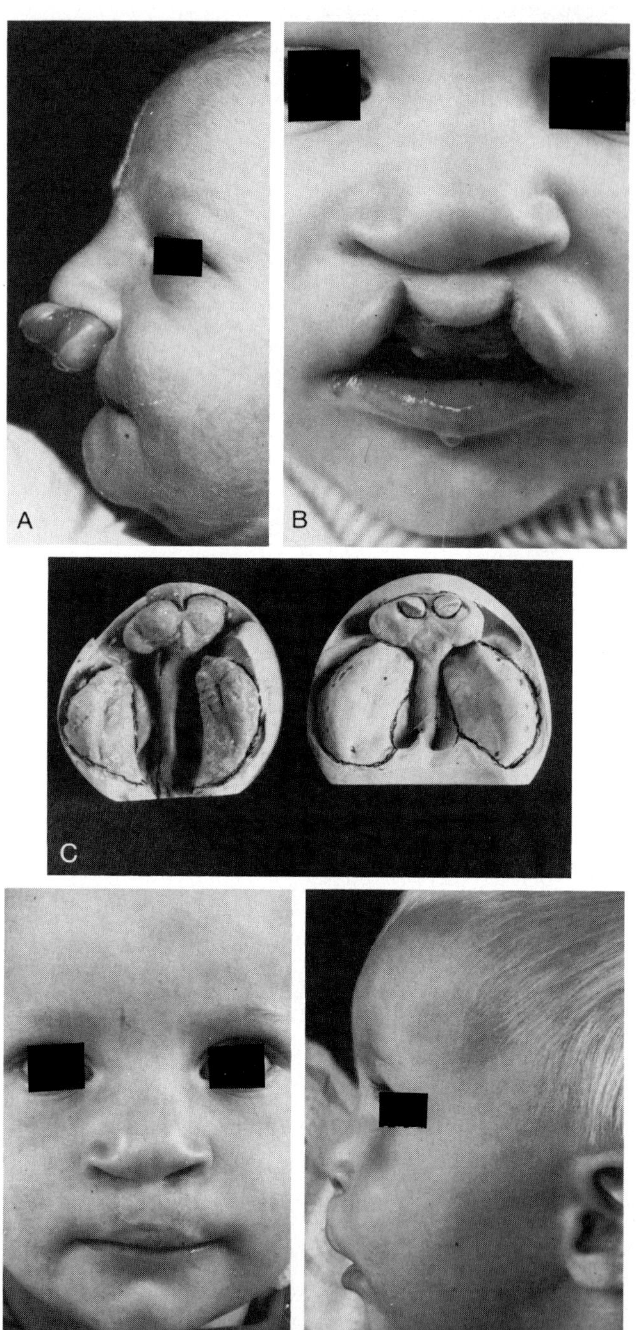

Figure 68–10 *A*, Newborn child with a wide bilateral cleft and protruding premaxilla. Impression taken for orthopedic plate. *B*, Bilateral partial lip adhesion according to Celesnik technique.[14] *C*, Under the influence of prosthetic plate and partial lip closure there is natural repositioning of the premaxilla and narrowing of bony gaps without maxillary compression. *D* and *E*, At the age of 18 months, before and after closure of the soft palate. Bilateral final lip closure according to the Veau technique.[21] Profile already almost normal.

age. Because the remaining cleft within the hard palate becomes narrower owing to bone apposition, closure of the remaining cleft in the hard palate can be performed easily between the ages of 5 and 6 years before the child begins school (Figs. 68–8, 68–9, and 68–10).

Conclusion

In surgical treatment of cleft lip, alveolus, and palate, all new ideas must be applied with the utmost care, and the results must be periodically reexamined.[18] We should also be prepared to change the sequence of surgical procedures as well as treatment strategies and techniques if the treatment produces adverse effects.

We still believe that Schmid's idea of using an autogenous bone graft for filling the bony defect is valuable.[19] However, this procedure should not be performed primarily, as it was for many years. There are indications that the best time for bone grafting is during the period of mixed dentition, as Bergland et al demonstrated in 1984.[20]

References

1. Schmid E: Die aufbauende Kieferkammplastik. Ost Z Stomat 51, 1954.
2. Schmid E: Die Annäherung der Kieferstumpfe bei Lippen-Kiefer-Gaumenspalten, ihre schadlichen Folgen und Vermeidung. Fortschr Kiefer u Ges Chir 1:37, 1955.
3. Reichert H: Surgical treatment of jaw deformities in patients with lip, alveolar and palate clefts. Transactions of Second International Conference on Oral Surgery, International Congressional Series 57. Amsterdam: Excerpta Medica, 1965, p 106.
4. Reichert H: Chirurgie der Lippen-Kiefer-Gaumenspalte heute. Deutsche Stomat 19, 1969.
5. Reichert H: Osteoplasty in complete clefts of the secondary palate. Br J Plast Surg 22:45, 1970.
6. Millard DR: Complete unilateral clefts of the lip. Plast Reconstr Surg 25:595, 1969.
7. Millard DR: Cleft Craft. Vol 1. The Unilateral Deformity. Boston: Little, Brown, 1976.
8. Reichert H: Forming the philtrum in primary lip cleft repair. Transactions of the Fifth International Congress of Plastic and Reconstructive Surgery. Australia: Butterworth, 1971, p 153.
9. Hotz M, Gnoinski W: Effects of early maxillary orthopedics in coordination with delayed surgery for cleft lip and palate. J Maxillofac Surg 7:201, 1979.
10. Hotz M, Gnoinski W, Perko M, et al: Early Treatment of Cleft Lip and Palate. Bern-Stuttgart: Hans Huber, 1986.
11. Pfeiffer G: Lippenkorrekturen nach früheren Spaltoperationen mit dem Wellenschnittverfahren. Dtsch Zahnarztl Z 25:569, 1970.
12. Pfeiffer G: Zehn Jahren Wellenschnittverfahren in der Lippenspaltchirurgie, in Wiederherstellung von Form und Funktion organischer Einheiten verschiedener Korperregionen. Stuttgart: Thieme-Verlag, 1977.
13. Pfeiffer G: Der Einflub der primaren Osteoplastik bei Lippen-Kiefer-Gaumenspalten, Behandlungskonzepte-Spatergebnisse, Teamwork und Fursorge, Teratologie. Stuttgart: Thieme, 1982.
14. Celesnik F: Notre procede de traitement chirurgical bec-de-lievre bilateral total. Rev Stomatol 63:386, 1962.
15. Widmaier W: Primary osteoplasty for gnathoschisis and palatoschisis. Third International Congress of Plastic Surgery, Washington, 1963.
16. Kriens O: An anatomical appraoch to veloplasty. Plast Reconstr Surg 43:29, 1969.
17. Schweckendiek W: Speech development after two-stage closure of cleft palate. In Kehrer B, et al (eds): Long Term Treatment in Cleft Lip and Palate. Bern: Hans Huber, 1981.
18. Reichert H: Experience and conclusions following primary osteoplasty. In Hotz M, Gnoinski W, Perko M (eds): Early Treatment of Cleft Lip and Palate. Bern-Stuttgart: Hans Huber, 1986.
19. Schmid E: Experience gathered and results obtained with primary osteoplasty. In Hotz M, Gnoinski W, Perko M (eds): Early Treatment of Cleft Lip and Palate. Bern-Stuttgart: Hans Huber, 1986.
20. Bergland O: The Oslo team approach to the rehabilitation of cleft anomalies. In Hotz M, Gnoinski W, Perko M (eds): Early Treatment of Cleft Lip and Palate. Bern-Stuttgart: Hans Huber, 1986.

CHAPTER 69

Surgical-Orthodontic Correction of the Protruded Premaxilla

Janusz Bardach,
William H. Olin,
and Kevin M. Kelly

The problems of management of the protruded premaxilla are complex and controversial. The complexity of the issue is based on the morphologic and functional changes associated with protrusion of the premaxilla. The controversies relate to the choice of treatment. Some specialists advocate presurgical orthopedic treatment followed by lip repair and further orthodontic management with no surgical repositioning of the premaxilla. Others prefer an approach in which there is no presurgical orthopedic treatment. Surgical retropositioning of the premaxilla is performed when the child is 4 to 6 years of age or older and is followed by orthodontic management. A few specialists use presurgical orthopedic treatment with subsequent lip repair. When the patient is older, closure of the oronasal and nasolabial fistulas with bone grafting is performed. In this treatment sequence, there is no surgical retropositioning of the premaxilla. In some centers treatment starts with the repair of the cleft lip followed at a later age by the premaxillary recession. The premaxilla, no matter how protruded and displaced it may be, is not dealt with until the patient is 7 to 8 years of age. At that time, bilateral bone grafting with subsequent orthodontic treatment is used. No surgical recession of the premaxilla is performed in this sequence of treatment. In the past, surgical treatment was limited to total resection of the premaxilla, a procedure that today is considered obsolete because it always leads to inhibition of midfacial growth.

In this chapter, discussion will focus on the severely protruded premaxilla because the premaxilla that is isolated from both maxillary segments but is positioned within the alveolar arch does not present a difficult clinical treatment problem. In such cases, bilateral bone grafting at 6 to 7 years of age or older and simultaneous closure of the oronasal and nasolabial fistulas provide highly satisfactory results. In contrast, the severely protruded premaxilla may present an extremely difficult management problem. Currently, there is no consensus on how to deal with it—that is, what constitutes the most successful treatment approach for this problem.

The protruded premaxilla in patients with complete bilateral cleft lip, alveolus, and palate may vary in size, shape, and position. It may be larger than the space between the maxillary segments, the same size, or smaller. The premaxilla may be positioned at the midline, deviated to the side, or rotated laterally and inferiorly. The maxillary segments may be closely approximated behind the premaxilla, or they may be evenly positioned on each side with enough space between them to move the premaxilla into the alveolar arch. In some patients, the maxillary segments are asymmetric with collapse of one side, usually that to which the premaxilla is deviated.

Because the premaxilla may be displaced in three dimensions—anteriorly, laterally, and inferiorly—use of pressure to distally reposition it may not be sufficient to achieve satisfactory results. Even when the premaxilla is displaced inferiorly, it may remain displaced in other dimensions as well. Displacement in the vertical dimension is difficult to correct by orthodontic treatment only.

When the protruded premaxilla is wider than the space between the maxillary segments in the alveolar arch, it cannot be retropositioned without expanding the maxillary segments to create adequate space in the anterior portion of the alveolar arch. However, during presurgical orthopedic treatment, it is impossible to control the occlusal relationships; therefore, many specialists avoid maxillary expansion at this early treatment stage. It is our experience that expansion of the maxillary segments prior to cleft lip repair may lead to overexpansion, creating an alveolar arch that is wider than that of the mandible, thus severely distorting the occlusal relationship and affecting balanced facial growth. When the premaxilla is the same size as, or smaller than, the gap between the maxillary segments, presurgical orthopedic treatment may effectively move the premaxilla close to or into the gap in the alveolar arch, using pressure induced by headgear or extraoral or intraoral appliances.

According to our experience, pressure of the repaired lip moves the premaxilla backward and downward, necessitating later orthodontic or surgical-orthodontic treatment to position it at the same level as the maxillary segments. The distortion in the vertical and lateral dimensions may be more difficult to correct than that in the anteroposterior dimension.

Another important issue that must be addressed when dealing with the premaxilla is its mobility and the presence of oronasal and nasolabial fistulas around it. The so-called floating premaxilla must be stabilized when it is placed within the alveolar arch. The best technique for stabilization is bilateral bone grafting. Leaving the premaxilla mobile, without stabilization, creates many problems including fistulas, possible fracture, and difficulty in dental rehabilitation.

Review of the literature indicates that numerous approaches have been advocated; however, there is no consensus as to which treatment technique is most successful.

Review of the Literature

Veau emphasized that "the premaxilla must never be taken away. The bone and the soft parts are indispensable to reconstruction of the lip. It would be rational to make a section, or better still, a resection of the septum."[1] Veau in France and Federspiel[2] in the United States were two of the first specialists to object strongly to total resection of the premaxilla. Both advocated resection of the vomer for moving the premaxilla into the alveolar arch.

Strong condemnation of excision of the premaxilla was presented by Ross, who considered this procedure mutilating and called for elimination of it from the practice.[3] Slaughter and Brodie indicated that cleft lip and palate surgery was the main cause of maxillofacial growth inhibition, which was directly proportional to injury of the growth centers and blood supply by such surgery.[4] Because one such center is the premaxillary-vomerine suture, injury to it may be detrimental to anteroposterior maxillofacial growth. Glover and Newcomb warned against resection of the premaxilla, indicating that severe growth disturbances occur following this operation.[5] Brauer and Cronin stressed the deleterious effects of injuring the premaxillary-vomerine suture.[6] They advocated presurgical orthopedic treatment to reposition the premaxilla prior to lip repair. Fara and Hrivnakova investigated 31 patients who underwent premaxillary recession.[7] In most patients, growth inhibition of the midface was evident. The authors considered this procedure harmful and not applicable in infants.

Cronin used excision of a rectangular segment of the vomer, posterior to the premaxillary-vomerine suture, to move the premaxilla backward and upward.[8] He used Kirschner wire to stabilize the premaxilla to the remaining portion of the vomer. Barsky et al used a similar approach, stabilizing the premaxilla with Kirschner wire and using mucoperiosteal flaps to close the fistulas around the premaxilla and improve its stability.[9] Matthews used a similar approach to retroposition the premaxilla.[10] Georgiade et al used oral-pin fixation and traction to retroposition the premaxilla prior to lip and palate repair.[11] Wilde used needles for fixation of the retropositioned premaxilla.[12]

Innis retropositioned the premaxilla surgically while simultaneously closing the bilateral cleft lip.[13] Monroe and his associates voiced their preference for surgical recession of the premaxilla.[14, 15] Twenty patients who underwent surgical premaxillary recession were studied. Following resection of the nasal septum, Kirschner wire was used to join the premaxilla with the posterior portion of the vomer. In evaluation of the long-term results, two of nine (22%) patients showed maxillofacial growth deficiency. The authors concluded that this operation was indicated in selected patients, especially when protrusion and downward rotation was severe and the gap between the maxillary segments was narrower than the premaxilla. Also, they indicated that when properly performed, with regard for the growth center (the premaxillary-vomerine suture), maxillofacial growth inhibition typically did not result.

Glass advocated presurgical orthopedic treatment; however, he objected to early bone grafting.[16] Instead, he favored recession of the premaxilla at a later age using vomerine resection combined with postsurgical orthodontic treatment. Muhler indicated the need for combined surgical-orthodontic treatment subsequent to presurgical orthopedic treatment with maxillary expansion.[17] Retropositioning of the premaxilla was achieved by resectioning the vomer and stabilizing the premaxilla with Kirschner wire. Friede and Pruzansky presented results of a longitudinal study of 54 patients with complete bilateral cleft lip, alveolus, and palate and protruding premaxilla.[18] In their opinion, protrusion of the premaxilla resulted from overgrowth of the premaxillary-vomerine suture. None of the patients had premaxillary recession. By the time the patients reached early adolescence, their facial profile was close to normal. The authors concluded that there was no indication in most patients for surgical treatment. They also warned that injuring the premaxillary-vomerine suture may be detrimental to maxillofacial growth.

Friede again emphasized the deleterious effects of injuring this area in his evaluation of the role of the premaxillary-vomerine suture in maxillofacial growth.[19] He concluded that this suture was essential to the anterior growth of the maxillary complex. In his opinion, a bone graft placed across the suture line may block growth completely, inhibiting development of the midface. He also indicated that closure of the palatal cleft may affect the premaxillary-vomerine suture, causing growth aberrations of various degrees of severity.

Despite the objection expressed by Pruzansky to surgical premaxillary recession, Motohashi and Pruzansky described three patients with severe bilateral cleft lip, alveolus, and palate with a protruded premaxilla in whom there were indications for removal of the premaxilla.[20] It is interesting that a similar opinion was expressed by Cosman, who stated that there were indications for resection of the premaxilla in some patients—not at the time of primary lip repair as typically performed but at 5 to 8 years of age.[21] He believed that early excision of the premaxilla would lead to maxillofacial growth inhibition. He reasoned that excision at a later age, when orthopedic treatment could be applied, would not influence maxillofacial growth to the same extent. In his experience, based on five patients operated on at 5 to 11 years of age, maxillofacial growth arrest did not occur. Cosman indicated a need for reevaluation of the indications for resection of the premaxilla.

In studies by Friede and Pruzansky[22] and Friede and Morgan,[23] the authors suggested that bilateral cleft lip repair in infants with a protruding premaxilla had a long-lasting effect in restricting growth of the maxillary complex. The significance of the premaxillary-vomerine suture was emphasized, especially in terms of its role in the growth of the midface.

Latham studied the morphology and development of the maxillary deformity in patients with bilateral clefts.[24] According to his findings, the premaxillary-vomerine suture was a site of active bone formation that elongated the premaxillary-vomerine stem. Rapid growth was stimulated by the normal forward growth tendency of the nasal septum. Georgiade et al emphasized that an infant ". . . with a bilateral cleft lip and associated premaxillary segments is the most challenging of problems."[25] In presurgical orthopedic treatment, they used a coaxial arch appliance, the Georgiade-Latham-Mark III appliance. After achieving proper positioning of the premaxilla, gingivoplasty was carried out bilaterally, followed by lip repair. Alignment of the orbicularis oris muscle and correction of the nasal deformity were performed at a later age.

Recently, several authors have advocated combined surgical-orthodontic treatment with secondary bone grafting. Browns and Egyedi described the need for surgical retropositioning of the premaxilla with bilateral bone grafting and closure of the fistulas followed by orthodontic treatment.[26] Hayward favored premaxillary recession performed between 8 and 14 years of age combined with bilateral bone grafting.[27] Deffez et al recommended surgical retropositioning of the premaxilla with simultaneous bone grafting at 10 years of age.[28]

Review of the literature indicates that there are serious controversies about the management of the protruding premaxilla. The basic controversy centers on orthodontic versus surgical-orthodontic management. When surgical management is suggested, most authors agree that resection of the protruding premaxilla should not be performed. However, other aspects of surgical treatment are still controversial. The problem of injuring the premaxillary-vomerine suture raises serious questions.

Another topic of debate is the timing and sequence of surgical procedures, that is, when to perform bone grafting and closure of oronasal and nasolabial fistulas. The techniques for retropositioning and stabilization of the premaxilla also remain controversial. The lack of recent studies precludes proper assessment of the validity of the surgical-orthodontic approach, which is currently used in several centers. More and better designated longitudinal studies are needed to evaluate the long-term results properly. Management of the protruding premaxilla is very difficult and requires greater effort to achieve better results.

There have been a number of experimental studies, which also present controversial data. However, most indicate that intervention on the septum, especially in the area of the premaxillary-vomerine suture, may cause growth aberrations.[29–38]

Surgical-Orthodontic Approach at the Iowa Cleft Palate Center

Several factors must be considered when planning treatment of an infant with complete bilateral cleft lip, alveolus, palate, and a protruding premaxilla. The following factors seem most important:

1. Width of the cleft lip
2. Symmetry of the cleft

3. Position of the maxillary segments
4. Distance between the maxillary segments
5. Size and shape of the premaxilla
6. Spatial relationship of the premaxilla
7. Severity of premaxillary protrusion and deviation in other dimensions
8. Relationship between the width of the premaxilla and the space between the maxillary segments
9. Size of the prolabium
10. Presence of Simonart's band

When evaluating the position of the premaxilla, it must also be noted whether or not it is protruded or rotated downward or laterally. Correction of the position of the premaxilla prior to lip repair may be extremely difficult, especially if the premaxilla is deviated in all three dimensions. Forceful manipulation of the premaxilla prior to lip repair is not feasible if there is a narrow space between the maxillary segments that cannot accommodate the premaxilla within the alveolar arch. In such patients, presurgical expansion prior to lip repair to create adequate space may result in overexpansion of the maxillary alveolar arch relative to the mandibular arch, resulting in subsequent malocclusion. Since we cannot control occlusion in infants and we want to avoid overexpansion, we do not use presurgical orthopedic treatment.

Furthermore, pressure applied to move the premaxilla backward has a tendency also to move it downward, producing a severe deviation of the nasal septum. It is our experience that external pressure, which may be applied by circumferential bands or other extraoral or intraoral appliances, is difficult to control in infants and may have a negative effect by transferring pressure to the maxillary segments, causing growth disturbances. Pressure from the repaired lip following lip adhesion or definitive lip repair moves the premaxilla backward and downward, so that the premaxilla remains displaced in the vertical dimension even when it is placed close to the arch. Usually pressure from the repaired lip approximates the premaxilla to the maxillary segments that remain behind it.

At the Iowa Cleft Palate Center, surgical-orthodontic treatment of the protruding premaxilla has been used on rare occasions when the premaxilla is severely displaced. If this condition persists when the child is 5 to 6 years of age, surgical recession of the premaxilla is performed to allow the child to enter school in a condition that will not cause mistreatment and teasing by peers. The method of surgical-orthodontic treatment used in the last 17 years is based on a protocol developed by the surgeon (J.B.) and orthodontist (W.H.O.). This protocol includes the following steps.

1. In patients with bilateral cleft lip, alveolus, and palate with a protruded premaxilla, two-stage lip repair is performed. During the first stage, one side (in asymmetric clefts, the wider side) is closed at 3 months of age; the other side is repaired 6 weeks later. At the time of lip repair, construction of the floor of the nose is performed using a mucoperiosteal flap from the lateral nasal wall and a mucoperichondrial flap from the nasal septum. In the anterior portion of the nasal floor the closure is done in two layers, the second layer consisting of two mucoperiosteal flaps, one from the vomer and the premaxilla and another from the lateral maxillary segment. At the same time the sulcus is created.

2. At 12 to 18 months of age, the cleft palate is repaired. Two-flap palatoplasty is used for closure of the palatal cleft. The anterior portion of the hard palate is not closed, leaving an approach to the vomer posterior to the premaxilla.

3. When there is severe collapse of the maxillary segments orthodontic treatment starts at 3.5 to 4 years of age. During this stage maxillary expansion allows retropositioning of the premaxilla and establishment of a proper occlusal relationship for surgical retropositioning of the premaxilla at 5 to 7 years of age.

4. Premaxillary retropositioning with partial excision of the vomer and in some cases ablation of the premaxillary-vomerine suture is combined with bilateral bone grafting to stabilize the premaxilla within the alveolar arch. During this operation, nasolabial and oronasal fistulas on both sides of the premaxilla are closed.

5. Following premaxillary retropositioning, sulcoplasty (if indicated) is performed 6 to 12 months later.

6. Secondary correction of the lip and nasal deformity is performed following premaxillary retropositioning and sulcoplasty.

7. Following premaxillary retropositioning, the patient remains under orthodontic treatment until 14 years of age or later depending on the age of tooth eruption.

The main objective of this protocol prior to surgical retropositioning of the premaxilla is to ensure undisturbed anteroposterior facial growth with the premaxilla manipulated only by pressure from the repaired lip.

Retropositioning of the premaxilla is performed at 5 to 7 years of age because we try to correct this severe deformity before the child starts school. The protruding premaxilla creates one of the most severe cleft deformities and may cause severe psychological problems if the child is teased and ridiculed by his or her peers. Surgical retropositioning is performed to:

1. Align the premaxilla within the alveolar arch in proper occlusion.

2. Stabilize the premaxilla with bone grafting and simultaneous closure of oronasal and nasolabial fistulas.

To achieve these goals proper planning and preparation are necessary with close collaboration between the orthodontist and surgeon. Prior to the operation, dental impressions are made, and the premaxilla is retropositioned on the dental models to determine the best occlusal relationship. After proper alignment of the premaxilla is achieved on the dental models, an acrylic appliance is prepared to stabilize the premaxilla in position following surgery. This appliance is wired to the existing teeth and left in place for 10 to 12 weeks following surgical retropositioning of the premaxilla, which is performed simultaneously with bilateral bone grafting and closure of the oronasal and nasolabial fistulas. The orthodontist determines whether any teeth must be extracted and prepares the appliance accordingly.

The operation starts with an incision at the midline

of the lower edge of the vomer, next to the premaxilla. This incision is made through the area left open in the anterior palate during palatoplasty. The incision is carried forward onto the lateral edges of the premaxilla, designing mucoperiosteal flaps that can be raised on the premaxilla. Then two incisions are carried along the edge of the alveolar ridge, posterior and inferior to the edges of the anterior palatal defect (Fig. 69–1).

Raising mucoperiosteal flaps is a most important part of this operation because the defects on the nasal side as well as on the oral side must be closed. Only after the nasal layer is closed precisely with mucoperiosteal flaps can cancellous bone grafts be placed successfully around the premaxilla. By raising the mucoperiosteal flaps, we also expose the vomer just behind the premaxilla, the lateral and posterior bony surfaces of the premaxilla, and the alveolar ridges on both maxillary segments. By means of this procedure, the vomer can be easily approached for partial resection and the proper conditions for the cancellous bone graft are created between the two bony surfaces on each side of the premaxilla. The only area where the mucoperiosteum remains attached to the premaxilla is on the prolabium. No undermining is perfomed in this area to ensure an adequate blood supply in the premaxilla.

On the premaxilla in the area behind the anterior incisors, a triangular flap is raised. This flap serves to close the anterior palatal defect following repositioning of the premaxilla. It is sutured to the mucoperiosteal flaps on the anterior hard palate. The vomer is transected approximately 5 mm behind the premaxillary-vomerine suture using a narrow osteotome. Following transection, the premaxilla with its attached part of the vomer is dislocated superiorly, exposing that portion of the vomer. Using a large cutting bur, part of the vomer is removed until the premaxilla can be placed within the alveolar arch on the same level as the maxillary segments.

This approach allows, with great ease and simplicity, elimination of the premaxillary displacement in all dimensions. That is, the premaxilla can be moved in whatever dimension is necessary to position it in the alveolar arch. In some cases, even after the mucoperiosteal flaps are raised, the bony premaxilla remains larger than the gap between the maxillary segments. In this situation, reduction in the width of the premaxilla or reduction of the bony edges of the maxillary segments may be indicated. The choice depends on the evaluation by the orthodontist, including clinical and radiographic evaluations, and on problems of dentition and occlusion.

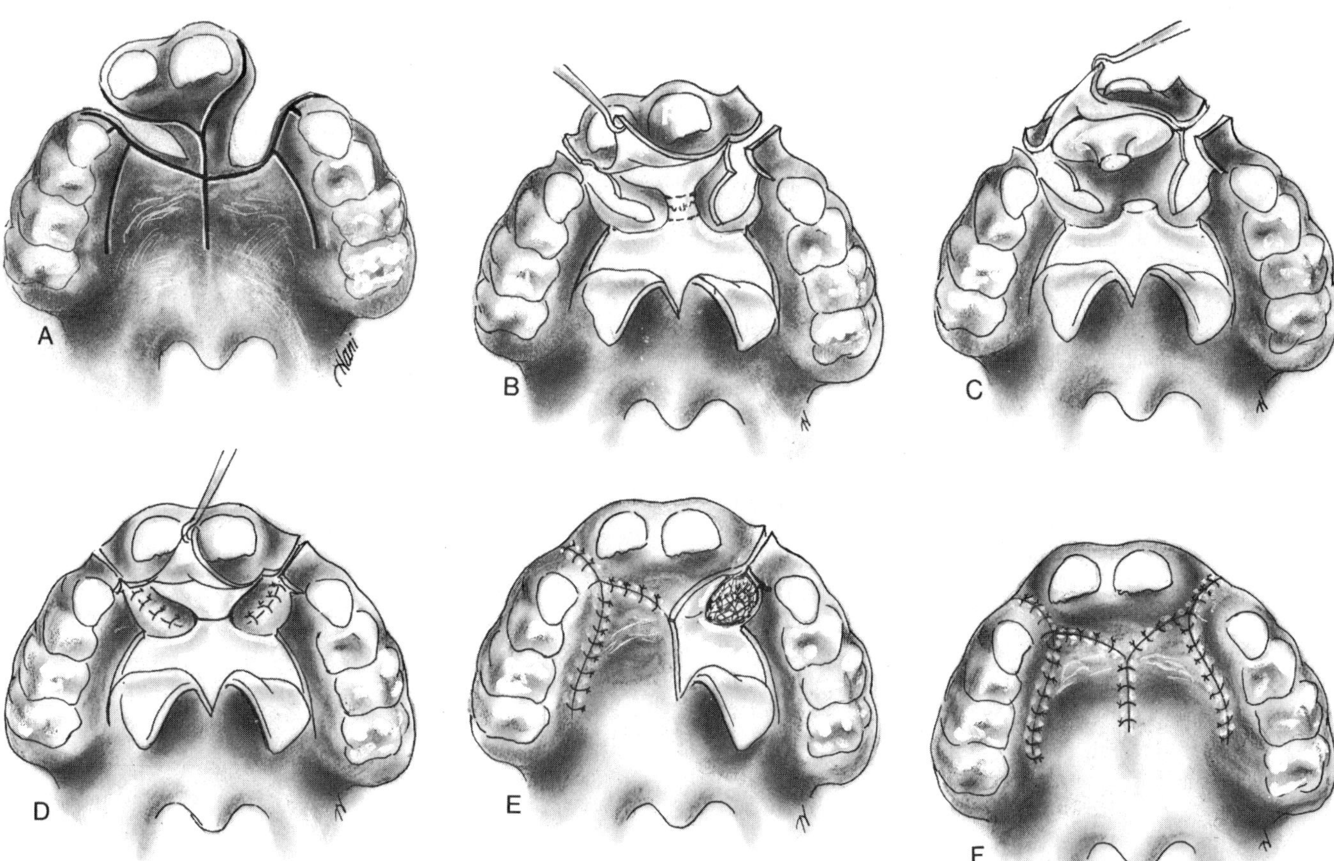

Figure 69–1 Premaxillary retropositioning. *A*, Design of the incisions on the hard palate, alveolus, and premaxilla. *B*, Turnover flaps raised on the hard palate on the vomer, edges of the alveolus, and premaxilla. The premaxillary-vomerine suture is shown. *C*, The portion of the vomer adjacent to the premaxilla is excised, including the premaxillary-vomerine suture. The amount of bone to be removed is determined by the protrusion of the premaxilla. *D*, Creation of the inner layers for closure of the oronasal fistulas. The space between the premaxilla, bony palate, and alveolus on each side of the premaxilla is filled with cancellous bone. *E*, On the right, cancellous bone is placed in the prepared pocket. On the left side, closure of the oronasal and nasolabial fistulas by suturing the mucoperiosteal flaps from the palate, premaxilla, and alveolus is shown. *F*, Both sides are closed, and the premaxilla is placed within the alveolar arch.

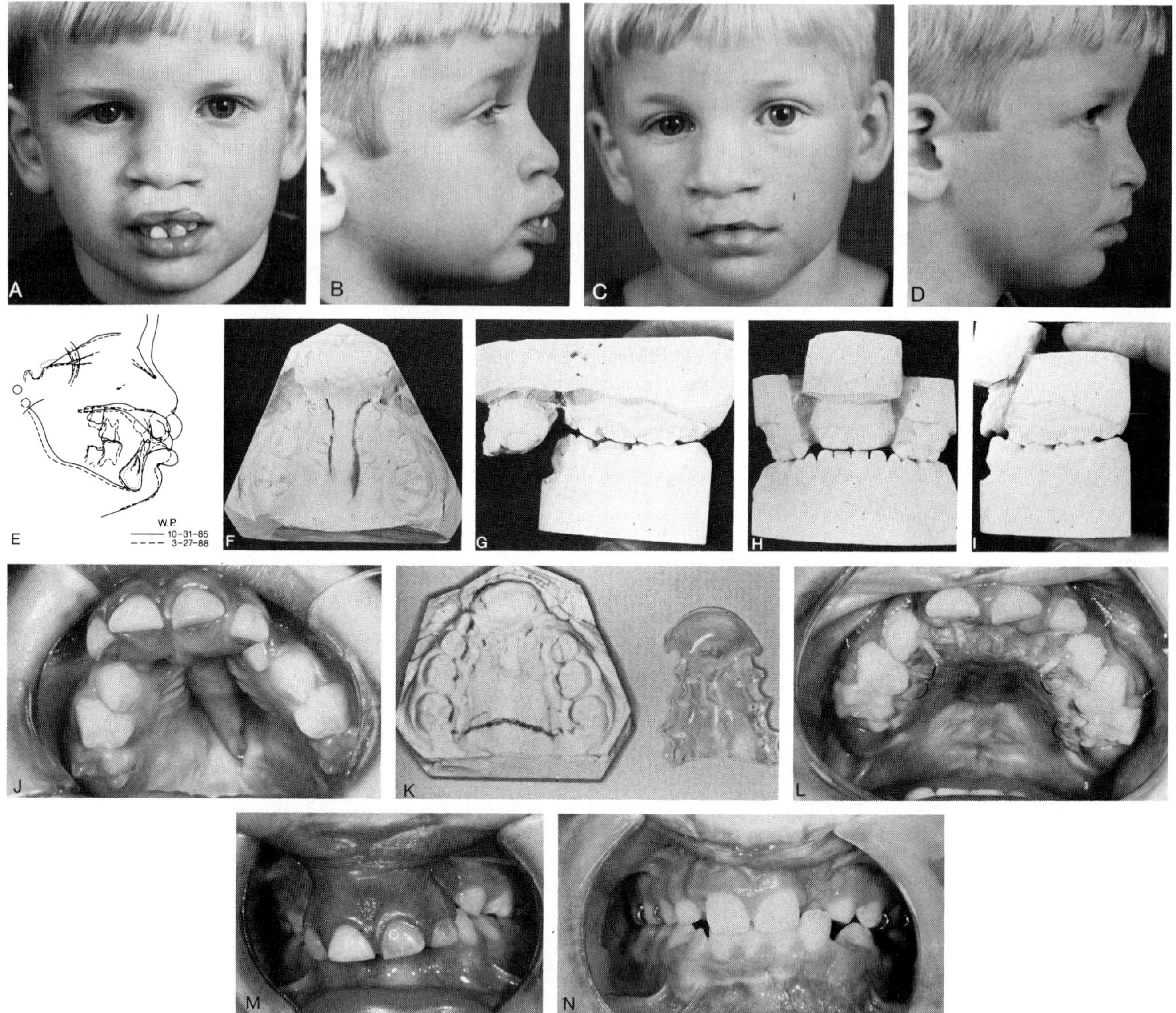

Figure 69–2 *A* and *B*, Patient at 5 years of age with severe protrusion of the premaxilla. *C* and *D*, Same patient 3 years after premaxillary retropositioning. *E*, Lateral cephalometric tracing before and after operation. *F* through *I*, Planning of the retropositioning of the premaxilla on a dental model. *J*, Preoperative status. *K*, Dental model used for preparation of the stabilizing appliance that is wired to the alveolus for 10 to 12 weeks after operation. *L*, Following retropositioning of the premaxilla with the appliance in place. *M* and *N*, Premaxilla before surgery and 2 years later.

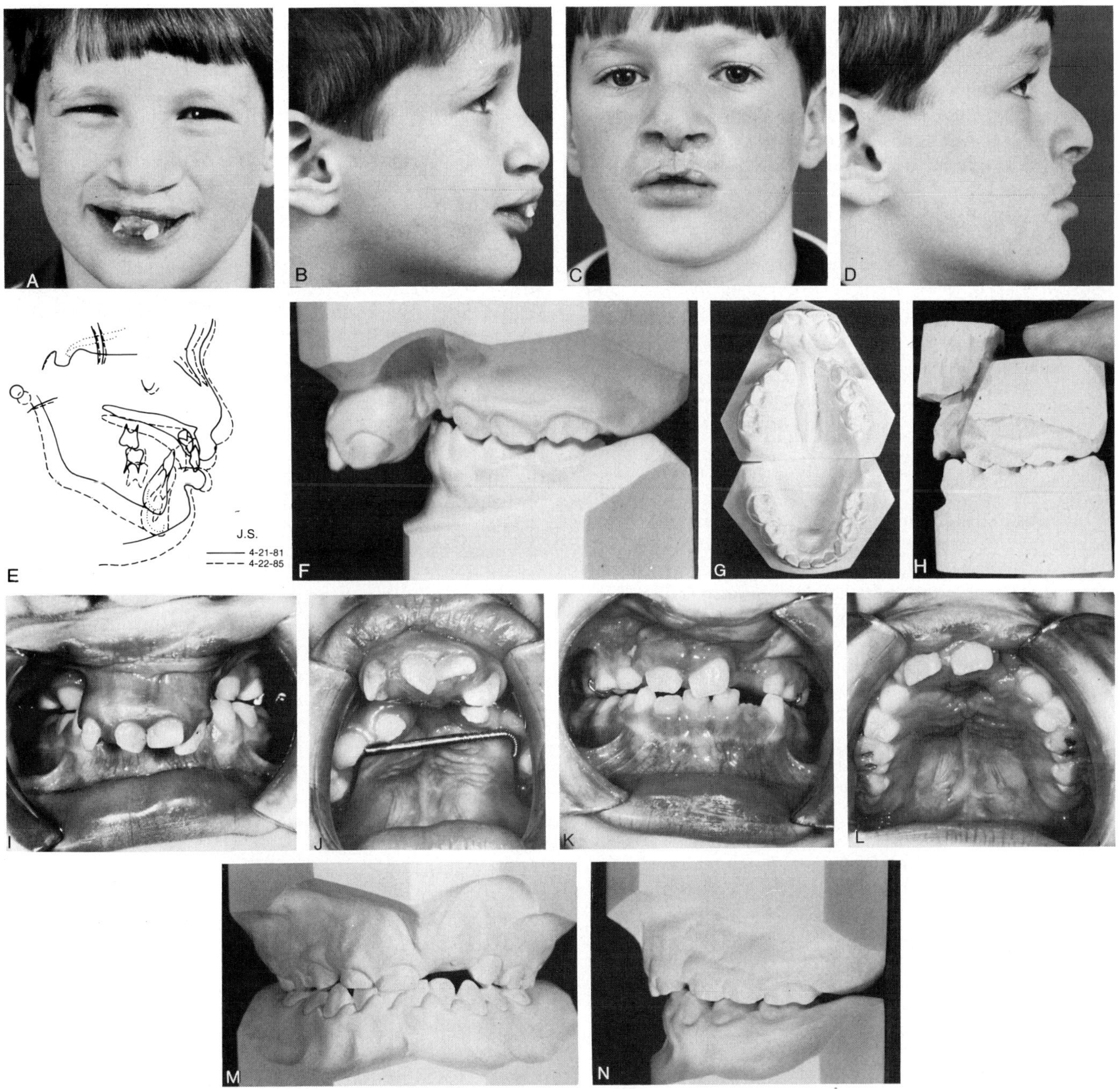

Figure 69–3 *A* and *B,* Patient at 5 years of age with severe protrusion of the premaxilla. *C* and *D,* Same patient following premaxillary retropositioning. *E,* Lateral cephalometric tracing before and after operation. *F–H,* Planning of the operation on dental models. *I* and *J,* Premaxilla before operation. Note the width of the premaxilla and the large defect in the anterior palate and in the alveolar area. *K–N,* After premaxillary retropositioning.

When the nasal layer is created prior to bone grafting there may be an excessive amount of mucoperiosteum owing to the reduction of space between the premaxilla and the hard palate. This excess must be removed to achieve good closure of the nasal layer and adequate protection for the bone grafts.

At this stage, the premaxilla is placed in the desired position to establish the occlusion as determined from the dental models. After closure of the oronasal fistulas on both sides, the only area that remains open is the alveolus on each side of the premaxilla. Cancellous bone is packed tightly through these openings. Cancellous bone grafts are obtained from the iliac crest using a split incision through its upper edge. Some surgeons may prefer to use cranial bone for the grafts. Following bone grafting, the mucoperiosteal flaps on the alveolus are sutured, closing the defects (Fig. 69–2).

In the final stage of the operation, the dental appliance, prepared prior to the surgery, is inserted and wired tightly to the alveolus and teeth. This appliance remains in place for 10 to 12 weeks, during which the patient must be placed on a soft diet.

Results of Surgical-Orthodontic Treatment

Our observations indicate that most patients who underwent this combined procedure for retropositioning of the premaxilla have had satisfactory facial growth. Thus, in general, our results have been quite acceptable.

Recently, 19 patients' records were examined to compare their facial growth and occlusion before and after surgical retropositioning of the premaxilla and bilateral alveolar bone grafting. At the time of surgery, these patients ranged in age from 4 years 5 months to 9 years 11 months; the majority were 5 to 6 years of age. Each of the 19 patients had undergone maxillary expansion when indicated prior to surgical retropositioning. The patients were examined 3 to 8 years following surgery (Fig. 69–3).

Twelve patients exhibited good occlusion with no crossbite. Four had only one canine in crossbite, two

Table 69–1. Postoperative Anteroposterior Occlusal Relationships of the Total Patient Sample Based on Cephalometric Analysis from Lateral Radiographs

Patient	SNA	SNB	ANB
1	80	70	10
2	82	76	6
3	82	76	6
4	70	68	2
5	75	75	0
6	81	79	2
7	78	69	9
8	73	77	−4
9	74	72	2
10	87	78	9
11	78	77	1
12	76	72	4
13	85	77	1
14	82	77	5

Table 69–2. Preoperative Summary of the Cephalometric Measures as Percentage Within Normal Limits (% WNL)

Measurement	No. Cases	% WNL
SNA	10	40
SNB	10	90
ANB	10	10
FH:NPog	10	90
MP:SN	10	100
MP:FH	10	70
NSGn	10	90
FH:SGn	10	80

had a posterior crossbite, and one had a complete maxillary crossbite. This patient was the only one who showed severe facial growth inhibition and malocclusion subsequent to the surgical retropositioning of the protruded premaxilla.

Results of the cephalometric analysis based on lateral radiographs are presented in Table 69–1. Of the 19 radiographic films available, we were able to measure only 14. On five of the films lead eye protectors occluded one of the major cephalometric points (nasion) necessary for tracing, so we were unable to measure these particular films. Tables 69–2 and 69–3 present the pre- and postoperative results of the cephalometric tracings for the ten male patients whose radiographs were not obstructed by lead eye protectors.

Analysis of these results indicated that facial growth of the entire group of patients was satisfactory with the exception of one patient. Four patients revealed an excessive ANB angle; due to the nature of the cleft deformity, the premaxilla remained a bit protruded. We believe that this condition will improve as the patient grows; if necessary, orthodontic treatment may be used later. However, the indications for correction will be clear only when the patient is older. Other patients may need no further revisions. We do not expect to find major growth problems because we have followed many of these patients for more than 6 years without observing any remarkable changes in the maxillofacial development (Fig. 69–4).

Surgical-orthodontic management of the severely protruded premaxilla according to the protocol used in the Iowa Cleft Palate Center is one of various approaches used in dealing with this difficult problem. We use this method when the displacement of the premaxilla is severe and the child is of preschool age. It is our intention to improve the position of the premaxilla and

Table 69–3. Postoperative Summary of the Cephalometric Measures as Percentage Within Normal Limits (% WNL)

Measurement	No. Cases	% WNL
SNA	10	90
SNB	10	100
ANB	10	60
FH:NPog	10	90
MP:SN	10	80
MP:FH	10	80
NSGn	10	80
FH:SGn	10	80

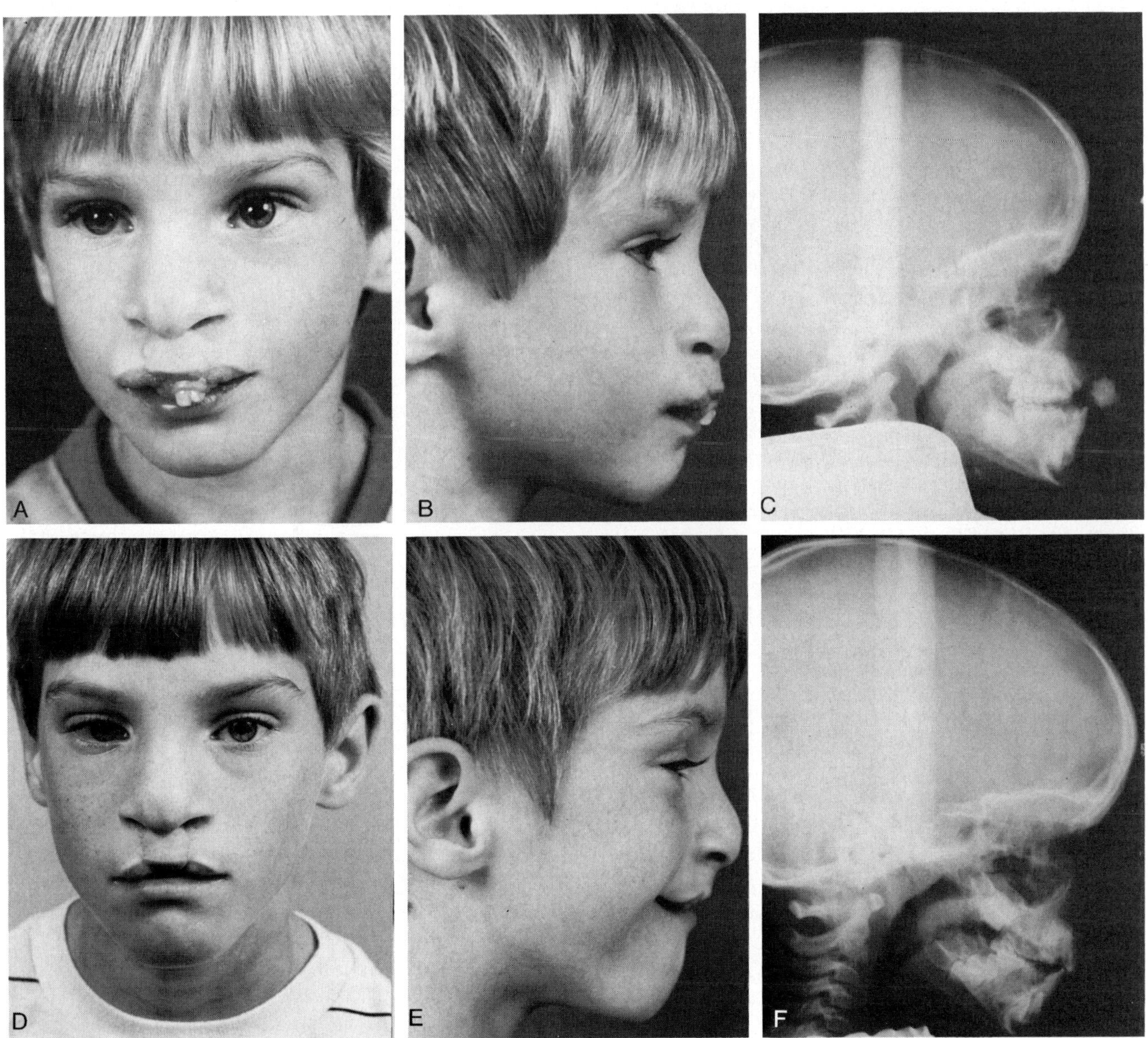

Figure 69–4 *A–C*, Five-year-old patient with severe protrusion of the premaxilla. *D–F*, After premaxillary retropositioning, 2 years later.

Illustration continued on following page

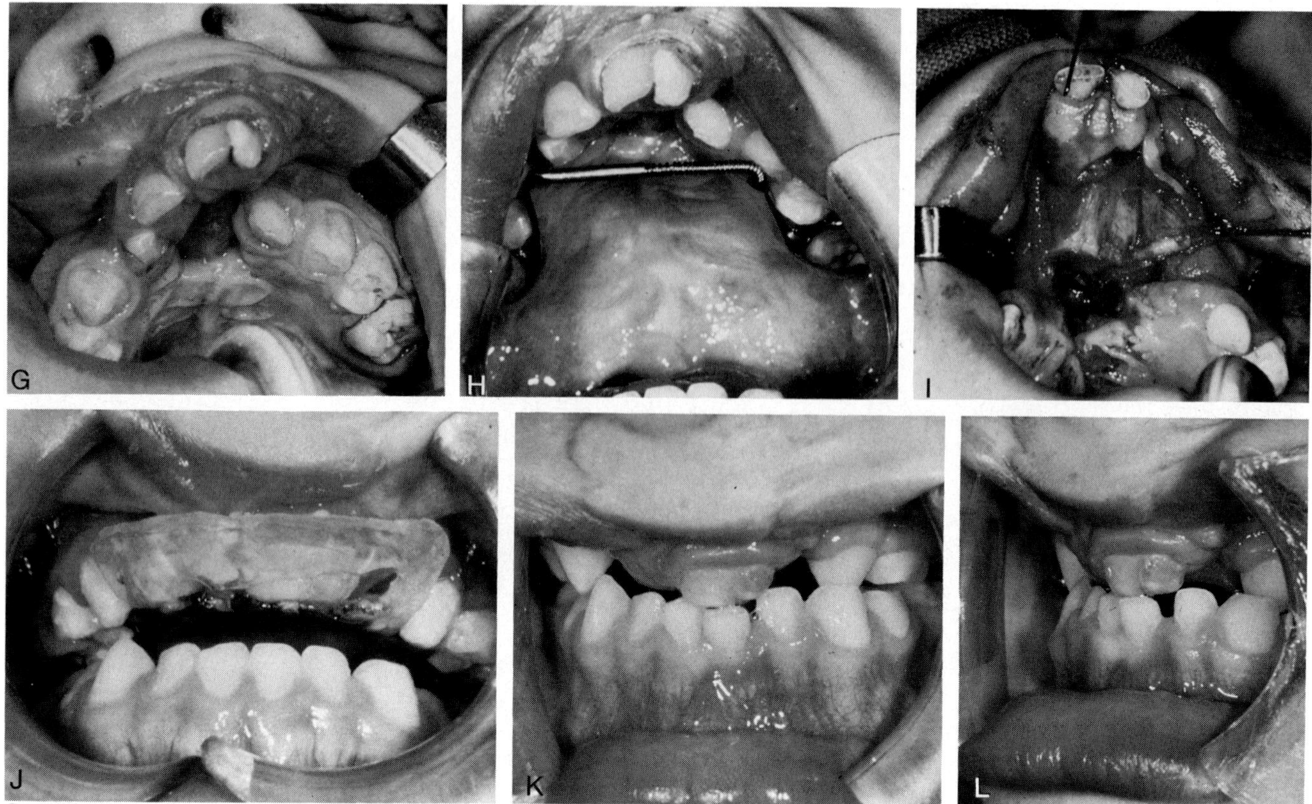

Figure 69–4 *Continued G,* Protruding premaxilla is severely tilted to the right side. Note the large defect in the anterior palate. *H,* Maxillary expansion prior to surgery. *I,* After partial excision of the vomer. The premaxilla is pulled backward. *J,* Stabilizing appliance wired in place. *K* and *L,* Occlusion after surgery.

the appearance of the patient prior to entering school. Because facial growth and occlusion in the group of patients followed for a longer period of time are quite satisfactory, we feel that this procedure is justified in light of our observations and results. We also understand that further studies are needed to draw conclusions on the long-term outcome of this procedure in terms of facial growth, dentition, and occlusion. There is also a need for studies comparing the long-term results of this approach with other methods of treatment of bilateral clefts with protruding premaxilla.

References

1. Veau V: Operative treatment of complete double hare lip. Ann Surg 76:156, 1922.
2. Federspiel MN: Harelip and cleft palate. Laryngoscope 32:909, 1922.
3. Ross B: A mutilating procedure? Cleft Palate J 19:148, 1982.
4. Slaughter WB, Brodie AG: Facial clefts and their surgical management in view of recent research. Plast Reconstr Surg 4:311, 1949.
5. Glover DM, Newcomb MR: Bilateral cleft lip repair and the floating premaxilla. Plast Reconstr Surg 28:365, 1961.
6. Brauer R, Cronin T: Maxillary orthopedics and anterior palate repair with bone grafting. Cleft Palate J 1–2:31, 1964–65.
7. Fara M, Hrivnakova J: The problem of protruding premaxilla in bilateral total clefts. Acta Chir Plast 7:125, 1965.
8. Cronin TD: Management of the bilateral cleft lip with protruding premaxilla. Am J Surg 92:810, 1956.
9. Barsky AJ, Kahn S, Simon BE: Early and late management of the protruding premaxilla. Plast Reconstr Surg 29:58, 1962.
10. Matthews DN: The premaxilla in bilateral clefts of the lip and palate. Br J Surg 5:77, 1952.
11. Georgiade NG, Mladick RA, Thorne FL: Positioning of the premaxilla in bilateral cleft lip by oral pinning and traction. Plast Reconstr Surg 41:240, 1968.
12. Wilde NJ: Repositioning of the premaxilla and its fixation. Br J Plast Surg 13:28, 1960.
13. Innis CO: Repositioning of the premaxilla and simultaneous closure of the bilateral cleft lip. Br J Plast Surg 14:153, 1961.
14. Monroe CW: Recession of the premaxilla in bilateral cleft lip and palate: A follow-up study. Plast Reconstr Surg 35:512, 1965.
15. Monroe CW, Griffith BG, McKinney P, et al: Surgical recession of the premaxilla and its effect on maxillary growth in patients with bilateral clefts. Cleft Palate J 7:784, 1970.
16. Glass D: The early management of bilateral cleft lip and palate. Br J Plast Surg 23:130, 1970.
17. Muhler VG: Zum problem des extrem vorstenenden burzels bei doppelseitigen lippen-kiefer-gaumen segel-spalten. Schilderung des eigene operativen verfahrensder rucklagerung. Zentralbl Chir 92(26):993, 1967.
18. Friede H, Pruzansky S: Longitudinal study of growth in bilateral cleft lip and palate from infancy to adolescence. Plast Reconstr Surg 49:392, 1972.
19. Friede H: The vomero-premaxillary suture—a neglected growth site in mid-facial development of unilateral cleft lip and palate patients. Cleft Palate J 15(4):398, 1978.
20. Motohashi N, Pruzansky S: Long-term effects of premaxillary excision in patients with complete bilateral cleft lips and palates. Cleft Palate J 18:177, 1981.
21. Cosman B: Premaxillary excision: Reasons and effects. Plast Reconstr Surg 73:195, 1984.
22. Pruzansky S, Friede H: Two sisters with unoperated bilateral cleft lip and palate, age 6 and 4 years. Br J Plast Surg 28:251, 1975.
23. Friede H, Morgan P: Growth of the vomero-premaxillary suture in children with bilateral cleft lip and palate. Scand J Plast Reconstr Surg 10:45, 1976.
24. Latham RA: Development and structure of the premaxillary deformity in bilateral cleft lip and palate. Br J Plast Surg 26:1, 1973.
25. Georgiade GS, Georgiade NG, Latham RA: The bilateral cleft lip. In Serafin D, Georgiade NG (eds): Pediatric Plastic Surgery. Vol 1. St Louis: CV Mosby, 1984.
26. Browns J, Egyedi P: Osteotomy of the premaxilla. J Maxillofac Surg 8:182, 1980.
27. Hayward JR: Management of the premaxilla in bilateral clefts. J Oral Maxillofac Surg 41:518, 1983.
28. Deffez JP, Allain P, Brethaux J, et al: Osteoplastie de reposition du borgeon median dan les fentes labio-maxillaires bilaterales. Rev Stomatol Chir Maxillofac 85:360, 1984.

29. Freng A: Growth in width of the dental arches after partial extirpation of the mid-palatal suture in man. Scand J Plast Reconstr Surg 12:267, 1978.
30. Freng A: Growth of the middle face in experimental early bony fusion of the vomeropremaxillary, vomeromaxillary and mid-palatal sutural system. Scand J Plast Reconstr Surg 15:117, 1981.
31. Latham RA, Deaton TG, Calabrese CT: A question of the role of the vomer in the growth of the premaxillary segment. Cleft Palate J 12:351, 1975.
32. Sarnat BG: Postnatal growth of the face: Some experimental considerations. In Broadbent TR (ed): Transactions of the III International Congress of Plastic Surgery. Amsterdam: Excerpta Medica, 1963.
33. Sarnat BG: Differential effect of surgical trauma to the nasal bones and septum upon rabbit snout growth. In Sanvanero-Rosselli G (ed): Transactions of the III International Congress of Plastic Surgery. Amsterdam: Excerpta Medica, 1967.
34. Sarnat BG, Wexler MR: Growth of the face and jaws after resection of the septal cartilage in the rabbit. Am J Anat 118:775, 1966.
35. Sarnat BG, Wexler MR: The snout after resection of nasal septum in adult rabbits. Arch Otolaryngol 86:129, 1967.
36. Sarnat BG, Wexler MR: Longitudinal development of upper facial deformity after septal resection in growing rabbits. Br J Plast Surg 22:313, 1969.
37. Siegel MI: Mechanisms of early maxillary growth—implications for surgery. J Oral Surg 34:106, 1976.
38. Siegel MI, Sadler D: An x-ray cephalometric analysis of premaxillary growth in operated and unoperated baboons (*Papiocynocephalus*). J Med Primatol 8:187, 1979.

Orthodontic Treatment of Cleft Lip and Palate

CHAPTER 70

Presurgical Orthopedic Treatment in Unilateral Cleft Lip and Palate

A. G. Huddart

Presurgical orthopedic treatment, as it is understood today, is undertaken to prepare an infant with a cleft for surgical repair of the lip and later, for repair of the palate. The technique derives from the work begun by Kerr McNeil in Glasgow, Scotland, in 1947 (Fig. 70–1). McNeil, a prosthetist, found that if he fitted a special kind of obturator plate that had stimulation pads on its palatal aspect in older cleft patients with a residual fistula, the cleft often diminished in size. When he applied the same type of treatment to newborn infants he saw a similar dramatic narrowing of the defect.

Looking back 30 or 40 years, it is perhaps difficult to appreciate the furor and disbelief these claims aroused. McNeil exacerbated the situation by claiming that the appliances "closed" the hard palate cleft (implying that soft tissue and perhaps bony continuity would be established) and that surgery would therefore be confined to repair of the lip and soft palate, ". . . or at the most, [the] soft palate and a minor defect of the hard palate."[1] Later, he was to protest that he had been misquoted, but the author personally heard him make the claim himself during the course of a lecture.[2] With the controversy at its height following various publications by McNeil,[3, 4] in 1955 the plastic and pediatric surgeons in the Liverpool area asked Dr. W. R. Burston, an orthodontist with a Ph.D. in embryology, to go to Glasgow to evaluate McNeil's claims.

Burston returned to Liverpool enthusiastically endorsing what he had seen in Glasgow, and because of his orthodontic and embryologic training he was able to rationalize what the treatment did and to begin explaining what at first sight had seemed inexplicable.[5, 6] As a result of his report, Burston was asked to start presurgical treatment in the Liverpool area. A special ward was provided for this purpose at the Children's Hospital in Heswell. There the author worked with Burston before leaving in 1957 to become consultant orthodontist at what is now the West Midlands Regional Plastic Unit.

McNeil believed that ". . . so long as there is arch asymmetry, anomalies of function with regard to respiration, swallowing and later mastication and speech present themselves. These abnormal functions influence development of the facial skeleton."[1] In the morphologic context, therefore, presurgical treatment aims at normalizing the maxillary arch by (1) aligning the displaced maxillary segments and (2) narrowing the cleft. Functionally, presurgical orthopedic treatment attempts to normalize feeding, tongue posture, and swallowing by obturating the cleft.

Although the original concept belongs to McNeil, Burston must be given credit for rationalizing the principles of the technique. It was he who continually emphasized the morphologic aspects of the cleft palate problem and the fact that ". . . at any given moment, a living organism will be in a state of dynamic equilibrium both within its own tissues and with its environment."[6] Perhaps because of his background, Burston tended to stress the importance of arch alignment more than McNeil, who placed greater emphasis on stimulating palatal closure.

During the next 20 years, more than 240 cleft specialists in the cleft palate field visited Liverpool to see Burston's work for themselves and to discuss the management of cleft palate patients with him. Following a terrible accident in 1973, Burston underwent 15 plastic surgery operations, and although he bravely returned to work afterward, his death in 1983 must have been a welcome release from suffering. The affection and respect with which friends, colleagues, and patients alike held him is commemorated by a window dedicated to his memory and to that of his colleague Peter Bush in the Chapel of Alder Hey Children's Hospital, Liverpool.[7] It is a unique tribute to a remarkable man. Since those days, 30 years ago, people have become much more restrained in their assessment of presurgical treatment. There is no longer the ". . . unbridled enthusiasm of innocent novices, misguided sheep and those who should know better," which stimulated Pruzansky to write his dissent. [8]

We now have a better appreciation of multidisciplinary management of clefts, but to understand what presurgical treatment actually does it is necessary to know how the maxillary arch of a unilateral cleft lip and palate patient differs from that of a normal child at birth (Fig. 70–2).[9–12] In such patients, the arch is too wide posteriorly because the absence of a functioning tensor

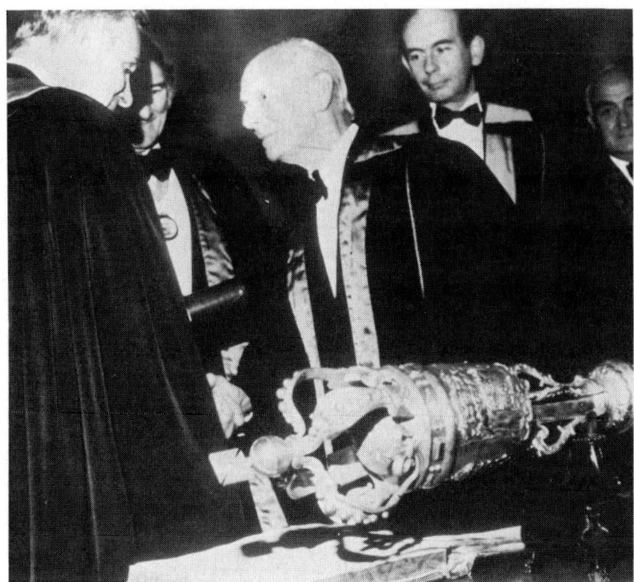

Figure 70–1 Kerr McNeil receiving an Honorary Fellowship from the University of Glasgow in 1986.

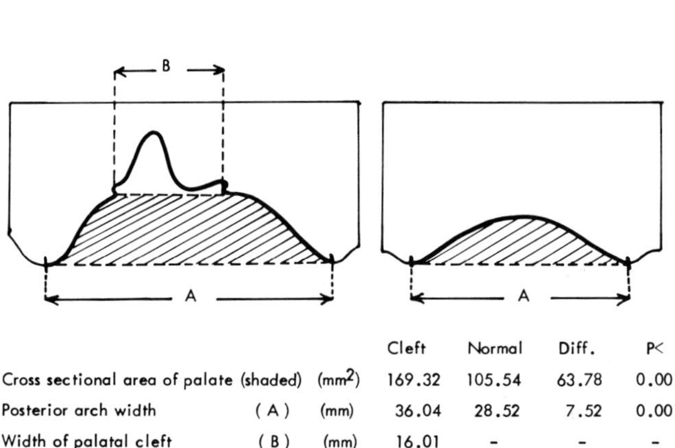

			Cleft	Normal	Diff.	P<
Cross sectional area of palate (shaded)	(mm²)		169.32	105.54	63.78	0.001
Posterior arch width	(A)	(mm)	36.04	28.52	7.52	0.001
Width of palatal cleft	(B)	(mm)	16.01	-	-	-

Figure 70–3 Transverse view of a unilateral cleft palate arch (left) and a normal arch (right) at birth. The place of section is 20 mm from the anterior dental papilla.[9] The posterior arch width (measurement A) is significantly greater in the cleft arch, as is the cross-sectional area of the palate (shaded). The sides of the palate also are steeper in the cleft patient compared with the normal. Wearing a presurgical appliance will reduce the cross-sectional area in the cleft subject to approximately the normal value and aid the development of normal tongue-tip behavior.

palati muscle leaves the outward pull of the pterygoids unopposed (Fig. 70–3). The center line is deviated to the intact side (Fig. 70–4) by a combination of muscle pull, the tongue's forcing its way into the cleft, and unilateral unrestrained growth of the cartilaginous nasal septum. This produces some distortion in the shape of the greater segment and perhaps some rotation as well, the axis of rotation being in the retromolar area. The lesser segment rotates with its posterior end displaced outward, and this defect may or may not be associated with some inward displacement of its anterior end as well (Fig. 70–2).

Because the sides of the palate slope more steeply upward than normal, the palate has nearly twice the normal cross-sectional area, giving the tongue a greatly increased space in which to work (Fig. 70–3). Finally, although the overall area of the arch is about 22% greater than normal, the area of palatal mucosa is about 16% less than that in a normal infant, suggesting that the maxilla is somewhat hypoplastic (Fig. 70–5).

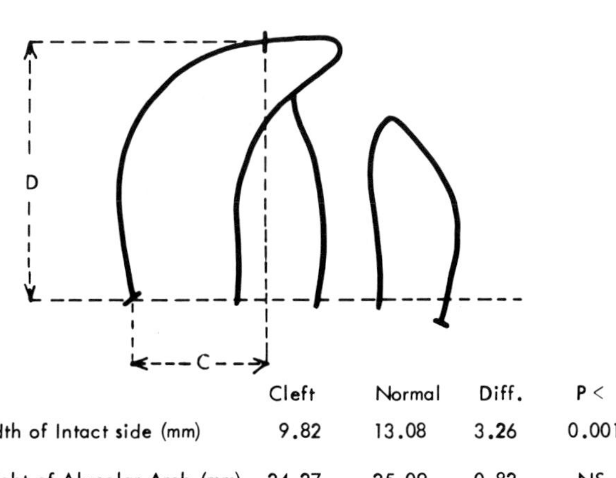

	Cleft	Normal	Diff.	P <
C = Width of Intact side (mm)	9.82	13.08	3.26	0.001
D = Height of Alveolar Arch (mm)	24.27	25.09	0.82	NS

NS = not significant

Figure 70–4 Greater segment at birth. The displacement of the center line to the intact side is shown by the smaller value of measurement C (width of the intact side) compared with that of a normal arch.[12] There is, however, no significant difference between cleft and normal subjects in the height of the alveolar arch (measurement D). From birth to 4 months of age, the increase in measurement D is almost identical in normal subjects and unilateral cleft palate subjects who did *not* receive presurgical treatment. The increase in the presurgical patients was slightly less (p < 0.05), probably because of the inhibiting effect of external strapping (From Huddart AG, Clark J, Thacker T: The application of computers to the study of maxillary arch dimension. Br Dent J 130:397–404, 1971).

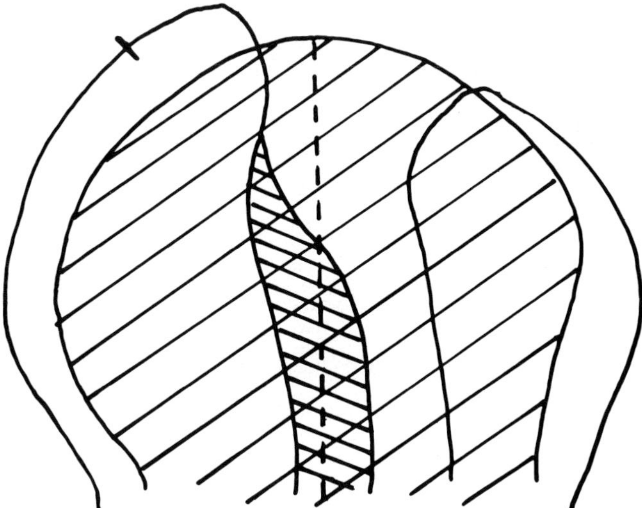

Figure 70–2 Outline of a normal (noncleft) maxillary arch superimposed on a unilateral cleft lip and palate arch at birth. The cleft arch is wider posteriorly, displacing the center line to the intact side. This may be associated with a rotation of the greater segment, the axis of rotation being located in the retromolar area. The lesser segment also is rotated, its tuberosity end displaced outward. There may be an inward displacement of its anterior end as well.

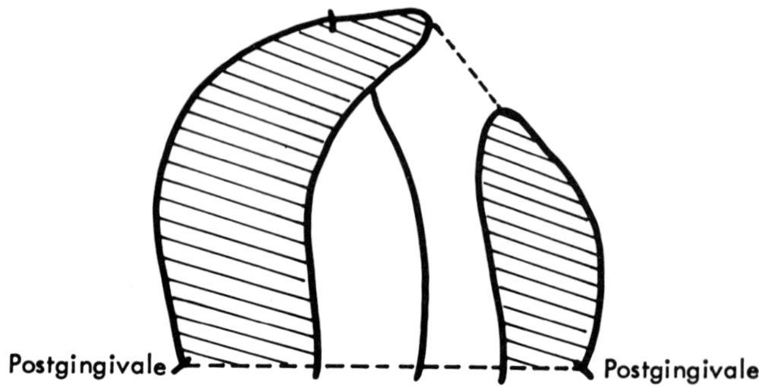

Figure 70–5 Overall area and area of palatal mucosa. The overall area, represented by the peripheral outline of the diagram, is a two-dimensional measurement. The area of palatal mucosa on the greater and lesser segments (shaded) is a three-dimensional concept involving depth. It can be measured accurately only by stereophotogrammetry or an equivalent method that takes depth into account.[11]

There are many different approaches to presurgical treatment,[5, 13–16] but ideally an impression should be taken as soon as possible after birth and an appliance inserted within the first 24 to 48 hours. Treatment may be carried out either with passive plates, which merely obturate the cleft, or with active appliances, that is, appliances that attempt to move the segments and reduce their displacement. In McNeil's original technique,[1] the active appliances were made by cutting the model along the line of the cleft and repositioning the lesser segment to reduce its displacement. The plate was then constructed on this modified model, so that when worn, it gradually corrected the position of the segment. In practice, a series of plates made on models, modified progressively toward normality, were used to achieve the desired segmental movement. These plates also carried stimulator pads that pressed gently on the palatal mucosa a short distance away from the margins of the palatal cleft. It was assumed that this pressure would stimulate growth of the underlying bone, thus reducing the width of the hard palate defect.

McNeil[3] put great emphasis on use of these stimulator plates (i.e., prepalatal repair) as a means of reducing the hard palate defect, stating that they should be worn up to the time of palate repair at about 18 months of age. The author, however, has found that it is very difficult to get babies to wear such appliances consistently much beyond the age of 4 to 6 months; this can be distressing for the parents because they feel that the failure in some way reflects on them personally.

In some centers external elastic strapping is also used in conjunction with the appliances to restrain the growth of the cartilaginous nasal septum and correct the center line.[5, 13] There are very few detailed reports of the results of presurgical treatment with active appliances,[17, 18] and in both the short term (up to the time of lip repair) and the long term, the results of using passive appliances appear to be equally as good.[12, 19–21]

The passive appliance the author has used for the past 30 years consists of a simple plate that merely covers the palatal cleft but does not extend into the nasal cavity. This serves to protect the underside of the nasal septum during feeding. The plate, however, does

extend well up into the buccal sulcus on each side to splint the segments and prevent them from moving farther apart (Fig. 70–6).

Two adjustable wire wings extend from the corners of the mouth and lie on the cheeks to prevent the baby from swallowing the appliance, and tape tied to the wings and stuck on the cheeks keeps the baby from pushing the appliance out of its mouth (Fig. 70–7). The plate is used in conjunction with external elastic strapping (Fig. 70–7), which in patients with unilateral clefts molds the anterior end of the greater segment to correct the center line displacement. To facilitate this result, the appliance is cut away anteriorly (Fig. 70–6).

A study of the effects of such treatment in the first 4 months of life revealed that the splinting action of the palate prevents the maxillary arch, which is already too wide at birth, from becoming wider as craniofacial growth proceeds.[12] In consequence, by 4 months of age the width of the arch approximates that of a normal child, whereas the palatal cleft is narrowed by up to 30% owing to the growth occurring at its margins. The treatment so reduces the width of the lip and alveolar clefts that the margins of the alveolar cleft may sometimes come completely into contact, although the author has never seen actual fusion of tissue as McNeil claimed. There is, however, a paradox: Although the defect is dramatically narrowed (Fig. 70–8), the treatment actually slightly reduces the rate of tissue growth on the margins of the palatal cleft. It certainly does not stimulate growth of hard or soft tissues, as McNeil claimed; instead, by reducing segmental displacement and preventing the arch from becoming any wider, it allows what growth there is to reduce the width of the cleft more effectively. As a result, the tissue shortfall (the width of the maxillary arch minus the width of palatal mucosa) is significantly improved, and surgical closure of the defect is facilitated.[22]

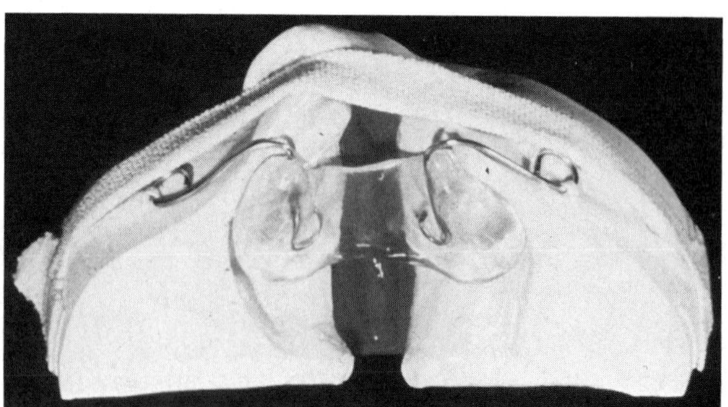

Figure 70–6 Model with passive presurgical appliance as used by the author. The plate bridges the palatal cleft and is 2 to 3 mm clear of the underside of the nasal septum to protect it from ulceration. It extends up into the buccal sulcus on each side to prevent the segments from moving apart as craniofacial growth proceeds. The plate is cut away anteriorly to allow the anterior end of the greater segment to be molded by the external strapping as the center line displacement is corrected. Projecting forward around the corners of the mouth, 1-mm hard-drawn, stainless steel, wire wings lie on the outside of the cheeks to prevent the plate being swallowed. Tape tied to the wings and attached to the cheeks with zinc oxide plaster keeps the baby from pushing the appliance out of its mouth.[14]

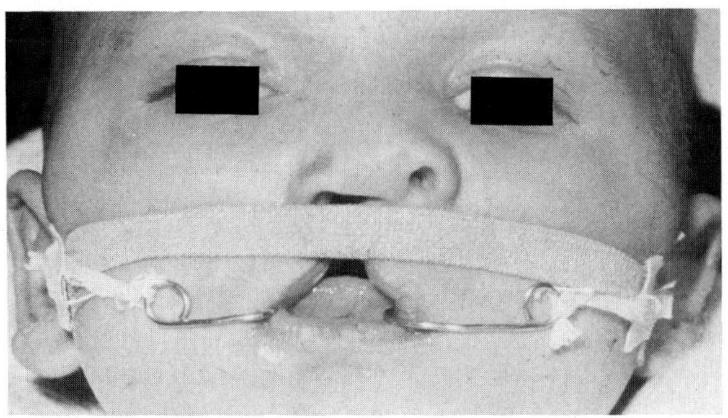

Figure 70–7 Baby wearing presurgical appliance and external elastic strapping. The wire wings on the outside of the cheeks keep the plate from being swallowed. The plate is inserted within 24 to 48 hours of birth, and the strapping is applied 2 to 3 days later. The appliance is worn continuously and is taken out for only a few minutes for cleaning after feeding. The strapping usually is changed once per day unless it becomes dirty.

Apart from correcting the center line, another effect of external strapping may be to restrict forward growth in the premaxillary area to reduce the height of the alveolar arch (Fig. 70–4). Ross, in an international multicenter study, commented that this restricted growth might encourage the formation of an increased class III incisor relationship in the older patient.[23]

Any adverse effect due to the strapping, however, would probably be relatively marginal compared to the benefits obtained by narrowing the lip and alveolar clefts to allow the surgeon to create a tension-free lip closure with minimal freeing of soft tissue from the surface of the maxilla. In the long term, the question of whether presurgical treatment results in a better facial aesthetic appearance because there is less postoperative segmental movement or a better dental occlusion because growth is normalized still remains to be answered. Unfortunately, it has not been possible to quantify and

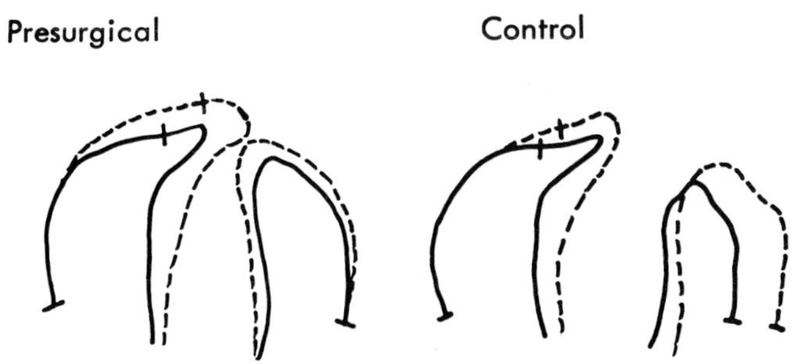

Figure 70–8 Maxillary arch changes from birth to 4 months. Effect of presurgical treatment (left) compared with a nonpresurgical (control) patient to whom no treatment was given (right). In the presurgical patient, the alveolar cleft is almost completely eliminated, but the posterior arch width has not increased because of the splinting action of the appliance (Fig. 70–6). There also is narrowing of the palatal cleft with a reduction in the tissue shortfall.[22] These changes were produced by one passive presurgical appliance and external strapping, as shown in Figure 70–6.

measure objectively the benefits of presurgical treatment separately from the total treatment received by a patient, and there appear to be no differences in appearance or occlusion between older patients who have received presurgical treatment and those who have not.

The case for presurgical treatment, therefore, must rest on subjective opinion, and in this respect people with long-term experience consider it a useful form of social medicine. It helps create a better working relationship with the parents and eases their acceptance of the child and his or her deformity. Presurgical orthopedic treatment facilitates feeding and, by narrowing the cleft, reduces the amount of muscle that must be freed to produce a tension-free repair (Fig. 70–8). Although the mother may harbor feelings of grief or guilt, she may not tell anyone. Her immediate involvement with the treatment—looking after the plate and strapping—almost certainly helps her come to terms with these feelings. The benefits obtained in this way, however, are impossible to quantify and measure objectively.

As far as skeletal pattern and occlusion in the older patient are concerned, no differences have been demonstrated between those with presurgical treatment and those without. The extravagant claims of Pruzansky's misguided sheep are false, therefore, at least in this respect. Ross came to a similar conclusion. "Presurgical orthopaedics in the neonatal period has no apparent long-term effect on facial growth in height and depth."[23] The treatment does have one benefit, however, and that is in relation to speech, because the abnormal swallowing pattern that a baby with a cleft lip and palate is forced to adopt could alter the motor action of the muscles common to speech and deglutition.

Stuffins found that 57% of older children who had received presurgical treatment had normal tongue-tip activity compared to 26% of children not treated in this way.[24, 25] The difference was significant at the 0.05% level and probably was due to the fact that the presurgical appliance reduces the excessive intraoral space found in cleft palate infants at birth to a more normal value and provides the semblance and feel of a normal intact palate to the mouth (Fig. 70–3). As a result, a more orthodox or normal pattern of tongue activity develops that, in Stuffins's view, leads to better speech. In the nearly 40 years of use of presurgical treatment, this is the only long-term benefit that can be specifically attributed to it. Everything else is speculation and opinion, but even so, this does not mean that such views should be dismissed.

Conclusion

With the perspective of hindsight, it is now possible to make a more balanced judgment of the benefits of presurgical treatment. The received opinion is that it is a useful adjunct to therapy—a useful preliminary measure that should be carried out whenever possible provided that it does not impose too much on the parents. We now better understand the role of presurgical orthopedic treatment in the total care of the cleft palate child, and in light of our increasing knowledge of the cleft condition, its application can be made a little more rational and perhaps a little less empirical than it was in the days of McNeil and Burston 40 years ago.

ACKNOWLEDGMENTS. I wish to thank Mr. T. Coote and the staff at the Photographic Department, Wordsley Hospital, and Mr. Nigel Beardsmore in the Photographic Department at the Royal Hospital, Wolverhampton, for the illustrations.

My grateful thanks also are due to Mr. G. McLennan and the University of Glasgow for permission to reproduce Fig. 70–1. In conclusion, I wish to express my appreciation and thanks to Mrs. K. Randle for her infinite patience in preparing the manuscript.

References

1. McNeil CK: Congenital oral deformities. Br Dent J 101:191–198, 1956.
2. McNeil CK: Orthopaedic principles in the treatment of lip and palate clefts. In Hotz R (ed): International Symposium on Early Treatment of Cleft Lip and Palate. Bern: Hans Huber, 1964, pp 59–67.
3. McNeil CK: Orthodontic procedures in the treatment of congenital cleft palate. Dent Rec 70:126–132, 1950.
4. McNeil CK: Oral and Facial Deformity. London: Pitman Medical Publishers, 1954.
5. Burston WR: The early treatment of cleft palate conditions. Dent Prac 9:41, 1958.
6. Forshall I, Osborne RP, Burston WR: Observations in the early orthopaedic treatment of cleft lip and palate conditions. In Hotz R (ed): International Symposium on Early Treatment of Cleft Lip and Palate. Bern: Hans Huber, 1964, pp 68–77.
7. Richards K: A unique tribute to two pioneers. Br Dent J 163:32–33, 1987.
8. Pruzansky S: Pre-surgical orthopaedics and bone grafting for infants with cleft lip and palate: A dissent. Cleft Palate J 1:164–187, 1964.
9. Huddart AG, MacCauley FJ, Davis MEH: Maxillary arch dimensions in normal and unilateral cleft palate subjects. Cleft Palate J 6:471–487, 1969.
10. Huddart AG, Clarke J, Thacker T: The application of computers to the study of maxillary arch dimensions. Br Dent J 130:397–404, 1971.
11. Huddart AG, Crabb JJ, Newton I: A rapid method of measuring the palatal surface area of cleft palate infants. Cleft Palate J 15:44–48, 1978.
12. Huddart AG: Presurgical changes in unilateral cleft palate subjects. Cleft Palate J 16:147–157, 1979.
13. Huddart AG: Presurgical dental orthopaedics. Trans Br Soc Orthod 107–117, 1961.
14. Huddart AG, Zilberman Y: Presurgical treatment in the newborn cleft palate infant. Is J Dent Med 26:15–25, 1977.
15. Robertson NRE: Oral Orthopaedics and Orthodontics for Cleft Lip and Palate. London: Pitman Medical Publishers, 1983.
16. Hotz M, Gnoinski W, Perko M, et al: The Zurich approach, 1964 to 1984. In Hotz M, et al: Early Treatment of Cleft Lip and Palate. Bern: Hans Huber, 1984, pp 42–48.
17. Robertson NRE, Hilton R: The changes produced by presurgical oral orthopaedics. Br J Plast Surg 24:57–58, 1971.
18. Shaw WC: Early orthopaedic treatment of unilateral cleft lip and palate. Br J Orthod 5:119–132, 1978.
19. Huddart AG: An analysis of the maxillary changes following presurgical dental orthopaedic treatment in unilateral cleft lip and palate cases. Trans Europ Orthod Soc 299–314, 1967.
20. Huddart AG: The application of computers to maxillary dimensional studies in cleft palate cases. Trans Europ Orthod Soc 363–371, 1971.
21. Sarnas K-V, Rune B, Jacobsson S: Changes in maxillary alveolar arch morphology in complete unilateral cleft lip and palate from birth to 19 months of age. In Hotz M, et al: Early Treatment of Cleft Lip and Palate. Bern: Hans Huber, 1984, pp 60–63.
22. Huddart AG, Crabb JJ: The effect of presurgical treatment on palatal tissue area in unilateral cleft lip and palate subjects. Br J Orthod 4:181–185, 1977.
23. Ross B: Treatment variables affecting facial growth in unilateral cleft lip and palate. Part 2: Presurgical orthopaedics. Cleft Palate J 24:24–32, 1987.
24. Stuffins GM: Speech and mental attitudes in the older presurgical child. In Kehrer B, et al: Long Term Treatment in Cleft Lip and Palate with Coordinated Team Approach. Proceedings of the First Symposium (1979). Bern: Hans Huber, 1981.
25. Stuffins GM: Tongue tip movement patterns in the unilateral cleft lip and palate child related to presurgical orthodontic treatment. Proceedings of the XIX Congress of the International Association of Logopaedics and Phoniatrics, August 14–18, 1983, University of Edinburgh, 1983.

CHAPTER 71

Infant Orthopedics and Later Orthodontic Monitoring for Unilateral Cleft Lip and Palate Patients in Zurich

Wanda M. Gnoinski

The use of plates or similar devices for covering the cleft palate in the newborn goes back at least to the turn of the century. The primary aim then was to render feeding feasible. Devices attached to a bottle were found to be of some help, but proper palatal plates were considered to be more effective because they gave some protection between meals as well.[1] Warnekros,[2] in the second edition of his monograph on cleft palate, advocated the routine use of soft rubber plates from the first days of life. Finding much similarity among the maxillae of unilateral, bilateral, and isolated palate clefts, War-

nekros intended to interest a manufacturer of rubber items in producing such devices. His effort waned, however, probably because of difficulties with material and lack of professional support. It is interesting that there is a distant parallel today.[3] An industrial anthropologist is now tackling the problem from the other end (in my opinion the wrong one) by designing a special nipple for cleft children that is meant to obturate the cleft *lip*.

Reintroduction of palatal plates for infants with clefts by McNeil[4] took place soon after the advent of acrylic resin in dentistry, which made procedures much simpler. Also, thermoplastic impression material had, in the meantime, replaced plaster, facilitating the task of taking an impression. A number of variations have developed from the McNeil technique.

Variation in Concepts and Appliances for Infant Orthopedic Treatment

"Active" McNeil-type approaches (Burston 1958, Brogan 1973, Huddart 1979, Roberston 1978) were modified in part but still actively approximate the maxillary segments to facilitate the surgeon's task of closing the lip.[5–7] Extraoral traction is sometimes still taken as an integral part of this procedure in patients with unilateral

clefts, although Burston[5] warned of its uncritical application. As a major exponent of the concept of active plates, Huddart[8, 9] repeatedly emphasized the need to restrain the maxillary segments in the transverse dimension, since the transverse distance between the pterygoid plates (and between the tuberosities) is excessive at birth. This influenced the design of his hard acrylic plate, which encompasses the maxilla to avoid an increase in width, thus taking into account the objections of Swoiskin[10] and Pruzansky,[11] derived from Subtelny's studies.[12] As a logical consequence, Huddart[9] also supported Malek and Psaume's concept of velar closure around the age of 3 months, which intends to reduce excessive pharyngeal width at an early age.[13]

An even more active device, the so-called T-traction, was advocated by Nordin et al in Stockholm.[14] By means of a T-shaped acrylic device and extraoral anchorage, lateral force is exerted on the anterior portion of the nasal septum in unilateral cleft patients with a severely deviated major maxillary segment. A plate may be used at the same time. This method does not seem to appeal to most professionals and has not come into widespread use.

Active, pin-retained plates[15, 16] have been the subject of much dissent. Although Jorgenson and his colleagues[17] have asserted the innocence of these plates in regard to damage of the developing teeth, the author cannot but consider them an overreaction to the problem in question.

"Passive" plates, used in conjunction with early lip repair and autogenous bone grafting, were introduced by the team from the Children's Memorial Hospital in Chicago after a trial period with the McNeil technique.[18–20] This specific approach has given rise to much controversy, but in the hands of those who developed it, it evidently works well.[21] Probably close cooperation between the orthodontist and surgeon as well as "surgical finesse" are the decisive factors.[22] Maintenance of the lateral maxillary dimension is a main concern in this method, and therefore the appliance ends at the height of the alveolar ridge and is unable to restrain transverse development of the maxilla.[19]

Passive plates used in conjunction with delayed surgical procedures[23] were introduced in Zurich in the mid-1960s after a frustrating 7-year period during which McNeil-type orthopedic treatment was applied along with "conventional surgery."[24] The current procedure is detailed below. In contrast to other types of plates, the "Zurich appliance" is a combination of both soft acrylic (which provides adaptability to the buccal side of the plate) and hard acrylic (which provides stability across the palatal vault). Although the plate penetrates into the cleft to some extent, stability is not provided by lining undercuts with soft material as in Rosenstein's technique,[18, 19] but by adhesion and functional adaptation as in complete dentures. Serving as a mold for the spontaneous relocation and growth of the maxillary segments after repositioning of the tongue in the oral cavity, such plates are worn continuously for about 16 months. They must be replaced after approximately 6 months. Grinding on the gingival side of the plate is performed every 3 to 8 weeks, depending on the child's growth rate; this gradually provides more space for development of the maxillary segments in the desired direction. A posterior extension to the tips of the cleft uvula is a specific feature of this appliance and renders swallowing more normal; proper adaptation of the posterior extension is, of course, a prerequisite. This adaptation seems to be a major obstacle for some clinicians who tried to adopt similar approaches.[25] The means needed to overcome this problem are a working knowledge of cleft palate muscle anatomy and repeated observation of soft palate function with the plate inserted. It has to be emphasized that the Zurich-type plate is meant to allow spontaneous development without the tongue or other mechanical interference in the cleft. No claim is made as to "stimulation" of growth.

A "growth stimulator" was proposed by Weil.[26] Although this device is very similar in appliance design to the Zurich plate, the basic intention is very different because, reverting to McNeil's original claim,[4] growth stimulation is postulated. Appliance therapy is continued subsequent to soft palate closure, and Weil states that ". . . usually no complementary surgical correction of the hard palate is necessary." This last statement is likely to elicit reactions of doubt and dissent from various sides.

This enumeration of the various concepts covers just the main lines and certainly is not complete, since individual variation is a keyword for clinicians dealing with cleft patients. A recent and rather comprehensive review of long standing was provided in a congress report;[27] more references are to be found in the state-of-the-art reviews by Spriestersbach et al[28] and Berkowitz et al[29] as well as in textbooks on cleft treatment.

The Zurich Approach to Treatment of Unilateral Cleft Lip and Palate

Hotz[30] described the first steps taken toward the current treatment routine, and Hotz and Gnoinski[23] provided a comprehensive review of the procedures used. The surgical procedures, intimately related to the orthopedic principles applied, were detailed by Perko,[31, 32] who also deals with them in his contribution to this book (Chap. 38). In summary, the procedures utilized consist in a modified Millard lip repair performed at 6 months of age, soft palate repair at around 18 months, and hard palate repair when the child is between 4 and 5 years. Hotz et al summarized the evolution of the therapeutic approach.[27]

Infant Orthopedic Treatment

Treatment is started in the first week of life and continues for 16 to 18 months. On an average, three plates are used, and 15 monitoring sessions are necessary during this period of time. The total cost of this treatment phase is equal to the base tariff for 8 days in the Zurich University Children's Hospital, or 50% of average orthodontic treatment of a class case with fixed appliances in Switzerland. ay be able to relate this to the possible effects of the procedure as requested by Berkowitz.[29]

Nursing. The plate's function in nursing is mentioned first because the primary concerns in dealing with a newborn cleft patient are pediatric more than orthodontic.[33] The dorsal extension of the plate (Fig. 71–1), as mentioned earlier, appears to allow a more normal pattern of deglutition. This conclusion is based on clinical observation of a number of patients coming to our clinic from abroad, where they were fitted with other types of plates that did not prevent massive aerophagia and the corresponding intestinal trouble. Within a day or two after we add a posterior extension to the child's plate and instruct parents in feeding technique, mothers report a striking improvement in the general condition of the child. This is a typical result.

In our routine cases, bottle-feeding is initiated by ourselves after adapting the plate, making sure that neither breathing nor velar movements are impeded. No breathing problems[25] have ever occurred in our 440 patients who had various types of palatal clefts and since 1969 have been fitted with the plates described. In addition, newborns readily accept the plates. This acceptance in turn facilitates matters for the parents and, together with solid clinical experience in adapting plates to the patient, prevents episodes of anxiety as described by Dorf et al.[34]

Children with a unilateral or bilateral cleft normally cope with the entire quantity of formula appropriate for their age after an adaptation period of 1 to 4 days and do not take more time per meal than noncleft babies. This seems preferable to the "hard work for nourishment" reported for children fed by means of plastic bottles with spoon like attachments.[35] Nasal regurgitation while drinking or aspiration between meals[36] has not occurred in our sample. By the time their mothers are dismissed from the hospital, babies can usually be

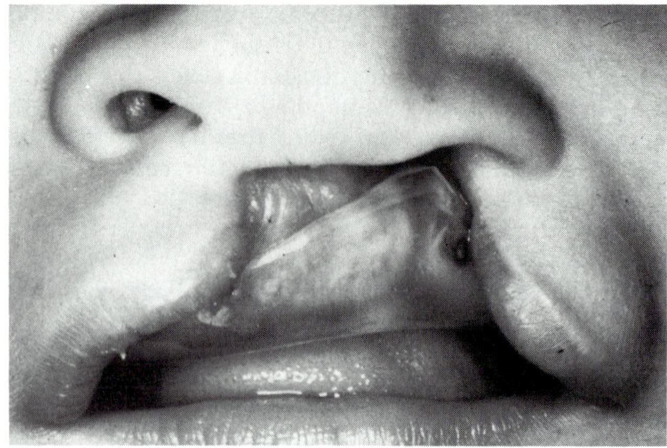

Figure 71–2 Zurich-type plate in situ. Note tongue posture.

dismissed as well; prolonged inpatient care is not necessary. In contrast to reports by Pashayan and Lichtenstein[37] and Jensen et al,[38] weight gain has never been a problem except for patients with rare syndromes. A statistical investigation of this issue is now under way. Breast feeding is the great exception; despite the plate, most children are not able to build up the vacuum necessary for efficient suckling.

Tongue Posture. In newborns with complete unilateral cleft lip and palate the anterior portion of the tongue is very often twisted vertically and positioned within the cleft. No one has investigated, to our knowledge, how long this habit persists and how it might also affect speech development. At any rate, it is eliminated by wearing a plate of appropriate design that also covers the anterior part of the cleft and provides near normal support for the tongue tip. One condition is that the acrylic material reach the level of the occlusal plane in the cleft area (Fig. 71–2). Dorsal displacement of the tongue, which Malek and Psaume[13] consider a regular feature in cleft patients, definitely does not occur in our patients (except for the initial situation in patients with the Pierre Robin anomalad). The tongue tip can be observed in its normal position above the lower alveolar process during feeding. One might hypothesize that extension of the plate down to the tips of the split uvula helps to prevent dorsal displacement of the tongue.

Position of the Maxillary Segments. In the newborn, both alveolar cleft width and the relative position of the maxillary segments are extremely varied (Table 71–1, Fig. 71–3). The most common configuration in our material (57 complete unilateral cleft patients documented from birth to at least age 5) was a rather large cleft in the alveolar area (9 to 16 mm) as well as in the palate (11 to 17 mm). When differentiating alveolar cleft width into anteroposterior and transverse components, we found that relationships between these components ranged between 1:3.5 and 1:1.3 in 65% of the patients (Fig. 71–3). Ratios of around 2:1 in wide clefts (over 13 mm), retrospectively, seem most likely to create problems (relative retroposition of the lesser segment) later on. Wood[39] observed the same thing. Fortunately, there are few (3%) clefts of this kind in our material. Otherwise, no simple pattern of reaction could be distin-

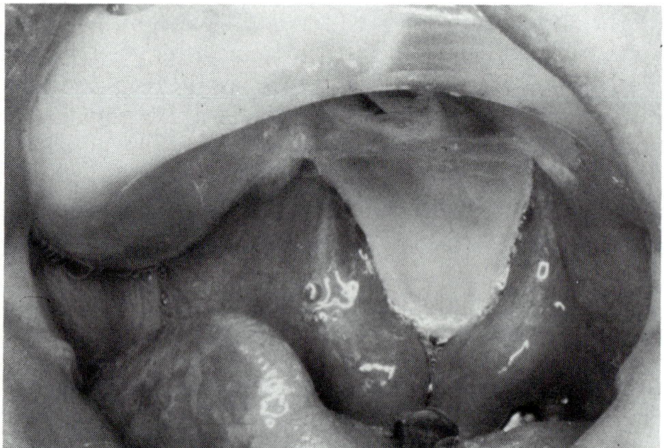

Figure 71–1 An infant orthopedic plate in situ according to the Zurich design. Note the posterior extension obturating also the velar cleft and the contour of the plate in the cleft area, where it follows the occlusal plane level, thus providing support for the tongue.

Table 71-1. Initial Cleft Width in Millimeters (N = 57)

	Minimum	Maximum	Mean/SD	75% Were Within
Alveolar cleft	3.6	19.0	11.97/3.25	9–16 mm
Palatal cleft	7.5	20.0	14.00/3.40	11–17 mm

guished, which seems to confirm Stockli's findings.[40] Further information might be gathered from the highly complex evaluation of infant casts proposed by Schwartz and his associates.[41]

With the plate described, a mold for spontaneous relocation and growth of the maxillary segments is created. Space is provided by periodically grinding material from the gingival side of the plate as development proceeds. Thus, optimal use can be made of the intrinsic tendency toward normalization that many authors have already described.

To solve a problem noted by Wood,[42] particular emphasis is put on relieving the anterior end of the major segment also in a vertical direction to permit downward development of this portion and eruption of the deciduous incisors into a normal vertical position without causing them to tip toward the cleft. Such tipping, considered typical for cleft patients,[43] rarely has been found in our sample. The "tissue deficiency from birth" in the anterior segment reported by Mapes et al,[44] might be a projection effect due to the initial problem mentioned.

Together with improvement of arch form, the difference in the level of the alar base on the cleft and noncleft sides is considerably reduced, providing a more favorable basis for surgical repair. This anteroposterior effect is considered much more important than the mere reduction of cleft width. The major changes in the alveolar area take place prior to lip repair (age 6 months) and right after. The plate is reinserted immediately after the operation and thus evenly distributes the action of the repaired orbicularis oris muscle; further approximation of the maxillary segments can be guided. The clinical effects are obvious, but objective assessment of segmental reactions is extremely difficult because of the lack of reference structures. Wada and Miyazaki's method[45] of reverting to higher cranial structures has its drawbacks, and even metallic implants cannot solve the problem completely.[46, 47]

In patients who are approximately 18 months of age, prior to the first step in palate repair (soft palate), we generally have found a good intermaxillary relationship and good arch form (40% abutment); another 35% showed good arch form but the alveolar segments were

still at some distance. The latter patients were usually those with extremely wide clefts initially in whom care had been taken not to let the arch collapse too fast. We found slight segmental overlap in 15% of the patients, i.e., in all patients with a supernumerary fissural tooth, and in some in whom a vestibularly based Burian flap had been used for closing the alveolar gap at lip repair.

As to the width of the palatal cleft, an average reduction of 45% of the initial width took place between birth and 18 months of age. This figure coincides with that of O'Donnell et al, who reported an overall reduction of 45.4% in mean posterior cleft width between birth and 13 to 18 months.[48] In 75% of our patients, maximum palatal cleft width as measured on the casts was between 5 and 10 mm (Table 71–2A). Direct measurement of the maximum distance between the bony shelves in the posterior portion of the hard palate performed during soft palate surgery showed a consistent difference of 2 to 3 mm between bone and cast measurements. This difference corresponded to the average total thickness of the soft tissue cover on both cleft margins.

Other Aspects of Infant Orthopedic Treatment. Many authors have claimed a positive psychological effect from early treatment. Pashayan and Lichtenstein,[37] on the other hand, were afraid that plates would give the parents, orthodontist, and physician a false sense of security. From our own experience, we can say that after early contact with clinicians who took time to explain the problem and its prospective solution honestly, concerned parents relaxed considerably and were able to deal with the situation on a team-approach basis. Acceptance of the plate is hardly ever a problem provided that the appliance is fitted as early as possible by an experienced and skilled clinician. Consequently, the parents' ability to cope is not particularly stressed; failure to accept the plate has never occurred in our sample. Within a week, babies learn how to feed without needing excessive time or conspicuous devices and thrive normally. This eases pressure on the family and facilitates acceptance of the child.

On reading the report by Dorf et al,[34] one might even be tempted to hope for a positive effect of the Zurich-type plate on the development of speech articulation. Because the plate provides two separate functional entities instead of a common oronasal cavity, it may be beneficial also for upper airway and middle ear conditions, as Oliver[49] and Oblak[50] have presumed.

Monitoring Development in the Deciduous Dentition Period

During the deciduous dentition period, the patient is seen once a year together with a speech clinician. Emphasis is on speech assessment and counseling of the parents. Orthodontic treatment is hardly ever performed during this period because there is no need, and most of its effects cannot be expected to last.

In our sample, arch form at 5 years of age was largely the same as that at 18 months. Altogether, 77% of patients showed good arch form, although 14% still had

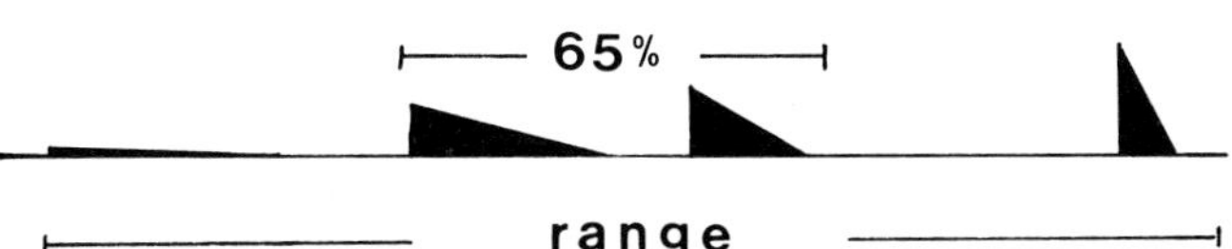

Figure 71–3 Schematic representation of segmental relationship in the alveolar cleft area showing the ratio of anteroposterior and transverse components in cleft width in complete unilateral cleft lip and palate patients (UCLP). N = 57.

Table 71–2. Maximum Width of the Palatal Cleft in Millimeters

	Minimum	Maximum	Mean/SD	80%
A. 18 months of age (N = 56)	2.3	12.9	7.7/2.4	Below 10 mm
B. 5 years of age (N = 46)	0.4	8.1	3.5/2.1	Below 5 mm

Note: The reduction in width between 18 months and 5 years is evident. Total reduction since birth (see Table 71–1) is about 75% of the initial width.

clinically irrelevant gaps of less than 2.5 mm. Maximum cleft width in the hard palate area was less than 5 mm in 80% of the sample (Table 71–2B). Other findings for the 5-year level were published earlier.[51, 52]

Change of Dentition

Monitoring of patients is intensified during the change of dentition. Patients are seen twice a year until all central incisors and 6-year molars have erupted. The main reason is early detection of possible undermining resorption of second deciduous molars by first permanent molars. However, this problem is now much less common than it was prior to the change in surgical approach. Unpublished data give us reason to assume that good functional results of lip surgery, permitting unhindered forward development of the maxilla, are the reason for this improvement. As to the incisors, our material cannot corroborate the findings of Ogidan and Subtelny[43]—that is, marked palatal inclination of the incisor germs is neither a problem on eruption nor does it increase with ongoing eruption. However, torsion and lateral tipping of the central incisors adjacent to the cleft do occur.

Orthodontic correction of incisor position at this stage is undertaken only in the few patients in whom malocclusion impedes occlusal function. If proper information is provided to patient and parents, it does not prove difficult, in our population, to postpone incisor correction to a later stage when it can be included in the comprehensive final treatment, thus reducing overall treatment time.

Extraoral forward traction on the maxillary arch for crossbite correction, as advocated for treatment of anterior crossbite at this stage by Delaire[53] and Rygh and Tindlund,[54] might not solve the problem in the long run. In light of experimental work done by Jackson et al,[55] one must suspect that there is a considerable tendency toward relapse, particularly the effect of forward fraction on the dentition. In addition, the excessive bone apposition in the tuberosity area, which is necessary for stabilization of the forward displacement of the maxilla, cannot take place for two reasons. On one hand, there is the counterpressure of a tight lip 24 hours a day, which has already brought about the condition to be treated by inhibiting normal forward/downward displacement of the maxilla with growth, and on the other hand, scarring in the pterygomaxillary region after extensive tissue mobilization for palate closure, which hampers bone apposition. Although the clinical effects of such forward traction were documented by a metallic implant study,[56] unfortunately not much information is available about the functional status prior to treatment, for example, premature contacts.

Among our patients, a few have a hereditary class III or a true maxillary tissue deficiency (congenital absence of one half of the premaxilla), in which the deformity clearly is so extreme that orthopedic treatment alone will not solve the problem. Their treatment is postponed until the time of permanent dentition and is then carried through in accord with maxillofacial surgery. The rest of our sample showed a good anteroposterior skeletal relationship at this stage.

Monitoring and Orthodontics in the Late Mixed and Permanent Dentition Period

If feasible, active therapy is postponed until the time of permanent dentition to reduce treatment time. The highest aim, of course, is a full complement of permanent teeth in both arches in good alignment on sagittally balanced skeletal bases. To this end, secondary alveolar bone grafting around the age of 10 years, as developed by the Oslo group (Bergland, Semb, and Abyholm 1986),[57] is very valuable if there is a fissural tooth of sufficient root diameter or a definite orthodontic indication for space closure in "extraction cases" with surplus tooth material in both the upper and lower arches.

For the following reasons, we find it difficult to share the general optimism regarding bone grafting prior to eruption of the canine on the cleft side. Bone in the alveolar area tends to resorb within 6 to 12 months unless teeth are moved into it, and certainly it is difficult to predict eruption of the canine. Our own experience in the late 1960s with less sophisticated grafting techniques showed that "postgrafting" eruption of canines did not necessarily occur in the graft area. El Deeb et al reported similar problems.[58] Our patients usually do not lack space in the lesser maxillary segment, and there is rarely a need to provide additional bone for the canine. Therefore, in most instances we prefer to have the teeth in question ready for fixed-appliance placement to start tooth movement 1 to 2 months after surgery, as Boyne originally suggested.[59]

Extractions for lack of space are preferably postponed until shortly before placement of the orthodontic appliance to take full advantage of the space gained for selective alignment. It should be stressed in this context that extractions in the lower arch are considered only when they are mandatory for correct alignment of the lower dentition per se relative to its skeletal base. With a view to long-term development, it is not considered wise to consider dental compensation for sagittal skeletal imbalance by extracting in the lower arch only. By doing so prior to cessation of pubertal growth, one may jeopardize the success of final treatment in patients in whom dental compensation ultimately proves insufficient, and maxillofacial surgery still is indicated for correction of the basic skeletal disharmony. Such patients do exist; the problem is to spot them early. One possible way of doing so has recently been developed (Gnoinski 1987)[60] but more data must be gathered.

Our experience with final orthodontic treatment in our patients according to the current approach is very limited because few patients are over 15 years old. Yet the success of their treatment has proved to be very similar to that of noncleft patients, and treatment results are almost always stable.

Results up to 10 Years of Age

After eruption of the central and lateral incisors, 72% of our sample presented with lack of space in the anterior portion of the maxillary arch, which exceeded 5 mm in 26% of patients. Frequently there also was lack of space in the mandibular arch.

Cephalometric results for the 10-year age group were published by Hotz et al.[27] Clinically, the most relevant fact was the good anteroposterior skeletal relationship found in 80% of the sample (Fig. 71–4). Maxillary arch measurements (Table 71–3) were made on standardized photographs of casts.[52] A sample of 19 complete unilateral cleft lip and palate patients was compared to a randomly selected group of 21 noncleft individuals of the same age provided from the collection of Prof. B. C. Leighton, King's College Hospital, London. A Wilcoxon test was performed to reveal significant differences. The intertuberosity width in the unilateral cleft group did not significantly differ from normal, but the total alveolar crest length (segmental measurements) and the anterior arch width (L–L')[40] were found to be significantly smaller in the unilateral sample. However, it should be noted that this sample included ten patients (53%) in which Burian flaps had been used for closing the alveolar gap at the time of lip repair. Such flaps obviously tend to push the lesser segment in a palatal direction.

Development up to 15 Years of Age

Eleven of the 19 patients mentioned above are now between 15 and 18 years of age. Contrary to what was often found in patients with "conventional" primary surgery, their anteroposterior facial pattern, as assessed

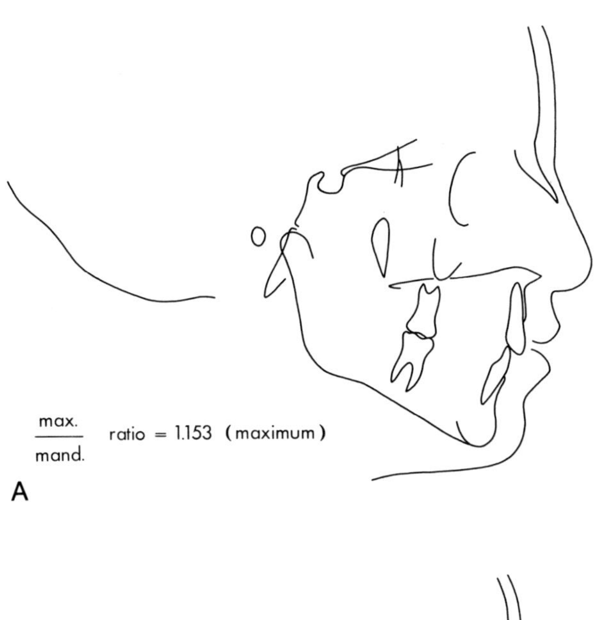

A

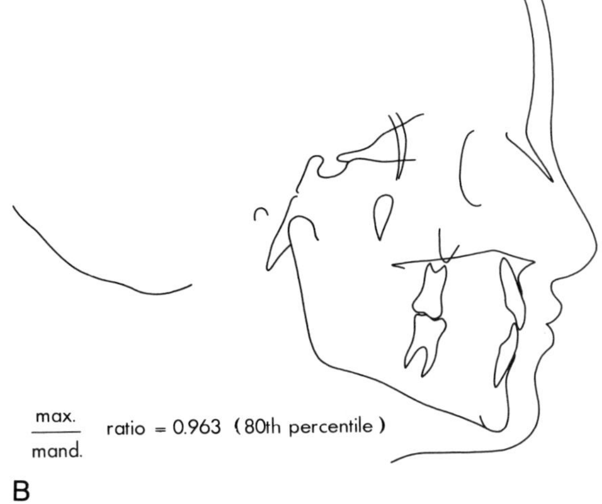

B

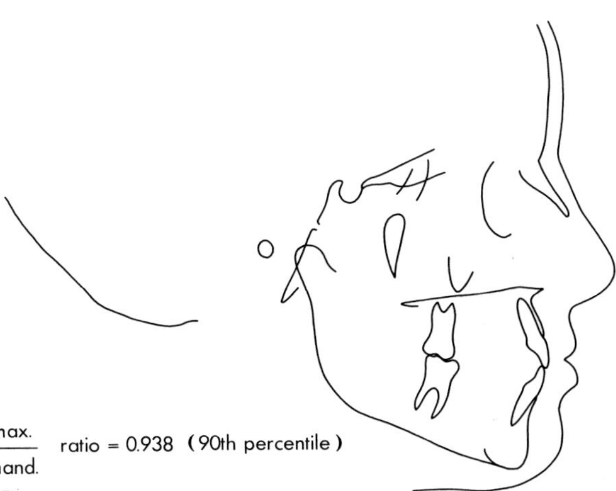

C

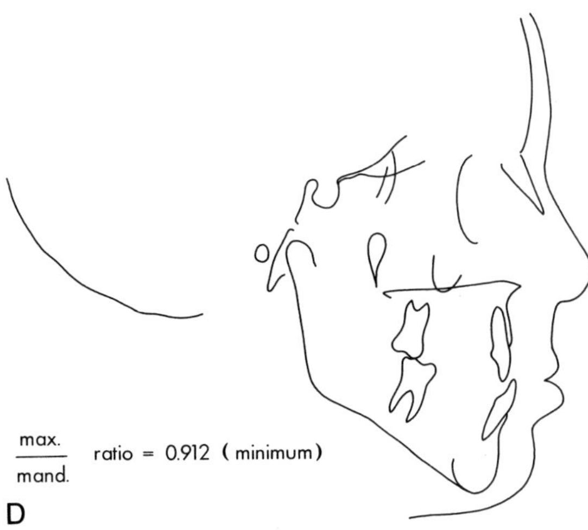

D

Figure 71–4 The range of anteroposterior facial balance in 10-year-old patients with complete cleft lip and palate. Individuals are classified according to their "upper to lower skeletal length ratio."[60–62] *A* and *B*, Of 18 UCLP patients, 80% have the range of facial balance illustrated by these two individuals. *C* and *D*, The two individuals delineating the worst 10% of UCLP profiles in the sample examined (consecutive patients born 1969 to 1974).

Table 71–3. Alveolar Arch Parameters (age 10 for noncleft [N = 21] and complete UCLP [N = 19])

	Total Crest Length		Tuberosity Width		Width at Level of Lateral Sulcus	
	Normal	*Cleft*	*Normal*	*Cleft*	*Normal*	*Cleft*
Minimum	98.74	93.63	36.71	37.65	29.85	26.32
Maximum	116.63	112.20	49.48	50.75	38.84	36.13
Mean	108.36	102.46[a]	41.76	43.23	34.11	30.03[a]
SD	5.67	5.68	2.81	4.06	2.79	2.72

Application of a Wilcoxon test ($2\alpha = 0.05$) revealed significant differences in total crest length and anterior width at the level of the anterolateral sulcus (points L–L′ according to Stockli[40]). Note: 10 UCLP patients (53%) had Burian flaps for closure of the alveolar gap at lip repair.

by the Enlow analysis,[61] did not show a relevant change between ages 10 and 15; their maxillae appeared to grow in proportion to the mandible.[62] Orthodontic treatment was started late and has been finished in only four patients.

No particular problems occurred in treatment, and retention appliances were not worn any longer than in noncleft orthodontic cases. Of course, growth has not yet ended in the males of this age, but all of these patients are past the maximum intensity of growth. If a prognosis of their ultimate sagittal skeletal balance is made on the basis of the Enlow analysis, we would expect 75% to 80% of them to end up with a good facial pattern.[62]

Conclusions

It now has been more than 30 years since various centers took up infant orthopedic treatment on a large scale, yet many questions have not been fully answered, or the critiques have not been completely rebutted on the basis of "documentary proof" as called for by Pruzansky.[11] The toughest question, regarding the influence of infant orthopedic treatment on the end result of cleft lip and palate treatment, will probably never be answered conclusively. The reason is that infant orthopedic methods are just one aspect of relatively short duration in a complex sequence of spontaneous development and treatment procedures acting on the orofacial structures over a period of about 20 years.

From all available information (e.g., Dahl 1981, Lennartsson and Friede 1984, Robertson 1973),[62a, 63, 64] it seems that variations in surgical procedures have a far stronger influence on orofacial development in cleft patients than do most other factors. In this context, the term *variation in surgical procedures* does not apply only to techniques characterized by keywords such as Millard, Tennison, Langenbeck, Wardill, Schweckendiek, or one-stage or two-stage palatal repair, nor to the timing of interventions alone. Even approaches carried out under the same label by different people yield rather divergent results (see Chapter 38 of this book).

Despite all the reservations, it now seems possible to make several statements concerning infant orthopedic methods. Orthopedic treatment certainly is not the panacea for which many people have taken it. Neither is it the procedure to be used when resources are scarce. It has, however, passed the test as a valuable ancillary measure in various basic approaches wherever surgeons were willing to cooperate and orthopedic clinicians were working long enough, with their eyes open for improvement, to acquire expertise. One hopes that good long-term documentation and interinstitutional exchange may shed more light on this aspect of cleft treatment. It should be borne in mind, however, that to evaluate a single procedure, no other factor in the sequence of events should be altered.[65] This seems obvious, but it rarely has been taken into account in past clinical research.

Our own experience and documentation show that in a suitable overall concept:

1. If proper adaptation is provided, the benefits of the plate as a feeding aid are self-evident to those most concerned—nursing staff and parents.

2. Excessive initial pharyngeal width will normalize without early application of force. Intertuberosity width in 5-year-old unilateral cleft lip and palate patients was found to correspond closely to normal after a primary treatment that exerted only limited transverse force through soft palate closure at 18 months of age, whereas the orthopedic plate had been designed to maintain maxillary width or even let it increase spontaneously.[52]

3. The growth potential of the cleft maxilla, often called into question, is close to normal. Our experience[66] and the evidence presented in this chapter indicate that under appropriate circumstances cleft maxillae develop surprisingly well in regard to both reduction in palatal cleft width during the first 18 months (while posterior arch width is maintained) and sagittal and vertical development as demonstrated in cephalometric measurements. Viscerocrania do tend to be smaller in cleft patients, but a harmonious facial pattern can still develop.

4. With the possibility that palatal cleft width will be significantly reduced prior to soft palate surgery, more tissue should be available to contribute to the length of the soft palate instead of using it for bridging cleft width. An indirect effect on velopharyngeal competence might be expected.

All things considered, we recommend infant orthopedics treatment when conditions are suitable. However, reports of good long-term results from centers with extremely different approaches have led to the conclusion that the decisive factor for success in the cleft field is a well-coordinated sequence of procedures carried out by a team of highly skilled specialists with the utmost consideration for developmental processes.

References

1. Martin C, Martin F: Prothese labio-palatine, permettant la succion chez le nouveau-ne atteint de gueule-de-loup compliquee de bec-de-lievre. Rev Stomatol 14:519–531, 1907.
2. Warnekros K: Gaumenspalten, 2nd ed. Berlin: Hirschwald, 1909.
3. Hummel S: Eine Saughilfe für Sauglinge mit Lippen-Kiefer-Gaumenspalte. Fortschr Kieferorthop 48:26–33, 1987.
4. McNeil CK: Congenital oral deformities. Br Dent J 101:191–198, 1956.
5. Burston WR: The early orthodontic treatment of cleft palate conditions. Dent Pract 9:41–56, 1958.
6. Brogan WF, McComb HK: The early management of cleft lip and palate deformities. Aust Dent J 18:212–217, 1973.
7. Robertson NRE: The orthodontic management of cleft lip and palate patients. Part 2. Pre-surgical oral orthopaedics. Br Dent J 145:236–240, 1978.
8. Huddart AG: Presurgical changes in unilateral cleft subjects. Cleft Palate J 16:147–157, 1979.
9. Huddart AG: The effect of form and dimension on the management of the maxillary arch in unilateral cleft lip and palate conditions. Scand J Plast Reconstr Surg 21:53–56, 1987.
10. Swoiskin BL: Discussion. Angle Orthod 33:135–137, 1963.
11. Pruzansky S: Pre-surgical orthopedics and bone grafting for infants with cleft lip and palate: A dissent. Cleft Palate J 1:164–187, 1964.
12. Subtelny JD: Width of the nasopharynx and related anatomic structures in normal and unoperated cleft palate children. Am J Orthod 41:889–909, 1955.
13. Malek R, Psaume J: Nouvelle conception de la chronologie et de la technique chirurgicale du traitement des fentes palatines. Resultats sur 220 cas. Ann Chir Plast Esthet 28:237–247, 1983.
14. Nordin KE, Larson O, Nylen B, et al: Early bone grafting in complete cleft lip and palate cases following maxillofacial orthopedics: I. The method and the skeletal development from seven to thirteen years of age. Scand J Plast Reconstr Surg 17:33–50, 1983.
15. Hagerty RF, Mylin WK, Hess DA: The pin-retained expandable prosthesis in cleft palate treatment. J South Carolina Med Assn 61:221–229, 1965.
16. Latham RA: Orthopedic advancement of the cleft maxillary segment: A preliminary report. Cleft Palate J 17:227–233, 1980.
17. Jorgenson RJ, Salinas CF, Hirsch H: The pin-retained palatal prosthesis and its influence on the dentition. J Dent Res 58:1570–1571, 1979.
18. Rosenstein SW: Early orthodontic procedures for cleft lip and palate individuals. Angle Orthod 33:127–137, 1963.
19. Rosenstein SW, Jacobson BN: Early maxillary orthopedics: A sequence of events. Cleft Palate J 4:197–204, 1967.
20. Monroe CW, Griffith BH, Rosenstein SW, et al: The correction and preservation of arch form in complete clefts of the palate and alveolar ridge. Plast Reconstr Surg 41:108–112, 1968.
21. Helms JA, Speidel TM, Denis KL: Effect of timing on long-term clinical success of alveolar cleft bone grafts. Am J Orthod Dentofac Orthop 92:232–240, 1987.
22. Jacobson BN, Rosenstein SW: Early maxillary orthopedics for the newborn cleft lip and palate patient: An impression and an appliance. Angle Orthod 54:247–263, 1984.
23. Hotz M, Gnoinski W: Comprehensive care of cleft lip and palate children at Zurich University: A preliminary report. Am J Orthod 70:481–504, 1976.
24. Hotz R: The indication for preoperative and postoperative orthopedic treatment of cleft lip and palate. In Hotz R (ed): Early Treatment of Cleft Lip and Palate. Bern/Stuttgart: Hans Huber, 1964, pp 78–82.
25. Björk G: Frühbehandlung von Kindern mit Lippen-Kiefer-Gaumenspalten. Technische Modifikation. Fortschr Kieferorthop 47:380–384, 1986.
26. Weil J: Orthopaedic growth guidance and stimulation for patients with cleft lip and palate. Scand J Plast Reconstr Surg 21:57–63, 1987.
27. Hotz M, Gnoinski W, Perko M, et al: The Zurich approach, 1964 to 1984. In Hotz M, et al (eds): Early Treatment of Cleft Lip and Palate. Toronto: Hans Huber, 1986, pp 42–48.
28. Spriestersbach DC, et al: Clinical research in cleft lip and cleft palate: The state of the art. IV. Pediatric and otologic aspects. Cleft Palate J 10:122–126, 1973.
29. Berkowitz S, et al: Cleft lip and palate research: An updated state of the art. Section III. Orofacial growth and dentistry. Cleft Palate J 14:288–301, 1977.
30. Hotz MM: Pre- and early postoperative growth—guidance in cleft lip and palate cases by maxillary orthopedics (an alternative procedure to primary bone grafting). Cleft Palate J 6:368–372, 1969.
31. Perko M: Two-stage closure of cleft palate. J Maxillofac Surg 7:76–78, 1979.
32. Perko M: Closure of the hard palate in unilateral cleft palate cases following previous closure of the soft palate according to the Widmaier-Perko technique. Chir Testa e Collo 1:9–13, 1984.
33. Scheuerle J, Olsen S, Guilford AM, et al: A survey of nursing care for parents and infants with cleft lip and palate. Cleft Palate J 21:110–114, 1984.
34. Dorf DS, Reisberg DJ, Gold HO: Early prosthetic management of cleft palate. Articulation development prosthesis: A preliminary report. J Prosthet Dent 53:222–226, 1985.
35. Asher C: Neonatal care of infants with clefts of the lip and palate. Br Dent J 160:438–439, 1986.
36. Pashayan HM, McNab M: Simplified method of feeding infants born with cleft palate with or without cleft lip. Am J Dis Child 133:145–147, 1979.
37. Pashayan HM, Lichtenstein GA: Growth pattern of infants with isolated cleft of the palate with or without cleft lip treated with presurgical orthopedics. Read before the 33rd meeting of the American Cleft Palate Association, New Orleans, February, 1975.
38. Jensen BL, Dahl E, Kreiborg S: Longitudinal study of body height, radius length and skeletal maturity in Danish boys with cleft lip and palate. Scand J Dent Res 91:473–481, 1983.
39. Wood BG: Maxillary arch correction in cleft lip and palate cases. Am J Orthod 58:135–150, 1970.
40. Stockli PW: Evaluation of Maxillary Arch Form in Complete Unilateral Cleft Lip and Palate Cases. Thesis. Chicago: Northwestern University, 1969.
41. Schwartz BH, Long RE, Smith RJ, et al: Early prediction of posterior crossbite in the complete unilateral cleft lip and palate. Cleft Palate J 21:76–81, 1984.
42. Wood BG: Three-dimensional arch correction in patients with unilateral cleft lip and palate. Am J Orthod 61:501–507, 1972.
43. Ogidan O, Subtelny JD: Eruption of incisor teeth in cleft lip and palate. Cleft Palate J 20:331–341, 1983.
44. Mapes AH, Mazaheri M, Harding RL, et al: A longitudinal analysis of the maxillary growth increments of cleft lip and palate patients. Cleft Palate J 11:450–462, 1974.
45. Wada T, Miyazaki T: Growth and changes in maxillary arch form in complete unilateral cleft lip and palate children. Cleft Palate J 12:115–130, 1975.
46. Rune B, Sarnas K-V, Selvik G: Oral orthopedics and movement of maxillary segments: A roentgen stereophotogrammetric study. Cleft Palate J 16:385–390, 1979.
47. Rune B, Sarnas K-V, Selvik G, et al: Movement of the cleft maxilla in infants relative to the frontal bone: A roentgen stereophotogrammetric study with the aid of metallic implants. Cleft Palate J 17:155–174, 1980.
48. O'Donnell JP, Krischer JP, Shiere FR: An analysis of presurgical orthopedics in the treatment of unilateral cleft lip and palate. Cleft Palate J 11:374–393, 1974.
49. Oliver HT: Neonatal orthodontics. Trans Eur Orthod Soc, 1973, pp 562–563.
50. Oblak P: Basic principles in the treatment of clefts at the University clinic for maxillo-facial surgery in Ljubljana, and their evolution in thirty years. In Hotz M, et al (eds): Early Treatment of Cleft Lip and Palate. Toronto: Hans Huber, 1986, pp 123–125.
51. Hotz MM, Gnoinski WM, Nussbaumer H, et al: Early maxillary orthopedics in CLP cases: Guidelines for surgery. Cleft Palate J 15:405–411, 1978.
52. Hotz MM, Gnoinski WM: Effects of early maxillary orthopaedics in coordination with delayed surgery for cleft lip and palate. J Maxillofac Surg 7:201–210, 1979.
53. Delaire J: La croissance maxillaire: Deductions therapeutiques. Trans Eur Orthod Soc, 1971, pp 81–102.
54. Rygh P, Tindlund R: Orthopedic expansion and protraction of the maxilla in cleft palate patients: A new treatment rationale. Cleft Palate J 19:104–112, 1982.
55. Jackson GW, Kokich VG, Shapiro PA: Experimental and postexperimental response to anteriorly directed extraoral force in young *Macaca nemestrina*. Am J Orthod 75:318–333, 1979.
56. Friede H, Lennartsson B: Forward traction of the maxilla in cleft lip and palate patients. Eur J Orthod 3:21–39, 1981.
57. Bergland O, Semb G, Abyholm FE: Elimination of the residual alveolar cleft by secondary bone grafting and subsequent orthodontic treatment. Cleft Palate J 23:175–205, 1986.
58. El Deeb M, Messer L, Lehnert MW, et al: Canine eruption into grafted bone in maxillary alveolar cleft defects. Cleft Palate J 19:9–16, 1982.
59. Boyne P: Use of marrow-cancellous bone grafts in alveolar and palatal clefts. J Dent Res 53:821–824, 1974.
60. Gnoinski W: Early identification of candidates for corrective maxillary osteotomy in a cleft lip and palate group. Scand J Plast Reconstr Surg 21:39–44, 1987.
61. Enlow DH, Moyers RE, Hunter WS, et al: A procedure for the analysis of intrinsic facial form and growth. Am J Orthod 56:6–23, 1969.
62. Gnoinski W: Orofacial development up to age 15 in UCLP cases treated according to the current Zürich approach. In Pfeifer G (ed): Craniofacial Anomalies and Clefts of Lip, Alveolus and Palate. Principles of Treatment, Long-Term Results; 4th Hamburg International Symposium. Stuttgart: G. Thieme, 1989.
62a. Robertson NRE: Early treatment—A critique. Trans Eur Orthod Soc 547–551, 1973.
63. Dahl E, Hanusardottir B, Bergland O: A comparison of occlusions in two groups of children whose clefts were repaired by three different surgical procedures. Cleft Palate J 18:122–127, 1981.
64. Lennartsson B, Friede H: Effect of post-surgical jaw-orthopedic treatment in unilateral cleft lip and palate patients. Scand J Plast Reconstr Surg 18:227–231, 1984.
65. Hellquist R: Discussion. In Hotz M, et al: Early Treatment of Cleft Lip and Palate. Toronto: Hans Huber, 1986, p 156.
66. Hotz MM: Orofacial development under adverse conditions. Eur J Orthod 5:91–103, 1983.

CHAPTER 72

Presurgical Orthopedic Treatment in Unilateral Cleft Lip and Palate

M. Fára, Ž. Müllerová, and Z. Šmahel

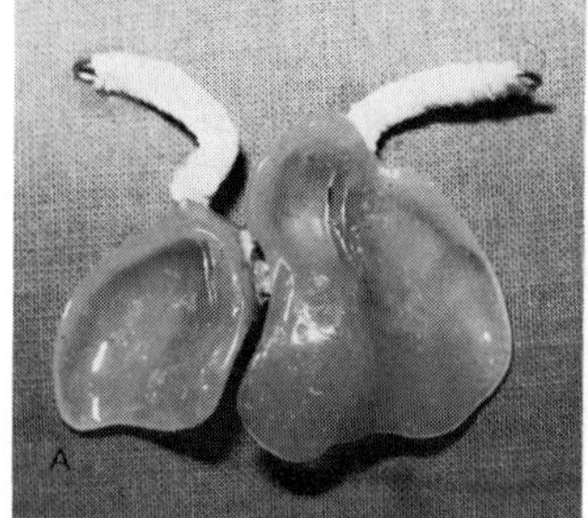
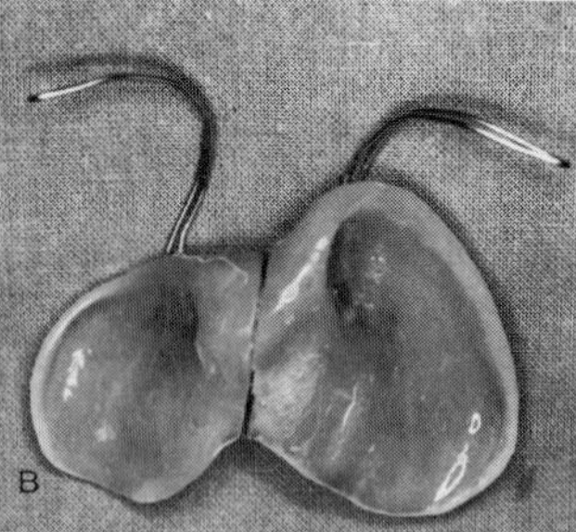

Figure 72–1 *A* and *B*, Upper appliance with a screw for preoperative orthopedic therapy of unilateral cleft lip and palate.

Correction of secondary maxillofacial deformities following cleft lip and palate repair presents a difficult problem. Every available means must be considered to prevent the development of these anomalies or to reduce their severity. Modern surgical techniques for cleft lip and palate repair have substantially reduced the frequency of secondary maxillofacial deformities. Presurgical orthopedic treatment presents an attractive alternative for establishing the proper position of the maxillary segments prior to cleft lip repair that avoids serious maxillofacial growth disturbances. Presurgical orthopedic treatment has attracted many clinicians and investigators. When the initial enthusiasm for this treatment subsided, critical reviews appeared in the literature expressing diverse opinions.

History

McNeil,[1] who originated the concept of presurgical orthopedic treatment, based it on early use of an intraoral appliance that in patients with unilateral complete clefts led to proper alignment of the maxillary segments in a relatively short time. This treatment resulted in a reduction of cleft width in both skeletal and soft tissues. Improvement of the position of the skeletal base led to marked improvement in the symmetry and balance of the nasal structures. Presurgical orthopedic treatment has an especially strong influence on the positioning of the base of the ala and on the shape of the ala and nostril on the cleft side.

Numerous observations have suggested that presurgical orthopedic treatment failed to prevent midfacial growth aberrations in the anteroposterior and vertical dimensions. Perhaps congenital dysmorphogenesis and various degrees of hypoplasia led to maxillary growth inhibition. Despite these observations, presurgical orthopedic methods gained popularity and were used in many cleft centers, including the Department of Plastic Surgery at Charles University in Prague. It was assumed that this treatment technique could provide better conditions for facial growth and occlusion and an improved skeletal base for surgical repair of the lip and palate (Figs. 72–1 to 72–4).

Among the first authors in the early 1950s who reported the results of presurgical orthopedic treatment with optimistic expectations were Nordin and Johanson,[2] Schmid,[3] Burston,[4] and Brauer, Cronin, and Reaves.[5] Georgiade[6] was the first to pin the appliance to the palatal segments. Latham[7] subsequently devised and described an intraoral appliance that appeared to exploit the anteroposterior adjustment potential of maxillary sutures. Hotz and Gnoinski[8] modified the procedure and continue to use it in the majority of their cases.

Starting in the mid-1960s, presurgical orthopedic treatment was frequently combined with primary bone grafting. Some investigators were critical of both procedures performed simultaneously, whereas others enthusiastically reported favorable results. In this respect, data reported by Pruzansky[9] were of considerable importance. Pruzansky was highly critical of combining presurgical orthopedic treatment with primary bone grafting. His paper was followed by numerous reports of failures recorded several years after presurgical orthopedic treatment and bone grafting had been used.[10–12]

Skoog[12] rejected presurgical orthopedic methods as unnecessary and not helpful, suggesting that the well-performed lip repair would mold and reposition the maxillary segments into proper alignment. Ross[13] pre-

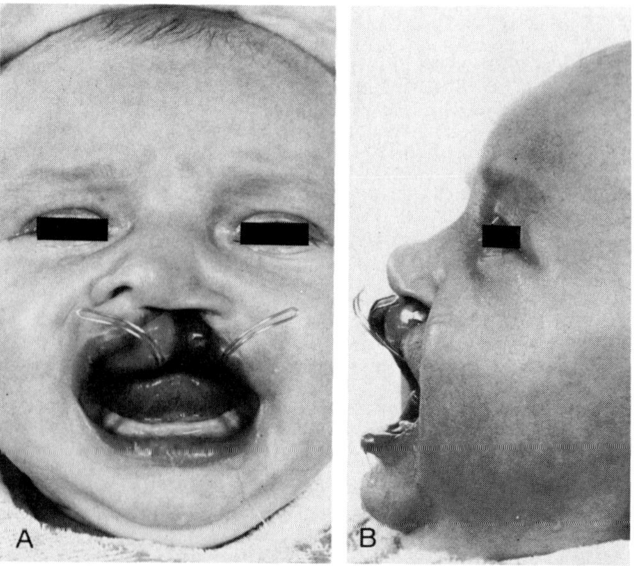

Figure 72–2 *A* and *B*, Unilateral cleft lip, alveolus, and palate. Preoperative orthopedic therapy with an upper appliance.

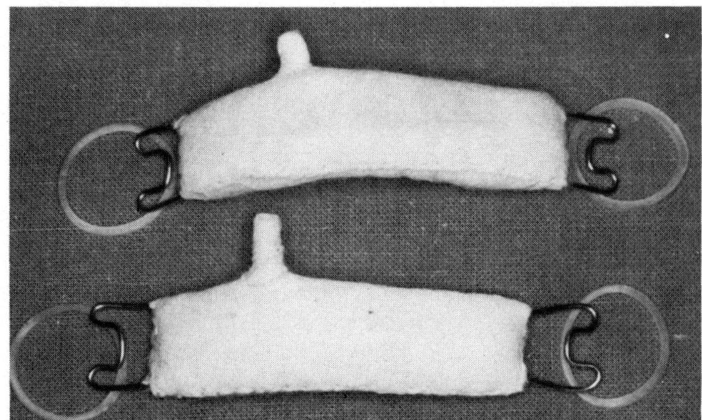

Figure 72–3 Traction bands for preoperative orthopedic therapy of unilateral cleft lip and palate with nostril plugs differing in height for correction of nasal asymmetry.

sented an objective and critical review of various means of achieving positive or negative effects in facial growth and development, among which he discussed the use of presurgical orthopedic treatment.

The Department of Plastic Surgery in Prague has used multidisciplinary treatment for many years. Every year 140 to 150 new patients have primary cleft lip repair, and a similar number have primary cleft palate repair. Between 1964 and 1973, patients with complete unilateral clefts of the lip, alveolus, and palate underwent primary bone grafting of the alveolar cleft. The rib was used as the source for the bone graft, and results were studied in a long-term follow-up report in 1983.[14] In the earlier period, patients who had alveolar bone grafting also had presurgical orthopedic treatment as a preparation for the bone grafting.

Facial growth and development following bone grafting was compared by means of lateral cephalometric measurement (Fig. 72–5) to that of patients with the same cleft form who had had primary periosteoplasty or had been treated without bone grafting and without a periosteal flap. In all patient series, palatoplasty consisted of a push-back procedure with a simultaneous pharyngeal flap when the child was about 4 to 5 years of age. Figure 72–6 shows a comparison of individuals with and without bone grafting at 10 years of age. Each group included 30 boys and 25 girls treated at our orthodontic department with removable appliances only. Presurgical orthopedic treatment was not used in the patients in these studies.

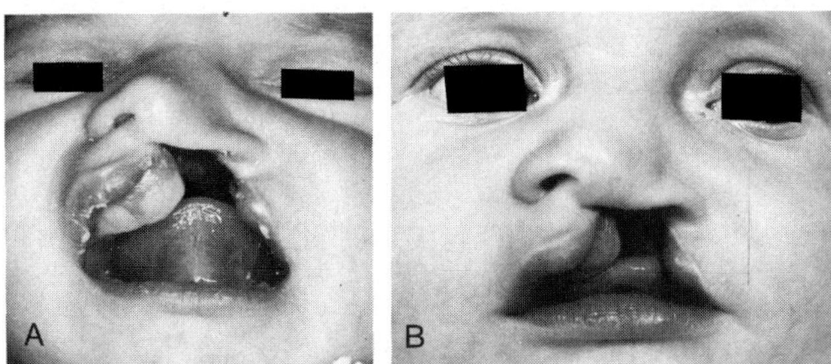

Figure 72–4 A and B, Unilateral cleft lip, alveolus, and palate. Before and after treatment using a traction band with a plug prior to cleft lip surgery.

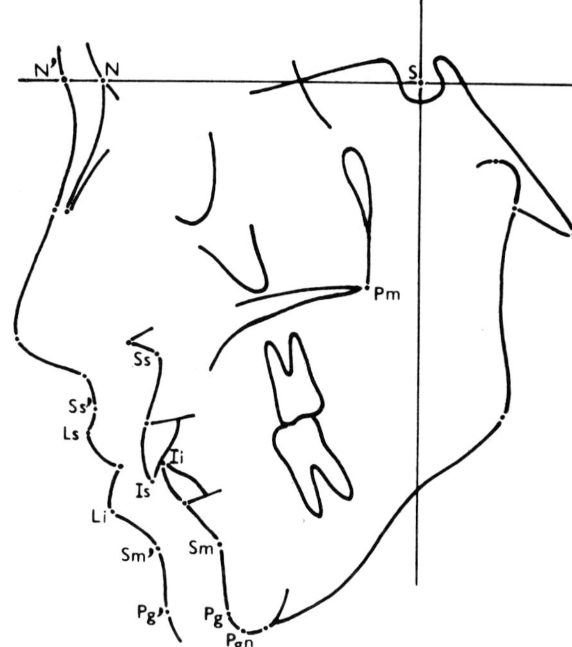

Figure 72–5 Cephalometric points. Point A′ = Ss′ (soft subspinale); point B′ = Sm′ (soft supramentale). Overjet Is–Ii (incisor superius to incisor inferius) was measured parallel to occlusion plane. Lip prominence was measured as projective distance between Ls (labiale superius) and Li (labiale inferius) perpendicular to the line connecting N (nasion) and Pg (pogonion).

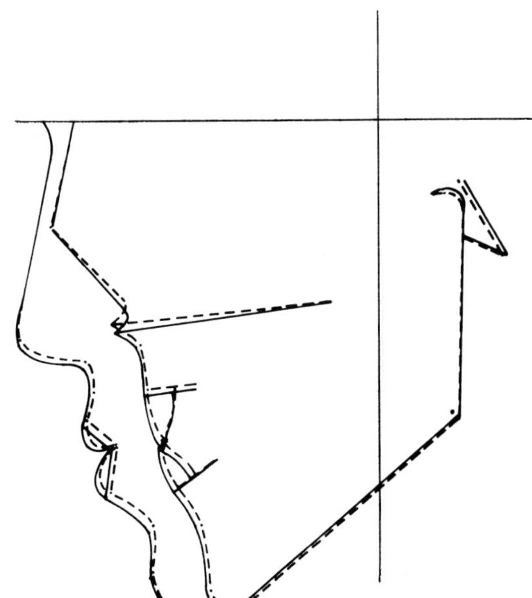

Figure 72–6 Craniograms for patients with complete unilateral cleft lip and palate, with and without primary bone grafting at the age of 10 years (30 boys and 25 girls in each group).

Individuals with bone grafts showed a marked deficiency in the vertical dimension of the midface and a marked retroinclination of the upper incisors. The deficiency of anterior maxillary growth, impairment of anteroposterior occlusal relations, and anterior crossbite were of a similar degree in both series. The width of the dentoalveolar arch measured on the dental models from birth to 15 years of age also failed to disclose any differences between individuals with and without bone grafts (Fig. 72–7). Following palatal surgery, both groups (boys and girls) showed a similar narrowing of the dentoalveolar arch, indicating that early bone grafting failed to prevent collapse of the maxillary segments. There also were no differences between the two groups at 15 years of age.

Periosteoplasty Versus Bone Grafting

Our investigation failed to prove that early bone grafting had a beneficial effect on maxillofacial growth. On the contrary, some parameters used in our study suggested a detrimental effect. These findings stimulated us to abandon early alveolar bone grafting in 1973 and use primary periosteoplasty at the time of primary cleft lip repair instead. Figure 72–8 presents the results recorded in 10-year-old patients (35 boys) who had periosteoplasty compared to those obtained in patients treated previously with early bone grafting (30 boys). Definite improvements following periosteoplasty compared to early bone grafting consisted in less retrusion of the maxilla and better prominence of the upper lip. A positive overjet was restored by orthodontic treatment.

Basic parameters for all three series are presented in Figure 72–8. The mean values indicated an improvement in anteroposterior occlusal relations (ANB) and in

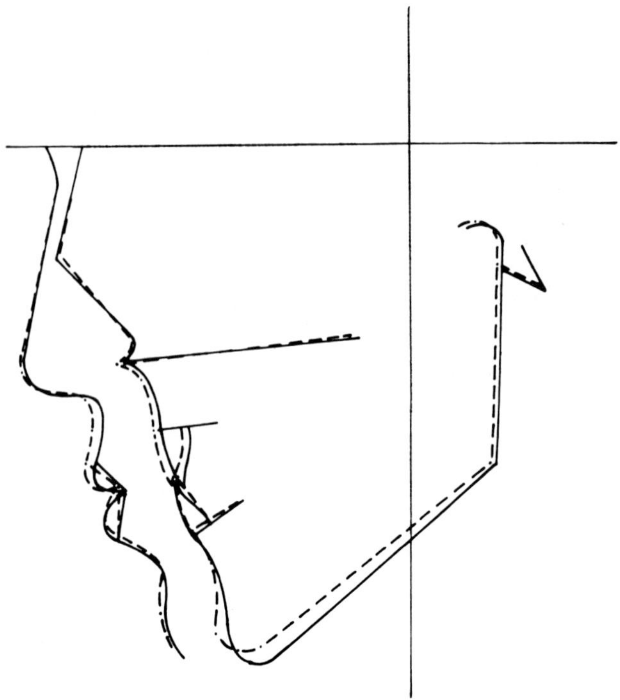

UCLP$_c$ – 10 years		ANB	Is – Ii	A'N'B'	Ls ⊥ Li
——	G	1.2	−0.9	4.5	0.5
	O	1.7	−0.8	5.5	1.0
− − −	P	2.3	+0.7^x	6.1^x	2.7$^{xxx}_{++}$

Figure 72–8 Craniograms for patients with complete unilateral cleft lip and palate (UCLPc) with primary osteoplasty (G) and primary periosteoplasty (P) at the age of 10 years. Mean values of basic parameters are presented, including values for individuals without graft or periosteal flap (0). There were 30 to 35 boys in each group ($\times$ = significant difference between P and G at $p < 0.05$; $\times \times \times$ = $p < 0.001$; $++$ = significant difference between P and O at $p < 0.01$.

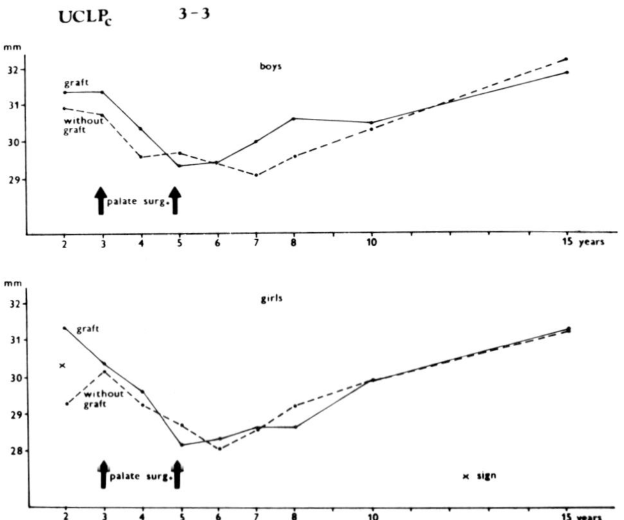

Figure 72–7 Growth curves of the distance between both cuspids in patients with complete unilateral cleft lip and palate, with and without primary osteoplasty (semilongitudinal study, each group containing 30 to 50 patients).

the overjet (Is–Ii). According to our findings, the best results were obtained in the group of patients in whom a periosteal flap was used to bridge the alveolar defect at the time of cleft lip repair. The next group included patients who had neither bone grafting nor a periosteal flap. The worst results relative to facial growth and occlusion occurred in patients who had early bone grafting.

Patients who had periosteoplasty showed improvement of the facial soft profile (A'N'B') and prominence of the upper lip (Ls–Li). This improvement was significant compared to results in two other groups. The favorable occlusion observed in these patients provided a basis for a subsequent adequate development of the mandible and for improved anteroposterior occlusal relations. It is important to understand that this improvement was the result not only of a surgical procedure but of orthodontic treatment as well.

Since the major growth problems occur during the pubertal spurt, one would expect the differences between the reported series to increase further during this time. Longitudinal growth studies confirmed an unsatisfactory developmental trend during this period in individuals between the ages of 10 and 15 who had had early bone grafts (Fig. 72–9). The anterior growth of the maxilla (measured at point Ss) was only half the value of mandibular growth (point Pgn); this resulted in a definite aberration of anteroposterior maxillomandibular relations (ANB). Yet in spite of this adverse trend, orthodontic treatment succeeded in maintaining the previously present level of occlusion of the incisors (Is–Ii).

Assessment of these patients indicated that anteroposterior occlusal relations did not improve but deteriorated during the above-mentioned period in 73% of the patients under study. In approximately 43% of the patients there was an improvement in the anterior occlusion, whereas another 43% of the patients displayed a deterioration of the occlusion. Our series of children with primary periosteoplasty is still younger than 15 years, and thus definite assessment is not yet possible.

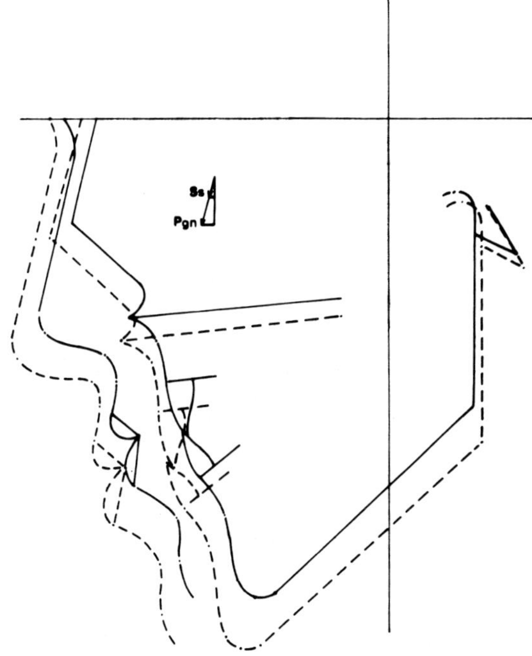

graft	ANB	Is–Ii	Ls ⊥ Li
—— 10 years	1.6	−0.7	0.5
- - - 15 years	−0.3	−0.8	0.2
better	0 %	43 %	33 %
the same	27	13	23
worse	73	43	43

Figure 72–9 Craniograms in patients with complete unilateral cleft lip and palate (UCLPc) with primary bone graft at age 10 and 15 years. Arrows indicate direction and amount of growth in Ss and Pgn points. Types of changes occurring between 10 and 15 years are expressed in percentages.

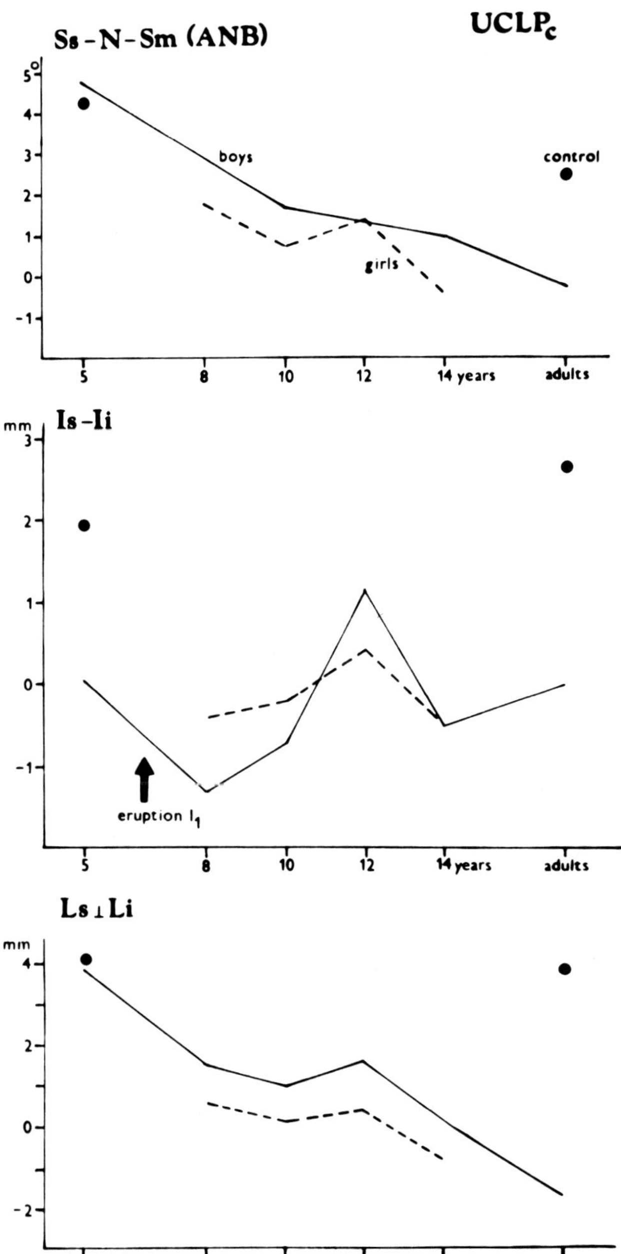

Figure 72–10 Growth curves in sagittal occlusal relations (ANB), overjet (Is–Ii, incisor superius–incisor inferius), and upper lip prominence (Ls–Li, labiale superius–labiale inferius) from the time of palate surgery up to adult age. Patients had neither bone graft nor periosteal flap (semilongitudinal study up to 14 years and including a group of adults). Individual age groups consisted of 20 to 30 boys and the same number of girls.

The third series of patients treated without bone grafts or periosteal flaps was followed at intervals of 2 years from the age of 5 years to 14 years. An analysis of the data in this series was supplemented with values obtained in another series of adults operated on using the same method during approximately the same period of time (1955 to 1963). The development of three clinically important characteristics is presented in Fig. 72–10.

Anteroposterior occlusal relations deteriorated gradually throughout the whole period, and thus after the age of 5 years the difference from controls gradually increased. In spite of this adverse growth trend, orthodontic treatment improved anterior occlusion from the condition of the anterior crossbite to an overjet by 12 years of age. During the pubertal spurt there was impairment of occlusion, and even intense orthodontic therapy failed to maintain the previously attained good results. This impairment occurred in all probability because of the maxillary growth inhibition combined with normal mandibular growth. This disproportion between maxillary and mandibular growth cannot be overcome by the compensation mechanism within the dentoalveolar components of both jaws. Prominence of the upper lip deteriorated simultaneously with anteroposterior occlusal relations. The slight improvement at the age of 12 years was due to the attained overjet.

These observations indicated that the main problems in facial growth developed only after surgical repair of the palatal cleft, particularly during puberty (Fig. 72–11). The effects of presurgical orthopedic treatment have no influence on maxillofacial growth and development during these periods. Table 72–1 shows a comparison of individuals with primary osteoplasty with and without presurgical orthopedic treatment as well as the group of patients treated without bone grafting or a periosteal flap. Each group included about 20–30 males with complete unilateral clefts.

In spite of the small differences in the ages of the patients in individual series, it is evident that the length and protrusion of the maxilla and anteroposterior occlusal relations were most favorable in patients who had not had bone grafting. The most unsatisfactory results were found in patients who had had early bone grafting combined with presurgical orthopedic treatment. However, the differences between individuals with or without presurgical orthopedic treatment and bone grafts were not significant. Because after the age of 15 years the impairment in maxillary protrusion and anteroposterior occlusal relations continued (see Fig. 72–10), one could expect equal values in adults with and without presurgical orthopedic treatment.

The other three characteristics (that is, facial convexity, anterior occlusion, and prominence of the upper lip) differed only slightly between individual series. These observations confirmed that during the long term

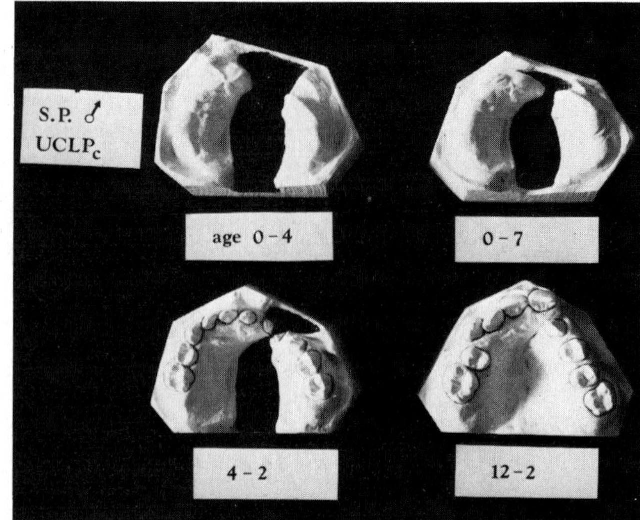

Figure 72–11 Complete unilateral cleft lip, alveolus, and palate. The initiation of preoperative orthopedic therapy at 4 months of age. Upper jaw casts at 4 and 7 months of age, prior to lip surgery; casts taken at 4 years 2 months of age, prior to palate closure; casts taken at 12 years 2 months, before initiation of orthodontic therapy. Preoperative orthopedic treatment failed to prevent subsequent upper jaw malformations.

facial growth and development was not affected by presurgical orthopedic treatment, and the final results of facial growth were no different from those found in individuals who had not had presurgical orthopedic treatment.

The effect of presurgical orthopedic methods is of rather short duration and thus in our opinion is completely eradicated by subsequent growth and development occurring in the postoperative period. We believe that the main developmental problem is deficient maxillary growth following palatoplasty. This obviously persists because of the adverse effects of certain factors that are impossible to control—e.g., bony cleft in the hard palate, congenital skeletal and soft tissue hypoplasia, altered anatomic and functional relations, and scar tension.

Assessment of maxillary models in 30 patients with unilateral cleft lip, alveolus, and palate (15 boys and 15 girls) obtained during the period between lip repair with alveolar bone grafting and palatoplasty (none had presurgical orthopedic treatment; Fig. 72–12) revealed

Table 72–1. Mean Values of X-ray Cephalometric Characteristics in UCLP_c Individuals Treated with Three Different Procedures

Treatment	Maxillary Length	Maxillary Protrusion	Sagittal Jaw Relations	Facial Convexity	Overjet	Lip Prominence
	Ss-Pm	*SNA*	*ANB*	*N-Ss-Pg*	*Is-Ii*	*Ls⊥Li*
Graft* + orthop† (18 years)	44.0	72.0	−1.0	184.3	−0.7	0.0
Graft only (15 years)	44.7	73.2	−0.3	182.7	−0.8	0.2
Without graft (14 years); without orthop	46.1	74.1	1.0	183.5	−0.4	0.1

*Graft = primary bone grafting
†Orthop = preoperative jaw orthopedics

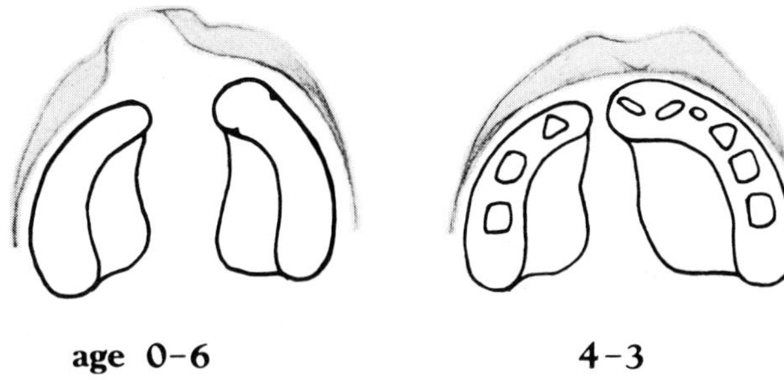

Figure 72–12 Schematic illustration of changes in maxillary segments in unilateral cleft lip and palate in the period between lip surgery and palate closure. Lip repair alone helped correct the position of maxillary segments without orthopedic and orthodontic therapy. The alveolar arch was rounded off, and the lateral segment of the maxilla was displaced anteriorly.

an increase of retrusion of the anterior alveolar process and anterior displacement of the lateral maxillary segment. The distance between the two cleft segments markedly decreased, and in numerous cases, full contact was established. The described changes can be documented by the position of the first pair of rugae palatinae. The distance between cuspids was reduced as well.

The dental model of the edentulous maxilla revealed marked asymmetry of maxillary segments prior to lip repair. Substantial improvement in position of the maxillary segments and contour of the alveolar arch was observed after lip repair (Figs. 72–13 and 72–14). Prior to palate surgery in our series of patients aged 4 years, anterior crossbite was demonstrated in 10% of cases. Lateral crossbite limited virtually to one cuspid was

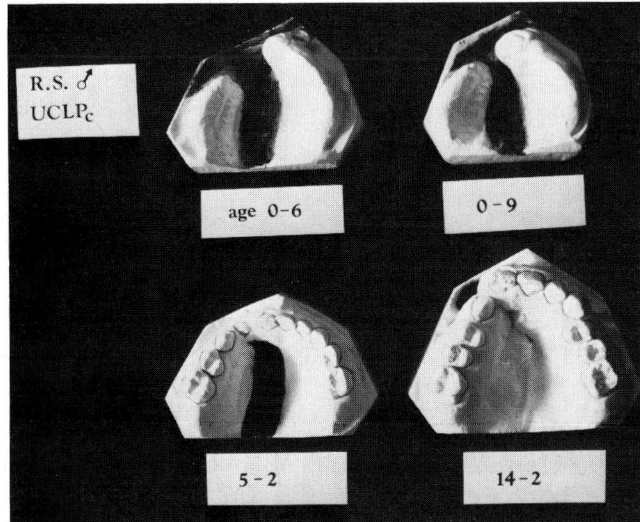

Figure 72–14 Complete unilateral cleft lip, alveolus, and palate without preoperative orthopedic treatment. Upper jaw casts taken at 6 and 9 months of age, prior to and after lip surgery; casts taken at 5 years 2 months prior to cleft palate closure; and casts taken at 14 years 2 months of age. Orthodontic therapy with removable appliances only.

found in 36%. Assessment of dental models indicated that "atraumatic" lip repair resulted in substantial improvement of the position of the maxillary segments without any orthodontic treatment.

We have tested various intraoral and extraoral appliances described in the literature that might be useful in very severe cases of malposition of the maxillary segments (Fig. 72–15). Our long-term studies indicate, however, that in the great majority of cases the surgical

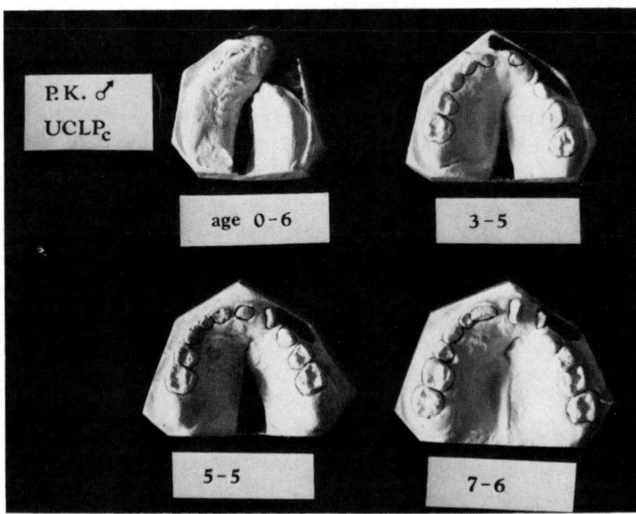

Figure 72–13 Complete unilateral cleft lip, alveolus, and palate without preoperative orthopedic treatment. Upper jaw casts taken at 6 months, prior to lip surgery; casts taken at 3 years 5 months, at 5 years 5 months, and at 7 years 6 months, without orthodontic therapy. Cleft palate closure is performed at age 5 years 2 months.

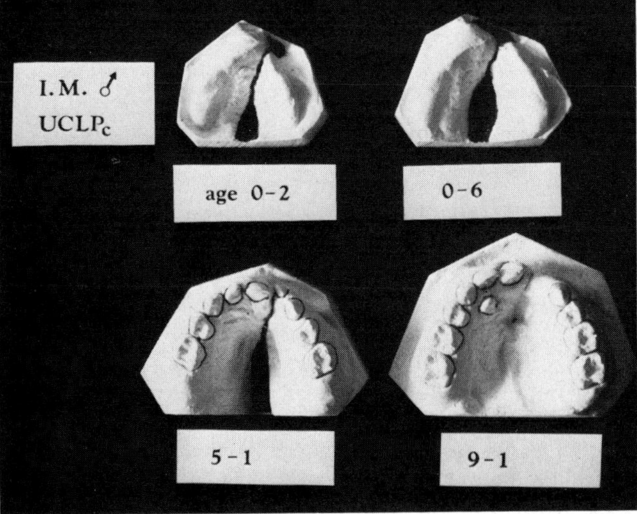

Figure 72–15 Complete unilateral cleft lip, alveolus, and palate. Initiation of preoperative orthopedic therapy at 2 months of age. Upper jaw casts taken at 2 and 6 months of age, prior to lip repair; casts taken at 5 years 1 month of age, prior to cleft palate closure; casts taken at 9 years 1 month of age, prior to the initiation of orthodontic therapy. The positive effect of preoperative orthopedic treatment on the configuration of maxillary segments is apparent.

technique of lip repair has been the means of creating normal alignment of the maxillary segments. Our investigations have revealed that presurgical orthopedic treatment has negligible clinical value because its effects are not permanent. For this reason, this treatment procedure has very limited application in our institution.

Conclusion

According to our studies and data from the literature, there are very limited indications for the use of presurgical orthopedic treatment. However, some authors still report beneficial effects of presurgical orthopedic treatment in preparation for alveolar bone grafting. In our opinion, future investigations should focus on studies of series of patients undergoing the same surgical and orthodontic treatment with and without presurgical orthopedic treatment. It is mandatory that both series of patients be treated in the same center and be operated on by the same surgeon or team of surgeons. A continuous assessment of the findings should begin as soon as the child is seen in the clinic. Long-term follow-up is necessary; however, results recorded subsequent to the pubertal spurt are the most important.

CHAPTER 73

Presurgical Maxillary Orthopedics

Haskell Gruber

From the examination of skulls found in archeological explorations in Peru, it is known that cleft palate has existed since the origins of mankind, and it is safe to hypothesize that this observation applies to cleft lip, too. The repair of a cleft lip is noted in an ancient monograph during the Ch'in dynasty (255–206 B.C.) and is the earliest report of such surgery anywhere in the world.[1] Both Jehan Yipperman, a Flemish surgeon (1295–1351), and LeMonnier, a French dentist (1753), described in detail the repair of a cleft lip and cleft palate. In the United States, Josiah Flagg, surgeon-dentist, advertised in a handbill in Boston in 1796, ". . . that among the many other things he does, he also sews up Hare Lip."[1]

Great strides have been made in the habilitation of the cleft patient owing to the realization that close cooperation among qualified specialists working as a team is essential and that treatment or patient monitoring should take place at centers specializing in cleft lip and cleft palate treatment (Fig. 73–1). These factors are

References

1. McNeil CK: Orthodontic procedures in the treatment of congenital cleft palate. Dent Rec 79:126, 1950.
2. Nordin KE, Johanson B: Freie Knochentransplantation bei Defekten im Alveolarkamm nach Kieferortopädischer Einstellung der Maxilla bei Lippen-Kiefer-Gaumenspalten. Fortschr Kiefer Gesichtschir 1:168, 1955.
3. Schmid E: Die Osteoplastik bei Lippen-Kiefer-Gaumenspalten. Langenbecks Arch Klin Chir 195:868, 1955.
4. Burston WR: The early orthodontic treatment of cleft palate condition. Dent Pract 9:41, 1958.
5. Brauer RO, Cronin TD, Reaves EL: Early maxillary orthopedics, orthodontia, and alveolar bone grafting in complete clefts of the palate. Plast Reconstr Surg 29:625, 1962.
6. Georgiade N: The management of premaxillary and maxillary segments in the newborn cleft patient. Cleft Palate J 7:411, 1970.
7. Latham RA: Orthopaedic advancement of the cleft maxillary segment: A preliminary report. Cleft Palate J 17:227, 1980.
8. Hotz M, Gnoinski WM: Comprehensive care of cleft lip and palate children at Zürich University: A preliminary report. Am J Orthod 70:481, 1976.
9. Pruzansky S: Pre-surgical orthopaedics and bone grafting for infants with cleft lip and palate: A dissent. Cleft Palate J 1:154, 1964.
10. Huddart AG, North JF, Davis MEH: Observations on the treatment of cleft lip and palate. Dent Pract 16:265, 1966.
11. Robertson NRE: The changes produced by pre-surgical oral orthopaedics. Br J Plast Surg 24:57, 1971.
12. Skoog T: Plastic Surgery: New Methods and Refinements. Stockholm: Almqwist-Wiksell International, 1974.
13. Ross RB: Treatment variables affecting facial growth in complete unilateral cleft lip and palate. Cleft Palate J 24:5, 1987.
14. Hrivnáková J, Fára M, Müllerová Ž: Maxillary development in facial clefts after primary bone implantation and after bridging the gap with a periosteal flap: A comparison. Acta Chir Plast 25:57, 1983.

all the more important because there is evidence that the incidence of cleft lip and palate may be on the rise throughout the world.[2,3]

Prior to 1954, a primary objective in the treatment of the child with cleft lip and palate was to repair the lip as soon as possible after birth, entirely in the interest of facial aesthetics. No thought was given to the relationship of the maxillary arch segments to each other and to the whole arch, or to the maxillomandibular spatial relationship.

Rationale

Surgical repair of the cleft lip causes a molding action to take place on the unfused arch segments. The molding action is caused by the tension of the repaired perioral musculature. Frequently this molding action changes the relationship of the maxillary arch segments present at birth to such an extent that a medial collapse of the smaller segment results as well as a total narrowing or constriction in the width of the maxillary arch. A portion of the maxillary arch may be in a lingual relationship to the mandibular arch. Furthermore, with a larger segment that includes the premaxilla protruding through the cleft, a great deal of undesirable undermining and stretching of the tissue occurs during repair of the lip. The molding effect of the lip can be controlled to rotate the larger segment medially to form a nicely contoured maxillary arch (Fig. 73–2).

In other instances, the infant may be born with a smaller arch segment collapsed palatally or caught under the larger arch segment. To repair the cleft lip without any regard for this poor relationship would only worsen

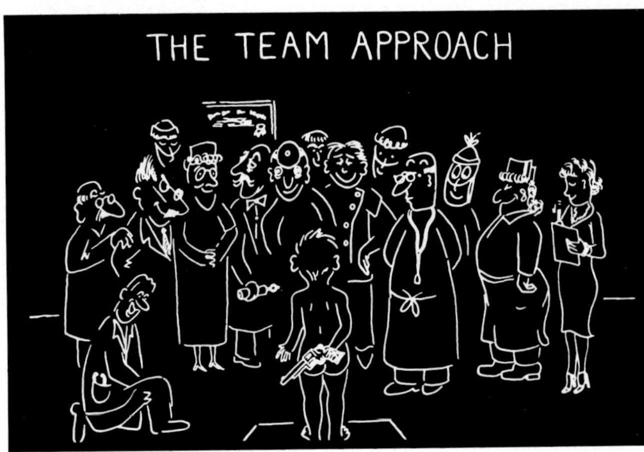

Figure 73–1 The cleft palate team.

the anatomic relationships (Fig. 73–3). When the lip is repaired without regard for the relationships of the maxillary arch segments and the maxilla to the mandible, the child is predestined to a malocclusion that includes not only maxillary incisor teeth in poor axial inclination and torsoversion but collapsed and crowded posterior or buccal segments as well. This narrow collapsed maxillary arch leads to poor masticatory function, perverted muscle habits, poor speech, poor respiration, and, no matter how well the lip is repaired, a poor facial aesthetic appearance.

Quoting the following excerpts from Pruzansky's article,[66] "Clinical Investigations of the Experiments of Nature":

"The skull is a community of bones and organ systems of diverse phylogenetic origin and variable patterns of development; altogether relating to several functions vital to the life and well-being of the organism. If, in the course of development, one member of this community is affected adversely, invariably other parts will suffer."[4] Thus, as a result of the insult to the lip and palate, some soft tissue or bony dysmorphology will

occur at some distant site in the craniofacial structures (Fig. 73–4).

The literature, both past and present, is replete with descriptions of techniques, treatment modalities, timing, and evaluation processes, all bemoaning the fact that no one technique has been accepted, whether it be surgery, orthodontics, or speech pathology. Should one treat early or late? Should one use maxillary orthopedic treatment or wait to treat in the late mixed or permanent dentition? Should the Tennison or Millard lip repair be used? Should the palate be repaired in one or two stages: soft palate, then hard palate, or vice versa; or early (6 months) or late (20 months), or in between? Should speech therapy begin at birth, or should it be delayed until the child can be evaluated at 3 to 4 years of age? Should pressure equalization tubes be placed routinely during the primary lip repair, or should one wait until the child has chronic otitis media? One can go on and on.

The essential nature of the cleft palate–craniofacial teams as a modus operandi for treatment of these children has been universally accepted.[5–7] Research on the gathering and evaluation of clinical materials has given the profession greater insight into and the ability to pinpoint some of the basic problems and to evaluate treatment modalities.[8] Use of tantalum implants and roentgenstereometry[9–11] has given the profession great insights into the segmental movement of the infant maxilla in the cleft lip and palate child after lip and palate surgery, maxillary orthopedic treatment, and expansion or secondary bone grafting. According to Rune et al the roentgenstereometric method gives information of great value in helping to improve the team's diagnostic and treatment abilities.[12]

It takes almost a professional lifetime to assess and evaluate a treatment modality and its results under the aegis of a scientific protocol. It is difficult to change techniques in midstream. Thus assessment of long-term results is a problem.[13] In assessing long-term surgical results, according to Saxby and Palmer, it is important to use a panel of laymen as judges, excluding anyone

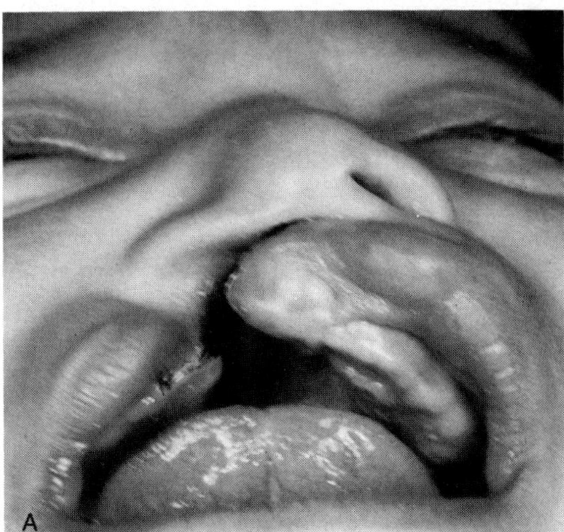
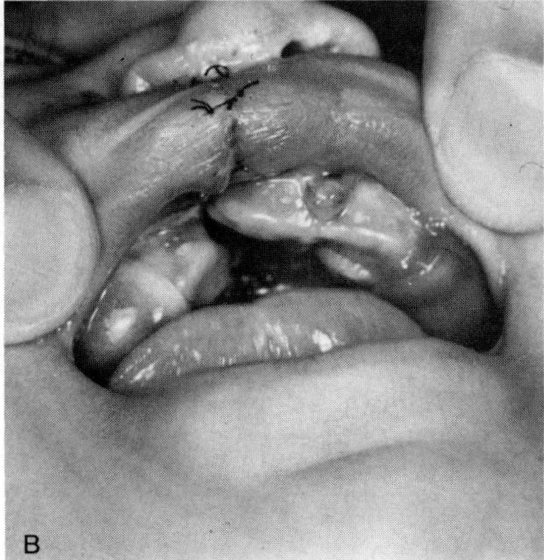
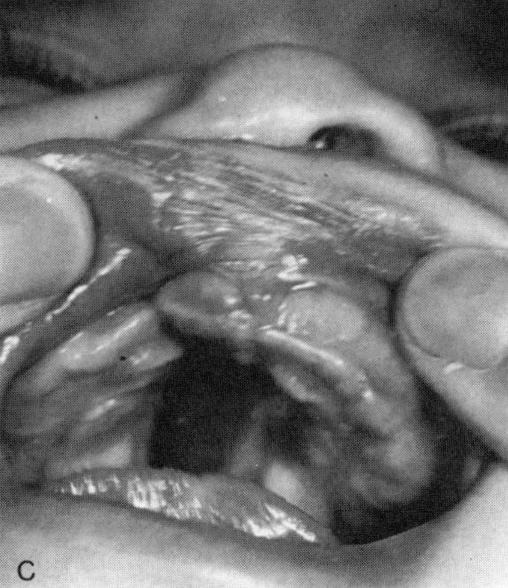

Figure 73–2 *A*, Patient prior to lip repair. Note larger segment protruding through nares. *B*, Same patient 3 days following lip repair. Note cut-back appliance and molding effect on larger segment. *C*, Eight weeks after lip repair. Nicely contoured maxillary arch has a good spatial relationship to the mandibular arch.

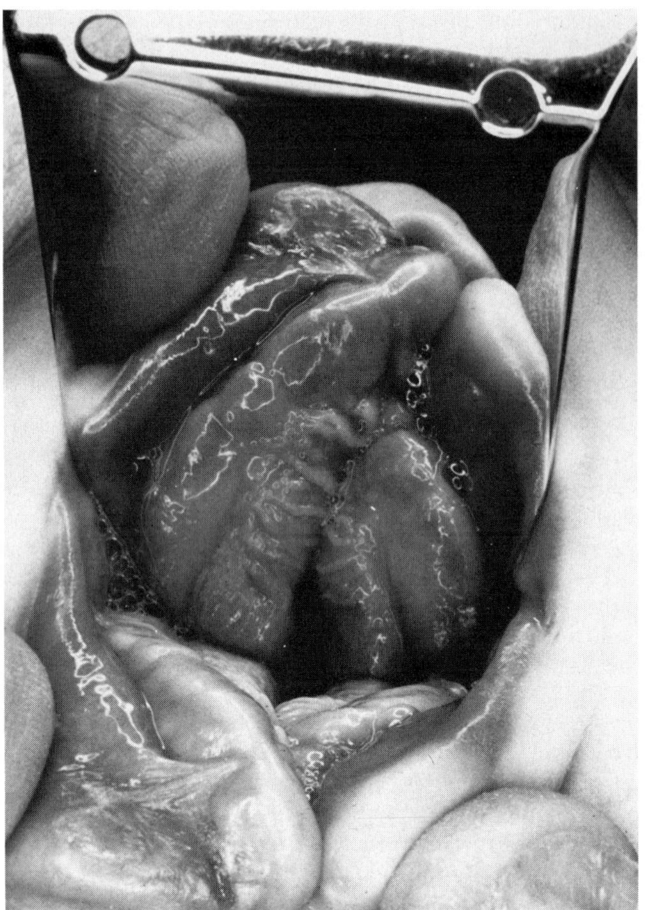

Figure 73–3 Patient at 3 months of age. Note collapsed smaller segment. No maxillary orthopedic treatment has been done.

with surgical training.[14] Surgeons have preconceived ideas of acceptable surgical outcomes and also have a tendency to make allowances for surgical problems in reconstruction.

Owing to the cleft lip and cleft palate deformity, disruption of the continuity of the soft tissue and underlying skeletal structures is present. This in turn affects facial growth and development. However, notwithstanding the presence of the anomaly, it appears that some children have an inherent lack of growth potential of the middle third of the face, no matter what is or is not done for them. The midfacial structures just do not grow as one would like them to. One need only look at a skull of an individual with complete cleft lip and palate to see the dysmorphology present on the cleft side, not only in the structures where the treatment has taken place but also quite distant from the lip and palate area and the site of the bone-grafted alveolus, where orthopedic surgery and orthodontics have been performed. It is felt that the combination of a distant untreated dysmorphologic area and an inherent lack of growth potential in the middle third of the face contributes to a failure of the patient to reach his or her full potential—namely, normal speech, a good and stable

masticatory function, and an acceptable aesthetic appearance (Fig. 73–4).

Treatment Protocol

Presurgical maxillary orthopedics was initiated by McNeil[15] and further developed by Burston[16] and his group. For the team at Texas Children's Hospital and Baylor College of Medicine, the primary goal of presurgical maxillary orthopedic treatment is to maintain a normal maxillary-mandibular gum pad relationship and arch form before and after lip repair, and to encourage normal growth and development. The parents and the newborn infant with cleft lip and palate are seen as soon after birth as practical. Literature is given to the parents, and all questions are discussed with them, including treatment modalities, prognosis, feeding, timing of surgeries, and so on. Every effort is made to put the parents at ease and to encourage them to feel comfortable with their newborn infant (Fig. 73–5).

The neonate's maxillary arch segments are evaluated as soon as possible after birth. If the segments are too wide, they are permitted to collapse under guidance to

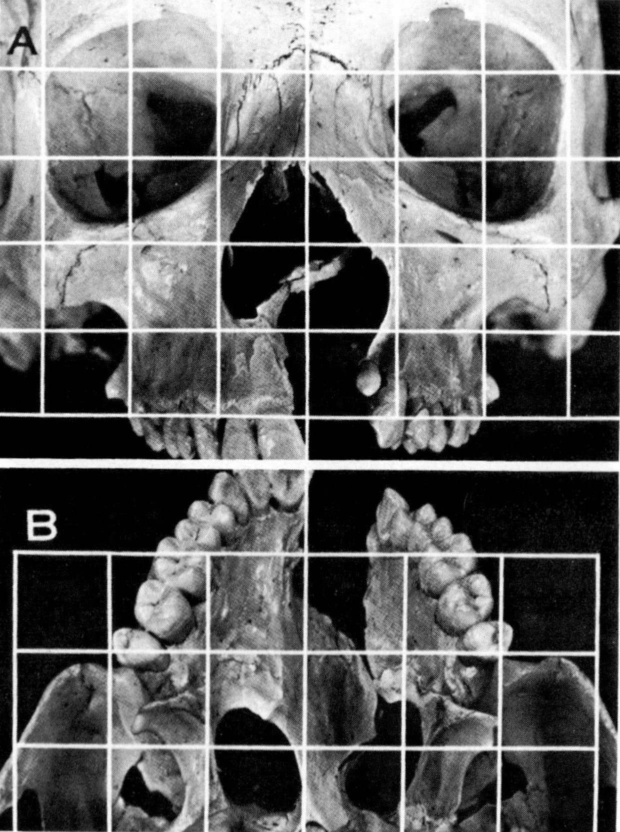

Figure 73–4 *A,* Note differences in size, shape, and position of the clefted side of the maxilla compared with the normal side. *B,* Inferior view. Note position of the vomer, the discrepancy in size between the anterior maxilla, the cuspid, and the first bicuspid area on the cleft side, and the pterygoid plates of the sphenoid bone. (Photographs courtesy of Ross and Johnson[25] and S. R. Atkinson.[26])

Table 73–1. Cleft Palate Protocol

	1–3 wk	6–12 wk	3 mo	6 mo	9 mo	2½–3 yr	5–6 yr	7–9 yr
Photographs, impressions for study casts and work models	*			*	*	*	*	*
Maxillary orthopedic appliance	Placed			Removed				
Lip adhesion		*						
Lip repair			*					
Cephalometric x-rays			*	*	*	*	*	*
Anterior palate repaired				*				
Secondary palate repaired					*			
Columella lengthening (bilateral cleft cases)						*		
Posterior crossbite corrected							*	
Autogenous bone graft								*

a normal maxillary-mandibular spatial relationship and are then held with a static appliance until lip repair is performed (Fig. 73–6). If the segments are in correct relationship to each other and to the mandibular gum pads, a static appliance is employed to maintain this relationship until the time of lip surgery (Fig. 73–7). If the maxillary arch segments are collapsed relative to the mandibular gum pads, an active dynamic expansion appliance is employed to move the smaller collapsed segment in a buccal direction to its normal maxillary-mandibular position (Fig. 73–8). Once this is accomplished, a static appliance is inserted until lip repair is done. The normal segmental arch relationship is such that the maxillary gum pads gently overlap the mandibular gum pads (Fig. 73–9).

It is necessary to answer the question: Why perform maxillary orthopedic treatment in the newborn infant with a unilateral complete cleft lip and palate? Difficulty is experienced in evaluating which complete cleft will have a collapsed arch pre- or postoperatively and which will maintain its integrity (Fig. 73–10). Therefore, to simplify the total treatment modality, all patients have

presurgical maxillary orthopedic treatment. Impressions are taken in an ambulatory surgery center. No premedication or anesthesia is employed in taking the alginate impressions of the jaws of the infant. Two sets of maxillary and mandibular impressions are taken. One set of orthodontic study casts is poured in white stone and becomes part of the permanent record of the infant. A maxillary orthopedic appliance is constructed and inserted as soon as possible after the impressions have been made.

Prior to lip repair and in close collaboration with the plastic surgeon, the appliance is adjusted to permit the larger segment to round out, forming a nicely contoured maxillary arch (Fig. 73–11). The appliance, in essence, acts as a fulcrum around which the larger segment will rotate or mold in response to the tension of the repaired perioral musculature (Fig. 73–2). Postoperatively, the appliance is not removed for some 7 to 10 days so as to not damage the suture line. The infant continues to wear the maxillary orthopedic appliance until the anterior palate is repaired, generally at 6 to 9 months of age.

The maxillary posterior segments in a newborn infant have normal relationships to the mandibular arch. Therefore, it is the team's preference to maintain this normal environment in the cleft patient. If one lets the segments collapse or intentionally brings them together, a skeletal crossbite will develop, usually on the cleft

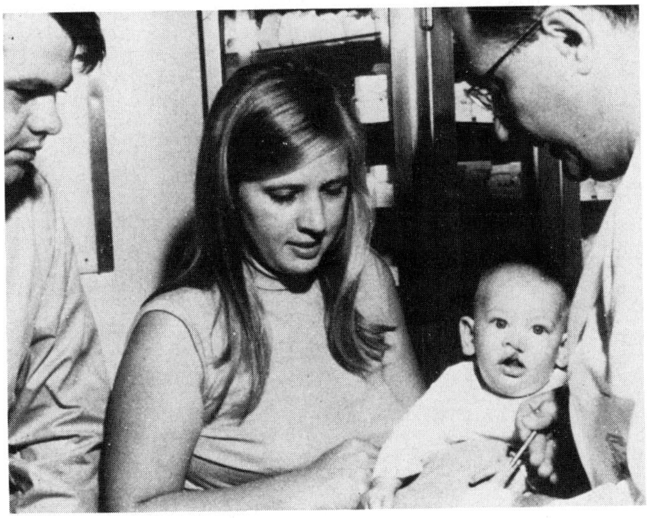

Figure 73–5 Discussing treatment modalities and prognosis with parents.

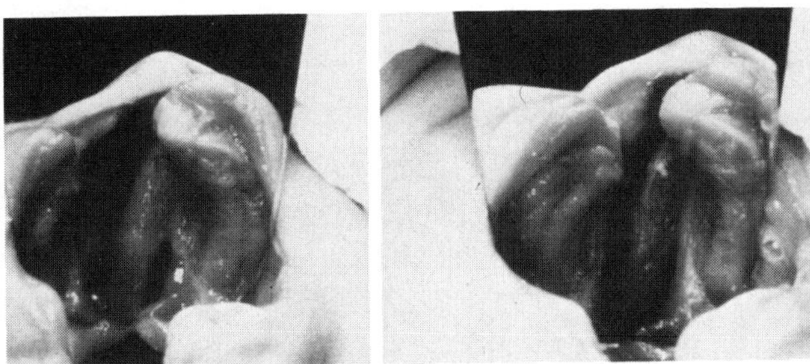

Figure 73–6 Cleft too wide. It was permitted to collapse to correct maxillomandibular spatial relationship. Time: 6 weeks.

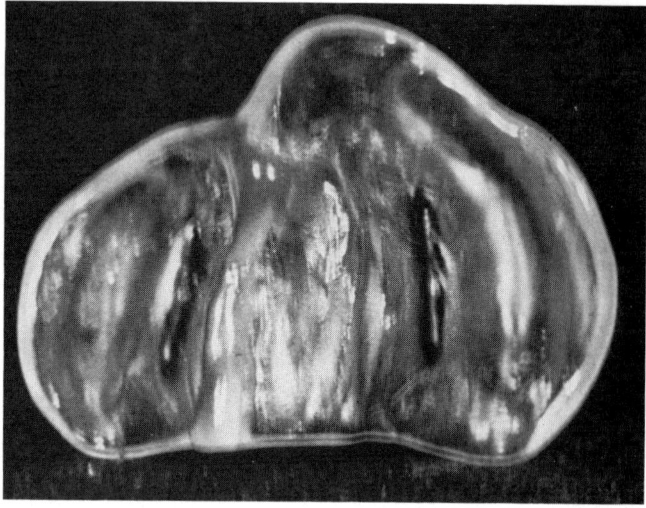

Figure 73–7 Static maxillary orthopedic appliance. Palatal view.

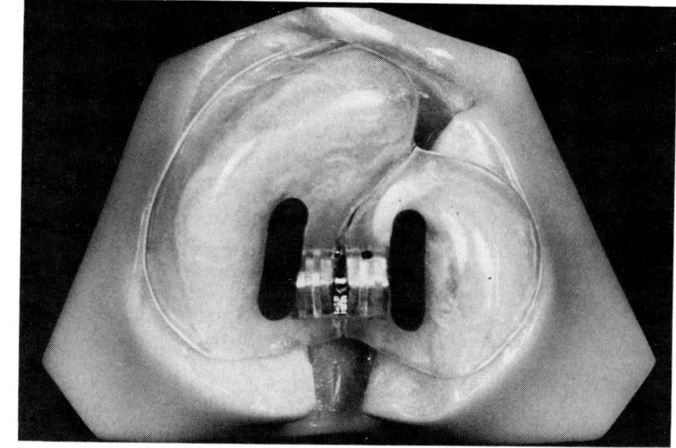

Figure 73–8 Dynamic active maxillary orthopedic appliance with spring-loaded expansion screw.

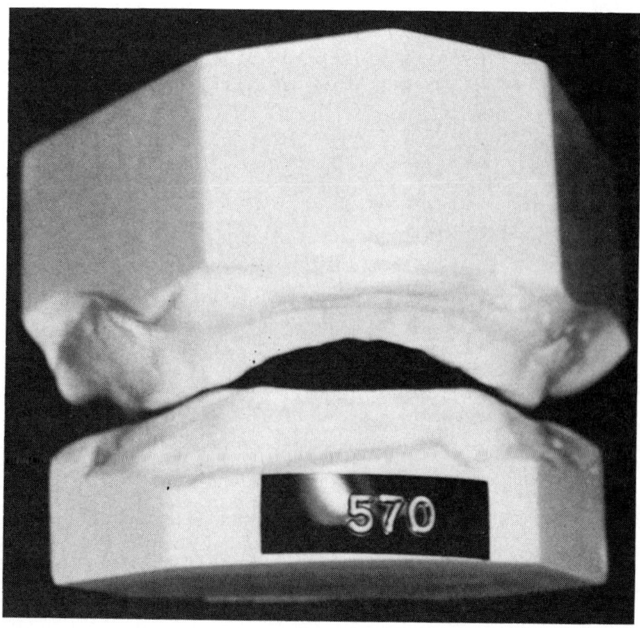

Figure 73–9 Normal maxillomandibular gum pad relationship in newborn.

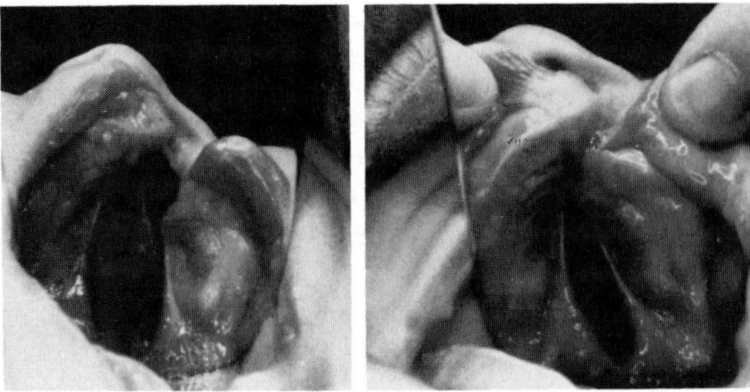

Figure 73–10 No maxillary orthopedic treatment. Smaller segment collapsed in 10 days.

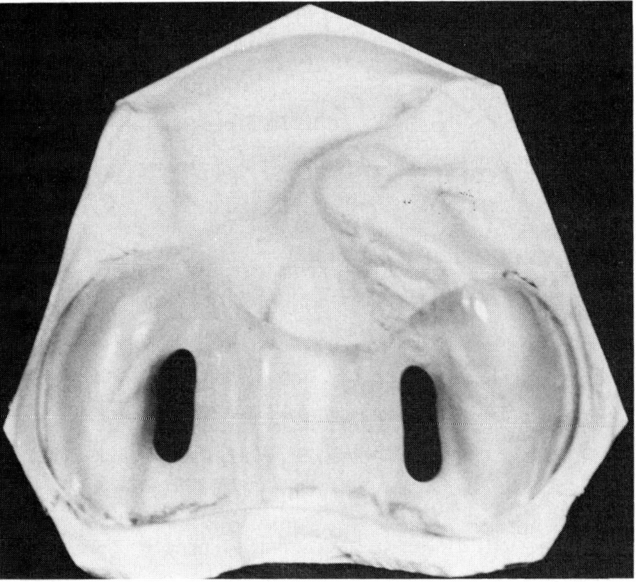

Figure 73–11 Appliance cut back just prior to lip repair to permit molding of larger segments.

side. On the other hand, as a result of presurgical maxillary orthopedic treatment, the width of the cleft can be decreased by medial rotation of the premaxillary part of the larger segment in response to the tension of the repaired orbicularis oris muscle after lip surgery; the rest of the maxillary arch maintains a normal maxillomandibular spatial relationship (Fig. 73–12).

Whenever possible, treatment is commenced during the first or second week of life. After determining that the spatial and segmental relationships are normal, a static or passive orthopedic appliance is fabricated and inserted as soon as possible after taking the impression. The appliance is constructed of clear acrylic.[17, 18] The parents are carefully instructed on:

1. How to place and remove the appliance.
2. How to clean and take care of the appliance.
3. What the normal mucous membrane should look like. This knowledge is necessary so that the parents can readily ascertain if the infant has developed thrush, *Candida albicans* infection, or irritation due to a high spot on the appliance.

After the appliance is inserted, the next visit is scheduled 1 week later, and thereafter every 4 to 5 weeks until lip repair. Of course, if any problems arise, the parents are instructed to call immediately. They are also instructed on how to use any one of the denture adhesive creams with the appliance. We want parents or caretakers to feel comfortable with inserting and removing the appliance.

In the operating room, prior to anterior palate repair, impressions are taken for a new set of study models. Cephalometric x-ray films are taken as well. The infant cephalometer is used for this purpose. This procedure is also repeated prior to posterior palate repair (Fig. 73–13).

The following is a summary of the protocol used for

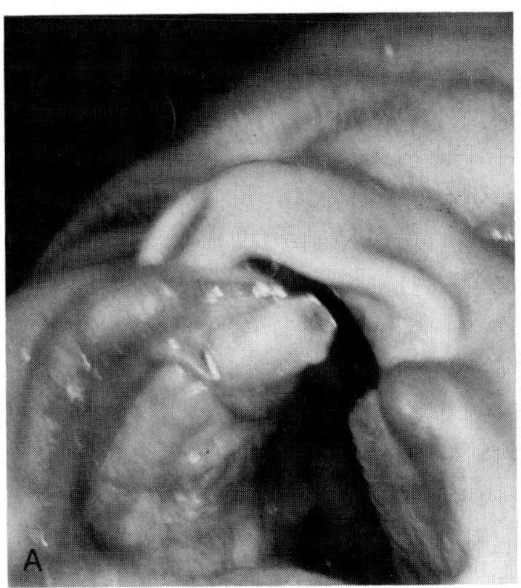
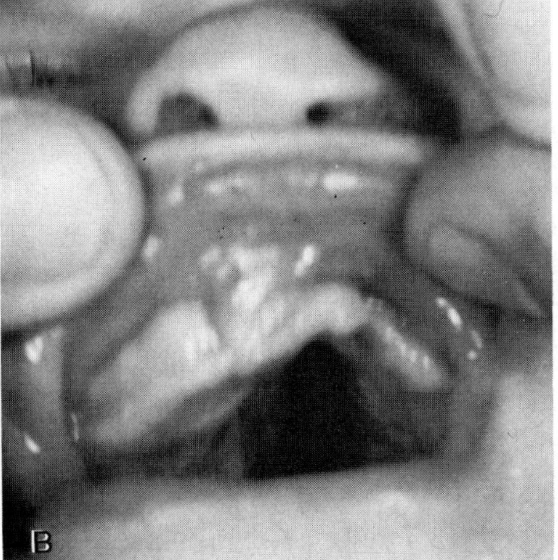
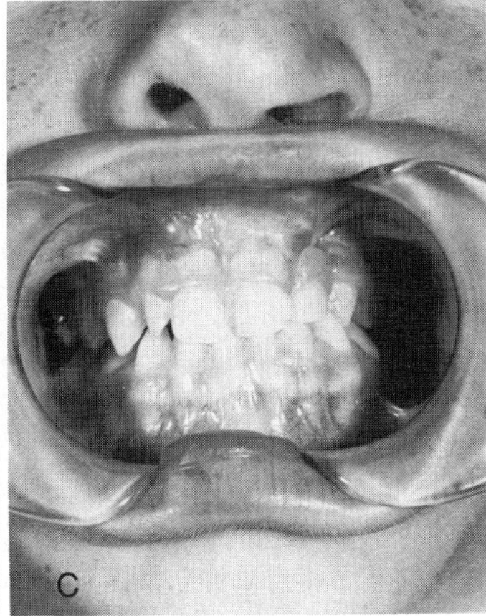

Figure 73–12 *A,* Prior to lip repair, note larger segment protruding through nares. *B,* Eight weeks following lip repair. Note nicely contoured maxillary arch with maxillary orthopedic treatment. *C,* Five years following maxillary orthopedic treatment. Left maxillary cuspid moved out of lingual crossbite. Missing maxillary deciduous lateral was replaced with pontic. Normal deciduous occlusion.

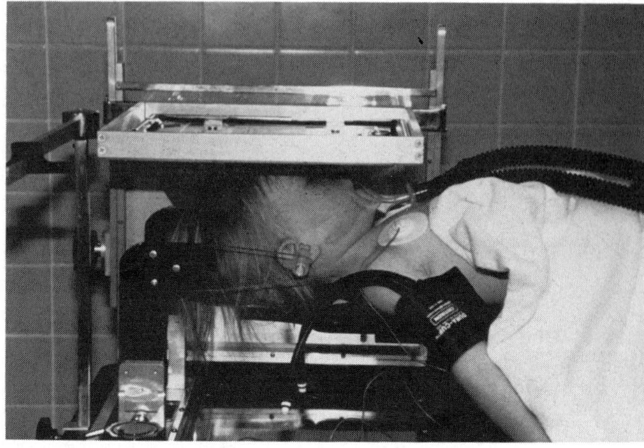

Figure 73–13 Infant cephalometer. Anteroposterior view being taken just prior to surgery.

maxillary orthopedic treatment in complete cleft lip and palate patients:

1. A static orthopedic appliance is used.

2. This appliance is adjusted to permit the tension of the repaired perioral musculature to round out the larger segment, forming a nicely contoured maxillary arch and a normal spatial relationship with the mandibular arch.

3. When necessary, one or two other appliances at 4-month intervals are fabricated to accommodate growth changes until the anterior palate is repaired at 6 to 9 months of age.

4. After anterior palate repair, the appliance is no longer worn.

5. Cephalometric radiographs are taken at birth when possible and prior to anterior and posterior palate closure. By 1 year of age, the infant may have three sets of radiographs and study models.

6. Following this, the patient is seen every 6 to 9 months, then at 24 months, and then on a yearly basis thereafter.

At one point, in a random selection in a double blind study, five patients with complete unilateral cleft lip and palate were selected; no maxillary orthopedic appliances had been used in this group. In all of these patients, the smaller segment collapsed medially before or after lip repair. This finding further strengthened the team's belief in the need for presurgical maxillary orthopedic treatment (Figs. 73–3 and 73–6).

During the early phases of orthopedic and orthodontic treatment, frequently a single tooth such as the deciduous cuspid may be in crossbite, or there may be a very mild, almost imperceptible posterior segmental edge-to-edge bite. These conditions are not treated unlike a full-blown posterior segmental crossbite, which is treated at the earliest possible time.[19, 20] Depending on the child's cooperation, this condition can be corrected at 2½, 3, 4, or 5 years of age. Correction is accomplished in a minimal amount of time with a fixed appliance followed by use of a fixed retention appliance consisting of two bands on the second deciduous molars, a transpalatal arch, and two horizontal projections on the lingual surfaces of the dental units up to and including the cuspids (Figs. 73–14 and 73–15).

Why is maxillary orthopedic treatment used for all of our neonate cleft lip and palate patients? The team members feel that one cannot precisely predict in which patients the smaller segment will collapse medially prior to or after lip repair, resulting in a skeletal crossbite; therefore, a static orthopedic appliance is fabricated for all patients. Among the attributes of this procedure are the following:

1. The neonate feeds better immediately.[21]

2. The appliance forces the tongue out of the cleft and into a more normal position.[22]

3. Normal intraoral volume is maintained.

4. There is more tongue space, and therefore better respiration.

5. Parents take an active part in the child's treatment.

6. Just prior to lip repair, the appliance is cut back on the larger segmental side, thus acting as a fulcrum to guide the rotation of the larger segment medially, forming a nicely contoured maxillary arch. This major bending takes place within 4 to 5 days following lip repair with the contouring finished by the eighth week. After lip repair, the appliance is not disturbed for 7 to 10 days.

The point is made that the maxillary segments are not being realigned but are being maintained in a normal, spatial relationship to the mandible. One may ascertain the normal relationship by viewing a noncleft neonate in a newborn nursery. For newborns with a medially collapsed smaller segment, an active orthopedic appliance is fabricated and placed as soon as possible. The appliance is constructed on a cast poured from an alginate impression and contains either a spring-loaded expansion screw or a two-piece fan and an arc-type expansion screw.[23] The lip is not repaired until the smaller segment has been repositioned buccally or laterally in a more normal relationship with the mandibular gum pads so that under the aegis of the repaired lip, a nicely contoured maxillary arch is formed.

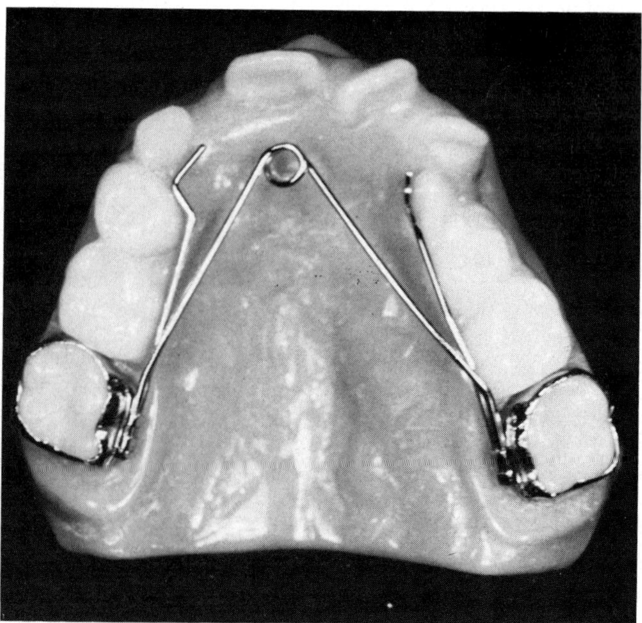

Figure 73–14 One type of appliance used to correct posterior crossbite.

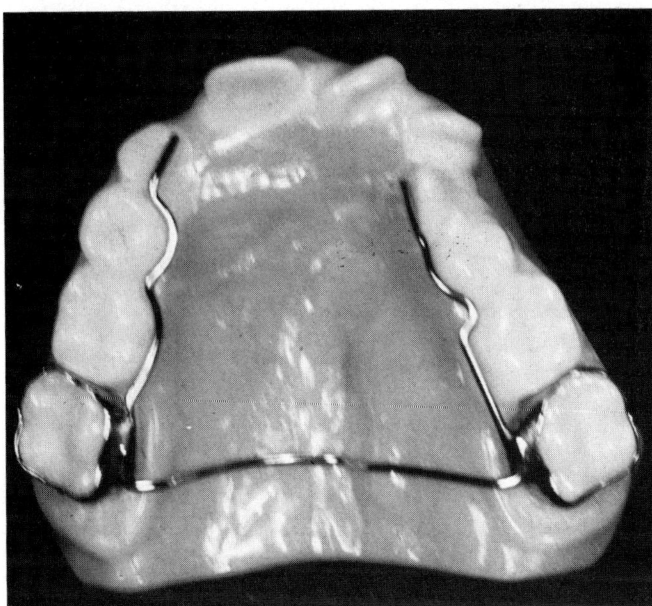

Figure 73–15 Fixed retention appliance used following crossbite correction.

Long-Term Analysis

By employing presurgical maxillary orthopedic treatment in the neonate with a cleft lip and palate, growth of the maxilla relative to the mandible is kept as near normal as possible. The team's goal is to maintain this normal relationship all through the deciduous, mixed, and adult dentitions. Of 106 patients, 80% of our treated cases have normal deciduous dentition (Fig. 73–16). The majority of the remaining 20% have either a mild to severe posterior segmental crossbite or a deciduous cuspid in lingual crossbite.

With the early restoration of normal maxillary arch form, normal maxillomandibular spatial relationships, normal function, and normal physiology in the orofacial region, an environment is achieved that encompasses not only a normal base for normal growth and development of the tongue, buccinator mechanism, and circumoral musculature but also a normal gross positioning of the bony skeletal parts (arch segments) and their dental units. Thus, with the bony scaffolding in a normal relationship, the other structures tend to develop normally too. Because a normally developing muscular environment is established early, there should be little tendency for a buccal crossbite or collapsed arches to occur in the deciduous, mixed, or adult dentition.

On the other hand, if one permits the collapsed arches to remain until 7 to 9 years of age (having performed a cheiloplasty and palatoplasty to reinforce the collapsed status of the arches), a skeletal crossbite will result. Thus, the muscular environment is predicated on a poorly positioned arch segment, growing and developing accordingly. Following expansion of these collapsed segments, whether fixed or removable appliances are employed or rapid or slow expansion, more often than not the expanded arch will collapse again and return to its original position. This does not usually occur if the musculature has been able to grow and develop on a more normal environmental base created by the employment of early maxillary orthopedic treatment.

Therefore, in patients who were treated with early maxillary orthopedic methods and continuous monitoring, occlusion is basically normal, with 20% of patients having either a mild to severe crossbite of perhaps one tooth (for example, the deciduous cuspid in lingual crossbite). These results are considered good and justify early maxillary orthopedic treatment in the infant. Given the results achieved the end result justifies the means. The majority of our patients have nearly normal occlusion considering the amount of surgery that has been done.

It is further believed that the most frequent causes of malocclusion, besides the inherent dysmorphology and lack of growth potential of the middle third of the face, are the scarred palate and the tight buccinator apparatus. If these problems can be overcome, one can establish a fairly good deciduous dentition, putting the patient well on the way to developing normal occlusion in the deciduous, mixed, and adult dentitions. One cannot wait until the patient is 11 to 13 years of age to correct a severe posterior skeletal crossbite and expect

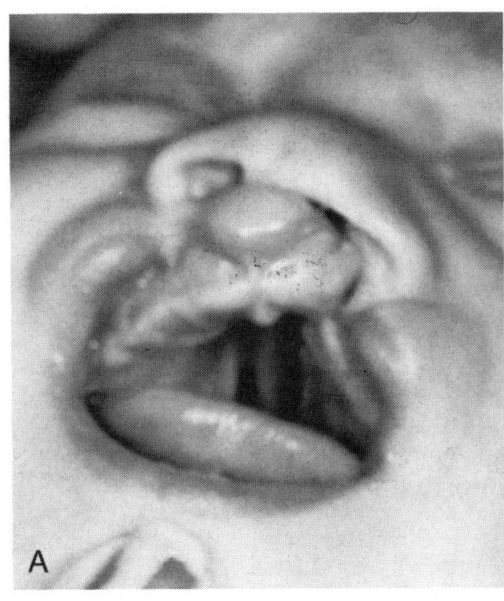

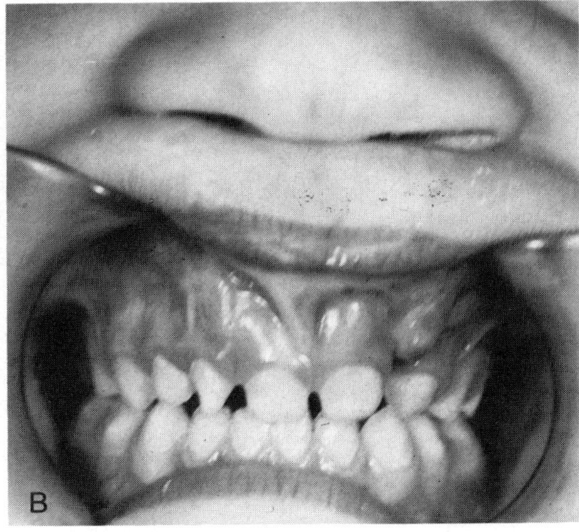

Figure 73–16 *A*, Age 3 months. Note collapsed smaller segment prior to its lateral or buccal repositioning. *B*, Age 6 years 6 months. Postmaxillary orthopedic treatment was continued until palate was repaired. No further treatment.

the correction to maintain itself in the presence of a scarred palate and tight buccinator or orbicularis apparatus.

In treating and correcting these skeletal crossbites at 10 to 13 years of age, the muscle systems are stretched into a new position. However, once retention is terminated, the muscles tend to pull back into their original position, and the posterior crossbite recurs. On the other hand, when the posterior segments are maintained in a normal relationship to the mandible, the normal growth environment for the buccinator apparatus and orbicularis oris muscle is preserved. With a normal skeletal framework and good occlusion all through the neonatal period and in the deciduous and mixed dentitions, all things being equal, the orthodontic end result should be stable.

Conclusion

The following two treatment principles will establish a stable orthodontic end result:

1. The maxilla should be kept growing in a normal relationship to the mandible at all times. When a posterior crossbite occurs, it should be corrected.

2. When teeth such as central and lateral incisors erupt in a poor axial inclination or in lingual crossbite, the malpositioning should be corrected as soon as possible. Retention and maintenance are the keys.

We do not subscribe to the early normalization of the maxilla and its segments only. This is only the beginning. The approach to the maxilla is one of aggressive and continuous treatment, stepping in and stepping out as the child continues to grow and develop. Following is a summary of our most salient treatment procedures.

1. In the neonate, hold the segments and allow them to be molded after lip repair.[24]

2. In the deciduous and mixed dentition periods, correct the posterior crossbites and the axial inclination and torsoversion of the incisors.

3. If the maxilla is hypoplastic, employ a face mask. This repositions the maxilla anteriorly and maintains normal maxillary-mandibular relationships.

4. Maintain all expansion and corrected tooth positions with retention devices, preferably fixed.

5. Definitive orthodontic treatment in the permanent dentition should require no more than ordinary orthodontic treatment.

6. If, on the other hand, a true hypoplastic maxilla is present and there is no hope of achieving a normal maxillary-mandibular relationship, one must discuss the option of performing orthognathic surgery (Le Fort I) at 14 to 17 years of age with the possibility also of placing onlay bone grafts in the malar regions.

The genesis of treatment begins in infancy, and the therapy that follows until definitive treatment occurs in the permanent dentition is a step-in and step-out type of treatment, each phase being as short as possible but keeping the original goal in mind: maintaining a normal growth environment for the maxilla in relation to the mandible. This is accomplished by whatever means are at our disposal.

For the team at Baylor College of Medicine–Texas Children's Hospital, presurgical maxillary orthopedic treatment is just the beginning of a treatment modality that will terminate some 16 to 17 years later. The team endeavors to integrate and channel all its efforts into achieving good aesthetics, good speech, and a properly functioning masticatory apparatus in a youngster who will enjoy a good quality of life, have a good self-image, and be capable of becoming an integral member of society. All of the team's efforts are geared to prepare this patient for "graduation."

References

1. Ring ME: In Abrams HE (ed): Dentistry: An Illustrated History. St. Louis: C V Mosby, 1985, pp 81, 191–192.
2. Personal communication with members of the Baylor College of Medicine–Texas Children's Hospital Craniofacial Cleft Lip and Cleft Palate Team.
3. Rintala A, Stegars T: Increasing incidence of clefts in Finland: Reliability of hospital records and central register of congenital malformations. Scand J Plast Reconstr Surg 16:35, 1982.
4. Pruzansky S: Clinical investigations of the experiments of nature. American Speech and Hearing Association Report 8:63, 1973.
5. Moran M, Savage D: Team management for cleft palate children. Ala Med 56:18, 1986.
6. Dalston R, Mason R: The team approach to cleft care in the state of North Carolina. North Carolina Med J 17:481, 1986.
7. Stueber K, Landis P: The role of cleft palate teams. Maryland Med J 35:587, 1986.
8. Ross R: Treatment variables affecting facial growth in complete unilateral cleft lip and palate. Cleft Palate J 24:5, 1987.
9. Rune B, Jacobsson S, Sarnas K, et al: A roentgen stereophotogrammetric study of implant stability and movement of segments in the maxilla of infants with cleft lip and palate. Cleft Palate J 16:267, 1979.
10. Rune B, Sarnas K, Selvik G: Oral orthopedics and movement of maxillary segments—a roentgen stereophotogrammetric study. Cleft Palate J 16:385, 1979.
11. Rune B, Sarnas K, Selvik G, et al: Movement of maxillary segments after expansion and/or secondary bone grafting in cleft lip and palate: A roentgen stereophotogrammetric study with the aid of metallic implants. Am J Orthod 77:643, 1980.
12. Rune B, Sarnas K, Selvik G, et al: Roentgen stereometry in the study of craniofacial anomalies—the state of the art in Sweden. Br J Orthod 13:151, 1986.
13. Perko M: The history of treatment of cleft lip and palate. Prog Pediatr Surg 20:238, 1986.
14. Saxby P, Palmer J: The use of an independent panel to assess the long-term results of cleft lip repair. Br J Plast Surg 39:373, 1986.
15. McNeil C: Oral and Facial Deformity. New York: Pitman, 1954.
16. Burston WR: The pre-surgical orthopaedic correction of the maxillary deformity in clefts of both primary and secondary palate. In Wallace AB (ed): Transactions of the Second International Congress on Plastic Surgery. Baltimore: Williams & Wilkins, 1960, p 28.
17. Rune B, Sarnas K, Selvik, G, et al: The effect of "passive" presurgical orthopaedic plates studied in terms of movement of maxillary bones. In Hotz M, Gnoinski W, Perko M, et al (eds): Early Treatment of Cleft Lip and Palate—Third International Symposium in Zurich. Lewiston: Hans Huber, 1986.
18. Asher C: Neonatal care of infants with clefts of the lip and palate: Report of a WHO study tour to West Germany and Scandinavia. Br Dent J 160:438, 1986.
19. McIntee R, Moore I, Yonkers A: A general review of maxillofacial cleft deformities with emphasis on dental anomalies. Ear Nose Throat J 65:286, 1986.
20. Moore R: Orthodontic management of the patient with cleft lip and palate. Ear Nose Throat J 65:356, 1986.
21. Balluff M, Udin R: Using a feeding appliance to aid the infant with a cleft palate. Ear Nose Throat J 65:316, 1986.
22. Huddart AG, Huddart AM: An investigation to relate the overall size of the maxillary arch and the area of palatal mucosa in cleft lip and palate cases at birth to the overall size of the upper dental arch at five years of age. J Craniofac Genet Devel Biol Suppl 1:89, 1985.
23. Jacobson B, Rosenstein S: Cleft lip and palate: The orthodontist's youngest patient. Am J Orthod Dentofac Orthoped 90:63, 1986.
24. Monroe C, Rosenstein S: Maxillary orthopedics and bone grafting in cleft palate. In Grabb W (ed): Cleft Lip and Palate: Surgical, Dental and Speech Aspects. Boston: Little, Brown, 1971, p 573–82.
25. Ross R, Johnson M: Cleft Lip and Palate. Baltimore: Williams & Wilkins, 1972, p. 117.
26. Atkinson SR: Jaws out of balance, Part II. Am J Orthod 52:371, 1967.

CHAPTER 74

Alveolar Molding Appliances in the Treatment of Cleft Lip and Palate Infants

Donald V. Huebener and Jeffrey L. Marsh

Rational choice of a habilitation program for the infant with the cleft lip and palate requires the evaluation of specific treatment regimes to determine the most favorable outcome. The deformity of complete cleft lip and palate challenges care providers with its combination of soft and hard tissue deficits. A number of combined maxillary orthopedic and surgical treatment protocols have been proposed for the initial phase of therapy for infants with complete cleft lip and palate. Among these protocols, three major variables can be identified: the type of maxillary appliance used, the specific surgical approach for the lip, and the timing between use of the appliance and performance of surgery with respect both to insertion and discontinuation.

Appliances inserted into the mouths of infants with clefts may be classified according to the dynamism of the appliance itself ("active" or "passive") and the intent for the appliance ("molding" or "feeding"). An *active maxillary appliance* is designed to move the cleft alveolar segments in specified directions using forces applied to (jackscrew) or contained within (springs) the appliance itself.[1–4] Active appliances vary from simplistic straps placed over a protrusive premaxilla to complex intraoral mechanical devices. A *passive maxillary appliance* delivers no force but acts as a palatal stabilizer on which the forces created by primary lip closure contour and mold the alveolar segments.[5–8] Although the passive molding appliance is a directional appliance, a *feeding appliance*, which also is passive in nature, is an obturator for the alveolar and palatal defect.[9] In fact, feeding appliances are usually contoured to prevent alveolar recontouring.

Surgically, the lip may be repaired either before or after placement of the maxillary appliance. Because restoration of soft tissue continuity across the cleft can cause unfavorable movement of the alveolar ridges, it seems logical that the appliance should be inserted prior to or immediately after the initial lip operation.

The operation may be an adhesion, followed by definitive cheiloplasty at a later date, or a definitive lip repair. The sequence of adhesion followed by definitive repair has the advantages of converting the complete cleft to a minimal incomplete one and of repositioning the protrusive and torqued premaxilla prior to definitive lip repair.

The question of timing between use of the appliance and the surgical procedure revolves around the philosophy of appliance usage. If the intent for the appliance is presurgical positioning of the alveolar segments, then the appliance must be inserted prior to lip surgery and maintained until the desired alveolar alignment is achieved. This is the case for active appliances. When a passive appliance is used, it must be retained past the time of surgical restoration of the lip continuously so that the soft tissues can mold the alveolar segments.

The use of either active or passive appliance therapy in cleft infants remains controversial. This is due in part to:

1. The difficulty of obtaining an accurate serial study of the alveolar and palatal spatial relationships before and after therapy.

2. The difficulty of accurately studying serial change from dental model analysis.

3. The absence of normative data for the maxillary alveolar arch form between birth and 18 months of age.

The first difficulty is partially overcome by cleft palate–craniofacial centers and team management, which have made populations for study more readily available. Second, a new methodology for dental model analysis involving spatial digitization to assess alveolar growth and change has been documented.[10] This recent development allows more precise study of the complexity of three-dimensional models. The absence of normative data remains an unresolved obstacle.

This chapter details our experience with passive alveolar molding appliances in 64 infants during the past 4½ years. The technique of appliance fabrication and usage is presented. We report quantified changes in alveolar relationships and maxillary and mandibular growth that have occurred during the first 4½ years following placement of a passive alveolar molding appliance in infants with complete cleft lip and palate.

Patient Management Protocol

Control of the alveolar segments of infants with complete unilateral or bilateral cleft lip and palate begins at an average age of 6 weeks. The plastic surgeon and pediatric dentist perform their initial procedures in concert to ensure a successful habilitation (Fig. 74–1). After the induction of general endotracheal anesthesia, the pediatric dentist obtains an alginate impression of the maxillary dental arch. The plastic surgeon then performs a surgical adhesion of the cleft lip. The infant is awaked, extubated, and returned to an inpatient room after postanesthestic recovery. During the intervening time, the pediatric dentistry department fabricates an acrylic passive alveolar molding appliance (Fig. 74–2). The pediatric dentist inserts the appliance into the infant's palatal cleft in the afternoon of the day of surgery. The infant is observed for respiratory problems, and the mother is instructed in lip care. The preoperative feeding regimen is reinstated on recovery from anesthesia. The infant is discharged home the morning after surgery.

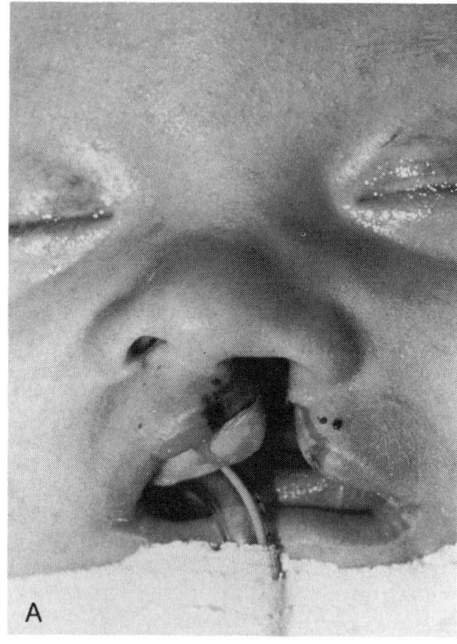
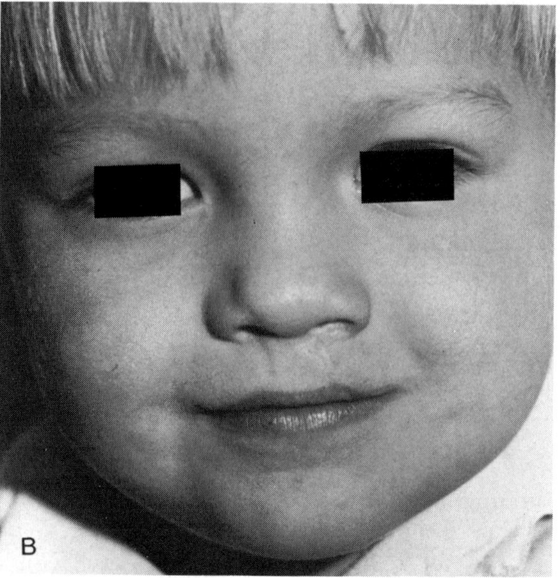

Figure 74–1 *A*, Six-week-old male with complete left cleft lip and palate. Note rotation of premaxilla and deformity of left nose. *B*, Same patient at 3 years of age after lip adhesion and placement of passive alveolar molding appliance (at 6 weeks of age), definitive lip repair (at 7 months), and palatoplasty (at 14 months).

These procedures, one surgical (lip adhesion) and the other nonsurgical (maxillary impression and fabrication of an alveolar molding appliance), permit dynamic tissue forces to move and contour the morphologically deficient alveolar segments in a controlled fashion. Without an alveolar molding appliance in position, lip closure alone can cause abnormal alveolar segment position. Utilizing a therapeutic regimen of both lip closure and a passive molding appliance, the alveolar segments can move in a predetermined fashion (Fig. 74–3).

Sequential maxillary alginate impressions are obtained during definitive lip repair at 7 months of age and during one-stage palatoplasty at 12 to 18 months of age (Table 74–1). All impressions are taken under general endotracheal anesthesia just prior to the surgical procedure. Dentstone models are made from the negative alginate impressions as permanent records. Maxillary and mandibular dental study models with wax-bite registration and lateral cephalograms are obtained between 3 and 4 years of age.

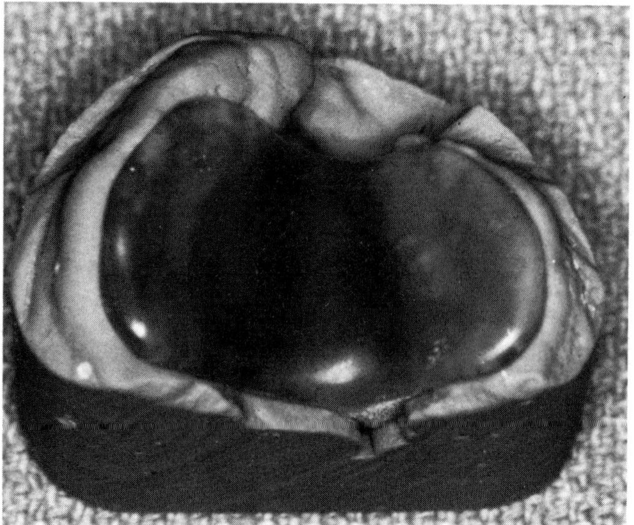

Figure 74–2 Unilateral cleft lip and palate dental model showing a finished passive alveolar molding appliance.

Maxillary Impression Procedure

The alginate impression procedure, which constitutes the beginning of the passive appliance therapy, is performed under general anesthesia just prior to surgical lip adhesion. After induction of anesthesia with an orotracheal tube, a small throat pack is placed in the posterior pharynx to prevent alginate material from migrating into the larynx. Next, a COE No. 17 (for small infants) or No. 15 (for larger infants) cleft palate impression tray is selected (Fig. 74–4). These specifically designed, perforated, rimmed trays should extend anteriorly from the maxillary frenum and cleft lip site posteriorly past the end of the alveolar ridges and laterally to include the lateral mucobuccal fold. Correct tray selection is necessary to enable the alginate to capture the important anatomic areas that are critical for appliance construction.

A fastset alginate impression material is used. Two scoops of powder to the recommended amount of water provides sufficient material for the tray and extra material for the cleft defect. Too thin a mix can result in tearing of the impression on removal; too thick a mix can prevent flow of the material into the undercut areas. Temperature of the water should be determined according to the manufacturer's recommendation.

The tray is loaded with part of the alginate mix, filled to the borders, and slightly mounded in the center. The alginate material should not be placed too high centrally in the tray because it would collect in the anterior labial cleft area of the infant's face on seating the impression.

Before insertion of the impression tray, a tongue blade is placed over the orotracheal tube and gentle pressure is applied to depress both the tube and tongue inferiorly away from the cleft site. This allows a maximum opening and an unobstructed working area. Next, the remaining portion of the alginate mix is placed on the index finger and gently pressed completely into the cleft defect. This is critical, especially for an impression of a bilateral cleft defect, in which the premaxilla may

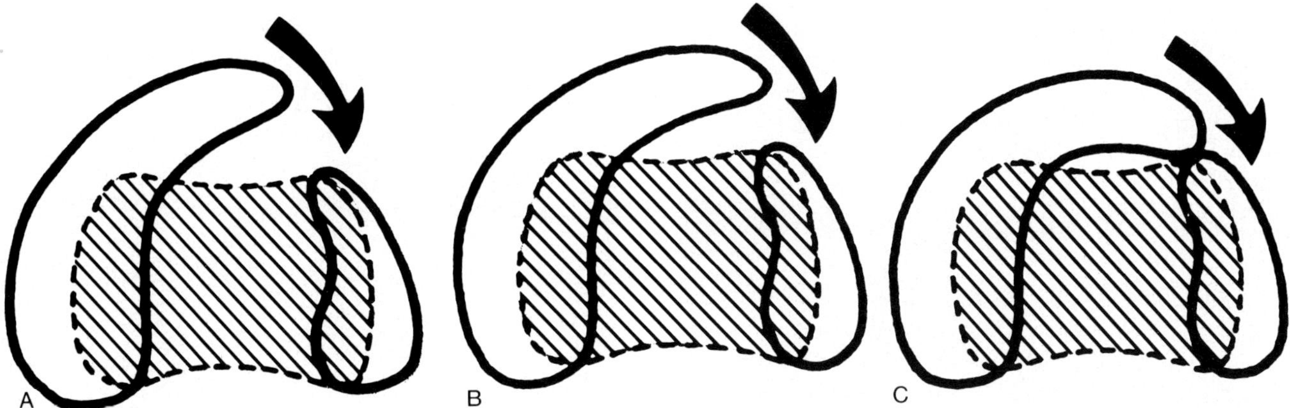

Figure 74–3 Schematic representation showing effect of unilateral passive alveolar molding appliance on alveolar segments. *A*, At 6 weeks of age at time of appliance placement. *B*, At 7 months of age. *C*, At 14 months of age at time of appliance removal.

prevent a good impression. The filled tray is then inserted into the oral cavity and guided gently into place.

The tray is removed carefully to avoid tearing of the nasal alginate extension of the impression. Examination of the impression is then made to determine whether all necessary landmarks and defective area have been captured (Fig. 74–5). Utilizing exactly the same impression procedure, a second tray is filled and seated, and a second impression is obtained. Finally, any residual particles of alginate are removed from the infant's mouth prior to removal of the oral pharyngeal throat pack.

The impression is poured with Dentstone, allowed to set, and then separated and trimmed. The finished models are inspected for accuracy. Because other researchers have noted that the success of appliance retention depends on the quality of the impression and undercuts in the palatal shelf area, the most accurate model is utilized for appliance construction.[8]

Technique of Appliance Construction

Undercuts utilized for retention purposes require the use of a soft autopolymerizing acrylic material to hold the appliance in position yet permit periodic removal for cleaning. The most prominent undercuts are those formed by the palatal shelves of the incomplete maxillary right and left segments. Hard autopolymerizing acrylic material is placed over the soft material to create palatal coverage.

The technique of appliance construction is modified after that of Rosenstein.[5, 8, 11] It begins with waxing out the anatomic areas on the construction model to prevent unwanted soft acrylic extension. This is usually necessary (1) in the superior aspect of the nasal airway and (2) in the anterior cleft area of the alveolus in both unilateral and bilateral cleft appliance construction.

Next, a separating medium is applied to the entire cleft and palatal area including the undercut retention areas. Pink, soft, autopolymerizing acrylic monomer and powder are alternately applied to the undercut cleft defect area. Application continues until the defect is filled with soft material and is continuous with the lateral palatal areas (Fig. 74–6). After the soft acrylic material has set, pink hard acrylic then is applied directly over the central soft acrylic, alternating monomer and powder in a "sprinkle" technique. The hard

Table 74–1. Cleft Palate Protocol

	6 wk	7 mo	12–18 mo	3–4 yr
Lip adhesion	*			
Maxillary dental model impression and study model	*	*	*	
Photographs	*	*	*	
Molding appliance	Placed	*	Removed	
Lip repair		*		
Palatoplasty			*	
Mandibular dental impression, study models, and bite registration				*
Lateral cephalogram				*

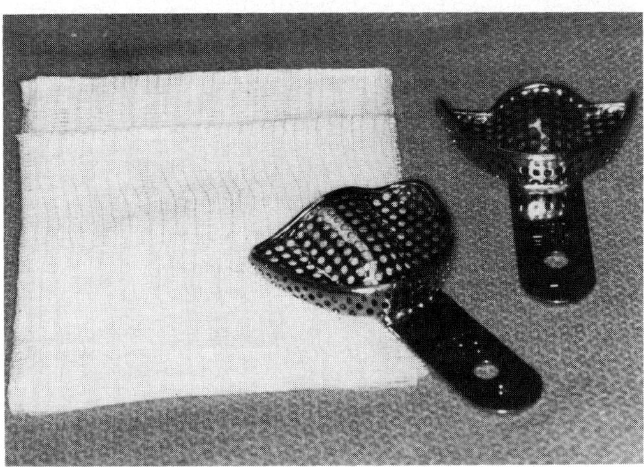

Figure 74–4 COE No. 15 and No. 17 cleft palate trays and 4 × 4 gauze throat pack.

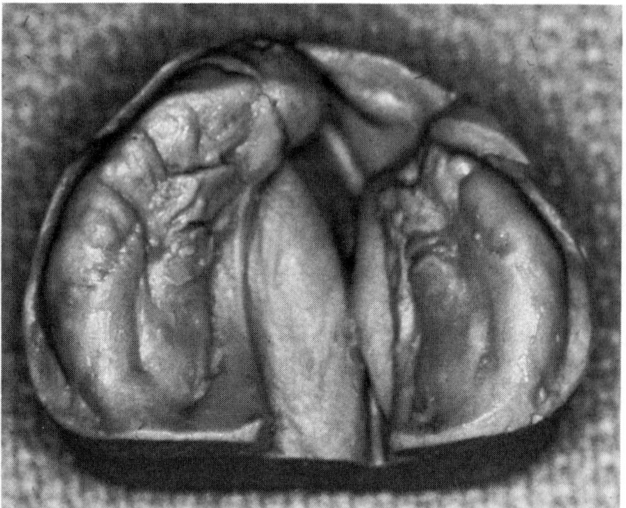

Figure 74–5 Unilateral cleft model showing detail of impression.

acrylic is carried to the crest of the alveolar ridges laterally, to the posterior border of the junction of the normal hard and soft palates, and anteriorly to the canine crest bilaterally. Care must be taken to prevent accumulation of the hard acrylic in the center of the palate during construction prior to setting. The palatal coverage should be smooth and of uniform thickness.

After the acrylics have completely set and prior to removal from the working cast, a finish line is drawn with a fine leaded pencil to mark the borders of the appliance (Fig. 74–7). In the unilateral cleft appliances,

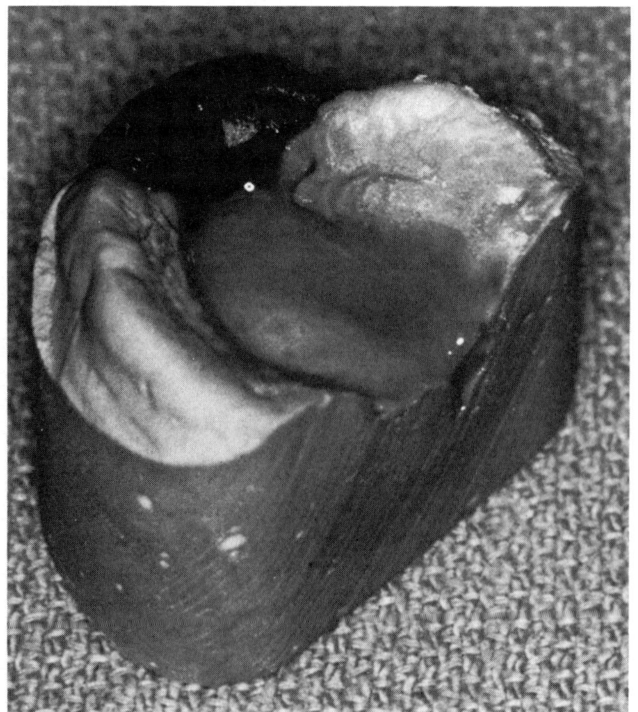

Figure 74–6 Unilateral cleft construction model showing placement of soft autopolymerizing acrylic in palatal cleft area.

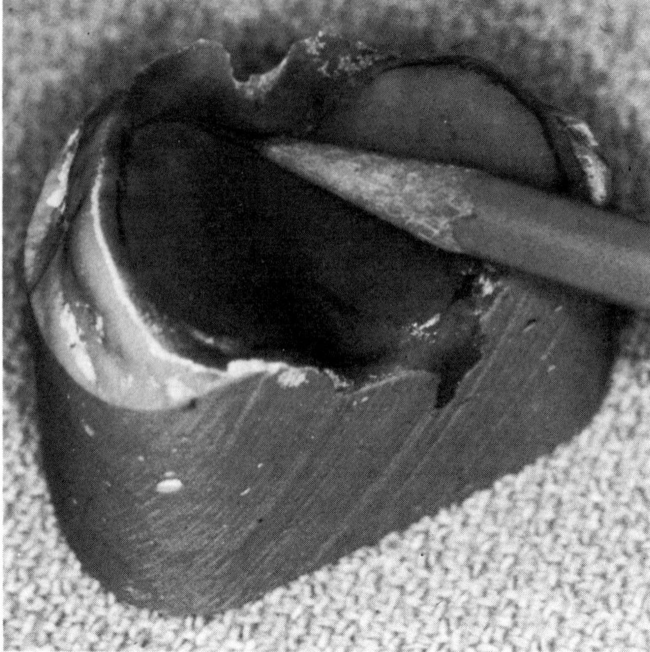

Figure 74–7 Unilateral cleft construction model and passive appliance showing placement of finish line.

the finish line is drawn on the appliance crest of the alveolar ridges laterally, contoured anteriorly to allow molding of the greater alveolar segment while preventing medial collapse of the lesser alveolar segment, and curved anteriorly from the posterior extent of the alveolar segments. In bilateral cleft appliances, the same finish line is placed except in the anterior area, where each bilateral segment is marked anteriorly and supported uniformly laterally, allowing the premaxilla to drift evenly posteriorly with lip pressure. One parameter of success in the construction of either a unilateral or bilateral appliance is the placement of the acrylic sufficiently anteriorly to prevent medial movement of the most anterior part of the lesser alveolar segment (or segments) during therapy. Such an omission could result in a later canine crossbite involving the lesser alveolar segment in the unilateral case and bilateral crossbite in the bilateral case.

The appliance is removed from the working model, trimmed with acrylic trimming burs, contoured appropriately anteriorly, finished with wet pumice and rag wheel, and cleaned prior to placement (Fig. 74–8).

Placement of the Appliance

The appliance is inserted into the infant's mouth late in the afternoon of lip adhesion surgery. The infant is placed in the supine position with the head near the operator. The appliance is warmed to allow the acrylic to reach body temperature and inserted gently to avoid disrupting the lip sutures. Then the infant is placed in a 45-degree position for several days to assist in the development of a more normal tongue posture. This position is helpful because during in utero development

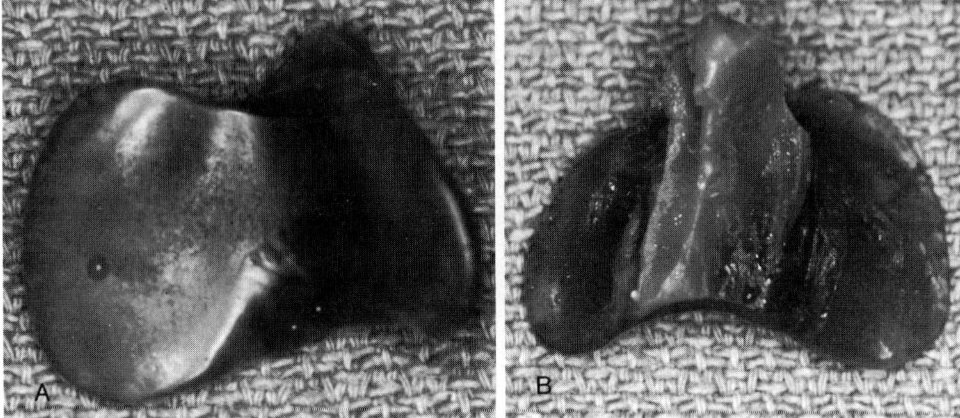

Figure 74–8 Unilateral passive alveolar molding appliance. *A*, Lingual surface. *B*, Palatal surface showing soft acrylic extension into the cleft area.

the tongue has acquired an abnormal position in the cleft site owing to the absence of an intact maxilla.

Most infants are discharged on the first day following surgery and placement of the appliance. If there are any airway complications, the patient is observed in the hospital until the problems are resolved. Appliances in two patients in our series of 64 infants had to be removed because of unacceptable airway problems. These two infants were neurologically compromised. The appliance is usually removed for the first time 2 to 3 weeks later when the parents and infant return for instructions and demonstration of cleaning. Thereafter, the appliance is worn continuously and removed for cleaning biweekly during the first several months of therapy. When baby foods are introduced into the infant's diet, more frequent removal and cleaning are necessary.

At an average age of 7 months, a definitive rotation-advancement lip repair is performed according to the protocol (Table 74–1). At that time the appliance is removed, a second dental model is obtained under general anesthesia prior to surgery, and the appliance is reinserted. Comparison of the model at 6 weeks of age with the one obtained at 7 months shows dramatic change in arch alignment (Fig. 74–9). The original appliance is worn continuously until 1 year of age when progress is reviewed by the entire cleft palate team. If the alveolar segments are abutting and arch alignment is approaching normalcy (Fig. 74–10), a one-stage palatoplasty procedure is scheduled. The average age of palatoplasty in our patients has been 14.2 months. If the alveolar segments are not abutting at the 1-year visit, appliance therapy continues, and the infant is reevaluated at 15 months of age. If the alveolar arch remains malaligned, regardless of the degree of arch alignment, molding appliance therapy is discontinued,

and palatoplasty is performed at 18 months to minimize negative effects on speech.

The alveolar molding appliance is discontinued at the time of palatoplasty. A third model is obtained under anesthesia just prior to palatoplasty. No alveolar osteoplasties or primary alveolar bone grafts are placed at any time during the infantile therapy period. No post-palatoplasty appliances are utilized.

The early maxillary orthopedic phase of treatment ends with the palate closure. Maxillary and mandibular dental study models with wax bite registration are obtained between 3 and 4 years of age along with lateral cephalometric and intraoral radiographs.

Maxillary Dental Study Model Analysis

As mentioned previously, a new methodology for assessing three-dimensional change in serial dental models has been developed at our facility. In preparation for this analysis, anatomic markings are drawn in pencil on the maxillary models obtained at all intervals. The alveolar ridge line, the maxillary frenum, the posterior alveolar end point, and the anterior extent of the cleft alveolar segments are identified and marked.

A single investigator digitizes these lines and end points utilizing the McDonnell-Douglas 3 Space System. This instrument utilizes a low-frequency, magnetic field technology to determine the position and orientation of a sensor in relation to a source. It provides the capability to capture the geometry of the three-dimensional dental model and transmit these data to a computer-aided design (CAD) system for measurements in three-dimensional space.

The anatomic areas measured on the CAD system include:

1. The alveolar ridge lengths of the greater and lesser segments (or both lateral segments in the bilateral cleft model).

2. The palatal distance between the posterior alveolar end points (baseline).

3. The perpendicular depth of the alveolar arch at the end point of the baseline.

4. The depth of the alveolar arch between the frenum and the midpoint of the baseline.

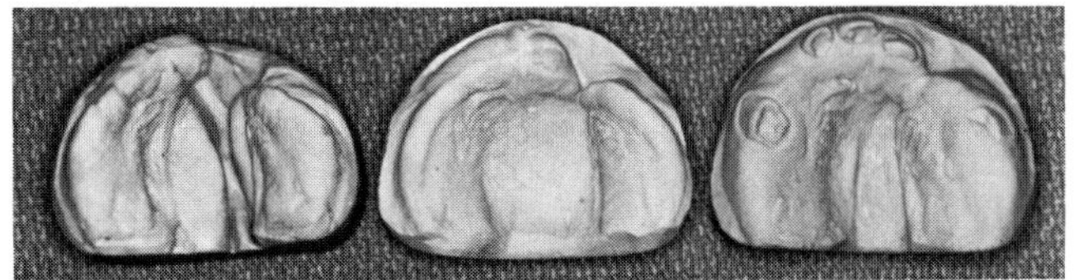

Figure 74–9 Unilateral cleft modal taken at 6 weeks of age (left); at 7 months (center); at 14 months (right).

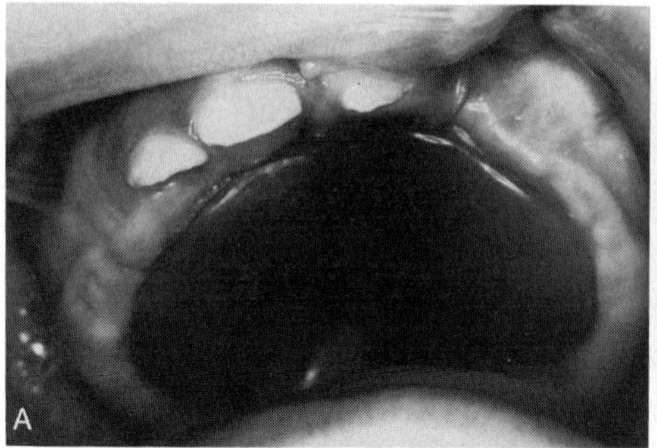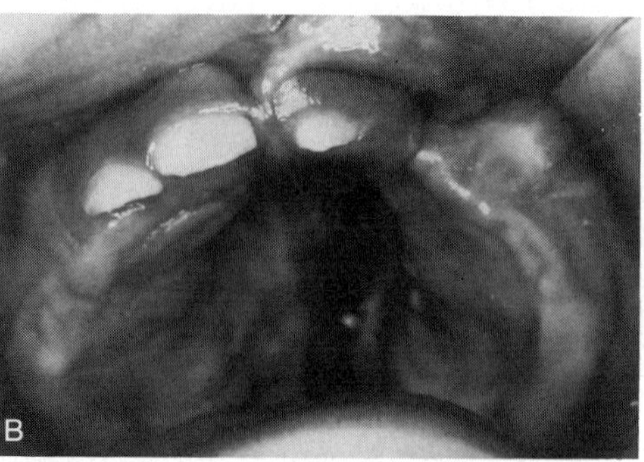

Figure 74–10 Configuration of maxillary alveolar arch immediately prior to palatoplasty. Note abutment of alveolar segment ends. *A,* With passive molding appliance in place. *B,* Without appliance.

5. The angle between the perpendicular depth and frenum depth.

Cephalometric Analysis

Standard lateral cephalometric radiographs have been obtained for the first seven unilateral cleft lip and palate children who have reached 3.5 to 4 years of age. Angular measurements of cephalometric tracings included SNA, SNB, ANB, ANa to GoGn, PoOr to GoGn, SNa to mandibular incisor, mandibular incisor to maxillary incisor, and GoGn to mandibular incisor. Male-female measured values (3 to 4 years) were compared to mean male-female pooled normal values of children (4 years, Bolton standards).

Results

For the first 22 unilateral complete cleft lip and palate cases analyzed with three-dimensional digitization, the total alveolar ridge length and perpendicular and frenum depths all increased significantly (p < .025) from 7 weeks to 14 months of age, the majority of the increase occurring between 7 weeks and 7 months. The ratio of ridge lengths of the lesser to greater segments of the alveolar ridge decreased significantly (p < .005). Angular deviation between the perpendicular and frenum depths decreased 59% during the course of treatment (p < .001).

Owing to the small number of bilateral cleft cases in our series, models of these infants have not been digitized. Qualitative evaluation suggested three distinct findings based on premaxillary segment position and lateral segment configuration. In the first type, when sufficient space between the lateral alveolar segments was available for posterior migration of the premaxilla, the premaxilla did become aligned between the anterior ends of the lateral alveolar segments in a relatively normal arch configuration. In the second type, when sufficient space was available for posterior migration but the premaxilla was torqued or rotated laterally, the premaxilla did become aligned between the ends of the lateral segments, the midline being reoriented toward the midsagittal plane. In the third configuration, when there was an existing medial position of the anterior ends of the lateral segments and insufficient space for posterior migration of the premaxilla, the premaxilla

remained anterior to the lateral segments with some reorientation of the midsagittal plane. In all patients, the lateral segments were maintained in position by the passive alveolar molding appliance while anterior premaxillary movement occurred.

The cephalometric results indicated no significant difference (p < .05) between cleft children managed with our protocol and normals in facial growth parameters: SNA, ANB, ANa–GoGn, and PoOr–GoGn. However, SNB for the cleft patients (73.8 degrees) was significantly less (p < .05) than that for normals (77.3 degrees). Dental relationships as measured by SNa to mandibular incisor, mandibular incisor to maxillary incisor, and GoGn to mandibular incisor also were not significant.

Conclusion

The present longitudinal study utilizing a passive alveolar molding appliance represents an attempt to control the segmental relationships in both unilateral and bilateral clefts by guiding the forces produced by lip adhesion. These forces can cause changes in the maxillary arch form and collapse of the alveolar segments if these are left unsupported.

The data suggest that the alveolar molding appliance prevents mesial migration of lateral segments during the early maxillary orthopedic phase of treatment. In unilateral cleft lip and palate infants, the lesser segment is held passively by the appliance while the greater segment rotates, ultimately abutting with the lesser segment. Qualitatively, in bilateral cleft lip and palate infants, both lateral segments are held passively while the forces of lip closure move the premaxillary segment posteriorly to abut and align in a relatively normal arch configuration. In both unilateral and bilateral cleft lip and palate infants, there is reorientation of the maxillary frenum toward the midsagittal plane. Cephalometric findings suggest that there is no restriction of anterior maxillary growth following the use of a passive alveolar molding appliance until at least 4 years of age. Facial growth parameters (except for SNB) appear normal, and dental parameters are not affected.

This prospective longitudinal study has provided some information on the early change in alveolar relationships. Later findings will document changes in the mixed and permanent dentition and facial growth patterns.

References

1. McNeil CK: Orthodontic procedures in the treatment of congenital cleft palate. Dent Rec 70:126, 1950.
2. Mylin WK: The pin-retained prosthesis in cleft palate orthodontics. Cleft Palate J 5:219, 1968.
3. Peat HP: Early orthodontic treatment for complete clefts. Am J Orthod 65:28, 1974.
4. Latham RA: Orthodontic advancement of the cleft maxillary segment: A preliminary report. Cleft Palate J 17:227, 1980.
5. Rosenstein SW: Early maxillary orthopedics: A sequence of events. Cleft Palate J 4:197. 1967.
6. Holz MM, Gnoinski WM: Effects of early maxillary orthopedics in coordi- nation with delayed surgery for cleft lip and palate. J Maxillofac Surg 7:210, 1979.
7. Gnoinski WM: Early maxillary orthopaedics as a supplement to conventional primary surgery in complete cleft lip and palate cases—long-term results. J Maxillofac Surg 10:165, 1982.
8. Jacobson BN, Rosenstein SW: Early maxillary orthopedic treatment of cleft lip and palate. Am J Orthod 55:765, 1969.
9. Jones JE, Henderson L, Avery DR: Use of a feeding obturator in infants with severe cleft lip and palate. Spec Care Dent 2(3):116, 1982.
10. Huebener DV, Marsh JL: Changes in alveolar segment relationships in infants with cleft lip/palate (Abstract). J Dent Res 67:280, 1988.
11. Rosenstein SW: A new concept in the early orthopedic treatment of cleft lip and palate. Am J Orthod 55:765, 1969.

CHAPTER 75

Stages of Orthodontic Treatment in Complete Unilateral Cleft Lip and Palate

Howard Aduss and Alvaro A. Figueroa

There is no single best treatment for complete uni- lateral cleft lip and palate. Although each patient with a complete unilateral cleft carries the same diagnostic label, individual differences in the morphology and spatial relationship of the cleft segments, the dynamics of growth, and the necessity of iatrogenic intervention all have a varied influence on form, function, and aesthetics (Fig. 75–1).

With this in mind, our approach to the orthodontic treatment of unilateral clefts is predicated on a series of developmental thresholds. These thresholds are deter- mined by factors related to the individual patient's craniofacial growth and dental development. The con- cept of developmental thresholds is based on the fact that girls mature at an earlier age than boys and dem- onstrate earlier dental eruption.[1] Additionally, there is a developmental or biologic range of normal for the exfoliation and eruption of teeth.[2, 3] Timing orthodontic treatment according to the individual patient's biologic readiness reduces overall treatment time.

The clinician's enthusiasm to make things whole as soon as possible has to be tempered by the fact that the child who has been in some type of orthodontic therapy through the primary and transitional dentition is less likely to be cooperative during the permanent dentition. This is particularly important for children with clefts in which dental eruption tends to be delayed. Instead of undergoing treatment in early adolescence, patients with clefts are more likely to be wearing appliances in late adolescence when most of their peers have had their treatment completed. Adolescence is difficult; wearing the facial scars of a repaired complete unilateral cleft lip and palate does not make it any easier. The superimposition of continuous orthodontic appliance therapy can make growing-up even more complicated.

A consideration of orthodontic treatment for children with clefts would be remiss if it did not emphasize that the child with a cleft is subject to all of the same orthodontic problems as the noncleft child as well as those associated with the complete unilateral cleft of the lip and palate. Although this chapter will stress the particular conditions that are related to the cleft, the orthodontist should not allow these to distort his usual and customary approach to care. Indeed, the treatment evaluation of a child with a cleft should begin with an assessment of the entire child. Because most children with clefts are associated with a cleft palate–craniofacial team, this assessment can be readily accomplished. Consultation with the team provides the orthodontist with the child's history, present status, and immediate and long-term needs. Working with the team, the orthodontist can most efficiently integrate his goals with those of other specialists involved in the patient's habi- litation.

Having established a working relationship with the child's team, the orthodontist's next step is to evaluate the individual's pattern of craniofacial growth and dental development and, finally, to define those problems specific to the cleft. For the orthodontist who does not treat large numbers of children with clefts, this approach to treatment allows a logical transition from noncleft or customary patient care to the unusual problems that may be associated with a unilateral cleft.

Historical Perspective

The role of the orthodontist in the evolution of treatment for children with clefts has been significant. It was only a few years ago that orthodontists demon- strated that palatal surgery interfered with maxillary growth. Surgeons were asked not to repair the palate until maxillary growth was complete so as to avoid midfacial deformity.[4–7]

In the years that followed, two important series of events took place. Orthodontists, in their role as mor- phologists, emphasized that clefts with the same diag- nostic label were not all alike.[8] At the same time, surgeons modified their techniques, the timing of sur- gery, and the number of palatal procedures that were

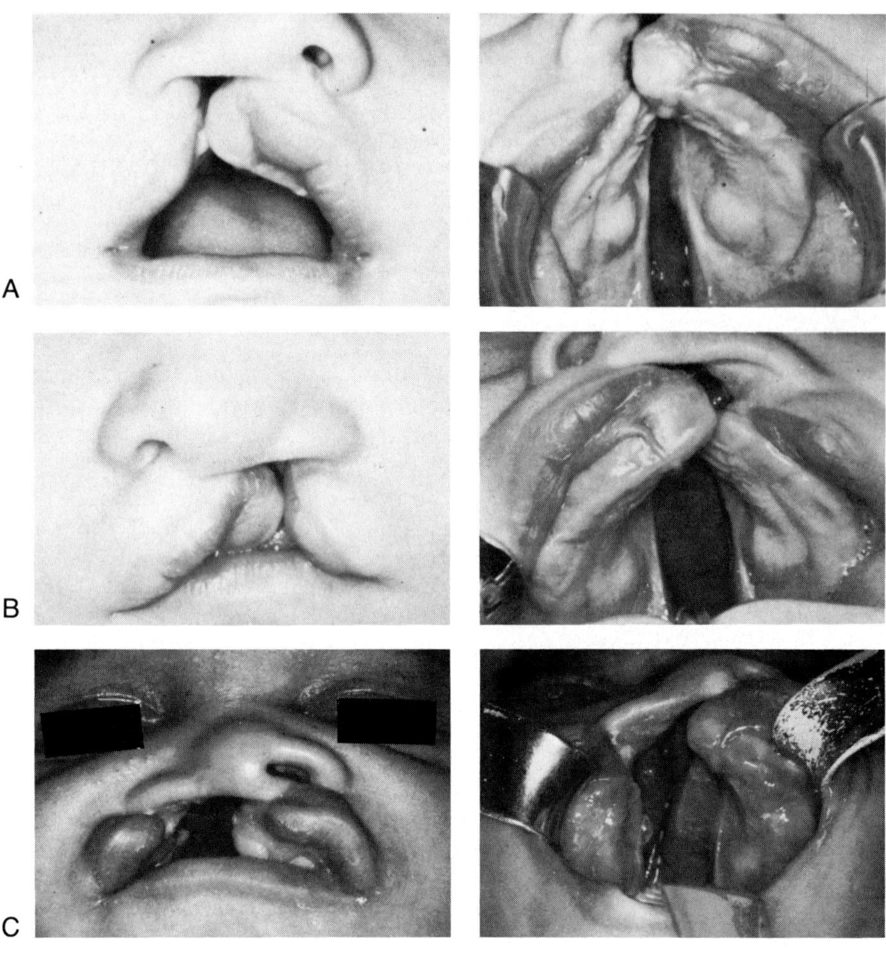

Figure 75–1 Variation in morphology in patients without surgical treatment of complete unilateral clefts of the lip and palate. *A*, A relatively narrow palatal cleft with contact of the cleft segments at the alveolar border. *B*, A moderately wide palatal cleft with contact at the level of the alveolus. *C*, A wide palatal cleft with marked separation of the cleft palatal segments.

performed. Subsequently, orthodontists, acting as roentgencephalometricians, documented craniofacial growth for these patients and revealed that iatrogenic aberration of midfacial growth was no longer a consequence of palatal surgery.[9–11] Indeed, most patients with clefts demonstrated the same pattern of growth as the noncleft population and reached their full craniofacial growth potential.

To further demonstrate the improvement in treatment that has taken place, Ross,[12] in discussing craniofacial growth in children with complete unilateral cleft lip and palate who had undergone surgery by a variety of techniques at different ages and in different parts of the world, wrote the following: "A millimeter less growth will not be an overwhelming inducement for most surgeons to change their operative procedures"; however, ". . . if it is possible to enhance the average growth pattern, even slightly, it is unquestionably worthwhile." Whereas the orthodontist once argued that treatment should prevent the inhibition of midfacial growth, improvements in treatment now revolve around differences as small as 1 mm. This does not mean that there are some cleft patients with intrinsically hypoplastic maxillas. Of course there are; however, there are a greater number of patients with complete unilateral clefts of the lip and palate in whom the size and growth of the maxilla more nearly approximate those of the noncleft population (Fig. 75–2).

An additional benefit that has emerged from our increased understanding of the cleft defect is improved function. A series of studies by Fara and associates[13–15] demonstrated how muscle was displaced along the margins of the cleft and emphasized the need to unite muscle bundles across the cleft to restore function. These studies combined the aesthetics of form with the dynamics of function.

Taken together, research concerned with craniofacial growth, with morphology and morphologic interrelationships of the cleft segments, and with muscle and the need to reorient it for improved function and aesthetics has resulted in greater latitude in the timing and success of surgery for the treatment of patients with complete unilateral clefts of the lip and palate. For example, narrow palatal clefts and thick muscular soft palates have been completely closed earlier than wide clefts and thin palatal tissues. The initial findings on patients in whom the palate has been completely closed before 12 months of age reveal no maxillary growth inhibition compared to those who have had complete palate closure after 12 months of age or have had early soft palate closure and subsequent hard palate repair (i.e., a two-stage repair) (H. A., unpublished data, 1988). In addition, in patients in the early complete palatal closure group (i.e., before 12 months of age) there was an absence of the compensatory speech articulation common to patients whose palates were completely repaired at a later time.[16]

This brief review began with the orthodontist asking

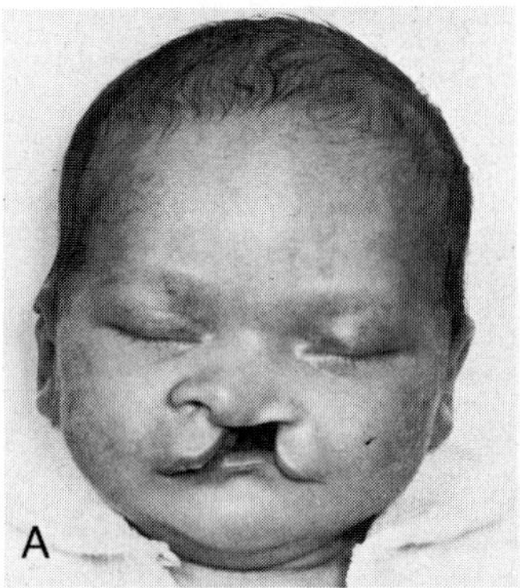 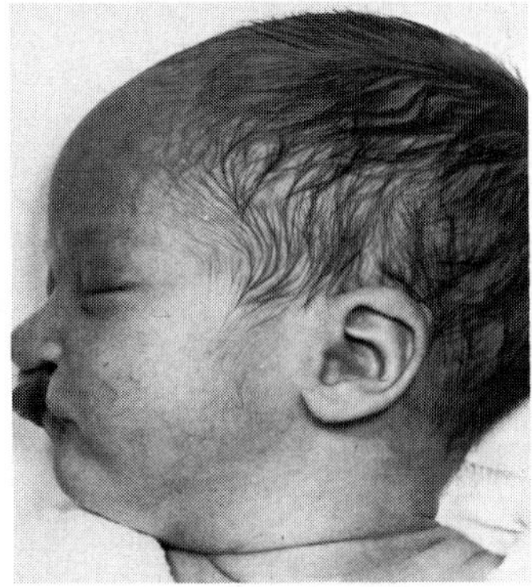 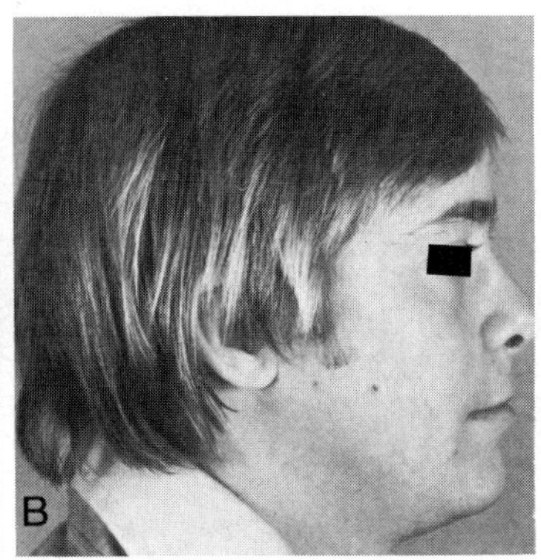 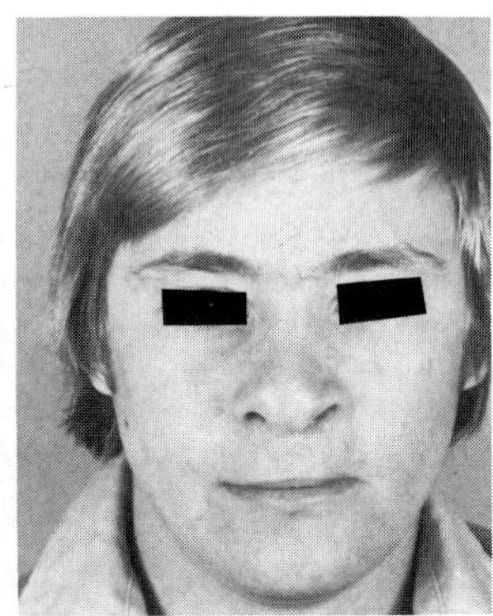

Figure 75–2 Complete unilateral cleft lip and palate. *A*, Newborn without operation. *B*, At age 21 years 6 months. This patient had only one surgical procedure on his palate and two on his cleft lip-nose deformity. He underwent 2 years of orthodontic treatment and is presently wearing a removable prosthesis to replace the congenitally missing lateral incisor in the line of the cleft. Present methods of treatment result in this type of face more often than the stereotypic facial cripple of earlier generations.

the surgeon not to operate before palatal growth was complete, and it ends with a request from the speech and language pathologist to operate early to prevent the development of compensatory mechanisms of articulation. At this time, advances in the treatment of children with clefts have resulted in a cleft population that is distinctly different from the facially crippled stereotypes of previous generations.

Orthodontic and Orthopedic Treatment

In this chapter, orthodontic treatment refers to the movement of teeth, whereas orthopedic treatment refers to the movement of the maxillary segments. There is little doubt that an orthopedic appliance moves the teeth along with the palatal segments, nor is there any question that an orthodontic appliance moves the cleft palatal shelves as well as the teeth. However, to distinguish between the two, orthopedic appliances are considered to be devices that are employed specifically to move the cleft segments (e.g., an infant intraoral appliance to control arch form) as opposed to orthodontic appliances that attach directly to the teeth specifically to control their movement (e.g., the edgewise appliance).

Orthodontic Treatment to Facilitate Surgical Intervention

Orthodontic treatment to facilitate surgery can take at least three forms: presurgical maxillary orthopedic methods; post–lip repair orthopedic methods; and orthodontic preparation for bony reconstruction of the anterior surface of the maxilla.

Presurgical maxillary orthopedics, once thought to be the treatment of choice for unilateral clefts, is now rarely performed.[17, 18] However, if a surgeon feels that orthopedic alignment of the cleft maxillary segments will facilitate repair of the lip, the procedure is justified.[19] With regard to facial growth, ". . . the findings are rather conclusive that presurgical orthopedics does not have an influence on facial growth and development."[12]

Maxillary orthopedic treatment following lip repair is designed to utilize the effect of the restored circummaxillary musculature to control arch form. It is usually followed by the placement of a bone graft to the anterior surface of the maxilla. A complete discussion of bone grafting in clefts is beyond the scope of this chapter but is beautifully presented by Witsenburg.[20]

In a study of the effects of bone grafting on facial growth performed in four centers in different parts of the world, Ross[12] concluded that, "Infant bone grafting, as represented by four centers in this sample, caused growth attenuation of the maxilla in the two planes of space analyzed" (i.e., the anteroposterior and the vertical). It should be noted that 16 children included in Ross' study came from a center that employs post–lip repair orthopedic treatment and early minimal bone grafting.[21] Of the more than 300 children who have "undergone this treatment regimen,"[22] the 16 included in the Ross study "had better overall proportions" than the children from the other three centers, "with none of the key measurement differences attaining statistical significance from the sample with unrepaired alveolus."[12] This raises the question, Why carry out an orthopedic/orthodontic and surgical procedure that does not appear to distinguish those who underwent the treatment from those who were untreated?

Orthodontic Treatment in the Primary Dentition

Orthodontic treatment in the primary dentition is utilized to correct a crossbite. This generally takes the form of the buccal maxillary teeth on the side of the cleft being palatal to the mandibular teeth to a varying degree. However, the incisors also may be in crossbite. The most obvious etiology of a buccal crossbite is a hypoplastic maxillary segment on the cleft side, which may be present in some patients with complete unilateral clefts.[23] Indeed, the earliest expression of an overall maxillary hypoplasia may be a crossbite in the primary dentition. It should be noted that crossbite is not a consistent finding in unilateral clefts. However, the canine adjoining the cleft will erupt palatally because of the displacement of its developing tooth bud. The tooth bud requires surrounding bone that is not present along the margins of the cleft. The canine tooth bud is therefore displaced palatally.

Correction of Crossbite Occlusion in the Primary Dentition

There are a number of factors to be considered before correcting a crossbite in the primary dentition. These include:

1. Patient cooperation. It makes no sense to overwhelm a young child with an appliance to align some teeth if this procedure can be carried out at a later time when the child is more mature and will more readily accept treatment.
2. Interference with function. Is the crossbite interfering with normal mandibular function? Are there occlusal interferences that are causing the abnormal mandibular movements? Can these abnormalities be corrected with occlusal equilibration (e.g., canine cusp reduction), thereby postponing the correction of the crossbite until the child is more mature? These are but a few of the questions that must be addressed in assessing function (Figure 75–3).
3. Interference with growth. Is the crossbite interfering with growth of the maxilla? If so, the crossbite should be corrected.
4. Interference with speech. Will expansion of the maxillary arch to correct a crossbite open the contact area between the unrepaired cleft segments at the alveolar level and create an anterior oronasal fistula that will interfere with speech or result in food and liquids being forced into the nose? If so, can the crossbite correction be delayed? If not, will an obturator be necessary until the fistula is permanently closed? In keeping with the philosophy that extended treatment is less than ideal, correction of a crossbite that results in the creation of even greater problems should be deferred.
5. Stability of treatment. If correction of a crossbite is to be completed in the primary dentition, the following points must be considered: How stable is the correction? Will retreatment be necessary in the transitional dentition? If so, can treatment be delayed until that time? If not, how much relapse can be expected? Will the degree of relapse necessitate a permanent type of retention?
6. Retention. Ideally, retention of the teeth and/or the maxilla after orthodontic or orthopedic treatment in the primary dentition should be avoided. However, should it be necessary, it should be designed so that it does not interfere with speech or increase susceptibility to caries.

In summary, it is not the purpose of this chapter to present a catalog of those conditions that require orthodontic or orthopedic treatment in the primary dentition.

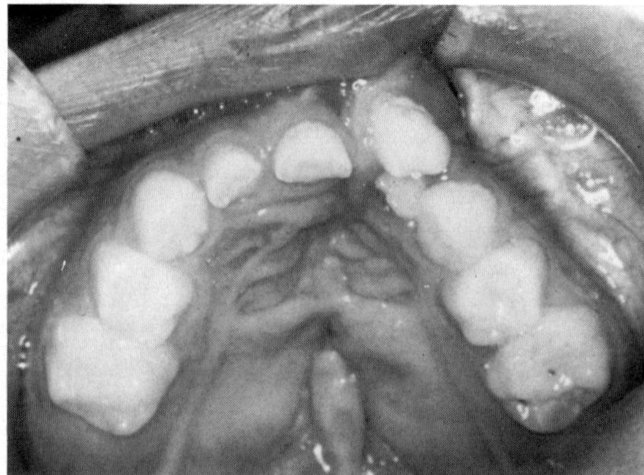

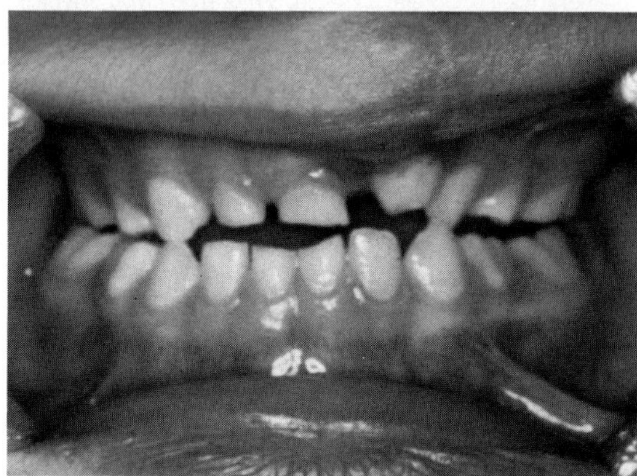

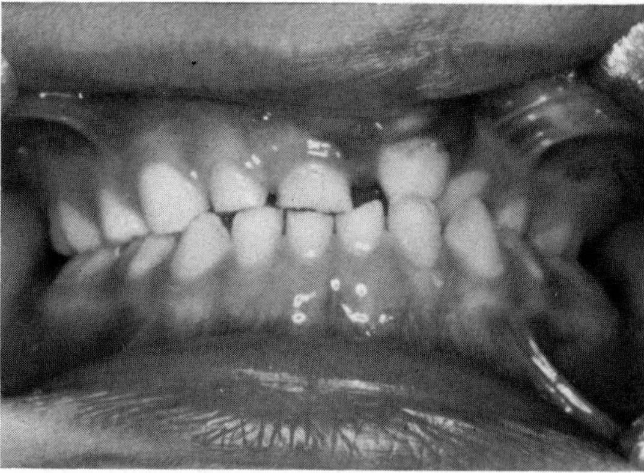

Figure 75–3 Contact between the palatally displaced primary canine on the cleft side with the mandibular canine causes a mandibular shift and subsequent crossbite occlusion *(A–C)*. Reduction of the cusps corrected the occlusion.

However, questions have been raised that can be used to develop criteria for treatment in a variety of situations. The major point to be emphasized is that treatment in the primary dentition should be limited to problems that demand resolution. Wherever possible, the clinician should think in terms of developmental thresholds that allow treatment to be combined—e.g., correction of a crossbite while at the same time aligning a rotated permanent central incisor adjoining the cleft. Both can be accomplished quite rapidly with an edgewise appliance in the transitional dentition. Most important, overtreatment should be avoided.

Orthodontic Treatment in the Transitional Dentition

Orthodontic treatment in the transitional dentition is primarily concerned with correction of rotated incisors adjoining the cleft; correction of maxillary crossbites to allow the dental arch to reach its full growth potential and to place the buds of the developing teeth in the best possible position for eruption; and attainment of the best possible arch form prior to bony reconstruction of the anterior surface of the maxilla (Figure 75–4). Alveolar and maxillary bone grafting facilitates closure of nasal fistulas, establishes a bony nasal sill on the side of the cleft, and provides bone for the eruption or movement of the lateral incisor (supernumerary incisor) and canine into the dental arch in the line of the cleft.

Orthodontic alignment of the maxillary arch (expansion) should precede bone grafting because there is evidence that once a bony bridge is established in this region, growth is inhibited.[12, 20, 21, 24] Additionally, placement of cancellous bone in the line of the cleft during the transitional dentition will allow the permanent lateral (or supernumerary) incisor and canine to erupt in a more normal position and will allow the lateral (or a supernumerary) incisor to be brought into a proper position in the dental arch.

In planning treatment in the transitional dentition, the most important consideration is timing. The timing of treatment is based on the threshold of development of the teeth or the development of the face.

Rotation of Incisors

Malposed or rotated incisors adjoining a cleft should not be corrected until the root of the tooth is completely formed. This avoids the risk of growth disruption or loss of the root. Alignment of the incisors is readily accomplished with a bonded edgewise appliance. This appliance is well tolerated and allows rapid correction of any malalignment and rotation. To retain the corrected rotation and prevent drifting of the incisor, a small piece of wire may be bonded across the lingual surfaces of the newly positioned tooth and the adjacent central incisor. This type of retainer can be maintained indefinitely or until a sufficient number of permanent teeth have erupted and the child is ready for definitive orthodontic treatment.

Crossbite Correction in the Transitional Dentition

The guidelines for crossbite correction that were previously presented in the discussion of treatment in the primary dentition also apply in the transitional

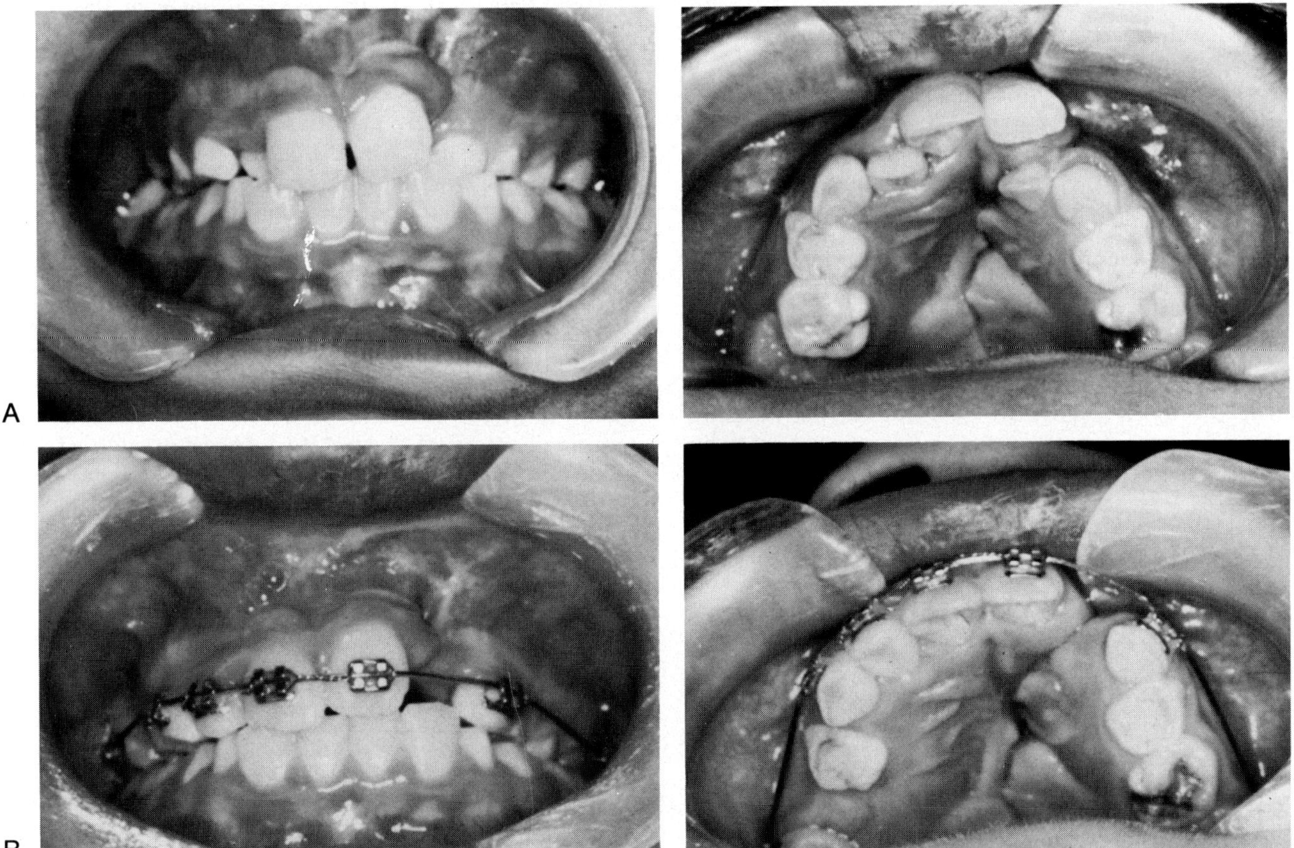

Figure 75–4 Frontal and palatal views in the early transitional dentition. *A*, The permanent incisors are malposed, and the canine on the cleft side is in crossbite occlusion. *B*, After 4 months of orthodontic treatment with a bonded edgewise appliance, the incisors are well aligned, the canine crossbite has been corrected, and the arch form is symmetric. Retention was accomplished with a wire bonded to the lingual surface of the central incisors. Note the small asymptomatic fistula in the anterior portion of the palate.

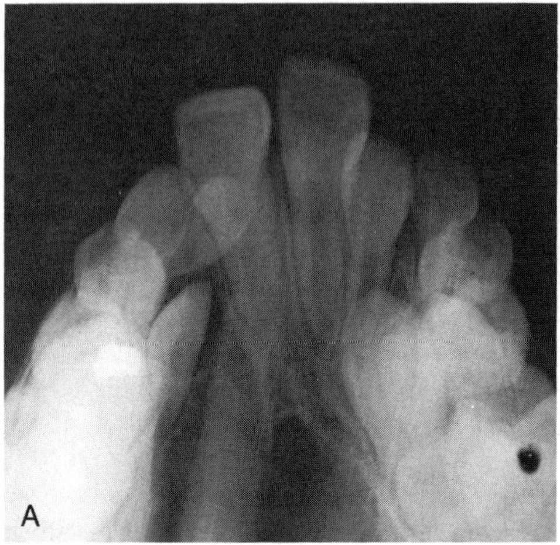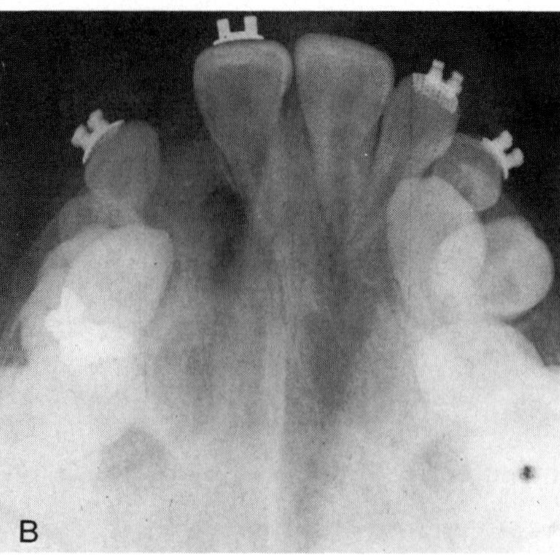

Figure 75–5 A, Pre- and (B) postorthodontic alignment and bone grafting in the transitional dentition. Supernumerary teeth in the line of the cleft were removed at the time the graft was placed. The tip of the cusp of the erupting canine is moving into the graft.

dentition. It is particularly important at this time to take advantage of those developmental thresholds that allow the patient's treatment needs to be combined.

Growth in width of the noncleft maxilla reaches its maximum during eruption of the canine. The same expression of growth occurs in children with complete unilateral clefts. It would therefore be most appropriate to time any orthodontic treatment to expand the maxilla to coincide with the active phase of eruption of the canine. This is particularly important if there is to be bony reconstruction of the anterior surface of the cleft maxilla. Maintenance of the cancellous bone used in reconstruction, particularly of the alveolar level, depends on eruption of the lateral or canine through the graft or movement of a tooth into the area.[25, 26]

An additional consideration in orthodontic treatment of unilateral clefts in the transitional dentition is the utilization of malformed incisors in the line of the cleft. Like the canine on the cleft side, supernumerary or malformed teeth usually develop palatally. If they are to become part of the dental arch, they have to be brought into the line of the cleft. The success of this procedure depends on selection of a tooth with adequate root length and, as previously mentioned, the presence of sufficient bone in the area of the cleft through which to move the tooth (Figure 75–5). With current bonding techniques, anomalous crowns can be covered, but the stability of the repositioned tooth depends on adequate root length. When more than one supernumerary tooth is present in the area of the cleft, the one with the best root should be retained.

Extraction in the Transitional Dentition

The question of arch length is managed in the child with a unilateral cleft in the same manner as it is with the noncleft child. For cleft children with inadequate arch length serial extraction can be initiated in the transitional dentition.[27] This does not preclude the need for appliance therapy with eruption of the permanent teeth but reduces the complexity of the malocclusion.

In cases in which there is inadequate arch length, (e.g., cases requiring the extraction of four first premolars), and there is congenital absence of the lateral incisor in the line of the cleft, there is always a tendency to retain the first premolar on the cleft side and to move the canine into the lateral incisor position. Although this procedure eliminates the need for a prosthesis to replace the missing lateral incisor, it does have certain functional disadvantages. The morphology of the canine, particularly its labiolingual diameter, does not permit ideal interincisor relationships, and the occlusion of the premolar with the mandibular canine may compromise the buccal occlusion on the cleft side (Fig. 75–6). With this in mind, and before a decision is made to retain the premolar, the morphology of the crowns of the canine and premolar and their final occlusal positions should be determined.

A final note with regard to treatment in the transitional dentition is: Do not start too early. Dental development and eruption can be readily monitored with panoramic radiography. By basing the initiation of active treatment on developmental thresholds, treatment be-

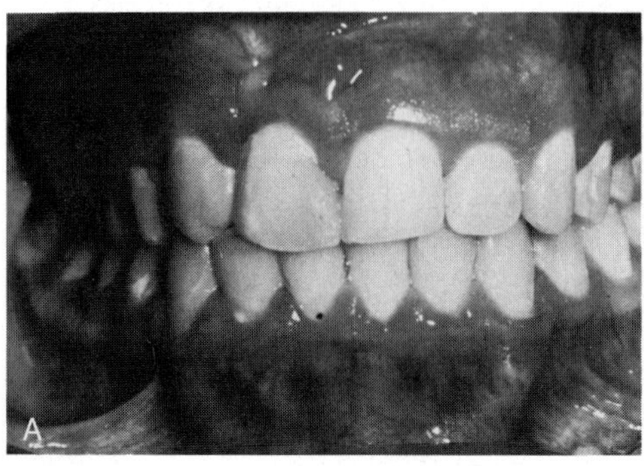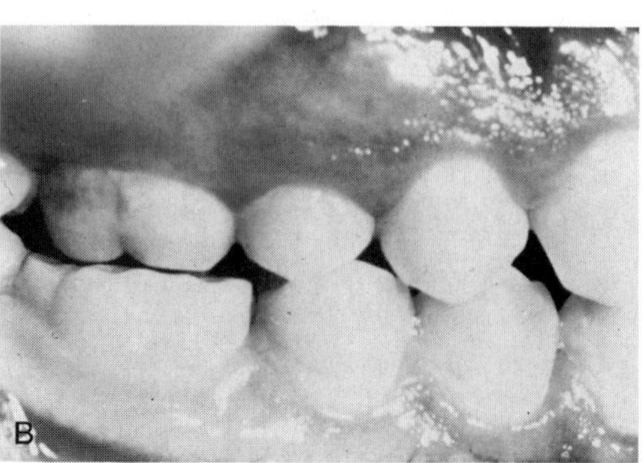

Figure 75–6 Frontal and buccal views of the occlusion. The canine has been brought into contact with the central incisor on the cleft side, resulting in a compromised buccal occlusion.

gun in the late transitional dentition can progress uninterrupted into the permanent dentition, thereby maximizing patient cooperation.

Orthodontic Treatment in the Permanent Dentition

For the patient with a complete unilateral cleft lip and palate, it would be most unusual for the first orthodontic contact to take place when all of their permanent teeth have erupted. The emphasis on interdisciplinary care (the cleft palate–craniofacial team) would more than likely have placed the patient in a program that, at a minimum, would have monitored craniofacial growth and dental development. With this in mind, the developmental threshold that would signal biologic readiness for final orthodontic treatment would be the complete, or almost complete, eruption of the permanent dentition.

As noted earlier, the time of the permanent dentition will find the orthodontist dealing with an older patient because there is a significant delay in tooth formation in children with clefts. During the 9- to 12-year age period, the canine and premolars on the cleft side are even more delayed than their antimeres on the noncleft side.[2]

For the patient who has been under the supervision of a cleft palate team and has had the coordinated care of an orthodontist and a surgeon, orthodontic treatment at the time of the permanent dentition is a fait accompli. A bone graft, if indicated, would have been placed. The lateral incisor and canine on the cleft side would have erupted through the bone graft in the line of the cleft. Questions related to arch length would have been resolved, and potential maxillomandibular disproportions would have been identified.

However, if the anterior surface of the maxilla has not been reconstructed prior to eruption of the lateral incisor or canine, the orthodontist has to address at least three questions: Is there sufficient alveolar bone to align the teeth? If so, bony reconstruction of the anterior surface of the maxilla for orthodontic purposes is not necessary. If there is insufficient bone to align the lateral incisor or canine, does bony reconstruction have to precede orthodontic treatment or can it be accomplished during treatment? In other words, can orthodontic alignment of teeth begin before bone grafting? As noted earlier, preservation of the alveolar portion of a bone graft is dependent on the eruption of teeth into the graft or the orthodontic movement of teeth into the area of the bone graft. Therefore, the orthodontist and the surgeon have a certain degree of latitude in timing this procedure. Orthodontic treatment can begin, and, following placement of the bone graft, the canine and lateral incisor can be brought into alignment in the arch.

At the time of the permanent dentition, the orthodontist who has monitored the patient's craniofacial growth will have to consider the question of maxillomandibular discrepancy. Recognizing that there will be patients with varying degrees of maxillary underdevelopment, a decision will have to be made about the degree of maxillary retrusion. Can it be resolved by orthodontic treatment alone, or will orthodontics have to be combined with orthognathic surgery? If orthognathic surgery is required, should bony reconstruction of the anterior surface of the maxilla precede the maxillary advancement? These questions can be partially answered by the need for bone to align the teeth as part of orthodontic treatment. However, if a bone graft has not been placed prior to surgical advancement of the maxilla, it is up to the surgeon to decide whether he would rather do the Le Fort I advancement with a one-piece maxilla or a two-piece maxilla. From the orthodontic perspective, at the time of the osteotomies, the two-piece maxilla permits greater latitude in positioning the cleft maxilla, particularly the anteroposterior movement of the cleft segment. From the surgical perspective, once the orthodontist has stabilized the position of the cleft segments and the occlusion, the surgeon is essentially dealing with a one-piece maxilla, and he has better access for soft tissue coverage of the area to be bone-grafted.

Points to be emphasized at this stage of treatment are as follows: It is the orthodontist who is responsible for determining readiness for orthognathic surgery. This decision is based on a longitudinal roentgencephalometric assessment of craniofacial growth as well as dental considerations. It is the orthodontist who is responsible for determining interocclusal and intermaxillary relationships. These may be modified by the limitations imposed by the patient—e.g., insufficient soft tissues to cover a graft, congenitally missing teeth. And finally, it is the orthodontist's responsibility to be in the operating room to position the cleft segments and place the teeth in their predetermined position. Acceptance of these responsibilities ensures the patient of the best possible orthodontic-surgical treatment.

A final consideration in the permanent dentition is retention (Figure 75–7). As with the noncleft patient, the greater the amount of tooth movement or maxillary expansion, the more critical is the type of retainer and the length of time retainers have to be utilized. For the patient with missing teeth, prosthetic placement of the teeth, particularly by means of a fixed prosthesis, provides excellent retention.

Conclusion

The stages of orthodontic treatment for the patient with a complete unilateral cleft lip and palate are based on a series of developmental thresholds. By assessing the individual's biologic readiness for treatment, orthodontic treatment can be accomplished in the shortest possible time.

Orthodontic treatment should not be carried out in isolation but should be coordinated with the patient's overall needs, as defined by a cleft palate–craniofacial team.

The individual patient's developmental threshold or biologic readiness for treatment can best be determined

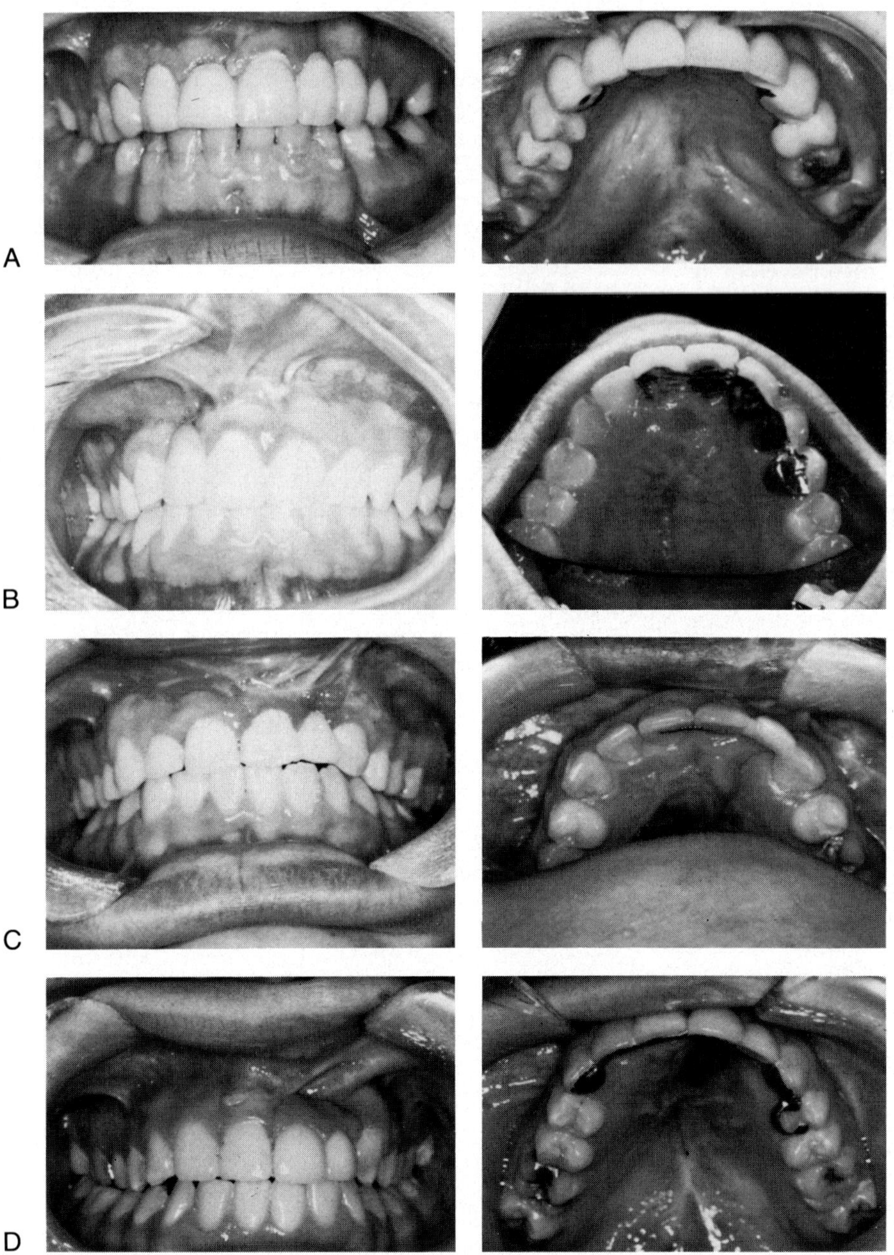

Figure 75–7 Four examples of fixed retention. *A,* Fixed prosthesis with full crowns extending from the canine on the noncleft side to the premolar on the cleft side. *B,* Bonded prosthesis replacing the congenitally missing lateral incisor on the cleft side. *C,* Temporary bonded prosthesis replacing the lateral incisor. *D,* Bonded prosthesis with a palatal extension for obturation of a fistula.

by the orthodontist using serial roentgencephalometry to assess craniofacial growth and panoramic radiography to evaluate dental development.

References

1. Nanda SK: Prediction of facial growth using different biologic criteria in females. In Carlson DS, Ribbens KA (eds): Craniofacial Growth During Adolescence. Monograph 20. Craniofacial Growth Series. Ann Arbor: Center for Human Growth and Development, University of Michigan, 1986.
2. Ranta R: A review of tooth formation in children with cleft lip and palate. Am J Orthod Orthop 90:11–18, 1986.
3. Loevy H, Aduss H: Tooth maturation in cleft lip and/or cleft palate. Cleft Palate J (in press, 1988).
4. Levin HS: A cephalometric analysis of cleft palate deficiencies in the middle third of the face. Angle Orthod 19:186–194, 1963.
5. Graber TM: Craniofacial morphology in cleft lip and cleft palate deformities. Surg Gynecol Obstet 88:359–369, 1949.
6. Graber TM: The congenital cleft palate deformity. J Am Dent Assoc 48:375–395, 1954.
7. Krogman WM: The problem of the cleft palate face. Plast Reconstr Surg 14:370–375, 1954.
8. Pruzansky S: Description, classification, and analysis of unoperated clefts of the lip and palate. Am J Orthod 39:590–611, 1953.
9. Aduss H: The nasal cavity in complete unilateral cleft lip and palate. Arch Otolaryngol 85:53–61, 1967.
10. Aduss H: The width of the cleft at the level of the tuberosities in complete unilateral cleft lip and palate. Plast Reconstr Surg 41:113–123, 1968.
11. Aduss H: Craniofacial growth in complete unilateral cleft lip and palate. Angle Orthod 41:202–213, 1971.
12. Ross RB: Treatment variables affecting facial growth in complete unilateral cleft lip and palate. Cleft Palate J 24:5–77, 1987.
13. Fara M, Chlumska A, Hrivanakova J: Musculus orbicularis in incomplete hare-lip. Acta Chir Plast 7:125–134, 1965.
14. Fara M, Smahel J: Postoperative follow-up of restitution procedures in the orbicularis oris muscle after operation for complete bilateral cleft of the lip. Plast Reconstr Surg 40:12–21, 1967.
15. Fara M: Anatomy and arteriography of cleft lips in stillborn children. Plast Reconstr Surg 42:29–36, 1968.
16. Dorf DS, Curtin JW: Early cleft palate repair and speech outcome. Plast Reconstr Surg 70:74–79, 1982.
17. Burston WR: The early treatment of cleft palate conditions. Dent Prac 9:41–52, 1958.

18. McNeil CK: Orthopedic principles in the treatment of lip and palate clefts. In Hotz RP (ed): International Symposium on Early Treatment of Cleft Lip and Palate. Berne: Hans Huber, 1964.
19. Hotz MM, Gnoinski WM, Nussbaumer H, et al: Early maxillary orthopedics in CLP cases: Guidelines for surgery. Cleft Palate J 15:405–411, 1978.
20. Witsenburg B: The reconstruction of the anterior residual bone defects in patients with cleft lip, alveolus and palate. J Maxillofac Surg 13:197–208, 1985.
21. Rosenstein SW, Monroe CW, Kernahan DA, et al: The case for early bone grafting in cleft lip and cleft palate. Plast Reconstr Surg 70:297–307, 1982.
22. Rosenstein SW: Early habilitation of the cleft lip and palate child. In Johnston LE (ed): New Vistas in Orthodontics. Philadelphia: Lea & Febiger, 1985.
23. Pruzansky S, Aduss H: Arch form and the deciduous occlusion in complete unilateral clefts. Cleft Palate J 1:411–418, 1964.
24. Jolleys A, Robertson NRE: A study of the effects of early bone grafting in complete clefts of the lip and palate—five year study. Br J Plast Surg 25:229–237, 1972.
25. Vig KWL, Turvey TA: Orthodontic-surgical inter-action in the management of cleft lip and palate. Clin Plast Surg 12:735–748, 1985.
26. Bergland O, Semb G, Abyholm F, et al: Secondary bone grafting and orthodontic treatment in patients with bilateral complete clefts of the lip and palate. Ann Plast Surg 17:460–474, 1986.
27. Aduss H, McDaniel RT, Pruzansky S, et al: Serial extraction. J Am Dent Assoc 95:573–582, 1977.

CHAPTER 76

Orthodontic Principles in Treatment of Cleft Lip and Palate

J. Daniel Subtelny

The present status of cleft palate rehabilitation is measurably improved compared to the situation three to four decades ago. At that time, few data existed, and clinical decisions were very difficult to make. Often the decision revolved around whether or not the appearance of the middle third of the face should be sacrificed to achieve surgical closure of the palate. The alternative question was, should the palate be left open and prosthetically treated to ensure good speech results? In the latter instance, the hope was that both facial appearance and speech would be equally good. The situation today is markedly improved—not yet optimal, but certainly better. Improvement in the clinical outlook is unquestionably the result of the interaction of many professional disciplines involved in the care of these individuals.

Orthodontists have played a measurable role, primarily through careful documentation and the compilation of records to evaluate favorable as well as adverse effects of many procedures employed over the years in the care of these individuals.[1–15] Further contributions have come through the application of knowledge of the growth and development of the skeletal craniofacial complex; other studies involving soft tissues of the face and the speech mechanism have added information in other dimensions facilitating the possibilities of more intelligent management procedures.[16–22] Contributions to the procedural principles of orthodontic treatment for cleft palate patients have also been made. Herein an attempt will be made to indicate the present status of the art of orthodontic rehabilitation of the cleft individual while maintaining a clinical focus on the implications of changes that occur with time and growth.

People who have worked in cleft palate rehabilitation with long-term interest acknowledge certain basic variables that influence judgment. The first relates to the heterogeneity involved in clefting; differences in cleft type and degree have been described and must be acknowledged (Fig. 76–1). As Pruzansky has stated, "All clefts are not alike."[23] Furthermore, he has emphasized that clefts and variables of clefting should be seen and recognized at the "time of beginning" to understand the differing progression to the time of maturity. Another significant variable influencing rehabilitation status is the stage of development at which judgments or measures of success are made. Orthodontists know well that things may look good at one stage of development and prove to be disappointing at a later stage. For this basic reason, the final status achieved in rehabilitation cannot be predicted until patients have reached maturity.

One of the fundamental controversies during the past has centered on the variable of whether a deficiency of tissue invariably exists in cleft palate patients. Some have expressed the opinion that the cleft itself represents a deficiency of hard palate tissue. Others believe that the hard palate shelves bordering a cleft are not deficient in structure but are displaced from the normal position.[6, 24–26] In one investigation, cephalometric laminography was used to compare the hard palate dimensions of 127 cleft palate children under 3 years of age without operation and 50 noncleft children of comparable age.[27] Bony palatal shelves were measured to determine the quantity of tissue. Comparison with measurements obtained from the noncleft children indicated the deficiency or adequacy of hard palate tissues in the cleft palate subjects. Distances between the right and left lateral walls of the nasal cavity were measured to determine whether the maxillary bones bordering the cleft were medially or laterally displaced compared to noncleft subjects.

These measurements revealed that, except for the cleft cases that involved only the lip and alveolar process, there was a definite tendency toward hard palate tissue deficiency in children with clefts involving the palate. However, the deficiency of hard palate tissue varied considerably in individual patients and according to cleft type. Subjects with bilateral clefts of the palate were most likely to have a deficiency of tissue and to show the greatest degree of deficiency followed by patients with posterior clefts and then by those with unilateral clefts.

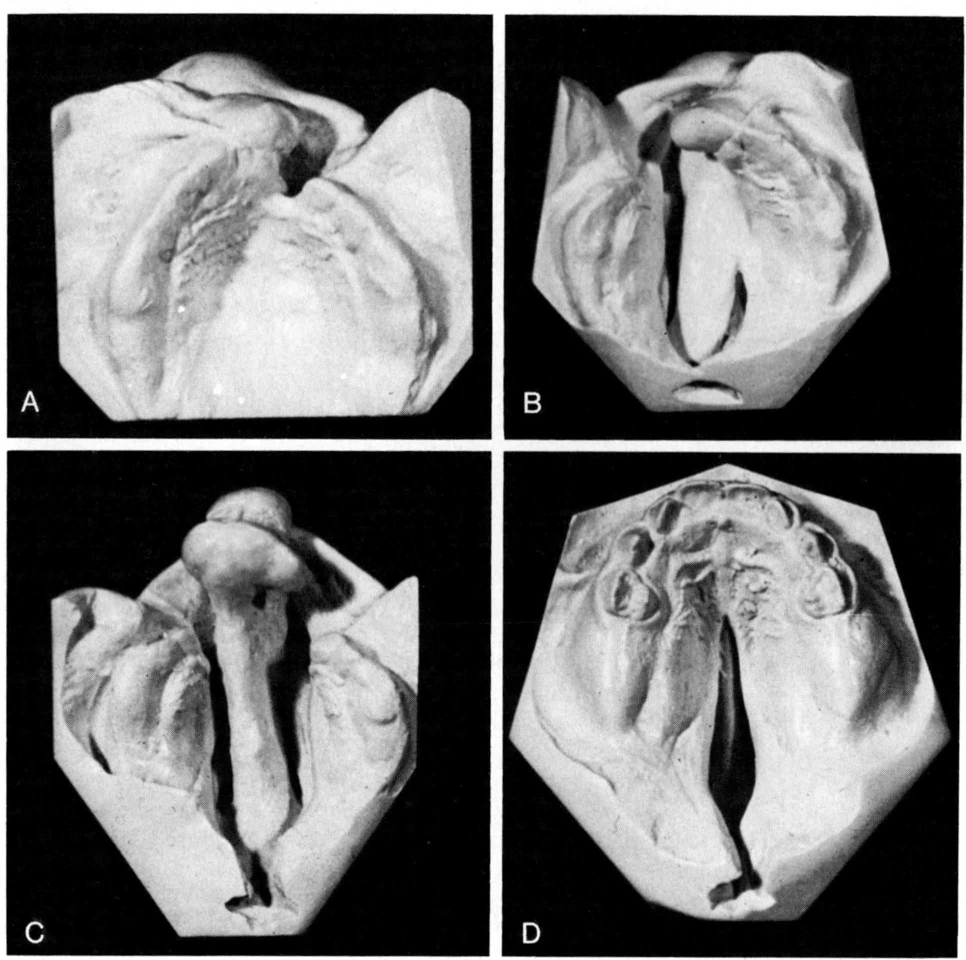

Figure 76–1 Dental casts depicting variation in cleft morphology. *A*, Left unilateral cleft of the lip and alveolar process. *B*, Right unilateral complete cleft of the lip and palate; the nasal septum is united with one of the palatal shelves. *C*, Complete bilateral cleft of the lip and palate; the nasal septum is not united with either of the palatal shelves. *D*, A posterior cleft of the hard and soft palates; the lip and alveolar process is not involved in cleftness.

Of particular significance to the present discussion was the finding of lateral displacement of the maxillary bones in the oronasal area of all cleft palate types. The greatest displacement as well as deficiency was found in patients with bilateral clefts. Although more deficiency of tissue was found in posterior clefts than unilateral clefts, a greater displacement of the maxillary bones was found in the subjects with unilateral clefts of the lip and palate. From all indications, lateral displacement of the maxillary bones as well as a deficiency of hard palate tissue can clearly exist in cleft palate subjects; it is not a matter of either/or—both can be present, and individually, neither may be evident.

Deficiency in dimension can be understood in terms of inadequacy or insufficiency in development. More difficult to comprehend are the developmental sequences leading to a displacement of the maxillary bones. It must be recognized that the spatial positions of the parts of the maxilla in a cleft lip and palate individual were developing long before birth. During prenatal development, muscle function is known to influence the configuration of developing bone and, subsequent to the formation of a complete cleft, can influence the spatial position of the bony parts closely related to the cleft. A cleft of the lip and palate is not solely a cleft of bony tissue; it is a cleft of muscle as well. A cleft of a muscular ring extends from the

posterior pharyngeal wall forward, encircling the maxillary and mandibular gum pads, and a cleft of the soft palate musculature is integrally related to the posterior aspect of the hard palate (Fig. 76–2).

Once a cleft of the lip is manifest, the fetal lip cannot function as an intact muscular structure. The cleft lip musculature, in close contiguity to an aberrant skeletal foundation, cannot surround the unfused bony maxillary structures. Not being able to exert its normal molding influence on the maxillary segments, the incomplete musculature acts in a disproportionate and asymmetric fashion on those structures. Aberrant muscle force vectors are exerted that tend to pull the bony cleft segments in a lateral direction (Fig. 76–3). Additionally, the cleft musculature is not capable of restraining the expansive forces exerted by the muscular tongue within the oral cavity and the maxillary complex. This inequality of muscle forces within and outside the maxillary gum pads results in the upward and outward positioning of the maxillary alveolar gum pads that is frequently evident at birth. It is surmised that this is the mechanism whereby the displacement of the bony maxillary segments takes place around the bony cleft, resulting in the increased width between the lateral nasal walls.[27]

This displacement of maxillary segments sometimes requires the surgeon to request early orthopedic intervention to facilitate lip closure. Usually surgical lip

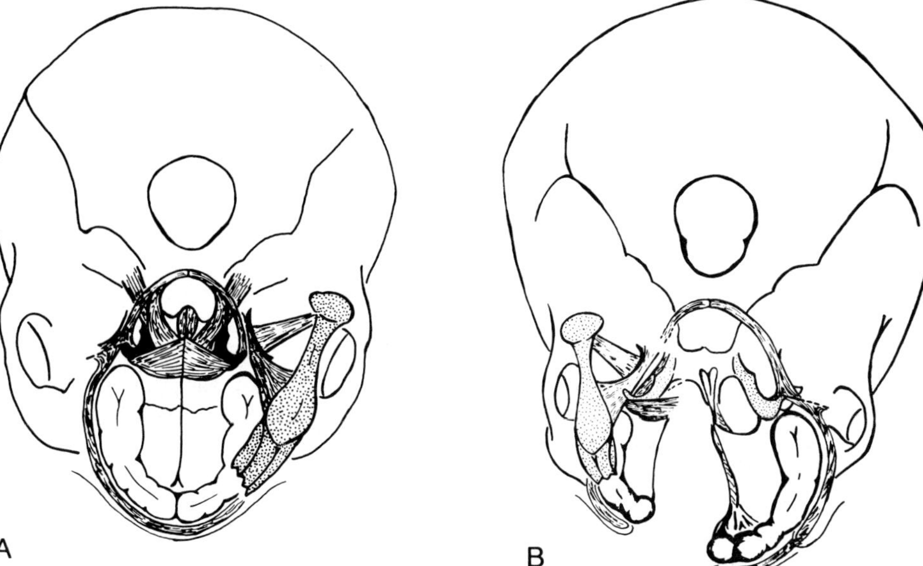

Figure 76–2 Diagrammatic representation of the inferior aspect of the nasomaxillary complex and the skull base illustrating the muscular ring from the posterior pharyngeal wall forward and encircling the maxillary gum pads. *A*, A normal, skull. *B*, A skull with a complete unilateral cleft of the lip alveolus and palate.

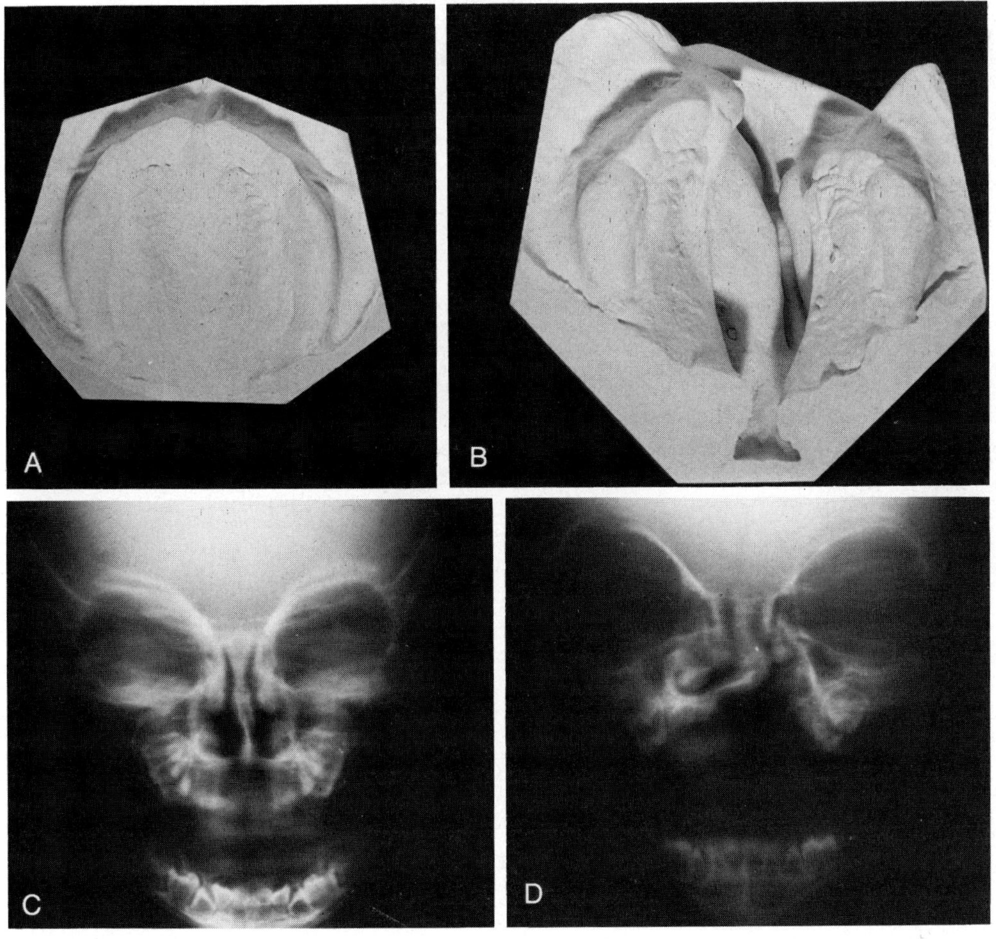

Figure 76–3 Dental cast registrations and frontal laminagraphs of normal and unilateral cleft individuals. *A*, Cast—normal sibling. *B*, Cast—complete unilateral cleft lip and palate sibling. *C*, Frontal laminagraph depicting the nasal cavity area of a normal individual. *D*, Frontal laminagraph depicting the nasal cavity area of a complete unilateral cleft of the lip and palate; distortion and displacement of parts are dramatic when compared to the noncleft individual *(C)*.

closure can be achieved without any need to reposition the parts to more closely approximate the lip segments. In fewer instances, adjunctive orthopedic molding forces may be necessary to more closely approximate the underlying nasomaxillary structures to allow surgical repair to be undertaken.[28–32] Aside from the occasional need to facilitate lip closure, in the author's orthodontic approach presurgical orthopedic treatment is not recommended nor are early bone grafting procedures following presurgical orthopedic methods. However, during the 1950s, 1960s, and 1970s, a number of surgeons and orthodontists recommended primary bone grafting following a period of presurgical orthopedic treatment.[33–37] Bone grafts from the rib or iliac crest were used to create a bony continuum from the premaxilla to the lateral segment. In other instances, periosteal transplants were performed to create a "boneless bone graft."[38]

After a period of time, the wave of enthusiasm for primary bone grafts began to decline when some researchers began to note undesirable changes in their grafted patients. With eruption of the permanent dentition, more crossbite relationships were noted along with inhibition of maxillary growth.[39–41] The actual graft sometimes decreased in dimension and eventually became too small to support teeth.[42] Additionally, presur-

gical orthopedic treatment and early bone grafting presuppose a deficiency of tissue, and this is not always the case.[27] Furthermore, from the orthodontic perspective, without the presence of mandibular dentition there are no visible clues on which to base a decision about where to position the maxillary parts. The only available structures are the tooth-bearing gum pads and part of the rapidly growing and repositioning mandible.

Cleft lip repair frequently changes the spatial relationship of the underlying nasomaxillary parts and the alveolar segments contiguous to the bony cleft. Just as the musculature was important in the prenatal positioning of parts, musculature also should be acknowledged in the development of malocclusion problems subsequent to surgical repair of the cleft lip.

The reconstructed lip musculature creates compressive forces on the displaced nasomaxillary bony segments, initiating a molding action that serves to bring the alveolar segments closer together. It has been shown that in some instances the molding effect of the lip pressure may cause the alveolar segments to approximate each other, forming an acceptable maxillary arch contour.[43] In other instances, the muscular forces may displace one or both of the maxillary segments medially while rotating and moving the premaxillary area posteriorly, potentially creating a constricted maxillary alveo-

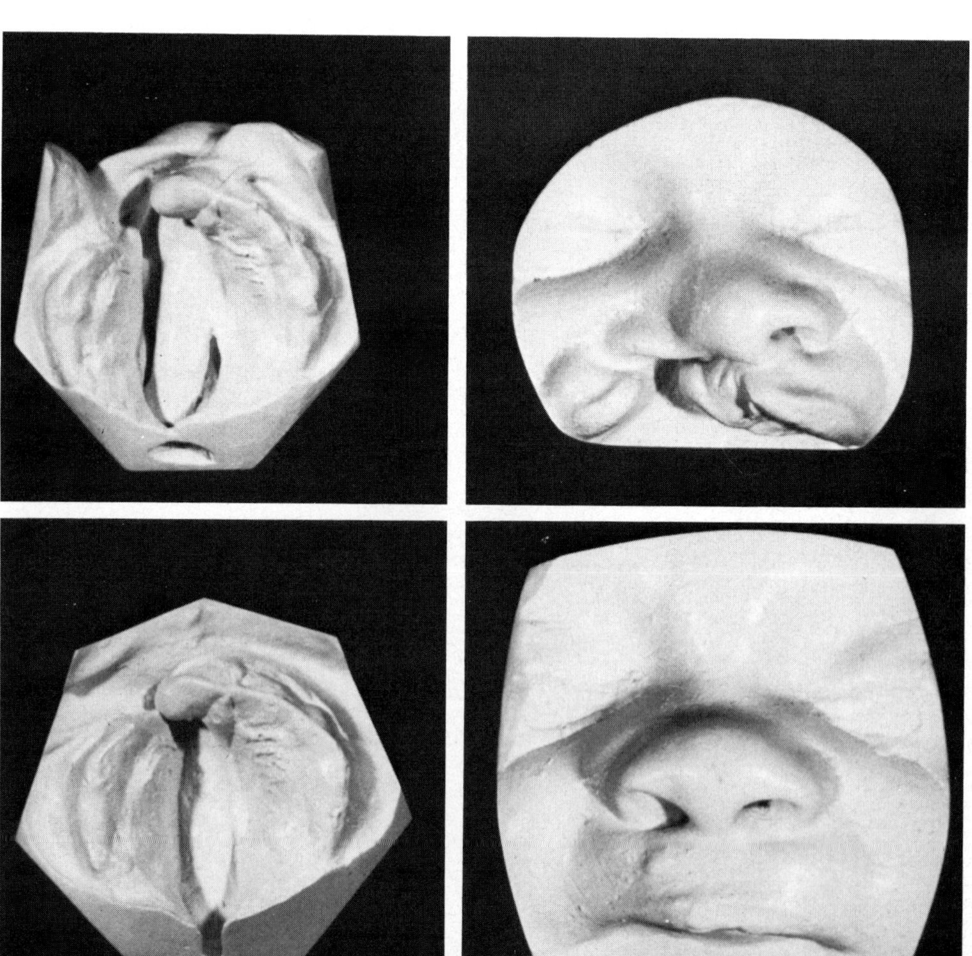

Figure 76–4 *A,* Facial and upper jaw casts of the same individual before and after lip repair. Muscle molding has moved segments, leading to approximation of the alveolar pads.

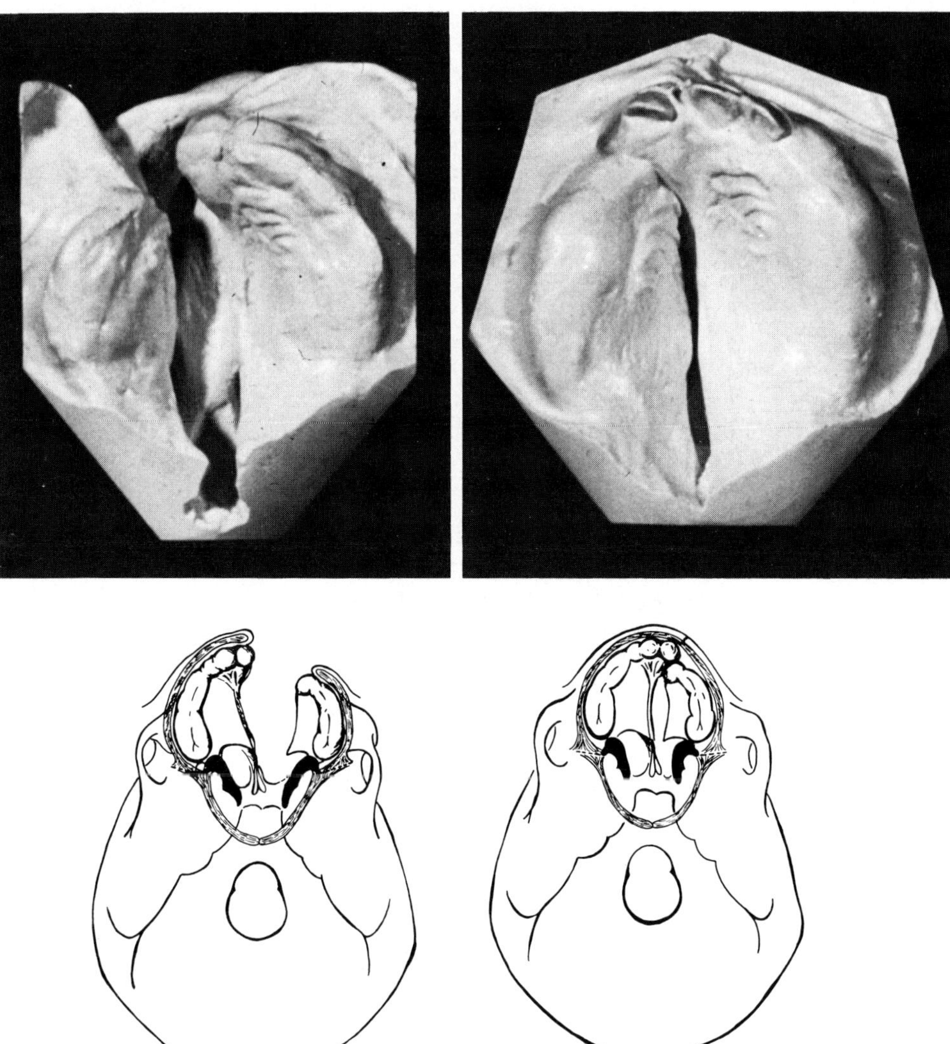

Figure 76–4 Continued B, Casts and illustrations indicating reconstruction of the muscular ring incidental to lip repair and movement of segments leading to an overlap of the premaxillary alveolar process over the gum pad of the smaller buccal segment.

lar arch. In individuals with complete unilateral cleft lip and palate the smaller bony segment sometimes can be displaced medially so that the deciduous cuspid region of that segment closely approximates the palatal process of the larger segment, while the premaxillary segment is being molded palatally to more closely approximate or even overlap the anterior portion of the alveolar process of the smaller maxillary segment (Fig. 76–4). Integral to the process of muscle molding is the original geometric relationship of the cleft bony segments. A medial overrotation can cause the alveolar process of the smaller maxillary segment to become contained within the premaxillary alveolar element of the larger segment.

It has been demonstrated that movement of segments, under the influence of lip muscle–molding forces, frequently results in a concomitant narrowing of the palatal cleft. From all indications, the effects of lip surgery on the unfused maxillary segments is not restricted to a constriction of the maxillary alveolar segments alone. Laminographic radiographs of children taken before and after surgical reconstruction of the lip indicate that the lip molding action can cause a nasomaxillary architectural rearrangement by moving the maxillary segments

(Fig. 76–5). Pruzansky and Aduss have shown that this movement can take place until contact between the inferior nasal turbinate and the nasal septum is achieved.[44] It should be emphasized that this medial displacement, in narrowing the palatal cleft, may enhance the possibility of a successful surgical correction of the palatal cleft if it occurs earlier than the time of optimal palatal surgical closure.

Concomitantly, this maxillary bony movement may be the precursor to a fairly typical orthodontic problem in the cleft lip and palate child even prior to palatal surgery. Incident to lip reconstruction, muscular forces may have moved the smaller maxillary segments into a lingual relationship with the corresponding mandibular segment, narrowing the maxillary arch more predominantly in the anterior region and resulting in a crossbite malocclusion in one or both of the posterior segments of the dental arches. Rather than the smooth curved alveolar arch, recognized as "normal" or acceptable, there may be a distortion toward the **V** shape with the apex pointed toward the lip in the premaxillary region. It has been observed that there are different degrees of reaction to the constricting effects of the surgically repaired lip.

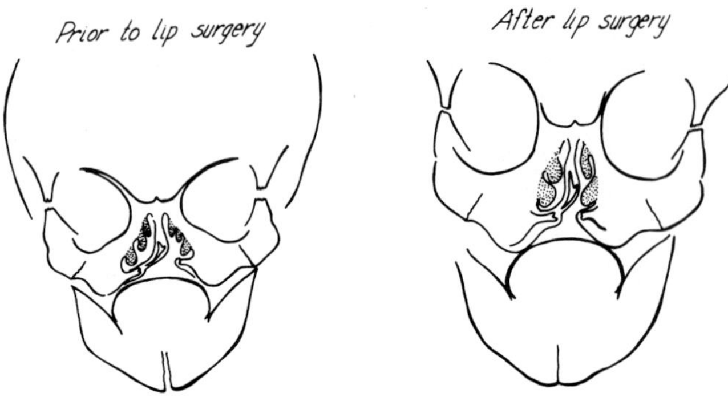

Figure 76–5 Frontal laminagraphs of the same (cleft lip and palate) individual before and after lip surgery; a 3-month interval existed between the radiographic registrations. Changes in the relationship of parts can be noted.

In a well-documented study, collapse of the maxillary arch was evident in only 40% of the patients.[45] In some of the patients only the deciduous cuspid was found to be in a crossbite relationship. This effect would be consistent with medial distortion of the anterior aspect of the posterior buccal segments. It is important to reemphasize that the muscle molding action can create the distorted and constricted maxillary alveolar arch and the potential for dental malocclusion prior to the undertaking of palatal surgery.[46] With age and growth, the continued influences of these forces and the potential for additional constrictive influences incidental to palatal surgery may lead to a more pronounced crossbite malocclusion in the deciduous dentition.

In years past, many centers reported a high percentage of maxillary constriction in complete cleft patients that was represented by crossbites in the deciduous dentition and was particularly noticeable after palatal surgery. Presently, presurgical orthopedic treatment and placement of a retentive stabilization appliance rather than bone grafts have been strongly advocated to hold the positioned bony segments after lip surgery and prior to palatal surgery.[47, 48] Delay of surgical closure of the hard palate has been recommended, with closure of soft palate tissue at an appropriate earlier time. A series of molding and retentive appliances are placed, obturating the hard palate cleft and guiding the bony segments and dentition into improved occlusion by preventing constriction of the bony parts.

Proponents who recommend that hard cleft palate closure be delayed, emphasize better midfacial and palate development until nasomaxillary growth sites are less active after 5 to 6 years of age. Schweckendiek introduced the two-stage procedure for surgical closure of the cleft of the palate.[49] Initially, surgical closure of the soft palate was undertaken at 18 to 24 months of age, and the oronasal fistula was occluded with a prosthesis until hard palate closure was undertaken at about 12 to 14 years of age. Other proponents of this procedure have usually recommended closure of the hard palate at about 5 to 6 years of age, considering that early completed growth of the hard palate may be possible.

By leaving the hard palate open, it was supposed that growth and development of the maxilla would not be impeded by scar tissue formation. Recent evaluation of patients who had undergone the delayed surgical procedure seems to indicate that, although the eventual occlusion might be improved and indeed might be quite adequate as far as crossbite malocclusion is concerned, speech results might be less than desirable.[50] As a consequence, the procedure is not without potential disadvantages.

Although much literature is devoted to the timing of cleft palate closure with many varying opinions, the conventional option still seems to be primary cleft palate closure prior to 2 years of age when feasible, with progressive review for future treatment modalities. To date, this timing has seemed to withstand the test of time and has most consistently withstood critical evaluation during late adolescence and adulthood. In essence, functional demands, the geometrics of the original cleft including soft tissue adequacy, the facial growth pattern, and the surgical procedure itself are the important factors that dictate the timing of palatal closure. It is acknowledged that palatal surgery prior to 2 years of age, because of the development of scar tissue, may add a constrictive influence to the maxillary complex. It is further acknowledged that this may lead to development of a partial or even total crossbite, usually on the side of the palatal cleft in the deciduous dentition. However, it also is emphasized that this malocclusion is amenable to orthodontic correction.

Treatment in the Deciduous Dentition

Orthodontic treatment in the cleft lip and palate child, if indicated, can be initiated after the eruption of the deciduous dentition. In most instances, this would be after the time of palatal closure, most probably around 3 to 4 years of age. As previously mentioned, in the development of the constricted and distorted maxillary arch, molding influences exerted by the repaired lip, with the superimposed constrictive action of the palatal repair, are not restricted to alveolar bone alone. They usually involve an architectural rearrangement of the different parts of the cleft maxilla. If the maxillary segments are malaligned the deciduous teeth frequently erupt into a crossbite malocclusion in one or both of the posterior segments of the dental arches. This crossbite relationship usually improves as it progresses posteriorly from the region of the deciduous cuspid to the region of the posterior (second) deciduous molar. Orthodontic therapy in cleft lip and palate cases must be directed toward counteracting the adverse influences that produced the maxillary constriction.

Whereas postoperative soft tissue forces constrict the maxillary arch and its supporting bone, orthodontic forces must expand and move the maxillary arch to a more normal configuration and positional occlusion. There is substantial evidence that orthodontic forces applied in children with a cleft of the lip and palate can actually move the unfused maxillary segments. Ordinarily, orthodontic treatment in the noncleft individual involves movement of individual teeth and changes within the alveolar bone surrounding the roots of these teeth. From all indications, orthodontic forces properly directed in a youngster with a repaired cleft lip and palate can actually move the unfused bony maxillary segments containing the erupted deciduous teeth as well as unerupted permanent teeth.[51, 52] In the latter instance, individual tooth movement might be minimal while the maxillary bones housing the teeth are repositioned.

This finding was substantiated by a cephalometric laminographic study of individuals with unilateral cleft lip and palate who were examined radiographically before and after orthodontic expansion.[52] Measurement of distances between the crowns of developing unerupted permanent teeth well encased within the maxillary bony segments showed an appreciable increase in width (Fig. 76–6). Additionally, the lateral walls of the nasal cavity formed by the maxillary bones were wider, and at times the inferior nasal turbinate had been moved away from contact with the nasal septum. This opening of the nasal cavity was most marked anteriorly.

In essence, this picture represents a movement of the bony segments to position the different parts of the maxillary arch into a more correct occlusal relationship to the mandibular arch. Awaiting full eruption of the deciduous dentition before initiating orthodontic treatment can be important because the mandibular arch affords an excellent basis for determining where to position the distorted maxillary parts and the dentition (Fig. 76–7).

Acknowledgment of bony movement rather than tooth movement at this early age may indicate the possible inadvisability of certain surgical procedures. The inadvisability of early bone grafts has already been shown because such grafts would preclude any future movement of bony parts. The desirability of bony movement may also contraindicate undertaking extensive vomer mucoperiosteal flaps or any other palatal periosteal flap as part of early age surgical reconstruction.

In a study undertaken at Eastman Dental Center on young male *Macaca mulatta* monkeys, autogenous periosteal transplants were placed in selected facial sutures.[53] As part of this study, autogenous periosteal transplants from the tibia were placed across the midpalatal suture. Cephalometric and occlusal radiographs as well as cast records were taken during a 6-month period. Subsequently, selected areas of interest were examined histologically. Examination revealed the formation of a bony bridge in the area of the palatal periosteal transplants. The palatal bony bridge formation affected palatal growth in that less than normal growth was manifested in the lateral and anteroposterior dimensions.

All of the surgical procedures seemed to affect growth in the lateral direction adversely, but the most significant effects occurred in the palatal transplant animals. Placing periosteum contiguous to the two osseous margins of a palatal defect might create a partial simulation of a vomer flap or periosteal flap in the palatal region. Unfortunately, the osteogenesis of new bone incident to the presence of periosteum across the suture could lead to reduced lateral growth and possibly to a reduction in nasomaxillary growth.[54]

Furthermore, it might preclude bony segmental

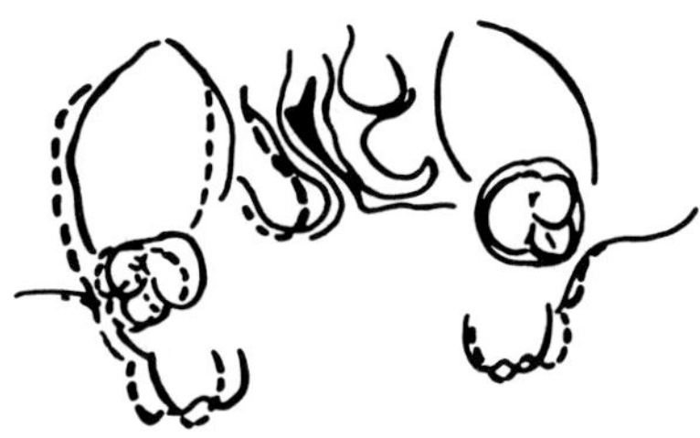

Figure 76–6 Frontal laminagraphic radiographs, sectioned in selected areas, indicating movement of the bony segments following orthodontic expansion in an individual with a repaired unilateral cleft of the lip and palate. Note the increase in width of the nasal cavities and changes in the position of unerupted permanent teeth indicating bony movement (solid line, before expansion; broken line, after expansion).

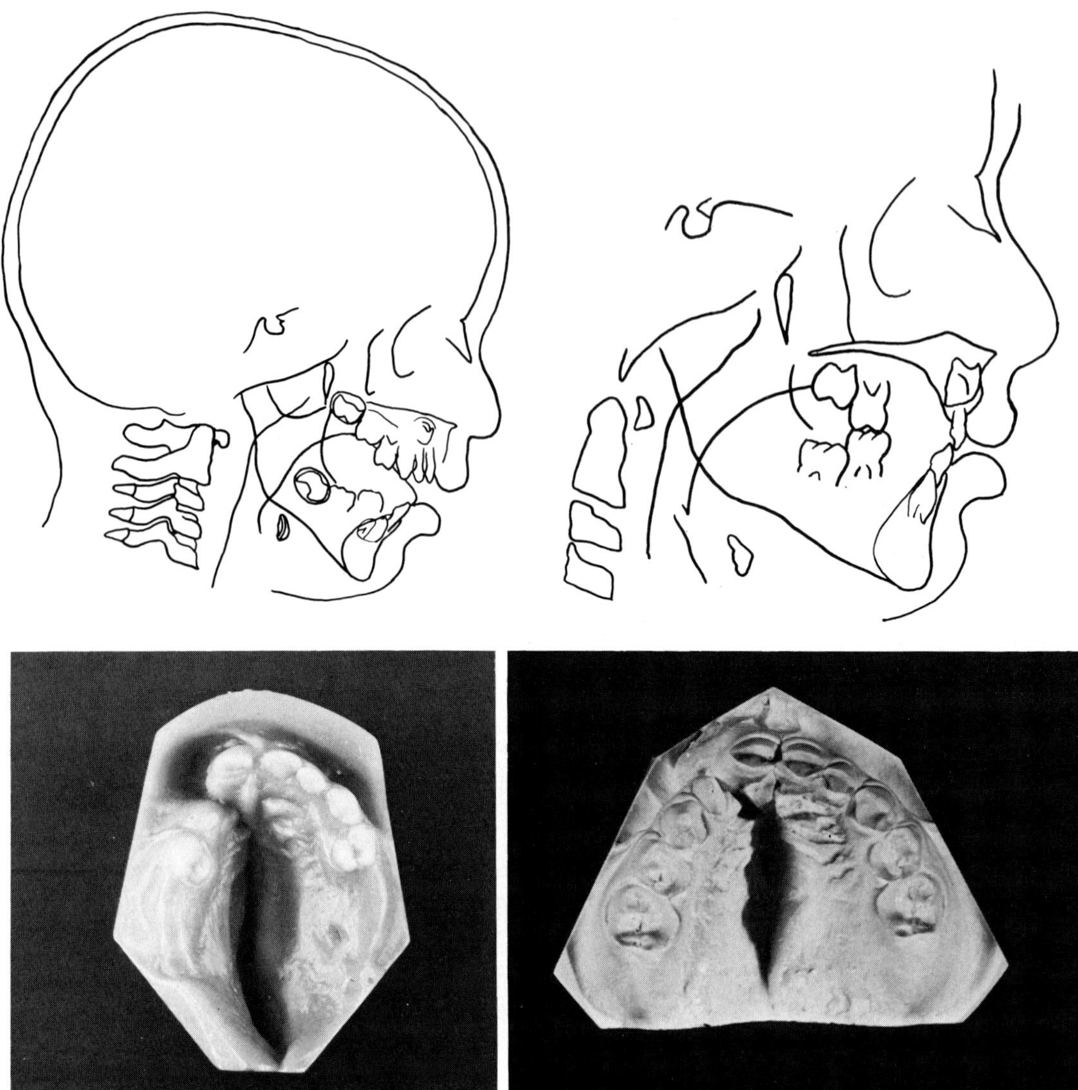

Figure 76–7 At 1 year 9 months the developing constriction of the maxillary arch is evident; lateral headplate denotes good facial development (right). Lateral headplate and cast at 5 years 4 months of age after orthodontic correction of the maxillary constriction; note opening in the anterior palatal region.

movement by means of orthodontic procedures at any age because the formation of a solid bony bridge makes it increasingly difficult to achieve crossbite correction as growth progresses. Until the later stages of growth, the orthopedic movement of bony segments is a very important aspect of orthodontic treatment of the individual with a cleft lip and palate.

To reiterate, it is recommended that the unfused bony segments be repositioned as early as possible after the eruption of deciduous teeth. The reorientation of the anatomy of the maxillary arch and palate may offer many benefits if it is accomplished effectively at an early age. First, it creates a more harmonious relationship between the maxillary bony architecture and the contiguous musculature. Segmental repositioning, if properly undertaken, creates a potentially more optimal foundation for the support and continued function of the reconstructed lip. Improved functional movements and lip posture and development may occur when the supporting maxillary bony segments are optimally po-sitioned because that musculature not only overlies the bone but is attached to the bone. Furthermore, the repositioning of the bony segments, in establishing a more normal scaffolding for the roof of the oral cavity, may enhance the probability that general tongue activity may more closely approximate normal function during mastication, speech, and deglutition. Compensatory adjustments of tongue activity dictated by abnormal palatal vault configurations as well as distorted and constricted dental arches may be avoided by this means.

Basic speech habits are established rapidly at early age levels. If the oral architecture is brought closer to the normal, it may be possible to reduce or prevent the development of misarticulations common to the cleft palate child. Aberrant anatomic and dental relationships can logically be considered to influence adversely the range and patterns of tongue movements and posture. Speech skills are acquired during a well-defined period of chronologic development; rapid growth in phonetic articulation occurs between 2½ and 4½ years of age, and a reasonably mature speech pattern is normally attained by 7 years of age. Thus, segmental repositioning during the early years may do the most good in regard to speech development.

Furthermore, by placing the bony segments in their proper positions the alveolar segments can be unlocked, enhancing the possibility of more normal vertical and anteroposterior development of the alveolar process in regions approximating the cleft.[52] Containment of one alveolar segment within another may keep the alveolar process from developing fully because one alveolar segment is buttressed within another, causing an impediment of alveolar growth and tooth eruption in the region of the cleft. When orthodontic forces have unlocked the alveolar segments, teeth erupt rapidly, and a concomitant increment in alveolar growth is noted. One can also assume that unlocking the alveolar segments may relieve the bony maxillary segments of their impaction and enhance the possibility of more normal maxillary growth, partially incident to providing better support for the upper lip. One can also hope that ventilation within the nasal cavity may improve. Nasal respiration in itself has been shown to improve the possibility of optimal maxillary growth.[55]

Any provision for the fullest expression of maxillary growth may vastly improve the potential for a more harmonious facial appearance. Optimal maxillary growth creates a more normal foundation for the support of the surgically repaired lip. Greater expression of potential alveolar growth also adds to the support of the lip. Added alveolar support helps to counteract adverse pressures from the reconstructed lip. Establishment of more normal geometric relationships and the fullest possible expression of nasomaxillary growth help to reduce any tendency toward depression of the middle third of the face. Unlocking the bony segments during the early stages of development when growth is rapid and when advantage may be taken of the greatest possible growth potential is all important.

It is emphasized that some form of prolonged, adequate retention is imperative because it may not be possible to stabilize the effects of the adverse muscular forces and soft tissue constrictive influences. Failure to place retentive appliances may permit orthodontically corrected structures to return rapidly to early undesirable segmental relationships and constricted maxillary dental arch positions, sometimes within a few days,

when many months have been needed for correction. Because retention appliances may be lost, a fixed or cemented, well-adapted, maxillary lingual arch appliance is recommended (Fig. 76–7). This can hold the maxillary arch in its optimal position and at the same time permits the tongue to remain in its natural posture in the region of the maxillary arch rather than in a low postural position.

In many instances, because of the medial displacement of the maxillary posterior segments, the smaller segment may approximate the palatal tissue of the larger segment in the more anterior regions of the hard palate. In such cases, when there is coaptation of soft tissue with soft tissue, the surgeon may decide not to introduce extensive undermining of tissue to achieve surgical closure and maintain a nonunited soft tissue fixation in the anterior region. Depending on the expansive movements of orthodontic forces, a re-opening of the nonunited soft tissue bordering the cleft may occur. This anterior opening may result in loss of intraoral air pressure during speech and may permit liquid to flow into the nasal cavity and from the nares during mastication and swallowing. It is recommended that removable, palatal coverage retention be constructed in addition to the fixed lingual arch retainer (Fig. 76–8) because the coverage can serve the added function of anterior obturation while the fixed retainer maintains the stability of the repositioned bony parts.

Treatment in the Transitional Dentition

Early orthodontic treatment in children with cleft lip and palate is a philosophy that is strongly favored. For reasons enumerated above, it is suggested that early orthopedic treatment be initiated after the eruption of the deciduous dentition. Early orthodontic repositioning of the bony segments and the establishment of acceptable occlusion of the deciduous dentition may permit the permanent teeth to erupt in a more favorable occlusal position; however, such treatment does not necessarily eliminate the need for orthodontic treatment at later stages of development.

The anterior permanent teeth, particularly those closely bordering the alveolar cleft, usually erupt excessively rotated, poorly inclined, and in undesirable positions. Longitudinal cephalometric lateral and frontal

Figure 76–8 Retainers used after orthopedic expansion during the deciduous dentition stage of development. *A*, Wire retainer, cemented into place (nonremovable). *B*, Palatal coverage, preferable when palatal openings are present, is removable. Note that this type of retainer can be used in conjunction with the fixed wire, nonremovable retainer.

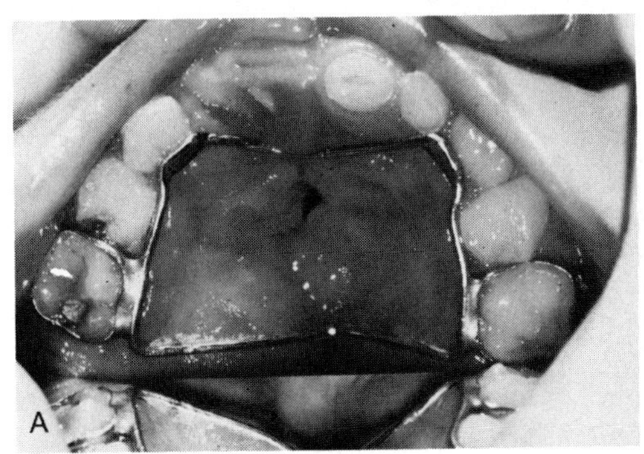
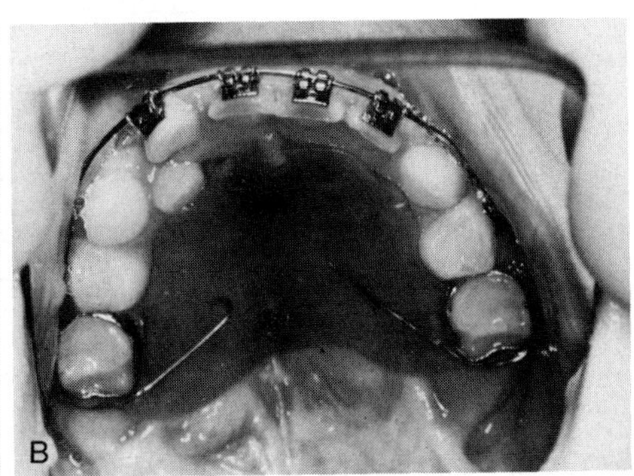

radiographs taken in individuals with complete unilateral and bilateral clefts of the lip and palate have been used to study the patterns of eruption of the permanent incisors and cuspid teeth.[56] It was found that the incisors bordering the cleft erupted downward and backward into a position more retroclined than normal and became more retropositioned with age. The incisor crowns approximating the cleft tipped progressively more toward the cleft with continued eruption. Vertical eruption of the maxillary cuspids approximating the cleft was significantly less than that observed in noncleft subjects, indicating the possibility of reduced dental-alveolar vertical development in this region.

Normally, the maxillary cuspid moves downward and forward as well as buccally as it erupts and gradually achieves an upright inclination by approximately 12 years of age. Although the same pattern was noted in the cleft subjects, the cuspids close to the cleft never showed the same amount of movement at comparable ages. Maxillary cuspids closely approximating the cleft were found to be positioned more palatally, and the crowns were tipped toward the cleft and the roots were more distally inclined and positioned compared to noncleft subjects.

It can be hypothesized that the differences may be due to some underdevelopment of the alveolar process on the cleft side as well as to potentially asymmetric soft tissue forces incident to the surgical correction. In this study it was found that the extent of the palatal cleft opening did not influence the eruption and position of the cuspid and incisor teeth adjacent to the cleft. It can be concluded that the position of the premaxilla and the buccal segments before and after surgical correction can influence the eruption and position of teeth adjacent to the cleft. This observation emphasizes the importance of early treatment to position the tooth-containing jaw

structures contiguous to the cleft but also acknowledges that treatment must be undertaken again following the eruption of the incisor teeth.

A renewed period of orthodontic treatment during the time of transitional dentition is usually necessary. Chronologically, this may occur at approximately 7 to 9 years of age or older because cleft palate children seem to be delayed in the timing of eruption of these teeth. The position of the permanent incisors by means of orthodontic procedures at this stage is accomplished in the context of individual tooth movement. If need be, orthopedic movement of bony segments can still be readily undertaken if no calcified unions have been created within the cleft areas. Most movements at the transitional dentition stage of development involve corrections of tooth malposition, poorly inclined teeth, undesirable rotations, and poor occlusal relationships. Correction of malpositioned incisors is best accomplished by using bands, brackets, and archwires to move those teeth into the desired positions. At this point, deciduous teeth also can be incorporated into the orthodontic manipulation to assist in tooth positioning and development of dental arch configuration and form (Fig. 76–9).

There are many advantages to be accrued from early correction of the position of the anterior teeth. Of course, in cleft patients there is always the need to improve the aesthetic appearance in the anterior region of the mouth. Well-aligned anterior teeth create an improved smile and a good dental aesthetic appearance as well as a desirable support for the surgically corrected cleft lip. Speech is a major consideration, and correcting incisor malalignment shortly after the eruption of the incisors may improve the potential for good tongue-tip contact and enhance the adequate development of skills needed in articulation. The adverse influences of rotated

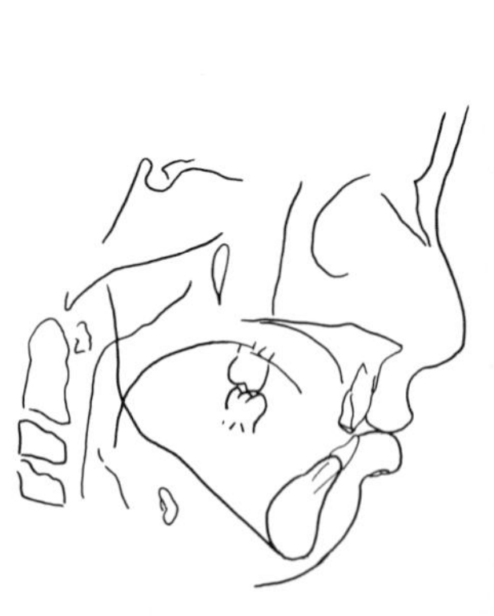
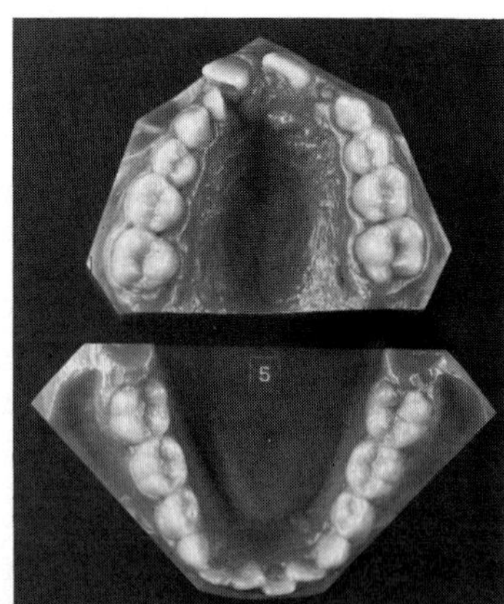
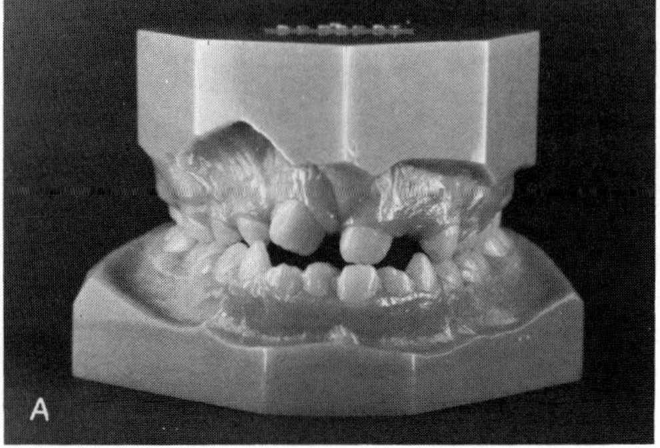

Figure 76–9 Same patient as shown in Figure 76–7. *A*, Lateral headplate tracing and cast indicate the extent of malocclusion and dental malposition at the transitional dentition stage of development.

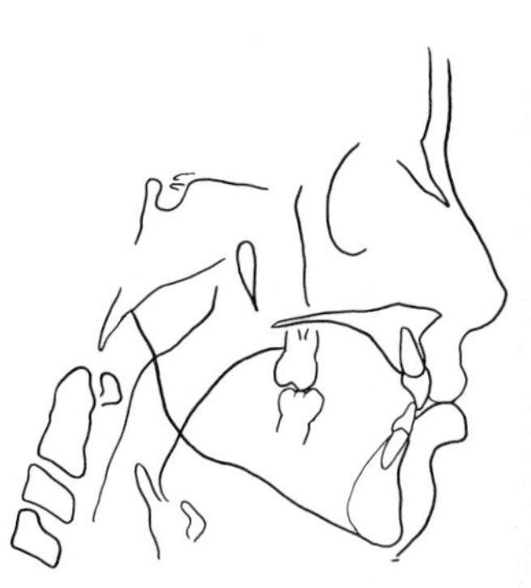

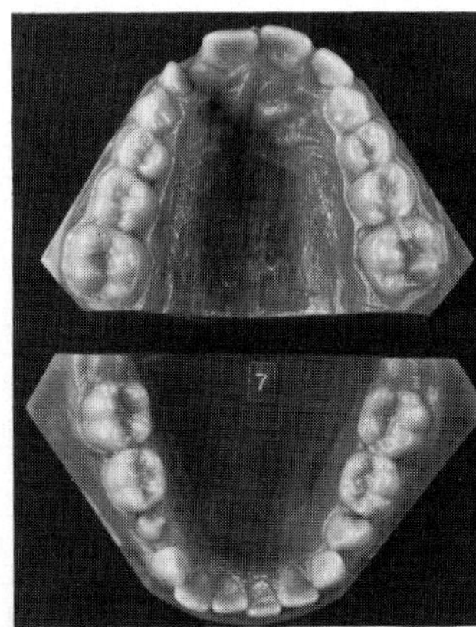

Figure 76–9 Continued B, Orthodontic correction of the maxillary dentition, both in alignment and position.

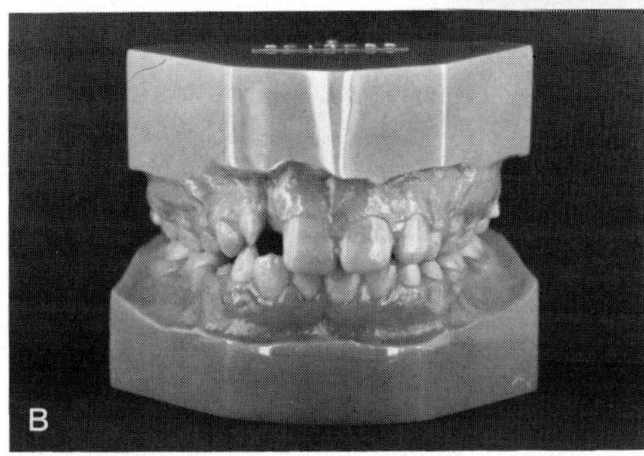

and malpositioned maxillary incisors on tongue-tip contact may be conducive to misarticulation of anterior dentoalveolar speech sounds. It is also realized that these alignments are more easily accomplished shortly after eruption and are more readily maintained subsequent to early correction.

Correction of severe tooth rotation seems to be more adequately retained and maintained if it is done before complete root formation occurs. Furthermore, resorption of the apical aspect of the root is less likely to occur if tooth movement is undertaken before completion of root formation. Controlled positioning of the permanent anterior teeth can aid in more adequate development of the surrounding alveolar process; the lingually locked maxillary incisor teeth can be moved into proper alignment with the mandibular incisors, and these teeth can be moved mesially and distally into a more adequate relationship with the mandibular teeth. Here a word of caution should be expressed. In cleft patients, a correct midline relationship of the maxillary arch to the mandibular arch may sometimes be impossible to achieve. It may not be possible to move an incisor adjacent to a cleft laterally in the direction of the cleft owing to the inadequacy of bone to maintain tooth support; this could lead to the exposure of the root surface and loss of dentition. Proximity of the cleft may preclude the establishment of desired maxillary midline positions.

After the most optimal possible alignment of the anterior dentition it may be appropriate to consider retention once again or to evaluate the possibility of alveolar bone grafting. If retention is decided on, it must be undertaken for a prolonged and continuous period. If this is not done, rapid collapse and constriction will recur under muscular influences; individual teeth can return to their original, undesirable positions. At

this time, artificial anterior teeth can be included on the retainer in areas where teeth are missing or unerupted, not only to enhance appearance but also to provide adjunctive help in ensuring continuous wear. Furthermore, if openings are still present in the hard palate region, retention appliances can adequately cover and obturate the openings.

At one time, secondary bone grafting into the cleft area was advocated after the completion of all orthodontic treatment and after the full eruption of the permanent teeth.[57] Grafting was recommended for many reasons but primarily to stabilize the bony segments. Currently, a secondary bone graft prior to the time of eruption of the permanent cuspids has been recommended, preferably when the unerupted permanent cuspid root is approximately two-thirds to three-fourths formed.[58] As of this date, cancellous bone taken from the iliac crest seems to afford the most desirable results. An attempt is made to enclose the bone graft completely with a palatal mucoperiosteal flap posteriorly and a gingivolabial flap anteriorly. It is recommended that the bone graft be placed well into the alveolar area as well as more superiorly at the level of the nasal floor.

Many advantages can be accrued from such a bone graft at this stage of development. A bony connection or union subsequent to graft placement will stabilize the moveable bony segments of the nasomaxillary complex and at the same time provide bony support for the lip, floor of the nose, and alar base. Concomitantly, it also may be possible to close all remaining palatal as well as sublabial oronasal fistulas.

If a bone graft is undertaken at this stage, it is advisable to fabricate a special "bone grafting" removable appliance (Fig. 76–10) to maintain the orthodontic correction achieved to that point. If the appliance is

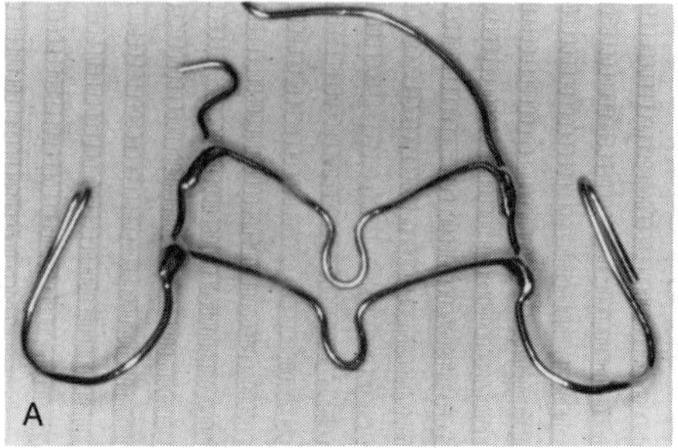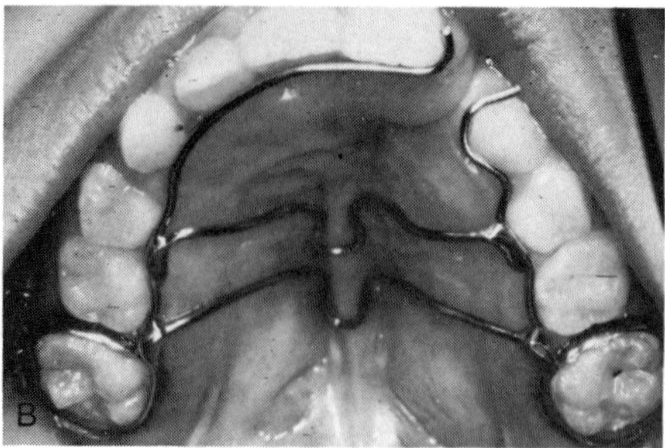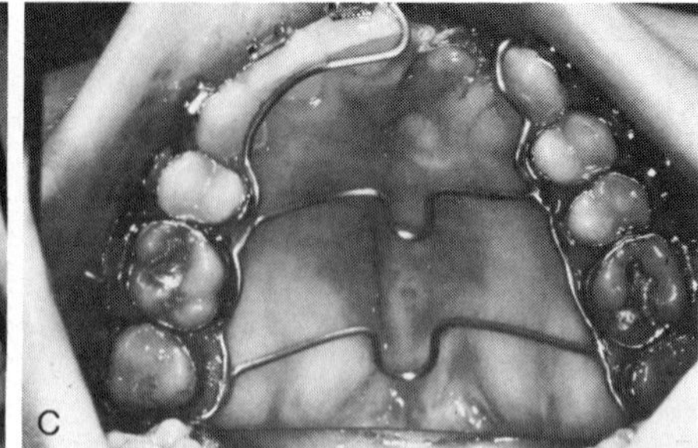

Figure 76–10 *A,* Removable, individually constructed bone graft appliance that can help stabilize the orthodontic result to this point and can be activated to help stimulate bone development. *B,* Appliance in place in a patient with transitional dentition, before permanent cuspid eruption. *C,* Appliance in place in a patient with permanent dentition.

fixed by cement, it should allow ready access for the bone grafting procedures. If removable, it should create no pressure at the site of the graft on placement. Pressure would cause undesirable bone resorption rather than bone development. It is recommended that the appliance be constructed so that tension forces are placed lightly on the bone graft in accordance with the concepts propounded by Chierici who placed bone grafts in surgically created clefts in rhesus monkeys.[59] In all of the animals in which a retention appliance was placed and activated to create tension across the graft, bone formed in the grafted area. If a retention appliance is not placed, constrictive pressure forces could reduce or even preclude bone formation.

After healing and removal of the appliance, orthodontic manipulation will facilitate maintaining the viability of the graft. Teeth such as cuspids can erupt into the graft with the periodontal fibers necessary to maintain the viability and existence of alveolar bone[60] and even induce alveolar bone formation.[58, 61] Supernumerary lateral incisor teeth, or teeth that were previously on the wrong side of the cleft and precluded movement into the cleft and were frequently extracted in the past, can be orthodontically moved into the graft. The new bone, much like alveolar bone, responds to physiologic orthodontic stresses and readily allows movement of teeth. Previously, canine and incisor teeth had minimal support on the side of the root adjacent to the cleft and were subject to periodontal problems. Now, with the support of new bone created by the graft, acceptable attachment levels that potentially improve periodontal health are possible and can increase the longevity of the dentition.

With the possibility of maintaining and moving teeth into the grafted area, the need for prosthetic replacement may be reduced. Turvey et al reported 24 patients who received secondary bone grafts.[62] Twelve patients subsequently required no prosthetic replacements after tooth movement, whereas 8 of the remaining 12 required minimal prosthetic bridge replacements. Even if bridgework cannot be eliminated, the bone graft in the alveolar area will provide more support for the artificial tooth replacement than would have been available with a nongrafted bony cleft. Bone grafting may not necessarily be recommended for every patient, but when applicable, it can aid in the rehabilitation of a cleft lip and palate individual.

Orthodontics—Adult Dentition

At an early age orthodontic treatment usually involves bony segmental repositioning. The later stages usually involve individual tooth movement, particularly if a successful bone grafting procedure has been undertaken. It must be understood that when no bony bridge has been created across a maxillary bony cleft, segmental movement is possible at any age. However, if several stages of orthodontic movement and retention have been successfully completed, with or without bone grafting, the later, adult stage should properly be confined to tooth movement and tooth alignment utilizing orthodontic forces.

By the time of eruption of the permanent dentition, it may be necessary to recommend the extraction of teeth, maxillary or mandibular, to achieve an acceptable occlusion (Fig. 76–11). Extractions, although undesirable in the upper arch, may be necessary because the bony segments may not be adequate to accommodate all of the maxillary teeth. If feasible, spaces should be developed in which to move malplaced maxillary teeth into the arch to minimize any reflection of skeletal deficiency or retrusion in the midfacial region. This is particularly true when underdevelopment of the maxilla relative to the mandible exists. In such patients, extractions should be avoided in the maxillary arch because they would further emphasize the undesirable retruded relationship of the maxillary complex.

During the adolescent stages of development, when maxillary retrusion is mildly evident, it may be advisable to extract the mandibular bicuspids to reposition the lower incisors lingual to the upper incisors to achieve adequate anterior overbite and overjet relationships and desirable lip contour and lip relationships.

At times during the later stages of growth, retrusion of the midface, which is particularly evident in the area of the upper lip, may become obvious owing to inadequate expression of skeletal growth. The lower portion of the face may continue to grow, and an anterior crossbite may begin to develop. In these instances, it becomes important to further the development of the maxillary region to improve the facial profile and facial appearance. To date, little consideration has been given to the potential of stimulating skeletal maxillary development in patients who have midfacial retrusion related to inadequate forward growth of the underlying maxil-

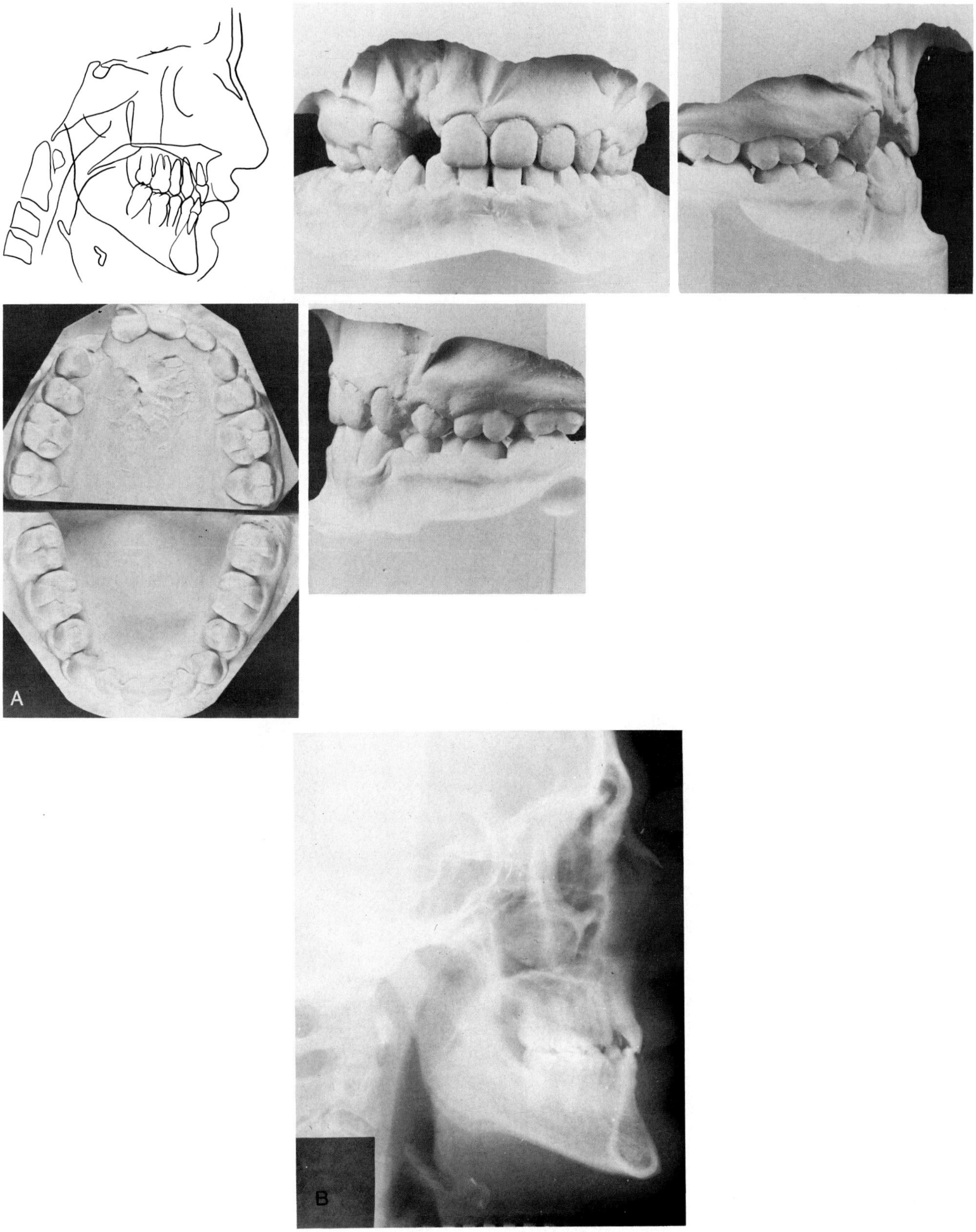

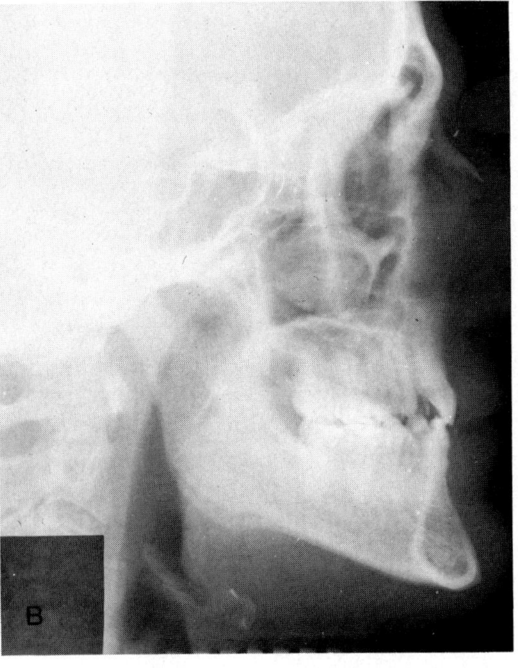

Figure 76–11 *A*, Cephalometric tracing and dental casts of patient shown in Figures 76–7 and 76–9 subsequent to the completion of all orthodontic treatment in the permanent dentition at approximately 15 years of age. *B*, Lateral cephalometric radiograph of the same individual at 33 years of age; the case is now in permanent retention, and the occlusion has maintained alignment.

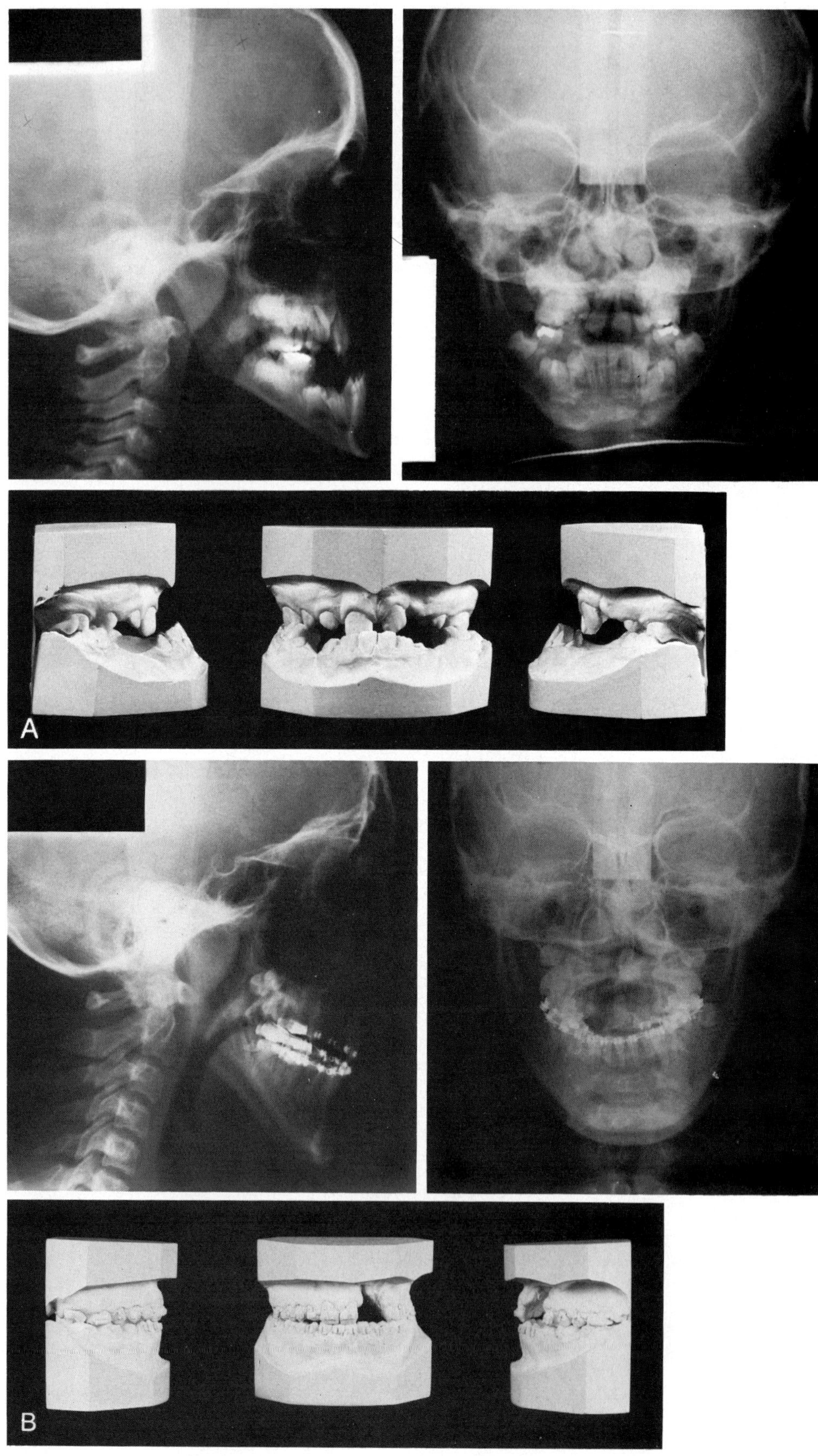

Figure 76–12 Cephalometric headplates and casts of an individual with a repaired unilateral cleft of the lip and palate who had successful results with face mask therapy in addition to other orthodontic appliances. *A,* Before treatment. *B,* Time of retention.

lary skeletal complex. In correcting this skeletal deficiency, relatively good success has been noted with the use of appliances similar to those advocated by DeLaire[63] and Verdon.[64]

The DeLaire face mask is an extraoral orthopedic device specifically designed to stimulate forward maxillary skeletal development. Structurally, it consists of a forehead rest and a chin cup for stabilization, with an intermediate wire framework located forward of the lip aperture and designed for attachment of elastics from the maxillary dental arch. Clinically, encouraging results have been noted, promoting continued clinical use, clinical investigation, and the introduction of certain modifications in treatment (Figs. 76–12 to 76–14).

After a period of use, it was found to be advantageous initially to develop the bone overlying the apices of the upper incisors prior to face mask use. First, advancing the incisors and primarily their root tips frequently made it possible to achieve sufficient arch length when it was obviously inadequate for permanent tooth eruption. Often, adequate arch length can be achieved for partially blocked out permanent cuspids, bicuspids, or even lingually blocked out maxillary lateral incisors, any of which are frequently observed in patients with skeletal maxillary retrusion. Incisor labial root torque and incisor advancement can promote observable development of bone in the anterior maxillary region; subsequently, face mask therapy is initiated to achieve anterior maxillary development. With the face mask resting against the forehead and the chin, heavy elastic bands are used to produce a downward- and forward-directed force on the maxillary complex.

Investigations have demonstrated that both the max-

illary dental arch and the maxillary skeletal complex can be advanced by means of face mask therapy, the extent of maxillary development being highly dependent on the stage of maturation.[65, 66] Younger patients, those who had not yet reached their peak of pubertal growth and who had much growth to look forward to, clinically showed the greatest amount of anteroposterior skeletal maxillary development and interarch correction. Patients in the transitional stage of dental development, approximately 9 to 10 years of age, demonstrated the most dramatic changes in enhancement of maxillary skeletal development. Concomitantly, the degree of facial convexity increased very much more than would normally be expected. Evaluation of this age group has led to the recommendation that, if possible, face mask therapy should be initiated at the beginning of the adolescent growth spurts because at this stage the greatest changes in development of the maxillary region might be anticipated. Skeletal maxillary development was observed in individuals past the peak of pubertal growth, but this development seemed to be more slowly achieved and was of lesser extent. At later age levels, in late adolescence and early adulthood, face mask therapy was helpful, but little enhancement of skeletal maxillary development could be anticipated, and changes seemed to be restricted to maxillary dental arch advancement.[55]

Face mask therapy can be undertaken at any age when the maxillary arch seems to be developing a retrusive relationship. It may be helpful when bone grafts have been undertaken at an early age and there is a noticeable reduction in maxillary growth (Fig. 76–15). Likewise, bone grafting at later ages, before the

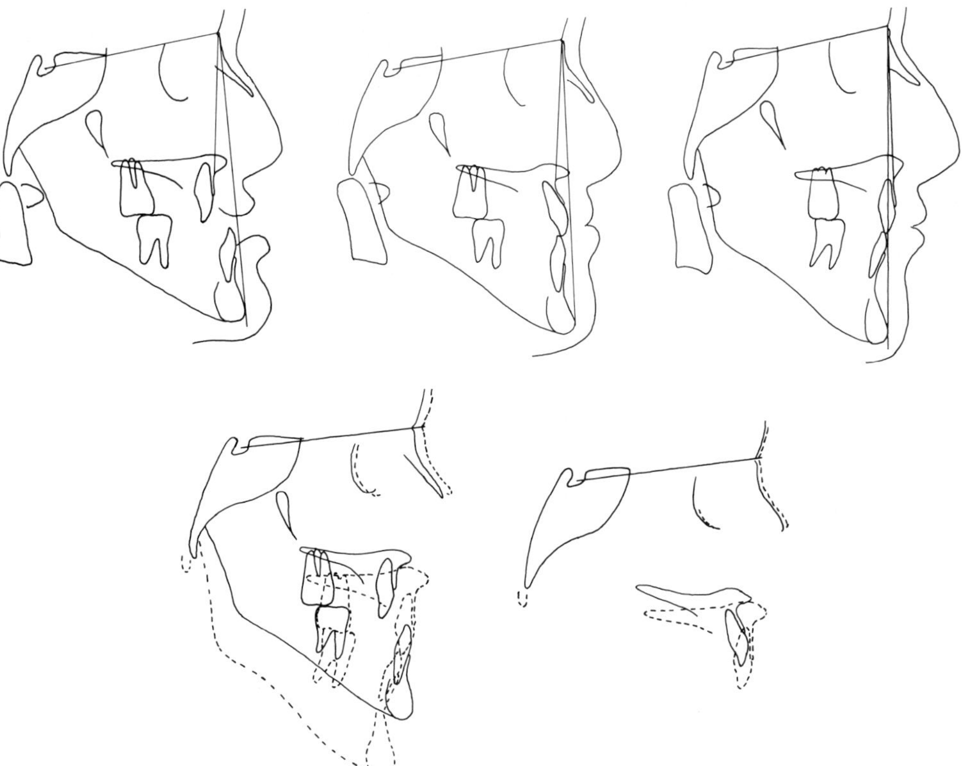

Figure 76–13 Tracings of lateral cephalometric radiographs of the patient depicted in Figure 76–12. Changes in skeletal relationships are evident. Below, the vertical direction of mandibular growth and positioning is evident, as well as notable maxillary advancement (broken line).

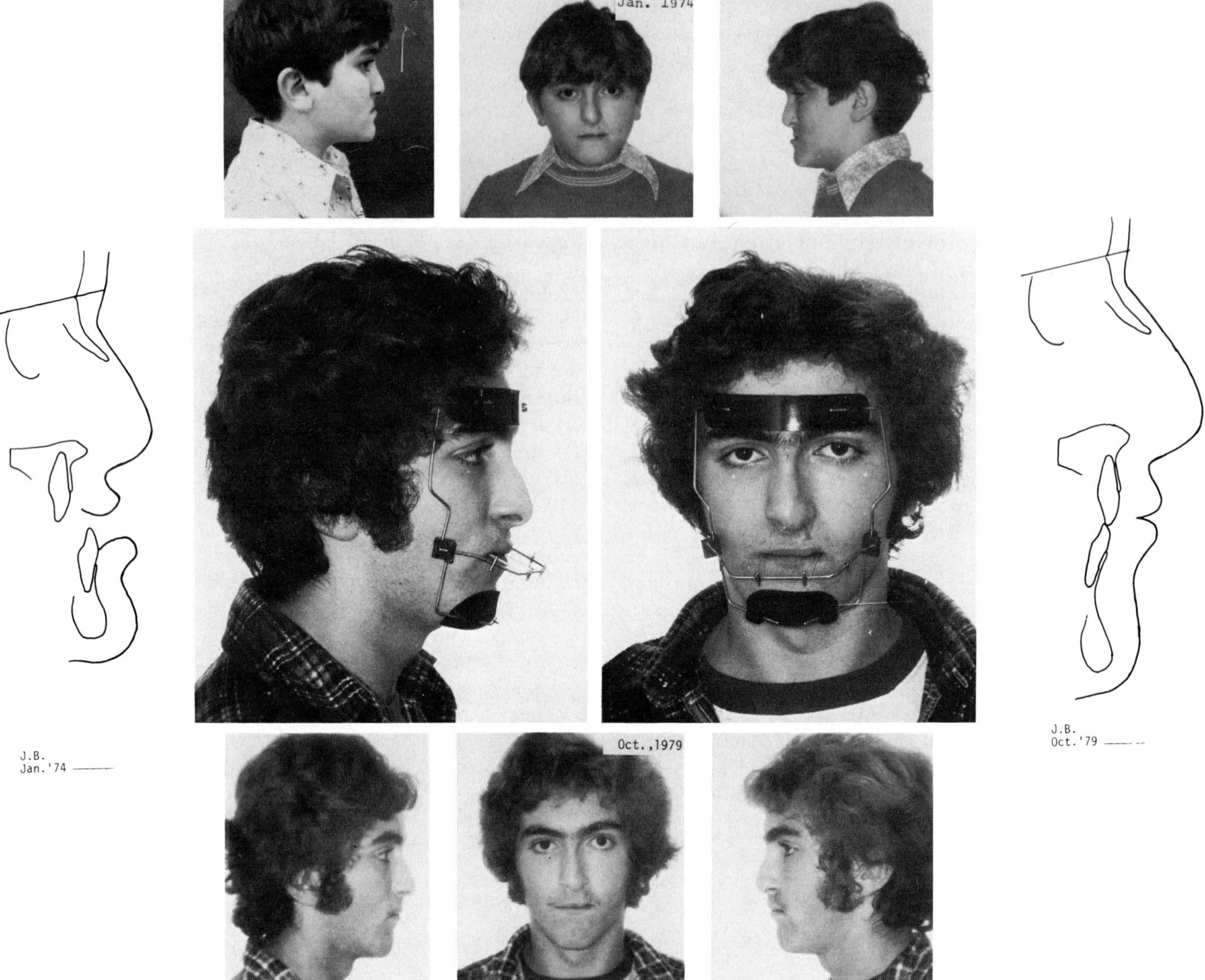

Figure 76–14 Patient shown in Figures 76–12 and 76–13. Changes in facial appearance and facial profile (1974 to 1979) resulting from orthodontic therapy with the adjunctive use of the DeLaire face mask (center photo).

eruption of the permanent cuspid, becomes a more feasible procedure because any retardation of maxillary growth due to grafting may be overcome with use of a face mask to keep the maxillary arch anterior to the mandibular arch.

Mandibular position was found to be a strong factor in the correction of the adverse influence of the maxillary retrusion on interarch relationships (Fig. 76–13). Cephalometric records clearly indicated that some of the correction occurred as a result of the change in the posture of the growing mandibular jaw. Under the influence of the chin cup of the face mask, a greater than normal increase in the lower anterior facial height was generally noted. Concomitant to this increase, a substantial increase in the convexity of the face was also noted. Much of the increment in lower facial height was the result of molar eruption. Although some variation was noted, the general trend of face mask influence on the lower jaw seemed to be a more downward and

comparatively less forward direction of the mandible during the process of midfacial advancement. The overall effect was helpful in creating an observable and notable improvement in facial appearance (Fig. 76–14).

It should also be mentioned that it may not be possible to correct excessive midface retrusion by face mask therapy alone. Correction by orthodontic means may be beyond the realm of possibility, and the adjunctive help of orthognathic surgery may be required. It has been noted that after forward maxillary development has been achieved by face mask use, the maxillary complex does not necessarily continue to express forward growth. With the maxillary position at a standstill, a decrease in facial convexity can again be observed. Thus, in the later stages, it may be necessary to institute face mask therapy again to further stimulate forward development.

To reemphasize a point, skeletal development of the maxillary complex by means of face mask therapy is strongly recommended at an early age during the transitional stage of dental development, when the orthodontist can take advantage of considerable potential growth. It is specifically recommended for patients who have skeletal maxillary retrusion, which must be differentiated diagnostically from skeletal mandibular prognathism. Both of these conditions may be similarly manifested as a developed or developing anterior crossbite in the dental occlusion, although the causative skeletal malrelationships are different and therefore require different therapies.

Following treatment of the full adult dentition, some form of permanent retention must be placed to maintain the orthodontic result. If no bone grafting has been undertaken up to the time of complete eruption and correction of the permanent dentition, it is recommended that, if feasible, this procedure be considered. A bony implant in the anterior region may help to stabilize the segments of the maxillary arch and reduce the adverse facial appearance of depressions at the level of the floor of the nose, adding support to the floor of the nose and the lip. Furthermore, a bone graft could add needed support to a prosthetic replacement if there is a need to replace missing dental units in the area of the cleft.

Lifetime retention may take the form of a fixed bridge, which serves as a stabilizing splint as well as a replacement for the missing dental units. A partial denture may serve equally as a lifetime retainer. It helps to stabilize the orthodontic correction, replace missing teeth, and add sublabial bulk under the upper lip, and it can also obturate sublabial and palatal fistulas if they remain. At any rate, retention and prolonged retention are necessary adjuncts to orthodontic treatment in cleft lip and palate individuals at all ages and stages of development.

Mandibular Growth and Orthodontic Correction

At one time it was observed that the facial deformity in a cleft lip and palate child became increasingly severe with progressive facial growth, in that growth of the upper face fell farther and farther behind relative to the forehead and the growing lower jaw. Inequality in the growth of the upper and lower jaws may occur and may become more evident with age and growth even if it is somewhat reflective of minimum reduction in maxillary growth and a continued expression of the genetic potential for the continued growth of the mandible. The visual effect of mandibular growth, whether orthodontic treatment is undertaken or not, may develop at any age, even during the later stages of growth and in adulthood.

In a contemporary growth study it was shown that facial growth continued in adults from 25 years to 55 years of age, albeit at a reduced rate and in an amount of 2 to 10% of jaw dimensions.[67] This growth explains the observation of a good facial appearance at a young age that subsequently develops into a less desirable facial appearance at a later age. In some instances, the amount and extent of mandibular growth exceeded maxillary growth, and the mandible continued to grow after the relative cessation of maxillary growth, leading

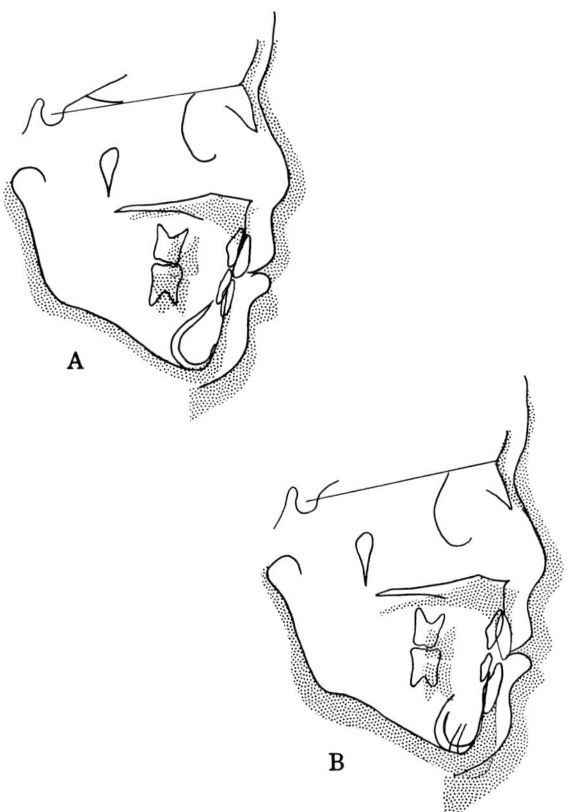

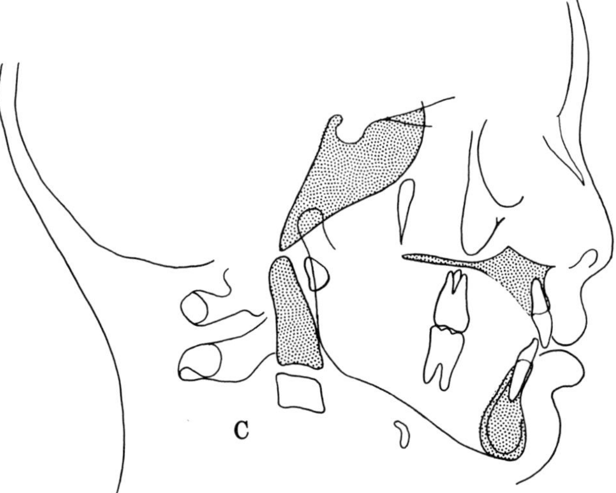

Figure 76–15 A young person with cleft lip and palate who had undergone presurgical oral orthopedic treatment and early bone grafting. A reduction in anticipated nasomaxillary growth was noted, and orthodontic treatment and face mask therapy were undertaken. *A*, Superimposed lateral headplate tracings 1980 to 1982 (dotted areas). *B*, Superimposed tracings 1982 to 1984. *C*, Tracing of lateral cephalometric radiograph taken in 1985.

to a relatively more forward position of the chin as well as the mandibular dentition and increasing difficulty in keeping maxillary incisors labial to the mandibular incisors. If face mask therapy is not feasible, then some variation of orthognathic surgery may be indicated.

Not only is the extent or amount of lower jaw growth important to the orthodontic result and facial appearance of the cleft lip and palate individual, but also the direction of mandibular growth is equally important and deserves equal consideration in considering what orthodontics can do to alter it.

A review of long-term observations on two young males born with bilateral clefts of the lip and palate may indicate how the amount and direction of mandibular growth can be important to the orthodontic result, the dental occlusion, and the adult facial configuration. At full maturity, both have had the same surgeon, orthodontist, and speech pathologist. Both had two-stage surgical repair of the lip, and 3 months before their second birthdays were readmitted for cleft palate repair. In one patient (D.J.), it was decided that the palatal cleft was too wide and should be repaired in two stages. The anterior portion was done first utilizing vomer flaps including mucous membrane and periosteum elevated from the vomer bone. Similar flaps were elevated from the palate. Nine months later, the remainder of the cleft of the palate was surgically repaired. In the other patient (G.E.), the palate was similarly repaired utilizing vomer flaps but in one procedure. Superiorly based pharyngeal flaps were surgically performed at age 10 to improve speech in both patients.

Orthodontic treatment was begun at age 8. In D.J.'s case, a forward position of the whole maxillary arch, consistent with a forward position of the premaxilla, with crossbites on both sides in the region of the cuspids was evident. The size of the premaxilla was judged to be large, moderately protruded, and positioned toward the mandibular sublabial sulcus. In G.E., an open bite relationship was noted anteriorly. The degree of crossbite at this age was considered mild. The size of the premaxilla was considered near normal and its position slightly retruded. The objectives of orthodontic treatment at that time were to (1) properly position the premaxilla; (2) expand the buccal segments; (3) align teeth; and (4) obturate the anterior fistulas.

In both patients, the philosophy of orthodontic treatment was similar; however, the mode of mandibular growth was quite dissimilar and led to varying orthodontic problems during the course of growth. Orthodontic treatment in each case was initiated at the time of the transitional dentition. Expansion of the maxillary buccal segments was undertaken during the initial phase of orthodontic treatment to correct buccal crossbites prior to attempting to reposition the premaxillary segment orthodontically. Once the expansion had been achieved, full banding of the permanent and deciduous dentition was undertaken, and appliance therapy was instituted to raise and retract the premaxillary element. In both cases, retraction, or at best, prevention of a more forward position of the premaxilla during development was maintained throughout the course of ortho-

dontic treatment. At intervals, temporary retainers were placed until the full permanent dentition could be banded to achieve proper dental alignment and good interarch relationships.

In D.J.'s case, the amount and direction of mandibular growth were favorable for achieving an adequate occlusion and a good profile result, whereas the direction and amount of mandibular growth in G.E.'s case were somewhat unfavorable for the ultimate occlusal result and profile relationships. In D.J.'s case (Figs. 76–16 and 76–17), considerable mandibular growth in an anteroposterior direction with a considerable increment in the vertical height of the ramus was evident. The premaxilla was raised and maintained in a anteroposterior position so that with the forward growth of the mandible the mandibular dentition was able eventually to approximate the premaxillary permanent dentition. Facial configuration changed from convexity to slight midface concavity in the facial profile (Fig. 76–18). Holding back the position of the premaxilla combined with the good fortune of mandibular growth in the desired direction made it possible to achieve a good profile and a good interarch relationship.

In the later stages of growth and treatment, it became impossible to maintain correction of the buccal dental crossbite. It is surmised that the vomer flap with periosteum placed across the cleft area led to bone formation underlying the periosteum. This procedure precludes a fibrous or sutural type adjustment area and seemed to preclude further development in width, preventing lateral movement of the bony maxillary segments. With continued forward growth of the mandible and forward positioning of the mandibular dentition, a wider part of the mandibular arch was progressively relating to a more narrow part of the maxillary arch, resulting in a crossbite that could not be orthodontically corrected. However, it was deemed to be functionally acceptable, and no further attempt was made at orthodontic correction. Despite growth, considerable alveolar tissue was missing on both sides of the premaxilla; the surgeon judged the area to be too large for safe placement of bone implants. Retention was achieved with a final removable prosthesis that maintained the altered position of the maxillary dentition and prosthetically replaced the alveolar tissue and dentition.

In G.E.'s case, the mode and amount of mandibular growth was considerably different and led to a different end result (Fig. 76–19). Once again, success was achieved in maintaining retropositioning of the premaxillary element despite continued growth and development. In his case it was possible to expand the buccal segments and maintain a correction in the width of the occlusal relationships. However, the direction of mandibular growth in this instance created some disadvantage despite the fact that the premaxilla was maintained anteroposteriorly and orthodontically was not permitted to assume a more forward position.

Mandibular growth was unfavorable, and considerable convexity in the facial profile of the patient resulted. Although growth did take place, much of it occurred in a vertical rather than an anteroposterior direction

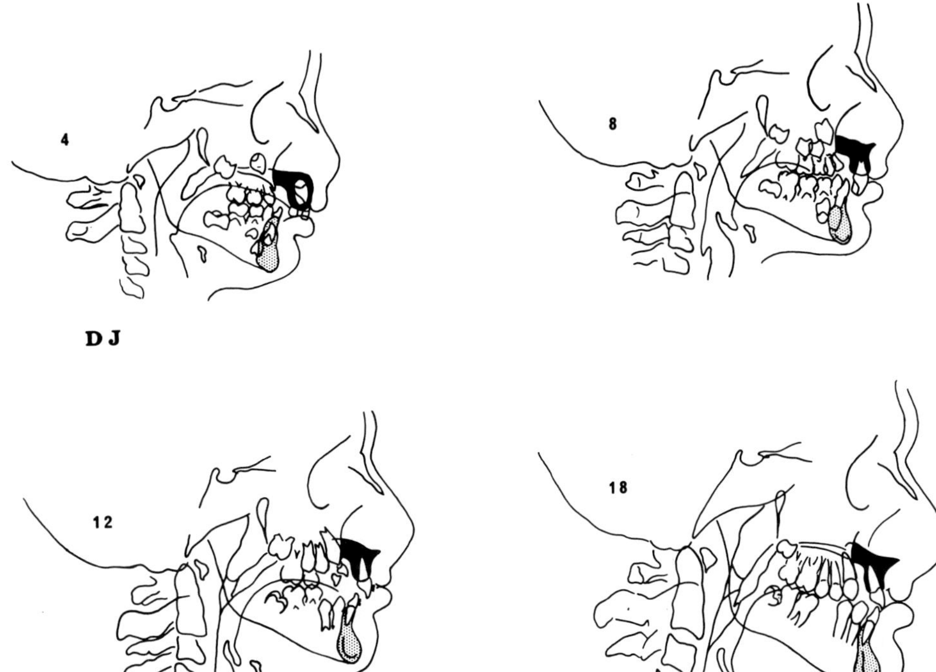

Figure 76–16 Tracings of cephalometric radiographs of D.J. taken progressively at 4, 8, 12, and 18 years of age. Growth and change with time are evident.

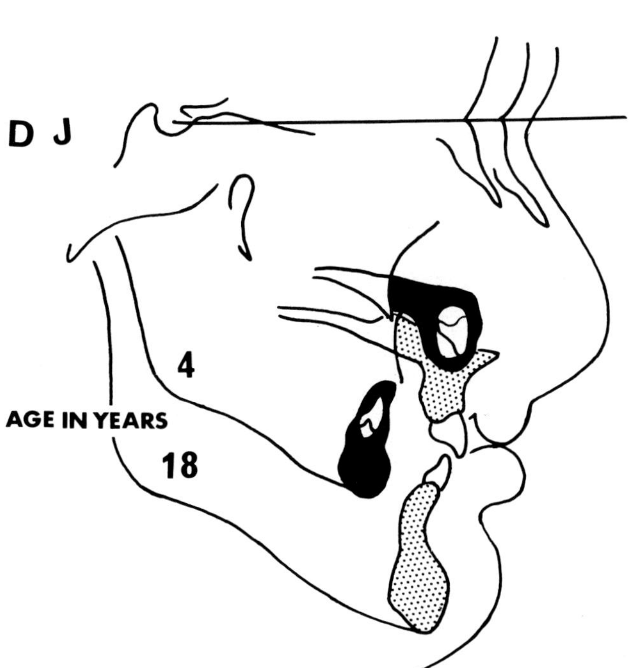

Figure 76–17 Superimposed tracings of the cephalometric radiographs of D.J. taken at 4 and 18 years of age. Note that the anteroposterior position of the maxillary jaw has been well maintained whereas the mandible has shown considerable forward growth.

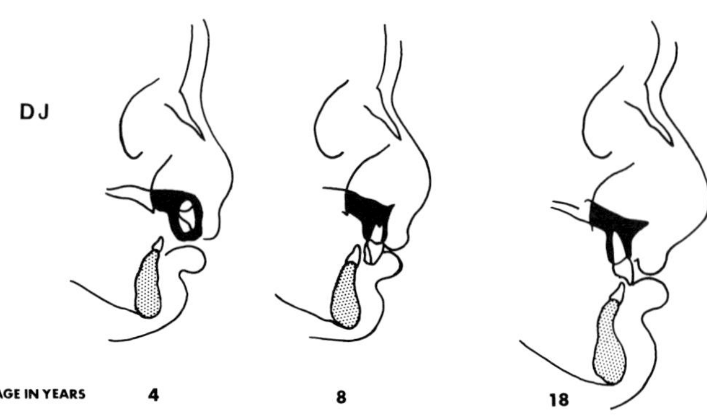

Figure 76–18 Profile tracings of D.J. obtained from cephalometric radiographs taken at 4, 8, and 18 years of age. Note the significance of forward mandibular growth to the profile and to the positional relationships of the anterior dentition.

(Fig. 76–20). Posterior facial height between the palate and the gonial region of the mandible did not increase as much as did the vertical height in the anterior facial region. Actually, the mandibular symphysis seemed to grow in a predominantly downward direction, which did not help to reduce the convexity of the facial configuration and appeared to accentuate the forward premaxillary position (Fig. 76–21). Although G.E. also had vomer flap surgery, a buccal crossbite did not develop during the later stages of growth. With decreased anteroposterior development and positioning of the mandible, relative forward progression of the mandibular arch did not take place, so that a narrower part of the mandibular arch could occlude with the maxillary dentition in a noncrossbite relationship.

It is obvious that the direction of mandibular growth is extremely important to the correction of facial disfigurement in bilateral cleft lip and palate patients and indeed, in all cleft palate individuals. In both instances, the ultimate mode and extent of mandibular growth dictated the final result despite strenuous orthodontic efforts. With a cleft of the lip and palate, the tendency is to concentrate on the growth of the maxilla and to forget that mandibular growth and its direction are equally important and may enhance or hurt efforts to achieve good facial profile relationships as well as desir-

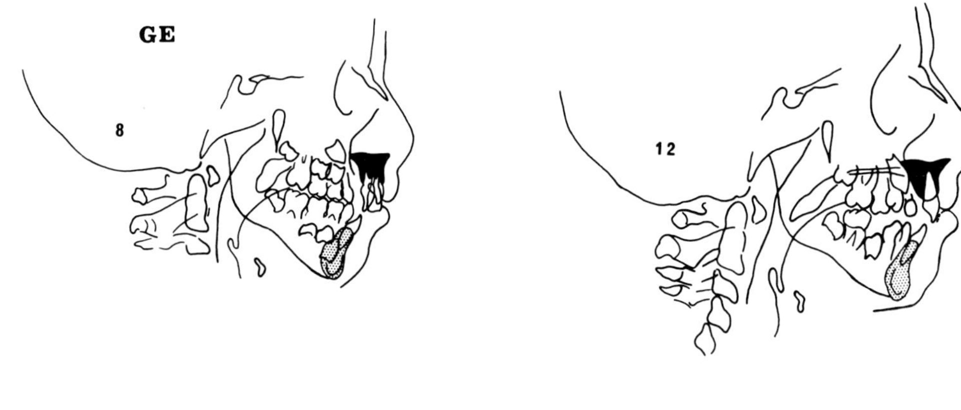

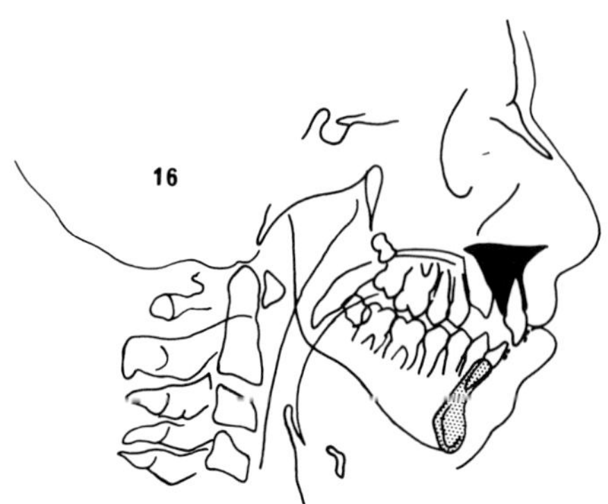

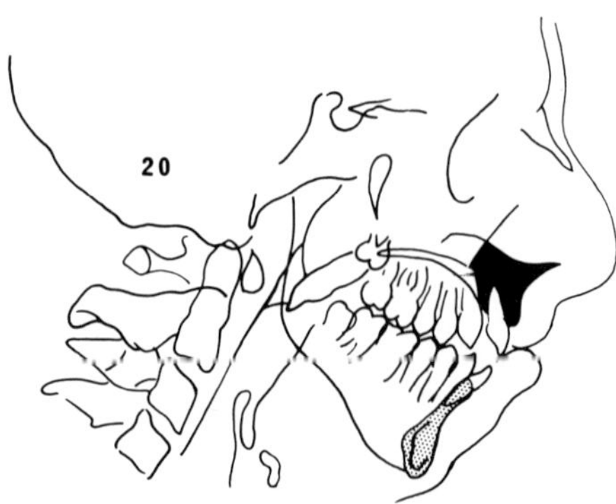

Figure 76–19 Tracings of cephalometric x-rays of G.E. taken progressively at 8, 12, 16, and 20 years of age.

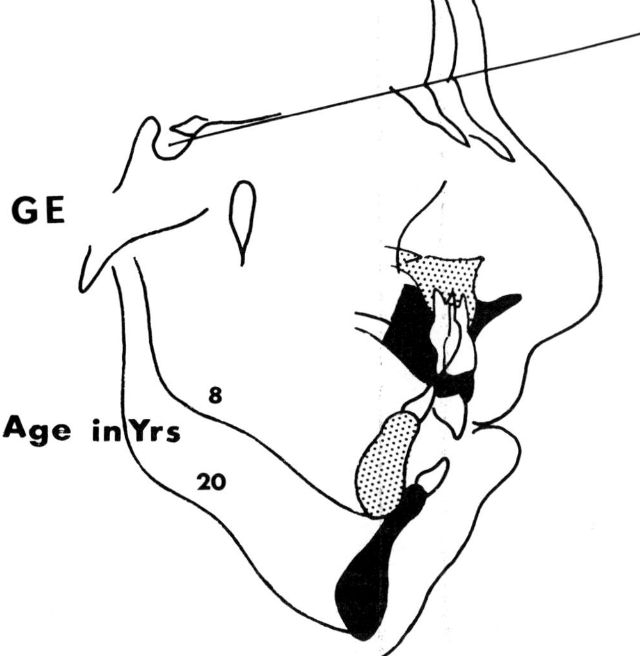

Figure 76–20 Superimposed tracings of radiographs of G.E. taken at 8 and 20 years of age. Note the considerable vertical growth of the mandible and the resultant open bite malocclusion.

able occlusal relationships. The position, growth, and configuration of the lower jaw are equally important to the aesthetic appearance of the face.

Environment itself may influence mandibular configuration and growth direction. In a longitudinal, cephalometric, radiographic study of individuals with unilateral cleft lip and palate and cleft palate only, comparative differences were found in mandibular position and direction of mandibular growth.[68] The unilateral cleft lip and palate patients had more retropositioned mandibles, and in general, their mandibles rotated more in a clockwise fashion during growth than was observed in the cleft palate only individuals, giving evidence of a more vertical direction of mandibular growth. In the unilateral cleft patients, a greater amount of nasorespiratory obstruction was noted, indicating a superimposed environmental influence, mouthbreathing, on the inherent pattern of mandibular growth. A similar influence was noted in a longitudinal study of individuals who had pharyngeal flap surgery, which, because of its anatomic location, partially obstructs the nasopharynx.[15] Clinically, such knowledge can be helpful in estimating the eventual mandibular position following growth and providing improved insight into treatment modalities that might be best suited for any individual patient.

Care for the individual with a cleft continues throughout the lifetime of that individual. A thorough knowledge of the anatomy and physiology of the naso-oropharyngeal cavities supplemented with knowledge of growth and age changes and how they relate to facial appearance and oropharyngeal function is pertinent to the reconstruction of the oral cavity and to the maintenance of the integrity of the results achieved through the efforts of many cooperating professional disciplines. Levels of clinical success have improved tremendously over the years, and achieving ideal results is becoming a more frequent possibility. Orthodontics, at all ages, plays a valuable role in striving to achieve ideal results in the rehabilitation of the cleft palate individual.

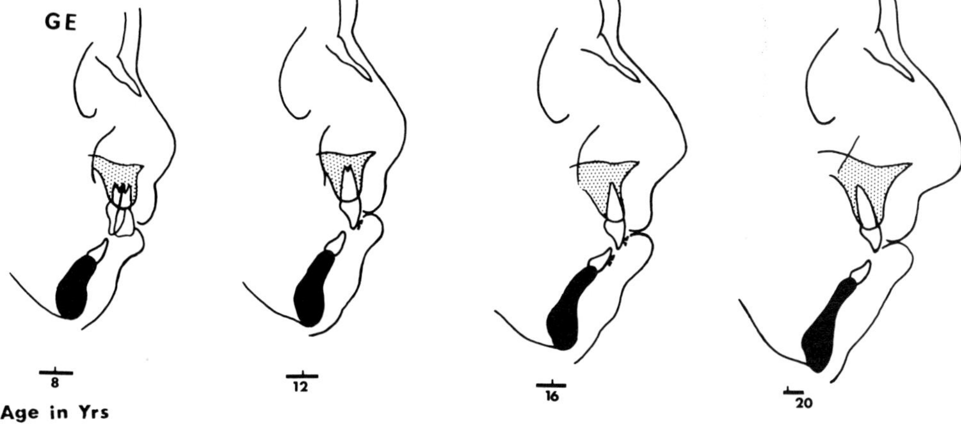

Figure 76–21 Profile tracings of cephalometric radiographs taken of G.E. at 8, 12, 16, and 20 years of age. The profile and anterior dental changes incident to the vertical growth are notable.

References

1. Graber TM: Craniofacial Morphology in Cleft Palate and Cleft Lip Deformities. Surg Gynecol Obstet 88:359, 1949.
2. Graber TM: The Congenital Cleft Palate Deformity. J Am Dent Assoc 48:375, 1954.
3. Slaughter WB, Brodie AG: Facial clefts and their surgical management in view of recent research. Plast Reconstr Surg 4:311, 1949.
4. Huddart AG: Presurgical changes in unilateral cleft palate subjects. Cleft Palate J 16:147, 1979.
5. Pruzansky S: Factors determining arch form in clefts of the lip and palate. Am J Orthod 41:827–851, 1955.
6. Harvold E: Cleft lip and palate. Morphologic studies of the facial skeleton. Am J Orthod 40:493, 1954.
7. Pruzansky S, Richmond JB: Growth of the mandible in infants with micrognathia. Am J Dis Child 88:29, 1954.
8. Pruzansky S: Factors determining arch form in clefts of the lip and palate. Am J Orthod 41:827, 1955.
9. Subtelny JD, Brodie AG: An analysis of orthodontic expansion in unilateral cleft lip and cleft palate patients. Am J Orthod 40:686, 1954.
10. Bishara SE, et al: Dentofacial relationships in persons with unoperated clefts: Comparisons between three cleft types. Am J Orthod 87:481, 1985.
11. Friede H, Pruzansky S: Long-term effects of premaxillary setback on facial skeletal profile in complete bilateral cleft lip and palate. Cleft Palate J 22:97, 1985.
12. Muir IF: Maxillary development in cleft palate patients with special reference to the effects of operation. Ann R Coll Surg 68:62, 1986.
13. Ross RB: Treatment variables affecting facial growth in complete unilateral cleft lip and palate. Parts I, V, VII. Cleft Palate J 24:5, 1987.
14. Siegel MI, et al: A comparison of craniofacial growth in normal and cleft palate rhesus monkeys. Cleft Palate J 22:192, 1985.
15. Subtelny JD, Nieto RP: A longitudinal study of maxillary growth following pharyngeal-flap surgery. Cleft Palate J 15:118, 1978.
16. Subtelny JD: A cephalometric study of the growth of the soft palate. Plast Reconstr Surg 19:49, 1957.
17. Subtelny JD: A longitudinal study of soft tissue facial structures and their profile characteristics, defined in relation to underlying skeletal structures. Am J Orthod 45:481, 1959.
18. Coccaro PJ: A Serial Cephalometric Study of the Growth of the Soft Palate in Cleft Palate Children. MS Thesis. Rochester NY: Department of Dentistry and Dental Research, University of Rochester, 1960.
19. Subtelny JD, Baker HK: The significance of adenoid tissue in velopharyngeal function. Plast Reconstr Surg 17:235, 1956.
20. Subtelny JD, Subtelny JD: Intelligibility and associated physiological factors of cleft palate speakers. J Speech Hear Res 2:353, 1959.
21. Subtelny JD, Koepp-Baker H, Subtelny JD: Palatal function and cleft palate speech. J Speech Hear Dis 26:213, 1961.
22. Subtelny JD, Worth JH, Sakuda M: Intraoral pressure and rate of flow during speech. J Speech Hear Res 9:498, 1966.
23. Pruzansky S: Description, classification and analysis of unoperated cleft lips and palate. Am J Orthod 39:590, 1953.
24. Peyton WT: The dimensions and growth of the palate in the normal infant and in the infant with gross maldevelopment of the upper lip and palate. Arch Surg 22:704, 1931.
25. Peyton WT: Dimensions and growth of the palate in infants with gross maldevelopment of the upper lip and palate. Further investigations. Am J Dis Child 47:1265, 1934.
26. Dorrance GM, Bransfield JW: Cleft palate. Ann Surg 117:1, 1943.
27. Coupe TB, Subtelny JD: Cleft palate—deficiency or displacement of tissue. Plast Reconstr Surg 26:600, 1960.
28. Georgiade N, Latham R: Intraoral traction for positioning the premaxilla in the bilateral cleft lip. In Georgiade NG (ed): Symposium on Management of Cleft Lip and Palate and Associated Deformities. St. Louis: C.V. Mosby, 1974, p 123.
29. Georgiade N, Latham R: Maxillary arch alignment in the bilateral cleft lip and palate infant, using the pinned coaxial screw appliance. Plast Reconstr Surg 56:52, 1975.
30. Hellquist R: Early maxillary orthopedics in relation to maxillary cleft repair by periosteoplasty. Cleft Palate J 8:36, 1971.
31. Rutrick R, Black PW, Jurkiewicz MJ: Bilateral cleft lip and palate: Presurgical treatment. Ann Plast Surg 12:105, 1984.
32. Reisberg DJ, Figueroa AA, Gold HO: An intra-oral appliance for management of the protrusive premaxilla in bilateral cleft lip. Cleft Palate J 25:53, 1988.
33. Backdahl MK, Nordin E: Replacement of the maxillary bone defect in cleft palate. A new procedure. Acta Chir Scand 122:131, 1961.
34. Georgiade NG, Pickrell KL, Quinn GW: Varying concepts in bone grafting of alveolar palatal defects. Cleft Palate J 1:43, 1964.
35. Johanson B, Ohlsson A: Bone grafting and dental orthopedics in primary and secondary cases of cleft lip and palate. Acta Chir Scand 122:112, 1961.
36. Rosenstein SW: Orthodontic and bone grafting procedures in a cleft lip and palate series: An interim cephalometric evaluation. Angle Orthod 45:227, 1975.
37. Stellmach R: Die funktionskieferorthopadische Behandlung der Kieferdeformitaten bei Lippen-Kiefer-Gaumenpalten im Sauglingsalter. Fortschr Kiefer Gesichtschir 1:247, 1955.
38. Skoog T: The use of periosteal flaps in the repair of the primary palate. Cleft Palate J 2:332, 1966.
39. Rehrmann A, Koberg WR, Koch H: Long term postoperative results of primary and secondary bone grafting in complete clefts of lip and palate. Cleft Palate J 7:206, 1970.
40. Rehrmann A: The effect of early bone grafting on the growth of upper jaw in cleft lip and palate children. Computer evaluation. Min Chirurgica 26:874, 1971.
41. Friede H, Johanson B: A follow-up study of cleft children treated with primary bone grafting I. Orthodontic aspects. Scand J Plast Reconstr Surg 8:88, 1974.
42. Robertson NRE, Jolleys A: An 11-year follow up of the effects of early bone grafting in infants born with complete clefts of the lip and palate. Br J Plast Surg 36:438, 1983.
43. Pruzansky S: Factors determining arch form in clefts of the lip and palate. Am J Orthod 41:827, 1955.
44. Pruzansky S, Aduss H: Prevalence of arch collapse and malocclusion in complete unilateral cleft lip and palate. Trans Europ Orthod Soc 1967, pp 1–18.
45. Pruzansky S, Aduss H: Arch form and the deciduous occlusion in complete unilateral clefts. Cleft Palate J 1:411, 1964.
46. Pruzansky S: The role of the orthodontist in a cleft palate team. Plast Reconstr Surg 14:10, 1954.
47. Hotz MM, Gnoinski WM, Nussbaumer H, et al: Early maxillary orthopedics in cleft lip and cleft palate cases: Guidelines for surgery. Cleft Palate J 15:405, 1978.
48. Schweckendiek W: Primary veloplasty: Long-term results without maxillary deformity. A twenty-five year report. Cleft Palate J 15:268, 1978.
49. Schweckendiek H: Zur zweiphosigen Gaumenspalten-Operation bei primarem Velumerschluss. Fortschr Kiefer Gesichtschir 1:73, 1955.
50. Bardach J, Morris HL, Olin WH: Late results of primary veloplasty: The Marburg Project. Plast Reconstr Surg 73:207, 1984.
51. Harvold E: Cleft palate: An experiment. Norske Tannlaegeforenings Tidende 3:105, 1949.
52. Subtelny JD, Brodie AG: An analysis of orthodontic expansion in unilateral cleft lip and cleft palate patients. Am J Orthod 40:686, 1954.
53. Waitkus AM: Histological and Cephalometric Evaluation of Autogenous Periosteal Transplants from the Tibia to Facial Sutures of *Macaca mulatta* with Regard to Their Efficacy and Effect on Facial Growth. MS Thesis. Rochester NY: Eastman Dental Center, University of Rochester, 1976.
54. Friede H, Johanson B: A follow-up study of cleft children treated with vomer flap as part of a three-stage soft tissue surgical procedure. Scand J Plast Reconstr Surg 11:45, 1977.
55. Subtelny JD: Oral respiration: Facial maldevelopment and corrective dentofacial orthopedics. Angle Orthod 50:147, 1980.
56. Ogidan O, Subtelny JD: Eruption of incisor teeth in cleft lip and palate. Cleft Palate J 20:331, 1983.
57. Subtelny JD: Orthodontic treatment of cleft lip and palate, birth to adulthood. Angle Orthod 36:273, 1966.
58. Abyholm FE, Bergland O, Semb G: Secondary bone grafting of alveolar clefts. A surgical/orthodontic treatment enabling a non-prosthodontic rehabilitation in cleft lip and palate patients. Scand J Reconstr Surg 15:127, 1981.
59. Chierici G: Experiments on the influence of oriented stress on bone formation replacing bone grafts. Cleft Palate J 14:114, 1977.
60. Boyne PJ, Sands NR: Combined orthodontic-surgical management of residual palato-alveolar cleft defects. Am J Orthod 70:20, 1976.
61. El Deeb M, Messer B, Lehnert MW, et al: Canine eruption into grafted bone in maxillary alveolar cleft defects. Cleft Palate J 19:9, 1982.
62. Turvey TA, Vig K, Moriarty J, et al: Delayed bone grafting in the cleft maxilla and palate: A retrospective multidisciplinary analysis. Am J Orthod 86:244, 1984.
63. DeLaire J: La croissance maxillaire: Deductions therapeutics. Trans Eur Orthod Soc 81, 1971.
64. Verdon P, Salognoc JM: Traitments originaux de quelques cas complexes. Utilisation successive des forces extra-orales (masque orthopedique et plaque de Stephenson) et des forces legeres (technique de mollia). Orthod Fr 47:802, 1977.
65. Simonsen RT: The Effects of Facemask Therapy: A Cephalometric Study. Thesis. Rochester NY: Department of Orthodontics, Eastman Dental Center, 1981.
66. Galletto LJ: Cephalometric Evaluation of Dentofacial Changes Incident to Facemask Therapy. Thesis. Rochester NY: Department of Orthodontics, Eastman Dental Center, 1988.
67. Behrents RG: Growth in the aging craniofacial skeleton. Monograph 17. Craniofacial Growth Series. Ann Arbor: Center for Human Growth and Development, University of Michigan, 1985.
68. Gonzalez, R: A Longitudinal Cephalometric Study of Growth of the Mandible in Relation to Nasorespiratory Airway Obstruction in Unilateral and Posterior Cleft Palate Patients. MS Thesis. Rochester NY: Eastman Dental Center, University of Rochester, 1984.

CHAPTER 77

Orthodontic Treatment Alternatives for Unilateral Cleft Lip and Palate Patients

Reijo Ranta

Facial Growth

Facial growth and development in individuals with cleft of the lip and palate are influenced by lip and palate surgery, either directly or through altered soft tissue function, respiration, tongue position, and speech. Some facial differences exist independently of the effects of surgery.[1-3]

Shortened depth, a posterior shift of the maxilla, and retroinclination of the alveolar process and the incisors are consistent findings.[4-11] Shortening of the mandibular body and ramus, an obtuse gonial angle, steeper slope of the body, posterior growth rotation and retrognathia of the mandible, elongation of the anterior mandibular height, and retroinclination of the incisors are widely accepted deviations.[4, 9, 12] Similar changes, but to a somewhat lesser degree, have been observed in children by the age of 5 years prior to palatoplasty.[10] The changes increase progressively with age. During the prepubertal growth period and following puberty, inadequate anterior growth is observed.[4, 12-24]

Ross concluded in his multicenter cephalometric investigations that early bone grafting of the alveolar cleft caused marked changes in the vertical development of the maxilla and in the facial proportions.[25] The type and timing of hard and soft palate repair did not cause an appreciable difference in facial growth.

In our cephalometric investigation of 38 adolescent patients with unilateral cleft lip and palate, the alveolar cleft was repaired using a primary maxillary periosteal flap or a tibial free periosteal graft.[22] A bony bridge over the cleft site was seen in about 70% of the patients. We compared the angles SNA and SNB, using them as indicators of maxillary growth in our series and in two primarily bone-grafted patient series. In the group with more radical repair,[26] both the alveolar and anterior palate clefts were grafted. In the conservative repair group,[21] only the alveolar cleft was grafted. Results revealed that conservative bone grafting seemed to provide better midfacial growth than radical grafting. However, growth was almost normal following periosteoplasty, which might be considered the most conservative procedure. Since all three series were otherwise treated similarly, one might conclude that the more conservative and less scar-producing the early primary repair, the less secondary growth retardation occurred.

We discontinued use of periosteoplasty in 1974 (Fig. 77–1).

Dentition

The prevalence of congenital absence of permanent teeth varies greatly in different populations.[27-29] Although more teeth are absent from the maxilla than the mandible, both jaws are affected. The prevalence of congenital absence of permanent teeth (excluding the cleft-side maxillary lateral incisor and the third molars) in Finnish children with unilateral cleft lip and palate is approximately 50%, and the same figure applies to the maxillary cleft-side lateral incisor alone. In children with the Van der Woude syndrome and a cleft, the prevalence of hypodontia is nearly double that of cleft children in general.[30, 31] At the age of mixed dentition, the formation of permanent teeth is delayed approximately 6 months.[28]

Recent Finnish studies have shown that the formation and eruption of the deciduous teeth as well as early development of the permanent maxillary incisors are close to the times reported for healthy children. Significant correlation was observed in timing of formation between the deciduous and permanent teeth.[32-37] Anomalies in the deciduous dentition outside the cleft area were more common in cleft than in noncleft children, and the prevalence of congenital absence of deciduous teeth was four times that of noncleft children.[32]

Dental Occlusion

At birth the maxillary segments are displaced outward, and the arch is wider than normal.[38-40] Following lip repair, the maxilla grows significantly in depth, in height, and in a forward direction, but the alveolar segments undergo rotation and approximation at the ends of the segments.[39, 41] After palate repair, the growth

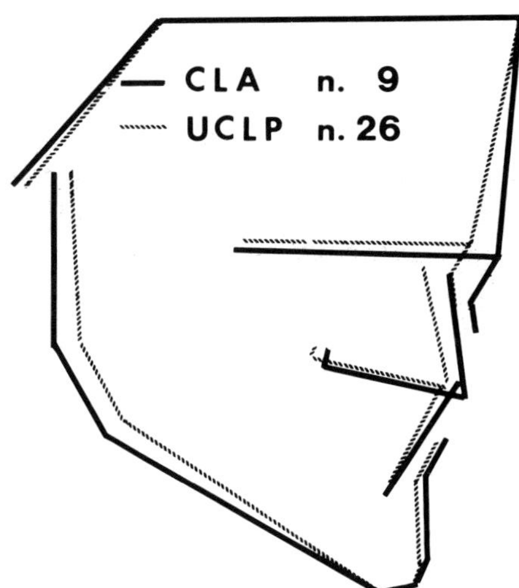

Figure 77–1 Mean facial diagrams for complete unilateral clefts (UCLP) and incomplete clefts (CLA) treated with maxillary periosteal flaps.

in height is significant but not the growth in depth and width. Changes in the size and shape of the arch occur quickly following lip and palate repair.[38, 39, 42–44] The effects of early maxillary orthopedic treatment are beneficial for a short period, but the long-term effect is minimal.[16, 45–48]

Prevalences of buccal and anterior crossbite are still high in the deciduous and early mixed dentition regardless of the timing and type of primary surgery. Buccal crossbite, especially in the region of the canine, is more prevalent than anterior crossbite.[18, 40, 48–53] Both anterior and posterior crossbite are due to a posterior shift of the shorter maxilla and to retroinclination of the alveolar process and teeth. With age, especially during and after the pubertal growth period, dental occlusion gradually worsens.[4, 5, 8, 9, 16, 17, 54, 55]

Goals and Timing of Orthodontic Treatment

The goals of orthodontic treatment are
1. Prevention of anatomic and functional growth aberrations of the jaws, teeth, and surrounding tissues.
2. Correction of the developing aberrations by transverse expansion of the maxilla, protraction of the maxilla, compensation for congenitally absent teeth, bone grafting of the alveolar cleft, or alignment of the teeth.
3. Permanent stabilization of harmonious dental occlusion and the facial profile.

In Helsinki and in many other cleft centers, the start of orthodontic treatment is delayed until the age of mixed dentition. This has several benefits. Many of the required orthodontic treatments can be combined at this age. Crowding or agenesis of the teeth, expansion and protraction of the maxilla, alignment of the incisors, and bone grafting of the alveolar cleft can be done step by step, one after the other, or simultaneously during the same active treatment period. The second active treatment period, if necessary, depends on the growth of the jaws and the development of their relationship and occurs during and after pubertal growth. Finally, retention or prevention of relapse after the active treatment is initiated.

Crowding and Agenesis of Teeth

Crowding of the teeth is common in both jaws in all dental stages, even at the age of 3 years, as our preliminary findings have indicated. With increasing age, crowding increases. Agenesis of the second premolars is common, especially in the maxilla.[27, 28] In our patients with unilateral cleft lip and palate, 32% of the maximum number of the maxillary second premolars were congenitally absent. Moreover, the development of the second premolars may be delayed for many years.[56, 57] Therefore, an absolute diagnosis of agenesis should be delayed until the age of 8 to 9 years.[57]

Transverse Expansion of the Maxilla

Expansion of the maxillary arch with conventional methods is restricted mainly to lateral dentoalveolar rotation of the cleft segment. Nearly all patients with a complete unilateral cleft need maxillary expansion at some period of growth.[43, 58] Lateral crossbite was observed in all our patients with complete unilateral clefts who were operated on with primary periosteoplasty. Anterior crossbite was noted in 85% of the subjects. The anterior crossbite was mostly dental and not skeletal. Orthodontic treatment with a fixed appliance was indicated in all patients. Those operated on without periosteoplasty had somewhat better dental occlusion.[22]

Treatment in the deciduous dentition is easy and rapid with the quad-helix appliance, but a new expansion is necessary in the later mixed dentition or in the permanent dentition. Regardless of the timing of maxillary expansion, lateral repositioning of the maxillary segments can be achieved in growing children and also in adult patients (Figs. 77–2 and 77–3).[11, 55, 59] Transverse expansion of the most collapsed arch is indicated in the deciduous dentition with simultaneous protraction of the maxilla.[60] Because of the prolonged treatment period, maxillary expansion should be delayed until mixed dentition. Relapse after expansion is always rapid if long-term retention is not in place.

Protraction of the Maxilla

The sagittal relationship of the maxilla may deteriorate progressively with age. During and after pubertal growth, dramatic worsening is not unusual.[5, 11, 16, 17, 22, 61] The following methods are available to correct the anterior crossbite or the sagittal relationship of the jaws:
1. Correction of dentoalveolar retroinclinations.
2. Orthodontic or orthopedic protraction of the maxilla and maxillary dentition.
3. Surgical advancement of the maxilla or surgical shortening of the mandible.

Orthodontic correction of the dentoalveolar retroinclination is indicated after the eruption of the permanent incisors. A removable plate, a fixed edgewise appliance, or the latter combined with a modified quad-helix

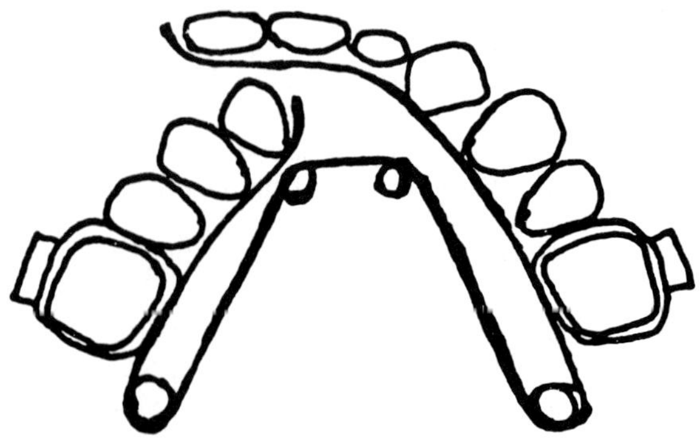

Figure 77–2 Modified quad-helix appliance.

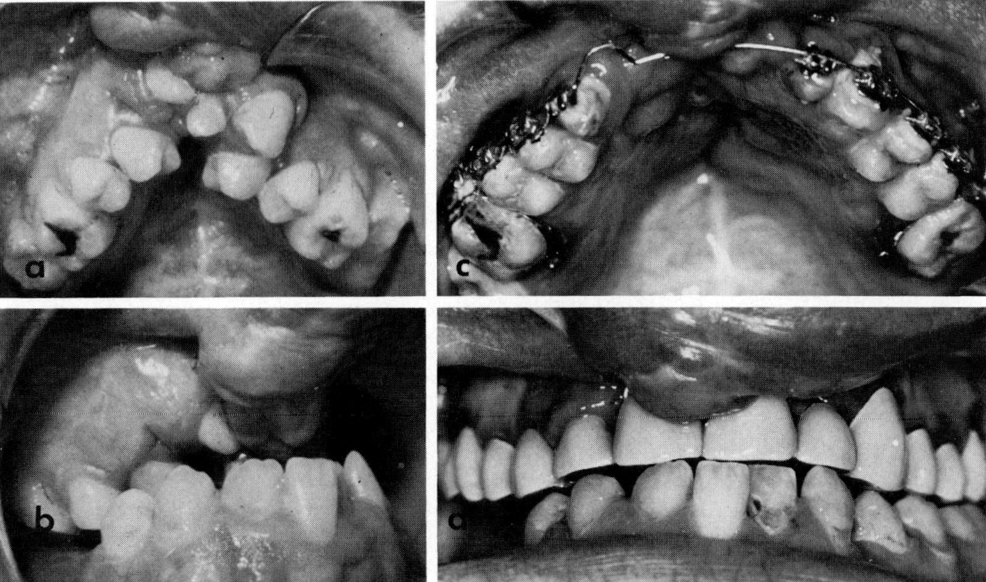

Figure 77–3 Male, aged 29 years, with bilateral cleft lip and palate. *A* and *B*, Dental occlusion and maxillary dental arch before orthodontic treatment. *C* and *D*, After 11 months of orthodontic-prosthodontic treatment.

expansion appliance may be used. In patients with extreme retrusion and collapse of the maxillary arch, it may be beneficial to start orthodontic treatment earlier. Then the transverse expansion and anterior protraction of the maxilla may be combined.

It is important to evaluate the future growth of the jaws and the demands of orthodontic treatment during the period of early permanent dentition. Useless orthodontic treatment should be avoided in patients who will later need surgical maxillary advancement. The cephalometric method of Enlow et al,[62] tested and described by Gnoinski,[16, 17] may help in detection of these patients.

Protraction of the basal maxilla with the face mask of Delaire is effective, at least during the deciduous and mixed dentition.[60, 61, 63–67] In the permanent dentition the skeletal changes may be restricted because of a bony or fibrous ankylosis of the maxilla.[64, 65] In our group of 14 patients with cleft lip and palate, traction on the maxilla was initiated between 9 and 15 years of age. Forward translation of the maxilla was observed only in 5- to 11-year-old patients, whereas no movement of this type was observed in nine patients over 11 years of age.

A slight retrusion of the mandible was observed in nine patients and was independent of age. In spite of the poor results of bringing the maxilla forward in the older patients, face mask therapy proved to be successful in correcting the anterior crossbite and the spacing of the dental arch, and as an anchor in widening the maxillary dental arch (Fig. 77–4).[61, 64–66] Further knowledge is needed about the skeletal effects of protraction of the maxilla on midfacial growth during and after pubertal growth and about its long-term results.

Bone Grafting and Periosteoplasty of the Alveolar Cleft

In patients with severe crossbite it is helpful to correct the anterior and posterior crossbite before bone grafting

and to continue orthodontic treatment after that. Secondary bone grafting, unlike infant bone grafting, has a minimal effect on growth and overall facial development. The canine will erupt into the grafted bone, but in some patients surgical exposure of a palatally impacted canine is required.[61, 68]

Various methods are used to reconstruct the continuity of the maxilla.[68–75] Neither early bone grafting nor infant or delayed periosteoplasty have prevented dental arch collapse or been satisfactory for maxillary growth.[5, 8, 18, 22, 27, 51, 76] Bone formation has not always occurred, and there rarely has been enough bone to render a

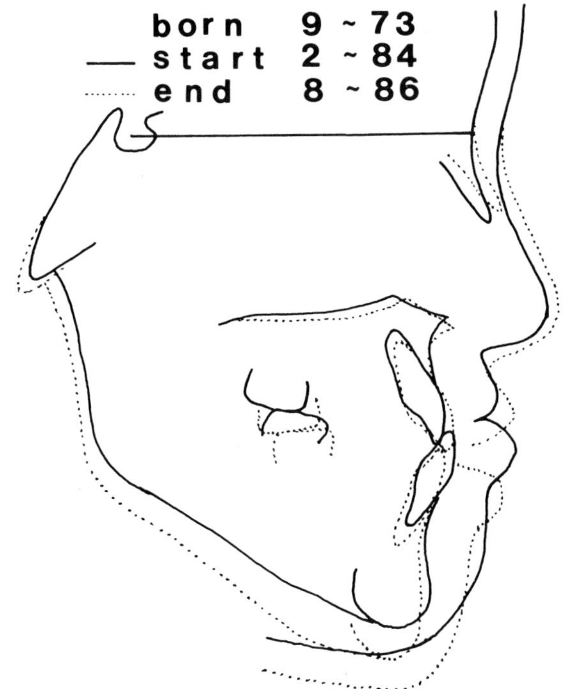

Figure 77–4 Lateral skull radiograph diagrams before and after 15 months of maxillary protraction. The patient is 10 years old.

complete secondary bone graft.[16, 21, 25] We found that a secondary bone graft was indicated and was performed in 72% of the patients with complete clefts who were operated on with primary periosteoplasty.[25] Secondary bone grafting in selected patients has proved to be better before eruption of the canine than afterward.[61, 75, 77]

The bone graft alone will not prevent transverse collapse of the dental arch, but it facilitates eruption and movement of the teeth toward the cleft and eliminates or facilitates later prosthodontic treatment. Bone grafting also supports the alar base and nasolabial counter.

Maxillary Osteotomies

Surgical advancement of the maxilla is necessary for patients with the most severe hypoplasia or retrusion of the midface. Friede and Johanson[26] reported that 50% of early bone-grafted patients also underwent maxillary osteotomy. Gnoinski[16] cephalometrically analyzed young adult patients who had undergone conventional surgery and showed that sagittal skeletal imbalance was present in more than 50% of them. The need for osteotomies is always determined individually and depends on several factors. Careful clinical examination of the patient is important before cephalometric analysis and before a decision is made to operate on the patient.[40, 71, 78–80]

Reported postsurgical results have shown a remarkable degree of relapse in the vertical direction and, to a lesser extent, anteroposteriorly. Varying degrees of relapse are observed with different methods of surgery and fixation; miniplate fixation seems to give the best results.[14, 78, 79, 81, 82]

Prevention of Postorthodontic Relapse

Postorthodontic relapse has scarcely been investigated. However, the stabilization of the maxillary arch and teeth is extremely important for the end result of overall treatment. The most important factors in preventing postorthodontic relapse appear to be good daily oral hygiene, prevention of segmental collapse, and prevention of the rotation, tipping, and crowding of each tooth.

Recommendations for the Directions of Future Research

The causal relationships of surgery, respiration, tongue position, and cleft-related intrinsic growth factors are still controversial. The physiologic role of tongue position and function in relation to nose versus mouth breathing has been overlooked in discussions of cephalometric results. Circumpubertal and postpubertal growth of the jaws and the relationship of the jaws to each other and to the cranial base should be investigated with different cephalometric methods according to the type and timing of surgery and the type of orthodontic treatment utilized.

The optimum age and methods for the transverse expansion and anterior protraction of the maxilla should be determined. Prognostic methods for early prediction of the need for later corrective osteotomies and the indications for osteotomies are still uncertain, and knowledge is scanty concerning postorthodontic long-term results of modern methods of preventing relapse of the teeth.

References

1. Berkowitz S: Cleft lip and palate research: An updated state of the art. Section III. Orofacial growth and dentistry. Cleft Palate J 14:288, 1977.
2. Berkowitz S: State of the art in cleft palate orofacial growth and dentistry. A historical perspective. Am J Orthod 74:564, 1978.
3. Maue-Dickson W: The craniofacial complex in cleft lip and palate: An updated review of anatomy and function. Cleft Palate J 16:291, 1979.
4. Bishara SE, Sierk DL, Huang K-S: Longitudinal changes in the dento-facial relationships of unilateral cleft lip and palate subjects. Cleft Palate J 16:391, 1979.
5. Friede H, Johanson B: Adolescent facial morphology of early bone-grafted cleft lip and palate patients. Scand J Plast Reconstr Surg 16:41, 1982.
6. Grayson BH, Bookstein FL, McCarthy JG, et al: Mean tensor cephalometric analysis of a patient population with clefts of the palate and lip. Cleft Palate J 24:267, 1987.
7. Goz G, Joos U, Schilli W: The influence of lip function on the sagittal and transversal development of the maxilla in cleft patients. Scand J Plast Reconstr Surg 21:31, 1987.
8. Robertson NRE, Jolleys A: An 11-year follow-up of the effects of early bone grafting in infants born with complete clefts of the lip and palate. Br J Plast Surg 36:438, 1983.
9. Smahel Z, Brejcha M: Differences in craniofacial morphology between complete and imcomplete unilateral cleft lip and palate adults. Cleft Palate J 20:113, 1983.
10. Smahel Z, Mullerova Z: Craniofacial morphology in unilateral cleft lip and palate prior to palatoplasty. Cleft Palate J 23:225, 1986.
11. Vargervik K: Growth characteristics of the premaxilla and orthodontic treatment principles in bilateral cleft lip and palate. Cleft Palate J 20:289, 1983.
12. Johnson GP: Craniofacial analysis of patients with complete clefts of the lip and palate. Cleft Palate J 17:17, 1980.
13. Cronin DG, Hunter WS: Craniofacial morphology in twins discordant for cleft lip and/or palate. Cleft Palate J 17:116, 1980.
14. Drommer R, Luhr H: The stabilization of osteotomized maxillary segments with Luhr miniplates in secondary cleft surgery. J Maxillofac Surg 9:166, 1981.
15. Enany NM: A cephalometric study of the effects of primary osteoplasty in unilateral cleft lip and palate individuals. Cleft Palate J 18:286, 1981.
16. Gnoinski W: Early maxillary orthopaedics as a supplement to conventional primary surgery in complete cleft lip and palate cases: Long-term results. J Maxillo-fac Surg 10:165, 1982.
17. Gnoinski W: Early identification of candidates for corrective maxillary osteotomy in a cleft lip and palate group. Scand J Plast Reconstr Surg 21:39, 1987.
18. Hellquist R, Svardstrom K, Ponten B: A longitudinal study of delayed periosteoplasty to the cleft alveolus. Cleft Palate J 20:277, 1983.
19. Hunter WS: Review: The Michigan cleft twin study. J Craniofac Genet Dev Biol 1:235, 1981.
20. Jorgenson RJ, Shapiro SD, Odinet KL: Studies on facial growth and arch size in cleft lip and palate. J Craniofac Genet Devel Biol 4:33, 1984.
21. Nordin K-E, Larson O, Nylen B, et al: Early bone grafting in complete cleft lip and palate cases following maxillofacial orthopedics: I. The method and the skeletal development from 7 to 13 years of age. Scand J Plast Reconstr Surg 17:33, 1983.
22. Rintala AE, Ranta R: Periosteal flaps and grafts in the primary cleft repair: A follow-up study. Plast Reconstr Surg 83:17, 1989.
23. Rygh P, Sirinavin I: Craniofacial morphology in 6-year-old Norwegian boys with complete cleft of lip and palate. Swed Dent J Suppl 15:203, 1982.
24. Smahel Z, Pobisova Z, Figalova P: Basic cephalometric facial characteristics in cleft lip and/or palate prior to the first surgical repair. Acta Chir Plast 27:131, 1985.
25. Ross RB: Treatment variables affecting facial growth in complete unilateral cleft lip and palate. Parts 1–7: Treatment affecting growth. Cleft Palate J 24:5, 1987.
26. Friede H, Johanson B: A follow-up study of cleft children treated with primary bone grafting. I. Orthodontic aspects. Scand J Plast Reconstr Surg 8:88, 1974.

27. Hellquist R, Linder-Aronson S, Norling M, et al: Dental abnormalities in patients with alveolar clefts, operated upon with or without primary periosteoplasty. Eur J Orthod 1:169, 1979.
28. Ranta R: A review of tooth formation in children with cleft lip/palate. Am J Orthod Dentofac Orthop 90:11, 1986.
29. Ranta R: Comparison of hypodontia in the region outside the cleft in different types of cleft lip and palate. Angle Orthod (in press, 1989).
30. Ranta R, Rintala A: Tooth anomalies associated with congenital sinuses of the lower lip and cleft lip/palate. Angle Orthod 52:212, 1982.
31. Ranta R, Stegars T, Rintala, AE: Correlations of hypodontia in children with isolated cleft palate. Cleft Palate J 20:163, 1983.
32. Poyry M, Ranta R: Anomalies in the deciduous dentition outside the cleft region in children with oral cleft. Proc Finn Dent Soc 81:91, 1985.
33. Poyry M, Ranta R: Emergence of deciduous teeth in children with oral cleft. Proc Finn Dent Soc 81:171, 1985.
34. Poyry M: Prenatal factors and tooth eruption in children with oral clefts. J Dent Child 53:436, 1986.
35. Poyry M, Ranta R. Formation of anterior maxillary teeth in 0 to 3-year-old children with cleft lip and palate and prenatal risk factors for delayed development. J Craniofac Genet Devel Biol 6:15, 1986.
36. Poyry M: Dental development in 0 to 3-year-old children with cleft lip and palate. Proc Finn Dent Soc Suppl XI:83, 1987.
37. Ranta R: Comparison of tooth formation in noncleft and cleft-affected children with and without hypodontia. J Dent Child 49:197, 1982.
38. Huddart AG: The effect of form and dimension on the management of the maxillary arch in unilateral cleft lip and palate conditions. Scand J Plast Reconstr Surg 21:53, 1987.
39. Wada T, Mizokawa N, Miyazaki T, et al: Maxillary dental arch growth in different types of cleft. Cleft Palate J 21:180, 1984.
40. Wada T, Yakushiji N, Tachimura T, et al: Late results of two-stage palatal closure in complete unilateral cleft lip and palate. J Osaka Univ Dent Sch 27:253, 1987.
41. Rintala A, Haataja J: The effect of the lip adhesion procedure on the alveolar arch with special reference to the type and width of the cleft and the age at operation. Scand J Plast Reconstr Surg 13:301, 1979.
42. Rune B, Jacobsson S, Sarnas K-V, et al: A roentgenstereophotogrammetric study of implant stability and movement of segments in the maxilla of infants with cleft lip and palate. Cleft Palate J 16:267, 1979.
43. Rune B, Sarnas K-V, Selvik G: Oral orthopedics and movement of maxillary segments. A roentgenstereophotogrammetric study. Cleft Palate J 16:385, 1979.
44. Rune B, Sarnas K-V, Selvik G, et al: Movement of the cleft maxilla in infants relative to the frontal bone. A roentgenstereophotogrammetric study with the aid of metallic implants. Cleft Palate J 17:155, 1980.
45. Hotz MM, Gnoinski WM: Effects of early maxillary orthopedics in coordination with delayed surgery for cleft lip and palate. J Maxillofac Surg 7:201, 1979.
46. Larson O, Ideberg M, Nordin K-E: Early bone grafting in complete cleft lip and palate cases following maxillofacial orthopedics. III. A study of the dental occlusion. Scand J Plast Reconstr Surg 17:81, 1983.
47. Lennartsson B, Friede H, Johanson B. Effect of post-surgical jaw–orthopaedic treatment in unilateral cleft lip and palate patients. Scand J Plast Reconstr Surg 18:227, 1984.
48. Weil J: Orthopaedic growth guidance and stimulation for patients with cleft lip and palate. Scand J Plast Reconstr Surg 21:57, 1987.
49. Dahl E, Hanusardottir B: Prevalence of malocclusion in the primary and early mixed dentition in Danish children with complete cleft lip and palate. Eur J Orthod 1:81, 1979.
50. Dahl E, Hanusardottir B, Bergland O: A comparison of occlusion in two groups of children whose clefts were repaired by three different surgical procedures. Cleft Palate J 17:122, 1981.
51. Hellquist R, Ponten B: The influence of infant periosteoplasty on facial growth and dental occlusion from 5 to 8 years of age in cases of complete unilateral cleft lip and palate. Scand J Plast Reconstr Surg 13:305, 1979.
52. Jonsson G, Stenstrom S, Thilander B: The use of a vomer flap covered with an autogenous skin graft as a part of the palatal repair in children with unilateral cleft lip and palate. Arch dimensions and occlusion up to the age of five. Scand J Plast Reconstr Surg 14:13, 1980.
53. Molsted K, Palmberg A, Dahl E, et al: Malocclusion in complete unilateral and bilateral cleft lip and palate. The results of a change in the surgical procedure. Scand J Plast Reconstr Surg 21:81, 1987.
54. Bishara SE, Sierk DL, Huang K-S: A longitudinal cephalometric study on unilateral cleft lip and palate subjects. Cleft Palate J 16:59, 1979.
55. Vargervik K: Orthodontic management of unilateral cleft lip and palate. Cleft Palate J 18:256, 1981.
56. Ranta R: Developmental course of 27 late-developing second premolars. Proc Finn Dent Soc 79:9, 1983.
57. Ranta R: Hypodontia and delayed development of the second premolars in cleft palate children. Eur J Orthod 5:145, 1983.
58. Dahl E. Transverse maxillary growth in combined cleft lip and palate. A longitudinal roentgen cephalometric study by the implant method. Cleft Palate J 16:34, 1979.
59. Markovic M: The role of the orthodontist in the treatment of adolescents with orofacial clefts. Int Dent J 36:131, 1986.
60. Rygh P, Tindlund R: Orthopaedic expansion and protraction of the maxilla in cleft palate patients: A new treatment rationale. Cleft Palate J 19:104, 1982.
61. Bergland O, Semb G, Abyholm FE: Elimination of the residual alveolar cleft by secondary bone grafting and subsequent orthodontic treatment. Cleft Palate J 23:175, 1986.
62. Enlow DH, Moyers RE, Hunter WS, et al: A procedure for the analysis of intrinsic facial form and growth: An equivalent-balance concept. Am J Orthod 56:6, 1969.
63. Delaire J, Verdon P, Kenesi M-C: Extraorale Zukrafte mit Stirn-Kinn-Abstutzung zur Behandlung der Oberkieferdeformierungen als Folge von Lippen, Kiefer, Gaumenspalten. Fortschr Kieferorthop 34:225, 1973.
64. Friede H, Lennartsson B: Forward traction of the maxilla in cleft lip and palate patients. Eur J Orthod 3:21, 1981.
65. Ranta R: Protraction of the cleft maxilla. Eur J Orthod 10:215, 1988.
66. Sarnas K-V, Rune B: Extraoral traction to the maxilla with face mask: A follow-up of 17 consecutively treated patients with and without cleft lip and palate. Cleft Palate J 24:95, 1987.
67. Subtelny JD: Oral respiration: Facial maldevelopment and corrective dentofacial orthopedics. Angle Orthod 50:147, 1980.
68. Enemark H, Krantz-Simonsen E, Schramm JE: Secondary bone-grafting in unilateral cleft lip palate patients: Indications and treatment procedure. Int J Oral Surg 14:2, 1985.
69. Abyholm FE, Bergland O, Semb G: Secondary bone grafting of alveolar clefts. A surgical/orthodontic treatment enabling a non-prosthodontic rehabilitation in cleft lip and palate patients. Scand J Plast Reconstr Surg 15:127, 1981.
70. Ames JR, Dyan DE, Maki KA: The autogenous particulate cancellous bone marrow graft in alveolar clefts. A report of 41 cases. Oral Surg 51:588, 1981.
71. Braun TW, Sotereanos GC: Orthognathic and secondary cleft reconstruction of adolescent patients with cleft palate. J Oral Surg 38:425, 1980.
72. Chierici G: Experiments on the influence of oriented stress on bone formation replacing bone grafts. Cleft Palate J 14:114, 1977.
73. Lilja J, Moller M, Friede H, et al: Bone grafting at the stage of mixed dentition in cleft lip and palate patients. Scand J Plast Reconstr Surg 21:73, 1987.
74. Nakasima A, Ichinose M: Characteristics of craniofacial structures of parents of children with cleft lip and/or palate. Am J Orthod 84:140, 1983.
75. Sindet-Pedersen S, Enemark H: Comparative study of secondary and late secondary bone-grafting in patients with residual cleft defects: short-term evaluation. Int J Oral Surg 14:389, 1985.
76. Larson O, Ideberg M, Nordin K-E: Early bone grafting in complete cleft lip and palate cases following maxillofacial orthopedics. IV. A radiographic study of the incorporation of the bone graft. Scand J Plast Reconstr Surg 17:93, 1983.
77. Turvey TA, Vig K, Moriarty J, et al: Delayed bone grafting in the cleft maxilla and palate: A retrospective multidisciplinary analysis. Am J Orthod 86:244, 1984.
78. Epker BN, Schendel SA: Total maxillary surgery. Int J Oral Surg 9:1, 1980.
79. Ward-Booth RP, Bhatia SN, Moos KF: A cephalometric analysis of the Le Fort II osteotomy in the adult cleft patient. J Maxillofac Surg 12:208, 1984.
80. Wylie GA, Fish LC, Epker BN: Cephalometrics: A comparison of five analyses currently used in the diagnosis of dentofacial deformities. Int J Adult Orthod Orthogn Surg 2:15, 1987.
81. James DR, Brook K: Maxillary hypoplasia in patients with cleft lip and palate deformity—the alternative surgical approach. Eur J Orthod 7:231, 1985.
82. Tideman H, Stoelinga P, Gallia L: Le Fort I advancement with segmental palatal osteotomies in patients with cleft palates. J Oral Surg 38:196, 1980.

CHAPTER 78

Orthodontic Treatment of Cleft Patients: Characteristics of Growth and Development/ Treatment Principles

Karin Vargervik

Orofacial growth and development in individuals with clefts of the lip and palate are influenced by irregularities in embryonic development causing tissue deficiencies and distortions, and by lip and palate surgery resulting in scar tissue. These influences on growth may act directly on developing structures or may affect growth patterns indirectly through deviant function and muscle activity. The commonly observed findings of irregularities in the nose, palate, and pharynx may affect speech, mastication, respiration, and the posture and movements of the tongue.

Appropriate treatment planning requires that distinctions be made between primary tissue defects and subsequent adaptations of normal structures to their altered environment. Therapy should focus on providing conditions for the optimal development of structures that have normal potential for development. Those structures that cannot develop sufficiently should be brought into positions that minimize the effect of their inadequacies.

Characteristics of Growth and Development in Cleft Patients

Clinical studies have demonstrated that characteristic abnormalities vary among individuals and change significantly during growth. It has been practical to distinguish four developmental stages: (1) infancy—before surgical closure of the lip; (2) deciduous dentition; (3) early mixed dentition; and (4) adolescence.

Infancy

The wide variation in tissue deficiencies and morphology in the newborn cleft infant will not be discussed here. The surgically closed lip and palate approximate the morphology of the normal lip and palate. However, the repaired lip and palate do not necessarily continue to develop favorably in either morphology or function because of neuromuscular abnormalities and scar tissue. The molding effect of the surgically restored lip on the protruding premaxillary region has been well documented.[1, 2]

Deciduous Dentition

Medial movement of the lateral segments subsequent to lip and palate closure is also a consistent finding. The maxillary segments usually contact each other in the alveolar region by 4 to 5 years of age.[3, 4] This contact counteracts further medial movement of the segments unless teeth are lost and alveolar bone in the cleft resorbs. The degree of maxillary width reduction is therefore closely related to the development of the alveolar processes; this in turn is determined to a large extent by the number, position, size, and shape of the teeth in that area.[1] Early removal of teeth in the cleft is, therefore, contraindicated.

The deciduous dentition is usually complete. Supernumerary teeth in the cleft occur more frequently than congenital absence of teeth. The alveolar processes are generally well developed and stable as long as the deciduous dentition is intact. Crossbite of one or more teeth on the cleft side is the most usual deviation from normal dental arch form during this stage.

In bilateral cleft lip and palate, the premaxilla is usually protrusive at birth and remains so during the first years of life if surgical intervention in this area is limited to lip closure. It has been shown that the rate of forward growth of the premaxilla from age 4 to adulthood is approximately one half of the rate recorded in noncleft controls, whereas the average mandibular growth rate is the same as that in control subjects. On the average, the mandible will catch up with the premaxilla at the age of 12 years.[5] In planning treatment for a child with a repaired bilateral cleft, it is therefore important to accept early prominence of the premaxilla and to take into account the fact that forward growth in this area is less than normal.[5]

Studies on skeletal morphology and size in children with unilateral cleft lip and palate have shown few differences from average values for normals in the late deciduous and early mixed dentition stages.[6–10] As part of a study of orthodontic treatment effects on subjects with unilateral cleft lip and palate in our center, pretreatment cephalometric head films of eight girls and eight boys with unilateral cleft lip and palate were studied.[11] The mean age was 8 years 1 month in girls and 7 years 2 months in boys. The mean values for these two groups did not differ significantly from the control values for any of the measurements that were selected to determine unit sizes of the maxilla and mandible and jaw relationship (Table 78–1).

Mixed Dentition

The transition from the deciduous to the mixed dentition is characterized by an increased discrepancy between maxillary and mandibular sizes and dental arches.[12–15] The permanent lateral incisor on the side of the cleft is frequently missing, and there is a high incidence of congenital absence of bicuspids.[16] The central incisor on the cleft side is on average 10% narrower than the other central incisor, and its shape is often abnormal.[3] The path of eruption of the central

Table 78–1. Minimum, Mean, and Maximum Values for Length of Jaws, Difference Between Upper and Lower Jaw Lengths and Lower Anterior Face Height in the Cleft Group Before Orthodontic Treatment and the Equivalent Values From the Burlington Control Subjects for the Same Age Group

	Group A—Boys Subjects with clefts before start of orthodontic treatment			Noncleft Controls		
Variables	Min.	Mean	Max.	Min.	Mean	Max.
TM-ANS	80	86	90	78	84	92
TM-PGN	102	105	108	93	102	111
TM-PGN—ANS	17	19	24	11	18	28
ANS-GN	56	65	72	53	60	73
	Group B—Girls Subjects with clefts before start of orthodontic treatment			Noncleft Controls		
Variables	Min.	Mean	Max.	Min.	Mean	Max.
TM-ANS	79	83	89	77	84	92
TM-PGN	101	105	109	92	103	111
TM-PGN—ANS	18	22	27	12	19	27
ANS-GN	56	62	67	49	59	69

Reprinted from Vargervik K: Orthodontic management of cleft lip and palate. Cleft Palate J 18:256–270, 1981.

incisors is lingual and toward the cleft, and these teeth usually are severely rotated as well.[17] Further medial displacement of the alveolar process on the cleft side and an increased incidence of anterior crossbite usually occur during this stage.

When the maxillary segments are displaced medially, the tongue cannot be accommodated in its normal position in the palate. The position acquired by the tongue becomes decisive for the pattern of further development of the maxilla as well as the mandible. If nasal respiration is adequate, the tongue may be positioned below and in contact with the occlusal surfaces of the maxillary teeth during rest. When this position occurs, alveolar height is inhibited even in the absence of restrictive scar tissue. If nasal respiration is impeded, the tongue may assume a low posture to facilitate oral respiration. If the tongue in this low position does not rest under the occlusal surfaces of the maxillary teeth, the alveolar height will increase, resulting in a progressive lowering of the mandible, a more open gonial angle, and a more retruded position of the chin.[1, 18]

Adolescent Growth Period

Progressive retrusiveness of the maxilla may occur during later growth.[1, 5, 19, 20] In noncleft children from 6 to 16 years of age there is a yearly average increase in mandibular length measured from condylion to pogonion of 2.5 mm. The corresponding figure for the maxilla is 1.5 mm.[21] Adjustments for this difference in growth in jaw length take place in the alveolar processes primarily by downward and forward development of the maxillary alveolar process. In persons with cleft lip and palate, this adjustment mechanism is often impeded[22] and becomes an important cause of jaw disproportion during active growth periods, particularly during adolescence.

A tight, scarred lip and scar tissue bands in the palate can impede the forward growth of the entire maxilla as well as the alveolar process. The retrusiveness of the maxilla and maxillary alveolar process generally becomes more pronounced during this stage.

Experimental Findings

Studies on young and adolescent rhesus monkeys have demonstrated that conditions similar to those usually observed in individuals with unilateral clefts are produced by spontaneous adaptations of normal tissues to a surgically produced cleft by loss of teeth in the cleft area and medial movement of the cleft segment.[23, 24]

Findings from these studies led to the conclusion that the palatal tilting of the maxillary incisors and the mandibular changes were adaptations to a lowered postural position of the mandible and tongue. This lower position was necessitated by tongue displacement, which was caused by the induced reduction of the palatal vault and arch width. These structural adaptations can be assumed to be reversible because they occurred in response to well-defined environmental changes. It was postulated that similar adaptations of normal structures occur in children with clefts and that these deviations from normal development can be prevented or corrected by properly designed treatment. This postulate has been further substantiated by clinical observations indicating that, in the absence of surgery, there usually is a potential for adequate development and forward growth of the segments in the cleft maxilla.[25–27]

Clinical Findings

A study was designed to test hypotheses based on the postulate that reversal of undesirable structural adaptations is possible by properly designed orthodontic treatment.[11] Some of the findings from this study are presented here.

Subjects

The subjects, whose ages ranged from 14 years 9 months to 18 years 3 months, were categorized into three groups:
1. Sixteen control subjects with good dental occlusion and no clefts.

Table 78–2. Distribution of Subjects According to Groups, Age, and Sex

	Group 1		Group 2	Group 3			
	Noncleft Controls		Subjects with Untreated Clefts	Subjects with Treated Clefts			
				Before Treatment		After Treatment	
Sex	F	M	M	F	M	F	M
Number	8	8	8	8	8	8	8
Mean age	16–3	16–6	16–2	8–1	7–2	16–2	16–0
Age range	14–9	15–1	14–10	7–0	6–1	14–9	14–2
	to	to	to	to	to	to	to
	17–5	17–5	17–8	10–3	8–7	18–3	17–3

Reprinted from Vargervik K: Orthodontic management of unilateral cleft lip and palate. Cleft Palate J 18:256–270, 1981.

2. Eight individuals who had complete unilateral clefts of the lip and palate who had not had any orthodontic treatment when the records were taken.
3. Sixteen individuals who had complete unilateral clefts of the lip and palate and who had received orthodontic treatment in our center. Records also had been obtained prior to the start of treatment. The distribution of ages and sexes in the three groups is shown in Table 78–2.

The orthodontically treated and untreated individuals with clefts of the lip and palate represented a variety of surgical techniques performed by different surgeons. They were referred to the center because they presented special treatment problems; therefore, they constitute biased samples. The major factors contributing to the special treatment problems were excessive scarring, a high incidence of missing teeth (either congenitally absent or prematurely lost), and maxillary deficiency. It was concluded that groups 2 and 3 were comparable, the main difference being orthodontic treatment. The criterion for inclusion in this study was the availability of records at the appropriate ages. The material from these patients was considered suitable for testing of the hypotheses. However, the cephalometric measurements may not be representative of the population of individuals with unilateral clefts of the lip and palate. The first group served as controls, whereas the second group demonstrated the development of craniofacial structures in the absence of orthodontic treatment. The third group was compared to the first and second groups to assess the effects of orthodontic treatment. The average age of the subjects in all three groups at the time of group comparisons was approximately 16 years. Standard statistical methods were applied.

Assessment of Records

Linear and angular measurements were obtained from tracings of lateral cephalometric head films. The presence or absence of teeth was evaluated from oblique cephalometric head films and from panoramic or periapical radiographs. Assessment of crossbite was made on dental casts, and evaluation of maxillary expansion was obtained from dental casts and anteroposterior cephalometric head films.

Cephalometric landmarks and planes are shown in Fig. 78–1.

Results

Pretreatment Data on the Cleft Palate Group that Received Orthodontic Treatment

Although data recorded on jaw size and relationship of the eight boys and eight girls treated at the center show no significant deviations from normal values (Table 78–1), the development and position of the anterior areas of the maxillary alveolar processes were impaired. The retruded position of the maxillary incisors relative to the mandibular incisors resulted in inadequate incisor overbite and overjet and in anterior crossbite. The

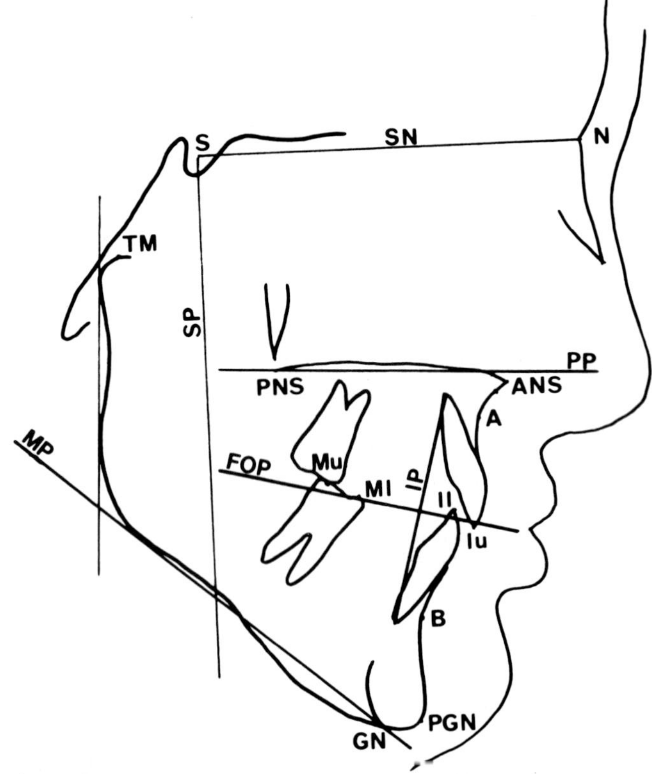

Figure 78–1 Tracing of a lateral head film demonstrating the reference points and planes used in this study. The following planes are drawn: SN = sella nasion plane; PP = palatal plane; FOP = functional occlusal plane; IP = incisor apex plane; MP = mandibular plane; SP = perpendicular to SN through S. (From Vargervik K: Orthodontic management of unilateral cleft lip and palate. Cleft Palate J 18(4):260, 1981. By permission of B C Decker Inc.)

Table 78–3. Distribution of Crossbite and Congenital Absence of Teeth

| | Group 1 | | Group 2
Subjects with
Untreated
Clefts | Group 3 Subjects with Treated Clefts | | | |
| | Noncleft Controls | | | Before Treatment | | After Treatment | |
Sex	F	M	M	F	M	F	M
Crossbite							
Cuspid only	0	0	0	0	0	0	0
Cuspid and molars	0	0	2	2	3	0	0
Incisors only	0	0	0	2	0	0	0
Incisors and cuspid	0	0	0	1	1	0	0
Incisors, cuspid and molar	0	0	6	1	4	0	0
Congenital Absence of Teeth							
Lateral incisor	0	0	6	8	7	—	—
Central incisor	0	0	0	1	0	—	—
Maxillary bicuspids	0	0	4	1	1	—	—
Mandibular bicuspids	0	0	0	1	0	—	—

Reprinted from Vargervik K: Orthodontic management of cleft lip and palate. Cleft Palate J 18:256–270, 1981.

reduction in transverse dimensions was demonstrated by the high incidence of lateral crossbite (Table 78–3).

Comparison of the Orthodontically Treated Cleft Group with the Noncleft Group

Data resulting from the comparison between the orthodontically treated cleft group and the control groups are shown in Table 78–4 for the girls and Table 78–5 for the boys. The distances from the maxillary incisor and the first molar to the sella perpendicular (Iu-SP and Mu-SP) were shorter in the male but not in the female cleft group. The distance from the lower incisor to the sella perpendicular (Il-SP) also was significantly shorter in the male cleft group.

The mean distance from the condyle to the anterior nasal spine was significantly shorter in both the male and the female cleft groups. All other dimensions and angles that were measured were not significantly different. Lateral repositioning of the medially rotated maxillary segment was achieved in all treated individuals. All dental crossbites were eliminated (Table 78–3).

Comparison of the Orthodontically Untreated Cleft Group with the Noncleft Group

Comparisons between normal subjects and those with orthodontically untreated clefts are shown in Table 78–6. All measurements of maxillary dimensions in the horizontal plane were significantly smaller in the cleft group than in the control group. All measurements of anteroposterior relationships between the jaws and the lips were also significantly different and indicated retrusiveness of the maxilla and maxillary dentition. The gonial angle was larger in the untreated cleft subjects. Vertical dimensions were not significantly different.

Comparison of the Orthodontically Untreated Cleft Group with the Treated Group

The results of the comparisons of the untreated with the treated cleft palate boys also are shown in Table 78–6. Maxillary arch length (Iu-Sp–Mu-Sp) was significantly smaller in the untreated group. The anterior nasal spine was significantly more retrusive relative to

Table 78–4. Means, Standard Deviations, and T Values for Group Comparison of Orthodontically Treated Cleft Subjects and Noncleft Controls, Girls

| Variables | Hypothesis | Noncleft controls | | Treated clefts | | t |
		Mean	S.D.	Mean	S.D.	
Max. post. alveolar height (Mu-PP)	1 + 3	23.3	4.4	26.4	2.2	.65
Max. ant. alveolar height (Iu-PP)	1 + 3	31.8	3.3	29.7	3.2	1.27
Anteroposterior pos. of max. molar (Mu-SP)	1 + 3	31.5	5.6	29.4	7.5	.64
Anteroposterior pos. of max. in. (Iu-SP)	1 + 3	60.7	7.2	58.5	8.0	.58
Max. dental arch length (Iu-SP—Mu-SP)	1	29.2	3.6	29.1	2.8	.04
Anteroposterior pos. of max. (TM-ANS)	2	94.3	2.8	88.4	5.4	2.72
Mandibular length (TM-PGN)	3	121.0	5.0	120.0	6.4	.48
Diff. in mand. and max. length (TM-PGN—TM-ANS)	3	26.8	3.4	31.2	4.4	2.06
Anteroposterior pos. of mand. inc. (Il-SP)	3	59.0	6.0	56.2	8.1	.81
Incisor relationship (Iu-SP—Il-SP)	3	2.1	.6	2.3	1.5	.20
Relative pos. of points A and B (ANB)	3	2.1	2.1	1.4	2.7	.52
Inclination of mand. plane (MP-SN)	3 + 4	32.9	4.1	36.6	7.9	1.19
Inclination of occlusal plane (FOP-SN)	3	16.9	5.6	14.6	4.9	.89
Occlusal plane angle (FOP-IP)	3	91.0	3.9	90.0	6.4	.38
Lower anterior face height (ANS-GN)	3	70.4	6.6	72.6	5.3	.73
Gonial angle	4	124.4	7.6	125.8	9.0	.35

Reprinted from Vargervik K: Orthodontic management of cleft lip and palate. Cleft Palate J 18:256–270, 1981.

Table 78–5. Means, Standard Deviations, and T Values for Group Comparison of Orthodontically Treated Cleft Subjects and Noncleft Controls, Boys

Variables	Hypothesis	Noncleft controls		Treated clefts		t
		Mean	*S.D.*	*Mean*	*S.D.*	
Max. post. alveolar height (Mu-PP)	1 + 3	27.3	2.3	28.2	2.6	.76
Max. ant. alveolar height (Iu-PP)	1 + 3	33.9	2.6	32.1	2.6	1.39
Anteroposterior pos. of max. molar (Mu-SP)	1 + 3	34.6	4.4	26.2	2.9	4.52[b]
Anteroposterior pos. of max. incisor (Iu-SP)	1 + 3	66.6	5.0	58.4	3.1	3.98[b]
Max. dental arch length (Iu-SP—Mu-SP)	1	32.0	1.7	32.2	1.9	.21
Anteroposterior pos. of maxilla (TM-ANS)	2	99.9	3.9	94.8	4.1	2.53[a]
Mandibular length (TM-PGN)	3	128.8	4.1	127.1	5.9	.64
Diff. in mand. and max. length (TM-PGN—TM-ANS)	3	28.9	3.7	32.1	4.6	1.52
Anteroposterior pos. of mand. inc. (Il-SP)	3	63.9	4.8	56.5	3.6	3.52[b]
Incisor relationship (Iu-SP—Il-SP)	3	2.7	.5	2.8	1.6	.10
Relative prominence of points A and B (ANB)	3	2.8	1.2	1.3	2.3	1.60
Inclination of mand. plane (MP-SN)	3 + 4	37.4	4.6	36.6	6.7	.26
Inclination of occlusal plane (FOP-IP)	3	15.6	3.7	16.4	5.6	.32
Occlusal plane angle (FOP-IP)	3	91.6	3.0	90.4	3.4	.75
Lower anterior face height (ANS-GN)	3	76.3	5.6	77.7	5.7	.51
Gonial angle	4	128.8	8.0	125.1	6.0	1.05

[a]P <0.005
[b]P < 0.001
Reprinted from Vargervik K: Orthodontic management of cleft lip and palate. Cleft Palate J 18:256–270, 1981.

the condyle (TM-ANS) and also to PGN (jaw length difference) in the untreated group. The average horizontal relationship between the maxillary and mandibular incisors (Iu-SP–Il-SP) was 2.6 mm in the treated group and −3.9 in the untreated group. This difference was larger in the untreated than in the treated group. Maxillary and mandibular alveolar heights were significantly smaller in the untreated than in the treated group.

It was concluded from the findings in this study that the following effects can be achieved when the treatment principles described here are followed:

1. Enlargement of the entire maxilla by repositioning the segments.
2. Counteraction of the inhibiting effects of scar tissue and dental irregularities on the forward development of the maxillary alveolar process and also partial counteraction of the forces inhibiting forward development of the maxilla as measured at the anterior nasal spine.
3. Enlargement of the palatal vault, allowing a higher tongue position and thereby contributing to a change in mandibular growth direction and a reduction in the gonial angle.

From this and other studies, it can be concluded that orthodontic treatment of most individuals with either unilateral or bilateral cleft lip and palate can achieve an acceptable occlusion and aesthetic facial appearance without surgery on the jaws other than alveolar bone grafting.

Table 78–6. Mean, Standard Deviations, and T Values for Group Comparisons of Orthodontically Untreated Cleft Subjects with Noncleft Controls and with Orthodontically Treated Cleft Subjects

Variables	Hypothesis	Noncleft controls		t	Untreated clefts		t	Treated clefts	
		Mean	*S.D.*		*Mean*	*S.D.*		*Mean*	*S.D.*
MU-PP	1 + 3	27.3	2.3	.24	27.5	1.9	.34	28.2	2.6
Iu-PP	1 + 3	33.9	2.6	1.47	32.1	2.3	.21	32.1	2.6
Mu-SP	1 + 3	34.6	4.4	2.19[a]	29.3	5.3	1.44	26.2	2.9
Iu-SP	1 + 3	66.6	5.0	4.82[b]	54.8	4.9	1.77	58.4	3.1
Iu-SP-Mu-SP	1	32.0	1.7	6.03[b]	25.5	2.5	6.00[b]	32.2	1.9
TM-ANS	2	99.9	3.9	4.89[b]	88.9	5.1	2.57[b]	94.8	4.1
TM-PGN	2 + 3	128.8	4.1	.46	127.7	5.1	.20	127.7	5.9
TM-PGN—TM-ANS	3 + 2	28.9	3.7	4.59[b]	38.8	4.9	2.86[a]	32.1	4.6
Il-SP	3	63.9	4.8	1.89	58.6	6.3	.83	56.5	3.6
Iu-SP—Il-SP	3	2.7	.5	3.80[b]	−3.9	4.9	3.66[b]	2.6	1.6
ANB	3	2.8	1.2	4.82[b]	−3.0	3.2	3.08[b]	1.3	2.3
MP-SN	3 + 4	37.4	4.6	1.08	40.1	5.6	1.14	36.6	6.7
FOP-SN	3	15.6	3.7	1.60	18.1	2.4	.82	16.4	5.6
FOP-IP	3	91.6	3.0	4.23[b]	79.9	7.3	3.73[b]	90.4	3.4
ANS CN	3	76.3	5.6	.20	77.0	4.5	.27	77.7	5.7
Gonial angle	4	128.8	8.0	1.22	133.6	8.0	2.43*	125.1	6.0

[a]P < 0.005
[b]P < 0.001
Reprinted from Vargervik K: Orthodontic management of cleft lip and palate. Cleft Palate J 18:256–270, 1981.

Orthodontic Treatment Procedures

The orthodontic treatment approach used for the subjects in this study represents our standard treatment for children with clefts.[5, 11] Treatment is usually started in the early mixed dentition stage before full eruption of the permanent incisors. Presurgical retraction of the premaxilla in children with bilateral clefts and of the anterior portion of the larger segment in those with unilateral clefts is done only in cases in which the cleft is too wide to achieve good lip repair.[5, 11]

The first phase of treatment involves lateral repositioning of the maxillary segment on the cleft side and correction of incisor position. A lingual wire (0.036 inch) is used to produce the main expansion force. This wire is attached to molar bands on either the second deciduous molars or the first permanent molars (Fig. 78–2). The distal ends of the wire are situated in vertical tubes with a diameter of 0.036 inch placed distolingually on the molar band. A loop is welded to the mesiolingual portion of the band and serves as a lock to prevent dislodging of the wire. A 0.018 inch wire is attached to the main wire and is adjusted to contact teeth in the segment to be moved. As the segment moves laterally, this spring follows and distributes the expansion forces to the teeth and bone anterior to the anchor tooth.

It is known that the fulcrum of rotation of the segment is located behind the tuberosity of the maxilla during the medial collapse of the segment as well as during lateral repositioning (Fig. 78–3). A 5- to 6-mm expansion between the molars is incorporated in the main wire to achieve segment rotation.

It should be noted that adequate segment repositioning cannot be achieved with a labial wire because this will always expand more in the molar area than in the cuspid area. Evidence for segment repositioning rather than tooth movements can be obtained from cephalometric radiographs in the posteroanterior view (Fig. 78–4).

Active extrusion of maxillary teeth may be indicated

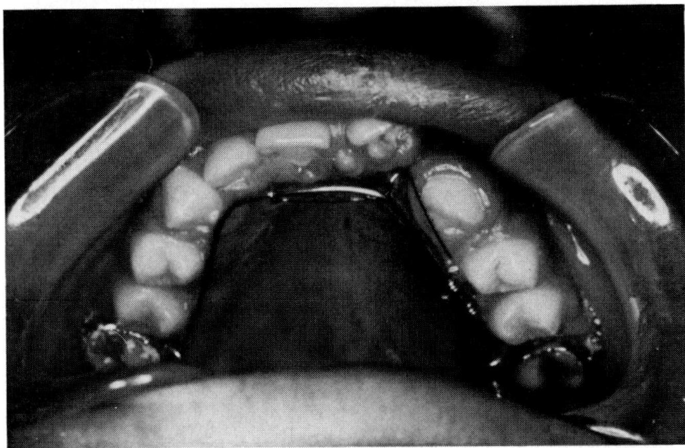

Figure 78–2 Conventionally used lingual wire with a lateral expansion spring for segment rotation is attached to the second deciduous molars in this 7-year-old child with a complete unilateral cleft. (From Vargervik K: Orthodontic management of unilateral cleft lip and palate. Cleft Palate J 18(4):260, 1981. By permission of B C Decker Inc.)

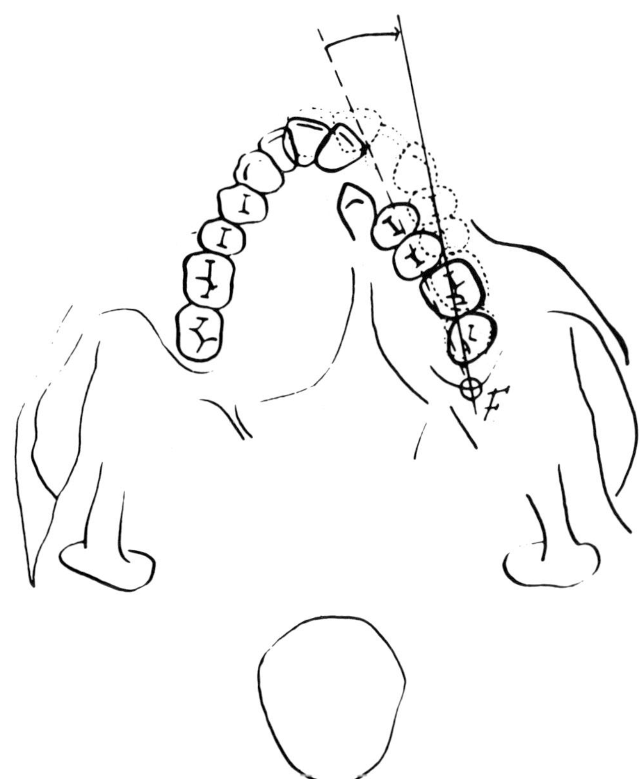

Figure 78–3 Medial rotation of the small maxillary segment, which is a common finding in unilateral clefts, has its fulcrum at the tuberosity of the maxilla. Lateral repositioning of the collapsed segment must be accomplished by rotation using the same fulcrum. (From Vargervik K: Orthodontic management of unilateral cleft lip and palate. Cleft Palate J 18(4):260, 1981. By permission of B C Decker Inc.)

if tongue position or scar tissue has inhibited vertical dentoalveolar development in the maxilla. Correction of incisor position usually consists of extrusion combined with protrusion and rotations. The extrusive and protrusive forces are generated from springs attached to the lingual wire and acting on individual teeth.

In some individuals, mandibular growth during adolescence exceeds maxillary growth to such an extent that it cannot be compensated for by correction of the maxillary deficiencies alone. In these cases, the mandibular prominence can be reduced by active overextrusion of maxillary teeth, which brings the chin farther down and back. This results in increased facial height, which can be aesthetically acceptable and is preferable to the appearance of a retruded midface.

The mandibular dental arch can be reduced in size when the above described procedures are not expected to result in a satisfactory incisor and lip relationship. If the mandibular second bicuspids are congenitally missing, the deciduous molars are extracted to allow closure of the bicuspid space. If all teeth are present but a crowding tendency is apparent, the mandibular bicuspids or first molars can be extracted. If extraction of the first molar is done before the second molar and bicuspids have erupted, the space is shared equally between mesial eruption of the second molar and distal eruption of the bicuspid.

Bone grafting of the alveolar clefts is almost always indicated and is beneficial for several reasons.[28–30] Ade-

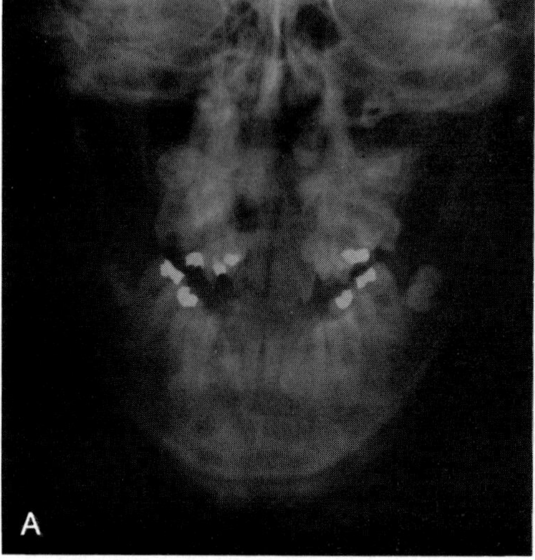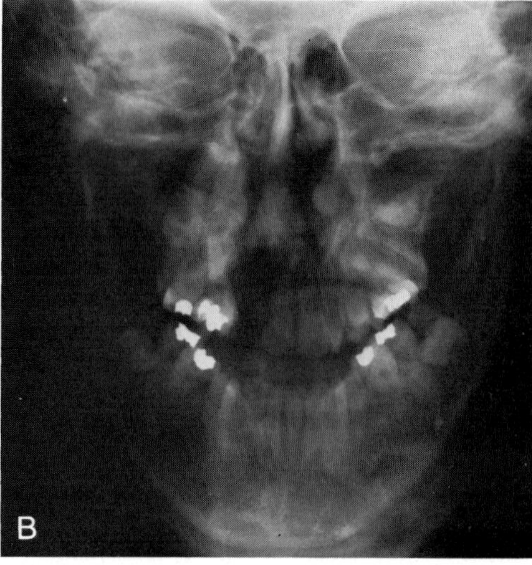

Figure 78–4 A, The maxillary segment on the side of the cleft is medially rotated, and there is contact between the cuspid and the central incisor. *B,* After 6 months of treatment, the segment has been moved laterally without changing the position of the teeth in the segment. (From Vargervik K: Orthodontic management of unilateral cleft lip and palate. Cleft Palate J 18(4):260, 1981. By permission of B C Decker Inc.)

quate width and position of the maxilla are secured before the maxillary segments are fused because after bony continuity has been established, segment repositioning cannot be done.[28]

The final phase of treatment consists of adjusting the alignment of teeth with conventional labial orthodontic appliances. If the lateral incisor is missing, a decision needs to be made whether to maintain space for prosthetic replacement or to move the cuspid and the rest of the teeth in the cleft segment forward to close the space. Subsequently, retainers are placed until the final prosthetic replacements can be made.

Conclusions

General agreement exists on overall treatment goals for the cleft lip and palate child. Results are generally good regardless of treatment approach and timing of the various treatment procedures such as palate closure, orthodontic treatment, and alveolar bone grafting.

Despite this, we still see compromised and difficult cases at various age levels. These difficult cases pose a particular challenge to our knowledge and ability to assess and treat them adequately. Certain factors may contribute to unfavorable growth and development and response to treatment. The most commonly observed unfavorable factors appear to be associated with the repair of the clefts and include:

1. Heavy scar tissue bands in the palate, particularly if they extend to the attached gingiva close to the teeth, thereby inhibiting alveolar development.
2. Scar tissue from the palate extending to the retromolar area.
3. A short, tight, low pharyngeal flap, particularly if created early in development.
4. A scarred, tight lip.

Factors not related to surgical repair are missing, malformed, and malpositioned teeth and factors associated with inherited growth patterns of the individual. These may be expressed in poor midfacial growth, excessive mandibular growth, or a combination of these

factors that are not infrequently seen in noncleft individuals as well. Treatment in these difficult cases may necessitate surgical advancement of the maxilla, reduction of the mandible, or a combination of these procedures.

Difficult patients in whom we have not been able to reach our treatment goals or those in whom the treatment time and procedures needed to achieve an acceptable result have been very extensive pose a particular challenge and require further study of the factors involved in both prevention and correction.

References

1. Harvold EP: Cleft lip and palate. Am J Orthod 40: 493–506, 1954.
2. Pruzansky S: Factors determining arch form in clefts of the lip and palate. Am J Orthod 41: 827–851, 1955.
3. Harvold EP: Observations on the development of the upper jaw in harelip and cleft palate. Odont Tidskr 55 3:289–305, 1947.
4. Pruzansky S, Aduss H: Arch form in the deciduous occlusion in complete unilateral cleft lip and palate. Europ Orthod Soc Trans 43:365–382, 1967.
5. Vargervik K: Growth characteristics of the premaxilla and orthodontic treatment principles in bilateral cleft lip and palate. Cleft Palate J 20:289–302, 1983.
6. Mazaheri M, Nanda S, Sassouni J: Comparison of mid-facial development of children with clefts with their siblings. Cleft Palate J 4:334–341, 1967.
7. Aduss, H: Craniofacial growth in complete unilateral cleft lip and palate. Angle Orthod 4:202–213, 1971.
8. Nakamura S, Savara BS, Thomas DR: Facial growth of children with cleft lip and/or palate. Cleft Palate J 9:119–131, 1972.
9. Mapes AH, Mazaheri M, Harding RL, et al: A longitudinal analysis of the maxillary growth increments of cleft lip and palate patients (CLP). Cleft Palate J 11:450–462, 1974.
10. Krogman WM, Mazaheri M, Harding RL, et al: A longitudinal study of the craniofacial growth pattern in children with cleft as compared to normal, birth to six years. Cleft Palate J 12:59–84, 1975.
11. Vargervik K: Orthodontic management of unilateral cleft lip and palate. Cleft Palate J 18:256–270, 1981.
12. Ross RB: The clinical implications of facial growth in cleft lip and palate. Cleft Palate J 7:37–47, 1970.
13. Bergland O, Sidhu SS: Occlusal changes from the deciduous to the early mixed dentition in unilateral complete clefts. Cleft Palate J 11:317–326, 1974.
14. Bishara SE, Sierk DL, Huang, D: A longitudinal cephalometric study on unilateral cleft lip and palate subjects. Cleft Palate J 16:59–71, 1979.
15. Bishara SE, Sierk DL, Huang, D: Longitudinal changes in the dentofacial relationships of unilateral cleft lip and palate patients. Cleft Palate J 16:391–401, 1979.
16. Bohn A: Dental Anomalies in Harelip and Cleft Palate. Oslo: Universitets Forlaget, 1963.
17. Subtelny JD: Orthodontic treatment of cleft lip and palate, birth to adulthood. Angle Orthod 26:273–292, 1966.

18. Harvold EP, Chierici G, Vargervik K: Experiments on the development of dental malocclusions. Am J Orthod 61:38–44, 1972.
19. Lande H: Size and Position of the Maxilla in Norwegian Boys with Complete Clefts of Lip and Palate. Thesis. Bergen: University of Bergen, 1970.
20. Hayashi E, Sakuda M, Takimoto K, et al: Craniofacial growth in complete unilateral cleft lip and palate: A roentgenocephalometric study. Cleft Palate J 13:215–237, 1976.
21. Harvold EP: Some biologic aspects of orthodontic treatment in the transitional dentition. Am J Orthod 49:1–14, 1963.
22. Ross RB, Johnston MC: The effect of early orthodontic treatment on facial growth in cleft lip and palate. Cleft Palate J 4:157–164, 1967.
23. Chierici G, Harvold EP, Vargervik K: Morphogenetic experiments in facial asymmetry: The nasal cavity. Am J Phys Anthrop 38:291–300, 1973.
24. Chierchi G, Harvold EP, Vargervik K: Morphogenetic experiments in cleft palate: Mandibular response. Cleft Palate J 10:51–61, 1973.
25. Ortiz-Monasterio F, Rebeil AS, Valderrama M, et al: Cephalometric measurements on adult patients with cleft palates. Plast Reconstr Surg 19:53–61, 1959.
26. Atherton JD: Morphology of facial bones in skulls with unoperated unilateral cleft palate. Cleft Palate J 4:18–30, 1967.
27. Bishara SE, Krause CJ, Olin WH, et al: Facial and dental relationships of individuals with unoperated clefts of the lip and/or palate. Cleft Palate J 13:238–252, 1976.
28. Vargervik K: New bone formation secured by oriented stress in maxillary clefts. Cleft Palate J 15:132–140, 1978.
29. Paulin G, Astrand P, Rosenquist JB, et al: Intermediate bone grafting of alveolar clefts. J Cranio Maxillofac Surg 16:2–7, 1988.
30. Abyholm FE, Bergland O, Semb G: Secondary bone grafting of alveolar clefts. J Plast Reconstr Surg 15:127–140, 1981.

CHAPTER 79

Orthodontic Treatment in Different Stages of Growth and Development

William H. Olin

Many changes have taken place in the orthodontic treatment of cleft patients during the last 40 years. During that time, the fabrication of appliances and the materials used have changed considerably. Techniques also have changed. Bands were once made individually for each tooth. This consumed a great amount of time and created space problems because each band circled the tooth and required space for the thickness of the band. Brackets were welded or soldered to each band, and in many cases small eyelets were attached to the band. Both stainless steel and precious metals were used for bands.

Wires were purchased in straight pieces, usually 12 inches in length, and the wires were fabricated for each individual patient. These also were made of stainless steel or precious metal. We changed from precious metal to stainless steel arch wires in the late 1940s.

In the 1960s preformed bands made their appearance, reducing greatly the amount of time necessary to fabricate a complete appliance. At this time preformed arch wires also were designed. Again, this reduced the amount of time involved in treatment.

In the 1970s bonds replaced bands. These allowed the orthodontist to maintain good control over the movement of the teeth and made it possible to close all spaces prior to removal of the appliance. Bonds are attached directly to the teeth and allow for better oral hygiene. In approximately 1976, nitinol wire was introduced to our profession. Nitinol wire gives superior performance, has an excellent "memory," and returns to its original form. This makes it especially valuable when working with cleft patients who have severely malpositioned and rotated teeth.

Today, two new products have appeared to make appliances more aesthetically acceptable. Tooth-colored nitinol wire and clear porcelain brackets are now being used experimentally. In our opinion, these will be used for many patients in the near future (Fig. 79–1).

Appliance therapy also has changed through the years. In the late 1940s several techniques were used, namely, Johnson twin wire, the labial lingual technique, and the edgewise appliance. Removable appliances were used mainly in Europe. Lingual orthodontic treatment was introduced in the early 1980s; however, it is not popular today and is rarely used in the treatment of cleft patients. Currently, many types of removable appliances are in use. The appliance most commonly used is the edgewise appliance, variations of which with the same rectangular wires are used by specialists. Very few, if any, orthodontists use the Johnson twin wire or the labial lingual technique today. The progress in appliance techniques has made significant improvements in the diagnosis and treatment of patients with facial clefts.

Growth and Development

Patients with clefts of the lip or palate have marked differences in their maxillofacial growth and development. Several factors may have an influence on growth, including the type and severity of the original cleft deformity, the surgical technique used for both the lip and palate, and timely and appropriate orthodontic treatment.

In the past, a distinguishing facial feature of an individual with a cleft of the lip and palate was a concave facial profile (Fig. 79–2). Foster, in 1962, reported that 34 of 200 patients with cleft lip and palate exhibited maxillary deficiency.[1] In 1963, Levin indicated that "an anterior-posterior deficiency" in the middle third of the face was observed in 29.6% of the cleft patients at the Northwestern Cleft Lip and Palate Institute.[2] Dahl found that 76% of 66 adult cleft patients had an anterior crossbite.[3]

Tables 79–1 through 79–6 present the cephalometric results from three different series of patients treated at the Iowa Cleft Palate Center: (1) patients born in 1947, 1948, 1956, 1957, and 1958, studied in 1964; (2) 45

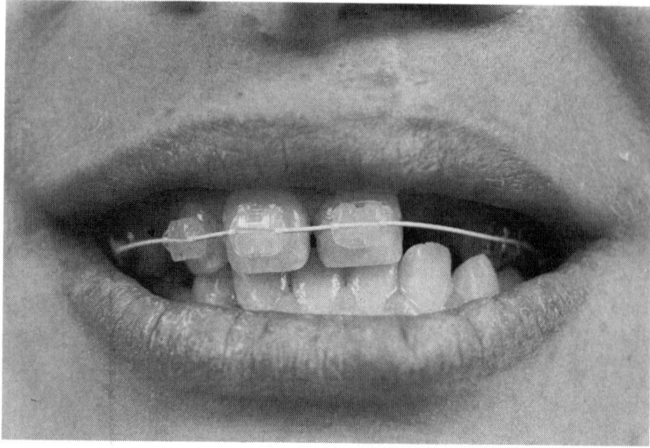

Figure 79–1 Clear porcelain brackets, clean elastics, and Teflon-coated arch wire.

Table 79–1. Unilateral Complete Clefts in Patients Born in 1946 and 1947 (Ages 12–14 at Time of Examination)

Patient	SNA	SNB	ANB
1	68.5	73.5	−05.0
2	78.0	77.0	01.0
3	80.5	82.0	−01.5
4	79.0	81.0	−02.0
5	78.0	77.5	00.5
6	81.0	78.0	03.0
7	71.5	77.0	−05.5
8	80.5	82.0	−01.5
9	73.0	76.0	−03.0
10	75.5	74.5	01.0
11	72.5	71.5	01.0
Mean	76.18	77.27	−01.09
sd	4.24	4.41	2.68
N	11	11	11

patients evaluated in 1984; and (3) 56 patients studied in 1988.

The early study indicated that a high percentage of patients born in 1946 and 1947 exhibited severe maxillofacial growth problems.[4] Six of eleven had a negative ANB, demonstrated clinically as severe facial growth inhibition. Those serious secondary maxillofacial deformities attributed to growth inhibition resulted from inadequate treatment techniques, both surgical and orthodontic. In 1984, Olin reported cephalometric results from 45 patients with complete cleft of the lip and palate (14 to 22 years of age).[5] Only 4 of the 45 had anterior crossbite; however, these four patients were still undergoing active orthodontic treatment at the time of our study.

We have just completed a study of 56 patients with unilateral cleft lip and palate, ranging in age from 5 to 17 years (see Chap. 12). Of this group of 56 patients, 7 were found to have a negative ANB or an anterior crossbite. The cephalometric data for patients who had completed treatment in our center were compared with standards derived from the Iowa Facial Growth Study.

The data from our patients revealed a slight retrusion of the middle third of the face and a slightly underdeveloped mandible compared to the Iowa norms. However, the relationship of the maxilla to the mandible, the ANB angle, was within normal limits.

In reviewing the patient data from our two most recent studies, done in 1984 and 1988, we found that most of our patients had satisfactory facial growth with reasonably good facial aesthetics (Chapter 12).[5] Today, the characteristic concave facial profile is rarely observed. Our results have improved significantly, due mainly to our increased knowledge of clefts, improved surgical and orthodontic techniques, better collaboration between surgeon and orthodontist, and continuous participation of the orthodontist in treatment of the cleft patient.

Objectives of Orthodontic Treatment

Orthodontic treatment for the cleft patient includes three main objectives:
1. To establish functional occlusion.

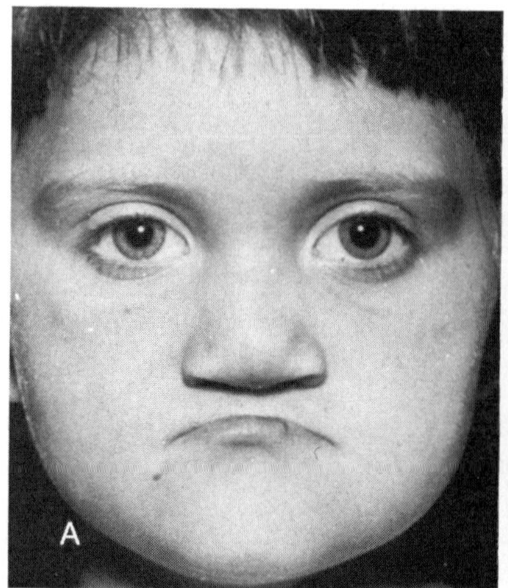
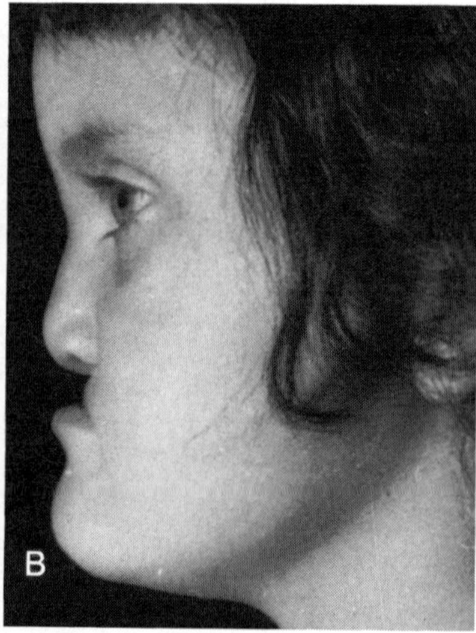
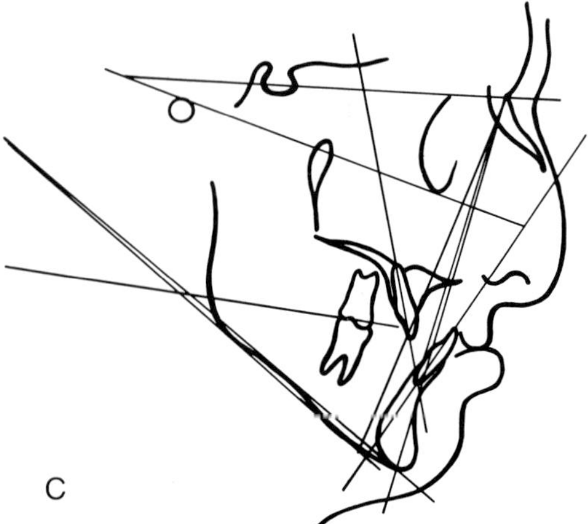

Figure 79–2 *A* and *B*, Patient exhibiting severe growth retardation of the middle third of the face. *C*, Cephalometric tracing indicating severe growth retardation.

Table 79–2. Unilateral Complete Clefts in Patients Born in 1956, 1957, and 1958 (Ages 12–14 at Time of Examination)

Patient		SNA	SNB	ANB
1		79.0	73.5	05.5
2		77.0	77.0	00.0
3		79.5	69.0	10.5
4		83.5	78.5	05.0
5		76.0	74.0	02.0
6		78.5	75.0	03.5
7		77.5	69.5	08.0
8		78.0	71.5	06.5
9		76.5	74.5	02.0
10		77.5	70.5	07.0
11		84.5	81.0	03.5
	Mean	78.86	74.00	04.86
	sd	2.75	3.79	3.05
	N	11	11	11

2. To give the patient the ability to communicate normally.
3. To achieve an acceptable appearance.

We attempt to reach these goals as early as possible. It is advisable for the orthodontist to see children with clefts shortly after birth to answer any questions the parents might have on growth and development and to observe conditions as the child grows. The collaboration between the orthodontist, the plastic surgeon, and other specialists on the cleft team is initiated during this period, and should continue throughout the treatment period which may extend into the patient's adult life.

Table 79–3. Late Results Study (1984) (Unilateral Complete Clefts— Finished Cases)

Patient		AGE	SNA	SNB	ANB
1.	A.	17.7	76.00	75.00	01.00
2.	B.	18.3	77.50	75.75	01.75
3.	DeH.	17.3	78.25	73.00	05.25
4.	E.	18.10	74.00	68.50	05.50
5.	E.	20.7	72.00	70.75	01.25
6.	F.	17.10	73.75	72.75	01.00
7.	H.	14.2	72.72	76.75	− 03.50
8.	H.	15.11	76.50	74.00	02.50
9.	H.	15.2	83.25	70.75	03.50
10.	H.	20.1	80.00	83.50	− 03.50
11.	H.	14.11	75.00	76.00	− 01.00
12.	J.	19.11	72.25	67.50	04.75
13.	K.	16.7	79.50	77.00	02.50
14.	L.	15.8	75.75	77.50	− 01.75
15.	M.	17.9	88.75	89.00	− 02.50
16.	M.	16.4	76.50	78.50	− 02.00
17.	M.	14.1	80.50	77.50	03.00
18.	R.	19.4	70.00	67.00	03.00
19.	S.	15.2	76.00	77.00	− 01.00
20.	T.	18.10	72.50	71.75	00.75
21.	T.	17.10	73.00	67.50	05.50
22.	T.	18.10	75.50	74.25	01.25
23.	V.	17.3	73.00	72.00	01.00
24.	V.	20.8	73.00	75.25	− 02.50
25.	W.	17.4	74.25	74.25	00.00
	Mean		75.98	74.85	01.03
	sd		4.07	4.97	2.76
	N		25	25	25

Table 79–4. Late Results Study (1984) (Unilateral Complete Clefts— Unfinished Cases)

Patient		AGE	SNA	SNB	ANB
1.	M.B.	15.2	79.75	81.00	− 01.25
2.	M.B.	17.7	70.00	67.75	02.25
3.	M.B.	17.11	76.00	74.50	01.50
4.	M.C.	14.1	68.75	70.50	− 01.75
5.	St.C.	16.5	71.25	73.00	− 01.75
6.	M.C.	19.7	72.50	70.50	02.00
7.	B.G.	14.1	78.50	76.75	01.75
8.	R.G.	14.11	73.00	75.50	− 02.50
9.	D.H.	17.1	75.50	71.00	04.50
10.	M.K.	15.5	72.00	74.00	− 02.00
11.	J.L.	19.3	73.50	79.00	− 05.50
12.	S.McC.	14.7	73.50	70.75	02.75
13.	B.O.	17.2	75.00	70.25	04.75
14.	J.P.	16.8	74.00	76.00	− 02.00
15.	T.P.	13.11	77.00	76.25	00.75
16.	S.P.	17.10	75.50	67.50	08.00
17.	T.S.	18.11	73.25	72.50	00.75
18.	L.S.	16.8	75.25	75.25	00.00
19.	R.S.	15.6	71.00	75.50	− 04.50
20.	D.V.	17.1	78.00	76.00	02.00
21.	J.W.	19.7	74.50	75.25	− 00.75
	Mean		74.18	73.75	00.43
	sd		2.81	3.49	3.19
	N		21	21	21

Presurgical Orthopedic Treatment

In the 1950s and early 1960s numerous articles appeared in the literature (mainly in the European journals) on presurgical orthopedic treatment. In 1954, McNeil, from the University of Glasgow, published a textbook on the treatment of clefts.[7] One technique he mentioned involved control of the alignment of the maxillary dental arch in early infancy (Fig. 79–3).

After reading McNeil's text and other papers, we

Table 79–5. Iowa/Hamburg Study (1987) Summary

	Males 5–10 Years Old Mean ± SD	Norms Mean ± SD
SNA	77.97 ± 2.84	80 ± 4.0
SNB	73.38 ± 3.88	76 ± 3.4
ANB	4.56 ± 3.07	4 ± 1.6
NAPog	8.62 ± 7.38	9 ± 3.8
SNPog	73.65 ± 4.20	76 ± 3.5
FHNPog	80.47 ± 4.43	83 ± 2.8
MPSN	37.00 ± 4.43	35 ± 4.6
MPFH	30.29 ± 5.18	27 ± 4.3
NSGn	69.70 ± 3.78	68 ± 2.8
FHSGn	62.91 ± 4.56	61 ± 2.6
	Males 10–17 Years Old Mean ± SD	**Norms Mean ± SD**
SNA	77.25 ± 3.73	81 ± 3.8
SNB	75.17 ± 2.29	78 ± 3.3
ANB	2.14 ± 2.55	3 ± 1.7
NAPog	1.33 ± 5.44	7 ± 4.3
SNPog	77.00 ± 2.61	78 ± 3.7
FHNPog	79.97 ± 4.59	83 ± 3.7
MPSN	35.14 ± 5.69	32 ± 5.2
MPFH	32.03 ± 7.79	28 ± 4.9
NSGn	69.30 ± 3.12	68 ± 3.2
FHSGn	66.14 ± 3.40	63 ± 3.3

Table 79–6. Iowa/Hamburg Study (1987) Summary

	Females 5–10 Years Old Mean ± SD	Norms Mean ± SD
SNA	78.12 ± 5.07	80 ± 4.0
SNB	75.54 ± 3.58	76 ± 3.4
ANB	3.33 ± 3.58	4 ± 1.6
NAPog	4.29 ± 10.64	9 ± 3.8
SNPog	76.83 ± 4.31	76 ± 3.5
FHNPog	83.42 ± 5.01	83 ± 2.8
MPSN	34.25 ± 5.64	35 ± 4.6
MPFH	27.71 ± 5.87	27 ± 4.3
NSGn	66.88 ± 4.53	68 ± 2.8
FHSGn	60.42 ± 5.24	61 ± 2.6

	Females 10–16 Years Old Mean ± SD	Norms Mean ± SD
SNA	77.67 ± 6.50	80 ± 3.8
SNB	76.11 ± 5.68	77 ± 3.3
ANB	1.56 ± 1.63	3 ± 2.1
NAPog	−1.22 ± 3.52	6 ± 5.6
SNPog	78.28 ± 5.37	77 ± 3.3
FHNPog	83.39 ± 7.21	84 ± 2.5
MPSN	34.44 ± 7.95	34 ± 4.2
MPFH	29.33 ± 9.46	28 ± 4.9
NSGn	68.11 ± 5.68	68 ± 3.0
FHSGn	62.94 ± 7.40	62 ± 2.9

incorporated presurgical orthopedic methods into our treatment plan at The University of Iowa Cleft Palate Center in the late 1950s (Fig. 79–4). A number of patients were treated with this procedure; however, we encountered several problems. One major problem was the complaint by families about the need to travel great distances from their homes to the treatment center and the expense involved. The Iowa Cleft Palate Center was the only treatment facility in the state using presurgical orthopedic methods, and some patients traveled 250 to 300 miles each way for this treatment procedure.

After treating a number of patients using presurgical orthopedic methods I went to Europe to visit the centers that were using these methods. Many surgeons believed that these procedures would facilitate a more successful lip repair. It was my intention to observe and examine

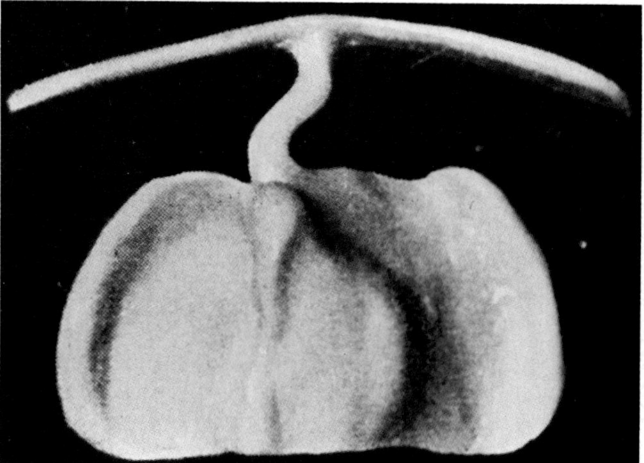

Figure 79–3 Presurgical orthopedic appliance used by McNeil in the 1950s.

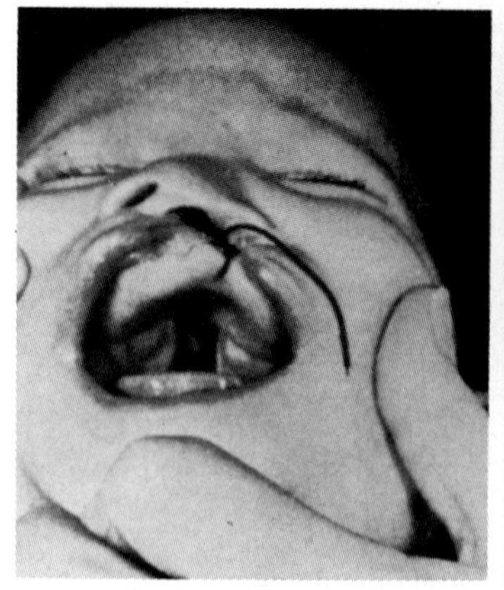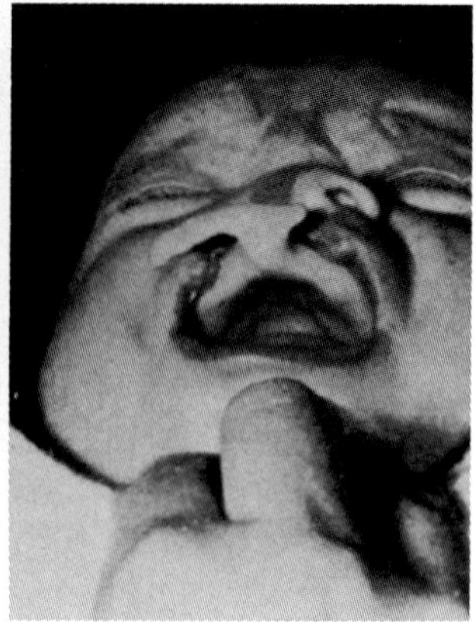

Figure 79–4 Presurgical orthopedic appliance used by Olin in the late 1950s.

cleft patients in different stages of orthodontic treatment. I was particularly interested in the appliances used for presurgical orthopedic treatment, its timing, sequence of procedures, and its influence on the alignment of the maxillary segments. The purpose of the visit was to assess the effectiveness of presurgical orthopedic treatment and compare patients who underwent the procedure to those who did not. On returning to the United States, I concluded that presurgical orthopedic treatment would not be incorporated into our treatment protocol.[8] I did not observe significant differences between the two groups of patients. Furthermore, this treatment was not cost-effective for patients who had to travel long distances to undergo the procedure.

Pruzansky wrote an article in the Cleft Palate Journal in 1964 entitled, Presurgical Orthopaedics and Bone Grafting for Infants with Cleft Lip and Palate: A Dissent.[9] Pruzansky was opposed to presurgical orthopedics and infant bone grafting and wrote, ". . . maxillary collapse is fully, quickly and economically correctable in the deciduous, mixed, or permanent dentition. The economics of the McNeil method, whether on an inpatient or an outpatient basis, pose an added disadvantage, except under government subsidy. There is no justification to date for the government or private support for such treatment, except for under the most carefully controlled experimental circumstances."

During the 1970s, several patients were again treated at the Iowa Cleft Palate Center with presurgical orthopedic procedures by another dentist (Fig. 79–5). The appliance used was called a "functional orthopedic appliance" and was fitted to the nipple of a feeding bottle. The appliance was used only during feeding and was designed so that the pressure exerted by the muscle forces at the time of feeding would move the maxillary segments into the desired position. Every 2 weeks, new impressions were made, and the appliance was refitted. The duration of the presurgical orthopedic treatment was 2 to 3 months.

Eighteen patients were randomly selected for study from this treated group. All had unilateral clefts of the lip, alveolus, and palate. The study was conducted after the primary teeth had erupted fully. Patients were between 3.5 and 6.5 years of age at the time of the

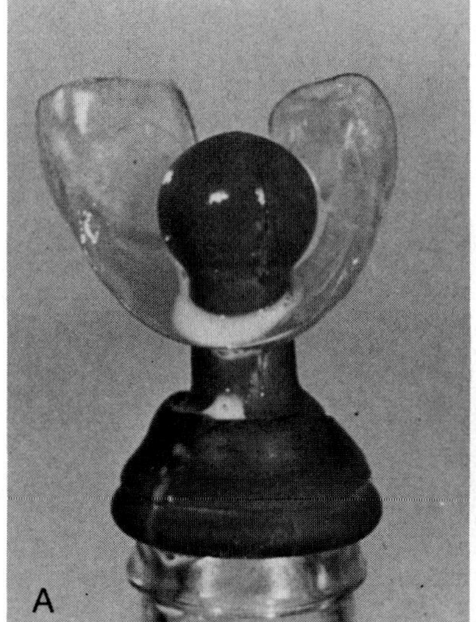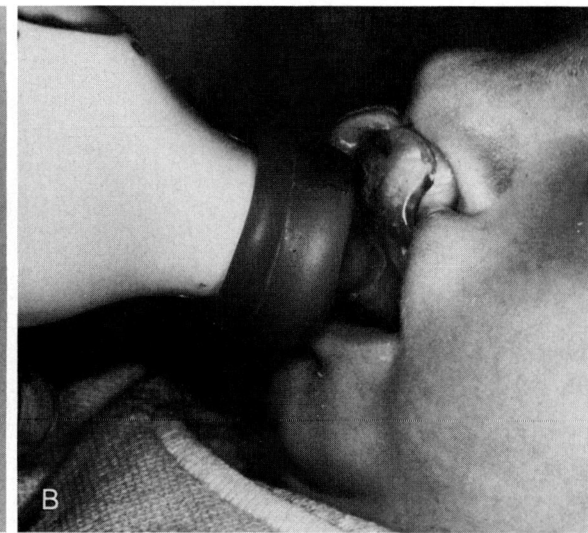

Figure 79–5 *A*, Presurgical orthopedic appliance used at the Iowa Cleft Palate Center in the 1970s and 1980s. *B*, The appliance is attached to the nipple and worn mainly when the child is feeding.

evaluation. Thirteen were found to have a complete crossbite, three had a crossbite of the canine only, and one had an anterior crossbite. One patient had no evidence of crossbite. These findings confirmed my impression that presurgical orthopedic treatment, in view of the long-term results, did not provide enough benefits to justify its use.

Presently, many cleft centers throughout the world, especially in Europe, continue to incorporate presurgical orthopedic methods into their treatment of unilateral and bilateral cleft patients. On the other hand, many outstanding centers do not use this technique. In 1984 I participated in a symposium in Zurich, Switzerland. Thirty-six centers from around the world were represented. Eighteen of these centers routinely used presurgical orthopedic treatment, five used it occasionally, and one rarely used it. Twelve centers did not use presurgical orthopedic treatment in their protocol. Five centers from the United States were represented at the meeting. Of these five, three did not use presurgical orthopedic treatment; one center routinely used it, and one center rarely employed the procedure (Table 79–7).

The controversy surrounding presurgical orthopedic treatment should be resolved through continued scientific investigations at various cleft centers using the same research protocol. Today, some highly regarded experts condone presurgical orthopedic treatment (Holtz, Gnoinski, Gruber), whereas others are critical of this technique (Huddart, Ross, Olin). In an article in the American Journal of Orthodontics I wrote, ". . .

many surgeons believe this procedure will enable them to obtain a more successful lip repair. Many patients have been treated with this technique; however, at the present time, we do not recommend it as a routine procedure."[8] At the Iowa Cleft Palate Center, I have not used presurgical orthopedics since that time.

At the First International Symposium in 1979 in Zurich, Ross presented a review of the proceedings. His opening remarks were in regard to presurgical orthopedic treatment. ". . . for a slightly cynical orthodontist, infant orthopedics thus appears to be something that you should do if it can be done on a convenient basis, but not too much can be expected of it in the long run."[10]

Figure 79–6 shows the results of treatment of a patient from the Iowa Cleft Palate Center who did not undergo presurgical orthopedic treatment. If maxillary collapse is observed in the primary dentition phase, it is corrected when the primary teeth are fully erupted (approximately 3.5 to 4 years of age).

General Dental Care

Each child with a cleft should be referred to a local dentist or pediatric dentist between 2.5 and 3 years of age. The primary teeth should be preserved and retained until they are shed physiologically except when the orthodontist recommends removal of certain teeth to aid in preventing abnormal eruption or crowding of the permanent dentition. Complete intraoral roentgenograms are recommended at 4 years of age. Early x-rays are valuable for the detection of dental caries, congenitally missing teeth, supernumerary teeth, and malformed and malpositioned teeth.

Congenitally Missing Teeth

A substantially higher incidence of congenitally missing posterior teeth in both the maxillary and mandibular arches has been reported in cleft children.[4, 5] Valinoti

Table 79–7. Zurich Conference, 1984 (36 Centers Represented)

18	routinely incorporate presurgical orthopedics
4	occasionally use orthopedics
1	uses orthopedics in 15% of patients
12	do not incorporate presurgical pretreatment into their treatment protocol
Five Centers from the United States Were Represented	
3	do not use orthopedics
1	rarely uses orthopedics
1	always uses orthopedics

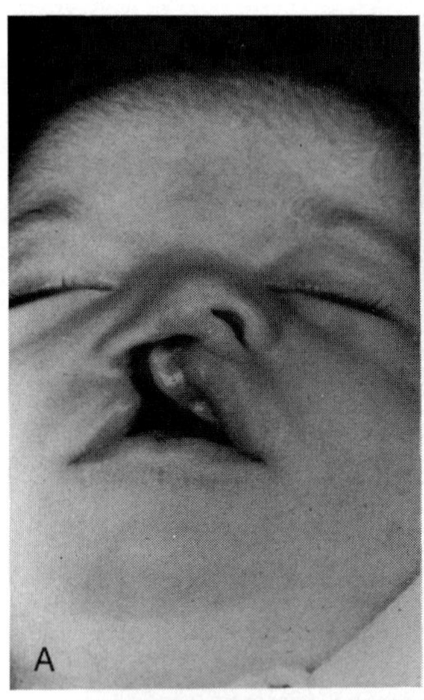
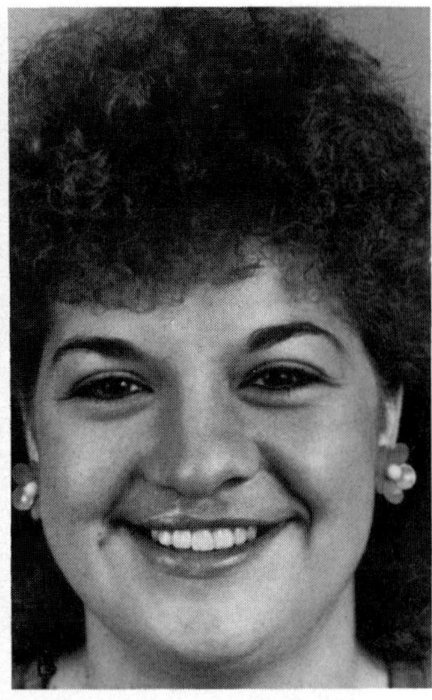
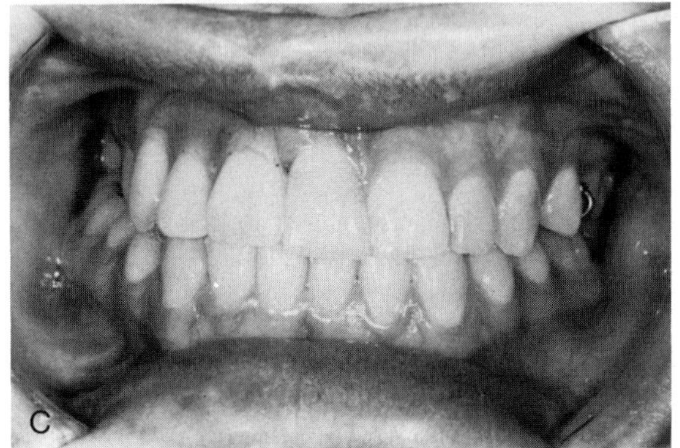

Figure 79–6 No presurgical orthopedic treatment. Right complete cleft lip and palate. A, Before surgery. B, Facial view following surgery. C, Final occlusion after treatment.

reported the incidence of missing premolars to be 6.6% in the general population.[11] Our 1964 study of patients with cleft lip and palate revealed an incidence of 24% (42 of 175 patients) with congenitally missing premolars.[4] In our recent examination of the Panorex films of 56 patients, 20 (35.7%) had one or more missing premolars (see Chap. 12). Mackey, in 1958 at the Northwestern University Cleft Palate Institute, reported that 49.6% of patients had one or more congenitally missing teeth.[12]

Supernumerary Teeth

Mackey also reported a greater incidence of supernumerary teeth in cleft children in his study. In his patient group, 21% had one or more supernumerary teeth. These teeth are most frequently found in the area of the cleft; however, they may be present in any area of the maxilla or the mandible. The lateral incisor in the area of the cleft is the most common supernumerary tooth. We must be aware of supernumerary teeth at an early age to allow for extraction when indicated and also to allow normal eruption of adjacent teeth.

Fused and Irregularly Shaped Teeth

Fused teeth present a diagnostic problem. The maxillary central incisor may be several millimeters larger

than normal. In some patients it may be permissible to reduce the size of these teeth and restore a more normal size and contour, whereas in others it is necessary to extract teeth. These teeth present problems related to arch length as well as aesthetics. Tooth size is probably determined by heredity. Irregularities of tooth size may also cause arch length discrepancies resulting in malocclusion. Tooth size varies within and between individuals. These variations should be carefully studied by means of x-rays, study models, and photographs. Direct measurements of the teeth should be taken as well.

Minor irregularities can be corrected either by stripping the larger teeth or restoring those of less than normal size. Malformed or irregularly shaped teeth usually are present adjacent to the cleft. The central incisor on the cleft side is especially susceptible. The tooth itself may be deformed, or the tooth structure may have been damaged during development. Extra thick marginal ridges and exaggerated singulum can force maxillary anterior teeth labially. The labial surface may be excessively convex, affecting the anterior aesthetic appearance. Cosmetic and functional restoration is necessary; if this cannot be accomplished, extraction may be indicated.

Delayed Eruption and Malpositioned Teeth

Delayed eruption of teeth frequently occurs in children with cleft lip and palate. This is especially true of the maxillary canine on the cleft side (Fig. 79–7). This delay may mean wearing appliances for an extended period while waiting for eruption. Furthermore, orthodontic treatment and prosthetic reconstruction may be difficult to complete. Many times the canine will fail to erupt because of the severity of the defect. Secondary bone grafting at 6 to 8 years of age may help to alleviate this problem and allow the teeth in the area to erupt into more favorable positions. Surgical exposure and attachment to the crown of the tooth may be required to move them into arch alignment. Malpositioned teeth may require extensive movement. In some patients, these teeth should remain where they are if they are in satisfactory arch alignment.

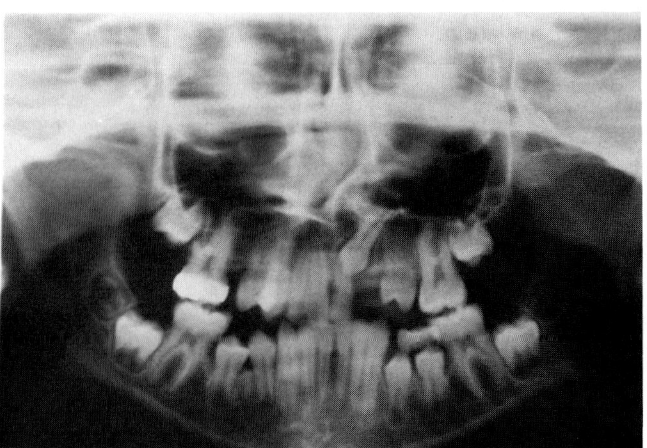

Figure 79–7 Panorex film showing delayed eruption of maxillary permanent canine.

Phases of Orthodontic Treatment

In my first publication concerning orthodontic treatment for cleft lip and palate children, I proposed that three phases of orthodontic treatment might be indicated for the cleft lip and palate patient.[13] I still follow these treatment phases today; however, we do not treat as many patients in the primary dentition phase as in the past, possibly due to improvements in surgical techniques, which result in less severe deformities with more normal growth patterns.

Early Treatment

The earlier a normal dental arch can be established, the more satisfactory the prognosis will be. By establishing normal dental arches in the primary dentition phase, we may eliminate later problems in the mixed and permanent dentitions. One of the most frequent problems in the primary dentition is that of crossbite. This may involve one tooth, the segment, or the entire maxillary arch. Crossbite may be unilateral or bilateral, and either anterior or posterior. If only one tooth is involved, treatment typically is not indicated. However, if the entire segment is in crossbite, we proceed with the appropriate treatment. This can be undertaken when the patient is 3 to 4 years of age.

The appliance of choice in our clinic is the Olin modification of the Arnold expander (Fig. 79–8). There are several other appliances that will accomplish the same goals (Fig. 79–9). For some patients with lingually locked maxillary, anterior, primary teeth, correction in the primary dentition may also be advantageous (Fig. 79–10). The decision for this treatment is based on the age of the patient, position of the teeth, and amount of resorption of the roots of the primary teeth. Occlusal interferences from the mandibular arch may make it impossible to obtain the desired expansion for these patients, and an acrylic bite plate should be constructed to be worn on the mandibular posterior teeth. The bite is open sufficiently to remove the occlusal interferences.

We also use a mandibular bite plate for anterior crossbite in both the primary and permanent dentition. Radiologic examination of the expansion obtained at an

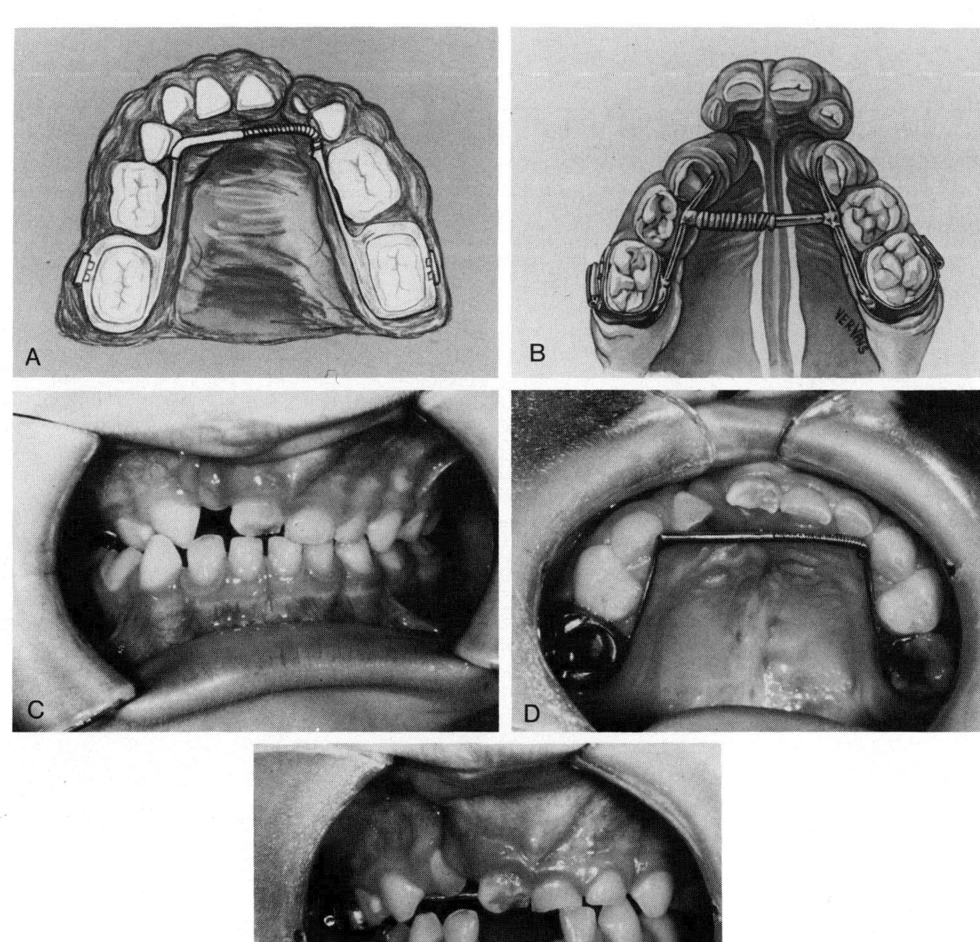

Figure 79–8 A and B, Olin-type expansion appliance. C–E, Early maxillary expansion.

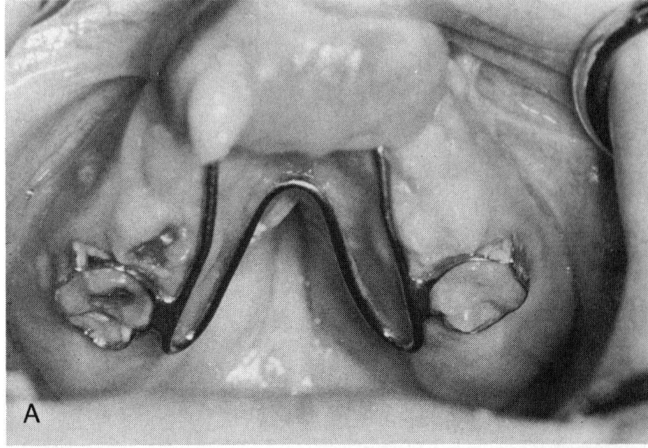

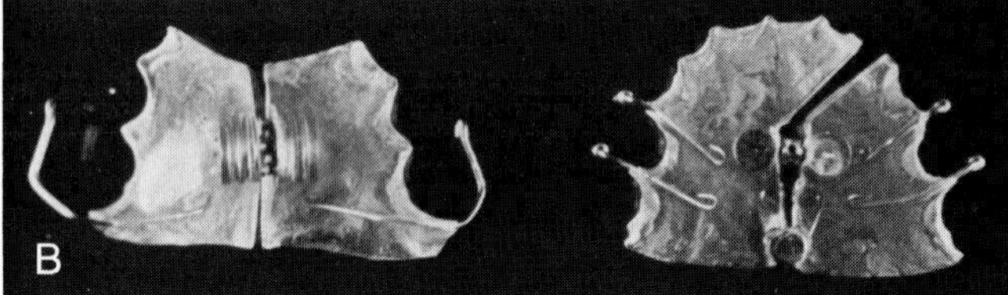

Figure 79–9 *A*, Arch wire for maxillary expansion. *B*, Split palate expansion appliance.

early age revealed that we can reposition the entire maxillary segment or segments if the cleft is bilateral. If the expansion is delayed past 6 to 7 years of age, the movement is confined to individual teeth rather than the entire segment (Fig. 79–11).

Management of the Premaxilla in Bilateral Cleft Patients

Management of the premaxilla in the bilateral cleft deformity has been a constant problem for the surgeon and the orthodontist. In our clinic, if the premaxilla is protruding, the following treatment procedures are undertaken:

1. Expansion of the maxillary segments at 3 to 5 years of age.
2. Surgical recession with cancellous bone graft just before the child starts school (bone is harvested from the iliac crest). Retropositioning of the premaxilla is fully explained in Chap. 69.

If the teeth in the premaxilla are not severely deformed, we attempt to move them to a normal position as soon as possible following their eruption. If this is not possible, we then resort to extraction and replacement with a prosthesis.

Mixed Dentition Treatment

The mixed dentition period represents an important time in the psychological development of the cleft child. A pleasing smile is important. When the permanent anterior teeth erupt they may be rotated or malpositioned. These conditions should be corrected as soon as the teeth are fully erupted (Fig. 79–12). We also must be aware that other dental–facial problems exist. As mentioned previously, many children with cleft lip and

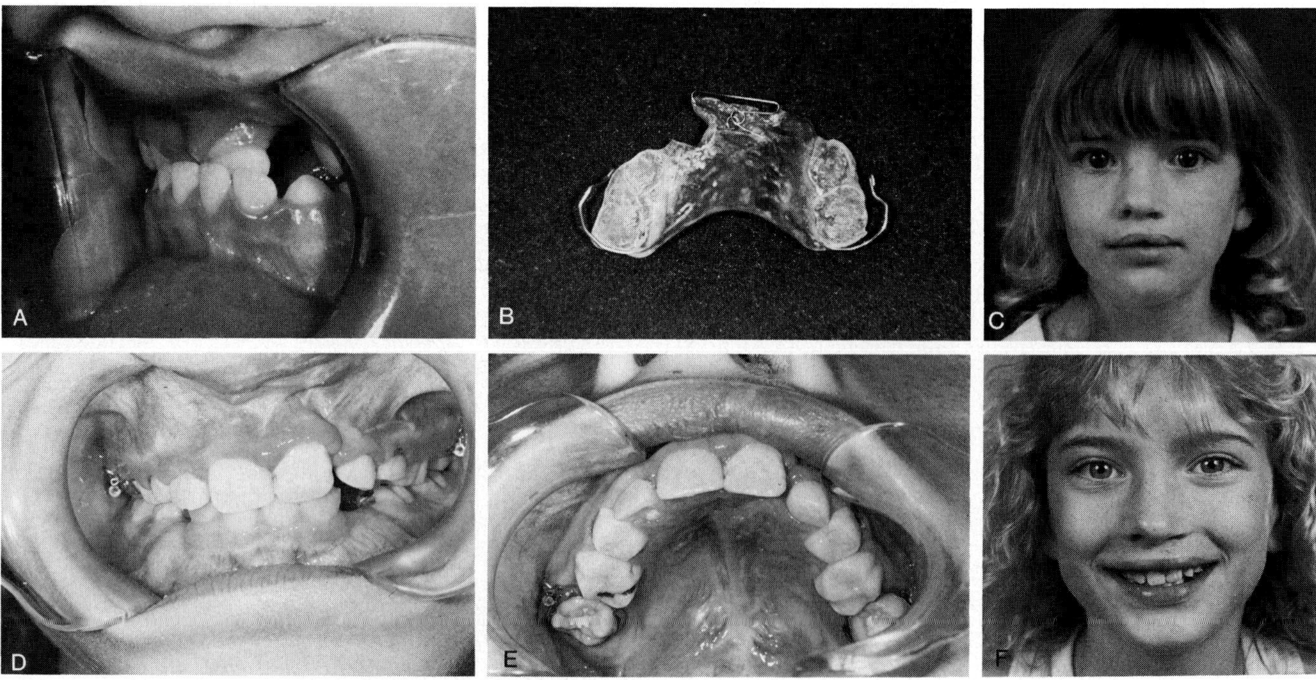

Figure 79–10 *A–C*, Patient with early maxillary anterior crossbite (primary dentition) corrected with removable appliance. *D–F*, After eruption of dentition and treatment of permanent anterior teeth. Mixed treatment of dentition consisted of 6 months of wearing bands to correct rotation.

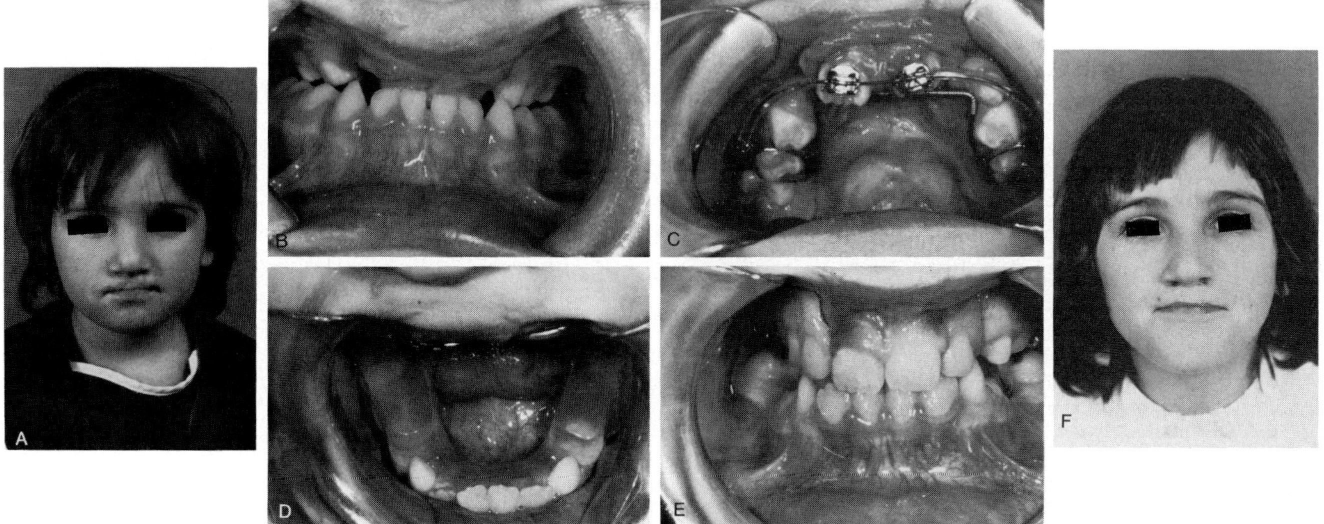

Figure 79–11 *A*, Before treatment. *B*, Occlusion with anterior and posterior crossbite. *C*, Appliances used to correct centrals in crossbite and posterior crossbite. Note tubing on arch wire to protect lips and cheek. *D*, Mandibular bite plate. *E*, Occlusion after correction of anterior crossbite. Temporary prosthesis; posterior expansion continues. *F*, Facial view after correction of anterior crossbite and insertion of temporary prosthesis.

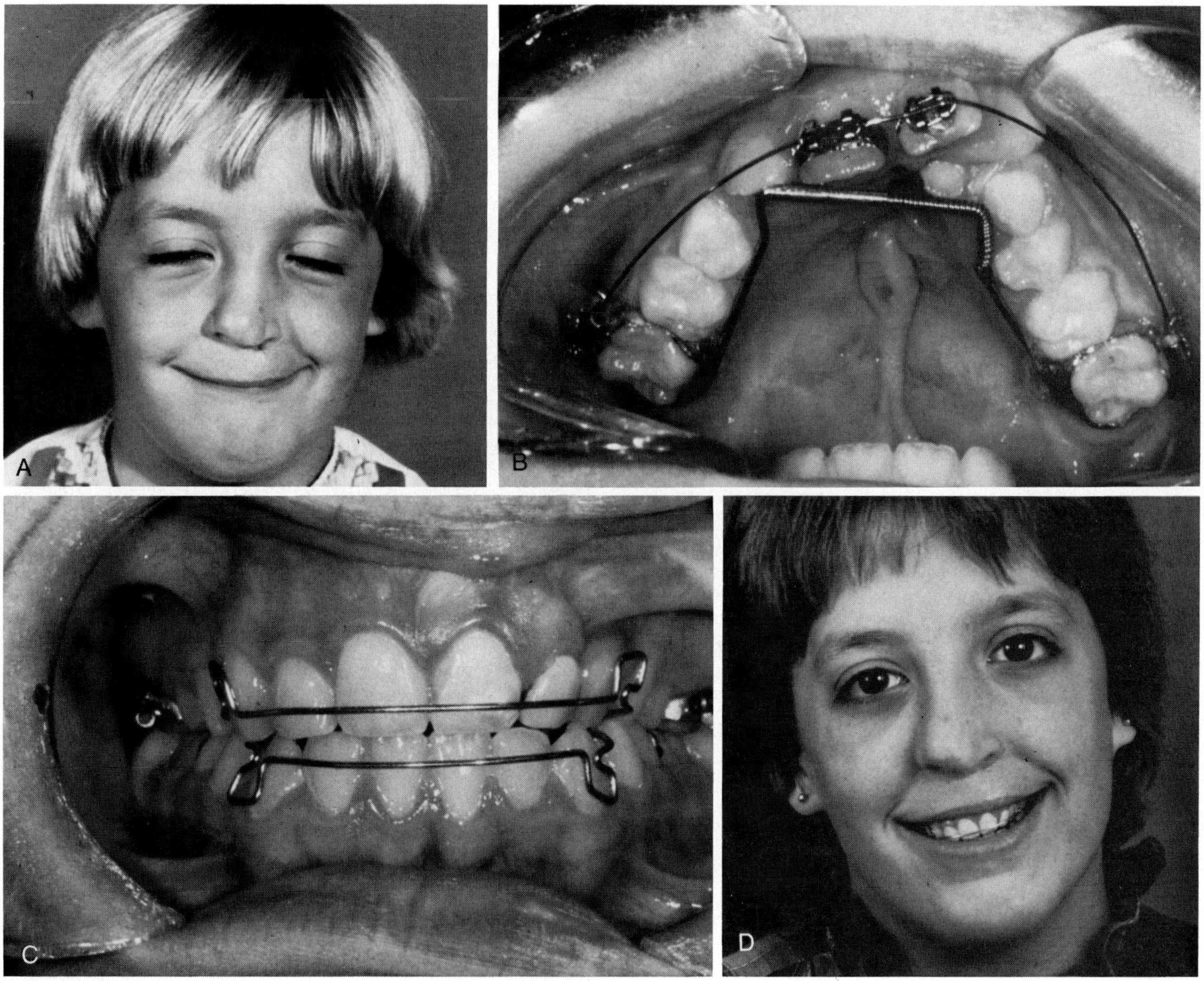

Figure 79–12 *A*, Before treatment. *B*, Treatment of rotated anterior segment and posterior expansion. *C*, Correction and insertion of temporary prosthesis and retainer. *D*, Facial view.

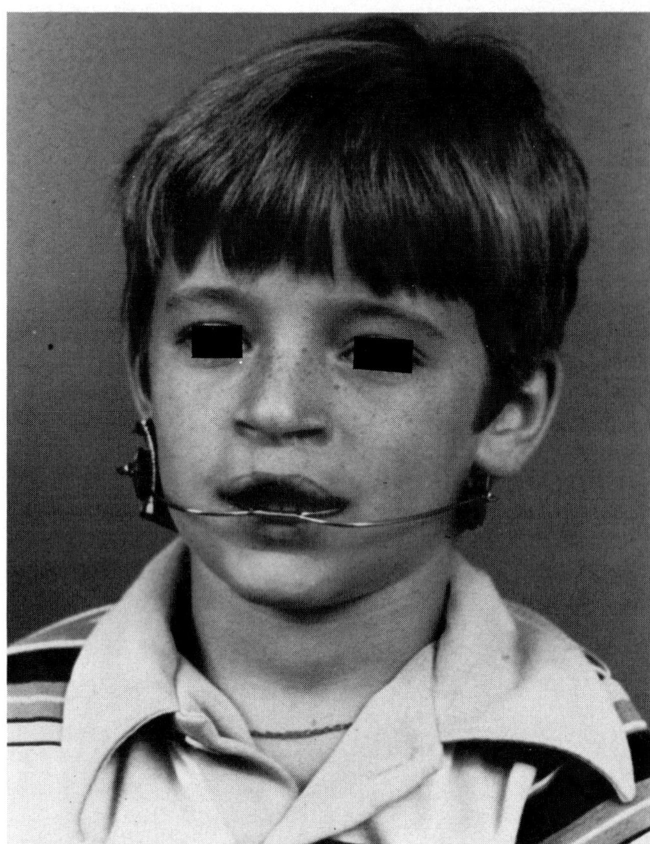

Figure 79–13 Headgear.

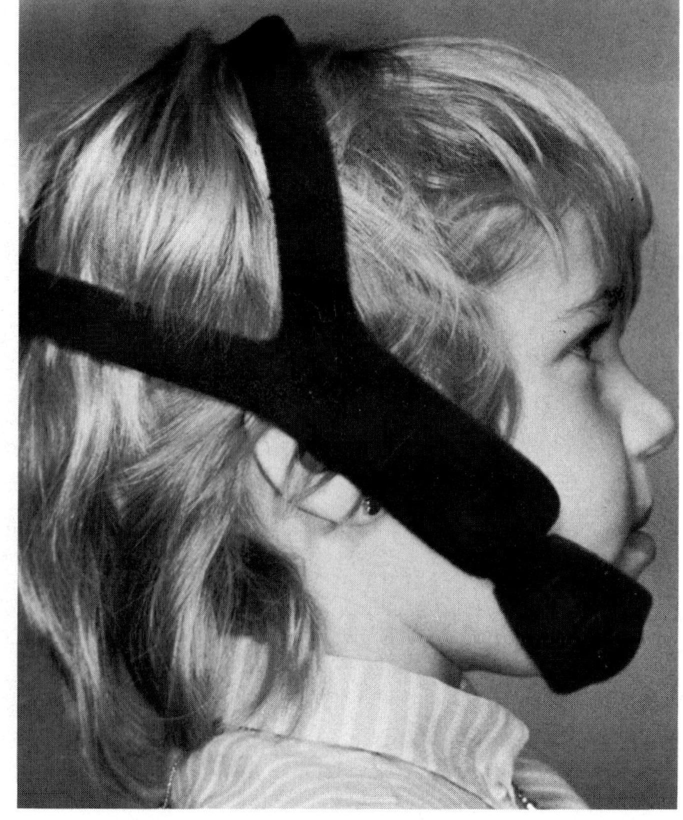

Figure 79–14 Chin cap.

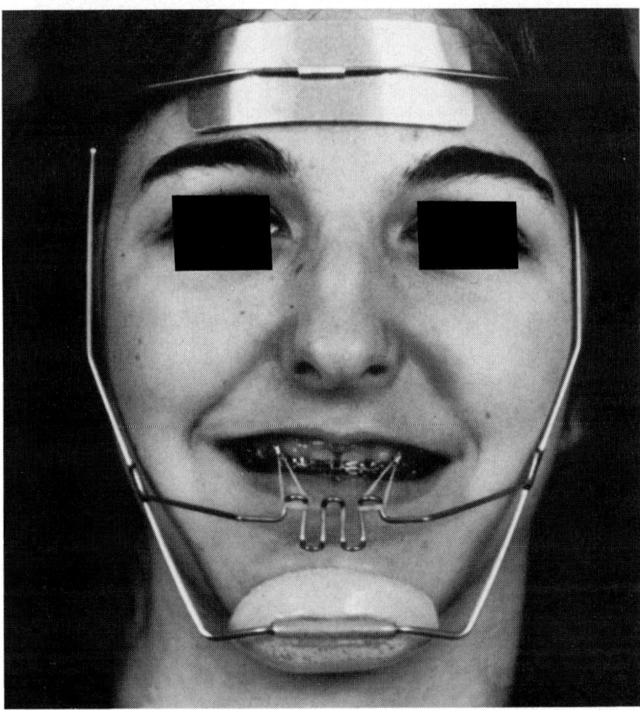

Figure 79–15 Reverse headgear.

palate have supernumerary or congenitally missing teeth. If it can be determined at this time that a supernumerary tooth is present or that there are congenitally missing teeth, we must plan our treatment taking these factors into consideration. These conditions complicate the treatment planning and should be dealt with as early as possible.

In the mixed dentition we also have observed class II occlusion, which may require the use of head gear (Fig. 79–13), or class III occlusion which may require chin cap therapy (Fig. 79–14) or, in the case of a deficient maxilla, a reverse head gear (Fig. 79–15). For some patients in the mixed dentition, we may recommend serial extraction (as first suggested by Dewell).[14] If it can be determined that there is insufficient arch length or a lack of width in the primary canine area, the timely removal of primary teeth, prior to the normal shedding, may allow erupting teeth to guide themselves to improved positions.

Treatment During the Permanent Dentition

The final stage of orthodontic treatment is usually undertaken during the later stages of eruption of the permanent dentition. This treatment ordinarily does not differ greatly from the routine orthodontic procedures used for children without clefts. We must be aware continuously that these patients may have, superimposed on their deviated structures, the same types of malocclusion and growth-development problems that affect the noncleft population. Severe growth inhibition may necessitate combined surgical and orthodontic intervention. The timing of these procedures should be carefully studied by the surgeon and the orthodontist.

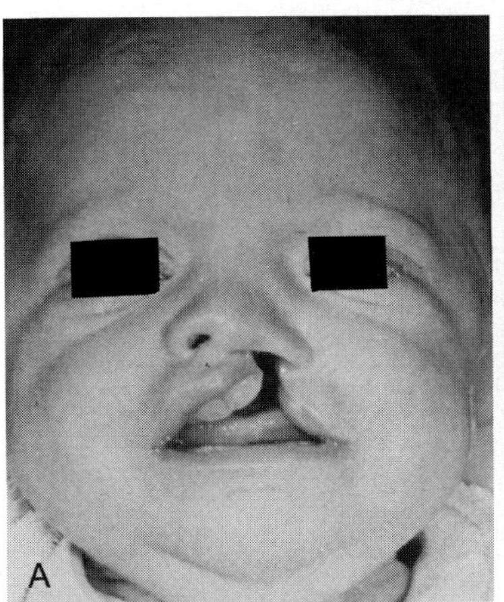
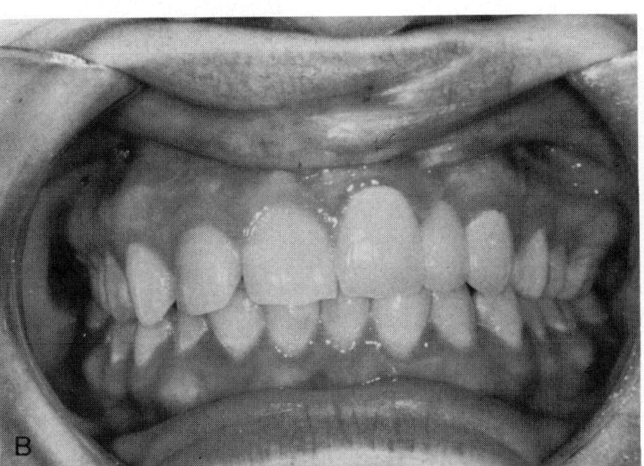
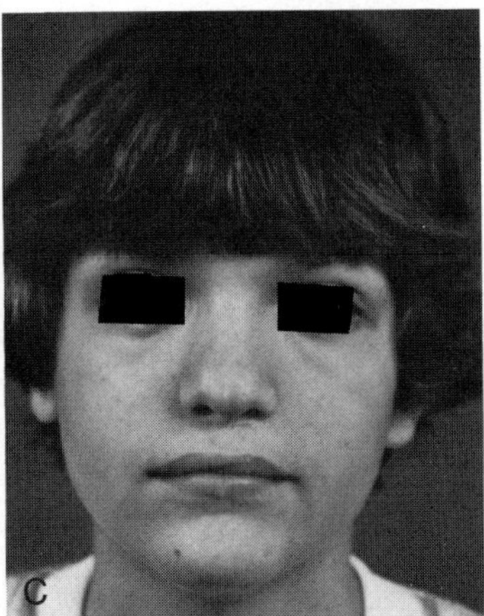

Figure 79–16 *A*, Preoperative view. *B*, Occlusion following three phases of orthodontic treatment. *C*, Facial view at completion of treatment. Facial view following treatment.

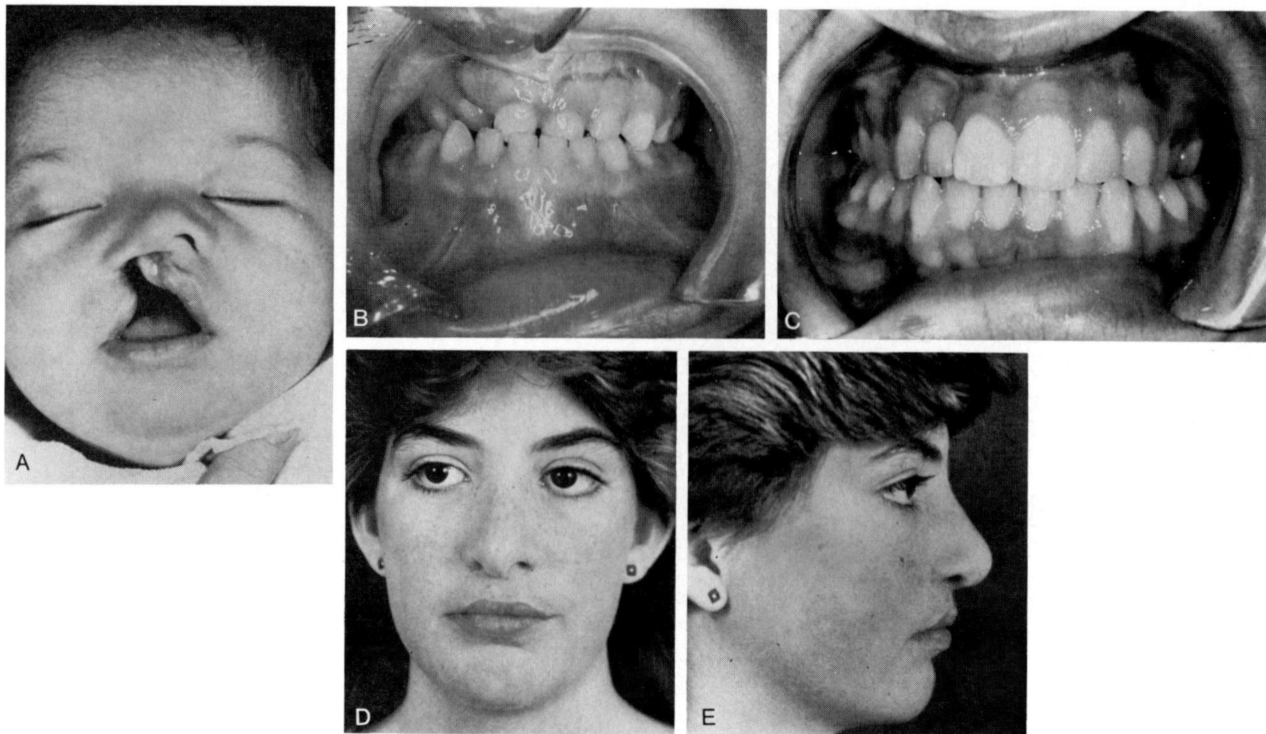

Figure 79–17 A, Preoperative view. B, Occlusion in primary dentition. C, Occlusion following three stages of orthodontic treatment. D and E, Facial and lateral view following treatment.

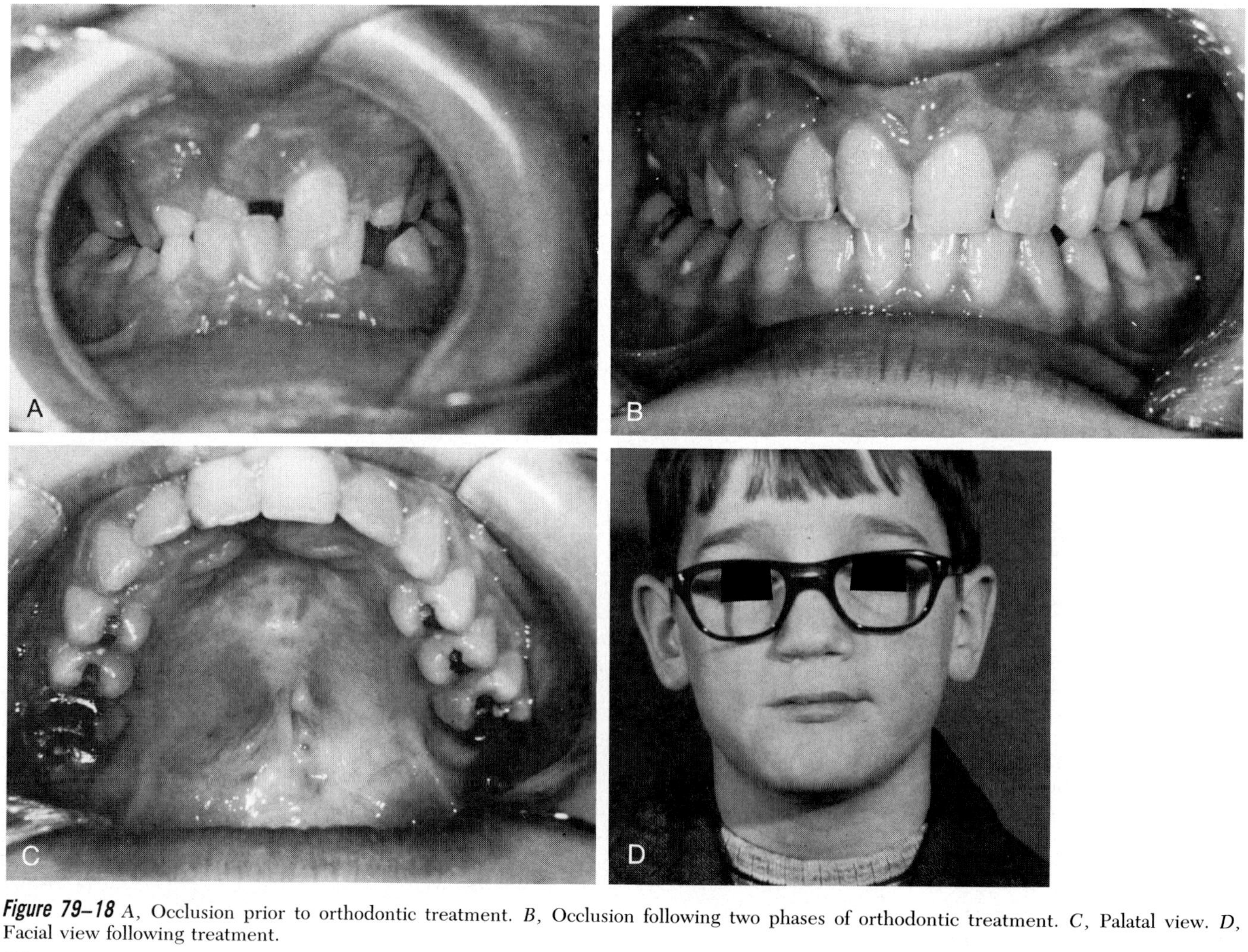

Figure 79–18 A, Occlusion prior to orthodontic treatment. B, Occlusion following two phases of orthodontic treatment. C, Palatal view. D, Facial view following treatment.

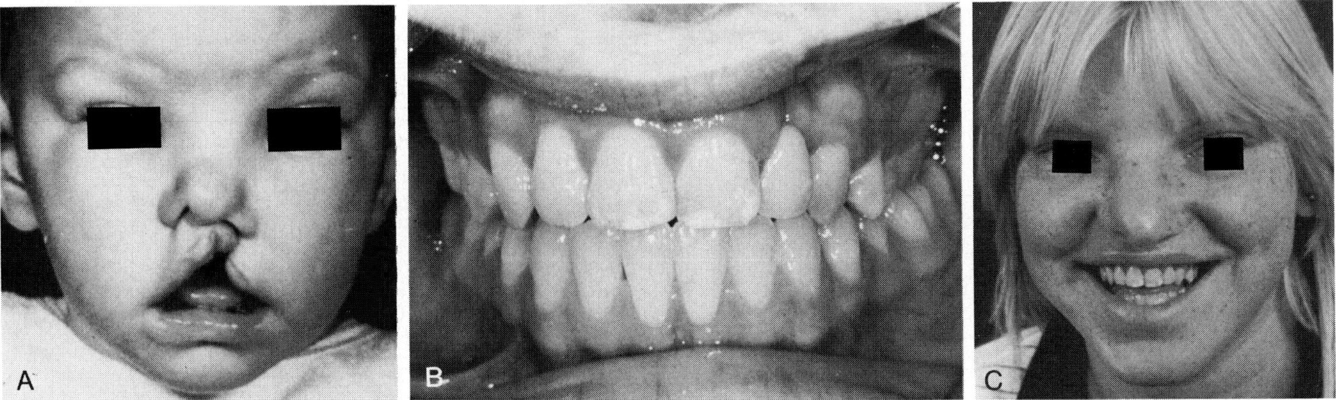

Figure 79-19 *A*, Preoperative view. *B*, Occlusion following three stages of orthodontic treatment. *C*, Facial view following completion of treatment.

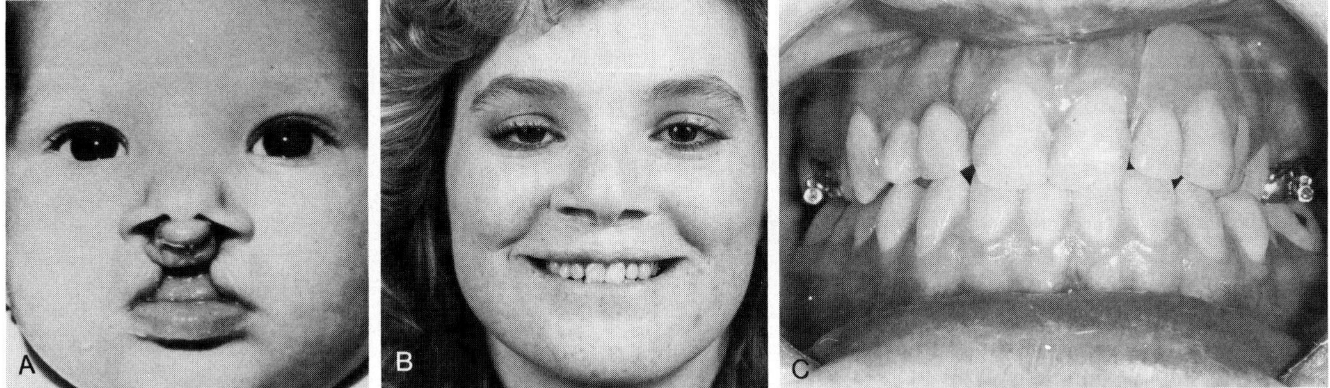

Figure 79-20 *A*, Complete bilateral cleft lip prior to surgery. *B* and *C*, Five years after treatment was completed.

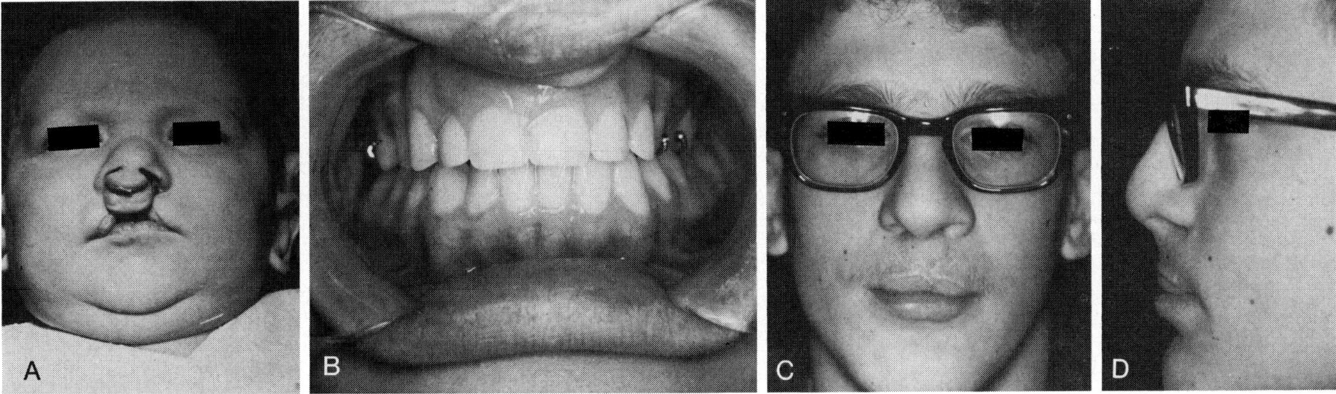

Figure 79-21 *A*, Complete bilateral cleft lip prior to surgery. *B*, Completion following orthodontic treatment and insertion of removable prosthesis. *C*, Facial view following treatment. *D*, Lateral view following treatment.

Teeth may erupt in abnormal positions. If they cannot be moved to their correct positions it may be necessary to extract them. If permanent canines fail to erupt, it may be necessary to expose these teeth, place attachments, and move them into the dental arch, provided adequate space exists.

It is important to maintain as many teeth as possible. We prefer to use fixed appliances; however, in a small percentage of our patients we do use various types of removable appliances. Retention following active orthodontic treatment must be observed closely. It may be necessary to use retention in some patients for life, depending on the amount of scar tissue present, tension from a tight lip, or lack of bony support.

In the majority of our patients with unilateral cleft lip and palate the treatment results are very acceptable functionally and aesthetically when the patients reach adulthood (Figs. 79–16 through 79–19). Unfortunately, the treatment results for the bilateral cleft lip and palate patient are not as successful, probably owing to the severity and initial conditions of the original cleft deformity (Figs. 79–20 and 79–21).

References

1. Foster TD: Maxillary deformities in repaired clefts of the lip and palate. Br J Plast Surg 15:182, 1962.
2. Levin HS: A cephalometric analysis of cleft palate deficiencies in the middle third of the face. Angle Orthod 33:186, 1963.
3. Dahl E: Craniofacial morphology in congenital clefts of the lip and palate. Acta Odontol Scand Suppl 57, 1970.
4. Olin WH: Dental anomalies in cleft lip and palate patients. Angle Orthod 34:119, 1964.
5. Bardach J, et al: Multidisciplinary management of cleft lip and palate. Ann Plast Surg 12:127, 1984.
6. Bishara SE: Longitudinal cephalometric standards from 5 years of age to adulthood. Am J Orthod 79:35, 1981
7. McNeil CK: Oral and Facial Deformity. London: Pitman and Sons, 1954.
8. Olin WH: Cleft lip and palate rehabilitation. Am J Orthod 52:126, 1966.
9. Pruzansky S: Pre-surgical orthopaedics and bone grafting for infants with cleft lip and palate: A dissent. Cleft Palate J 1:154, 1964.
10. Ross RB: Treatment variables affecting growth in complete unilateral cleft lip and palate. Cleft Palate J 24:5, 1988.
11. Valinoti JR, Jr: The congenitally absent premolar problem. Angle Orthod 28:36, 1958.
12. Mackey R.: Incidence of congenital anomalies in cleft palate patients vs. Public Health Service. Undergraduate Research Fellowship Study, Northwestern University, 1958.
13. Olin WH: Cleft Lip and Palate Rehabilitation. Springfield, IL: Charles C Thomas, 1960.
14. Dewell BF: Serial extraction in orthodontics: Indications, objections, and treatment procedures. Int J Orthod 40:906, 1954.

CHAPTER 80

Development of the Maxillary Arch in Cleft Patients Treated by the Schweckendiek Technique

Miluse Brousilová and Miroslav Fára

The purpose of this longitudinal study was to assess the positive or negative influence of the two-stage palatoplasty performed according to the Schweckendiek technique[1] on development of the alveolar arch. Patients in this study were compared to a control sample of patients who underwent one-stage palate repair.

Forty-six patients from a pool of 70 were regularly followed from the time of palatoplasty to adulthood. They were divided into four groups (Figs. 80–1 and 80–2).

Group 1. Total bilateral cleft patients operated on in one stage (TBC-controls).

Group 2. Total bilateral cleft patients operated on in two stages (TBC-Schweckendiek).

Group 3. Total unilateral cleft patients operated on in one stage (TUC-controls).

Group 4. Total unilateral cleft patients operated on in two stages (TUC-Schweckendiek).

Repair of the soft palate in the Schweckendiek groups

was performed at the time of primary lip repair when the patient was 5 months old; repair of the hard palate was done at 6 to 7 years of age. In the control groups one-stage palate repair was performed at 3 to 4 years of age. Early results of this series indicated that one-stage

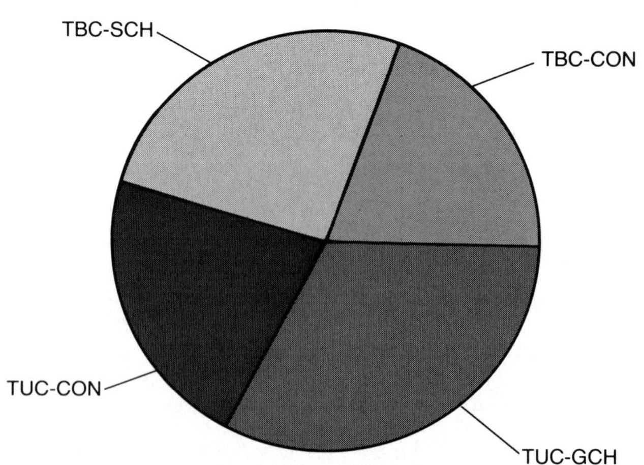

Figure 80–1 Division of the four study groups according to cleft type and procedure for palate repair.

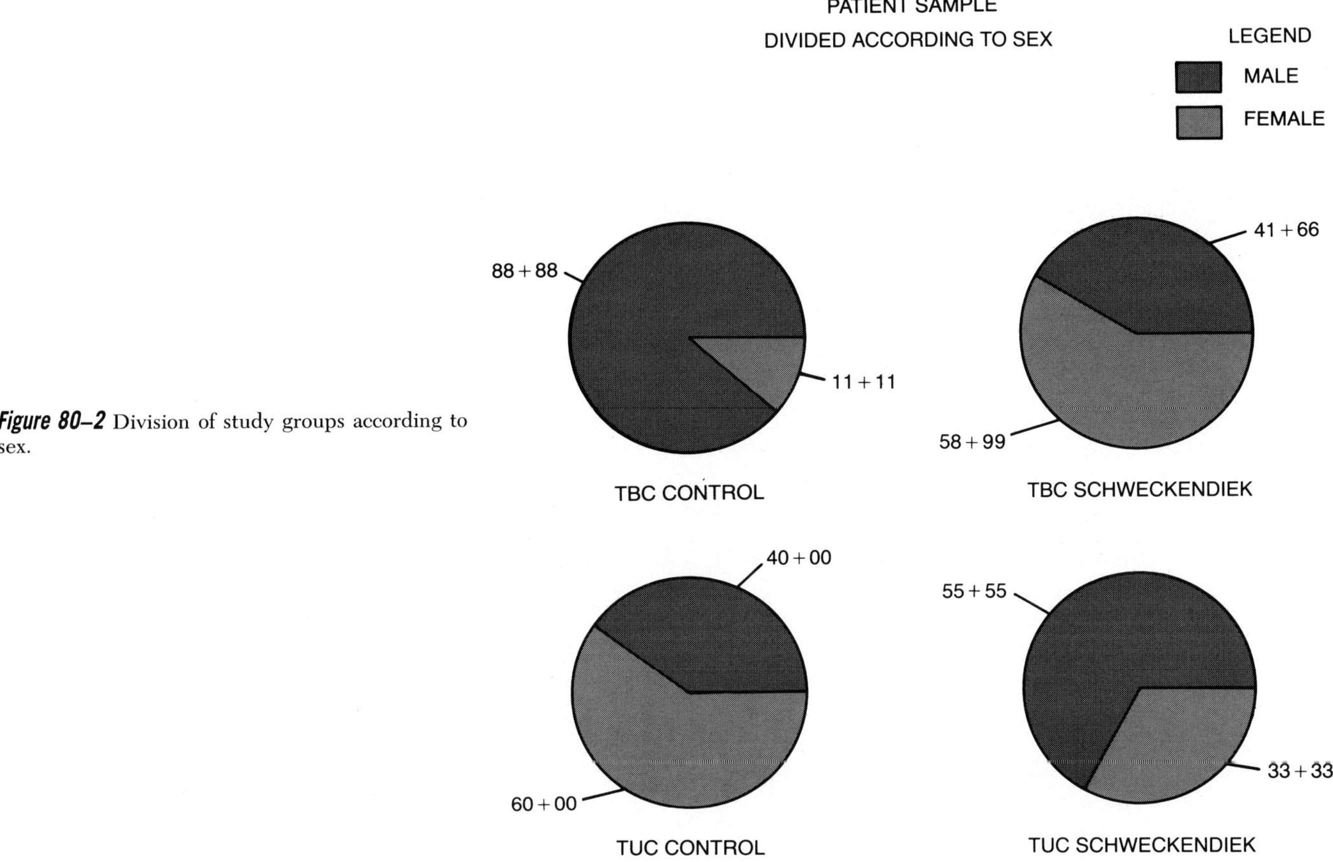

Figure 80–2 Division of study groups according to sex.

closure of the palate at approximately 3 years of age was more beneficial to the patients than the two-stage closure.[2] Currently, two-stage closure is performed only in selected cases.

Three dental impressions were taken in all patients: one was obtained before lip repair, one prior to palate repair, and one when the patients were 15 to 18 years of age.

Results

Width of the cleft was evaluated from the first two dental casts. Results are presented in Fig. 80–3. Although the cleft width in the control groups stayed constant or was slightly increased, the width of the cleft was significantly reduced in the Schweckendiek groups.

The growth dynamics of the palate are illustrated in Fig. 80–4. It is evident that the type of operation has no influence on the growth rate of the palate. Similar results were found when the growth dynamics of the alveolar segments were studied (Fig. 80–5).

Changes in width of the alveolar defect are represented in Fig. 80–6. Although the type of operation had no influence on the width of the defect in the bilateral cleft group, the two-stage procedure resulted in a larger alveolar defect in the unilateral cleft group.

Evaluation of the alveolar arch at the final stage shows that the type of operation had no significant influence

with the exception of narrowing in the area of the canines in patients operated on in two stages (Fig. 80–7).

Because the sex representation was not comparable in all groups of patients, the dental casts obtained after the patients were 15 years of age were evaluated separately for males and females (Fig. 80–8). No significant differences were found.

Discussion

Wolfram Schweckendiek must be credited for the popularization of the two-stage palatoplasty. However, acceptance of this method presently is not unanimous. This is due in part to the controversial results of longitudinal evaluation of the growth and development of the maxilla and speech. There also are social reasons that make acceptance of this method difficult.

Results obtained are in agreement with those in the literature. That is, the Schweckendiek two-stage palate repair contributes to reduction of the cleft width during the period between both operations. On the other hand, there is no evidence that this technique contributes to normal growth of the maxillary complex.

From the orthodontic point of view, both types of palate repair, one-stage and two-stage procedures, basically create the same conditions for final configuration of the dentoalveolar arch of the cleft maxilla. The

Text continued on page 671

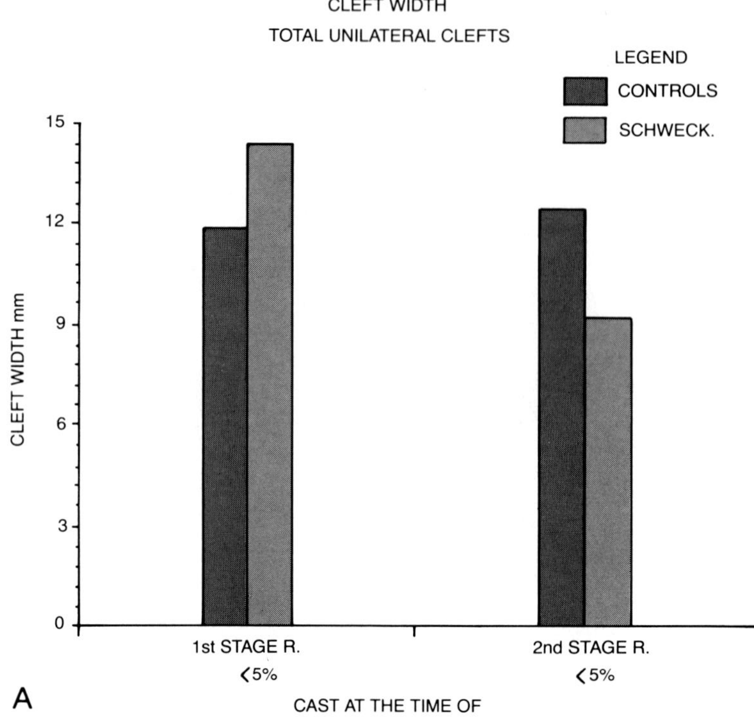

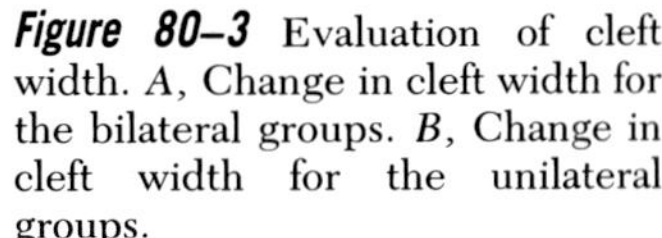

Figure 80–3 Evaluation of cleft width. A, Change in cleft width for the bilateral groups. B, Change in cleft width for the unilateral groups.

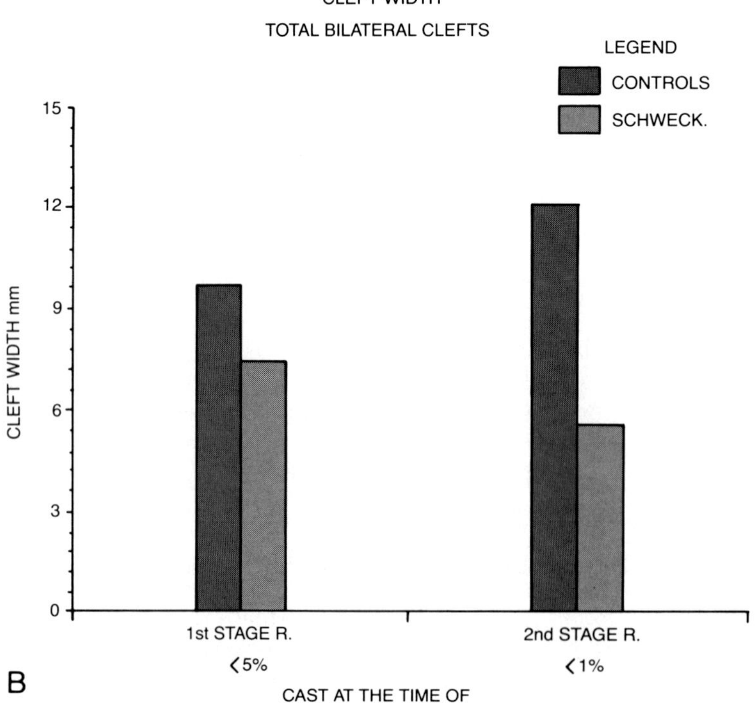

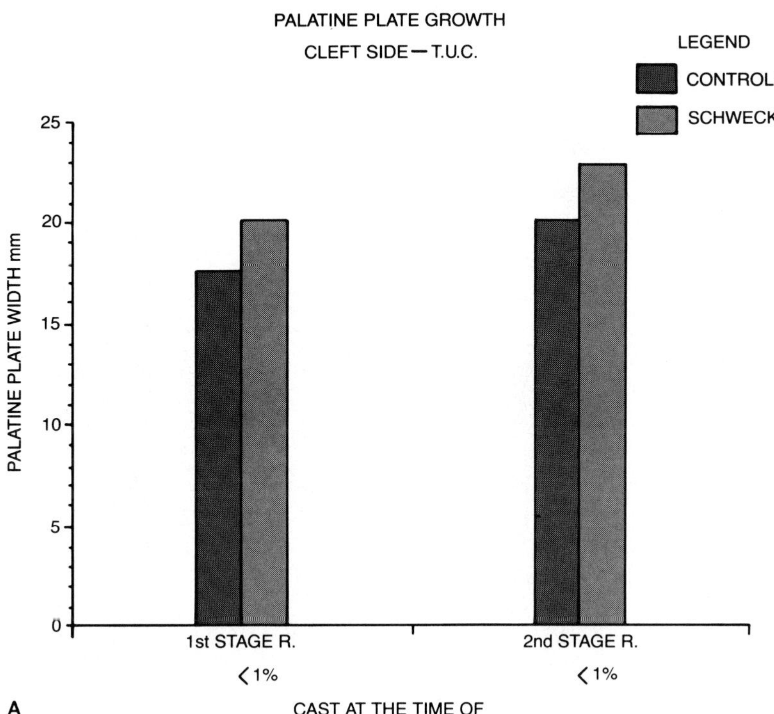

Figure 80–4 Growth dynamics of the palatal plates for the unilateral groups. *A*, Growth as measured on the cleft side. *B*, Growth as measured on the intact side.

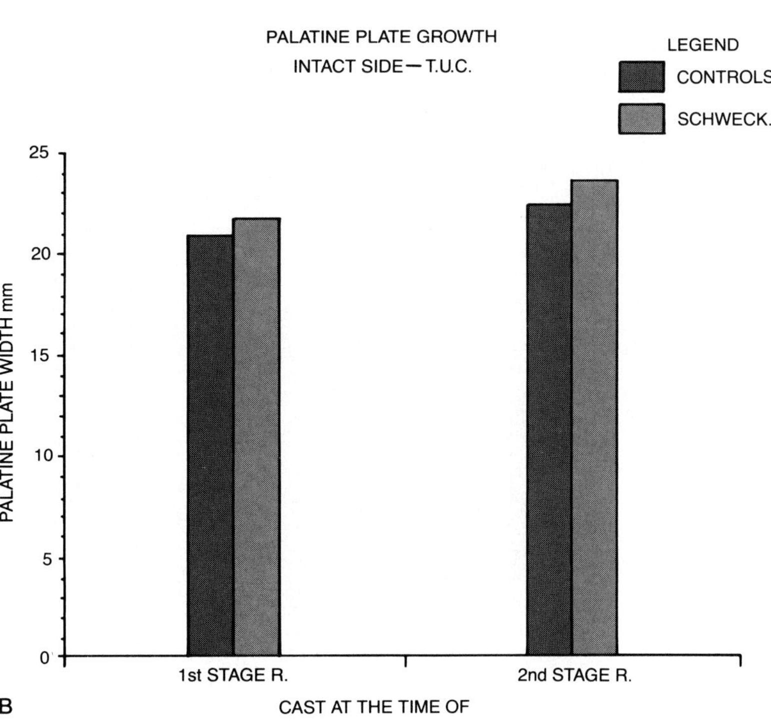

Orthodontic Treatment of Cleft Lip and Palate

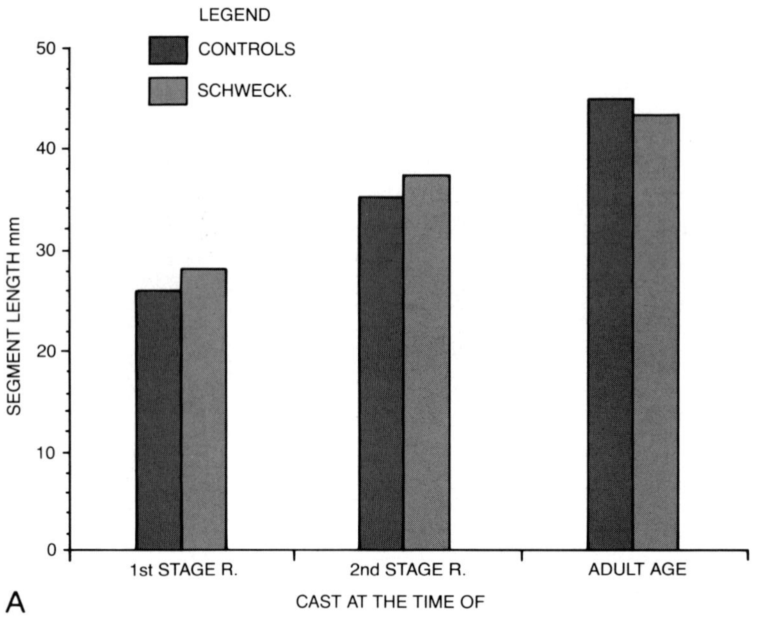

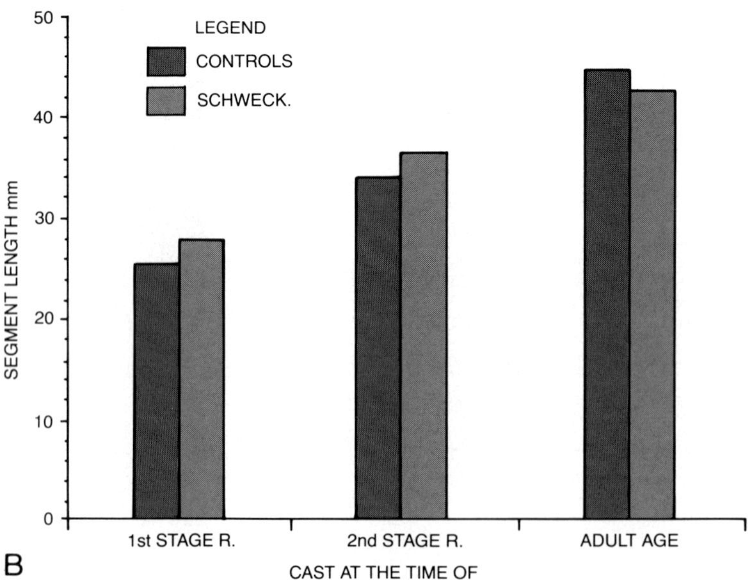

Figure 80–5 Growth dynamics of the alveolar segments. *A* and *B*, Comparison of the right and left segments in bilateral groups.

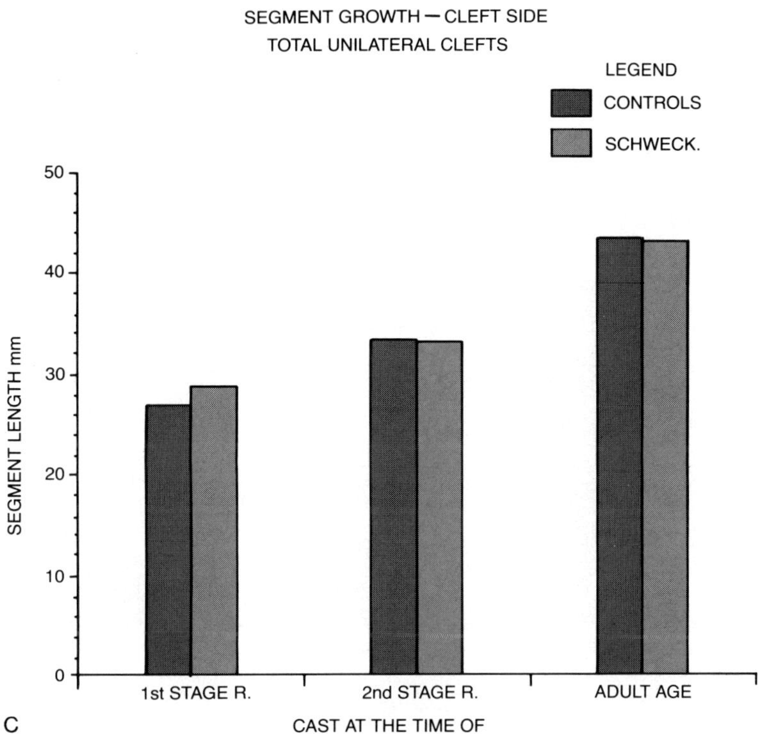

Figure 80–5 *Continued* C and D, Comparison of the cleft/intact sides in the unilateral groups.

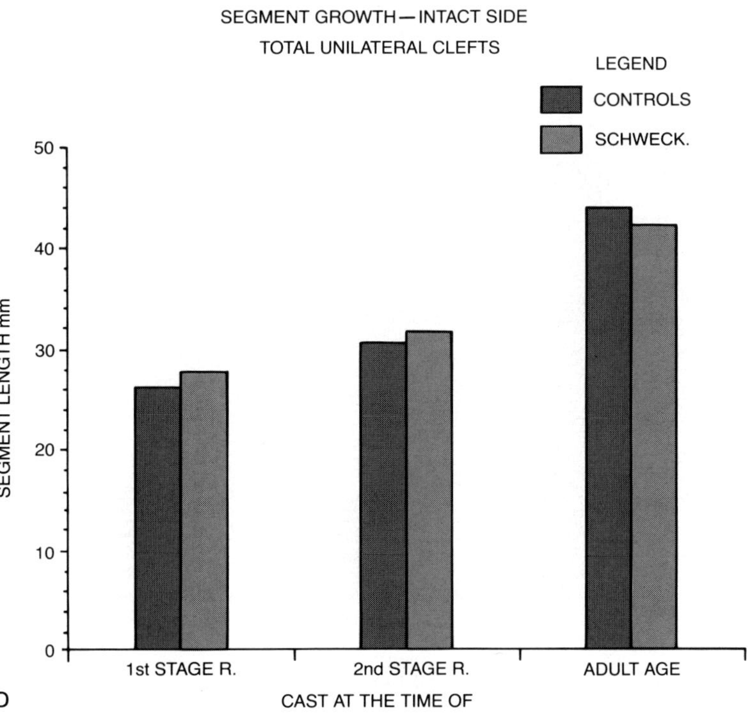

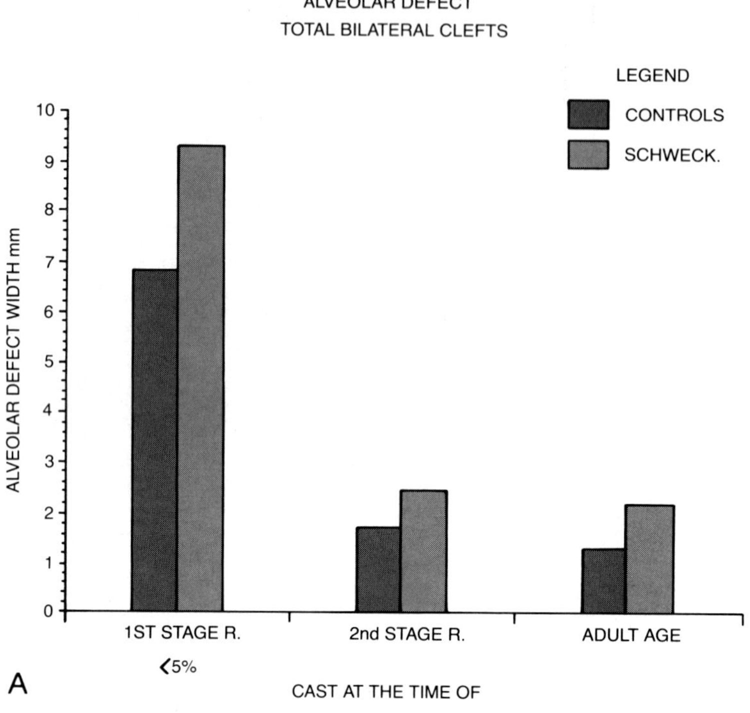

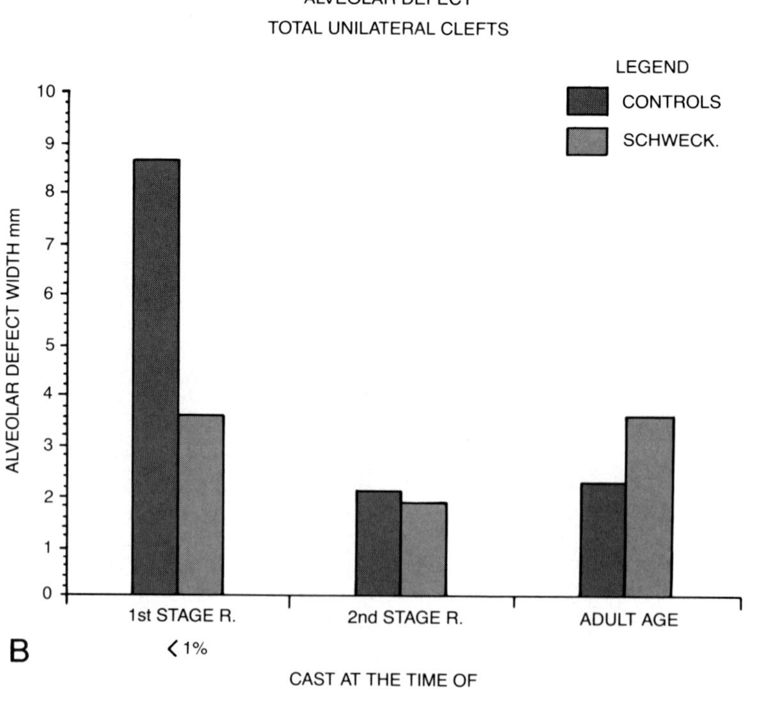

Figure 80–6 Changes in width of the alveolar defect as a function of type of repair. *A*, Changes for the bilateral groups. *B*, Changes for the unilateral groups.

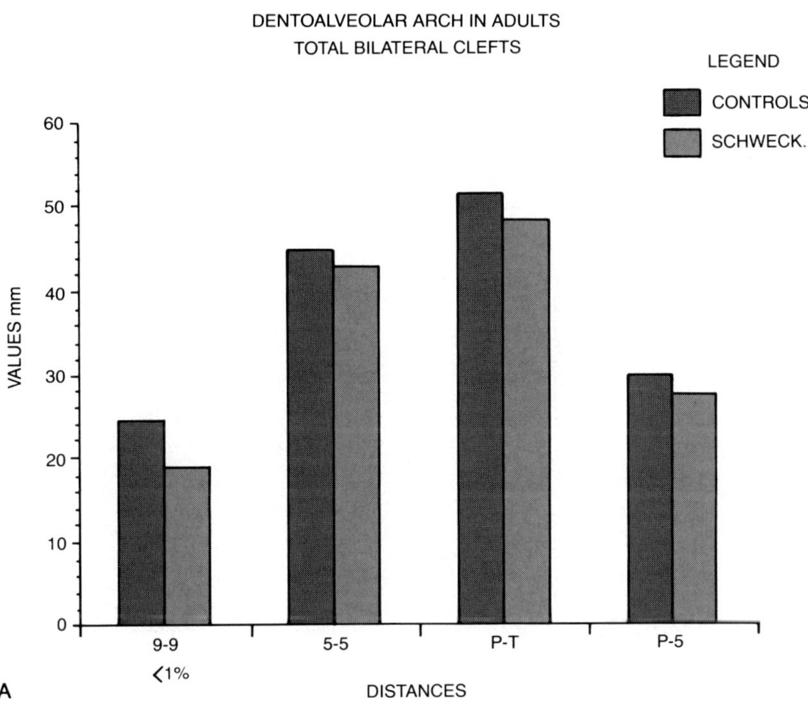

Figure 80–7 Evaluation of alveolar arch during the final phase of the study. *A*, Changes in the bilateral groups. *B*, Changes in the unilateral groups.

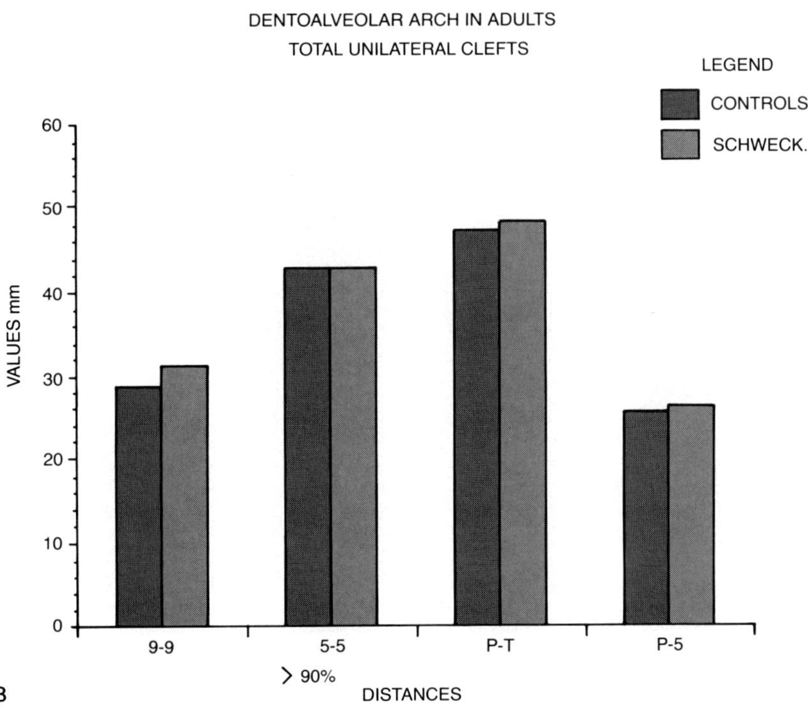

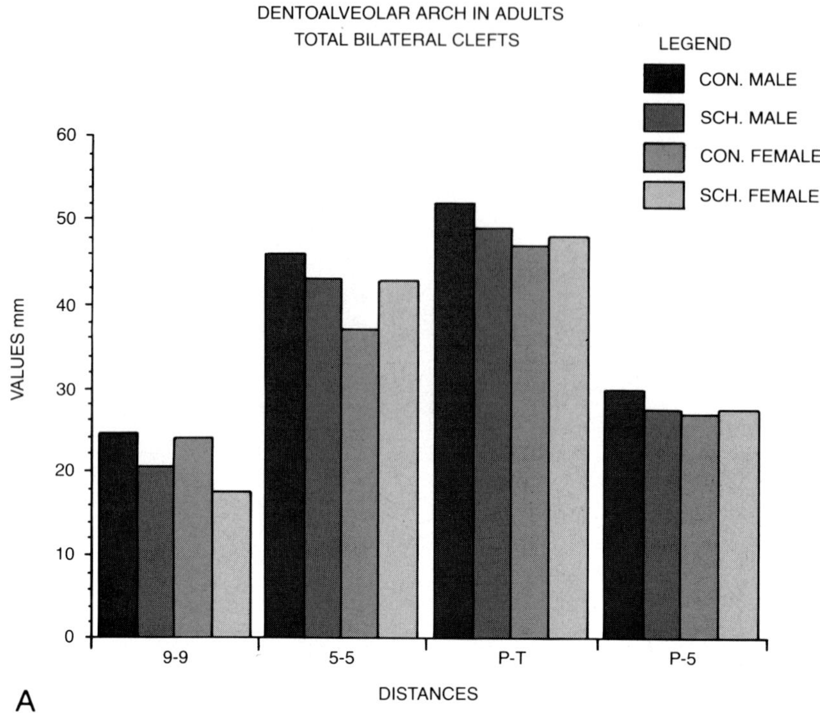

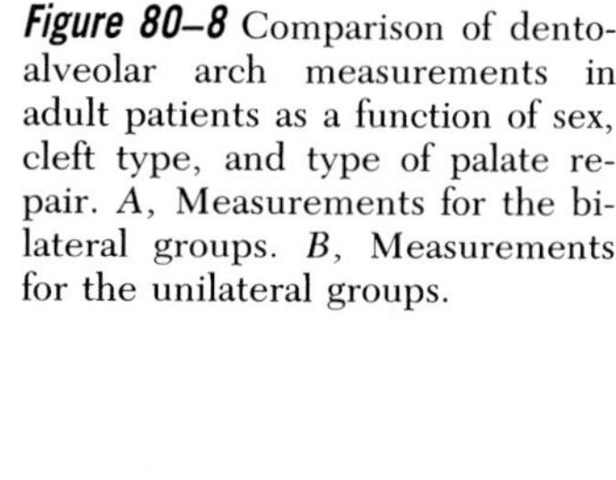

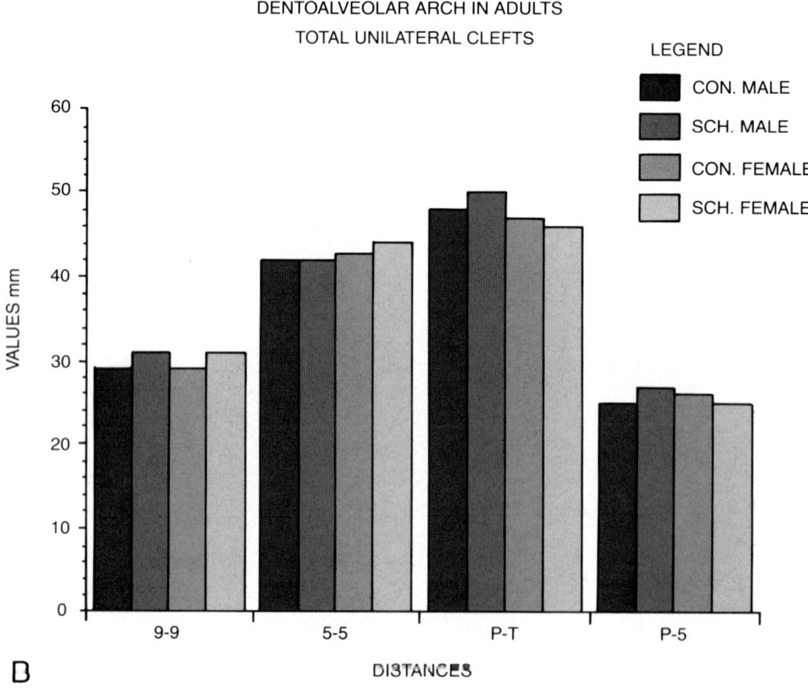

Figure 80–8 Comparison of dento-alveolar arch measurements in adult patients as a function of sex, cleft type, and type of palate repair. *A*, Measurements for the bilateral groups. *B*, Measurements for the unilateral groups.

Schweckendiek repair in patients with complete bilateral clefts contributes to narrowing of the transverse dimensions of the maxilla between the canines. In children with complete unilateral clefts, the repair extends the alveolar defect. This results in the same width of the alveolar defect at adulthood as prior to surgery. Following one-stage palatoplasty, the width of the alveolar defect is reduced during growth and development.

Slower reduction of the width of the alveolar defect may be observed even before the second stage of repair. At that time, the defect width was reduced to 24.1% of its original size in the control samples, whereas reduction was 51.9% in the Schweckendiek samples. Changes in cleft width were assessed during the same period of time. Whereas cleft width increased in the control groups by 25.8%, the cleft in the Schweckendiek groups was reduced by 25% owing to the influence of the repaired soft palate.

Patients were treated with the same orthodontic routine, so it appears that the Schweckendiek repair does reduce the cleft width following the one-stage palatoplasty, although there is limited reduction of the alveolar defect. Orthodontic appliances that support the normal relations between the maxilla and mandible and correct the configuration of the maxillary dentoalveolar arch act also as a support for levers represented by both parts of the maxilla.

The traction that acts on the distal ends of these levers following simultaneous repair of the lip and soft palate causes an extension of the alveolar defect on their proximal ends. The premaxilla that is fixed to the segment on the normal side is shifted by these forces on its cleft side proximally. This mechanism does not exist in bilateral clefts, in which the premaxilla is not fixed to any segment.

Conclusion

From our data on 46 patients operated on by one surgeon in 1961 and 1962 who were regularly examined up to adulthood, it may be concluded that the growth results of the two-stage palatoplasty, when the second stage is done before the patient is 7 years of age, are almost identical to the results of one-stage palate repair performed at the age of 3 to 4 years. However, a greater orthodontic effort is needed to achieve a properly aligned dentoalveolar arch with the two-stage palatoplasty.

References

1. Schweckendiek W: Die Technik der primaren Veloplastik und ihre Ergebnisse. Acta Chir Plast 8:188, 1966.
2. Fára M. Brousilová M: Experiences with early closure of velum and later closure of hard palate. Plast Reconstr Surg 44:134, 1969.

Nasal Airway, Otologic, and Audiologic Problems Associated with Cleft Lip and Palate

CHAPTER 81

Evaluation and Management of Nasal Airway Obstruction in the Cleft Patient

Dennis M. Crockett and Robert M. Bumsted

During the past decade, clinicians involved in the treatment of patients with cleft lip and palate have become increasingly aware of the importance of adequate nasal respiration. This awareness has resulted from knowledge of applied nasal physiology in the normal human as well as from studies showing a high prevalence of increased nasal airway resistance and mouth breathing in the cleft population.[1-4]

Several relevant considerations support the idea that nasal breathing is vital and physiologic for most mammalian species including man.[5-8] Nasal breathing through normal nasal passageways is asymptomatic, while restricted nasal breathing may produce unpleasant symptoms. The nose functions as a variable resistor to airflow, providing humidification, heating, and filtration of inspired air through contact with mucosa covering the septum, nasal floor, and turbinates.[7] Unconditioned inspired air (mouth breathing, tracheotomy) results in mucociliary dysfunction[9] and squamous metaplasia of normal ciliated pseudostratified epithelium in the respiratory tract.[10]

Nasal breathing is an important factor in pulmonary physiology.[11, 12] Clinical and experimental data postulate the existence of a rhinosinobronchial or nasopulmonary reflex.[13, 14] This reflex is initiated through stimulation of neurochemical receptors (H_1 histamine, cholinoceptor, and irritant receptors) located in the mucosa lining the nasal cavity, nasopharynx and sinuses. Afferent impulses are carried in the trigeminal, facial, and glossopharyngeal nerves to the medulla oblongata. Short neural arcs connect the impulse to the vagal nucleus, resulting in efferent impulses along the vagus nerve to the tracheobronchial tree, causing bronchoconstriction. The complexities of the nasopulmonary reflex are poorly understood, and additional cardiopulmonary reflex pathways associated with the nose may result in bradycardia and apnea.[14]

Clinical evidence for the nasopulmonary reflex is provided by observations that functional lung compliance in human subjects improves following use of mucosal vasoconstrictors in the nose and operative procedures to relieve nasal obstruction.[15-17] Medical or surgical treatment of chronic nasal and sinus disease in asthmatic patients has resulted in improved pulmonary function with concomitant decrease in the requirement for corticosteroid medication.[18-22] Conversely, complete nasal obstruction produced by posterior nasal packing results in a significant increase in pulmonary airway resistance, as shown in at least two studies.[16, 17, 23] However, a third study was unable to replicate this observation in young healthy subjects.[24]

The significance of impaired nasal respiration with resultant mouth breathing in terms of facial growth in the noncleft population has been debated for more than a century. Abnormal and inadequate dentofacial growth has been associated with high nasal resistance and mouth breathing. A cause-and-effect relationship has been suggested but not proved.[25] The so-called adenoid facies has become associated with mouth breathing and consists of an open mouth posture, short lip–nasal tip complex with flattened alae and small nostrils, enlarged lower lip and, as a result of the open mouth posture, a dull, vacant facial expression.[25-34] Dental and facial skeletal abnormalities include a high palatal arch with a V-shaped maxillary arch, increased vertical dimension of the maxilla, a class II occlusal relationship, a retrognathic mandible, and proclined upper incisors.[25-34]

Other investigators postulate that genetic factors predestine some individuals to narrow or hypoplastic facial morphology with increased nasal resistance as a natural consequence (for example, those with Crouzon's syndrome).[25, 35, 36] Adenoid hypertrophy in an individual with a narrow nasopharynx will cause a relatively greater obstruction of nasal airflow than the same degree of adenoid hypertrophy in another individual with a wide nasopharynx.

Because dentofacial growth and development are important to patients with cleft lip and palate, ideas linking nasorespiratory function and facial growth have naturally been extrapolated to the cleft population.[25] There is a high prevalence of increased nasal resistance and mouth breathing in cleft patients, presumably because of both intranasal (septum, turbinate, and nasal valve obstructions) and extranasal abnormalities and maxillary deficiencies that persist following primary lip and palate repair.[1–4] Certain secondary aesthetic rhinoplasty procedures and operations to correct velopharyngeal incompetence may further inhibit nasorespiratory function.[2, 37] The result is a child with a cleft lip and palate who spends the first decade of his or her life with significant nasal obstruction. A significant number of children with cleft lip and palate develop maxillary retrusion and hypoplasia as they approach the second decade of life, and much attention has been focused on lip and palate repair as the etiology of this growth disturbance.[38–41] Perhaps an additional hypothesis is that chronic increased nasal resistance with resultant mouth breathing (and open mouth posture) in cleft children may affect dentofacial development. It is possible that earlier correction of intranasal abnormalities causing nasal airway obstruction may result in more normal midfacial growth.

Inadequate nasal respiration may be associated with obstructive sleep apnea syndrome. Besides apnea, sleep disturbance and cor pulmonale,[42, 43] other symptoms of this syndrome include hypersomnolence, enuresis, somnambulism, nightmares, generalized fatigue, poor school academic performance, and inhibited social interaction.[44] Children with impaired nasal breathing but without obstructive sleep apnea as demonstrated by polysomnography may exhibit varying degrees of any of these symptoms.[45] Children with facial clefts may be at risk for academic and social conduct problems. A reasonable thought is that school and social problems in some cleft children might improve following medical or surgical treatment of their nasal airway obstruction.

The purpose of this chapter is twofold:

1. To present, from the rhinologic surgeon's point of view, an evaluation and assessment of the cleft nasal airway.
2. To discuss principles, goals, and details of surgery of the cleft nasal septum, turbinates, and nasal valve area.

In contrast to Warren's discussion in Chap. 83, in which quantitative data on the physiology of the cleft nasal airway are presented, most of the information presented in this chapter is retrospective and is based largely on clinical experience. Although quantitative information is available documenting improvement in the obstructed nasal airway following surgical intervention in noncleft adult patients,[46] these data have yet to be replicated in the cleft population. All of the cleft patients operated on by the authors have achieved marked subjective improvement in nasal breathing and are quite happy. This is probably not, in our opinion, a reflection of the surgeons' expertise but rather evidence that the problem

of nasal obstruction in the cleft patient is so significant that improvement in the airway is inevitable with any attempt at surgical intervention.

Clinical Evaluation

The Cleft Nasal History

The obvious anatomic abnormalities causing nasal obstruction in the cleft patient do not preclude the performance of a careful history. Apart from their lip and nasal deformities, nonsyndromic cleft children are normal, and, as in the general population, more than one-fourth may have symptoms consistent with seasonal or perennial allergic rhinitis and vasomotor rhinitis.[47] However, obtaining an allergic history in cleft children can be taxing and problematic. Surprisingly, many cleft children think that they breathe normally through the nose and will not admit to nasal airway obstruction even when questioned very carefully.[48] We have found this to be the case even for mature 12- to 16-year-olds.

A plausible explanation for this apparent contradiction between what the physician observes and the patient perceives is the fact that cleft children have breathed abnormally through their noses all their lives and therefore are not aware that a problem exists. They have no basis for comparison and do not know what normal breathing is. The parents are usually aware of the increased nasal resistance because they may note constant nasal congestion, mouth breathing, and nocturnal snoring. Only after surgical intervention that results in nasal airway improvement do the children realize that significant preoperative nasal obstruction existed.

Nasal obstruction and rhinorrhea associated with morning sneezing and itching of the eyes, nose, and pharynx are important elements in the history that suggest allergic rhinitis.[49] Additional evidence includes any history of eczema, bronchospasm, or asthma, as well as any familial history of allergy. Seasonal allergic rhinitis is suggested by correlating the timing of symptomatology with exposure to allergens.[50] Symptoms that are worse outdoors in the early morning or evening hours and correlate with a particular season or time of year strongly suggest an allergic cause. Allergic symptoms may be intermittent or continuous, depending on the nature of exposure to allergies.

Pollen allergies tend to occur seasonally during spring to late summer. The most common perennial allergies are house dust and animal dander which cause symptoms throughout the year. Patients with perennial allergic rhinitis present a greater diagnostic challenge. Laboratory confirmation of allergic rhinitis may be provided by skin end-point titration tests and by the radioallergosorbent (RAST) immunoassay test.[49–51]

Vasomotor rhinitis is a poorly understood clinical entity and has been observed in a small percentage of patients with cleft lip and palate. Vasomotor rhinitis is a manifestation of hyperfunction of the neurovascular and neurosecretory mechanisms in the nasal mucosa that are regulated by the parasympathetic nervous system.[52] The result is a hyperplastic mucosa overlying the turbinates and lateral nasal wall that secretes a diffuse watery discharge, resulting in partial or total nasal obstruction. Symptoms may be intermittent but are usually perennial. Possible etiologies or aggravating factors include emotional stimuli (especially anxiety), temperature changes (cold air exposure), fatigue, stress, and endocrine (thyroid) dysfunction.

Nasal obstruction aggravated by chronic infection and sinusitis, prolonged use and abuse of nasal sympathomimetic nose drops or sprays (rhinitis medicamentosa), and systemic illness is less common, although possible, and therefore should be sought for in the history.[50] One must not forget that the adult female cleft patient may become pregnant and suffer from rhinitis of pregnancy secondary to nasal mucosal engorgement caused by increased estrogen levels.

The Cleft Nasal Physical Examination

The nose acts as a variable resistor to airflow, and a basic understanding of this concept is important when performing an intranasal examination to determine the cause or causes of nasal obstruction. The nose should not be considered a static or passive conduit of airflow because a certain amount of dynamic resistance is necessary for the nose to accomplish its functions of olfaction, filtration, heating, humidification, and maintenance of physiologic harmony with the lungs.[6, 53] Any medical or surgical attempts to alter nasal airflow must be tempered by this understanding.

Presently, evaluation of nasal obstruction, especially in the cleft patient, relies considerably on the patient's subjective assessment (although, as stated, this can be difficult in the cleft child), and the rhinologist's view through the nasal speculum. Rhinomanometry can be an objective assessment of nasal obstruction, and only recently have attempts been made to use this method to quantitate changes in airflow following surgical correction of obstructive elements in the noncleft adult nose.[45, 54–57] In the future, rhinomanometry can be used to evaluate intranasal cleft surgery as well.

Functional regulation of nasal airflow is accomplished by means of three sets of paired valves and a midline septal valve.[58] The valves form dynamic constrictions along the length of the nasal fossae from the external nares to the posterior choanae. During respiration, airflow through the nose is primarily laminar; however, turbulent flow occurs posterior to intranasal constrictions and is favored as the respiratory rate increases. Poiseville's law governs the relationship between resistance to airflow and the effective cross-sectional area of the intranasal vault: Resistance increases inversely proportional to the fourth power of the diameter.[6, 58] The four regulatory valves consist of the septum, turbinates, external nasal valve, and internal nasal valve.[58]

The nasal septum includes the cartilaginous septum and the premaxillary crest anteriorly, the vomer, and the perpendicular plate of the ethmoid bones. There are three nasal turbinates in each nasal vault—the inferior, middle, and superior turbinates. The inferior turbinate is the most important regulator of airflow and

is one component of the nasal valve area. The inferior turbinate is the primary regulator of airflow of all the nasal valves in the platyrrhine (wide) nose. The internal nasal valve is *the nasal valve* and is defined as the space between the caudal edge of the upper lateral cartilage and the septum.[59, 60] The *nasal valve* is the primary airflow regulator in the leptorrhine (narrow) nose. The nasal valve is dynamic, narrowing with inspiration and widening with expiration. An important concept is the nasal valve area, defined as the cross-sectional area bounded by the nasal valve superiorly, the septum medially, the upper lateral cartilage and head of the inferior turbinate laterally, and the floor of the nasal vault inferiorly.[61] Finally, the external nasal valve is formed by the lower lateral cartilage laterally and superiorly, the vestibule, the columella medially, and the nasal sill inferiorly.

Physical examination of nasal obstruction in the cleft patient begins with careful observation of the nose with quiet breathing and forced inspiratory and expiratory respirations. Especially important is observation of the nose from the base view. Alar collapse may be viewed on the side of the cleft secondary to any one or a combination of anatomic problems typical of the secondary cleft deformity. Careful anterior rhinoscopy is performed with the aid of a nasal speculum and adequate illumination and may be augmented by the use of rigid fiberoptic telescopes or flexible fiberoptic scopes. The nasal septum, floor of the nasal vault, superior aspect of the nasal cavity including the nasal valve and nasal valve area, and the lateral wall of the nose including the turbinates are inspected.

Inspection and palpation (with a cotton-tipped applicator) is performed on all cartilaginous, bony, and mucosal elements of the internal nose. Movement of the internal nasal valve is observed during quiet breathing and forced inspiration. In the cleft patient, performance of the classic Cottle sign test to assess function of the nasal valve is generally not helpful in most cases secondary to consistent "false positive" results generated by alar collapse or excess soft tissue in the lateral vestibule. Posterior rhinoscopy is always performed to rule out other causes of nasal obstruction such as adenoid hypertrophy, polyps, and tumors present in the nasopharynx.

Anterior rhinoscopy is always repeated following shrinking of the nasal mucosa with the application of 5% cocaine-soaked cotton pledgets placed in the nose. Significant relief of nasal obstruction may indicate mucosal disease of the turbinates secondary to allergic or vasomotor rhinitis. The degree of bony turbinate hypertrophy is better visualized following shrinking of the mucosa. A decision about whether or not to perform turbinate reduction and cryotherapy may then be made after proper assessment.

The Cleft Nasal Septum. The detailed anatomy of the cartilaginous and bony nasal septum was studied in a group of 140 cleft patients who underwent secondary correction of external nasal deformities, including nasal-septal reconstruction, at The University of Iowa.[62] Of the 140 patients, 135 were operated on between the ages of 12 and 16, and five younger children underwent nasal-septal reconstruction between the ages of 8 and 12 for severe nasal obstruction.

Four general categories of cartilaginous septal deformities were discernible by careful preoperative clinical evaluation and intraoperative findings (Fig. 81–1). Although the anatomy of the cartilaginous septal deformity for each patient was unique, it generally could be categorized as one of the four anatomic types (I, II, III, or IV). Types I, II, and III were associated with unilateral cleft lip nasal deformities, whereas the type IV septal deformity was associated with the bilateral nasal deformity. The most common cartilaginous septal abnormality was the type I septum (found in 61% of the unilateral clefts), which consisted of the following features:

1. Deflection of the anterior nasal spine into the noncleft side of the nose.
2. Deviation of the caudal end of the cartilaginous septum to the noncleft side.
3. Either deviation of the wing of the premaxilla (Fig. 81–1a) or deflection of the inferior cartilaginous septum (Fig. 81–1b) into the noncleft nasal vault.
4. Bowing of the superior portion of the cartilaginous septum with the convexity toward the cleft side of the nose, resulting in consistent constriction of the nasal valve on the cleft side.

The type II septum (found in 6% of the unilateral clefts) is similar to the type I septum except that significant obstruction in the noncleft nasal vault secondary to either a projecting wing of the premaxilla or the inferior cartilaginous septum is absent. The type II septum is characterized by:

1. Deviation of the anterior nasal spine into the noncleft nasal vault.
2. Deflection of the caudal border of the cartilaginous septum into the noncleft side.
3. Deviation of the caudal end of the cartilaginous septum to the cleft side as opposed to the noncleft side as found in type I and II deformities.

In patients with bilateral clefts, the septal deformity (type IV) consisted of a general bowing of the entire cartilaginous septum, perpendicular plate of the ethmoid bone, and vomer bone into either the right or the left side. The inferior border of the cartilaginous septum was attached to the crest of the premaxilla and was not deviated.

In septum types I, II, and III, the bony septum (perpendicular plate of the ethmoid and vomer bone) was deviated toward the cleft side in 80% of the cases. Twenty percent of patients had bony septa that were in the midline and were nonobstructive. In general, significant deviation of the bony septum into the noncleft nasal vault was not observed.

The Cleft Nasal Turbinates. The turbinates, especially the inferior turbinates, play a significant role in the regulation of nasal airflow. The nasal cycle is a phenomenon that occurs in approximately three-fourths of normal individuals and involves a rhythmic congestion and decongestion of turbinate mucosa.[63] The nasal cycle is balanced and alternates between the two nasal cavities, one side opening and secreting mucus while the other side closes. The overall nasal airflow remains constant, and most individuals are unaware that the phenomenon is occurring. A full cycle between the two sides takes 3 to 4 hours to complete. The nasal cycle is affected by temperature (cold air), humidity, allergy, physical, activity, emotional state, and medications.

For the rhinologist, the nasal cycle is important because it must be recognized and taken into account when evaluating a patient for nasal obstruction. Related to the nasal cycle is the fact that the turbinates become hypertrophic or hyperplastic in response to a greater volume in the nasal vault. In other words, the turbinates enlarge to fill the gap afforded them to provide physiologic resistance to airflow. Turbinate hypertrophy is typical of the majority of patients with cleft lip and palate.

In the 140 patients studied, intranasal examination revealed that turbinate enlargement characteristically occurred on the side with the larger volume between the septum and the lateral nasal wall in the floor of the nasal vault.[62] Accordingly, in patients with types I and II septal deformities, compensatory hypertrophy of the anterior portion of the inferior turbinate occurred on the cleft side, whereas in type III septal deformity, turbinate hypertrophy occurred on the noncleft side. In type IV septal deformity, compensatory hypertrophy of the inferior and middle turbinates occurred on the concave side of the septal deformity. In any of the unilateral cleft patients, however, if deviation of the vomer toward the cleft side was marked, turbinate hypertrophy occurred on the noncleft side.

Cleft patients with mucosal disease (seasonal or perennial allergic rhinitis, vasomotor rhinitis) have pale, boggy-appearing turbinates with a thickened overlying mucosa that shrinks readily following administration of a topical vasoconstrictor agent. However, longstanding, end-stage mucosal disease may not respond to decongestants.

The Cleft External Nasal Deformity. Depending on the particular method of primary lip repair done in infancy as well as the degree of attention paid to surgical details, nasal airway obstruction in the patient with a unilateral cleft may be caused by a relatively small nostril on the cleft side, if present, as well as by any hooding of the superior portion of the ala. Depending on the resiliency of the existing nasal cartilages, alar collapse may occur with nasal breathing on the cleft

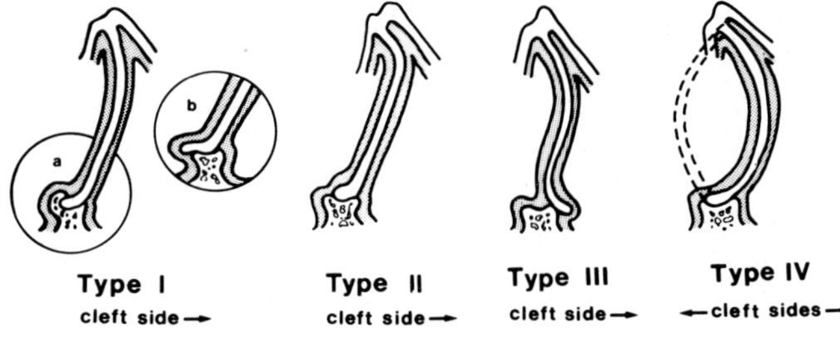

Figure 81–1 The four types of cleft septa are shown in schematic cross-section planes through the anterior cartilaginous septum at its point of fusion with the upper lateral cartilages and its point of contact with the crest of the premaxilla.

side secondary either to displacement of the lower lateral cartilage in the frontal and horizontal (backward and downward) planes or to excessive soft tissue and skin in the lateral vestibule on the cleft side. These problems may or may not be corrected at the time of secondary nasal surgery. The relative contribution of the external nasal deformity to nasal airway obstruction in the cleft patient is incompletely understood. Further clinical evaluation and objective rhinomanometric data are needed in this area.

The Cleft Nasal Valve and Nasal Valve Area. The nasal valve angle ranges from 10 to 15 degrees in the unobstructed leptorrhine nose.[61] The nasal valve and the nasal valve area represent the primary regulators of intranasal airflow; the nasal valve cross-sectional area measures between 55 and 64 mm.[2, 59, 64] The nasal valve changes inspiratory air currents from a column to a sheet of moving air, thus controlling its direction, velocity, and shape.[65] The nasal valve functions as a Starling resistor subject to Bernoulli's principle, according to which velocity of air increases and pressure decreases as the conduit diameter decreases.[59] The nasal valve does not move with quiet respiration and constricts slightly as airflow increases with increased respiration. With increased airflow, the pressure difference between the nasopharynx and the nasal vestibule reaches a critical point, and collapse of the nasal valve occurs, obstructing airflow (Starling resistor). With expiration, the nasal valve opens again.

Airflow obstruction at the nasal valve and nasal valve area can be caused by any pathologic condition involving any of the cutaneous, mucosal, cartilaginous, or bony elements in these areas. For the patient with cleft lip and palate, depending on the method of primary lip repair performed in infancy (and whether or not any primary nasal reconstruction was done) as well as on whether or not secondary nasal surgery has been performed, any one or a combination of the following anatomic problems may be observed:

1. Deflection of the cartilaginous septum into the cleft side superiorly in the unilateral cleft, resulting in constriction of the nasal valve.
2. Scarring and blunting of the sharp nasal valve angle secondary to any previous surgical incisions.
3. Flaccidity of the upper lateral cartilage, producing alar collapse with inspiration.
4. Obstruction of the nasal valve area in the noncleft nasal vault by the premaxillary wing and anterior nasal spine in types I and II septa, or obstruction of the cleft nasal vault in the type III septum.
5. Obstruction of the nasal valve area by the inferior border of the cartilaginous septum.
6. Obstruction of the nasal valve area by the anterior portion of the inferior turbinate.
7. A relative stenosis of the nasal vault just anterior to the nasal valve on the cleft side, caused by a bowstring contracture of skin from the apex of the vestibule following the upper border of the lateral crus of the lower lateral cartilage to the piriform aperture laterally.

Surgical Management

Cleft Nasal Septum

Cottle described the maxilla-premaxilla approach to surgery of the nasal septum that emphasized reconstruction of existing cartilage and bone rather than simple submucous resection of septal cartilage.[66] The maxilla-premaxilla approach to the nasal septum allows:

1. Complete access to all cartilaginous and bony portions of the septum as well as the anterior nasal spine, premaxilla, maxilla, and upper lateral cartilages.
2. Direct visualization of the obstructive components that require correction to improve nasal function.
3. Good surgical exposure for mobilization, reshaping, and repositioning of septal cartilage and bone to improve the nasal airway.

Reconstruction of the cleft septum may be accomplished alone or may be combined with tip rhinoplasty and osteotomies to correct the external cleft nose deformity.[67] In many cases, correction of the external cleft nasal deformity cannot be accomplished unless reconstruction and straightening of the septum is performed concomitantly. If ancillary corrective procedures such as turbinate reduction or cryotherapy are anticipated, these procedures are combined with septoplasty and external rhinoplasty performed 6 months to 1 year later.

Nasal septoplasty in the cleft patient may be performed with local anesthesia and analgesia or under general anesthesia depending on the age and cooperation of the patient. General anesthesia is usually required for 13- and 14-year-old teenagers undergoing external rhinoplasty and nasal septal reconstruction. Mucosal analgesia and vasoconstriction are accomplished with neurosurgical cottonoid strips soaked in 5% cocaine solution placed in each nasal vault. The mucoperichondrium on both sides of the septum, the nasal floors, and the soft tissues surrounding the anterior nasal spine are injected with 0.5% lidocaine with epinephrine 1:200,000. A full 10 minutes is allowed to ensue before the initial incision is made.

The Cottle maxilla-premaxilla approach to the nasal septum is begun with a hemitransfixion incision made approximately 1 mm from the caudal end of the cartilaginous septum (Fig. 81–2A). The hemitransfixion incision and subsequent dissection of the anterior tunnel in the types I and II cleft septum is performed on the noncleft side. In the type III cleft septum it is easier to begin the initial incisions on the cleft side because this facilitates dissection and mobilization of the inferior border of the cartilaginous septum. In the type IV cleft septum, dissection is usually commenced on the concave side of the cartilaginous septum. If preferred, access to the nasal septum may be achieved through a marginal external rhinoplasty incision.

Dissection of the anterior tunnel posteriorly to include the bony septum is accomplished between the overlying mucoperichondrium and septal cartilage with a Cottle elevator (Fig. 81–2B). A second incision is completed

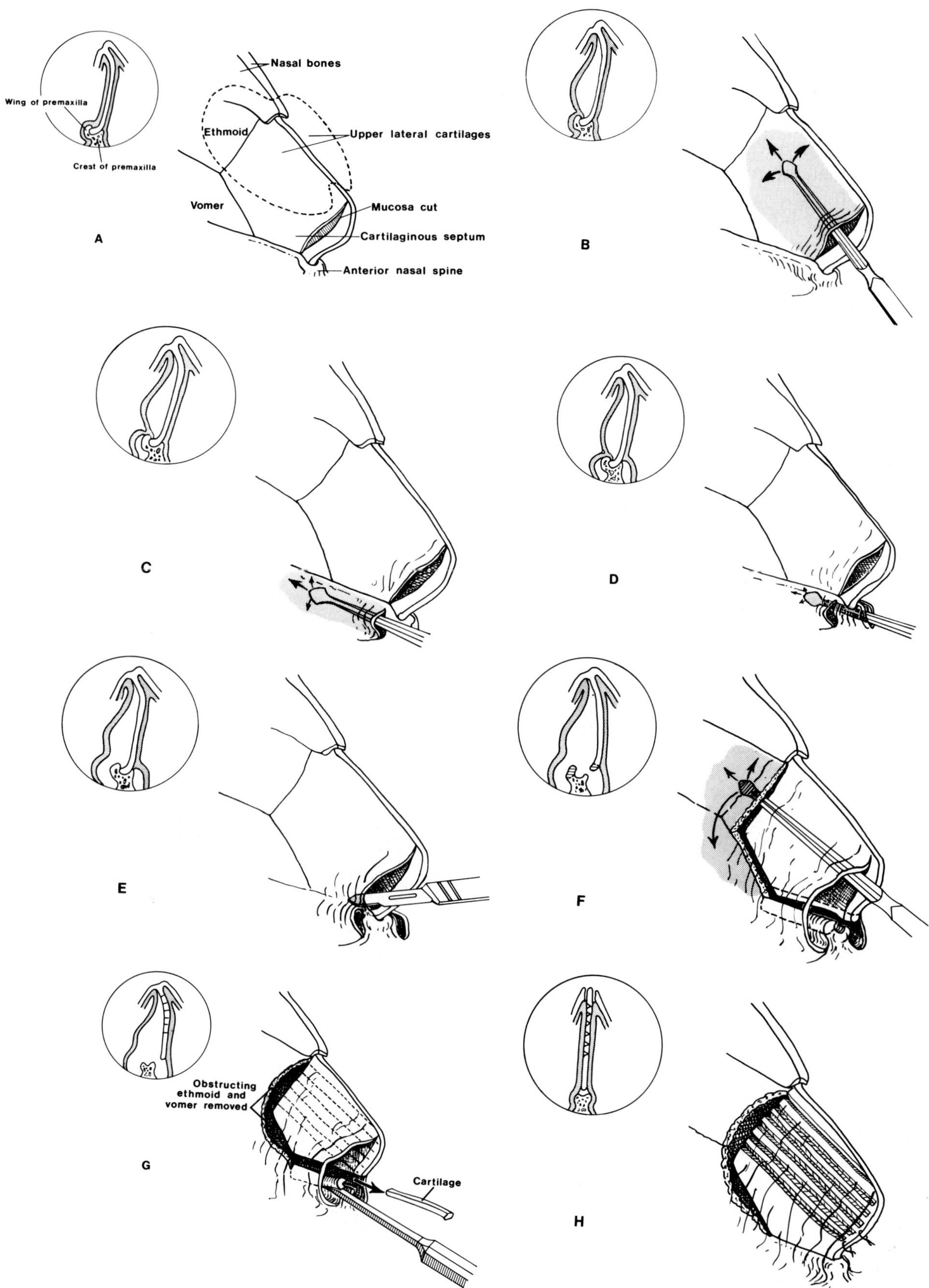

Figure 81–2 *A–H*, Adaptation of the Cottle maxilla-premaxilla approach to the cleft nasal septum (illustrated for the type I septum).

in the anterior floor of nose, and an inferior tunnel is completed between the overlying mucoperiosteum and the underlying anterior nasal spine and the wing of the premaxilla (Fig. 81–2C). An inferior tunnel in the nasal floor of the cleft side is then created in a similar fashion (Fig. 81–2D). This dissection must be done carefully to avoid disrupting the soft tissue layers spanning the bony cleft in the floor of the nasal vault. Dissection may be difficult if previous bone grafting has been done in the area.

The anterior tunnel and the inferior tunnel on the noncleft side are joined by a sharp division of the decussating fibers at the junction of cartilage and bone in the crest of the premaxilla (Fig. 81–2E). A vertical incision is completed through the posterior portion of the septal cartilage, and the mucoperichondrium and mucoperiosteum are dissected free of the underlying posterior septum and vomer and perpendicular plate of the ethmoid on the cleft side (Fig. 81–2F). The inferior border of the cartilaginous septum is dissected free from the anterior nasal spine, crest of the premaxilla, and vomer bone.

The performance of these maneuvers allows complete exposure of the cartilaginous septum including its caudal end as well as the anterior nasal spine and the wing of the premaxilla. Figure 81–2G illustrates the maneuvers that may now be accomplished to eliminate the obstructive elements of the abnormal septum. The obstructing inferior margin of the cartilaginous septum may be excised. A 2-mm osteotome is used to remove the obstructing wing of the premaxilla. Obstructing portions of the vomer and ethmoid plate may be resected under direct visualization. The freed portion of the cartilaginous septum is then scored with the incisions made completely through the cartilage but not transecting the mucoperichondrium on the opposite or cleft side. The cuts may be oriented vertically or horizontally depending on the judgment of the surgeon as to which orientation will best straighten the particular septal deformity. The upper lateral cartilages may be completely separated from the superior border of the septum to increase mobility (Fig. 81–2H). This maneuver, in combination with a medial osteotomy, will open the nasal valve to a significant degree. The caudal end of the septum may be swung to the midline and sutured to a pocket created in the soft tissues of the columella or to the skin of the columella by means of through-and-through sutures tied over bolsters.

All incisions are closed with absorbable sutures. Transmucoperichondrial-septal through-and-through sutures are placed throughout the septum to hold the septal flaps in place (Fig. 81–2H). Silastic splints are used only if turbinate reduction and cryotherapy are to follow. The nasal cavities are lightly packed with Telfa gauze that is removed 24 hours postoperatively.

The operating scheme presented for the type I septum is also applicable to types II and IV cleft septa. For the type III cleft septum, we have found it easier to complete the hemitransfixion incision and anterior tunnel on the cleft side of the nose.

The Cottle maxilla-premaxilla approach as outlined will correct the majority of cleft septal deviations. Oc-

casionally the septal deflection is so severe that an anterior tunnel on the cleft side must be raised, and the septal cartilage must be removed in toto, straightened, and put back into place. Occasionally the caudal end of the septum resists straightening and requires creation of an anterior tunnel (on the convex side) with resection of a vertical wedge of cartilage at the septal angle so that the caudal septum may be swung toward the midline as a "swinging door."[68] Resection of any portion of the superior caudal border of the cleft septum or removal of the anterior nasal spine are avoided because this may have a negative effect on tip projection.

Cleft Nasal Turbinates

The method of turbinate reduction is varied for each patient depending on the degree and location of obstruction as determined by the clinical examination as well as on any history of allergic or vasomotor rhinitis (mucosal disease). Patients with marked turbinate hypertrophy without mucosal disease undergo turbinate reduction through a "turbinoplasty" technique.[69–71] Anterior turbinate resection followed by cryotherapy is performed for patients with evidence of mucosal disease.[72]

Turbinoplasty may be performed immediately following nasal septal reconstruction (Fig. 81–3). Mucosal analgesia and vasoconstriction are accomplished in the same manner as that used for septoplasty. The inferior

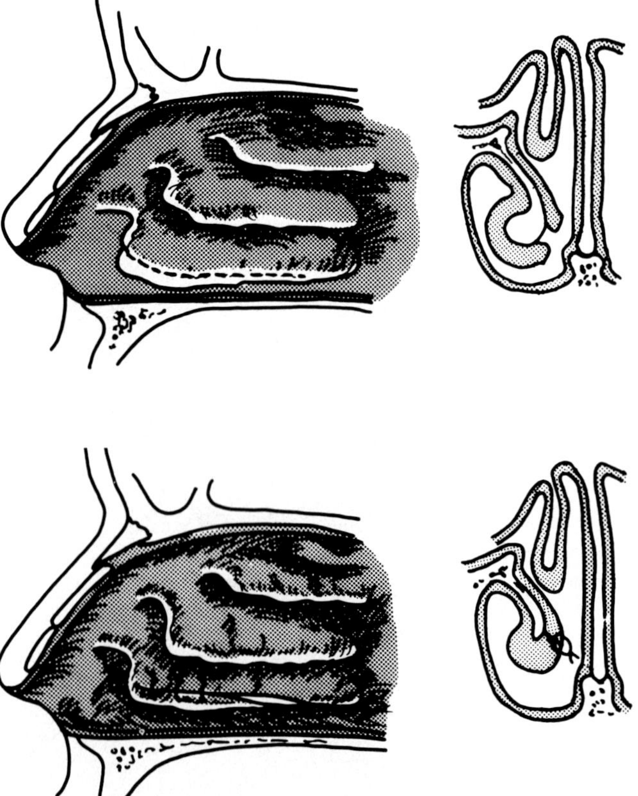

Figure 81–3 Technique of turbinoplasty for reduction of hypertrophied turbinates. The underlying bony concha is resected and the overlying mucosa trimmed and sutured.

turbinate is infractured medially for better exposure, and an incision is accomplished through the mucoperiosteum to bone along the anterior two-thirds of the inferior edge and the anterior edge of the turbinate. An elevator is used to dissect the mucoperiosteum from the medial and lateral surfaces of the bony concha. The obstructing underlying bony concha is resected, and the overlying mucosa is trimmed and sutured. The cut through the bony concha is beveled appropriately to remove preferentially the anterior portion of the inferior turbinate that obstructs the nasal valve area. Ointment-impregnated packs are placed and removed 24 hours postoperatively.

Turbinate resection is similar to turbinoplasty but includes removal of a portion of the diseased mucosa (Fig. 81–4). Most of the anterior portion of the turbinate is resected, leaving the posterior portion intact. Following turbinate resection, cryotherapy is accomplished. Reinforced Silastic sheets are shaped to approximate the nasal septum and are sutured together on each side of the septum. The Silastic sheets protect the septum from inadvertent freezing during the cryotherapy procedure that could lead to necrosis and subsequent perforation. The probe of the cryotherapy unit is applied to the cut surface of the resected inferior turbinate as well as to the mucosa overlying the superior aspect of the base of the turbinate. The cryotherapy probe is also applied to the medial surface of the middle turbinate. Particular care is taken to avoid application of the probe to the middle meatus, which contains the ostia of several paranasal sinuses. The freeze time for each area is 30 seconds. Ointment-impregnated gauze packs are placed and are removed 48 hours postoperatively.

Thus far, none of 56 patients that have undergone turbinate procedures with or without cryotherapy have experienced long-term nasal crusting, dryness, or any symptoms associated with atrophic rhinitis. Significant

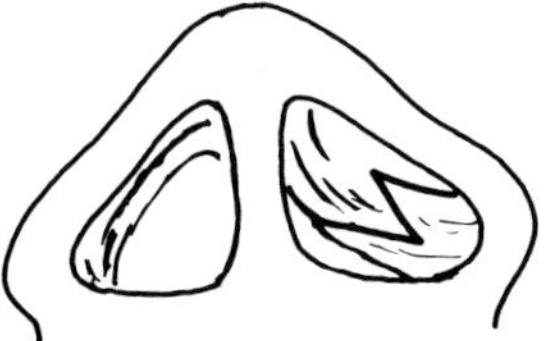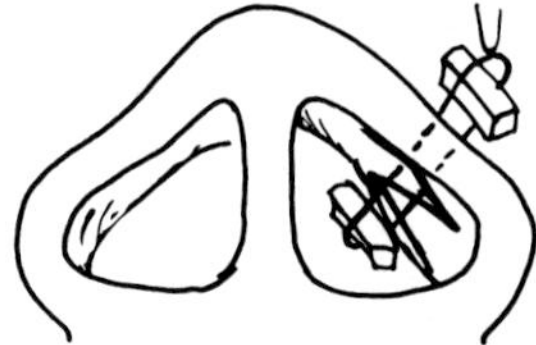

Figure 81–5 Z-plasty technique for correction of contracture in the lateral vestibule.

bleeding that required repacking was observed in three patients. The packing was eventually removed in all three without sequelae.

Cleft External Nasal Deformity

As stated, the relative contribution of the external cleft nasal deformity to nasal airway obstruction is incompletely understood. Conceptual and technical advances have been accomplished in both primary and secondary correction of the cleft nasal deformity for aesthetic reasons.[73] Little attention has been given to the external cleft nose as a modifier of nasal airflow. Presumably, as surgical advances allow the cleft nose to approach the aesthetic form of the noncleft nose, nasal airway function will also improve. Attention to surgical details must be the rule during primary lip repair and nasal reconstruction to ensure nasal airway function as well as the obvious aesthetic results.

Cleft Nasal Valve and Nasal Valve Area

In general, attention to surgical correction of the cartilaginous and bony septum components and turbinates that obstruct the nasal valve and nasal valve area has resulted in marked airway improvement in the majority of patients. Our experience with opening and widening the nasal valve angle by means of Gray's technique, which involves surgery of the upper lateral cartilages, is minimal in the cleft nose, although extensive in the noncleft nose.[74] We have utilized a Z-plasty technique with good success in eight cleft patients to correct the cutaneous bowstring contracture along the cephalic border of the lateral crus of the lower lateral cartilage from the apex of the vestibule to the lateral piriform aperture (Fig. 81–5).

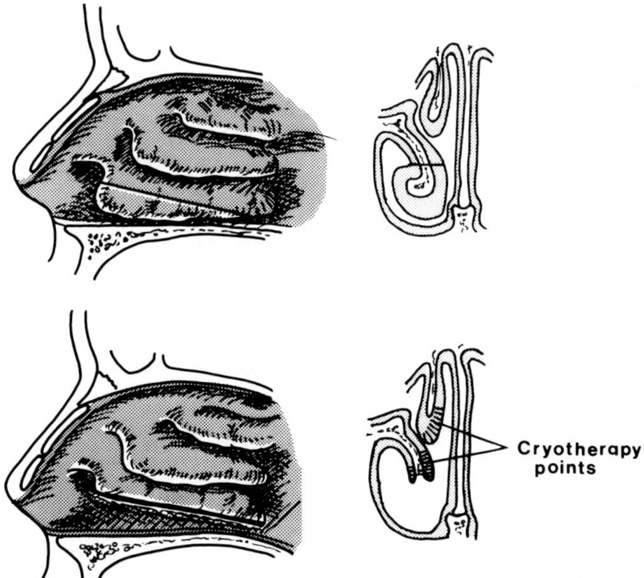

Figure 81–4 Technique of turbinate resection. Most of the anterior portion of the turbinate is resected, leaving the inferior portion intact.

References

1. Warren DW, Duany LF, Fisher WD: Nasal pathway resistance in normal and cleft lip and palate subjects. Cleft Palate J 6:134–140, 1969.
2. Warren DW, Trier WL, Bevin AG: Effect of restorative procedures on the nasopharyngeal airway in cleft palate. Cleft Palate J 4:367–373, 1974.
3. Warren DW: Aerodynamic studies of the upper airway—implications for growth, breathing and speech. In McNamara JA (ed): Nasorespiratory Function and Craniofacial Growth. Ann Arbor; University of Michigan, Center for Human Growth and Development, 1979, pp 41–86.
4. Turvey TA, Hall DJ, Warren DW: Alterations in nasal airway resistance from superior repositioning of the maxilla. Am J Orthod 85:109–120, 1984.
5. Proctor DF: The upper airways. Nasal physiology and defense of the lungs. Am Rev Respir Dis 115:97–129, 1977.
6. Abramson M, Harker LA: Physiology of the nose. Otolaryngol Clin North Am 6:623–635, 1973.
7. Hilger JA, Hilger PA: Physiology of the nose and paranasal sinuses. In Goldman JL (ed): The Principles and Practice of Rhinology. New York: Wiley, 1987.

8. Mygind N: Applied physiology of the nose. In Mygind N (ed): Nasal Allergy, 2nd ed. Oxford: Blackwell Scientific Publications, 1979.

9. Mecklenburg CV, Mercke U, Hakansson CH, et al; Morphological changes in ciliary cells due to heat exposure. Cell Tiss Res 148:45–56, 1974.

10. Mygind N, Bretlau P, Sorensen H: Scanning electron microscopic studies of nasal polyps. Acta Otolaryngol (Stockholm) 78:436–443, 1974.

11. Drettner B: Pathophysiological relationship between upper and lower airways. Ann Otolaryngol 79:499–505, 1970.

12. Settipane GA (ed): Rhinitis. Providence. NER Allergy Proceedings, 1984.

13. Settipane GA: Rhino-sino-bronchial reflex. Immunol Allergy Prac 7(12):29–32, 1985.

14. Olsen KD: Sleep and breathing disturbance secondary to nasal obstruction. Otolaryngol Head Neck Surg 89:804–810, 1981.

15. Ogura JH, Nelson JR, Dammkoehler R, et al: Experimental observations of the relationships between upper airway obstruction and pulmonary function. Trans Am Laryngol Assoc 85:40–64, 1964.

16. Ogura JH, Togawa K, Dammkoehler K, et al: Nasal obstruction and the mechanics of breathing. Physiologic relationship and effects of nasal surgery. Arch Otolaryngol 83:135–150, 1966.

17. Ogura JH, Unno T, Nelson JR: Nasal surgery. Physiological considerations of nasal obstruction. Arch Otolaryngol 88:288–295, 1968.

18. Slavin RG: Relationship of nasal disease and sinusitis to bronchial asthma. Ann Allergy 49:76–79, 1982.

19. Rachelefsky G, Siegel S, Katz R: Chronic sinus disease with associated induced reactive airways disease in children. J Allergy Clin Immunol 71(Pt 2):156, 1983 (abstract).

20. Slavin RG, Linford PA, Friedman WH: Sphenoethmoidectomy (SE) in the treatment of nasal polyps, sinusitis and bronchial asthma. J Allergy Clin Immunol 71 (Pt 2): 156, 1983 (abstract).

21. Friedman R, Ackerman M, Wald E, et al: Bacterial sinusitis exacerbating asthma. J Allergy Clin Immunol 71 (Pt 2): 155, 1983 (abstract).

22. Crockett DM. Unpublished data.

23. Wyllie JW, III, Kern EB, O'Brien PC, et al: Alteration of pulmonary function associated with artificial nasal obstruction. Surg Forum 27:535–537, 1976.

24. Jacobs JR, Levine LA, Davis H, et al: Posterior packs and the nasopulmonary reflex. Laryngoscope 91:279–283, 1981.

25. Linder-Aronsen S: Naso-respiratory function and craniofacial growth. In McNamara JA (ed): Nasorespiratory Function and Craniofacial Growth. Ann Arbor: University of Michigan, Center for Human Growth and Development, 1979, pp 121–147.

26. Ricketts RM: Respiratory obstruction syndrome. Am J Orthod 54:495–507, 1968.

27. Linder-Aronsen S: Effects of adenoidectomy on the dentition and facial skeleton over a period of five years. Trans Eur Orthod Soc 1973, pp 177–187.

28. Quinn GW: Airway interference and its effect upon the growth and development of the face, jaws, dentition and associated parts. NC Dent J 60:28–31, 1978.

29. Quinn GW: Are dentofacial deformities a preventable disease? NC Dent J 61:5, 1978.

30. Schulhof RJ: Consideration of airway in orthodontics. J Clin Orthod 12:440, 1978.

31. Linder-Aronsen S: Adenoids: Their effect on mode of breathing and nasal airflow and their relationship to characteristics of the facial skeleton and the dentition. Acta Otolaryngol Suppl 265:1–24, 1979.

32. Ricketts RM: An early treatment, Part I.J.C.O. interviews. J Clin Orthod 13:23–28, 1979.

33. Rubin RM: Mode of respiration and facial growth. Am J Orthod 78:505–517, 1980.

34. Harold EP: Neuromuscular and morphological adaptations in experimentally induced oral respiration. In McNamara JA (ed): Nasorespiratory Function and Craniofacial Growth. Ann Arbor: University of Michigan, Center for Human Growth and Development, 1979, pp 149–164.

35. Watson RM, Warren DW, Fisher ND: Nasal resistance, skeletal classification and mouth breathing in orthodontic patients. Am J Orthod 54:367–379, 1968.

36. Vig PS, Sarver DM, Hall DJ, et al: Quantitative evaluation of nasal airflow in relation to facial morphology. Am J Orthod 79:263, 1981.

37. Hairfield WM, Warren DM, Hinton VA, et al: Inspiratory and expiratory effects of nasal breathing. Cleft Palate J 24:183–189, 1987.

38. Bardach J, Mooney MP: The relationship between lip pressure following lip repair and craniofacial growth in beagles. Plast Reconstr Surg 73:544–555, 1984.

39. Bardach J, Bakowska J, McDermott-Murray J, et al: Lip pressure changes following lip repair in infants with unilateral clefts of the lip and palate. Plast Reconstr Surg 74:476–479, 1984.

40. Bardach J, Roberts DM, Klausner EC: Influence of two-flap palatoplasty on facial growth in rabbits. Cleft Palate J 16:402–411, 1979.

41. Bardach J, Mooney M, Bardach E: The influence of palatoplasty on facial growth in beagles. Plast Reconstr Surg 69:927–936, 1982.

42. Bluestone CD: The role of tonsils and adenoids in the obstruction of respiration. In McNamara JA (ed): Nasorespiratory Function and Craniofacial Growth. Ann Arbor: University of Michigan, Center for Human Growth and Development, 1979, pp 251–273.

43. Yonkers AJ, Spaur RC: Airway obstruction and pharyngeal lymphoid tissue. Otolaryngol Clin North Am 20:235–239, 1987.

44. Healy GB: Personal communication.

45. Crockett DM: Unpublished data.

46. Mertz JM, McCaffrey TV, Kern EB: Objective evaluation of anterior septal reconstruction. Otolaryngol Head Neck Surg 92:308–311, 1984.

47. Hagy GW, Settipane GA: Bronchial asthma, allergic rhinitis and allergy skin tests among college students. J Allergy 44:323, 1969.

48. Bumsted RM: Unpublished data.

49. Nalebuff DJ: Allergic rhinitis. In Cummings CW, et al (eds): Otolaryngology—Head and Neck Surgery. St. Louis: C.V. Mosby, 1986.

50. Mullarkey MF, Hill JS, Webb DR: Allergic and nonallergic rhinitis: Their characterization with attention to the meaning of nasal eosinophilia. J Allergy Clin Immunol 65:122–129, 1980.

51. Nalebuff DJ, Fadal RG, Ali M: The study of IgE in the diagnosis of allergic disorders in an otolaryngology practice. Otolaryngol Head Neck Surg 87:351, 1979.

52. Goldman JL: Vasomotor rhinitis and sinusitis. In Goldman JL (ed): The Principles and Practice of Rhinology. New York: Wiley, 1987.

53. Goode RL: Diagnosis and treatment of turbinate dysfunction. Acad Otolaryngol, 1977.

54. McCaffrey TV, Kern EB: Clinical evaluation of nasal obstruction: A study of 1000 patients. Arch Otolaryngol 105:542–545, 1979.

55. Pallanch JF, McCaffrey TV, Kern EB: Normal nasal resistance. Otolaryngol Head and Neck Surg 93:778–785, 1985.

56. McCaffrey, TV, Kern EB: Rhinomanometry. In Mackay I (ed): Facial Plastic Surgery, Rhinoplasty and Airway, New York: G. Thieme, 1986, pp 217–223.

57. Santiago-Diez de Bonilla J, McCaffrey TV, Kern EB: Normal nasal resistance. Ann Otol Rhinol Laryngol 95:229–232, 1986.

58. Beeson WH: The nasal septum. Otolaryngol Clin North Am 20:743–767, 1987.

59. Bridger GP: Physiology of the nasal valve. Arch Otolaryngol 92:543–553, 1970.

60. Haight JSJ, Cole P: The site and function of the nasal valve. Laryngoscope 9:349–355, 1983.

61. Kasperbauer JL, Kern EB: Nasal valve physiology. Implications in nasal surgery. Otolaryngol Clin North Am 20:699–719, 1987.

62. Crockett DM, Bumsted RM, Bardach J. Unpublished data.

63. Hasaqawa M, Kern EB: The human nasal cycle. Mayo Clin Proc 52:28, 1977.

64. Masing H: Experimentelle Untersuchungen über die Stromung im Nasenmodell. Arch Klin Exp Ohren Nasen Kehlkopfheilk 189:59–70, 1967.

65. Hinderer KH: Surgery of the valve. Int Rhinol 8:60–67, 1970.

66. Cottle MH, Loving RM, Fisher GG, et al: The "maxilla-premaxilla" approach to extensive nasal septum surgery. Arch Otolaryngol 60:301–313, 1958.

67. Bardach J, Salyer KE: Surgical Techniques in Cleft Lip and Palate. Chicago: Year Book, 1987.

68. Rees TD: Aesthetic Plastic Surgery. Vol. I. Philadelphia: Saunders, 1980, p 315.

69. Courtiss, EH, Goldwyn RM, O'Brien JJ: Resection of obstructing inferior turbinates. Plast Reconstr Surg 62:249–257, 1978.

70. Mabry RL: Inferior turbinoplasty. Laryngoscope 92:459–461, 1982.

71. Martinez SA, Nissen AJ, Stock CR, et al: Nasal turbinate resection for relief of nasal obstruction. Laryngoscope 93:871–875, 1983.

72. Bumsted RM: Cryotherapy for chronic vasomotor rhinitis: Technique and patient selection for improved results. Laryngoscope 94:539–544, 1984.

73. Salyer KE: Primary correction of the unilateral cleft lip nose: A 15-year experience. Plast Reconstr Surg 77:558–569, 1986.

74. Gray VD: Physiologic returning of the upper lateral cartilage. Int Rhinol 8:56–59, 1970.

CHAPTER 82

The Importance of Nasal Airways in Cleft Patients

Peter Oblak

Our actions in everyday life depend to a great extent on our basic views of the world and the events in it. Only to a certain degree are we aware of these views. To a greater extent, they can be discerned in our behavior and actions. The same fact applies to our professional work. Basic views in a profession are a result of our upbringing more than of our own experiences and comprehension. In the field of medicine this fact is obvious from its own history.

Treatment of clefts is no exception to the rule. In our early treatment of patients we are constantly guided by our basic views of cleft characteristics, of mechanisms regulating their growth and development of the affected areas, and by basic views of the influence of therapeutic procedures on growth and development. These views have been imparted to us and adopted by us during the years of our professional education, and we firmly believe in them, although often not with full awareness. In our later work we usually try to use our experiences to confirm the accuracy of our basic views rather than change and adjust them to new findings.

Progress in the treatment of clefts lies, however, in the elucidation of basic views, adoption of the correct ones, and the conscious transfer of these views into daily routines. It is even more difficult to master and adopt the evolving basic views than it is to pursue them. A basic view is like an old habit—an armor narrowing and limiting us in our actions.

Clefts of lip, alveolus, and palate are looked on as clefts of the oral cavity. Our goal in the early treatment of patients is to reconstruct a functionally and anatomically perfect oral cavity to give the face a normal appearance. We also try to shape the nose adequately, usually neglecting to bear in mind the importance of the nasal cavity as a functional space. It is, in fact, handicapped more than the oral cavity. Typical deformation of cleft-affected areas in some cleft forms is a result of intrauterine functional adaptation of the cleft oral cavity to the nasal cavity.[1]

In reconstruction and functional restoration of the oral cavity after birth, we try to take into consideration its relatively well known and complicated activities as well as its less recognized role in facial development. In reconstruction of the nasal cavity we do not give enough consideration to two extremely important facts:

1. The nasal cavity is a very important and complex component of the respiratory tract.

2. The cleft nasal cavity is typically deformed at the time of birth, depending on the cleft form.

The Complex Role of the Nasal Cavity

Air passes from the environment into the lungs through the airway. The anatomic structure and physiologic significance of the airway are well known. The classic physiology book, Samson Wright's *Applied Physiology*,[2] states that during breathing, air enters the lungs through the nose and mouth. This is a generalized statement covering all manner of breathing.

Nasal breathing is characteristic of quiet respiration. Nearly 5000 years have passed since this characteristic was described in the Memphis theologic tractate as one of the first written observations on the functions of the human body.[3] Quiet nasal respiration appears to be taken for granted as an inborn premise required for olfaction and undisturbed use of the oral cavity for digestive purposes. This endowment, however, is not unconditional. It has its own developmental path with both objective and subjective causes of diversity. The most notable diversity is quiet oral respiration.

The pharynx as an air switch is shared by the digestive tract and the airway. A number of mechanisms are required to make possible its alternate uses for breathing and feeding. The epiglottis closes the airway in the laryngeal part of the pharynx every time a bolus passes into the esophagus. In the oral part, the closed oral cavity directs airflow through the nose. Movements of the thorax and diaphragm result in the passage of air along the airway. The rhythm of respiratory movements is regulated by the respiratory centers, namely, their inspiratory, expiratory, and apneustic components located in the central nervous system. The respiratory centers base their programmed activity on individual airway specifications as well as factors well known in physiology. Duration of a particular phase of respiration is also affected by established and quantitatively defined physical airway properties. The most important among these are airflow resistance and turbulence capacity.

Airflow resistance depends on the length and diameter of the airway. Resistance is modified by the moving parts narrowing or widening their respective segments. Vocal cords can change the diameter of the lower airway; the pharyngeal constrictors, tongue, and soft palate perform the same function in its middle and upper regions; and the nasal valve does the same at the end (or beginning) of the nasal airway. Airflow resistance is further influenced by widening and narrowing of the airway lumen due to mucosal congestion and decongestion.[4]

Air turbulence increases the airway airflow resistance and causes air to stand still in regions of turbulence. Turbulence and stagnation of air along the airway allow for moistening, warming, and cleansing of the inspired air and for perception of its scent. Turbulence intensity depends on lengths of straight airway as opposed to the curved parts of the airway, on the shape of its surface, and on the volume rate of airflow. Air turbulence is emphasized more at the airway curves. It is increased by the rugged surface of the nasal cavity and its turbinates and, as a rule, is increased above a given surface by an increased volume rate of airflow in deeper breathing.

Duration of the inspiratory, expiratory, and apneic phases of a respiratory cycle can be correlated with the described physical properties of the upper airway when other known factors of breathing are accounted for. The programmed individual respiratory rhythm of quiet breathing, once established, can be observed in a respirator-treated patient, whose respiratory centers must be depressed if the respiratory rhythm differs from the one enforced.

Quiet nasal respiration is, therefore, a part of the adopted individual respiratory program. The program is based on the individual's established needs. It functions through several feedback mechanisms and controls any changes without conscious support. Changes arising outside the adaptational frame request conscious support of quiet respiration, thus causing discomfort. For instance, should the nasal cavity become entirely or partially obstructed, the oral cavity must be used in respiration, leading to unease of the individual accustomed to nasal respiration.

The essential condition of quiet nasal respiration is the airtightness of the oral cavity. An experiment showed that nasal airflow is significantly reduced by the mouth being held open, even a little.[5] The airtightness of the anatomically well-built oral cavity is maintained by the correct resting posture of the oral cavity and the resultant negative air pressure. Correct resting posture of the oral cavity is characterized by a balanced posture of otherwise antagonistic muscles enclosing and filling the oral cavity as well as by those opening, closing, and moving it laterally.[6–8]

The correct resting posture of the airtight, closed oral cavity, directing air through the nose (Fig. 82–1), can be distinctly discerned in a sleeping newborn[9] and even in a cross-section of a newborn.[10] The newborn's oral cavity takes up much more than the third of a proportionally developed face it occupies in adulthood. Muscles of the oral cavity are much better developed at

birth compared with the other skeletal muscles[11] owing to the intensive pumping of amniotic fluid that occurs during the fetal period.[1] The newborn's little nose does not yet take up the whole middle third of the face as it does in the properly developed face of an adult. The nasal cavity does not take part in the intrauterine transplacental gas exchange, yet it is a channel through which respiratory movements of the thorax and diaphragm drive the inspired amniotic fluid, mixed with the expired lung secretion, back to the amniotic cavity.

Respiratory movements appear very early in fetal life and play a significant role in differentiation and maturation of the lung tissue,[13] at the same time training the respiratory system for its postnatal functions. Prenatal assay of lung functional maturity is based on analysis of amniotic fluid ingredients of lung origin. Since digestive flow through the oral cavity is strictly unidirectional,[14] it seems highly probable that in the healthy fetus, fluid driven by respiratory movements of the thorax and diaphragm into the lungs and back into the amniotic cavity flows through the nose. One can therefore conclude that the separation of functions of the airway and digestive tract has already taken place before birth.

A healthy child thus is born with a neuromuscular pattern of the correct oral cavity posture that secures quiet nasal respiration. It can be stated that the child is born with a habit of quiet nasal respiration with the mouth shut. Three consequences should be noted:

1. Air enters lung by the nose, whose role as an airway section is obvious and has already been described.
2. The oral cavity is always at disposal for digestive purposes.
3. The habit of quiet nasal respiration with the correct resting posture of the oral cavity supports the proper function of the growth and development mechanisms of the facial areas pertaining to the nasal and oral cavities.

It was stated at the beginning of this chapter that nasal breathing, along with other physiologic facts, gives the impression of an inborn premise; therefore, the correctness of such respiration is never denied. Nobody denies the other fact that food can only be chewed well with simultaneous nasal breathing. Opinions on the third consequence of nasal breathing differ significantly.

Numerous researchers have recently become aware of the great importance of the oral cavity posture in facial development, demonstrating the importance of nasal breathing.[15–20] Nasal breathing alone renders possible the correct oral cavity posture, and consequently the correct growth and development of the middle and lower thirds of the face. Such breathing only makes the correct oral cavity posture possible but does not ensure it.

Oral cavity posture can differ greatly despite nasal breathing.[21] Both quiet nasal breathing that is possible only with the mouth shut and the correct resting posture of the oral cavity in the child's growth and development are encouraged by nature in the newborn. A newborn with bilateral choanal atresia is imperiled by acute suffocation.[22] Bilateral nasal obstruction from trivial upper respiratory infection in the small sleeping infant who does not instinctively or voluntarily breathe

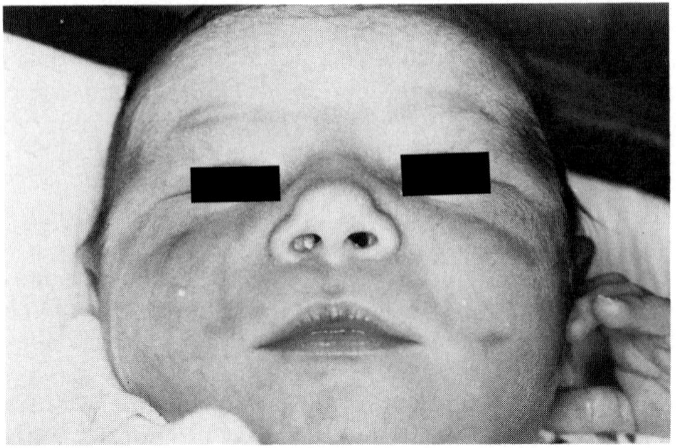

Figure 82–1 Normal newborn breathing quietly through the nose with the mouth shut.

through the mouth is a significant factor in sudden unexpected death of infancy.[23] The infant opens the mouth and uses it for breathing only when crying, which is certainly not an eupneic condition. Interestingly, no noteworthy problem is caused by unilateral choanal atresia.[24]

The behavior of the newborn with complete bilateral choanal atresia seems to contradict the intrauterine establishment of the airway described before. It is obvious, though, that nature, in its pursuit of individual survival, employs other solutions beside the customary ones. Clefts of the lip, alveolus, and palate present an example.

Nasal Cavity in Newborns with Clefts

Clefts of the lip and palate almost inevitably affect the nasal cavity; cleft forms affecting only the lip or uvula are an exception to the rule. The nasal cavity is affected at birth in different ways that share a common denominator: functional adaptation of the cleft nasal cavity to efficient pumping of amniotic fluid by the oral cavity. Deformity in various cleft forms originates morphogenetically from this adaptation.[1] Morphogenesis of the cleft confirms the theory that the active morphogenetic factor is a function of a space and whatever characterizes it.[25] This factor is predominantly musculature in the case of the oral cavity[26] and not skeletal structures with intrinsic growth forces,[27, 28] as was earlier suggested.[29, 30]

In the cleft palate, the tongue functions and rests in the oral cavity in destroyed balance with the surrounding musculature, exerting great influence on the oral cavity, which is fused with the nasal cavity. The nasal cavity responds only to mechanical stimulation. The purpose of the transformation of the nasal cavity in a cleft is its sealing. In a sealed nasal cavity, amniotic fluid cannot flow from the oral cavity through the nose back to the amniotic cavity instead of into the digestive tract. Should that happen, the peroral nutrition of the fetus would be ineffective, impairing functional development of the fetal digestive system and imperiling its survival after birth.[1]

The nasal cavity deformity consequently depends on the form and extent of the cleft. Especially important for treatment are the facts that (1) at birth, the nasal and oral cavities are fused into a functional entity of the oral cavity, and (2) the nasal cavity, as an airway, is sealed.

Careful observation of the nasal cavity immediately after the birth of a cleft infant provides a means of diagnosing some of the basic types of its transformation. The nasal cavity on the noncleft side in an infant with a unilateral complete cleft is obstructed by a compressed septum in the hard palate region and oblique columella at the cavity entrance. The cleft nasal cavity is functionally a part of the oral cavity with a common orifice. The airway is not separated at birth. A newborn breathes through the upper part of the functional oral cavity (Fig. 82–2). The nasal cavity in a baby with a unilateral

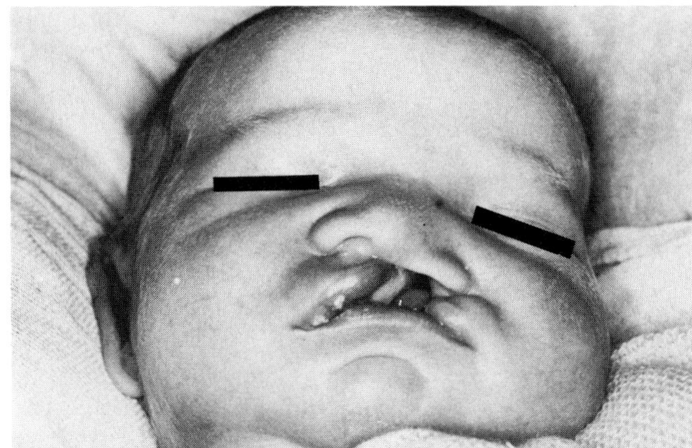

Figure 82–2 Newborn with complete unilateral cleft lip, alveolus, and palate breathing through the common oronasal cavity. Nasal cavity of the unaffected side is sealed. Resting mouth posture is correct.

complete cleft with a Simonart's band is obstructed at birth just as is that without a band. The difference is that the band fits the nostril of the affected side tightly, closing the opening above it that could possibly cause functional disturbances (Fig. 82–3).

The shape of the nasal cavity is different in infants with a complete bilateral cleft. The nasal cavity in the symmetric form is sealed by the premaxilla positioned in the middle and protruded. The nostrils lean against it tightly with the mobile part of the nasal valve. The functional oral cavity, consisting of the anatomic oral and both nasal cavities, is closed by the lateral parts of the lip on the sides and the premaxilla in the middle, compensating for the missing middle part of the lip (Fig. 82–4). The septum is straight, and the nasal cavity is deep, spacious, and sealed at the entrance (Fig. 82–5).

The asymmetric bilateral cleft more or less resembles the unilateral complete cleft in functional compensation (Fig. 82–6). One side of the nasal cavity is not incorporated into the functional entity of the oral cavity and is closed by the premaxilla. The nasal septum is pushed

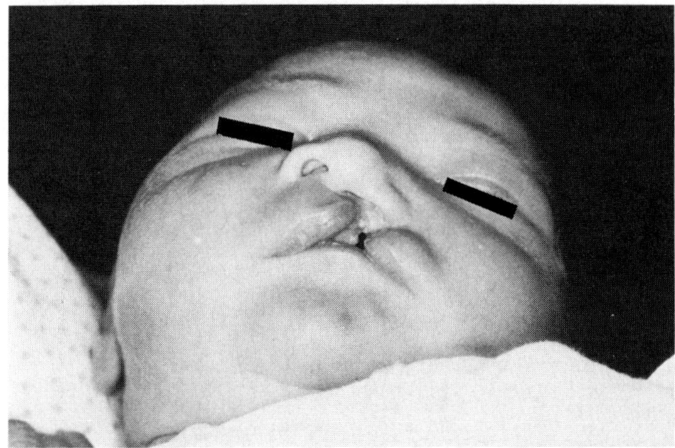

Figure 82–3 Newborn with complete unilateral cleft with a Simonart's band. Exceptionally small orifice suffices for quiet breathing through the common oronasal cavity. Nasal cavity of the unaffected side is sealed. Resting mouth posture is correct.

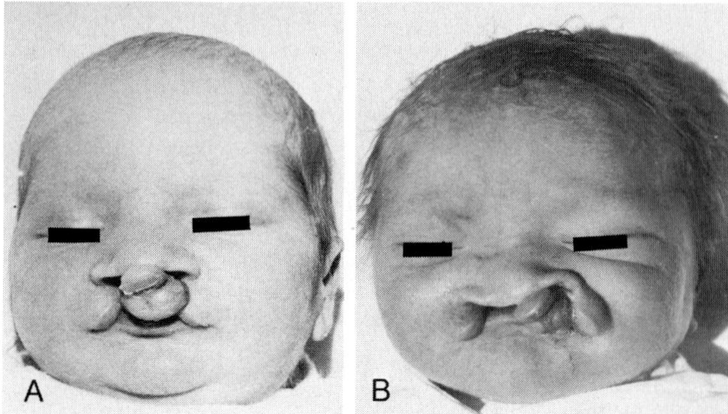

Figure 82–4 Two newborns with different types of complete bilateral clefts. *A*, Symmetric bilateral cleft lip, alveolus, and palate. Nasal cavity is sealed at the entrance by the nasal valves. The infant breathes through the opening on the right side. Resting mouth posture is correct. *B*, Asymmetric bilateral cleft lip, alveolus, and palate. Premaxilla and prolabium are shifted to the left. Resting mouth posture is correct. The child breathes through the common oronasal opening. Nasal cavity of the left side is blocked.

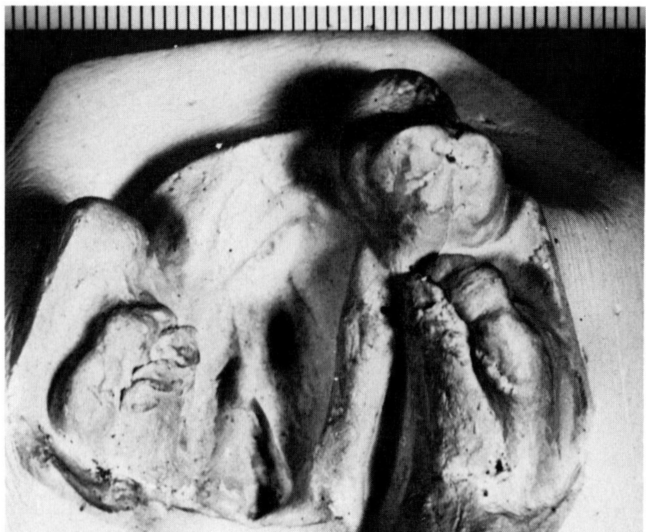

Figure 82–6 Nasal cavity in the complete asymmetric bilateral cleft lip, alveolus, and palate. Septum and premaxilla are shifted to the left, blocking the left nasal cavity (same child shown in Fig. 82–4).

aside. The open side is fused into the space of the oral cavity. Models and photographs of 89 infants with complete bilateral clefts without operation, taken immediately after birth or in the first months following, were examined by the author. Symmetric compensation of the first form was found in 40 patients, and lateral compensation of the second form was found in 49. Twenty of the latter functionally resembled the right complete unilateral cleft, and 29 resembled the left unilateral cleft. A thin skin band appeared in some cases, usually on the closed side.

In clefts of the palate, the nasal cavity can be seen on models only partially, if at all. The ability to see the nasal cavity depends on the extent of the cleft. The patency and shape of the nasal cavity in clefts that extend only into the soft palate do not differ much from

patency and shape in healthy children because the oral cavity is sealed by the soft wings of the cleft palate. The situation is different in clefts that extend into the hard palate. In these, the nasal cavity is compressed from the oral side. The palate has a higher arch than it does in healthy children,[1] and patency of the nasal cavity is reduced by the enlarged nasal turbinates. These can sometimes be seen in the cleft palate or on a model of this part of the oral cavity, and sometimes they can be palpated when the patency of the nasal cavity is tested on the operating table.

In other cleft forms it is also apparent how function in the intrauterine period adapts the shape of the cleft for greater efficiency in the described ways. Compensation is most difficult in the bilateral cleft in which skeletal continuity in the alveolar ridge is preserved.

Following birth, children with complete unilateral or bilateral clefts breathe through the functional oral cavity. Since the airway leads through the upper part of the functional oral cavity, which anatomically represents the nasal cavity, the newborn breathes at least partially through the cleft nasal cavity. The air and food entrances are one, at least in the first moments after birth. It is the opening into the functional oral cavity. An exceptionally small opening is sufficient for quiet breathing (Fig. 82–3). Further development of a separated respiratory opening and airway depends on the cleft form and method of treatment.

The sealed nasal cavity in patients with a complete unilateral cleft starts opening on the unaffected side in the first month after birth. Its patency at first, however, is not yet sufficient even for quiet breathing. Obstruction of the common oronasal orifice on the cleft side provokes respiratory crisis in the infant. This occurs mainly in infants with complete bilateral clefts, which are laterally compensated as described above. In centrally compensated symmetric complete bilateral clefts, a closed nasal valve opens enough soon after birth to

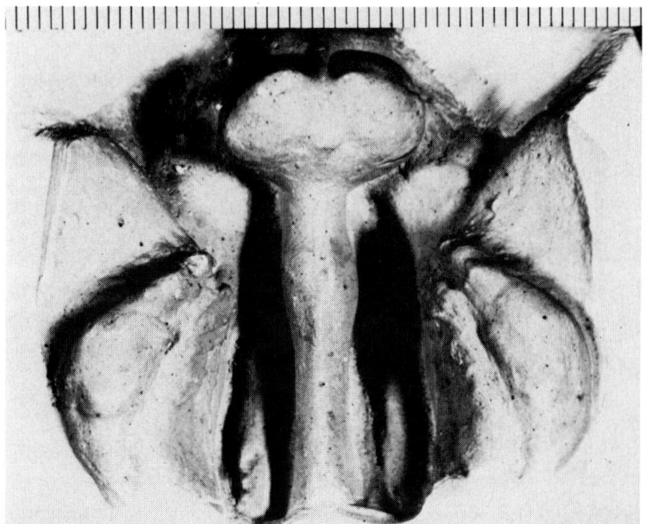

Figure 82–5 Nasal cavity in complete symmetric bilateral cleft with a protruded premaxilla (plaster model). Nasal cavity is deep, spacious, and sealed at the entrance by the nasal ala.

allow quiet nasal breathing. Although infants with clefts actually breathe through the functional oral cavity, the airway runs in such a way that it does not exert any influence on the correct resting posture of the oral cavity.

Taking into account the special importance of a correct resting posture of the oral cavity in proper facial growth and development, it could be stated that the oral and nasal cavities develop correctly. Unless treatment interferes with the further course of events, the middle and lower thirds of the face develop relatively harmoniously, a fact known from analyses of adults without operation. The position of the premaxilla in bilateral clefts is an exception, because it remains functionally a part of the upper lip, not of the alveolar ridge. Thus, its position after birth is constantly aggravated by growth of the oral cavity.

In accordance with the concept of programmed respiratory rhythm, property parameters of the infant's virtual airway through the fused oral and nasal cavities are entered into the program. This programmed rhythm can be noticed from the infant's reactions when the airway entrance is experimentally obstructed. The infant does not open his mouth to mouth breathe quietly but struggles instead against the changes enforced, trying to retain the conditions he is accustomed to.

Risks in Cleft Treatment

Treatment begins soon after birth. Although there is stress on the functional restitution of the cleft region, this is often secondary to formative restitution. Use of an active, preoperative, maxillary orthopedic device attempts to reform the alveolar ridges into a more proper position, whereas a plate made for this purpose often obstructs the nasal cavity, through which the airway could be, or even has been already, established. Because of its construction it can even change the established correct oral cavity posture by pushing the jaws apart. If too wide, the strapping can impair nasal breathing. A passive plate with retention stretching inside the nasal cavity can obstruct or stop the airway through the cleft nasal cavity as well.

Some references not quoted include several figures that clearly show that the authors, their well-intentioned zeal undisputed, have concentrated solely on the function and form of the oral cavity. It is clear, however, that the "treated" nose-breathing infant will eventually become a mouthbreather despite the marked initial discomfort. It is fortunate that an infant can be compelled to carry a plate only with great difficulty because it is not to its liking. Mothers know this better than doctors.

In the past, in particular the German surgeons (Axhausen, Wassmund, Schuchardt) and their successors advocated the simultaneous repair of the lip and alveolus (up to the incisive foramen) at the age of about six months. It was my experience[31] that in most cases the closure of the alveolar ridge at that time stopped the airflow through the clefted nasal cavity. When the lip

repair was performed, the entrance in the unaffected nasal cavity was widened, but the patency was not improved because of the deviated septum in the region of the hard palate. The result was mouth breathing, with all its consequences for further growth and development. In cases of seemingly more extensive anomaly, in which in addition to the unilateral complete cleft the hard palate was clefted on both sides, the effect of closing the alveolar ridge was not detrimental. After straightening the columella during the lip repair, the airway on the nonclefted side was opened widely. I have had a patient with this problem, who grew and developed well after this treatment. The treatment has been successful even with a more extensive anomaly, as is found in a unilateral complete cleft.

Patency of the established nasal airway is gravely impaired by closure of the cleft in the hard palate region. Due to the characteristic differences in nasal cavity shape, this risk is more imminent in children with complete unilateral clefts and in those with isolated clefts of the palate than in those with complete bilateral clefts. Airway patency is significantly changed by tissue mobilization. The initial discomfort then compels the infant to open its mouth, with all consequences for further growth and development. In the child with a complete unilateral cleft, such a possibility is more likely if the nasal cavity is insufficiently patent on the unaffected side.

In two-stage palatoplasty, closure of the most problematic region can be postponed until a later time, when nasal airway patency is increased. However, this brings about the possibility and risk of different airway courses and different oral cavity postures. The first and only proper possibility is for air to enter through the nose with the mouth shut, flowing along the partially separated nasal cavity. The second possibility is for air to enter through the nose, although the airway leads through the remaining opening in the hard palate into the oral cavity and through the oropharynx. The third possibility is breathing through the open mouth and the remaining opening in the hard palate through the nasopharynx. The airflow is stopped at the oropharynx if the tongue touches the soft palate. The fourth possibility, which is the worst, is for air to enter exclusively through the oral cavity. Ascertaining the actual course of the upper airway in an infant is difficult except in the fourth case. It is a fact that the width of the cleft in the hard palate in infants can differ greatly during growth and development.

Fundamental Principles of Correct Treatment

Proper nasal cavity reconstruction and adoption of quiet nasal breathing as well as proper oral cavity reconstruction and adoption of its correct resting posture are fundamental conditions of normal growth and development of the oral and nasal cavities and the associated facial parts. The aim of treatment, therefore, is reconstruction of the cleft cavities to support adoption of the required proper habits or their preservation should they already have been adopted.[33] Taking into account the mutual interdependence of both cavities on the one hand and the described habits on the other is of fundamental importance in successful treatment. The correct resting posture of the oral cavity is only possible as a habit when it is associated with the adopted habit of quiet nasal breathing. Quiet nasal breathing, again, can only take place when the mouth is shut tightly, a characteristic of the correct posture of the oral cavity.

The concept, required conditions, and significance of quiet nasal breathing were defined earlier in this discussion. These were only briefly mentioned because more detailed descriptions exceed the scope of this chapter. It is rather curious that clefts are typically omitted when mechanisms of growth and development (so important in the formation and treatment of dentofacial anomalies) are being researched or discussed. It seems as if different rules were followed in cleft phenomena. However, it is the very observation of cleft phenomena, particularly morphogenesis and treatment effects, that provides valuable insight into the general rules. That is, findings about the growth and development of cleft-related regions and their dependence on treatment procedures provide important information about the theories of general growth and development mechanisms so eagerly sought by researchers.

It has been mentioned in the preceding paragraphs that the duration of a respiratory rhythm phase is also correlated with the physical properties of the airway. This probably poses the biggest difficulty in the early treatment of clefts: how to close the oral cavity airtight and change only the airway's physical properties to which quiet nasal breathing has been adapted within the permissible tolerance.

In patients with extensive clefts in which the entire nasal cavity, or a large part of it, is fused with the oral cavity, complete reconstruction of the nasal and oral cavities in compliance with the demands postulated may not be feasible owing to habits inborn or adopted immediately after birth. Depending on the cleft form, separation of the nasal cavity from the oral cavity, in most cases, can be performed only gradually to meet the stated demands.

In infants with a complete unilateral cleft, the first means of separation can be an acrylic plate. If the plate is made correctly, the airway through both nasal cavities develops underneath it during the first months after birth. The cleft nasal cavity is deepened by straightening the compressed septa, thereby making the unaffected side of the nasal cavity patent also. Shifting the anterior part of the alveolar ridge causes the obstructed nasal entrance of the unaffected side to open as well (Fig. 82–7). Without the plate, conditions remain unchanged after birth in spite of growth-enlarged structures (Fig. 82–8).[34] The infant not only acquires a chance to breathe nasally but also the habit of quiet nasal breathing. Permanence of this habit is, however, uncertain. It depends primarily, although not entirely, on further surgical treatment.

The different course of growth and development in two patients with the same type of cleft and the same treatment procedure but a different way of breathing is shown in Figures 82–9 and 82–10. The successful patient has been a 100% nasal breather from birth with the correct adopted posture of the oral cavity. The unsuccessfully treated child, now an adult, was a mouth breather all the time. In spite of identical surgical treatment, he never adopted nasal breathing and, therewith, the correct oral cavity posture.[35]

Conclusion

It is a common practice when evaluating the results of a treatment to try to establish a link between the results and the type of orthopedic plate or incision used in the cutaneous or mucosal cleft region. The sequence of procedures and the age of the operated infant are taken into account as well. A method (a distinct plate, eponymic incision, or defined sequence) is only useful and can be successful only insofar as it meets the demands cited. It should be borne in mind that any given method has only two alternatives: it either meets the demands and supports proper growth and development, or it does not meet them and does not allow proper growth and development. Unfortunately, no method currently used can vouch for proper growth and development.

Growth and development of cleft-affected regions depend primarily on the infant's habits, which lead into either the proper course of development or the improper one. A successful method of treatment must

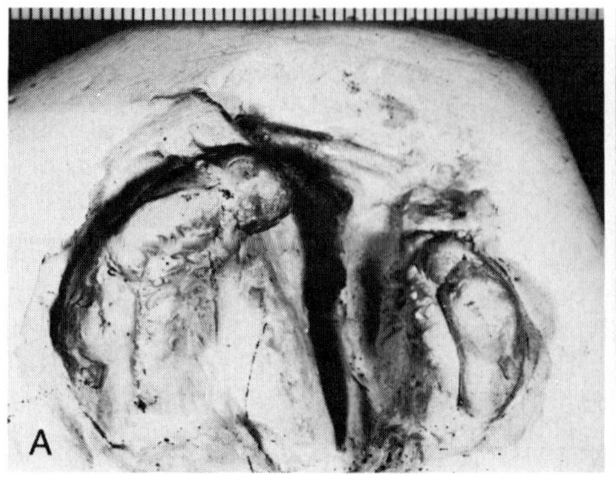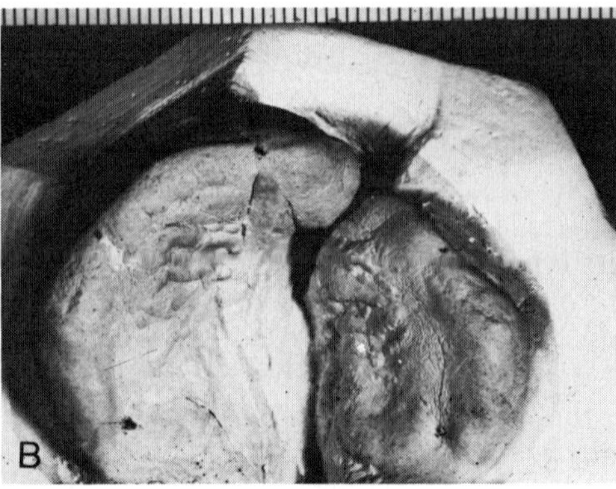

Figure 82–7 Complete unilateral cleft lip, alveolus, and palate. *A,* Note distance between maxillary segments and wide opening of the nasal cavity. *B,* Same patient at 6 months of age after surgical maxillary orthopedics. Note changes in the alveolar ridges and approximation of maxillary segments with partial sealing of the nasal cavity.

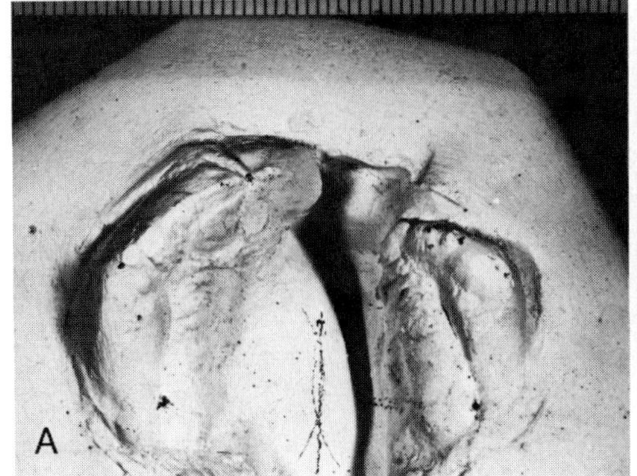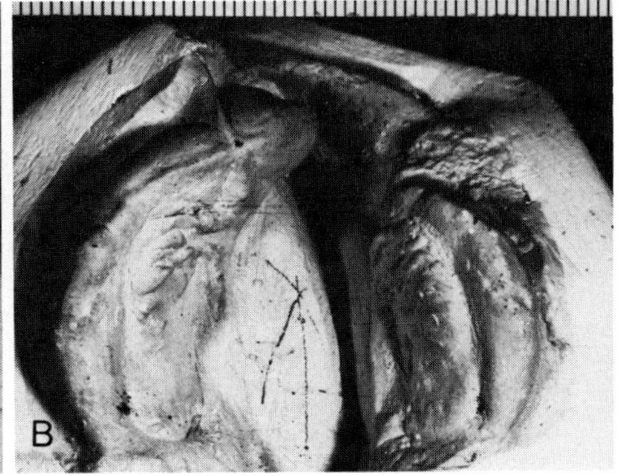

Figure 82–8 Newborn with complete unilateral cleft lip, alveolus, and palate. *A*, Note wide space between maxillary segments and wide opening of the nasal cavity. *B*, Patient 6 months later. No presurgical orthopedic treatment or lip repair was performed. Note that the relationship of the maxillary segments did not change and the side opening of the nasal cavity remains.

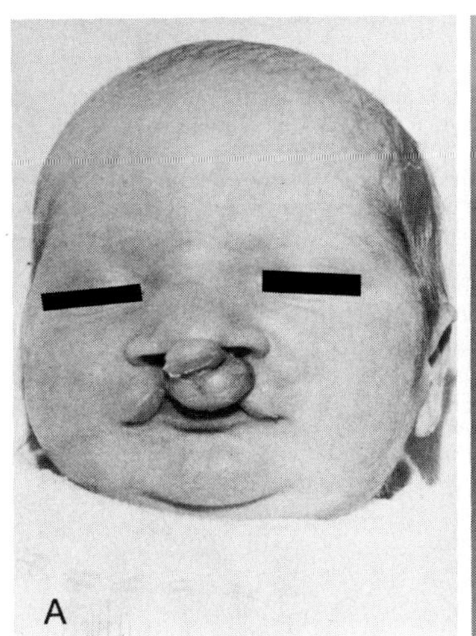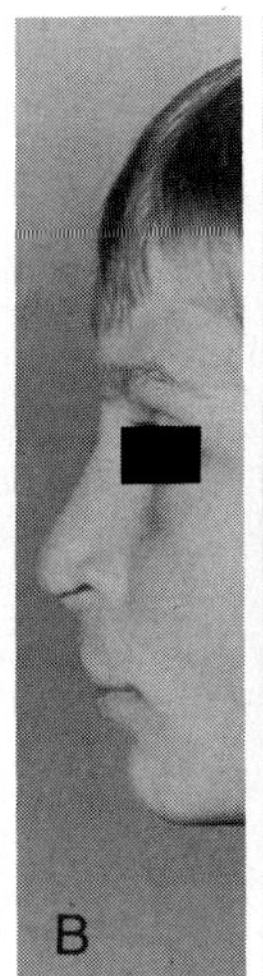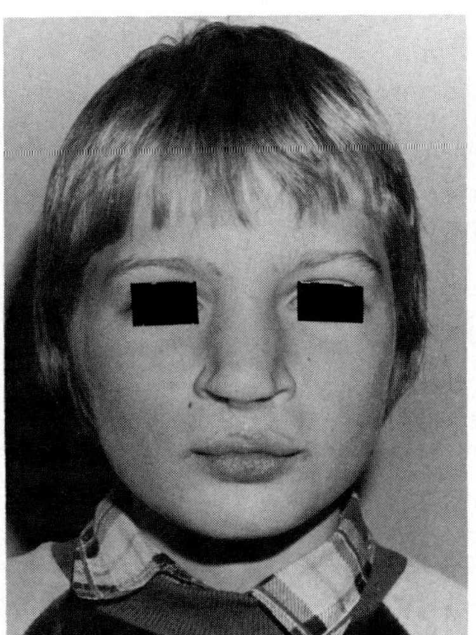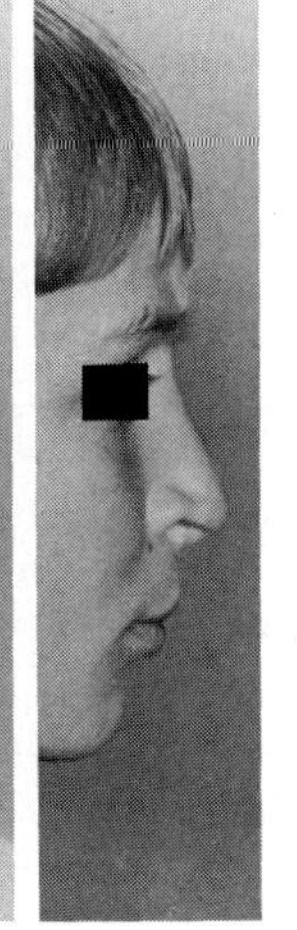

Figure 82–9 *A* and *B*, An example of successful complete bilateral cleft treatment. The child has always been a nose breather and has retained the correct resting mouth posture.

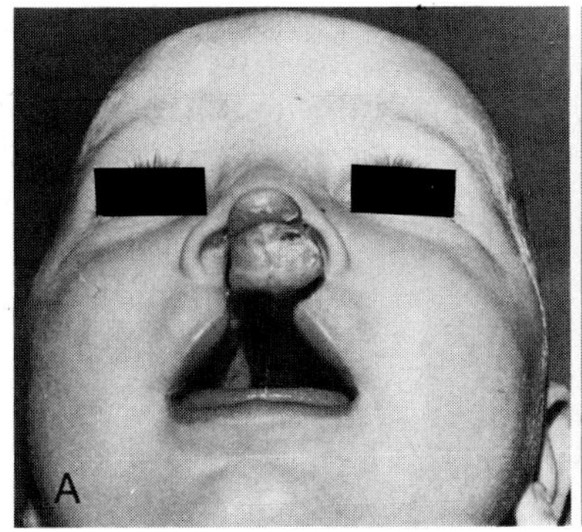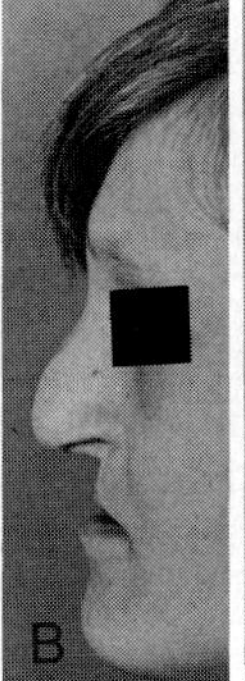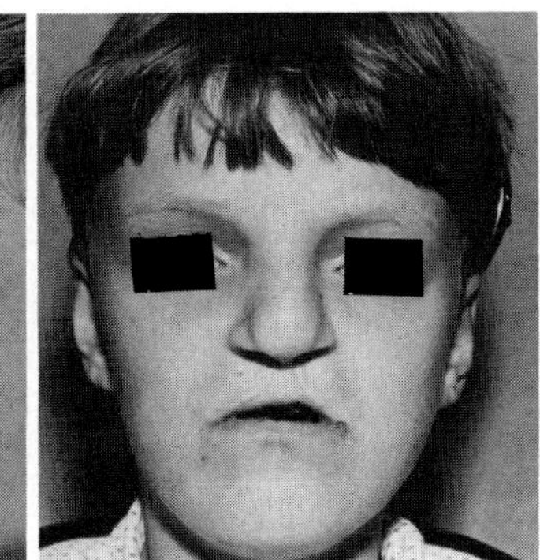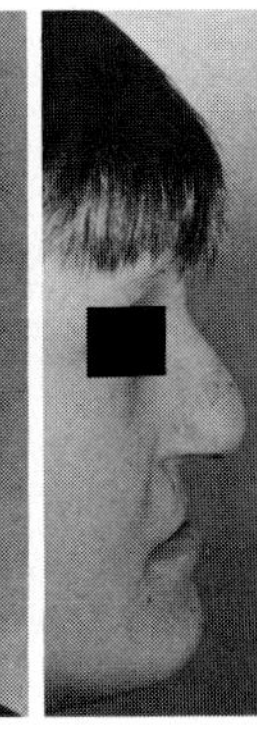

Figure 82–10 *A* and *B*, Unsuccessful complete bilateral cleft treatment. The child has always been a mouth breather and has never adopted the correct resting mouth posture. Surgical treatment in this patient was identical to that given to the patient shown in Figure 82–9.

enable and support the proper course; however, it is the operated child who must set the course by adopting the proper habits. At our current level of knowledge, no sure way of encouraging the child to do so has yet been devised. And therein lies the whole complexity and ambiguity of even the most proper treatment.

References

1. Oblak P: New concept of morphogenesis of clefts in the lip, alveolus and palate. J Maxillofac Surg 3:182–187, 1975.
2. Neil E, Keele C (eds): Wright's Applied Physiology, 13th ed. New York: Oxford University Press, 1982.
3. Posener G: Dictionnaire de la Civilisation Egyptienne. Paris: Fernand Hazan, 1959, p 60.
4. Hairfield WM, Warren DW, Hinton VA, et al: Inspiratory and expiratory effects of nasal breathing. Cleft Palate J 24:183–189, 1987.
5. Warren DW, Ryon WE: Oral port constriction, nasal resistance and respiratory aspects of cleft palate speech: An analog study. Cleft Palate J 4:38–46, 1967.
6. Peat JH: A cephlometric study of tongue position. Am J Orthod 54:339–351, 1968.
7. Ricketts RM: Respiratory obstruction syndrome. Am J Orthod 54:495–507, 1968.
8. Oblak P: Das physiologische Wechselspiel der Mundhoehlenmuskeln und seine Wirkung auf die Entwicklung der Spaltregion. In Pfeider G (ed): Lippen-Kiefer-Gaumenspalten. Stuttgart: Thieme Verlag, 1982, pp 121–123.
9. Bosma JF: Maturation of function of the oral and pharyngeal region. Am J Orthod 49:94–104, 1983.
10. England MA: A Colour Atlas of Life Before Birth. London: Wolfe Medical, 1983, p 63.
11. Schwarz AM: Lehrgang der Gebissregelung. Bd I. Wien-Insbruck: Urban und Schwarzenberg, 1961, p 389.
12. Jenkins PA, Baum JD: Respiratory distress syndrome. In Wald NJ (ed): Antenatal and Neonatal Screening. Oxford: Oxford University Press, 1984, pp 298–313.
13. Koskinen-Moffet L, Moffet B: Influence of prenatal jaw function on human facial development. Birth Defects 20:47–64, 1984.
14. Russel JGB: Radiology in obstetrics and antenatal paediatrics. London: Butterworths, 1973, p 12.
15. Harvold EP, Tomer BS, Vargervik K, et al: Primate experiments on oral respiration. Am J Orthod 79:359–372, 1981.
16. O'Ryan FS, Gallagher DM, LaBlanc JP, et al: The relation between nasorespiratory function and dentofacial morphology: A review. Am J Orthod 82:403–410, 1982.
17. Vargervik K, Miller AJ, Chierici G, et al: Morphologic response to changes in neuromuscular patterns experimentally induced by altered modes of respiration. Am J Orthod 85:115–124, 1984.
18. Vig PS, Showfety KJ, Phillips C: Experimental manipulation of head posture. Am J Orthod 77:258–268, 1980.
19. Warren DW, Hinton VA, Hairfield WM: Measurement of nasal and oral respiration using inductive plethysmography. Am J Orthod 89:480–484, 1986.
20. Wenzel A, Henriksen J, Melsen B: Nasal respiratory resistance and head posture: Effect of intranasal corticosteroid (Budesonide) in children with asthma and perennial rhinitis. Am J Orthod 84:422–426, 1983.
21. Lowe AA, Takada K, Yamagata Y, et al: Dentoskeletal and tongue soft-tissue correlates: A cephalometric analysis of rest position. Am J Orthod 88:333–341, 1985.
22. Williams HJ: Posterior choanal atresia. Am J Roentgenol Rad Ther Nucl Med 112:1–11, 1971.
23. Shaw EB: Sudden unexpected death in infancy syndrome. Am J Dis Child 119:416–418, 1970.
24. Diner PA, Andrieu-Guitrancourt J, Dehesdin D: Unilateral congenital choanal atresia and maxillary sinus development. J Maxillofac Surg 14:285–288, 1986.
25. Moss ML: Functional cranial analysis and the functional matrix. In Schumacher GH (ed): Morphology of the maxillo-mandibular apparatus, Leipzig: VEB Thieme, 1972, pp 160–165.
26. Graber TM: The three M's: Muscles, malformation and malocclusion. Am J Orthod 49:418–450, 1963.
27. Stenstrom SJ, Thilander BL: Effects of nasal septal cartilage resections on young guinea pigs. Plast Reconstr Surg 45:160–170, 1970.
28. Bergland O, Borchgrevink H: The role of the nasal septum in midfacial growth in man elucidated by the maxillary development in certain types of facial clefts. Scand J Plast Reconstr Surg 8:42–48, 1974.
29. Scott JH: Dentofacial development and growth. Oxford: Pergamon Press, 1967, p 86.
30. Latham RA: The pathogenesis of the skeletal deformity associated with unilateral cleft lip and palate. Cleft Palate J 6:404–414, 1969.
31. Oblak P: New guiding principles in the treatment of clefts. J Maxillofac Surg 3:231–239, 1975.
32. Celesnik F: Notre procede de traitement chirurgical du bec-de-lievre bilateral total. Rev Stomat 63:386–388, 1962.
33. Oblak P, Kozelj V: Basic principles in the treatment of clefts at the University clinic for maxillo-facial surgery in Ljubljana, and their evolution in thirty years. In Gnoinski W (ed): Early Treatment of Cleft Lip and Palate. Toronto: Hans Huber, 1986, pp 123–127.
34. Kozelj V: Maxillary arch dimensions in patients with clefts of lip, alveolus, and palate with or without presurgical orthodontic treatment. In Pfefer G (ed): Craniofacial Anomalies and Clefts of Lip, Alveolus, and Palate. Stuttgart: Thieme Verlag, in press.
35. Oblak P: An essay in evaluating the Celesnik method in treatment of bilateral clefts (in Slovene). Research report. Research Communities of Slovenia, Ljubljana, 1987.

CHAPTER 83

The Nasal Airway in Cleft Palate

Donald W. Warren and W. Michael Hairfield

Clefts of the lip and palate frequently produce significant nasal deformities, such as a deviated septum, vomerine spurs, atresia of the nostrils, and maxillary growth deficits that alter the nasal floor.[1–3] These abnormalities tend to reduce the size of the nasal airway.

Review of the Literature

Drettner reported that septal deformities, atresia of the nostrils, and turbinate hypertrophy diminish airway size and increase airway resistance.[1] Interestingly, in studies previously performed in our laboratory, otolaryngologic examination revealed that about 60% of the "normal" subjects demonstrated clinical evidence of septal defects, vomerine spurs, or turbinate hypertrophy in spite of the fact that their nasal airways were judged to be normal.[2] Approximately 70% of the cleft lip and palate subjects also presented with similar nasal defects, although these defects were usually more severe. Those with cleft lip and palate had a greater incidence of nasal deformities than those with cleft palate alone. We determined that nasal resistance in the cleft population is about 20% to 30% higher than that in the normal population.[2, 3]

There is evidence that airway deficiency in individuals

with unilateral cleft lip and palate is present in utero. Siegel et al recently observed that the fetal septum appeared to be enlarged and distorted and was flanked laterally by reduced nasal airway passages at 17 weeks.[4] They suggested that reduced nasal size may be a function of both nasal capsule deficiency and nasal septum hypertrophy.

We recently reported that the nasal airway of an adult with a cleft lip or palate is generally about 25% smaller than that of a normal adult.[3] The normal adult nose is about 0.62 cm² in its smallest cross-sectional area compared with about 0.47 cm² in cleft subjects.[3, 5] Evidence that the cleft airway is narrow implies that the airway is impaired and that mouth breathing is common. Indeed, a recent study by Hairfield et al confirms this.[6] Mode of breathing was assessed in 85 children and adults using a pneumotachograph to measure nasal volumes and an inductive plethysmograph to measure tidal volumes. Breathing mode was defined as follows: 80% to 100% were nasal breathers; 60% to 79% were predominantly nasal; 40% to 59% were mixed oral-nasal; 20% to 39% were predominantly oral; 0% to 19% were mouth breathers.

Results

Figure 83–1 illustrates the findings according to group. The largest number of subjects (37%) were oral breathers. Sixty-eight percent of the sample fell within groups that were more oral than nasal. Only 32% of the subjects were either predominantly nasal or nasal breathers.

Figure 83–2 illustrates the findings according to age. The adult group comprised those 15 years and older, whereas the children's group consisted of those less than 15 years of age. Justification for these age categories is based on our previous studies, which have demonstrated that internal growth of the nose generally ceases by age 15. There were 22 subjects in the adult group and 63 subjects in the children's group.

Figure 83–3 illustrates the findings for those subjects who had received posterior pharyngeal flaps. A total of 32 belonged to this subgroup. Fifty percent of this subgroup were oral breathers, 22% were predominantly oral breathers, and 6% were mixed oral and nasal breathers. Only 22% were nasal or predominantly nasal breathers.

Published data on mouth breathing in the normal population indicate that the prevalence is approximately 15%.[7–9] Our own continuing studies suggest that about 30% of the normal population breathes through the mouth to some extent. Most habitual mouth breathers in the noncleft population are mixed oral-nasal breathers or predominantly nasal breathers rather than predominantly oral or oral breathers. The cleft population presents an almost complete reversal of those patterns. About 70% of the subjects in the Hairfield study were oral, predominantly oral, or mixed oral-nasal breathers.[6]

Another unexpected finding in the Hairfield[6] study was that the prevalence of mouth breathing in adults was the same as that in children. We previously reported that the nasal airway in children with cleft palate improves somewhat with growth.[2, 10] Therefore, a lower prevalence of mouth breathing was expected in adults. Since the prevalence of mouth breathing did not change, it appears that the improvement with growth is not sufficient to induce a change in breathing mode. Another possibility is that once the pattern of mouth breathing is established, change does not rapidly occur even when

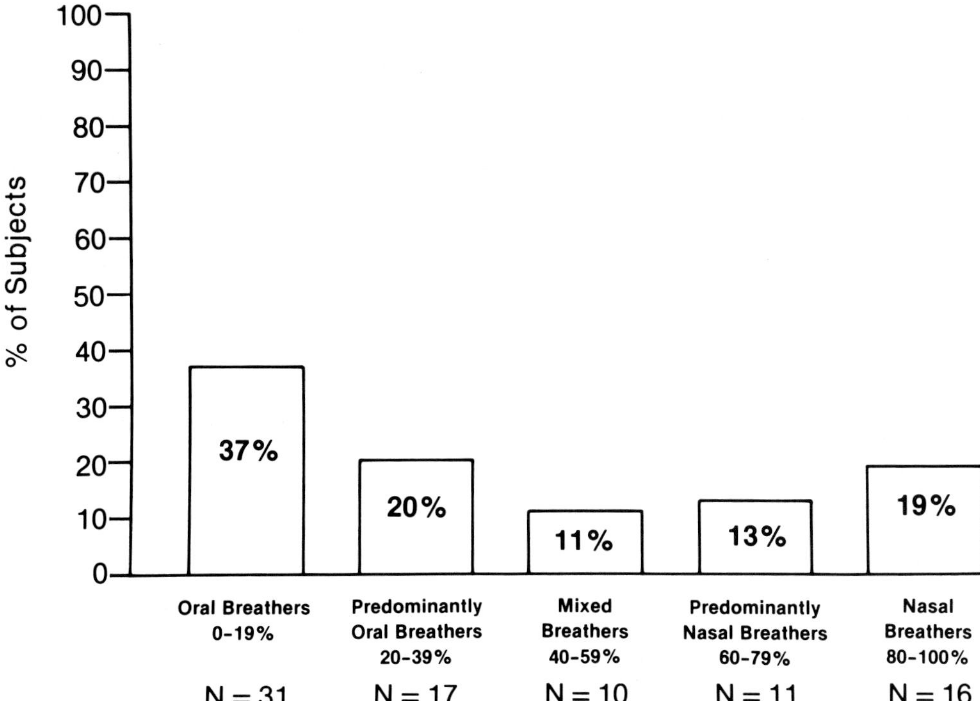

Figure 83–1 Percentages and number of individuals according to respiratory classification.[6]

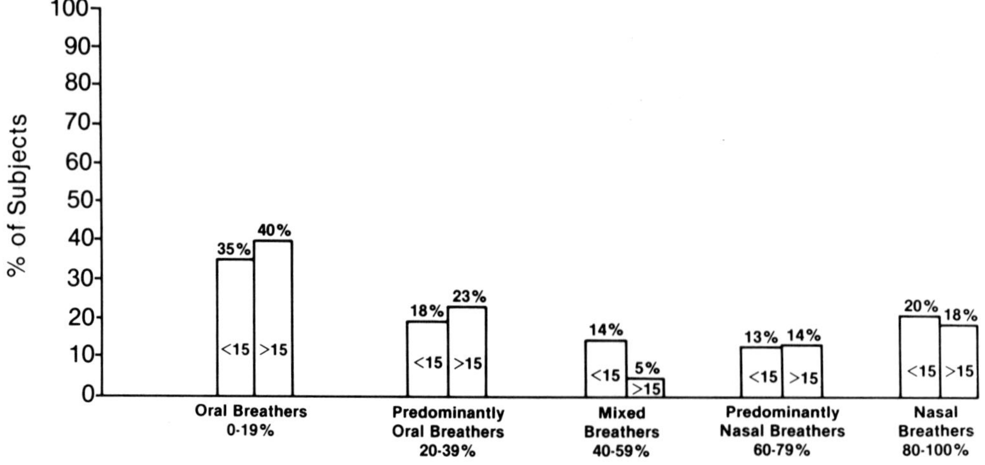

Figure 83–2 Percentages of individuals according to age and respiratory classification. Adults were defined as being 15 years or older.[6]

the airway improves. That is, obligatory mouth breathing is replaced by habitual mouth breathing rather than by nasal breathing. There is evidence in the literature that mouth breathing can become a learned behavior.[11, 12]

There is only one report at variance with previous findings. Sandham and Solow did not find any difference in nasal airway resistance between cleft subjects and a normal control group.[13] The authors suggest that the differences between their results and those of others may be due to their using a decongestant prior to taking measurements. Although this procedure undoubtedly affected their results, Sandham and Solow also studied groups that were not well matched by age. The median age for the controls was 12 years, whereas the median age for the unilateral cleft lip and palate group was 16. This important difference may account for their findings because the nose continues to grow in cross-sectional size until the child is about 15 years of age.[2, 10]

Warren et al recently reported that the type of cleft affects the nasal airway in children.[14] Table 83–1 presents data on nasal airway size during inspiration and expiration according to type of cleft. Normative data also are shown for comparison. The differences among cleft types are readily apparent. The bilateral cleft lip

and palate group and the unilateral cleft lip group have nasal cross-sectional areas that are significantly larger than those in individuals with the other cleft types. Indeed, nasal size in the bilateral cleft lip and palate group is slightly larger than that in the normal group.

Although a reduced nasal airspace for subjects with cleft lip and palate was expected, the difference between the unilateral and bilateral cleft lip and palate subjects was not anticipated. Previously, only differences between cleft lip and palate and cleft palate have been noted. Drettner reported that individuals with cleft lip and palate had a narrower nasal airspace than those with cleft palate alone.[1] Sandham and Solow, although not directly comparing the two groups, did show a slight but not statistically significant difference between them.[13]

Otolaryngologic examination of cleft subjects in the study by Warren et al revealed that septal deformities occurred most frequently in the subjects studied.[14] However, stenosed nasal apertures, thickened nasal mucosa, and hypertrophied turbinates were also observed. Similarly, the collapsed nasal ala associated with the typical cleft lip–nasal deformity was frequently observed, especially in the group with unilateral cleft lip and palate.

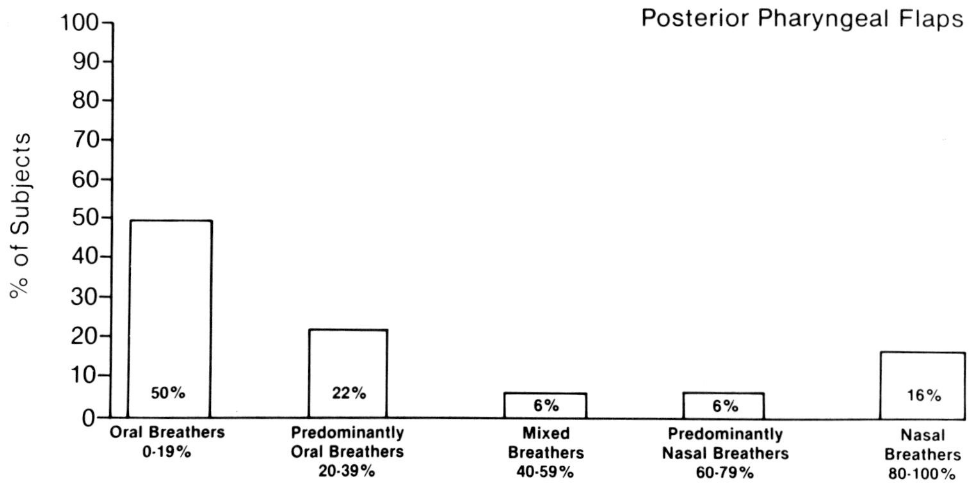

Figure 83–3 Findings for subjects who had received posterior pharyngeal flaps.[6]

Table 83–1. Nasal Airway Size (cm²) and Standard Deviation by Type of Cleft

	UCL	UCLP	BCLP	CHP	CSP	Normal
Inspiration	.37 ± .22	.21 ± .13	.40 ± .15	.26 ± .14	.26 ± .05	.36 ± .18
Expiration	.36 ± .20	.22 ± .12	.41 ± .14	.27 ± .15	.23 ± .05	.34 ± .17

UCL = Unilateral cleft lip; UCLP = unilateral cleft lip and palate; BCLP = bilateral cleft lip and palate; CHP = cleft hard palate; CSP = cleft soft palate.

(From Warren DW, Hairfield WM, Dalston ET, et al: Effects of cleft lip and palate on the nasal airway in children. Arch Otolaryngol Head Neck Surg 114:987–992, 1988.)

Discussion

The validity of equating subjective clinical observations of nasal deformities with objective measurements is open to question. However, some comment is appropriate. There is evidence that conditions or procedures that alter the shape or function of the nasal valve also affect the nasal cross-sectional area. Hall et al[17] and Guenthner et al[18] demonstrated that superior repositioning of the maxilla increases the nasal area, presumably by changing the shape of the nasal valve. Cosmetic procedures that inappropriately scar or cause collapse of the upper lateral cartilage may narrow the airway.[19] In fact, any morphologic changes within the critical nasal valve region may influence the mode of breathing. Individuals with bilateral cleft lip and palate usually undergo surgery that lengthens the columella. Presumably, this procedure has a positive effect on alar shape and widens the nasal valve. It is quite possible that the difference in airway size between those with bilateral cleft lip and palate and those with unilateral cleft lip and palate stems from this surgery.

Data on the percentage of nasal breathers by cleft type pose other interesting clinical questions (Table 83–2). Specifically, all groups involving clefts of the palate, including the bilateral cleft lip and palate group, contained more oral than nasal breathers. The bilateral cleft lip and palate group should have had a higher mean percentage of nasal breathers based on airway size. In fact, a percentage of nasal breathers similar to that observed in the unilateral cleft lip group would be expected. Although this is only conjecture, we suggest that distortion of the nasal valve and alar collapse, which are so frequently associated with bilateral cleft lip and palate prior to the initial repair and columellar lengthening, resulted in high nasal resistance. Because there is open communication between the nose and mouth at birth, a normal nasal breathing pattern is not established. In addition to the high airway resistance, this open communication may produce a persistent pattern of mouth breathing that remains even after surgical repair.

It should be noted that these findings vary from those in the noncleft population. Linder-Aronson reported that children with adenoidal obstruction return to a nasal breathing mode after adenoidectomy.[20, 21] Perhaps this difference in results arises from the fact that individuals with adenoid obstruction were nasal breathers at birth, whereas the cleft subjects were not.

If obligatory mouth breathing becomes habitual mouth breathing in this population and the precipitating factor is early airway impairment, then a change in surgical approach might be considered. That is, clinicians might want to consider the possible advantages of early surgical intervention to reduce airway impairment. Elimination of nasal deformities, especially those septal defects that interfere with nasal valve function, might prove beneficial. This approach must be balanced, of course, with the need to provide treatment that does not interfere with nasomaxillary growth.[22]

Secondary procedures for velopharyngeal inadequacy frequently compromise the nasopharyngeal airspace, especially in children.[10] Table 83–3 lists the data on nasal size and percentage of nasal respiration in children who received flaps compared to children with clefts and no flaps and normal controls. Comparisons within cleft types reveal that the flap has very little effect on those with unilateral cleft lip and palate and cleft palate alone. On the other hand, the nasal airway is reduced approximately 35% by the flap in the bilateral cleft lip and palate group. The group of normal controls consisted of predominantly nasal breathers. On the other hand, the flap groups were predominantly oral or mixed oral-nasal breathers. The pharyngeal flap obviously impairs the airway and produces obligatory mouth breathing in most individuals. Although this procedure is very successful in moderating velopharyngeal inadequacy for speech, it is the great equalizer in terms of airway impairment. That is, all cleft types become almost equally compromised after the flap. The flap appears to have little effect on the already compromised airway of the unilateral cleft lip and palate and cleft palate only groups, but it has a significant effect on the bilateral cleft lip and palate group. These findings are disturbing and lead us

Table 83–2. Percentage of Nasal Breathing and Standard Deviation by Type of Cleft

UCL	UCLP	BCLP	CHP	CSP	Normal
66 ± 28	41 ± 37	43 ± 32	50 ± 32	53 ± 14	69 ± 35

UCL = Unilateral cleft lip; UCLP = unilateral cleft lip and palate; BCLP = bilateral cleft lip and palate; CHP = cleft hard palate; CSP = cleft soft palate.

(From Warren DW, Hairfield WM, Dalston ET, et al: Effects of cleft lip and palate on the nasal airway in children. Arch Otolaryngol Head Neck Surg 114:987–992, 1988.)

Table 83–3. Comparison Among Cleft Types With and Without Pharyngeal Flap

	UCLP Flap	UCLP No-flap	BCLP Flap	BCLP No-flap
Area (cm^2)	.19 ± .05	.22 ± .13	.28 ± .10	.41 ± .15
% nasal breathing	38	41	21	43
	CP flap	CP no-flap	UCL no-flap	Normal
Area (cm^2)	.24 ± .14	.27 ± .15	.37 ± .22	.34 ± .17
% nasal breathing	46	52	66	69

UCLP = Unilateral cleft lip and palate; BCLP = bilateral cleft lip and palate; CP = cleft palate; UCL = unilateral cleft lip. (From Seaton D, Warren DW, Hairfield WM, et al: The posterior pharyngeal flap: Effects on airway size and breathing. J Dent Res 67:259, 1988.)

to conclude that primary palatoplasty must be improved so that secondary procedures such as the pharyngeal flap will be unnecessary. Earlier reports indicate that flaps and prosthetic speech appliances that obturate the nasopharyngeal airspace impair breathing in adults as well.[10]

Studies at present suggest that clinicians should focus greater attention on airway compromise, especially in a population that already has tissue deficiencies, tissue distortions, and tissue displacement problems. Clinicians have been concerned primarily with aesthetic appearance and speech in the cleft population, not with airway patency. In rare instances, respiratory behaviors may have life-threatening implications, and in other instances there may be morphologic consequences affecting dentofacial growth.

ACKNOWLEDGMENT. This study was supported by grants DE 06957, DE 07105, and DE 00129 from the National Institute of Dental Research.

References

1. Drettner B: The nasal airway and hearing in patients with cleft palate. Acta Otolaryngol 57:131, 1960.
2. Warren DW, Duany LF, Fischer ND: Nasal airway resistance in normal and cleft palate subjects. Cleft Palate J 6:134, 1969.
3. Warren DW: A quantitative technique for assessing nasal airway impairment. Am J Orthod 86:306, 1984.
4. Siegel MI, Mooney MP, Kimes KR, et al: Analysis of the size variability of the human normal and cleft palate fetus nasal capsule by means of three-dimensional computer reconstruction of histologic preparations. Cleft Palate J 24:190, 1987.
5. Hairfield WM, Warren DW, Hinton VA, et al: Inspiratory and expiratory effects of nasal breathing. Cleft Palate J 24:183, 1987.
6. Hairfield MA, Warren DW, Seaton DL: Prevalence of mouthbreathing in cleft lip and palate. Cleft Palate J 25:135, 1988.
7. Uddstromer M: Nasal respiration. Acta Otolaryngol 42:3, 1940.
8. Saibene F, Mognoni P, Lafortuna CL, et al: Oronasal breathing during exercise. Pflügers Arch 378:65, 1978.
9. Niinimaa V, Cole P, Mintz S, et al: Oronasal distribution of respiratory airflow. Respir Physiol 43:69, 1981.
10. Warren DW, Trier WC, Bevin AG: Effect of restorative procedures on the nasopharyngeal airway in cleft palate. Cleft Palate J 11:367, 1974.
11. Polgar G, Kong GP: The nasal resistance of new born infants. J Pediatr 67:557, 1965.
12. Bouhuys A: The Physiology of Breathing. A Textbook for Medical Students. New York: Grune & Stratton, 1977.
13. Sandham A, Solow B: Nasal respiratory resistance in cleft lip and palate. Cleft Palate J 24:278, 1987.
14. Warren DW, Hairfield WM, Dalston ET, et al: Effects of cleft lip and palate on the nasal airway in children. Arch Otolaryngol Head Neck Surg 114:987–992, 1988.
15. Foster TD: Maxillary deformities in repaired clefts of the lip and palate. Br J Plast Surg 15:182, 1962.
16. Aduss H, Pruzansky S: The nasal cavity in complete unilateral cleft lip and palate. Arch Otolaryngol 85:75, 1967.
17. Hall DJ, Turvey TA, Warren DW: Alterations in nasal airway resistance from superior repositioning of the maxilla. Am J Orthod 85:109, 1984.
18. Guenthner TA, Sather AH, Kern EB: The effect of Lefort I maxillary impaction on nasal airway resistance. Am J Orthod 85:308, 1984.
19. Kern EB: Surgery of the nasal valve in plastic and reconstructive surgery of the face and neck. In Sisson GA, Tardy ME (eds): Rehabilitative Surgery. Vol. 2, New York: Grune & Stratton, 1977, p 43.
20. Linder-Aronson S: Effect of adenoidectomy on the dentition and facial skeleton over a period of five years. Trans Eur Orthod Soc, 1973, p 177.
21. Linder-Aronson S: Adenoids: Their effect on mode of breathing and nasal airflow and their relationship to characteristics of the facial skeleton and the dentition. Acta Otolaryngol Suppl 265:1, 1979.
22. Delaire J, Precious D: Influence of the nasal septum on maxillonasal growth in patients with congenital labiomaxillary clefts. Cleft Palate J 23:270, 1986.
23. Seaton D, Warren DW, Hairfield WM, et al: The posterior pharyngeal flap: Effects on airway size and breathing. J Dent Res 67:259, 1988.

CHAPTER 84

Cleft Septorhinoplasty: Free Septum Replantation for Secondary Correction

Wolfgang Gubisch and Heinz Reichert

Contemporary surgical treatment of patients with cleft lip and palate leads, in general, to more satisfactory aesthetic and functional results than surgical techniques used only a generation ago. Better results have markedly decreased the need for many secondary corrective operations and have resulted in less severe secondary maxillofacial deformities. Surgical repair of cleft lip and palate has definitely improved in recent years, although correction of the nasal deformity associated with clefting still presents a difficult problem. Careful examination of patients with unilateral cleft of the lip, alveolus, and palate following cleft lip and palate repair reveals that most have marked nasal deformities characterized by asymmetry, deviation of the septum, and some degree of airway obstruction. The existing nasal deformity may require the combined efforts of an otolaryngologist, maxillofacial surgeon, and plastic surgeon working on one team to achieve optimal results in the secondary correction.

Surgical Rationale

A typical nasal deformity in patients with unilateral cleft lip and palate usually is characterized by a flat, sometimes depressed ala, an asymmetric nasal tip, misplaced alar base (usually repositioned), and a deviated septum (Figs. 84–1 and 84–2). The oblique position of the columella may result from a muscle imbalance when the orbicularis oris has not been united precisely at the base of the columella during primary lip repair. At the time of primary lip repair, we always attempt to create continuity of the orbicularis oris by attaching the upper portion of the muscle fibers to the anterior nasal spine. This maneuver, which has become routine in our practice, may preclude malpositioning of the columella. To determine whether this technique is as effective as we expect, we must examine the patients operated on this way after they have become adolescents.

The malpositioned and misshapen ala on the cleft side, combined with medial shortening of the alar cartilage and downward rotation and flattening of its lateral component, can be corrected by a three-dimensional Z-plasty. We mobilize and lift the medial part of the alar cartilage, filling the triangular-shaped defect that is created following an incision of the lining on the cleft side of the columella with a web-shaped triangle of skin in the dome of the depressed nostril. Alternatives

that we have also found useful are the techniques described by Straight[1] and the so-called reversed U-flap described by Taijima and Maruyama.[2]

We would like to highlight one detail that facilitates the obtainment of optimal results while correcting the depressed ala. This involves the use of two flap pieces of silicone (Fig. 84–3); one is fixed on the skin and the other on the inner lining of the lifted nostril. The pieces of silicone are sutured together with mattress sutures to stabilize the ala in the desired position. This prevents dead space, hematoma, and displacement of the nostril in the postoperative period.

It is our opinion that the major problem in the secondary cleft lip–nasal deformity is the deviated septum. Therefore, straightening the septum becomes paramount in correcting the secondary nasal deformity. Because the anterior nasal spine is dislocated, the lower portion of the septum may be deviated (usually to the noncleft side). Sometimes the lower edge is deviated so severely that it almost completely obstructs the nasal passage. Furthermore, traction of the misplaced muscle fibers may lead to a more or less severe dislocation of

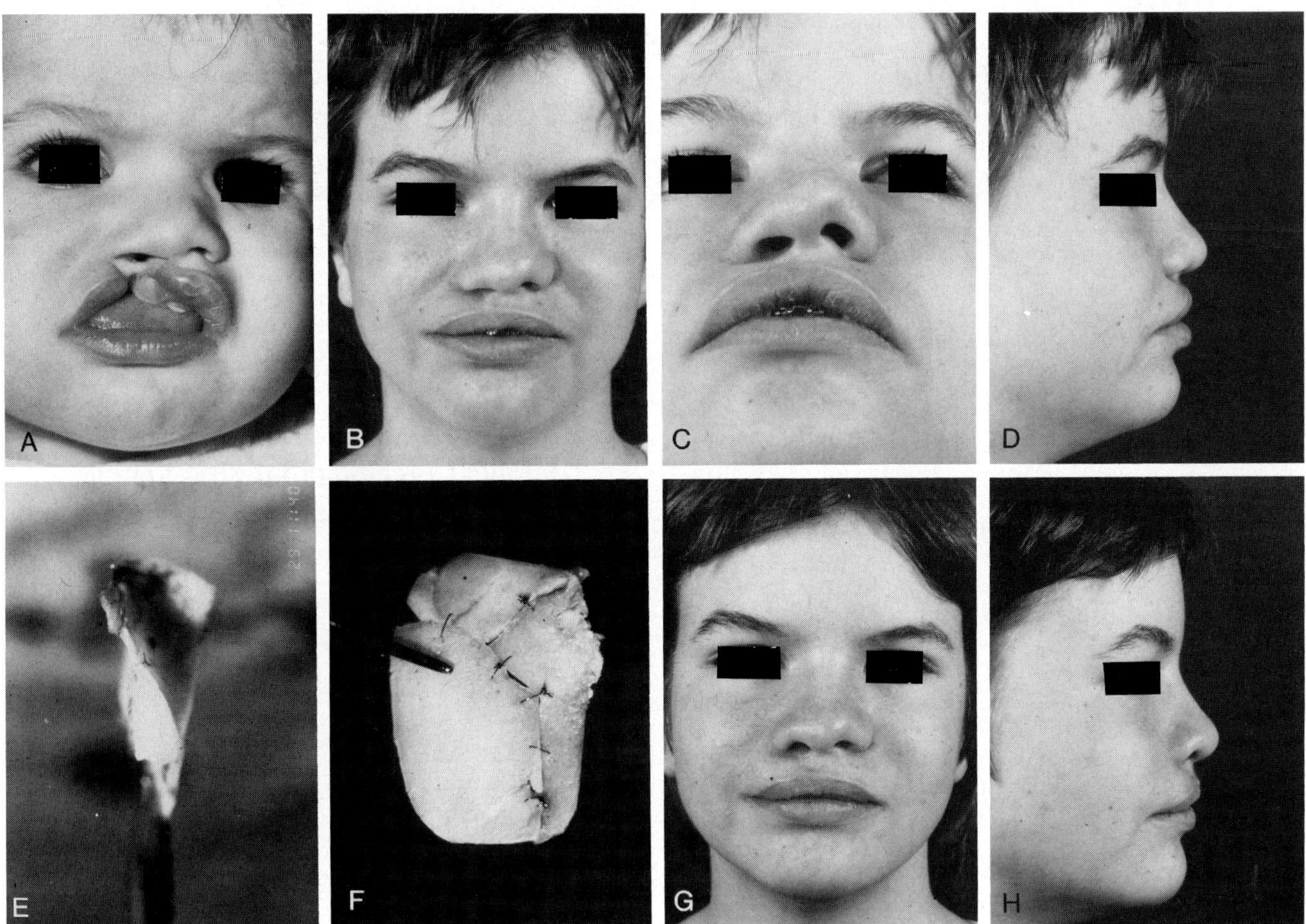

Figure 84–1 A, Girl at age 6 months with incomplete lip and palate before first operation. *B,* Visible asymmetry of nose 14 years later, after primary closure of lip and palate. *C,* Flat right ala and deformed septum. *D,* Well-rounded upper lip due to the Millard technique but depressed base of columella. *E,* Septal cartilage after total mobilization, showing marked deformities. *F,* Straight parts of septal cartilage joined and ready for replantation. *G,* Symmetric nose with unobstructed airways after replantation of straightened septal cartilage. *H,* Improved profile with correct nasolabial angle.

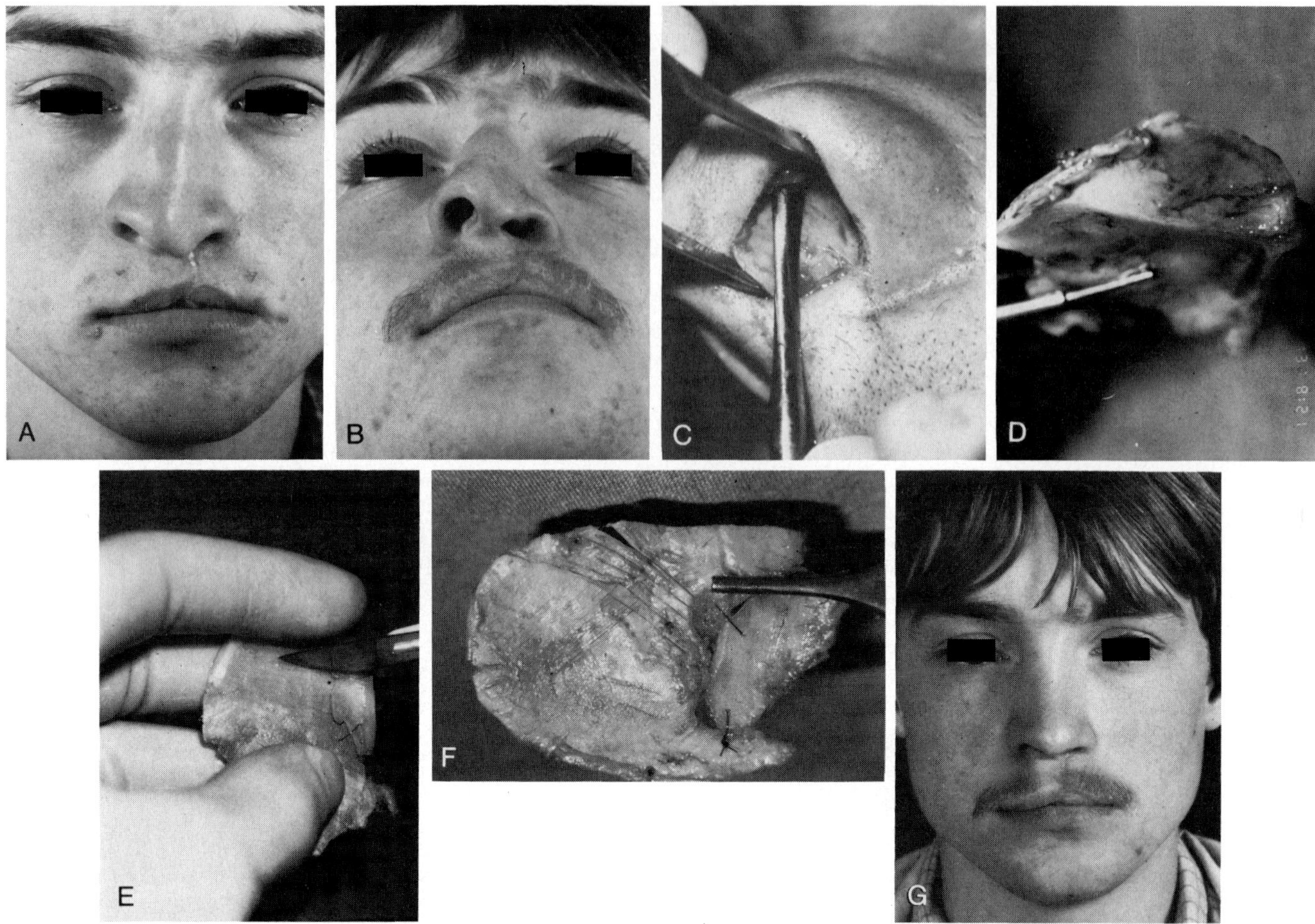

Figure 84–2 *A,* Seventeen-year-old male with surgically treated left cleft lip and palate, very asymmetric and depressed nose, and blocked air passage. *B,* View from below, showing marked deformation of septum. *C,* Beginning the total mobilization of the septal cartilage. *D,* Deformed septal cartilage totally mobilized, ready for extracorporeal correction. *E,* Correcting the shape of the septal cartilage by removing bent parts and changing the balance of tension in the cartilage through planned small incisions on the concave surface. *F,* Corrected and reunited septal plate ready for replantation. *G,* Improved symmetry of nose and free airways after replantation of straight septum (in combination with lateral osteotomy).

the lamina quadrangularis to the noncleft side. The deviation of the septum in the majority of our patients was directed toward the cleft side, contradicting many observations reported in the literature of septal deviations directed toward the noncleft side. We have not been able to explain whether this tendency of the growing septum to deviate toward the cleft side is associated with formation of the cleft itself or if it is caused by lip repair and correction of the nasal deformity.

In any case, very extensive deformities of the septum are present in almost all patients with unilateral cleft lip, alveolus, and palate. Septal deviation may result in secondary deformities of the columella, asymmetry of the external nose, and a narrow or completely obliterated nasal passage. In most of these patients, we now correct the deviated septum using the technique described by Gubisch.[4] Perret proposed some aspects of this procedure in 1958,[5] and Rees presented the idea again in 1986.[6]

Surgical Technique for Free Septum Replantation

The technique designed by Gubisch consists of maximum mobilization of the septum, its removal and straightening, and subsequent replacement of the straightened septum into its natural bed. This technique, called free septum replantation, has been performed in more than 450 patients, of whom 132 were patients with cleft lip and palate.

The surgical procedure starts with a hemitransfixation incision that is extended laterally as an intercartilaginous incision. One can also use a Rethi incision, which facilitates the open approach to the lower lateral cartilage and nasal septum. We prefer the intranasal approach. To free the deviated septum from its attachments, the mucoperiosteum on both sides must be undermined carefully. Attention should be directed to elevating the mucoperiosteum without perforations,

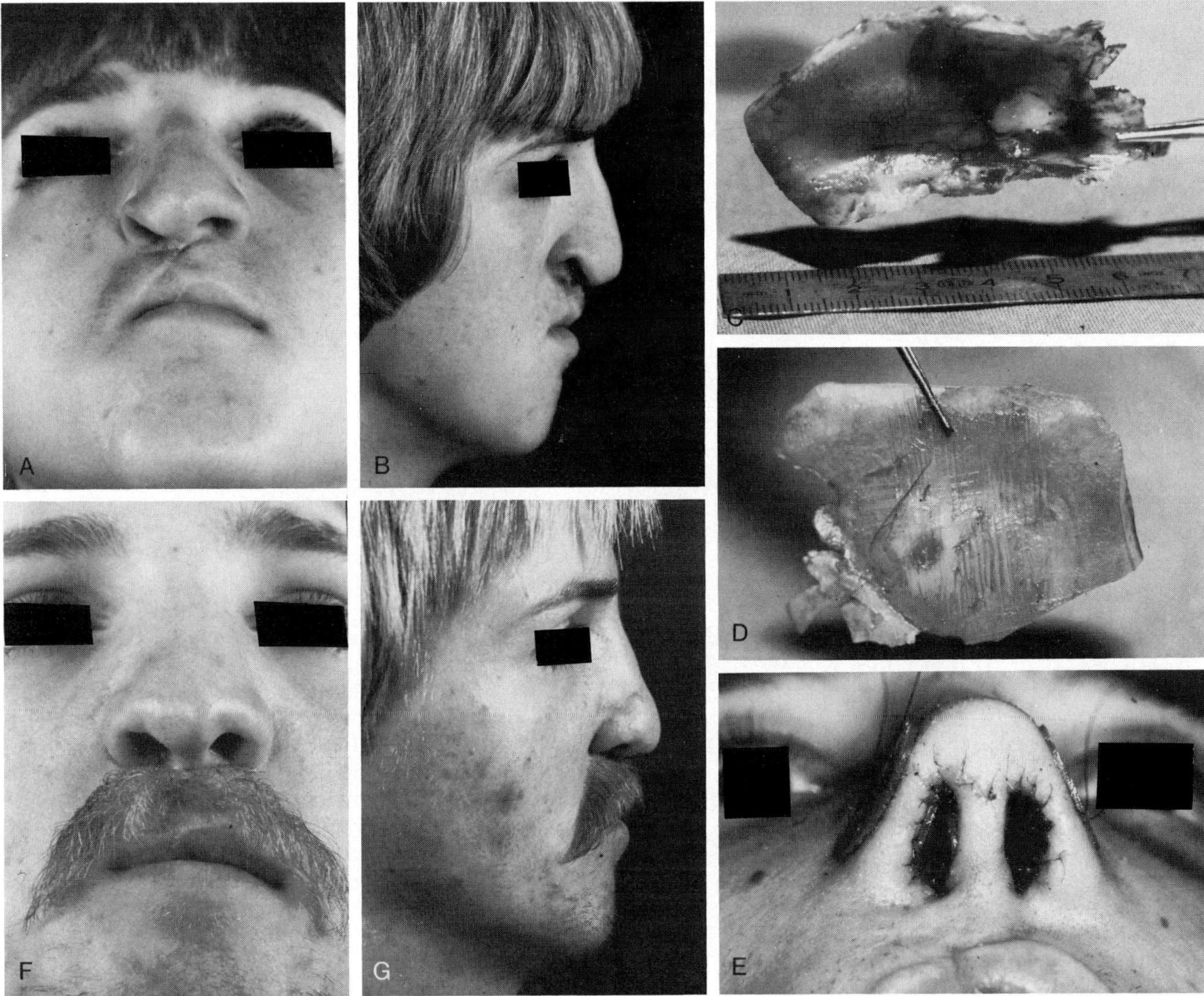

Figure 84–3 *A*, Very poor result of unsatisfactory closure of cleft lip and palate in 21-year-old male. *B*, Marked depression of tip of nose, flat cleft-side nasal wing, and blocked airway arising from extremely deformed septum. *C*, Septal cartilage after removal and ready for correction. *D*, Straightened part of septal cartilage before replantation. *E*, Corrected cartilage-support of nose, stabilized by silicone plates on both sides of septum as well as on inner and outer surfaces of both alae. *F*, Improved symmetry and shape of frontal part of nose with unobstructed air passage. *G*, Profile corrected by supporting tip of nose with replanted septal cartilage (in connection with small Z-plasty to lower alar base on the cleft side).

which in some patients can be extremely difficult. Absence of perforations creates safer conditions for replantation and uncomplicated healing.

The next step involves separation of the upper lateral cartilage from the anterior edge of the septum, followed by separation of the posterior edge of the septal cartilage from the dislocated premaxilla, and finally fracture of the bony septum. After this, the septal cartilage, with the attached bony cartilage, is removed in one piece, and all deformities of these structures are corrected at the operating table. We usually select the larger, flat, even parts of the septal cartilage, remove the twisted irregularities, and join the straight layers in the same plane using fine, atraumatic sutures.

When the entire cartilage is twisted and bent and there are not enough large areas of straight cartilage, we change the shape by well-planned scarifications on the convex side. By so doing, we rely on our long-term experience in reshaping ear cartilage, using Reichert's technique.[8] This technique is completely different from cross-hatching of the cartilage because the balance of tension within the cartilage is changed but not destroyed.

After repositioning the nasal spine, we replant the straightened septum and fix it with sutures. With the help of two so-called pilot threads, we pull the cartilage as far as possible anteriorly into the pocket of the columella. During this procedure, the angle between the upper lip and columellar base can be exactly adjusted. Additional transseptal sutures hold the septum in position and prevent hematomas between cartilage and mucosal lining.

Conclusions

Despite definitive advances in the surgical treatment of patients with unilateral cleft lip and palate, correction of the nasal deformity remains a difficult problem. Our surgical technique of free septum replantation following straightening of the septum provides optimal conditions for establishing an unobstructed nasal airway and an aesthetically pleasing appearance of the nose.

In our opinion, this technique has the following advantages:

1. Exposure of the entire septal cartilage facilitates its straightening.
2. The straightened septal cartilage is reimplanted, creating a normal nasal airway.
3. Straightening improves the nasal aesthetic appearance.
4. This technique facilitates the change of the nasolabial angle.

5. Subsequent to free septum replantation, secondary correction can be performed if necessary.

References

1. Straight CL: Reconstructions about nasal tip. Gynecol Obstet 62:73, 1936.
2. Taijima S, Maruyama M: Reverse U-incisions for secondary repair of cleft lip nose. Plast Reconstr Surg 60:256, 1977.
3. Tolhurst DE: Secondary correction of the unilateral cleft lip–nose. Br J Plast Surg 36:449, 1983.
4. Gubisch W: Aesthetic and functional reconstruction after nose trauma by septum replantation. Ind J Otolaryngol 36:1, 1984.
5. Perret P: Correction chirurgicale des nez devies. Pract Oto-Rhino-Laryngol (Basel) 20:114, 1958.
6. Rees TD: Surgical correction of the severely deviated nose by extra mucosal excision of the osseo-cartilaginous septum and replacement as a free graft. Plast Reconstr Surg 78:320, 1986.
7. Reichert H: Plastic surgery of the nose in children. Plast Reconstr Surg 31:51, 1963.
8. Reichert H: Correction of protruding ears by making use of the natural elasticity of the cartilage. Transactions of the Fifth International Congress for Plastic and Reconstructive Surgery, Australia. Butterworths, 1971, p 422.

CHAPTER 85

Ear Disease in Children with Cleft Palate: State of the Art

Sylvan E. Stool

The high prevalence of otitis media in infants and young children has been documented in numerous publications during the last 20 years. Prior to that time, a high incidence of hearing loss and otorrhea had been observed in older children and adults as a major sequel of the cleft palate deformity.

The initial observations of ear disease in infants were stimulated by the development and use of the operating microscope. Further technologic developments such as auditory brainstem response testing, the acoustic bridge, and endoscopic optical systems are now providing more information about anatomic and functional abnormalities associated with clefting. The purpose here is to review the diagnostic methods to be used with these patients and to describe briefly the research findings from the University of Pittsburgh about the general problem of ear disease in children with cleft palate.

The Pneumatic System

The ear is intimately related to the airway and is part of a system that contains air; therefore, it is pneumatized (Fig. 85–1). Abnormalities of the nose and palate, such as those that occur in cleft palate children, may have a secondary effect on the development of the air-containing cavities (pneumatization) of the middle ear and the air cell system that by convention has been called the mastoid. It is therefore important when considering factors that may influence the development of ear disease to include a complete examination and evaluation of these adjacent structures. However, for the purposes of this chapter, we will concentrate on the methods of diagnosis and specific findings of the middle ear.

Observations of the Tympanic Membrane

The diagnostic otoscope is a primary tool used in the physician's evaluation, and it is important that the health care provider who examines children with cleft palates be familiar with the principle of pneumatic otoscopy because middle ear effusions are frequent and will decrease the mobility of the tympanic membrane (Fig. 85–2). The external canal should be free of debris because many cleft palate children have cranial and facial abnormalities associated with small external canals, and small amounts of cerumen may obscure the tympanic membrane.

The operating microscope has been an important advance in visualization of the ear because it provides a powerful light source and enables the physician to clean the external canal and visualize the tympanic membrane. Recent optical advances, including rod and lens telescopes, have improved our ability to examine, photograph, and document the tympanic membrane structures.

The rationale and procedures for audiologic evaluation are presented in some detail in Chapter 86. In general, pure tone testing is used in children who can give

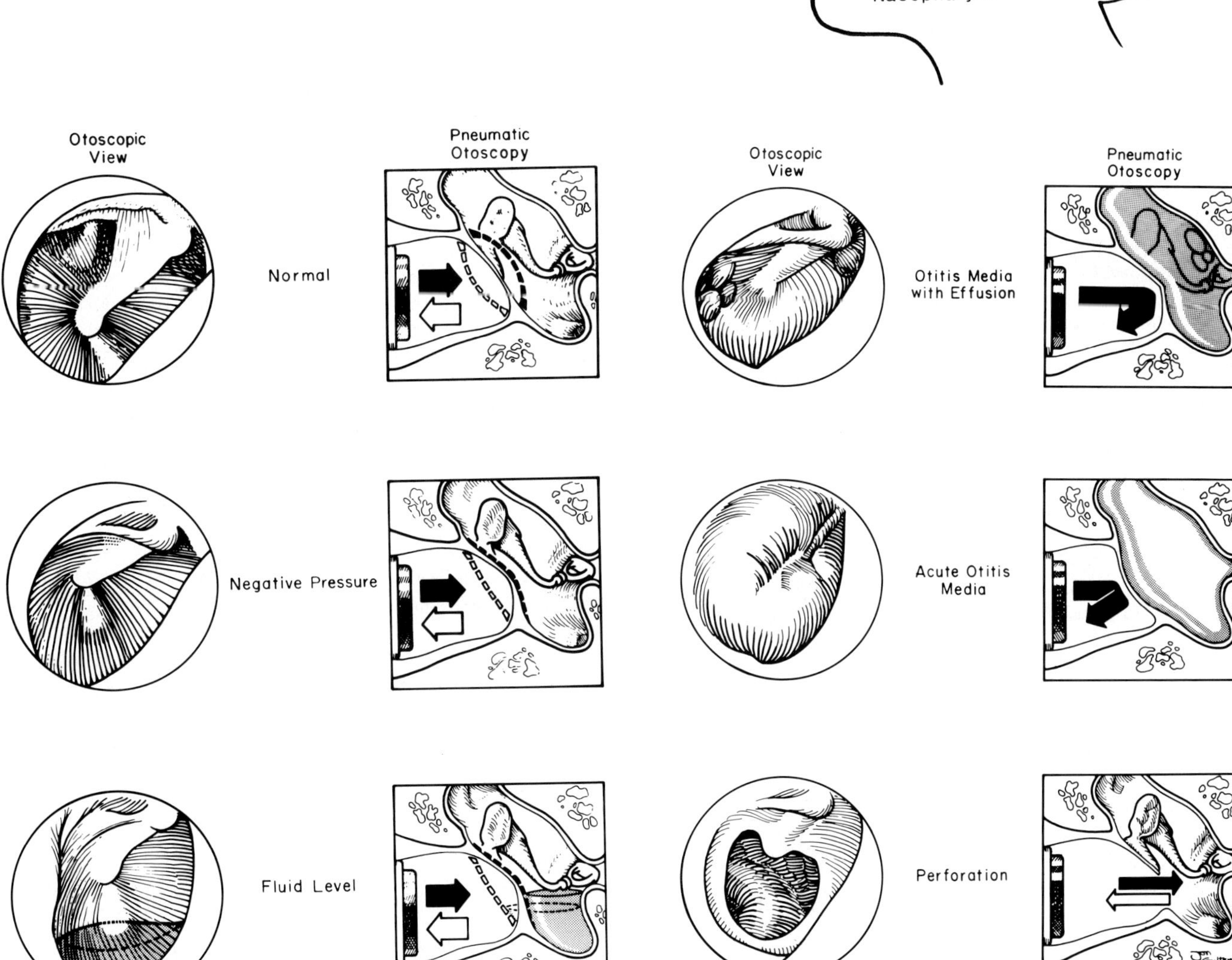

Figure 85–1 The pneumatic system of the ear. Abnormality of the nose, nasopharynx, mastoid, or eustachian tube may affect the middle ear.

Figure 85–2 *A,* Normal ear. The tympanic membrane has a neutral position and moves crisply with small amounts of applied or negative pressure. It is translucent.

Negative pressure. The tympanic membrane is retracted toward the medial wall of the middle ear. It moves more on applied negative pressure than on positive pressure because it is already retracted.

Fluid level. The tympanic membrane is usually slightly retracted. Fluid levels can be seen to move on application of positive or negative pressure. The color may vary with the thickness of the tympanic membrane and the color of the fluid.

B, Otitis media with effusion is a frequent finding in the child with cleft palate. The tympanic membrane is slightly retracted, and there is very little movement on applied positive or negative pressure. The color may vary from amber to blue, reflecting the contents of the middle ear.

Acute otitis media. The tympanic membrane may bulge and is usually opaque. There is little mobility, and the color may be yellow or red.

Perforation. There is no movement of the tympanic membrane because the opening prevents pressure from building up in the external auditory canal. There may be a small or large perforation, or a tube may be present in the tympanic membrane, giving similar results.

voluntary responses and is important in serial evaluation of patients. Nonvoluntary responses with auditory brainstem testing have enabled us to demonstrate that young infants with cleft palates have a conductive hearing loss. Fria et al tested 23 infants with cleft palates and demonstrated that 18 had mild or moderate hearing loss in both ears, and four had similar loss in one ear.[1] Some of these children were tested immediately and postoperatively; most of them had improved. This study confirms that even in the very young, a hearing loss can be demonstrated.

Tympanometry or impedance testing is of great value in the cleft palate population because it is very reliable in the detection of middle ear effusion. In addition, this technique may be used to evaluate eustachian tube patency in the child who has an opening in the tympanic membrane. There are some techniques that can be used on the intact tympanic membrane to show eustachian tube function.

Eustachian Tube

Dysfunction of the auditory tube has been postulated as a major cause of middle ear disease in children with cleft palate. The major functions of the tube are ventilation and pressure equalization, drainage, and protection (Fig. 85–3). Although cleft palate may affect all of these functions, its effect on ventilation is probably the most important. As stated previously, the middle ear must be ventilated if the air cell system is to develop in the temporal bone. The middle ear is filled with fluid at birth, and if the eustachian tube does not function properly and the ear is not ventilated, pneumatization will be decreased. Several years ago we demonstrated that the child with a cleft palate had less pneumatization than normal controls. This finding was achieved by examining cephalometric films measuring the pneumatized region with a planimeter and comparing the findings with those in normal controls.[2]

The auditory tube is located in the skull base, which includes an osseous portion and a neuromuscular portion (Fig. 85–4). The latter has a cartilaginous support that is attached to the tubal musculature (Fig. 85–5). The tensor veli palatini's primary function is to open the tube when it contracts (Fig. 85–6). The lumen of the tube is lined with a mucosal epithelium. There has been much speculation about the relationship of the cranial base and the eustachian tube. However, it seems probable that a relatively flat cranial base and a horizontal position of the eustachian tube are both important etiologic factors in the increased prevalence of otitis media in both the cleft palate and the normal populations. Various alterations in the morphology of the cranial base have been described in the cleft palate patient, and it is obvious that these also may contribute to abnormal eustachian tube function.

Several mechanisms may result in middle ear effusion owing to tubal dysfunction. The tube may be obstructed or abnormally patent. In the event of tubal obstruction, the middle ear space becomes atelectatic and can subsequently fill with sterile fluid (Fig. 85–7). This fluid may become infected if bacteria are insufflated into the middle ear. The tube also may be semipatulous or floppy, a condition that is thought to be prevalent in children and that makes the tube likely to become dysfunctional. In some instances, the tube is patent, and secretions may reflux from the nasopharynx to the middle ear. We have seen children with cleft palate who have a perforation of the tympanic membrane and have observed milk passing from the nasopharynx to the middle ear and out through the perforation to the external canal. Although these instances are rare, they do demonstrate the possibility of this anatomic connection and dysfunction.

PHYSIOLOGY OF EUSTACHIAN TUBE

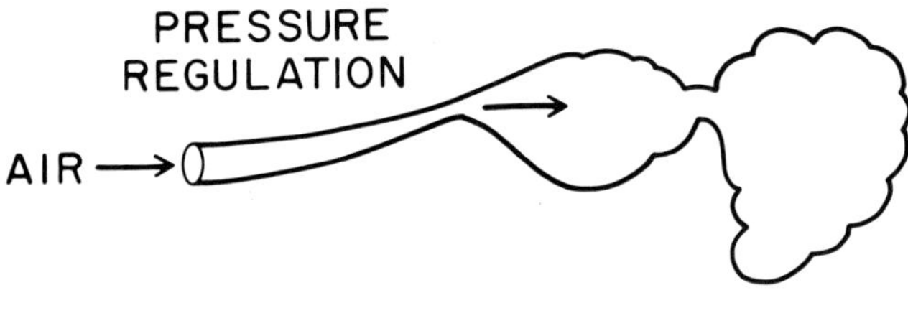

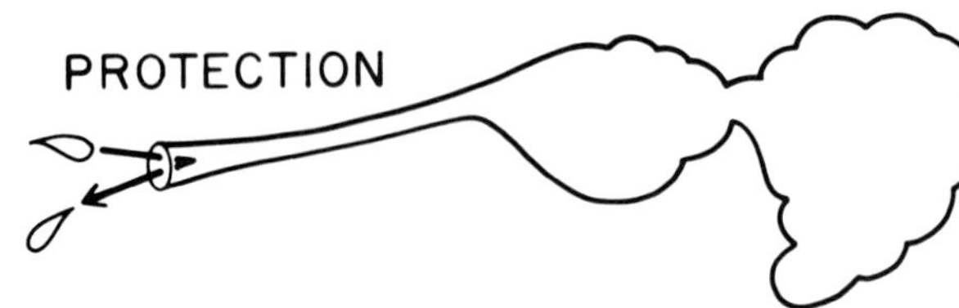

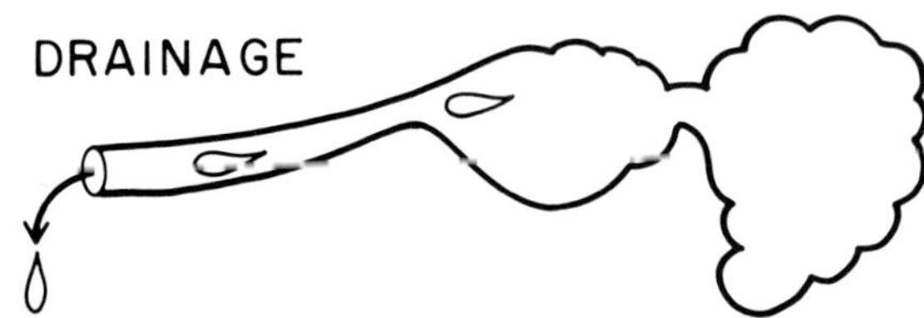

Figure 85–3 The functions of the eustachian tube include ventilation, which provides pressure regulation and protection from secretions and sound, and drainage of secretions that may develop in the middle ear.

Eustachian Tube Function Test

Because the eustachian tube is believed to be responsible for most of the middle ear effusions that occur in cleft palate patients, it is obvious that evaluation of its function is an important component in contemporary etiologic care. Researchers have expended considerable effort on developing methods of tubal evaluation. In general, the methods of evaluation fall into two categories: tests performed on the intact tympanic membrane, and tests performed on the perforated tympanic membrane.

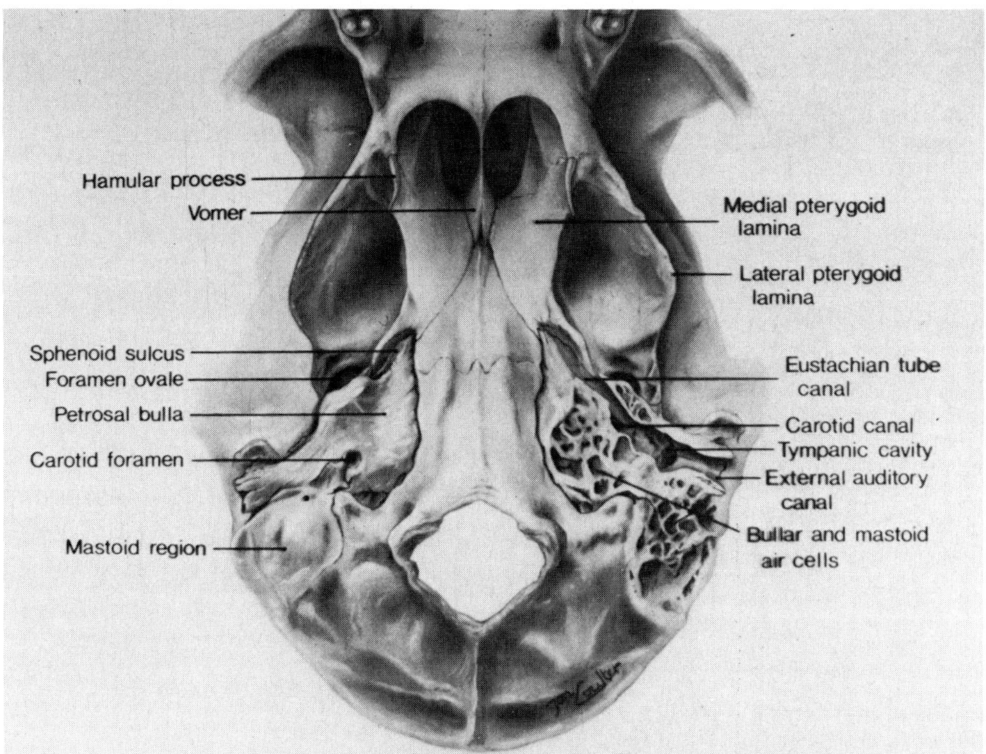

Figure 85–4 External base of the skull showing landmarks pertinent to the auditory tube. (From Stool S, Rood, SR: Cleft palate and related disorders. Otolaryngol Clin North Am 14(4):867, 1981.)

Tests on the intact tympanic membrane show changes in tympanometric measurements or demonstrate opening of the tube when sound or light passes through it. Examples are sonometry, which utilizes sound, and light-carrying bundles inserted into the tube to be detected in the external auditory canal.

Tests on the perforated tympanic membrane are the most frequently used in clinical practice. Positive pressure is applied to the middle ear, and the amount of pressure that causes the tube to open is ascertained. Then positive pressure is applied below this threshold and the patient is asked to swallow. This active swallowing should equalize the middle ear pressure in about five swallows. Failure to do so indicates tubal malfunction.

The forced response test is performed by forcing a constant flow of air through the external auditory canal. This test requires the presence of a perforation or tympanostomy tube in the tympanic membrane. This flow of air opens the eustachian tube. The subject is then instructed to swallow; the action of the musculature of the eustachian tube then opens the tube further, and a decrease in pressure is noted. In the normal subject the pressure falls when the tube dilates. In the abnormal individual there may not be active function, or the tube may constrict, causing the pressure to rise. These tests have been performed on a number of children with cleft palate. In the infant with an unrepaired palate, there was a higher forced opening pressure than in the infant with a repaired palate, and there were poor active dilating pressures.[3] The same group of children was tested following repair of the palate, and improvement in the passive functions was found; that is, with the eustachian tube open, the pressures were closer to those characteristic of the normal population. However, during active function, that is, changes occurring during swallowing, the pressures were not significantly improved. There was a subgroup of children with very active ear disease in whom the eustachian tube constricted instead of opening during swallowing. These tests ultimately may have predictive value for identifying children who will develop severe ear disease (Fig. 85–8).

Experimental work on primates may be of value in understanding the relationship of the cleft to middle ear effusion. Casselbrant studied tubal function in the rhe-

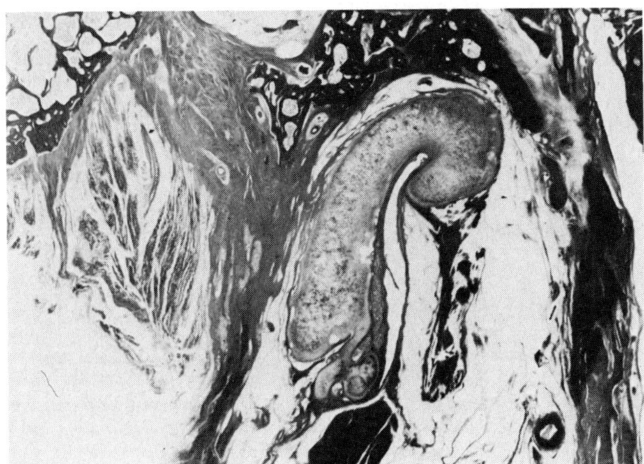

Figure 85–5 Cross section of the auditory tube showing the cartilage and muscular attachments. Courtesy of Steward Rood, Ph.D.

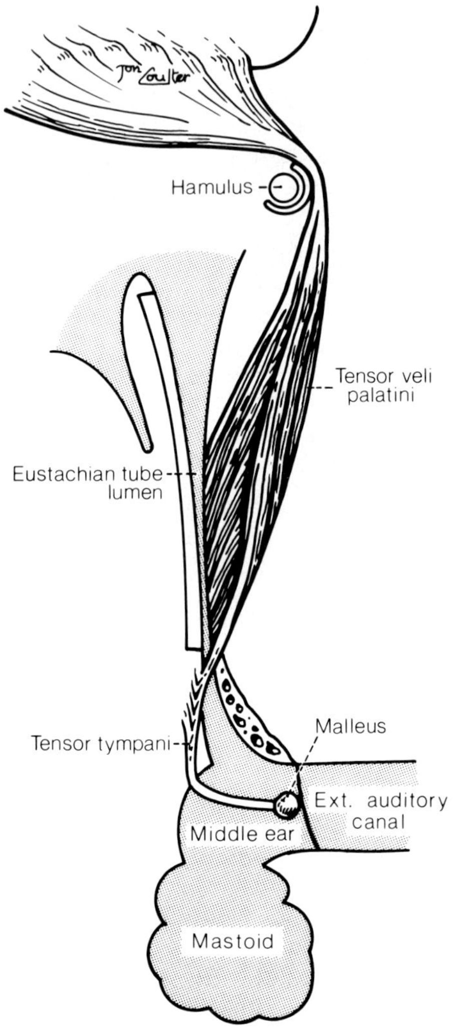

Figure 85–6 The major muscle that controls the opening of the eustachian tube is the tensor veli palatini, which is attached to the tubal cartilage and inserts into the palate.

sus monkey with a surgical cleft.[4] Using the eustachian tube test discussed previously, she showed that active tubal function was severely compromised by the cleft but was reversible with spontaneous healing of the cleft.

A series of histopathologic studies on eight individuals with cleft by Shibahara and Sando produced several characteristic findings.[5] These findings suggest that the individual with cleft palate not only lacks anchorage of the tensor veli palatini muscle and the soft palate but also demonstrates abnormalities of the eustachian tube and its cartilage and abnormal anatomic relationships of these structures to the tensor veli palatini.

Bacteriology of the Middle Ear

Surprisingly few reports have been made about the bacteriology of the fluid of the middle ear in children with cleft palate considering the frequency of this disorder. One probable reason is that in the past, many otologists did not culture the fluid removed from the

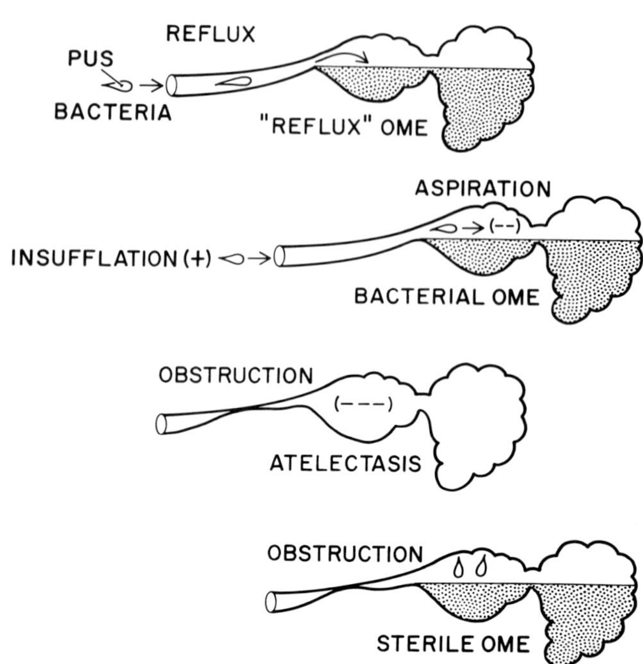

Figure 85–7 The concept of the tubal malfunction that may result in otitis media; pus or bacteria in children with cleft palate may reflux into the tube and into the middle ear. The tube may be "floppy," and the middle ear may be insufflated. When the tube has become obstructed, atelectasis may develop, and a sterile effusion may occur; this effusion may subsequently become infected.

middle ear, and in cultures that were made, there was not a high rate of positive findings. We also had a low incidence of positive cultures before a program was introduced in which a microbiologist came to the operating room and made a culture of the specimen immediately after it was removed from the middle ear. Using this technique, we have found that the most frequently encountered organisms were *Haemophilus influenzae*, *Streptococcus pneumoniae*, *Branhamella catarrhalis*,

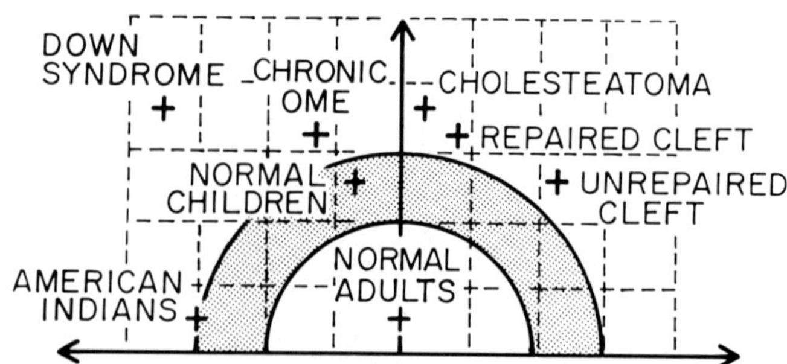

Figure 85–8 Eustachian tube function in various groups of patients. The child with cleft palate is usually outside the normal range and is similar to the child who has cholesteatoma. (From Cantekin E: State of the art: Physiology and pathophysiology of the eustachian tube. In Lim DJ, Bluestone CD, Klein GO, Nelson JD, eds: Recent Advances in Otitis Media with Effusion. Toronto: B. C. Decker, 1984, pp. 45–48. With permission.)

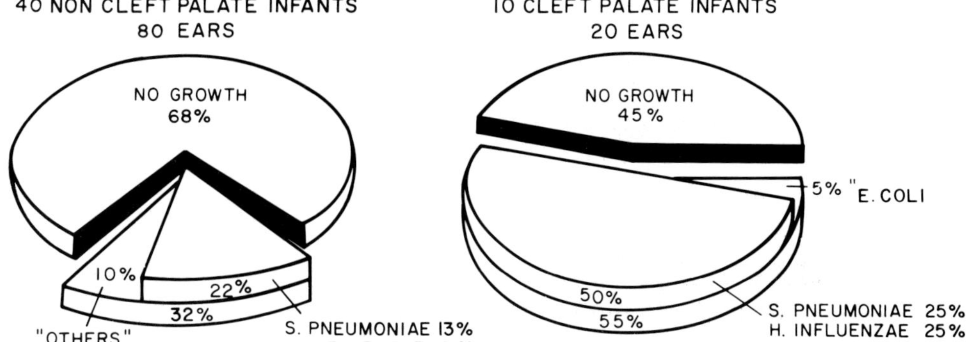

Figure 85–9 Bacteriologic findings from ears of infants with cleft palate compared to those in a group of normal infants. The pathogens in both groups are similar.

and *Staphylococcus aureus*, coagulase-positive. These are the same pathogens found in the normal noncleft population and in about the same proportions. We also noted that when children with clefts had received antibiotics prior to the time of surgery, there were fewer positive cultures. This information seems highly significant for the treatment of otitis media in the cleft palate population. It shows that the organisms are not unusual and are susceptible to the same drugs used in the normal population (Fig. 85–9).

The Sequelae of Middle Ear Effusion in the Cleft Palate Child

Chronic otitis could adversely affect the development of any child. However, there is a special concern about the child who has a cleft palate because he or she is expected to have some difficulty with speech development owing to the cleft. As a result, the long-term effect of middle ear effusion or middle ear infections with suppuration obviously is more important in this group. Hubbard et al addressed this question recently by comparing 24 closely matched pairs of children with repaired cleft palate whose otologic treatment had been very aggressive with a group of children who had not had myringotomy with tube placement at an early age.[6] The children were studied at ages 5 to 7 years, and both groups were found to be similar in regard to physical and chronologic findings. In both groups there was scarring of the tympanic membrane, and hearing was slightly affected. Although the articulation problems were essentially the same in the two groups, they were more substantial in the group that underwent later myringotomy. Verbal performance and IQ scores were essentially the same in both groups. The authors concluded that children with cleft palate do have some lasting adverse effects from otitis media during early life. However, it was not felt that this abnormality extended to the cognitive and language problems.

The anatomic alterations in the tympanic membrane and middle ear structures of children with cleft palate remain a constant finding. Although there has been increased interest in the problem, and in many instances aggressive therapy utilizing myringotomy tube place-

ment early in life has been performed, there still remains a group of children who develop unrelenting middle ear disease and irreversible changes such as cholesteatoma. The pathogenesis of the development of acquired cholesteatoma is illustrated in Figure 85–10.

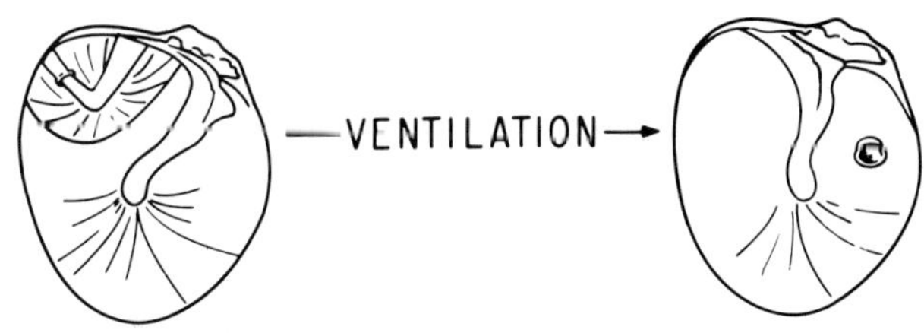

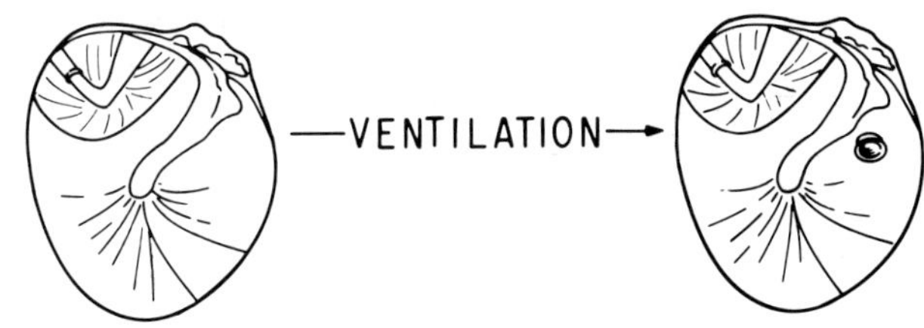

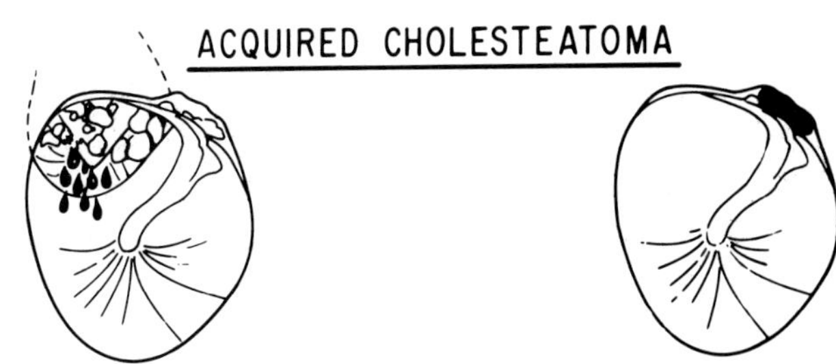

Figure 85–10 The pathogenesis of acquired cholesteatoma. There is faulty ventilation with development of atelectasis, and a retraction pocket is present posterosuperiorly. This pocket fills with debris, and a cholesteatoma then forms that may destroy the structures of the middle ear. The effect of ventilation with a tube is illustrated. With atelectasis the tympanic membrane may recover; however, when the membrane becomes adhesive, it remains the same and cholesteatoma may develop.

References

1. Fria TJ, Paradise JL, Sabo DL, et al: Conductive hearing loss in infants and young children with cleft palate. J Pediatr 3:84, 1987.
2. Stool SE: Pneumatization of the temporal bone in children with cleft palate. Cleft Palate J 6:154, 1969.
3. Doyle WJ, Reilly JS, Stool SE, et al: Eustachian tube function in children with unrepaired cleft palates. In Lim DJ, Bluestone CD, Klein JO, Nelson JD (eds): Recent Advances in Otitis Media with Effusion. Philadelphia: B C Decker, 1984, p. 59.
4. Casselbrant, M: Personal communication, 1988.
5. Shibahara Y, Sando I: Histopathologic study of eustachian tube in cleft palate patients. Ann Oto Rhinol Laryngol 97:403–408, 1988.
6. Hubbard TW, Paradise JL, McWilliams BJ, et al: Consequences of unremitting middle-ear disease in early life: Otologic, audiologic, and developmental findings in children with cleft palate. N Engl J Med 312:1529, 1985.

CHAPTER 86

Audiologic Considerations for Cleft Patients

Ruth A. Bentler

Cleft Palate and Hearing Loss

The frequency and effects of hearing loss associated with cleft palate were first described by Gaines.[1] The ever present middle ear effusion is known to produce chronic middle ear (conductive) hearing loss in as many as 90% of children with clefts.[2] More recently, sensorineural losses (found in up to 15% of children with clefts) have been ascribed to pathologic changes in the cochlea resulting from chronic middle ear effusion and presumably mediated through the round window.[3–6] Sensorineural deficits may also be present with certain syndromes.[7, 8] Extended high-frequency impairment has been documented as well.[9, 10] These reports of incidence of hearing loss in children with cleft palate (with or without cleft lip) are significantly higher than those occurring in the noncleft population.[11, 12] (In the noncleft population, Berg[11] reports incidences of 0.9%, 0.5%, and 0.05% for losses of 26 to 40 dB, 41 to 55 dB, and more than 71 dB, respectively. Based on a survey of 3197 children between 0 and 5 years old, Klein[12] estimates that the occurrence of middle ear disease ranges between 8.3% and 25.3%.) However, by adulthood, the incidence of hearing impairment is apparently similar for both groups.[13, 14]

The major audiologic or otologic difference between the cleft population and the noncleft population is that the frequency of middle ear disease is greater in the cleft group, particularly during infancy and early childhood. Another difference between the two populations may be the underlying mechanisms in etiology, although that also may be more in degree than in kind (see Chap. 85). The major implication of these differences, or lack of differences, is that audiologic principles and procedures to be used with patients with clefts are identical to those used with other patients with suspected or known hearing impairment. As a consequence, the major portion of the following discussion is general in nature, with emphasis on the assessment and management of the cleft palate child.

Audiologic Intervention

The deleterious effects of reduced auditory sensitivity in children in general have been delineated by numerous investigators; these include deficits in vocabulary acquisition, articulation skills, receptive and expressive language skills, use of grammar and syntax, auditory memory skills, auditory processing, auditory visual integration, reading disorders, and spelling skills.[15–20] When this depressed auditory sensitivity is superimposed on an impoverished auditory environment, the effects are even more disastrous—that is, in addition to hearing loss, locomotor limitations, frequent respiratory illnesses, and multiple hospitalizations may reduce the communicative opportunities of the child with cleft. The physical presence of the cleft may influence the manner and extent of parent-child interaction, which is important to the learning process involved in speech and language acquisition. Speculations about pathogenics include emotional reactions to the deformity and the abnormal interpersonal relationships that may result.[21]

The role of the audiologist extends well beyond early and expert audiologic evaluation into rehabilitative planning (including amplification considerations) and appropriate referral for related educational, psychological, and emotional impairments. The audiologist is cognizant of the impact of hearing impairment during the early formative years of speech, language, and psychosocial development. In addition, the technical skills of this specialist in assessment procedures and amplification options must be adept for the successful management of the child or adult with cleft.

The need for documentation of hearing deficits has become more apparent in recent years. To obtain and sustain nonmedical remediation services for the child with cleft, many educational and service-funding agencies require painstakingly thorough documentation of the child's hearing status. Thus, although philosophically the audiologist or speech pathologist may have no difficulty in justifying implementation of rehabilitative measures for any child with cleft, on a more esoteric level, ongoing proof (in terms of numbers) of actual degree of hearing impairment often becomes necessary. Consequently, great attention has been focused on improving the methods for identifying hearing impairment in children. The techniques most commonly used in audiometric assessment of the child with cleft include pure tone air- and bone-conduction audiometry, electroacoustic immittance measurements, and (more recently) measurement of auditory brainstem response. Using information from these current assessment tools, reliable frequency-specific hearing sensitivity can often be obtained with children as young as 7 months of age.[22]

Assessment

Rosenberg[23] has described the case history as the "first test" in audiometric evaluation. We must view the child and not just his or her ears. "Knowledge of the youngster's background and behaviors and his or her parents' attitude and concerns is absolutely essential" if we are to evaluate (primarily) his or her receptive communication skills and assist him or her and his or her family to remediation or compensation for the auditory deficits.[24]

Pure Tone Audiometry

The degree of hearing loss associated with middle ear effusion varies considerably and can range from levels of normal sensitivity to hearing loss as great as 50 dB HL.[25] The amount of information obtained during the audiologic assessment of the child with a cleft will vary, depending on a number of factors, including:[26]

1. Mental age—a determinant of the child's ability to learn new responses as well as an indicator of the responses already present (for example, the language requisite for speech audiometry).
2. Chronologic age—primarily adequate neuromuscular coordination plus limiting factors specific to disabilities that cause a difference between chronologic age and mental age.
3. Neurologic status—both motor and perceptual ability to make the required response.
4. Hearing level—an important determinant of experience in auditory response and the ease with which the child learns to respond to new auditory signals.
5. Willingness to perform—influenced by the child's motivation, fears, the rapport established by the clinician, and the skill with which the clinician operates.
6. Prior experience—with auditory testing on the child's part.
7. Test environment—the quality and flexibility of the equipment, the appearance of the room, and the toys or other motivational devices that are available to interest the child.

As a result, there will be variations in the amount of information that can be obtained during a given evaluation. For some children, frequency-specific information can be obtained for air conduction and bone conduction across frequencies using hand-raising techniques or play audiometry (e.g., dropping blocks, placing rings on a peg). For other children behavioral observation or visual reinforcement techniques are necessary.

Behavioral Observation Audiometry

Behavioral observation audiometry involves a stimulus-response paradigm whereby the child is closely observed for alterations in behavior (e.g., head turning, eye blinking, cessation of movement, vocalization, or breathing) following the presentation of some auditory stimulus. Stimuli of various (and known) intensities and frequencies should be used in an attempt to obtain the best estimate of auditory function. Northern and Downs[27] provide a comprehensive summary of the responses and levels that can be expected from infants and small children.

Visual Reinforcement Audiometry

Liden and Kankkonen[28] first coined the term visual reinforcement audiometry (VRA) based on a technique described by Suzuki and Ogiba[29] and termed by them conditioned orientation reflex (COR) audiometry. Their procedure involved lighted transparent toys that were flashed on simultaneously with the presentation of the auditory signal during a conditioning period. During the testing phase the light was flashed on immediately following a response (looking toward the light). Pure tones, warble tones, and speech stimuli have been employed in a sound field as well as under ear phones. Matkin[30] estimated that 12 to 30 months of age was the most successful age for using this technique.

Even when VRA audiometry is employed, behavioral observations must be employed as well. No matter how attractive the visuals or play, the young child may lose interest in the game. Consequently, behavioral observations must be incorporated throughout. Lloyd and coworkers[31] described a technique of systematic reinforcement audiometry for use with mentally retarded children. This technique, TROCA (tangible reinforcement operant conditioning audiometry), also is favored among clinicians for testing young normal children.[30] The TROCA procedure provides a positive reinforcement (candy, cereal, or trinket) for appropriate responses and a mild punishment (withholding the reinforcement or time out for inappropriate responses).

Electroacoustic Immittance

Since 1970, when Jerger[32] detailed the clinical application of immittance audiometry with a variety of disorders and populations, electroacoustic immittance (tympanometry, acoustic reflex, or static compliance measurements) has become a relatively standard component of the audiologic test battery. In terms of objectivity (no overt response is necessary from the child) the test requires no more than minimal cooperation from the child with a cleft. As a single test, the effectiveness of tympanometry in detection of middle ear effusion is limited. Inclusion of static immittance measures and acoustic reflex measures provides additional diagnostic information when the relationships between the three tests are considered. Schwartz[33] performed retrospective analysis on electroacoustic immittance data obtained from more than 2500 children in nine studies that have been conducted since 1976. Although test sensitivity averaged 94% across the nine studies, test specificity was only 57%.

Inclusion of immittance audiometry within a battery of tests can provide confirmation of results and continues to be a widely used supplement to pure tone audiometry for detection of the middle ear effusion that is so commonly present with cleft defects.

Auditory Brainstem Response

Use of the auditory brainstem response (ABR) is gaining widespread acceptance as a tool for determining the presence and extent of conductive hearing impairment. Its use in the diagnosis of degree and type (conductive versus sensorineural) of hearing loss requires considerable skill and judgment on the part of the examiner.

Auditory brainstem response waveforms are fairly similar among individuals and are highly stable and reproducible in any single individual, being almost unaffected by attention, sleep, medications, and most other metabolic factors. Normal ABR results consist of 5 to 7 msec following the presentation of an abrupt acoustic stimulus (click). Evidence suggests that waves I through V of the ABR represent activity in or around the eighth cranial nerve, cochlear nucleus, superior olivary complex, lateral lemniscus, and inferior colliculus.[34] Typically, wave V is the most robust component, and latency (as a function of stimulus intensity) approximates normal adult values by 18 to 24 months of age.[35]

With a conductive hearing loss the amount of stimulus energy that reaches the cochlea is reduced. As a result, the wave V latency-intensity function parallels that of the normal ear but is displaced by an amount estimated to be the amount of hearing loss. Fria and Sabo[34] have suggested that wave I rather than wave V should be used for making predictions of the degree of hearing impairment. It should be noted that the ABR is most sensitive to high frequency hearing loss (over 2000 Hz).

Habilitation

Although considerable attention has been focused on means of accurate identification of hearing impairment in children with clefts, auditory (re)habilitation is equally important. Because of the known deleterious effects of reduced or intermittent auditory sensitivity, it is obvious that medical, psychological, and speech-language referrals may be necessary. Preferential seating in the classroom or other group situations should be considered. In addition, because audition is the normal route through which speech and language develop, early and appropriate selection and use of amplification may be an important habilitative tool. Seewald and Ross[36] suggest that although we need to know as much as possible about the child's auditory sensitivity, what we do not know should not preclude early intervention with appropriate amplification. Their comment, "the major problem of most hearing impaired children is that they have trouble hearing," is not as trite as it may first appear. Auditory input needs to be provided early and consistently.

Although it is outside the scope of this chapter to provide an overview of amplification considerations such as the style and type of device, electroacoustic considerations, and hearing aid evaluation procedures, some general guidelines can be provided.

Style and Type of Aid

There are three basic styles of aids that can be considered for the child with a cleft: body-worn, postauricular, and in-the-ear (ITE). The body-worn aid, with its transistor radio appearance and cord to the ear(s), is rarely utilized in contemporary amplification fittings. Equivalent gain and power can be obtained from head-worn (postauricular) aids, which have significantly greater aesthetic appeal. In-the-ear hearing aids are typically not the aid of choice for two major reasons: Chronic middle ear involvement frequently entails drainage, which has high potential for damaging the internal components of an inserted hearing aid, and the proximity of the microphone to the receiver often precludes sufficient gain before feedback occurs.

It is somewhat difficult to discuss style of aid without considering type of aid: bone-conduction or air-conduction. Since the prevalence of hearing impairment consistent with cleft palate is conductive in nature, the bone-conduction hearing aid could provide ample gain and power without necessitating use of an earmold, which is often contraindicated with middle ear involvement or drainage. A newer style of bone-conduction hearing aid, which is completely encased in a "headband," may be preferable to the more traditional body-worn aid with a headband transducer.

Electroacoustic Considerations

There are a number of threshold-based approaches to selecting frequency-gain characteristics that can be useful with young children as well as adults.[37-39] In addition, Seewald and Ross[36] have outlined a speech spectrum-based approach for selecting frequency-gain characteristics for children. Their goal is to place the long-term average speech spectrum at levels that are sufficiently above threshold to be useful for the widest possible frequency range. With the advent of probe tube (microphone) technology, direct measurements of hearing aid output and gain at the tympanic membrane improve the fitting procedures for hearing aids.

Evaluation of Amplification

There is no one single preferred method for evaluating the performance of children with clefts with hearing aids. Because of the (frequently) fluctuating nature of the hearing loss, the (often) young age of the child involved, and the multiple communication environments traversed in a single day, actual evaluation of amplification for appropriateness can be accomplished best by a combination of clinical and nonclinical approaches.

Within the "clinical" dimension, aided sound field threshold measures are the primary method for evaluating the provision of appropriate gain. These measurements can be obtained regardless of the response mode employed (visual reinforcement audiometry, conditioned play audiometry, and so on). More recently, probe tube (microphone) technology has provided a means for assessing gain and measuring output levels without the overt cooperation of the aided child.

Outside of the clinical setting, the audiologist must rely on observational reports of the child's behavior in various situations provided by parents, teachers, speech-language pathologists, and other managing adults. By keeping a daily log of their child's adjustment to and performance with amplification, the parents become more actively involved in the child's habilitative program while providing insightful and useful information to the managing audiologist.

Conclusion

On the basis of present information, it seems reasonable to suppose that the *nature* of audiologic-otologic disorders and diseases shown by children and adults with cleft palate (with or without cleft lip) is identical to that shown by the general population (that is, individuals without cleft palate). The major difference between the two groups is that the frequency of middle ear disease is greater in the cleft palate group, and therefore audiologic-otologic considerations of that kind are important in the care of such patients, especially during infancy and early childhood. The deleterious effects of reduced auditory sensitivity in the first years of life have been delineated by numerous investigators. The audiologist can supply information about the child's hearing acuity and sensitivity, recommend and implement (re)habilitative measures within the speech-language-hearing realm, and direct the family appropriately for other help as needed. The advent and subsequent widespread application of physiologic measures of hearing such as the auditory brainstem response and immittance measures have significantly reduced the uncertainty of the auditory status in the young child. Documentation of degree and level of hearing impairment can be made with accuracy at a young age.

Early and consistent provision of auditory input by means of amplification, if necessary, may be one of the most effective (re)habilitative procedures. Upfold[40] has identified two new trends in amplification: (1) an "upsurge in the number of children fitted with hearing aids as a result of middle ear disease"; and (2) an "increase in the number of children with mild hearing impairment who are being fitted with hearing aids." He attributes these (interrelated) trends to changes in audiologic and otologic methods as well as developments in hearing aids, and increased awareness of the severity of impairment associated with chronic middle ear involvement.

As Rood and Stoole[41] aptly stated, the cleft palate patient "presents a continuing complex diagnostic and treatment challenge to a wide range of professionals," including the audiologist. A multidisciplinary team must provide and receive information in an ongoing effort to derive a management scheme that is progressive, flexible, and tailored to each individual child's needs. The audiologist is a key member of that specialty management team for the cleft palate patient, especially when that patient is a child.

References

1. Gaines FP: Frequency and effect of hearing losses in cleft palate cases. J Speech Hear Disord 52:141–147, 1940.
2. Fria TJ, Paradise JL, Sabo DL, et al: Conductive hearing loss in infants and young children with cleft palate. J Pediatr 110:86–87, 1987.
3. Bennett M: Symposium on ear diseases III. The older cleft palate patient (a clinical otologic audiology study). Laryngoscope 82:1217–1221, 1972.
4. Paparella MM, Oda M, Hiraide F: Pathology of sensorineural loss in otitis media. Ann Otol 81:632–637, 1972.
5. Watson DJ, Rohrich RJ, Poole MD, et al: The effect on the ear of late closure of the cleft hard palate. Br J Plast Surg 39:190–192, 1986.
6. Webster JC: Middle ear function in the cleft palate patient. J Laryngol Otol 94:31–37, 1980.
7. Cohen MM: An etiologic and nosologic overview of craniosynostosis syndromes. In Bergsma D (ed): Malformation Syndromes. Amsterdam: Excerpta Medica, 1975.
8. Cohen MM: Syndromes with cleft lip and cleft palate. Cleft Palate J 15:306–328, 1978.
9. Ahonen JE, McDermott JC: Extended high-frequency hearing loss in children with cleft palate. Audiology 23:467–476, 1984.
10. McDermott JC, Fausti SA, Frey RH: Effects of middle ear disease and cleft palate on high frequency hearing in children. Audiology 25:136–148, 1986.
11. Berg FS: Definition and incidence. In Berg FS, Fletcher SG (eds): The Hard of Hearing Child. New York: Grune & Stratton, 1970.
12. Klein JO: Epidemiology of otitis media. In Harford ER, Bess TH, Bluestone D (eds): Impedance Screening for Middle Ear Disease in Children. New York: Grune & Stratton, 1978.
13. Swigart E: Hearing sensitivity of adults with cleft lip and/or palate. Cleft Palate J 16:72–80, 1979.
14. Yules RB: Hearing in cleft palate patients. Arch Otolaryngol 91:319–323, 1970.
15. Hoffman-Lawless K, Keith RW, Cotton RT: Auditory processing abilities in children with previous middle ear effusion. Ann Otol Rhinol Laryngol 90:543–545, 1981.
16. Holm VA, Kunze LH: Effect of chronic otitis media on language and speech development. Pediatrics 43:833–839, 1969.
17. Masters L, Marsh GE: Middle ear pathology as a factor in learning disabilities. J Learn Disabil 11:103–106, 1978.
18. Ventry IM: Effects of conductive hearing loss: Fact or fiction. J Speech Hear Disord 45:143–156, 1980.
19. Webster DB: Effects of peripheral hearing losses on the auditory brainstem. In Lasky EZ, Katz J (eds): Central Auditory Processing Disorders. Problems of Speech, Language and Learning. Baltimore: University Park Press, 1983.
20. Zinkus PW, Grottlieb MI, Shapiro M: Developmental and psychoeducational sequelae of chronic otitis media. Am J Dis Child 132:1100–1104, 1978.
21. Wylie HL, McWilliams BJ: Mental health aspects of cleft palate: A review of literature intended for parents. ASHA 8:31–34, 1966.
22. Wilson WR, Thompson G: Behavioral audiometry. In Jerger J (ed): Pediatric Audiology. San Diego: College Hill Press, 1984.
23. Rosenberg P: The test battery. In Katz J (ed): Handbook of Clinical Audiology. Baltimore: Williams & Wilkins, 1972.
24. Ehrlich CH: A case history for children. In Katz J (ed): Handbook of Clinical Audiology. Baltimore: Williams & Wilkins, 1988.
25. American National Standards Institute: Specifications for Audiometers (S3.6). New York: American National Standards Institute, 1969.
26. Hodgson WR: Testing infants and young children. In Katz J (ed): Handbook of Clinical Audiology. Baltimore: Williams & Wilkins, 1988.
27. Northern J, Downs M: Hearing in Children. Baltimore: Williams & Wilkins, 1974.

28. Liden G, Kankkonen A: Visual reinforcement audiometry. Acta Otolaryngol 67:281–292, 1961.
29. Suzuki T, Ogiba Y: Conditioned orientation audiometry. Arch Otolaryngol 74:192–198, 1961.
30. Matkin ND: Some essential features of a pediatric audiologic evaluation. Read before the Eighth Danovox Symposium, Copenhagen, Denmark, 1973.
31. Lloyd L, Spradlin J, Reid M: An operant audiometric procedure for difficult to test patients. J Speech Hear Disord 33:236–245, 1968.
32. Jerger J: Clinical experience with impedance audiometry. Arch Otolaryngol
33. Schwartz DM: Current status of techniques for screening and diagnosis of middle ear disease in children. In Workshop on Controversies in Screening for Hearing Loss and Middle Ear Disease. Pediatrics 77:57–70, 1986.
34. Fria TJ, Sabo DL: Auditory brainstem responses in children with otitis media with effusion. Ann Otol Rhinol Laryngol 89:200–206, 1980.
35. Finitzo-Hieber T, Friel-Patti S: Conductive hearing loss and the ABR. In Jacobsen TJ (ed): The Auditory Brainstem Response. San Diego: College Hill Press, 1985.
36. Seewald RC, Ross M: Amplification for young hearing impaired children. In Pollack MC (ed): Amplification for the Hearing Impaired, 3rd ed. Orlando: Grune & Stratton, 1988.
37. Berger KW: Prescription of hearing aids: A rationale. J Am Audiol Soc 2:71–78, 1976.
38. Byrne D, Tonnison W: Selecting the gain of hearing aids for persons with sensorineural hearing impairments. Scand Audiol 5:51–62, 1976.
39. McCandless GA, Lyregaard P: Prescription of gain/output (POGO) for hearing aids. Hear Instruments 34:16–21, 1983.
40. Upfold LJ: Children with hearing aids in the 1980s: Etiologies and severity of impairment. Ear Hear 9:75–80, 1988.
41. Rood SR, Stool SE: Current concepts of the etiology, diagnosis, and management of cleft palate related otopathologic disease. Otolaryngol Clin North Am 14:865–884, 1981.

CHAPTER 87

Approaches to the Study of Speech Production

John W. Folkins and Jerald B. Moon

This chapter reviews the experimental procedures available to the investigator who wishes to study speech production. The scope of the review is broad in the sense that the approaches apply to normal speech as well as disordered speech. However, when discussing the measurement of speech disorders our emphasis is directed toward those disorders related to clefts of the lip and palate.

One goal of this chapter is to inform the reader who is not familiar with research in speech production about the existence of different approaches and how each one can be applied. Many of the approaches covered involve electronic instrumentation. However, we have organized the chapter according to the advantages and disadvantages of each approach, the types of information about speech to be obtained, and the articulators that each approach applies to (Table 87–1) and not according to the different kinds of instruments. No attempt is made to describe how the various instruments or procedures work or to explain how the procedures are performed.

Anatomy

Anatomic methods fall into the general categories of dissection and histology. Dissection can be further divided into gross dissection (done with the unaided eye) and microdissection (done with a dissecting microscope). Histology can be divided into light techniques and electron techniques. Light techniques include macroscopic analyses (using only a simple camera lens) and microscopic analyses (using a microscope). Electron microscopy can be either transmission or scanning.

Dissection

In the dissection of a cadaver or cadaveric material, structures are reflected and removed to expose underlying structures. The results are often quite dependent on the skill of the anatomist to recognize and isolate structures. Dissection, unlike other anatomic techniques, has an order effect—that is, the manner in which the first structures are removed influences the view of later structures. Dissection usually progresses from superficial to deep structures, and therefore the order effect is biased from superficial to deep. However, one can do complete midline sections and then dissect from deep to superficial, or the same structure can be approached from different directions in different specimens.

Table 87–1. Approaches to the Study of Anatomy and Physiology Related to Speech Production

	Structure						Type of Information			
Approach	Lips	Jaw	Tongue	Velum	Lateral Pharyngeal Wall	Larynx	Structural Outline	Point Displacement	Area	Regional Muscle Activity
Dissection	xx	xx	xx	xx	xx	xx	xx		x	
Histology	xx	xx	xx	xx	xx	xx	xx		x	
Electromyography	xx	xx	xx	xx	x	xx				xx
High-speed x-ray	xx	xx	xx	xx	xx		x	xx		
X-ray microbeam	x	x	x	x				x		
Strain gauge	xx	xx		x				xx		
Optical transduction	xx	xx	xx	xx	xx	x		xx	xx	
Ultrasound			xx		x	xx	x	xx		
Magnetometry	x	x	x	x				x		
Endoscopy				xx	xx	xx	x		x	
Pressure-flow[a]	x		x	xx	xx				xx	

xx = Commonly used; x = occasionally used or proposed.
[a]Warren and Dubois technique; see reference 37.

Dissection is a useful method when one has strong a priori evidence for the existence and accurate identification of discrete structures such as bone, organs, and (usually) muscles. Dissection allows measurement of the size and shape of different structures and shows the relations among different three-dimensional structures. Examples include observing the attachments of muscles and tracing the course of major bundles of peripheral nerves. Some of the structures used in speech, such as the muscles of the lips and velum, are difficult to dissect because it is difficult (in some areas perhaps arbitrary) to identify discrete muscles.[1, 2]

Microdissection is done with a microscope that has relatively low power (from $4\times$ to $100\times$ magnification) and a large depth of field. Of course, when anatomic structures are quite small, microdissection is preferable to gross dissection. However, increased acuity is gained at the expense of both the size and depth of the observed field. The anatomist's skill in making small incisions is often a limiting factor in microdissection. Unlike histologic procedures, microdissection does not require the staining, sectioning, and mounting of tissue, and therefore the shrinkage and artifact introduced with these techniques are avoided. However, the embalming procedures used prior to dissection and storage of the specimens may produce other artifacts. Microdissection gives a much clearer perspective of the three-dimensional shape and orientation of many structures than does light microscopy. Its disadvantages are that it is often difficult to make accurate measurements from dissected preparations, and one cannot stain selectively for tissue types.

Histology

Histology is the study of different tissue types in the body. However, the term is often applied to procedures used to allow such study, which include

1. Removing small sections of tissue from the body
2. Placing them in a fixative to preserve, dehydrate, and harden them
3. Embedding the fixed specimens in paraffin, gelatin, or plastic
4. Slicing them very thinly with a microtome
5. Mounting them on glass slides
6. Applying stains that adhere selectively to different tissue types.

Such specimens are typically analyzed with a high-power light microscope.[3]

Histologic techniques are suited for making measurements that are determined by changes in tissue type not easily dissected, such as layering within the palatal mucosa. A major disadvantage is that all information becomes essentially two-dimensional (limited by the thickness of the tissue slice, usually 5 to 7 μm). Three-dimensional information can be obtained by reconstructing information from slides taken in series. This often involves laborious analytic procedures, and often it is still difficult for an investigator to gain an accurate three-dimensional perspective of the material. It also is quite difficult to align the slices in the standard anatomic

planes (or even in planes that are consistent across specimens), and, of course, the alignment of any one slice will greatly influence any dimensional measurements taken on the slide.

Large sections of tissue do not fit on standard 3-inch by 1-inch glass slides. One can use oversized glass slides, although such macrospecimens are especially sensitive to artifact from tissue separation and breakage. Camera lenses can be used for analyses requiring much wider fields than are available from even low-power microscopes. Oversized slides are not very common histologic procedures; however, the large size of many speech structures may require them.

Electron microscopy is useful for showing the detail of tiny structures, those beyond the resolution of the light microscope. Transmission electron microscopy provides a two-dimensional view of sections analogous to that of light microscopy, but the magnification is much greater (up to $200,000\times$). Scanning electron microscopy provides a photographic image that appears three dimensional, and again, provides magnifications that give extraordinary resolution of very fine detail. Although electron microscopy has had many applications in the study of human anatomy, including the study of the inner ear, the majority of anatomic questions related to speech do not involve measurements that are this small (down to about 100 Å for scanning microscopy and 5 Å for transmission microscopy).

Anatomical Specimens

Virtually all of the anatomic procedures discussed above involve cadaveric material. A major limitation of anatomic work is that most of the human material is either from fetuses or from people who were quite old when they died. It is difficult to obtain material from young adults and even more difficult to get material from children. Consequently, very little research has been published based on these age groups. For most purposes, one must extrapolate between measurements taken from individuals who died in the seventh decade and fetal material. A related difficulty is that the precise age and past history of the material is usually unknown.

Much of the anatomic study of the structures used in speech has been conducted for the purpose of obtaining a general understanding of the structures rather than focusing specifically on the role of the structures in speech. This is certainly an advantage to the speech scientist in that it makes available a vast amount of data. However, very often the anatomist who may not be directly concerned with how structures function in speech will not ask the questions that are most important to the speech scientist.

A large amount of the current work done by basic anatomists is based on animal material. The use of animals rather than human cadavers has a number of advantages to the anatomist, especially in that he or she can complete various experimental procedures or injections prior to sacrifice (for example, horseradish peroxidase can be injected into nerve fibers to allow later histologic tracing of individual fibers) that allow more powerful analysis of the material. The anatomist also has more control of the age and history of the experimental animal than would be the case with human material; however, this can still be a problem with animal specimens.

As indicated earlier, it is especially difficult to obtain infant cadavers for anatomic study. Infant material with naturally occurring clefts of the lip or palate is even more difficult to find. With the exception of a study of 18 stillborn infants with palatal clefts completed by Fara and Dvorak,[4] the few reported anatomic studies of infant cadavers with clefts involve single cases.[5-7] Obviously, the collection of enough data in this area to make definitive generalizations will take prolonged searches of many sources of material.

Physiology

In the study of speech, physiologic techniques have the great advantage over anatomic procedures in that the former can be used in live humans and during speech. However, data from physiologic procedures cannot be substituted for anatomic information. We need to know the size, shape, and location of various structures as we use physiologic approaches to develop theories of how they function. Beyond the need for basic anatomic descriptions, anatomic evidence is often used as the basis of theories relating to function, which are beyond the reach of present physiologic techniques or which lead to subsequent physiologic tests.

A large number of physiologic techniques are not specific to speech but can be used in either acute or chronic experiments with animals. Animal procedures have the advantage that the experimenter can record information directly from many deep structures in the body and can perform follow-up anatomic procedures. The disadvantages of physiologic procedures with animals are similar to those of anatomic procedures used with animals. There are structural differences among species, and animals do not talk in the same way humans do. On the other hand, we can often build theories about speech functions from more general information about anatomic and physiologic principles that has been derived from experiments not related to speech. Furthermore, some animal behaviors may provide us with valuable insights into human speech processes. For example, it has been possible to do physiologic experiments during vocalization in the monkey[8] and cat.[9]

Physiologic procedures used in humans during the production of speech include the measurement of muscle activity by means of electromyography, movements of the various speech articulators, locations or pressures of articulatory contact, and speech aerodynamics (low-frequency pressures and flows of air in the respiratory system, larynx, or vocal tract). In general, the procedures have different advantages and disadvantages related to their application. However, the fundamental distinction to be stressed here is that the various procedures are designed to provide different information about many aspects of speech production. Some of these distinctions are presented in Table 87-1.

Electromyography

Electromyography is a procedure of great value in that it allows us to measure the activity of muscle fibers during speech production. Loeb and Gans provide an excellent explanation of the basic procedures used in electromyography.[10] By using fine wires (usually about 100-μm diameter), muscle activity can be measured without appreciably interfering with the performance of the speaker. The wires can be placed in virtually any muscle of the body. Although electromyography provides a window into the physiology of the cooperating human that has tremendous potential, it has a number of limitations.

Most important, the signals measured by electromyography may reflect muscle activity, but they do not indicate the force of muscle contraction. They can be used as a substitute for measures of muscle force only under very exceptional circumstances. The force produced by muscle action potentials varies with both the length of the muscle and the velocity of shortening. During speech, muscles are constantly changing length and velocity. It is only in very restricted paradigms that an investigator knows both how the muscle fibers are changing in length when force is estimated from electromyographic data and the specific relations between movement and force for that particular electrode pair. Generally, during speech one can observe electromyographic data to determine when muscle fibers in a particular location are active and to obtain a rough idea of the overall amount of activity, but one cannot infer that higher muscle forces are associated with the higher levels of activity.

It is routine to use anatomic criteria to place electrodes within a muscle and then to infer that one has a sample that is representative of the muscle as a whole. However, one should be cautious in drawing inferences because we are seldom able to

1. Confirm that the electrodes are actually in the vicinity of muscle fibers that would be defined as belonging to the muscle intended.[1]
2. Define the extent of the region sampled by the electrodes and demonstrate that other regions of the same muscle are not acting differently.
3. Ensure that activity from muscle fibers of what would be considered a nonintended muscle is not also being measured.[11]

These considerations are of special concern for speech muscles because many of the muscles are relatively small, often are divided into different compartments that may or may not function separately, and are not necessarily made up of homogeneous muscle fiber types or fibers with parallel orientations. The situation is further exacerbated in the muscles of the face and tongue, in which there is a large amount of interdigitation among muscle fibers identified with different muscles.[12]

In addition to these concerns about the validity of the signals in relation to anatomic concepts of a muscle, one needs to consider the reliability of the signals obtained from different pairs of electrodes. The size of the electromyographic signal depends on the distance between the muscle fibers and the electrodes and on the number of muscle fibers sampled. These factors depend not only on the precise placement of the electrodes but also on the distance between electrodes, the size of the electrodes, the material used to make the electrodes, and the orientation of a line drawn between electrodes relative to the direction of travel of the muscle action potentials.

Concerns about the reliability of electromyographic procedures can be minimized by taking precautions to define electrode placement criteria explicitly and in detail, and to control such factors as depth and angle of needle insertion, state of the tissue during needle insertion, and the distance and orientation between electrodes. When the target muscles are relatively large, reliability can be improved by increasing the size of the region sampled by using widely spaced electrodes with large exposed surfaces. Also, two electrode pairs can be used to obtain signals from the same region simultaneously to measure reliability.[13, 14]

In general, hooked-wire electrodes are hardly noticeable to the subject when in place. However, there is some discomfort when the hypodermic needles are inserted to place the wires. The discomfort is slightly greater around the vermilion of the lips than in many other locations and greater in the upper lip than in the lower lip. Some subjects also report a slight discomfort when the electrodes are removed by tugging on the wires to straighten the hooked ends. Because of the discomfort and the generally invasive nature of the procedure, investigators have been reluctant to place hooked wire electrodes in children.

Small nonobtrusive surface electrodes have been fabricated to record electromyographic activity from the lips.[15] There are a number of differences in use and application between hooked-wire electrodes and surface electrodes. The most important differences are that surface electrodes are limited to measuring muscle activity just below the skin and also are not well suited to intraoral placement. One cannot vary the depth of the placement of surface electrodes. For measurement of muscle activity during speech, the lips provide the only area of musculature suited to their use.

Some studies have used electrodes placed closely together to record activity from single motor units in the speech musculature.[16] Such procedures are cumbersome. For most purposes a large amount of analysis is required for each motor unit sampled, and a large number of motor units should be sampled. It is difficult to continue sampling from a single unit with a very selective electrode pair during speech.[17] For most speech gestures the contraction of the muscle or the movement of the structures will influence the electrodes, and therefore either the unit under analysis is lost or the recruitment of new units makes it impossible to measure the units separately.

Measurement of Speech Movements

There are a wide variety of systems available for measuring the movements of speech structures. Many of the systems are designed to measure laryngeal or respiratory movements. However, this review will be limited to describing the procedures for measuring movement of upper airway articulators. Procedures for measuring articulatory displacement include analysis of high-speed x-rays,[18] the use of small lights (such as light-emitting diodes) attached to structures from which the movements of the lights are transduced,[19] the use of stiff wires attached between moving structures and bendable cantilevers, allowing measurement of the bend of the cantilever with a strain gauge,[20] the use of a computer-controlled x-ray beam to track pellets attached to the articulators (called an x-ray microbeam),[21] pulsing ultrasound between a source and a tiny receiver attached to an articulator,[22] and measuring the changes in magnetic flux between a stationary and a moving magnetic coil.[23, 24] These procedures differ greatly in their ease of use, accuracy, applicability to different structures (see Table 87–1), interference with movements, acceptability by subjects, and availability of data for online analysis or training. A description of all of these procedures and their specific advantages is beyond the scope of this chapter; however, a number of detailed reviews are available.[25–27]

When measuring speech movements, one of the most fundamental questions concerns not just what articulators to measure, but where on the articulator to make the measurements. Some of the earliest studies of speech movements traced the structures observable in lateral-view x-ray motion pictures.[18] Criteria were developed to define specific points on the traced structures so that movements of the points could be tracked from frame to frame. Kent explains that a useful refinement in x-ray analysis occurred when investigators began attaching radiopaque markers to the midline of the moving structures prior to filming.[28] Not only did this eliminate tracing contours of structures that were never interpreted but it also automated analysis. However, it also changed the analysis in a fundamental way. Previously, criteria such as the most superior point on the tongue body or lower lip, or the most posterior point on the velum would have been used. The tissue corresponding to the reference point might shift as the shape of a structure was modified during speech. Attaching radiopaque markers ensured not only that the same fleshpoints were traced from frame to frame but also that the points of interest were at the midline. This is an important consideration for x-ray analyses, in which all sagittal planes influence the size and clarity of the image, so that tissue closer to the x-ray source appears much smaller than tissue farther away.

The points chosen for movement analysis often correspond to articulators involved in traditional phonetic taxonomies (for example, a point on the superior surface of the tongue tip, one or two points further back on the superior surface of the tongue body, a point on the anterior surface of the vermilion of the lower lip and a corresponding point on the upper lip, a point on the inferior surface of the velum often in the region of the velar knee, and a point on the mandible). In all of these cases, it is assumed that the movement of one point reflects an overall change of the shape of the vocal tract that has either acoustic or aerodynamic significance. In some cases it has been inferred by the investigators that the motor system actually controls the movement of the articulator during speech and that this control is directly reflected in the movement of the chosen point.

There are other systems in use that scan a contour of the tongue. These include scanning ultrasound in which both the transmitter and the receiver are located on the underside of the chin,[29] and photoelectric systems that use an artificial palate both to transmit light and to receive the light reflected from the tongue.[30, 31] Like the older procedures for measuring x-rays, data from these procedures can be analyzed over a period of time, but there should be no expectation that the same fleshpoint is being analyzed. However, in some theoretical applications it may be preferable to base the analyses on criteria such as the point of highest elevation rather than on a fleshpoint.

In general, little attention has been given to measurements that are not along the midline, such as the contour of the lips as they filter the sound exiting the vocal tract, even though this has acoustic significance and is represented in traditional phonetic taxonomies (see the studies by Folkins[32] and Fromkin[33] for exceptions). Movements of the lateral pharyngeal walls also have received less attention than some other speech structures. This may be due in part to the nonsagittal plane of their movements but also to their deep location and the difficulty of attaching markers to specific fleshpoints on the lateral pharyngeal walls.

In mastication, movements occur in three dimensions. Movements made in speech are somewhat easier to transduce in that most articulatory movements can be characterized well in two dimensions.[34] For most articulators, these dimensions are inferior-superior and anterior-posterior. Again, the exceptions are movements that do not occur in the midsagittal plane, movements of the corner of the mouth, grooving of the sides of the tongue tip, and medial movements of the lateral pharyngeal walls.

Transduction systems are often aligned to measure displacement within either the sagittal, coronal, or transverse planes. However, most speech movements do not occur within the standard anatomic planes, and a full description of any displacement thus requires inclusion of a third dimension. If a movement is truly two-dimensional, this requirement can be avoided by changing the transduction system to measure the two dimensions that capture most of the movement regardless of the anatomic plane.[32]

A further dimensional simplification is common for some articulatory movements, such as the movements of the lips. It is often adequate to measure and analyze inferior-superior movement across time and to ignore any anterior-posterior component of the movement. Although this procedure greatly simplifies analysis and may not influence the way in which some data may address a particular theory, it is important for investigators to keep in mind the differences in both displacement and velocity that occur between movement measurements in a maximal dimension and in the largest of two standard anatomic dimensions.

Another general category of measurement systems does not track a fleshpoint during time or even the distance across the vocal tract at specific points, but rather the cross-sectional area of a minimum construction of the vocal tract. One way of doing this is to measure the light passing through a constriction, such as the photodetector system described by Dalston[35] and Moon and Lagu.[36] Such systems have been used to measure the cross-sectional area of the velopharyngeal port and can be applied also to measure the glottal area or the area of maximum oral constriction.

A related but somewhat different approach is offered by the Warren and DuBois[37] system for estimating minimum area from measures of oral pressure and nasal flow, to be discussed below. Like the photodetector systems, this system is designed to estimate the minimum cross-sectional area across a constriction in a tube, regardless of where in the tube the minimum occurs. This may give very different information than that obtained from systems measuring the cross-sectional area at fixed points along the tract. It is also important to note that pressure-flow procedures do not give an accurate indication of minimum area over time, and measurements should be restricted to the instances of maximum airflow.

Articulatory Contact

There is often theoretical interest in the pressure, force, or extent of contact between two articulators. For example, the amount of pressure involved in a bilabial seal relative to the resistance to oral air pressure has often been discussed. We also would like to know the factors that affect the seal of the velopharyngeal port. However, very little work has been done generally to develop systems to measure bilabial pressure or the pressure that occurs during closure of the velopharyngeal port. Proffit et al have attempted to develop an artificial palate with embedded strain gauges that measure the force of contact between the tongue tip and the alveolar ridge.[38] Linville and associates attempted to develop procedures for measuring the contact pressure of the velopharyngeal seal.[39] However, much work remains before this method can be used as a viable experimental procedure.

In contrast to concern about the force or pressure of articulatory contact, a number of systems have been developed to measure the spatial configuration of tongue contact along the hard palate.[40] In general, these systems involve an artificial palate embedded with an array of contacts that sense the presence or absence of lingual contact. The systems must be fabricated separately for each subject, and the analysis of the data can be cumbersome if 32 to 64 data points are analyzed over time; however, a more important consideration is that the spatial location of tongue tip contact may not have the same theoretical utility as many other possible measurements.

Aerodynamic Measurements

Different measurements of the pressure and flow of air in the vocal and nasal tracts may be used to provide information about speech that is useful for a variety of purposes. They can be used to explore how aerodynamic phenomena are used in the production of acoustic phenomena and to study the nervous system's control of speech aerodynamics. In some cases, measures of air pressure and airflow during speech can be used to try to extrapolate information about movements of the upper airway, laryngeal movements, and respiratory movements.[41] Air pressures are typically measured with either a gauge or a differential pressure transducer. A number of electronic approaches may be applied. These include variable capacitance, variable resistance, variable reluctance, and piezoresistance systems. All accept a pressure signal, usually from a small tube placed in the vocal tract, and produce a voltage measurement with magnitude related linearly to the difference in pressure within the tube and a reference pressure.

Airflows are typically transduced by measuring the pressure drop across a resistance placed in the air stream. The pressure drop across a constant resistance will be linearly related to the laminar flow through the resistance. The most common type of resistance employed is a fine-wire mesh screen, although a honeycomb of narrow tubes has also been used. The air inlet, air outlet, resistance component, and pressure-sensing ports are incorporated into a device called a pneumotachograph. The pneumotachograph is coupled to the subject with a mask of some type, or with a tube placed in the mouth or nose. Although pneumotachographs are the most common instrument used to measure airflow, one can also measure flow by measuring respiratory volume and inferring airflow from its rate of change.[27] It has also been suggested that hot-wire anemometers have potential for measuring airflow during speech.[42]

Unlike many other techniques, aerodynamic measures may be applied easily in both research and clinical situations. They are relatively noninvasive, requiring only a small tube to be placed in the oral or nasal cavity, or a mask covering the nose, mouth, or both nose and mouth. The systems are relatively inexpensive, they are easy to use and calibrate, and data are often available immediately.

However, a number of precautions must be taken into account regarding the instrumentation, its use, and the interpretation of data. Exhaled air is humidified, and pneumotachographs are prone to a buildup of condensation. Condensation may alter the resistance of the pneumotachograph, affecting calibration. Although some pneumotachographs are equipped with heated mesh screens to obviate this problem, others are not. Some investigators feel that the time spent breathing through the device and the amount of condensation are

not significant enough to make this precaution necessary. Others blow heated air through the pneumotachograph periodically to evaporate any condensation.

The length and inside diameter of the tubing connected to the pressure transducer of the pneumotachograph will limit the frequency response of the system.[43] One must also be careful to prevent clogging of the pressure tube with saliva. Hardy[44] and Fritch and Saxman[45] have discussed the artifacts that are possible with inadequate placement of the pressure tube in the mouth. Placement of a mask against the face for measurement of nasal or oral airflow may produce an alteration in the shape or function of the face. A tight nasal mask might pinch the nasal ala, artificially increasing the nasal airway resistance and reducing the flow. A large nasal mask impinging on the upper lip may impede its movement. A face mask covering the nose and mouth may be expected to affect mandibular movement during speech. In some cases it may be possible to minimize these artifacts by using a restricted speech sample. Finally, the seal of the mask against the face is extremely important. Anything less than an airtight seal will produce large artifacts.

Some of the procedures used to measure the physiologic aspects of speech production have been used to study speakers with a repaired cleft of the lip or palate.[46] However, experimental studies of measurements of electromyographic or articulatory movements over time in cleft palate speakers are extremely rare.[47, 48] Much of what we know about the physiologic processes of speakers with a cleft is derived either from clinical data or by extrapolating data from experimental measures made in normal subjects. There are a number of reasons for this situation. Most important, many of the procedures are invasive, uncomfortable, and sometimes associated with greater than minimal risk. We have been reluctant to use them with patients, especially children. In many cases, we have been able to ask the experimental questions needed to understand the disordered speakers by studying the flexibility and plasticity of physiologic processes in normal speakers.[49]

In contrast to other physiologic tools, measurements of airflows and air pressures have long been used in the study of velopharyngeal dysfunction in speakers with cleft palate, both in research and in clinical situations. For example, Warren and his colleagues have employed measures of oral pressure, nasal pressure, and nasal flow on a routine basis. The Warren and DuBois system mentioned above uses airflow and air pressure differences across the velopharyngeal port to estimate the cross-sectional area of the port during speech.[37, 50] The accuracy of Warren's procedure continues to be debated and scrutinized,[51] but numerous reports support its use and have attempted to assess its accuracy.[52, 53]

Acoustic Analyses

Traditionally, speech acoustics have been analyzed using the sound spectrograph. The spectrograph uses a filter system to produce a frequency by time display, with the intensity at any frequency-time point represented by the darkness of the display. Spectrographs have been replaced during the last two decades by inexpensive yet fast and powerful computer systems for acoustic analysis. Some computer systems emulate the type of display traditionally provided by the spectrograph. Others provide a much wider variety of display and analysis options. It should be stressed that all systems are designed to allow accurate analysis of the features of sound that are thought to be most important in the perception of speech; however, to do so requires the distortion of other characteristics of the acoustic signal.[54, 55]

Only a microphone placed in front of a speaker and a quiet environment are required to transduce the acoustics of speech production. Furthermore, the acoustic signal carries most of the information important to a listener. Considering also the ready availability of present computer systems, it would seem that acoustic analyses should provide ideal instrumental procedures in that they are entirely noninvasive and the data are relatively easy to collect and analyze. Indeed, there are many important uses for acoustic analyses of speech production; however, acoustic measures of disordered speech have often been difficult to interpret in a meaningful manner. This is especially the case for acoustic measures of the speech of speakers with a repaired palatal cleft.

Coupling the nasal cavity to the oral cavity alters the resonance of the vocal tract and hence the spectrum of the speech output. A number of studies have addressed the acoustic consequences of coupling the nasal tract to the oral tract.[56–60] The primary characteristics of this procedure are a reduction in the intensity of the first formant, the addition of one or two antiresonances, the addition of one or two small resonances, and a shift of the center frequency of the formants. The effects differ according to the size of the oral-to-nasal coupling and the size of the oral opening.

Although the acoustic effects of oral to nasal coupling are well understood in theory, in practice they are combined with many other factors that influence the speech signal. In typical circumstances, we cannot analyze a speech signal and discern with any certainty whether or not nasal coupling is present. Bjork and Nylen have shown that the acoustic features of nasality are not evident in disordered speakers until an extreme level of perceptually identified nasality is present.[61] Dickson also showed that none of the traditional spectral measures can be used to differentiate between normal and hypernasal speakers consistently.[58]

One approach to circumventing the difficulties with traditional acoustic procedures is to use both oral and nasal microphones with a horizontal sound separator between them. The signals are rectified and smoothed, and a ratio (referred to as nasalance) is determined by dividing the amplitude of the nasal signal by the sum of the oral and nasal amplitudes. Much of the developmental work for this type of system has been conducted

by Fletcher.[62, 63] The system has been marketed as TONAR (The Oral Nasal Acoustic Ratio) and TONAR II. It is now commerically available as the Nasometer.™ Both Fletcher[64] and Dalston and Warren[65] have shown significant positive correlations (r = 0.91 and r = 0.76, respectively) between nasalance scores and group ratings of nasality in disordered speakers.

The acoustic energy present in the nasal cavity not only will be propagated outward through the nares but will also vibrate the hard and soft tissues of the nose. A second alternative to traditional acoustic transduction involves using an accelerometer placed over the nasal bone to measure the vibration of the tissues.[66, 67] A simultaneous signal is measured either from a standard microphone or from a second accelerometer placed on the neck over the thyroid lamina.[68] The two signals are rectified and smoothed, and a ratio is determined through one of a variety of procedures such as HONC (Horii Oral Nasal Coupling),[67] NAVI (Nasal Accelerometric Vibrational Index),[69] or the Nasal Resonance Index.[68] Only a few comparative studies have been conducted to compare accelerometric ratios to perceptual ratings of nasality. Horii used normal speakers who simulated hypernasal speech and found an average correlation of 0.92 between mean HONC measurements and perceived nasality.[70] Redenbaugh and Reich obtained moderate to high correlations between NAVI scores and objective nasality judgments in 12 speech-disordered children and three normal-speaking children.[69, 71]

Although nasalance measures and accelerometric ratios provide scores that often correlate with perceptual judgments, it is also clear that the different procedures do not always match each other well. If one wishes to obtain accurate measures of nasality, one should use objective perceptual procedures (to be discussed below). Neither nasalance nor accelerometric ratios can be expected to provide a good substitute for objective perceptual measurements. One advantage of both nasalance and accelerometric measurements is that both signals can be computed throughout the time course of voicing during speech. Therefore, when used in conjunction with perceptual measures, procedures may eventually be developed to help us understand what factors during the time course of speech production contribute most to perceptions of disordered nasality.[72]

Perceptual Measures

Auditory judgments have a long history in the study of speech production. They form the standards for normal and disordered performance that are central to the interpretation of all other levels of analysis. Auditory judgments can take the form of informal clinical assessment, a score made within the structure of a formal test battery (such as a standardized articulation test), or a measure obtained from application of a psychophysical scaling procedure. Specific judgments have been made for overall defectiveness, defective articulation, intelligibility, nasality, bizarre speech, stress patterning, loudness, and other descriptive parameters.

There are three common psychophysical procedures that have been studied and refined extensively: direct magnitude estimation, interval scaling, and paired comparisons. Direct magnitude estimation involves assigning a number to each sample so that the numbers represent the ratio of the sample to a standard reference. For interval scaling, the listener assigns each sample a position on a linearly partitioned scale. For paired comparisons, the listener does not choose one reference but compares all stimuli with others in sets of two.

The advantages and appropriateness of one psychophysical procedure compared with another have been evaluated many times. Paired comparisons can be quite laborious and are not very applicable to speech judgments. Direct magnitude estimation is sometimes more reliable than interval scaling. However, the differences between the two procedures may not always justify the extra work required to perform direct magnitude estimation procedures. The choice of procedure may depend also on the characteristics of the parameter to be scaled.

Categorical decisions such as those involved in standard phonetic transcriptions are not only important in the definition of many independent and dependent variables in speech experiments, they also form the basis of both diagnostic and therapeutic approaches to many speech disorders. It has been shown that transcriptional procedures can be quite reliable if standard procedures are carefully applied;[73] however, when used in a clinical setting many factors may make the reliability of the measures difficult to assess. These factors include variations in the listening conditions,[74] variation in any preestablished standard,[75, 76] the articulation skill of the speaker,[50, 77] vocal pitch and intensity,[78] and the past experience or skill of the listener.[50]

In addition to auditory judgments, some procedures require relatively broad visual judgments to be made by an experimenter or clinician. For example, these procedures may involve assessment of velopharyngeal movement or function as observed through nasal endoscopy,[79] velopharyngeal activity as viewed in two dimensions from videofluorographic films,[80] velopharyngeal activity as viewed in three dimensions from videofluorographic films,[81] vocal fold movement observed through stroboscopy,[82] and facial gestures.[83] As with many auditory judgments, the reliability of many visual judgments is difficult to estimate. Many factors, such as the consistency of a preestablished standard, past experience of the examiner, the method of visualization, the size of the visual image, and the distortion inherent in the visual display used, have an obvious impact. Some attempts have been made to assess the reliability of visual judgments that might be used for experimental purposes,[84] but many of these factors present serious theoretical or practical barriers that hinder the evaluation of their importance. For example, it has not been practical to perform experiments that compare judgments by different clinicians on a scale that would make them most meaningful.

How Approaches Combine

It is clear that a wide variety of procedures are available to the investigator wishing to study speech production. The procedures differ in many ways that are related to the practical considerations of their use. Some procedures are invasive; some cannot be used easily with children; and some involve awkward or expensive data analysis.

Perhaps even more important than the practical considerations in the application of the procedures are the theoretical distinctions among the measurements on any level of the system. The different procedures often provide distinctly different information about the various aspects of speech production. Physiologic measurements are not a substitute for anatomic analyses of articulatory structure. By using electromyographic procedures in various ways, one can study different aspects of motor control of speech (for example, the timing of single motor units versus the timing of gross muscle activity). Measurements of any articulatory movement depend on the point of the structure that is tracked and the dimensions in which they are tracked. Different measures of tongue movement result if fleshpoints on the surface of the tongue are tracked instead of the distance between the closest part of the tongue to a reference point on the palate. Movement of a point on the inferior surface of the velum may look very different from a measurement of the minimum cross-sectional area of the velopharyngeal port during the same time span.[85] There are many other examples.

The dependency of the information on the procedures employed underscores the importance of keeping the general levels of analysis separate. One can measure muscle activity, force, movement, aerodynamics, acoustics, or perceptually defined effects. A measurement on one level is not necessarily more objective than a measurement on another level. One level is not to be preferred to another level unless the preference is based on a theoretical distinction. Only under very restricted conditions can one hope to use a measurement on one level as a substitute for a measurement on another level.

It is sometimes possible to extrapolate information on one level to another level. For example, in the Warren and DuBois procedure aerodynamic measurements are extrapolated to give the minimum cross-sectional area.[37] But the adequacy of the assumptions involved in this estimate have been the subject of continuous study (and some controversy). It is clear that extrapolating from one level to another is seldom, if ever, straightforward.

Extrapolations between levels typically require a computer simulation, a large amount of data on the level analyzed, a number of limiting assumptions, and a tolerance for large errors. For example, if one were to model an articulatory motion it would require information about the anatomic orientation of muscles acting on the articulator, including the directions of the muscle forces, the biomechanics of the tissues, the activity of the muscle fibers, and a model of the force across different muscle lengths and shortening velocities. The data available for use in such a simulation would be difficult to obtain, and the circumstances of measurement would undoubtedly limit the range of the model. In spite of such limitations, some computer simulations have been developed to allow one to predict articulatory movement during speech from anatomic or physiologic measurements. For example, there are models of vocal fold motion,[86] tongue movement,[87] and lip movement.[88]

Models of aerodynamic and acoustic phenomena are usually better when they are based on knowledge of speech movements; however, these models still require large amounts of information and work only under limited circumstances.[51] Furthermore, the type of information necessary, such as the three-dimensional contour of the vocal tract and the manner in which it changes over time, is seldom available. Some attempts have been made to start from acoustic measurements and work upstream to model movements that could have been used to produce them.[89, 90] Such models often work in a general sense; however, one must be careful to remember the limits of the model in relation to its underlying assumptions.

It is also important to stress that specific measurements at each level of the speech production system can be related to many different combinations of events at preceding levels. The downstream mapping of events generally proceeds in a many-to-one fashion. Therefore, even if a large amount of acoustic information is available, it may often be necessary to know a good deal about the factors limiting the movement of the vocal tract before one can work upstream to model accurately the speech movements that produced the acoustic events.

Conclusion

We have reviewed the procedures used for gathering anatomic, physiologic, acoustic, and perceptual data related to speech production. It is clear that the general areas, as well as the specific procedures within each area, have different methodologic advantages and disadvantages and provide the investigator with very different information. In our opinion, the important question is not "What type of analysis is best?" but rather, "What combination of different measurements and assumptions will provide the most insight about any particular experimental or clinical question?"

References

1. Kennedy J, Abbs J: Anatomic studies of the perioral motor system: Foundations for studies in speech pathology. In Lass N (ed): Speech and Language: Advances in Basic Research and Practice. Vol. 1. New York: Academic Press, 1979.
2. Kuehn D, Azzam N: Anatomical characteristics of palatoglossus and the anterior faucial pillar. Cleft Palate J 15:349, 1978.
3. Bloom W, Fawcett D: A Textbook of Histology. Philadelphia: Saunders, 1975.
4. Fara M, Dvorak J: Abnormal anatomy of the muscles of palatopharyngeal closure in cleft palates. Plast Reconstr Surg 46:288, 1970.
5. Wynn SK, Lynch KL: Gross and microscopic anatomical studies of palate structure and osteotomy site. Ann Plast Surg 3:406, 1979.
6. Doyle W, Kitajiri M, Sando I: The anatomy of the auditory tube and paratubal musculature in a one month old cleft palate infant. Cleft Palate J 20:218, 1983.
7. Latham R, Long R, Latham E: Cleft palate velopharyngeal musculature in a five month old infant: A three dimensional reconstruction. Cleft Palate J 17:1, 1980.
8. Larson C, Sutton D, Lindeman R: Cerebellar regulation of phonation in Rhesus monkey (*Macaca mulatta*). Exp Brain Res 33:1, 1978.
9. Garrett J: The response of laryngeal mechanoreceptors innervated by the superior laryngeal nerve during evoked phonation in the cat. Ph.D. thesis. Iowa City: University of Iowa, 1986.
10. Loeb G, Gans C: Electromyography for Experimentalists. Chicago: University of Chicago Press, 1986.
11. Blair C, Smith A: EMG recording in human lip muscles: Can single muscles be isolated? J Speech Hear Res 29:256, 1986.
12. Blair C: Interdigitating muscle fibers throughout orbicularis oris inferior: Preliminary observations. J Speech Hear Res 29:266, 1986.
13. Kewley-Port D: EMG signal processing for speech research. Haskins Lab Status Rep Speech Res SR–50, 123, 1977.
14. Cooper D, Folkins J: Comparison of electromyographic signals from different electrode placements in the palatoglossus muscle. J Acoust Soc Am 78:1530, 1985.
15. Cole K, Konopacki R, Abbs J: A miniature electrode for surface electromyography during speech. J Acoust Soc Am 74:1362, 1983.
16. Sussman H, MacNeilage P, Powers R: Recruitment and discharge patterns of single motor units during speech production. J Speech Hear Res 20:613, 1977.
17. Smith A, Zimmermann G, Abbas P: Recruitment patterns of motor units in speech production. J Speech Hear Res 24:567, 1981.
18. Moll K: Photographic and radiographic procedures in speech research. ASHA Reports 1:129, 1965.
19. Lindblom B, Bivner P: A method for continuous recording of articulatory movement. Speech Transmission Laboratory, Quarterly Progress and Status Report, Stockholm: Royal Institute of Technology, 1966, p. 14.
20. Muller E, Abbs J: Strain gauge transduction of lip and jaw motion in the midsagittal plane: Refinement of a prototype system. J Acoust Soc Am 65:481, 1979.
21. Abbs J, Nadler R: User's Manual for the University of Wisconsin X-ray Microbeam. Madison, WI: University of Wisconsin, 1987.
22. Watkin K, Zagzebski J: On-line ultrasound technique for monitoring tongue displacements. J Acoust Soc Am 54:544, 1973.
23. Hixon T: An electromagnetic method for transducing jaw movements during speech. J Acoust Soc Am 49:603, 1971.
24. Sonoda Y: A high sensitivity magnetometer for measuring tongue point movements. In Sawashima M, Cooper F (eds): Dynamic Aspects of Speech Production. Tokyo: University of Tokyo Press, 1977, p. 145.
25. Folkins J, Kuehn D: Speech production. In Lass N, McReynolds L, Northern J, et al (eds): Speech, Language and Hearing. Vol I. Philadelphia: Saunders, 1982.
26. Borden G, Harris K: Speech Science Primer, 2nd ed. Baltimore: Williams & Wilkins, 1984.
27. Baken R: Clinical Measurement of Speech and Voice. Boston: College-Hill, 1987.
28. Kent R: Some considerations in the cinefluorographic analysis of tongue movements during speech. Phonetica 26:16, 1972.
29. Sonies B, Shawker T, Hall T, et al: Ultrasonic visualization of tongue motion during speech. J Acoust Soc Am 70:683, 1981.
30. Chuang C, Wang W: Use of optical distance sensing to track tongue motion. J Speech Hear Res 21:482, 1978.
31. Smith H, Fletcher S, McCutcheon M: Progress in optical transduced measurement and tracking of tongue height. In Saha S (ed): Proceedings of the Fifth Southern Biomedical Engineering Conference. New York: Pergamon Press, 1986, p 66.
32. Folkins J: Lower lip displacement during in vivo stimulation of human labial muscles. Arch Oral Biol 23:195, 1978.
33. Fromkin V: Parameters of lip position. UCLA Working Papers in Phonetics 1:15, 1964.
34. Gibbs C, Messerman T: Jaw motion during speech. ASHA Reports 7: 104, 1972.
35. Dalston R: Photodetector assessment of velopharyngeal activity. Cleft Palate J 19:1, 1982.
36. Moon J, Lagu R: Development of a second-generation phototransducer for the assessment of velopharyngeal activity. Cleft Palate J 24:240, 1987.
37. Warren D, DuBois A: A pressure-flow technique for measuring velopharyngeal orifice area during continuous speech. Cleft Palate J 1:52, 1964.
38. Proffit W, Palmer J, Kydd W: Evaluation of tongue pressure during speech. Folia Phoniatr 17:115, 1965.
39. Linville R, Scherer R, Folkins J: Study of velopharyngeal kinetics. Presented at the annual convention of the American Speech Language Hearing Association, San Francisco, 1984.
40. Fletcher S, McCutcheon M, Wolf M: Dynamic palatometry. J Speech Hear Res 18:812, 1975.
41. Muller E: The effects of laryngeal articulation during stop consonant

production on the time-course of supraglottal air pressure. In Bless D, Abbs J (eds): Vocal Fold Physiology: Contemporary Research and Clinical Issues. San Diego: College-Hill Press, 1983, p 176.

42. Quigley L, Shiere F, Webster R, et al: Measuring palatopharyngeal competence with the nasal anemometer. Cleft Palate J 1:304, 1964.

43. Edmonds T, Lilly D, Hardy J: Dynamic characteristics of air-pressure measuring systems used in speech research. J Acoust Soc Am 50:1051, 1971.

44. Hardy J: Techniques of measuring intraoral air pressure and rate of airflow. J Speech Hear Res 10:650, 1967.

45. Fritch E, Saxman J: Dental appliance for support of intraoral air pressure sensors. J Dental Res 50:980, 1971.

46. McWilliams B, Morris H, Shelton R: Cleft Palate Speech. Philadelphia: B. C. Decker, 1984.

47. Karnell M, Folkins J, Morris H: Relationships between the perception of nasalization and speech movements in speakers with cleft palate. J Speech Hear Res 28:63, 1985.

48. Li C, Lundervold A: Electromyographic study of cleft palate. Plast Reconstr Surg 21:427, 1958.

49. Folkins J: Issues in speech motor control and their relation to the speech of individuals with cleft palate. Cleft Palate J 22:106, 1985.

50. Dalston R, Warren D: The diagnosis of velopharyngeal inadequacy. Clin Plast Surg 12:685, 1985.

51. Muller E, Brown W: Variations in the supraglottal air pressure waveform and their articulatory interpretation. In Lass N (ed): Speech and Language: Advances in Basic Research and Practice. Vol 4. New York: Academic Press, 1980.

52. Smith B, Weinberg B: Prediction of modeled velopharyngeal orifice areas during steady flow conditions and during aerodynamic simulation of voiceless stop consonants. Cleft Palate J 19:172, 1982.

53. Smith B, Moon J, Weinberg B: The effects of increased nasal airway resistance on modeled velopharyngeal orifice area estimation. Cleft Palate J 21:18, 1984.

54. Wakita H: Instrumentation for the study of speech acoustics. In Lass N (ed): Contemporary Issues in Experimental Phonetics. New York: Academic Press, 1976, p 3.

55. Rabiner L, Schafer R: Digital Processing of Speech Signals. Englewood Cliffs NJ: Prentice-Hall, 1978.

56. Bloomer H, Peterson G: A spectrographic study of hypernasality. Cleft Palate J 5:5, 1955.

57. Hattori S, Yamamoto K, Fujimura O: Nasalization of vowels in relation to nasals. J Acoust Soc Am 30:267, 1958.

58. Dickson DR: An acoustic study of nasality. J Speech Hear Res 5:103, 1962.

59. Curtis J: The acoustics of nasalized speech. Cleft Palate J 6:380, 1968.

60. Schwartz M: Acoustic measures of nasalization and nasality. In Grabb W et al (eds): Cleft Lip and Palate: Surgical, Dental, and Speech Aspects. Boston: Little, Brown, 1971.

61. Bjork L, Nylen B: Cineradiography with synchronized sound spectrum analysis: A study of velopharyngeal function during connected speech in normals and cleft palate cases. Plast Reconstr Surg 27:397, 1961.

62. Fletcher S: Theory and instrumentation for quantitative measurement of nasality. Cleft Palate J 7:601, 1970.

63. Fletcher S: Contingencies for bioelectric modification of nasality. J Speech Hear Dis 37:329, 1972.

64. Fletcher S: Nasalence vs listener judgments of nasality. Cleft Palate J 13:31, 1976.

65. Dalston R, Warren D: Comparison of Tonar II, pressure-flow, and listener judgments of hypernasality in the assessment of velopharyngeal function. Cleft Palate J 23:108, 1986.

66. Stevens K, Kalikow D, Willemain T: A miniature accelerometer for detecting glottal waveforms and nasalization. J Speech Hear Res 18:594, 1975.

67. Horii Y: An accelerometric approach to nasality measurement: A preliminary report. Cleft Palate J 17:254, 1980.

68. Edgerton M, Sandove M, Comptom M, et al: Nasal vibration analysis: A noninvasive objective technique to evaluate the speech of patients with palatopharyngeal disorders. Plast Reconstr Surg 68:153, 1981.

69. Redenbaugh M, Reich A: Correspondence between an accelerometric nasal/voice amplitude ratio and listeners' direct magnitude estimations of hypernasality. J Speech Hear Res 28:273, 1985.

70. Horii Y: An accelerometric measure as a physical correlate of perceived hypernasality in speech. J Speech Hear Res 26:476, 1983.

71. Redenbaugh M, Reich A: Perceptual validation of nasal/voice accelerometry using equal appearing interval scaling. Presented at the annual convention of the American Speech Language Hearing Association, Washington, 1985.

72. Jones D: Effect of speech production time on perception in disordered nasality and measures of nasal accelerometry. Ph.D. thesis. Iowa City: University of Iowa, 1987.

73. Oller K, Eilers R: Phonetic expectation and transcription validity. Phonetica 31:288, 1975.

74. Moller K, Starr C: The effects of listening conditions on speech ratings obtained in a clinical setting. Cleft Palate J 21:65, 1984.

75. Counihan D, Cullinan W: Reliability and dispersion of nasality ratings. Cleft Palate J 7:261, 1970.

76. Kuehn D: Assessment of resonance disorders. In Lass N, McReynolds L, Northern J, et al (eds): Speech, Language and Hearing. Vol II. Philadelphia: Saunders, 1982.

77. Spriestersbach D: Assessing nasal quality in cleft palate speech of children. J Speech Hear Dis 20:266, 1955.

78. Hess D: Pitch, intensity, and cleft palate voice quality. J Speech Hear Res 2:113, 1959.

79. Pigott R: Assessment of velopharyngeal function. In Edwards M, Watson A (eds): Advances in the Management of Cleft Palate. London: Churchill Livingstone, 1980.

80. Eisenbach C, Williams W: Comparing the unaided visual exam to lateral cinefluorography in estimating several parameters of velopharyngeal function. J Speech Hear Res 49:136, 1984.

81. Croft C, Shprintzen R, Rakoff S: Patterns of velopharyngeal valving in normal and cleft palate subjects: A multi-view videofluoroscopic and nasendoscopic study. Laryngoscope 91:265, 1981.

82. Kitzing P: Stroboscopy—a pertinent laryngological examination. J Otolaryngol 14:151, 1985.

83. Philips B: Perceptual evaluation of velopharyngeal competency. Annals Otol Rhinol Laryngol, Suppl 69:153, 1980.

84. Karnell M, Ibuki K, Morris H, et al: Reliability of the nasopharyngeal fiberscope (NPF) for assessing velopharyngeal function: Analysis by judgment. Cleft Palate J 20:199, 1983.

85. Zimmermann G, Dalston R, Brown C, et al: Comparison of cineradiographic and photodetection techniques for assessing velopharyngeal function during speech. J Speech Hear Res 30:564, 1987.

86. Titze I, Talkin D: A theoretical study of the effects of various laryngeal configurations on the acoustics of phonation. J Acoust Soc Am 66:60, 1979.

87. Kakita Y, Fujimura O, Honda K: Computation of mapping from muscular contraction patterns to formant patterns in vowel space. In Fromkin V (ed): Phonetic Linguistics: Essays in Honor of Peter Ladefoged. New York: Academic Press, 1985.

88. Muller E, Milenkovic P, McLeod G: Perioral tissue mechanics during speech production. In DeLisi C, Eisenfeld J (eds): Proceedings of the Second IMAC International Symposium on Biomedical Systems Modeling, Amsterdam: North Holland, 1985.

89. Fant G: Acoustic Theory of Speech Production. The Hague: Mouton, 1960.

90. Ladefoged P, Harshman R, Goldstein L, et al: Generating vocal tract shapes from formant frequencies. J Acoust Soc Am 64:1027, 1978.

CHAPTER 88

Early Speech Development in Cleft Palate Babies

*Mary M. O'Gara and
Jerilyn A. Logemann*

When an infant is born with craniofacial anomalies, including cleft palate, it is anticipated that routine multidisciplinary treatment planning will be provided throughout the child's growing years. Early team referral of such infants to a speech-language pathologist is desirable because it allows an opportunity to assess speech and language acquisition longitudinally, thereby providing therapy intervention as soon as it is judged necessary. Just as important, the team speech-language pathologist attempts to provide the parents and family members with guidelines for their role in maximizing the natural progression of the infant's speech and language development. During the first year of their baby's growth, the parents should be provided with information about the role of the velopharyngeal mechanism in speech production and the detrimental role of untreated conductive hearing loss in language learning. Because they have an active and primary role in the daily activities of their child, the parents are natural facilitators for the development of normal communication skills and should be equipped with sufficient information to stimulate and positively reinforce vocalizations appropriate to the child's age and status of the cleft palate (that is, unrepaired or repaired).

This chapter defines the phonetic productions we have observed in the earliest stages of phonologic development of children with cleft palate aged 3 to 36 months in an ongoing longitudinal study of speech sound productions. The implications of these data in parental counseling and clinical management of this aspect of speech development are also discussed.

Normal Development of Vocalizations and the Theory of Continuity

First, let us briefly examine the phonetic patterns observed in the vocalizations of normally developing babies and consider a proposed theoretical relationship between prelinguistic vocalizations and early linguistic development.

Investigators have recently and strongly argued in favor of a theory of continuity of phonetic productions beginning with infant babbling and extending to early speech development and later speech development.[1–5] According to Locke, the theory of discontinuity comprises the premise that in babbling infants produce the sounds of all languages, resulting in a large quantity of phones that must necessarily occur with low frequencies.[3] However, in reviewing the data from three studies of the babbling of 11- to 12-month-old American infants,[6–8] he found that a small number of phones (only 12) accounted for nearly 95% of the consonant productions in the babbling repertoire at that age. These included the six oral stops [p], [b], [t], [d], [k], [g], two glides [w], [j], two nasals [m], [n], and the fricatives [h], [s]. Finding these marked similarities across the three studies, Locke argued that, "the infant has a segmental repertoire that is phonetically highly patterned and selective." In reviewing cross-linguistic studies of babbling and the babbling of normally developing hearing-impaired and Down's syndrome babies, he concluded that phonologic development is a "continuous process whose beginnings predate the child's first words. . . . The infant's variegated babbling is intimately related to his early speech patterns."[3]

Stoel-Gammon also provided evidence for a model of continuity between babbling and speech production.[9] She studied the phonetic inventories of 34 normally developing children aged 15 months through 24 months and found that early phonetic inventories consisted predominantly of oral stops, nasals, and glides, which were voiced and anterior in placement and consisted of either labial or alveolar productions. By 24 months of age, phonetic inventories had expanded to include voiced and voiceless velars and voiceless fricatives. Finding similarities between her data and the reviews of Irwin,[6] Fisichelli,[7] and Pierce and Hanna[8] provided by Locke,[3] Stoel-Gammon reported that these findings support a model of continuity between the phonetic inventories of prelinguistic speech at 11 to 12 months and the early meaningful speech of 15- to 24-month-olds. She also stated that the phonetic inventories of the 24-month-old subjects in her study contained consonant productions similar to those reported by Sanders,[10] as those consonants that were correctly produced 50% of the time across word positions by 3-year-olds. Stoel-Gammon concluded that continuity is also evident between the phonetic inventories at the first word level and the later phonetic inventories that are directly related to, and targeted to, the adult language.[9]

Smith and Oller studied the consonant production of nine normally developing infants from birth through 12 to 15 months of age.[11] Back velars predominated over labial and alveolars until 6 months of age. However, from 6 to 9 months of age, alveolars occurred more frequently than labials and velars. With later extension of the data to include phonetic transcription of meaningful speech from 15 to 21 months of age for these same infants, Smith noted no changes in the relative frequency of occurrences of these three place features: Alveolars were always more frequent than labials, which were always more frequent than velars.[5] He concluded that these results suggest continuity between the use of phonetic place features noted in the prelinguistic babbling at 6 to 9 months of age and those noted in early meaningful speech at 15 to 21 months of age.

The Development of Vocalizations in Infants with Cleft Palate

If babbling and early linguistic speech sound production are continuous "events" within phonologic development, how does babbling in the presence of an unrepaired cleft palate affect the speech sound productions in the early meaningful speech of these infants with cleft palate? The literature abounds with descriptions of the compensatory articulations noted to occur in the meaningful speech of individuals with cleft palate,[12–18] but few data are available on the phonetic inventories of the babbling and early meaningful speech of infants with cleft palate.

In a first report of the results of ongoing longitudinal studies of phonetic productions, we transcribed longitudinally the comfort-state vocalizations of 23 infants with cleft palate from 3 to 36 months of age.[19] Place and manner features produced by all 23 babies were examined. These features were also evaluated for the same babies grouped according to the nonrandomized age of palatoplasty. In this latter analysis, phonetic productions of babies with sufficient intraoral tissue to permit palatoplasty at or before 12 months of age (that is, the earlier/greater tissue group) were compared with those of babies with lesser amounts of tissue that did not allow for palatal repair until after 12 months of age (the later/lesser tissue group). Results revealed that none of the cleft babies in either group exhibited the "alveolar takeover" noted to occur at 6 to 9 months in the normally developing and Down's syndrome subjects of the Smith and Oller[11] study. Also, despite a mean age of 9.3 months at palatoplasty, which was prior to the onset of meaningful speech, the infants in the earlier/greater tissue group did not produce oral place features at the frequencies produced by the normally developing and Down's syndrome babies, as reported by Smith and Oller. Given the evidence for continuity between babbling and early meaningful speech,[1–5, 9, 11] our data on babbling in these infants with cleft palate suggest that the structural constraint of unrepaired cleft palate during the prelinguistic period could delay the early use of the high intraoral pressure targets, particularly [p], [b], [t], [d], [k], and [g] in early meaningful speech, even when palatoplasty is accomplished prior to the onset of meaningful speech. Our data on the speech sound productions of these infants during early meaningful speech support this hypothesis. Infants in both groups studied (earlier/greater tissue and later/lesser tissue) revealed a low-frequency use of high intraoral pressure consonants until they were at least 18 to 19 months of age.

There were, however, some interesting differences in the phonetic repertoires between the two groups of infants. The earlier/greater tissue group evidenced a greater frequency of occurrence of oral stops than nasal stops [m], [n], and [ŋ] or glottal stops [ʔ] for the first time at 18 to 19 months and maintained this oral stop predominance over glottal and nasal stop productions through 35 to 36 months of age (Fig. 88–1). With a mean age of palatoplasty of 16.1 months, the later/lesser

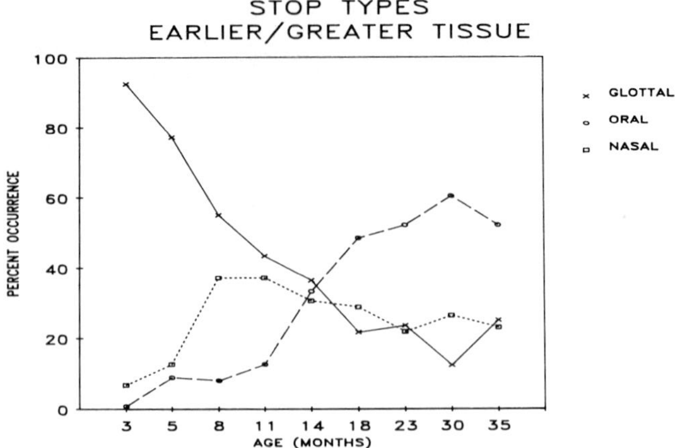

Figure 88–1 Frequency of occurrence (percent) of glottal, oral, and nasal stops as a function of age (months) for the earlier or greater tissue group. (From O'Gara MM, Logemann JA: Phonetic analysis of the speech development of babies with cleft palate. Cleft Palate J 25(2):122–138, 1988. With permission.)

tissue group never showed evidence of oral stop predominance over nasal or glottal stop production through 35 to 36 months of age. Instead, the later/lesser tissue group evidenced glottal stop [ʔ] predominance through 23 to 24 months of age, after which nasal stops predominated in the phonetic repertoire (Fig. 88–2). Although neither group evidenced consistent predominance of oral fricatives over glottal and nasal fricatives, the earlier/greater tissue group demonstrated a greater frequency of oral fricatives from 11 to 12 months of age through 23 to 24 months of age (Fig. 88–3) than the later/lesser tissue group (Fig. 88–4). The differences in oral stop emergence between the two groups may be due to:

1. Different rates of expansion of the restricted phonetic repertoire during variegated babbling.
2. Actual tissue difference between the two groups that dictated the timing of palatoplasty and resulted in

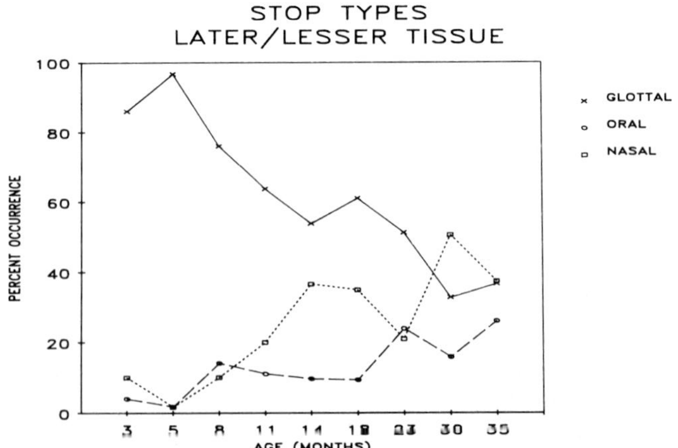

Figure 88–2 Frequency of occurrence (percent) of glottal, oral, and nasal stops as a function of age (months) for the later or lesser tissue group. (From O'Gara MM, Logemann JA: Phonetic analysis of the speech development of babies with cleft palate. Cleft Palate J 25(2):122–138, 1988. With permission.)

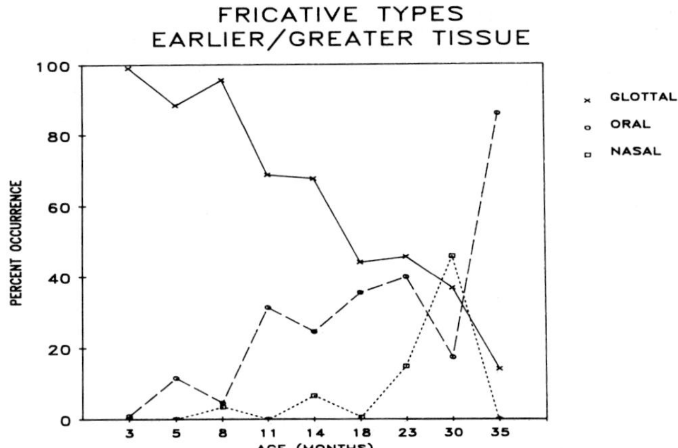

Figure 88–3 Frequency of occurrence (percent) of glottal, oral, and nasal fricatives as a function of age (months) for the earlier or greater tissue group. (From O'Gara MM, Logemann JA: Phonetic analysis of the speech development of babies with cleft palate. Cleft Palate J 25(2):122–138, 1988. With permission.)

reduced success in establishing primary velopharyngeal sufficiency in the later/lesser tissue group.

3. Both. Greater differences may be hypothesized to exist between the two groups for oral stops rather than oral fricatives because of the relative ease of learning the stop versus the fricative manner following repair of the velopharyngeal mechanism.

Stops appear at earlier ages than fricatives in normally developing children, so it may be expected that children with cleft palate will follow the same sequence, albeit in the context of already delayed emergence of oral articulations.

Interestingly, both groups displayed a marked increase in production of nasal fricatives at 30 to 31 months of age (30% to 40% frequency of occurrence), with only a low frequency of occurrence of this non-English consonant articulation immediately prior to this age level (Figs. 88–3 and 88–4). It should be noted, however,

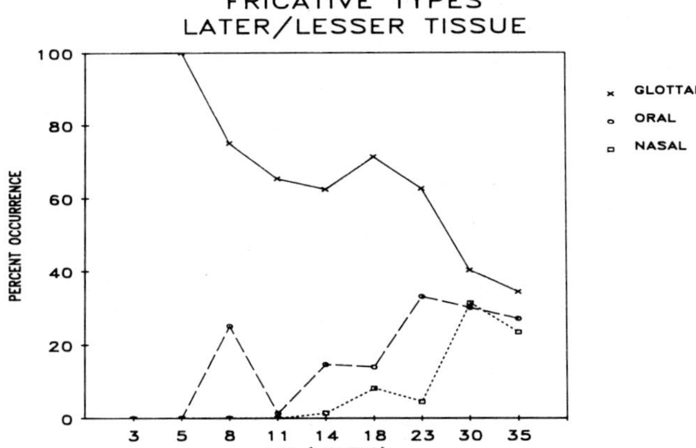

Figure 88–4 Frequency of occurrence (percent) of glottal, oral, and nasal fricatives as a function of age (months) for the later or lesser tissue group. (From O'Gara MM, Logemann JA: Phonetic analysis of the speech development of babies with cleft palate. Cleft Palate J 25(2):122–138, 1988. With permission.)

that phonetic transcription alone of the nasal frication or posterior nasal fricative does not clarify whether this phone occurred unintentionally as a consequence of velopharyngeal insufficiency or whether it is an articulatory event that is phonemically substituted for adult oral fricatives. In the former instance, the presence of posterior nasal frication suggests the need for longitudinal monitoring of velopharyngeal function to maintain the oral path of emission for the stops, fricatives, and affricates, particularly during the later peak resorption of the adenoid mass. In the latter case, speech therapy intervention is warranted because the feature of nasal path of emission is a learned articulation pattern and is not indicative of velopharyngeal sufficiency versus insufficiency. In our clinical judgment, posterior nasal *frication* is that which occurs intermittently and unpredictably on production of any of the targeted oral stops, fricatives, and affricates in the presence of borderline incomplete velopharyngeal closure. With the high oral impedance that is present during these productions, a small velopharyngeal gap results in this pressure leak into the nasal cavity. In some cases, however, this unintentional posterior nasal frication has been noted to undergo development toward the volitional, learned posterior nasal *fricative* as a substitution for the oral fricative targets /s/, /z/, /ʃ/, /ʒ/, and frequently, the affricates /tʃ/, /dʒ/. We have learned that when posterior nasal *frication* is perceived at these early stages of phonologic development, close monitoring is warranted to prevent development into the posterior nasal *fricative*.

Facilitating Normal Oral Articulations in Infants with Cleft Palate

These data from our ongoing longitudinal study begun in 1982 have since enabled us to develop a set of guidelines for our role as speech-language pathologists in facilitating normal oral articulations for the infant born with cleft palate. As stated at the beginning of this chapter, early team referral is desirable to permit longitudinal assessment of the earliest speech vocalizations, preferably prior to the age when the baby is engaged in reduplicative or variegated babbling. We believe that during this stage of the baby's development, the speech-language pathologist should assist the parents in establishing a home program aimed at enriching the babbling repertoire of the infant, at a time when the cleft palate is not yet likely to be repaired. Hahn[20] maintained that "parents are going to teach speech and language consciously or unconsciously, whether or not they are being advised; they need information on normal language development and specific suggestions on practical ways to start."

From this early referral and longitudinal involvement with the team speech-language pathologist, the parents should ultimately understand that they play an active, daily role in facilitating their child's speech and language skills. More specifically, parents need to be informed about:

1. The role that the normal noncleft hard and soft palates play in normal speech sound acquisition.
2. The restrictions imposed by the unrepaired cleft hard or soft palate on the variety of consonant phones produced by their child during babbling and perhaps first word productions.
3. The avoidance of positive reinforcement of consonant constrictions that involve backed glottal and pharyngeal place features.

Also, although the focus of this chapter has centered on facilitation of speech articulation, we use every opportunity to remind parents that routine otologic care and audiologic monitoring are paramount to the facilitation of normal language learning.

We recently have begun encouraging parents to stimulate actively phonetic features that are potentially capable of later shaping into phonemic development, explaining that production of high intraoral pressure consonant constrictions (that is, the oral stops, fricatives, and affricates) need to await palatoplasty. Prior to palatoplasty, features that could be encouraged include the following:

1. Consonant place features anterior to the velum for which little or no intraoral pressure buildup is required, including the nasals [m] and [n], glides [w] and [j], and variations of liquid [ɫ].
2. Tongue tip up articulation to alveolar, dental, or labial articulators, potentially resulting in tongue tip up lateral liquid [ɫ] or tongue tip nasal [n] (rather than always "accepting" tongue tip down, which could encourage backing of place features with elevation of the back of the tongue).
3. The full range of English vowels.

These sound productions may be elicited with repetitive sound play with direct visual cueing and social-verbal reinforcement for any close approximations to the target.

In addition to the stimulation of these types of desirable articulatory features, the parents should be informed when early, excessive use of backed place features is observed, which may encourage later development of these same place features into compensatory articulations. For example, although normally developing infants have been noted to produce exuberant vocalizations, such as "squealing," "growling," "yelling," and "ingressive-egressive sequences" from approximately 4 to 6 months of age,[2] we consider the persistent and abundant use of rough laryngealizations, including rough, tense ingressive and egressive productions and playful posterior nasal fricatives, to be early, undesirable features that parents should be instructed not to reinforce positively with imitation or provision of immediate visual attention.

Following the completion of palatoplasty, the parents need to be counseled that expansion of the phonetic repertoire to include oral stops (and later, oral fricatives and oral affricates) will likely not take place immediately nor emerge instantaneously with the degree of intraoral pressure buildup exhibited by noncleft peers. The parents must be instructed to listen for the acceptable approximations of anterior place features with attempts at intraoral pressure buildup, positively reinforcing and

shaping these articulations in the acquisition of new vocabulary items. Clinically, it has been our experience that first words learned in the presence of unrepaired velopharyngeal insufficency frequently remain "frozen forms" and are the most difficult to change.[9] The task then becomes one of incorporating new vocabulary items for which little or no previous production experience interferes with the articulations constituting the word shape. Occasionally, sound play using oral place features and intraoral pressure buildup, without reference to a phonemic target, must precede that phonetic event into meaningful speech attempts.

With this type of home program, we have found it necessary to provide the parents routinely with written goals for stimulation, with follow-up appointments approximately every 3 to 4 months after primary palate repair to assess speech and language growth. We currently use several guidelines to determine the need for more formal therapeutic intervention strategies after surgical repair of the cleft palate is accomplished. First, we look for emergent forms of the oral stops, typically the voiced stops, within the first 6 to 8 months postpalatoplasty when the type of home program previously described has been maintained. By emergent forms, we mean articulatory use of place features at or anterior to the velum, with some attempt at intraoral pressure buildup. Second, we look for stabilization of the low intraoral pressure consonant constrictions, including the nasals [m] and [n] and glides [w] and [j] used in conjunction with a rich variety of differentiated vowels. Should the child not meet these two production criteria within the first 6 to 8 months postpalatoplasty, we recommend that weekly sessions be provided by the speech-language pathologist.

Conclusions

Our data provide descriptions of the patterns of phonetic productions used by infants born with cleft palate from 3 to 36 months of age as revealed by longitudinal assessment. Given a model of continuity between prelinguistic and linguistic behavior, infants with cleft palate may benefit from early speech-language intervention, even prior to surgical repair of the cleft palate. Enrichment of the phonetic features of variegated babbling prior to primary palate repair and shaping of acceptable orally targeted consonants during the early months after palatoplasty may be important to later, more normal, phonemic development of oral articulations. Our ongoing analyses should continue to provide important information about the possible continuous link between babbling and early phonologic development in babies with cleft palate.

References

1. Oller D, Wieman L, Doyle W, et al: Infant babbling and speech. J Child Lang 3:3–12, 1976.
2. Oller D: The emergence of the sounds of speech in infancy. In GH Yeni-Komshian GH & Ferguson CA (eds): Child Phonology. Vol 1. Production. New York: Academic Press, 1980, pp 93–112.

3. Locke J: Phonological Acquisition and Change. New York: Academic Press, 1983.
4. Vihman M, Macken M, Miller R, et al: From babbling to speech: A reassessment of the continuity issue. Language 61:397–446, 1985.
5. Smith B: The emergent lexicon from a phonetic perspective. In Smith MD, Locke JL (eds): The Emergent Lexicon: The Child's Development of a Linguistic Vocabulary. San Diego: Academic Press, 1988, pp 75–106.
6. Irwin O: Infant speech: Consonantal sounds according to place of aritculation. J Speech Hear Dis 12:397–401, 1947.
7. Fisichelli R: An experimental study of the prelinguistic speech development of institutionalized infants. Unpublished doctoral dissertation, Fordham University, 1950.
8. Pierce J, Hanna I: The development of a phonological system in English speaking American children, Portland, OR: HaPi Press, 1974.
9. Stoel-Gammon C: Phonetic inventories, 15–24 months: A longitudinal study. J Speech Hear Dis 28:505–512, 1985.
10. Sanders E: When are speech sounds learned? J Speech Hear Dis 37:55–63, 1972.
11. Smith B, Oller D: A comparative study of the pre-meaningful vocalizations produced by normally developing and Down's syndrome infants. J Speech Hear Dis 46:46–51, 1981.
12. Olson D: A descriptive study of the speech development of a group of infants with unoperated cleft palate. Unpublished doctoral dissertation, Northwestern University, 1965.
13. Morris H: Velopharyngeal competence and primary cleft palate surgery, 1960–1971: A critical review. Cleft Palate J 10:62–71, 1973.
14. Peterson S: Nasal emission as a component of the misarticulation of sibilants and affricates. J Speech Hear Dis 40:106–114, 1975.
15. Van Demark D, Morris H: Patterns of articulation abilities in speakers with cleft palate. Cleft Palate J 16:230–240, 1979.
16. Trost J: Articulatory additions to the classical description of the speech of persons with cleft palate. Cleft Palate J 18:193–203, 1981.
17. Dorf D, Curtin J: Early cleft repair and speech outcome. Plast Reconstr Surg 70:74–79, 1982.
18. McWilliams BJ, Morris H, Shelton R: Cleft Palate Speech. Philadelphia: B.C. Decker, 1984.
19. O'Gara M, Logemann J: Phonetic analyses of the speech development of babies with cleft palate. Cleft Palate J 25:122–134, 1988.
20. Hahn E: Directed home training program for infants with cleft lip and palate. In Bzoch KR (ed): Communicative Disorders Related to Cleft Lip and Palate, 2nd ed. Boston: Little, Brown, 1979, pp 311–317.

CHAPTER 89

Communicative Competence in Children with Cleft Lip and Palate

Kathy L. Chapman and Mary A. Hardin

Until recently, descriptions of children's language acquisition and disorders have focused on linguistic competence (knowledge of linguistic rules). With the current emphasis on the use of language in a social context, however, researchers and clinicians have broadened their focus to encompass not just linguistic competence but communicative competence as well.

Communicative competence* is defined as the ability of a speaker to convey information to a listener in an effective and efficient manner.[1] In the development of communicative competence, a child acquires knowledge about the various components of language (such as syntax, semantics, and phonology) and the ability to use this knowledge in socially appropriate contexts (i.e., sociocommunicative competence).

Traditionally, the study and management of communication disorders in children with cleft lip and palate have focused almost exclusively on articulation or aspects of linguistic form. Little attention has been directed toward the child's use of language in sociocommunicative contexts. In light of the facial deformities and speech proficiency deficits that these children exhibit, they are at risk for long-term sociocommunicative difficulties. The response of the child as well as that of

his or her communicative partners to the clefting experience may significantly affect the acquisition and expression of these skills. Therefore, any attempt to describe the communicative competence of these children must consider sociocommunicative as well as articulatory and linguistic aspects of communication.

The purpose of this chapter is threefold. First, it is a discussion of selected factors that may influence the development of communicative competence in children with cleft lip and palate. A second purpose is to describe what is known about the communicative competence of children with cleft lip and palate. Finally, a model for examining the sociocommunicative skills of children with cleft lip and palate will be presented.

Selected Factors Influencing Communicative Competence

A number of factors may contribute to the communication problems evidenced by children with cleft lip and palate (for a review see McWilliams et al[2]). In this section we will restrict our discussion to two factors that have received limited attention in the literature but have direct bearing on the child's acquisition of language, particularly sociocommunicative skills.

Mother-Child Interaction

Current models of language acquisition view interaction between the infant and primary caregiver (typically the mother) as the context through which language is acquired. Mother-infant interactions during the first years of life provide foundational support for the development of language. It is what the infant learns about communication, before the onset of spoken language, that provides the basis for later language acquisition.

In interactions with the mother, the infant is portrayed as an active and competent participant.[3–5] The infant is endowed with a number of behaviors that elicit positive social responses from the mother that are in turn rewarding to the child. Likewise, the mother elicits

---

*Although articulation proficiency undoubtedly affects a child's communicative competence, the term communicative competence is used in this context to refer to aspects of language usage.

responses from the child that are satisfying to the mother. This reciprocal responding and matching of infant behavior and caregiver responses facilitate positive patterns of caregiver-child interaction.[3] However, if there are limitations in the infant skills or adult responses, the development of a positive cycle of interaction may be disrupted, thus interfering with normal development. One such limitation might be the structural deficits characteristic of children with cleft lip and palate. These deficits or abnormalities may preclude the normal expression of some of these skills. Among some of the infant skills that serve the development of cycles of interaction are reflexive behaviors associated with feeding, for example, sucking and rooting, and social behaviors useful in maintaining contact between the infant and caregiver (smiling and vocalizing).

Goldberg emphasized the importance of feeding in this context by describing it as a "cooperative effort in which adults use infant behavior as a guide for their own."[3] Infants with cleft lip or palate are at high risk for feeding problems. If infants are not able to perform these behaviors satisfactorily, adults may not be easily able to modify their own behaviors so that interactions during the feeding period are positive. Rather than providing a pleasant experience for the caregiver, feeding becomes stressful for both mother and infant.

Early forms of social behavior such as smiling and vocalizing are important for initiating and maintaining social interaction between infant and caregiver. Because of the facial deformity caused by a cleft lip, mothers of children with cleft lip may have difficulty reading their infant's smile behavior. This causes them to be less attuned to the infant's early social-communicative behaviors. Furthermore, children with cleft lip and palate are reported to vocalize less frequently than their noncleft peers, and so there may be fewer opportunities for contingent responding by mothers.[6]

Some preliminary data have revealed patterns of interaction between mothers and children with cleft lip and palate that are different from those observed between mothers and normal children during the first year of life. A greater degree of maternal detachment was shown by mothers of infants with facial anomalies than was shown by mothers of infants with other handicapping conditions.[7] Field and Vega-Lahr also found that mothers of infants with craniofacial anomalies showed less frequent smiling, vocalizing, imitative behavior, contingent responding, and game playing than did mothers of normal infants.[8] These are among some of the early caregiver behaviors that have been shown to relate to early language development.

Another aspect of interaction, maternal language input, has been implicated as a variable that may affect the acquisition of language skills in children positively or negatively. Mothers of normally developing children modify their speech in ways that seem to aid children in the language acquisition process. Furthermore, these modifications are related to the language level of the child.[9] Studies examining the maternal language addressed to other populations of language-impaired children (developmentally delayed, specific language im-

paired, and so on) have identified problematic patterns of interaction. In summarizing the data obtained from a number of studies, the most consistent findings indicate that parents of language-impaired children use their speech to direct their children more often[10] and also produce fewer semantically contingent utterances than do parents of normal children.[11-13]

To date, there has only been one study examining maternal language input to children with clefts. Chapman and Hardin examined the maternal language addressed to two groups of children: 13 children with cleft lip and palate and 13 noncleft children (eight 1-year-olds, ten 2-year-olds, and eight 3-year-olds).[14] Of the 18 input variables examined, only two differentiated the two groups of mothers: conversational devices and modeling. Both of these features were used more frequently by the mothers of children with cleft lip and palate. We viewed these differences not as negative strategies but as necessary adjustments mothers make to maintain conversational interaction with their children.

In summary, mothers and their cleft palate infants are at risk for problems in early interaction. During the child's first year, aspects of interaction such as social and verbal responsiveness—that is, smiling, vocalizing, imitative behavior, and game playing—may be disrupted. Early interaction contexts provide the foundation for the development of early language and sociocommunicative skills; therefore, problems in interaction may contribute to the language impairment evidenced by some children with cleft lip and palate.

Peer Interaction

As children move into the preschool years, interaction contexts expand to include peers and other less familiar people. Like mother-child interaction, peer interaction also influences the child's acquisition of communicative competence. As indicated by Muma, the role of peer interaction in the language acquisition process has not been clearly delineated.[15] However, Owens suggests that interaction with peers provides a context for the refinement of conversational skills in young children.[16] In the case of children with cleft lip and palate, the response of peers to the child's speech or facial appearance may influence long-term sociocommunicative successes or failures. Although negative peer interactions are not expected to influence linguistic development directly, they may lead a child to avoid situations that require interpersonal exchanges, thus reducing the number of opportunities for "practice" and improvement of sociocommunicative skills.

At least two investigations have been conducted that suggest that children with cleft lip and palate may receive less favorable responses from peers and other adults on the basis of speech and facial scarring. Blood and Hyman examined the reactions of 120 noncleft kindergarteners, first graders, and second graders to audiorecordings of four females with cleft palate who exhibited varying degrees of hypernasality.[17] The children were asked if they liked the speaker, liked the way the speaker talked, and would like to talk to the speaker.

The children's responses became increasingly negative as the severity of hypernasality increased. Results of a second study indicate that adults may respond differentially to the speech of cleft palate children on the basis of facial scarring. Podol and Salvia had speech-language pathologists rate the speech of a female child with cleft lip and palate.[18] Half of the judges viewed a photograph of a child with a lip scar while listening to a tape-recorded speech sample. The remaining judges listened to the same tape recording but were shown a retouched photograph with the lip scar removed. Judges who viewed the child with the lip scar present were more likely to recommend speech therapy.

The impact of negative peer reactions on the development of sociocommunicative skills of children with cleft lip and palate is not well understood. However, it is likely that these negative reactions may lead a child to view himself or herself as a poor communicator. Requests by adults and peers to repeat a message signal communicative failure to a child. Although the child may modify the message to accommodate the listener's needs, he may begin to question his or her effectiveness as a communicator. There are data to suggest that at least some of these children show a reduction in expressive language as they mature.[19] It is likely that this reluctance to initiate and foster interpersonal communication stems not from inadequate knowledge of conversational conventions but rather from behavioral inhibition related to the child's poor social image or self-image as a communicator. Later acquisition of age-appropriate phonologic and linguistic skills may yield intelligible speech but have little impact on the child's self-perceived competence as a speaker.

Few investigations have been conducted to examine the perceptions of children and adolescents with cleft lip and palate toward their speech and facial appearance. Data reported by Richman have indicated, however, that adolescents with clefts who express moderate-to-great concerns about their facial appearance tend to demonstrate greater social introversion than their cleft peers who express satisfaction with facial appearance.[20] Richman's findings warrant further investigation, particularly because behavioral inhibition has frequently been noted in the cleft palate population.[20-24] These children perform lower on measures of self-esteem than noncleft children and tend to view themselves as less socially acceptable than their noncleft peers.[25] Consequently, one might expect these children to exhibit deficits in conversational skills or a reluctance to participate in conversation.

Communicative Competence in Children with Cleft Lip and Palate

To review, a number of different skills make up communicative competence. These include knowledge of linguistic rules as well as knowledge of sociocommunicative conventions, such as the ability to use language to express different purposes (that is, communicative intentions) and skills in conversational initiation and maintenance. Children described as "delayed in language" may exhibit difficulty with some of these skills but not with others. For example, some children show deficits in linguistic form (their sentences may be grammatically incorrect or their vocabulary limited), yet they may use their limited linguistic skills very effectively in communicative interactions. Other children, regardless of their level of skill with the linguistic code, may have difficulty in establishing and maintaining social contact. Like all children, children with cleft lip and palate are equally heterogeneous in these ways. However, because of the factors cited above, these children seem particularly susceptible to certain profiles of impairment. In the section below, we will review some of the available information about the communication skills of children with cleft lip and palate, specifically linguistic competence and sociocommunicative competence. In the next section, we will propose a sociocommunicative framework, borrowed from Fey,[26] that should be considered in the further study and management of the communication problems of children with cleft lip and palate.

Linguistic Competence

Studies of linguistic competence in children with cleft lip and palate have examined syntactic, morphologic, and semantic components of language during the preschool and school-aged years. With some exceptions,[2] the majority of data published to date suggest that these children exhibit a number of linguistic deficits. Early delays in lexical acquisition have been reported.[27] In addition, reduced vocabulary usage, utterance length, structural complexity, and psycholinguistic abilities have been noted.[19, 27-31]

Although few authors question the prevalence of linguistic delays in preschoolers and young school-aged children with cleft lip and palate, little agreement exists about the long-term status of linguistic functioning in this population. Several authors have suggested that although the language skills of children with cleft lip and palate may initially lag behind those of their noncleft peers, they "catch up" by mid-childhood and demonstrate comparable skills.[2, 32, 33] Others have argued that the linguistic deficits noted in childhood may persist and become more apparent as the child gets older.[29, 34]

Limited data are available to characterize the linguistic proficiency demonstrated by adolescents and adults with cleft lip and palate. Recent findings by Scorfield et al suggest that early language delays exhibited by these children do not resolve by adolescence.[35] These investigators administered the Test of Adolescent Language (TOAL)[36] and the Sentence Combining Subtest of the Test of Language Development—Intermediate (TOLD-I)[37] to 40 adolescents with cleft lip and palate. Their findings indicated that, as a group, the subjects performed significantly poorer than age-matched controls who composed the normative population of the TOAL. Additional evidence of the persistence of linguistic deficits in this population was provided in an earlier study by Pannbacker.[38] She examined the oral language skills of 20 adults with cleft palate and compared them to 20 age-matched controls. Although differences between the groups in syntax and vocabulary knowledge were not noted, the cleft palate adults tended to use shorter responses and employed fewer different words. A correlation between speech intelligibility and oral language skills also was noted. Pannbacker concluded that adults who demonstrate speech that is difficult to understand may sacrifice response length to facilitate speech intelligibility.

The findings of the aforementioned studies support a need for further investigation of the long-term linguistic status of individuals with cleft lip and palate. The nature of linguistic deficits noted in adolescence and adulthood is of paramount concern because they may not reflect performance deficits per se but rather attempts by the speaker to achieve effective communication. It is of interest to note that although many linguistic deficits noted in the young child with a cleft tend to disappear by adulthood, a commonly reported finding across all age levels is reduced utterance length. Although this clinical finding may be interpreted as a linguistic delay in the very young child, it is important to recognize that structural complexity and utterance length may be sacrificed by individuals of all ages in an effort to promote speech intelligibility.[38] Furthermore, many of the linguistic deficits seen in these children may be the result of articulatory or phonologic limitations. The child may possess knowledge of the appropriate syntactic or morphologic rules but may not use the correct form because of limits on the speech production mechanism. With these cautions in mind, assessment of linguistic functioning in children with cleft lip and palate must differentiate between competence and performance-based problems.

Sociocommunicative Competence

Only a few investigations have been conducted to examine the sociocommunicative skills of children with cleft lip and palate. In an early study, Shames and Rubin[39] examined communicative intent and other conversational skills demonstrated by 75 children with cleft palate and 75 noncleft children matched for age. Subjects ranged in age from 18 months to 5 years 3 months. A standardized interview, composed of 135 stimulus episodes, was employed to elicit a variety of verbal responses such as greeting, questioning, answering, and commenting. The children with cleft palate demonstrated a 12- to 18-month delay in "the frequency with which they emit the response expected to be evoked by the prearranged stimuli" until the age of 3 years 9 months.[39] After that time, the performance of the two groups was comparable.

Long and Dalston compared the early communicative intentions (i.e., showing, refusal, showing-off) of two groups of children—ten cleft lip and palate children and ten normal children.[6] The results indicated that although the children with cleft lip and palate were delayed in their ability to pair a vocalization with their communicative intentions, there was no difference between the two groups in the number of communicative intentions

expressed through gesture alone. Another point of interest in the Long and Dalston study concerned the frequency of occurrence of the different communicative intentions studied. There was only one intention, refusal, that occurred more frequently in the cleft group. The other communicative intentions, all of which could be classified as intentions used to establish social interaction with a conversational partner (showing, pointing, giving, showing off), were used less frequently by the children with cleft lip and palate.

More recently, Warr-Leeper et al[40] examined the communicative intentions (e.g., informing, requesting, naming, answering) used by 27 preschool and school-aged cleft lip and palate children on the Test of Pragmatic Skills.[41] These investigators found no difference between the preschool children with cleft lip and palate and their age-matched noncleft peers on the test. However, the school-aged children with clefts were less competent than their peers without clefts on this same task. The authors hypothesized that the lower scores for the school-aged children with cleft lip and palate may have been related to a tendency seen in older cleft speakers to communicate with "minimal verbal output." Interpretation of these data with regard to the sociocommunicative abilities of children with cleft lip and palate is difficult because only a few intentions were examined and pragmatic usage was confounded by utterance length. A child may have obtained a higher score for a particular test item because she or he communicated the target intention using a longer utterance. Therefore, the lower scores seen in the older cleft lip and palate group may have been related to shorter utterance length rather than to limitations in communicative intentions.

The limited data available about the sociocommunicative skills of children with cleft lip and palate are inconclusive to date. The findings of Shames and Rubin suggest that early delays in these skills disappear by school age.[39] In contrast, Warr-Leeper and her colleagues did not note differences between the cleft and noncleft groups until school age.[40] Further investigation is needed to delineate the nature of the sociocommunicative problems noted in these children. Early delays in these skills may be related to difficulty in the acquisition of rules for sociocommunicative interaction. Older children may have knowledge of the appropriate conversational conventions, but their experience with negative listener reactions may lead them to limit their conversational participation. Because it may be in the dimension of conversational participation that some children and adolescents with cleft lip and palate differ from their noncleft peers, we propose use of a scheme developed by Fey[26] for classifying children's abilities with regard to sociocommunicative skills.

Model for Assessment of Sociocommunicative Competence with Cleft Lip and Palate

Fey's model was originally proposed to capture the differences noted among specific language-impaired children in their ability to use language for communication, but it has direct application to describing the language problems of children with cleft lip and palate.[26] Furthermore, although some of the patterns may be better than others for characterizing the conversational skills of the cleft lip and palate child, all profiles will be presented because of the range of individual differences noted among children with cleft lip and palate.

The model evaluates two components of the child's conversational participation: conversational assertiveness and conversational responsiveness. Conversational assertiveness is defined as the "ability or willingness (or both) to take a conversational turn when none has been solicited by a partner."[26] Conversational responsiveness measures how well the child responds to a conversational turn initiated by their partner (e.g., answering questions, maintaining or elaborating the topic). Children may vary in their abilities with regard to these two components. Therefore, four different patterns of conversational participation can be described. Children who fit the first pattern are described as "active conversationalists." They initiate conversation frequently and are responsive to conversations initiated by their partners. These children may have difficulty with linguistic form but are effective communicators nevertheless. Obviously, for these children, management should focus on developing the form components of language.

The second group of children are labeled "passive conversationalists." The children who fit this profile are "aware of the social nature of conversation" and are responsive to the initiations of their conversational partners. They do not, however, tend to initiate conversations on their own. Furthermore, their responses to partner initiations usually serve to maintain rather than extend the topic. These children also may exhibit problems with other components of language (e.g., syntax and morphology) that may mask their deficits in socioconversational skills. To fully understand the nature and extent of this type of communicative impairment, it is essential that evaluation extend beyond examination of linguistic form to include an analysis of conversational skills. A passive conversational style may not be responsible for all the communication problems noted in these children; however, it may serve to maintain the problem. When a child does not initiate interactions with other children or adults, he or she is perhaps excluded from those experiences that facilitate language learning. For children with such patterns of conversational style, Fey suggests that intervention should focus on increasing the frequency of conversational initiations.

The third group is composed of children who rarely initiate interactions and are not very responsive to partner's initiations. These children are described by Fey as "inactive communicators." Children who fit into this category are often children with unintelligible speech. This group of children, more than either of the two groups previously described, usually possesses a limited repertoire of communicative intentions. For these children, therapy should focus on facilitating social interaction and appropriate responding as well as developing intelligible speech.

The final group of children described by Fey are those who initiate conversation frequently but are not very responsive conversational partners. They seem to be assertive but unresponsive in social situations. These children, who were labeled "verbal noncommunicators," talk a lot but do not modify their speech to take into account listener needs. Their speech is often unrelated to the topic initiated by their conversational partner or to their own prior utterances. For such a child, Fey suggests that therapy focus on developing a more responsive style of interaction, that is, producing utterances related to his or her conversational partners or to the child's own prior speech.

Our clinical experience suggests that the second and third profiles might prove to be the most useful in describing the language performance of children with cleft lip and palate. It is not uncommon in cleft palate clinics to identify children who appear reticent and reluctant to engage in lengthy interactions. For some children with cleft lip and palate, this reluctance to talk is likely related to speech intelligibility problems or to the child's poor perception of himself or herself as a speaker. Or it may be related to the child's lack of knowledge about conversational rules. Finally, it is important to recognize that some children may simply limit the extent of their verbal output as a result of individual personality styles.

Conclusions

A number of recent advances in the study of child language acquisition and disorders have important implications for understanding and describing the language problems of children with cleft lip and palate. These children are at risk for delays not only in linguistic development but in sociocommunicative skills as well. The caregiver's response to the clefting condition, including anxiety about facial scarring, early feeding difficulties, and speech-language development, may disrupt early interaction with the child. Since early caregiver-child interaction provides the context for acquisition and practice of conversational rules, disruptions in early interactions may interfere with the child's acquisition of socially appropriate conversational conventions. As the child matures, she or he is exposed to other conversational partners such as peers and teachers. Negative peer reactions and negative self-perceptions about facial appearance and communicative effectiveness may lead a child to withdraw from the verbal limelight and avoid verbal interactions when possible.

Traditionally, management programs for children with cleft lip and palate have focused on establishing "normal" articulation and linguistic rules. Although they may have been successful in achieving these goals, the ability to produce correct sounds and grammatic forms does not necessarily yield a good communicator. Unless management also focuses on the development of sociocommunicative skills, the end result may yield a proficient speaker but an ineffective communicator.

References

1. Wilcox MJ: Developmental language disorders: Preschoolers. In Costello JM, Holland AL (eds): Handbook of Speech and Language Disorders. San Diego: College-Hill Press, 1986.
2. McWilliams BJ, Morris HL, Shelton RL: Cleft Palate Speech. Philadelphia: B. C. Decker, 1984.
3. Goldberg S: Social competency in infancy: A model of parent-infant interaction. Merrill-Palmer 23:163, 1977.
4. Lewis M, Rosenblum L: The Effects of the Infant on Its Caregiver. New York: Wiley, 1974.
5. Trevarthen C: Descriptive analysis of infant communicative behavior. In Schaffer HR (ed): Studies in Mother Infant Interaction. London: Academic Press, 1977.
6. Long N, Dalston R: Paired gestural and vocal behavior in one-year-old cleft lip and palate children. J Speech Hear Dis 47:403, 1982.
7. Wasserman GA, Allen R: Maternal withdrawal from handicapped toddlers. J Child Psychol and Psychiat 28:381, 1985.
8. Field T, Vega-Lahr N: Early social interaction and language acquisition. In Schaffer HR (ed): Studies in Mother Infant Interaction. London: Academic Press, 1977.
9. Snow C: Mothers' speech to their children learning language. Child Devel 43:549, 1972.
10. Nienhuys TG, Cross TG, Horsborough KM: Child variables influencing maternal speech style: Deaf and hearing children. J Comm Dis 17:189, 1984.
11. Cross TG: Mother's speech adjustments: The contribution of selected child listener variables. In Ferguson CE (ed): Talking to Children: Language Input and Acquisition. Cambridge: Cambridge University Press, 1977.
12. Cross TG: Mother's speech and its association with rate of language acquisition in young children. In Waterson N, Snow C (eds): The Development of Communication. London: Wiley, 1978.
13. Laskey EZ, Klopp K: Parent child interactions in normal and language-disordered children. J Speech Hear Dis 47:7, 1982.
14. Chapman KL, Hardin MA: Mother-child interaction patterns in children with cleft palate. Paper presented at the American Speech-Language-Hearing Association Annual Convention, New Orleans, 1987.
15. Muma J: Language Acquisition. Austin TX: Pro-Ed, 1986.
16. Owens RE: Language Development. Columbus OH: Charles Merrill, 1987.
17. Blood G, Hyman M: Children's perception of nasal resonance. J Speech Hear Dis 42:446, 1977.
18. Podol J, Salvia J: Effects of prepalatal cleft on the evaluation of speech. Cleft Palate J 13:361, 1976.
19. Morris HL: Communication skills of children with cleft lip and palate. J Speech Hear Res 5:79, 1962.
20. Richman LC: Self-reported social, speech, and facial concerns and personality adjustment of adolescents with cleft lip and palate. Cleft Palate J 20:108, 1983.
21. Spriestersbach DC: Psychosocial Aspects of the "Cleft Palate Problem." Iowa City: University of Iowa Press, 1973.
22. Richman LC: Behavior and achievement of cleft palate children. Cleft Palate J 13:4, 1976.
23. Richman LC, Harper DC: School adjustment of children with observable disabilities. J Abnormal Child Psychol 6:11, 1978.
24. Richman LC, Harper DC: Self-identified personality patterns of children with facial or orthopedic disfigurement. Cleft Palate J 16:256, 1979.
25. Kapp-Simon K: Self-concept of the cleft lip and/or palate child. Cleft Palate J 16:171, 1979.
26. Fey ME: Language Intervention in Young Children. San Diego: College-Hill Press, 1986.
27. Bzoch KR: An investigation of the speech of preschool cleft palate children. Thesis (Ph.D.). Evanston IL: Northwestern University, 1956.
28. Spriesterbach DC, Darley FL, Morris HL: Language skills in children with cleft palate. J Speech Hear Res 1:279, 1958.
29. Smith RM, McWilliams BJ: Psycholinguistic abilities of children with clefts. Cleft Palate J 5:238, 1968.
30. Nation J: Vocabulary comprehension and usage of preschool cleft palate and normal children. Cleft Palate J 7:639, 1970.
31. Nation J, Wetherbee MA: Cognitive-communicative development of identical triplets, one with unilateral cleft lip and palate. Cleft Palate J 22:38, 1985.
32. Zimmerman JD, Canfield WH: Language and speech development. In Stark RB (ed): Cleft Palate: A Multidisciplinary Approach. New York: Harper & Row, 1968.
33. Musgrave R, McWilliams BJ, Matthews H: A review of the results of two different approaches for the repair of clefts of the soft palate only. Cleft Palate J 12:281, 1975.
34. Phillips BJ, Harrison RJ: Articulation patterns of preschool cleft palate children. Cleft Palate J 6:245, 1969.
35. Scorfield DM, Warr-Leeper GA, Leeper HA, McCann KK: Language abilities of selected cleft lip and palate adolescents (In press, 1989).
36. Hammill DD, Brown VL, Larsen SC, et al: Test of Adolescent Language. Austin TX: Pro-Ed, 1980.
37. Hammill DD, Newcomer PL: Test of Language Development—Intermediate. Austin TX: Pro-Ed, 1980.
38. Pannbacker M: Oral language skills of adult cleft palate speakers. Cleft Palate J 12:95, 1975.
39. Shames G, Rubin H: Psycholinguistic measures of language and speech. In Bzoch KR (ed): Communicative Disorders Related to Cleft Lip and Palate, 2nd ed. Boston: Little, Brown, 1979.
40. Warr-Leeper G, Crone L, Carruthers A, et al: A comparison of the performance of preschool children with cleft lip and/or palate on the test of pragmatic skills. Paper presented at the Annual Convention of the American Cleft Palate Association, Williamsburg, Virginia, 1988.
41. Shulman BB: Test of Pragmatic Skills. Tucson: Communication Skill Builders, 1985.

CHAPTER 90

Early Speech Development: The Interaction of Learning and Structure

Karlind T. Moller

In an infant born with cleft lip and palate we can predict with certainty that there will be concerns about developing communication skills, hearing, dental relationships, and appearance. Optimal interdisciplinary management for persons with cleft lip and palate requires treatment decisions and intervention that are correlated with physical and behavioral growth and development. For example, surgical revision of the lip and nose or orthognathic procedures to the jaws are indicated when growth and development factors are favorable and when there is agreement among the patient and family and the interdisciplinary team that a decided functional and aesthetic benefit will result.

Decisions to proceed with physical treatment to improve speech performance are made with a similar rationale: Growth and development factors are favorable, and there is a functional and aesthetic benefit. However, it is frequently more difficult to make the decision that physical management of the speech structures is required to improve speech. There is little the child can do to mask the real appearance and function of the lip and nose and dental occlusion, yet certain speech compensations associated with cleft palate can mask the child's ultimate potential for acceptable speech. Certainly, we all share the common challenge of improving and optimizing the end result to obtain acceptability (aesthetically and functionally) as early as possible. To meet that challenge for speech, early observation of emerging speech productions and efforts to communicate are strongly encouraged.

This chapter will present a view of how learning

factors and structural capabilities interact with potential effects on early speech attempts and perhaps speech performance for years to come. In this context, we define *early* as before 36 months of age. After this age, more standardized assessment of speech and physiologic function can be carried out to arrive at clinical management decisions about the integrity of the structure.

The Task of the Speech-Language Pathologist

In the main, as speech and language pathologists committed to following these children over time, our task has been to describe, from a diagnostic point of view, the vocalizations and speech characteristics and to determine the relationship between speech production and structure. The major structural issue following initial palatal surgery is velopharyngeal closure. There would be little argument that inadequate velopharyngeal closure remains the primary causal factor of speech problems in individuals with cleft palate. As diagnosticians and hands-on clinicians, we focus on the questions, "What *is* this child doing with the present structure?" and, more importantly, "What *can* this child do with the present mechanism?" That is, is this child's physical mechanism potentially adequate to produce acceptable speech? If it is, then our task is to encourage and help the child use that potentially adequate mechanism consistently for speech. If it is not, our task is to require improvement of velopharyngeal closure for improved speech.

Of course we want to make that decision as early as possible. However, this is not always a simple task. We do know that following the initial palatal repair a substantial number of children develop normal speech with no intervention, yet many do not. It is a well-established finding that speech problems are more prevalent in this group than in persons born without clefts. These same data indicate that the range of speech skills among children with clefts varies extensively and that some children develop normal speech. In an effort to understand this variability, investigators have looked at a variety of factors associated with clefting that are assumed to be related to speech production.

Historically, the early (birth to age 3 years) focus of attention in children born with cleft palate has been on the physical mechanism. There has been limited attention to detail on emerging speech and language performance. In a real sense, we have continued to play the "waiting game" to see how speech develops following primary palatal surgery until we are able to elicit a large enough sample of utterances. This examination is usually carried out in a clinical environment and frequently in an all too short period of time. However, by that time, we may have missed some important information about the child's early efforts: information about what the child is attempting to do with the physical mechanism and how the child is organizing productive efforts at speech to match the more mature adult model. As Menn has suggested, the task that any child faces is to sound like others when communicating with them.[1]

We need to appreciate in the full sense that speech is *learned* behavior and that those factors that affect speech can and do vary from child to child. When children with no physical deviations have speech problems, we assume they are the products of faulty learning. When clefts are present we often behave as though the physical factors are the *sole* cause of the problems. In the presence of physical deviations such as clefts, learning factors, such as strategies employed to compensate for those deviations, may play an even more significant role in the acquisition of speech. Knowledge of the interactions between learning and physical deviations should be increased by systematic study of children's behavior and physical factors present *during* the time they are acquiring sounds. Sound production patterns learned early, desirable or undesirable, may have a significant impact on speech performance following primary surgery and on the communication level that is eventually attained.

Speech Characteristics of Children with Cleft Palate

Clearly, most of the information we have about speech characteristics in children with cleft palate is based on descriptions of older children. Descriptions of articulation performance have been related to type of cleft,[2–5] surgical procedures and techniques of primary palate repair,[2, 6] age at time of testing,[3, 4, 7–10] and the influence of physiologic factors such as velopharyngeal competence and dental variations on performance.[6, 9, 11, 12] Studies typically have been cross-sectional; however, more recently, longitudinal data have been reported.[13–15]

For the most part, articulation performance has been analyzed from a *phonetic* standpoint, according to the number (or percentage) of correct versus incorrect speech productions; type of errors; manner, place, and voicing distinctions; consistency of productions (error consistency as well as consistency of correctness); phonetic complexity; and descriptions of *compensatory* or nonstandard productions. The latter description has led some people to talk about "cleft palate speech"; however, we know very well that this is not appropriate for any given speaker. The clear fact remains that individuals with cleft palate represent a highly heterogeneous group in terms of speech performance and, indeed, in terms of the structural mechanism. The decision about whether an improved velopharyngeal closure mechanism will be required for any given child may be confounded by speech patterns learned, perhaps before primary palatal surgery, in an attempt to compensate for an inadequate mechanism. We know also that many children develop normal speech following initial palatal repair with no subsequent physical or behavioral intervention.

Compensatory Articulation

The possibilities for unacceptable speech following initial palatal repair may fall into two broad and probably oversimplified categories. First, these children may demonstrate normal placement skills but cannot meet the requirements for manner of production for nasalization to an acceptable degree. In this situation, we often believe that the diagnosis is clear and recommend improvement of velopharyngeal closure by physical management. That is, we infer that the child is demonstrating what the velopharyngeal closure mechanism is capable of doing. Second, these children may be honoring manner requirements (that is, constricting the airstream at some point along the vocal tract) but not the requirements for placement. In this situation, our recommendation is considerably less clear, at least regarding the *potential* adequacy of velopharyngeal closure. This latter pattern of articulation is well known to clinicians involved in cleft palate assessment and treatment.

Very simply, we *talk* about this pattern as inappropriate placement and *describe* the pattern as glottal stops, pharyngeal fricatives, velar fricatives, mid-dorsum stops, pharyngeal stops, and so on. We explain it as a "compensatory" articulation pattern that presumably develops in response to inadequate velopharyngeal closure, with onset occurring perhaps even before the hard and soft palates were initially repaired. Clearly, we recognize it as a problem for basically two reasons:

1. These patterns are inconsistent with the acquisition of normal speech and, once habituated, may be difficult to modify.
2. These patterns frequently confound the decision-making process of whether or not velopharyngeal closure is potentially adequate for acceptable speech.

In the presence of this so-called posterior pattern, the potential adequacy of velopharyngeal closure for speech is often unclear because the speaker is attempting to constrict or restrict the airstream at points nearer the respiratory system than the velopharyneal port. In other words, during such speech patterns, the child does not demonstrate what his or her velopharyngeal closure mechanism can, or cannot, do for speech. There is evidence that velopharyngeal movements are not the same (that is, they are less normal) when glottal placement is utilized.[16] Although in general terms compensatory patterns of this type are considered undesirable, we usually talk about compensatory phenomena as desirable. Some persons with cleft palate and, therefore, deviant structures, develop desirable compensations from a structural point of view that are beneficial to and consistent with normal speech. Examples include extensive medial movement of the lateral pharyngeal walls and extensive anterior movement of the posterior pharyngeal wall. For many speakers, perhaps these kinds of movement provide adequate velopharyngeal closure.

The problem of maladaptive or undesirable compensatory articulation has been recognized in the literature for many years by researchers and clinicians.[3, 17–20] Philips and Kent have for years written encouragingly about the appropriateness of early recognition and early intervention to intercept the development of this pattern.[10] Peterson has cautioned us that there are important individual differences between speakers with similar structures and that we must be aware that persons with questionable velopharyngeal closure may adopt different neuromuscular patterns in attempting to produce speech.[21] We often ask why some speakers adopt the strategy of compensatory articulation, which is considered inconsistent with acceptable speech, and others do not. Trost has taught us that there may be a whole range of inappropriate placements, not just the classic glottal stops and pharyngeal fricatives.[22] Warren has suggested that compensatory strategies develop because of a "need" to regulate pressures and flows in the vocal tract even at the expense of undermining speech performance.[23] His data were derived from patients who are older and who have known velopharyngeal dynamics. Ideally, it would be desirable to obtain aerodynamic information on very young children; however, at the very least we should have perceptual details of speech performance.

The Need to Observe Early Development

Earlier attention to and detailed descriptions of emerging speech productions are necessary to better understand the prevalence, nature, and development of this problem. As speech and language pathologists we should not be content to say, for example, that we will reevaluate at about 3 years of age. We may be losing important information that will be helpful to management if we do.

There is also a need for more parent education and involvement in speech development in these children. Too often we are content to explain to the parents something about our concerns for speech development and hope that they will do a good job of following through. As speech-language pathologists, we may counsel the parents shortly after primary palatal repair, and perhaps before, and discuss the role of the normal speech structures for producing speech. We describe the soft palate in relation to the back wall of the throat and how it needs to move up and back to contact the back wall of the throat for most speech sounds. That is, velopharyngeal closure is an important requirement for normal vowels and consonants with the exception of the nasals. We explain the effect of an unrepaired cleft palate on speech so that they can understand that velopharyngeal closure cannot be accomplished in this situation. We guide them to an understanding of the possible effect of a repaired cleft palate on speech, noting that there is a possibility that the soft palate in some individuals might be too short or lack sufficient mobility to obtain adequate velopharyngeal closure.

We then make our move about the problem at hand and superimpose our judgment about what is good and what is not good. We say something like, "As your child starts to talk, be tolerant of nasal air emission and hypernasality if it occurs, but be less tolerant of inappropriate placement. Let's make sure that when the /p's/ and /b's/ are being attempted, the two lips are coming together," and so on. In that sense, we tell them what to prefer.

More than 15 years ago a state-of-the-art conference on cleft palate[24] called for "the need for procedures describing the development of articulation skills and for accurately identifying variations in articulation behavior in children with cleft palate." Four years later, an updated state-of-the-art report suggested that we had not progressed significantly in describing variations in articulation behavior but had some new ways of looking at development.[25] Several models of speech acquisition in children with normal speech structures have been proposed during the last 15 to 20 years. In general, each of these models has attempted to describe more adequately the normal acquisition of speech. Examples include the learning of distinctive features or contrast sounds,[26, 27] a set of phonologic rules that relate the child output to the adult model,[28–32] or learning to suppress natural processes that act together to simplify speech.[33–35] As more longitudinal data about speech acquisition become available, it is increasingly evident that no single model explains, in a powerfully predictive way, speech acquisition of normal children. What is evident is that children are different. They may take different paths (creative errors) as they master speech. For the most part, children do master speech. On the other hand, the mastery of speech for a particular child is based on that child's experiences, speech-producing capabilities, and insights and perceptions into the structure of language. However, the models referred to above serve primarily to describe in more detail the productive speech attempts at earlier and earlier ages; they provide not just a listing of errors, but patterns of errors that suggest where the child was coming from and, perhaps, the direction in which she or he was headed.

Moving Toward a Phonologic Focus

We have moved from looking at articulation performance from a phonetic orientation to a more *phonologic* orientation. There has been confusion about what is meant by phonology and how it differs from articulation. We have become accustomed to the word *articulation* referring to the correct or incorrect production of individual consonant or vowel sounds. We have talked about sound substitutions, distortions, or omissions characterizing speech. We have talked about these in the context of what is there and what is not there, and how articulation patterns affect speech intelligibility. Articulation observations for individual speakers are thus on a peripheral level, showing where and how speech sounds are made.

Phonology can be defined as a representation of the higher processes of speech, referring to the speaker's knowledge and perception of the sound system and the patterns of errors. Phonetics is a part of phonology. As Locke has noted, what had previously been called multiple articulation errors could also be described as sound class problems.[36, 37] The meaning conveyed by the word *phonologic* to many was organizational. Phonology encompasses the total speech and language process, ranging from the more central and cognitive aspects to the peripheral or motor aspects. It is not suggested that we are any better at explaining what is going on but rather that what we describe coming out of the mouths of our very young patients with cleft palate may tell us more and be more helpful in determining more appropriate intervention.

There is now sufficient evidence to suggest that normal children (with no structural deviations) are active and creative in the process of acquiring phonologic skills and that no one single order of acquisition exists for all children.[32, 38, 39] All children initially lack sufficient motor control to produce accurate speech, and their early productions may reflect only the sounds and words that they are capable of producing.[1, 30–33, 38] There is also evidence that the prelinguistic behavior we call babbling may be an important forerunner of early speech and that a continuum exists from prelinguistic to early meaningful speech.[1, 36, 37, 40, 41]

The Child with Cleft Palate: A Special Structure-Learning Interaction

It is in this context that we approach the very young child with cleft palate. Consider the very young child going about the process of acquiring normal speech. From a learning standpoint, we assume that she or he behaves similarly to children without cleft palate in the sense of possessing the capability of learning the complex speech and language system. Now superimpose on that process an inadequate velopharyngeal mechanism for a varying period of time before the hard and soft palates are repaired, and possibly after the initial repair; superimpose the very high probability of middle ear problems and subsequent hearing loss; and superimpose the frequent modified dental and occlusal conditions that in some children may present hazards along the way. Clearly, compared with the child born with normal structures, children with cleft palate have their own set of complicating factors that potentially affect the acquisition of normal speech.

With the perspective that children with cleft palate are, for the most part, normal children learning to produce speech with an imperfect mechanism, the compensatory speech productions that have been described are more reasonable. Also, one would expect to find as much variability from child to child as is found in the normal population, plus the added variability that results from variations in the physical mechanism. However, the productions of an individual child may be as *systematic* as those of normal children. Perhaps we have focused on the problems of the cleft palate child for too long and have failed to recognize that the child is a normal child trying like any other to master the language, that is, to sound like others.

There are very few studies in the literature on early productions and vocalizations of children with cleft palate before 2 years of age, although interest and productivity in this area appear to be increasing.[10, 42–49] To date, numbers of patients have been relatively small. Compensatory pharyngeal and glottal patterns may be an early strategy for some, even before the palate is repaired. This proposal is almost speculation in search of data because we know very little about the onset or course of development of these productions or the factors that may contribute to their development. What has not been appreciated is that these patterns may be creative attempts by the child to organize a productive phonologic system.

We certainly do know that very young children develop prelinguistic and linguistic capabilities at varying ages. Some are precocious. Dorf and Curtin[48] and Randall et al[50] provide information suggesting that early palatal repair may result in better speech performance later. Philips and Kent provide examples of the contribution of acoustic analyses as it applies to early identification of words, patterns of prelinguistic utterances, and compensatory productions to supplement and perhaps validate what listeners perceive.[10] Detailed transcription-based studies with the aid of acoustic analysis when appropriate now allow us to look further back (earlier) at the developing phonologic system. The results may have an important implication for the timing of intervention, whether surgical, functional, parental, or any combination thereof.

Preliminary studies carried out at the University of Minnesota by Ebert[51] and Garcia[52] indicate that it is possible to secure samples of vocalizations from 6- to 12-month old children and to describe consonantlike productions according to place and manner. Transcriber agreement levels of 85% to 95% can be expected with trained listeners. Estrem and Broen followed five children with cleft palate and five normal children longitudinally during the time they were acquiring their first 50 words.[43] Transcription-based analysis of their productions reveals that the cleft children selected words that contained sounds that they were capable of producing, and that they selected and produced more posterior sounds and also more labial sounds than the normal children.

In the Estrem and Broen study, individual children with cleft palate differed from one another. One child selected words that began with nasals and approximants and produced them correctly. Ultimately, this child required physical management to improve velopharyngeal closure. Another child selected words beginning with stops and fricatives but substituted glottal stops for oral stops. The potential adequacy of this child's closure mechanism remained questionable. Interestingly, this was the one child who produced her first words before primary palatal surgery.

In several respects, the cleft children were like the normal children. Syllable structure was similar for the two groups. Data such as these have important implications for the timing of primary palatal surgery and perhaps for early identification of those children requiring secondary improvement of velopharyngeal closure, and merit expansion.

We have always attempted to predict, based on speech and other factors, which children will need secondary improvement for velopharyngeal closure.

Much of the weight of that decision is based on speech performance. Increased knowledge of the speech characteristics that distinguish the very young child with inadequate closure from a child with adequate closure is needed. Van Demark analyzed retrospective speech data that suggested that inability to produce certain phonemes correctly at age 4 years was a factor distinguishing those who needed improved closure from those who did not.[53]

Broen and coworkers examined speech characteristics of children who had been followed longitudinally until a decision could be reached about the need for improved closure.[54] Analysis of data at 30 months of age revealed that children who ultimately required further physical management made significantly more errors on pressure consonants and substituted nasals and approximants for these phonemes. Furthermore, the substitution of nasals and approximants for stop consonants appeared to be the most potent predictor of the need for improved closure.

Responses to the early speech patterns of these children by parents, peers, and others also may be important in the early development and maintenance of compensatory articulation. Studies examining listener preferences of peers, parents, and others suggest strongly that the compensatory pattern is preferred to the pattern of correct placement when the latter is accompanied by excessive hypernasality and audible nasal air emission.[55–58] This suggests that parents may need increased understanding of speech development and more appropriate responses to early speech attempts.

O'Gara and Logemann studied the speech development of 23 babies with cleft palate at 6-month intervals from age 3 months to 36 months.[42] Occurrence of consonant and vowel place features, consonant manner features, types of stops and fricatives, and vowel height features were observed. During the time these children were followed, initial palatal repair occurred. Data were analyzed for those children whose cleft palate was repaired before and after 12 months of age. Findings suggested that oral place features were produced less frequently in cleft children than noncleft children. However, the data indicated that more frequent pressure consonant production and a reduction in the frequency of posterior compensatory placement occurred in the children who had primary palatal repair before 12 months of age.

Longitudinal data, which are now limited in availability, should provide the opportunity to study timing factors and sequential events. Studies of learning variables and their effect on speech have been limited for the most part to studies of normal children. If such variables are truly significant and powerful, their influence should be apparent in studies of children with a high potential for developing articulation problems such as children with cleft lip and palate. Therefore, we need more information about the process by which children learn compensatory behavior and factors associated with its etiology.

Conclusions

In summary, our goal as speech-language pathologists, shared certainly by parents and the interdisciplinary team, is to facilitate acceptable communication skills for the cleft palate child as early as possible. The infant born with cleft palate brings to the task of acquiring normal speech a significantly altered mechanism. The process of learning speech and language begins early, the proficiency varies from child to child, and each child may demonstrate a somewhat unique and creative way of attempting to master the sound system given their particular structural capability. It is hoped that, if more attention is paid to the emerging phonologic development, that structural capability or lack of it can be determined early, thereby increasing the number of younger and younger individuals with cleft palate who are effective communicators.

References

1. Menn L: Development of articulatory, phonetic, and phonological capabilities. In Butterworth B (ed): Language Production. Vol 2: Development, Writing and Other Language Processes. New York: Academic Press, 1983.
2. Byrne MD, Shelton RL, Diedrick W: Articulatory skills, physical management and classification of the children with cleft palates. J Speech Hear Dis 26:326–333, 1961.
3. Bzoch KR: Articulatory proficiency and error patterns of pre-school cleft palate and normal children. Cleft Palate J 2.340–349, 1965.
4. Counihan DT: Articulation skills of adolescents and adults with cleft palates. J Speech Hear Dis 25:181–187, 1960.
5. Spriestersbach DC, Moll KL, Morris HL: Subject classification and articulation of speakers with cleft palates. J Speech Hear Res 4:362–372, 1961.
6. Spriestersbach DC, Powers GR: Articulation skills, velopharyngeal closure, and oral breath pressures of children with cleft palates. J Speech Hear Res 2:318–325, 1959.
7. Morris HL: Communication skills of children with cleft lips and palates. J Speech Hear Res 5:79–90, 1962.
8. Olson DA: A descriptive study of the speech development of a group of infants with cleft palate. Thesis (Ph.D. unpublished). Evanston IL: Northwestern University, 1965.
9. Starr CD: A study of the characteristics of the speech and speech mechanisms of a group of cleft palate children. Thesis (Ph.D.). Evanston IL: Northwestern University, 1956.
10. Philips BJ, Kent RD: Acoustic-phonic descriptions of speech production in speakers with cleft palate and other velopharyngeal disorders. In Lass N (ed): Speech and Language: Advances in Basic Research and Practice. New York: Academic Press, 1984.
11. Subtelny J, Koepp-Baker H, Subtelny JD: Palatal function and cleft palate speech. J Speech Hear Dis 26:213–224, 1961.
12. Van Demark DR, Van Demark AH: Misarticulations of cleft palate children achieving velopharyngeal closure and children with functional speech problems. Cleft Palate J 4:31–37, 1967.
13. Riski JE: Articulation skills and oral-resonance in children with pharyngeal flaps. Cleft Palate J 16:421–428, 1979.
14. Riski J, Delong E: Articulation development in children with cleft lip/palate. Cleft Palate J 21(2):57–62, 1984.
15. Van Demark DR: Predictability of velopharyngeal competency. Cleft Palate J 16:429–435, 1979.
16. Henningsson GE, Isberg AM: Velopharyngeal movement patterns in patients alternating between oral and glottal articulation: A clinical and cineradiographical study. Cleft Palate J 23(1):1–9, 1986.
17. Morris HL: Etiological bases for speech problems. In Spriestersbach D, Sherman D (eds): Cleft Palate and Communication. New York: Academic Press, 1968.
18. Morris HL: Evaluation of abnormal articulation patterns. In Grabb W, Rosenstein S, Bzoch K (eds): Cleft Lip and Palate. Boston: Little, Brown, 1971.
19. Morley ME: Cleft Palate and Speech. Baltimore: Williams & Wilkins, 1970.
20. Bzoch KR: Etiological factors related to cleft palate speech. In Grabb W, Rosenstein S, Bzoch K (eds): Cleft Lip and Palate. Boston: Little, Brown, 1971.
21. Peterson S: Velopharyngeal function; some important differences. J Speech Hear Dis 38:89–97, 1973.
22. Trost JE: Articulation additions to the clinical description of persons with cleft palate. Cleft Palate J 18:193–203, 1981.
23. Warren D: Compensatory speech behaviors in cleft palate: A regulation/control phenomenon? Cleft Palate J 23(4): 251–260, 1986.
24. Spriestersbach D, et al: Clinical research in cleft lip and palate: The state of the art. Cleft Palate J 10:113–164, 1973.
25. Fletcher S, et al: Cleft lip and palate research: An updated state of the art. Cleft Palate J 14:261–321, 1977.
26. Jakobson R: Child Language, Aphasia, and Phonological Universals. The Hague: Mouton, 1968.
27. Menyuk P: The role of distinctive features in children's acquisition of phonology. J Speech Hear Res 11:138–146, 1968.
28. Compton AJ: Generative studies of children's phonological disorders. J Speech Hear Dis 35:315–339, 1970.
29. Dinnsen DA: Methods and empirical issues in analyzing functional misarticulation. In Elbert M, Dinnsen DA, Weismer G (eds): Phonological Theory and the Misarticulating Child. ASHA Monograph No. 22. Rockville MD: American Speech-Language-Hearing Association, 1984.
30. Ingram D: Phonological rules in young children. J Child Language 1:49–64, 1974.
31. Ingram D: Fronting in child phonology. J Child Language 1:233–241, 1974.
32. Smith NV: The Acquisition of Phonology. Cambridge: Cambridge University Press, 1973.
33. Stampe D: The Acquisition of Phonetic Representation. Chicago Linguistic Society, 5th Regional Meeting, 1969, pp 443–454.
34. Ingram D: Phonological Disability in Children. New York: Elsevier, 1976.
35. Shriberg LD, Kwiatkowski J: Natural Process Analysis. New York: Wiley, 1980.
36. Locke JL: Clinical phonology: The explanation and treatment of speech sound disorders. J Speech Hear Dis 48(4):339–341, 1983.
37. Locke JL: Phonological Acquisition and Change. New York: Academic Press, 1983.
38. Ferguson CA, Farwell CB: Words and sounds in early language acquisition: English initial consonants in the first fifty words. Language 51:419–439, 1975.
39. Fey M, Gondour J: Rule discovery in early phonological acquisition. J Child Language 9:71–82, 1982.
40. Lieberman P: On the development of vowel production in young children. In Yeni-Komshian GH, Kavanaugh JF, Ferguson CA (eds): Child Phonology. Vol 1: Production. New York: Academic Press, 1980.
41. Oller DK, Wieman L, Doyle W, et al: Infant babbling and speech. J Child Language 3:1–11, 1975.
42. O'Gara M, Logemann JA: Phonetic analysis of speech development of babies with cleft palate. Cleft Palate J 25(2):122–135, 1988.
43. Estrem T, Broen PA: Early speech productions of children with cleft palate. J Speech Hear Res 32:12–23, 1989.
44. Trost-Cardemone JE: Speech development and the timing of primary palatoplasty. Presented at the Annual Meeting of the American Cleft Palate Association, Williamsburg, Virginia, April 1988.
45. Moller KT, Broen P: Early phonological development in children with cleft palate. Study session presented at the American Cleft Palate Association Annual Meeting, Seattle, Washington, May 1984.
46. Moller KT, Broen P, Schwartz R: Early phonological development: The normal and cleft palate experience. Miniseminar presented at the American Speech-Language-Hearing Association, New Orleans, Louisiana, 1987.
47. Lynch J, Fox D, Brookshire B: Phonological proficiency of two cleft palate toddlers with school-age follow-up. J Speech Hear Dis 48:274–285, 1983.
48. Dorf D, Curtin SW: Early cleft palate repair and speech outcome. Plast Reconstr Surg 70:74–79, 1982.
49. Grunwell P, Russell J: Vocalizations before and after cleft palate surgery: A pilot study. Br J Dis Comm 22:1–17, 1987.
50. Randall P, LaRossa DD, Fakhrace SM, et al: Cleft palate closure at 3 to 7 months of age: A preliminary report. Plast Reconstr Surg 71:264, 1983.
51. Ebert S: Babbling patterns in infants. Thesis. In process, personal communication.
52. Garcia S: Comparing the vocalizations of children with cleft palate to the vocalizations of children without cleft palate. Thesis. In process, personal communication.
53. Van Demark D: Predictability of velopharyngeal competency. Cleft Palate J 16:429–435, 1979.
54. Broen P, Felsenfeld S, Kittelson-Bacon C: Predicting from phonological patterns observed in children with cleft palate. Paper presented at the Symposium on Research in Child Language Disorders, Madison, WI, May 1986.
55. Paynter E, Kinard M: Perceptual preferences between compensatory articulation and nasal escape of air in children with velopharyngeal incompetence. Cleft Palate J 16:262–266, 1979.
56. Paynter E: Parental and child preference for speech produced by children with velopharyngeal incompetence. Cleft Palate J 24:112–118, 1987.
57. Diegel C: Parental preferences and severity ratings for hypernasal and compensatory patterns of articulation in the speech of children with cleft palate. Thesis (Master's, unpublished). Minneapolis: University of Minnesota, 1984.
58. Persoon J: Unsophisticated listener judgments for hypernasal and compensatory patterns of articulation in the speech of children and adults. Thesis (Master's, unpublished). Minneapolis: University of Minnesota, 1986.

CHAPTER 91

Early Speech Management

Betty Jane Philips

The attainment of normal speech by children born with cleft palate is a primary goal of the cleft palate team. Provision of speech-language services at an early age has been advocated for attaining this goal. The rationale for early services is derived from a knowledge of phonologic and linguistic development and also from the influence of palatal dysfunction on speech and language. Rapid progression from infant vocalizations toward increasingly complex verbal communication occurs during a child's first 3 years. As early as the first 12 months and well before the emergence of words, infants are developing control that elicits contrasts in pitch, voice quality, resonance, and timing (Table 91–1).[1] Constraints imposed by palatal clefting are reflected in infant vocalizations.[2,3] Differences in phonetic development between children with cleft palate and noncleft peers were reported by Olson.[4] He also reported delay in use of first words. Estrem and Broen indicated that the words used by children with cleft palate were more frequently composed of sonorants than of phonemes, which require control of intraoral air pressure and airflow.[5] Acquisition of atypical speech patterns, such as the pharyngeal and glottal replacements that are frequently seen in the speech of those who have had cleft palate, is a concern because once habituated, these patterns are likely to persist.

All children with cleft palate are at risk for speech-language problems. Surgical closure of the palate may not provide a competent mechanism for speech production. Until normal development can be ascertained, the assistance of the speech-language pathologist is needed. Three types of early speech-language programs are advocated (Table 91–2). The first is a program of parent education; the second, a program of stimulation; and the third, a program of remediation. These can be viewed as levels within a continuum of services. The level of service will vary over time in relation to the needs of the child and the parents.

Level One: Parent Education

The objectives of the first level program, parent education, are to
1. Provide information about expectations for speech-language development during the first 12 to 18 months.
2. Encourage the parents in facilitating their child's speech and language development.
3. Obtain the parents' assistance in monitoring and reporting the child's progress.

This program can be accomplished by providing counseling sessions at the time of visits to the cleft palate clinic and by telephone follow-up. The parents should be given information about early phonologic and linguistic development, particularly stages they will encounter in the near future. For example, a parent should be informed about the types of phonation, such as growling and squealing, that are likely to occur at the age of 4 to 6 months and be assured that this is normal and is observed in many children with or without cleft palate. They need information on the effects of a cleft palate on speech development. For example, children with cleft palate will demonstrate the repetitive vocalization associated with babbling, but the parents may not recognize it as babbling because of the absence of common consonantal markers such as /z/ and /d/.

Similarly, they may need to understand that at 12 to 18 months a production such as /mɑmɑ/, when accompanied by the appropriate gesture, is bye bye, and to know why the child isn't producing sounds such as /b/ and /d/. The information needed by the parents will depend on the child's development and their reaction to it. Parents can be helped by the assurance that children progress at different rates and that although their child's vocalizations may be different, these differ-

---

Table 91–1. Stages of Development in Phonetic Control (Modified from Oller DK: The emergence of sounds of speech of infancy. In Yeni-Komshian GH, Cavanaugh JF, Ferguson CA [eds]: Child Phonology. Vol. I: Production. New York: Academic Press, 1980.)

Age in Months	Speech-Language Programs
3	Parent Education
6	
12	Speech-Language Stimulation
18	
24	
30	Speech-Language Remediation Intensive Stimulation - Remediation
36	

Table 91–2. Type and Timing of Early Speech-Language Management

Age in Months	Stage	Contrasts
0 - 1	Phonation stage	Nonreflexive vocalization
2 - 3	Goo stage	Vocal tract opening and closure
4 - 6	Expansion stage	Resonance, place, pitch amplitude
7 - 10	Canonical stage	Syllabic timing
11 - 12	Variegated babbling	Vocalic-consonantal, stress

ences are to be expected when there is a cleft palate. Parents also may need assistance at the time of surgery because they sometimes expect immediate, positive changes in speech and are disappointed or think the surgery has failed when these expected benefits do not immediately occur.

Parents should be encouraged to provide stimulation and feedback by babbling, talking, and singing to their child, playing simple games such as "peek-a-boo," and naming objects, people, and activities. Although most parents naturally will encourage their child's vocal play and early speech, there are those that benefit from direction and demonstration. Hahn has provided suggestions for such assistance.[6]

A journal should be kept by the parents as a record of their child's developing communication skills. They should note and describe occurrences such as babbling, specific speech sounds, unusual sounds, and words—written as the child said them. This record helps the clinician to monitor development that is not always demonstrated when the child is seen, and it promotes parental awareness of progress. Depending on the composition of the cleft palate team, the speech-language pathologist may be the person who is responsible for providing instruction to the parents on feeding and information about middle ear disease and hearing. If so, this information should be incorporated into the parent education program.

Level Two: Language Stimulation

The second level, a speech-language stimulation program, was advocated by Philips.[7] This level should begin at approximately 12 months, the age at which children begin to use first words. The objectives are to
1. Support and promote the child's phonologic and linguistic development.
2. Minimize the development of atypical speech-language problems.
3. Assess the competence of the velopharyngeal mechanism for speech.

This program and the parent education program are merged. Both the child and parents are participants. The sessions should be conducted in the clinical environment, preferably a playroom with toys selected by the clinician to provide the desired stimulation.

Services for this program should be scheduled on a weekly or biweekly basis for periods of 30 to 45 minutes and at a time when the child will not be fatigued. The proposed structure provides a stable environment that soon becomes familiar and secure for the child and is free of distractions that could occur if the program were conducted in the child's home. The child's play, and thus verbalizations, can be influenced to some extent by the toys and pictures that are in the room. The clinician is responsible for shaping the child's activities toward accomplishment of goals for the session. The parent is given information about the child's progress and also direction in recognizing, stimulating and reinforcing the child's attempted productions. Opportu-

nities are provided for parents to participate so that the clinician may observe, direct, and assist the parents in facilitating the child's speech-language development.

For children who have an unrepaired cleft, the clinician should
1. Encourage vocabulary development by repetitive modeling of names of objects, activities, and people.
2. Identify the child's word attempts, e.g. /mɑ/ for ball, /nʌn/ for sun.
3. Provide positive reinforcement by recognizing attempted word productions, but make no attempt to elicit the plosive, fricative, and affricate phonemes.

Some parents have considerable anxiety about their child's speech and language development under these circumstances and seek assurance and explanation of the acceptability of productions such as /mɑ/ for ball.

For the child whose cleft has been surgically repaired, the procedures for stimulation of speech-language development are different. Effort is made to elicit plosives and fricatives, to encourage their production in words, and to promote their occurrence in spontaneous speech using expanded language forms. Procedures such as visual and tactile stimulation, modeling, and paired stimuli are useful.

The stimulation program should continue advancing the child's speech-language until the phonologic and linguistic development is within normal limits for the child's age. In some children, however, indications of velopharyngeal dysfunction will appear. For them, the stimulation program provides close monitoring that will assist in identification of indicators of a need to consider surgical or prosthetic management. When surgical repair of the cleft has not been completed and speech-language development is proceeding rapidly or when nasal, pharyngeal, or glottal phonemes occur in words as replacements for oral plosives or fricatives, the speech-language pathologist should encourage the surgeon to schedule closure as soon as possible.

For children whose clefts have been repaired, inability to obtain oral production of plosives in at least some contexts strongly suggests an incompetent velopharyngeal mechanism. Van Demark demonstrated that inability to produce plosives by age 4 was indicative of velopharyngeal dysfunction.[8] Broen et al suggested that by the age of 30 months the use of sonorants (nasals, liquids, glides, including /h/, and glottal onset of voiceless consonants and vowels) as substitutes for oral plosives was a good predictor of velopharyngeal incompetence.[9] This conclusion was based on retrospective study of the speech of two groups of children who had surgically repaired palates. At 30 months, the group that had been identified as incompetent substituted sonorants for nonsonorants 69.1% of the time. In contrast, the group identified as competent used the sonorant substitution pattern in 8.4% of cases. Sonorant substitutions occurred in the speech of noncleft controls 1.7% of the time. These data suggest that inability to achieve plosive productions with speech-language stimulation following surgical closure of the palate is a matter of concern for the cleft palate team. When surgical management is not an option for any period of time, stimulation should not include promotion of plosives and fricatives because it is important to avoid the acquisition and habituation of the atypical nasal, pharyngeal, and glottal phonemes as far as possible.

Level Three: Remedial Services

The program at the third level is one of remedial services. This program is for children who have developed phonologic patterns of nasal, pharyngeal, glottal, or other atypical replacements for oral plosive, fricative, and affricate productions but who show evidence of a potential for development of good valving—that is, with stimulation, productions of at least one pressure consonant can be elicited. The objectives of the program are to

1. Develop oral productions of plosives, fricatives, and affricates, eliminating compensatory patterns that have been established prior to attainment of competence.
2. Promote use of the oral productions in spontaneous speech.

An intensive remedial program is recommended because this is preferable to traditional weekly services. In an intensive program the child is placed in a group play program and may be there for a half or a full day. The child is then available for individual remedial sessions that are provided two to four times daily. In addition, the playroom staff (the ratio is no lower than one adult to two children) are directed in monitoring, assisting, and reinforcing the child in using productions learned in the individual sessions. The opportunity to adjust the frequency and length of individual remedial sessions and the constancy with which stimulation can be maintained accommodate the attention span of the preschool child and assist the child in incorporating newly learned productions into spontaneous speech. The parents should be invited to observe the individual sessions and participate with the staff in the group sessions when and if they are able to do so. This increases their understanding of their child's phonologic problems and helps to develop their skills in stimulating, modeling, and reinforcing. This participation will not be appropriate if it is disruptive for the child or the group, as occasionally happens.

Procedures are selected from among those used for articulation disorders such as direction for articulatory placement, visual and tactile stimulation, modeling, and paired stimuli. The first step is to provide direction that will elicit oral airflow and achieve oral approximation of pressure consonants that will gradually be shaped toward acceptable productions. When modeling, caution is taken to use slow speech and also to avoid exaggeration of airflow and air pressure. Language patterns and expansion are modeled for the child in both the individual and group settings.

Promotion of expressive language development does not receive the emphasis that is given to phonologic development. Although delays in language development are reported for children with cleft palate, these reports require careful interpretation. Evaluation of expressive language is difficult when intelligibility of speech is poor and when atypical phonemes are used. Evaluation should begin with careful assessment of the child's phonologic capacities and consideration of the applications as well as the constraints they impose. The clinician must recognize that compensatory linguistic patterns (such as shortening of length of utterances, omissions of syntactic markers and words, use of temporal and suprasegmental variations, and use of atypical phonemes as syntactic markers) may be embedded in the expressive language as a result of the child's efforts to communicate in the presence of velopharyngeal dysfunction. Table 91–3 illustrates the use of atypical phonemes, by two children who had postsurgical velopharyngeal dysfunction, for accomplishment of syntactic markers as well as an omission that may have been a response to the constraints imposed by these atypical phonemic productions. Improvement in phonologic development along with simple modeling of expressive language patterns usually is sufficient to remedy patterns such as those described in Table 91–3 unless a child is found to have language disabilities independent of the phonologic difficulties.

When a child is unable to progress to oral production of a plosive or fricative within the first 2 weeks, the intensive program should be discontinued. Two weeks in an intensive program is equivalent to approximately 20 individual half hour remedial speech sessions. The child should then be referred to the cleft palate team for further evaluation and planning for appropriate management of the problems.

Those children who have a competent palatovelopharyngeal mechanism can be expected to make rapid

Table 91–3. Transcription Illustrating Productions That Served as Syntactic Markers in the Speech of Children with Velopharyngeal Incompetence

---

N, age 35 months

    here's mama /ɪɣmʌmə/

    where's my mommy / wə–mɛʔmʌmɪ/

    don't know /nʊʔnʌo/

    mommy put this here /mɑmɪ p̆ʊ̆t jɪɣhɪjʌo/

M, age 36 months

    bear /meɚ/

    bears /meɚ̃/

    knocks /nɑʔh/

    baby's bed /memɪš mɛ·/

    he wants /hɪ wã̰/

Key: velar fricative /ɣ/, glottal stop /ʔ/, nasal airflow /◌̃/, omission —

progress in the intensive remedial program. Tables 91–4 and 91–5 illustrate the progress made by one child in an intensive remedial speech program. The boy had a submucous cleft palate that was surgically repaired when he was 28 months old. Intensive remedial speech services were initiated 2 months postsurgery. He participated in the program for 4 weeks and then received an individual remedial program twice a week for an additional 4 weeks. Following this, his progress was both continued and sustained, although he received no additional speech-language remediation. This was a typical pattern of progress for young children who participated in an intensive remedial speech-language program when there was potential for development of adequate velopharyngeal function for speech.

An intensive remedial speech program appears to be advantageous for the preschool child. The concentrated stimulation maximizes and speeds the learning of new patterns and their carry-over to spontaneous speech. As soon as the child learns to use oral airflow in production of pressure consonants, rapid generalization can be expected. Frequent practice coupled with constant monitoring and reinforcement helps to establish the new patterns quickly. When remedial sessions are scheduled only once or twice a week, these too can be beneficial; however, generalization and habituation probably will be slower than in an intensive program. Children are highly motivated to communicate effectively. The intensive program capitalizes on this motivation and helps to maintain it.

Summary

Some children for whom competence is established at very early age levels do very well without any of the speech-language services that have been described. Nevertheless, prudence dictates the provision of these speech-language programs rather than waiting to see if problems develop and persist. Some children will be

Table 91–4. Progress of a Child, Aged 30 Months, Receiving Intensive Remedial Speech Services Initiated 2 Months Following Surgery

Phoneme	Pattern Week 1	Percent Correct Week 1	Percent Correct in Context Week 8
p	m/p	50	100, phrase
b	-/b	59	100, phrase
t	n/t	0	100, word
d	n/d	0	100, word
f	m/f	0	90, word
s	n/s	0	80, word
ʃ	m/ʃ	0	80, word
tʃ	-/tʃ	0	69, word

Table 91–5. Correct Productions of Phonemes (Underlined) Evidenced in Spontaneous Speech of a Child, Aged 32 Months, After 8 Weeks in an Intensive Remedial Speech Program

Phoneme	Words Produced In Spontaneous Speech			
p	pig	open	soup	purple
b	bear	baby		blue
t	table		tight	tractor
d	ducks	Adam spider	head	
f	found		off	frog
s	some	house	moose	horse
ʃ	shoe		push	
tʃ	choo choo	Archie	watch	
dʒ	giraffe		huge	

followed in the stimulation program for only a few weeks, during which time need for the program is not evidenced. Such children can then be monitored periodically. The types of programs described provide a range of services for the infant and toddler with cleft palate and should be used selectively in relation to the timing of surgical procedures and to the child's development. Regardless of the age at which surgical closure of the palate is completed, continuous monitoring of speech development is important in determining velopharyngeal competence. Monitoring is best accomplished in an environment in which the child is comfortable and secure. Repeated observations yield more information than can be obtained in single sessions. Response to stimulation provides important information that assists in evaluation of velopharyngeal competence. Nearly all children with cleft palate have the potential to achieve speech and language skills appropriate for their age level. Provision of early speech-language programs helps to ensure that by the age of 36 months, or earlier for most children, the transition from speech-language patterns influenced by clefting to those used by noncleft children will be accomplished. Those who do not have this potential need to be identified early and referred for appropriate services.

There is a great need for continuing education and informational materials for public school personnel who will provide services for children with cleft palate at early ages. The average speech-language pathologist has relatively little knowledge about cleft palate and very limited experience in its management, as do primary providers in all professions. Continuing education programs and information will assist in ensuring that appropriate effective and timely speech-language services are provided.

References

1. Oller DK: The emergence of sounds of speech of infancy. In Yeni-Komshian GH, Cavanaugh JF, Ferguson CA (eds): Child Phonology. Vol. I: Production. New York: Academic Press, 1980.

2. Bzoch KR: An investigation of the speech of pre-school cleft palate children. Dissertation (Ph.D.). Evanston IL: Northwestern University, 1956.
3. Philips BJ, Kent RD: Acoustic-phonetic descriptions of speech problems in speakers with cleft palate and other velopharyngeal disorders. In Lass MJ (ed): Speech and Language: Advances in Basic Research and Practice. Vol. II. Orlando: Academic Press, 1984.
4. Olson DA: A descriptive study of the speech development of a group of infants with unoperated cleft palate. Dissertation (Ph.D.). Ann Arbor: University of Michigan, 1965.
5. Estrem T, Broen PA: Early speech production of children with cleft palate. J Speech Hear Res 32:12, 1989.
6. Hahn E: Directed home training program for infants with cleft lip and palate.
In Bzoch KR (ed): Communicative Disorders Related to Cleft Lip and Palate. Boston: Little, Brown, 1979.
7. Philips BJ: Stimulating syntactic and phonological development in infants with cleft palate. In Bzoch KR (ed): Communicative Disorders Related to Cleft Lip and Palate. Boston: Little, Brown, 1979.
8. Van Demark DR: Predictability of velopharyngeal competency. Cleft Palate J 16:429, 1979.
9. Broen PA, Felsenfeld S, Bacon CK: Predicting from phonological patterns observed in children with cleft palate. Read before the Symposium on Research and Child Language Disorders, University of Wisconsin, Madison, WI, 1986.

CHAPTER 92

Speech Development and the Timing of Primary Palatoplasty

Susan I. Kemp-Fincham, David P. Kuehn, and Judith E. Trost-Cardamone

The timing of primary cleft palate surgery has been viewed historically in relation to two opposing factors, speech acquisition and maxillofacial growth potential. Proponents of speech and language acquisition argue for early surgery so that speech structures will be in a more favorable position to function normally, thereby avoiding compensatory behavior. In contrast, those concerned about maxillofacial development argue for late surgery at an age closer to physical maturation because they fear that surgery may retard maxillofacial growth.

As a compromise, some surgeons performed early surgical repair of the velum, to provide an intact structure for speech, and then performed late surgical closure of the hard palate to avoid growth retardation.[1–3] This approach is often referred to as primary veloplasty. Unfortunately, speech results using this approach have not been gratifying.[4–8] Moreover, the benefits of delaying hard palate closure in relation to midfacial growth remain somewhat questionable.[9, 10]

In an extensive study, Ross analyzed 538 cephalometric radiographs of males with unilateral cleft lip and palate to determine the effect of the timing of primary surgery on maxillofacial growth.[11] He found that growth was least adversely affected if the hard palate was never closed, or if closure was delayed until the teenage years. Interestingly, however, the next best results in terms of maxillofacial growth parameters were found in patients in whom surgery had been completed by 11 months of age or earlier. The worst results were found in those in whom surgery had been performed after 20 months of age, including primary veloplasty procedures with hard palate closure performed at 4 to 9 years of age.

Even if primary surgery is not delayed until the teenage years, the optimal time for such surgery remains to be determined. That is, how early is "early" and how late is "late" for optimal speech development? Convincing answers to these questions await a larger data base than is presently available. It will be important to compare speech development in the cleft palate population to that of normal individuals. Clearly, without any surgical management most cleft palate individuals would develop speech that eventually becomes different from normal. When does such divergence occur? Are early speech precursors (vegetative sounds, cooing, babbling, and so on) different in cleft palate and noncleft palate babies? Do such differences perhaps exist from birth? What is the nature of primary surgery in changing the course of abnormal speech development toward a more normal development? In the absence of an adequate data base one can only argue from a theoretical perspective. Thus, inferences about the timing of primary surgery can be made in relation to the comparatively greater body of knowledge about developmental trends in normal infants. Our primary purpose is to address the issue of timing of primary palatoplasty in regard to factors associated with speech development.

It is not our intention to debate the technical merits and limitations of specific surgical procedures. However, because speech development is a physical process, anatomic and physiologic factors logically must be taken into consideration. We support those procedures that reasonably provide the best possible anatomic mechanism with which optimal functioning could develop. An example of this is levator veli palatini (LVP) muscle reconstruction. It is assumed in the remainder of this chapter that primary palatoplasty incorporates LVP reconstruction and that the hard and soft palates are closed surgically in one stage—that is, during the same operation.

It is often assumed that there are rather well delineated periods that are identifiable as children grow and develop. In particular, such periods may be crucial in terms of development in the areas of speech motor control, cognitive-linguistic skills, and psychosocial adjustment. The more salient aspects of development in these areas relevant to primary surgery are reviewed in the following sections. In this chapter the term *sensitive period*, as opposed to *critical period*, will be used because it implies that there are times at which owing to biologic maturation, many physiologic systems are attuned to encourage certain types of learning. However, it appears that these periods in motor learning may be neither absolute nor discrete. Rather, it is assumed that the acquisition of skills follows a continuum along which learning is cumulative in nature and in which earlier skills form the building blocks for later learning. It has been argued by Netsell that sensitive periods for the acquisition of speech motor control occur during periods of "nonlinearity" along the developmental continuum when changes in a number of areas of development coincide.[12] Thus, if a sensitive period is somehow "missed" or if learning during this period is hampered, later skills building on this earlier learning may be affected negatively. The concept of sensitive period is implicit in all of the following sections that deal with developmental trends.

Developmental Factors Related to Primary Palatoplasty

Motor Development

During the first 2 months of life, the infant's motor behavior is primarily reflexive.[12-14] It is during the following 2 months (that is, between 2 and 4 months of age) that the infant achieves increasing head control and sits with support.[15] These postural changes are associated with changes in the oral cavity shape, which in turn allow greater mobility of the tongue. In addition, Thelen observed that at this time the onset of "rhythmical stereotypes" using the limbs and torso occurs, involving quite rapid repeated rhythmic movement of the body part involved (Table 92–1).[13] These movements occur in a variety of contexts and cannot therefore be considered reflexive. Indeed, Thelen argues that such movements constitute a transition behavior between uncoordinated activity and complex, coordinated voluntary control. Thus, Thelen claims that these repeated rhythmic movements may predict the appearance of motor milestones involving the same muscle groups.

Interestingly, the infant's behavioral repertoire is dominated by rhythmic movements at around 6 months of age.[13] As can be seen in Table 92–1, it is at this time that the infant sits without support, begins "canonical" or reduplicated babbling (e.g., vocalizations such as babababa)[16] and may even begin rocking back and forth on hands and knees in preparation for crawling.[15, 16] Langlois and colleagues observed that postural control in the sitting position at about 6 months postnatally facilitated a decrease in breathing rate owing to increased chest expansion.[17] This decrease allows a longer expiration phase, which is necessary for the production of reduplicated babble sequences. Kent has suggested a possible correspondence between rhythmic stereotypes in body movement and reduplicated babbling.[18] If Thelen's thesis on the role of such movements in the gradual emergence of functionally mature neuromuscular pathways is correct, then this period, which begins at about 6 months of age and is dominated by repeated cyclical movements, may assume considerable importance in the development of speech motor control. Kent has suggested that rhythmic or cyclic patterns form the natural basis for the organization of movement systems.[19] Thus, babbling may play a vital organizational role in the development of motor control systems for the spatiotemporal dimensions of speech. Consequently, it may be important for palatal closure to be achieved prior to the onset of this potentially significant period, that is, prior to about 6 months of age.

The motor precursors of this period of intense rhythmic activity appear to be

1. Momentary head control in ventral suspension.[15]
2. Diminished head lag when pulled from the supine to a sitting position.

Table 92–1. Relationship Between Phonetic, Anatomic-Physiologic, and Motor Development in the First Year of Life

Age (months)	Phonologic Development	Anatomic-Physiologic Development	Motor Development
0–2	Quasi-resonant nuclei, vegetative sounds, glottal attack	Engaged larynx and nasopharynx. Tongue fills the oral cavity, moving along the anterior-posterior plane	Primitive reflexes
2–4	Quasi-resonant nuclei, velar and uvular or pharyngeal constrictions; cooing, gooing, and laughter	Change in oral cavity shape. Increased mobility of the tongue, but tongue is still restricted by larynx-nasopharynx engagement	Increased head control. Sits supported. Onset of rhythmic stereotypes using legs, torso, and arms
4–6 "expansion phase"	Fully resonant nuclei. Yelling, growling, squealing, prolonged vocalizations, raspberries, trills, repetition of vowels, marginal babbling, whispering, shouting	Onset of disengagement of the larynx and nasopharynx. Better coordination of the respiratory system and the larynx	Sits without support. Onset of rocking on hands and knees
6–9	Reduplicated or canonical babbling. Cyclicity or rhythmicity of repeated utterances		Crawls, pulls himself to standing position. Peak in rhythmic movements of limbs and torso
9–12	Variegated babbling, first words		Decline in rhythmic movements. Walks without support

Data drawn from references 13, 20, and 25.

3. Control of the torso when sitting supported.
4. Onset of rhythmic stereotypes involving the limbs and torso.

Frequent monitoring of the cleft palate infant would facilitate observation of these motor behaviors, which occur prior to the possible sensitive period of 4 to 6 months of age.

Speech Development

Speech Motor Control. The development of speech motor control relative to the timing of cleft palate closure will be discussed in terms of an integrated motor approach as opposed to a coarticulation approach.[20–22] The latter approach assumes a serial ordering of the segments (phones or syllables) that constitute the targets of speech production. The appeal of the integrated motor approach lies in the assumption that parallel rather than serial motor processes interact to achieve holistic behavioral goals (a multisyllabic phonetic unit or a phrase). These may be perceptual goals consisting of multiple integrated parts rather than a series of discrete phonetic units. They may also be aerodynamic goals achieved by finely tuned interacting regulatory behaviors throughout the vocal tract.[22] Both perceptual and aerodynamic goals may occur together. Indeed, it is highly likely that a number of behavioral goals are achieved at the same time. Thus, movements of the oral, pharyngeal, laryngeal, and thoracic musculature become components integrated into motor systems. These systems of coordinated structures have various behavioral outcomes determined by the way in which component structures are integrated. An example of a mechanism involving coordinated structures is the positioning of the velum by the LVP, palatoglossus, and palatopharyngeus muscles.[23] The way in which this mechanism is integrated depends in part on the characteristics of the behavioral goal as a whole (an entire phrase) rather than the individual segments (phones or syllables) comprising the target production.

A certain amount of flexibility is built into motor systems in the form of free or forced variation and adaptation of movements.[21] Variation in movement that depends on phonetic context or timing factors may be considered free variation (assimilation of one or more of the features of a preceding or succeeding segment in connected speech), whereas forced variation involves flexibility within the system of coordinated structures when certain elements are physically constrained. In forced variation the perceptual goal is attained by varying the role of unconstrained elements in the system. This kind of variation is observed in bite block studies, in which the size of the oral aperture is mechanically determined and subjects adjust their articulatory movements to achieve a perceptually acceptable outcome.[21, 22, 24]

Environmental changes that threaten to exceed the degrees of freedom of a particular physiologic system require adaptation of the coordinated structures within that system. This would appear to be necessary to attain the same behavioral goals that were achieved prior to the environmental changes. For example, the LVP, palatoglossus, and palatopharyngeus may interact in a certain way within a particular environment (oronasal opening) to achieve velopharyngeal closure adequate for the production of pressure consonants (obstruents). If a radical change occurs in the environment within which this motor system functions (a change from oronasal opening to surgical closure of the hard and soft palates), then the muscles comprising the motor system may have to interact in a very different way to achieve the original goal of velopharyngeal closure. Thus, adaptation entails molding the rule system over time to reintegrate the component movements of coordinated structures. It may even involve the addition or subtraction of certain component structures. Adaptation may also be called plasticity and represents the means whereby the coordinated structures evolved in the first place.[21, 22] This plasticity is characteristic of any homeostatic mechanism and is essential for learning.

Given the complex organization of speech motor control, with numerous subcomponents at different levels, it seems plausible that development of these highly sophisticated coordinated structures requires a great deal of practice or experience. Appropriate conditions are facilitated by musculoskeletal and neuromotor maturation, which are themselves influenced by experience or use.[12, 14, 18, 19] The infant's earliest vocalizations, vegetative sounds, and cry patterns may serve as the early building blocks for later speech motor control because they provide opportunities for integration of some low level subcomponents. This integration is probably highly flexible because of the rapidly changing physical dimensions of the vocal tract at this time. The impact of abnormal structures at this stage within the first 4 months of life may therefore be transient as long as the inappropriate interactions between structures are not allowed to become stable or automatic. However, once the infant enters the "expansion stage" of phonetic development, at about 4 to 6 months, early subcomponents of speech motor control may begin to be used in a more stable fashion as she or he appears to test the limits of the vocal tract and its related structures.[25]

During this expansion phase of phonetic development the infant with a cleft palate may discover that particular coordinated structures give rise to certain behavioral outcomes. For example, she or he may achieve adequate aerodynamic control for the production of a velar pressure consonant by integrating movements of the tongue and velopharyngeal mechanism in a certain way. This movement system is then integrated continuously in the same way to achieve a repetition of the original behavioral outcome. With repetition, the mechanism of motor control for that particular goal (be it perceptual, aerodynamic, or both) becomes stabilized. However, this system of coordinated structures is functional only in terms of the infant's current abnormal oropharyngeal environment. Once this environment is altered surgically, the subcomponent of speech motor control that had been approaching stabilization is rendered inappropriate.

The mechanisms underlying speech motor control

during this expansion stage are probably still quite plastic, given the dramatic anatomic and physiologic changes occurring at this time. If surgery is provided early enough, that is, before 6 months of age, the effects of surgery on these evolving mechanisms may be minimized. The sudden anatomic changes brought about by primary palatoplasty probably require complete remodeling of the pattern of systems governing the integration of underlying components of speech motor control. There is little doubt that the infant is capable of such adaptive behavior. However, this adaptation process may detract from the resources necessary for the following developmental phase in speech motor control, thereby possibly delaying the developmental process and ultimately the onset of meaningful speech. "Corrected" structures, therefore, may be especially important at the time of phonetic expansion (between 4 and 6 months of age).

Sensorimotor Feedback. Sensorimotor feedback is essential to the infant's exploratory learning processes, disruption in any modality having potentially detrimental effects. Both Kent and Oller and Eilers maintain that auditory feedback is of primary importance in early speech development.[14, 16] However, the developmental sequence of the different sensory systems suggests that this need not necessarily be so. Gottlieb claims that the vestibular and tactile sensory systems are the first to develop, followed by the kinesthetic system.[26] On the other hand, both the auditory and visual systems develop later and continue to develop throughout the first 2 years of life. Therefore, given the likely assumption that tactile and kinesthetic feedback are used in early speech development, it would seem more plausible for these two modalities to be at least as important as the auditory system in the first few months of life. The auditory system would presumably assume greater importance with increasing central nervous system development.

Indeed, Warren suggests that aerodynamic performance rather than acoustic accuracy receives priority in the development of speech motor control.[22] The development of aerodynamic regulatory systems must rely heavily on tactile-kinesthetic feedback and evolve gradually, incorporating changes in anatomy and the general shape of the vocal tract over time. The tactile-kinesthetic feedback derived from an unrepaired cleft palate may give rise to aberrant motor control systems aimed at aerodynamic regulation. These in turn may become incorporated in control mechanisms aimed at achieving specific perceptual goals. The extent to which such mechanisms can be adapted once the structural environment is "corrected" depends on the plasticity of the systems involved.

A Sensitive Period for Speech Motor Control. Kent refers to a number of anatomic, neurologic, and motor developments that occur together during the first year of life.[14, 19] Indeed, until 3 months of age, the neonate has primarily subcortical function and consequently largely reflexive behaviors, with head and neck anatomy characteristic of adult nonhuman species.[14, 27] During this period, a short pharynx with a gradually sloping nasopharynx results in engagement of the larynx and nasopharynx. That is, the larynx is situated high in the neck with the epiglottis approximating the velum. This is clearly illustrated in Figure 92–1A. Consequently, oral and pharyngeal cavities are coupled into one fairly continuous tube, which severely constrains the possible phonetic output of the vocal tract.[14] The tongue completely fills the oral cavity at this time, allowing lingual movement along the anteroposterior plane only.[28] Thus, restricted tongue movement provides a further constraint on the possible phonetic output of the vocal tract.

Onset of disengagement of the larynx and nasopharynx, the disappearance of many primitive reflexes, increased myelination, increased dendritic branching of cortical cells, and significant advances in motor control all occur between 4 and 6 months of life.[12, 14, 19, 29] This time period also constitutes the expansion stage of babbling, culminating in the onset of "canonical" or "reduplicated" babbling. This development in turn heralds the onset of the production of more mature phonetic sequences, which may well function as the "phonetic

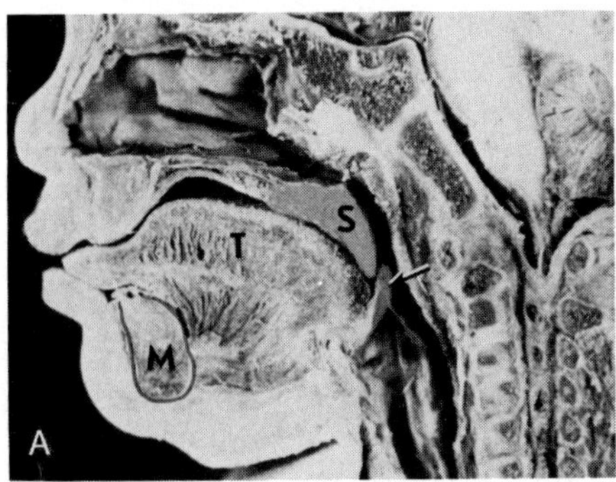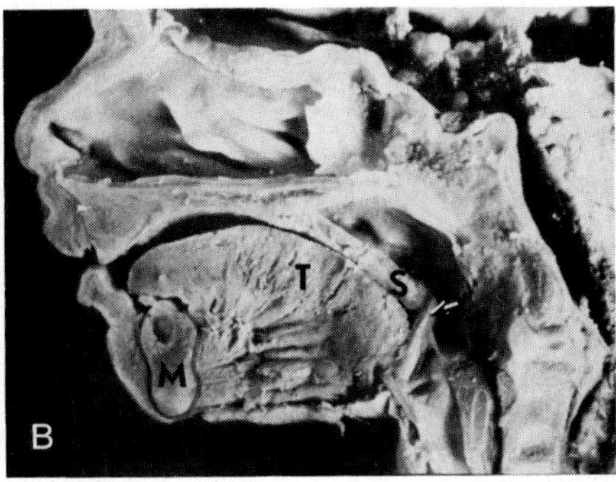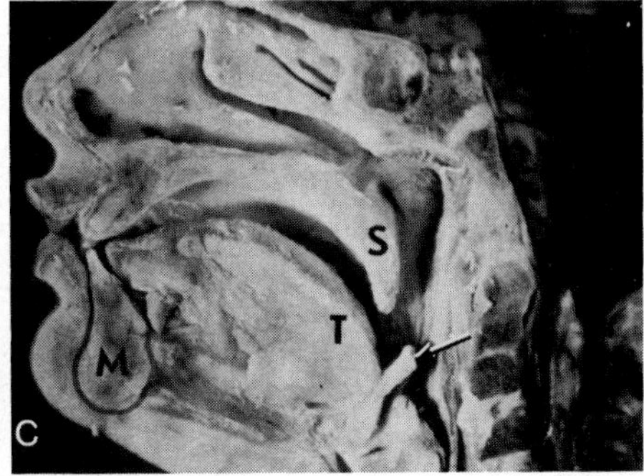

Figure 92–1 Gradual descent of the larynx within the pharynx.[27] *A,* Saggital surface of the head of a full-term newborn infant. The epiglottis (arrow) is in direct contact with the soft palate (S). The tongue (T) is located entirely in the oral cavity. *B,* Sagittal surface of the head of a 2-year-old child. The epiglottis (arrow) is in direct contact with the soft palate (S). However, the angle between the pharynx and the oral and nasal cavities has become less obtuse than it is in the neonate. *C,* Sagittal surface of the head of a 6-year-old child. The epiglottis (arrow) is not in contact with the soft palate (S). The pharynx now runs perpendicular to the nasal and oral cavities. The posterior third of the tongue (T) forms the anterior wall of the oropharynx. (From Crelin ES: The Human Vocal Tract: Anatomy, Function, Development, and Evolution. New York: Vantage Press, 1987. With permission.)

building blocks of words."[16] All these concurrent and highly significant developments in different areas may well indicate the onset of a sensitive period for the development of the precursors of meaningful speech.

As the larynx begins to descend in the pharynx and contact between the epiglottis and velum becomes less pronounced, two essential properties of speech are facilitated. The infant is now capable of exclusively oral vocalizations for vowel-like utterances and impounding oral air pressure for consonantlike utterances by virtue of the separation between the oral and nasopharyngeal cavities. The lengthening of the pharynx and a change in the relationship between the cavities to a less obtuse angle (Fig. 92–1B)[27] contribute to this decoupling of the confluence of the pharyngeal-oral-nasal cavities. Thus, the remodeled vocal tract can now produce a consonant vowel (CV) syllable, which forms the basic element of reduplicated or canonical babbling. The completion of the velar-laryngeal disengagement process by the age of 6 years is illustrated in Figure 92–1C.[27]

If the co-emergence of certain structural and functional mechanisms between 4 and 6 months of age does indeed represent a sensitive period of development, surgery may need to be performed in advance of this time to ensure that structures are intact and feedback mechanisms are functional once this stage is reached. Another reason for completing surgery prior to the onset of this sensitive period may be that certain interactions between related structures need to be stabilized for optimal learning to occur.

The first year of life represents a period of progressively more cortical control over voluntary behavior. Both Kent[19] and Netsell[12] argue that a substantial amount of general cortical control over vocalization occurs between 6 and 12 months of age. Thus, the interval between 4 and 6 months of age may represent a sensitive period for the development of certain basic speech motor control mechanisms in anticipation of the more cortically controlled succeeding period and the onset of meaningful speech.

Early Vocalizations. A number of researchers maintain that meaningful speech is shaped by premeaningful vocalizations.[16, 20, 30–32] The complexity and acoustic patterns of these vocalizations are constrained by the physical limits of the vocal tract and the developing neuromotor system. As these constraints are reduced and the infant progresses from one developmental stage to another, new elements are added to the existing repertoire while old elements are incorporated into an increasingly complex system.

During the first 2 months of life the infant produces vegetative and comfort sounds (Table 92–1) that have glottal attack (glottal stops) and "quasi-resonant nuclei."[16] These early precursors of vowels acquired their name by virtue of their acoustic features, which are remarkably similar to those associated with nasal coupling in adult populations.[20] The most consistent effect of nasal coupling is the decreased intensity of the first formant due to acoustic damping in the nasal cavity.[33] Extra formants occur owing to the bifid and asymmetric nature of the resonating chamber. These antiresonances

resulting from a side-branching chamber attenuate the formant transitions into and out of neighboring segments, reducing the spectral contrasts that differentiate vowels.[20] A low-frequency resonance or nasal formant is also observed. These features of nasalization are evident in the infant's earliest vocalizations because of the nature of the neonatal vocal tract.

Between the second and the fourth months of life quasi-resonant nuclei are accompanied by velar, uvular, and pharyngeal constrictions (Table 92–1) rather than glottal attack.[20] A reduction in frequency of glottal attack in association with the onset of velar, uvular, and pharyngeal constrictions may therefore signify a readiness for the onset of phonetic expansion and the production of "fully resonant nuclei."[16] If a large oronasal opening (unoperated hard palate) persists beyond this stage of phonetic expansion, compensatory motor control mechanisms may be developed to achieve the resonant nuclei essential to the following canonical stage of babbling. Onset of the expansion stage of babbling (Table 92–1) may therefore signal an important cut-off period for cleft palate infants, after which their different oronasal structures have a greater impact on later speech development. Interestingly, Oller and Eilers have described this period between 4 and 6 months in a similar manner in deaf infants, whose canonical babbling appears to be both delayed in onset and deviant in nature.[16] In addition, preliminary data of Trost-Cardamone suggest that such a delay and deviancy may occur in cleft palate babies as well.[34] Babbling in the babies studied by Trost-Cardamone was slower in onset and contained fewer true consonant segments. Consequently, appropriately timed palatoplasty may encourage both an enlarged consonant inventory and the emergence of true consonants because hard and soft palate closure would facilitate the babies' production of pressure consonants.

The Transition Between Babbling and Speech. The CV syllable structure forms the basic element of reduplicated or canonical babbling. This structure is then elaborated in nonreduplicated or "variegated" babble between 9 and 12 months and is a common exponent of meaning during the emergence of the first 50 words.[25] Inappropriate nasal coupling at the stage of canonical babbling most likely reduces the acoustic contrasts between CV syllables. This potential lack of perceptual-acoustic differentiation may subsequently impede the expression of semantic contrasts in the oral mode, resulting in a possible delay in the onset of meaningful speech. If acoustic contrasts are maintained by compensatory speech motor control systems, these control mechanisms may become part of the developing phonologic system (in the form of maladaptive articulations) and therefore are far less amenable to later change than the control mechanisms of early vocalizations.[35]

The first year of life is generally described as the "prelinguistic period" of speech and language development, with the first true words beginning to emerge at about 12 months of age.[36, 37] In the production of the first 50 words, babbling-like sounds are used meaningfully, forming a link between the earlier babbling period and the emergence of a rule-governed phonologic system.[38] These "transitional items"[30] or "proto-words"[38] cannot be classified as either babbling or speech and are initially strictly context bound. For example, "bye-bye" may be uttered only in association with hand waving and on exiting, whereas "all gone" may be used only at meal times once the child has finished his or her food. During the first 50-word phase of language acquisition proto-words gradually lose their semantic-pragmatic constraints. That is, the child gradually begins to use these words in a variety of situations. Furthermore, proto-words, words, and variegated babble may appear concurrently. At this stage individual speech sounds (phones) are not the units of development; rather, the entire word appears to function as a phonetic unit. Thus, individual words are produced as holistic elements that cannot be divided into smaller, permutable elements.[38, 39]

Ferguson and Farwell provide an example of a child who produced the word "pen" in ten different ways within a half hour period.[40] The features of nasality, bilabial and alveolar approximation, and voicelessness had emerged in the child's physiologic (or phonetic) repertoire but were not firmly associated with any particular phone segment (as they would be in a phonemic repertoire). A set of phonetic (physiologic) features had not yet been bound to individual speech sounds, and consequently relevant phonologic contrasts had not yet been established. Thus, in the case of the child with an unrepaired cleft palate, maladaptive place features such as [+ glottal] and [+ pharyngeal] may begin to emerge in the production of stop and fricative consonants during the first 50-word stage of phonologic development. However, such maladaptive features may not be firmly established until a child's phonologic system develops further.

Development of Phonologic Contrasts. Ingram argued that a child's phonologic development may parallel his or her cognitive development.[41] With the onset of the "period of concrete operations" at about 18 months, the child gains the ability to use symbolic representation.[42] It has also been observed that children's rate of lexical acquisition increases rapidly at the point when about 50 words have been acquired.[30] Thus, Ingram argued that the child's ability to manipulate symbols mentally in association with a rapidly expanding vocabulary enables her or him to develop a rule-governed phonologic system.[41] This rule-governed system becomes necessary because the number of holistic word elements otherwise required would be excessively large. Therefore, it appears more efficient for the child to develop a smaller inventory of permutable sound segments that can be merged in many different combinations for the construction of a very large word inventory.

If sound segments (phones) are indeed permutable and identifiable in different contexts, a unique set of stable features appears to be necessary to serve as a signature for individual sound segments used contrastively in the child's native language. Thus, the less stable features of the first 50-word stage must become more robust and more firmly attached to individual

speech sounds as the child develops phonologic rules. For example, a set of phonetic features associated with glottal attack (− voice, + back, + glottal) that have begun to emerge during the first 50-word stage (or sooner) may become intrinsic features of stop phonemes such as /p/, /t/, and /k/. Consequently, as the child's phonologic system evolves and phonemic contrasts are established, maladaptive features such as [+ glottal] and [+ pharyngeal] may become more firmly associated with stop and fricative phonemes and hence more difficult to eradicate with speech therapy.

Primary palatoplasty prior to the first 50-word stage (prior to about 12 months of age) appears to be important to avoid the emergence of maladaptive features within the developing phonologic system. However, surgery prior to the onset of rule-governed phonologic behavior, at about 18 months, may be critical in avoiding long-term entrenchment of these maladaptive features.[43, 44]

Developmental Milestones. There is individual variation in the onset of developmental milestones. Thus, careful monitoring of the cleft palate infant's motor, phonetic, cognitive, and social behavior may provide a more reliable index of developmental readiness than chronologic age alone.

Precursors of the phonetic expansion stage of babbling, that is, (1) reduced glottal attack; (2) velar, uvular, and pharyngeal constriction; and (3) possible production of resonant nuclei (Table 92–1) appear to be the significant phonetic features that need to be monitored in the cleft palate infant. This monitoring may be both perceptual and acoustic, forming an important aspect of the postnatal management of such infants. However, these features may not arise when expected or may be diminished in the cleft palate infant. Development of cognitive-linguistic and psychosocial parameters as well as of gross and fine motor skills may then provide additional information about the development status of individual infants.

Cognitive-Linguistic Development

The timing of palatal closure may have effects on cognitive-linguistic development beyond the realm of phonologic acquisition. For example, the infant's earliest explorations of objects in the environment are oral. This early mouthing behavior is an essential component of the processes underlying object recognition and concept formation.[45] Thus, intact oral structures and unimpeded sensory receptors at these sites may be vital to the infant's construction of perceptual gestalts.

Early parent-child interaction patterns play an important role in communicative-interactive development. Precursors of turn-taking and a shared communicative responsibility are seen even at the early prelinguistic stage.[46] Furthermore, optimal parent-child interaction facilitates language acquisition in general by providing a rich verbal and emotional environment within which incidental language learning can take place. An improvement in this relationship has been reported after palatal closure has been completed.[47] Thus, early closure may be important for development in this area as well.

Psychosocial Development

Evans and Renfrew raise the very important issue of the effect of hospitalization on the development of cleft palate children.[48] They claim that in their experience admission to the hospital prior to 7 months of age is seldom associated with distress, whereas hospitalization between 7 months and 4 years can result in disturbed behavior and emotional problems. These emotional problems can seriously affect both the acquisition of speech and language and general development itself. The effect of hospitalization may be minimized if care is taken in monitoring the infant's emerging awareness of strangers (Mahler's phase of differentiation), which usually signals the onset of separation anxiety between 5 and 10 months.[49] Ideally, it would be most appropriate to perform surgery prior to the onset of stranger awareness. Although this may not always be possible, every effort should be made to perform surgery before the onset of separation anxiety.

Development of Communicative Competence

A cleft palate child eventually may develop speech that is indistinguishable from that of his or her peers. Yet the possible long-term effects of an earlier communication deficit may persist. A communication deficit may not be signaled by abnormal speech patterns per se but rather by behavioral signs such as an unwillingness to initiate verbal interaction, or "shyness." It is difficult to determine with certainty that later communicative deficits are related to early delays in physical or behavioral development. However, justification of late surgery on the basis of eventual normal speech patterns would miss the point of total communication habilitation. Effective communication may be a cumulative process that also undergoes sensitive periods of development. If a child's inappropriate early speech patterns interfere with the sensitive stage of communicative development, a communication deficit may persist whether or not the child's speech patterns are eventually normalized.

Determining the Timing of Primary Palatoplasty

The Decision Process

The timing of primary palatoplasty involves consideration of factors in addition to those related to the cleft palate infant's developmental status or progress. These factors include (1) surgical and postoperative facilities that should meet the criteria necessary for early surgery; (2) an orofacial morphology that is amenable to early surgery; and (3) general health robust enough to sustain major surgery.

This decision process becomes relevant only if the available surgical, postoperative, and management facilities meet the requirements for early surgery. An individualized treatment program requires a multifaceted, interdisciplinary team approach to the management of the child with cleft palate. Consequently, all members of the interdisciplinary craniofacial team should be involved in this decision process. Of primary concern is the medical feasibility of early surgery. Once life-threatening risk factors have been accounted for, the nature of the orofacial morphology will determine whether the benefits of early surgery for the purpose of speech outweigh the limitations of possible tissue deficiencies. If structural considerations favor a developmental approach, the team should then consider the results of assessments in the areas of motor, speech, cognitive-linguistic, and psychosocial development.

Louw and Uys provide a protocol applicable to such an evaluation of cleft palate babies.[50] They recommend the use of formal standardized tests, acoustic analyses, and detailed observation to evaluate the following factors in the cleft palate infant:
1. Orofacial morphology.
2. Cognitive development.
3. Auditory abilities.
4. Feeding abilities.
5. Cry patterns.
6. Vocalizations.
7. Receptive and expressive language abilities.
8. Communicative-interactive abilities.
9. Motor development.

Ideally, cleft palate babies are monitored from birth in all appropriate developmental areas to obtain an accurate gauge of the child's developmental status. A developmentally appropriate time for primary palatoplasty can then be determined on the basis of these assessments.

A Template for the Timing of Primary Palatoplasty

Figure 92–2 provides a schematic representation of the broad framework within which the timing of primary palatoplasty may be determined. The possible benefits and hazards of surgery at different ages are considered in terms of (1) physical or medical risks, (2) developmental catalysts, and (3) possible socioemotional constraints. The height of the curve in Figure 92–2 represents a weighted measure of relevant medical, developmental, and socioemotional factors. This weighted measure determines the relative strength with which surgery is recommended during the different age ranges represented. It should be noted that the different age ranges represent developmental stages along a developmental continuum in which chronologic age represents merely an approximate margin of the various developmental stages. Hence, the cleft palate infant's developmental stage is more important than his or her chronologic age in determining the appropriate time for primary palatoplasty.

Proponents of the most radical approach to the timing of primary palatoplasty advocate hard and soft palate surgery during the neonatal period up to 2 months of age to provide an intact mechanism as soon as possible

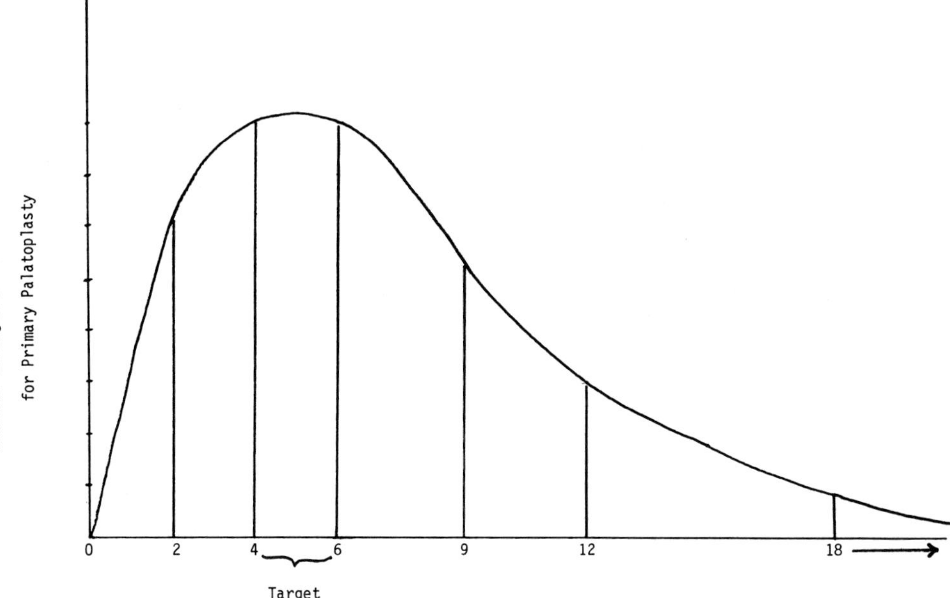

Figure 92–2 Broad framework within which the timing of primary palatoplasty may be determined.

without unduly disrupting the parent-infant relationship. Such a decision would be based on purely developmental and socioemotional factors. However, physical or medical risks such as airway obstruction, blood loss, and possible anesthesia errors far outweigh developmental concerns. Given the magnitude of the risks attached to surgery at this early age, 0 to 2 months of age is considered too early for the performance of primary palatoplasty.

The convergence of developmental events between 4 and 6 months of age suggests that this age range may represent a sensitive period for the development of speech motor control. It appears, therefore, that the period between 2 and 4 months postnatally may be a developmentally optimal time for the performance of primary palatoplasty. This strategy would provide intact structures at the onset of this significant period of development. Furthermore, hospitalization would occur well before the onset of separation anxiety and possibly even before the onset of stranger awareness. However, the risk factors associated with surgery at this early age may again outweigh socioemotional and developmental considerations. Craniofacial teams would have to assess the feasibility of surgery at this stage in terms of both their own capacity to deal with the demands of such early surgery and the needs of the individual cleft palate infants in their care. Thus, this period between 2 and 4 months of age may be considered questionably early for the performance of primary palatoplasty.

Three positions may be adopted regarding the performance of primary palatoplasty between the ages of 4 and 6 months. No matter when surgery is performed, it will be disruptive. However, it could be argued that surgical intervention at this stage would constitute a major disruption of the maturational processes converg-

ing at this time. Intervention could result in delayed onset of certain functions that depend on these overlapping maturational events. Consequently, it might be more appropriate to delay closure until after 6 months of age to avoid the possible disruptive effects of surgery at this critical time.

On the other hand, it may be developmentally more beneficial to risk the possible effects of surgery on the maturational processes than to place the infant in a position where she or he needs to remold the underlying motor control systems acquired during this period. That is, structural components may be integrated in systems that are functionally incompatible with the repaired oropharyngeal environment. In this case, delayed onset of relevant functions might also be expected.

A third possibility is that the convergence of developments in different areas may mark the 4- to 6-month period as one of heightened plasticity in the development of motor control. This heightened plasticity could enable the infant to deal with naturally occurring environmental changes at this time. Thus, the infant may be better equipped to deal with surgery at this point than at a later stage. Consequently, delays might be minimized according to this third viewpoint. Thelen suggests that rhythmic stereotypes provide the infant with a means of incorporating the temporal dimensions of motor control within his or her evolving motor systems in anticipation of later goal-directed motor behavior.[13] This claim is supported by her observation that such behaviors peak at around 6 months of age and decline in the last third of the first year (between 9 and 12 months) when goal-directed behavior gains precedence. A period of high plasticity may well precede the onset of a period dominated by rhythmic behaviors. Therefore, primary palatoplasty prior to 6 months of age may allow the infant to benefit maximally from his or her reduplicated babbling experience. Furthermore, the effects of hospitalization on socioemotional development may be minimized if the infant has not yet developed separation anxiety. On the basis of these considerations it is suggested that surgery between 4 and 6 months of age be viewed as the target age for primary palatoplasty.

There may be circumstances that preclude surgery before 6 months of age (general health considerations or a very wide cleft). In such cases, the craniofacial team must determine the most appropriate time for surgery within the constraints of the special circumstances of each case. Between 6 and 9 months of age the infant engages in canonical or reduplicated babbling, emphasizing the cyclicity and rhythmicity of repeated utterances. The baby also crawls and pulls himself or herself to a standing position during this time. Furthermore, separation anxiety becomes fully developed. Given the substantial strides being made in a number of areas of development, primary palatoplasty may be contraindicated at this time. However, it may be preferable to intervene during this period prior to the onset of variegated babbling, the appearance of the first words, and the onset of unsupported locomotion, all of which normally occur between 9 and 12 months of age. Grunwell and Russell, in a pre- and postoperative study of the vocalizations of three cleft palate children (aged 11, 13, and 14 months at the time of surgery), found that all three subjects had recovered from the effects of surgery within 21 days postoperatively.[51] Thus, it appears that the negative effect of primary palatoplasty on the vocalization behavior of these subjects, although substantial, was of short duration.

Once the infant enters the phase of increasingly goal-directed vocalizations and the onset of meaningful speech (after about 12 months of age), the maladaptive motor control systems acquired in the uncorrected environment may be stabilized, even if structures are corrected at this time. Stated in phonologic terms, the functionally inappropriate motor control systems may give rise to maladaptive articulatory features that in turn may become incorporated into the phonology of the first 50 words and ultimately into the child's evolving phonologic system.

During the 12- to 18-month period when the child completes the first 50-word phase of phonologic development, his or her phonologic system gradually becomes increasingly rule governed. Phonemic segments begin to assume greater importance at this time, and the child may actively avoid or select words containing certain segmental sound types.[32, 38, 40, 52] Indeed, Estrem and Broen found that cleft palate toddlers in the first 50-word phase of phonologic development avoided words beginning with coronal sounds (i.e., sounds produced by contact between the tongue and the hard palate).[53] These children demonstrated a preference for words beginning with not only velar and glottal phonemes but also labial phonemes. Furthermore, the cleft palate children, in addition to using sounds produced at the periphery of the oral tract, also substituted noncoronal sounds for coronal sounds. Thus, intact palatal structures

at the onset of the first 50-word stage of phonologic development may be important. The urgency of palatal closure would appear to increase as the child progresses through the first 50-word stage.

Greater attention to phonemic segments (as opposed to whole words) may result in far less opportunity for adaptation of underlying motor control mechanisms. Toward the end of this period between 12 and 18 months the child becomes able to manipulate symbols mentally, and individual speech sounds gain a symbolic identity. Maladaptive articulatory features may thus become inherent elements of individual speech sounds and consequently part of the rule-governed phonologic system. Once these maladaptive features become part of the child's phonologic system they are far more resistant to therapeutic intervention. Furthermore, Paden and colleagues found that children with a history of recurrent otitis media with effusion (OME) who were not in remission from OME between 10 and 16 months had a higher prevalence of later phonologic disorders than a similar group of children who were in remission during this period.[54] These data suggest that 10 to 18 months of age may well represent a sensitive period for phonologic development. Thus, delaying primary palatoplasty until the latter part of this period may be too late if entrenched maladaptive articulatory patterns are to be avoided.

Beyond 18 months of age the child is not only involved in the elaboration of his or her phonologic rule system and the expansion of his or her lexicon but also makes substantial syntactic and pragmatic gains as the first sentences are formed to express a variety of communicative intents. At this time the child begins to use language for a number of purposes as she or he learns to use verbal skills to manipulate the environment. An unrepaired cleft palate at this stage may lead to considerable frustration because maladaptive phonetic features that have become deeply entrenched in the child's phonologic system may result in poor intelligibility. This frustration may in turn cause avoidance of communicative situations, thereby jeopardizing the child's development of communicative competence. In addition, this period is one of increased separation anxiety as the child enters a phase of individuation.[49] Consequently, performing primary palatoplasty after 18 months of age should be avoided.

Conclusions

In this chapter we have attempted to provide support for a flexible developmental approach to the timing of hard and soft palate closure. Technical advances have made early surgery a viable option, and professionals involved in the management of cleft palate children should now seriously consider an earlier surgery schedule.

There seems to be a sensitive period for development in a number of areas, including the development of speech motor control and consequently phonetic development, that occurs between 4 and 6 months of age. It may be important to close the palate prior to or during this period if the infant is to benefit optimally from this state of readiness. Furthermore, if the onset of meaningful speech is not to be delayed and if maladaptive articulations are to be avoided completely, oronasal structures may need to be intact during this period between 4 and 6 months of age. Similarly, the potentially adverse effects of hospitalization may be minimized if surgery is performed during the 4- to 6-month period.

The ideal of developmentally determined surgical intervention may not always be possible. The size of the cleft, general health considerations, or limitations of surgical facilities available for pediatric surgery may preclude palatal closure during the 4- to 6-month period. The management of children with cleft lip and palate, therefore, requires an individualized treatment program in which all of the above factors are considered. The degree of plasticity in evolving speech motor control mechanisms has not yet been determined. However, clinical data suggest that a substantial amount of adaptation may be possible prior to 12 months of age. Thus, a flexible developmental approach to the timing of palatal closure, taking into account all pertinent variables of patient well-being, will best serve the individual needs of the child with cleft lip and palate.

References

1. Gillies HD, Fry WK: A new principle in the surgical treatment of congenital cleft palate and its mechanical counterpart. Br Med J 1:335, 1921.
2. Slaughter WB, Pruzansky S: The rationale for velar closure as a primary procedure in the repair of cleft palate defects. Plast Reconstr Surg 13:341, 1954.
3. Schweckendiek W: Primary veloplasty: Long-term results without maxillary deformity. A twenty-five year report. Cleft Palate J 15:268, 1978.
4. Cosman B, Falk AS: Delayed hard palate repair and speech deficiencies: A cautionary note. Cleft Palate J 17:27, 1980.
5. Jackson IT, McLennan G, Scheker LR: Primary veloplasty or primary palatoplasty: Some preliminary findings. Plast Reconstr Surg 72:153, 1983.
6. Bardach J, Morris HL, Olin WH: Late results of primary veloplasty: The Marburg project. Plast Reconstr Surg 73:207, 1984.
7. Hotz M, Gnoinski W, Nussbaumer H, et al: Early maxillary orthopedics in cleft lip and palate cases: Guidelines for surgery. Cleft Palate J 15:405, 1978.
8. Witzel MA, Salyer KE, Ross RB: Delayed hard palate closure: The philosophy revisited. Cleft Palate J 21:263, 1984.
9. Walter JD, Hale V: A study of the long term results achieved by the Gillies Fry procedure. Br J Plast Surg 40:384, 1987.
10. Friede H, Moller M, Lilja J, et al: Facial morphology and occlusion at the stage of early mixed dentition in cleft lip and palate patients treated with delayed closure of the hard palate. Scand J Plast Reconstr Surg 21:65, 1987.
11. Ross RB: Treatment variables affecting growth in unilateral cleft lip and palate. Part 5: Timing of palatal repair. Cleft Palate J 24:54, 1987.
12. Netsell R: A Neurobiologic View of Speech Production and the Dysarthrias. San Diego: College-Hill Press, 1986.
13. Thelen E: Rhythmical behavior in infancy: An ethological perspective. Dev Psychol 17:237, 1981.
14. Kent RD: Sensorimotor aspects of speech development. In Aslin R, Alberts J, Peterson M (eds): Development of Perception: Psychobiological Perspectives. New York: Academic Press, 1981.
15. Egan DF, Illingworth RS, MacKeith RC: Developmental screening 0–5 years. Clinics in Developmental Medicine 30. London: Spastics International Medical Publications, Heinemann Ltd, 1969.
16. Oller DK, Eilers RE: The role of audition in infant babbling. Child Dev 59:441, 1988.
17. Langlois A, Baken RJ, Wilder CN: Pre-speech respiratory behavior during the first year of life. In Murry T, Murry J (eds): Infant Communication: Cry and Early Speech. Houston: College-Hill Press, 1980.
18. Kent RD: Converging principles in phonologic development and motor development. Paper presented at the Child Phonology Conference, University of Illinois at Urbana-Champaign, May 6–7, 1988.
19. Kent RD: The psychobiology of speech development: Co-emergence of language and a movement system. Am J Physiol 246:R889, 1984.
20. Philips BJ, Kent RD: Acoustic-phonetic descriptors of speech production in speakers with cleft palate and other velopharyngeal disorders. In Lass NJ (ed): Speech and Language: Advances in Basic Research and Practice. New York: Academic Press, 1984.
21. Folkins JW: Issues in speech motor control and their relation to the speech of individuals with cleft palate. Cleft Palate J 22:106, 1985.
22. Warren DW: Compensatory speech behaviors in individuals with cleft palate: A regulation/control phenomenon. Cleft Palate J 23:251, 1986.
23. Kuehn DP, Folkins JW, Cutting CB: Relationship between muscle activity and velar position. Cleft Palate J 19:25, 1982.
24. Cole KJ, Abbs JH: Intentional responses to kinesthetic stimuli in orofacial muscles: Implications for the coordination of speech movements. J Neurosci 3:2660, 1983.
25. Oller DK: Infant vocalizations and the development of speech. Allied Hlth Behav Sci 1:523, 1978.
26. Gottlieb G: Conceptions of prenatal development: Behavioral embryology. Psychol Rev 83:215, 1976.
27. Crelin ES: The Human Vocal Tract: Anatomy, Function, Development, and Evolution. New York: Vantage Press, 1987.
28. Bosma JF: Anatomic and physiologic development of the speech apparatus. In Tower DB (ed): The Nervous System. Human Communication and Its Disorders. New York: Raven Press, 1975.
29. Sasaki CT, Levine PA, Laitman JT, et al: Postnatal descent of the epiglottis in man. Arch Otolaryngol 103:169, 1977.
30. Menyuk P, Menn L: Early strategies for the perception of words and sounds. In Fletcher P, Garman M (eds): Language Acquisition: Studies in First Language Development. Cambridge: Cambridge University Press, 1979.
31. Smith BL: Implications of infant vocalizations for assessing phonological disorders. In Lass NJ (ed): Speech and Language: Advances in Basic Research and Practice. New York: Academic Press, 1984.
32. Vihman MM, Macken MA, Miller R, et al: From babbling to speech: A reassessment of the continuity issue. Language 61:395, 1985.
33. Kuehn DP: Assessment of resonance disorders. In Lass NJ, McReynolds LV, Northern JL, et al: Speech, Language and Hearing. Philadelphia: Saunders, 1982.
34. Kuehn DP, Trost-Cardamone JE: Speech development and the timing of primary palatoplasty. Paper presented at the Annual Meeting of the American Cleft Palate Association, Williamsburg, Virginia, 1988.
35. Trost JE: Articulatory additions to the classical description of the speech of persons with cleft palate. Cleft Palate J 18:193, 1981.
36. Bullowa M: Prelinguistic communication: A field for scientific research. In Bullowa M (ed): Before Speech: The Beginning of Interpersonal Communication. Cambridge: Cambridge University Press, 1979.
37. Schwartz RG: The phonological system: Normal acquisition. In Costello J (ed): Speech Disorders in Children. San Diego: College-Hill Press, 1984.
38. Ferguson CA: Learning to pronounce: The earliest stages of phonological development in the child. Papers and Reports on Child Language Development (Stanford) 11:1, 1976.
39. Waterson N, Snow CE: The Development of Communication: Social and Pragmatic Factors in Language Acquisition. New York: Wiley, 1978.
40. Ferguson CA, Farwell CB: Words and sounds in early language acquisition: English initial consonants in the first fifty words. Language 51:419, 1975.
41. Ingram D: Phonological Disability in Children. London: Edward Arnold, 1976.
42. Piaget J: The Language and Thought of the Child, 3rd ed. London: Routledge Kegan Paul, 1959.
43. Kuehn DP, Dalston RM: Cleft palate and studies related to velopharyngeal function. In Winitz H (ed): Human Communication and Its Disorders: A Review 1988. Vol 2. Norwood NJ: Ablex, 1988.
44. Trost-Cardamone JE: Speech in the first year of life: A perspective on early acquisition. In Kernahan DA, Rosenstein SW (eds): Cleft Lip and Palate: A System of Management. Baltimore: Williams & Wilkins (In press, 1989).
45. Gibson EJ, Spelke ES: The development of perception. In Mussen PH (ed): Handbook of Child Psychology, 4th ed. Vol 3. New York: Wiley, 1983.
46. Bateson MC: The epigenesis of conversational interaction: A personal account of research development. In Bullowa M (ed): Before Speech: The Beginning of Interpersonal Communication. Cambridge: Cambridge University Press, 1979.
47. Kaplan I, Ben-Bassat M, Taube E, et al: Ten-year follow-up of simultaneous repair of cleft lip and palate in infancy. Ann Plast Surg 8:227, 1981.
48. Evans D, Renfrew C: The timing of primary cleft palate repair. Scand J Plast Reconstr Surg 8:153, 1974.
49. Harter S: Developmental perspectives on the self-system. In Mussen PH (ed): Handbook of Child Psychology, 4th ed. Vol 4. New York: Wiley, 1983.
50. Luow B, Uys IC: Critical review of evaluation techniques applicable to cleft lip and palate infants. S Af J Comm Dis 33:28, 1986.
51. Grunwell P, Russell J: Vocalizations before and after surgery: A pilot study. Br J Dis Comm 22:1, 1987.
52. Menn L: Evidence for an interactionist-discovery theory of child phonology. Papers and Reports on Child Language Development (Stanford) 2:169, 1976.
53. Estrem T, Broen PA: Early phonological and lexical choices of children with cleft palate. Miniseminar presented at the Annual Meeting of the American Speech Language Hearing Association, San Francisco, California, 1984.
54. Paden EP, Novak MA, Beiter AL: Predictors of phonological inadequacy in young children prone to otitis media. J Speech Hear Dis 52:232, 1987.

CHAPTER 93

Communication Skills of Children with Cleft Lip and Palate: A Status Report

Rodger M. Dalston

The intent of this chapter is to provide a broad range of information about the communicative capabilities of a large number of patients treated at the Oral-Facial and Communicative Disorders Program Clinic at the University of North Carolina at Chapel Hill. The standard protocol for surgical intervention at this clinic involves palate repair at 14 to 16 months of age. Despite this avowed protocol, a large number of our patients are not operated on between 14 and 16 months of age for a variety of reasons. As indicated elsewhere (see Chap. 92), there may be a range of ages that constitutes the optimal time for surgical intervention. Therefore, patients were included for study here if they underwent primary closure of the palate anywhere between 12 and 18 months of age.

All patients were operated on using either a Von Langenbeck or a V-Y push-back palatoplasty. Separate analyses were not employed in the current investigation to differentiate the relative efficacy of these two techniques.

The data reported below are taken from a computerized data base that has been described elsewhere.[1] As of May 1988, this data base contained 1597 speech-language evaluations for 877 patients. In an attempt to study a reasonably well defined subset of this total population, only children in two age groups were included here. Patients in the first group were between the ages of 4 years 0 months (4–00) and 5 years 11 months (5–11), whereas those in the second group were between 14–00 and 15–11 years of age. The latter group was chosen because several authors have suggested that the articulation skills of cleft palate youngsters continue to improve well beyond the age at which noncleft children have attained adultlike articulation proficiency.[2, 3]

In both groups included for study here, patients were excluded if they manifested any of the following characteristics: clefts involving only the primary palate, palatal clefting in the context of a syndrome, dysarthria, phone-specific nasal emission and no palatal cleft, diagnosed mental retardation, or ablative surgery involving any part of the speech mechanism. Finally, as noted above, all patients underwent primary palatoplasty between 12 and 18 months of age. Since many of the older patients had not been managed under this protocol, the number of older patients that met this criterion was comparatively small (Table 93–1). Of those included for study, 38.8% had had secondary surgical management for residual velopharyngeal impairment. In all cases, this treatment involved surgical placement of a superiorly based pharyngeal flap.

Information about the communicative skills of the two patient groups reported here is considered useful. However, it is fully acknowledged that caution must be exercised in interpreting data from a retrospective, cross-sectional, descriptive study of this sort in which a number of important variables could not be controlled.

The patient population is described in Table 93–1. As can be seen in that table, 49% of the 4- to 5-year-olds and 55% of the 14- to 15-year-olds had primary and secondary clefts, whereas 51% of the 4- to 5-year-olds and 45% of the 14- to 15-year-olds had clefts of the secondary palate only.

The overall prevalence of communicative disorders in the two subject groups is recorded in Table 93–2. For comparative purposes, normative data on 4- to 5-year-olds are presented in column 1 of this table. These prevalence data for the general population were extrapolated from published reports that specifically excluded cleft palate youngsters and nonspeaking deaf children.[4, 5]

Based on information provided by the parents, the patients, or professionals working with the patients, 35.5% of the 4- to 5-year-olds were receiving speech or language therapy at the time of their last team evaluation. An additional 17.7% had received treatment that had been terminated. Thus, 46.8% of the 4- to 5-year-olds had not received therapy. Among the 14- to 15-year-olds, 30.6% were receiving therapy, 44.4% had received it at some time in the past, and 25% had never received either speech or language intervention.

Table 93–1. Primary Diagnosis of the 99 Patients Included in the Present Study

Diagnosis	4–0- to 5–11-year-olds		14–00- to 15–11-year-olds	
	Frequency	*Percent*	*Frequency*	*Percent*
Left unilateral complete	7	11.1	4	11.1
Right unilateral complete	15	23.8	8	22.2
Bilateral complete	9	14.3	8	22.2
Soft palate only	4	6.3	7	19.5
Hard palate and velum	26	41.3	9	25.0
Submucous	1	1.6	—	—
Incomplete primary/secondary	1	1.6	—	—
Total	63	100.0	36	100.0

Table 93–2. Prevalence of Communicative Disorders

Disorder	General Preschool Population	4- to 5-year-olds (N = 63)	14- to 15-year-olds (N = 36)
All types	9	75	25
Velopharyngeal inadequacy	N/A	10	11
Language	3.3	21 (rec.)	— (rec.)
		26 (exp.)	3 (exp.)
Hearing	0.6	22	12
Articulation	3.5	74	14
Voice	3.0	13	14
Stuttering	0.8	3	—

This table shows the prevalence of communicative disorders among the patients investigated here. Velopharyngeal inadequacy was determined by clinical assessment. Language data for the younger group are based on formal test results on 19 of the 63 patients (see text). All table values are percentages.

Velopharyngeal Adequacy

As can be seen in Table 93–2, 10% of the 4- to 5-year-olds and 11% of the 14- to 15-year-olds manifested velopharyngeal inadequacy at the time of their last speech and language evaluation. This assessment was a subjective one made by the team speech-language pathologist. Such assessments represent a compound judgment transcending individual assessments of hypernasality, hyponasality, nasal emission, and vocal intensity.[6]

In patients 5 years of age and older, aerodynamic testing also was performed during each clinic visit.[7] Among the 61 patients for whom pressure-flow data were available, the instrumental findings corroborated the clinical judgments in that only 6 (10%) were considered to have velopharyngeal inadequacy.

Expressive and Receptive Language Skills

Although the differences tend to be small, research results suggest that the language abilities of cleft palate individuals are somewhat impaired compared with their noncleft peers.[8-11] The data presented in Table 93–2 support this contention. However, due to time constraints or other extenuating circumstances, language assessment for most of the 4- to 5-year-olds was a clinical evaluation made without benefit of formal test results. Therefore, the percentages reported in Table 93–2 pertain only to those nineteen 4- to 5-year-old children for whom formal language test results were available. These results were obtained using the Test of Language Development—Primary (TOLD-P).

Virtually all language assessments of the adolescent patients reported in Table 93–2 were clinical in nature. Among the teens whose language was judged normal on clinical evaluation, none were enrolled in language treatment. Nevertheless, it is conceivable that routine administration of standardized tests of language performance might have revealed some patients with language impairments. This potential limitation certainly needs to be taken into account when interpreting these data.

Hearing Loss

It is generally accepted that virtually all cleft palate children are born with middle ear effusions that place them at high risk for conductive hearing loss. In addition, regardless of the nature and timing of otologic treatment provided youngsters with palatal clefts, and perhaps in spite of such treatment,[12] it appears that auditory function does improve with age.[13] Nevertheless, impaired auditory tube function and conductive hearing loss seems to persist into adolescence and adulthood.[14, 15] The cross-sectional data presented in Tables 93–3 and 93–4, based on both tympanometric and pure tone testing, suggest that both groups of patients were typical in that hearing loss was high in childhood and tended to persist despite aggressive treatment.

In accordance with protocol that has prevailed at our clinic for many years, children manifesting evidence of otitis media with effusion (OME) that is resistant to medication typically undergo pressure-equalization (PE) tube placement at the time of palate repair. They are followed closely by our otolaryngologists both pre- and postoperatively.

A recurrent problem in studies of auditory function among cleft palate individuals is that they have assessed hearing on only one occasion or on repeated but infrequent occasions. Such reports have obvious limitations because conductive hearing losses manifest dramatic day-to-day fluctuations.[16] The present report is no exception. The data concerning hearing problems reported in Tables 93–3 and 93–4 were obtained at the time of biannual evaluations. Although follow-up testing was provided for those patients with abnormal test results, those data are not part of the speech data base records reported here. Therefore, Tables 93–3 and 93–4 are presented solely for the purpose of describing the prevalance of hearing loss in our patients on the day they were last seen for team evaluation.

Articulation

Glottal stops and pharyngeal fricatives undoubtedly are the best known forms of compensatory articulation

Table 93–3. Prevalence of Hearing Loss by Type

Type of Loss	4- to 5-year-olds (N = 63)	14- to 15-year-olds (N = 36)
All types	22	12
Conductive	20	6
Sensorineural	—	6
Mixed	2	—

All table values are percentages.

manifested by speakers with impaired velopharyngeal function. However, Trost[17] has described three additional types of compensatory articulation patterns that are useful in identifying the phonetic repertoire of these individuals: pharyngeal stops, middorsum palatal stops, and posterior nasal fricatives.

Although numerous studies published prior to 1975 speak of the high prevalence of glottal stop and pharyngeal fricative substitutions in the speech of cleft palate patients, at least two reports since that time seem to suggest that these errors are now found less frequently in this population.[3, 18] It is tempting to suggest that this apparent reduction is the result of improved patient care. However, the current evidence is not sufficient to warrant such a conclusion.

Data presented in Table 93–5 indicate that nearly half the 4- to 5-year-olds produced at least one articulatory error typically associated with compensatory adjustments to velopharyngeal impairment. However, that number is reduced to 26% if only patients with glottal stops or pharyngeal fricatives are included. In marked contrast to the 4- to 5-year-olds, the overall frequency of compensatory misarticulations is notably lower in the older group (Table 93–5). Unfortunately, owing to the cross-sectional nature of the data, it is not possible to determine the extent to which the differences between groups is a function of maturation.

Voice

McWilliams et al[19] note that there has been confusion in the literature about terms such as *voice quality* and *voice disorders*. Some authors consider that resonance phenomena such as hypernasality and phonatory consequences of laryngeal activity belong under the rubric of *vocal* quality. This seems inappropriate and unnecessarily vague. Therefore, in keeping with the terminology suggested by McWilliams and her colleagues, the term *voice disorders* will be used here to refer specifically to disturbances arising from abnormal laryngeal activity.

Table 93–4. Prevalence of Hearing Loss by Extent

Extent of Loss	4- to 5-year-olds (N = 63)	14- to 15-year-olds (N = 36)
WNL (10–26 dB)	78	88
Mild (27–40 dB)	22	12
Moderate (41–55 dB)	—	—
Moderate/severe (56–70 dB)	—	—
Severe (71–90 dB)	—	—
Profound (91+ dB)	—	—

WNL = within normal units
All table values are percentages.

Table 93–5. Prevalence of Articulation Errors Typically Associated with Compensatory Adaptations Made by Speakers with Velopharyngeal Inadequacy

Articulation Error Type	4- to 5-year-olds (N = 63)	14- to 15-year-olds (N = 36)
All types	48	11
Glottal stops	26	3
Pharyngeal fricatives	8	7
Pharyngeal stops	—	—
Dorsum midpalatal stops	21	7
Posterior nasal fricatives (incl. flap fricatives)	23	—

All table values are percentages.

Numerous studies appearing before 1975 indicated that there was an increased prevalence of voice disorders among individuals with impaired velopharyngeal function. A few reports appearing since then seem to substantiate these findings.[20–22] There appear to be at least two possible reasons why patients with velopharyngeal inadequacy may be at increased risk for voice disorders. One is that oronasal coupling through the incompletely closed velopharyngeal port could cause a reduction in overall speech intensity for which the patient might attempt to compensate by increasing vocal effort.[23]

A more probable basis for voice disorders among patients with impaired velopharyngeal function is that increased laryngeal muscle tension may occur owing to a spread of activity that results from increased muscular efforts to close the velopharyngeal port. This possibility has been reiterated recently by McWilliams et al.[19] However, no empiric evidence of such synkinetic activity was found in the literature reviewed for this chapter.

The data provided in Table 93–2 certainly suggest that the cleft population manifests a fairly substantial increase in the prevalence of voice disorders compared with that observed in the general population. Information in Table 93–6 suggests that the predominant type of voice disorder observed among the patients reported here was hoarseness. This finding is in keeping with the discussion above. However, perusal of the clinic files for these patients revealed that 75% of the eight 4- to 5-year-olds with hoarseness had a cold at the time of their evaluation or were known to manifest obvious vocal abuse. In addition, the only 14- to 15-year-old with hoarseness had been smoking more than a pack of cigarettes a day for almost 2 years prior to her last evaluation. Therefore, the hoarseness in these patients may have been totally unrelated to the status of their velopharyngeal mechanism. Indeed, none of the patients with voice disorders manifested velopharyngeal inadequacy at the time of their last evaluation.

Stuttering

The stuttering prevalence reported in Table 93–2 seems to suggest that cleft palate individuals are at

Table 93–6. Prevalence of Voice Disorders by Type

Voice Disorder Type	4- to 5-year-olds (N = 63)	14- to 15-year-olds (N = 36)
All types	13	8
Breathiness	3	5
Hoarseness	10	3
Pitch breaks	—	—
Glottal fry (pervasive)	—	—
Abnormal pitch	—	—

All table values are percentages.

increased risk for this speech impediment. In fact, available evidence in the literature suggests the opposite.[24] In that retrospective study of 534 patients, only one individual was found to have speech characterized by stuttering. Since that article was published, two more stutterers have been seen at our clinic, and both of them were in the 4–00 to 5–11 year group reported here. As noted in the original research on this topic, it will be necessary for clinicians working in a number of craniofacial centers to pool their observations to determine the true relationship between velopharyngeal impairment and speech dysfluency.

Summary

The most unique aspect of the current investigation concerns the breadth of information obtained on the speech, language, and hearing abilities of the children studied. Such information should be of considerable interest to those wishing to obtain a more complete picture of the communicative skills of children born with clefts.

As might be expected, the cleft palate patients investigated here performed more poorly than their noncleft peers in virtually every facet of communication. Nevertheless, within the limits imposed by the cross-sectional nature of the current study, the data tend to suggest that because the communicative skills of these patients may be expected to improve dramatically as they mature and progress through the habilitation process. To the extent that patient care has improved during the past 10 years, the performance of the 14- to 15-year-olds may grossly underestimate the performance

to be expected of the current 4- to 5-year-olds when they grow into adolescence.

References

1. Dalston RM: Computer-generated reports of speech and language evaluations. Cleft Palate J 20:227–237, 1983.
2. Van Demark DR, Morris HL, Vandehaar C: Patterns of articulation abilities in speakers with cleft palate. Cleft Palate J 18:193–203, 1981.
3. Karnell MP, Van Demark DR: Longitudinal speech performance in patients with cleft palate: Comparisons based on secondary management. Cleft Palate J 23:278–288, 1986.
4. Fein DJ: Population data from the U.S. Census Bureau. Am Speech Hearing Assoc 25(3):47, 1983.
5. Punch J: The prevalence of hearing impairment. Am Speech Hearing Assoc 25(4):27, 1983.
6. Kuehn D, Dalston R: Cleft palate studies related to velopharyngeal function. In Winitz H (ed): Human Communication and Its Disorders: An Annual Review, Vol 2. Norwood, NJ: Ablex, 1989.
7. Warren DW, DuBois, AB: A pressure-flow technique for measuring velopharyngeal orifice area during continuous speech. Cleft Palate J 1:52–71, 1964.
8. Pannbacker M: Oral language skills of adult cleft palate speakers. Cleft Palate J 12:95–106, 1975.
9. Shames G, Rubin H: Psycholinguistic measures of language and speech. In Bzoch KR (ed): Communicative Disorders Related to Cleft Lip and Palate, 2nd ed. Boston: Little, Brown, 1979.
10. Leeper HA, Jr, Pannbacker M, Roginski J: Oral language characteristics of adult cleft palate speakers compared on the basis of cleft type and sex. J Commun Disord 13:133–146, 1980.
11. Richman LC: Cognitive patterns and learning disabilities in cleft palate children with verbal deficits. J Speech Hear Res 23:447–456, 1980.
12. Freeland AP, Evans DM: Middle ear disease in the cleft palate patient: Its effect on speech and language development. Br J Plast Surg 34:142–143, 1981.
13. Webster JC, Edis F: Ear disease in relation to age in the cleft palate child and adolescent. Clin Otolaryngol 3:455–461, 1978.
14. Caldarelli DD: Incidence and type of otologic disease in the older cleft palate patient. Cleft Palate J 12:311–314, 1975.
15. Swigart, E: Hearing sensitivity of adults with cleft lip and/or palate. Cleft Palate J 16:72–80, 1979.
16. Tos M, Holm-Jensen S, Sorensen CH, et al: Spontaneous course and frequency of secretory otitis in 4-year-old children. Arch Otolaryngol 108:4–10, 1982.
17. Trost JE: Articulatory additions to the classical description of the speech of persons with cleft palate. Cleft Palate J 18:193–203, 1981.
18. Cohn ER, McWilliams BJ: Early cleft palate repair and speech outcome (letter). Plast Reconstr Surg 71:442–443, 1983.
19. McWilliams BJ, Morris HL, Shelton RL: Cleft Palate Speech. Philadelphia: B. C. Decker, 1984.
20. Musgrave RR, McWilliams BJ, Matthews HP: A review of the results of two different surgical procedures for the repair of clefts of the soft palate only. Cleft Palate J 12:281–290, 1975.
21. Bzoch, KR: Measurement and assessment of categorical aspects of cleft palate speech. In Bzoch KR (ed): Communicative Disorders Related to Cleft Lip and Palate, 2nd ed. Boston: Little, Brown, 1979.
22. Dixon VL, Bzoch KR, Habal MB: Evaluation of speech after correction of rhinophonia with pushback palatoplasty combined with pharyngeal flap. Plast Reconstr Surg 64:77–83, 1979.
23. Bernthal JE, Beukelman WR: The effect of changes in velopharyngeal orifice area on vowel intensity. Cleft Palate J 14:63–77, 1977.
24. Dalston, RM: Stuttering prevalence among patients at risk for velopharyngeal inadequacy: A preliminary investigation. Cleft Palate J 24:233–239, 1987.

CHAPTER 94

A Cross-Sectional Analysis of Speech Results Following Palatal Closure

Sally J. Peterson-Falzone

In 1973 Morris undertook a literature survey of the results of primary palatal surgery with specific regard to estimates of velopharyngeal function as published in the years 1960–1971, inclusive.[1] For purposes of that review, no restrictions were placed on type of cleft, type of surgical approach, age at surgery or at time of assessment, criteria used in assessment, or qualifications of those making the assessment. Notwithstanding the amorphous nature of the papers reviewed, Morris concluded that velopharyngeal competence had been achieved in roughly 75% of the cases reported.

Since 1971, numerous studies have examined the speech-velopharyngeal function results of primary palatal surgery, but none have been conducted from a general perspective comparable to that attempted by Morris. For example, investigators have studied the speech results of specific types of surgical procedures,[2–15] compared results across types of palatoplasty,[16–20] or specifically addressed effects of timing of repair.[8, 21–34]

Clearly, the key question in studies such as those cited above has been what surgical strategy produces the best speech results? Although cleft palate teams use such data to devise their own treatment approaches, most teams also must deal with secondary or tertiary cases—that is, cases in which the initial surgery was performed elsewhere. To the extent that this is true, a broader question emerges: In general, what speech results are we apt to see in children following palatal closure? This retrospective study was undertaken to provide data related to that question, expanding on and updating the information provided by Morris in 1973.

Method

Clinical files from three cleft palate treatment centers were reviewed to identify children who met the following criteria:

1. Isolated cleft palate or unilateral or bilateral cleft lip and palate, with no known syndrome other than Van der Woude syndrome.
2. Ages 4 years to 10 years 11 months, a range chosen to correspond to the early school years.
3. Hard and soft palates closed in a single procedure (no primary veloplasty).
4. No secondary surgical procedures performed on the velopharyngeal system; no velopharyngeal prostheses.
5. No patent oronasal fistulas.
6. No known history of hearing loss classified by the testing audiologist as moderate or worse in the better ear.
7. No known developmental delay.
8. No less than two speech evaluations performed by the author, at least one of which was performed no less than 1 year postoperatively.
9. Full team evaluations performed on postoperative clinic visits.
10. Daily usage of conversational English if English was not the primary language.

Because this project was intended as a general assessment of speech results following palatal closure, no attempt was made to control for surgeon, specific type of surgical procedure, age at closure, or site of treatment. For many of these children, the palatal closure had been performed outside the United States.

A total of 240 children who met the criteria listed above were found. Subject distribution by sex and cleft type may be found in Table 94–1; mean ages are given in Table 94–2. Figure 94–1 is a graphic representation of the distribution by cleft type.

All speech evaluations included administration of a standardized articulation test devised specifically for use with children with cleft palate[35] plus a sample of conversational speech. The clinical evaluations were coded for reports of

1. Perceptual stigmata of velopharyngeal inadequacy (VPI): nasal emission, posterior nasal frication, or hypernasal resonance; phoneme-specific nasal emission and posterior nasal frication were excluded.[36]
2. Hyponasality.
3. Presence of compensatory articulations used in identifiable patterns as consistent or predominant substitutions for, or produced simultaneously with, pressure consonants.[36]
4. Other phonologic or phonemic sound production differences.

Both hypernasal resonance and nasal emission or posterior nasal frication were coded only into a binary classification—"sporadic-infrequent" versus "predominant-consistent"—rather than along a rating scale of mild–moderate–severe. The binary classification was felt to be a more easily replicable judgment.

Intraexaminer and interexaminer reliability were determined for 20 of the children. Live versus tape-recorded judgments yielded intraexaminer reliability figures of 0.96 for the stigmata of velopharyngeal inadequacy, 0.95 for compensatory articulations, and 0.92

Table 94–1. Distribution of Subjects by Sex and Cleft Type

	UCLP	BCLP	CPO
Male	70	46	22
Female	62	17	23
Totals	132	63	45

UCLP = Unilateral cleft lip and palate; BCLP = bilateral cleft lip and palate; CPO = cleft palate only.

Table 94–2. Mean Ages for Male, Female, and Combined Subjects in Each Cleft Type

	UCLP	BCLP	CPO
Males	6:9	7:4	6:9
Females	6:11	6:6	6:6
Combined	6:10	7:2	6:7

UCLP = Unilateral cleft lip and palate; BCLP = bilateral cleft lip and palate; CPO = cleft palate only.

for other errors. Judgments obtained from another speech pathologist (experienced in the area of cleft palate) who listened to the recorded articulation tests and samples of conversational speech yielded interexaminer reliability figures of 0.91 for the stigmata of velopharyngeal inadequacy, 0.90 for compensatory articulations, and 0.94 for other errors.

Nasopharyngoscopic studies had been obtained for a total of 86 of the children who met the selection criteria for this report.

Results

Overview of Speech Results

Table 94–3 gives an overview of the speech results by cleft type. Only 3.3% of the children were found to be entirely asymptomatic in speech, with the highest percentage in the cleft palate only (CPO) group. More than 90% of the entire group of 240 subjects exhibited articulation errors (errors of place or manner of production, judged separately from nasal emission or posterior nasal frication). Predominant or consistent evidence of velopharyngeal inadequacy was found in 16.6%, with similar percentages in the unilateral cleft lip and palate (UCLP) and cleft palate only (CPO) groups and a lower percentage in the bilateral cleft lip and palate (BCLP) group. The relative prevalence of specific types of articulation problems and types of evidence of velopharyngeal inadequacy (VPI) are discussed below.

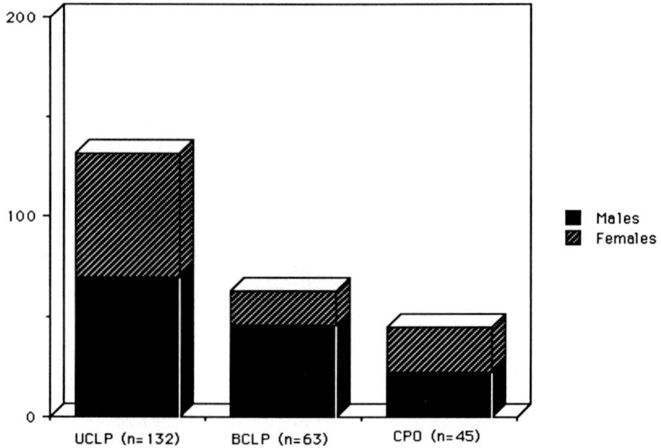

Figure 94–1 Cleft types of the 240 patients.

Nasal Air Loss and Resonance

Tables 94–4 and 94–5 tabulate the occurrence of audible nasal emission or posterior nasal frication and hypernasal resonance in the three cleft types. It should be noted that in this particular sample all seven children who had been judged to exhibit sporadic or infrequent nasal resonance also showed sporadic audible nasal air loss; similarly, the 24 with consistent hypernasal resonance were among the 40 with consistent nasal air loss. Thus, the numbers should not be added to obtain the total number with consistent perceptual stigmata of velopharyngeal inadequacy.

Approximately 24% of the entire group showed infrequent or sporadic audible nasal air loss (and inconsistent hypernasal resonance in seven of these), with a somewhat higher percentage of occurrence in the children with bilateral clefts than in the other two groups. Interestingly, in the 16.6% with consistent audible air loss and hypernasal resonance, the children with bilateral clefts had the lowest percentage of occurrence.

Four children exhibited chronic hyponasal resonance; all had either unilateral or bilateral clefts of the lip and palate, and all had some degree of intranasal obstruction on otolaryngologic examination.

Articulation Problems

Table 94–6 shows the prevalence of two general types of articulation problems (not mutually exclusive) in the three groups of children. The main focus of interest was on the use of articulations judged to be compensatory.[36, 37] Speech sound production differences that were deemed to be related to the child's level of phonologic development, to his linguistic background, or to structural factors such as missing teeth or malocclusion were tabulated separately from the notorious maladaptive articulatory gestures so often seen in children with clefts.[36, 37] Although children could and did exhibit misarticulations in both general categories, the percentage of those with noncompensatory articulation errors far outweighed the percentage demonstrating compensatory errors (Table 94–6). Furthermore, it should be noted that 22 of the 52 children who did have compensatory errors showed mid-dorsum palatal stops only, not glottal stops, pharyngeal stops, or fricatives or any of the other gestures described by Trost.[36] If these children were eliminated, the percentage exhibiting compensatory errors would be reduced to 12.5%.

Table 94–7 allows comparison of the number of children in each cleft type who showed compensatory articulations with the overall number exhibiting such behaviors. In either case, the highest percentages are associated with the children with bilateral clefts.

No trend could be identified with regard to the percentages of children in each yearly age group who showed compensatory articulations (Table 94–8).

Table 94–9 and Figures 94–2 and 94–3 allow comparison of the numbers of children who showed compensatory articulations with no evidence of velopharyngeal inadequacy, compensatory articulations with sporadic or infrequent evidence of velopharyngeal in-

Table 94–3. Overview of Speech Results by Cleft Type

	UCLP	BCLP	CPO	Totals
Asymptomatic	2/132 = 1.5%	0	6/45 = 13.3%	8/240 = 3.3%
Articulation problems	131/132 = 99.2%	55/63 = 87.3%	32/45 = 71.1%	218/240 = 90.8%
Consistent evidence of VPI	26/132 = 19.6%	6/63 = 9.5%	8/45 = 17.8%	40/240 = 16.6%

UCLP = Unilateral cleft lip and palate; BCLP = bilateral cleft lip and palate; CPO = cleft palate only; VPI = velopharyngeal inadequacy.

Table 94–4. Incidence of Audible Nasal Emission or Posterior Nasal Frication Among Cleft Types

	UCLP	BCLP	CPO	Totals
Inaudible or sporadic/infrequent audible nasal emission or posterior nasal frication	30/132 = 22.7%	18/63 = 28.6%	9/45 = 20.0%	57/240 = 23.8%
Predominant or consistent audible nasal emission/posterior nasal frication	26/132 = 19.6%	6/63 = 9.5%	8/45 = 17.8%	40/240 = 16.6%

UCLP = Unilateral cleft lip and palate; BCLP = bilateral cleft lip and palate; CPO = cleft palate only.

Table 94–5. Incidence of Hypernasal Resonance Among the Three Cleft Types

	UCLP	BCLP	CPO	Totals
Sporadic or infrequent hypernasality	4/132 = 3.0%	3/63 = 4.7%	0	7/240 = 2.9%
Predominant or consistent hypernasality	14/132 = 10.6%	4/63 = 6.3%	6/45 = 13.3%	24/240 = 10.0%

UCLP = Unilateral cleft lip and palate; BCLP = bilateral cleft lip and palate; CPO = cleft palate only.

Table 94–6. Types of Articulation Errors

	UCLP	BCLP	COP	Totals
Noncompensatory (developmental, dialectal, and/or structural)	127/132 = 96.2%	52/63 = 82.5%	31/45 = 68.6%	224/240 = 87.5%
Compensatory	20/132 = 15.1%	24/63 = 38.1%	8/45 = 17.8%	52/240 = 21.7%

Note: Developmental errors are currently viewed as the result of naturally occurring "phonologic processes" that the child gradually eliminates as he matures. The terms *dialectal* and *structural* also imply etiology. Compensatory articulations were those described by Trost (1981). It should be noted that the occurrence of these two major groups of errors was *not* mutually exclusive.
UCLP = Unilateral cleft lip and palate; BCLP = bilateral cleft lip and palate; CPO = cleft palate only.

Table 94–7. Two Perspectives on the Occurrence of Compensatory Articulations in Each Cleft Type

Incidence of Compensatory Articulations in Each Cleft Type (Total 52/240 = 21.7%)	Representation of Cleft Types in Children Exhibiting Compensatory Articulations
UCLP 20/132 = 15.1%	UCLP 20/52 = 38.4%
BCLP 24/63 = 38.1%	BCLP 24/52 = 46.1%
CPO 8/45 = 17.8%	CPO 8/52 = 15.4%

Note: On the left, the percentage of children in each diagnostic category who exhibited compensatory articulations is tabulated. The figures on the right show the relative contribution of each cleft type to the total number of children exhibiting these behaviors.
UCLP = Unilateral cleft lip and palate; BCLP = bilateral cleft lip and palate; CPO = cleft palate only.

Table 94–8. Percentage of Children in Each Yearly Age Group Exhibiting Compensatory Articulations

4 years	9/52	17.4%
5 years	11/32	34.4%
6 years	11/46	23.9%
7 years	8/36	22.2%
8 years	3/28	10.7%
9 years	6/22	27.3%
10 years	4/24	16.6%
Totals	52/240	21.7%

Table 94–9. Summary Information about Numbers of Subjects Exhibiting Compensatory Articulations (CA) According to Velopharyngeal Status, for 240 Subjects

Velopharyngeal Status
Of the 240, 142 demonstrated no evidence of velopharyngeal incompetence
Of the 240, 98 showed evidence of velopharyngeal incompetence
Of the 98 with velopharyngeal incompetence:
    50 showed sporadic evidence
    40 showed consistent evidence

Compensatory articulations
Of the 240, 188 showed no compensatory articulations
Of the 240, 52 showed no compensatory articulations
Of the 52 with compensatory articulations:
    29 demonstrated no evidence of velopharyngeal incompetence
    23 showed evidence of velopharyngeal incompetence
    Of the 23 with velopharyngeal incompetence:
        7 showed sporadic evidence
        16 showed consistent evidence

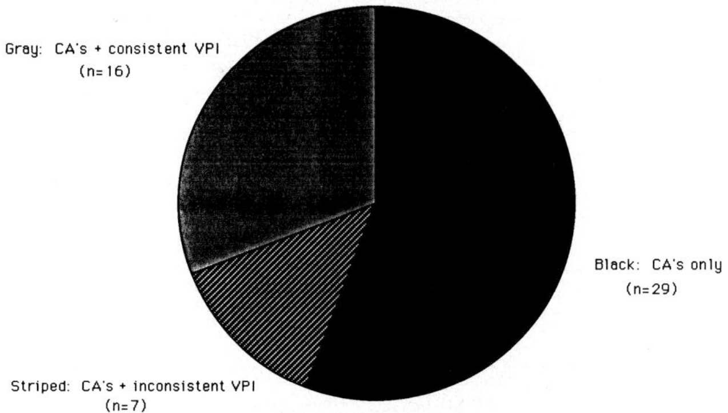

Figure 94–3 Relationship between compensatory articulations and VPI.

adequacy, and compensatory articulations with predominant or consistent evidence of velopharyngeal inadequacy. There appeared to be a stronger relationship of compensatory articulation with consistent evidence of velopharyngeal inadequacy, although over half (29/52) showed no nasal emission or hypernasality. Of these 29, it is of interest that 16 showed mid-dorsum palatal stops only.

Although reliable information about age at palatal closure was not a criterion for inclusion of a child in this study, such information was in fact available for 90 children. The range in age at time of closure was 2 months to 9 years 3 months, with a mean age of 24.55 months. For purposes of comparison to a previous study on the relationship of age at closure to the occurrence of compensatory articulations,[27] these 90 children were segregated into those in whom closure occurred at or before 1 year of age and those in whom closure occurred at a later age (Fig. 94–4). As can be seen in Table 94–10, the percentage of children who exhibited compensatory articulations was higher in the early closure group, although this difference was not statistically significant (chi square = 0.329) and the disparity in group sizes (17 versus 73) must be taken into account. In Table 94–11, it can be seen that the mean age of closure for those children with compensatory articulations was less than 3 months later than the mean age for those who did not exhibit them. These results will be discussed in greater detail below.

Selected Physical Findings

Nearly 74% (177/240) of the children had dental or occlusal problems that would have been judged a possible hazard to speech production; however, 27 of these children showed no problems with sibilants or affricates. The most common problems were anterior and buccal crossbites, missing teeth, and everted teeth.

Nasopharyngoscopic studies were carried out in 42 of the children who showed inconsistent nasal emission or hypernasality, 35 of those with consistent evidence of velopharyngeal inadequacy, and nine children with no subjective evidence of residual velopharyngeal inadequacy. The results were basically in agreement with those reported by previous investigators: The majority of the children, regardless of their speech results, showed a coronal pattern of closure or movement toward closure. Results are tabulated in Table 94–12. There was virtually no disagreement between the perceptual

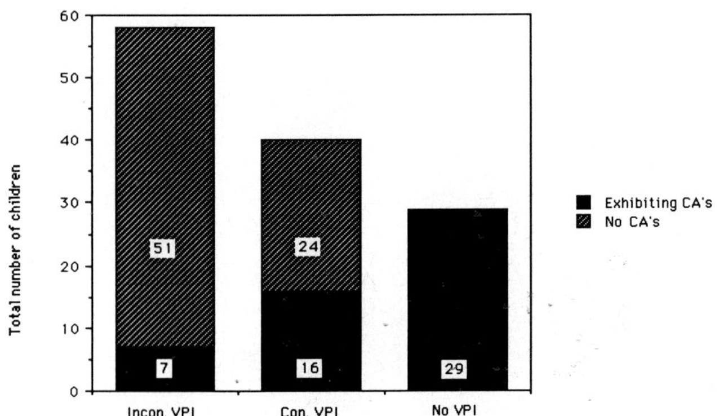

Figure 94–2 Relationship between compensatory articulations and velopharyngeal inadequacy (VPI).

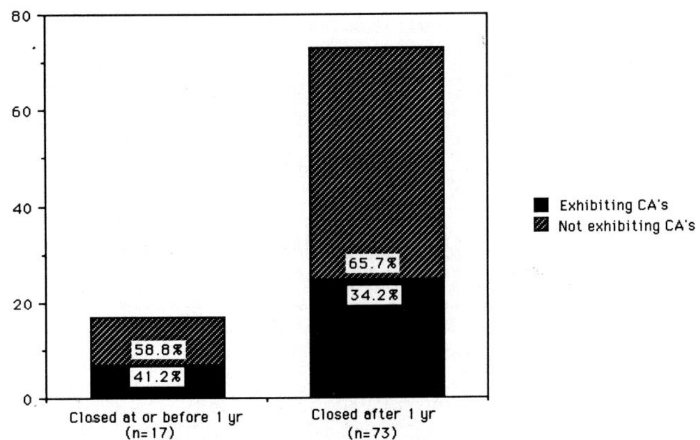

Figure 94–4 Children with and without compensatory articulations, closed before and after 1 year of age.

Table 94–10. Presence or Absence of Compensatory Articulations in the 90 Children for Whom Age at Palatoplasty Was Known

	With Compensatory Articulations	Without Compensatory Articulations	Totals
Closed at or before 1 year of age	7 (41.2%)	10 (58.8%)	17
Closed after 1 year of age	25 (34.2%)	48 (65.7%)	73
			90

Table 94–12. Patterns of Closure or Movement Toward Closure Seen On Nasopharyngoscopic Examination of 86 Children

	No VPI (N = 9)	Inconsistent VPI (N = 42)	Consistent VPI (N = 35)
Coronal	6	19	18
Circular	2	12	7
Circular with Passavant's ridge	1	8	8
Sagittal	0	3	2

For description of these patterns, see reference 37.
VPI = Velopharyngeal inadequacy.

categories of presence or absence of nasal air loss in speech and the consistency of closure seen on nasopharyngoscopy; however, the author was involved in making both judgments.

Discussion

If the success of palatoplasty is judged solely on the basis of absence of consistent perceptual evidence of velopharyngeal inadequacy, the average rate of that success was somewhat higher in this cross-sectional sample than in the reports reviewed by Morris in 1973: Of the 240 children 83.4% met this criterion. This figure is similar to those found in many reports submitted by individual surgeons or teams practicing only one or possibly two surgical approaches on clinical populations for whom critical independent variables are typically under better control than was possible in this study.[2, 11, 16, 20, 25]

If the more demanding criterion of no occurrence of nasal emission or hypernasality in speech were applied, the success rate among these children would drop to approximately 60%, with the percentages varying from 57.7% to 62.9% across cleft types (see Table 94–4). In the clinical judgment of the author, sporadic or infrequent audible nasal air loss has not been considered indicative of immediate need for further physical management of the velopharyngeal system. However, other clinicians may consider sporadically audible nasal air loss indicative of surgical failure.

Of particular interest in the data analysis was the question of the prevalence of so-called compensatory articulations. The presence of such behaviors is not necessarily indicative of current inadequacy of the velopharyngeal mechanism because these patterns often persist after an adequate system has been provided.[36, 37] Nonetheless, their presence or absence may be related to the age at which the palate was closed,[27] presuming that such closure did in fact result in a functional velopharyngeal mechanism. The results of the present study did not concur with those of Dorf and Curtin in regard to the following items:[27]

1. For the total group of 240 subjects, the overall percentage of children exhibiting these behaviors was much lower (21.7% versus 66.2%).
2. Among the 90 children in this study for whom age at palatal closure could be reliably identified, the total number showing compensatory articulations was again much lower than that reported by Dorf and Curtin (32/90 = 35.5% versus 53/80 = 66.2%).
3. When these 90 children were segregated into those with closure at or before 1 year of age and those with closure later, the percentage exhibiting compensatory articulations was higher in the early closure than in the late closure group. Also, in the late closure group, 65.7% were free of these behaviors as opposed to 13.5% in the earlier study.

Table 94–13 and Figures 94–5 and 94–6 provide a more detailed comparison between the Dorf and Curtin data and those of the present study. Apart from the fact that the bilateral cleft groups in both studies showed the highest number of children exhibiting compensatory articulations, there are few other similarities. In some instances, the percentages of children exhibiting compensatory articulations in the early versus later closure groups appear to be virtually reversed. Comparison must be undertaken with caution, however, for a variety of reasons:

1. The proportion of subjects in each cleft type is not

Table 94–11. Mean Ages at Closure for Children With and Without Compensatory Articulations

	With Compensatory Articulations (N = 32)	Without Compensatory Articulations (N = 58)	Totals (N = 90)
Mean age at closure	24.2 months	21.3 months	24.09 months

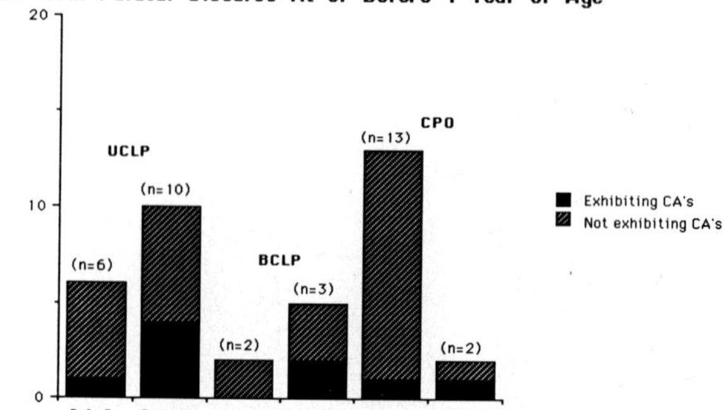

Figure 94–5 Comparison between the Dorf and Curtin data (1982) and the current study on children who were operated on at or before 1 year of age.

Table 94–13. Comparisons of the Percentages of Children Exhibiting Compensatory Articulations by Cleft Type and Age at Closure Between the Dorf and Curtin Data (1982) and the Current Study

	UCLP				BCLP				CPO				Totals			
	< 1 yr		*> 1 yr*		*< 1 yr*		*< 1 yr*		*> 1 yr*		*> 1 yr*		*< 1 yr*		*> 1 yr*	
	(N = 6)		*(N = 24)*		*(N = 2)*		*(N = 12)*		*(N = 13)*		*(N = 23)*		*(N = 21)*		*(N = 59)*	
	CA +	*CA−*	*CA+*	*CA−*	*CA+*	*CA−*	*CA+*	*CA−*	*CA+*	*CA−*	*CA+*	*CA−*	*CA +*	*CA−*	*CA+*	*CA−*
N =	*1*	*5*	*21*	*3*	*0*	*2*	*11*	*1*	*1*	*12*	*19*	*4*	*2*	*19*	*51*	*8*
Dorf and Curtin (1982)	16.7%	83.3%	87.5%	12.5%	0%	100%	91.6%	8.4%	7.7%	92.3%	82.6%	17.4%	9.5%	90.5%	86.4%	13.5%
Total percentage of CA + for each cleft type	22/30 = 73.3%				11/14 = 78.6%				20/36 = 55.5%				53/80 = 66.2%			

	UCLP				BCLP				CPO				Totals			
	< 1 yr		*> 1 yr*		*< 1 yr*		*< 1 yr*		*> 1 yr*		*> 1 yr*		*< 1 yr*		*> 1 yr*	
	(N = 10)		*(N = 36)*		*(N = 5)*		*(N = 21)*		*(N = 2)*		*(N = 16)*		*(N = 17)*		*(N = 73)*	
	CA +	*CA−*	*CA+*	*CA−*	*CA+*	*CA−*	*CA+*	*CA−*	*CA+*	*CA−*	*CA+*	*CA−*	*CA +*	*CA−*	*CA+*	*CA−*
N =	*4*	*6*	*7*	*29*	*2*	*3*	*15*	*6*	*1*	*1*	*3*	*13*	*7*	*10*	*25*	*48*
Current study	40.0%	60.0%	19.4%	80.6%	40.0%	60.0%	71.4%	28.6%	50.0%	50.0%	18.8%	81.2%	41.2%	58.8%	34.2%	65.7%
Total percentage of CA + for each cleft type (for these 90 subjects)	11/46 = 23.9%				17/26 = 65.3%				4/18 = 22.2%				32/90 = 35.5%			

UCLP = Unilateral cleft lip and palate; BCLP = bilateral cleft lip and palate; CPO = cleft palate only; CA+ = compensatory articulations.

similar between the two studies (Table 94–14). Approximately half of the subjects in the subset of 90 for whom age at surgery was known in the present study had unilateral clefts, whereas in the earlier study unilateral clefts accounted for 37.5%. It is of interest that the overall percentage of children with unilateral cleft lip and palate exhibiting compensatory articulations in the earlier study was more than three times what it was in the present study. It is also of interest that in the present study the percentages of children exhibiting compensatory articulations were similar in the unilateral cleft lip and palate and cleft palate only groups despite the disparity in group sizes. In both studies, the lowest percentage of occurrence was in the cleft palate only groups, although the percentage in the earlier study was more than twice that found in the current study.

2. Both studies suffer from the virtually universal limitation of having to classify subjects by cleft type alone rather than by other measures of severity such as width, tissue deficiency, and so on.

3. The earlier study does not specify the age(s) at which evaluations were made, although the theoretical impact of this factor is unclear. No trend could be identified in the present study regarding occurrence of compensatory articulations in yearly age groups (Table 94–8), but these are cross-sectional data. It is clear that longitudinal data are needed to delineate changes through time in each child, although the gathering of such data would pose an obvious ethical problem because any child who demonstrates compensatory behaviors should be enrolled in therapy.

4. In segregating subjects according to time of palatal closure (before or after 1 year of age),* both studies made the questionable assumption that an intact, functional velopharyngeal mechanism was in fact provided by the palatoplasty. Very few of the children in the current study who were operated on at or before 1 year of age were seen by the author immediately following palatal closure; the Dorf and Curtin report makes no specifications regarding this point.[27] In any case, assessing velopharyngeal closure for speech in a child of 14 or 16 months requires that that child be producing anterior pressure con-

---

*It should be noted that the cut-off age in the Dorf and Curtin study[27] was actually 12 months 15 days; for purposes of consistency, the same age was used in the current study.

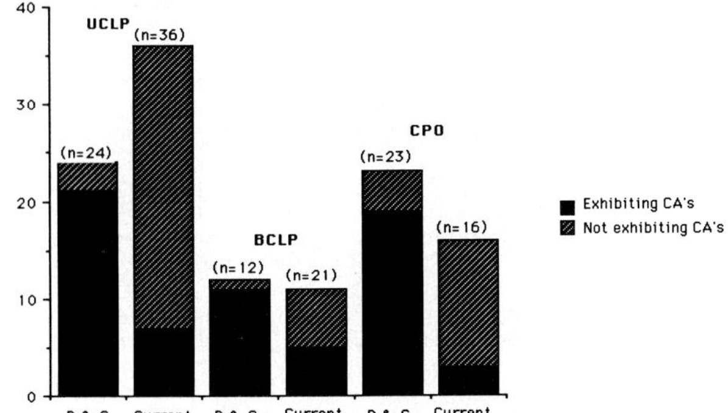

Figure 94–6 Comparison between Dorf and Curtin data (1982) and current study on children who were operated on after 1 year of age.

Table 94–14. Comparison of Subject Distribution Between Dorf and Curtin and the 90 Subjects in the Current Study for Whom Age at Palatal Surgery Was Known

	UCLP	BCLP	CPO	Totals
Dorf and Curtin (1982)	30 (37.5%)	14 (13.5%)	36 (45.0%)	80
Current study	47 (52.2%)	26 (28.9%)	17 (18.9%)	90

UCLP = Unilateral cleft lip and palate; BCLP = bilateral cleft lip and palate; CPO = cleft palate only.

sonants (consonants requiring the impounding of intraoral air pressure) in vocal play and early words. Because a number of factors besides velopharyngeal function may determine whether a toddler is using or attempting to use these consonants, sample size becomes a problem for clinicians trying to assess velopharyngeal adequacy at this age. In fact, Dorf and Curtin made the point that it is not chronologic age that should be considered in planning palatal closure but "articulation age."[27]

5. In neither study are the variables of speech therapy, stimulation in the home, health history, and so on documented. Even the variables of significant hearing loss and developmental delay were essentially categorized in both studies as present or absent. All of these factors can be extremely difficult to specify even in a prospective, single clinical center study. This author found it impossible to identify or quantify them reliably in a retrospective study of a patient sample that was diverse in cultures as well as in treatment centers.

Taking the above limitations into account, it is nevertheless clear that the results of the two studies are dissimilar and that the effect of the age at palatoplasty on the prevention of compensatory articulations needs continued investigation.

Within the current study, it is of interest that nearly half (22/52) of the children who exhibited compensatory articulations were using only mid-dorsum palatal stops. The question arises as to whether these articulations occur in children with no history of palatal problems— that is, although we hear them in children with clefts, are they truly compensatory?

It may be argued that the high prevalence of compensatory articulations in the children with bilateral clefts may have contaminated judgments of the occurrence of nasal air loss: Fourteen of these children exhibited compensatory articulations in the absence of demonstrable nasal emission or posterior nasal frication. However, seven of these children were using mid-dorsum palatal stops only, an articulatory gesture that does not prevent the airstream from escaping through an open velopharyngeal port. Only two children were using glottal stops and pharyngeal fricatives so consistently that adequacy of velopharyngeal function could not be judged perceptually. Neither cooperated for nasopharyngoscopy, a procedure that in itself can be invalidated if the child is simply bypassing use of the velopharyngeal stream.

The high numbers of children exhibiting noncompensatory articulations is not surprising, given the ages of the children, the diversity of linguistic backgrounds, and the high prevalence of dental or occlusal anomalies. The results do suggest that a closer look at dental problems as possible causative factors of speech problems in children with clefts may be warranted.

Conclusions

In this survey of speech results in 240 children aged 4 years to 10 years 11 months who had undergone primary palatoplasty with no secondary procedures, the percentage exhibiting adequate velopharyngeal closure for speech was approximately 84% if the criterion is the absence of predominant or consistent nasal air loss; 60% if sporadic, infrequent air loss is considered indicative of a physically inadequate system. Depending on the criterion accepted, the percentage of "success" is thus either about 14% better or 15% worse than that in the Morris survey of 1973. The percentage of children exhibiting compensatory articulations was remarkably lower than was expected, based on the earlier work of Dorf and Curtin.[27] In addition, the current data did not support the dramatic difference in numbers of children showing these behaviors between those in whom closure had occurred at or before 1 year of age and those who had had closure at a later age. Although the numbers of children in each diagnostic category were dissimilar between the two studies, the present results do suggest that the question of the effect of age at palatal closure on the development of compensatory articulations deserves reexamination.

References

1. Morris HL: Velopharyngeal competence and primary cleft palate surgery, 1960–1971: A critical review. Cleft Palate J 10:62, 1973.
2. Aaronson S, Fox D, Cronin T: The Cronin push-back palate repair with nasal mucosal flaps: A speech evaluation. Plast Reconstr Surg 75:805, 1985.
3. Blocksma R, Leuz C, Mellerstig K: A conservative program for managing cleft palates without the use of mucoperiosteal flaps. Plast Reconstr Surg 55:160, 1975.
4. Butow KW, Steinhauser E: Follow-up investigation of palatal closure by means of a one-layer cranially based vomer-flap. Int J Oral Surg 13:396, 1984.
5. Coston G, Hagerty R, Jannarone R, et al: Levator muscle reconstruction: Resulting velopharyngeal competency—a preliminary report. Plast Reconstr Surg 77:911, 1986.
6. Kaplan E: Soft palate repair by levator muscle reconstruction and a buccal mucosal flap. Plast Reconstr Surg 56:129, 1975.
7. Kaplan I, Labandter H, Ben-Bassat M, et al: Long-term follow-up of clefts of the secondary palate repaired by von Langenbeck's method. Br J Plast Surg 31:353, 1978.
8. Koberg W, Koblin I: Speech development and maxillary growth in relation to technique and timing of palatoplasty. J Maxillofac Surg 1:44, 1973.
9. Lewin M, Heller J, Kojak D: Speech results after Millard island flap repair in cleft palate and other velopharyngeal insufficiencies. Cleft Palate J 12:263, 1975.
10. Luce E, McClinton J, Hoopes J: Long-term results of the island flap palatal pushback. Plast Reconstr Surg 58:332, 1976.
11. Marks S, Wynn S: Speech results after bilateral osteotomy surgery for cleft palate: A review of 413 patients. Plast Reconstr Surg 86:230, 1985.
12. Noordhoff MS, Kuo J, Cheng W: Results of the Widmaier-Perko palatoplasty in clefts of the secondary palate. Ann Acad Med (Singapore), 12:359, 1983.
13. O'Riain S, Hammond B: Speech results in cleft palate surgery: A survey of 249 patients. Br J Plast Surg 25:380, 1972.
14. Randall P, LaRossa D, Solomon M, et al: Experience with the Furlow double-reversing Z-plasty for cleft palate repair. Plast Reconstr Surg 77:569, 1986.
15. Zeng XH: Speech improvement following cleft palate repair. Chung Hua Kou Chiangkotsa Chin 4:241, 1981.
16. Dreyer T, Trier W: A comparison of palatoplasty techniques. Cleft Palate J 21:351, 1984.
17. Holtmann B, Wray R, Weeks P: A comparison of three techniques of palatorrhaphy: Early speech results. Ann Plast Surg 12:514, 1984.
18. Krause C, Tharp R, Morris H: A comparative study of results of the von Langenbeck and the V-Y pushback palatoplasties. Cleft Palate J 13:11, 1976.
19. Musgrave R, McWilliams B, Matthews J: A review of the results of two different surgical procedures for the repair of clefts of the soft palate only. Cleft Palate J 12:281, 1975.
20. Witzel MA, Clarke J, Lindsay W, et al: Comparison of results of pushback or von Langenbeck repair of isolated cleft of the hard and soft palate. Plast Reconstr Surg 64:347, 1979.
21. Ainoda N, Yamashita K, Tuskada S: Articulation at age 4 in children with early repair of cleft palate. Ann Plast Surg 15:415, 1985.

22. Bardach J, Morris H, Olin W: Late results of primary veloplasty: The Marburg project. Plast Reconstr Surg 73:207, 1984.
23. Blijdorp P, Muller H: The influence of the age at which the palate is closed on speech in the adult cleft patient. J Maxillofac Surg 12:239, 1984.
24. Cosman B, Falk A: Delayed hard palate repair and speech deficiencies: A cautionary report. Cleft Palate J 17:27, 1980.
25. Daniller A, Shprintzen R, Strauch B: Nasopharyngoscopic investigation of the results of primary palate repair completed by 18 months of age. Presented before the Fourth International Congress on Cleft Palate and Related Craniofacial Anomalies, Acapulco, May 7, 1981.
26. Desai S: Early cleft palate repair completed before the age of 16 weeks: Observations on a personal series of 100 children. Br J Plast Surg 36:300, 1983.
27. Dorf D, Curtin J: Early cleft palate repair and speech outcome. Plast Reconstr Surg 70:74, 1982.
28. Egyedi P: Timing of palatal closure. J Maxillofac Surg 13:177, 1985.
29. Evans D, Renfrew C: The timing of primary cleft palate repair. Scand J Plast Reconstr Surg 8:153, 1974.
30. Kaplan E: Cleft palate repair at three months? Ann Plast Surg 7:179, 1981.
31. Perko M: Two-stage closure of cleft palate. J Maxillofac Surg 7:76, 1979.
32. Randall P, LaRossa D, Fakhraee S, et al: Cleft palate closure at 3 to 7 months of age: A preliminary report. Plast Reconstr Surg 71:624, 1983.
33. Robertson N, Jolleys A: The timing of hard palate repair. Scand J Plast Reconstr Surg 8:49, 1974.
34. Schweckendiek P: Primary veloplasty: Long-term results without maxillary deformity. A twenty-five year report. Cleft Palate J 15:268, 1978.
35. Van Demark DR, Tharp R: A computer program for articulation tests. Cleft Palate J 10:378, 1973.
36. Trost JE: Articulatory additions to the classical description of the speech of persons with cleft palate. Cleft Palate J 18:194, 1981.
37. Croft CB, Shprintzen RJ, Rakoff SJ: Patterns of velopharyngeal valving in normal and cleft palate subjects: A multiview videofluoroscopic and nasoendoscopic study. Laryngoscope 91:265, 1981.

CHAPTER 95

Clinical Assessment by the Speech Pathologist

Hughlett L. Morris

The purpose of this chapter is to review the kind of information about speech production that can be obtained from a clinical speech pathology examination of a patient with a cleft palate or a related disorder, and to comment about how that information can be interpreted in management decisions. The discussion focuses specifically on clinical assessment and is intended to supplement discussions in other chapters about various aspects of speech diagnosis and management. The discussion will be relatively brief, since more detailed and technical descriptions of various procedures, their rationale, and the interpretation of the obtained findings are available elsewhere.[1, 2]

Purpose of the Assessment

In general terms, clinical assessment of the cleft palate patient by the speech pathologist is designed to answer several questions, including the following:

1. Does the patient have a communication disorder of clinical significance? This question is answered on the basis of the clinical experience of the speech pathologist, although results from tests with norms and reports by the family members of the community can be highly useful also. The latter information is needed especially when the disorder is marginal in degree of severity, and the speech pathologist must determine whether any variation from the normal that is demonstrated during the examination is perceived also by the people with whom the patient interacts. In all cases, the speech pathologist must take special care to consider the public standard in making the judgment. If the disorder is only in the speech pathologist's ear, then *disorder* is quite probably the wrong term.

2. If there is a disorder, what is its nature? The speech pathologist must have expertise in differential diagnosis because the etiology of communication disorders shown by cleft palate patients is generally multifactorial in nature. Some very important clues about the various factors and their relative influence can be easily obtained from the clinical speech pathology examination.

3. What previous relevant treatment has the patient had and what can we learn from it? In the case of cleft lip and palate, certainly the speech pathologist needs some information about previous physical management of the cleft (surgical, dental, other), both completed and planned. Information is needed also about otologic and audiologic status, especially if the patient is a young child. Finally, information is needed about any other health problems and birth anomalies, and their treatment.

Information about previous speech and language therapy, the nature and duration of the therapy, and its judged outcome is also significant. This information is particularly important for patients for whom the question is whether behavioral therapy has been adequately tried, unsuccessfully, and whether other treatment methods (primarily physical management) should be considered. In other words, the results of therapy, positive or negative, are frequently the best available evidence in planning future treatment.

4. Does it seem reasonable to suppose that additional behavioral therapy will result in further improvement in speech and language and, if so, what changes can be expected? This is a primary question for the speech pathologist because the treatment considered is the one offered by speech pathologists. If behavioral therapy seems indicated, the speech pathologist must be specific in identifying the changes expected and when they may be observed.

Recommendations for other types of treatment, such as surgical or dental treatment, are made when there is sufficient reason to believe that structural limitations prevent behavioral therapy from being effective. If the clinical findings indicate that other types of treatment are needed for improvement of speech and language, the speech pathologist must have evidence for making the recommendation. Further, the recommendation must be made *for consideration of* other types of management to avoid the perception that management decisions are being made by the speech pathologist for other specialists (just as speech pathologists do not want other specialists to make such decisions for them!).

Methods of Assessment

As indicated above, the focus of the following discussion is on clinical assessment by the speech pathologist, using conventional procedures. Procedures for obtaining physiologic observations, particularly about velopharyngeal function during speech, are described elsewhere in this text and will not be repeated here. Information of that type supplements but cannot be used in place of the clinical assessment. Physiologic measures that are imaging in nature, such as endoscopy and radiography, are also particularly useful to the surgeon or dentist in planning physical management.

Clinical History

We have already considered several items from the clinical history that are useful to the speech pathologist in the clinical assessment. They include a description of the problem by the patient, the family, and other members of the community. In this regard, information is needed specifically about the degree to which any speech and language problems are reported to have social, educational, and vocational significance, and by whom such judgments are made.

Also needed is information about the original (untreated) defect or disorder and about any treatment that has been given. As indicated above, information about treatment by speech therapy is especially important, more so perhaps to the speech pathologist than is extensive detail about previous palatal surgery. Obviously, questions must be asked also about health and educational and vocational status (if the patient is an adult) because that status is relevant to matters of speech and language.

Clinical Examination

The speech pathologist needs to accomplish several purposes within the practical limits of a clinical examination of reasonable duration. One purpose is to formulate a description of general communication effectiveness. A second is to obtain a somewhat detailed itemization of specific errors (if any) and the circumstances under which they occur. Generally, we can accomplish the first by means of clinical judgments about connected speech observed during the examination, and the second by use of some kind of word articulation test.

A third purpose is to obtain information about variability of the level of skills, and about factors that seem to influence variability. We can do this by examining observed performance and by stimulability. Information about variability is particularly useful in predicting whether speech therapy may be useful in further improvement.

A fourth purpose is to make some working hypotheses about etiologic factors for the observed disorders and to make plans for further treatment. As we shall see, this phase of clinical assessment requires clinical judgment, made on the basis of all available clinical findings.

Parameters for Examination

The speech-language pathologist in contemporary practice is prepared to deal with aspects of communication that relate to speech production, language, and voice. Since cleft lip and palate and related disorders are primarily structural defects that affect the articulators and the mechanisms for controlling oronasal resonance, speech production and voice are of prime concern. Of these two, it frequently is more expedient and efficient to focus on speech production. That will be the main consideration in this discussion. Certainly nasal vocal tone is characteristic of "cleft palate speech," but that problem is usually resolved when sufficient velopharyngeal function has been achieved for normal aerodynamic patterns during "pressure" consonant production.

There are considerable data to indicate that children with cleft palate may be somewhat delayed in language performance skills in early childhood; however, any remaining delay after entrance to school is usually not clinically significant. As a result, it seems unjustified to conduct diagnostic language tests routinely for every cleft palate child. For most purposes, a screening procedure will suffice. Chapman and Hardin (Chap. 89) and Eliason (Chap. 105) consider these issues in greater detail than is warranted here. For these reasons, the focus of this discussion will be on speech production.

The Word Articulation Test

There are a number of word articulation tests constructed for general use that can be adapted for use with cleft palate patients.[2] Two have been devised specifically for that purpose: the Iowa Pressure Articulation Test[3] and the Bzoch Error Pattern Diagnostic Articulation Tests.[1] Regardless of which test is selected, or whether a new one is constructed for a special purpose, certain characteristics seem highly desirable.

1. The test must contain a fair number of so-called pressure consonants (plosives, fricatives, affricatives) because these speech sounds require (1) the buildup of intraoral air pressure in an amount greater than atmospheric, and (2) the oral release of that air pressure. This buildup and release of oral air pressure is possible only if the palate serves properly as a partition between the oral and nasal cavities. A palate with a physical cleft, a postsurgical fistula of substantial size, or a residual anterior cleft cannot serve as a proper partition. Nor can a palate serve as a

partition when the velopharyngeal opening cannot be closed during speech even though, anteriorly, the structure is intact. It follows, then, that performance on these test items provides information about the degree to which partitioning is effective during speech. Further, in the general case, if partitioning is not effective during speech in the presence of a physically intact palate, the likelihood is that the problem is with the velopharyngeal mechanism.

2. The test must contain a fair number of fricatives and affricates that are sibilants (/s/, /z/, /sh/, /zh/, /ch/, /j/) because these sounds may be distorted in articulation when there is dental malocclusion. Such errors are oral, not nasal, in character (although obviously a patient can show both nasalization and imprecise articulation on a sibilant at the same time). The imprecision may be due to either dental malocclusion factors, tongue tip placement factors, or both—and frequently, we cannot determine which!

3. The test must contain a fair number of glides (/r/,/l/) because many of our cleft palate patients are children, and children frequently have difficulty in mastering glides. There is one data set that indicates that some cleft palate children have more trouble with glides than normal children, even though typically we consider the glides to be unassociated with the structural deficits of cleft lip and palate.[4]

4. The test must contain a fair number of nasals (/m/, /n/, /ng/). In this case, the interest is not on whether the velopharyngeal opening can be properly closed during speech but whether it can be properly opened. If it cannot, nasals will be heard as plosives (/b/ or /d/), or at least plosivelike, and the overall speech will be regarded as denasal or hyponasal. That could be the finding in the presence of enlarged adenoids or a very wide pharyngeal flap.

5. The test must be long enough to contain a sufficient number of these items to reflect, in a reasonable manner, the variability of the patient's speech production patterns. At the same time, the test must be short enough to hold everyone's attention to the task. It must be economically realistic. For example, when can we justify a 2-hour-long word articulation test that costs the family $200?

The Importance of Error Type

Regardless of the word articulation test selected, provision must be made in the scoring procedure for the careful notation of error type. Specifically, the examiner must indicate in the scoring procedure whether speech production errors are oral or nasal in character. The distinction is important in regard to the apparent etiology of the error patterns: Errors that are nasalized raise questions about velopharyngeal function; errors that are oral indicate that velopharyngeal function is within normal limits but articulation placement is not. Obviously, cleft palate patients frequently show both error types on the same sound production, and the scoring procedure must be sufficiently flexible to reflect that as well.

The scoring procedure also must reflect use of "unusual" speech sound substitutions. Two examples are the glottal stop and the pharyngeal fricative, reported for cleft palate speakers as early as 1945,[5] and by many authors since then.[6–12] Trost has suggested others as well: the pharyngeal stop, the mid-dorsum palatal stop, and the posterior nasal fricative.[13]

The presumption is that these substitutions are adopted because of deficits of the oral structures. Specifically, the suggestion is that the glottal stop and the pharyngeal fricative compensate for velopharyngeal dysfunction because the plosiveness or fricativeness can be obtained by a buildup of air pressure "posterior" (in this case, below) to the velopharyngeal mechanism. Because these sound substitutions are learned behavior, they may persist after the physical deficit (velopharyngeal dysfunction) has been resolved. For that reason, the occurrence of substitutions like the glottal stop does not always yield useful information about velopharyngeal function during speech. Speech therapy is clearly required to teach more "anterior" articulation patterns. Additional discussions about these compensatory speech production patterns are provided in Chapters 44 and 91 to 94.

Finally, the scoring procedure must allow observations of facial movement, generally involving nares constriction, during production of pressure consonants. Such movements of the nares, midface, or even brow can usually be taken to indicate velopharyngeal dysfunction. That is, the patient is attempting to prevent nasal emission of air at the level of the nares that cannot be prevented by the velopharyngeal mechanism. Clinical experience indicates that not all patients with velopharyngeal dysfunction demonstrate nares constriction but, with rare exceptions, the presence of nares constriction is a reliable indicator of velopharyngeal dysfunction. The exceptions are patients who have recently had physical management of the velopharyngeal mechanism.

Testing for Stimulability of Performance

The importance of obtaining information about variability of performance has been emphasized earlier. One source of such information is the word articulation test; the examiner evaluates the degree of consistency of performance among the test items. How consistent are the error patterns? Are the pressure consonants always nasalized, or are some judged to be oral? Is there variability in precision of the sibilants among test items?

Another source of information about variability can be obtained from a comparison between performance on the word articulation test and performance during connected speech. For example, some patients with a velopharyngeal mechanism that appears only marginally normal perform well on a word test but show nasalization during connected speech.

A third source of information about variability of performance can be obtained from results of auditory-visual stimulation. As reported in McWilliams et al,[2] the notion of stimulability was introduced by Milisen and associates[14] and was considered further by Carter and Buck in an attempt to determine the use of such a measure in predicting whether "normal" children would benefit from therapy.[15] Later, Harrison applied the theory to cleft palate children and found that stimulability was a predictor of improvement in both treated and untreated children.[16] Since then, information about stimulability has been used as part of a clinical protocol for evaluating the speech results of patients undergoing cleft palate surgery in a variety of clinical populations.[17–21] In particular, this concept provides important information for distinguishing between two hypothesized subgroups within the diagnostic classification of marginal velopharyngeal function.[2, 22, 23] The two subgroups are:

1. The almost-but-not-quite (ABNQ) subgroup, who show highly consistent but minimal nasalization of speech.
2. The sometimes-but-not-always (SBNA) subgroup, who show marked variability in performance that ranges from normal to clinically significant nasalization, depending on the task according to the model.

The former subgroup (ABNQ) is neither variable or stimulable, but the latter subgroup (SBNA) is both.

The response to stimulation by a cleft palate patient (or a patient with any other structural deficit suspected as being a detriment to speech production) is especially useful because it yields information about the extent to which both physiologic and behavioral variability is possible. For example, if a child shows relatively consistent nasalization of pressure consonants during most verbal activities but is stimulable to oral production of any of them, the examiner can hypothesize that the desired response (an oral pressure consonant) is in both the physiologic and behavioral* repertoire of the child and that articulation therapy for the purpose of generalization is a reasonable treatment. If, on the other hand, stimulation results in persistent nasalization, the possibility of velopharyngeal dysfunction must be considered.

Evaluations of Connected Speech

The various kinds of findings obtained from word articulation tests are highly useful for the purpose of examining speech production patterns with a kind of dissecting microscope. There is also great need to evaluate the patient's typical conversational connected speech in purposeful conversation. This, after all, is what the public hears and reacts to. Usually, the speech pathologist uses a scale (for example, *one* for normal, *five* for severely abnormal) or categorical system (for example, *normal, mildly disordered, moderately disordered, severely disordered*) to describe the connected speech of the individual in relation to the clinical population that the patient represents. Scales like this can be applied to any aspect of speech. For the cleft palate patient, aspects of nasal voice quality, normalcy of articulation skills, and overall defectiveness are usu-

ally considered. Evaluation of nasal voice quality is important in decisions about velopharyngeal function. The emphasis on articulation skills focuses on the precision of speech production patterns. Finally, a judgment about overall defectiveness (or normalcy) is intended to reflect the same kind of skills that a speaker uses in dealing with the general public.

Performance on Nonspeech Tasks

There is considerable information about the marked differences that occur in oral function patterns between speech and nonspeech tasks. For example, rarely does a patient with even severe velopharyngeal dysfunction during speech show nasal regurgitation during swallowing. In the same way, patients can be "taught" to demonstrate extended movement of the palate or pharyngeal wall during isolated tasks but do not generalize those extended movements during connected speech.

On the other hand, sometimes one can learn about the potential for velopharyngeal activity from performance on a nonspeech task. Sometimes a small child can perform an oral blowing task (blowing a very small paper "boat" held in the palm of the hand) when she cannot or will not perform a similar speech task orally. The ability to blow the tiny boat without nasal emission of the airstream can be an important, and is certainly a simple, diagnostic finding.

In contrast, the act of sucking is not generally useful diagnostically. Buccal pressure is used initially to suck liquid into the mouth, without the help of the velopharyngeal mechanism, and then the liquid is swallowed in the usual manner. As a result, the act of sucking tells the examiner little about the normalcy of velopharyngeal function.

Physical Examination

Usually clinical assessment of a cleft palate patient includes a physical examination of the oral structures. Certainly it is relatively easy to conduct such an examination with gloves, a tongue blade, a flashlight, and the unaided eye, but interpretation of some of the findings is more difficult.

For example, one can find out from such an examination whether the palatal structures are intact or whether there is an unrepaired cleft or a postsurgical fistula. Judgments can be made also about dental occlusion, especially the degree to which the occlusion may be a hazard to normal speech production. Judgments can also be made about other oral structures, such as the height of the palatal vault, relative size and mobility of the tongue, tonsillar size, palatal length, and amount and symmetry of velar elevation, but these judgments must be interpreted with caution because of variability in the normal and the imperfect relationship between these structures and the associated patterns of function. Finally, it is common knowledge that one cannot learn much about movement of the velopharyngeal structures during speech because they are hidden from view during such an examination.

---

*Behavioral in the sense that the child can demonstrate appropriate articulator placement for the speech sound in question.

Issues of Reliability

On occasion, clinical judgments such as those just reviewed are referred to in a disparaging manner because they are "subjective" and are inherently of unknown or unsatisfactory reliability. Certainly these judgments are subjective because the very nature of clinical assessment is subjective—that, indeed, is the value of clinical judgment. It is the process by which the clinician attempts to collate all available information about the patient in judgments about clinical status and decisions about management. Further, judgments about speech are obviously valid, because the bottom line is how the patient sounds to her or his family and friends and to the public in general.

On the other hand, the question about reliability is a fair one. Clinicians have the obligation to examine and describe the basis for their clinical judgments, to calibrate their standards with colleagues, and to report steps taken in this direction in clinical papers.

Making Decisions About Management

In simplest terms, the speech pathologist examines the variety of clinical data from the examination described above with one question in mind: Is it reasonable to suppose that speech and language therapy will be productive in assisting the patient to gain more normal verbal communication skills? We ask this question because our findings are most pertinent to what we do, behavioral therapy. If the answer to the question is yes, behavioral therapy should be provided. If the answer is no, we must consider what other kinds of treatment may be needed to achieve our goals of better speech and language, such as surgical reduction of the velopharyngeal space or orthodontics.

Following are several hypothetical patients, descriptively labeled, to be considered as examples in relating speech pathology findings to therapy planning.

1. Patient DWQ (doing well, but quiet), 6 years of age.
   a. Speech pathology findings
      (1) Only a few nasal distortion errors on the word articulation test, and those are stimulable.
      (2) Oral distortion of most sibilants is due to dental factors.
   b. Treatment planning
      (1) Continue to observe.
      (2) Consider whether language testing and treatment are needed.
      (3) Watch, learn about the need for orthodontic attention.
2. Patient NMH (not much hope), age 7 years.
   a. Speech pathology findings
      (1) Nasalized connected speech, moderate extent.
      (2) Nasal distortion during most pressure consonants on the word articulation test; only a few single plosive items seem to be oral.
      (3) Some plosives are stimulable (or are produced with such little nasal distortion that it is not audible, but fricatives, affricates are not).
   b. Treatment planning
      (1) Limited experimental therapy to determine the generalization of oral plosives, but the outlook is not good. If no improvement occurs after 4 hours of therapy, or if patient begins to show nares constriction earlier than that, discontinue therapy. Refer for consideration of physical management.

Patient CCS (clear case for surgery), age 9 years.

3. a. Speech pathology findings
      (1) Nasal emission on all pressure consonants during the word articulation test and connected speech.
      (2) Not stimulable.
      (3) Had trial therapy for 6 months last year that was not successful.
      (4) Nares constriction.
   b. Treatment planning
      (1) Speech therapy for nasalization contraindicated.
      (2) Refer for consideration of physical management.

Patient TYTS (too young to say), age 3 years.

4. a. Speech pathology findings
      (1) Connected speech has limited intelligibilty.
      (2) Moderate number of glottals.
      (3) Voice quality minimally nasal.
      (4) A few good plosives, appropriately used.
      (5) Nasal distortions, /s/, /z/.
      (6) Stimulable for nearly all plosives.
      (7) Can do blowing tasks without audible or observable nasal emission.
      (8) Probably language delayed.
   b. Treatment planning
      (1) Language testing and therapy if needed.
      (2) Maybe speech therapy for the purpose of generalizing the available oral responses.
      (3) Observe closely at 2-month intervals.

Patient MPH (maybe perhaps), age 5 years.

5. a. Speech pathology findings
      (1) Mostly oral during the word articulation test and connected speech, but an occasional sibilant distorted nasally.
      (2) Sibilants are stimulable.
      (3) Considerable difficulty with glides /r/, /l/; not stimulable.
   b. Treatment planning
      (4) Retest in 3 months. Might do some experimental therapy for sibilants and glides.

Patient SOS (same old story), age 8 years.

6. a. Speech pathology findings
      (1) Nasal distortion on pressure consonants, but inconsistent.
      (2) Connected speech more nasal than the word articulation test.
      (3) Errors are stimulable.
      (4) These findings also obtained last year and the year before that; child has had speech therapy during those 2 years also.

b. Treatment planning
  (1) Probably a problem of timing.
  (2) More therapy? Not unless past therapy seems silly or not effective for a specific reason.
  (3) Refer to a specialty team, with a comprehensive report, for their consideration about physical management.
  (4) Prognosis is guarded because physical reduction in size of the velopharynx will not resolve motor incoordination; however, such management may be justified to minimize the effect of the incoordination.
7. Patient NBB (not bad but), age 8 years.
  a. Speech pathology findings
    (1) Consistent nasalization of speech during both the word articulation test and connected speech, but to a minimal degree.
    (2) Not stimulable.
    (3) Findings similar to those from past 2 years; child also had therapy during that period.
  b. Treatment planning
    (1) Probably a problem of minimal structural deficit.
    (2) More therapy? Probably not, unless considered a special case. Even then, treatment should be given on a limited basis.
    (3) Refer to a specialty team, with a comprehensive report, for their consideration for physical management.
    (4) Issue here: Is disorder sufficiently severe to warrant surgery or other physical management?

Both patients SOS and NBB can be considered by most standards to demonstrate marginally normal velopharyngeal function, or velopharyngeal dysfunction that is only marginally severe. As indicated earlier, Morris suggests there may be two subgroups of patients in the marginal category: one a disorder of timing, which he labels SBNA (sometimes but not always), the other a disorder of structure, ABNQ (almost but not quite).[22, 23] In such a scheme, SOS is SBNA, and NBB is ABNQ.

Conclusion

The speech pathologist experienced in cleft palate and related disorders has the clinical tools available to gather enough information for intelligent treatment planning. The important questions are:

1. What are the nature and severity of the oral communication disorder?
2. What is the extent of variability in speech production patterns?
3. Has behavioral therapy been provided and did it result in improvement?
4. If behavior therapy is not productive, what alternatives are available?

By such examination of the findings, diagnosis and treatment by speech pathologists can be effectively and efficiently planned for a large majority of these patients.

ACKNOWLEDGMENT. This paper was critically read by David L. Jones, Ph.D.; I thank him for his assistance.

References

1. Bzoch KR (ed): Communicative Disorders Related to Cleft Lip and Palate, 3rd ed. Boston: Little, Brown, 1989.
2. McWilliams BJ, Morris HL, Shelton RL: Cleft Palate Speech. Toronto: B.C. Decker, 1984.
3. Morris HL, Spriestersbach DC, Darley FL: An articulation test assessing competency of velopharyngeal closure. J Speech Hear Res 4:48, 1961.
4. Pitzner JH, Morris HL: Articulation skills and adequacy of breath pressure ratios of children with cleft palate. J Speech Hear Dis 31:26, 1966.
5. Morley ME: Cleft Palate and Speech. Edinburgh: E & S Livingstone, 1945.
6. Sherman D, Spriestersbach DC, Noll JD: Glottal stops in the speech of children with cleft palates. J Speech Hear Dis 24:37, 1959.
7. Bzoch KR: Articulatory proficiency and error patterns of preschool cleft palate and normal children. Cleft Palate J 2:340, 1965.
8. Moll KL: Speech characteristics of individuals with cleft lip and palate. In Spriestersbach DC, Sherman D (eds): Cleft Palate and Communication. New York: Academic Press, 1968, p 62.
9. Bzoch KR: Categorical aspects of cleft palate speech. In Grabb WC, Rosenstein SW, Bzoch KR (eds): Cleft Lip and Palate: Surgical, Dental, and Speech Aspects. Boston: Little, Brown, 1971, p 713.
10. Morris HL: Abnormal articulation patterns. In Grabb WC, Rosenstein SW, Bzoch KR (eds): Cleft Lip and Palate: Surgical, Dental and Speech Aspects. Boston: Little, Brown, 1971.
11. Wells CG: Cleft Palate and Its Associated Speech Disorders. New York: McGraw-Hill Book, 1971.
12. Edwards M, Watson ACH: Advances in the Management of Cleft Palate. Edinburgh: Churchill Livingstone, 1980.
13. Trost JE: Articulatory additions to the classical description of the speech of persons with cleft palate. Cleft Palate J 18:193, 1981.
14. Milisen RA: A rationale for articulation disorders. J Speech Hear Dis Monograph, Suppl 4, 1954.
15. Carter ET, Buck M: Prognostic testing for functional articulation disorders among children in the first grade. J Speech Hear Dis 23:124, 1958.
16. Harrison RJ: A demonstration project of speech training for the preschool cleft palate child. Final report, Project No. 6–1101, Grant No. DE6–2–6–061101–1553. Washington: U.S. Office of Education, 1969.
17. Morris HL: Velopharyngeal competence and the Demjen W/V-Y technique. In Morris HL (ed): The Bratislava project: Some Cleft Palate Surgical Results. Iowa City: University of Iowa Press, 1978.
18. Bardach J, Morris HL, Olin WH: Late results of primary veloplasty: The Marburg project. Plast Reconstr Surg 73:207, 1984.
19. Bardach J, Morris HL, Olin W, et al: Late results of multidisciplinary management of unilateral cleft lip and palate. Ann Plast Surg 12:235, 1984.
20. Hardin MA, Morris HL, VanDemark DR: A study of cleft palate speakers with marginal velopharyngeal competence. J Commun Dis 19:461, 1986.
21. VanDemark DR, Gnoinski W, Hotz H, et al: Speech results of the Zurich approach in treatment of unilateral cleft lip and palate. Plast Reconstr Surg 83:605, 1989.
22. Morris HL: Cleft palate. In Weston AJ (ed): Communication Disorders: An Appraisal. Springfield: Charles C Thomas, 1972.
23. Morris HL: Marginal velopharyngeal incompetence. In Winitz H (ed): For Clinicians by Clinicians: Articulation and Language. Baltimore: University Park Press, 1984.

CHAPTER 96

Methods of Assessing Velopharyngeal Function

Mary Anne Witzel and David A. Stringer

The formation of speech is a complex, coordinated task involving interaction of the structures of respiration and mastication. These structures generate, shape, and direct the airstream needed to produce voice and speech. After the airstream passes through the glottal opening of the larynx, it enters the pharynx and is directed through the nasal or oral cavities by the opening and closing of the velopharyngeal valve. It is then narrowed or stopped and released by the movements of the tongue and lips to produce individual speech sounds. Thus, control of the airstream is possible at five sites: larynx, velopharyngeal valve, nasal valve, tongue, and lips. The entire area, including the laryngopharynx, velopharynx, nasal cavity, and oral cavity, is known as the vocal tract. In this chapter, we focus on the velopharyngeal valve, its function, and its effect on the vocal tract during speech.

The degree of closure of the velopharyngeal valve is related to the sound being produced. High vowel sounds (/i/ [key], /u/ [two], /I/ [kit]) combined with oral sibilant-fricative consonants (/s/, /z/, /sh/) require the most complete closure, whereas low vowels (/a/ [knock], /o/ [ball], /æ/ [man]) combined with nasal consonants (/m/, /n/, /ng/) are produced with the valve open. Normal velopharyngeal function comprises the opening and closing of the velopharyngeal valve consistently and appropriately during correctly articulated speech.

Incomplete closure of the velopharyngeal valve often causes speech problems such as hypernasality, nasal air emission, and certain articulation errors. It has also been implicated in voice problems such as hoarseness[1, 2] and restricted resonance due to the hyperfunctional alterations to the vocal tract such as constriction of the hypopharynx and oral pharynx.[3] During formation of non-nasal speech, incomplete velopharyngeal closure allows sound waves emanating from the vocal folds to enter both the oral and nasal cavities. The two cavity chambers vibrate and enhance the sound waves, often resulting in hypernasal resonance. Hypernasal resonance is perceived in vowels and in consonants such as /w/, /j/ (yes), /r/, and /l/.[4] Incomplete closure of the valve also may produce nasal air emission, which may or may not be audible. Nasal air emission may occur throughout speech or selectively with specific consonants. In the latter case, sometimes referred to as phoneme-specific or sound-specific velopharyngeal insufficiency, the emission usually occurs only during formation of the sibilant-fricative and affricate sounds,

particularly /s/ and /z/.[5–7] Hypernasality and nasal air emission, the most common manifestations of velopharyngeal insufficiency, often coexist and may be interrelated, but they are not synonymous.

Incomplete closure also may affect the formation of speech sounds, specifically, the features of voicing, place of articulation, and manner of formation. Sounds such as /b/, /d/, /g/, and /z/ are referred to as voiced sounds because they are produced by adduction and vibration of the vocal folds during exhalation of air, sending sound waves into the pharynx and oral cavity to be shaped by the tongue and lips. Voiceless sounds such as /p/, /t/, /k/, and /s/ result when the vocal folds abduct as the air-stream passes through the larynx, where it is stopped or narrowed by the tongue and lips. If velopharyngeal closure is incomplete, some patients compensate for lack of control of the airstream at the velopharyngeal valve by hyperfunction of structures at the other sites of air control within the vocal tract (larynx, tongue, lips, and anterior nasal valve).

Place of articulation refers to the location within the vocal tract where two articulators occlude or are approximated to form a specific sound. For example, bilabial sounds (/p/, /b/, /m/) are produced when the lips contact each other, and lingual alveolar sounds (/t/, /d/, /n/, /s/, /z/) are produced when the tongue contacts or approximates the alveolar area of the palate.

A distinctive category of errors of place of articulation in patients who do not or cannot close the velopharyngeal valve during speech is commonly known as compensatory articulation. These errors of place of articulation were described by Morley[8] as "compensatory adjustments," and by Bzoch[9] as "laryngeal and pharyngeal gross substitution errors." The most detailed description has been provided by Trost.[6, 7] Compared with normal oral consonants, these erroneous sounds, which presumably occur in an attempt to shape the airstream below the velopharyngeal valve, are produced more posteriorly and inferiorly in the vocal tract by posterior positioning of the tongue (pharyngeal stop, fricative, or affricate), associated vocal fold adduction (glottal stop), or abnormal positioning of the arytenoid cartilage and epiglottis (laryngeal fricative or affricate).[10] For example, the pharyngeal fricative, which may be substituted for sibilant-fricative sounds, occurs when the dorsum of the posterior tongue approximates the posterior pharyngeal wall to give frication to the airstream. Because frication occurs below the velopharyngeal valve, velopharyngeal closure is unnecessary to produce this sound. Although compensatory articulation is sometimes a consequence of velopharyngeal insufficiency, velopharyngeal insufficiency may be a consequence of compensatory articulation because limited movements of the velopharyngeal valve occur during production of these sounds.[10–14] Reports by these authors have described increased movements of the components of the velopharyngeal valve after correction of compensatory articulation. In some cases, complete velopharyngeal closure results from correction of these misarticulations.

Manner of formation refers to the degree of narrowing or constriction of the oral or pharyngeal cavity to impede or give frication to the airstream flowing through the vocal tract. It also refers to the direction of the airstream through the mouth (over the sides of the tongue) or through the nose. In velopharyngeal insufficiency, the airstream escapes into the nasal cavity and cannot be impeded orally to create sounds requiring oral air pressure. This is often described as weak production of pressure sounds. In some cases, sounds such as /p/, /b/, /t/, and /d/ are perceived as /m/ and /n/. The child attempts to produce pressure sounds in the correct places in the mouth, but manner is altered when the airstream cannot be prevented from entering the nose through the velopharyngeal valve.

Velopharyngeal insufficiency may also affect speech intelligibility and acceptability. Intelligibility is an overall judgment of speech influenced by many variables including resonance, nasal air emission, voice, rate and fluency of speech, stress, accent, and intonation.[15] Articulation errors appear to influence intelligibility more directly than does hypernasality.[16–18] Acceptability is the subjective impression of the pleasingness of speech. Research is scant in this area; however, two studies suggest that single words produced with compensatory articulation are more acceptable to both children and their parents than single words produced with audible nasal air emission.[19, 20]

Mechanism of Velopharyngeal Valving

The velopharyngeal valve includes the soft palate, the lateral pharyngeal walls, and the posterior pharyngeal wall. Each component has tissue mass, elasticity, innervation, shape, size, and muscle force.[21] The muscles thought to control velopharyngeal closure are the *levator veli palatini, musculus uvulae,* and *superior constrictor.* However, the role of the superior constrictor muscle appears to be controversial, and the contribution of the musculus uvulae has not been well defined.[22]

During speech, four distinct patterns of movement of velopharyngeal valve components have been observed both in subjects achieving complete velopharyngeal closure and in those with incomplete closure.[23–26] The patterns are coronal, circular, circular with a Passavant's ridge, and sagittal. Identification of the pattern is believed to be helpful in planning surgical[27] or prosthetic treatment in velopharyngeal insufficiency.

The velopharyngeal valve is three-dimensional.[28–30] In many cases, the size and shape of gaps in the valve differ at varying points in the height of the valve,[28, 29] and this difference may be influenced by the pattern of muscle movements within the vocal tract.[31]

Velopharyngeal function is influenced directly and indirectly by many factors. Direct factors include the anatomy of velopharyngeal valve components including tissue mass and elasticity, nerve supply, size and location of tonsil and adenoid tissue, presence of a palatal fistula,[32] nasal anatomy and function, and laryngeal anatomy and function. Indirect factors include the child's age, hearing, intelligence, articulation (specifically tongue positioning), respiratory efforts, tension in the vocal tract, timing and coordination of velopharyn-

geal valving, and degree of mouth opening during speech. Complete assessment of velopharyngeal function should address these factors for differential diagnosis of velopharyngeal insufficiency.

Assessment of Velopharyngeal Function

Patients with speech manifestations of velopharyngeal insufficiency should be assessed by a cleft palate or craniofacial team. The patient's hearing, facial growth, dentition, associated anomalies, intelligence, and family environment may all contribute to the etiology, diagnosis, and treatment planning of velopharyngeal insufficiency.

Evaluations of speech characteristics assess velopharyngeal function only indirectly, whereas imaging techniques provide observations of the anatomy and dynamic movements of the velopharyngeal valve and vocal tract during speech. Complete assessment requires both types of evaluation to ascertain the interaction between the velopharyngeal anatomy and function and the speech outcome and to plan appropriate treatment.

Common methods of evaluating speech characteristics include detailed articulation analysis and listener judgments of resonance, nasal air emission, articulation, intelligibility, and acceptability. Many forms of instrumentation have been used to support clinical evaluations of speech characteristics. The mirror test indicates the presence of nasal air emission during speech.[33] The TONAR system, developed by Fletcher, measures the resonant frequency of the oral and nasal chambers during speech.[34] The findings from this system correlate well with listener judgments of hypernasality.[35] The accelerometer,[36] which measures vibrations on the surface of the nose, also reportedly correlates with ratings of hypernasality.[37, 38]

Aerodynamic studies measure nasal airflow and differences in air pressure above and below the point of maximum constriction of the velopharyngeal port during specific speech tasks as well as resistance to airflow through the nose.[39–45] These measures allow calculation of changes in the relative size of the velopharyngeal valve over time. As applied to the assessment and treatment planning of velopharyngeal insufficiency, this technique has several limitations—namely, an inability to determine the location and etiology of the defect and the pattern of muscle movements in the velopharyngeal valve.[28–30, 46] These factors are believed to be important in the type and design of surgical or prosthetic treatment. The aerodynamic technique may be most useful in assessing the timing and coordination of velopharyngeal movements during speech and the regulation of airflow through the vocal tract.[47, 48] This information is helpful in both diagnosis and treatment planning, specifically, in planning speech therapy.

Another recently developed system that has potential for assessing the timing of velopharyngeal movements during speech is the use of the photodetector.[49] This procedure, which may be combined with nasendoscopy,[50, 51] records variations in the amount of intensity of light passing through the velopharyngeal valve at specific time intervals. This system allows observation of changes in the relative size of the velopharyngeal valve over time. It may have potential as a biofeedback tool for speech therapy[52] and for documentation of consistency of velopharyngeal movements.[50]

Methods providing direct visualization of the valve during speech include lateral still cephalometry, multiview videofluoroscopy, ultrasonography, tomography, computed tomography scanning, and fiberoptic endoscopy. Of these, only multiview videofluoroscopy and fiberoptic endoscopy permit continuous observation of the dynamic activity of the velopharyngeal valve over time.

In our experience, planning effective and efficient treatment of velopharyngeal valving problems with speech manifestations requires the following information:

1. The type and severity of speech manifestations of velopharyngeal insufficiency (abnormal nasal resonance or other aspects of voice quality, nasal air emission, articulation, intelligibility, and acceptability).
2. Articulation analysis with particular emphasis on compensatory articulation, weak pressure sounds, and substitution of nasal sounds for oral pressure sounds.
3. The anatomy of the velopharyngeal valve; movement of velopharyngeal valve components; presence, location, size, and consistency of the velopharyngeal gap; timing of velopharyngeal movements; and tongue function.
4. The presence, location, size, and effect on velopharyngeal function of a palatal fistula.
5. Presence, size, location, and effect on velopharyngeal function of tonsil and adenoid tissue.
6. Anatomy and function of the laryngeal structures.
7. The patient's ability to change voluntarily any speech manifestation and velopharyngeal function.

To meet these criteria the assessment of velopharyngeal function at The Hospital for Sick Children, Toronto, Ontario, incorporates information obtained from the clinical speech assessment with the imaging techniques of multiview videofluoroscopy and flexible fiberoptic videonasopharyngoscopy.

Clinical Speech Assessment

The evaluation of velopharyngeal function begins with the clinical speech assessment. The information from the clinical assessment forms the basis for interpreting the findings from the imaging assessments and is crucial in the selection of treatment.

Patient History

Important aspects of the patient's history include age at onset of the speech problem; sucking, swallowing, and drooling problems; family history of craniofacial anomalies or hypernasal speech; tonsillectomy or adenoidectomy; hearing problems; developmental delay; learning disabilities; physical anomalies; duration and type of speech therapy; sleeping or breathing difficulties; and patient and family concerns.

Examination of Oral Structures

Important aspects of the oral structures include occlusion, maxillary collapse, size and location of any fistulas, soft and hard palate anatomy, bifid uvula, size and location of tonsils, pharyngeal flap, tongue anatomy and mobility, and symmetry of structures. Although the relative size of the soft palate and its movement when the patient says "ah" are noted, they often do not correlate well with velopharyngeal function during connected speech production.[33] Because /a/ is a low vowel produced with the tongue held on the floor of the mouth and the mandible open, this vowel does not require complete closure of the velopharyngeal valve, and its usefulness in diagnosis is limited.

Listener Judgments

Judgments of perceived hypernasality, nasal air emission, and overall speech intelligibility and acceptability are crucial to the decision to pursue treatment. Severity of these factors is often rated by one or more speech pathologists using interval scales. However, these judgments remain subjective and may vary from examiner to examiner. Although some clinicians reportedly recommend specific forms of treatment (surgery, dental prosthesis, therapy) on the basis of listener judgments only, this guesswork does not permit accurate treatment planning.[53] The most effective treatment may not be chosen, and sometimes an entirely inappropriate treatment is used. Listener judgments are important in the assessment of velopharyngeal function but are most effective when used in conjunction with other aspects of the clinical speech assessment and imaging techniques.

Articulation Analysis

For consistency and completeness, an articulation test such as the Templin-Darley tests of articulation or the Fisher Logemann test is beneficial. Any test may be used, but particular attention should be paid to the nature, type, and consistency of articulation errors; the use of compensatory articulation; weak production of pressure sounds; and nasal substitutions. Some patients with compensatory articulation respond to speech therapy either alone[14] or combined with a temporary prosthetic obturator or videonasopharyngoscopic biofeedback.[54, 55] Therefore, these possibilities must be investigated to ensure selection of effective treatment.

Stimulability Testing

Stimulability testing refers to assessment of the patient's ability or potential to improve abnormal nasal resonance, nasal air emission, or articulation with instruction and awareness. Patients who are easily stimulated to improve their speech patterns are excellent candidates for speech therapy.

Imaging Techniques

Multiview Videofluoroscopy

Multiview videofluoroscopy is a radiologic technique that allows evaluation of the velopharyngeal valve in several planes during the production of speech. Early descriptions of the technique included the lateral, base, and frontal views.[56, 57] Recently, the Towne's,[58–60] oblique,[61] and Waters' views[62] have been shown to be useful additions to the technique (Fig. 96–1). Not all views are used during each examination. The number of views taken depends on the information needed and the anatomy of the skull and vocal tract.

At The Hospital for Sick Children, all examinations are now conducted with over-table tube fluoroscopy equipment (Fig. 96–2) and evaluated by both a radiologist and a speech pathologist. The examinations are recorded and maintained on videotape with audio recording.

Videofluoroscopy is preferred to cinefluoroscopy because a much lower radiation dosage is used to transfer the image to videotape than to film. Radiation dosage is kept to a minimum by coning the x-ray beam to the smallest area, shielding the patient with lead sheets except in the region of interest, and ensuring that the

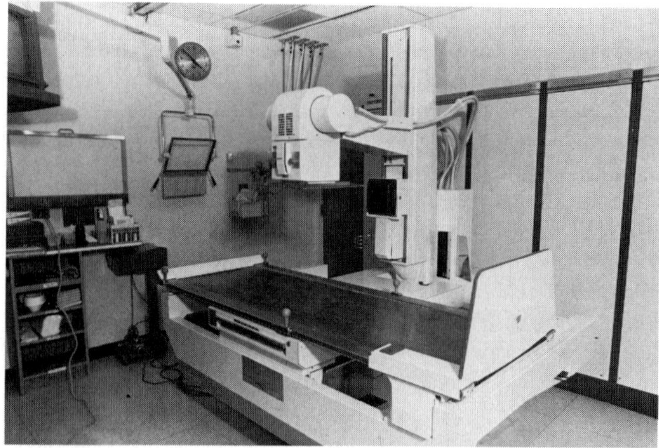

Figure 96–2 Over-table tube fluoroscopy equipment currently used at The Hospital for Sick Children, Toronto.

equipment is emitting the minimum radiation necessary to produce a diagnostic image. Rare earth filters such as erbium, ytterbium, holmium, or gadolinium fixed on the x-ray tube not only increase the tube-to-patient distance but also reduce the dose of radiation absorbed by the skin. The dose can be further reduced by using recently available digital fluoroscopic units with last image hold and digital photospot capability. With these units, the fluoroscopic image and the photospot images are frozen on the television monitor for immediate inspection, reducing the need for repeated or prolonged exposure. Spot images are usually unnecessary because diagnosis is best made directly from the video recording.

In the future, the use of stimulable phosphorus (photostimulable luminescent device) technology may further reduce the radiation dosage of radiographic exposures. Three-dimensional computer tomography reconstruction is another technologic advance that may be helpful in the investigation of velopharyngeal insufficiency; however, this technical method is likely to continue to be more expensive and to generate a higher radiation dose than fluoroscopic techniques.

Some clinicians are reluctant to refer patients with speech symptoms suggestive of velopharyngeal insufficiency for multiview videofluoroscopic examination of the vocal tract because of the patient's exposure to radiation. Obviously, patients should be carefully selected for this procedure. However, the information provided by the technique is not yet obtainable by other methods and is often crucial in the diagnosis and treatment planning, particularly if surgery is required for speech problems related to velopharyngeal insufficiency.

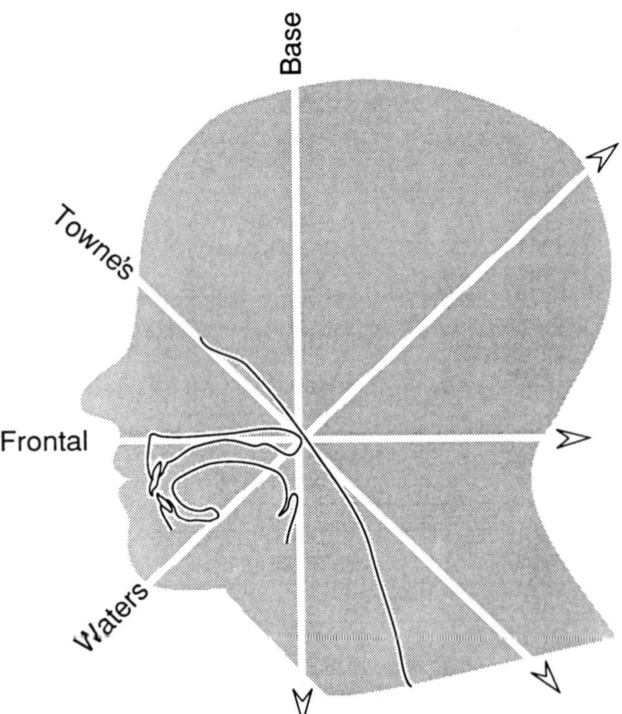

Figure 96–1 Schematic drawing of the direction of the x-ray beam through the velopharyngeal valve for the base, Towne's, frontal, and Waters' views.

Technique

High-density barium is instilled into each nostril using a syringe with a plastic tip. About 1 to 2 ml of barium is used, and the patient is instructed to sniff this back into the nasopharynx (Fig. 96–3). The patient is then positioned to obtain the various views necessary to assess the movements of the velopharyngeal valve completely

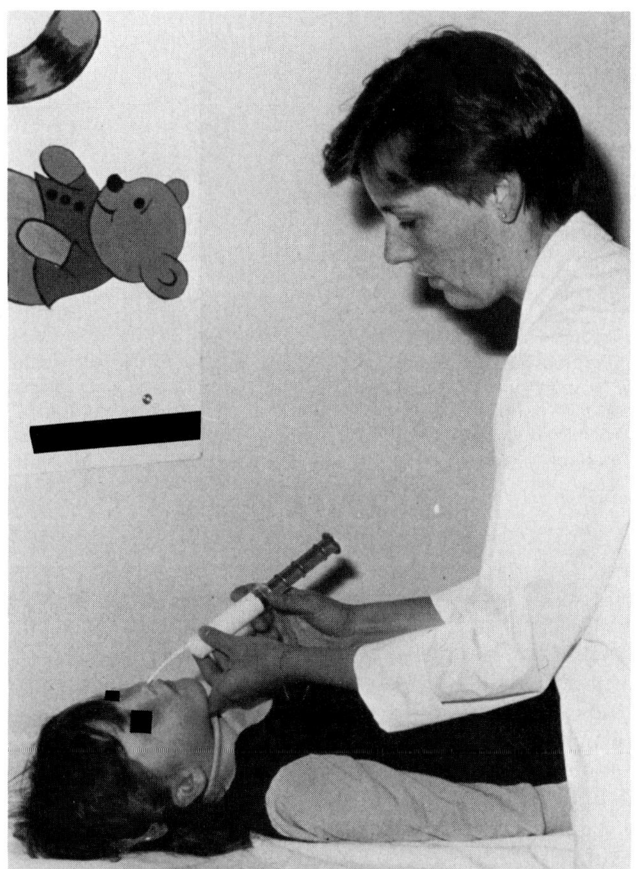

Figure 96–3 Instillation of high-density barium into both nostrils of a 4-year-old child.

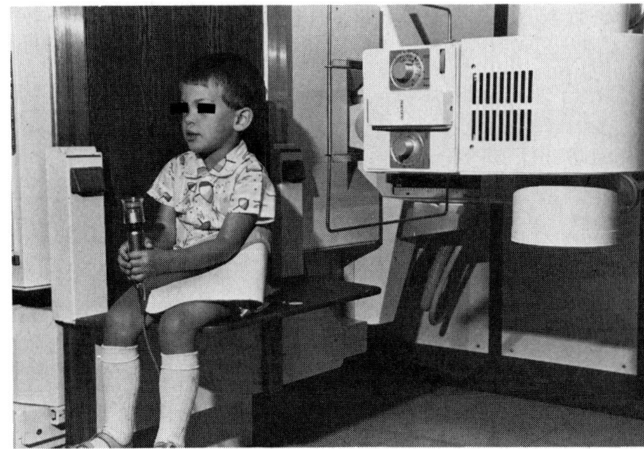

Figure 96–4 Patient in position for the lateral view.

during speech. A standard speech sample is used for each view. The patient counts from 1 to 10 and repeats the "Pittsburgh" sentences: "Put the baby in the buggy," "Give Gary the chocolate cake," "Susie sees the sun in the sky," and "My name is ________," and also forms the isolated sounds /s/, /sh/, and /ooh/.

The Lateral View

The lateral view is taken first, with the patient sitting upright (Fig. 96–4). It provides information about the relative length and thickness of the soft palate and the depth of the pharynx. The position and size of the adenoid and tonsillar tissue are noted. During speech, the excursion of the soft palate is observed (Fig. 96–5), and evidence of a Passavant's ridge or more generalized pharyngeal wall movement is noted. The level and inferosuperior area of contact between the soft palate and the adenoid or posterior pharyngeal wall are observed. This view also allows detection of any interference with soft palate excursion due to posterior displacement of hypertrophied tonsils.[63, 64]

Abnormal movements of the posterior and anterior aspects of the tongue during speech are also readily visualized. Barium coating of the tongue may help to enhance the image of tongue function during speech.[32] In some cases, the tongue attempts to raise the soft

palate to effect velopharyngeal closure, particularly for the velar stop sounds /k/ and /g/, or approximates the soft palate to form the compensatory articulation sound known as the velar fricative.[6, 9] In other cases, the posterior tongue approximates or contacts the posterior pharyngeal wall to produce the pharyngeal fricative, pharyngeal affricate, and pharyngeal stop. In some patients who have a palatal fistula, the blade of the tongue is often elevated to occlude the fistula for production of the stop sounds /t/, /d/, /k/, and /g/ (mid-dorsum palatal stop)[6, 7] or fricative sounds (mid-dorsum palatal fricative).[13] The abnormal movements of the epiglottis and larynx during formation of the laryngeal fricative can also be observed from this view.[10]

The lateral view assesses the depth of the valve and demonstrates approximation of the soft palate and the pharynx, but it is not sufficient to determine velopharyngeal adequacy because it does not confirm closure of the valve along its width.[60, 65] Irregularities in the border of the soft palate or the adenoid tissue[26] that allow air to escape through the velopharyngeal valve often cannot be detected, and small gaps in velopharyngeal closure may be missed if there is too little barium to demonstrate bubbling of air through the valve during speech (Fig. 96–6). Other views are required to assess the

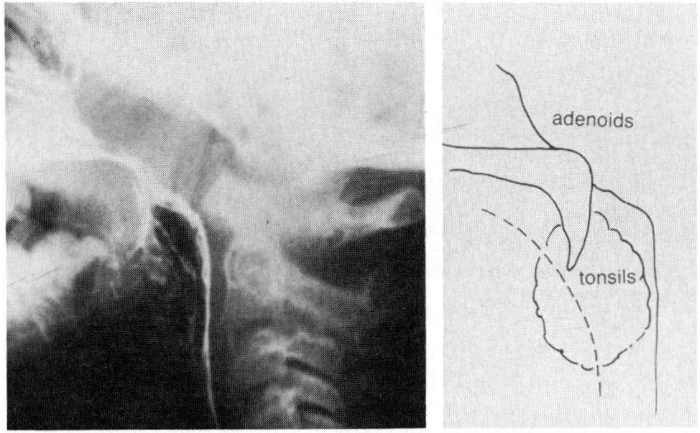

Figure 96–5 Lateral view multiview videofluoroscopy showing velopharyngeal closure against the adenoid. Note the large tonsillar mass.

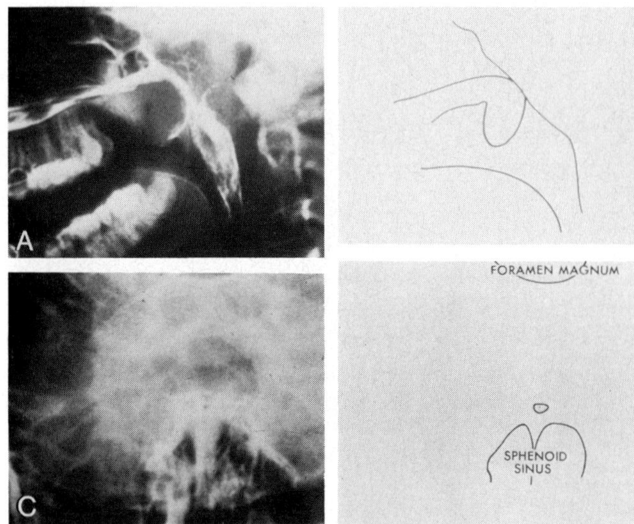

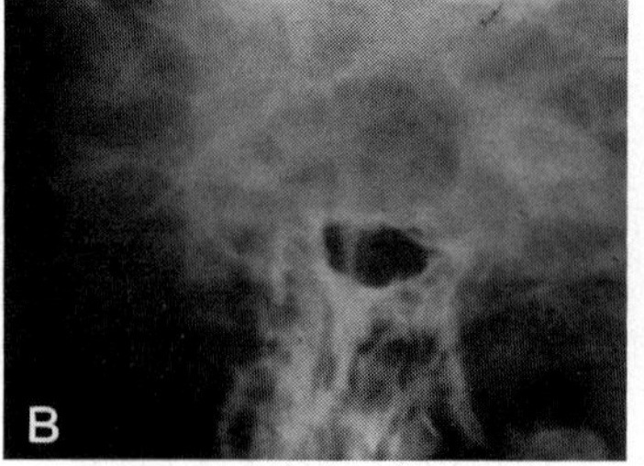

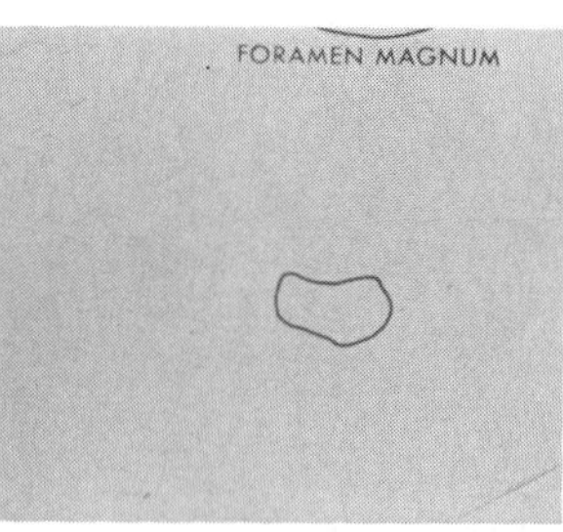

Figure 96–6 *A,* The lateral view showing contact of the soft palate and posterior pharyngeal wall. *B,* Towne's view of the same patient with the velopharyngeal valve open. *C,* During speech a small circular velopharyngeal gap is observed that was not detected in the lateral view.

shape, size, and location of the defect and lateral pharyngeal wall movements.

The Base View

In the base view, the patient lies prone in a sphinx-like position with the head and neck hyperextended so that the inferior border of the mandible is parallel to the table. We have found it helpful to place a Styrofoam wedge under the patient's mandible for stability (Fig. 96–7). This view has three drawbacks: the presence of overlying levels of tissue or rings of barium in the pharyngeal tube or adenoids that may compromise the view,[29] the presence of abnormal retrusive tongue positions that may be mistaken for the posterior border of the soft palate, and the necessity for hyperextension of the neck. Hyperextension of the head and neck is often difficult for adults and those with vertebral anomalies and may actually cause velopharyngeal insufficiency that is not apparent when the patient's head is in a more normal position.[66] The posterior positioning of the tongue in patients with pharyngeal fricative, pharyngeal affricate, and pharyngeal stop articulation errors may be mistaken for soft palate approximation or closure with the pharynx. In a child with adenoid tissue, velopharyngeal valving is often velar adenoidal and is at an oblique angle to the nasopharynx, necessitating extreme hyperextension to view the actual valve en face. In addition, accurate visualization of the velopharyngeal ports after pharyngeal flap surgery may be difficult, particularly if the ports are small or oblique to the vertical axis, as may occur in patients with a "tubed" flap.

In many patients, the base view helps to evaluate the velopharyngeal valve (Fig. 96–8); however, it is the most difficult view from which to obtain reliable information.[29, 67]

Towne's View

Towne's view is a useful alternative to the base view and is used when adenoid tissue approximates the palate during valving, causing an oblique axis of velopharyngeal closure. With over-table tube fluoroscopy equipment, the patient is seated upright and the camera is rotated (Fig. 96–9) until the velopharyngeal valve is visualized en face (Fig. 96–6B and C). With more standard equipment, the patient is positioned sitting or supine with the head lowered toward the chest. This view eliminates many of the overlying structures that obscure the valve in the base view and provides information about the shape of the valve, location of the gap, pattern and symmetry of velopharyngeal valving, and consistency of velopharyngeal movements. Findings on Towne's view correlate well with nasopharyngoscopic evaluations of velopharyngeal function.[67]

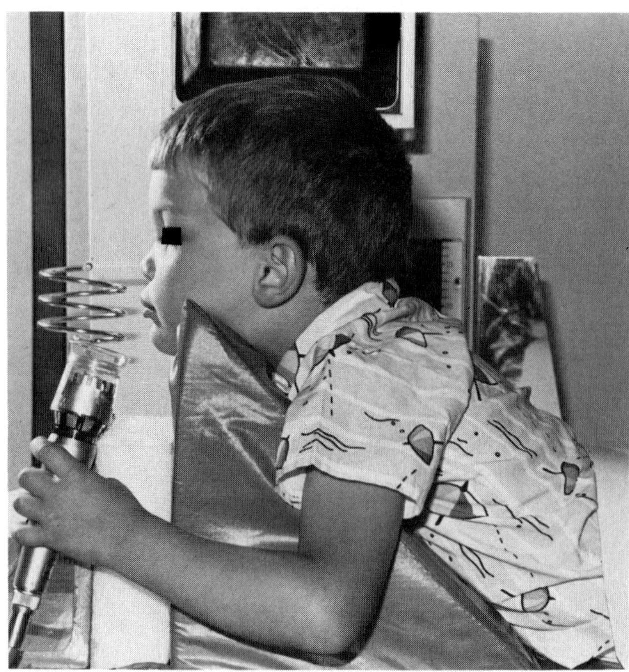

Figure 96–7 Patient in position for the base view.

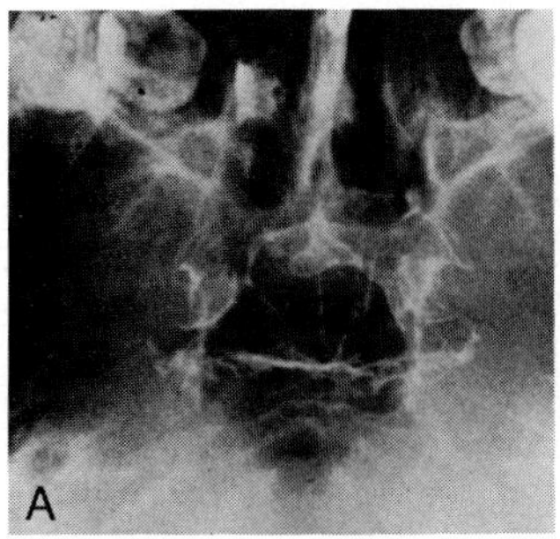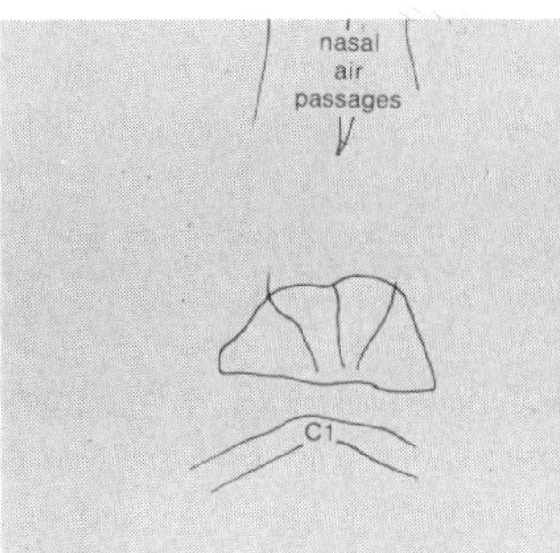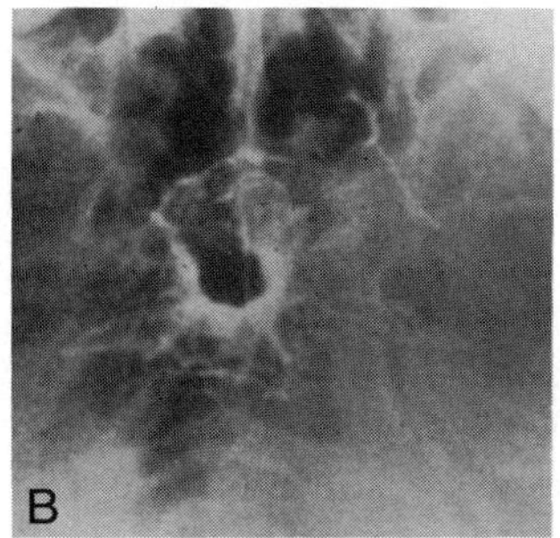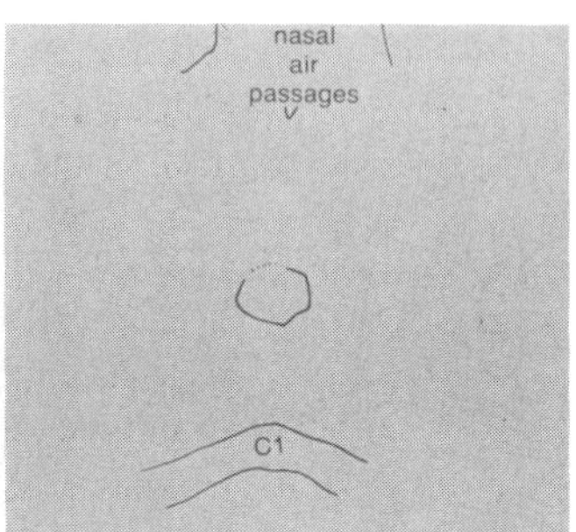

Figure 96–8 *A*, The lateral view showing the velopharyngeal portal at rest and *(B)* during maximum closure.

The Frontal and Waters' Views

The frontal and Waters' views permit visualization of the location of the lateral pharyngeal walls and their excursion during speech. This information is believed to be crucial in planning pharyngeal flap surgery[27] or designing a dental prosthesis to treat velopharyngeal insufficiency. An adequate barium coating of the nasopharynx is essential.

For the frontal view the patient is seated with the head in the Frankfurt horizontal plane facing the image intensifier (Fig. 96–10). Lateral pharyngeal wall movements may occur along an extensive area of the velopharyngeal tube (Fig. 96–11) or may be localized (Fig. 96–12). The Waters' view is a helpful alternative when the overlying bony structures obscure the lateral pharyngeal walls in the frontal view.[62] For the Waters' view the head is tilted upward about 45 degrees from the Frankfurt horizontal (Fig. 96–13). Hyperextension of the neck in this view may uncover unsuspected velopharyngeal insufficiency[66] or may be difficult for patients with limited neck mobility. Shprintzen recommends rotation of the head to the right and left along the X axis when asymmetric movement of the lateral walls is observed to more clearly identify the extent of movement.[61]

Selection of Views

In most patients, only two or three views are used. All patients undergo the lateral view initially. When velopharyngeal valving is oblique (Fig. 96–6A), the Towne's projection is chosen rather than the base view. When the lateral pharyngeal walls are obscured by bony structures in the frontal view, the Waters' view is used. Oblique projections of the frontal view are reserved for patients with asymmetric lateral wall movements.

Figure 96–9 Patient in position for Towne's view.

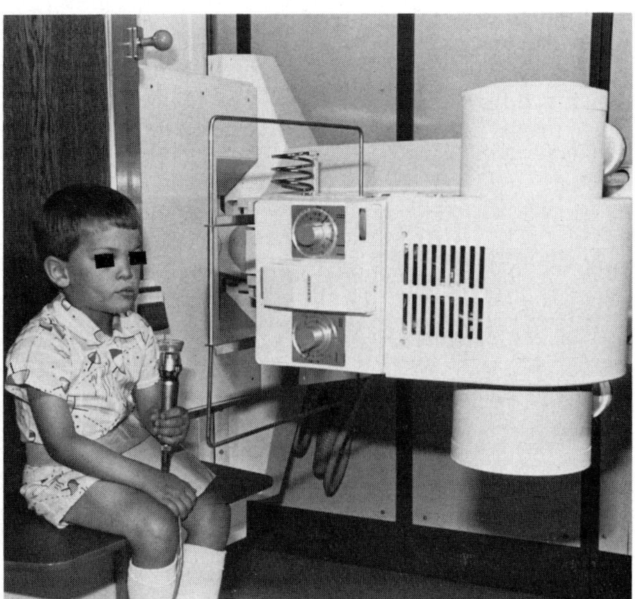

Figure 96–10 Patient in position for the frontal view.

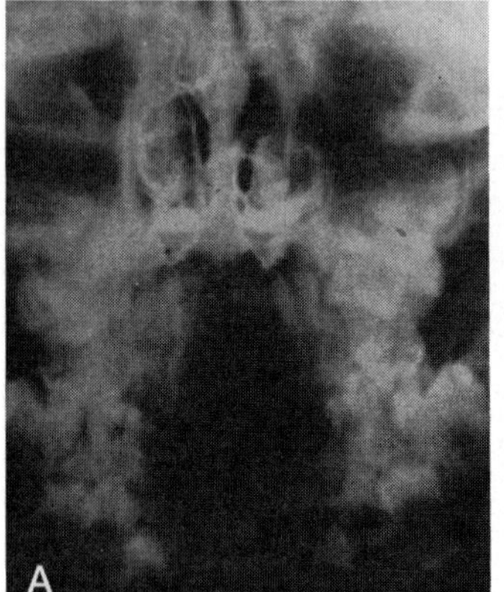
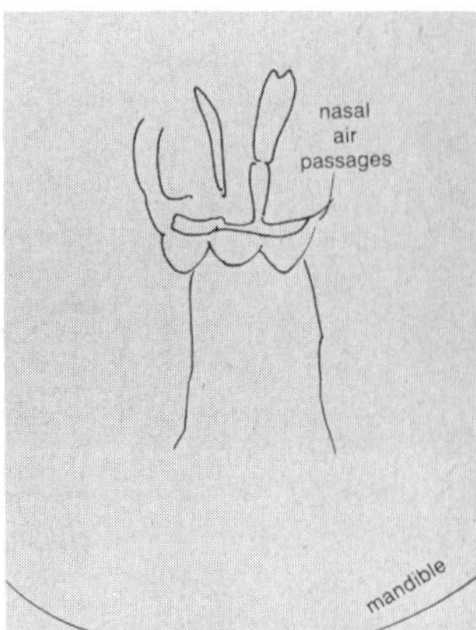
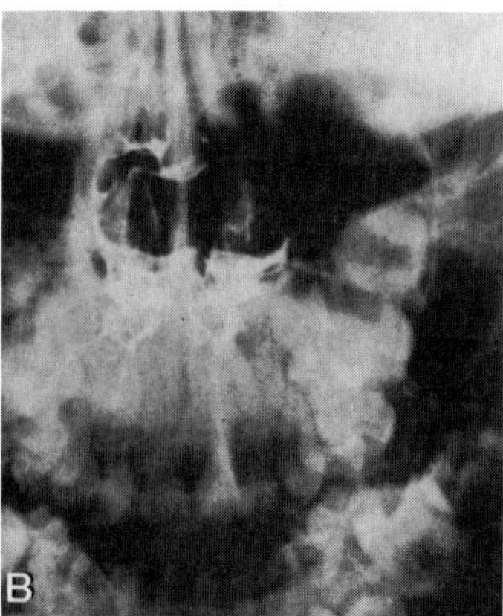
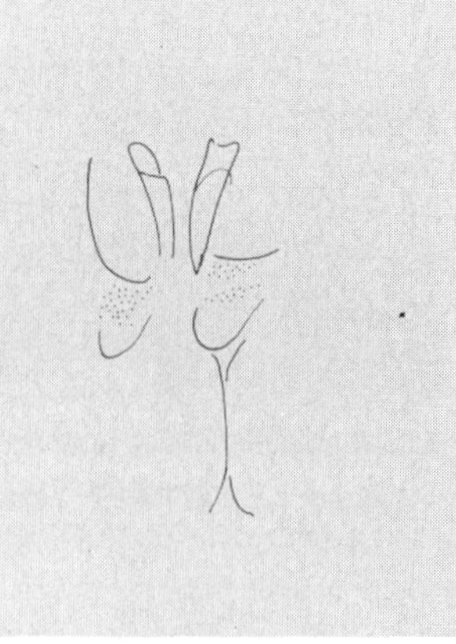

Figure 96–11 A, The lateral view showing lateral pharyngeal walls at rest and *(B)* during maximum mesial movement in speech showing extensive area of contact.

Analysis of Information and Reporting

At the end of the examination, the videotapes are reviewed jointly by the radiologist and the speech pathologist, and judgments of anatomy and function are recorded on a standard form, providing the basis for a written report. This information is used in conjunction with the clinical speech assessment and nasopharyngoscopic findings to formulate treatment recommendations.

Video Nasopharyngoscopy

The technique of nasopharyngoscopy for assessing velopharyngeal function was described in the late 1960s.[68] The procedure provides information on the anatomy of the velopharyngeal valve, closure of the valve during speech, relative size and location of velopharyngeal gaps, consistency of movements, movement of the specific components, function of the dorsum of the posterior tongue during speech, and anatomy and function of the laryngeal structures. It gives a direct superior view of the velopharyngeal valve. Three types of endoscopes are available: side-viewing rigid, side-viewing flexible, and end-viewing flexible. Most clinicians prefer end-viewing flexible scopes (Figs. 96–14 and 96–15) because all aspects of the velopharyngeal

tube, including the larynx in patients with large adenoids, may be examined by passing the scope through the velopharyngeal valve.[29] In general, the flexible endoscopes have a smaller diameter than the rigid scopes, allowing examination in younger children.

At The Hospital for Sick Children, the Olympus ENFP flexible 3.7-mm end-viewing endoscope is used. Illumination is provided by a CUDA M2 300 fiberoptic video light source. All examinations are recorded on a ¾-inch video cassette machine (Sony Umatic Recorder) with audio recording by a high-resolution video camera (Sony Dx 1850). Other excellent flexible endoscopes and ancillary equipment are available, and the size and quality of equipment are constantly being improved. The use of audio-video recording allows the examiner, patient, and accompanying family members to view the velopharynx and laryngopharynx simultaneously on a television monitor throughout the examination and permits maintenance of a permanent record that can be reviewed and compared with previous and subsequent examinations and with videofluoroscopy.

A topical anesthetic is used before the endoscope is inserted. One side of the patient's nasal cavity is sprayed with 2% tetracaine hydrochloride and 0.5% phenylephrine mixed in equal parts.[69] The nasal cavity is further anesthetized with direct application of 2% tetracaine

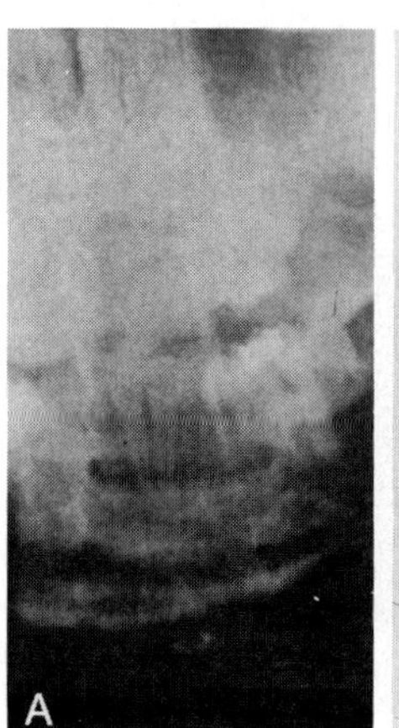
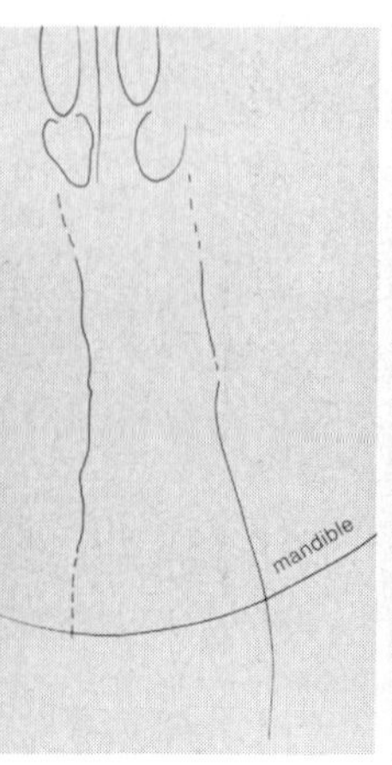
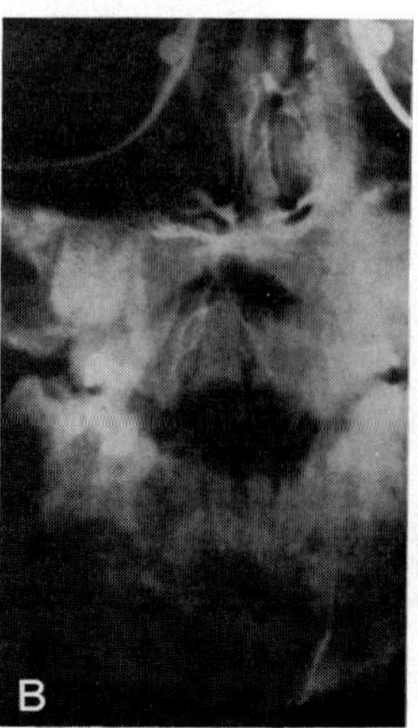
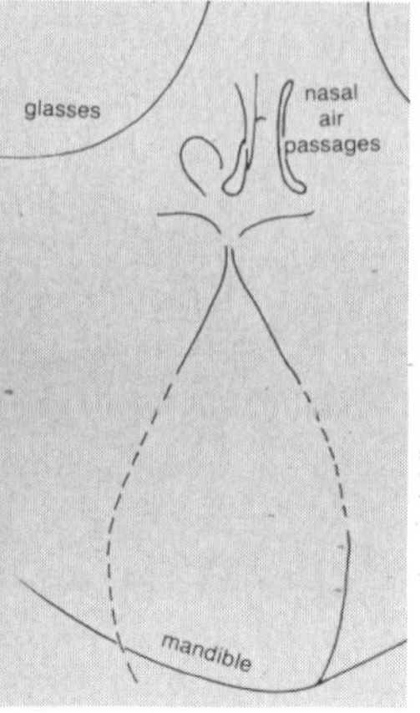

Figure 96–12 A, The lateral view showing lateral pharyngeal walls at rest and *(B)* during speech showing a localized area of contact.

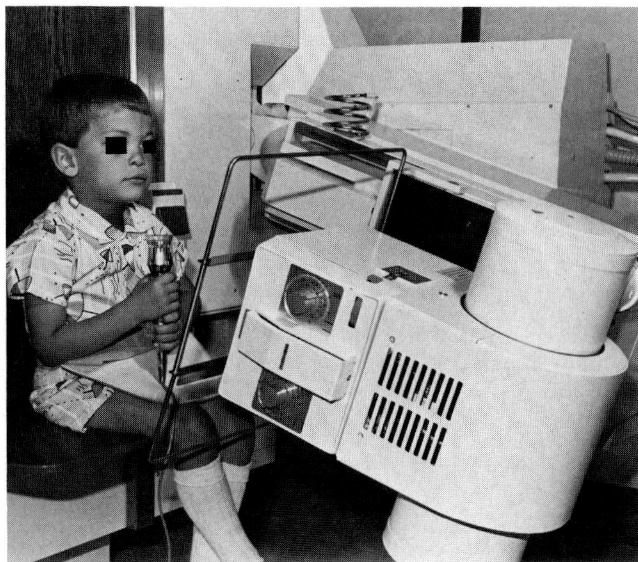

Figure 96–13 Patient in position for the Waters' view.

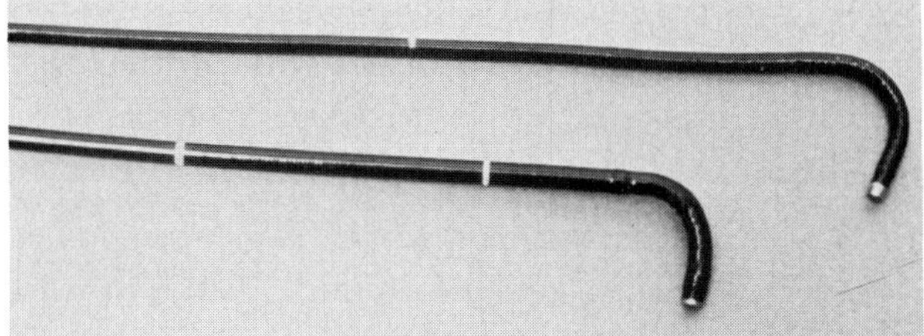

Figure 96–15 Downward flexion 90 degrees of the flexible nasopharyngoscopes.

hydrochloride by a cotton swab or nasal packing. In general, the nostril that allows easier breathing is chosen; in a patient with unilateral cleft lip and palate this is usually the noncleft side. The anesthetic may be applied with the patient sitting or lying prone. The prone position is preferred, especially in young children who require steadying. The topical anesthetic is applied in less than 5 minutes in a cooperative patient.

The endoscope is inserted through the nasal passage with the patient sitting upright in a chair (Fig. 96–16). Once the scope is inserted and the velopharyngeal port is visualized, the patient repeats the speech sample used in the videofluoroscopy examination. This provides a consistent sample for comparison of patients and permits data collection for clinical research. The patient is asked to perform other speech tasks as necessary to complete the examination, with particular emphasis on his ability to change velopharyngeal movements voluntarily during speech either as a result of observing his

movements on the TV monitor (biofeedback) or by altering formation of specific speech sounds.[13, 55, 70–73]

Care is taken during the examination to ensure adequate visualization of the anatomy of the superior surface of the soft palate, the eustachian tube orifices,[74] and the anatomy of the pharynx including the relative size and shape of the adenoid tissue (Fig. 96–17). The presence or absence of pulsations suggestive of a medially displaced carotid artery,[75] the size and position of the tonsils (Fig. 96–18), and the anatomy and function of the epiglottis (Fig. 96–19) and laryngeal structures are noted. The viewing end of the endoscope is positioned directly above the velopharyngeal valve to allow visualization in the horizontal and vertical planes. This may be difficult if the adenoid pad is excessively large or the musculus uvulae is particularly prominent during function, dislodging the scope. A false-positive or false-negative impression of velopharyngeal closure will be obtained if the scope is not positioned directly above the valve (Fig. 96–20). The scope should be passed through the valve during speech to appreciate lateral and posterior wall movements occurring below the upper surface. This procedure is particularly useful in patients with a pharyngeal flap. The anatomy of the velopharyngeal ports on either side of a pharyngeal flap and the function of each port during speech can be observed (Fig. 96–21). Passing the scope into the valve also allows observation of the movements of the dorsum of the posterior tongue (Fig. 96–22), attempts to elevate

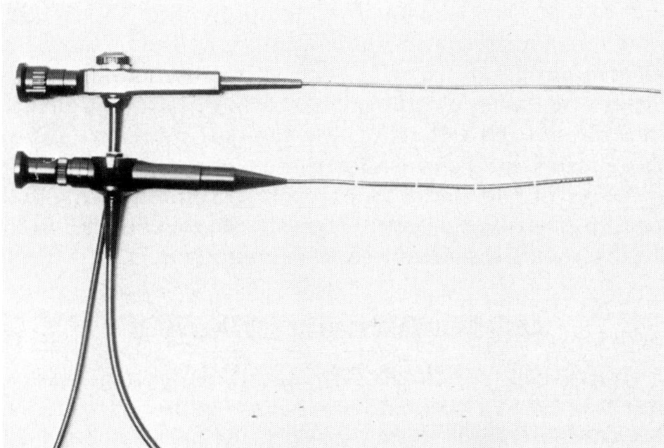

Figure 96–14 Machinda ENT 3L (upper) and Olympics ENFP (lower) nasopharyngoscopes.

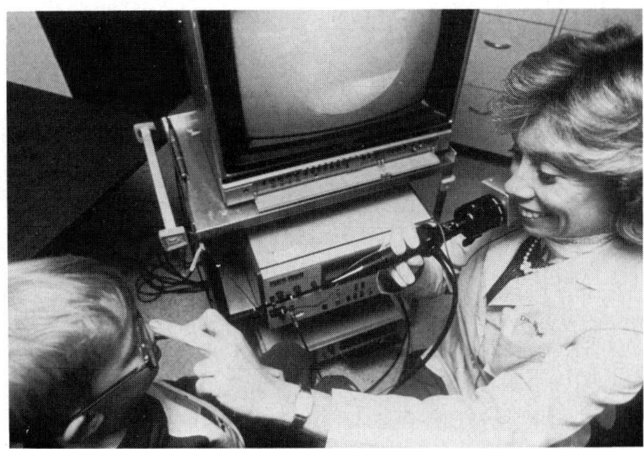

Figure 96–16 Nasopharyngoscope in the child's nose. The fiberoptic scope is connected to a TV camera to allow visualization of the port on the TV monitor.

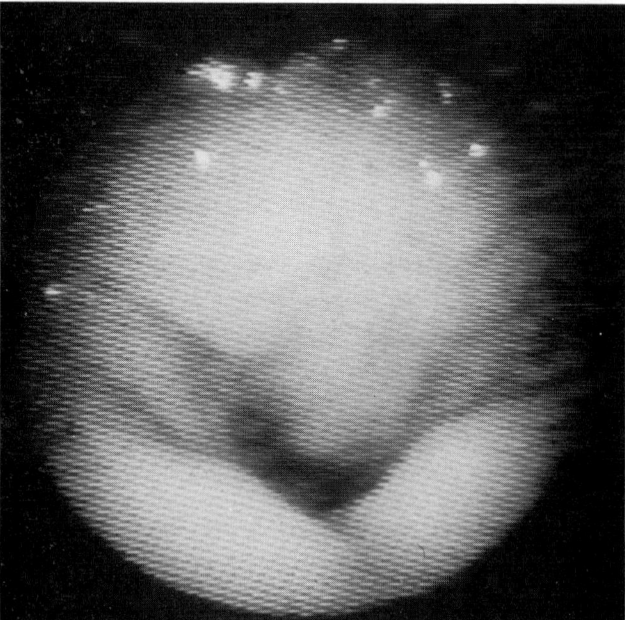

Figure 96–17 The velopharyngeal valve as viewed from above. The adenoid tissue is located in the upper part of the photograph, and the soft palate is shown in the lower aspect.

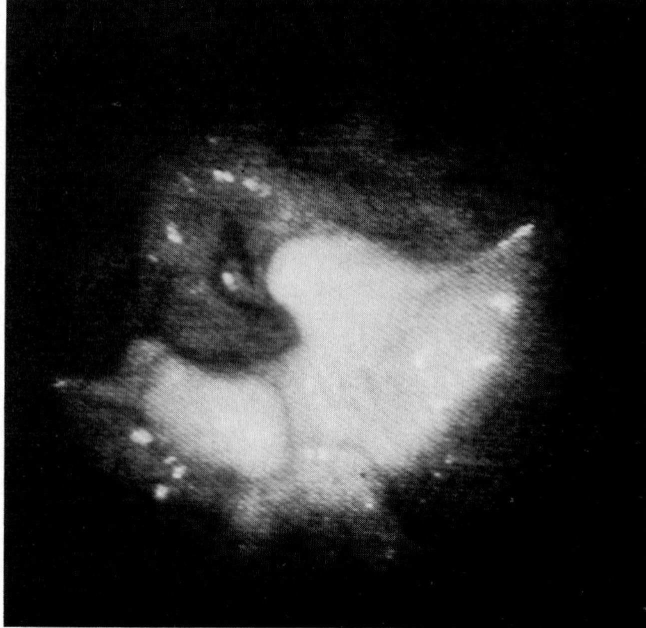

Figure 96–19 Cleft of the epiglottis in a child with cleft palate and Stickler syndrome.

the palate with the tongue, and compensatory articulation gestures such as the pharyngeal stop, pharyngeal fricative, or affricate. We recommend that the examination also include routine visualization of the laryngeal structures to screen for such findings as vocal nodules or polyps (Fig. 96–23), laryngeal granulomas, or abnormal use of the larynx (glottal stop articulation) and the larynx and epiglottis (laryngeal fricative and affricate articulation).[10]

Patient Cooperation

In general, adults and children over 8 years of age have no difficulty with the test. However, some children 3 to 8 years old may be apprehensive or frightened, particularly if they have had any negative hospital experiences or if their parents are anxious. In such cases, the parents and child are reassured, adequate anesthesia is used, and a relaxed and fun atmosphere is created. We have found techniques such as describing the scope as an elephant's trunk, claiming to be searching the nose for the "Cookie Monster" or other favorite childhood characters, and using small rewards such as stickers and balloons to be useful. The more relaxed the patient is, the more reliable the findings are. Children and parents are usually fascinated by the TV image. When a gentle approach emphasizing fun is used, a failed examination is rare, even in a preschool child.

Because some anesthetic may drip onto the laryngeal area and affect swallowing, the patient is advised not to eat or drink for 1 hour after the examination. Although insertion of the endoscope rarely results in intranasal bleeding, antibiotic prophylaxis should be considered in children with significant cardiac anomalies.

Analysis of Information and Reporting

The speech pathologist and attending surgeon review the videotaped examination results together and record their judgments of anatomy and function on a standard form, providing the basis for a written report.

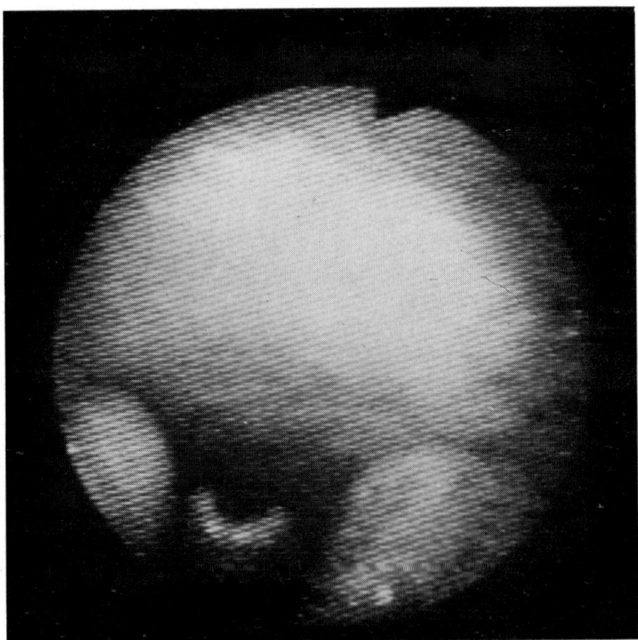

Figure 96–18 View of palatine tonsils and epiglottis from nasopharyngoscopy.

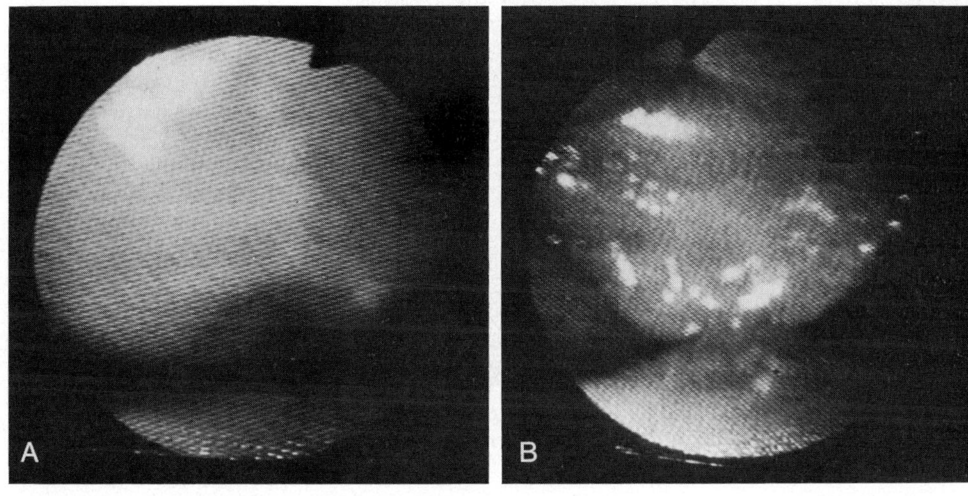

Figure 96–20 Child with a submucous cleft palate. *A*, Velopharyngeal closure appears complete just below the adenoid. *B*, On closer inspection, bilateral gaps were noted even though the soft palate contacted a Passavant's ridge in the midline.

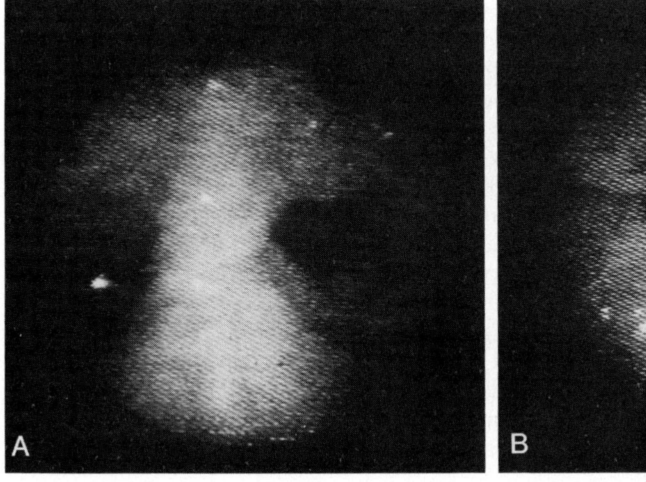
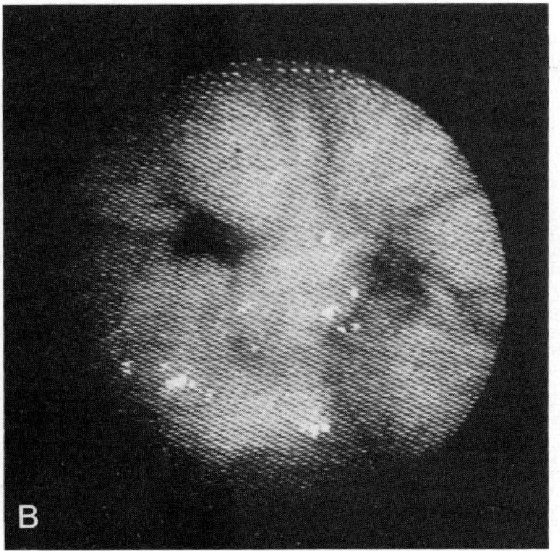

Figure 96–21 Patient with a pharyngeal flap. *A*, Ports open. *B*, Partial closure of both velopharyngeal ports during speech.

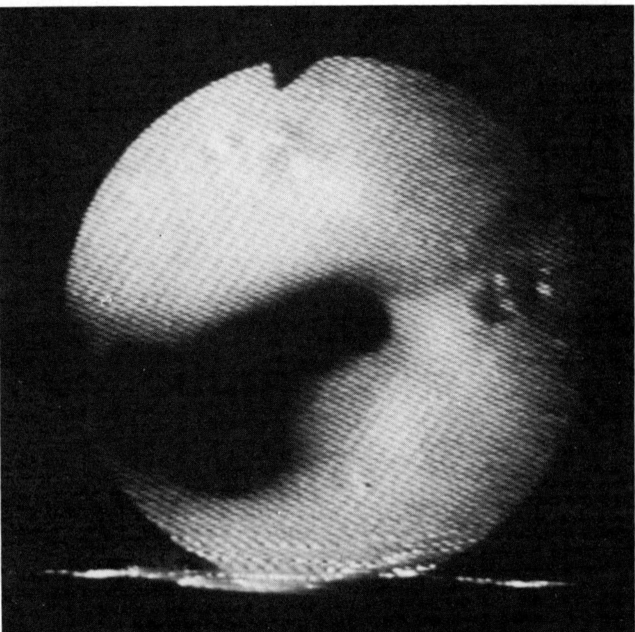

Figure 96–22 The nasopharyngoscope has been positioned to observe posterior tongue function through the velopharyngeal gap in a patient with velopharyngeal insufficiency.

Age of Assessment of Velopharyngeal Function

Clinical speech assessment can begin at any age, and children who are at risk for velopharyngeal insufficiency should be evaluated by clinical speech assessment regularly after the onset of speech to monitor speech and language development and ensure that therapy is provided when necessary. Imaging of velopharyngeal function during speech is most reliable when the child is mature enough to cooperate throughout the examination and has sufficient speech development and consistency in speech to allow evaluation of velopharyngeal valving during all classes of speech sounds. Therefore, except in a child who matures early, imaging assessments are not undertaken until 4 to 5 years of age.

Conclusions

The results of the clinical speech assessment and observations of the anatomy and function of the velopharyngeal valve are used to select the most appropriate treatment of the patient's speech characteristics. Abnormalities in anatomy and function of the structures of the vocal tract are not always responsible for speech outcome. The conditions of cleft lip and palate or other craniofacial anomalies are often complex, and the coexistence of speech problems and abnormalities in anatomy and function of the vocal tract are often assumed to be related. The correlation may truly exist, or the findings may be coincidental. Herein lies the challenge of diagnosis.

Treatment of speech problems related to velopharyngeal insufficiency usually involves speech therapy, surgery to the velopharyngeal valve, a dental prosthesis, or a combination of these procedures. During the past 25 years, clinicians have been concerned with assessing the dynamic aspects of velopharyngeal movements, but few actively use this information to adapt treatment to the specific needs of the patient.[29, 46, 53] However, we believe that careful, detailed assessment of velopharyngeal function combining clinical speech assessment with imaging techniques greatly increases the likelihood of selecting appropriate, efficient, and effective treatment. Some clinicians have already identified the need to develop methods to assess palatal bulk and elasticity, tension in the vocal tract, strength of the seal of the velopharyngeal valve during speech, timing of velopharyngeal movements during speech,[21, 46, 47, 52] size and shape of the resonating cavities,[76] and three-dimensional reconstruction of the velopharyngeal movements during speech. Furthermore, we believe that complete assessment of velopharyngeal function and its effects on speech should include evaluation of the entire vocal tract including tongue function and laryngeal anatomy and function.[73] As clinicians become more adept at assessing and interpreting the various components of the vocal tract that affect speech outcome, further refinements in treatment will be forthcoming.

ACKNOWLEDGMENT. This manuscript was prepared with the assistance of the Medical Publications Department and the Department of Visual Education, The Hospital for Sick Children.

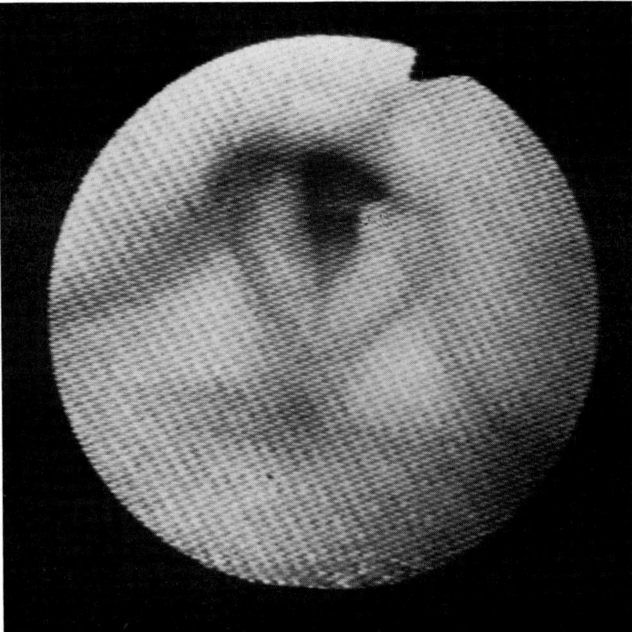

Figure 96–23 A polyp on the left vocal cord in a patient with inconsistent velopharyngeal closure.

References

1. McWilliams BJ, Bluestone CD, Musgrave RH: Diagnostic implications of vocal cord nodules in children with cleft palate. Laryngoscope 79:2072, 1969.

2. McWilliams BJ, Lavorato AS, Bluestone CD: Vocal cord abnormalities in children with velopharyngeal valving problems. Laryngoscope 83:1745, 1973.

3. Brodnitz FS: Vocal Rehabilitation. Rochester, MI: American Academy of Ophthalmology and Otolaryngology, 1971.

4. Ladefoged P: A Course in Phonetics. New York: Harcourt Brace Jovanovich, 1975.

5. Peterson SJ: Nasal emission as a component of the misarticulation on sibilants and affricates. J Speech Hear Dis 40:106, 1975.

6. Trost J: Articulatory additions to the classical description of the speech of persons with cleft palate. Cleft Palate J 18:193, 1981.

7. Trost-Cardamone JE: Effects of velopharyngeal incompetence on speech. J Child Commun Dis 10:31, 1986.

8. Morley ME: Cleft Palate and Speech, 7th ed. Baltimore: Williams & Wilkins, 1970.

9. Bzoch KR: Categorical aspects of cleft palate speech. In Bzoch KR (ed): Communicative Disorders Related to Cleft Lip and Palate. Boston: Little, Brown, 1971, pp 109.

10. Kawano M, Isshiki N, Harita Y, et al: Laryngeal fricative in cleft palate speech. Acta Otolaryngol (Suppl) 419:180, 1985.

11. Golding-Kushner K: The effect of articulation therapy on velopharyngeal closure. Paper presented at the Fourth International Congress on Cleft Palate and Related Craniofacial Anomalies, Acapulco, 1981.

12. Henningsson GE, Isberg AM: Velopharyngeal movement patterns in patients alternating between oral and glottal articulation: A clinical and cineradiographical study. Cleft Palate J 23:1, 1986.

13. Hoch L, Golding-Kushner K, Siegel-Sadewitz VL, et al: Speech therapy. Semin Speech Lang 7:313, 1986.

14. Shprintzen RJ: Surgery for speech. In Huddart AG, Ferguson M (eds): Cleft Lip and Palate—Long Term Results and Future Prospects. Manchester: Manchester University Press, 1988.

15. Fletcher SG: Diagnosing speech disorders from cleft palate. New York: Grune & Stratton, 1978.

16. Philips BR: An experimental investigation of the relationship between ratings of speech intelligibility based on auditory and visual cues and on auditory cues alone in a group of cleft palate adults. Masters thesis. Pittsburgh: University of Pittsburgh, 1954.

17. Subtelny JD, Van Hattum RJ, Myers BB: Ratings and measures of cleft palate speech. Cleft Palate J 9:18, 1972.

18. Moore WH, Sommers RK: Phonetic contexts: Their effects on perceived intelligibility in cleft-palate speakers. Folia Phoniatr 27:410, 1975.

19. Paynter ET, Kinard MW: Perceptual preferences between compensatory articulation and nasal escape of air in children with velopharyngeal incompetence. Cleft Palate J 16:262, 1979.

20. Paynter ET: Parental and child preference for speech produced by children with velopharyngeal incompetence. Cleft Palate J 24:112, 1987.

21. Folkins JW: Issues in speech motor control and their relation to the speech of individuals with cleft palate. Cleft Palate J 22:106, 1985.

22. Dickson DR: The normal velopharyngeal mechanism: Recent findings. J Child Commun Dis 10:5, 1986.

23. Skolnick ML, Shprintzen RJ, McCall GN, et al: Patterns of velopharyngeal closure in subjects with repaired cleft palate and normal speech: A multiview videofluoroscopic analysis. Cleft Palate J 12:369, 1975.

24. Croft CB, Shprintzen RJ, Rakoff SJ: Patterns of velopharyngeal valving in normal and cleft palate subjects: A multiview videofluoroscopic and nasendoscopic study. Laryngoscope 91:265, 1981.

25. Siegel-Sadewitz VL, Shprintzen RJ, Daniller AI: Multiview videofluoroscopic analysis of velopharyngeal closure in normals. Videotape produced by the Center for Craniofacial Disorders, Montefiore Medical Center, Bronx, New York, 1985.

26. Witzel MA, Posnick JC: Patterns and location of velopharyngeal valving problems: Atypical findings on video nasopharyngoscopy. Cleft Palate J 26:1, 1989.

27. Shprintzen RJ, Lewin ML, Croft CB, et al: A comprehensive study of pharyngeal flap surgery: Tailor made flaps. Cleft Palate J 16:46, 1979.

28. Shprintzen RJ: An invited commentary on the preceding article by Ibuki, Karnell and Morris. Cleft Palate J 20:105, 1983.

29. Shprintzen RJ: Evaluating velopharyngeal incompetence. J Child Commun Dis 10:51, 1986.

30. Siegel-Sadewitz VL, Shprintzen RJ: Changes in velopharyngeal valving with age. Int J Pediatr Otorhinolaryngol 11:171, 1986.

31. Osberg PE, Witzel MA: The physiologic basis for hypernasality during connected speech in cleft palate patients: A nasendoscopic study. Plast Reconstr Surg 67:1, 1981.

32. Isberg A, Henningsson G: Influence of palatal fistulas on velopharyngeal movements: A cineradiographic study. Plast Reconstr Surg 79:525, 1987.

33. McWilliams BJ, Morris HL, Shelton RL: Cleft Palate Speech. St. Louis: C. V. Mosby, 1984.

34. Fletcher SG: Theory and instrumentation for quantitative measurement of nasality. Cleft Palate J 7:601, 1970.

35. Fletcher SG, Bishop ME: Measurement of nasality with TONAR. Cleft Palate J 7:610, 1970.

36. Stevens KN, Kalikow DN, Willemain TR: A miniature accelerometer for detecting glottal waveforms and nasalization. J Speech Hear Res 18:594, 1975.

37. Stevens KN, Nickerson RS, Boothroyd A, et al: Assessment of nasalization in the speech of deaf children. J Speech Hear Res 19:393, 1976.

38. Reich AR, Redenbaugh MR: Relation between nasal/voice accelerometric values and interval estimates of hypernasality. Cleft Palate J 22:237, 1985.

39. Warren DW: Velopharyngeal orifice size and upper pharyngeal pressure-flow patterns in normal speech. Plast Reconstr Surg 33:148, 1964.

40. Warren DW, DuBois AB: A pressure-flow technique for measuring velopharyngeal orifice area during continuous speech. Cleft Palate J 1:52, 1964.

41. Warren DW, Devereux JL: An analog study of cleft palate speech. Cleft Palate J 3:103, 1966.

42. Warren DW: Nasal emission of air and velopharyngeal function. Cleft Palate J 4:148, 1967.

43. Warren DW, Ryon WE: Oral port constriction, nasal resistance, and respiratory aspects of cleft palate speech: An analog study. Cleft Palate J 4:38, 1967.

44. Warren DW: The determination of velopharyngeal incompetency by aerodynamic and acoustical techniques. Clin Plast Surg 2:299, 1975.

45. Warren DW: Perci: A method for rating palatal efficiency. Cleft Palate J 16:279, 1979.

46. McWilliams BJ: Unresolved issues in velopharyngeal valving. Cleft Palate J 22:29, 1985.

47. Warren DW, Dalston RM, Trier WC, et al: A pressure-flow technique for quantifying temporal patterns of palatopharyngeal closure. Cleft Palate J 22:11, 1985.

48. Warren DW: Compensatory speech behaviors in individuals with cleft palate: A regulation/control phenomenon. Cleft Palate J 23:251, 1986.

49. Dalston RM: Photodetector assessment of velopharyngeal activity. Cleft Palate J 19:1, 1982.

50. Karnell M, Seaver EJ, III, Dalston RM: A comparison of photodetector and endoscopic evaluation of velopharyngeal functions. J Speech Hear Res 31:503, 1988.

51. Seaver EJ, Karnell MP: Consistency of photodetector/endoscopic assessments of velopharyngeal activity (poster). The Cleft Palate Foundation 14th Annual Meeting. American Cleft Palate Association, Williamsburg, Virginia, April 26–29, 1988.

52. Zimmermann G, Dalston RM, Brown G, et al: Comparison of cineradiographic and photodetection techniques for assessing velopharyngeal function during speech. J Speech Hear Res 30:564, 1987.

53. Pannbacker M, Lass NJ, Middleton GF, et al: Current clinical practices in the assessment of velopharyngeal closure. Cleft Palate J 21:33, 1984.

54. Witzel MA, Tobe J, Salyer K: The use of nasopharyngoscopy biofeedback therapy in the correction of inconsistent velopharyngeal closure. Int J Pediatr Otorhinolaryngol 15:137, 1988.

55. Witzel MA, Tobe J, Salyer KE: The use of video nasopharyngoscopy for biofeedback therapy in adults after pharyngeal flap survery. Cleft Palate J 26:129, 1989.

56. Skolnick ML: Video velopharyngography in patients with nasal speech, with emphasis on lateral pharyngeal motion in velopharyngeal closure. Radiology 93:747, 1969.

57. Skolnick ML: Videofluoroscopic examination of the velopharyngeal portal during phonation in lateral and base projections—a new technique for studying the mechanics of closure. Cleft Palate J 7:803, 1970.

58. Quattromani FL, Benton C, Cotton RT: The Towne projection for evaluation of the velopharyngeal sphincter. Radiology 125:540, 1977.

59. LaRossa D, Brown A, Cohen M, et al: Video-radiography of the velopharyngeal portal using the Towne's view. J Maxillofac Surg 8:203, 1980.

60. Stringer DA, Witzel MA: Velopharyngeal insufficiency on videofluoroscopy: Comparison of projections. AJR 146:15, 1986.

61. Shprintzen RJ: Palatal and pharyngeal anomalies in craniofacial syndromes. Birth Defects 18:53, 1982.

62. Stringer DA, Witzel MA: Waters' projection for evaluation of lateral pharyngeal wall movement in speech disorders. AJR 145:409, 1985.

63. MacKenzie-Stepner K, Witzel MA, Stringer DA, et al: Velopharyngeal insufficiency due to hypertrophic tonsils. A report of two cases. Int J Pediatr Otorhinolaryngol 14:57, 1987.

64. Shprintzen RJ, Sher AE, Croft CB: Hypernasal speech caused by tonsillar hypertrophy. Int J Pediatr Otorhinolaryngol 14:45, 1987.

65. Williams WN, Eisenbach CR: Assessing VP function: The lateral still technique vs. cinefluorography. Cleft Palate J 18:45, 1981.

66. McWilliams BJ, Musgrave RH, Crozier PA: The influence of head position upon velopharyngeal closure. Cleft Palate J 5:117, 1968.

67. Stringer DA, Witzel MA: Comparison of multi-view videofluoroscopy and nasopharyngoscopy in the assessment of velopharyngeal insufficiency. Cleft Palate J 26:88, 1989.

68. Pigott RW, Bensen JF, White FD: Nasendoscopy in the diagnosis of velopharyngeal incompetence. Plast Reconstr Surg 43:141, 1969.

69. Shprintzen RJ, Schwartz RH, Daniller A, et al: Morphologic significance of bifid uvula. Pediatrics 75:553, 1985.

70. Miyazaki T, Matsuya T, Yamaoka M: Fiberscopic methods for assessment of velopharyngeal closure during various activities. Cleft Palate J 12:107, 1975.

71. Yamaoka M, Matsuya T, Miyazaki T, et al: Visual training for velopharyngeal closure in cleft palate patients: A fibrescopic procedure (preliminary report). J Maxillofac Surg 11:191, 1983.

72. Siegel-Sadewitz VL, Shprintzen RJ: Nasopharyngoscopy of the normal

velopharyngeal sphincter: An experiment of biofeedback. Cleft Palate J 19:194, 1982.
73. Witzel MA, Zuker RM, Crysdale WS: Velopharyngeal and laryngeal function: Essentials of the endoscopic examination. Paper presented at the Annual Meeting of the Society for Ear, Nose and Throat Advances in Children, New York, NY, 1988.
74. Shprintzen RJ, Croft CB: Abnormalities of the eustachian tube orifice in individuals with cleft palate. Int J Pediatr Otorhinolaryngol 3:15, 1981.
75. MacKenzie-Stepner K, Witzel MA, Stringer DA, et al: Abnormal carotid arteries in the velocardiofacial syndrome: A report of three cases. Plast Reconstr Surg 80:347, 1987.
76. MacKenzie-Stepner K, Hoffstein V, Witzel MA, et al: Measurement of pharyngeal and glottal area in craniofacial patients using the acoustic reflection technique. Program, The Cleft Palate Foundation 14th Annual Meeting. American Cleft Palate Association, Williamsburg, Virginia, April 26–29, 1988.

CHAPTER 97

Measurement Problems in Estimating Velopharyngeal Function

Michael P. Karnell and Earl J. Seaver

In this chapter issues that have been raised about various techniques for assessing velopharyngeal function will be examined and discussed. First, four specific measurement criteria or goals will be proposed for determining the applicability of techniques for assessing velopharyngeal adequacy for speech. Next, a brief description of *validity* and *reliability* will be provided as these terms are defined for the purposes of assessing velopharyngeal adequacy. The limits of clinical efficacy will be acknowledged. Some phonetic and physiologic aspects of velopharyngeal function will be discussed in relation to the manner in which they may contribute to measurement problems and complexity. We offer a summary of various techniques that have been used along with a discussion of the reliability, validity, and clinical efficacy of each. A perspective will be presented throughout the discussion regarding the role of instrumentation in the assessment of velopharyngeal adequacy for speech.

Goals of Velopharyngeal Measurement

Any discussion about problems associated with evaluation of velopharyngeal closure should include a discussion of the parameters of interest. It is imperative that there be a clear understanding about what aspects of velopharyngeal closure are important enough to include in our assessment techniques. We suggest that techniques used in the assessment of velopharyngeal closure for speech must meet some basic technical criteria. Any such technique should include provisions for obtaining information about any or all of four basic parameters of velopharyngeal closure: structure, movement, extent of closure, and timing.

Structure

The velopharyngeal structure is complex even in normal individuals.[1, 2] Although there are similarities among individuals, the absolute dimensions of and interrelationships among the velopharyngeal structures depend in part on age, sex, and other idiosyncratic variables that are not yet clearly understood.

The extent of normal variability is overshadowed by the variability that exists in individuals who have been born with palatal clefts.[3] Such variability complicates surgical treatment of structural deficits and may account for a considerable portion of the variability that occurs in surgical results.

Movement

The complexities of structural variability are accompanied by variability of velopharyngeal movement.[4–6] This aspect of velopharyngeal function has special relevance to those who attempt to evaluate the nature of velopharyngeal valving for speech. The resting configuration has little significance as long as there is sufficient movement of the structures to achieve velopharyngeal closure for oral speech sounds and velopharyngeal opening for nasal speech sounds and respiration.

Assessment of velopharyngeal movement includes assessment of each potential component of closure. These components are usually limited to the velum, the lateral pharyngeal walls, and the posterior pharyngeal wall. The results of evaluation of each component of velopharyngeal closure have important clinical significance. Some have advocated that the choice of treatment of velopharyngeal insufficiency should be contingent on the findings of a thorough physiologic examination of the relative contribution of each component of closure.[7, 8] The normal intersubject variability of the relative contribution to closure from each component has been demonstrated.[9, 10] Failure of any of these components to contribute adequately to closure can result in velopharyngeal insufficiency.[17]

Extent of Closure

This parameter imposes the most direct influence on perceived speech production. Indeed, it seems obvious that individuals with complete velopharyngeal closure should have no hypernasality or perceived nasal emission of air during speech production. Some studies have described in detail the relationship between various degrees of opening and oral or oronasal valving of air for speech.[1, 12] However, the presence of opening does not necessarily guarantee perceived evidence of velopharyngeal inadequacy. For example, Osberg and Witzel found that 13 of 19 patients with speech described as nonhypernasal failed to achieve complete velopharyngeal closure by videoendoscopic assessment.[11]

Some reports suggest that other variables interact with the extent of closure to produce perceived speech characteristics.[13-16] Although extent of closure is clearly important, consideration of this variable to the exclusion of others will result in limited understanding of the physiologic correlates of normal and abnormal speech production.

Timing

Finally, there is growing evidence that timing of velopharyngeal movement and closure must be considered, particularly in individuals with so-called borderline or marginal velopharyngeal adequacy.[16-20] The dynamic nature of speech production requires that movements of the palate be coordinated closely with movement of the lips, jaw, tongue, and larynx. Failure to achieve velopharyngeal closure at the right time, even though ability to achieve closure may have been demonstrated in some context, means that the patient does not have adequate velopharyngeal function for speech.

Validity and Reliability

Validity

Validity, in the context of velopharyngeal assessment, is generally considered the extent to which an assessment technique genuinely and accurately represents some aspect of the intended measurement parameter. Stated more concisely, validity is the extent to which a technique actually measures what the users of the technique intend it to measure.

Frequently, the validity of a measurement procedure seems so obvious that little if any attention is given to assessing it. In other procedures, validity is vague, less accepted, and more regularly assessed. Dalston and Warren have suggested that the validity of listener judgments, spectrography, Tonar II, pressure-flow, phototransduction, lateral cine- or videofluorography, multiview videofluorography, and oral and nasal endoscopy is acceptable when used for diagnosis of velopharyngeal inadequacy.[21]

In the context of diagnosing velopharyngeal insufficiency, one important outside criterion for establishing the validity of a measurement technique is the extent to which the findings agree with perceived judgments of oral-nasal resonance for speech. This approach was taken by McWilliams and her colleagues.[22] They found that pressure-flow data tended to misdiagnose most patients who were considered to have borderline velopharyngeal inadequacy (VPI) by perceptual judgments. Multiview videofluorography was found to agree with

perceived judgments in 100% (23/23) of borderline cases and in 87% (13/15) of incompetent cases. The authors infer that videofluorography findings are more valid than aerodynamic findings in diagnosis of velopharyngeal insufficiency. It seems probable that carefully obtained perceived and instrumental findings are both equally valid, each measuring different, yet related, phenomena. Incongruous findings may be central to the goal of further illuminating the complex relationship between perceived speech and its physiologic correlates.

Reliability

Reliability specifies the extent to which results of a technique are reproducible and therefore credible. The examination of reliability is particularly important for techniques that require clinical judgment. This obviously includes judgments of audible speech quality but also should include visual judgments about radiographic and endoscopic records and signal measurement techniques in which the measurement depends on investigator identification of specific signal characteristics (such as voice onset and offset). Any technique applied to the evaluation of velopharyngeal insufficiency must have measurable reliability.

Clinical Efficacy

Clinical efficacy refers to the extent to which a procedure or instrument is appropriate for a specific task, given the constraints of patient tolerance, time, cost, space, training, and other practical considerations that are characteristic of the patient population and clinical facility. Discussion of these considerations will be emphasized in the critical review that follows for only those procedures that seem to press the limits of clinical efficacy. Special consideration will be given to patient tolerance, ease of use, and expense.

Phonetic and Physiologic Considerations that Influence Measurement

A general finding of the research involving observations of the velopharyngeal mechanism during the production of speech is that the status of the mechanism varies according to both the phonetic and nonphonetic properties of the utterances used. These variations need to be carefully considered in any evaluation of the status of the velopharyngeal mechanism before analysis techniques are examined in detail.

A great deal of research involving phonetic influences on velopharyngeal function has focused on velar positioning. With few exceptions, the activity of the posterior and lateral pharyngeal walls is generally believed to be strongly correlated with the activity of the velum. Observations of velar positioning during speech production have revealed consistent differences in velar height between oral consonants, vowels, and nasal consonants. Consonants that require increases in intraoral air pressure are generally associated with higher velar positions than are consonants that require relatively little intraoral air pressure.[23] Several investigators have demonstrated that vowels with higher tongue positioning are associated with greater velar height than are vowels produced with lower tongue positioning.[24–28] Interestingly, Moore and Sommers reported that a hierarchical order of perceived intelligibility for vowels may exist in speakers with cleft palate.[29] In that study, intelligibility decreased from low to high vowels.

Differences in velar positioning also have been observed when voiceless consonants are compared with voiced consonants, although there is disagreement about those findings.[30–32] Studies of velar positioning also have resulted in the finding that various nonphonetic properties, such as rate of utterance and effort level, may be associated with variations in velar height.[25, 28, 33] Finally, phonetic effects of a given speech sound are often spread across phonetic boundaries to neighboring speech sounds. This is the phenomenon described as coarticulation.

Initial attempts to describe these variations in velar positioning focused on mechanical interconnections between the tongue and velum[24, 25] and on differences in palatal levator activity.[26, 27, 34] However, results from more recent studies have led investigators to broaden their perspective to view the velopharyngeal mechanism as a complex system, with active and passive components that all have the ability to affect velar positioning.[28, 35]

Although rarely reported directly, considerable inter- and intrasubject variation has been noted in the velopharyngeal activity of normal speakers. Velar height or pharyngeal wall displacements reported in most studies represent central tendency measurements with associated degrees of variability. This variability can be attributed to differences between individual speakers and the flexibility within a speaker to achieve velopharyngeal movements, in addition to the phonetic and nonphonetic speech influences summarized above. Obviously, this variability from subject to subject has to be taken into account when the adequacy of the velopharyngeal mechanism is evaluated.

Critical Review of Analysis Techniques of Velopharyngeal Insufficiency

It seems useful to estimate how assessment techniques measure up regarding the criteria described above. Table 97–1 includes a list of those techniques along with the authors' judgments about the extent to which each is acceptable with regard to the measurement criteria of structure, movement, closure, and timing. Judgments on reliability and validity as well as patient tolerance and expense are also provided. A critical discussion of each technique follows.

Perceptual Judgments of Speech Quality

Perceived hypernasality, nasal emission of air, and related articulation errors are widely considered primary symptoms of velopharyngeal insufficiency.[11, 13, 14, 22, 36–44] In fact, as indicated earlier, these attributes may be considered the outside criteria for judging the validity of instrumentation-based assessment techniques and for determining the need for treatment. Surveys indicate that judgments of perceived speech quality (nasality judgments, articulation testing, and so on) are the techniques most frequently used for assessing velopharyngeal insufficiency.[45, 46] For these reasons, the importance of an examination by a speech-language pathologist with appropriate credentials, including expertise on the speech characteristics of individuals with orofacial and craniofacial anomalies, cannot be overstated.

Table 97–1. Summary of Techniques Used to Assess Velopharyngeal Adequacy for Speech with Estimates of Applicability

Technique	Structure	Movement	Closure	Timing	Reliability	Validity	Patient Tolerance	Expense
Perceptual Judgments								
Speech quality	N	N	Y	N	Y	Y	Good	Low
Visualization/Imaging								
Transoral	Y/N	Y/N	N	N	Y	Y	Good	Low
Fluoroscopy	Y	Y	Y	Y[a]	Y	Y	Good	High
Endoscopy	Y	Y	Y	Y[a]	Y	Y	Fair	High
Ultrasound	Y	Y	N	Y[a]	N	Y	Good	High
Signal processing								
Spectrography	N	N	N	N	Y	Y	Good	High
Nasometry	N	Y[b]	Y	Y	Y	Y	Good	Moderate
Accelerometry	N	Y[b]	Y	Y	Y	Y	Good	Low
Aerodynamics	N	Y[b]	Y	Y	Y	Y	Good	Moderate
Mechanical	N	Y[b]	N	Y/N	Y	Y	Poor	Moderate
Photodetection	N	Y[b]	Y/N	Y	Y	Y	Fair	Low

N = No, technique is inadequate or does not apply; Y = yes, technique is adequate; Y/N = technique provides some data in this area but is generally inadequate.

[a]Usual video frame rate inadequate for most timing comparisons between velum and tongue or voicing. This problem can be resolved through the use of more expensive high-speed recording equipment.

[b]Movement can be detected but the specific contribution of individual structures cannot be differentiated.

Perceived speech judgments are fundamentally important for determining the need for additional testing and the need for treatment. They may or may not be useful for determining the type of treatment. For example, it is not possible to decide on the basis of perceived speech information alone whether a pharyngeal flap is the most appropriate treatment approach. Physiologic information is necessary before that decision can be made with confidence. However, if the degree of perceived symptoms of velopharyngeal inadequacy are quite variable in an individual, particularly if the individual shows some ability to eliminate or significantly reduce those symptoms under some controllable and repeatable circumstances, perceived observations may well be the basis for choosing speech therapy over surgery as an indicated treatment approach.

One limitation of judgments of perceived speech quality is that such judgments provide no objective information on structure, movement, or timing. The findings of McWilliams et al support the general belief that perceived hypernasality or nasal emission of air is a valid indication of inadequate closure, assuming the absence of other routes, such as a fistula, of air transmission to the nasal passages.[22] If this is true, such observations may relate to at least one of the four physiologic criteria we have considered important for assessment techniques. However, perceived speech characteristics do not linearly relate to the size of the velopharyngeal opening.[14] The finding of such characteristics suggests velopharyngeal insufficiency and indicates that confirming physiologic testing is warranted.

Reliability of judgments of perceived speech characteristics associated with velopharyngeal function generally has been good. This seems to be true for judgments of velopharyngeal competence,[22, 47, 48] speech intelligibility,[29] articulation defectiveness,[49–51] and nasalization.[16]

Van Demark reported an average of 75% agreement about the degree of judged velopharyngeal competence by four experienced clinicians based on 35 tape recorded samples of conversation produced by 108 children with cleft palate from Denmark.[47] Morris reported reliability of judged velopharyngeal competence based on perceived speech production of 101 patients with cleft palate who spoke Slovak.[48] Agreement among seven trained English-speaking American judges was 76.2%. Agreement was reported as 85.7% between those judgments and similar judgments made by a single trained speech pathologist who included in his rating radiographic, manometric, and oral-peripheral examination data.

McWilliams et al placed 48 subjects with repaired palatal clefts into nine categories differentiated on the basis of perceived speech production.[22] Those categories were then used to further categorize the subjects as competent, borderline, or incompetent. Their decisions were based on speech articulation, nasal escape of air, nasality, and vocal hoarseness. They reported 94% agreement among categorizations provided independently by two participating speech pathologists.

Reliability of speech intelligibility ratings when applied to patients with clefts has been shown to be quite

good under controlled conditions. For example, Moore and Sommers reported a correlation coefficient of 0.978 among average intelligibility ratings made by three trained judges of 16 cleft palate speaker's vowel-consonant-vowel syllable productions.[29]

Van Demark reported a correlation coefficient of 0.95 on the reliability of average ratings of articulation defectiveness provided by a group of 22 observers on 154 subjects with cleft palate.[49] Bardach and associates reported 85% to 95% agreement among trained American judges when rating articulation of 43 German children with repaired cleft palate.[50] Agreement was slightly lower, 65%, between untrained German judges and trained American judges. Agreement was high regarding ratings of severity of nasality. On a six-point scale, mean differences were less than one point. Riski and DeLong reported 97% agreement between two trained judges when evaluating articulation performance of 108 subjects with cleft palate.[51]

Reliability of nasalization ratings also has been shown to be acceptable. Karnell et al reported a correlation coefficient of 0.82 for test–retest agreement of ratings of nasalization on 50 consonant-vowel-consonant and consonant-vowel-nasal samples produced by four cleft palate speakers.[16]

Three observations can be made about the reliability of perceived speech characteristics based on the studies reviewed above. For most purposes, judgments of adequate reliability can be made about various perceived speech characteristics associated with cleft palate speech and about estimates of velopharyngeal competence based on such characteristics. Agreement seems to approximate 80% or higher in most cases. However, this finding must be considered in light of two additional observations. All of the studies used multiple judges. Test–retest agreement is likely to be higher when ratings of perceived speech characteristics are acquired from a single judge, but the credibility of such judgments is questionable. The importance of training must be emphasized also. Judging the presence and severity of characteristics of speech disorders associated with velopharyngeal insufficiency requires experience and sophistication. Given these and other sources of variability and error that can affect judgments of perceived speech quality, it seems imperative that reports of studies that use such judgments should routinely include evidence of reliability.

Visualization and Imaging

Transoral Observation. After judgments of perceived speech quality, the most clinically utilized method of obtaining information about velopharyngeal movement for speech is transoral observation.[45, 46] This technique is appealing because it is quick and simple, requiring only patient cooperation, a flashlight, and a tongue blade. It provides a direct view of the oral surface of the palate and velum and allows some limited observation of structure and movement. When movement is observed, judgments about movement symmetry may be possible.

However, it is not possible to observe directly the velopharyngeal mechanism by transoral observation because the plane of closure is almost always obscured by the mass and shape of the soft palate. Moreover, given the limits of speech sound production imposed by the presence of a firmly held tongue blade against the tongue dorsum or, in the absence of a tongue blade, extremely lowered jaw and tongue position, it is not possible to make inferences about velopharyngeal sufficiency. Transoral observation is a good starting place for evaluation of the velopharyngeal structure. However, if speech quality is judged to be hypernasal during conversational speech, additional testing beyond the transoral observation is always necessary.

Fluorography. Video or motion picture fluorographic examination of velopharyngeal structures and movements provides a visual means of viewing velopharyngeal function on selected planes of observation. Observation on multiple planes has been recommended to obtain information about the sphincteric function of the velopharyngeal mechanism.[5, 52] When properly performed, multiview fluorographic records of velopharyngeal function can provide information about all four basic aspects of velopharyngeal function: structure, movement, extent, and timing. Fluoroscopic diagnostic techniques are more frequently used than any other instrumentation-based technique for assessing velopharyngeal insufficiency.[45, 46]

The expense of the equipment required, the special expertise required to operate the equipment safely, and the inherent risks of radiation exposure require that fluorographic evaluation of velopharyngeal function be thoroughly justified and carefully performed. Because the equipment needed is imposing and is generally found in an intimidating setting, adequate patient cooperation must not be automatically assumed. The need for application of liquid contrast material further complicates the technique and jeopardizes young patient compliance. Limited image resolution and the necessity to limit total observation time to minimize patient radiation exposure may compromise precise observation of details such as the location of small, inconsistent breaches of closure. In spite of these limitations, fluorographic imaging of velopharyngeal function generally meets all of the technical criteria for an adequate velopharyngeal examination.

With few exceptions, the great majority of reports that use fluoroscopic techniques to assess velopharyngeal closure make no direct mention of validity. Some reports address validity indirectly. For example, Astley appeared to argue for the validity of his interpretation of frontal view cinefluorographic images of lateral wall movement because the configuration of the barium-coated pharyngeal outline appeared as expected in more than one fluorographic view.[53] Astley wrote, "Comparison of the disposition of the barium in the frontal and lateral pictures left no doubt that it was coating the nasopharyngeal walls." Skolnick included a comparison of cadaver material with videofluorographic images of the velopharyngeal area in the lateral and base views.[52] The comparison helped to establish the validity of videofluorographic imaging for evaluation of velopharyngeal configuration. Some investigators advocated the use of multiple radiographic perspectives (lateral, frontal, and base views) for videofluorographic evaluation of velopharyngeal closure in cleft palate patients.[5, 54] Use of multiple views in this manner provides some cross validation among the various views employed. Kuehn and Azzam used comparisons of dissections and radiographic views to demonstrate the validity of their findings.[55]

Sinclair et al directly compared videofluorographic and nasopharyngoscopic findings from 100 videotape records made of patients suspected of velopharyngeal insufficiency.[56] They also examined the effects of age and the presence of a pharyngeal flap on the quality of lateral and base view videofluorographic records and videoendoscopic records. Their findings generally indicated that percentage of videoendoscopic records considered "good" or "very good" dropped from 79% in patients 8 years and older to 57% in younger patients. Videofluorographic records of the lateral views were consistent at approximately 85% "good" or "very good," and records of the base view were consistent at 58% to 65% "good" or "very good." The presence of a pharyngeal flap reduced image quality in videofluorographic records but had no negative effect in videoendoscopic records.

Comparisons of anterior-to-posterior estimates of velopharyngeal gap indicated that basal view videofluorographic images showed a slightly larger gap than videoendoscopic records and lateral videofluorographic records. Anteroposterior gaps viewed from lateral videofluorographic records appeared slightly larger than those viewed by means of videoendoscopy. Comparison of basal view videofluorography and videoendoscopy regarding lateral wall movement indicated that the basal view yielded larger estimates of lateral wall movement.

It seems evident from this review that the validity of videofluoroscopy applied to the evaluation of velopharyngeal adequacy is acceptable when used with caution and interpreted by clinicians experienced in reading radiographic records. Reports employing videofluorographic data should routinely provide evidence of reliability, a measure that is easily accomplished by reporting the extent of agreement among multiple interpreters or repeated measurements.[22]

Endoscopy. Results of endoscopic examinations, like those of fluorography, have gained a considerable degree of acceptance among those who are charged with the task of assessing velopharyngeal closure for speech. This technique makes use of a variety of medical-grade periscopes, called endoscopes, that are designed specifically for examining internal body parts. It allows observation of the structure, movement, timing, and closure of the velopharyngeal area. Application of video cameras to the endoscopic technique provides the examiner with a relatively inexpensive method of producing permanent video records of endoscopic images for immediate playback and review. In spite of these advantages, videoendoscopy is reported to be used much less frequently than fluorographic techniques.[45, 46]

With the advent of advanced fiberoptics, the endoscopes used for observation of velopharyngeal closure are becoming smaller and therefore less invasive and presumably more tolerable for the patient. Such advances have made obsolete early endoscopes such as the Taub Oral Panendoscope with its large outside diameter and heat-producing incandescent light.[57, 58]

Several approaches to endoscopy have been described in the literature and are routinely used for velopharyngeal assessment. Oral endoscopy requires the use of a rigid endoscope with a lens configured so that a view can be obtained nearly parallel to the plane of the observation lens.[59, 60] It provides a view of the oral surfaces of the velopharyngeal area. When used appropriately, oral endoscopy can provide information about structure, movement, and timing. It is somewhat less invasive than nasal endoscopy and therefore poses fewer risks to the patient. Therefore, it continues to hold a place among the various approaches to endoscopy currently in use. In 1980, Schneider and Shprintzen reported that 22% of speech pathologists relied on oral endoscopy for evaluation of velopharyngeal insufficiency.[45]

Oral endoscopy does have several important limitations, however. Most important, the presence of the oral endoscope on the tongue causes inherent limitations to lingual movement during speech. Examiners attempt to sidestep this problem by limiting the speech sample used so that only sounds that do not require tongue elevation are necessary. Samples consisting of low vowels and bilabial consonants are most frequently used. Maximum velar elevation is not usually achieved during production of consonants in context with low vowels, a phenomenon that has been well documented in several studies. Moreover, the presence of the scope on the surface of the tongue may indirectly impose a mechanical load on the palate through the palatoglossus-palatopharyngeus and levator muscular linkage. Such a load may further inhibit velar movement. Oral endoscopy frequently causes stimulation of the gag reflex, which is clearly inconsistent with patient comfort and optimal speech production.

Nasal endoscopy is reported to be used less frequently than oral endoscopy.[45] However, it has certain advantages compared with oral endoscopy. By inserting the endoscope nasally and positioning it above the level of the soft palate, the examiner can observe the nasal surfaces of the velopharyngeal structures without influencing their movements directly or indirectly. Also, the movements of the oral articulators are uninhibited. Both rigid and flexible endoscopes have been advocated for nasal examination of velopharyngeal function. Of these, flexible fiberoptic endoscopes have enjoyed much wider acceptance, particularly in the United States, because they are easier to insert and more comfortable for the patient.

Another advantage of flexible nasal endoscopy is maneuverability. The flexible nature of the endoscope coupled with the tendon-wire tip control system included with all but the smallest of flexible scopes allows the examiner considerable freedom of movement in the nasopharynx and, when indicated, the oropharynx and hypopharynx. Such maneuverability has been shown to be very useful for observing lateral wall movement that may be obscured by palatal movement.

Karnell and Morris (1985) compared findings from oral and nasal endoscopic examinations in 15 normal adult individuals.[10] They reported that some of the data gave evidence that oral endoscopy may tend to underestimate posterior wall movement. They further suggested that the differences in observed pattern of closure between the two techniques were more likely differences in perspective rather than limitations in either procedure. Sinclair et al found that nasal endoscopic evaluation tended to underestimate lateral wall movement compared to base view videofluorography.[56]

Like fluoroscopy, endoscopy has traditionally enjoyed acceptance of so-called face validity. That is, there is common acceptance that if velopharyngeal insufficiency exists, it will be visible during an adequate endoscopic examination. Although this may be true for most clinical situations, considerable variability and subjectivity are involved, as is evident when attempts are made to correlate endoscopic data with acoustic or perceived data. This variability is particularly important when temporal considerations are being examined. Like fluorographic images, the complexity of endoscopic images requires that the images undergo substantial data reduction before they are used for either clinical or research purposes. This process of data reduction has most frequently been a matter of making visual judgments about the images, and such judgments are by their very nature inherently subjective. Moreover, the quality of the images is variable, particularly in younger patients.[56] Thus, just as with other techniques, there is a strong need to examine the reliability and validity of endoscopic images, and several reports with that intent have been published.[56, 61–63]

Sinclair and associates compared rigid and flexible nasal videoendoscopic records with lateral and base view videofluorographic records.[56] Those findings were described above in the discussion of fluorographic imaging techniques. Ibuki and his colleagues compared measurements from simultaneously recorded photoendoscopic and cinefluorographic images.[61] Agreement between measurements involving velar displacement was good, with correlation coefficients ranging from 0.87 to 0.99. Interjudge reliability of measurements of velar displacement from the endoscopic and fluorographic images was high (for endoscopy, r = 0.98; for fluorography, r = 0.95). Reliability of endoscopic measurements involving the lateral walls varied depending on the nostril through which the endoscope was inserted. Interjudge reliability was significantly better for the lateral wall on the side ipsilateral to endoscope insertion (r = 0.86) compared with the side contralateral to insertion (r = 0.09).

Clinical application of endoscopic techniques typically involves judgments of endoscopic images rather than measurements. For that reason, Karnell et al[62] examined agreement between judgments based on the same endoscopic and fluorographic images measured by Ibuki et al.[61] Agreement was high between endoscopic and fluorographic images regarding judgments about velar movement and diameter of the velopharyngeal port. Interjudge reliability was also high (r = 0.74 to 0.92) for those parameters but was considerably lower (r = 0.32 to 0.66) for judgments of lateral wall movement based on endoscopic images.

The data in the Ibuki et al and the Karnell et al reports described above were based on photographic, not video data and therefore were not influenced by observation of real-time velopharyngeal movement.[61, 62] Also, the endoscope they used, a flexible nasal endoscope with a side-mounted lens, is not commonly used for assessment of velopharyngeal closure outside Japan. Therefore, caution should be exercised when extending those data to videoendoscopic data derived through the use of rigid scopes or flexible scopes with end-mounted lenses.[64]

D'Antonio and her colleagues investigated the reliability of clinical judgments of end-view flexible endoscopic images of velopharyngeal closure observed in 95 videorecorded segments. This investigation considered differences among so-called "expert" raters as well as "novice" raters.[63] The data indicated that experience and expertise influence interpretation of endoscopic images of velopharyngeal closure. Moreover, in spite of the seemingly objective nature of the data, there is considerable variability of agreement about the extent of movement of the components of velopharyngeal closure, even among experts!

Ultrasound. A few studies have examined the use of ultrasound for noninvasive, nonradiographic assessment of lateral pharyngeal wall movement. Originally, this technique employed a single ultrasonic transducer that provided data about movement at a single point on the tissue-air interface of the lateral pharyngeal walls.[65-68] In that form, ultrasound is probably better described as a signal processing technique rather than an imaging technique. Skolnick et al described the application of a multi-element ultrasonic transducer that provides a radiographlike two-dimensional image of the lateral pharyngeal walls.[69] It is this latter technique that enjoys broad application today for various medical diagnostic purposes.

Ultrasonic data appear to reflect accurately the expected movements of the lateral pharyngeal wall being tested compared with the acoustic speech signal,[65-67] intraoral air pressure data,[68] and cineradiographic data.[66] The validity of the technique, therefore, appears to be adequate. Zagzebski pointed out that transducer placement below the external auditory canal posterior to the ramus of the mandible was necessary to obtain lateral pharyngeal wall data pertinent to velopharyngeal closure.[68] Kelsey et al pointed out that ratings of ultrasonic reflections of lateral wall movement can be made reliably and appeared to have some predictive value regarding speech outcome after pharyngeal flap surgery.[66]

Ultrasound application to assessment of velopharyngeal function has not gained wide acceptance as a diagnostic or research tool despite the promise it appeared to hold when it was first introduced. Difficulties

in obtaining useful ultrasonic data include problems in identifying the lateral wall with confidence and "multi-layered" signals that make interpretation subject to error. The latter of these problems appeared to be resolved by the introduction of multi-element transducers.[69] However, owing to the difficulty and subjectivity associated with positioning the transducer and the variable quality of the data provided, ultrasound has not been found to be an adequate replacement for radiographic imaging of the lateral pharyngeal walls.[70]

Signal Processing Techniques

The assessment techniques to be described below all involve the processing of some signal that has been produced by activity in the velopharyngeal mechanism. None of these techniques involve the direct observation of the structures of the mechanism, and therefore they have frequently been described as indirect assessment procedures. None of these techniques will provide information about the particular structures involved in closure and hence cannot provide detailed information about how those structures move. Therefore, these variables will not be discussed with each procedure.

Spectrography. Variations in velopharyngeal closure during speech lead to acoustic changes that may be perceived by listeners. Judgments about nasal versus non-nasal speech in normal subjects and judgments about abnormal speech characteristics (hypernasality, nasal distortion of consonants) discussed above are a result of the acoustic changes in the speech signal brought about by coupling of the oral and nasal cavities.

A number of investigators have attempted to describe the spectral changes associated with velopharyngeal opening.[71-75] Most of these studies have agreed on only two variables that appear to be related to the existence of hypernasality in speakers: a reduction in the amount of energy present in the first format, and the existence of antiresonances in the spectrum. Considerable inter- and intraspeaker variations have been observed. These forms of variability have been attributed to the complexity of the interactions between the opening into the nasopharynx (velopharyngeal opening), which can vary from speech sound to speech sound, and the nature of the oral cavity shape, which also can vary from speech sound to speech sound.[73, 74, 76, 77] This complex interaction between two variables, which can vary simultaneously during speech, has generally been thought to be the reason why spectrography is ineffective in quantifying the perceptual judgments of hypernasality.

Acoustic analyses of patients with velopharyngeal incompetence may have more potential in the investigation of timing of aberrations in speech motor control. Forner utilized spectrographic analyses to study various timing relationships in children with and without cleft palates.[78] By measuring speech segment durations, she was able to demonstrate differences in timing variables that may be significant in understanding the production problems imposed by an inadequate mechanism.

Dalston and Warren[21] point out that acoustic analyses may be useful in the further delineation of the acoustic characteristics associated with the production of various compensatory articulation behaviors that develop in response to velopharyngeal incompetence.[79, 80]

Without question, the spectrographic analysis of speech has face validity in determining the spectral distribution of energy. However, if validity is defined as the ability to measure the nasalization of speech, spectrography is quite lacking in this quality. Reliability, as determined by remeasurement of acoustic data, has generally been high.

Nasometry. TONAR (the oral-nasal acoustic ratio) was developed by Fletcher and his colleagues as an attempt to quantify judgments about the degree of perceived nasality of speech.[81] The most recent version of this device (Nasometer, Kay Elemetrics Corp) uses microphones placed in front of the oral cavity and nasal cavity openings. The microphones are separated by a sound isolator that rests against the upper lip. The outputs from both microphones can be input to a computer, which calculates the ratio between oral and oral plus nasal cavity output (nasalance).

Fletcher reported a correlation coefficient of 0.91 between listener judgments of hypernasality and nasalance scores derived from TONAR.[15] This high degree of relationship between the perceptual judgment and TONAR data makes nasometry an appealing method for the instrumental quantification of perceived nasality.

Dalston and Warren investigated the interrelationships among listener judgments, nasalance scores, and pressure-flow analysis in 124 clinical subjects.[21] They found a "reasonably high degree of correlation" among the data from these three procedures. If treatment decisions (no treatment, trial therapy, physical management) had been made using nasometry data alone, three patients would have been diagnosed as adequate when clinical judgments indicated that physical management was the treatment choice. Ten patients would have been recommended for trial therapy when physical management was the recommendation of the clinical judgments. When pressure-flow analysis data were incorporated into the decision process, the "instrumental error" would have been reduced to involve only 6 of the 188 patients for whom speech data were available. Clearly, these data provide additional support for the ability of nasometry to assist in the verification of clinical judgments.

Recent studies have resulted in data that suggest that nasometry can be used to assess velopharyngeal closure and timing. Dalston compared the changes in nasalance values from a nasometer and velopharyngeal opening using phototransduction (see below).[82] An average difference of 1 msec was found on comparison of the outputs of both devices when they indicated velopharyngeal opening maxima and minima. In addition, Dalston and colleagues found that velopharyngeal reaction times, as measured using simultaneous nasometry and phototransduction, were different by an average of less than 20 msec.[83] Therefore, when coupled to an output device (computer monitor), nasometry can provide time-varying information that may be useful in the study of speech motor control in clinical subjects. Certainly, the time-varying output may prove useful for biofeedback therapy.

Accelerometry. Several investigators have attempted to use miniature accelerometers placed on the surface of the nose to measure the vibrations associated with nasalized speech.[84–87] When the output from the nasal transducer is compared to the output from a laryngeal contact microphone, to account for variations in loudness, the resulting signal is felt to vary with the degree of nasalization exhibited by the patient.

To date, no studies have reported on the relationship between accelerometric output and physiologic measurements of velopharyngeal opening, so it is not clear to what extent one predicts the other.

Stevens et al published data on the use of the accelerometer to study nasalization in deaf children.[54] The authors presented some data depicting changes in accelerometer output as a function of time that appeared to indicate the presence of timing control problems in the subjects. However, to date no systematic comparisons have been made between changes in accelerometric output and changes in velopharyngeal activity monitored by other assessment techniques.

A number of studies have been conducted to compare the output from various modifications of the basic accelerometric instrumentation to listener judgments of hypernasality.[85, 88] In general, these studies have resulted in correlation coefficients ranging between 0.70 and 0.91, indicating a moderately strong relationship. However, these relationships were tested using normal subjects simulating nasality. Redenbaugh and Reich compared accelerometric data derived from their instrumentation and listener judgments (equal-appearing interval scale) of nasality in 12 hypernasal and three normal-speaking children.[87] The reliability of their accelerometric system was found to be high, as indicated by the strong positive correlation coefficient of 0.99. Moderate to strong correlation coefficients were found from the relationships between accelerometric output and ratings of sentences containing all obstruents and sentences containing glides. Better correlation coefficients were obtained for the obstruent sentences. No correlation was found for comparisons involving sentences containing only vowels and nasal consonants.

Jones et al found no relationship between temporal-magnitude accelerometric data and perceived ratings of nasalization in 20 speakers with cleft palate.[89] They qualified their findings owing to methodologic factors, however. For example, measures were taken from single word productions only. Different findings may have resulted from average measures obtained from longer samples.

Accelerometric devices are appealing from the clinician's point of view because of their relatively low cost and the noninvasive nature of the technique. Certainly the technique could be useful in the quantification of listener judgments of hypernasality.

Aerodynamic Measurements. Warren and his colleagues have reported on the effects of velopharyngeal inadequacy on oral-nasal air pressure and oral-nasal airflow relationships.[12, 43, 90, 91] Measurements of oral-nasal pressure differential and nasal flow can be placed in a hydrokinetic formula to estimate the area of opening in the velopharyngeal orifice at the moment of peak pressure of a stop consonant. These measurements attempt to relate various degrees of velopharyngeal opening to classifications of velopharyngeal incompetence (0 to 9 mm^2 indicates velopharyngeal competence; 10 to 19 mm^2, marginal or borderline incompetence; 19 mm^2 and above, incompetence). Although these categories can be used as guidelines for patient behavior, the speech characteristics exhibited by a particular patient will depend not only on the size of the velopharyngeal opening but also on the amount of nasal resistance and oral cavity configuration during the act of production.

The major advantage of the use of pressure-flow data in the assessment of velopharyngeal function is its ability to provide, in a minimally invasive fashion, quantifiable data that are reliable. Recent investigations by Smith and Weinberg have raised several questions about the validity, or accuracy, of the procedure in making "exact" measurements of velopharyngeal opening.[92–94] However, their results have generally indicated that the derived area measurements are reasonable estimates of openings in bench models (6% overall error estimate) and appear to be acceptable if clinicians do not attempt to overinterpret the measurements of velopharyngeal opening in the absence of perceptual judgments. The technique provides information during stop consonant production about the extent of closure. Obviously, this is true in the absence of significant nasal resistance that would be greater than the resistance provided by the approximated velopharyngeal mechanism. This caveat probably suggests that measurements using this technique should be accompanied by measurement of nasal resistance as well.

Although the reliability of pressure-flow analysis has not been tested directly, one would assume from bench-model studies that it would be very acceptable. However, the inherent variability of speech production indicates that multiple measurements should be made on each patient.

Warren et al reported on the use of pressure-flow analysis to study the timing relationships between nasal flow and transvelar pressure differential.[20] Their results led them to suggest that timing measurements could be made from production of the word *hamper* that would differentiate patients with differing degrees of velopharyngeal adequacy. Therefore, it would appear that pressure-flow analysis is capable of providing timing information within a limited context.

Mechanical Methods. Horiguchi and Bell-Berti have reported on the Velotrace, which consists of two levers connected to a light-emitting diode (LED) by way of a push rod.[95] The internal lever is inserted transnasally so that it rests upon the superior surface of the velum. This internal lever is connected to an external lever for support and to the push rods that transfer the movements of the internal lever to the external lever. The external lever houses a light-emitting diode, allowing velar movements to be transferred to light variations that can be displayed for analysis. The authors reported

two evaluation studies. One utilized endoscopic data from one subject and Velotrace data from another subject. Ensemble averages from the devices and for the two separate subjects appeared to display similar patterns of movement. A second evaluation study utilized simultaneous cineradiographic and Velotrace data collected from a single subject. Comparisons of the position of the Velotrace and the vertical position of the velum resulted in correlation coefficients ranging from 0.982 to 0.995 for the 12 tokens produced. Questions of validity and reliability appear to have been addressed by these two studies.

Therefore, it appears that this device is capable of tracking changes in velar height as seen in cineradiographic studies and has application to the study of timing changes in the position of the velum. However, no information is obtainable from this device about the extent of velopharyngeal closure.

Phototransduction. Dalston reported on using phototransduction to monitor changes in velopharyngeal opening.[96] A small pick-up probe attached to a photocell is inserted transnasally through the velopharyngeal orifice into the oral pharynx. Light from a nasally positioned probe is transmitted through the velopharyngeal port and is sensed by the pick-up probe. The amount of light transmitted through the velopharyngeal portal is directly proportional to the size of the opening. Dalston reported finding a correlation coefficient of 0.91 between openings measured using phototransduction and pressure-flow analysis in normal-speaking subjects simulating various degrees of velopharyngeal incompetence. Moon and Lagu reported finding a correlation coefficient of 0.998 between phototransduction output and cross-sectional area in a bench model.[97] These two studies indicate that phototransduction can be used to monitor the extent of velopharyngeal closure.

Comparisons have been made also between the output of the phototransduction system and observations of velopharyngeal movement using cineradiography[98] and nasal endoscopy.[99] In general, phototransduction was found to agree with these two procedures in determining onsets and offsets of velopharyngeal opening and closing gestures. Large disagreements (greater than 30 to 40 msec) between the procedures were considered to be due to imaging problems associated with either the radiographic or endoscopic procedures. The results from these studies and others[82, 83] indicate that phototransduction can be useful in studying the timing of velopharyngeal closure.

The reliability of phototransduction in measuring velopharyngeal opening is reported to be excellent, as indicated by bench-model testing. In addition, Dalston presented data in figure form that demonstrated the repeatability of phototransduction in monitoring changes in velopharyngeal opening.[96] It is assumed that any variability in performance observed within subjects would be due to variability in the subject, not the instrumentation.

Although initial bench-model testing[97] and comparisons with pressure-flow analysis[96] are encouraging with regard to validity, some questions have been raised about the effects of variables of tissue reflectivity and translucency and the presence of mucus and velopharyngeal configuration on the ability of phototransduction to monitor the extent of closure and timing. However, the consistently acceptable comparisons of the results of this technique with the results of cinefluorography,[98] nasal videoendoscopy,[99] and nasometry[21, 82, 83] indicate that the influence of these effects may be minimal. Specific criteria for determining the presence of complete velopharyngeal closure from phototransduction data alone have yet to be identified.

Conclusion

It is clear that the complexities of the velopharyngeal mechanism have induced complexities in the development of assessment techniques and procedures. It is also clear that no single technique is superior to the exclusion of all others. Flexibility is necessary to fit the appropriate assessment techniques to the patient in order to elicit the maximum amount of useful information.

It has not been the purpose of this chapter to determine the best assessment technique for the evaluation of velopharyngeal function. Rather, we have reviewed various procedures in light of the information these procedures provide about structure, movement, closure, and timing of velopharyngeal function, the validity and reliability of each procedure, and, finally, the constraints placed on each by clinical efficacy.

It is anticipated that the information discussed above will serve as a reference for clinicians and investigators in determining the procedures that may work best in any given assessment situation. Specific applications must then proceed with caution and with a clear vision of the strengths and limitations of the chosen techniques. Most important, the clinician must always recognize that instrumentation serves to assist, never to replace, sound clinical judgment.

References

1. Bjork L: Velopharyngeal Function in Connected Speech. Uppsala: Appelbergs Boktryckeri AB, 1961.
2. Bjork L, Nylen BO: Cineradiography with synchronized sound spectrum analysis: A study of velopharyngeal function during connected speech in normals and cleft palate cases. Plast Reconstr Surg 27:397, 1961.
3. Maue-Dickson W, Dickson DR: Anatomy and physiology related to cleft palate: Current research and clinical implications. Plast Reconstr Surg 65:83, 1980.
4. Moll KL: A cinefluorographic study of velopharyngeal function in normals during various activities. Cleft Palate J 2:112, 1965.
5. Skolnick ML, McCall GN, Barnes M: The sphincteric mechanism of velopharyngeal closure. Cleft Palate J 10:286, 1973.
6. Shprintzen RJ, Lencione RM, McCall GN, et al: A three dimensional cinefluoroscopic analysis of velopharyngeal closure during speech and nonspeech activities in normals. Cleft Palate J 11:412, 1974.
7. Shprintzen RJ, Rakoff SJ, Skolnick ML, et al: Incongruous movements of the velum and lateral pharyngeal walls. Cleft Palate J 14:148, 1977.
8. Jackson I: Sphincter pharyngoplasty. Clin Plast Surg 12:711, 1985.
9. Croft CB, Shprintzen RJ, Rakoff SF: Patterns of velopharyngeal valving in normal and cleft palate subjects: A multiview videofluoroscopic and nasendoscopic study. Laryngoscope 91:265, 1981.
10. Karnell MP, Morris HL: Multiview videoendoscopic evaluation of velopharyngeal physiology in 15 normal speakers. Ann Otol Rhinol Laryngol 94:361, 1985.
11. Osberg PE, Witzel MA: The physiologic basis for hypernasality during connected speech in cleft palate patients: A nasendoscopic study. J Plast Reconstr Surg 67:1, 1981.
12. Warren DW, Dubois AB: A pressure-flow technique for measuring velopharyngeal orifice area during continuous speech. Cleft Palate J 1:52, 1964.
13. Shelton RL Jr, Brooks AR, Youngstrom KA: Articulation and patterns of palatopharyngeal closure. J Speech Hear Res 29:390, 1964.
14. Brandt SD, Morris HL: The linearity of the relationship between articulation errors and VPI. Cleft Palate J 2:176, 1965.
15. Fletcher S: Theory and use of Tonar II - a status report. Biocommunication Res Rep 1:1, 1970.
16. Karnell MP, Folkins JW, Morris HL: Relationships between perceived and kinematic aspects of speech production in cleft palate speakers. J Speech Hear Res 28:63, 1985.
17. D'Antonio LL: An investigation of speech timing in individuals with cleft palate. Unpublished dissertation. San Francisco: University of California, 1982.
18. Kuehn DP: A cineradiographic investigation of velar movement variables in two normals. Cleft Palate J 13:88, 1976.
19. Zimmermann GN, Karnell MP, Retalliata P: Articulatory coordination and the clinical profile of two cleft palate speakers. J Phonetics 12:297, 1984.
20. Warren DW, Dalston RM, Trier RW, et al: A pressure-flow technique for quantifying temporal patterns of palatopharyngeal closure. Cleft Palate J 22:11, 1985.
21. Dalston RM, Warren DW: Comparison of Tonar II, pressure flow and listener judgments of velopharyngeal function. Cleft Palate J 23:108, 1986.
22. McWilliams BJ, Glaser ER, Philips BJ, et al: A comparative study of four methods of evaluating velopharyngeal adequacy. J Plast Reconstr Surg 68:1, 1981.
23. Moll KL, Daniloff RG: Investigation of the timing of velar movements during speech. J Acoust Soc Am 50:678, 1971.
24. Moll KL: Velopharyngeal closure on vowels. J Speech Hear Res 5:30, 1962.
25. Moll KL, Shriner T: Preliminary investigation of a new concept of velar activity during speech. Cleft Palate J 4:58, 1967.
26. Lubker JE: An electromyographic-cinefluorographic investigation of velar function during speech production. Thesis (Ph.D.). Iowa City: University of Iowa, 1967.
27. Fritzell B: The velopharyngeal muscles in speech: An electromyographic-cineradiographic study. Acta Otolaryng Suppl 250, 1969.
28. Seaver EJ, Kuehn DP: A cineradiographic and electromyographic investigation of velar positioning in non-nasal speech. Cleft Palate J 17:216, 1980.
29. Moore WH, Sommers RK: Phonetic contexts: Their effects on perceived intelligibility in cleft palate speakers. Folia Phoniatr 27:410, 1975.
30. Kent RD: Vocal-tract characteristics of the stop cognates. MA Thesis. Iowa City: University of Iowa, 1969.
31. Perkell JS: Physiology of Speech Production: Results and Implications of a Quantitative Cineradiographic study. Cambridge: MIT Press, 1969.
32. Bell-Berti F, Hirose H: Velar activity in voicing distinctions: A simultaneous fiberoptic and EMG study. Status Reports Speech Research. Haskins Lab, SR–31/32, 223, 1972.
33. Tucker LT: Articulatory variations in normal speakers with changes in vocal pitch and effort. MA Thesis. Iowa City: University of Iowa, 1963.
34. Bell-Berti F: An electromyographic study of velopharyngeal function. J Speech Hear Res 19:225, 1976.
35. Kuehn DP, Folkins JW, Cutting CB: Relationships between muscle activity and velar position. Cleft Palate J 19:25, 1982.
36. McWilliams BJ: Some factors in the intelligibility of cleft palate speech. J Speech Hear Dis 19:524, 1954.
37. Morris HL: Etiologic bases for speech problems. In Edwards M, Watson ACH (eds): Advances in Cleft Palate. New York: Academic Press, 1968.
38. Morris HL, Smith JK: A multiple approach for evaluating velopharyngeal competency. J Speech Hear Dis 27:218, 1962.
39. Curtis JF: Acoustics of speech production and nasalization. In Spriestersbach D, Sherman D (eds): Cleft Palate and Communication. New York: Academic Press, 1968.
40. Subtelny JD, Subtelny JD: Intelligibility and associated physiological factors of cleft palate speakers. J Speech Hear Res 2:353, 1959.
41. Weinberg B, Shanks G: The relationship between three oral breath pressure ratios and ratings of severity of nasality for talkers with cleft palate. Presented at the Annual Convention of the American Cleft Palate Association, Pittsburgh, 1970.
42. Carney PJ, Morris HL: Structural correlates of nasality. Cleft Palate J 8:307, 1971.
43. Warren DW: The determination of velopharyngeal incompetence by aerodynamic and acoustic techniques. Clin Plast Surg 2:299, 1975.
44. Moller KT, Burzynski C, Garber S, et al: Self-perception of hypernasality in speakers wearing speech appliances. Paper presented at the American Speech Language Hearing Association, Los Angeles, California, 1981.
45. Schneider E, Shprintzen RJ: A survey of speech pathologists: Current trends in the diagnosis and management of velopharyngeal insufficiency. Cleft Palate J 17:249, 1980.
46. Pannbacker M, Lass NJ, Middleton GF, et al: Current clinical practices in the assessment of velopharyngeal closure. Cleft Palate J 21:33, 1984.
47. Van Demark DR: Assessment of velopharyngel competency for children with cleft palate. Cleft Palate J 11:310, 1974.

48. Morris HL: Velopharyngeal competence and the Demjen W/V-Y technique. In Morris HL (ed): The Bratislava Project. Iowa City: University of Iowa Press, 1978.

49. Van Demark DR: Misarticulations and listener judgments of the speech of individuals with cleft palates. Cleft Palate J 1:232, 1964.

50. Bardach J, Morris HL, Olin WH: Late results of primary veloplasty: The Marburg Project. Plast Reconstr Surg 73:207, 1984.

51. Riski JE, DeLong E: Articulation development in children with cleft lip/palate. Cleft Palate J 21:57, 1984.

52. Skolnick ML: Videofluoroscopic examination of the velopharyngeal portal during phonation in lateral and base projections—a new technique for studying the mechanics of closure. Cleft Palate J 7:803, 1970.

53. Astley R: The movements of the lateral walls of the nasopharynx: A cineradiographic study. J Laryngol 72:325, 1958.

54. Iglessius A, Kuehn DP, Morris HL: Simultaneous assessment of pharyngeal wall and velar displacement for selected speech sounds. J Speech Hear Res 23:429, 1980.

55. Kuehn DP, Azzam NA: Anatomical characteristics of palatoglossus and the anterior faucial pillar. Cleft Palate J 15:349, 1978.

56. Sinclair SW, Davies DM, Bracka A: Comparative reliability of nasal pharyngoscopy and videofluorography in the assessment of velopharyngeal incompetence. Br J Plast Surg 35:113, 1982.

57. Taub S: The Taub oral panendoscope: A new technique. Cleft Palate J 3:328, 1966.

58. Willis CR, Stutz ML: The clinical use of the Taub oral panendoscope in the observation of velopharyngeal function. J Speech Hear Dis 37:495, 1972.

59. Zwitman DH, Sonderman JC, Ward PH: Variations in velopharyngeal closure assessed by endoscopy. J Speech Hear Dis 39:366, 1974.

60. Beery QC, Aramny MA, Katzenberg B: Oral endoscopy in prosthodontic management of the soft palate defect. J Prosthet Dent 54:241, 1985.

61. Ibuki I, Karnell MP, Morris HL: Reliability of the nasopharyngeal fiberscope (NPF) for assessing velopharyngeal function. Cleft Palate J 20:97, 1983.

62. Karnell MP, Ibuki I, Morris HL, et al: Reliability of the nasopharyngeal fiberscope (NPF) for assessing velopharyngeal function: Analysis by judgment. Cleft Palate J 20:199, 1983.

63. D'Antonio LL, Marsh JL, Province MA, et al: Reliability of flexible fiberoptic nasopharyngoscopy for evaluation of velopharyngeal function in a clinical population. Paper presented at the Annual Meeting of the American Cleft Palate Association, Williamsburg, Virginia, April 27–28, 1988.

64. Karnell MP: The nasopharyngeal fiberscope. Cleft Palate J 20:260, 1983.

65. Kelsey CA, Minifie FD, Hixon TJ: Applications of ultrasound in speech research. J Speech Hear Res 12:564, 1969.

66. Kelsey CA, Evanowski SJ, Crummy AB, et al: Lateral pharyngeal wall motion as a predictor of surgical success in velopharyngeal insufficiency. N Engl J Med 287:64, 1972.

67. Minifie FD, Hixon TJ, Kelsey CA, et al: Lateral pharyngeal wall movement during speech production. J Speech Hear Res 12:584, 1970.

68. Zagzebski JA: Ultrasonic measurement of lateral pharyngeal wall motion at two levels in the vocal tract. J Speech Hear Res 18:308, 1975.

69. Skolnick ML, Zagzebski JA, Watkin KL: Two dimensional ultrasonic demonstration of lateral pharyngeal wall movement in real time—A preliminary report. Cleft Palate J 12:299, 1975.

70. Skolnick ML: Personal communication. 1988.

71. Curtis JF: An experimental study of wave-composition of nasal voice quality. Thesis (Ph.D). Iowa City: University of Iowa, 1942.

72. Hattori S, Yamanoto K, Fujimura O: Nasalization of vowels in relation to nasals. J Acoustical Soc Am 30:267, 1958.

73. Fant G: Acoustic Theory of Speech Production. The Hague: Mouton, 1960.

74. Dickson DR: An acoustic study of nasality. J Speech Hear Res 5:103, 1962.

75. Andrews JA, Rutherford D: Contribution of nasally emitted sound to the perception of hypernasality of vowels. Cleft Palate J 9:147, 1972.

76. House AS, Stevens KN: Analog studies of the nasalization of vowels. J Speech Hear Dis 21:218, 1956.

77. Schwartz MF: Acoustic measures of nasalization and nasality. In Bzoch KR (ed): Communicative Disorders Related to Cleft Lip and Palate, 2nd ed. Boston: Little, Brown, 1979.

78. Forner LL: Speech segment duration production by 5- and 6-year-old speakers with and without cleft palates. Cleft Palate J 20:185, 1983.

79. Honjow I, Isshiki N: Pharyngeal stops in cleft palate speech. Folia Phoniatr 23:347, 1971.

80. Weinberg B, Horii Y: Acoustic features of pharyngeal /s/ fricatives produced by speakers with cleft palate. Cleft Palate J 12:12, 1975.

81. Fletcher S: Theory and instrumentation for quantitative measurement of nasality. Cleft Palate J 7:601, 1970.

82. Dalston RM: Using simultaneous photodetection and nasometry to monitor velopharyngeal behavior during speech. J Speech Hear Res 32:195–202, 1989.

83. Dalston RM, Seaver EJ, Keefe MJ: Nasometric and phototransductive measurement of reaction times among normal adult speakers. Cleft Palate J (in press).

84. Stevens KN, Nickerson RS, Boothroyd A, et al: Assessment of nasalization in the speech of deaf children. J Speech Hear Res 19:393, 1976.

85. Edgerton MT, Sadove M, Compton M, et al: Nasal vibration analysis: A noninvasive objective technique to evaluate the speech of patients with palatopharyngeal disorders. Plast Reconstr Surg 68:153, 1981.

86. Horii Y: An accelerometric measure as a physical correlate of perceived hypernasality in speech. J Speech Hear Res 26:476, 1983.

87. Redenbaugh MA, Reich AR: Correspondence between an accelerometric nasal/voice amplitude ratio and listeners' direct magnitude estimations of hypernasality. J Speech Hear Res 28:273, 1985.

88. Horii Y, Lang JE: Distributional analyses of an index of nasal coupling (HONC) in simulated hypernasal speech. Cleft Palate J 18:279, 1981.

89. Jones DL, Folkins JW, Morris HL: Speech production time and judgments of disordered nasalization in speakers with cleft palate. J Speech Hear Res (In press, 1989).

90. Warren DW: Velopharyngeal orifice and upper pharyngeal pressure-flow patterns in cleft palate speech: A preliminary study. Plast Reconstr Surg 34:14, 1964.

91. Warren DW: Velopharyngeal orifice size and upper pharyngeal pressure-flow patterns in normal speech. Plast Reconstr Surg 33:148, 1964.

92. Smith BE, Weinberg B: A re-examination of model experimentation. Cleft Palate J 17:277, 1980.

93. Smith BE, Weinberg B: Prediction of modeled velopharyngeal orifice areas during steady flow conditions and during aerodynamic simulation of voiceless stop consonants. Cleft Palate J 20:1, 1982.

94. Smith BE, Weinberg B: Velopharyngeal orifice area prediction during aerodynamic simulation of fricatives. Cleft Palate J 20:1, 1983.

95. Horiguchi S, Bell-Berti F: The velotrace: A device for monitoring velar position. Cleft Palate J 24:104, 1987.

96. Dalston RM: Photodetector assessment of velopharyngeal activity. Cleft Palate J 19:1, 1982.

97. Moon JB, Lagu RK: Development of a second generation phototransducer for the assessment of velopharyngeal activity. Cleft Palate J 24:240, 1987.

98. Zimmermann G, Dalston RM, Brown C, et al: Comparison of cineradiographic and photodetection techniques for assessing velopharyngeal function during speech. J Speech Hear Res 30:564, 1987.

99. Karnell MP, Seaver EJ, Dalston RM: A comparison of photodetector and endoscopic evaluations of velopharyngeal function. J Speech Hear Res 31:503, 1988.

CHAPTER 98

Oronasal Fistulas and Speech Production

Gunilla Henningsson and Annika Isberg

Oronasal fistulas in cleft palate patients are a well-known residual condition that occasionally occurs after cleft palate repair. Of the symptoms mentioned in the literature, regurgitation of fluid into the nasal cavity is the most commonly noted. It also is known that an oronasal fistula can influence speech, mainly by means of an extra acoustic component caused by air leakage through the fistula. In patients with large fistulas, the associated nasalization has been presumed to result from a major airflow through the oronasal passage. Some authors have expressed the opinion that a small palatal fistula has no effect at all on resonance.[1, 2] However, it has recently been demonstrated that both small and large oronasal fistulas can impair velopharyngeal function and result in hypernasality.[3, 4] As indicated later, documenting the size and location of an oronasal fistula and evaluating its influence on speech and resonance are very important in the choice of treatment.

Incidence and Location of Oronasal Fistulas

The reported incidence of fistulas following surgery for cleft lip and palate varies between 9% and 47% and is influenced by the surgical technique used.[5–8] Fistulas are more frequent in patients with cleft lip and palate than in those with a cleft palate only.[9] A fistula may be found anywhere along the midline of the former cleft, from the buccal sulcus through the alveolar ridge into the hard palate and occasionally involving its whole length into the velum, but the most frequent location is the area of the incisive foramen or at the conjunction of the hard and soft palate.

Clinical Examination of the Fistula

The examination of a suspected fistula can be performed in several ways. For example, a thin, stiff, but soft rubber stick can be smoothly inserted into the passage; some children do react negatively, however. Another technique is to illuminate the area from above by means of a nasopharyngoscope, inspecting the palate from below. To examine the possible influence of a documented fistula on speech, the fistula must be temporarily covered. The most common material for this is dental wax or chewing gum. An advantage of

using chewing gum is that the child is usually familiar with it and can use his or her own tongue to place it correctly over the fistula. If this fails, the examiner must help. Regardless of the material used, it stays in place better if the surrounding mucosa is dried carefully before covering the fistula.

The speech material is repeated by the patient with the fistula covered and open, respectively. If the "uncovered" findings indicate nasalization and the "covered" findings do not, the inference can be made that the fistula is the main contributor to the nasalization disorder. If nasalization occurs in both conditions, the inference must be made that the nasalization is the result of dysfunction of the velopharyngeal mechanism. Sealing of the fistula is sufficiently accomplished when a difference in speech and resonance is noticed with the fistula uncovered and covered. If no difference in speech and resonance is perceivable, the fistula has no influence on velopharyngeal function, but the possibility also exists that the fistula has been improperly sealed. The whole fistula covering procedure should then be repeated to minimize the risk of misinterpretation. Efficiency of obturation must be determined in examining the effect of a fistula videofluoroscopically and can be regarded as complete only when no evidence of air bubbles can be seen in the contrast medium outlining the fistula area.

Efficiency of the covering plate also should be checked when fistula sealing in children is achieved by means of a covering plate that has been in use for any length of time. Covering plates have a tendency to lose their fitness relatively quickly owing to the dental and bony developmental changes in growing patients. An additional examination is recommended with the covering plate replaced by chewing gum over the fistula.

Speech Symptoms and Fistula Size

The critical limit of fistula size for influencing speech quality has been discussed. Stark suggested that an area exceeding 5 mm^2 is necessary for a fistula to interfere with speech.[10] Henningsson and Isberg found that a fistula of 4.5 mm^2 has a definite impact on speech and resonance, resulting in hypernasality, audible nasal escape, and weakness of pressure consonants.[4] The effect was evaluated by comparing the examination results with the fistula open versus results with the fistula temporarily covered by chewing gum. In their limited sample, no significant correlation was found between any of the characteristics: fistula length, width, and area, and the speech parameters examined. Our clinical experience is that fistulas of only a few square millimeters can affect speech and resonance. Figure 98–1 illustrates two small and one large fistula, all three of which affected speech and resonance significantly.

Speech and Resonance Symptoms

Speech and resonance deviations associated with a palatal fistula can be identified as (1) symptoms gener-

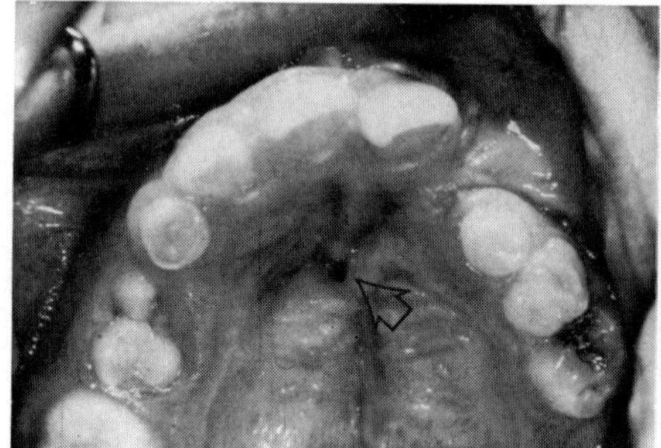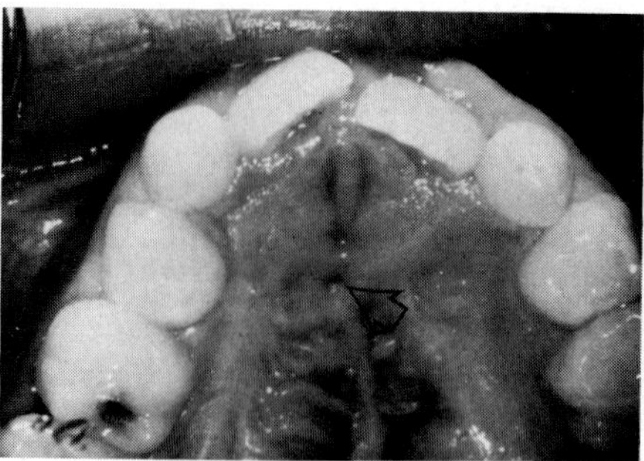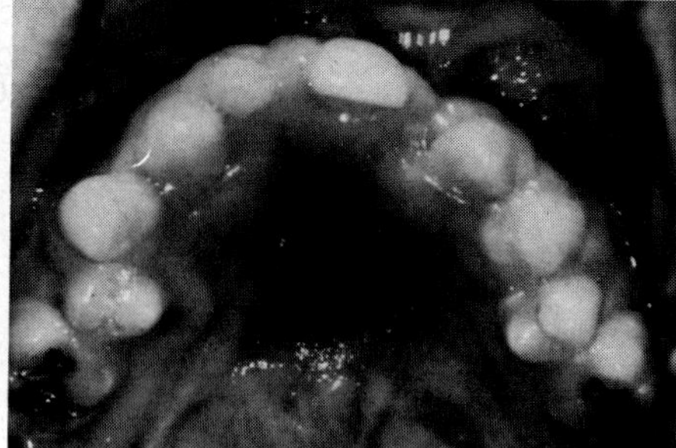

Figure 98–1 Small and large fistulas, all of which affected speech and resonance significantly.

ated at the fistula, and (2) symptoms occurring secondary to impaired velopharyngeal sphincter function induced by the fistula.

Symptoms Generated at the Fistula

Air leakage through the fistula during speech that is articulated anterior to it often gives rise to an extra acoustic component associated with the speech sound. This component is a bubbling sound or, more frequently, a high-frequency fricative sound with a slight whistling quality. There is intraindividual variation with respect to the occurrence and intensity of the symptom, and it is usually heard only when the fistula is small. The authors' experience is that this deviant sound is more pronounced if the fistula is circular in shape than if it has a slitlike appearance, other factors being equal. The whistling component should not be confused with the velar snort sound originating from the velopharyngeal sphincter region. However, distinguishing between the two intruding sounds is particularly difficult when they occur simultaneously.

Morley claimed that large fistulas are a great hindrance to the development of good speech, and she mentioned production of weak pressure consonants in association with large fistulas.[11] This observation was later supported by Perko.[12] Accordingly, Shelton and Blank registered a loss of intraoral air pressure for large fistulas but not for small ones.[13] In addition, audible nasal escape in association with fistulas has been mentioned by several authors.[14–18]

Fistulas, however, do not necessarily influence speech, presumably because speech behavior varies between individuals, especially when oronasal anatomy is deviant during the period of speech and language development.

Some nonsymptomatic oronasal fistulas need to be closed following velopharyngeal flap surgery. A fistula that originally has had no influence, either on speech or on resonance, can sometimes become a site for generating the extra acoustic components mentioned above after velopharyngeal flap surgery. This is presumably the result of increased intraoral air pressure because the air no longer escapes through a velopharyngeal insufficiency.

Symptoms Due to Secondary Velopharyngeal Insufficiency

Following cleft palate surgery some patients have both an oronasal fistula and insufficient velopharyngeal sphincter function. The importance of separating the speech symptoms due to the fistula from those caused by insufficient sphincter function has been pointed out.[13, 15, 19, 20] In line with this reasoning, a fistula and velopharyngeal insufficiency occurring in the same patient have been regarded as two independent factors causing speech and resonance deviation. However, in 1987 Isberg and Henningsson showed that the presence of a fistula correlated with the occurrence of velopharyngeal insufficiency in patients with morphologic prerequisites for sphincter closure.[4] They also found that a residual velopharyngeal insufficiency could be further impaired by the presence of a fistula. This impairment was more pronounced for the lateral pharyngeal walls than for the velum.

Since a palatal fistula may impair velopharyngeal activity, it may be associated with any kind of speech or resonance deviation related to velopharyngeal insufficiency such as hypernasality, weakness of pressure consonants, audible nasal escape, and velar snort sounds. The importance of determining whether hypernasality or other speech and resonance problems are exclusively a result of fistular influence on velopharyngeal function is obvious. If the symptoms disappear after temporary covering of the fistula, surgical or prosthetic closure is the proper treatment, and treatment procedures directed at the sphincter area are not justified. If hypernasality is increased by a fistula's influence on velopharyngeal function, the contribution of the fistula should be determined. One difference between speech and resonance symptoms related to a primary velopharyngeal insufficiency compared to a fistula is that only the latter is influenced by the place of speech articulation in relation to the fistula location. Thus, the deviant speech and resonance is heard only during speech articulation anterior to the fistula. The improvement of velopharyngeal function and of speech and resonance that can be achieved by covering the fistula is thus a combined effect of the elimination of air leakage through the fistula and increased velopharyngeal activity.

The impairment of velopharyngeal movement and speech quality related to an oronasal fistula does not depend on aerodynamic factors alone. We do not know which aspect of the velopharyngeal function is the most important one for speech or how much flexibility or plasticity normal speakers and speakers with a cleft palate have in their velopharyngeal movements.[21] It may be that when normal intraoral pressure cannot be maintained, the speech motor control system does not strive for complete velopharyngeal closure. In patients with a fistula it is reasonable to assume that when the fistula is covered, the motor strategy will be modulated. When the fistula is open, there is no point where velopharyngeal muscles can be fully active.

Speech Symptoms Associated with a Prealveolar Fistula

Differences in fistula location are related to various speech symptoms. A prealveolar fistula is rarely associated with serious speech symptoms and does not influence resonance. By its natural pressure against the alveolar ridge the upper lip usually covers any fistula in this region well and thus prevents speech symptoms. When air leakage occurs, an extra acoustic component concomitant with the articulated speech sound can be heard. This usually happens when the fistula is large or the lip is short or stiff, resulting in air leakage through the fistula during articulation of high-pressure bilabial consonants such as /p/ and /b/. Other speech sounds that might be influenced are labiodental speech sounds such as /f/ and /v/ and interdentally produced speech sounds such as /θ/ and /ð/.

Speech and Resonance Symptoms Associated with a Hard Palate Fistula

When the fistula is located in the hard palate, both speech and resonance are likely to be affected even when the fistula is small.[4] A fistula that is more like a slit in the midline may be clinically difficult to discover. The symptoms may be significant or discrete. In some patients, the mucosa surrounding such a fistula plugs the slit until the intraoral pressure becomes high enough to open the oronasal passage, resulting in air leakage.

When the fistula occurs in the hard palate only, the region of the incisive foramen is the most common location. An examination for a possible influence of a fistula on speech and resonance must include speech articulated both anterior to ("prefistula"—e.g., *pop*) and posterior to the fistula ("postfistula"—e.g., *cook*). The speech quality for words or short phrases including vowels in combination with bilabial, labiodental, interdental, or dental pressure consonants should be compared with words and phrases including palatal or velar pressure consonants followed by vowels.

The speech evaluation should be performed with and without temporary covering of the fistula. The quality of speech and resonance produced during prefistula speech with the fistula covered should correspond with speech quality produced during postfistula speech. If there are deviations during speech with the fistula covered they are thus an effect of a primary velopharyngeal insufficiency and are not influenced by the fistula. One pitfall to be aware of is that when a fistula is temporarily covered with dental wax or chewing gum, the articulation pattern may change because of the unaccustomed situation; tongue tip sounds may unconsciously be articulated posterior to the inserted material. This temporarily eliminates the evaluation possibilities for the speech pathologist, but the displacement can be overcome with some practicing. Some patients, mostly children, spontaneously develop a compensatory articulation pattern. They articulate dental pressure consonants as palatal, that is, behind the fistula.

If the deviant speech quality is heard only during prefistula articulation and only when the fistula is open, it is exclusively an effect of the fistula; that is, even a hypernasal quality is the result of the fistula's influence on velopharyngeal function. This was shown in a cineradiographic study of velopharyngeal activity during speech in hypernasal patients with and without fistula covering.[3] The velopharyngeal movements for prefistula speech were registered with the fistula open and temporarily covered, respectively. At comparison, the velopharyngeal movements were found to improve in all ten patients when their fistulas were covered (Fig. 98–2). The improvement of sphincter function was consistently correlated with an improvement in speech and resonance quality.[4] In four of the ten patients examined, speech and resonance were fully normalized when the fistula was covered. Two of these four patients had previously been subjected to velopharyngeal flap surgery but with no effect on hypernasality. A conclusion drawn was that a palatal fistula influencing speech and resonance should always be closed surgically or with a dental covering plate before any velopharyngeal surgery is carried out.

Speech and Resonance Symptoms Associated with a Residual Cleft in the Hard Palate

In some surgical habilitation programs for cleft palate patients the cleft in the hard palate is intentionally left open during the primary repair to be closed at a later age. Until the final closure, a covering plate is sometimes used (with varying results) in an attempt to reduce temporarily the effects of the open cleft on speech. There are similarities in pathological anatomy between such a residual cleft in the hard palate and a palatal fistula, and the same speech and resonance symptoms are likely to occur. In patients with residual clefts, an early surgical closure of the soft palate has usually been carried out to achieve velopharyngeal sphincter closure. Hypernasal quality in speech is common in these patients, presumably because of the air leakage through

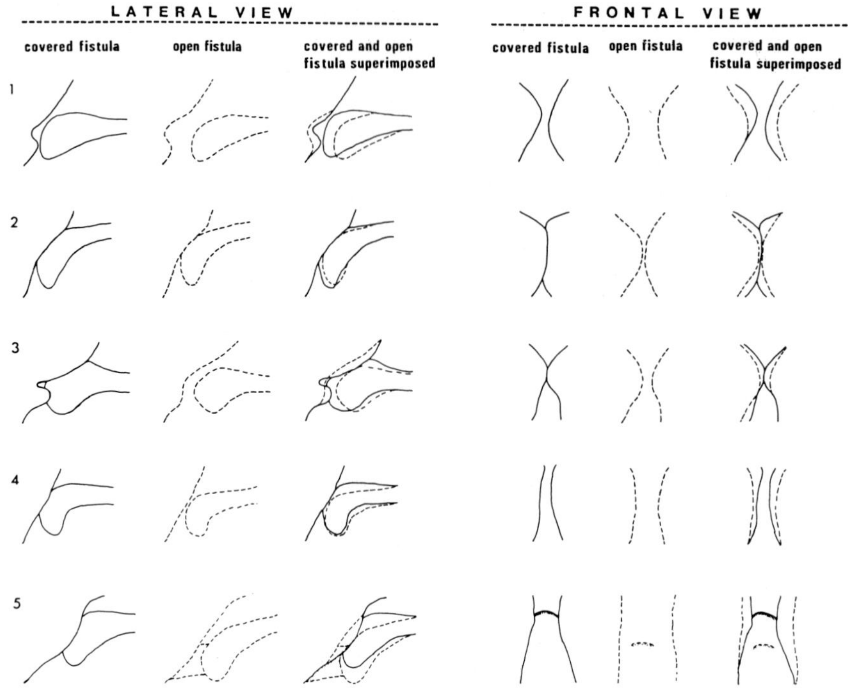

Figure 98–2 Tracings of velopharyngeal movements from cineradiographic frames in lateral and frontal projections during anterior articulation of pressure consonants with the fistula covered and open, respectively. Shadowed areas represent velopharyngeal flap. Superimposition of tracings for speech with covered fistulas (continuous lines) and for speech with open fistulas (dashed lines) shows improvement of velopharyngeal movements during speech with the fistulas covered. (From Isberg A, Henningsson G: Influence of palatal fistulae on velopharyngeal movements. A cineradiographic study. Plast Reconstr Surg 79(4):525–530, 1987. With permission.)

the cleft. However, as long as the residual cleft is left open, the velopharyngeal activity can be expected to be impaired in accordance with the influence of an open fistula on velopharyngeal activity.[3] Not until the oronasal passage is covered can maximal velopharyngeal activity be expected.

There are reports of specific articulatory problems related to residual clefts that are due to posterior displacement of dental pressure consonants.[22–24] The child displaces the articulation with the tip of the tongue to a position behind the cleft, where the back of the tongue can make full palatal contact. Since a residual cleft is usually larger than a fistula, at least initially, the articulatory problems are more common in these patients, but the compensatory misarticulation is in principle the same.

In patients with a consistent posterior displacement of dental and labiodental pressure consonants, the negative influence of the residual cleft on the velopharyngeal function is inhibited. After speech training when the child becomes capable of producing pressure consonants anterior to the residual cleft, hypernasality sometimes occurs because of an impairment of velopharyngeal function induced by the oronasal passage.

Speech and Resonance Symptoms Associated with a Soft Palate Fistula

The speech deviations associated with a soft palate fistula are the same as those described for a hard palate fistula. The fistula often has the shape of a slit and is frequently obscured by the surrounding soft tissue, resulting in underdiagnosis of the condition. During videofluoroscopic examination of velopharyngeal function, bubbles of contrast medium at the location of the fistula can sometimes reveal its presence. The fistula's influence on speech is sometimes difficult to evaluate. It can be difficult to cover the fistula without discomfort to the patient, and a temporary cover will easily be displaced by the velar movement.

Speech Material

The speech material should be composed to facilitate evaluation. Because only syllables and words articulated anterior to the fistula are affected by it, they should be grouped together to facilitate a comparison with words and syllables articulated posterior to the fistula. Moreover, our experience is that reduplications of sounds such as /pi:pi:pi:/ are very useful in the examination of small children. Most of them are usually capable of producing such syllables correctly after a few minutes of practice even though they would normally use compensatory articulation or demonstrate phonematic problems in spontaneous speech. Their success in the use of three-syllable repetitions seems to be due to the fact that these syllables have no linguistic meaning either in Swedish or English.

If the fistula is placed at the conjunction of the premaxilla and the maxilla, the following speech material could be used for examination of speech anterior to the fistula (isolated words or short phrases):

/ma-ma-ma/	Suzy sees Sally
/pi-pi-pi/	Suzy eats fish
/pu-pu-pu/	Suzy watches TV
/ti-ti-ti/	Popeye plays baseball
/si-si-si/	Stop the bus
	Peter has a puppy
	The baby has a doll
	Peter eats potatoes.

The following syllables and phrases could be used for the examination of speech posterior to a hard palate fistula:

/ki-ki-ki/	Give Gary a cookie
/ka-ka-ka/	Kay, call Guy quick!
/ku-ku-ku/	

Even though the presence of a fistula would be considered as unpleasant for most of us, the child gets adjusted to it. Now and then children with an acquired oronasal passage, especially those with a residual hard palate cleft, respond negatively to having the oronasal communication covered. They sometimes say that they cannot breathe properly.

It is also noteworthy that some types of deviant speech behavior sometimes make an evaluation of the fistula's influence on speech impossible. For example, the production of compensatory speech sounds such as glottal substitutions[25] and pharyngeal substitutions of high-pressure consonants is already accomplished at the glottis and in the pharynx, respectively. Because the oral cavity with the fistula is thus never involved in the speech act, no fistular influence on speech quality can be evaluated. The perceived hypernasality usually found in these patients is at least partly a result of the compensatory speech behavior. However, patients who use compensatory glottal articulation do have hypernasal speech, which can be mistakenly regarded as an effect of the patient's fistula. Only when a clinical examination has been performed by a speech pathologist with knowledge about the relationship between the place of articulation and the location of the fistula can the possible influence of the fistula on speech and resonance be evaluated.

Conclusions

Oronasal fistulas are a well-known residual condition that can occur after cleft palate repair and can be found anywhere along the midline of the former cleft. In addition to symptoms such as regurgitation of fluid into the nasal cavity, fistulas also may generate speech and resonance problems, even if fistula size is small. These symptoms are:
1. Extra acoustic, whistling component associated with the speech sound.

2. Weak pressure consonants in patients with a large fistula.
3. Audible nasal escape.

A palatal fistula also may impair velopharyngeal activity, causing velopharyngeal insufficiency. A fistula may then be associated with any kind of speech or resonance deviation related to velopharyngeal insufficiency such as hypernasality, weakness of pressure consonants, audible nasal escape, and velar snort sounds. To evaluate any possible influence of a fistula on speech quality, examination must be performed with the fistula both open and temporarily covered. To facilitate evaluation of speech quality, the speech sample should be grouped according to fistula location, that is, speech articulated anterior to ("prefistula") and posterior to the fistula ("postfistula"). If speech and resonance symptoms disappear after a temporary covering of the fistula, surgical or prosthetic closure of the fistula is the proper treatment, and treatment procedures directed at the velopharyngeal sphincter area are not justified. An improvement of velopharyngeal function and of speech and resonance that can be achieved by covering the fistula is thus a combined effect of the elimination of air leakage through the fistula and increased velopharyngeal activity.

References

1. Oneal RM: Oronasal fistulas. In Grabb WC, Rosenstein SW, Bzoch KR (eds): Cleft Lip and Palate. Boston: Little, Brown, 1971.
2. Krause CJ, Tharp RF, Morris HL: A comparative study of results of the von Langenbeck and the V–Y pushback palatoplasties. Cleft Palate J 13:11–19, 1976.
3. Isberg A, Henningsson G: Influence of palatal fistulae on velopharyngeal movements. A cineradiographic study. Plast Reconstr Surg 79:525–530, 1987.
4. Henningsson G, Isberg A: Influence of palatal fistulae on speech and resonance. Folia Phoniatr 39:183–191, 1987.
5. Peer LA, Hagerty RF, Hoffmeister FD, et al: An evaluation of the Warren Davis osteoplastic technique in the cleft palate repair. Plast Reconstr Surg 14:1–9, 1954.
6. Lindsay WK: Von Langenbeck palatorraphy. In Grabb WC, Rosenstein SW, Bzoch KR (eds): Cleft Lip and Palate. Boston: Little, Brown, 1971.
7. Van Demark DR: A comparison of articulation abilities and velopharyngeal competency between Danish and Iowa children with cleft palate. Cleft Palate J 11:463–470, 1974.
8. Abyholm FE, Borchgrevink HH, Eskeland G: Palatal fistulae following cleft palate surgery. Scand J Plast Reconstr Surg 13:295–300, 1979.
9. Drillien CM, Ingram TT, Wilkinson EM: The Causes and Natural History of Cleft Lip and Palate. Edinburgh: E & S Livingstone, 1966.
10. Stark RB: Cleft palate. In Converse JM (ed): Reconstructive Plastic Surgery. Philadelphia: Saunders, 1964.
11. Morley ME: The assessment of speech. Cleft Palate and Speech, 6th ed. Edinburgh: E & S Livingstone, 1966.
12. Perko MA: Two-stage closure of cleft palate. J Maxillofac Surg 7:76–80, 1979.
13. Shelton RL, Blank JL: Oronasal fistulas, intraoral air pressure and nasal air flow during speech. Cleft Palate J 21:91–99, 1984.
14. Jackson IT: Closure of secondary palatal fistulae with intra-oral tissue and bone grafting. Br J Plast Surg 29:295–296, 1979.
15. Jackson MS, Jackson IT, Christie FB: Improvement in speech following closure of anterior palatal fistulas with bone grafts. Br J Plast Surg 29:295–296, 1976.
16. Leonard MS: Repair of oronasal fistula with mucoperiosteal island flap: Report of case. J Oral Surg 37:511–512, 1979.
17. Rintala AE: Surgical closure of palatal fistulae. Scand J Plast Reconstr Surg 14:235–238, 1980.
18. Pigott RW, Rieger FW, Moodie AF: Tongue flap repair of cleft palate fistulae. Br J Plast Surg 37:285–293, 1984.
19. Bless DM, Ewanowski SJ, Dibbell DG: A technique for temporary obturation of fistulae. Clinical note. Cleft Palate J 17:297–300, 1980.
20. Thompson RPJ, Ferguson JW, Barton M: The role of removable orthodontic

appliances in the investigation and management of patients with hypernasal speech. Br J Orthodont 12:70–77, 1985.
21. Folkins JW: Issues in speech motor control and their relation to the speech of individuals with cleft palate. Cleft Palate J 22:106–122,1985.
22. Cosman B, Falk AS: Delayed hard palate repair and speech deficiencies: A cautionary report. Cleft Palate J 21:263–269, 1984.
23. Witzel MA, Salyer KE, Ross RB: Delayed hard palate closure: The philosophy revisited. Cleft Palate J 21:263–269, 1984.
24. Henningsson G, Karling J: A comparison of speech in 4-year old cleft palate children operated with early or late hard palate surgery. In Huddart AG, Ferguson MWJ (eds): Cleft Lip and Palate: Initial Surgery; Speech, Surgery and Growth. Manchester: Manchester University Press, 1989.
25. Henningsson G, Isberg A: Velopharyngeal movement patterns in patients alternating between oral and glottal articulation: A clinical and cineradiographical study. Cleft Palate J 23:1–9, 1986.

CHAPTER 99

Treatment by Therapeutic Exercises

Clark D. Starr

Muscle Training Programs and Velopharyngeal Closure

Background

The use of muscle training programs to improve velopharyngeal closure and decrease hypernasality has a long and tumultuous history. Judicious use of these programs has been advocated by respected and experienced speech pathologists.[1–4] Equally qualified persons have expressed strong doubts about the efficacy of this approach.[5–8] The former group has relied on reasoned assumptions that muscle training leads to development of muscle functions similar to those needed for velopharyngeal closure, and on their clinical experiences, which suggest that these programs work, at least in some cases. The latter group has stressed the paucity of systematic research that supports the effectiveness of muscle training in persons with inadequate velopharyngeal mechanisms and has questioned the likelihood that changes developed through muscle training programs are comparable to those used in speech or, if they are comparable, that they can be incorporated into speech activities. Although this point of view appears to be widely accepted by authors of texts and essays about this issue, it is interesting that a survey of speech pathologists who treat persons with cleft palate and hypernasality indicates that 54% use muscle exercises as a part of their treatment programs for some patients.[9]

Why does this situation exist? Is one group wrong, or is there still insufficient information to allow us to decide the question? In this chapter some assumptions are offered that appear to be basic to our efforts to understand the potential benefits of muscle training, and some studies of attempts to use muscle training to resolve velopharyngeal closure problems are reviewed. Finally, several tentative conclusions are drawn about the state of our knowledge in this area, and some suggestions are made about the implications of this understanding to our clinical management efforts.

Some Assumptions

When confronted with a person who has excessive nasality in speech, we tend to make one or more of the following assumptions:

1. The person has a normal speech mechanism but does not use it appropriately.
2. The person has an abnormal mechanism but has muscles that will compensate for the abnormality if he or she can learn to use them.
3. The person has a mechanism that has the potential to achieve velopharyngeal closure, with or without the use of compensatory muscles, but muscle strength, mass, endurance, or range of motion has not developed to the point where closure can be attained and maintained.
4. The person has adequate anatomic structures and muscle function but is unable to use them effectively because of central or peripheral problems with motor control, motor planning, or sensory feedback.
5. The person has inadequate anatomic structures or muscle function potential to accomplish velopharyngeal closure for speech.

There is still debate about the extent to which our diagnostic tools allow us to determine which of these assumptions is valid for an individual patient.

Some More Assumptions

If muscle training is to be one of our treatment tools, we must understand the assumptions underlying this type of training. For example, discussions by Krusen et al[10] and Fox[11] indicate that training programs can increase muscle strength, mass, endurance, and length; improve sensory feedback and motor control; develop coordinated patterns needed to accomplish specific tasks; and, under certain circumstances, help nerves regain lost capacities.

If we decide that a patient has a velopharyngeal closure problem that might be helped by muscle training, we still face the task of deciding what to do and how to do it. Again, we must be aware of another set of assumptions, as indicated by the discussion of Krusen et al[10] and Fox.[11] For example, it is assumed that, to increase strength and mass, a muscle must be exercised in such a manner that it contracts near its maximum potential while working against high resistance and that this can be accomplished with relatively few repetitions on a daily basis. A muscle exercised by numerous daily contractions against low resistance will improve its endurance. Increasing muscle length or contractability usually involves stretching exercises. Attempts to increase or modify sensory function rely on procedures that involve electrical, tactile, and other types of stimulation. Improvement in coordination must be learned and practiced repeatedly before it can be incorporated into daily living activities.

If programs of muscle training are to be effective, they must be planned with these assumptions in mind. We must be able to identify the nature of a patient's velopharyngeal closure problem as completely as possible. We must formulate a reasonable hypothesis about the effects of specific changes in muscle state or function. Finally, we must figure out ways to accomplish the needed change. These are not easy tasks. The measurement tools and exercise procedures needed are not readily available, and even their nature is not well understood. As pointed out by Shelton,[12] few clinicians are in a position to make judgments based on those that are available.

Nevertheless, some investigators have attempted to determine whether and how muscle training programs can contribute to our efforts to provide appropriate clinical management to persons with velopharyngeal closure problems, as indicated in the following discussion.

The Evidence

There are not many previously reported systematic studies about the effectiveness of muscle training programs on velopharyngeal closure. In addition, the obtained findings are not in agreement and may even be regarded as discouraging. As in several previous reviews,[6, 7, 13] in this review we will take another look at selected studies in an attempt to identify assumptions made in their execution and to determine the extent to which the findings indicate that further investigations might be warranted. We have divided the studies into three categories. Those in the first category focus directly on attempts to modify velopharyngeal closure outside of the speech context; in the second category are studies that attempt to modify closure in the speech context; and in the third group are studies that make direct attempts to modify speech in the expectation that this improvement will have an effect on the mechanism. Since several studies include multiple procedures, we have arbitrarily assigned them to the category that appears to reflect their major focus.

Studies That Focus on the Velopharyngeal Mechanism Outside of the Speech Context

Massengill et al[14] have reported the most extensive study of this type. They examined the effects of traditional blowing, sucking, and swallowing exercises on velopharyngeal closure. All of their subjects had surgically repaired clefts. Five were assigned to a swallowing group, four to a blowing group, and four to a sucking group. Twice a day for 27 days each group performed

exercises for 20 minutes. Each group also received articulation therapy during this period. Pre- and post-training lateral cinefluorographic films were made to obtain measures of velopharyngeal gap on sustained vowels. Analysis of these data indicated that patients in the swallowing group were the only ones that significantly decreased the velopharyngeal gap. No evaluations of speech were made. However, three subjects reduced their gaps to 2 mm or less, an amount that seems, on the basis of other reported findings, to be within the range of some persons with acceptable nasality levels.

Powers and Starr[15] carried out a similar study. They had four subjects with surgically repaired clefts and clinically significant hypernasality perform blowing, sucking, swallowing, and gagging exercises four times a day for 6 weeks. Their subjects were rewarded for progressively greater effort on these tasks. Lateral x-rays of sustained vowel productions and tape recordings of connected speech were obtained before and after muscle training. Neither measurements of velopharyngeal gap nor listeners' judgments of nasality indicated that any change had occurred.

In neither of these studies were direct attempts made to modify speech. One did look at the effects of muscle training on speech and found none. Both studies evaluated the midsagittal velopharyngeal gap, and one found a significant change, in that regard, for subjects who did swallowing exercises. In the earlier study, Massengill et al[14] reported that subjects did not achieve closure on the vowels tested prior to therapy, but they did not determine whether closure occurred in other speech contexts or nonspeech activities. In the other study, Powers and Starr[15] reported that their subjects did not achieve closure on vowels but did achieve it on a blowing task. In neither study did the investigators include conjectures or hypotheses about the nature of the subjects' closure problems, nor did they suggest what types of muscle change was needed or indicate what changes might be brought about with the exercises used. In retrospect, it appears that in both studies the exercises used might be expected to lead to increases in muscle strength and mass and possibly endurance. Because none of these variables was measured directly, the effectiveness of the exercises in this regard cannot be determined. Because only limited change in velopharyngeal gap was found, one can only conclude that if the exercises did increase strength and mass, these changes were not the ones needed to improve closure. The use of a view of the velopharyngeal gap on lateral films as a measure of change is a limiting factor in both studies.

Studies That Focus on Modifying the Velopharyngeal Mechanism in the Context of Speech

One of the most frequently quoted studies of this type was done by Yules and Chase.[16] Twenty subjects with surgically repaired cleft palate and other velopharyngeal problems underwent 2- to 6-week therapy regimes of electrical stimulation. Electrodes were placed on the posterior pillars, and muscle function was stimulated during a series of speechlike and speech tasks. Stimulation was withdrawn as subjects learned to do the tasks voluntarily. Next, an acoustic feedback device was used to teach subjects to control nasality in speech activities while using their newly learned ability to achieve closure. While all this was going on, a home training program of tactile stimulation and visual feedback was used to aid subjects in practicing their new closure patterns. Based on pre- and post-therapy cinefluorographic films and airflow measures, the authors concluded that 24 of the 30 subjects had learned to control velopharyngeal closure on speech tasks. They noted that hypertrophy of the pharyngeal muscles developed in two patients and that nasality in these two became normal without increased contraction of the pharyngeal walls. The 24 subjects who appeared to have learned to control closure were enrolled in speech therapy. According to the authors, 60% of these attained normal nasality, 30% showed some improvement, and 10% did not change.

Weber et al[17] replicated this study using 34 subjects who had cleft palate or other closure problems. They report using the same therapy procedures and the same pre- and post-therapy measures. Eighteen of their subjects dropped out of the study because they were not making progress, and nine of the remaining 16 did not return for post-therapy testing. According to the authors, the remaining seven subjects had little difficulty learning to produce velopharyngeal closure voluntarily but had difficulty transferring this activity to connected speech. Only one of the seven showed a significant decrease in nasality on post-therapy tests.

Neither report provided detailed information about the nature of the subjects' velopharyngeal problems or why electrical stimulation was judged an appropriate procedure for modifying muscle function. Apparently it was assumed that all subjects had the physical potential to accomplish closure with increased use of the pharyngeal constrictor muscles and that the training task would demonstrate this potential and possibly increase sensory functions so that subjects could achieve voluntary control over closure. Unfortunately, the procedures used for stimulation and measurement in these studies were not sufficiently well described to allow careful assessment of the reported results. Also, the variety of approaches used in the study make it difficult to determine cause and effect relationships.

Peterson[18] also studied the effect of electrical stimulation and reported findings contrary to those reported by Yules and Chase,[16] that is, she found that electrical stimulation did not produce palatal elevation on a consistent basis. She also documents the difficulties associated with the placement of pharyngeal electrodes, the determination of patterns of reaction to electrical stimulation, and the problems associated with gaining subject cooperation for this type of task.

In another study of the effects of sensory stimulation, Tash et al[19] used a cotton swab to stimulate directly the palate and pharyngeal walls of two children without clefts who had normal velopharyngeal closure and two with clefts who had inadequate closure. Therapy continued until the subjects completed 30 training sessions or were able to demonstrate voluntary mesial movement of the lateral pharyngeal walls and anterior movement of the posterior walls on speech tasks. Pre- and post-therapy cinefluorographic films and audio recordings were made during phonation of vowels, with and without voluntary movement, and while the subjects read sentences. According to the authors, both normal subjects learned to produce voluntary wall movement during speech tasks, one cleft subject learned to do it inconsistently during speech tasks, and the other could do it consistently but only in nonspeech tasks. These findings are similar to those of Yules and Chase[16] in that they suggest that subjects can learn to control some velopharyngeal behaviors in response to stimulation; the results are different in that they do not show that this change can be incorporated into speech. Although the purpose of the Tash et al[19] study was to examine the effects of stimulation, the task set for the subjects appears to involve a certain amount of muscular exercise as well.

Again, neither the nature of the subjects' velopharyngeal problems nor the reason why the authors believed that stimulation was an appropriate treatment procedure for them was described in any detail. It is of interest that the authors reported that clinicians' visual observations of the subjects' pharyngeal movements did not appear to indicate accurately what was actually happening.

Three studies in this category have used designs in which endoscopes are attached to videorecorders and monitors. This instrumentation provides subjects with visual feedback of their velopharyngeal activity in three dimensions and offers a chance to reassess the observations made during treatment.

Shelton et al[20] used such instrumentation to train two subjects. They used an orally placed rigid endoscope and observed velopharyngeal activity from below. One of their subjects had a cleft palate and a pharyngeal flap. His speech was hypernasal and he had multiple articulation errors. The other subject did not have a cleft but had hypernasal speech related to velopharyngeal insufficiency. Therapy involved asking subjects to make voluntary efforts to modify closure during speech and nonspeech tasks while observing their velopharyngeal mechanisms on a video screen. Analyses of pre- and post-therapy videotapes and speech indicated that the cleft subject learned to modify his closure pattern in some contexts but could not do so consistently. His articulation did not change. The noncleft subject modified her closure pattern more consistently but not in all contexts.

This study offers further evidence that subjects can learn to modify velopharyngeal closure but does not show that learned closure activities can be transferred to speech. Again, it would appear that the tasks used in this study provided some degree of muscle exercise, although this was not evaluated.

Siegel-Sadewitz and Shprintzen[21] used similar instrumentation with a noncleft subject who had normal speech. A flexible fiberendoscope was inserted in the subject's nose, allowing her to observe her velopharyngeal mechanism from above. The subject's task was to modify the relative contributions of the pharyngeal walls and the soft palate to velopharyngeal closure. Visual feedback was provided as she learned the tasks and was then gradually withdrawn until she mastered the tasks without it. According to the authors, she learned the tasks with relative ease and could use different closure patterns during speech without feedback. Little information about the reliability of these observations is reported.

Yamaoka and associates[22] also used a nasally placed fiberendoscope as a feedback device in a training program administered to 59 subjects with surgically repaired clefts. All subjects had persistent hypernasality despite long-term speech therapy. Their training program involved observations of the velopharyngeal mechanism through the endoscope and voluntary efforts to create closure in speech and nonspeech activities. Training sessions were conducted every other week for a period of nearly 1 year. Some subjects also received articulation therapy. Articulation testing and endoscopic records were obtained pre- and post-therapy. Before training, subjects were categorized on the basis of the amount of closure they obtained during vowel phonation, consonant production, blowing, and swallowing.

Post-training observations indicated that the 23 subjects who demonstrated complete closure on blowing and some speech tasks during pretraining observations were the ones most likely to improve the consistency with which they obtained closure on speech tasks. Thirty-six subjects did not obtain complete closure on blowing or speech tasks before training. Twelve of these showed improvement in velopharyngeal closure, but only seven showed significant improvement in speech. Articulation test analyses suggested to the authors that vowel nasality and consonant distortion decreased after training.

Although this study suggests that visual feedback training may be of value for some subjects, the procedures used to evaluate the changes that occurred preclude an adequate evaluation of their clinical significance. However, the authors did attempt to categorize subjects in relation to their ability to accomplish selected closure tasks and to use a system for making endoscopic observations.

These three endoscopic studies suggest that velopharyngeal closure patterns and the consistency of closure can be improved for some subjects. The changes that occur appear to be related to increased involvement of the pharyngeal constrictors in closure. Although it appears that this new pattern can be incorporated into the speech of a normal subject, the extent to which this can occur in cleft subjects remains questionable. Perhaps the two most significant insights to be gained from these studies are that visual feedback helps subjects to modify their closure patterns and that those who begin training with the ability to obtain closure in some speech or speechlike tasks are the ones most likely to profit from this type of training.

In a single subject study, using a different methodology, Moller et al[23] provided visual feedback of palatal function during speech by a palatal sensing device. The device was placed on the oral surface of the soft palate and held in place with a dental appliance. The subject had a repaired cleft palate, a midsagittal velopharyngeal gap on sustained production of vowels, and a moderate degree of hypernasality. The subject observed his palatal movements during speech tasks and made an effort to increase palatal elevation. The data indicated that the subject did learn to increase palatal elevation while he received feedback. However, x-rays and speech recordings taken before and after training indicated that the velopharyngeal gap did not change and hypernasality did not decrease.

This study is of interest primarily because it suggests that subjects can learn to increase palatal elevation with this type of training program. Why the increase did not lead to improved velopharyngeal closure of this subject is not clear. Again, it appears that the training tasks had the potential to increase muscle strength and endurance as well as contractability. However, these changes were not measured.

Studies That Attempt to Modify Speech on the Assumption That This Will Lead to Modification of the Velopharyngeal Mechanism

The most frequently quoted study of the effects of articulation therapy on velopharyngeal closure was conducted by Shelton and colleagues.[24] They examined velopharyngeal closure in subjects who were participating in a companion study on the effectiveness of an approach to articulation therapy.[25]

Their subjects were 6 to 12 years of age, had repaired cleft palate or palatal insufficiency, and made errors on at least three phonemes in an articulation test. Eight were assigned to an experimental group, in which they received up to 48 therapy sessions, and eight were assigned to a control group. Lateral cinefluorographic films of two sentences and isolated phonemes were obtained before and after therapy to provide measures of the midsagittal velopharyngeal gap, frequency of posterior wall movements, and the type of closure pattern used. Subjects who received therapy showed improved articulation but no significant changes in velopharyngeal gap, frequency of their pharyngeal wall movements, or closure patterns.

According to these data, articulation improvement can occur with no apparent change in velopharyngeal function. It seems unlikely that articulation therapy would provide the type of muscle training that would lead to changes in strength, mass, or endurance. However, this type of training might be expected to provide some sensory stimulation and possibly improve coordinated closure movements.

Several studies that focus directly on speech have used some form of instrumental feedback to aid subjects in their efforts to improve closure. Most often visual feedback based on acoustic output or nasal airflow is used. Fletcher[26, 27] and Daly and Johnson[28] used an acoustic feedback device called Tonar (a new version of this device is called a Nasometer) in programs designed to reduce nasality. Tonar measures selected frequencies of acoustic output at the mouth and the nares and provides a computed ratio of the energy emitted nasally to the sum of the energy emitted nasally and orally. This ratio is called nasalance and has been shown to be related to listeners' ratings of nasality.[27]

In one report, Fletcher[26] described his use of Tonar with two subjects. The speech of one became nasal after a tonsillectomy and adenoidectomy. She had palatal push-back surgery but remained hypernasal and did not respond to traditional speech therapy. Her pretherapy nasalance ranged from 70% to 80% on speech tasks. Fletcher reported that after speech training with Tonar the subject's nasalance decreased to 5% and her perceived nasal resonance was judged to be normal. This change became generalized to spontaneous speech after 16 sessions, and the change was maintained when the subject was rechecked 3 months later.

A speech bulb was placed in a second subject with a surgically repaired cleft palate, and she was given speech therapy using Tonar. Reportedly, she began with nasalance readings of 80%. After a week of intensive therapy her progress was erratic, and her bulb was enlarged. Subsequently, her nasalance was reduced to 10%, and she was able to generalize this gain across therapy tasks. No long-term effects of this change were reported. Fletcher did not determine whether the two subjects changed their closure patterns or whether they extended the use of existing closure patterns.

Daly and Johnson[28] used Tonar to explore nasalance reduction potential in three mentally retarded subjects, one of whom had a cleft palate. Their training sessions lasted 3 weeks and resulted in nasalance decreases of 15%, 20%, and 28% on criterion speech tasks. The authors did not report on efforts to generalize these reductions to spontaneous speech.

The most extensive use of feedback devices in therapy is described in a lengthy report by Fletcher[27] of a study in which 13 sessions of Tonar-based training were administered to 19 subjects with surgically repaired clefts. Prior to training all subjects had nasalance ratios of 20% or more on a series of sentences used to evaluate training progress. After training eight of the subjects had reached and maintained a preset goal of 15% or less nasalance on 85% of the test sentences; five subjects reached the goal but were unable to maintain it, five performed in an erratic manner, and one could not decrease his nasalance. These results indicate that nasality can be modified through training, but they contribute little information about the nature of the change when it occurs.

Shprintzen and colleagues[29] performed a study that employed feedback procedures as well as blowing and whistling activities to modify nasality and velopharyngeal function. Although it could be classified as a study that focuses on modification of the velopharyngeal mechanism in the context of speech, the authors' description suggests that blowing and whistling activities were used for demonstration purposes rather than as exercises.

Based on their observations that velopharyngeal closure in normal persons is similar during speaking, whistling, and blowing tasks, these authors hypothesized that subjects who demonstrated normal closure on either of the latter tasks would be able to learn closure for speech. They tested this hypothesis on four subjects, all of whom had normal closure on blowing and whistling tasks and deficient closure on speech tasks. Normal and abnormal classifications were based on observations made from videofluoroscopic tapes. All subjects had failed to modify nasality through traditional speech therapy. The method required that subjects attempt to combine phonation with whistling and blowing while observing nasal air escape on a device called a Scape-Scope. As training progressed, whistling and blowing activities were eliminated, and the subjects worked on speech tasks. These tasks were organized so that subjects began with sustained vowels, moved on to consonant-vowel productions, and then to words and phrases. Subjects were urged to be aware of kinesthetic and auditory sensations accompanying correct productions and were rewarded or punished for adequacy of response as noted on the Scape-Scope. Judgments of nasality and observations made from the Scape-Scope were used to evaluate the training program.

The first subject, a 19-year-old youth, had a pharyngeal flap. Prior to training his speech was judged to be severely hypernasal, and Scape-Scope observations showed frequent nasal air emission during the reading of a standard paragraph. Videofluoroscopic evaluation showed gaps at both lateral portals and restricted velar elevation. Maximal pharyngeal wall approximation occurred above the level of the flap. After 36 training sessions during a 15-week period, his speech was judged to be normal, and infrequent instances of nasal air emission were observed on the reading passage. Videofluoroscopy tapes indicated that after training, velar height, velar posterior wall contact, and closure of the lateral portals increased during the reading task. According to the authors, these gains were still present at a 4-month recheck.

The second subject, a 4-year-old boy, had a surgically repaired cleft palate. His speech was judged to be slightly hypernasal, and he had infrequent instances of nasal air emission. Videofluoroscopy showed touch velar-pharyngeal wall closure on production of vowels and inconsistent closure during connected speech. After 26 therapy sessions, his speech was judged to be normal, and no instances of nasal air emission were noted. Videofluoroscopy showed a tight velar-pharyngeal wall contact during speech.

The third subject, a 6-year-old boy, had a pharyngeal flap. His speech was judged to be severely hypernasal, and he had nearly continuous nasal airflow during speech. Videofluoroscopy indicated limited velar elevation and a slight narrowing of lateral ports during speech. After 22 training sessions, he could control nasality in conversational speech. Videofluoroscopy showed good velar-pharyngeal wall contact and complete closure of the lateral ports during speech.

The fourth subject, a 10-year-old girl, had a severe hearing loss. She developed a speech problem after an adenoidectomy. Judgments of nasality were not reported; however, there were frequent instances of nasal air emission during speech. Videofluoroscopy indicated a somewhat short velum that elevated extensively during speech but missed the posterior wall by about 2 mm. After 24 training sessions, she produced non-nasal phrases but could not monitor her nasality in connected speech. Videofluoroscopy indicated that velar-pharyngeal wall contact increased after training but that she did not consistently attain closure during speech.

This is one of the few studies that provides detailed information on the subjects' velopharyngeal mechanisms pre- and post-training. It is possible that the training activities used increased muscle strength, mass, or endurance; however, it seems more likely that they served to generalize existing closure patterns to new tasks.

Summary

This discussion began with a statement that the use of muscle training programs to improve velopharyngeal closure is a controversial issue. Further, it seemed probable that investigators who study this problem make assumptions regarding the nature of subjects' velopharyngeal closure problems, the muscle changes that will be needed to resolve the problems, and the training procedures that will lead to the needed changes. Finally, it appears that procedures for testing these assumptions are limited but that we must make full use of those available.

In an effort to evaluate the state of our knowledge of the effects of training programs on velopharyngeal closure, several relevant studies were categorized and reviewed. Two of the studies subjected patients to muscle exercise programs and attempted to determine the effect of these programs on velopharyngeal closure during speech. One reported changes in the midsagittal velopharyngeal gap in a few subjects, and the other failed to find change. Neither reported details of the subjects' pretraining closure mechanisms, indicated what changes were needed, or suggested what changes the training was designed to produce. Both studies measured the velopharyngeal gap during speech tasks, but neither incorporated speech tasks in the training programs. Perhaps the most reasonable conclusion to be drawn from this approach is that the studies demonstrate that the traditional training procedures used have limited applicability if the clinician's goal is to reduce the velopharyngeal gap during speech. Although it is not possible to understand fully the effects of the training tasks used on the function of individual muscles, it appears most likely that the primary effect would be on the pharyngeal constrictors. Changes in these muscle functions, if they occurred, would be more easily observed from velopharyngeal measures other than those used in the studies. Furthermore, it seems unlikely that clinicians would anticipate that the results of training activities done in nonspeech tasks would be transferred spontaneously to speech.

Seven of the studies reviewed used some form of muscle training to modify velopharyngeal closure during speech activities. Some form of palatal stimulation was used in three of the studies. All three provided some evidence that subjects with closure problems learned to modify closure patterns in isolated speech tasks, but only one found that the new closure patterns were transferred to complex speech tasks. Again, these studies did not attempt to analyze subjects' closure patterns, determine what specific changes were needed, or indicate how stimulation training would lead to the desired changes. In spite of these limitations, the successes reported in one study appear impressive.

Three studies used endoscopes to provide subjects with visual feedback of velopharyngeal function in speech and speechlike tasks. Again, all three showed that subjects could modify their closure patterns under some study conditions. The apparent ease with which a normal subject was able to modify the contributions of the pharyngeal constrictor muscles to speech is impressive. Similarly, the extent to which subjects with velopharyngeal problems were able to modify their closure mechanism suggests that this approach holds some promise. The use of this procedure requires more extensive study to determine the conditions under which it may be of value.

Three studies used acoustic feedback to modify hypernasality and velopharyngeal function. All three reported success with some subjects. Unfortunately, none of the studies provided pre- or post-training descriptions of subjects' velopharyngeal functioning. Without additional information, one can only conjecture about whether the subjects who met success experienced changes in their muscles, in their closure patterns, or in the consistency with which they attained closure.

One study used nasal airflow feedback to help subjects reduce nasality and reported success with some subjects. Velopharyngeal patterns of these subjects were documented and showed that training changed palatal elevation and pharyngeal wall activity. The authors of this study suggest that subjects had learned to use existing closure patterns.

Although several of the studies reviewed in this chapter suggest that velopharyngeal function and nasality can be modified with functional training programs, they offer limited information about the nature of the changes that occur as a result of training or about the type of problem that is most likely to change with training. A liberal interpretation of the information provided by these studies suggests that subjects in whom nasality decreased tended to demonstrate an ability to accomplish velopharyngeal closure under some circumstances prior to their involvement in training. This conclusion suggests the possibility that speech improvement came about when the subjects increased the consistency of their use of available closure potential or when they transferred closure potential from one task to another. Another tentative interpretation is that an increase in the use of pharyngeal wall movement is the closure change most often associated with speech change. Also, it appears that training conducted in the speech context is most likely to be effective. Although studies using sensory stimulation and acoustic, airflow, or visual feedback all report some successes, those that rely on feedback procedures seem to be the most popular and easiest to carry out.

If one views the studies reported in relation to the assumptions underlying muscle training programs, it appears that these assumptions received limited consideration by the investigators. With the exception of studies that used subjects with pharyngeal flaps who needed to improve pharyngeal constrictor muscles, little attention was paid to determining which muscles were to be trained or how specific training activities would affect individual muscles. Also, there were few attempts to make direct measurements of change in muscle strength, endurance, mass, contractability, or motor control. The authors appear to assume that if any of these changes occurred, they would be reflected in general measures of velopharyngeal closure or in speech.

Two questions can be asked in light of the above discussion:

1. Should clinicians use muscle training programs to treat velopharyngeal closure problems? A tentative answer would be yes, under certain conditions. Although we cannot yet specify all of these conditions, there are some possibilities to consider. A clinician may consider the use of muscle training programs when:

    a. There is documented evidence that the patient can produce speech with acceptable levels of nasality in some contexts.

    b. There is documented evidence that the patient can accomplish velopharyngeal closure in speech or other contexts, in addition to swallowing.

    c. The clinician has access to instrumentation that provides visual, acoustic, or airflow feedback that can be used in training activities.

    d. The patient and the clinician are willing to devote at least 1 year to this approach.

    e. The clinician and the patient are willing and in a position to document their procedures.

    f. The patient is well aware that there is no certainty that training will be successful.

    g. The patient is aware of other approaches to the management of velopharyngeal closure problems.

2. Should further study of the issue be encouraged? The answer is yes. However, further studies will have to be more comprehensive than those now available if the findings are to provide information needed to determine the conditions under which muscle training may serve persons with velopharyngeal problems. They will have to include extensive evaluations and descriptions of subjects' velopharyngeal mechanisms and speech. Multiview videofluoroscopy and endoscopy appear to be promising ways of carrying out these evaluations, although the validity and reliability of measurements made with these procedures have not been fully established. Acoustic and perceptual evaluations of speech must include appropriate tasks to determine whether there are circumstances in which nasality and articulation show evidence of closure potential. Training programs must be based on needs and potentials revealed by these evaluations, and training tasks must be designed to accomplish specific goals. Without this attention to detail, it appears unlikely that additional studies will provide the information needed to make clinical management decisions.

References

1. Kantner CE: The rationale of blowing exercises for patients with repaired cleft palate. J Speech Dis 12:281, 1947.
2. Berry M, Eisenson J: Speech Disorders: Principles and Practices. New York: Appleton-Century-Crofts, 1956.
3. Westlake H, Rutherford D: Cleft Palate. Englewood Cliffs, NJ: Prentice-Hall, 1966.
4. Morley M: Cleft Palate and Speech. Baltimore: Williams & Wilkins, 1970.
5. McDonald ET, Koepp-Baker H: Cleft palate speech: An integration of research and clinical observation. J Speech Hear Dis 16:9, 1951.
6. Cole R: Direct muscle training for the improvement of velopharyngeal activity. In Bzoch K (ed): Communicative Disorders Related to Cleft Lip and Palate. Boston: Little, Brown, 1979.
7. McWilliams BJ, Morris H, Shelton R: Cleft Palate Speech. St. Louis: C. V. Mosby, 1984.
8. Shelton RL, Morris H, McWilliams BJ: Assessment of speech. In Speech, Language and Psychosocial Aspects of Cleft Lip and Cleft Palate: The State of the Art. American Speech and Hearing Association Reports, No. 9. Washington: American Speech and Hearing Association, 1973.
9. Schneider E, Shprintzen R: A survey of speech pathologists: Current trends in the diagnosis and management of velopharyngeal insufficiency. Cleft Palate J 17:249, 1980.
10. Krusen F, Kottke F, Ellwood P: Handbook of Physical Medicine and Rehabilitation. Philadelphia: Saunders, 1982.
11. Fox S: Human Physiology. Dubuque, IA: William C. Brown, 1987.
12. Shelton RL: Therapeutic exercise and speech pathology. Asha 5:855, 1963.
13. Ruscello D: A selected review of palatal training procedures. Cleft Palate J 91:181, 1982.
14. Massengill R, Quinn D, Pickrell K, Levinson C: Therapeutic exercises and velopharyngeal gap. Cleft Palate J 5:44, 1968.
15. Powers G, Starr C: The effects of muscle exercises on velopharyngeal gap and nasality. Cleft Palate J 11:28, 1974.
16. Yules R, Chase R: A training method for reduction of hypernasality in speech. Plast Reconstr Surg 43:180, 1969.
17. Weber J, Jobe R, Chase R: Evaluation of muscle stimulation in the rehabilitation of patients with hypernasal speech. Plast Reconstr Surg 46:173, 1970.
18. Peterson S: Electrical stimulation of the soft palate. Cleft Palate J 11:72, 1974.
19. Tash E, Shelton R, Knox A, et al: Training voluntary pharyngeal wall movements in children with normal and inadequate velopharyngeal closure. Cleft Palate J 8:277, 1971.
20. Shelton R, Beaumont K, Trier W, et al: Videoendoscopic feedback in training velopharyngeal closure. Cleft Palate J 15:6, 1978.
21. Siegel-Sadewitz V, Shprintzen R: Nasopharyngoscopy of the normal velopharyngeal sphincter: An experiment of biofeedback. Cleft Palate J 19:194, 1982.
22. Yamaoka M, Matsuya T, Miyazaki T, et al: Visual training for velopharyngeal closure in cleft palate patients: A fiberscopic procedure. J Maxillofac Surg 11:191, 1983.
23. Moller K, Werth L, Christianson P: The modification of velar movement. J Speech Hear Dis 38:323, 1973.
24. Shelton R, Chisum L, Youngstrom K, et al: Effect of articulation therapy on palatopharyngeal closure, movement of the pharyngeal wall, and tongue posture. Cleft Palate J 6:440, 1969.
25. Chisum L, Shelton R, Arndt W, et al: The relationship between remedial speech instruction activities and articulation change. Cleft Palate J 6:57, 1969.
26. Fletcher S: Contingencies for bioelectronic modification of nasality. J Speech Hear Dis 37:239, 1972.
27. Fletcher S: Diagnosing Speech Disorders from Cleft Palate. New York: Grune & Stratton, 1978.
28. Daly D, Johnson H: Instrumental modification of hypernasal vocal quality in retarded children: Case Reports. J Speech Hear Dis 39:508, 1974.
29. Shprintzen R, McCall G, Skolnick L: A new therapeutic technique for the treatment of velopharyngeal incompetence. J Speech Hear Dis 40:69, 1975.

CHAPTER 100

Speech Therapy for the Child with Cleft Lip and Palate

D. R. Van Demark and Mary A. Hardin

Children with cleft lip and palate are at high risk for speech production disorders. Although many of these children undoubtedly exhibit age-appropriate skills, descriptive findings obtained from numerous investigators suggest that as a group these children demonstrate poorer articulation and phonologic performance than their noncleft peers.[1] The etiology of articulation and phonologic errors noted in this population is multifactorial, and successful therapy will be contingent on the speech pathologist's ability to recognize and address the nature of the errors noted. These errors may be attributed to developmental delays, poor dental-occlusal status, or velopharyngeal incompetence. In addition, some children may develop aberrant patterns of articulation that seem to have been learned in response to (or to compensate for) presurgical velopharyngeal incompetence.

The goal of speech therapy for any child is to establish age-appropriate speech production patterns through behavioral modification. In addition to addressing any developmental articulation deficits that the child may demonstrate, therapy for the child with cleft lip and palate is typically directed toward the objectives of eliminating or reducing inappropriate patterns of nasalization, oral distortions, and "compensatory" articulation gestures. For the first two of these objectives, therapy may be employed on a trial basis to test the adequacy of physical structures for speech production, including velopharyngeal function and dental-occlusal status.

The purposes of this chapter are:

1. To review available data regarding the efficacy of speech therapy for children with cleft lip and palate.
2. To describe procedures that may be employed in therapy to treat the speech production disorders of these children.
3. To explore directions for future research.

Review of the Reported Research Findings

Few systematic investigations have been conducted to examine the efficacy of speech therapy for children with cleft lip and palate. The majority of findings that are available stem from descriptive accounts of therapy that employed limited experimental control and utilized subjects that were heterogeneous for factors such as velopharyngeal function and dentition. Regardless of the treatment protocol employed, the primary purpose of the bulk of this research has been to examine the relationship between behavioral management and changes in speech production.

In this chapter, we will review the use of articulation therapy, muscle training exercises, and biofeedback. Obturator reduction has also been used as a treatment method but is discussed elsewhere in this text in considerable detail.

Articulation Therapy

Schneider and Shprintzen[2] reported that articulation therapy is the most commonly employed training procedure used to treat velopharyngeal valving disorders. The popularity enjoyed by this procedure is interesting in light of the available experimental data, which cast doubt on the relationship between articulation therapy and modification of velopharyngeal function. One of the earliest studies conducted to examine the effectiveness of articulation therapy was reported by Chisholm and her associates.[3] Eleven subjects received conventional articulation therapy twice weekly for an average of 7 months. Improvement in articulation performance for these subjects, as measured by a 233-item articulation test, was compared with spontaneous improvement in articulation performance for 12 children who had no therapy and served as controls. The subjects ranged in age from 6 to 12 years and demonstrated hypernasality, audible nasal emission, or both. In addition, each subject misarticulated a minimum of three phonemes and evidenced six or more errors on the articulation test prior to study. Each subject was diagnosed as having borderline velopharyngeal competence. Although both groups demonstrated improved articulation on follow-up examination, greater improvement was evidenced by the group that received therapy.

Shelton and his associates examined the impact of conventional articulation therapy on measures of velopharyngeal function taken from lateral cinefluorographic films for 17 subjects with borderline velopharyngeal competence.[4] Improvement in articulation performance was noted; however, modifications in velopharyngeal activity were not observed. Although these findings suggest that conventional therapy alone does not appear to influence velopharyngeal function directly, the findings of several descriptive studies suggest that promoting correct articulatory placement can decrease the perception of hypernasality and audible nasal emission.

Van Demark examined the responses of 11 school-aged children with cleft palate to an intensive articulation therapy program.[5] Each subject received 1 hour of individual therapy and 1½ hours of group therapy daily for a period of 6 weeks. As a group, the subjects demonstrated less severe articulation defectiveness and hypernasality in connected speech and improved articulation test scores following therapy.

In a later study, Van Demark contrasted the articulatory changes in a group of 31 Danish children who had received speech therapy with the changes in a comparable group of 36 children who had not received therapy.[6] Fourteen of the 31 therapy subjects exhibited marginal velopharyngeal competence, and nine subjects were judged to demonstrate incompetence. The remaining eight subjects demonstrated velopharyngeal competence. In the control group, 23 subjects were judged to have velopharyngeal competence, 12 had marginal competence, and one was judged to exhibit incompetence. All subjects were administered the Danish Pressure Articulation Test (DPAT) at a mean age of 63 months. Follow-up examination was conducted at a mean age of 83 months. The findings of this study revealed that the children who received therapy demonstrated significant improvement on the DPAT. The nontherapy group demonstrated no significant difference in the averaged pre- and post-therapy test scores.

More recently, Van Demark and Hardin[7] examined the response of 13 children with cleft palate to an intensive 6-week articulation therapy program. Subjects enrolled in the program were judged to exhibit velopharyngeal competence or marginal velopharyngeal competence. Prior to enrollment in therapy, each subject was administered the Iowa Cleft Palate Articulation Test (ICPAT). In addition, severity ratings of articulation defectiveness and nasality in connected speech were obtained. Each subject was seen for two 1-hour sessions of individual therapy and two 1-hour sessions of group therapy 5 days a week for the 6-week period. Conventional articulation therapy was employed using the systematic multiple-sound approach described by McCabe and Bradley.[8] Following the intervention program, the pretherapy assessment protocol was administered to each subject. The assessment protocol was then administered 9 months later to examine maintenance of post-therapy articulation performance. Articulation proficiency on word articulation tests improved significantly for all subjects in the post-therapy condition. Test scores obtained immediately following therapy were not significantly different from those obtained during the follow-up examination, even though 11 of the 13 subjects had received speech therapy in the public schools in the interim. Severity ratings of articulation defectiveness in connected speech improved for 8 of the 13 subjects immediately following therapy. On the 9-month follow-up examination, all subjects were judged to demonstrate improved articulation performance in conversational speech. Severity ratings of nasality improved for 7 of the 13 subjects following therapy. It should be noted that of the six subjects for whom improvement was not noted, four had evidenced normal resonance prior to therapy, and so improvement would not have been expected.

In the aforementioned studies, Van Demark and his colleagues examined the effectiveness of articulation therapy in modifying the perceptual consequences of velopharyngeal valving deficits in children with cleft palate. Changes in velopharyngeal function were not assessed in these studies; rather, changes in perceived hypernasality and audible nasal emission were examined. The findings of these studies suggest that although the number of errors attributed to nasal distortion may not always decrease with articulation therapy, severity of both hypernasality and audible nasal emission does, at least for some children. This improvement, along with concomitant improvement in articulation, may facilitate speech intelligibility for select children and minimize the need for secondary surgical management.

Muscle Training Exercises

Early attempts to "train" velopharyngeal closure in patients with a marginally adequate mechanism involved the use of muscle training exercises. An excellent review of palatal training procedures was provided by Ruscello.[9] Blowing, sucking, gagging, and swallowing tasks were traditionally employed by some clinicians on the premise that these activities would strengthen the palatopharyngeal musculature and facilitate range of motion.[10–14] Other investigators have utilized tactile and electrical stimulation to enhance voluntary control of the velopharyngeal musculature.[15–18] Although greater range of movement following introduction of these palatal training procedures has been reported, there is little evidence to indicate that these procedures result in improved velopharyngeal closure or diminished hypernasality and nasal airflow in conversational speech.

Although palatal exercises do not appear to promote velopharyngeal closure during speech production, there are data to suggest that closure obtained during selected nonspeech activities may be used to facilitate velopharyngeal closure for speech. Shprintzen and his colleagues examined closure patterns during speech and nonspeech activities in normal subjects and found that patterns of closure achieved during speech, blowing, and whistling were highly similar.[19] Subsequently, Shprintzen et al described a therapy technique that they had developed and employed with four subjects, all of whom showed velopharyngeal closure on multiview videofluoroscopy during whistling and blowing but not during speech.[20] Two of the four subjects evidenced hypernasality and audible nasal emission after pharyngeal flap surgery. One subject demonstrated velopharyngeal incompetence after an adenoidectomy, and the remaining subject had incompetence following a primary palatoplasty. All subjects had received previous uneventful speech therapy. The subjects were taught to phonate while whistling or blowing. Nasal emission was monitored by the subjects using a Scape-Scope. Once the subjects could produce both activities simultaneously, the nonspeech activity was gradually eliminated.

According to the investigators, each subject demonstrated improved velopharyngeal function during speech following termination of the program. Two of the four subjects had normal conversational speech on 4- to 6-month follow-up. Mild hypernasality and infrequent nasal emission were noted on follow-up for the remaining two subjects. Shprintzen and his colleagues hypothesized that patients who have closure of the velopharyngeal port during whistling and blowing but not during speech probably have "functional" incompetence. Although these data are encouraging and suggest that closure obtained during nonspeech acts may be carried over to speech for some patients, further study of this procedure is warranted.

Biofeedback

Information feedback (or biofeedback) devices have also been employed in therapy to provide children with direct or indirect information on velopharyngeal function. Simple (yet effective) tools, such as the nasal mirror and the See Scape, are clinical tools that have long been used by practicing clinicians. Both devices are inexpensive and provide visual evidence of nasal airflow. More sophisticated tools, originally developed to evaluate velopharyngeal function, have also been employed to treat valving disorders. Aeromechanical devices (such as TONAR), nasendoscopes, and photodetectors have all been cited as valuable instruments in feedback therapy for velopharyngeal valving disorders.[21–27]

Kunzel described a photoelectric device, the velograph, consisting of a cold light probe and a photocell inserted transnasally to monitor closure of the velopharyngeal port.[28] He reported positive results in training purposeful movement of the velum in four subjects with repaired palatal clefts who exhibited velopharyngeal insufficiency. The period of training ranged from 3 weeks to 5 months, with one or two training sessions per week. Velar movement increased for all subjects with training; however, untrained listeners indicated that speech performance had improved in only two of the four subjects. Kunzel asserted that velographic results may be more positive when employed with subjects who demonstrate inconsistent velopharyngeal closure.

Although instrumental procedures of this type are becoming more frequently accepted as clinical training tools, some are expensive and require the application of a topical anesthetic for transnasal placement. Consequently, they may be of little practical value to the practicing clinician who must develop and implement treatment programs on limited budgets in schools or centers that do not offer medical assistance. It is pertinent, nonetheless, to recognize that instrumental feedback may be a powerful adjunct to conventional therapy and is a treatment option that should be examined more carefully in future research. At present, little information is available to characterize the type of patient that may benefit from biofeedback devices. The usefulness of these devices in promoting velopharyngeal closure appears most promising for the patient who exhibits borderline or marginally inconsistent valving problems.

Speech Therapy

In many children with cleft lip and palate, a multiplicity of factors may contribute to the speech problem. Unfortunately, the speech clinician in general practice may have little concrete information available on which to establish a therapy program. Information may be available on the surgery performed, history of hearing loss, and the child's dental status, but often the adequacy

of velopharyngeal function remains questionable. The importance of these factors has been discussed in other chapters, and parents should be informed about their influence on speech and language therapy.

When a child with cleft lip and palate is initially referred for speech therapy, more often than not a definitive diagnosis of the adequacy of the velopharyngeal mechanism has not been made. There may be several reasons why the diagnosis has not been made, but the predominant factors may be the child's age and the child's ability to cooperate for physiologic assessment of velopharyngeal function. Additionally, therapy may be recommended when physiologic assessment of velopharyngeal function has been conducted but the cleft palate team remains uncertain about the adequacy of the mechanism. In many cases, the results of therapy are important in this regard. More often than not, therapy is a combination of both diagnosis and treatment, and it is the speech pathologist's task to sort out those speech attributes that are related to learning from attributes that are related to the structural or functional integrity of the velopharyngeal mechanism.

It is not uncommon on initial evaluation for the preschool child to exhibit some hypernasality, audible nasal emission, other articulatory or phonologic errors, depressed expressive language skills, slight hoarseness, and irregular dentition. Although the speech pathologist who works in a cleft palate clinic may be quite familiar with children who exhibit varying degrees of problem associated with the above factors, the speech pathologist in general practice is not. The speech pathologist should be aware that although behavioral therapy may be needed to stimulate language development and facilitate age-appropriate articulation or phonologic skills for these children (as with the noncleft child), speech therapy may also be needed to determine the adequacy of the velopharyngeal mechanism for normal speech production. Instrumental assessment of velopharyngeal function may well be performed to assess the functional potential of the mechanism; however, information derived from such an assessment alone may not adequately predict the child's ability to use the mechanism for speech, particularly when marginal or borderline incompetence is present.

Because information about the changes (or lack thereof) resulting from the therapeutic process is often considered in decisions to pursue secondary surgical management for velopharyngeal incompetence, it is essential that the speech pathologist carefully document any changes noted. Dramatic changes can be demonstrated by tape recordings of conversational speech or imitative tasks but only if the clinician records a sample of the child's speech before therapy is initiated. Documentation need not be complex but should be obtained in a descriptive, systematic fashion.

Pre- and postarticulation test scores are often employed to assess improvement in therapy. The astute speech pathologist recognizes, however, that although information derived from such testing will reveal *some* of the progress a child has made, test scores alone do not account for many changes in the child's repertoire that are revealed in daily therapy sessions. Test scores are not, for example, descriptive of the child who eliminates nasal distortion of a consonant but who continues to exhibit oral distortion of that same consonant. Nor are test scores descriptive of the child who initially is unable to produce a consonant with stimulability testing and then successfully learns to produce the consonant in consonant-vowel combinations.

Since some children with velopharyngeal valving disorders will be considered for secondary surgical management when changes are not evidenced in behavioral therapy, it is essential that the speech pathologist provide the cleft palate team with definitive information about changes that do or do not occur.

Articulation Therapy for Children with Velopharyngeal Competence

The primary goal of conventional articulation therapy is to establish correct articulatory placement. The goals and procedures of articulation therapy for children with cleft lip and palate do not differ from those of therapy for the noncleft child. The child with a cleft, however, may evidence articulation problems that are not typically seen in their noncleft peers, including phoneme-specific nasalization and compensatory articulation patterns. Both types of articulation errors may develop (in all probability) prior to primary palatal surgery and persist as learned behaviors. The latter types of errors also may have developed in response to behavioral attempts to modify errors related to velopharyngeal incompetence.

Phoneme-specific nasalization is generally easily eradicated in therapy. Auditory training should be employed to help the child identify the nasal distortion. If the child is unable to eliminate nasal emission during production of the error sound, oral pressure achieved during production of another consonant may be used to stimulate oral production of the target phoneme. Consider, for example, the child who consistently produces /s/ with nasal emission and achieves oral production of other pressure consonants that share the same place of articulation and voicing characteristics (e.g., /t/). Rapid successive productions of the latter consonant followed by the target phoneme (i.e., asking the child to say "t . . . t . . . t . . . ts") can be used to promote oral production of /s/. When available, biofeedback devices may be used to provide the child with visual feedback about nasal emission (See Scape) or velopharyngeal closure (nasendoscope).

The majority of compensatory articulation patterns noted in children with cleft lip and palate involve errors in place of production and typically represent posterior articulation patterns.[29] The goal in therapy designed to eliminate these aberrant patterns of production is to move the place of articulation more anteriorly in the vocal tract. According to Trost, attempts to modify these patterns will probably be unsuccessful with auditory modeling alone.[29] She advocates the use of diagrams to help the child contrast faulty and correct articulatory placements. She also recommends that therapy be directed initially only toward establishing correct placement of production. If manner of production is also in error, modification of that error should be attempted only following correct placement.

Although we have found it rather easy to modify these compensatory articulation patterns in young children, we have noted that maintenance of these patterns in conversational speech is not easily accomplished. Consequently, we recommend that the speech pathologist carefully monitor these children after they have been dismissed from therapy.

Articulation Therapy for Children with Borderline Velopharyngeal Competence

The practice of employing speech therapy to modify velopharyngeal valving deficits has long been a controversial issue in cleft palate management. Although patients who exhibit gross velopharyngeal incompetence are usually referred for surgical management, trial speech therapy is likely to be recommended for the child who evidences marginal or borderline incompetence, that is, mild or inconsistent nasalization of speech. These children are typically referred for trial therapy in the hope that behavioral management will:

1. Maximize the range of velar or pharyngeal wall movement when small portal openings are evident.
2. Generalize oral responses obtained during simple speech tasks (single word production) to more complex tasks (connected speech) when inconsistent closure is demonstrated.

Proponents of behavioral therapy have argued that a patient who evidences marginal closure should be able to enforce purposeful movement of the velopharyngeal structures. Opponents have pointed out, however, that despite clinical case reports of success, limited data are available to support the notion that velopharyngeal competence can be taught.

The speech pathologist who has worked with children who have articulation or phonologic delays should not find the cleft palate child who has marginal velopharyngeal valving problems perplexing. Generally, the same therapeutic principles apply. Therapy for these children should focus on establishing age-appropriate phonology and correct articulatory placement as well as enhancing precision of articulation. In addition to the developmental articulation disorders that may be present, some of these children, as indicated earlier, will exhibit compensatory articulation patterns that will require intervention. Considerations for the modification of these atypical patterns of articulation were described earlier in this chapter. There may also be dental deviations (that is, missing lateral incisors or canines) that influence the precision of articulation for sounds such as /s/ and /z/. Articulation therapy for these children is appropriate. However, the speech pathologist should recognize that children with severe dental anomalies may not always achieve the articulation proficiency expected in therapy, particularly if therapy is initiated during prosthetic or orthodontic treatment. Although attention to phonology and articulation placement may not eliminate audible nasal emission during speech, improvement in intelligibility typically will be noted, and a reduction in perceived nasalization should occur.

The speech pathologist should, on enrolling the child in therapy, make note of the patterns and consistency of audible nasal emission. To initiate therapy without this information may be fruitless because the majority of children referred for therapy will not show nasal distortion of all pressure consonants in all phonetic contexts. For example, it is not uncommon for a child to produce /p/ correctly in one phonetic context but experience audible nasal emission when /p/ is produced in another context. To say simply that the child evidences "inconsistent" audible nasal emission is not sufficient for planning therapy. The speech pathologist should scrutinize the child's spontaneous speech sample (or articulation test when whole word transcription has been performed) to determine if audible nasal emission is indeed occurring inconsistently or randomly across all phonetic contexts or if the behavior is context dependent. Such information will minimize the amount of therapy time needed to determine the efficacy of behavioral treatment because the target behaviors for therapy will have been well identified.

All too often, a child who has been referred for "trial" therapy remains in therapy for extended periods of time without success because the speech pathologist interprets correct production of a consonant in one context to be predictive of correct production in all other contexts. The physiologic demands placed on the velopharyngeal mechanism, however, will vary with both the phonetic context and the complexity of the speech task. A child who may easily achieve oral production of /s/ in the word "sock" may be unable to achieve velopharyngeal closure during that same phoneme when it is adjacent to a nasal consonant ("smoke") because the latter task will necessitate rapid and careful timing of velar movement. Likewise, oral production of a sound in an isolated word may not always be predictive of production characteristics in connected speech because the latter task will place greater demands on rate and timing of velar and pharyngeal movement.

We would like to add a note of caution here. Several authors have asserted that children with velopharyngeal valving disorders who correctly produce plosives but demonstrate audible nasal emission of fricatives are good therapy candidates.[30] We support the notion that these children should be enrolled in trial therapy, and efforts should be made to reduce or eliminate nasal distortion. However, we do not agree with the premise that an ability to impound oral pressure for production of plosives is necessarily predictive of a child's ability to impound *and maintain* oral pressure for production of sibilants and fricatives in conversational speech. When therapy is unsuccessful in reducing audible nasal emission, the clinician should feel obligated to refer the child back to the cleft palate team.

After correct articulatory placement has been achieved and the child's patterns of nasalization have been identified, the speech pathologist may attempt to modify nasal distortion of pressure consonants. As a first step, we recommend auditory training. The child's ability to distinguish between oral and nasal productions is, in our opinion, essential if behavioral modification is to be successful. For the young child, activities designed to teach oral direction of airflow may be beneficial. Some activities include: displacing a cotton ball or tissue while blowing gently, using a straw to blow bubbles in water, and so on. A nasal mirror, See Scape, or other simple device may then be employed to augment ear training and provide the child with visual feedback of nasal emission during production tasks.

Finally, if the child is unable to reduce or eliminate audible nasal emission with auditory or visual feedback alone, the clinician may attempt to minimize the perception of nasal distortion by

1. Decreasing oral resistance.
2. Encouraging light articulatory contacts.
3. Manipulating rate of speech production.

These strategies may be considered "compensatory" because they do not affect velopharyngeal closure per se but rather influence other variables that affect the perception of audible nasal emission. Oral resistance can be decreased by having the child employ a larger mouth opening during speech. As indicated by McWilliams et al ". . . in the presence of small velopharyngeal openings, increase in mouth opening results in speech that is perceived as more oral."[1] Procedures to promote oral openness have been described by Morley[31] and Boone and McFarlane.[32]

The use of light articulatory contacts (that is, touch pressure contact) also may be used as a "compensatory" strategy to decrease the listener's perception of speech nasalization.[33, 34] Although this technique appears to be useful clinically, little is known about the variables that are affected that result in differences in perception. It has been suggested that the use of light articulatory contacts involves a reduction in both speech rate and expiratory effort.[1]

Modification of speech rate to decrease the perception of speech nasalization is a somewhat controversial issue. Surgical repair of a palatal cleft typically results in a scarred velum that, for some children, moves somewhat sluggishly. Clinicians have hypothesized that decreasing the rate of production will decrease nasalization because the velum will have more time to produce an articulatory gesture. Although this is an attractive clinical hypothesis, researchers investigating the effect of speaking rate on perceived nasalization have found little systematic relationship between the two.[35, 36] Nevertheless, some children may benefit from changes in speech rate.

Some children with borderline valving deficits may show evidence of nasal grimacing. Constriction of the nasal alae may accompany nasal emission during production of pressure consonants in conversational speech, and this may persist for some children after adequate velopharyngeal valving has been established. Apparently, these movements are compensatory in nature and arise as the child attempts to valve the air, lost through the velopharyngeal port, at the anterior nares. Fortunately, the visual distraction caused by nasal grimacing is easily modified in most children with visual feedback (use of a mirror).

Articulation Therapy for Children with Velopharyngeal Incompetence

Articulation therapy to eliminate nasalization of speech is not advised for the child who exhibits gross velopharyngeal incompetence; articulation errors related to structural or physiologic incompetence can be eliminated only through surgical or prosthetic management. Attempts to establish correct articulatory placement in the presence of velopharyngeal incompetence may, however, be deemed necessary at times when physical management is delayed for a child who produces unintelligible speech.

Therapy to promote correct articulatory placement will enhance speech intelligibility and facilitate good postoperative speech production. The speech pathologist must recognize, however, that attempts to establish correct sound production in the presence of an incompetent velopharyngeal mechanism may lead a child to develop aberrant posterior patterns of articulation if emphasis is placed on elimination of nasalization rather than on placement alone. The clinician should avoid the temptation to stress "oral" speech when velopharyngeal incompetence is clearly evident. Attempts to reduce or eliminate audible nasal emission through behavioral therapy should be restricted to the child who evidences velopharyngeal competence or marginal velopharyngeal competence.

Therapy for Resonance Disorders

As with most speech therapy, resonance therapy for the individual with cleft palate necessarily involves some diagnostic evaluation. Good therapy is a process that helps clarify and describe the problem. Thus, diagnosis is a continual process and should be considered part of the therapy process. Because children and adults with cleft palate are heterogeneous, categorization of voice quality and voice problems may provide a simplistic approach to the problem, yet for clarity it seems best to divide our discussion into several areas.

Certainly, the resonance of the speech of individuals with cleft palate is probably the most common feature people respond to when they attempt to describe the speech problems of individuals with cleft palate. Diagnostically, a sizable number of individuals have some difficulty distinguishing between hypernasality and hyponasality.

Hypernasality, or excessive nasal resonance, is perceived primarily during production of vowels and dipthongs. It may occur in individuals with adequate velopharyngeal competence or in those with varying degrees of velopharyngeal incompetence. Those individuals with some degree of velopharyngeal incompetence may have concomitant nasal emission of air on pressure consonants, but the two terms are not interchangeable. Nasal emission of air implies some inadequacy of the velopharyngeal closure mechanism, which may occur on a consistent or inconsistent basis. It is our opinion that when severe nasal emission occurs it is questionable that therapy for nasal resonance is appropriate.

Hyponasality, or a reduction of normal nasal resonance, is perceived primarily during production of vowels, dipthongs, and nasal consonants. It is generally assumed that hyponasality occurs because of a physical blockage (such as a pharyngeal flap or hypertrophied adenoidal tissue) that reduces coupling between the oral and the nasal cavities for normal resonance. Thus, therapy for hyponasality involves medical or surgical management to decrease nasal resistance (that is, medication for allergies, adenoidectomy, and revision of pharyngeal flap).

Mixed nasality is a combination of both hypernasality and hyponasality. It may occur in individuals with cleft palate because the timing and structure of the mechanism at times allows too much nasal resonance, whereas in other situations there is insufficient resonance on nasal consonants to provide an acceptable balance.

When initiating therapy, it is appropriate first to establish an overall rating of the patient's hypernasality in conversational speech. We employ a seven-point clinical severity scale (1 = mild, 7 = extremely severe). It is also appropriate to have the patient read a passage to allow comparison of the degree of hypernasality to conversational speech. Preferably, these samples should be recorded so that they can be used in post-therapy comparisons.

If it is difficult to determine which vowels and dipthongs are nasalized and the context in which they are nasalized, a closed nostril test is appropriate.[37] Generally, the speech pathologist will find that nasality occurs on specific vowels but not all vowels. For example, early research indicated that for functionally nasal individuals, words like "cat" and "father" tended to be more nasal, whereas in individuals with cleft palate, high vowels such as /i/ and /u/ tended to be more nasal. Likewise, considering coarticulatory effects, the speech pathologist should not be surprised to find that many individuals exhibit nasality with a combination of consonant phonemes. Again, it is important to observe whether the patient exhibits just hypernasality or also shows nasal emission on such combinations. If nasal emission occurs to any degree, it is quite probable that the patient may not be able to alter nasality on the production of vowels.

After those vowels and dipthongs with excessive nasal resonance are identified, several therapeutic procedures may be of assistance to the patient. Auditory discrimination between nasalized vowel production and non-nasalized production is appropriate; however, if the patient or speech pathologist has difficulty in discriminating between these productions, closing the nares often gives both additional cues. Increased mouth opening or the concept of orality as described by Boone and others may also decrease the perception of nasality.[32] However, if there is tension in the oral cavity extra nasal resonance may be perceived.

If nasality is perceived on several vowels, low vowels should be approached first. A step-by-step approach from simple to more complex will help both the speech pathologist and the patient evaluate the success of the behavioral management program. A program similar to the one proposed by Lang, and cited by Sommers,[38] is appropriate. Basically, one should first work in simple contexts with glides followed by plosives, and finally work in fricatives and affricates. The vowel context should be varied both preceding and following consonants. It is particularly helpful to establish a normal resonance pattern on simple tasks before nasal consonants are included in the therapy program.

It should be noted here that some of the problems in setting a goal for a client to decrease hypernasality are as follows:

1. The patient does not have an adequate velopharyngeal closure mechanism to decrease hypernasality.
2. Often the speech pathologist's goal is vague.
3. The speech pathologist's listening skills are not strong enough to be consistent in reinforcing appropriate responses, and therefore the client does not know when she or he is doing something different or when she or he is producing the correct response.

Therapy Postsecondary Management

As was stated earlier, secondary surgical management for velopharyngeal incompetence does not guarantee that a child's speech will change. Although changes may be dramatic for some children, we have observed numerous children who show little change following pharyngeal flap surgery. That may be because secondary management did not provide an adequate mechanism. Conversely, surgery may have yielded an adequate or near adequate mechanism, but the child simply has not learned to use it in production of speech sounds. For example, if a child has consistently said "mamy" for "baby," adequate pharyngeal flap surgery does not ensure that the child will automatically change his or her articulatory behavior for the targeted word, but it may provide the physiologic potential to change behavior.

Thus, postoperative pharyngeal flap speech therapy attempts to determine the adequacy of the mechanism by the behavioral changes the child can make. Because both behavioral and physiologic changes must occur concurrently, it may be some time before those changes are evident. It is not uncommon for a child to need up to 1 year to develop the potential for velopharyngeal closure effectively in conversational speech, and speech therapy is entirely appropriate to help accomplish those changes. When changes in speech production are not accomplished, physiologic measures may be needed to help assess the adequacy of the mechanism. If necessary, a revision of the flap (or other secondary management procedure) may be indicated.

When articulation has been normalized in individuals with pharyngeal flaps, attention is often given to voice quality. Some hypernasality may persist, or, in other cases, hyponasality may be present. Therapeutic measures to determine whether the hyponasal child can achieve nasal resonance are appropriate. As with nasal emission, hyponasality is related to structural components that do not respond to behavioral treatment. Quite often the patient has other complaints such as snoring, mouth breathing, and discomfort. It is our opinion that these factors must be weighed in considering further management, and the patient's preferences should be part of that decision. In our experience, the majority of postpharyngeal flap patients with hyponasality tend to reject surgical revision of the flap, preferring slightly hyponasal speech to the risk of hypernasality.

Recommendations for Future Research

Although speech therapy has undoubtedly assisted in the acquisition of normal or improved speech for many individuals with cleft palate, essentially no research is available to support or refute many aspects of therapy. One would suspect that there is an optimal time when a child can change behavioral patterns more easily, yet the age at which therapy is initiated is usually determined by the availability of speech pathology services rather than by research findings. Likewise, the type of therapy administered has not been studied to any degree and is usually related to the same type of therapy used for children who have articulatory or phonologic delay.

Although diagnosticians in speech pathology who work directly with individuals who have cleft palate are aware that some children and adults can easily modify physiologic movements and do so appropriately, research efforts to teach such movements have been ineffective. Again, the age of the child, the method used, and the reinforcement given have not been thoroughly investigated.

It is possible that in the future methods will be developed to determine the potential of a given velopharyngeal mechanism. The ability to teach a person to use the mechanism to its maximum potential, however, seems now to lie far in the future, and thus the study of the dynamics of the normal mechanism and the variability of the mechanism seem entirely appropriate to allow further understanding of the capabilities of the abnormal mechanism. Although it is apparent that speech therapy is beneficial to individuals with cleft lip and palate, research evidence to demonstrate its effectiveness is very sparse. It is not surprising that this is the case because research controlling all variables is essentially impossible to conduct. The behavioral or learned aspects can be studied, but the concomitant physical variability of the mechanism and the possibility of change within the mechanical structures with growth contribute to the lack of documentation of the therapeutic process.

Thus, it is essential that future research be directed not only to understanding the therapeutic process but also to determining the most efficacious way in which to make behavioral and physiologic changes in the patient with cleft palate. Such research is important not only in encouraging cost-effective treatment but also in helping the patient eliminate a most psychologically frustrating experience: attempting to do something that physically cannot be done or expecting a behavioral change without being told how to change the behavior.

References

1. McWilliams BJ, Morris HL, Shelton RL: Cleft Palate Speech. Philadelphia: B. C. Decker, 1984.
2. Schneider E, Shprintzen RJ: A survey of speech pathologists: Current trends in the diagnosis and management of velopharyngeal insufficiency. Cleft Palate J 17:249–253, 1980.
3. Chisum L, Shelton RL, Arndt WB, et al: Relationship between remedial speech instruction activities and articulation change. Cleft Palate J 6:57–64, 1969.
4. Shelton RL, Chisum L, Youngstrom KA, et al: Effect of articulation therapy on palatopharyngeal closure, movement of the pharyngeal wall, and tongue posture. Cleft Palate J 6:440–448, 1969.
5. Van Demark DR: Clinical research methodology in evaluating the therapeutic process. Cleft Palate J 8:26, 1971.
6. Van Demark DR: Some results of speech therapy for children with cleft palate. Cleft Palate J 11:41, 1974.
7. Van Demark DR, Hardin MA: Effectiveness of intensive articulation therapy for children with cleft palate. Cleft Palate J 23:215–224, 1985.
8. McCabe RB, Bradley DP: Systematic multiple phonemic approach to articulation therapy. Acta Symbolica 6:1, 1975.
9. Ruscello DM: A selected review of palatal training procedures. Cleft Palate J 19:181–193, 1982.
10. Kanter CE: The rationale of blowing exercises for patients with repaired cleft palates. J Speech Dis 12:281, 1947.
11. Kanter CE: Diagnosis and prognosis in cleft palate speech. J Speech Hear Dis 13:211, 1948.
12. Massengill R, Quinn GW, Pickrell KL, et al: Therapeutic exercise and velopharyngeal gap. Cleft Palate J 5:44–48, 1968.
13. Powers GL, Starr CD: The effects of muscle exercises on velopharyngeal gap and nasality. Cleft Palate J 11: 28–35, 1974.
14. Cole RM: Direct muscle training for the improvement of velopharyngeal activity. In Bzoch KR (ed): Communicative Disorders Related to Cleft Lip and Palate, 2nd ed. Boston: Little, Brown, 1979.
15. Yules RB, Chase RA: A training method for reduction of hypernasality in speech. Plast Reconstr Surg 43:180–185, 1969.
16. Weber J, Jobe RP, Chase RA: Evaluation of muscle stimulation in the rehabilitation of patients with hypernasal speech. Plast Reconstr Surg 46:173–174, 1970.
17. Tash EL, Shelton RL, Knox AW, et al: Training voluntary pharyngeal wall movements in children with normal and inadequate velopharyngeal closure. Cleft Palate J 8:277–290, 1971.
18. Peterson SJ: Electrical stimulation of the soft palate. Cleft Palate J 11:72–86, 1974.
19. Shprintzen RJ, Lencione RM, McCall GN, et al: A three-dimensional analysis of velopharyngeal closure during speech and nonspeech activities in normals. Cleft Palate J 11:412–428, 1974.
20. Shprintzen RJ, McCall GN, Skolnick ML: A new therapeutic technique for the treatment of velopharyngeal incompetence. J Speech Hear Dis 40:69–83, 1975.
21. Fletcher SG: Contingencies for bioelectronic modification of nasality. J Speech Hear Dis 37:329–346, 1972.
22. Daly DA, Johnson HP: Instrumental modification of hypernasal voice quality in retarded children. J Speech Hear Dis 39:500–507, 1974.
23. Nishio J, Yamaoka M, Matsuya T, et al: How to exercise the velopharyngeal movement by the velopharyngeal fiberscope. Jap J Oral Surg 20:450–457, 1974.
24. Miyazaki T, Matsuya T, Yamaoka M: Fiberscopic methods for assessment of velopharyngeal closure during various activities. Cleft Palate J 12:107–114, 1974.
25. Siegle-Sadewitz VL, Shprintzen RJ: Nasopharyngoscopy of the normal velopharyngeal sphincter: An experiment of biofeedback. Cleft Palate J 19:194–200, 1982.
26. Dalston RM: Photodetector assessment of velopharyngeal activity. Cleft Palate J 19:1–8, 1982.
27. Yamaoka M, Matsuya T, Miyazaki T, et al: Visual training for velopharyngeal closure in cleft palate patients: A fibroscopic procedure (preliminary report). J Maxillofac Surg 11:191–193, 1983.
28. Kunzel HJ: First applications of a biofeedback device for the therapy of velopharyngeal incompetence. Folia Phoniatr 34:92–100, 1982.
29. Trost JE: Articulatory additions to the classical description of the speech of persons with cleft palate. Cleft Palate J 18:193–203, 1981.
30. Hirshberg J: Velopharyngeal insufficiency. Folia Phoniatr 38:221–276, 1986.
31. Morley ME: Cleft Palate and Speech. Baltimore: Williams & Wilkins, 1962.
32. Boone DR, McFarlane SC: The Voice and Voice Therapy. Englewood Cliffs, NJ: Prentice-Hall, 1988.
33. Wells CG: Cleft Palate and Its Associated Speech Disorders. New York: McGraw-Hill, 1971.
34. Shelton RL, Hahn E, Morris HL: Diagnosis and therapy. In Spriestersbach DC, Sherman D (eds): Cleft Palate and Communication. New York: Academic Press, 1968.
35. D'Antonio LL: An investigation of speech timing in individuals with cleft palate. Thesis. San Francisco: University of California at San Francisco, 1982.
36. Jones DL, Folkins JW: The effect of speaking rate on judgments of disordered speech in children with cleft palate. Cleft Palate J 22:246–252, 1985.
37. Bzoch KR: Measurement and assessment of categorical aspects of cleft palate speech. In Bzoch KR (ed): Communicative Disorders Related to Cleft Lip and Palate. Boston: Little, Brown, 1979.
38. Sommers RK: Articulation Disorders. Englewood Cliffs, NJ: Prentice-Hall, 1983.

CHAPTER 101

The Conceptual Framework for Pharyngeal Flap Surgery

Robert J. Shprintzen

The literature describing pharyngeal flap surgery reaches back into the nineteenth century and includes hundreds of reports. The emphasis in clinical research on pharyngeal flap surgery falls into two broad categories: surgical technique and speech results. A careful review of the literature, however, fails to show much agreement on the conceptual decisions that serve as indications for the procedure. Even less agreement is found in the judgments of success of the operation. Although claims of success consistently approach 100%, the appearance of additional reports of "new" pharyngeal flap techniques or other "new" pharyngoplasties continues unabated. Obviously, if so many procedures have 100% success, there would be little reason to invent new ones.

It is the contention of this author that one essential component is missing in the approach to pharyngeal flap surgery: a sound conceptual framework. The conceptual framework should take into account the goal of the procedure, indications for the operation, and definitions of "success." It is the purpose of this chapter to suggest such a conceptual framework. Because it is the goal of this chapter to be critical of the evolution of the scientific endeavors relating to the pharyngeal flap, it will be free of direct references to publications about pharyngeal flap surgery to avoid singling out any particular author for what is perceived to be faulty research. We all share the blame equally.

Goal

The first step is to ask the question, What is the goal of pharyngeal flap surgery? Perhaps a simpler and more appropriate way of asking the same question is, Why is this operation done? The answer that comes immediately to mind is that pharyngeal flap surgery is done to improve speech in patients with velopharyngeal insufficiency. This answer is, of course, absolutely incorrect. Just as the goal of coronary artery bypass surgery is not to make a cardiac cripple run faster, the goal of pharyngeal flap surgery is not to improve speech. Pharyngeal flap surgery is performed only when an individual displays a velopharyngeal insufficiency that results in hypernasal resonance or audible nasal air escape during speech. The goal of the operation is to eliminate the insufficiency and therefore give the patient normal resonance balance. Therefore, it is fair to say that the success of the procedure should be based on what the operation is designed to do. Normal speech is not the goal. The elimination of velopharyngeal insufficiency and its resulting symptom of hypernasality is the goal.

Indications

The indications for pharyngeal flap surgery need to be consistent with the goals of the operation. Therefore, if the elimination of velopharyngeal insufficiency and hypernasal resonance is the goal of the operation, the confirmation of insufficiency and the determination that resonance is abnormal is the indication for the procedure. The first step is for a speech pathologist to confirm the presence of abnormal hypernasal resonance. Without the clinical confirmation of an abnormal degree of hypernasal resonance, surgery of any type is obviously contraindicated, regardless of the physical findings. However, once hypernasal speech has been diagnosed, it becomes essential to confirm the presence of the insufficiency and to describe it with sufficient accuracy to provide evidence that the problem can be surgically eliminated. This obviously involves instrumentation and diagnostic tests, which will be described later.

Previous Research Approaches

The postoperative speech assessments reported in the literature to date have been so variable that any meaningful comparison from study to study is impossible. Only a few studies have utilized direct visualization techniques to ascertain data on the postoperative prevalence of velopharyngeal insufficiency in relation to acoustic judgments of nasal resonance. The overwhelming majority of studies have described postoperative results according to some type of rating scale of "speech." The following terms are only a few selected ones that have been used by authors to describe the results of pharyngeal flap surgery: socially acceptable, significant improvement, satisfactory speech, improved speech, average speech, reduced hypernasality, or intelligible speech. None of these assessments represents a valid way of determining the success or failure of a pharyngeal flap.

First, as pointed out earlier in this chapter, the purpose of pharyngeal flap surgery is not to improve speech, but rather to eliminate only one pathologic feature of speech, velopharyngeal insufficiency. If velopharyngeal insufficiency is eliminated successfully, hypernasal resonance will no longer be a factor. However, there are many other features of abnormal speech in individuals with clefts that will confound judgments. Articulatory compensations, vocal quality, language impairment, rate of speech, dysarthria, and even the speech sample used for the judgment can affect the postoperative assessment. Because all of these confounding features are also a part of speech, assessments of how satisfactory, improved, socially acceptable, or intelligible speech is after surgery cannot possibly judge the change in resonance alone. A review of the many reports about the pharyngeal flap procedure will show that very few studies have attempted to hold the other aspects of speech constant. To truly assess the effect of the operation, hypernasality should be the only speech abnormality present prior to the operation.

A large number of the studies assessing pharyngeal flap surgery have used rating scales to assess the operation's results, such as ratings of no improvement, some improvement, or marked improvement, or severely impaired, moderately impaired, mildly impaired, or normal. Another term that consistently appears in the literature is *borderline*. Authors operationally define success as marked improvement, acceptable, or borderline. Such rating scales are invalid because hypernasality is either present or absent. It may be present in degrees, but it cannot be absent in degrees. Because the operation is designed to eliminate velopharyngeal insufficiency, the only valid definition of success should be normal with regard to resonance. If even mild hypernasality or borderline nasality is present, the operation cannot be considered successful. In other words, the success or failure of an operation must be determined by what the operation is supposed to do in the first place. The reader of the reports in question should be asking, "If a patient has improved from severely hypernasal to mildly hypernasal, will that patient be exempt from further treatment?" Or even more appropriately, "Why should a curable condition merely be improved to a lesser degree of impairment?"

Valid research approaches to pharyngeal flap should include the following:
1. Direct three-dimensional visualization of the velopharyngeal valve both before and after surgery.
2. Acoustic assessments of speech resonance characteristics both before and after surgery.
3. The ability to filter out any confounding speech disorders.
4. Long-term postoperative assessment (at least 1 year, though 2 or more years is preferable).
5. Documentation.

Perspectives and Recommendations

The purpose of this next section is to summarize some thoughts on pharyngeal flap surgery that, to the best of my knowledge, have not been addressed sufficiently in the literature to date. The following perspectives and recommendations are based on my personal observations of hundreds of pharyngeal flap procedures performed by many surgeons at a number of institutions. They are also based on a large number of observations (more than 200) of patients with failed pharyngeal flaps from other institutions referred to our center specifically for nasopharyngoscopy and multiview videofluoroscopy. Although we have frequently published data from our observations, we have not really addressed the more philosophical questions pertinent to the operation. Some of these perspectives are summarized below.

When Should the Operation Be Done?

Age is a factor that has received little attention in previous reports. Pharyngeal flap surgery should not be performed in children below the age of approximately 4½ years. There are four reasons for waiting until just before school age before considering the operation.

Language Development. It is generally recognized that a child's language does not really become "adultlike" until approximately 4½ years of age. Prior to complete language development, intelligibility is more difficult to assess. Many parts of speech are omitted, and the complexity of utterances is reduced. In order to perform acoustic assessment of a child's speech, sufficient language must be available for an accurate analysis. The normal language development of the preschool child should be undisturbed by surgical trauma until clinicians have been able to determine conclusively that surgery is unavoidable.

Articulation Development. Articulation development prior to 5 years of age also is incomplete. There are many sounds that have not yet entered into the child's phonemic repertoire. The close relationship between articulatory errors and velopharyngeal insufficiency has recently been demonstrated.[1, 2] The resolution of articulation errors in children with cleft palate has been shown to result in a corresponding resolution of the velopharyngeal insufficiency in many cases.[2] It is unlikely that appropriate speech therapy could be completed in very young children (2 or 3 years old) to determine if surgery might be avoided.

Assessment of Velopharyngeal Insufficiency. I am still incredulous that some clinicians have not grasped the importance of obtaining definitive, direct observations of velopharyngeal insufficiencies prior to operating to relieve them. Surgeons especially should appreciate the value of seeing their operative field and the defect they are trying to correct prior to treatment planning. As of this writing, there are only two diagnostic tools that completely describe velopharyngeal insufficiencies three-dimensionally when used in combination: multiview videofluoroscopy and nasopharyngoscopy.[3] Both techniques are of equal importance for the physiologic and anatomic description of the velopharyngeal mechanism. Having personally performed over 4000 fluoroscopic and endoscopic examinations, I can state with some certainty that it is a very rare child under the age of 4 who will be compliant for these examinations. At

our institution, we would not think of recommending surgery without these assessments because of our technique of varying flap width according to velopharyngeal gap size.[4–6] Therefore, surgery must be deferred until the operation of choice can be specified.

Compliance and Morbidity. Pharyngeal flap surgery can hardly be considered a benign procedure. Patients are typically quite uncomfortable for several days after the operation. Adequate hydration is very important after surgery to prevent other complications and provide relief for the retropharyngeal pain from the donor site. Because the surgery is in the upper airway, the potential for upper airway obstruction and obstructive sleep apnea exists.[7] The smaller the airway at the time of surgery (the airway is smaller when the child is young), the greater the risk of obstructive episodes. Two- and three-year-old children are, as a rule, very noncompliant. They are behaviorally immature and less likely to follow instructions with regard to drinking postoperatively. It is difficult to explain to them why they are in the hospital and why they are going to have, at the very least, a bad sore throat. It is not until after the fourth birthday (when receptive language is more intact) that explanations can be offered and assurances of compliance can be obtained. The trauma and ordeal of the surgical event will be far more difficult at 3 years of age than at 4 or 5.

Syndromes and Pharyngeal Flap Surgery

Three recent publications have shown that the frequency of congenital multiple anomaly syndromes associated with clefting of the palate or lip and palate is far higher than previously thought.[8–10] Some syndromes associated with clefting present increased risk for both postoperative failure and postoperative complications. For example, congenital airway narrowing is a common finding in Stickler syndrome, one of the more common syndromes of clefting.[10, 11] The potential for obstructive sleep apnea in children with this syndrome is much higher than that in the nonsyndromic cleft population.[7] In the velocardiofacial syndrome, pharyngeal hypotonia not only increases the risk of obstructive sleep apnea but also results in generally poor lateral pharyngeal wall motion.[7, 12] The absence of adequate lateral pharyngeal wall motion will result in flap failure unless the flap is extremely wide in the postoperative period. These or similar factors are operative for many other syndromes associated with clefting, and such patients may make up almost half the population of children with clefts.[9, 10]

Decision Makers

Perhaps the most controversial philosophic issue is that of who decides what to do and when. It could be argued that because pharyngeal flap surgery is an operation, it is the surgeon who should shoulder the responsibility of the final decision. But because the operation is performed to improve speech, the speech pathologist could make a strong case for the proposal that the surgeon should share or defer much of the decision making to the communication specialist. Perhaps the final word should come from the pediatrician because of the medical risks incurred with the operation. Other specialists who perform the endoscopic, fluoroscopic, and other diagnostic tests might also feel they should have a major influence in the recommendation.

In centers which function in a truly interdisciplinary way (which is different from a multidisciplinary center), the decision should obviously be made as a unit. All of the information should be integrated and interrelated so that unanimous agreement can be achieved. But in the real world, it is understood that some personalities tend to be stronger than others, and decisions may be influenced by the presence of a particularly "strong" individual. In such cases, truly cooperative decisions may not be reached. The so-called bottom line, however, is that surgeons are generally not properly equipped to make the decision unilaterally, nor are speech pathologists. The goals and indications for the operation should be followed, and if they are, it should be obvious that more than one professional and preferably many professionals should be consulted prior to reaching a decision about surgery.

The difficulty encountered in reaching perfectly objective decisions is perhaps the major reason why certain principles regarding the implementation of pharyngeal flap surgery need to be established. Perhaps we need "standards of practice" on which we can all agree to prevent unnecessary surgery, untoward complications, and unrealistic assessments of the results of the procedure. Unfortunately, even though there is a 100-year history of publications about pharyngeal flap surgery, we are no closer today to any agreement about any aspect of this commonly used operation. A combination of more rigorous science and more practical common sense is urgently needed.

References

1. Henningsson GE: Velopharyngeal movement patterns in patients alternating between oral and glottal articulation: A clinical and cineradiographical study. Cleft Palate J 23:1–9, 1986.
2. Hoch L, Golding-Kushner K, Sadewitz VL, et al: Speech therapy. Semin Speech Lang 7:311–323, 1986.
3. Shprintzen RJ: Evaluating velopharyngeal insufficiency. J Childh Commun Dis 10:38–50, 1986.
4. Argamaso RV: Physical management of velopharyngeal incompetence. J Childhood Commun Dis 10:67–74, 1986.
5. Argamaso RV, Shprintzen RJ, Strauch B, et al: The role of lateral pharyngeal wall motion in pharyngeal flap surgery. Plast Reconstr Surg 66:214–219, 1980.
6. Shprintzen RJ, Lewin ML, Croft CB, et al: A comprehensive study of pharyngeal flap surgery: Tailor made flaps. Cleft Palate J 16:46–55, 1979.
7. Shprintzen RJ: Pharyngeal flap surgery and the pediatric upper airway. Int Anesthesiol Clin 26:79–88, 1988.
8. Jones M: Etiology of facial clefts: Prospective evaluation of the 428 patients. Cleft Palate J 25:16–20, 1988.
9. Rollnick BR, Pruzansky S: Genetic services at a center for craniofacial anomalies. Cleft Palate J 18:304–313, 1981.
10. Shprintzen RJ: Palatal and pharyngeal anomalies in craniofacial syndromes. Birth Defects Orig Art Series 18(1):53–78, 1982.
11. Sher AE, Shprintzen RJ, Thorpy MJ: Endoscopic observations of obstructive sleep apnea in children with anomalous upper airways. Predictive and therapeutic value. Int J Pediatr Otorhinolaryngol 11:135–146, 1986.
12. Shprintzen RJ, Goldberg RB, Lewin ML, et al: A new syndrome involving cleft palate, cardiac anomalies, typical facies, and learning disabilities: Velocardio-facial syndrome. Cleft Palate J 15:56–62, 1978.

CHAPTER 102

Prosthetic Treatment of Velopharyngeal Incompetence

Carl O. McGrath and Marc W. Anderson

Prosthetic treatment of velopharyngeal incompetence is an old concept that has been renovated in recent years. The basic concept of treating velopharyngeal incompetence prosthetically was introduced in 1860 by McGrath and advanced by Suersen in 1867.[1] The appliance was all but abandoned late in the nineteenth century but was revived in the twentieth century.[2] Prior to 1970 the management of appliances was limited to an empiric trial and error process. This process involved sequential modification of the appliance until symptoms of velopharyngeal incompetence were eliminated. During the past 20 years, visualization techniques that utilize multiview fluoroscopy and fiberoptic nasendoscopy have been developed. These techniques allow more precise fitting of appliances in a dramatically shorter time period. In view of these technologic advances and highly controllable results, it is surprising that appliances do not have more universal acceptance.

This chapter presents a rationale for prosthetic treatment, criteria for patient selection, the role of the speech-language pathologist, and the role of the dental specialist. The technical and dental aspects of appliance treatment and long-term management are specified. Uses of fluoroscopic and endoscopic data are discussed in relation to defining the nature of velopharyngeal incompetence, selecting a prosthesis type, and modifying the prostheses as velopharyngeal structure and function change over time. The discussion is limited to patients with symptoms of velopharyngeal incompetence associated with overt or covert cleft palate.

Rationale for Prosthetic Treatment

Symptoms of velopharyngeal incompetence can be controlled prosthetically with a pharyngeal bulb or palatal lift. Potential candidates for this treatment include anyone over 2 years of age.

In sharp contrast to the initial use of a secondary surgical procedure to manage velopharyngeal incompetence, considerable treatment flexibility exists when velopharyngeal incompetence is first brought under control with a temporary prosthesis. When velopharyngeal incompetence is controlled, its symptoms no longer contribute to impaired speech. Subsequently, the patient, the family, and the cleft palate team are not pressured into premature decision making but can decide about definitive prosthetic or surgical resolution of the problem in a more deliberate fashion.

With a prosthesis the relative value of treating velopharyngeal incompetence for the individual patient can be tested. This step is particularly useful when it is questionable whether control of velopharyngeal incompetence makes enough difference in speech to warrant surgery. If not enough difference in speech results, the patient has avoided surgery and can simply discontinue prosthetic treatment. Grames referred to this approach as a "reversible trial" and advocated it for patients in whom it is uncertain whether physical management will be sufficiently beneficial.[3] However, in their patients and also in ours, obturated speech is typically found to be significantly better than unobturated speech, even when the extent of the disorder seems relatively slight.

Temporary control of velopharyngeal incompetence is especially important in children under the age of 4 years, in whom velopharyngeal incompetence threatens primary articulation development. Gaining control of velopharyngeal incompetence in these children can prevent or reverse the development of compensatory misarticulations, thereby minimizing or eliminating the need for later speech therapy.

There are indications that wearing a prosthesis can serve to stabilize velopharyngeal function and increase muscle motion.[4–10] Patients frequently have varying degrees of velopharyngeal motion on different non-nasal syllables before prosthetic treatment. The extremes of this variability result in what has been termed minimum versus maximum velopharyngeal incompetence.[11] Prosthetically obturating the maximum velopharyngeal incompetence for several months can increase velopharyngeal motion, sometimes to such an extent that a competent system is acquired. These patients have avoided surgery and no longer need the appliance. Other patients appear to relax their velopharyngeal muscles, allowing air and sound to escape around the appliance. In these patients the velopharyngeal port needs to be totally obstructed temporarily until the patients "learn" to articulate without relaxing the velopharyngeal musculature. This temporary obstruction causes no sleep disturbance because the appliance is not worn during sleep.

Many patients who demonstrate little or no velopharyngeal motion prior to prosthetic treatment begin to exhibit muscle motion after wearing an obstructive prosthesis. When that happens, the prosthesis can subsequently be modified to minimize nasal airway obstruction. Continued modification of the prosthesis in relation to changes in function can result in stabilization of velopharyngeal motion. When patients have had velopharyngeal motion activated or stabilized in this fashion, they are in theory better candidates for procedures of surgical obturation that rely on adequate muscle motion.

This increase in velopharyngeal muscular activity is not a universal finding, however. For some patients the velopharyngeal system remains immobile, and virtually total prosthetic or surgical obstruction is required to control velopharyngeal incompetence. A removable prosthesis has the advantage in such cases of allowing the patient periodic respite from nasal airway obstruction; there is no such temporary relief from surgical obstruction.

In the child patient, anatomic change occurring within the velopharyngeal system is another reason to prefer the flexibility afforded by temporary prosthetic treatment of velopharyngeal incompetence. These changes occur with growth and also as a consequence of adenotonsillar hypertrophy and subsequent atrophy. Patients require varying degrees of obturation as anatomic relationships change. Orthognathic surgeries, such as maxillary advancement, can also produce changes in velopharyngeal relationships that have ramifications for planning definitive surgical treatment of velopharyngeal incompetence.[12] A temporary prosthesis can be readily modified to accommodate any changes that occur in the velopharyngeal system as a consequence of these factors. Thus, the best time to consider surgical obturation is after growth changes and optimum velopharyngeal muscle motion have been determined and stabilized.

Unfortunately, the emphasis of prosthetic effect on muscle function became the dominant and controversial issue in the literature, as summarized by McWilliams et al.[13] This emphasis neglected the undisputable and practical fact that speech appliances can control the symptoms of velopharyngeal incompetence, thereby making normal speech possible.

In summary, this rationale challenges the assumption that surgery is the better first approach to managing velopharyngeal incompetence. Whenever possible, surgical obturation of velopharyngeal incompetence should be considered only after velopharyngeal incompetence symptoms have been successfully controlled with a prosthesis.

Criteria for Patient Selection

1. There are perceived speech differences that can be attributed to symptoms of velopharyngeal incompetence and that are identified as a problem by the patient and the family.
2. Velopharyngeal incompetence is not phoneme specific, nor is the patient stimulable for eliminating velopharyngeal incompetence symptoms.
3. The patient has the mental capacity for and is compliant with requests to imitate speech.
4. Patient or parent prefers a nonsurgical treatment.
5. The oral cavity is in a healthy state.
6. The goal of treatment has been explained to the patient and parent and they are committed to its implementation.
7. The patient and parent will take responsibility for maintaining good oral hygiene and keeping the appliance clean.
8. The patient must be able to cooperate for treatment;

a skilled, child-oriented practitioner can usually start treatment shortly after the child's second birthday.

Selecting the Appliance

Two types of appliances are available, the palatal lift and the pharyngeal bulb. Traditionally, the palatal lift has been selected when there is a long but dysfunctional palate; the palate is lifted by the appliance to facilitate closure of the velopharyngeal port. Pharyngeal bulb appliances have been used when velopharyngeal incompetence is associated with a short palate. Bulbs are also effective when lateral pharyngeal motion is minimal. Because of their passive nature, bulb appliances are easier to retain than lifts.

Some clinicians use a combination of these two appliances. If the lift does not result in control of velopharyngeal incompetence symptoms, lateral extensions are added to the lift, producing a "bulb-lift" appliance. It remains unclear whether one type of appliance is more effective than another for a given patient.

Speech-Language Pathologist's Role

A speech evaluation is done to diagnose velopharyngeal incompetence and to determine whether its symptoms are making an important contribution to defective speech. Then the speech-language pathologist conducts a velopharyngeal examination for the purpose of defining the nature of velopharyngeal incompetence. This examination includes dynamic views of the velopharyngeal system obtained from frontal and lateral videofluoroscopic imaging and from fiberoptic videonasendoscopic examination. From these videotapes diagrams are developed for sagittal, coronal, and transverse views (Fig. 102–1). These diagrams show the anteroposterior, vertical, and horizontal configurations of the velar, lateral, and posterior pharyngeal aspects of the velopharyngeal system during minimum and maximum motion.[11] These diagrams are used by the dental specialist and the speech pathologist to select the prosthesis type and to determine the optimal positioning of the prosthesis. Viewing the diagrams and videotapes also enables the

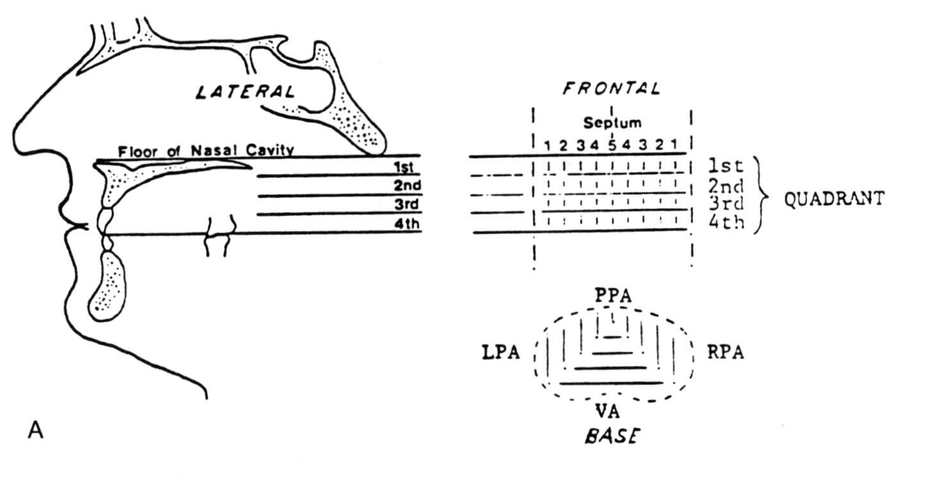

Figure 102–1 A, Form utilized for diagramming velopharyngeal function in sagittal, coronal, and transverse views.[11] *B,* Diagram of velopharyngeal function, showing level of maximum muscle motion (first quadrant), and minimum and maximum velopharyngeal incompetence.

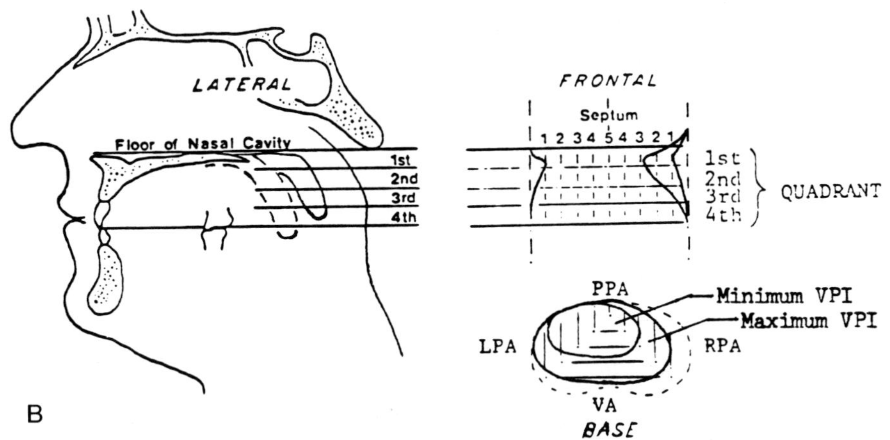

parents to readily understand velopharyngeal incompetence and the objectives of treatment.

Dental Specialist Role

During the initial consultation the parents' motivation and attitude are evaluated as well as the child's behavior. Approaches vary depending on the age of the patient. Parents of preadolescent patients are told that they must be committed to appliance therapy so that the child will accept and wear the appliance. Wearing the appliance is not an issue when the child understands that there is no choice. Adolescent and adult patients make this commitment for themselves. Prosthetic treatment is reviewed with the patient and parent to facilitate a thorough understanding of the treatment process and its objectives. Treatment time and costs are explained. Oral hygiene practices are reviewed in relation to appliance wear. The patient is examined to ensure that the oral cavity is free of disease. It is also emphasized that routine dental visits must be maintained with the patient's own dentist.

The procedure is begun at the next visit with the placement of retentive lugs on the buccal surface of posterior teeth in the maxillary arch. In the very young child, the first primary molars or canines can be used; in older children and adults the preferred location is the most posterior tooth. The retentive lugs are a bonded hybrid composite mass about 1.5 mm in width and 6 mm long. These lugs are typically placed in the occlusal one-third of the tooth (Fig. 102–2). Many cleft patients have posterior cross-bite that requires alternate placement. An alternative method of gaining retention is the use of orthodontic bands. A fitted band has a piece of 0.055 wire welded to the buccal surface and covered with solder (Fig. 102–3).

An alginate impression is taken with the lugs in place, and a palatal appliance is made (Fig. 102–4). The clasps are made of 0.036 wire for pharyngeal bulb obturators and 0.040 to 0.045 wire for palatal lifts. This palatal

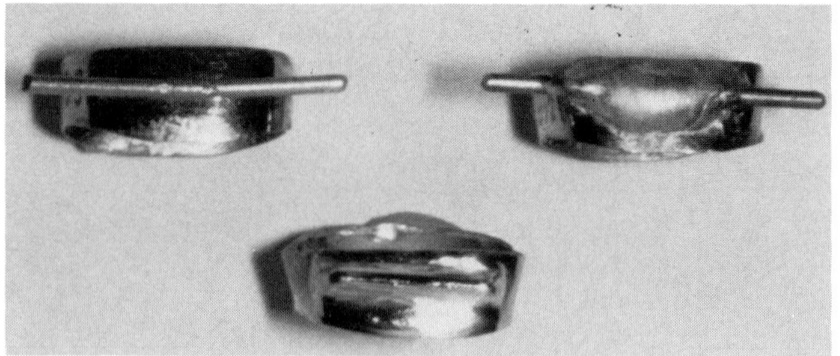

Figure 102–3 Buccal lug—soldered band.

appliance is worn for 1 or 2 weeks so that the patient can accommodate himself to an intraoral device. The steps and sequence of appointments shown in Figure 102–5 are identical for lift and bulb appliances through step three.

After step three, one method of creating the lift is to add modeling compound to the posterior aspect of the palatal appliance. The compound is added until the lift is extended to the patient's tolerance or until velopharyngeal incompetence symptoms are eliminated. The compound is converted to acrylic by taking an alginate impression of this addition. The compound is removed, and the appliance is returned to the impression. Acrylic is poured into the impression and cured in a pressure pot. This step can usually be completed in one or two visits (Fig. 102–6).

After step three, for the pharyngeal bulb appliance a tail is added that conforms to the passive contour of the soft palate and extends to the base of the uvula. The tail addition is usually completed in two visits. The first addition extends to or past the vibrating line as tolerated by the patient (Fig. 102–7). Beeswax is used to form the tail addition. To ensure that the addition is in passive contact with the soft palate, the beeswax should be 1 mm away from tissue. Mouth temperature wax is added to make contact with the soft palate. The appliance is left in place for a few minutes, and passive contact is obtained as the mouth-temperature wax is molded by tissue contact. The wax is converted to acrylic by taking an alginate impression of the wax addition. The wax is removed, and the appliance is returned to the impression. Acrylic is poured into the impression and cured in a pressure pot. This process is carried out on subsequent visits until the tail extends to the base of the uvula (Fig. 102–8).

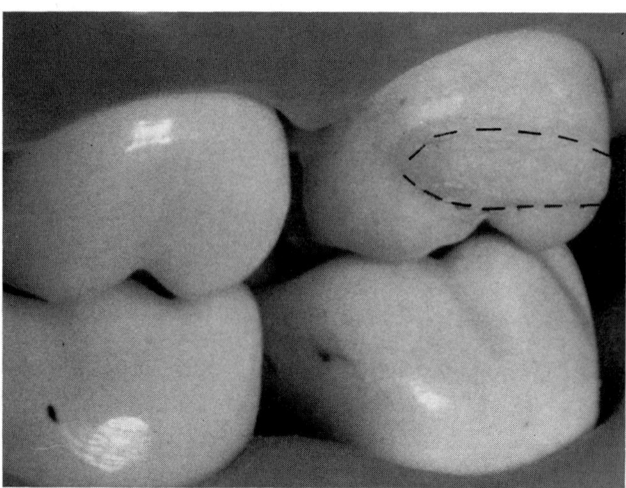

Figure 102–2 Buccal lug—hybrid composite.

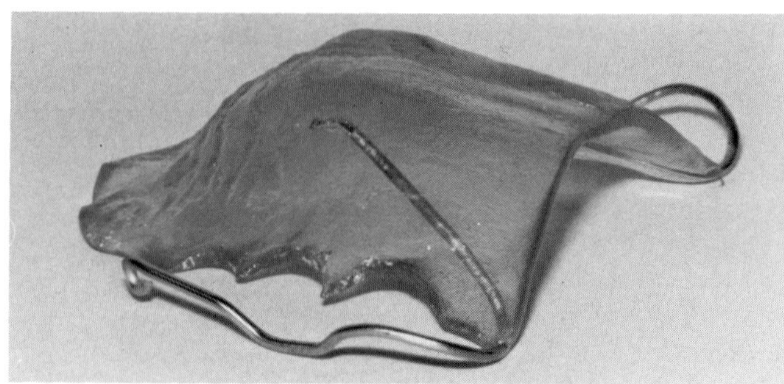

Figure 102–4 Palatal appliance—maxillary portion.

1. Evaluation of patient for program
   a. Explanation of program to parent or patient
   b. Desensitization of young child to office
   c. Examination of patient
2. Placement of buccal lugs and maxillary impression
3. Insertion of palatal appliance
4. Palatal extension (tailpiece) added
5. Extension of tailpiece
6. Placement of wire and mini-bulb
7. Additions to bulb
8. Additions to bulb (appliance complete)
9. through 16. Evaluation of bulb and appliance

Figure 102–5 Sequence of appointments.

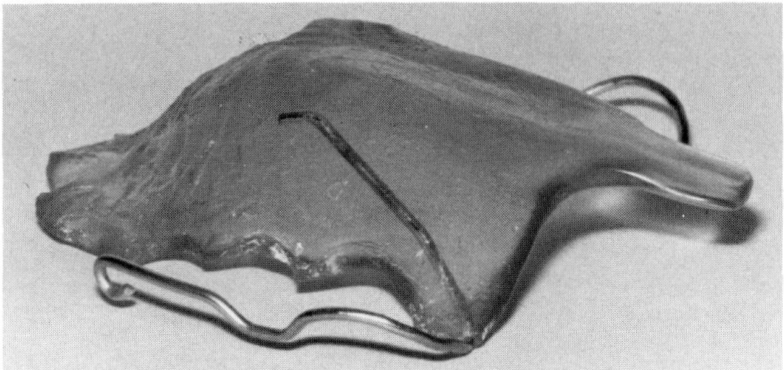

Figure 102–7 Tailpiece extended to vibrating line.

At the next visit, an 0.055 wire is bent to conform to the contour of the tail, maintaining passive contact with the soft palate. This wire is extended up behind the soft palate to the level of greatest velopharyngeal narrowing as defined in the patient's velopharyngographic diagram described above. The wire is attached to the appliance with acrylic, and a small ball of clear acrylic is applied to the pharyngeal portion of the wire to create a mini-bulb (Fig. 102–9). Bulb expansion and subsequent modifications are accomplished with the aid of videonasendoscopy. As the effective portion of the appliance is developed and subsequently modified, its effects on speech and oral tissues must be evaluated and monitored (Fig. 102–10). This can be done most effectively when the speech-language pathologist and dental specialist see the patient together. Patients are seen once every 4 months to evaluate hypernasality, nasal air loss, velopharyngeal motion, and adequacy of appliance fit. In our experience, technical difficulties in constructing and wearing a prosthesis have usually been minimal and quite varied. These various difficulties are resolved by the dental specialist.[14]

Initially, successful management of velopharyngeal incompetence with a prosthesis depends on the patient and parent being committed to wearing the appliance. This commitment is reinforced when the patient realizes that speech is improved.

Most practitioners have a preference for either bulbs or lifts. We use mainly the bulb obturator. Our description of long-term management is based on our experience with bulbs, although the principles are much the same when a lift is used.

Long-Term Management

Periodic visits are essential. Each visit is begun by asking the parent or patient if there have been any problems with wearing the appliance. This is done to reinforce the idea that the appliance must be worn all day every day and removed at bedtime, similar to wearing glasses. The patient or parent is asked whether the appliance has continued to make a significant positive difference in speech. Appliance fit is always checked and the oral tissues are examined to ensure optimal health. Hygiene is reviewed, including a reminder to brush the appliance each night and to cleanse it periodically overnight with a denture cleaner. Speech is assessed by the speech pathologist with the appliance in place to ensure that hypernasality is controlled.

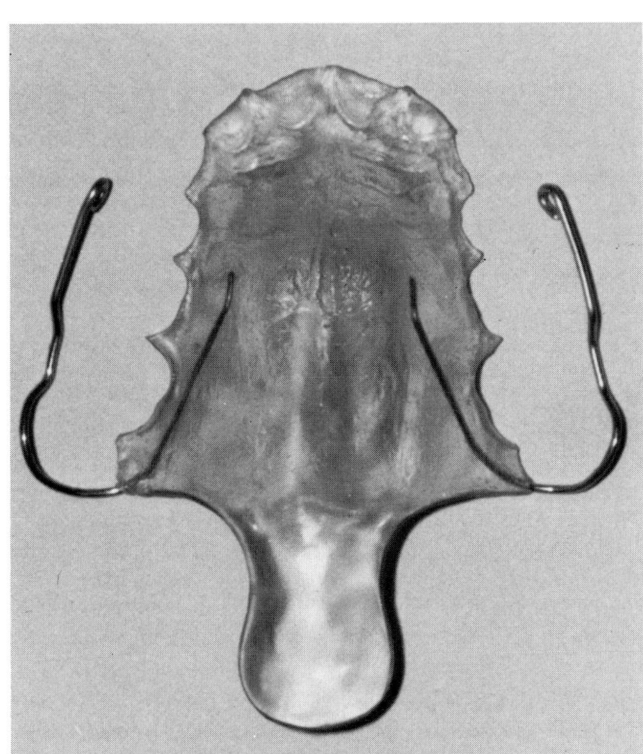

Figure 102–6 Palatal lift.

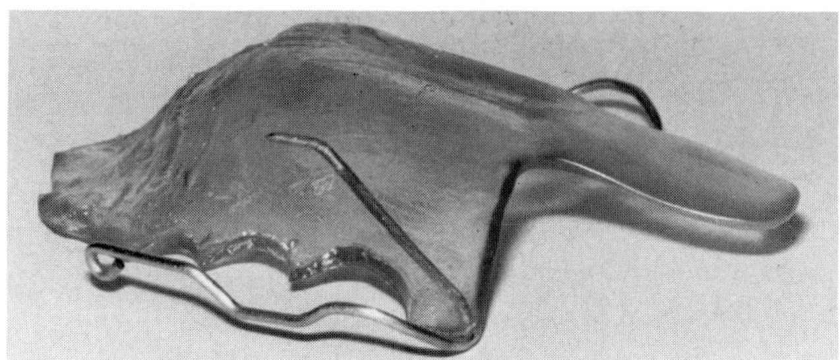

Figure 102–8 Tailpiece extended to base of uvula.

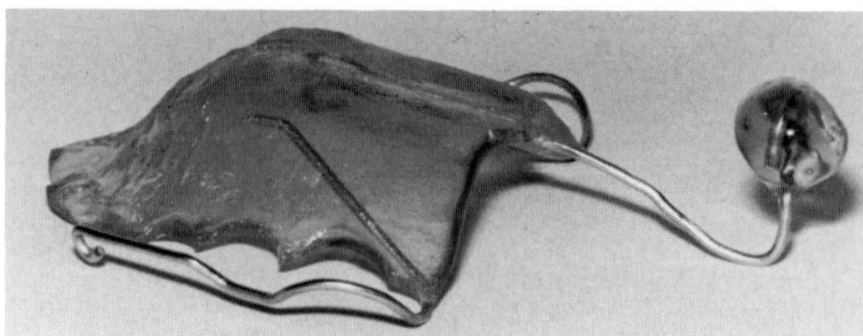

Figure 102–9 Mini-bulb.

Videonasendoscopic examination is done to inspect velopharyngeal function visually with the appliance in place and with it removed. Both lifts and bulbs may need periodic modification to maintain control of velopharyngeal incompetence.

With a bulb, the goal is to establish minimal impact on velopharyngeal tissues and minimal interference with its motion. This goal is most readily established with the use of videonasendoscopy. When muscle motion is seen to be greater with the bulb removed, the bulb is modified to make it less obstructive and to allow greater motion. This modification is repeated until the mucosa appears just barely to make contact with the bulb. The patient is then scheduled for a visit in 4 months for reevaluation. This process is repeated until no further modifications of the bulb are needed. The result of this process is an appliance that has been gradually made less obstructive to accommodate increased muscle motion until the motion is stabilized. We tell patients and parents to expect this process to take place over a minimum of 3 years. This process has been termed *obturator reduction*, but the term *obturator modification* more accurately describes the therapeutic process. It must be emphasized that although muscle motion frequently increases or stabilizes velopharyngeal function, *the primary purpose of treatment is control of symptoms of velopharyngeal incompetence.*

The velopharyngeal system of a growing child cannot be considered stabilized until facial growth is nearly complete at about 8 to 10 years of age. In most growing children, the bulb must be modified periodically. When modification involves an increase in bulb size, it is emphasized to the patient or parent that this is not a *setback* but rather merely a modification needed to accommodate growth. These periodic visits continue until velopharyngeal function has been stabilized, and for observation thereafter.

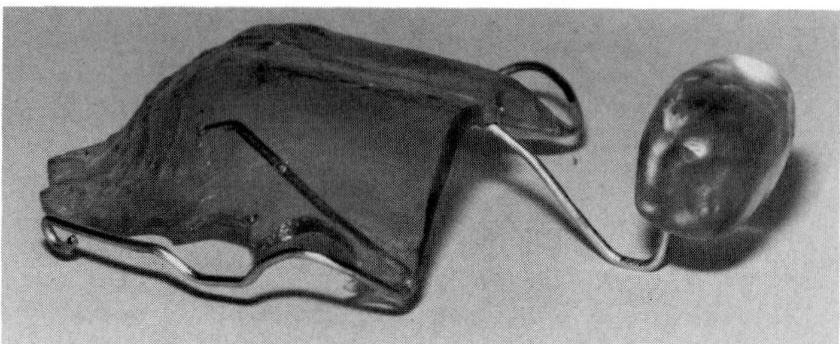

Figure 102–10 Completed bulb.

Clinical Results

During the past 12 years our success rate in controlling velopharyngeal incompetence symptoms in 200 patients has been 95%. In addition, 15% have no longer needed physical management of velopharyngeal incompetence following prosthetic treatment. In an effort to compare our experience with that of other clinicians, a questionnaire on prosthetic treatment of velopharyngeal incompetence was sent to 11 centers in North America. Nine responses were received. All respondents were speech-language pathologists involved with team management of velopharyngeal incompetence. There was considerable variability in the responses with regard to patient selection criteria, treatment protocols, long-term management, and length of clinician experience. Types of prostheses used were bulbs, lifts, and bulb-lift combinations. Although each center reported use of all three types, the majority (70%) preferred bulbs. The success rate reported in controlling velopharyngeal incompetence symptoms ranged from 75% to 100% and was not related to the type of appliance used.

Patients treated ranged in age from 2 years to adult, the majority being between 5 and 10 years of age. The current trend is to initiate treatment earlier, prior to 5 years of age. The percentage of patients who no longer need physical management following prosthetic treatment ranged from 3% to 60%. This variability was not related to prosthesis type but could be a function of patient selection criteria and length of patient follow-up. The results from this survey emphasized the need for standardizing our methods of patient selection and treatment protocols to obtain data that are comparable.

Conclusions

This chapter has presented our rationale for treatment, patient selection criteria, treatment protocol, plan for long-term management, and the basis for our preference for bulb appliances. Also presented were comments about the value of fluoroscopy and endoscopy, and the clear advantages of having both a speech pathologist and a dental specialist examine and treat patients concurrently. Our experiences and those of others indicate that symptoms of velopharyngeal incompetence can be controlled prosthetically for children over 2 years of age and for adults. Control of velopharyngeal incompetence symptoms is especially beneficial during the time of primary speech acquisition. In some patients, use of these appliances eliminates the need for physical augmentation of the velopharyngeal system. Estimates of patients not needing physical management of velopharyngeal incompetence following prosthetic treatment range from 3% to 60%. Patients with continued need can wear the appliance until circumstances warrant consideration of other options. These options include a permanent appliance, surgical implants, and pharyngoplasties. To receive comprehensive, quality care, patients with velopharyngeal incompetence need access to prosthetic treatment.

ACKNOWLEDGMENT. Photography by Pamella Cox.

References

1. Suersen W: Am J Dent Sci. 1(8), 1867.
2. Harkins CS, Harkins WR, Harkins JF: Principles of Cleft Palate Prosthesis. New York: Columbia University Press, 1960.
3. Grames LM: Personal communication, May 1988.
4. Harkins CS, Baker HK: Twenty-five years of cleft palate prosthesis. J Speech Hear Dis 13:23, 1948.
5. Blakeley RW: Temporary speech prosthesis as an aid in speech training. Cleft Palate Bull 10:63, 1960.
6. Blakeley RW: The complementary use of speech prostheses and pharyngeal flaps in palatal insufficiency. Cleft Palate J 1:194, 1964.
7. Blakeley RW: The rationale for a temporary speech prosthesis. Br J Comm Dis 4:214, 1969.
8. Blakeley RW, Porter DR: Unexpected reduction and removal of an obturator in a patient with palate paralysis. Br J Comm Dis 6:33, 1971.
9. Shelton RL, Lindquist AF, Arndt WB, et al: Effect of speech bulb reduction on movement of the posterior wall of the pharynx and posture of the tongue. Cleft Palate J 5:195, 1968.
10. Weiss CE: Success of an obturator reduction program. Cleft Palate J 8:291, 1971.
11. McGrath CO: Diagramming velopharyngeal inadequacy from video-fluoroscopy and nasopharyngoscopy. Poster presented at The American Cleft Palate Association Meeting, 1987, San Antonio, Texas.
12. Watzke I, Turvey T, Warren D: Maxillary advancement in the presence of cleft palate: Its effect on velopharyngeal function. Paper presented at the American Cleft Palate Association Meeting, 1988, Williamsburg, Virginia.
13. McWilliams BJ, Morris HL, Shelton RL: Cleft Palate Speech. St. Louis: C.V. Mosby, 1984.
14. Mazaheri M, Mazheri EH: Prosthodontic aspects of palatal elevation and palatopharyngeal stimulation. J Prosth Dent 35:319, 1976.

CHAPTER 103

The Long-Term Speech Results of Primary and Secondary Surgical Correction of Palatal Clefts

Betty Jane McWilliams

Data on the speech outcome of palatal surgery are incomplete, but they permit discussion of issues that should be addressed when planning for the future. The results of primary procedures and then of secondary surgery will be presented in this chapter.

Speech Results Following Primary Surgery

Speech results following primary palatal repair are affected by many closely related variables including evaluational methodologies. Reports from the eighteenth and nineteenth centuries indicate that speech was marked by velopharyngeal incompetence and that Passavant and Shoenborn in the mid–1800s even attempted pharyngeal flaps.[1] Defective speech was typical well into the 1950s.[2–5] Reports from England were more encouraging,[6, 7] and speech outcome gradually improved in this country as well. Children with clefts began to demonstrate better speech than adults who had been treated earlier.[8, 9]

During the past 25 years success rates have ranged from 21% to 94%;[10] however, these percentages are not necessarily representative of *final* outcome. Most studies have dealt with children or with nonrandomized subjects over a wide age range because adults were often lost to follow-up.

Variability in Results

There has always been wide variability in speech results achieved from one clinic, one surgeon, and one procedure to another and indeed, within the same procedure as reported by different investigators. The reasons for this variability are difficult to document, but there are suggestions that cannot be ignored.

Surgical Skill. The skill of the surgeon must be a factor. Deficient speech is the rule in some clinics. In others, the results are usually superb. However, estimates of outcome are based on a limited number of patients treated in particular ways by specific clinicians. We know little of the results obtained for the many patients who are never studied, and we are unlikely to collect the data necessary to demonstrate the extent to which outcome is influenced by surgeons.

Surgical Procedure. The surgical procedure is another source of variability. The role of the surgeon is unclear in this regard, but it is questionable that any two surgeons perform a given procedure in precisely the same way or even if the same surgeon does so consistently. Conditions differ, and slight changes may be required. For these reasons, comparative studies of surgery are the despair of biostatisticians, and there are always concerns about generalization. Despite these reservations, the evidence is that different procedures probably do result in different success rates with considerable overlapping in reported ranges.

For example, a range from 21% to 95% with a mean of 71% has been reported for the V–Y procedure.[10] Five of the 13 studies reviewed showed success rates of between 80% and 95%. Data for the von Langenbeck procedure, on the other hand, showed a success rate of 51% to 73% with a mean of 60%.

Four studies comparing the two techniques performed in the same setting also yielded varying results. Musgrave et al had a success rate of 89% with the V–Y and of 73% with the von Langenbeck.[11] Witzel et al[12] and Dreyer and Trier[13] found no differences between the two procedures, but Dreyer and Trier achieved consistently better results when they combined the von

Langenbeck with the intravelar veloplasty. Holtmann et al reported no differences among the V–Y, the von Langenbeck, and the von Langenbeck with pharyngeal flap except that complications were fewer with the von Langenbeck.[14] In a study by Van Demark and Hardin, 26% of patients treated with the Wardill procedure required pharyngeal flaps as opposed to 43% of those having the von Langenbeck.[15] For most surgeons then, but not all, the V–Y procedure yielded somewhat better results than the von Langenbeck.

Delayed hard palate closure has also been studied.[16–19] The hard palate has either been left open or closed prosthetically until major maxillary growth has occurred. Hagerty and Mylin inserted a pin-retained appliance until hard palate repair was performed at about age 7.[20]

Speech results following this procedure have been discouraging (McWilliams and Garrett).[30] Schroder[21] and Fara and Brousilova[22] concluded that most of their patients required pharyngeal flaps. Cosman and Falk reported "normal" speech in only 34% of the patients they treated.[23] Bardach et al found velopharyngeal competence in only 16% of their cases.[24] Witzel et al concluded that the assumptions on which the method is based have never been proved and that the deleterious effects on speech have not been appropriately studied.[25]

On the other hand, Van Demark et al reported that only 2 of 37 patients (5%) in their series of patients undergoing hard palate repair required secondary management and that only 1.1% had compensatory articulation.[26] Coston and McWilliams evaluated children who had had the procedure and found fewer articulation errors than in matched controls.[27] However, the errors in the two groups also differed; there were more gross errors and fewer dentally related errors in the children whose hard palates had been closed prosthetically until about age 7. Thus, surgical management influenced both the nature and the extent of articulation problems. Data on this topic continue to be accumulated, but studies to date have not been sufficiently well controlled to provide final answers.

Furlow introduced a procedure designed to improve speech and enhance maxillary growth.[28] He reported that only 2 of 18 babies who had had the procedure showed any evidence of velopharyngeal incompetence. Randall used the Furlow procedure to close 106 soft palates.[29] He predicted that secondary procedures would be reduced from 50% to 20%. Detailed speech examinations of 22 of Randall's patients at 3 or 4 years of age revealed a mean composite speech score of 2, indicating a competent to borderline competent valving mechanism. Thirty-six percent were unquestionably competent, and 36% were borderline. None was grossly incompetent.[30] No final assessment is possible until the children are older.

The pharyngeal flap as a primary procedure, has been associated with excellent speech by Stark et al,[31] Bingham et al,[32] and Dalston and Stuteville.[33] Riski et al, however, noted that 27% of 15 children had velopharyngeal inadequacy following Orticochea procedures and that at least 57% might never have required flaps, a potent argument against primary flaps.[34]

All surgical procedures have both champions and detractors, and there is no consensus about which is best or how its effectiveness may be altered by the nature of the defect. There is not even agreement about whether palatal surgery should be performed in one or two stages, although it appears that an increasing number of surgeons are closing the hard and soft palates in one operation.

Age at Closure. The age of primary closure of the palate also has been implicated in outcome. Although specific data are still missing, evidence now available suggests that earlier repairs yield better speech results than late repairs.[6, 35–40] Just how late is too late is still controversial. Age of surgery interacts with all of the other variables, so it is unrealistic to discuss age apart from other considerations. In fact, language age may be more relevant than chronological age. However, 12 to 18 months is still a common target even though more and more surgeons are repairing palates much earlier, sometimes as early as 3 months.

Assessment Standards

Understanding outcome is limited by our systems for describing speech and for making judgments about it. Moll stressed the importance of listener judgments because of the perceptual nature of speech.[41] That position is still accepted, but the variability in such judgments can limit their usefulness, particularly for research purposes. Although it is possible to objectify listener judgments,[42, 43] it is clear that what one listener hears as severe hypernasality may seem mild to another and that such judgments are often contaminated by other speech characteristics, many of which are also related to velopharyngeal incompetence. Another significant problem is that many studies have not used measurements at all but have resorted to such imprecise statements such as "socially acceptable speech," "needed a pharyngeal flap," or "improved following a flap." Thus, studies cannot be interpreted or compared. For this reason, it is impossible to say that one center reporting a success rate of 75% is any more or less satisfactory than others reporting rates of 60% or 90%. Different criteria may have been used for making decisions. Greater reliance on instrumentation, on objective methods of assessing speech, on establishing reliability when judgments are made about speech or the results of endoscopy or videofluoroscopy[10] should provide replicable data for making clinical decisions, measuring change after secondary procedures, and conducting research. Universal standards or criteria for reporting treatment results are required. Dalston et al addressed this issue in an effort to establish minimal standards for reporting surgical results.[44] It would be valuable to use the same rigid standards to assess randomly selected patients from a number of different centers, clinics, and private practices to determine success rates. However, such data are unlikely to be generated.

Rigorous criteria for describing original defects, associated abnormalities including cranial base and cervical deformities, surgical procedures, timing of intervention, and other variables also are needed. Controlled clinical trials taking those variables into account can provide data about specific outcomes and help to define "success" and the conditions under which less than "normal" speech might be considered a positive rather than a negative outcome. Presently, we can do no more than draw cautious conclusions from a compilation of studies that are not truly comparable.

Average Outcome

Although the prevalence of normal speech will differ from clinic to clinic, it appears that roughly 25% of all patients with palatal clefts eventually will have secondary management. How many more might profit from such treatment is unknown, but it is probable that the number is substantial given the poor agreement on criteria for determining need. This probability is supported by the report of Bardach et al.[45] They concluded that velopharyngeal valving competence was achieved in only 46% of their patients following primary palatoplasty. While we continue to generate increasing amounts of data, outcome for the patient has probably not improved significantly, although it is to be hoped that more and more treatment programs are now achieving a success rate of 75% or better.

Once a secondary procedure is decided on, some version of the pharyngeal flap is usually chosen, although other approaches also are used.[10] Augmentation of the posterior pharyngeal wall, the intravelar veloplasty, the so-called push-back, the Hynes pharyngoplasty, the Orticochea procedure, and various prosthetic appliances are all possibilities. This paper will discuss only the pharyngeal flap.

Pharyngeal Flaps

There are many types of pharyngeal flaps, but approximately 95% of the training programs in plastic surgery use variations of traditionally described flaps,[46] and most recommend that they be superiorly based, even though Randall et al[47] made a case for inferiorly based flaps in some patients. When Yules and associates[1] reviewed the state of the art in 1971, nine reports included both superior and inferior flaps, eight stressed superior flaps, and seven, inferior flaps. Today, the superiorly based flap is more commonly used because speech results associated with it appear to be better.

Variables Related to Successful Outcome

Several variables are probably related to successful outcome, but supportive data are sparse and conflicting. **Type of Cleft.** The type of cleft may be one factor. Tuttle found that flaps were less effective for bilateral than for other types of clefts.[48] Riski reported a higher success rate for clefts of the lip and palate than for isolated palatal clefts.[49] Most other studies have either not looked at cleft type or have reported equivocally.

The extent and nature of the valving deficit and concomitant skeletal deviations may be more relevant to outcome than the severity of the original cleft.

The Nature of the Valving Problem. Success has been consistently higher when the motor system was not impaired.[48] Although subjects with motor impairment of palatal and pharyngeal structures improve following pharyngeal flaps, most do not achieve completely normal speech. Limited, poorly timed, or uncoordinated movements are negative prognostic factors and are associated with less than ideal results.

Better results have been attributed to small rather than large deficits,[48] and the shape of the orifice may also play a role. Small, midsagittal openings springing from deficiency in the musculus uvulae have a positive outlook, whereas very wide openings associated with limited movement in the lateral walls are less satisfactory even when the design of the flap has taken both anatomy and physiology into account. Studies specifying the nature of the deficit are needed. Velopharyngeal incompetence is not a helpful designation because the condition has a variety of etiologies requiring different treatment strategies.

Type of Surgery. The type of surgery often has not been specified. Those who have described their procedures usually have reported improved results when the needs of the patient were taken into account.[50, 51] Kapetansky wrote that different problems may require different solutions, and he found his transverse pharyngeal flap to be useful.[52, 53] Hathaway, on the other hand, reported no differences in results with transverse or vertical flaps.[54]

Although "tailor-made" flaps that survive healing without alteration may not be possible, predetermining the position and width of the flap and its relationship to orifice shape and motor deficits is helpful. Preoperative diagnosis using one of several visualization and measurement techniques leads to improved outcome; undertaking pharyngeal flaps without such evaluations is a questionable practice.

Shprintzen et al found that all their subjects who had push-back procedures combined with pharyngeal flaps developed normal speech, whereas only 77% of those who had the split-return and 72% who had the sandwich flap reached that level.[50] Hyponasality was never a problem with the push-back, but it was the primary speech complication of the other two procedures. These authors expressed the need to plan surgery designed to correct the preoperative deficit.

Which procedures are best, when they should be used, or in whose hands they are most effective, are questions that remain unanswered.

Age for Pharyngeal Flap Surgery. The most desirable age for pharyngeal flaps is another confusing issue. Moran[55] and Moll et al[56] reported that normal speech is achieved less often after age 15, whereas Tuttle[48] found greater success before age 8 years, although age was more relevant to articulation than to resonance. Riski noted that children who had had flaps before age 7 acquired "acceptable" resonance.[49] Van Demark and Hardin concluded that age was not a critical factor, although few subjects in their series had pharyngeal flaps after 8 years of age.[43]

Pharyngeal flaps are probably more successful in children who are still developing speech than they are in those who have established speech patterns. Thus, children will, on the average, do better than adults.

Karnell and Van Demark[57] concluded that children who had velopharyngeal incompetence at age 4 but were treated later did not do as well as children who had pharyngeal flaps when their incompetence was first discovered. This conclusion supports the contention that valving deficits should be managed as early as they can be diagnosed. The age at which velopharyngeal incompetence can be accurately assessed will differ from child to child. Obviously, speech must be well enough developed to permit evaluations. The problem of diagnosis may be reflected in the findings of Van Demark and Hammerquist to the effect that children who had pharyngeal flaps before age 4 did less well than those treated later.[58] Although this conclusion is not a universal experience, it does suggest that caution is necessary in managing little children.

Closure Mechanism. The closure mechanism following pharyngeal flaps is controversial. Data differ on how closure is achieved and on which patterns of closure are most effective. There is no dispute about the need for closure of the lateral ports during demanding speech tasks. The issue is whether the lateral pharyngeal walls are responsible as they interact with a nondynamic palato-flap structure[50, 59, 60] or whether the palato-flap structure is a dynamic one.[48, 61, 62] Tuttle identified five different closure patterns, of which the dynamic ones were associated with better speech.[48] Multi-institutional research is required, but the final conclusion is likely to be that there are many possible combinations of movements, some more effective than others,[63] and that movement that occurs with one surgical approach may not result from another.

Speech Therapy. The role of speech therapy after flaps is another unknown factor. Some patients never require it, and others do not improve after years of work. Still others benefit quickly from techniques recommended to change articulation, and some are able to decrease nasal resonance through biofeedback techniques when portal closure is variable. How well these new patterns are maintained is not known. It is known that speech usually improves spontaneously after the pharyngeal flap procedure[15, 48] and continues to do so for some time with or without speech therapy. Determining which patients should have therapy, when it should begin, which therapy under which circumstances is most likely to be helpful, and at what point it should be terminated are unanswered questions.

Discussions of outcome often do not state whether the results were achieved by surgery alone or in conjunction with speech therapy. When therapy was part of the protocol, the type, timing, and effects are often not specified. Research to answer these questions is overdue.

Speech Outcome

It is unclear how pharyngeal flaps turn out in general and whether or not results are improving. Yules et al[1] reported success rates of from 61% to 100% with a mean of 85% for 18 studies published between 1951 and 1967.

Because of the highly variable criteria used for assessing outcome, it is impossible to compare these percentages. However, it is probable that results have not changed substantially, especially when the best results of today are compared with the best of the past, and the worst with the worst.

Van Demark and Hardin reported a success rate of 79% with another 16% showing marginal incompetence.[15] Only two of their 129 subjects retained hyponasality for the entire period of this longitudinal study. These rates compare with those reported by Shprintzen et al[50] for the split-return and the sandwich flap but fall short of the 100% reported for the push-back combined with the pharyngeal flap. Hyponasality is seen as a significant postflap problem.[15, 50, 64] Smith et al, basing outcome on aerodynamic measurements, concluded that only 52% of their subjects had successful results.[65] Although only 13% had velopharyngeal inadequacy, 35% had substantial obstruction of the nasal airway. Trier reported velopharyngeal competence in 92% of his cases as measured by aerodynamic factors.[66] In how many past studies has hyponasal speech been counted with the successes? How severe was it? How long did it last? Was it associated with any other symptoms? Answers to these questions are unavailable. Thus, today's success rates, although comparable with those of the past, may or may not mean what they did in 1971.

Looking to the Future

A major obstacle to predicting future outcomes lies in our inability to assess results as they relate to current treatment modalities. When the speech of adults or even children is evaluated, the effects of management carried out in the past is under scrutiny. Research of this type tells us little about what can be expected of today's babies when they reach adulthood unless the same type of management in the hands of the same treatment team is being provided. Studies of outcome must always be directed toward events of the past, whereas clinical concerns are for today and for future outcomes. To test the validity of any treatment theory, it must first be applied, ideally in clinical trials, and the results evaluated over time. That takes years of careful and consistent follow-up using rigidly defined assessment criteria, and it demands methodological rigor that is still largely ignored today. For these reasons, there is always a considerable lag between what is believed and what can be demonstrated with data. For the same reasons, many short-lived treatment fads appear from time to time, and endless arguments about the merits of one procedure over another continue. It is unlikely that these problems will be solved in the near future. Attempts can be made, however, to improve future research by using better and more consistent criteria and methodologies for determining success.

References

1. Yules RB, Chase RA, Blocksma R, et al: Secondary techniques for correction of palatopharyngeal incompetence. In Grabb WC, Bzoch K, Rosenstein S (eds): Cleft Lip and Palate. Boston: Little, Brown, 1971, p 451.

2. McWilliams BJ: An experimental study of some of the components of intelligibility of the speech of adult cleft palate patients. Thesis (Ph.D.). Pittsburgh: University of Pittsburgh, 1953.

3. McWilliams BJ: Some factors in the intelligibility of cleft palate speech. J Speech Hear Dis 19:525, 1954.

4. McWilliams BJ: Articulation problems of a group of cleft palate adults. J Speech Hear Res 1:68, 1958.

5. Spriestersbach DC, Darley FL, Rouse V: Articulation of a group of children with cleft lips and palates. J Speech Hear Dis 21:436, 1956.

6. McWilliams BJ: Cleft palate management in England. Speech Pathol Ther 3:3, 1960.

7. Braithwaite F: Cleft palate repair. In Gibson T (ed): Modern Trends in Plastic Surgery. London: Butterworth, 1964, p 30.

8. Counihan DT: A clinical study of the speech efficiency and structural adequacy of operated adolescent and adult cleft palate persons. Unpublished thesis (Ph.D.). Evanston, IL: Northwestern University, 1956.

9. Van Demark DR, Morris HL, Vandehaar C: Patterns of articulation abilities in speakers with cleft palate. Cleft Palate J 16:230, 1979.

10. McWilliams BJ, Morris HL, Shelton RL: Cleft Palate Speech. Burlington, Canada: Brian C. Decker, 1984.

11. Musgrave RH, McWilliams BJ, Matthews HA: A review of the results of two different surgical procedures for the repair of clefts of the soft palate only. Cleft Palate J 12:281, 1975.

12. Witzel MA, Clarke JA, Lindsay WK, et al: Comparison of results of pushback or Von Langenbeck repair of isolated clefts of the hard and soft palate. Plast Reconstr Surg 64:347, 1979.

13. Dreyer TM, Trier WC: A comparison of palatoplasty techniques. Cleft Palate J 21:251, 1984.

14. Holtmann B, Wray RC, Weeks PM: A comparison of three techniques of palatorrhaphy: Early speech results. Ann Plast Surg 12:514, 1984.

15. Van Demark DR, Hardin MA: Longitudinal evaluation of articulation and velopharyngeal competence of patients with pharyngeal flaps. Cleft Palate J 22:163, 1985.

16. Slaughter WB, Pruzansky S: The rationale for velar closure as a primary procedure in the repair of cleft palate defects. Plast Reconstr Surg 13:341, 1954.

17. Schweckendiek W: Primary veloplasty. In Schuchardt K (ed): Treatment of Patients with Clefts of Lip, Alveolus and Palate. Stuttgart: G. Thieme, 1966, p 85.

18. Friede H, Lilja J, Johanson B: Cleft lip and palate treatment with delayed closure of the hard palate. Scand J Plast Reconstr Surg 4:49, 1980.

19. Dingman RD, Argenta LC: The correction of cleft palate with primary veloplasty and delayed repair of the hard palate. Clin Plast Surg 12:677, 1985.

20. Hagerty RF, Mylin WK: Facial growth and arch symmetry in the surgical prosthetic treatment of cleft lip and palate. Plast Reconstr Surg 5:682, 1981.

21. Schroder F: Operation der Spalte in harten Gaumen in Auschluss an Velumplastik nach Schweckendiek. Acta Chir Plast (Prague) 8:257, 1966.

22. Fara M, Brousilova M: Experiences with early closure of velum and later closure of hard palate. Plast Reconstr Surg 44:134, 1969.

23. Cosman B, Falk AS: Delayed hard palate repair and speech deficiencies: A cautionary report. Cleft Palate J 17:27, 1980.

24. Bardach J, Morris HL, Olin WH: Late results of primary veloplasty: The Marburg project. Plast Reconstr Surg 73:207, 1984.

25. Witzel MA, Salyer KE, Ross RB: Delayed hard palate closure: The philosophy revisited. Cleft Palate J 21:263, 1984.

26. Van Demark DR, Hotz M, Perko M, and Nussbaumer H: Speech results of the Zurich approach in treatment of unilateral cleft lip and palate. Plast Reconstr Surg 83:605, 1989.

27. Coston GN, McWilliams BJ: Articulation skills in children with cleft palate: Two different treatment protocols. Fifth International Congress on Cleft Palate and Related Craniofacial Anomalies, Monte Carlo, September, 1985.

28. Furlow LT: Cleft palate repair by double opposing Z-plasty. Plast Reconstr Surg 78:724, 1986.

29. Randall P, LaRossa D, Solomon M, et al: Experience with the Furlow double-reversing Z-plasty for cleft palate repair. Plast Reconstr Surg 77:569, 1986.

30. McWilliams BJ, Garrett WS: Speech results in primary veloplasty as compared to the V–Y. In preparation, 1989.

31. Stark RB, Dehaan CR, Frileck SP, et al: Primary pharyngeal flap. Cleft Palate J 6:381, 1969.

32. Bingham HG, Suthunyara P, Richards S, et al: Should the pharyngeal flap be used primarily with palatoplasty? Cleft Palate J 9:319, 1972.

33. Dalston RM, Stuteville OH: A clinical investigation of the efficacy of primary nasopalatal pharyngoplasty. Cleft Palate J 12:177, 1975.

34. Riski JE, Georgiade NG, Serafin D, et al: The Orticochea pharyngoplasty and primary palatoplasty: An evaluation. Ann Plast Surg 18:303, 1987.

35. Peet E: The Oxford technique of cleft palate repair. Plast Reconstr Surg 28:282, 1961.

36. Evans D, Renfrew C: The timing of primary cleft palate repair. Scand J Plast Reconstr Surg 8:153, 1974.

37. Kaplan I, Dresner J, Gorodischer C, et al: The simultaneous repair of cleft lip and palate in early infancy. Br J Plast Surg 27:134, 1974.

38. Kaplan I, Taube E, Ben-Bassat M, et al: Further experience in the early simultaneous repair of cleft lip and palate. Br J Plast Surg 33:299, 1980.

39. Kaplan EN: Cleft palate repair at three months. Ann Plast Surg 7:179, 1981.

40. Randall P, LaRossa D, Fakhraee SM, et al: Cleft palate closure at 3 to 7 months of age: A preliminary report. Plast Reconstr Surg 71:624, 1983.

41. Moll KL: "Objective" measures of nasality. Cleft Palate J 1:371, 1964.

42. McWilliams BJ, Philips BJ: Velopharyngeal Incompetence. Audio Seminars in Speech Pathology. Philadelphia: Saunders, 1979.

43. Van Demark DR, Bzoch K, Daly D, et al: Methods of assessing speech in relation to velopharyngeal function. Cleft Palate J 22:281, 1985.

44. Dalston RM, Marsh JL, Vig KW, et al: Minimal standards for reporting the results of surgery on patients with cleft lip, cleft palate, or both: A proposal. Cleft Palate J 25:3, 1988.

45. Bardach J, Morris HL, Olin W, et al: Late results of multidisciplinary management of unilateral cleft lip and palate. Ann Plast Surg 12:235, 1984.

46. Osborn JM, Kelleher JC: A survey of cleft lip and palate surgery taught in plastic surgery training programs. Cleft Palate J 20:166, 1983.

47. Randall P, Whitaker LA, Neone RB, et al: The case for the inferiorly based pharyngeal flap. Cleft Palate J 15:262, 1978.

48. Tuttle GA: A teleradiographic investigation of the correlates of normal voice quality in patients having pharyngeal flaps. Thesis (Ph.D.). Pittsburgh: University of Pittsburgh, 1969.

49. Riski JE: Articulation skills and oral-nasal resonance in children with pharyngeal flaps. Cleft Palate J 16:421, 1979.

50. Shprintzen RJ, Lewin ML, Croft CB, et al: A comprehensive study of pharyngeal flap surgery: Tailor made flaps. Cleft Palate J 16:46, 1979.

51. Albery EH, Bennett JA, Pigott RW, et al: The results of 100 operations for velopharyngeal incompetence—selected on the findings of endoscopic and radiological examination. Br J Plast Surg 35:118, 1982.

52. Kapetansky DI: Bilateral transverse pharyngeal flaps for repair of cleft palate. Plast Reconstr Surg 52:52, 1973.

53. Kapetansky DI: Techniques in Cleft Lip, Nose and Palate Reconstruction. Philadelphia: J.B. Lippincott, 1987.

54. Hathaway RR: A comparison of transverse and vertical pharyngeal flaps using electromyography and judgments of nasality. Cleft Palate J 17:305, 1980.

55. Moran RE: The pharyngeal flap operation as a speech aid. Plast Reconstr Surg 7:202, 1951.

56. Moll KL, Huffman WC, Lierle D, et al: Factors related to the success of pharyngeal flap procedures. Plast Reconstr Surg 32:581, 1963.

57. Karnell MP, Van Demark DR: Longitudinal speech performance in patients with cleft palate: Comparisons based on secondary management. Cleft Palate J 23:278, 1986.

58. Van Demark DR, Hammerquist PJ: Longitudinal evaluation of articulation and velopharyngeal competency of patients with pharyngoplasties. Paper presented to the American Cleft Palate Association, Atlanta, Georgia, 1978.

59. Skoog T: The pharyngeal flap operation in cleft palate. Br J Plast Surg, 18:3, 1965.

60. Harrington J: A cinefluorographic study of the posterior pharyngeal flap mechanism. Paper presented to the International Cleft Palate Congress, Houston, 1969.

61. Uchiyama T: Studies on speech sound changes before and after pharyngeal flap operation. 1. Cephalometric radiographic measurements of articulatory organs. J Jap Cleft Palate Assoc 5:53, 1980.

62. Zwitman DH: Velopharyngeal physiology after pharyngeal flap surgery as assessed by oral endoscopy. Cleft Palate J 19:36, 1982.

63. Morris HL, Spriestersbach DC: The pharyngeal flap as a speech mechanism. Plast Reconstr Surg 39:66, 1967.

64. Thurston JB, Larson DL, Shanks JC, et al: Nasal obstruction as a complication of pharyngeal flap surgery. Cleft Palate J 17:148, 1980.

65. Smith BE, Skef Z, Cohen M, et al: Aerodynamic assessment of the results of pharyngeal flap surgery: A preliminary investigation. Plast Reconstr Surg 76:402, 1985.

66. Trier WC: The pharyngeal flap operation. Clin Plast Surg 12:697, 1985.

Psychosocial Aspects of Cleft Patients

CHAPTER 104

Psychosocial Adjustment to Cleft Lip and Palate

Joyce M. Tobiasen

In the last 40 years there have been numerous social-psychological studies of adjustment to chronic disabilities in adults[1] and in children.[2] Researchers in the field have typically distinguished two essential elements of a physical disability: the functional disability and the disability associated with deviations from regular expectations and potential social rejection.[3]

The World Health Organization[4] has developed specific definitions for the International Classification of Impairment, Disabilities, and Handicaps. This classification scheme defines an *impairment* as "any loss or abnormality of psychological, physiological, or anatomical structure or function." A *disability* is defined as "any restriction or lack of ability to perform an activity in a manner or within the range which is considered normal." A *handicap* is defined as a "disadvantage for a given individual, resulting from an impairment or a disability that limits or prevents the fulfillment of a role that is normal (depending on age, sex, social and cultural factors) for the individual." A handicap represents the potential consequences for the individual and society resulting from an impairment or a disability consisting of psychosocial, cultural, environmental, and economic dimensions.[5] The goal of habilitation is to minimize the disability and impairment and to prevent the development of psychosocial and physical handicaps.

Clefts of the lip and palate are a chronic disability throughout infancy, childhood, and young adulthood. An infant with a cleft of the lip and palate experiences problems from the moment of birth: feeding, family adjustment, and surgical problems. From early childhood to adulthood there are often speech, dental, surgical, medical, and psychosocial problems. Treatment of the speech, dental, and medical-surgical problems is often completed by early adulthood, but the facial impairment is rarely completely repaired, speech problems may linger, and the individual may spend a lifetime coping with a psychosocial handicap that influences the quality of life for affected individuals and their families. Issues concerned with long-term adjustment to cleft lip and palate, life quality, psychosocial coping, and functional independence are clearly key concerns of the field.

Stress from Cleft Lip and Palate

Chronic disabilities, especially those that are present from birth, share a myriad of stressors. Other stressors are unique to the particular disability. There are two general areas of stress for individuals with cleft lip and palate: adjustment to the physical disability of the cleft and the societal reaction to the facial appearance.

Stress Related to Adjustment to the Disability

For persons with clefts of the lip and palate there is a recurrent need for intrusive medical and surgical procedures beginning in the first year of life and extending throughout childhood and young adulthood. Speech and dental problems may emerge as the child grows older. No one has attempted to study the number and quality of stressors experienced by cleft lip and palate children and their families, but a core set has been described clinically.[6, 7] Some of the more salient stressors are early feeding problems, hospitalization for surgery, separation from the family, recurrent ear infections, absences from school (which can make it difficult to keep up with academic responsibilities), restrictions of physical activity following surgery, and regular interruptions in peer relationships.

The family with a cleft lip and palate child is likely to experience numerous stressors, due to both the chronic nature of the disability and its unique properties. Parents may experience guilt for producing a child with a congenital anomaly that may have a genetic basis. Feeding problems may be frustrating and frightening to new parents and may interfere with the development of the parent-child relationship. Explanations to friends and family may be painful. The child will probably require surgery in both the first and second years of life. Questions about the child's "future" may plague some parents. Finally, the direct financial costs of treatment and the indirect costs must be absorbed by the parents (e.g., babysitting for siblings when the child must go for the treatment, or the need to take time off from work).

Societal Reaction to Facial Impairments

In the pioneer study by MacGregor and her colleagues,[8, 9] extended interviews with facially impaired patients revealed the serious social and psychological difficulties that were often encountered by them in everyday life. These difficulties included staring, remarks, curiosity, questioning, pity, rejection, ridicule, whispering, nicknames, and discrimination.[8] The social rejection of these facially disabled patients extended to ". . . their attempts to obtain jobs, attract members of the opposite sex, or make friends. Set apart as different from others and even regarded as social outcasts, they frequently developed psychological disturbances which often became more grave than the physical impairment."[8]

The empiric data support MacGregor's observations.[8, 9] People find cleft-related facial impairments to be less socially acceptable than the absence of impairment. Richardson[10] asked children to rank drawings of children who were either normal or had various physical handicaps (in a wheelchair, amputated leg, obese, and cleft lip) in the order in which they best liked them. Both English and American children consistently ranked children who had a cleft lip or who were obese as least liked.

In a similar study, Landsdown and Polak[11] asked children 9 to 11 years old to rank, in order of "best liked," drawings of children with a normal face, "bat ears," eye squint, protruding teeth, cleft lip, and misshapen nose. Drawings of children with a cleft lip or misshapen nose were consistently ranked as least liked. Glass et al,[12] using Identikit sketches, asked adults to judge which of two sets were most preferred—a set showing faces with clefts of the lip or a set showing faces without clefts of the lip. Impairments of the lip were least preferred by raters.

Podol and Salvia[13] asked speech pathology students to rate the hypernasality of children with visible cleft-related impairments and those with cleft palate only. Children with visible scars received more negative speech evaluations than those with cleft palate only.

Tobiasen[14] examined personality and ability judgments associated by peers with cleft-related impairments. Children were shown either photographically corrected versions of children with congenital facial clefts or uncorrected versions. Children and adolescents, males and females, aged 7 through 16 years, rated individuals with cleft impairments as less popular, friendly, smart, and a less likely choice as a friend.

Summary

Clinical observations and research suggest that children with clefts of the lip and palate and their families experience significant chronic physical, emotional, and social stress. Our understanding of the impact of the disability would be enhanced if the presence and effect of these and other stressors could be empirically identified. Clinical observation and existing research on social reactions to facial impairment raise serious concerns about the psychosocial adjustment of the cleft lip and palate child and family.

Psychosocial Adjustment

Epidemiologic studies show that about 30% of all children with chronic disabilities may be expected to develop psychosocial maladjustments.[15] These surveys did not report separate results for cleft lip and palate children. The existing research in this area suggests difficulties in two areas: 1) academic performance and intelligence; and 2) socialization and social behavior.

Academic Performance and Intelligence

In general, individuals with clefts tend to score at significantly lower levels than normal children on standardized tests of achievement and on teachers' and parents' ratings of achievement.[16–19] The reasons for these findings are multivariate and include factors such as the high incidence of middle ear pathology and resultant hearing impairment[20] and increased absences from school; speech and language problems and reduced verbal output,[19, 21, 22] teacher expectations associated with facial impairment,[23] and peer expectations associated with facial impairment.[14] However, children with clefts of the lip and palate do tend to finish high school as often as their noncleft siblings.[24–26]

Numerous studies have examined the intellectual abilities of cleft lip and palate children. Most recent studies have found that the distribution of general intelligence in the cleft population falls within the normal range (i.e., IQ = 90 to 109).[27] Other studies suggest that verbal intelligence may be impaired whereas nonverbal intelligence tends to be within normal limits.[28] Richman and colleagues[28, 29] have conducted numerous studies in the area of cognitive strengths and weaknesses and learning disabilities in children with clefts. They have reported that children with cleft palate only[29] often have verbal expressive deficits associated with problems in verbal comprehension and developmental disabilities in language, whereas children with clefts of the lip and palate are significantly less likely to have these problems. Other work has shown that children with cleft palate only tend to have more severe reading disabilities than children with both cleft lip and palate,[29] whereas children with cleft lip and palate are more likely to have verbal expressive deficits and milder reading problems.[29]

In summary, achievement in school does appear to be lower in children with congenital clefts. The reasons for the achievement problems are not well understood but appear to be related to hearing, speech, social, emotional, and specific diagnostic factors. It is not known what the effects of achievement problems are on children's self-esteem, peer relationships, and long-term ability to obtain employment. Cleft lip and palate children are not routinely screened for potential learning problems,[30] and therefore, specific interventions have not been developed for their specific needs. Whether or not children with cleft lip and palate can be helped to improve their overall academic achievement is unknown.

Socialization and Social Behavior

There are few existing laboratory or naturalistic studies of how facial clefts affect socialization and social behavior. There are a small number of studies of parents' reactions to the birth of a child with a facial cleft. Field and Vega-Lahr[31] conducted a laboratory study of mothers' behavioral reactions to children with craniofacial anomalies, not exclusively cleft lip and palate. They found that these mothers smiled and vocalized at their infants less than mothers who were interacting with normal infants. The quality of the interaction for infants with craniofacial anomalies also was different. Their mothers engaged in less imitative behavior, game playing, and responsivity contingent on the infants' behavior than the mothers of normal children.

Brantley and Clifford,[16, 32] Clifford,[33] and Richman and Harper[34] found that parents believed that their acceptance of a child with a facial defect was more difficult than their acceptance of a normal child. However, these same parents asserted that the cleft child was eventually integrated into the family and that the initial tension subsided. Descriptive work by MacGregor and her colleagues[9] suggests that families do not easily recover from the shock of parenting a congenitally deformed child. Richman and Harper[34] reported that children with orofacial clefts described their birth and infancy as far more difficult for their parents than did children who were either normal or born with cerebral palsy.

Parents of older children with congenital facial clefts (ages 2 to 12 years) stated that they were more tolerant of several kinds of conduct problems in their children than were parents of normal children.[35] These data suggest that parents of children with facial clefts may be more permissive about misbehavior than parents of normal children. Wasserman et al[36] reported that mothers of children with clefts and related craniofacial anomalies behaviorally compensated for their children's interactional deficits. If their children were socially withdrawn, they were more active than mothers of noncleft children who were withdrawn. These findings suggest that not only do parents of children with clefts and related craniofacial anomalies expect less from their children, they may also overcompensate for their child's defect. The sum of these findings suggests that a congenital facial anomaly may have significant effects on the development of the parent-child relationship.

Other studies suggest that children with clefts suffer in peer relations. Heller and associates[37] reported that cleft lip individuals with poor cosmetic repair believed that they had fewer opportunities to date and make friends compared with those judged to have good cosmetic repair. Teachers[38] and parents,[19, 39] rated children with clefts of the lip and palate as shy and more socially withdrawn than normal children. Results from personality testing,[34, 40] psychiatric interviews,[39] and archival analysis[41] are consistent with this view. Individuals with facial clefts tend to marry later and less frequently than their normal siblings,[25, 42] participate in fewer social activities, and depend more on the immediate family for social activities and support.[43] Finally, no one has reported significant psychopathology in cleft lip and palate samples.[44]

The behavioral disturbances of children with facial clefts seem to be dominantly social in nature. They tend to be socially withdrawn. Shyness may seem to be a trivial problem, but it is one of the main reasons why people enter counseling.[45, 46] The ability of children to make friends and to be liked by others is considered by most parents, teachers, and child development specialists to be a major development milestone.[47] Social acceptance and being liked by others in young children predicts later adult social competence and positive mental health.[48–50] Therefore, a better understanding of the ways in which facial impairment may interfere with the development of effective social skills seems essential.

Psychosocial Interventions

Psychosocial interventions for children with clefts of the lip and palate and their families are derived from the broad fields of clinical child psychology and family therapy. Psychosocial factors must be treated comprehensively in that the focus of treatment includes both child and family, begins at birth, and may need to be available throughout the school years.

Treatment of the Child: Overview of Evaluation, Diagnosis, and Treatment

Evaluation of emotional, social, and cognitive development can begin as early as the age of 2 with standardized measures of intellectual functioning, observational techniques such as diagnostic play,[51] and standardized measures of parent reports of child behavior.[52, 53] More sophisticated techniques are available for other children including projective measures to evaluate personality functioning.[54] At the very least, a child with cleft of the lip and palate should have a comprehensive psychological evaluation prior to entering elementary school. Children with cognitive and potential social-emotional problems could be identified and treatment made available before the stress of school adjustment is imposed on the developing child; such evaluations could be performed every 2 to 3 years after the beginning of school.

Older children and their parents should consult routinely with a psychologist prior to and after major surgery. Surgery is often an anxiety-provoking experience for the child. Preparation and follow-up by a psychologist may be critical to maximizing the patient's and parents' satisfaction with surgery.[55]

Noncompliance with medical regimens, especially those that require the use of oral appliances, may compromise the result of surgical interventions. Psychological interventions with medical compliance problems have been moderately successful.[56]

Group therapy and education can be an essential element to the overall treatment of cleft lip and palate. Social skills, assertiveness training, and social support groups may be particularly useful to adolescents with clefts of the lip and palate.[57]

Finally, some children may require individual psychotherapy. Some children with clefts of the lip and their families may need to be helped to understand that a major disability often requires considerable social-psychological adjustment and that counseling to assist with that adjustment is critical to the comprehensive care of the disability.

Treatment of the Family

The first psychological intervention begins with the family at the birth of the child. Parents often need supportive counseling to help them cope with the feelings of shock, guilt, anger, and helplessness they may experience after having a child with a congenital anomaly.[7] When the emotional crisis subsides, family education can begin. Parents need to know the correct descriptions of the condition, and its etiology. Myths about parent responsibility for the congenital anomaly need to be addressed and dispelled. Other family education issues include an outline of the specific surgical steps necessary to modify the impairment. Hope for amelioration should be encouraged, but parents may need assistance in understanding that total amelioration is unlikely.

Parents may need help in understanding that early breathing, feeding, and hearing problems are not uncommon for cleft lip and palate children and that ongoing assessment for developmental delays (e.g., motor, speech, or visual delays) as well as potential learning disabilities may be useful.[29]

Throughout the child's growth and development families may need to be encouraged to become involved in decisions about hospitalization and treatment for their child. They also may need to be reminded that their child is "normal" except for the cleft lip and palate and therefore needs the same kind of attention, social stimulation, and discipline and limit-setting that any other child needs. Parents also benefit by being prepared for the social reactions of strangers to their child. Parents may see strangers "freezing" in front of their children and feel inhibited in their response to the child. They may need to be encouraged to continue to allow the child to have regular opportunities for social exchange and not restrict the child to the home or other non-threatening situations. In fact, parents often benefit from open discussions of how to improve their child's appearance (e.g., clothing, hair style).

Parents may need to be encouraged to expose the child as early as possible to regular peer activities. In this way, children will have opportunities to learn age-appropriate social skills, gain self-confidence, and desensitize themselves as well as others to the socially negative aspects of appearance and speech. The earlier children develop peer relationships, the sooner they learn to deal with questions of teasing and staring.

Children can be taught when they are 2 to 4 years old how to answer simple questions about their appearance (e.g., "I was born with a split in my lip and the doctors had to fix it when I was a baby"). Play therapy is often useful in helping children become more comfortable with their appearance as well as in counseling them about their feelings and educating them about societal misconceptions about physical impairment.[51]

Not only do children and families need education and counseling about clefts, teachers and schools often benefit as well. Parents can be encouraged to educate teachers about clefts. There are many opportunities to educate classmates about clefts in report writing and science projects. Members of cleft palate teams can visit classrooms and provide teacher workshops. Education of this kind can promote empathy and sensitivity in an open and honest atmosphere and minimize teasing and gossip.

Future Directions

From this review of the current body of psychosocial research and treatment of clefts of the lip and palate, several recommendations are offered for future directions.

Multifactorial Approach

Previous research has employed relatively simple approaches to psychosocial adjustment. One or two variables may be manipulated. It is far more likely that a range of psychosocial, medical-surgical, and speech factors mediate adjustment. Researchers must consider factors such as severity of physical handicap, socioeconomic status, social support, developmental delays, coping style,[58] and marital and family factors when studying psychosocial adjustment of children with cleft lip and palate.

Measurement Problems: Severity of Facial Impairment

Little is known about how the severity of cleft impairment influences social-psychological adjustment. Common sense suggests that the more severe the impairment, the more difficult the social-psychological adjustment. Anecdotal data suggest the opposite.[8] Standard measures of severity of cleft impairment are needed to address this question.[59]

Measures of severity of cleft impairment also are needed to allow evaluation of the benefits of surgical and dental treatment. The decision to seek secondary surgical repair is often based on improving the aesthetic acceptability of appearance. Yet, there are almost no data to show that an individual's quality of life is improved following secondary surgical repair and long-term treatment of dental and speech problems for children with clefts of the lip and palate.[60]

Stress

There is almost no empiric understanding of the stressors impinging on cleft lip and palate children and their families. This knowledge is essential to permit effective intervention and subsequent improvement of the psychological prognosis for these children and their families.

Conclusions

The purpose of this chapter was to describe the central role of psychosocial factors in the habilitation of patients with clefts of the lip and palate. The importance of psychosocial factors has been relatively neglected in practice[30] and in theory and research[61] by cleft lip and palate investigators. The evidence and conclusions presented in this chapter suggest not only that this attitude of neglect is changing but also that it must change. The goal of habilitation is to reduce disability and impairment and thus minimize handicaps. This means that in the broadest sense, treatment of cleft lip and palate is a psychosocial developmental adjustment process involving multispecialty interventions whereby patients are helped to become more competent and independent as they meet and overcome surgical, dental, speech, and psychosocial problems during a period of many years.

ACKNOWLEDGMENT. The preparation of this chapter was supported in part by R. L. Smith Research Center, National Institutes of Health Grant HD02528, Sutherland Institute of Facial Rehabilitation Endowment Fund No. 83652, and National Institute of Dental Research Grant No. R29 DE08153-02.

References

1. Livneh H: On the origins of negative attitudes toward people with disabilities. Rehab Lit 43:338–347, 1982.
2. Varni JW, Wallender JL: Pediatric chronic disabilities: Hemophilia and spina bifida as examples. In Routh DK (ed): Handbook of Pediatric Psychology. New York: Guilford Press, 1988.
3. Wright B: Physical Disability: A Psychosocial Approach. New York: Harper and Row, 1983.
4. World Health Organization. International Classification of Impairments, Disabilities, and Handicaps. Geneva, WHO, 1980.
5. Symington DC: The goals of rehabilitation. Arch Phys Med Rehabil 65:427–430, 1984.
6. Clifford E: The cleft experience: New perspectives on management. Cleft Palate J 6:235–243, 1987.
7. Goin JM, Goin MK: Changing the Body: Psychosocial Effects of Plastic Surgery. Baltimore: Williams & Wilkins, 1981.
8. MacGregor FC: Some psychosocial problems associated with facial deformities. Am Soc Rev 16:629–638, 1951.
9. MacGregor FC, Abel TM, Bryt A: Facial Deformities and Plastic Surgery: A Psychosocial Study. Springfield, IL: Charles C Thomas, 1953.
10. Richardson SA: Research report: Handicap, appearance and stigma. Soc Sci Med 5:621–628, 1971.
11. Landsdown R, Polak L: A study of the psychological effects of facial deformity in children. Child Care Health Dev 1:85–91, 1975.
12. Glass L, Starr C, Steward C, et al: Identikit model II—A model tool for judging cosmetic appearance. Cleft Palate J 18:147–151, 1981.
13. Podol J, Salvia J: Effects of visibility of a prepalatal cleft on the evaluation of speech. Cleft Palate J 13:361–366, 1976.
14. Tobiasen JM: Social judgments of facial deformity. Cleft Palate J 24:323–327, 1987.
15. Pless IB, Rohmann KJ: Chronic illness and its consequences: Observations based on three epidemiologic surveys. J Pediatr 79:351–359, 1971.
16. Brantley HJ, Clifford E: Cognitive, self-concept, and body image measures of normal cleft palate and obese adolescents. Cleft Palate J 1:177–182, 1979.
17. Kommers MS, Sullivan MD: Written language skills of children with cleft palate. Cleft Palate J 16:81–85, 1979.
18. Richman LC: Behavior and achievement of cleft palate children. Cleft Palate J 10:4–10, 1976.
19. Spriesterbach DC: Psychological Aspects of the Cleft Palate Problem, Vols 1 and 2. Iowa City: University of Iowa Press, 1973.
20. Paradise JL, Bluestone CD, Felder H: The universality of otitis media in 50 infants with cleft palate. Pediatrics 44:35–42, 1968.
21. Morris MP: Oral language skills of adult cleft palate speakers. J Speech Hear Res 5:79–90, 1962.
22. Pannbacker MP: Oral language skills of adult cleft palate speakers. Cleft Palate J 12:95–106, 1975.
23. Richman LC: The effects of facial disfigurement on teachers perception of ability in cleft palate children. Cleft Palate J 15:155–160, 1978.
24. Lahti A, Rintala A, Soivio AL: Education level of patients with cleft lip and palate. Cleft Palate J 11:36–40, 1974.
25. McWilliams BJ, Paradise LP: Educational occupational and marital status of cleft palate adults. Cleft Palate J 10:223–229, 1973.
26. Peter JP, Chinsky RR: Sociological aspects of cleft palate adults: II. Education. Cleft Palate J 11:443–449, 1974.
27. McWilliams BJ, Matthews H: A comparison of intelligence and social maturity in children with unilateral complete clefts and those with isolated cleft palates. Cleft Palate J 16:363–372, 1979.
28. Richman LC, Eliason M: Psychological characteristics of children with cleft lip and palate: Intellectual, achievement, behavioral, and personality variables. Cleft Palate J 19:251–257, 1982.
29. Richman LC, Eliason MJ, Lindgren SD: Reading disability in children with clefts. Cleft Palate J 25:21–25, 1988.
30. Broder H, Richman L: An examination of mental health services offered by cleft/craniofacial teams. Cleft Palate J 24:158–162, 1987.
31. Field TM, Vega-Lahr N: Early interactions between infants with craniofacial anomalies and their mothers. Infant Behav Dev 7:527–530, 1984.
32. Brantley HJ, Clifford E: Maternal and child locus of control and field-dependence in cleft palate children. Cleft Palate J 16:183–187, 1979.
33. Clifford E: Parental ratings of cleft palate infants. Cleft Palate J 6:235–243, 1969.
34. Richman LC, Harper DC: Observable stigmata and perceived maternal behavior. Cleft Palate J 15:215–219, 1978.
35. Tobiasen JM, Hiebert JM: Parents' tolerance for the conduct problems of cleft palate children. Cleft Palate J 21:82–85, 1984.
36. Wasserman GA, Allen R, Solomon CR: At-risk toddlers and their mothers: The special case of physical handicap. Child Dev 56:73–83, 1985.
37. Heller A, Tidmarsh W, Pless IB: The psychosocial functioning of young adults born with cleft lip or palate. Clin Pediatr 20:459–465, 1981.
38. Richman LC: Parents and teachers: Differing views of behavior of cleft palate children. Cleft Palate J 153:360–364, 1978.
39. Simonds JF, Heimberger RE: Psychiatric evaluation of youth with cleft lip-palate matches with control group. Cleft Palate J 15:193–201, 1978.
40. Harper DC, Richman LC: Personality profiles of physically impaired adolescents. J Clin Psychol 34:636–642, 1978.
41. Gluck A, Wylie H, McWilliams G, et al: Comparison of clinical characteristics of children with cleft palate and children in a child guidance clinic. Percept Motor Skills 27:806–810, 1965.
42. Peter JP, Chinsky RR: Sociological aspects of cleft palate adults. Cleft Palate J 11:443–449, 1974.
43. Peter JP, Chinsky RR, Fisher MJ: Sociological aspects of cleft palate adults: III. Vocational and economic aspects. Cleft Palate J 12:193–199, 1975.
44. McWilliams BJ: Social and psychological studies of plastic surgery. In MacGregor FC (ed): Clin Plast Surg 9:317–326, 1982.
45. Eisenberg S, Patterson LE: Helping Clients with Special Concerns. Chicago: Rand-McNally, 1979.
46. Zimbardo PG: Shyness: What It Is; What To Do About It. Reading, MA: Addison-Wesley, 1977.
47. Caplan T, Caplan F: The Early Childhood Years: The 2 to 6 Year Old. New York: Bantam Books, 1983.
48. Roff M: Childhood social interactions and young adult bad conduct. J Abnorm Soc Psychol 63:333–337, 1961.
49. Roff M: Childhood social interaction and young adults psychosis. J Clin Psychol 19:152–157, 1963.
50. Roff M, Sells SB, Golden MM: Social Adjustment and Personality Development in Children. Minneapolis: University of Minnesota Press, 1972.
51. Schaefer CE, O'Connor KJ: Handbook of Play Therapy. New York: Wiley, 1983.
52. Achenbach TM: The child behavior profile: I. Boys aged 6–11. J Consult Clin Psychol 46:478–488, 1978.
53. Achenbach TM, Edelbrock CJ: The child behavior profile: II. Boys aged 12–16 and girls aged 6–11 and 12–16. J Consult Clin Psychol 47:223–233, 1979.
54. Haworth MR: The Cat: Facts About Fantasy. New York: Grune & Stratton, 1966.
55. Johnson JE: Psychological interventions and coping with surgery. In Baum A, Taylor SE, Singer JE (eds): Handbook of Psychology and Health. Hillsdale, New Jersey, Lawrence Erlbaum, 1984.
56. DiNicola DD, DiMatteo MC: Practitioners, patients, and compliance with

medical regimens: A social psychological perspective. In Baum A, Taylor SE, Singer JE (eds): Handbook of Psychology and Health. Hillsdale, New Jersey: Lawrence Erlbaum, 1984.

57. Bull R, Rumsey N: The Social Psychology of Facial Appearance. New York: Springer-Verlag, 1988.

58. Cohen F, Lazarus RS: Coping and adaptation and health professions. In Mechanic D (ed): Handbook of Health, Health Care and the Health Professions. New York: Free Press, 1983.

59. Tobiasen JM, Hiebert JM: Reliability of aesthetic judgments of cleft improvement. Cleft Palate J 25:313–317, 1988.

60. Bardach J, Morris H, Olin W, et al: Late results of multidisciplinary management of unilateral cleft lip and palate. Ann Plast Surg 12(3):235–242, 1984.

61. Clifford E: The state of what art? Cleft Palate J 25(2):174–175, 1988.

CHAPTER 105

Neuropsychological Perspectives of Cleft Lip and Palate

Michele J. Eliason

The study of neuropsychological development in children with cleft lip and palate is a relatively new endeavor. In the past, more emphasis has been placed on social adjustment factors for the individual with a cleft and the family. Variables such as adaptation to the birth of a child with a birth defect, social effects of facial disfigurement, influence of multiple ear infections on later language development and behavior, and other equally important topics have been the focus of study.

Neuropsychology is the study of brain-behavior relationships. Cleft lip and palate, as a deviation of craniofacial development, is a highly appropriate area for neuropsychological study. Research on other physical and developmental disorders has demonstrated the influence of neuropsychological development on many aspects of life, such as social interaction, academic achievement, and vocational attainment. It has been suggested that deviant neuropsychological development can directly influence social skill development and grades in school, which then indirectly affect other aspects of life such as peer relationships, family harmony, vocational choices, and so on. With cleft lip and palate, delays in or deviations of neuropsychological development may interact with facial appearance and speech and hearing impairments to affect adult functioning and adaptation. This chapter will review the limited literature available on neuropsychological development in individuals of all ages with clefts, because the effects may vary according to differing expectations by chronologic age. It should be kept in mind that children with syndromic clefts may differ considerably on neuropsychological profiles from children with isolated clefts. This review is concerned only with individuals with nonsyndromic clefts.

Possible Brain-Behavior Correlates in Cleft Lip and Palate

Clefts of the lip and palate result from a failure of neural crest cells to migrate properly from the forebrain to the frontonasal process and the maxillary process. In normal development, the frontonasal cells unite with the lateral maxillary processes at about 6 weeks to form the lip, at about 7 to 9 weeks to form the hard palate, and at about 10 to 12 weeks to form the soft palate and uvula.[1, 2]

Most structural birth defects occur during this early stage of prenatal development. Perhaps the underlying cause of this failure of cells to migrate to the facial area may also disrupt the migration of cells to higher brain structures. For example, in the fetal alcohol syndrome, both facial clefts and disruptions of the migratory pattern of cells in the cortex have been identified.[3] Also, microscopic studies of dyslexic individuals have identified deviations in cell migration.[4] Thus far, there are no reports in the literature of studies that have examined brains of individuals with cleft lip and palate for subtle microscopic differences. However, there appears to be ample reason to conduct noninvasive neuropsychological studies of individuals with clefts to determine whether subtle cognitive deficits might suggest underlying brain differences.

Introduction to Neuropsychology

Neuropsychologists differ in their approach to defining and identifying neuropsychological functions. Child or developmental neuropsychology, in particular, is a relatively new field and still draws heavily from adult neuropsychological methods and research. This can create problems because the child's brain is in a state of development, and brain-behavior relationships that are fairly clearly defined for adults may not apply in children. Thus, child neuropsychologists must be careful in assigning the origins of deviant performance to specific brain loci.

Developmental neuropsychology can be defined as the study of normal and abnormal development in people of all ages as it relates to the development of the central nervous system.[5] Considerable progress has been made in the last ten years in describing both normal and abnormal neuropsychological development.

There are at least two commercially available neuropsychological batteries of tests for children and several for adults (Luria-Nebraska and Halstead-Reitan batteries, among others). These tests are widely used in settings in which children or adults with identified brain lesions are seen but are less often used for evaluating individuals with unknown or unidentified brain anomalies or developmental delays.

Most researchers in child neuropsychology develop hypotheses and then administer a battery of tests aimed at addressing their hypotheses. Although this leads to difficulty in comparing studies that have used different measures, there appears to be some consistency in the general areas that are considered important to assess. The most commonly identified neuropsychological functions include the following broad areas:[6] general intelligence, verbal-language, memory, nonverbal functions, and cognitive style.

General intellectual ability serves as a measure of global neuropsychological functioning. Specific subtests of individual intelligence tests are often examined for patterns, such as verbal-performance discrepancies, or deviations on Kaufman's factors of verbal comprehension, perceptual organization, and freedom from distractibility.

Language development can be viewed from a number of perspectives, depending on the orientation of the researcher. Language is discussed in detail in other chapters of this volume from the perspective of the speech and language pathologist. In this discussion, it is viewed from the neuropsychological standpoint with a specific focus on receptive language, expressive language, and verbal mediation (the executive function of language, often thought to be a frontal lobe function). Like the speech-language pathologist, the neuropsychologist also considers language in terms of syntax (form), semantics (meaning), and pragmatics (social use of language).

Memory abilities are another important aspect of neuropsychological development. Memory skills can be considered in terms of modality (auditory versus visual versus intersensory), span versus sequence, and rote versus meaningful memory. Short-term memory is generally directly assessed in a neuropsychological evaluation by means of repetition of strings of numbers, sentences, word lists, or drawings. Long-term memory is assessed by asking general information questions and by delayed memory tests.

Nonverbal functions include visual-perceptual or spatial skills (the ability to perceive and interpret visual information in the environment), motor coordination and planning, constructional abilities, and often, tactile perception (perceiving and interpreting information by touch).

Cognitive style differences, such as impulsivity versus reflectivity and field dependence or independence, may reflect either personality style or neuropsychological functioning and may or may not be assessed in a formal neuropsychological evaluation. Attentional capacity is evaluated by use of observation techniques, behavior rating scales, or vigilance tasks. Finally, personality and emotional functions, such as inhibition, anxiety, general mood quality, and social interactional patterns are assessed.

Early Studies: Intellectual Functioning

Prior to the initiation of more sophisticated studies of neuropsychological functioning, many researchers examined general intellectual development in children with cleft lip and palate. These early studies found that the average IQ of cleft population samples fell below that of the general population.[7–11] Certainly, there were design problems in these early studies that were not well addressed. For example, many of these studies did not include control groups, had samples containing children with multiple congenital anomalies or syndromic clefts, used several different IQ tests within one study, or reported a single IQ score. However, in the majority of studies, one consistent finding emerged, that the average IQ in cleft samples was just a few points lower than the normative mean of 100.

In addition, studies that utilized the Wechsler Intelligence Scales for Children (WISC), with its separate verbal and nonverbal scales, found that the lower overall IQ in cleft samples could be attributed almost exclusively to deficits on verbal subtests.[12, 13] This verbal deficit has been blamed on numerous factors, including lack of verbal stimulation in the home,[11] hearing loss,[8] speech deficit,[14] type of cleft,[12, 15] age,[16] and specific neuropsychological deficit.[17, 18]

Lamb and associates suggested that a sex-by-cleft type interaction may be identified in differences in intellectual development.[19] In their sample of 73 children with clefts, the least frequent sex-by-cleft type groupings (i.e., females with cleft lip and palate and males with cleft palate only) were the groups most likely to display language deficiencies on the WISC and Peabody Picture Vocabulary Test (PPVT). In a sample of over 200 children with cleft,[20] no such differences were noted on the WISC. However, the cleft sample as a whole displayed more low verbal–high performance discrepancies than did the general population. More than 30% of the children with clefts had splits of 12 points or greater favoring the performance scale, compared to 16% of the normative sample. Heineman-De Boer also failed to find a sex-by-cleft type interaction in a sample of 150 children.[21]

Research investigations of language disorders or low verbal patterns in children without clefts have determined that these problems are associated with school learning deficits, especially in the area of reading achievement. Studies of cleft samples also have identified achievement deficits. For example, Richman found that males with clefts scored, on the average, 1 year lower than their classmates on group achievement tests.[22] In a later study, Richman found that 50% of a group of children with clefts and a lower Verbal IQ were significantly below age and grade expectations on the reading and math subtests of an individually administered achievement test.[17] Kommers and Sullivan found deficits in written language that became more pronounced with age.[23]

Spriestersbach interviewed parents of 175 cleft and 175 control children on a variety of topics, including school achievement.[24] Twice as many of the parents of children with clefts reported holding their children back a year from starting school, repeating a grade, or demonstrating delays in school achievement. Parents of the cleft children tended to have lower expectations for their children than parents of controls. Kapp found that children with clefts also considered themselves less successful in school.[25]

The consistent findings of lower Verbal IQ and school achievement deficits provide a rationale for searching for underlying neuropsychological deficits in children with cleft lip or palate.

Infant and Preschool Children with Cleft

The few studies that have examined infants with clefts have found average infant scale scores[26, 27] and normal levels of receptive language development with mild expressive language delays.[28]

Neuropsychological functions are in a state of rapid development in the normal preschooler and thus are difficult to measure reliably. Preschoolers are difficult to assess for behavioral reasons as well, and the preschooler with a cleft is also plagued by speech difficulties, increased behavioral inhibition, fluctuating hearing, and sometimes fear of or reluctance to interact with medical professionals.

Fox and colleagues compared scores in a sample of preschoolers with clefts to those in a control group on 11 cognitive measures and found the cleft group's scores significantly lower on six of the subtests.[29] Five of these were language measures, and one assessed fine motor skills. Nation found that cleft preschoolers scored lower on vocabulary comprehension and usage than noncleft controls.[30]

Data relevant to the question also came from a preliminary report by Eliason and Richman based on a large study of language development in young children with cleft lip or palate.[31] The authors reported cross-sectional data on the first 65 children enrolled in the study. Subjects did not include those with syndromic clefts or other congenital anomalies. Children with a moderate or greater degree of mental retardation also were excluded because of the difficulties inherent in attempting to study specific cognitive functions in the young child with generalized intellectual deficits. The sample included 29 children with cleft lip and palate (21 males and 8 females) and 36 children with cleft palate only (15 males and 21 females). By age, there were 23 four-year-olds, 24 five-year-olds, and 18 six-year-olds.

The test battery included two language reasoning tasks: Picture Association[32] and Auditory Association,[33] a vocabulary definition task Wechsler Preschool and Primary Scale of Intelligence (WPPSI Vocabulary),[34] and a memory-for-colors task (Color Span).[35]

In the preliminary report, the 65 children were studied as a group because the sample was not yet large enough to examine sex-by-cleft type relationships. Compared to normative standards on the measures administered, children in the cleft group displayed average vocabulary development, could solve verbal analogies (Auditory Association), and had a normal verbal memory span. However, they showed significant deficits on visual categorization (Picture Association) and three of the memory-for-colors trials (visual memory, auditory-visual, and visual-auditory trials). These tasks appear to require verbal mediation skills, that is, the ability to select an efficient problem-solving strategy. Normal children appear to develop this skill between the ages of 5 and 6 years, as suggested by the change in their pattern of responding on the Color Span test between those ages. At age 5, they show poor memory span for the first three trials, which require a verbal rehearsal strategy. On the fourth trial this strategy is given to them by the examiner labeling the colors for them. Figure 105–1 shows the performance of children in the normative sample and the cleft sample at age 5 years, indicating little or no difference in the pattern of responding on the four trials.

By 6 years of age, noncleft children are equally efficient on all four trials. Children with clefts, however, continue to show the pattern of poor performance on the first three trials at age 6. Figure 105–2 displays the performance of 6-year-old children with clefts compared with that of children from the normative sample.

Verbal mediation deficits may affect performance on a number of tasks, all of which require some cognitive strategy for effective performance. Thus, conflicting

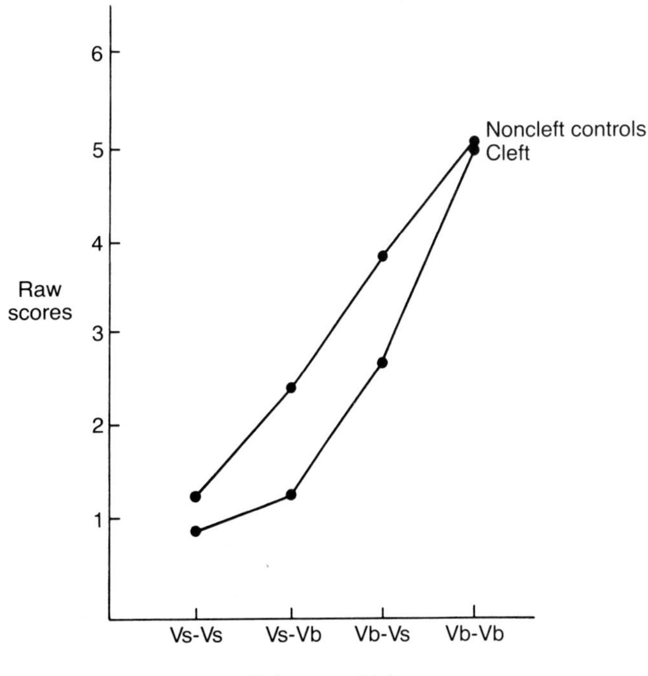

Figure 105–1 Five-year-old cleft group and controls performance on the Color Span test, four trials: Visual-Visual (Vs-Vs), Visual-Verbal (Vs-Vb), Verbal-Visual (Vb-Vs), and Verbal-Verbal (Vb-Vb).

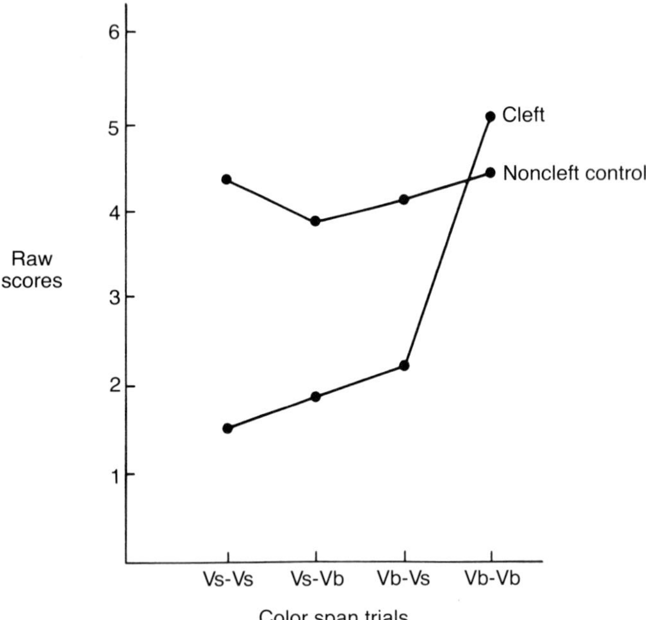

Figure 105–2 Six-year-old cleft group and controls performance on the Color Span test, four trials: Visual-Visual (Vs-Vs), Visual-Verbal (Vs-Vb), Verbal-Visual (Vb-Vs), and Verbal-Verbal (Vb-Vb).

evidence on the language development of children with clefts may be related to task requirements, with cleft children performing well on tasks that do not require strategies and poorly on tasks that do require strategies.

In summary, in spite of the difficulties in assessing young children, there is some evidence that specific cognitive deficits exist in cleft children, primarily in verbal language development. It is still not clear whether children with clefts have a long-term deficit in verbal mediation skills or a delay in acquiring these skills. The longitudinal aspect of the Eliason-Richman study (in progress) will address this question and will also examine sex-by-cleft type interactions, perceptual motor development, and predictors of reading performance.

School-Aged Children with Clefts

Following reports of lowered Verbal IQ and poor school achievement, Richman studied 57 children with cleft lip or palate who displayed a Verbal IQ that was 15 points or more below their Performance IQ.[17] Two patterns of cognitive deficits were identified in these children. Twenty-six of the fifty-seven children showed a verbal expressive deficit (poor verbal fluency and naming skills) but normal performance on the Hiskey-Nebraska Test of Learning Aptitude[32] (a nonverbal measure of intellectual functioning developed for use with hearing-impaired children), and average scores on reading and arithmetic achievement subtests. The remaining 31 children were classified as general language disability and showed deficits on the language subtests of the Hiskey-Nebraska Test and were characterized by significant reading and math underachievement. It was noted that 77% of the group with verbal expressive deficits had clefts of the lip and palate (CLP), whereas 58% of the general language disability group had palate only clefts (CPO). Richman concluded that there were at least two distinct neuropsychological patterns associated with clefting and that cleft-type differences in cognitive patterns were likely.

A follow-up study examined the possibility of cleft-type differences directly.[18] Twenty-four children with CLP were compared to 24 age-, IQ-, and speech-matched children with CPO. A low verbal–high performance IQ test pattern was present in both groups. A battery of language, memory, and nonverbal measures was administered. Children with CPO, as a group, had lower scores than the CLP group and normative standards on measures of memory and language association but not on the nonverbal measures. Table 105–1 shows the weighted scores on the neuropsychological measures.

The groups also differed in regard to type of reading errors. The CPO group displayed primarily a pattern of sight word errors (guessing based on initial consonant, shape of word), suggesting poor development of phonics skills. Children with CLP made errors related to ineffective phonetics, suggesting poor pronunciation, possibly due to peripheral speech deficits.

In a recent study Richman and associates examined reading achievement by cleft type and age in an unselected sample of elementary school-aged children with cleft lip or palate.[36] As before, children with syndromic clefts, other congenital anomalies, or placement in special education classrooms were excluded. The sample included 94 children with CLP and 78 children with CPO (100 males and 72 females). Results suggested no sex differences but revealed significant age differences and a trend toward cleft type differences (Table 105–2).

Children with CPO had a higher overall rate of reading disability at all ages, with 53% reading more than one grade level below grade placement at ages 6 to 7, 38% at age 8 to 9, and 33% at ages 10 to 13. Children with CLP tended to have a high rate of reading problems in the early grades, but the frequency of problems dropped to about 8% by grade six, about the same rate as the general population. No significant sex or sex-by-cleft type effects were identified.

Table 105–1. Neuropsychological and Reading Subtest Performance (means or percents and significance levels)

Variable	CLP	CPO	p
Auditory memory	103.1	81.0	.001
Language	99.9	74.8	.001
Visual-perceptual	97.8	93.5	NS
Word recognition	79.4	78.7	NS
Reading comprehension (grade level scores)	4.21	2.81	.01
Sight word errors[a]	21%	74%	.001
Phonetic errors[a]	69%	26%	.001

CLP = cleft lip and palate; CPO = cleft palate only; NS = nonsignificant
[a]Chi square analysis

Table 105–2. Percentage of Children with Reading Disability by Age Group and Cleft Type

Age in Years	CLP	CPO
6–7	49%	53%
8–9	23%	38%
10–13	9%	33%

CLP = cleft lip and palate; CPO = cleft palate only.

A hypothetic model derived from the results of the three studies summarized above suggests the following picture. The child with CLP is likely to experience mild verbal expressive deficits and a delay in verbal mediational skills in the early school grades, compounded by speech deficits, hearing loss, and behavioral inhibition. This pattern of behavioral and neuropsychological deficits may result in difficulty with early reading activities that focus on sound-symbol relationships and decoding and blending tasks. This child slowly learns phonics skills but may not have the mechanism to produce all the speech sounds accurately. As hearing and speech improve and secondary management of the cleft is completed as needed, the child displays catch-up growth in reading and finishes elementary school with grade-level reading skills.

The same model suggests that the child with CPO also has early verbal expressive, verbal mediational, medical and behavioral difficulties that impede early progress. However, a significant number of CPO children continue to have neuropsychological deficits in language reasoning skills. Their reading problems persist throughout elementary school and presumably, throughout life. They make sight word errors in reading similar to those made by dysphonetic dyslexic children without clefts.[37] The long-term academic course for these children is similar to that of noncleft children with a language-based learning disability. That is, they generally require some remedial services in school and may require more intensive planning for college or vocation.

Thus far, this review of school-aged children has focused on verbal-language development. There is also some evidence of a higher frequency of perceptual-motor disabilities in children with clefts. Smith and McWilliams found that a sample of children with clefts performed poorly on the visual subtests of the ITPA (Illinois Test of Psycholinguistic Abilities).[38] They interpreted this finding as evidence of perceptual-motor disability. However, the ITPA is a language test, and the visual subtests are heavily loaded with language content, and it therefore does not represent a pure measure of nonverbal functioning.

Brennan and Cullinan presented pictures of objects on a tachistoscope and measured recognition, naming ability, and response time.[39] Children with clefts were slower and less accurate in naming objects than controls. The authors proposed that these children showed a deficit in visual processing. However, these results also can be interpreted as slower language processing time because the task required verbal naming. In contrast, studies by Richman and Eliason[18] and Lamb et al[13] failed to find perceptual-motor deficits in samples of children with clefts.

In summary, neuropsychological studies of school-aged children with clefts suggest that at least two types of language impairment can be identified, and these are related to cleft type. Cleft lip and palate appear to be associated with a milder expressive type of deficit or delay, and CPO with a general language disability similar to that seen in language-learning disabled children. There has been little evidence to suggest problems with nonverbal development in cleft children. Patient studies will identify children with clefts and nonverbal deficits by chance only, because these learning disabilities occur in the general population and can coincide with a cleft. Alternatively, studies that find a significant frequency of nonverbal deficits may have included children with syndromic cleft conditions or other congenital anomalies in addition to clefts.

Adolescents and Adults with Cleft

Few studies have examined intellectual or neuropsychological variables in adolescents or adults with cleft. Brantley and Clifford compared a measure of cognitive style (field dependence-independence) and locus on control in 51 cleft, 22 obese, and 100 normal adolescents.[40] The cleft group was more field dependent (influenced by context). It is difficult to interpret this finding in terms of neuropsychological functions. It may be that children with verbal deficits depend on context cues to aid their comprehension because they cannot rely on their own language skills. Thus, verbal mediational skills may be involved in situations that require interpretation of the environment and reflective thinking skills.

Indirect evidence of continuing neuropsychological deficits may be gleaned from studies of adult educational attainment and vocation. For example, Peter and Chinsky found that individuals with CLP were more likely to complete college than those with CPO, offering some support for the finding of greater impairment in the CPO group.[41] Also, Heller et al studied psychological adjustment in 96 adults with repaired cleft lip or palate.[42] When questioned about schooling, 25% of these reported that they had had school achievement difficulties, and 40% had repeated a grade. The majority were employed, although 30% reported difficulty in finding a job and 55% were not enthusiastic about their current job. It is difficult to determine the factors involved in these adult employment problems. Variables such as facial disfigurement, speech deficits, lowered self-esteem, and others may be as important as continued neuropsychological deficits. It is apparent that further investigation of adult development is needed.

Conclusions and Implications

Although there is clear evidence of neuropsychological deficits within the broad area of verbal-language development in preschool and school-aged children with clefts, the etiology of these deficits is unknown. Furthermore, the role of other factors such as middle ear disease, differences in parenting skills and verbal stimulation in the home, experience with early language activities (verbal games in infancy), and type and severity of speech deficits has not been elucidated. Two diametrically opposed hypotheses can be raised regarding neuropsychological deficits in cleft lip or palate children:

1. Neuropsychological deficits are caused by a deviation in prenatal brain development, resulting from the same agent that caused the cleft lip or palate.
2. Neuropsychological deficits arise as a result of environmental influences such as early hearing loss, lack of verbal stimulation, difficulties with the adult speech and language system, and so on.

It is likely that the answer will be some combination of the two hypotheses, and considerable research is needed to address several relevant issues:

1. There is a pressing need for longitudinal studies to determine long-term outcomes of neuropsychological deficits and to determine predictors of school achievement deficits and vocational adjustment.
2. The role of verbal mediation on the behavior and achievement of young children with clefts needs to be examined.
3. Children with school achievement deficits and clefts need to be compared with noncleft learning-disabled students to determine whether the same remedial interventions are appropriate. For example, intensive phonics programs are often recommended for the learning disabled. Can children with clefts benefit from phonics even if they are unable to produce all the sounds correctly?
4. Environmental factors that may contribute to neuropsychological deficits have not yet been explored. The role of early experience may prove crucial. The notion of a critical period for language development is controversial, but it does appear that some children with early hearing loss develop later language disabilities. Children with cleft lip and palate may serve as a good study group for addressing the issue of critical periods for language. Many cleft children have consistent and aggressive ear care, well documented in their medical records when they are treated in cleft palate specialty clinics, compared to care in children who are treated by family doctors or individual specialists not associated with a team. Thus, the two groups (aggressive ear care versus nonaggressive ear care) could be compared in regard to later language development and school achievement.
5. Children with syndromic clefts (such as velocardiofacial syndrome and Sticklers' syndrome) need to be studied from a neuropsychological perspective and compared with children with nonsyndromic clefts.

In conclusion, children (and perhaps adults) with nonsyndromic cleft lip or palate have been found to exhibit neuropsychological deficits, primarily in language-related skill areas. Further research is needed to specify the types and frequency of these deficits and to examine the effectiveness of different types of educational intervention.

References

1. Johnston MC: The neural crest in abnormalities of the face and brain. In Bergsma D (ed): Morphogenesis and Malformations of the Face and Brain. New York: Alan Liss, 1975.
2. Krogman WM: Craniofacial growth: Prenatal and postnatal. In Cooper HK, Harding RL, Krogman WM, et al: Cleft Palate and Cleft Lip. Philadelphia: W. B. Saunders Co., 1979.
3. Clarren SK: Neuropathology in fetal alcohol syndrome. In West JR (ed): Alcohol and Brain Development. New York: Oxford, 1986.
4. Galaburda AM, Kemper TL: Cytoarchitectonic abnormalities in developmental dyslexia: A case study. Ann Neurol 6:94–97, 1979.
5. Spreen D, Tupper D, Risser A, et al: Human Developmental Neuropsychology. New York: Oxford, 1984.
6. Lezak MD: Neuropsychological Assessment, 2nd ed. New York: Oxford, 1983.
7. Billig AL: A psychological appraisal of cleft palate patients. Proc Pennsylvania Acad Sci 29:31, 1951.
8. Means B, Irwin J: An analysis of certain measures of intelligence and hearing in a sample of the Wisconsin cleft palate population. Cleft Palate Newsletter 4:2–4, 1954.
9. Munson S, May A: Are cleft palate persons of subnormal intelligence? Educ Res J 48:617–622, 1955.
10. Lewis R: A survey of the intelligence of cleft palate children in Ontario. Cleft Palate Bull 11:83–85, 1961.
11. Estes R, Morris H: Relationship among intelligence, speech proficiency, and hearing sensitivity in children with cleft palates. Cleft Palate J 7:763–773, 1970.
12. Goodstein L: Intellectual impairment in children with cleft palates. J Speech Hear Res 4:287–294, 1961.
13. Lamb M, Wilson F, Leeper H: A comparison of selected cleft palate children and their siblings on the variables of intelligence, hearing loss, and visual-perceptual motor skills. Cleft Palate J 9:218–228, 1972.
14. McWilliams BJ, Musgrave R: Psychological implications of articulation disorders in cleft palate children. Cleft Palate J 9:294–303, 1972.
15. Cervenka J, Drabkova H: The intelligence quotient in cleft lip and palate. Acta Chir Plast 7:58–61, 1965.
16. Musgrave R, McWilliams BJ, Matthews H: A review of the results of two different surgical procedures for the repair of clefts of the soft palate only. Cleft Palate J 12:281–290, 1975.
17. Richman LC: Cognitive patterns and learning disabilities in cleft palate children with verbal deficits. J Speech Hear Res 23:447–456, 1980.
18. Richman LC, Eliason MJ: Type of reading disability related to cleft type and neuropsychological patterns. Cleft Palate J 21:1–6, 1984.
19. Lamb M, Wilson F, Leeper H: The intellectual function of cleft palate children compared on the basis of cleft type and sex. Cleft Palate J 10:367–377, 1973.
20. Eliason MJ, Richman LC: Sex and cleft type influences on intellectual development in children with cleft. Read before the American Cleft Palate Association, Miami, Florida, 1985.
21. Heineman-De Boer JA: Cleft Palate Children and Intelligence. Lisse: Swets and Zeitlinger, 1985.
22. Richman LC: Behavior and achievement of cleft palate children. Cleft Palate J 13:4–10, 1976.
23. Kommers M, Sullivan M: Written language skills of children with cleft palate. Cleft Palate J 16:81–85, 1979.
24. Spriestersbach DC: Psychosocial Aspects of the "Cleft Palate Problem." Iowa City: University of Iowa Press, 1973.
25. Kapp K: Self-concept of the cleft lip and/or palate child. Cleft Palate J 16:171–176, 1979.
26. Plotkin RR, Wirls CJ, Finney BJ: Developmental evaluation of the cleft infant. Read before the Annual Meeting of the American Cleft Palate Association, Portland, Oregon 1970.
27. Starr P, Chinsky R, Canter H, et al: Mental, motor, and social behavior of infants with cleft lip and/or palate. Cleft Palate J 14:140–147, 1977.
28. Long NV, Dalston RM: Comprehension abilities of one-year-old infants with cleft lip and palate. Cleft Palate J 20:303–306, 1983.
29. Fox D, Lynch J, Brookshire B: Selected developmental factors of cleft palate children between two and thirty-three months of age. Cleft Palate J 15:239–245, 1978.
30. Nation JE: Vocabulary comprehension and use of preschool cleft palate and normal children. Cleft Palate J 7:639–644, 1970.
31. Eliason MJ, Richman LC: Language and memory development in preschool children with cleft lip and palate. Read before the Annual Meeting of the American Cleft Palate Association, San Antonio, Texas, 1987.
32. Hiskey MS: Hiskey-Nebraska Test of Learning Aptitude. Lincoln: Union College Press, 1966.

33. Kirk SA, McCarthy JJ, Kirk WD: Illinois Test of Psycholinguistic Ability. Urbana, IL: University of Illinois, 1968.
34. Wechsler D: Manual for the Wechsler Primary and Preschool Scale of Intelligence. New York: Psychological Corp, 1969.
35. Richman LC, Lindgren SD: The Color Span Test. Iowa City: University of Iowa, Department of Pediatrics, 1978.
36. Richman LC, Eliason MJ, Lindgren SD: Reading disability in children with cleft lip and/or palate. Cleft Palate J 25:21–25, 1988.
37. Boder E: Developmental dyslexia: A diagnostic approach based on three atypical reading-spelling patterns. Dev Med Child Neurol 15:663–687, 1973.
38. Smith R, McWilliams BJ: Psycholinguistic abilities of children with clefts. Cleft Palate J 5:238–249, 1965.
39. Brennan D, Cullinan W: Object identification and naming in cleft palate children. Cleft Palate J 11:188–195, 1974.
40. Brantley H, Clifford E: Cognitive, self-concept, and body image measures of normal, cleft, and obese adolescents. Cleft Palate J 16:177–182, 1979.
41. Peter J, Chinsky R: Sociological aspects of cleft palate adults: education. Cleft Palate J 12:443–449, 1974.
42. Heller A, Tidmarsh W, Pless IB: The psychosocial functioning of young adults born with cleft lip or palate. Clin Pediatr 20:459–465, 1981.

CHAPTER 106

Psychological and Sociocultural Aspects of Cleft Lip and Palate

Ronald P. Strauss and Hillary Broder

This chapter presents an overview of relevant psychosocial theory and research pertaining to cleft rehabilitation and examines relationships between the individual and the social environment. Research on social learning, self-concept, and physical attractiveness using a developmental and sociologic perspective will be summarized.

Emotional and social development occurs in normative stages that influence how a child, including one with a cleft lip or palate, will respond to his world. The neonate is solely focused on his own physical needs to survive and is dependent on his caretakers. Initially, he has no awareness of his parents' emotions; however, by the first month babies do respond to positive (smiling) and negative signals.[1] At 2 months of age infants focus on the mother's eyes and mouth and by 3 months have control over their visual system. By the third month children reflect the moods of the people with whom they interact, and the social smile emerges.[2] Social interaction begins, and the infant becomes an effective partner.[3] Between 3 and 6 months positive affect is observable.[4] Between 7 and 9 months of age, children initiate and participate in social interactions (peek-a-boo) and avoid situations that lead to negative emotions.

At 1 year of age attachment to the mother is present, and separation anxiety is observed. Children will be happy in the presence of the significant caretakers and unhappy in their absence.[2] At this time, psychological assessment of the child's developmental skills is typically conducted with the parent present. During the attachment period, children are wary of strangers and have a strong preoccupation with the primary caregiver. Evidence suggests that early separations or adverse experiences are overcome in time by normal care;[5] however, family interaction and stability, cultural factors, and the child's temperament and cognitive development are important variables in emotional and social development.[6]

The stage of exploring and practicing emotions in the child's world is observed between 12 and 18 months of age. The self-concept emerges in toddlers by 3 years of age, and parental expectations then become manifest in their child's behaviors. The young child develops a repertoire of emotional reactions indicating his own emotional states and inferring those of others.[3] Preschool-age children see events as strictly outcome dependent and are happy if the outcome is positive. If the caretaker is pleased with the results of surgery the child notes satisfaction and will be pleased. During the child's elementary school years, patient satisfaction becomes more complex. In the preschool-age or younger child, fears are expressed to tangible and immediate stimuli. These fears stem from not having enough information (loud noises). The elementary school-age child develops fears of less tangible situations and has more realistic fears based on a wider range of social experiences. An individual's behavior develops along with cognitive and social environmental changes, as in the case of angry behaviors and tantrums.[7] At 2 years temper tantrums peak. At 3 years of age the child is angry that "no one will play with me." At age 6 the child makes causal attributions—that is, the child may still be angry with the outcome but seeks to explain why.[8]

Relationships with peers become increasingly important as the child develops ties outside of the family that depend on a child's ability to connect, exchange information, resolve conflict, and share "private" information.[9] By mid-childhood the importance of belonging to a group and achieving increases in importance. Popularity and success are more easily attained if one is attractive. Children prefer to play with and like children that are more attractive.[10, 11] Our styles of interacting and learning are based on feedback from others, trial and error, observational learning, modeling, and reinforcement contingencies.[12] The child's ability to form close relationships with others depends on his self-concept and his perception of his physical appearance. Children also mimic parental perceptions as well as parental styles of relating to others.[13] Thus, they learn attitudes toward a facial scar, defect, or facial asymmetry. Honest self-disclosure is more likely if a person feels that no danger will follow.[14]

Persons with birth defects, physical disfigurations, or speech disabilities have altered social experiences. Being different implies being perceived by others as less than complete, as handicapped, or otherwise reduced. The bodily signs of being different, known as stigma, carry a moral evaluation, usually a negative one. Goffman's classic work *Stigma* has provided a theory of stigmatization and handicap that is useful in understanding the social responses to human difference[15] and health conditions.[16] Initial interactions with strangers are based on observations of attributes that become "transformed into normative expectations" and then into "righteously presented demands."[15] Persons with clefts of the lip or palate may be seen as deviant when judged by cosmetic norms or when prejudices operate about the cause and impacts of congenital deformities.[17] Some generalizations about the relationship between appearance and behavior are:

1. Physical appearance is a social stimulus.
2. It arouses expectations for behavior.
3. It is one of the criteria for assigning a person to a social role.
4. It influences a person's perception of himself by comparison with others and through others' expectations of him.[18]

Social stereotyping and behavioral expectations associated with facial attractiveness provide one of the most consistent and robust research findings in social science.[19] Deviant facial appearance is readily noticeable and central. The face is the primary focus of attention in interpersonal interaction. A large body of research indicates that attractiveness has an important effect on psychological development and social relationships.[20] The research into physical appearance examines how being an attractive or unattractive child influences social life and personal adaptations. One study examined the role of physical attractiveness on childhood social expectations by testing how school teachers evaluated educational potential when given school records and facial photographs.[21] Attractive students were judged to have higher educational potential and social ability than unattractive students. This finding has been replicated in various school settings and grade levels; thus there is strong support for the hypothesis that teachers of attractive children expect them to perform better[11] and probably offer them greater opportunity to excel.[22]

The "beauty is good" hypothesis is confirmed across age, race, and varying situations.[23] There is evidence that infants may be able to differentiate between pretty and ugly images.[24] By age 7, children are able to differentiate between attractive and unattractive children and use consistent judgments about attractiveness,[25] although there is controversy about whether preschool children operate with a facial attractiveness stereotype.[26, 27] Nurses, parents, school teachers, and peers rate the attractive infant, child, and adult more positively— nicer, more cooperative, more likeable, and better adjusted.[28–31] In addition to the attribution of positive qualities to attractive infants, children, and adults, the attractive also receive preferential treatment—that is, more attention from caretakers.[22] Since expectations for behavior are shaped from feedback, the individual with a facial birth defect may not be expected to achieve to the same levels as attractive infants and children.[21, 32]

The positive impact of appearance has been demonstrated in dating and mating, and one study documented that physical appearance increased in importance as the partners became fully acquainted during the period of five dates.[33] The role of physical attractiveness in marital satisfaction is evident regardless of the length of marriage or the ages of the couples.[34] There is evidence that expectations about appearance affect both the person who is viewed as well as the viewer. In one study, phone callers were shown a fictitious picture of a potential date and were asked to evaluate the person based on the phone call that was also taped and independently rated.[35] The callers were found to bring out behaviors in the recipients of the calls that were consistent with their supposed, not actual, appearance. Such studies suggest that physical attractiveness is a major determinant of social expectation.

Appearance has been shown to affect legal proceedings, hiring, promotion, and psychotherapeutic prognosis. In a simulated jury study, college students on a mock jury were exposed to attractive and unattractive defendants.[36] For certain crimes, such as nonviolent burglary, unattractive defendants were more likely to be found guilty and got longer sentences than attractive defendants. For other crimes, such as engaging in a swindle or con game, attractive defendants were more likely to receive a long sentence. One might interpret the stringent sentencing on the latter crime as a reaction to the abuse of the gift of beauty. Indeed, attractive persons are not always seen in uniformly positive terms. Attractive people may be seen as egotistic, vain, and snobbish.[37] Unattractive persons may receive the compensation of being seen as more honest and moral.[38]

In work settings, personnel decisions are usually positively influenced by attractiveness,[39] and attractive persons may be viewed as better employees in spite of their sometimes poor actual performance.[40] One study assessed how psychologists rate new patient prognosis.[41] In the psychologist's office, new patients were rated independently for attractiveness. After the initial psychologist's session, the professional was asked to evaluate the patient's likelihood of receiving benefit from therapy. The attractive clients were predicted to have a better prognosis than unattractive patients. The implication of this body of research is that appearance judgments globally affect the social expectations of persons and that even professionals are influenced by these values.

The self-concept is formed by a trial-and-error learning process by which values, attitudes, roles, and identities are learned.[42] The "looking glass theory" postulates that we come to see ourselves as others see and value us.[43] Through internal regulation, conscious and unconscious, our behavior is guided. Self-concept has been held to be predictive of academic achievement, social expectations, and vocational aspirations.[44, 45] If an individual has a poor self-concept, behavior is shaped to avoid situations that are anxiety-producing or make one feel inferior.[46] The patient with a cleft palate who has a poor self-concept may thus avoid seeking treatment and avoid challenging social interactions.

Self-concept is a dynamic, evaluative, and emotional construct that defines the way a person sees and feels about himself.[46] It entails:

1. Self-image. What the person sees when he looks at himself.
2. How strongly the person feels about his physical, intellectual, and social self-images.
3. Whether the person has a favorable or unfavorable opinion of the various self-image factors.
4. What the person is likely to do in response to his evaluation of himself.[47]

Thus, coping strategies, problem-solving skills, and behavior are directed. The perceptions of self depend on social experiences, attitudes, the setting of interactions, and the cultural milieu. Self-concept theory lacks explanations of how changes in self-concept, perception, and behavior occur.

Humanists have sometimes criticized the high value society places on attractiveness and the degree to which appearance influences opportunity. Controversy surrounding the surgical normalization of the faces of children with Down's syndrome has been based on the belief that the values of the society should change, not the faces of the affected children.[48] Indeed, even when this set of surgical procedures is studied, it is clear that children who look more normal are judged more positively by school-aged peers.[49] Parents and advocates of active approaches to remediation of appearance argue that social values are difficult to change and that each person must adapt to the cultural context and stereotypes. Health education interventions in school settings have been shown to alter attitudes on a short-term basis,[50] but pervasive advertising and mass media images bolster the desirability of physical attractiveness.

Facial surgery has often been used to alter social experience. Reports of the use of rhinoplasty in Jewish patients[51] and of alterations of ethnic features in black patients[52] suggest that patients may strive to accommodate to social norms rather than struggle against discrimination or stigmatization. Even when the cosmetic blemish is erased, persons may still retain their different identity. Naturally, surgery cannot change racial nor ethnic origins, nor can it really alter the reality of Down's syndrome. The search for aesthetic change is based on the hope that a change in appearance may, in part, create opportunities for other changes. Improvement in appearance has been shown to change social perceptions. One study of "before" and "after" plastic surgery photographs, drawn from texts and journals, revealed that observers uniformly found postoperative views more attractive.[53] The postoperative photographs were seen as belonging to people who were kinder, more sexually appealing, and better marriage partners than were the preoperative views. The benefits of appearance change due to surgery were apparent to the viewers.

Persons who have had long-standing defects that are repaired late in life may be especially aware of the ways in which defects may be used. For some patients, the defect provides an accessible explanation for their failures and difficulties. When a correction occurs, the explanation drops away, and the person may have the troubling realization that even so-called "normals" have dissatisfactions and difficulties in living. The benefits of sickness, known as "secondary gains," are well documented as contributing to the difficulty that some persons have in relinquishing their identity as "different."[15]

Persons with scars, disabilities, or defects that cannot be effectively repaired may be deeply aware of the social unacceptability of being different. They feel the uncertainty of how others perceive them and have concerns about whether others will honestly reveal their reactions to them. The polite avoidance of contact with physically or otherwise different persons serves to isolate them. Furthermore, it is clear that people with deviant characteristics realize that others do not accept them, and they may respond with anger, denial, or shame. The perception of oneself as reduced or defiled, elements of shame, can lead to bitterness or withdrawal. For some people, the experience of being different presents a challenge and an opportunity for positive growth. Activists for handicapped persons' rights have been able to present a social and political critique based on their different viewpoint and experience. The ability to stand outside dominant social perspectives may allow for many realizations and insights not available to others.[54]

How society treats the unattractive or deformed person raises many questions. Clinicians may find themselves having to decide if the goal of plastic surgical care is the attainment of perfection in appearance and function. Surgeons may find themselves wondering if an almost normal result or a socially acceptable result is sufficient. The surgeon is charged with the actualization of social and aesthetic values, yet surgical activism itself may alter how deviance is perceived. What may have once been an acceptably unusual appearance when treatment was not possible, may become an unacceptably deviant appearance when a repair is possible. This tension, as found in the case of malocclusion and orthognathic surgery,[55] may result in a high degree of surgical activism and high rates of per capita surgery. The physician's role as an ethical gatekeeper is an important element in preserving the balance between marketplace forces, the surgeon's desire to be productive, and society's need to provide health care of real benefit to patients.

The social devaluation of persons with deformities is related to the anxiety with which they are generally perceived. Myths, fiction, and legends reveal a cross-culturally shared distress with difference.[56] Does the universal threat of bearing a child with a defect cause the avoidance and fear that permeate the social attitudes about physical deformities? Is there a human need for conformity that dictates that there will always be someone who is an outcast?

Studies of international groups suggest that cultural mores and values provide the criteria for treatment decisions.[57] Infanticide, considered a cruel and primitive practice by Westerners, has been used in many cultures as a means of limiting family size,[58] coping with economic or demographic conditions,[59] or dealing with birth defects.[60] African case studies reveal that a minor physical handicap may result in malnourishment of the child, making the child a beggar or seeing him as a family embarrassment.[61] In some contexts, the difference between infanticide and child maltreatment may be slight. Facial clefts have been described as the basis of infanticide, and according to one author some traditional feeding practices are "certain to kill a child with cleft palate."[62] Other studies suggest that child neglect and concealment of the defective person are responsible for the small numbers of children that receive surgical care for birth malformations in some locations.[63] Reports from China[64] and Brazil[65] support the continued occurrence of infanticide to date.

In cultures where infanticide is considered nonexistent, activism about treatment and understanding of the defect may vary. Religious fundamentalism has been found to be a determinant of how birth defects are understood and of how decisions regarding treatment and prevention are made.[66] Economic status influences attitudes, and studies in Israel find that as groups achieve greater economic and educational attainments, they become more positive toward the care of the disabled.[67] The greater the society's reliance on Western biomedical technology and paradigms, the more likely are they to encourage treatment and medical remediation of birth defects. In developed nations, the combination of economic resources, professional manpower, and Western activism has resulted in wide acceptance of the multidisciplinary team-based model for cleft palate care.

The medical, dental, speech, and psychosocial complexities of treating persons with clefts of the lip and palate have mandated that groups of professionals participate in the planning and delivery of care. This specialization may lead to a situation in which individual professionals direct their efforts to a part of the patient's total treatment. Specialization of care raises the risk that fragmentation of care will occur, in which the global needs of the patient will not be recognized while specific treatment needs are addressed. Health teams provide an excellent way of avoiding this pitfall because they allow coordinated and rational planning of care while drawing from the resources of specialists.[68] Team meetings provide the opportunity to coordinate actions and communicate findings. Teams have chosen other organizational strategies, such as shared medical charts, centralized offices, and rotating team leadership, to develop a common identity and encourage communication.

The team-based cleft lip and palate care delivery model is especially helpful in ensuring that the psychosocial needs of the patient are addressed.[69] Team discussion allows identification of psychosocial concerns and adjustment of treatment plans to meet patient needs. Teams in large treatment centers may have psychologists, social workers, or other mental health professionals who are specifically interested in psychological and social issues.[70] Although some have questioned the need for psychological services because of the relatively low rates of psychopathology among patients with clefts,[71] clinical observations and research findings suggest that children with clefts of the lip and palate are at increased risk for psychosocial problems.

Recent studies of self-concept,[72, 73] psychoeducational development,[74, 75] social perception by peers,[76, 77] parents and teachers,[78, 79] and the public[80] clarify the psychosocial risks among school-age children with clefts. Studies of adolescents with cleft lip and palate have established that appearance and speech may remain problematic[81, 82] even in patients who have had extensive surgical and team-based care.[83] Studies of parental tolerance of conduct problems[84] and school experience with children who have clefts[85] suggest that there is an association between cleft lip and palate and the increased reporting of conduct problems at home and behavioral and learning problems at school.

Studies of cognitive function and intellectual status within the cleft population report slightly lower mean IQ scores than those in normative data.[75, 86] Lower verbal IQ scores and language deficiencies are observed more frequently in children with clefts.[87] Children with cleft lip and palate are more likely to have verbal expressive deficits and reading problems that resolve with increased age,[75] and children with isolated cleft palate sometimes demonstrate more severe reading disabilities.[88] Children with clefts tend to underachieve relative to their intellectual ability.[89] These students' academic problems may be associated with verbal or language deficiencies.[90, 91] Teachers tend to underestimate the intellectual ability of children with more severe, cleft-related facial deformities.[32] Lower academic expectations are expressed by parents for their children with clefts.[72]

In general, there exists no distinctive personality type or pattern of psychopathology among cleft subjects. Self-concepts in children with clefts appear to be lower than those in noncleft cohorts.[72, 77] Subjects with facial clefts are reported to be more concerned about their physical self-concepts.[92] Children with facial clefts and intelligibility problems may be at higher risk for poor self-concepts. Additional congenital malformations increase the likelihood of school and home behavior problems. Females tend to express more concern about their appearance than males.[72] Inhibition and shyness are observed more frequently among individuals with clefts.[84] Adjustment and achievement problems are noted among adolescents with clefts.[81, 83] One study found a cleft lip to be judged more acceptable in a work partner than in a marriage partner (80% versus 8%).[93] Adults with clefts report less dating experiences and marry later in life.[94]

The absence of high rates of significant psychopathology among persons with cleft lip or cleft palate as studied in United States samples,[95] suggests that patients learn to cope with being different and usually are able to make appropriate adaptations and learn to participate in the social life of the community. Most researchers in this area conclude that this coping occurs in spite of a variety of social, educational, and personal challenges. The need to cope with these challenges in this population provides a rationale for the presence of psychological and social work inputs into team-based cleft palate care.

Several interventions have been identified as helpful in the prevention of psychosocial problems related to cleft lip and palate. The team can encourage parents to follow consistent behavior-management techniques. Team professionals can routinely assess the patient's developmental skills, thus allowing the team to note and address changes in the person and family system over a period of time. Parents can be helped to confont fear-provoking stimuli (for example, needles) and thereby allow the child to understand his fears. The team can effectively time treatments to address the concerns of the patient and family and may encourage more patient involvement in decisions as the child's verbal ability develops. Teams can be helpful by articulating professional expectations for behavior (for example, oral hygiene).

Adolescents must be encouraged to express their feelings and become involved in clinical decisions and the timing of treatment. Because adolescence is often marked by rebellious behavior with parents and increased need for autonomy,[96] members of the treatment team should interview the parent and patient separately. Issues, such as unresolved parent guilt or patient shame with their facial appearance are more readily expressed during private interviews with the parents. In addition, self-disclosure is more honest if it is done in private. Children are apt to express the same views as their parents, especially in their presence.[97]

During adolescence, body image is of critical importance.[98] Addressing the individual's wishes and aspirations is essential; however, the ideal self may not be reality-based. The young adult faces the psychosocial task of being attractive to the opposite gender, which places renewed emphasis on the physical self. If surgery is carried out without a thorough assessment of patient expectations, postoperative depression and devaluation may result.

The authors emphasize that each individual's life experiences vary. Furthermore, the degree of facial disfigurement is not predictive of the degree of psychic distress.[17, 99] Multidisciplinary team assessments are made to develop the patient's treatment plan, which must be tailored to the patient's physical and psychological status. The psychosocial assessment must not lead to stereotyped inferences about needs, abilities, and support systems based on the type of defect. The psychosocial assessment can include evaluation of developmental skills in the preschool child, intellectual and aptitude testing, personality factors (for example, self-concept), and the function of the family system.

Presurgical counseling is important to ascertain the expectations of treatment and anxiety associated with surgery. Postsurgery evaluations can assess the patient's level of satisfaction with treatment. This counseling is considered preventive in nature. The counselor may describe procedures that could increase patient motivation. If counseling or special education or vocational needs are identified, referrals to local schools or agencies are made. Psychological therapy for children and parents

experiencing particular problems is a common recommendation of team-based cleft palate programs.

Parent and patient groups organized along the mutual aid or self-help model provide peer support and newborn counseling in a nonprofessional context. An elaborate network of such organizations has been developed in the United States, furthered by the formation of a national cleft palate parent and patient organization in 1984. The provision of genetic counseling and information has been suggested as an important factor in the prevention of family guilt and psychosocial dysfunction.[100] Genetic counseling can be directed toward building a patient's understanding of the causes of a defect as well as family planning and decisions about prenatal screening and diagnosis.

Social workers, team coordinators, and nurses have been helpful in accessing resources that may relieve the financial burden felt by lower income families of children with clefts. In the United States, state-funded agencies (Crippled Children Programs, Childrens' Special Health Services Agencies) offer funding for cleft lip and palate team-based care for families unable to afford the high costs of treatment.[101] Customarily, families qualify for such coverage when their income falls at or below the poverty line, adjusted for family size. Social workers and related personnel can arrange for such treatment coverage and are helpful at locating transportation, nutrition, and community assistance. Vocational rehabilitation counselors can provide specific assistance to adults or students who aspire to improve their employability and vocational potential through further rehabilitation.

In the United States, the financial burden of care may fall particularly hard on the family that does not qualify for low income assistance but has either inadequate or no health insurance coverage. The combined costs of cleft lip and palate therapy may be prohibitive to such families, and they require assistance in arranging for treatment. Recent initiatives in cost control and prepaid health care have sometimes posed a barrier to paying for team-based cleft care. Parent and patient support group advocacy has led to some state legislation ensuring the coverage of team-based cleft palate care. The organization of health services and the mechanisms for payment are actively changing and probably will provide a challenge to families and cleft teams seeking to ensure comprehensive payment for the full course of cleft remediation.

References

1. Brazelton TB: Precursors for the development of emotions in early infancy. In Plutchik R, Kellerman H (eds): Emotion: Theory, Research and Experience. Vol 2. New York: Academic Press, 1983.
2. Sroufe LA: Socioemotional development. In Osofsky JD (ed): Handbook of Human Development. New York: Wiley, 1979.
3. Murphy LB: Issues in the development of emotion in infancy. In Plutchik R, Kellerman H (eds): Emotion: Theory, Research and Experience. Vol 2. New York: Academic Press, 1983.
4. Sroufe LA: The coherence of individual development: Family care, attachment and subsequent developmental issues. Am Psychol 34:834, 1979.
5. Maccoby EE: Social Development: Psychological Growth and the Parent-Child Relationship. New York: Harcourt Brace Jovanovich, 1980.
6. Damon W: Social and Personality Development: Infancy Through Adolescence. New York: Norton, 1983.

7. Weiner B: Human Motivation. New York: Holt, Rinehart, & Winston, 1980.

8. Weiner B, Graham S: An attributional approach to emotional development. In Izard CE, Kagan J, Zazonc RB (eds): Emotions, Cognition, and Behavior. New York: Cambridge University Press, 1984.

9. Gottman J: How children become friends. Monographs for Research in Child Development 48:2, 1983.

10. Sigelman CK, Miller TE, Whitworth LA: The early stigmatizing reactions to physical differences. J Appl Dev Psychol 7:17, 1986.

11. Adams GR, Crane P: An assessment of parents' and teachers' expectations of preschool and children's social preference for attractive or unattractive children and adults. Child Dev 5:224, 1980.

12. Hartup WW: Peer relations. In Hetherington EM (ed): Handbook of Child Psychology. Vol 4. Socialization, Personality, and Social Development. New York: Wiley, 1983.

13. Jourard SM, Remy RM: Perceived parental attitudes, the self, and security. J Consult Psych 19:364, 1955.

14. Freud A: The role of bodily illness in the mental life of children. In The Psychoanalytic Study of the Child. Vol 7. 1952, p 69.

15. Goffman E: Stigma—Notes on the Management of Spoiled Identity. Englewood Cliffs, NJ: Prentice-Hall, 1963.

16. Ablon J: Stigmatized health conditions. Soc Sci Med 15B:5, 1981.

17. Macgregor FC: Transformation and Identity—The Face and Plastic Surgery. New York: Quadrangle/New York Times, 1974.

18. Meyerson L: Somatopsychology of physical disability. In Cruikshank WM (ed): Psychology of Exceptional Children and Youth. Englewood Cliffs, NJ: Prentice-Hall, 1955.

19. Langlois JH, Roggman LA, Casey RJ, et al: Infants' preferences for attractive faces: Rudiments of a stereotype? Dev Psych 23:363, 1987.

20. Bersheid E: Overview of the psychological effects of physical attractiveness. In Lucker GW, Ribbens KA, McNamara JA (eds): Psychological Aspects of Facial Form. Craniofacial Growth Series Monograph, No 11. Ann Arbor: Center for Human Growth and Development, University of Michigan, 1980.

21. Clifford M, Walster E: The effect of physical attractiveness on teacher expectations. Soc Educ 46:248, 1973.

22. Adams GR, LaVoie JC: Teacher expectations: A review of the student characteristics used in expectancy formation. J Instruct Psycho Mono 4:1, 1977.

23. Cunningham MR: Measuring the physical in physical attractiveness. J Pers Soc Psych 58:618, 1986.

24. Boukydis ZC: Infant attractiveness and the infant-caretaker relationship. Read before the International Conference on Love and Attraction, Swansea, Wales, 1977.

25. Cross JF, Cross J: Age, sex, race, and the perception of facial beauty. Dev Psych 5:433, 1971.

26. Dion KK: Young children's stereotyping of facial attractiveness. Dev Psych 9:183, 1973.

27. Cavior N, Lombardi DA: Developmental aspects of judgment of physical attractiveness in children. Dev Psych 8:67, 1973.

28. Byrne D: The Attraction Paradigm. New York: Academic Press, 1971.

29. Boukydis Z: Infant attractiveness and the infant-caretaker relationship. Pediatrics 61:373, 1978.

30. Corter C, Trehub S, Boukydis C, et al: Nurses' judgments of the attractiveness of premature infants. Infant Behav Dev 1:374, 1978.

31. Nida SA, Williams JE: Sex stereotypes traits, physical attractiveness and interpersonal attraction. Psych Reports 41:1311, 1977.

32. Richman LC: The effects of facial disfigurement on teachers perception of ability in cleft palate children. Cleft Palate J 15:155, 1978.

33. Mathes EW: The effects of physical attractiveness and anxiety on heterosexual attraction over a series of five encounters. J Marriage Fam 37:768, 1975.

34. Weiszhaar O: Sex drive, accentuation of physical attraction and marital satisfaction. Thesis (Ph.D). Minneapolis: University of Minnesota, 1978.

35. Snyder M, Tanke ED, Bersheid E: Social perception and interpersonal behavior: On the self-fulfilling nature of social stereotypes. J Pers Soc Psych 35:956, 1977.

36. Sigall H, Ostrove N: Beautiful but dangerous: Effects of offender attractiveness and nature of the crime in juridic judgement. J Pers Soc Psych 31:410, 1975.

37. Dermer M, Thiel DL: When beauty may fail. J Pers Soc Psych 31:1168, 1975.

38. Dipboye RL, Fromkin HL, Wiback K: Relative importance of applicant sex, attractiveness and scholastic standing in evaluation of job applicant resumes. J Appl Psych 60:39, 1975.

39. Scheuerle J, Guilford AM, Garcia S: Employee bias associated with cleft lip/palate. J Appl Rehab Couns 31(2):6, 1982.

40. Landy D, Sigall H: Beauty is talent: Task evaluation as a function of the performer's physical attractiveness. J Pers Soc Psych 29:299, 1974.

41. Barocas R, Vance FL: Referral rate and physical attractiveness in third-grade children. Percept Motor Skills 39:731, 1974.

42. Rogers CR: On Becoming a Person. Boston, Houghton Mifflin, 1961.

43. Videbeck R: Self-conception and the reaction of others. Sociometry 23:351, 1960.

44. Purkey WW: Self Concept and School Achievement. Englewood Cliffs, NJ: Prentice-Hall, 1970.

45. Fitts WH: The Self-Concept and Behavior. Nashville, TN: Counselor Recordings and Tests, 1972.

46. Sullivan HS: Interpersonal Theory of Psychiatry. New York: Norton, 1953, p 165.

47. Rosenberg M: Society and the Adolescent Self Image. Princeton: Princeton University Press, 1965.

48. Mearig JS: Facial surgery and active modification approach for children with Down's syndrome: Some psychological and ethical issues. Rehab Lit 46:72, 1985.

49. Strauss RP, Mintzker Y, Feuerstein R, et al: Social perceptions of the effects of Down's Syndrome facial surgery: A school-based study of ratings by normal adolescents. Plast Reconstr Surg 81:841, 1988.

50. Arndt EM, Lefebre AM, Klaiman P, et al: The impact of two educational programs on normal high school students' impressions of those with craniofacial anomalies. Paper read to the American Cleft Palate Association, Williamsburg, Virginia, April 26, 1988.

51. Macgregor FC: Social and cultural components in the motivations of persons seeking plastic surgery of the nose. J Health Soc Behav 8:125, 1967.

52. Munro IR: The psychological effects of surgical treatment of facial deformity. In Lucker GW, Ribbens KA, McNamara JA (eds): Psychological Aspects of Facial Form. Craniofacial Growth Series Monograph No. 11. Ann Arbor: Center for Human Growth and Development, University of Michigan, 1980, p 173.

53. Bersheid E, Gangestad S: The social psychological implications of facial physical attractiveness. Clin Plast Surg 9:198, 1982.

54. Zola IK: Ordinary Lives—Voices of Disability and Disease. Cambridge Mass: Apple-wood Books, 1982, p 12.

55. Strauss RP: Ethical and social concerns in facial surgical decision making. Plast Reconstr Surg 72:727, 1983.

56. Shaw WC: Folklore surrounding facial deformity and the origins of facial prejudice. Br J Plast Surg 34:237, 1981.

57. Strauss RP: Culture, rehabilitation and facial birth defects: International case studies. Cleft Palate J 22:56, 1985.

58. Williamson L: Infanticide: An anthropological analysis. In Kohl M (ed): Infanticide and the Value of Life. Buffalo: Prometheus Books, 1978, p 61.

59. Dickeman M: Demographic consequences of infanticide in man. Ann Rev Ecol Sys 6:107, 1975.

60. Sheper-Hughes N: Child Survival—Anthropological Perspectives on the Treatment and Maltreatment of Children. Dordrecht, Holland: D. Reidel Pub, 1987, p 11.

61. Oyemade A, Olugbile A: Barriers to the rehabilitation of the handicapped in Nigeria. London: Public Health, 95:82, 1981.

62. Oluwasanmi J, Adelunkle O: Congenital clefts of the face in Nigeria. Plast Reconstr Surg 46:245, 1970.

63. Gupta B: The incidence of congenital malformations in Nigerian children. W Afr Med J 18:22, 1969.

64. Mosher SW: The Broken Earth: The Rural Chinese. New York: Free Press, 1983, p 194.

65. Sheper-Hughes N: Culture, scarcity and maternal thinking: Mother love and child death in Northeast Brazil. In Sheper-Hughes N (ed): Child Survival—Anthropological Perspectives on the Treatment and Maltreatment of Children. Dordrecht, Holland: D. Reidel, 1987, p 187.

66. Strauss RP: Genetic counseling in the cross cultural context: The case of highly observant Judaism. Pat Educ Couns 11:43, 1988.

67. Florian V, Katz S: The impact of cultural, ethnic and national variables on attitudes towards the disabled in Israel. Int J Intercult Rel 7:167, 1983.

68. Nagi SZ: Teamwork in health care in the US: A sociological perspective. Milbank Mem Fund Q 53:75, 1975.

69. Strauss RP, Broder H: Interdisciplinary team care of cleft lip and palate: Social and psychological aspects. Clin Plast Surg 12:543, 1985.

70. Broder HL, Richman LC: An examination of mental health services offered by cleft craniofacial teams. Cleft Palate J 24:158, 1987.

71. Clifford E: The state of what art? Cleft Palate J 25:174, 1988.

72. Kapp K: Self-concept of the cleft lip and/or palate child. Cleft Palate J 16:171, 1979.

73. Kapp-Simon K: Self-concept of primary school-age children with cleft lip, cleft palate or both. Cleft Palate J 23:24, 1986.

74. Richman L, Eliason M: Psychological characteristics of children with cleft lip/palate: Intellectual achievement, behavioral and personality variables. Cleft Palate J 19:249, 1982.

75. Richman L, Eliason M: Type of reading disability related to cleft type and neuropsychological patterns. Cleft Palate J 21:1, 1984.

76. Schneiderman CR, Harding JB: Social ratings of children with cleft lip by school peers. Cleft Palate J 21:219, 1984.

77. Tobiasen JM: Social judgments of facial deformity. Cleft Palate J, 24:323, 1987.

78. Schneiderman CR, Auer KE: The behavior of the child with cleft lip and palate as perceived by parents and teachers. Cleft Palate J 21:224, 1984.

79. Mitchell CK, Lott R, Pannbacker M: Perceptions about cleft palate held by school personnel: Suggestions for in-service training development. Cleft Palate J 21:308, 1984.

80. Middleton GF, Lass NJ, Starr P, et al: Survey of public awareness and knowledge of cleft palate. Cleft Palate J 23:58, 1986.
81. Richman L, Holmes C, Eliason M: Adolescents with cleft lip and palate: Self-perceptions of appearance and behavior related to personality adjustment. Cleft Palate J 22:93, 1985.
82. Richman L: Self-reported social, speech and facial concerns and personality adjustment of adolescents with cleft lip and palate. Cleft Palate J 20:108, 1983.
83. Strauss RP, Broder H, Helms R: Perceptions of appearance and speech in adolescent patients with cleft lip and palate and their parents. Cleft Palate J 25:335, 1988.
84. Tobiasen JM, Hiebert JM: Parent's tolerance for the conduct problems of the child with cleft lip and palate. Cleft Palate J 21:82, 1984.
85. Tobiasen JM, Levy J, Carpenter MA, et al: Type of facial cleft, associated congenital malformations, and parent ratings of school and conduct problems. Cleft Palate J 24:209, 1987.
86. Smith R, McWilliams BJ: Psycholinguistic abilities of children with clefts. Cleft Palate J 5:238, 1968.
87. Richman LC: Cognitive patterns and learning disabilities in cleft palate children with verbal deficits. J Speech Hear Res 23:447, 1980.
88. Richman LC, Eliason MJ, Lindgren SD: Reading disability in children with clefts. Cleft Palate J 24:21, 1988.
89. Richman LC, Harper DC: Observable stigmata and perceived maternal behavior. Cleft Palate J 15:215, 1978.
90. Richman LC: Behavior and achievement of the cleft palate child. Cleft Palate J 13:4, 1976.
91. Richman LC, Lindgren SD: Patterns of intellectual ability in children with verbal deficits. J Abnorm Child Psych 8:65, 1980.
92. Tobiasen JM, Levy J, Carpenter C, et al: Type of facial cleft, associated congenital malformations, and parents' ratings of school and conduct problems. Cleft Palate J 24:205, 1987.
93. Shears LM, Jensema CJ: Social acceptability of anomalous persons. Except Child 36:91, 1969.
94. Peters JP, Chinsky RR: Sociological aspects of cleft palate adults: I Marriage. Cleft Palate J 11:443, 1974.
95. Clifford E, Crocker E, Pope B: Psychological findings in the adulthood of 98 cleft lip-palate children. Plast Reconstr Surg 50:234, 1972.
96. Erickson EH: Childhood and Society. New York: Norton, 1963.
97. Helper MM: Learning theory and self concept. J Abnorm Soc Psych 51:184, 1955.
98. Coleman JS: Relationships in Adolescence. New York: Routledge-Kegan Paul, 1974.
99. Broder H: Perceptions of children with visible or invisible oral-facial defects. Thesis (Ph.D). Durham, NC: Duke University, 1980.
100. Broder HL, Trier WD: The effectiveness of genetic counseling for families with craniofacial disorders. Cleft Palate J 22:22, 1985.
101. White RB: Services for children with congenital facial clefts through a state Crippled Children's service program. Cleft Palate J 18:116, 1981.

CHAPTER 107

Psychosocial Aspects of Cleft Lip and Palate: The Family

Marcy T. Rogers, R. Christopher Barden, and Stan A. Kuczaj, II

Although psychosocial problems have been documented for children and adults with craniofacial deformities, little has been written suggesting any means of management or prevention. Similarly, medical schools, residency programs, and the curriculum of most allied health programs continue to be deficient in providing courses dealing with the management of the craniofacial patient. Due to this lack of attention, many pediatric residents may complete their training without the benefit of treating or even examining a child with an unrepaired cleft lip and palate. In some programs, even though residents may see one or two of these problems during their training, owing to the lack of an interdisciplinary team approach in their institution, these patients may be inappropriately referred to an individual practitioner for management of this complicated problem. Consequently, many pediatric residents report feeling ill-equipped to deal adequately with the emotionally charged issues families experience as a consequence of facial deformity. These same professionals are later called on to advise families in delicate and complicated treatment decisions.

Although an interdisciplinary team approach to treatment has been advocated,[1] standards for what comprises a team approach have yet to be agreed on. Treatment teams continue to be diverse in composition; some advocate strong psychosocial programs, others have no such programs, and still others emphasize individual specialties versus an integrated team approach. For example, the timing of a family's contact with a team varies greatly from center to center. This is true even though self-report information obtained from surveys of parents done at several treatment institutions and freestanding parent groups uniformly indicates a need for early education and emotional support in the first hours following the birth of a child with a cleft lip, cleft palate, or craniofacial deformity.[2] In that study, interview data obtained from institutions providing outreach programs to families within the first 24 to 48 hours of the birth of affected infants indicated a reduced rate of failure to thrive. Furthermore, parents who participated in such programs said they not only felt less anxious about taking their infant home but were also better informed about impending treatments. Overall, these families reported feeling less overwhelmed by the birth defect and its ramifications and better prepared to cope with the emotional strains of repeated hospitalizations and surgeries.

Psychosocial Issues for Families of Children with Cleft Lip and Palate

The psychosocial sequelae associated with children born with cleft deformities are only now becoming understood. Some of these problems seem inevitable given our society's orientation toward physical beauty. Findings that the social stigma affiliated with craniofacial deformities may lead to psychosocial disadvantage are prevalent in the literature, reflecting the recognition that others' reactions to a craniofacial deformity may be more damaging psychologically than the deformity itself.[3–7]

Psychosocial difficulties resulting from cleft defects may appear as early as infancy. For example, because some degree of feeding difficulty is experienced by most families of infants with cleft palate or craniofacial disorders, early maternal-infant interaction processes may be adversely affected. Poor feeding coupled with the usual feelings of isolation, guilt, anxiety, and denial faced by most parents of infants with birth defects does little to foster good infant-maternal interaction. In addition, support from other parents who have faced similar problems may be rejected at this critical early phase in the socialization process because of the emotional stages of denial and later acceptance that parents typically experience.[8–10] Field and Vega-Lahr[11] and Barden et al[12] have noted that mothers of cleft lip and palate and craniofacially deformed infants tend to engage in less frequent smiling, vocalizing, imitative behaviors and game playing with their infants than do mothers of normal infants and also tend to be unaware of their unnurturant behavior. Careful longitudinal research is needed to further specify the developmental implications that may result from the types of mother-child interactions that seem to characterize the early development of the cleft lip and palate infant.

In addition to these demonstrated deficiencies in the quality of early mother-infant interaction, the arrival of a cleft lip or palate child may create an array of difficulties for the family as an integrated unit. For example, the birth of such a child has been reported potentially to divide the family into two groups: the mother and the child with the cleft or craniofacial deformity, and the father and other children.[13] This division may isolate the deformed child from family members other than the mother, thereby potentially limiting important family socialization experiences. Furthermore, as noted above, interactions between these mothers and their infants also may be deficient. If the mother is the family member providing the major part of the child's early social interactions, the cleft child is likely to receive less than optimal social stimulation, thus potentially leading to later problems of social development. Additional research is needed in this area to specify both the factors that may produce the potential schism of the family, the consequences of such a division for the development of a cleft or craniofacially deformed child, and sources of social support that may ameliorate such difficulties.

The importance of early psychosocial support and corrective surgery is exemplified by other findings in the literature. For example, a long-term follow-up investigation of young adults with bilateral cleft lip and palate revealed many psychosocial problems, especially among males.[14] The females in this group had married early, raised children, and reported few serious psychosocial problems. In contrast, fewer than half of the 30 male patients reported being married, and 2 of the 30 had committed suicide. Similarly, other research indicates that young adults with cleft lip and palate may have significantly lower incomes, marry later in life, have more childless marriages, and are almost three times as likely as noncleft lip and palate young adults to be unmarried.[15]

In contrast to these findings is a large body of research that has found little if any psychosocial disability associated with cleft lip and palate families or patients of any age.[16–18] Such conflicting research findings have left us without an empiric foundation for a psychosocial prevention or treatment regimen. The absence of investigations on the effects of cleft lip and palate on familial functioning is even more striking.

One consistent conclusion that is reported in the research literature is that cleft lip and palate patients, parents, and siblings do not appear to be at high risk for psychosocial problems that fit into traditional diagnostic categories of psychopathology.[15] This may be due to the fact that current reconstructive surgical procedures are capable of bringing many patients into the low-normal range of physical attractiveness at an early age.[7, 19, 20]

In addition to these potential problems, parental emotional and behavioral reactions to their child's deformity also may influence the child's level of adaptation. Parents who are anxious or depressed about their child's appearance may visually or verbally convey their averse reactions to their child.[7, 21] With age, this may lead to decreased opportunities for modeling by the parents and heightened risk for a variety of behavior problems (e.g., aggression, dependency, inhibition) that are associated with some older cleft patients. In an effort to reduce socialization deficits and prevent potential behavior problems, some medical teams have recommended that corrective surgery be performed as early as medically possible.[11, 12, 22]

Successful medical intervention involves not only corrective surgery but also adequate psychosocial preparation of the family and the patient for such surgery.[23] The appropriately prepared family and patient are more likely to feel comfortable with and remain in treatment, thus decreasing the risk that potentially problematic psychosocial consequences associated with a cleft or craniofacial deformity will be manifested. Appropriate education and preparation of family members for the psychosocial stresses of medical treatments for cleft lip and palate are the major tasks of the psychosocial members of the medical team.

Role of the Psychosocial Specialists on a Multidisciplinary Team

The major clinical task of the psychologist or other psychosocial specialists on a craniofacial or cleft lip and palate team is to ensure that patients and their families have clearly heard and understood what the multidisciplinary team has attempted to communicate to them and vice versa. In such an emotionally laden situation, the clear communication of sometimes complicated medical information is not always an easy task. To further complicate matters, the cleft lip and palate population tends to be a very psychologically heterogeneous one.[24] Many patients have additional deformities or problems, and there is a large degree of variability in the cleft, speech, or hearing problems they may present. Patient families also are very heterogeneous and present with varying degrees of inter- and intrafamilial support, different coping styles such as philosophic or religious beliefs, and varying levels of stress due to concerns about financial resources. In addition, families and patients arrive with a wide variety of preconceptions about cleft patients, medical teams, and mental health professionals. It is the psychosocial teams' task to quickly assess these factors and prevent potential problems in patient-team interaction.

In many cases, accurate communication is the most critical element of team management. For example, the psychosocial staff must decipher such psychologically sensitive questions as: Are the parents' goals and fears realistic and are they compatible with the teams' goals and prognoses? Do the parents understand the nature of the problem, the medical risks involved in treatment, and the long-term implications, if any, for socioemotional and educational functioning of the child? Are there family, economic, or religious issues that may affect treatment? By sensitively and accurately exploring these issues and portraying information in a way that will not engender fear or reactance from the family, the psychosocial team members can avert emotional trauma, fear, and even anger from patients and families. By deciphering and averting communication obstructions, the psychosocial team can also expedite the work of the other team professionals while increasing the families' inclination to remain in treatment and abide by often stringent treatment regimens.

At times, more traditional assessment and psychotherapeutic efforts also are required to improve family functioning and maximize the resources available to the patient. Psychotherapeutic needs vary tremendously, depending on such factors as the severity of the clefting and other biologic disorders, the socioeconomic level of the parents, the cohesion or functioning of the family, the developmental level of the patient, and the satisfaction of the family with their medical care. The psychological support staff must be particularly sensitive to these variables and communicate potential problems to the team before they affect the effectiveness of other modalities of treatment.

Two assessment procedures that seem increasingly necessary for effective therapeutic efforts as the patient develops are individual interviews and validated self-report data. Recent research evidence indicates that patients and families are not always able to provide an accurate account of their psychosocial status. The pressures of medical settings also can contribute to potential misinformation gathered through simple questionnaires, self-report tests, and interviews.[12] To combat these sources of error, other sources of information such as school records, teacher questionnaires, and observational in vivo data should be obtained whenever possible. Similarly, much more accurate and thorough assessments of family functioning are obtained when family members are interviewed separately as well as together. Adolescent patients are especially reluctant to discuss their personal problems in front of parents or medical staff. In sum, efforts to combat anxiety, depression, family strife, unrealistic expectations, and social withdrawal are all important components of the psychosocial teams' role.

Finally, there is increasing evidence that a means for providing both professional and parent outreach and support within the first 24 to 48 hours of an affected infant's birth could profitably become an active part of the services provided by parent groups and treatment providers. Perhaps some of the early maternal-infant interaction problems documented in these families could be reduced by instituting aggressive newborn outreach and education programs. The craniofacial treatment community could take a more active role in educating the public and the staffs of birthing hospitals in an attempt to reduce some of this potentially avoidable early psychosocial trauma. With a coordinated effort combining resources from research projects, treatment teams, and public or medical education, the potential psychosocial tribulations faced by cleft lip and palate patients may be at least partially ameliorated.

ACKNOWLEDGMENT. This project was supported by grants from the National Craniofacial Foundation and a Faculty Scholar Award from the William T. Grant Foundation to R. Christopher Barden.

References

1. Cooper H, Harding R, Krogman W, et al: Cleft Palate and Cleft Lip: A Team Approach in Clinical Management and Rehabilitation of the Patient. Philadelphia: W.B. Saunders Co., 1979.
2. Sterken S, Strong J: Challenge: Providing immediate and accurate information to parents of children born with cleft lip and palate. Read before the Annual Meeting of the American Cleft Palate Association, Williamsburg, Virginia, 1988.
3. Baker W, Smith L: Facial disfigurement and personality. JAMA 112:301, 1939.
4. Edgerton M, Jacobson E, Mayer C: Surgical-psychiatric study of patients seeking plastic (cosmetic) surgery. Br J Plast Surg 13:136, 1960.
5. Kalick S: Toward an interdisciplinary psychology of appearances. Psychiatry 4:243, 1978.
6. *Harvard Law Review*, Facial discrimination: Extending handicap law to employment discrimination on the basis of physical appearance. 100:2035–2052, 1988.
7. Barden RC, Ford ME, Wilhelm WM, et al: Emotional and behavioral reactions to facially deformed patients before and after craniofacial surgery. Plast Reconstr Surg 82:409, 1988.
8. Ramsey J, Rogers-Salyer M, Barden RC, et al: Patient/parent support groups: Why they fail and how we can help them succeed. Read before the American Cleft Palate Association, Annual Meeting, New York, 1986.
9. Field T: The three R's of infant-adult interactions: Rhythms, repertoires and responsivity. J Pediatr Psychol 3:131, 1978.
10. Goldberg S: Premature birth: Consequences for the parent-infant relationship. Am Sci 67:214, 1979.
11. Field T, Vega-Lahr N: Early interactions between infants with cranio-facial anomalies and their mothers. Infant Behav 7:527, 1984.
12. Barden RC, Ford ME, Jensen GA, et al: Effects of infant facial deformity on mother-infant interaction. Child Dev 60:819–824, 1989.
13. Richardson SA, Hastorf A, Dornbusch S: Effects of physical disability on a child's description of himself. Child Dev 35:893, 1964.
14. Ross RB, Johnston MC: Cleft Lip and Palate. Baltimore: Williams & Wilkins, 1972, p 96.
15. Starr P, Pearman W, Peacock JL: Cleft Lip and/or Palate: Behavioral Effects from Infancy to Adulthood. Springfield, IL: Charles C Thomas, 1983.
16. Clifford E: Role of the psychologist on the cleft palate team. *In* Georgiade N (ed): Symposium on Management of Cleft Lip and Palate and Associated Deformities. St. Louis: C. V. Mosby, 1974.
17. Clifford E, Crocker E, Pope B: Psychological findings in the adulthood of 98 cleft lip/palate children. Plast Reconstr Surg 50:234, 1972.
18. Pickrell K, Clifford E, Quinn G, et al: Study of 100 cleft lip-palate patients operated upon 22 to 27 years ago by one surgeon. Plast Reconstr Surg 49:149, 1972.
19. Barden RC, Ford ME, Wilhelm WM, et al: The physical attractiveness of facially deformed patients before and after craniofacial surgery. Plast Reconstr Surg 82:229, 1988.
20. Barden RC, Ford ME, McCarty S, et al: The effectiveness of craniofacial surgery across diagnostic and age groups: An empirical study. Read before the American Cleft Palate Association, San Antonio, Texas, 1987.
21. Lefebvre A, Munro I: The role of psychiatry in a craniofacial team. Plast Reconstr Surg 61:564, 1979.
22. Edgerton M, Jane J, Berry F: Craniofacial osteotomies and reconstructions in infants and young children. Plast Reconstr Surg 54:13, 1974.
23. Peterson L, Ridley-Johnson R, Tracy K, et al: Developing cost effective presurgical preparation: A comparative analysis. J Pediatr Psychol 9:439, 1984.
24. Barden RC: Psychological interventions for craniofacial anomlies. *In* Lahey B, Kazdin A (eds): Advances in Child Clinical Psychology. New York: Plenum Press. (In preparation, 1989).

Nursing Care for Cleft Patients

CHAPTER 108

Comprehensive Nursing Care for Cleft Patients

Linda Chase, Deb Starr, Cindy Tvedte, and Bonnie Wagner

Management of cleft lip and palate patients offers a unique challenge for nursing specialists and necessitates a multidisciplinary approach for provision of optimal care. As a vital member of the cleft palate team, the nurse's role is established immediately after the birth of an infant with a cleft deformity. Initial nursing intervention is related to feeding techniques and the provision of emotional support to the family. The nurse maintains this role throughout the years of treatment by providing continuous teaching and support.

Care of the patient with cleft lip and palate requires a sound knowledge base in pediatric-surgical nursing, genetic counseling, growth and development, and family dynamics. Such a background enables the nurse to provide preoperative and postoperative management and assist the patient and family with their psychosocial needs.

The nursing care described in this chapter reflects the procedures followed at The University of Iowa Hospitals and Clinics. Other health care institutions may vary in their approach to nursing care of cleft patients.

Emotional and Social Adjustment

The birth of a cleft lip or palate child can be a traumatic event for parents, and supportive care from health professionals is essential. The nurse is an important member of the cleft team—a group of specialists involved in the multidisciplinary management of children born with cleft deformities.

After a child is born with a cleft defect, the nurse is notified by telephone or written referral. Basic information is obtained to formulate a care plan for the child. Information about the child's birth date, type and severity of the cleft, family financial status, and the home situation is useful to have before initial contact is made with the parents. All information is retained in a file to be used for future reference in preparation for surgery.

After initial contact has been made by telephone from an outside referring institution, the nurse continues to serve as a resource person. The nurse is available both to the medical professionals who take care of the cleft child and to the parents. Consultation regarding feeding techniques and appointments can be provided by telephone, and instructional materials are sent to the family. A follow-up telephone call is made to the parents after the child is discharged to see if any problems have developed (especially with feeding) and to answer questions about home care of the child.

When a child is born within a hospital setting that has a cleft team, the nurse is able to perform the initial nursing assessment to determine the type and severity of the cleft. Other congenital defects, if present, must be noted also because these will be important in making decisions about surgery and feeding techniques, and in assisting with long-term expectations of the parents.

The nurse makes contact with the parents after the initial assessment to determine their level of understanding of the child's cleft defect. Often it is the nurse's responsibility to interpret and clarify the information given to the parents. Typically, parents experience grief or disappointment and are not ready for detailed information at this point. Also, it is important to determine the parent's perceptions of the child and allow ample time for them to cope with and adjust to the situation. Dealing with the unknown often results in feelings of anxiety for the parents, especially when faced with questions from friends and relatives concerning the nature and cause of the cleft defect.[1] Parents need to know that these feelings are natural. The nurse should display an accepting attitude toward the infant and emphasize the positive aspects of the child's physical appearance.

Parents may be reassured by seeing pictures of children with similar cleft deformities before and after surgery. Involvement of other family members promotes communication and understanding within the family and strengthens relationships.[2] The parents should be encouraged to bring other family members on return visits and to allow siblings and grandparents to assist in the physical care and handling of the infant when possible.

While in the hospital, the parents are expected to participate in the care of their child. They should hold and feed the child and examine the cleft. Parents need to be allowed to express their feelings and ask questions. When the parents take the baby home from the hosptial, they should have received enough information and support to have developed a positive feeling toward the child and be able to deal adequately with the many attitudes of our society toward individuals with deformities.[1]

Feeding

Feeding the infant with a cleft prior to repair offers a special nursing challenge. Feeding fulfills the important functions of providing the nourishment necessary for growth and strengthening the parent-infant bond. Maintaining nutrition is the first priority in feeding an infant with a cleft lip or palate. A second priority is finding a viable feeding technique that is as close to normal as possible.[3] A variety of feeding devices are available to parents of children with clefts depending on the type and severity of the cleft. Infants with an isolated cleft lip most often feed normally by bottle or breast. Nipples with a broad base work well with regular bottles. Children with clefts of the lip and palate or palate only generate negative pressure when sucking and may tire easily, resulting in unfinished feedings and possibly failure to thrive. A feeding device is needed that will deliver formula into the mouth to conserve the infant's energy. Soft, premature nipples tend to conform more readily to the defect than hard nipples. Cross-cut nipples allow for easier flow of formula. Lamb's nipples are successful for feeding infants with cleft palates owing to the additional length of the nipple. A squeezable, soft, plastic bottle allows the caregiver to squeeze the formula into the infant's mouth if the sucking reflex is weak. A bulb syringe is used as a method of delivering formula without requiring the infant to suck.

If the mother prefers to breastfeed the cleft child, this can be attempted. Infants who have clefts of the lip only should not experience problems except for leaking of milk when the baby is sucking.[4] This is due to the inability of the child to form a seal on the breast. Instruct the mother to experiment with various positions, using the areola to fill the defect and form a seal.[5] If the cleft is unilateral and involves the alveolus, the nipple should be pointed to the unaffected side. The seal also can be improved by placing a finger over the lip defect as the baby nurses.[5]

Infants with clefts of the soft or hard palate or both have more difficulty with breastfeeding because they cannot position the nipple and maintain the necessary vacuum. Instruct the mother to position the nipple to the side of the cleft palate. Supporting the breast with the mother's fingers during feeding also assists the infant to hold on to the nipple and prevents loss of suction.[5] Chin support is necessary also for effective breastfeeding. The mother can be instructed to place her hand under the chin of the infant to help hold the jaw steady and to press the nipple and areola between the infant's gums.[5]

After a feeding technique has been selected, several further modifications can be made to make feeding an infant with a cleft easier. Feeding the infant in a semi-upright position minimizes nasal regurgitation. Feedings should be relaxed and unhurried, allowing adequate time. Initially, feeding the infant may take more time, but length of the feeding time should shorten as the parent and child adjust to the technique. If feeding consistently takes longer than 45 minutes, the infant may be working too hard and the feeding technique should be reevaluated. After feeding is completed, the cleft should be cleansed of mucus and formula using an oral swab dipped in water to prevent irritation and possible infection.

Parents must practice feeding techniques in the hospital prior to discharge. Adequate nutrition and hydration are essential for the infant and for preparation of upcoming surgery. Subsequent to discharge, it is important that these infants be followed to ensure that feeding is going well and that the infant is growing and developing normally. Introduction of solid foods is the same for infants with clefts as for those without cleft defects. Growth and development of the child should be monitored closely by a pediatrician. If the child does not gain weight as desired, the feeding technique should be reevaluated or nutritional supplements added. Nasal or oral gastric tube feedings may be necessary if the infant fails to gain adequate weight. However, these feeding routes should be considered only after all possible oral feeding methods have been tried. In extreme cases, gastrostomy tube placement may be considered if feeding problems are extensive.

Presurgical Management and Preoperative Teaching

Approximately 2 weeks after discharge, an appointment is made for the surgeon to examine the child and schedule future surgery. At this time, the parents also meet with the other members of the cleft team, which may include a surgeon, orthodontist, speech pathologist, audiologist, genetic counselor, and psychologist. At that time, the parents are given a program for overall management that includes information about the timing of various surgical procedures, associated problems, length and type of therapy, estimate of costs, and so on. The nurse facilitates meetings with the professionals on the team and helps the parents recognize and understand their role in the child's future treatment.

Feeding techniques are reviewed again with the parents, and problems, if any, are discussed. At this point, general information is given to the parents regarding cleft lip repair, hospitalization, anesthesia, admission procedures, preoperative laboratory tests, photographs, general anesthesia, items to bring to the hospital, length of hospital stay, and postoperative care. The usual time for cleft lip repair is 3 months of age. By this time, the infant should show a steady weight gain and a satisfactory hemoglobin level. The nurse can recommend that the parents feed the infant using the bulb syringe method one to two times a day for 2 weeks prior to lip surgery. This helps the infant become accustomed to the bulb syringe because this is the feeding technique that will be used for 3 weeks after surgery. Pacifiers may be used preoperatively to strengthen the infant's sucking reflex; however, use of pacifiers is not allowed after surgery for 3 weeks.

Because the prone position is not allowed for 3 weeks after lip surgery, the parents should be encouraged to accustom the infant to lying on his or her back or sitting in an infant seat. This helps to reduce irritability associated with change of the infant's routine. The parents also are instructed on the use of arm cuffs postoperatively for both lip and palate surgery to keep the child from placing his hands or objects in the mouth.

Timing of cleft palate repair is based on many factors, including the type and severity of the cleft and the child's general health development. The goal of cleft palate repair is to close the cleft so that the palate will perform its normal function for eating and speech production. The palate usually is closed when the child is between 12 and 18 months of age.

Parents should be instructed that only a liquid diet is allowed for 3 weeks postoperatively. To help the child adjust to this type of diet, recommend that the parents slowly wean the child from the bottle and accustom him to a cup prior to surgery. This makes the postoperative course easier for both parent and child. As with lip surgery, use of a pacifier is restricted after palatoplasty, and arm restraints are used to keep the child's hands away from his mouth.

At the time of surgery the parents are given further instruction on what can be expected during the postoperative period. Parents usually have several questions about their child's appearance and may find it helpful to talk with other parents and to see a child who has recently had similar cleft surgery. An explanation of what the child will look like helps parents anticipate the appearance of suture lines, drainage, and swelling. Nursing care during the postoperative period should be discussed. This may include intravenous therapy, positioning, restraints, feeding methods, and diet restrictions. Information about these nursing interventions increases the parent's knowledge and allows them to become more involved in the care of the child during hospitalization.

Parents also should be aware of the potential discomfort that the child may experience after surgery and the availability of pain medications. Parents can be a valuable resource is assessing signs of discomfort and communicating this to the nurse. Postoperative discomfort is greater after palatal and pharyngeal surgeries than after lip repairs, so initially narcotics may be required.

Any other specific precautions related to surgery should be described to the parents so that they are aware of things the child can or cannot do in the immediate postoperative period. These precautions include no nose blowing, restricted eating utensils, and limiting the child's activity. This knowledge assists parents in helping their child cooperate with these precautions and precludes accidental trauma to surgical areas due to innocent actions on the part of the parents.

For obvious reasons, toddlers and preschool-age children usually do not comprehend explanations of surgical techniques. Because separation anxiety is a primary problem with this age group, teaching should stress continuity of care, and the mother should be encouraged to help care for her child.[6] If the child is able to understand the preoperative teaching, the nurse should include him or her as much as possible. The nurse should assess the child's emotional and cognitive development and use language that is consistent with the child's developmental level.[2]

In most cases, school-age children will comprehend basic teaching explanations. Visual aids or pictures facilitate teaching this age group.[6] School-age children also benefit from tours of hospital playrooms or units and from discussions in which they can learn about their surgery and treatment plans. Use of medical play techniques increases their understanding of intravenous therapy, suture lines, and arm restraints.

When teaching teenagers about surgery, the procedures should be explained fully, allowing adequate time for questions. This age group typically is concerned with self-image; thus teenage patients often have several questions about personal appearance and care. With this age group, it also is important to stress compliance with restrictions and the fact that improved appearance is not seen immediately.

Postoperative Care and Teaching

Postoperative Care Following Cleft Lip Repair

Primary lip repair is performed at approximately 3 months of age. Exact timing is determined by the infant's weight and general state of health. The cleft patient is admitted to the inpatient unit for 2 to 4 postoperative days.

The length of surgery for a primary lip repair is typically 1 to 1½ hours. The patient is then taken to the post anesthesia care unit (PACU) to recover from the general anesthetic. It is beneficial for both patient and parent if the institution has a parent visitation policy in the PACU. The presence of a parent is calming to the infant as he awakens from the general anesthesia and also helps to relieve parental anxiety. The average length of time spent in the PACU is one hour.

The initial role of the nurse on the inpatient unit as the infant arrives from the PACU is to stabilize and monitor the new surgical patient. The frequency with which vital signs are taken is determined by the unit policy. The patient is positioned supine with the head of the bed elevated to 45 degrees. The infant may be held by the parent or restrained in an infant seat or car seat to maintain this position. During hospitalization, the infant should not be allowed to assume a prone position because the integrity of the surgical site could be compromised if the infant rubs his face into the bed.

The infant's arms should be restrained in a manner that prevents him from getting his hands to his mouth. Restraints are available that fit from the axilla to the wrist. Such restraints prevent the patient from bending the arm at the elbow and should be worn at all times for a 3-week postoperative period, except when removed by the nurse for range of motion exercises approximately every 4 hours.

The infant is given continuous intravenous therapy for 8 to 12 hours subsequent to surgery. Broad-spectrum antibiotics may be instilled through the intravenous (IV) line, followed by oral doses after IV therapy has been discontinued.

When the patient's condition is stabilized and he or she is positioned and restrained, the nurse cleanses the suture line. This is done using cotton-tipped applicators saturated in normal saline followed by application of an antibiotic ointment. The nurse should cleanse the incision in a proximal to distal fashion taking care to cleanse both the floor of the nose and the underside of the lip and alveolar ridge if it is closed at the time of the cleft lip repair. After the incision is cleansed of drainage and debris, it is dried in the same manner and a thin film of antibiotic ointment is applied. This ointment also may be applied to the remaining areas of the upper and lower lips to moisten and protect them. The primary lip repair patient may have a small amount of active sanguineous drainage for 12 to 24 hours after surgery.

The first postoperative feeding usually consists of a sterile glucose solution and may be initiated by the nurse when the infant is awake and alert and appears hungry. Subsequent feeding consists of the patient's routine formula or expressed breast milk. Caution is taken to avoid tension on the suture line, which could occur while the infant is sucking on a nipple. Feeding the infant with a bulb syringe accomplishes this purpose.

The infant is held securely in a semi-upright position with arm restraints in place throughout the feeding. The bulb syringe is positioned in the patient's oral cavity on the side opposite the incision. Constant gentle pressure is maintained on the bulb during the feeding. The infant swallows a significant amount of air with this feeding method and should be burped in an upright position after every 1 to 2 ounces. Most infants generally take 2 to 3 ounces of the glucose solution.

The patient's alveolar ridge and mouth are rinsed with sterile or distilled water using the bulb syringe after feeding. The infant is positioned in an upright and slightly forward position during rinsing and should not be expected to swallow the water. The infant is fed in this manner for approximately 2 to 3 weeks. It is helpful if the patient has been accustomed to the bulb syringe feeding method prior to surgery. These patients tend to have a smoother postoperative course, and the parents experience less stress than those who have not familiarized their infant with this feeding method.

Intravenous therapy generally is discontinued after the first formula feeding. Cleansing of the suture line, as previously described, is performed after each formula feeding. Oral antibiotics should be administered in accordance with the infant's feeding schedule. They are best tolerated if given after the formula but prior to rinsing the mouth. The infant should be held or positioned in a supine, upright position for 30 to 45 minutes after each feeding to decrease the potential for aspiration should regurgitation occur.

Postoperative pain subsequent to cleft lip repair usually is controlled with non-narcotic oral analgesics. Pain medication typically is not required for more than 2 postoperative days. Patients have significant discomfort from flatus on the operative day due to a combination of general anesthesia and air swallowed during bulb syringe feeding. This subsides by postoperative day one.

The nurse's role during the patient's remaining hospital course is to observe and support the patient and to facilitate parent education in preparation for discharge. Assignment of primary nursing caretakers allows a consistent approach when teaching cleft care to parents. Spending sufficient time with parents enhances the learning environment. Notify the parents that after the child has had surgery, the nurse will demonstrate cleft care to them and any other family members. After the initial demonstration, the parents do the actual care with nursing support. Reassure the parents that someone will stay and observe them until they feel comfortable with the procedure. Repetition of information is valuable in teaching cleft care. Visual aids, such as booklets, also enhance the parent's learning. Table 108–1 summarizes postoperative care and parent education tips.

The most concentrated teaching is done at the time of primary cleft lip repair. Usually this is the first surgical procedure the child has had, and it is an anxious time for parents. When teaching bulb feeding, mouth rinsing, and suture care, it is beneficial if both parents are present. Show the parents what equipment is needed for performing cleft care so that they can become acquainted with the routine they will be following.

Initiate the teaching session by demonstrating correct positioning for feeding. Give tips about positioning—for example, a pillow can be placed under the feeder's arm and the infant to make him or her more comfortable. Instruct the parents that bulb syringe feedings may take longer and they should not rush. Place the bulb syringe in the infant's mouth making sure to demonstrate correct placement of the bulb tip on the tongue of the infant. Parents frequently are concerned about how fast to give the formula and whether the infant might choke. Tell the parents to squeeze the bulb with a gentle, constant pressure. Also, the infant should be burped frequently because of the amount of air ingested when using a bulb syringe. A guideline for parents is to burp the infant after every 2 ounces of formula or after the amount in each bulb has been given. If the child is unaccustomed to the bulb syringe, the parents may be worried about the infant's discontent with this method of feeding. Reassure the parents that within a few days the child will adapt to the bulb syringe and take the feedings readily. Parents also are instructed to rinse the child's mouth with water following the bulb syringe feeding.

Suture care is demonstrated next because it must be done after each feeding. Most parents will not be thorough enough when cleaning the suture line. Also, parents must be instructed on cleaning drainage from the nostril and under the upper lip. Parents often forget these difficult areas or perhaps are uneasy about performing the task.

Other points to be highlighted with parents include use of arm restraints and correct positioning. Correct application of restraints is essential and tricks to keep

Table 108–1. Postoperative Care and Parent Teaching After Cleft Lip Repair

Postoperative Care	Rationale	Parent Education Tips
Positioning: Patient not allowed to lie prone. Do not burp infant over the shoulder.	Prevent trauma to suture line.	Use of an infant seat is a safe and secure method of maintaining correct position.
Elbow restraints (arm cuffs): Need to be worn unless patient is under direct supervision. Use for 3 weeks from the day of surgery.	Prevent infant from putting hands to mouth.	Secure arm cuffs from axilla to wrist and use a safety pin placed horizontally at the top of the arm cuff to prevent slipping. Parents may launder arm cuffs at home.
Feeding: Bulb syringe feedings are used for 3 weeks from the day of surgery. No bottle or breast feedings or pacifiers are used after surgery.	Prevention of sucking is necessary to decrease tension on the suture line.	Allow enough time for bulb feedings—about 30 to 45 minutes. Place infant in semi-upright position for feeding. Position bulb syringe in the mid to posterior oral cavity on the side opposite the defect. Burp frequently (after every 2 ounces) owing to the large ingestion of air during bulb feedings. If choking occurs, stop feeding until airway is clear, reposition, and resume feeding slowly.
Oral care: Follow each feeding with sterile water given per bulb syringe.	Mouth rinsing removes formula from the oral cavity and suture lines. Residue formula can be a medium for bacterial growth.	A small amount of sterile water will cleanse the oral cavity. If the child is taking oral antibiotics, rinse the mouth with water after giving the medication.
Suture care: Cleanse the suture line after each feeding with normal saline followed by application of an antibiotic ointment.	Removal of wound drainage and exudate promotes healing and prevents infection.	Extra care must be taken with sutures under the upper lip and in the nares. These areas are easily missed. Apply only a thin film of antibiotic ointment.

restraints secure often are welcomed by parents. For arm splints, it helps to pin the cuff to a sleeve so it will not slide. Positioning is important so that the parents know how to position the child correctly after each feeding. Stress that proper positioning is essential for preventing injury to the suture line and that close observation at home is important.

Repetition of important points and positive support makes teaching most successful. Allow sufficient time for both parents to participate in learning. Parents welcome explanations of reasons for procedures performed. Their increased understanding improves compliance of care at home. Verbally questioning the parents and having them give return demonstrations are the best methods for ensuring that parents can perform the care correctly. Give constructive criticism or positive reinforcement in response to their efforts.

The patient is discharged from the hospital on postoperative day three to five. The parents should be supplied with the following: bulb syringes, normal saline, cotton-tipped applicators, antibiotic ointment, two sets of arm restraints, and a prescription for antibiotics. All discharge teaching should be provided in written form for home use. Include all instructions using step-by-step, lay terminology, and provide telephone numbers if questions should arise. Parents must receive guidelines for observing signs of suture line dehiscence and infection. Indicate clearly any follow-up appointments. The sutures used for lip repair are nondissolvable, and an appointment should be made for approximately 1 week later for suture removal.

Postoperative Care for Lip Revision Patients

Secondary lip revisions are performed on some cleft lip patients to improve the function or appearance of the lip. Revisions may be performed at any age during childhood or adolescence and are often done in combination with other cleft repairs, such as palatoplasty or cleft rhinoplasty.

Nursing care of secondary lip revision patients is similar to that of primary lip repair; however, this procedure is generally less stressful for both the patient and parents. Hospitalization typically is required for 1 day following the procedure.

When the patient is admitted to the nursing unit following surgery, he or she is positioned in a side-lying position with the head of the bed elevated. The patient should not be allowed to lie prone. The patient's temperature must be taken by the axillary or rectal route because intraoral probes are contraindicated. If the patient is under 3 to 4 years of age, arm restraints should be maintained at all times when the patient is not under direct observation. Older patients require arm restraints until they are fully awake and should be applied for naps and bedtime. Iced normal saline gauze may be applied to the surgical site for a maximum of 24 hours to minimize edema. Postoperative pain generally is controlled with non-narcotic oral analgesics. Intravenous therapy is maintained until the patient is free of nausea and tolerates clear liquids.

Patients who have secondary lip revisions usually are taking a solid diet prior to the procedure. Their diet must be restricted to a soft diet high in calories and protein for approximately 1 week after surgery. A registered dietician can provide helpful instruction to parents about this type of diet. If the patient is young enough to be taking a bottle, a bulb syringe must be used for feeding for 1 week postoperatively.

Care of the incision, as previously described, is performed three to four times per day. Oral care is restricted to rinsing with water or normal saline after meals and snacks for 1 week, when gentle toothbrushing may be performed by the parent or by the patient, if he or she is old enough.

When teaching the required physical care subsequent to secondary cleft lip revision, the nurse uses some of the same techniques as those used for primary lip repair. Again, assignment of a primary nurse promotes patient-nurse-parent interaction. The parents already should be familiar with the principles of cleft care, but it is important to assess their present knowledge base before initiating further instruction. Use demonstrations and return demonstrations to help parents master the required physical care. Teaching about cleft care includes suture care, diet restrictions, and oral rinses after meals.

If the child is old enough, include him or her in the instruction and ensure his or her understanding. Written releases from physical education classes and contact sports for 1 month postoperatively should be given if the child is of school age.

On discharge from the hospital, the patient should be supplied with incisional care supplies, a prescription for antibiotics (if indicated), and an appointment for suture removal approximately 1 week from surgery.

Postoperative Care of the Palatoplasty Patient

Palatoplasty is performed on patients who are usually under 2 years of age. The child may or may not be admitted to the inpatient unit the day prior to surgery. The patient remains hospitalized for approximately 3 to 5 postoperative days. The actual surgical time for performing a palatoplasty is approximately 1½ hours. Following a 1- to 2-hour stay in the PACU, the patient returns to the inpatient unit.

Palatoplasty patients require close observation of the airway and should be positioned in a side-lying or prone position with the head of the bed elevated to 45 degrees to help minimize edema of the airway. The patient is expected to have sanguineous oral or nasal drainage for 12 to 24 hours. Suctioning of the oral cavity should be avoided because it may cause trauma to the surgical incision. The patient may receive one to two doses of corticosteroids intravenously to prevent or reduce airway edema. The surgeon should be notified if the patient exhibits any signs of respiratory distress.

Intravenous therapy is continued until the patient is free from nausea and is taking adequate oral fluids. The patient usually takes sufficient fluids 24 to 48 hours postoperatively. Palatoplasty patients usually require narcotic analgesics for 1 to 2 postoperative days for control of pain. Then non-narcotic analgesics may be needed for several additional days.

The patient's diet is restricted for 3 weeks to liquids high in protein and calories. The nurse must pay close attention to the child's oral intake and fluid balance. Because patients may resist taking fluids, it may be helpful to administer a mild analgesic prior to meals and snacks to facilitate this effort. The bulb syringe method, as previously described, may help to obtain adequate oral fluid intake. This method is useful particularly if the patient has been taking a bottle up to the time of surgery. Bottles, pacifiers, and eating utensils of any form are contraindicated postoperatively because they can traumatize the surgical site.

Oral hygiene consists of rinsing the patient's mouth with water after meals and snacks. Commercial mouthwashes should be avoided. Gentle toothbrushing can be performed by the parent 1 week after surgery. Arm restraints should be maintained continuously for 3 weeks postoperatively; however, they should be removed every 4 hours for range of motion exercises.

Parent education subsequent to palatoplasty focuses on maintaining the nutrition and fluid intake requirements for the patient. Usually on the first postoperative day a liquid diet using a cup is initiated. At this time, review with the parents that the child is not allowed to use a bottle or eating utensils to avoid injury to the palate. Parents may be concerned if their child has not been weaned from a bottle prior to palatoplasty. If that is the case, a bulb syringe or a cup with a small rim can be used. Give parents guidelines for how much fluid their child should take. Use understandable terminology to describe the need for 1 to 1½ quarts of fluid per day. Instruct the parents that the child may experience discomfort while eating and that a mild analgesic such as Tylenol can be given 20 to 30 minutes before meals. Usually it is beneficial to have a registered dietician speak with the parents about blending soft foods at home in a blender or food processor so that the patient's nutritional and caloric needs are met. The dietician can also give parents ideas about how to add variety to the liquid diet.

Parents should demonstrate that they know how to apply arm restraints and provide oral hygiene. Emphasize safety precautions when teaching the parents. The palatoplasty patient usually is in the toddler age range and will be very active and compulsive, necessitating close supervision.

As for the surgical procedures mentioned earlier, the parents should receive written instructions on the signs of postoperative complications such as dehydration, infection, and dehiscence of the incision. Discharge supplies include two pairs of arm restraints and a prescription for antibiotics. The sutures used to repair a cleft palate are dissolvable. A return appointment to see the surgeon is generally made for 1 month after discharge.

Postoperative Care of the Pharyngeal Flap Patient

A pharyngeal flap is a surgical procedure to correct the hypernasal speech that is characteristic of some cleft palate patients. The procedure is reserved for patients who have not obtained adequate speech production subsequent to palatoplasty and speech therapy. The pharyngeal flap procedure reduces the amount of air allowed into the nasal cavity, resulting in a more orally resonant voice. Some patients who do not have a previous history of a cleft palate may also be candidates for this procedure. This surgical procedure typically is performed at 4 to 6 years of age.

Nursing care of a child undergoing a pharyngeal flap

procedure is similar to that for the palatoplasty patient; however, these patients are at greater risk for airway compromise. The nurse should observe the patient closely during the early postoperative period for signs of respiratory distress and notify the surgeon immediately should this occur. Because these patients are at such high risk, two nasopharyngeal stents are placed during the surgical procedure to provide for an adequate airway and facilitate drainage. The stents remain in place 24 to 48 hours after surgery. The nurse should suction these stents to maintain their patency, taking precautions to avoid dislodging them. Arm restraints prevent the patient from removing the stents prematurely.

Intravenous therapy is maintained until the patient is taking adequate oral fluids. Pain management is of greater concern for the pharyngeal flap patient than for the previously addressed surgical groups; therefore, the pharyngeal flap patient requires IV or intramuscular narcotic analgesics for 24 to 48 hours, followed by several more days of periodic oral narcotics. It is a challenge to get these patients to take adequate oral fluids owing to the postoperative pain and edema. Their diet, like that of the palatoplasty patient, is restricted to liquids high in calories and protein for 3 weeks after surgery. Eating utensils are contraindicated.

Discharge generally occurs on the fourth or fifth postoperative day. Discharge supplies and parent instructions are identical to those for palatoplasty patients. The patient and parents should be told that immediate improvement in speech quality is not to be expected. Improvement is a gradual process that occurs as the surgical site heals, edema subsides, and speech therapy is resumed.

Postoperative Care of the Cleft Rhinoplasty or Septoplasty Patient

Many children with cleft deformities require nasal surgery. Such surgery generally is performed after the age of 8 years, most often during adolescence. Nasal reconstruction is done for two major reasons: to enhance aesthetic appearance (cleft rhinoplasty) and to relieve obstructed nasal breathing (septoplasty, turbinectomy). Septal reconstruction and cleft rhinoplasty can be performed simultaneously if indicated.

Nasal surgery can be done on an outpatient basis; however, some patients may be admitted to a nursing unit for 1 or 2 days. Anesthesia can be general or local with IV sedation, depending on the age and maturity of the patient. The length of the procedure is 1 to 2 hours.

During the immediate postoperative period, vital signs are taken according to the recovery unit policy. The patient requires narcotic analgesics administered orally or intramuscularly for the first 24 to 48 hours to control discomfort, which can be compounded by the presence of nasal packing. Increased pain can cause hypertension, exacerbating bleeding, so it is essential to keep the patient comfortable.

The patient is positioned supine with the head of the bed elevated to decrease edema and facilitate breathing.

Supplemental bedside humidity delivered through a face mask keeps the oral cavity moist and the patient more comfortable because he is restricted to mouth breathing. Additionally, frequent oral care with adequate fluid intake will maintain a moist oral mucosa.

The type of nasal packing varies with the surgeon's preference. The packing must remain in place. If displacement occurs anteriorly (from the nares) or posteriorly (seen in the posterior oropharynx), notify the surgeon immediately.

Observe the type and amount of nasal drainage. During the immediate postoperative period, bright red drainage can be expected, which gradually subsides and turns to serosanguineous and then mucoid drainage. The patient wears a nasal "dripper" (small 3- by 3-inch gauze folded in thirds) taped under the nose, similar to a moustache, to collect nasal drainage. If active bleeding occurs (four to six saturated nasal drippers in 1 hour), examine the oropharynx for bleeding, note symptoms of frequent swallowing and increased nausea, and call the surgeon immediately.

Blood swallowed during surgery may cause nausea with coffee-ground emesis for the first 4 to 6 hours postoperatively. Intravenous therapy should be maintained until the patient tolerates clear liquids. For persistent vomiting of bright red emesis, check the oropharynx and notify the surgeon.

In cleft rhinoplasty patients a cast or splint is placed over the nasal dorsum. This cast must be kept dry and

Table 108–2. Instructions Following Nasal Surgery Procedures

1. Do not blow your nose for 2 to 3 weeks after surgery to protect it from injury.
2. If sneezing cannot be avoided during the first 2 to 3 weeks, try to sneeze with your mouth open. Avoid nasal irritants such as smoke and dust.
3. You may have swelling and discoloration of your eyelids for several days. Apply cold compresses to eyes for the first 24 hours. Sleep with your head elevated on two pillows.
4. Do not take aspirin or aspirin-containing medication. It can cause an increase in bleeding.
5. If you have packing or Silastic sheets in your nose, you will be scheduled for return appointments to have them removed. A room humidifier helps to decrease dryness in your mouth.
6. Propylene glycol nasal spray should be used after the packing is removed to prevent crust formation. To use this nasal spray, insert tip of atomizer, inhale, hold breath, spray, and exhale. DO NOT INHALE THIS MEDICATION. It contains oil and could cause lung inflammation.
7. If a case or stent is placed over the nose, keep it dry. Do not add or remove tape because it may alter the position of the cast or stent and affect the results of surgery.
8. A gauze dressing (dripper) may be worn under your nose to absorb nasal drainage. Tape dripper to cheeks. Do not tape dripper over the cast or stent.
9. You may not participate in contact sports or vigorous exercise until these are cleared by your physician. Resume school or work as indicated by your physician.

Notify your physician if any of the following occur:
Persistent bleeding (four to six saturated nasal drippers in 1 hour).
Persistent fever.
Persistent pain.
Cast becomes displaced.
Displaced nasal packing or Silastic sheets.
Foul or yellow-green drainage (pus) from nose.
Injury to the nose.

not altered in any way, or else the aesthetic results of surgery may be affected. Do not tape the nasal dripper over the cast or add tape to the cast. If skin sutures are present, incision care is indicated. To minimize eyelid edema, iced normal saline compresses are applied to the eyes for the first 24 hours after surgery. Care must be taken not to place compresses over the cast or splint.

With septal reconstruction, Silastic sheeting is sutured with one stitch on both sides of the septum to prevent adhesions postoperatively. This causes no discomfort, and the stitches can be removed in 7 to 10 days. Nasal packing is removed on postoperative day one, and a nasal spray is used to prevent crusting. Patients are constantly reminded not to blow their nose and to sneeze with their mouth open to prevent injury to the nose.

Nasal surgery patients are discharged with written instructions (Table 108–2), incision care supplies, gauze and tape for nasal drippers, prescriptions for nasal spray, antihistamine, or decongestant, antibiotics, oral analgesics, and a return appointment scheduled for 1 week after discharge.

On the first postoperative visit, the Silastic sheeting, cast, and sutures are removed after spraying the nose with a topical anesthetic. The nose is gently cleansed, and the surgeon replaces the cast with paper tape to maintain the redraped skin for 1 to 2 weeks. Again, it is crucial to reinforce the prohibition on nose blowing and not to remove the tape if it is reapplied.

Three months after surgery the patient's nose should be well healed, and the final cosmetic or functional result should be apparent. Further nasal revisions may be necessary depending on the severity of the cleft deformity. Such decisions are made as the child continues to grow and develop.

Coordination of Follow-Up Care

Coordination of follow-up care is extremely important for children who have had cleft repairs. Depending on the severity of the initial deformity, these children need to be followed closely by specialists from birth through adulthood. Frequent outpatient evaluations and hospital admissions may become a strain for some families. This strain can be lessened if an effort is made to coordinate visits to the various members of the cleft team. The nurse may be the individual to implement this, that is, to coordinate appointments with the surgeon, orthodontist, speech pathologist, and so on. Encouraging and assisting the family in making and keeping these appointments results in less frustration and better care for the patient.

References

1. Spriestersbach DC: Counseling parents of children with cleft lips and palates. J Chronic Dis 13:244–252, 1961.
2. Whaley L, Wong D: Nursing Care of Infants and Children. St. Louis: C. V. Mosby, 1987, pp 193–194.
3. Clarren SK, Anderson B, Wolf LS: Feeding infants with cleft lip, cleft palate, or cleft lip and palate. Cleft Palate J 24:244–249, 1987.
4. Dunning Y: Feeding babies with cleft lip and palate. Nurs Times 82:46–47, 1986.
5. Danner S: Nursing Your Baby with a Cleft Palate or Cleft Lip (pamphlet). Cleveland: Childbirth Graphics, 1984.
6. Redman B: The Process of Patient Education. 5th ed. St. Louis: C. V. Mosby, 1984, pp 102–105.

CHAPTER 109

Directions for Future Research

Hughlett L. Morris and Janusz Bardach

The present book, which reflects the state of the art in treatment techniques and strategies for cleft lip and palate, clearly indicates that tremendous progress has been made in the last 25 years. However, the effectiveness of contemporary treatment is not as complete as one would expect. This conclusion indicates that further clinical and experimental research is necessary to improve treatment techniques and advance management strategies to achieve better and more consistent results.

Many cleft palate centers and many individuals pursue research related to various aspects of cleft lip and palate. Diversified directions and topics, along with a lack of criteria for establishing priority problems, led us to an attempt to establish a list of high-priority research issues. The initial attempt was made in October 1987 at the international conference in Iowa City on multidisciplinary management of unilateral cleft lip and palate. Leading clinicians in their fields, chosen on a worldwide basis, participated in this meeting. With assistance from the conference participants, a list of high-priority research issues pertaining to cleft lip and palate was compiled and has been reported for further consideration and discussion.[1] We expand that list in this chapter on the direction of future research, adding our personal perspectives as academicians and clinicians with specific interest in clinical research. In indicating these directions of high priority for future research, we limit ourselves to introducing subject areas for such research, leaving the specific topics to the invention of individual researchers.

The Issues

Embryologic and Fetal Development of the Oral, Facial, and Cranial Structures. Because cleft lip and palate and related disorders are structural and developmental anomalies, there is continued need to better understand the processes by which the structures are formed in both the normal and the pathologic fetus.
Etiologic Factors for Cleft Lip and Palate and Related Disorders. More information is needed about the factors that cause cleft lip or palate birth defects. There is a special need for additional information about possible genetic etiologic factors because the public finds it so difficult to deal satisfactorily with our present uncertain knowledge about the problem. One of the very great challenges that we as clinicians face is helping the parents of a new baby with a cleft deal with this problem of etiology. This is a very human need and one that deserves high priority.

Prevention. We think there is universal agreement about the necessity for further research about prevention. For obvious reasons, this research objective should receive highest priority.

Anatomy and Physiology. There is a continued need for better understanding of the anatomy and physiology of the facial, oral, nasal, pharyngeal, and associated structures, not only in the patient with a cleft or related disorder but also in situations of normal development. This information is vital in approaching aspects of the disorder that are both physical and functional. It is especially relevant to the surgeon in planning and performing procedures to reconstruct the lip, alveolar, nasal, palatal, and pharyngeal structures to normal status, or as near normal as possible. Careful attention is clearly needed to the anatomic diversity among patients with clefts and to the implications to the surgeon of this diversity. Further consideration of the influence of various surgical procedures on maxillofacial growth and development and on the function of the lip, nose, and palate is essential to modify present surgical techniques for achieving better results. It is also imperative to investigate further the effects of wound healing and its influence on reconstructive procedures. More research is necessary to understand the correlation between anatomic structures and function in the velopharyngeal region.

Surgical Treatment. Several variables in lip and nose surgery warrant further study: the most efficient surgical techniques for correction of cleft lip and nose deformity; the effect of cleft lip and palate surgery on subsequent maxillofacial growth and development; the effects of early correction of nasal deformity on growth and development; the improvement of surgical techniques for early and late correction of nasal deformities; and methods of improvement of secondary lip and nose revisions. Certainly the need for investigations leading to better understanding and management of the bilateral cleft lip, alveolus, and palate is of highest priority; these cleft types continue to present the most difficult treatment problem.

There continues to be ample evidence that in contemporary practice cleft palate surgery should yield velopharyngeal function that is within normal limits in at least 75% of patients in random series, and with very few postsurgical fistulas, if any. Further, although we favor a two-flap palatoplasty technique, equally good results could probably be obtained by the careful use of other techniques. The challenge is to identify the remaining 25% of patients before surgery and to devise new methods for palatoplasty that are more effective with these problem cases than conventional techniques.

Coordination of surgical treatment with the work of the orthodontist and speech pathologist is important in designing and timing various surgical procedures. More attention must be focused on surgical-orthodontic treatment and the planning of these procedures. Close cooperation between surgeon and speech pathologist is of high priority to ensure proper diagnosis and timing for surgical intervention.

Further investigation of the available secondary procedures for correction of velopharyngeal dysfunction is needed as well as development of new secondary procedures. Also, more information is needed about surgical techniques that can be used to provide normal velopharyngeal function while avoiding chronic stenosis of the velopharyngeal port. Further attention must also be given to the refinement of methods such as pharyngeal implants. Better investigation is necessary to assess the value of prosthetic management of patients with palatal clefts or velopharyngeal incompetence.

Physical Growth and Development, Specifically of the Face, Mouth, and Head. One major sequel of cleft lip and palate and related disorders is a disturbance of orofacial growth patterns (and craniofacial growth patterns, depending on the disorder considered.) In our opinion, there is ample evidence that severe growth disturbances occur less frequently now than they did 25 years ago. However, we think all clinicians doing this kind of work continue to see patients with such severe growth problems that successful management is difficult. For this reason, there is continued need for research dealing with all phases of oral, facial, and dental growth, including growth of both soft tissue and bone. Since treatment of cleft lip and palate includes surgical and orthodontic procedures at different stages of growth and development, more information is required about the effects of various treatment procedures and the interactions between treatment and growth and development.

Orthodontic Treatment. Additional information is needed about the relative effectiveness of various techniques for orthodontic treatment and particularly about indications for surgical orthodontics. Further investigation of the biologic mechanisms that underlie malocclusion and its treatment is also urgently needed. Additional attention is warranted to more clearly identify the limitations of orthodontic treatment and the interaction between treatment and cleft lip and palate surgery. Finally, there is need for further development of criteria, particularly with regard to cosmetic appearance, by which to evaluate the need for and success of orthodontic treatment of cleft lip and palate patients.

Speech and Language Development. Another major sequel of the disorder is disturbance of normal speech acquisition. As before, we interpret present findings to indicate that more children with this disorder talk more normally than they did 25 years ago. However, also as before, we see patients not infrequently who have such unusual speech patterns that either intelligibility is at risk or, at best, their speech is so unusual that it is a social hazard. Thus, the task of speech research is by no means completed. Of special interest here are problems of speech proficiency, for which there seems to be close interaction between oral structural hazards and the process by which speech is normally learned. The same story applies to aspects of language: Although many of these children show language development that is essentially normal, others deserve more careful study.

Speech and Language Therapy. There appears to be nearly universal agreement that present speech therapy techniques are not effective in the treatment of physiologic velopharyngeal dysfunction. However, we can hardly discourage further investigation of the idea because by all standards, behavioral therapy, if effective, would be preferable to surgical treatment or even dental prosthetic management.

There is continued need for research about the relative effectiveness of speech therapy for patients with disordered speech and indications of normal velopharyngeal function. Of special interest is the patient with marginal velopharyngeal function who seems to show a disorder in timing rather than of structure. The question here is to discover when the patient has made as much progress as possible toward normal oral speech and when physical management of the velopharyngeal mechanism should be considered. The possible neuromotor basis for these apparent timing disorders warrants careful investigation both to understand the nature of the problem and to devise effective treatment.

More information is needed as well about the effectiveness of early language therapy for assisting the young child to learn normal speech and language patterns, even before structural deficits are resolved. Of particular interest would be the development of intervention methods that could be used satisfactorily by the family or child care worker.

Psychosocial Aspects. There is a continued need for descriptions of the impact of the cleft lip and palate on the psychosocial and educational-vocational status of the individual. Such data about the adult must always be placed in historical perspective—e.g., the status of a forty-year-old patient is influenced greatly by treatment regimens used 30 to 40 years ago. For children, additional information is needed about interactions among cosmetic appearance, speech proficiency, and psychosocial and educational status.

Issues of Research Design and Strategy

1. We see a great need for clinical treatment research designed to report the results of various treatment techniques. Such investigations are not easy to design or conduct. In addition, there are always important variables that are not satisfactorily measurable or controllable. However, data of this sort, carefully reported, are often our best means of evaluating treatments, and we owe it to our patients and to the public to continue these efforts. Sometimes clinical studies are best per-

formed on a retrospective basis, making as full use as possible of existing records. Certainly, prospective designs frequently yield more reliable and more relevant findings, but they are also expensive and, in addition, may be obsolete in methodology before the study is completed.

It seems best to keep an open mind about the various types of clinical investigations, collecting relevant data about an issue wherever it is available.

2. Continued attention to experimental models is needed. Animal models are clearly preferable to other strategies for many purposes, especially in studying growth mechanisms. However, in the final analysis, it is a matter of informed judgment whether and how the animal model approximates the human patient. The same qualification is true for computer and other types of models.

3. It seems highly probable that the multicenter strategy could be used more effectively than it has been in the past to provide data for comparison of treatment regimens. Such a strategy frequently requires suspension of some rules of scientific rigor, but the benefits from such attempts can easily outweigh the hazards.

4. There is a strong need for clinical investigations that are comprehensive in describing the outcome of treatment. For example, for the best assessment of surgical method for palatal surgery, data about both speech-velopharyngeal function and dento-occlusion status should be reported for the same group of patients.

5. There are a number of indicators of increasing concern about the issue of reliability of data in clinical investigations. We take the position that in research of this type, clinical judgments are frequently the most valid measures of clinical status, but we agree that the reliability of those judgments, including both intrajudge and interjudge measures, ought to be estimated and reported.

6. One feature of this book we are proud of is the group of reports about clinical programs in a number of countries around the world. Our interest in international exchange is long-standing, and we have experienced great professional and technical growth, as well as personal satisfaction, from these opportunities.

7. Several of the issues identified above, notably those concerning embryology, etiology, and prevention, require the attention of experimental scientists working in the areas of developmental, cellular, and molecular biology. More research programs in cleft lip and palate investigations that include their participation, especially cooperative efforts with clinicians, are very much needed.

Conclusion

The above list of research issues is not intended to be comprehensive, but instead to identify the range of topics that we think deserve careful attention. Listed below are seven of the issues judged by us to be of highest priority for consideration by individuals in the clinical and scientific community interested in the problems posed by patients with cleft lip and palate:

1. Prevention of cleft lip and palate and related disorders.
2. More efficient methods of primary management to lessen the need for secondary techniques to improve aesthetic appearance and function of orofacial structures, speech and language, and dental occlusion.
3. Greater efficiency in predicting problem cases so that they can be identified early and receive careful, expert assistance.
4. Continued evaluation of single treatments and of treatment systems on as comprehensive a basis as possible.
5. Better methods for secondary management of residual problems, aesthetic appearance, function of orofacial structures, speech and language, dental occlusion, and nasal airway maintenance.
6. Better understanding of anatomic, physiologic, and behavioral mechanisms and the interactions of these that underlie cleft birth defects and their resulting disorders.
7. Continued attention to the patient and his or her family so that the patient's personal development will be hampered as little as possible by the birth defect.

ACKNOWLEDGMENTS. We gratefully acknowledge the contributions to this chapter by participants in the October 1987 Iowa City Conference on the identification of research issues and their priority, and specifically to Betty Jane McWilliams, Howard Aduss, and Peter Randall, who served as discussion leaders.

Reference

1. Morris HL, Bardach J: Cleft lip and palate and related disorders: Issues for future research of high priority. Cleft Palate J 26:141–144, 1989.